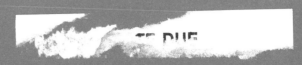
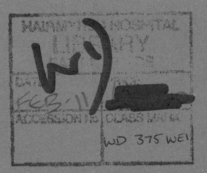

Enzinger and Weiss's

SOFT
TISSUE
TUMORS

Enzinger and Weiss's
SOFT TISSUE TUMORS

FIFTH EDITION

Sharon W. Weiss MD

Professor and Vice Chair
Department of Pathology and Laboratory Medicine
Associate Dean
Emory University School of Medicine
Atlanta, Georgia
USA

John R. Goldblum MD

Professor of Pathology
Chairman, Department of Anatomic Pathology
Cleveland Clinic Lerner College of Medicine
Cleveland, Ohio
USA

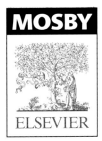

MOSBY

ELSEVIER

MOSBY
ELSEVIER

Mosby is an affiliate of Elsevier Inc

First edition 1983
Second edition 1988
Third edition 1995
Fourth edition 2001
© 2008, Mosby, Inc., an affiliate of Elsevier, Inc. All
rights reserved.

The content of Chapter 3 is derived from the Armed
Forces Institute of Pathology and is therefore in the
public domain.

978-0-323-04628-2

British Library Cataloguing in Publication Data
A catalogue record for this book is available from the
British Library

Library of Congress Cataloging in Publication Data
A catalog record for this book is available from the
Library of Congress

Notice

ELSEVIER your source for books,
journals and multimedia
in the health sciences
www.elsevierhealth.com

Working together to grow
libraries in developing countries

www.elsevier.com | www.bookaid.org | www.sabre.org

ELSEVIER | BOOK AID International | Sabre Foundation

The
publisher's
policy is to use
paper manufactured
from sustainable forests

Commissioning Editor: William Schmitt
Development Editor: Sheila Black
Editorial Assistant: Liz MacSween
Project Manager: Alan Nicholson
Designer: Erik Bigland
Illustration Manager: Bruce Hogarth
Marketing Managers:
Kathleen Neely (US); John Canelon (UK)

Printed in China

Last digit is the print number: 9 8 7 6 5 4 3 2 1

CONTENTS

LIST OF CONTRIBUTORS

Fadi W. Abdul-Karim MD
Professor of Pathology and Orthopedics
Director, Anatomic Pathology
University Hospitals – Case Medical Center
Cleveland, OH, USA

Cristina R. Antonescu MD
Associate Professor
Department of Pathology
Memorial Sloan-Kettering Cancer Center
New York, NY, USA

Paola Dal Cin PhD
Associate Professor of Pathology
Cytogenetics Laboratory
Brigham and Women's Hospital
Boston, MA, USA

Andrew L. Folpe MD
Professor of Laboratory
Medicine and Pathology
Division of Anatomic Pathology
Mayo Clinic
Rochester, MN, USA

Kim R. Geisinger MD
Professor of Pathology
Director, Surgical Pathology and Cytology
Department of Pathology
Wake Forest University School of Medicine
Winton-Salem, NC, USA

Allen M. Gown MD
Medical Director and Chief Pathologist
PhenoPath Laboratories
Seattle, WA, USA

Mark J. Kransdorf MD
Professor of Radiology
Mayo Clinic College of Medicine
Rochester, MN
Consultant
Department of Radiology
Mayo Clinic
Jacksonville, FL, USA

Marc Ladanyi MD
Attending Pathologist and Chief
Molecular Diagnostics Service
Department of Pathology
Member, Human Oncology and Pathogenesis Program
Memorial Sloan-Kettering Cancer Center
New York, NY, USA

Mark D. Murphey MD
Chief, Musculoskeletal Radiology
Department of Radiologic Pathology
Armed Forces Institute of Pathology
Washington, DC
Professor of Radiology
Department of Radiology and Nuclear Medicine
Uniformed Services University of the Health Sciences,
Bethesda, MD, USA

Peter W.T. Pisters MD FACS
Professor of Surgery
Chief, Sarcoma Service
Department of Surgical Oncology
University of Texas M.D. Anderson Cancer Center
Houston, TX, USA

PREFACE TO FIFTH EDITION

Twenty five years have passed since the first edition of this book—a Silver Anniversary for those who like to reckon time by precious metals and gemstones. But what seems most precious to us are our colleagues who continue to share their fascinating cases that ever enhance our experience and understanding of soft tissue tumors, our outstanding – and largely new – co-authors who have crafted several masterful chapters, our superlative assistants, Ms. Kathleen Ranney and Ms Susan Raven, who tirelessly shouldered the typing, and our dedicated young faculty, Drs. Andrea Deyrup, Erinn Downs-Kelly, and Raj Patel, who expunged the flaws from the final proofs. We thank all of you!

Sharon W. Weiss   *John R. Goldblum*
November 2007

PREFACE TO THE FIRST EDITION

Since the publication of the *AFIP Fascicle on Soft Tissue Tumors* by A.P. Stout in 1957 and the revised edition by A.P. Stout and R. Lattes in 1967, there have been numerous advances and changes both in the diagnosis and treatment of soft tissue tumors. This book combines traditional views, which have stood the test of time, and newer concepts and observations accrued over the past 20 years. Because a precise diagnosis is essential for planning of treatment and assessment of prognosis, emphasis has been placed throughout the book on clear and concise descriptions and differential diagnoses of the tumors discussed. Each chapter has been freely illustrated, and comprehensive references have been added with emphasis on recent publications.

The WHO Classification of Soft Tissue Tumors provided the basis for the classification in this book. However, since its publication in 1969 several modifications have become necessary. Fibrohistiocytic and extraskeletal cartilaginous and osseous tumors have been included as separate groups, and a number of changes have been made, especially in the classification of fibrous, vascular, and neural tumors. The role of histochemistry, electron microscopy, and immunohistochemistry has been noted when applicable. Relatively less emphasis, however, has been placed on the specifics of therapy because of the rapidly changing nature of this discipline. It is our hope that this blending of old and new will make this book valuable not only as a reference book for those specifically interested in soft tissue tumors but also as a diagnostic aid for the practicing general pathologist.

In many areas the contents of this book reflect our personal experience derived from approximately 5000 cases reviewed annually in the Department of Soft Tissue Pathology of the Armed Forces Institute of Pathology. The large number of cases has afforded us a unique opportunity for which we are extremely grateful.

We also wish to express our appreciation and gratitude to the many contributing pathologists who not only shared their interesting and problematic cases with us but also provided additional teaching material in the form of photographs, roentgenograms, and electron micrographs. We also owe thanks to our professional colleagues for their advice and support in this endeavor, to the photographic staff of the Institute, especially Mr. C. Edwards and Mr. B. Allen, for their skill and assistance in preparing the photographs, and to Mrs. P. Diaz and Mrs. J. Kozlay for typing the manuscript. We are also greatly indebted to our publishers for their cooperation and help throughout the production of this book. We are particularly indebted to our families for their patience and tolerance.

Franz M. Enzinger   Sharon W. Weiss

DEDICATION

To Bernie and Francine

Sharon W. Weiss MD

This book is dedicated to my wife Asmita, my dearest companion for 27 years, to my four incredible children Andrew, Ryan, Janavi and Raedan, my dear mother Bette Jean and my late father Raymond, and the rest of the Goldblum and Shirali families whom I also cherish.

John R. Goldblum MD

GENERAL CONSIDERATIONS

Soft tissue can be defined as nonepithelial extraskeletal tissue of the body exclusive of the reticuloendothelial system, glia, and supporting tissue of various parenchymal organs. It is represented by the voluntary muscles, fat, and fibrous tissue, along with the vessels serving these tissues. By convention it also includes the peripheral nervous system because tumors arising from nerves present as soft tissue masses and pose similar problems in differential diagnosis and therapy. Embryologically, soft tissue is derived principally from mesoderm, with some contribution from neuroectoderm.

Soft tissue tumors are a highly heterogeneous group of tumors that are classified on a histogenetic basis according to the adult tissue they resemble. Lipomas and liposarcomas, for example, are tumors that recapitulate to a varying degree normal fatty tissue; and hemangiomas and angiosarcomas contain cells resembling vascular endothelium. Within the various histogenetic categories, soft tissue tumors are usually divided into benign and malignant forms.

Benign tumors, which more closely resemble normal tissue, have a limited capacity for autonomous growth. They exhibit little tendency to invade locally and are attended by a low rate of local recurrence following conservative therapy.

Malignant tumors, or *sarcomas*, in contrast, are locally aggressive and are capable of invasive or destructive growth, recurrence, and distant metastasis. Radical surgery is required to ensure total removal of these tumors. Unfortunately, the term sarcoma does not indicate the likelihood or rapidity of metastasis. Some sarcomas, such as dermatofibrosarcoma protuberans, rarely metastasize, whereas others do so with alacrity. For these reasons it is

important to qualify the term sarcoma with a statement concerning the degree of differentiation or the histologic grade. "Well differentiated" and "poorly differentiated" are qualitative, and hence subjective, terms used to indicate the relative maturity of the tumor with respect to normal adult tissue. Histologic grade is a means of quantitating the degree of differentiation by applying a set of histologic criteria. Usually, well-differentiated sarcomas are low-grade lesions, whereas poorly differentiated sarcomas are high-grade neoplasms. There are also borderline lesions for which it is difficult to determine the malignant potential.

INCIDENCE

The incidence of soft tissue tumors, especially the frequency of benign tumors relative to malignant ones, is nearly impossible to determine accurately. Benign soft tissue tumors outnumber malignant tumors by a wide margin. The fact that many benign tumors, such as lipomas and hemangiomas, do not undergo biopsy makes direct application of data from most hospital series invalid for the general population, however.

Malignant soft tissue tumors, on the other hand, ultimately come to medical attention. Soft tissue sarcomas, compared with carcinomas and other neoplasms, are relatively rare and constitute fewer than 1% of all cancers, with an estimated 9500 new soft tissue sarcomas diagnosed in 2006 (Table 1–1).[1]

There seems to be an upward trend in the incidence of soft tissue sarcomas, but it is not clear whether this represents a true increase or reflects better diagnostic capabilities and greater interest in this type of tumor. Data from the National Cancer Institute's Surveillance, Epidemiology and End Results Program (SEER) showed a marked increase in the age-adjusted incidence of soft tissue sarcomas between 1981 to 1987.[2] However, when patients with Kaposi sarcoma were eliminated from this analysis, the rates remained relatively unchanged throughout that time period. Judging from the available data, the incidence and distribution of soft tissue sarcomas seem to be similar in different regions of the world. Soft tissue sarcomas may occur anywhere in the body, but most arise

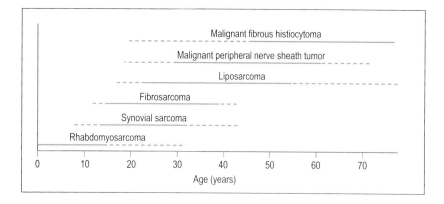

FIGURE 1–1 Approximate relation of age to incidence of various types of sarcoma. Continuous line indicates peak incidence of tumor. Dotted line indicates reduced incidence of tumor.

TABLE 1–1	ESTIMATED NEW CASES OF CANCER BY SITE (UNITED STATES, 2006)
Site	**No. of cases**
Prostate	234 460
Breast	214 640
Lung	174 470
Colon and rectum	148 610
Soft tissue	9 530
Bone and joints	2 760

Data from Jemal A, Siegel R, Ward E, et al. CA Cancer J Clin 2006; 56:106.

from the large muscles of the extremities, the chest wall, the mediastinum, and the retroperitoneum. They occur at any age and, like carcinomas, are more common in older patients; about 15% affect persons younger than 15 years, and about 40% affect persons 55 years or older.

Soft tissue sarcomas occur more commonly in males, but gender and age-related incidences vary among the histologic types (Fig. 1–1).[1] For instance, embryonal rhabdomyosarcoma occurs almost exclusively in young individuals, whereas pleomorphic undifferentiated sarcoma (malignant fibrous histiocytoma) is predominantly a tumor of old age and is rare in children younger than 10 years. There is also no proven racial variation.

PATHOGENESIS

As with other malignant neoplasms, the pathogenesis of most soft tissue tumors is still unknown. Recognized causes include various physical and chemical factors, exposure to ionizing radiation, and inherited or acquired immunologic defects. Evaluation of the exact cause is often difficult because of the long latent period between the time of exposure and the development of sarcoma, as well as the possible effect of multiple environmental and hereditary factors during the induction period. Origin of sarcomas from benign soft tissue tumors is exceedingly rare, except for malignant peripheral nerve sheath tumors arising in neurofibromas, which are nearly always in patients with the manifestations of type 1 neurofibromatosis (von Recklinghausen's disease).

Environmental factors

Trauma is frequently implicated in the development of sarcomas. Many of these reports are anecdotal, however, and the integrity of the injured part was not clearly established before injury. Consequently, trauma often seems to be an event that merely calls attention to the underlying neoplasm. Occasionally, there is reasonable evidence to suggest a causal relation. Rare soft tissue sarcomas have been reported as arising in scar tissue following surgical procedures or thermal or acid burns, at fracture sites, and in the vicinity of plastic or metal implants, usually after a latent period of several years.[3,4] Kirkpatrick et al. studied the histologic features in capsules surrounding the implantation site of a variety of biomaterials.[5] Interestingly, these authors noted a spectrum of change, from focal proliferative lesions through preneoplastic proliferations to incipient sarcomas and suggested a model of multistage tumorigenesis akin to the adenoma–carcinoma sequence.

Environmental carcinogens have been related to the development of sarcomas, but their role is largely unexplored, and only a few substances have been identified as playing a role in the induction of sarcomas in humans. A variety of animal models exist to induce sarcomas, including the subcutaneous implantation of methylcholanthrene-induced sarcoma in Fischer rats[6] and the induction of angiosarcomas in mice using dimethylhydrazine.[7]

Asbestos, a hydrated silicate, is the most important known environmental carcinogen. Exposure to this substance, principally in the form of crocidolite or chrysotile, occurs in asbestos miners and industrial workers who process, install, or repair electrical and thermal insulation, brake linings, cement tiles, or pipes. Inhaled as a microscopic particle, asbestos ultimately reaches the pulmonary parenchyma and pleural surface, where after many years it may be associated with the development of pleural and peritoneal mesotheliomas or pulmonary carcinomas. Important risk factors are the intensity and duration of asbestos exposure, the type of asbestos, and the submicroscopic fiber diameter.[8] The risk is greatest with crocidolite, the blue asbestos mined in South Africa;

the risk is much less with chrysotile, the white asbestos chiefly found in Canada and Russia, which accounts for more than 95% of the asbestos used commercially (see Chapter 28).[9]

Phenoxyacetic acid herbicides, chlorophenols, and their contaminants such as 2,3,7,8-tetrachlorodibenzo-para-dioxin (dioxin) have been linked to sarcomagenesis.[10–14] A series of case–control studies from Sweden from 1979 to 1990 reported an up to sixfold increased risk of soft tissue sarcoma associated with exposure to phenoxyacetic acids or chlorophenols in individuals exposed to these herbicides in agricultural or forestry work.[15–19] Similar reports of an increased risk of sarcoma associated with these herbicides were reported from Italy,[20] Great Britain,[21] and New Zealand.[22] Although a study by Leiss and Savitz linked use of phenoxyacetic acid lawn pesticides with soft tissue sarcomas in children,[23] several other studies with more detailed exposure histories did not confirm this association.[24] These inconsistencies may be due in part to the predominant phenoxyacetic herbicide used in different locations. In the United States, 2,4-dichlorophenoxyacetic acid is the primary phenoxyacetic herbicide used, whereas in Sweden the main herbicides contain 2,4,5-trichlorophenoxyacetic acid and 2-methyl-4-chlorophenoxyacetic acid, both of which are more likely contaminated with dioxin.[25,26] High levels of dioxin exposure due to accidental environmental contamination near Seveso from an explosion at a chemical factory was followed by a threefold increased risk of soft tissue sarcomas reported among individuals living near this factory.[20,27] In addition, the possibility of an increased incidence of sarcomas was claimed for some of the 2 million soldiers stationed in Vietnam between 1965 and 1970 who were exposed to Agent Orange, a defoliant that contained dioxin as a contaminant.[28,29] However, in several case–control and proportional mortality studies, no excess risk of soft tissue sarcoma was reported among those Vietnam veterans who were directly involved with the spraying of Agent Orange.[26]

Vinyl chloride exposure is clearly associated with the development hepatic angiosarcoma.[30,31] There are also rare reports of extrahepatic angiosarcoma associated with this agent.[32]

Radiation exposure has been related to the development of sarcomas; but considering the frequency of radiotherapy, radiation-induced soft tissue sarcomas are quite uncommon. The incidence of postradiation sarcoma is difficult to estimate, but reports generally range from 0.03% to 0.80%.[33] Much of the data regarding the incidence of postradiation sarcomas are derived from large cohorts of breast cancer patients treated with postoperative radiation therapy.[34] To qualify as a postradiation sarcoma, there must be documentation that the sarcoma developed in the irradiated field, histologic confirmation of the diagnosis, a period of latency of at least 3 years between irradiation and the appearance of tumor, and documentation that the region bearing the tumor was normal prior to administration of the radiation.[35] Nearly all postradiation sarcomas occur in adults, and women develop these tumors more frequently, an observation that reflects the common use of radiation for treatment of breast and gynecologic malignancies.

Postradiation sarcomas do not display the wide range of appearances associated with sporadic non-radiation-induced tumors. The most common postradiation soft tissue sarcoma is pleomorphic undifferentiated sarcoma (malignant fibrous histiocytoma), which accounts for nearly 70% of cases, followed by osteosarcoma, fibrosarcoma, malignant peripheral nerve sheath tumor, chondrosarcoma, and angiosarcoma. Unfortunately, most postradiation sarcomas are high-grade lesions and are detected at a relatively higher stage than their sporadic counterparts. Thus, the survival rate associated with these lesions is quite poor.

The prognosis of postradiation sarcomas is most closely related to anatomic site, which in turn probably reflects resectability. Patients with radiation-induced sarcomas of the extremities have the best survival (approximately 30% at 5 years), whereas those with lesions arising in the vertebral column, pelvis, and shoulder girdle generally have survival rates of less than 5% at 5 years.[34,36]

The total dose of radiation seems to influence the incidence of postradiation sarcoma; most are reported to occur at doses of 5000 cGy or more.[37,38] Mutations of the *p53* gene have been implicated in the pathogenesis of these tumors.[39] Extravasated Thorotrast (thorium dioxide), although no longer used for diagnostic or therapeutic purposes, has induced soft tissue sarcomas, particularly angiosarcomas, at the site of injection.[40,41]

Oncogenic viruses

The role of oncogenic viruses in the evolution of soft tissue sarcomas is still poorly understood, although there is strong evidence that the human herpesvirus 8 (HHV8) is the causative agent of Kaposi sarcoma (see Chapter 24).[42–44] In addition, there is a large body of literature supporting the role of the Epstein-Barr virus in the pathogenesis of smooth muscle tumors in patients with immunodeficiency syndromes or following therapeutic immunosuppression in the transplant setting.[45] Aside from these settings, there is no conclusive evidence that human-transmissible viral agents constitute a major risk factor in the development of soft tissue sarcomas.

Immunologic factors

As mentioned above, immunodeficiency and therapeutic immunosuppression are also associated with the development of soft tissue sarcomas, particularly smooth muscle tumors. In addition, acquired regional immunodeficiency, or loss of regional immune surveillance, may also be the underlying mechanism in the development of the relatively rare angiosarcomas that arise in the setting of chronic lymphedema,[46] secondary to radical mastectomy (Stewart-Treves syndrome),[47] or congenital or infectious conditions.[48,49]

Genetic factors

A number of genetic diseases are associated with the development of soft tissue tumors, and the list will undoubtedly lengthen as we begin to understand the molecular underpinnings of mesenchymal neoplasia. Neurofibromatosis 1, neurofibromatosis 2, and familial adenomatous polyposis (FAP)/Gardner syndrome are classic examples of genetic diseases associated with soft tissue tumors. Familial cancer syndromes associated with soft tissue sarcomas are more fully described in Chapter 4.

CLASSIFICATION OF SOFT TISSUE TUMORS

Development of a useful, comprehensive histologic classification of soft tissue tumors has been a relatively slow process. Earlier classifications have been largely descriptive and have been based more on the nuclear configuration than the type of tumor cells. Terms such as "round cell sarcoma," "spindle cell sarcoma," may be diagnostically convenient but should be discouraged because they convey little information as to the nature and potential behavior of a given tumor. Moreover, purely descriptive classifications do not clearly distinguish between tumors and tumor-like reactive processes. More recent classifications have been based principally on the line of differentiation of the tumor, that is, the type of tissue formed by the tumor rather than the type of tissue from which the tumor arose.

Over the past three decades there have been several attempts to devise a useful, comprehensive classification of soft tissue tumors. The classification used herein is similar but not identical to the 2002 WHO classification, a collective effort by pathologists throughout the world.[50,51]

Each of the histologic categories is divided into a benign group and a malignant group. In addition, for several tumor categories, some tumors are classified as being of intermediate (borderline or low malignant potential) malignancy, implying a high rate of local recurrence and a small risk of metastasis. Most tumors retain the same pattern of differentiation in the primary and recurrent lesions, but occasionally they change their pattern of differentiation or may even differentiate along several cellular lines.

Pleomorphic undifferentiated sarcoma (malignant fibrous histiocytoma) and liposarcoma are the most common soft tissue sarcomas of adults; together they account for 35–45% of all sarcomas. In the series by Markhede et al., the three most common sarcomas were malignant fibrous histiocytoma (28%), fibrosarcoma (14%) and liposarcoma (9%).[52] Rhabdomyosarcoma, neuroblastoma, and the extraskeletal Ewing sarcoma/primitive neuroectodermal tumor (ES/PNET) family of tumors are the most frequent soft tissue sarcomas of childhood. A histologic classification of soft tissue tumors is presented in Table 1–2.

GRADING AND STAGING SOFT TISSUE SARCOMAS

With a few notable exceptions, histologic typing does not provide sufficient information for predicting the clinical course of a sarcoma and, therefore, must be accompanied by grading and staging information. *Grading* assesses the degree of malignancy of a sarcoma and is based on an evaluation of several histologic parameters, whereas *staging* provides shorthand information regarding the extent of the disease at a designated time, usually the time of initial diagnosis. Many variables affect the outcome of a sarcoma. Their relative importance may vary with time and with the sarcoma subtype. Mitotic activity, for example, is important when grading leiomyosarcomas but is of much less significance when grading the various subtypes of malignant fibrous histiocytoma. Congenital/infantile fibrosarcoma, on the other hand, is a tumor of relatively low-grade malignancy despite its cellularity and prominent mitotic activity. Grading and staging systems of necessity simplify these variables and emphasize the most important ones that seem to have the most universal applicability for all sarcomas. Extensive discussions related to grading systems and issues have been published by Kilpatrick[53] and Deyrup and Weiss.[54]

GRADING SYSTEMS

Grading of soft tissue sarcomas was first proposed in 1939 by Broders, who used a combination of mitotic activity, tumor giant cells, and fibrous stroma in assigning a grade to fibrosarcomas.[55] Broders also acknowledged the importance of cellular differentiation in grading. He suggested that fibrosarcomas could be divided into several subtypes (fibrous, fibrocellular, and cellular) and that those that were highly cellular should be considered grade 4 regardless of the level of mitotic activity. These principles persist in grading systems today, namely that certain parameters (e.g., mitotic activity) should be evaluated in sarcomas, that some histologic subtypes

TABLE 1–2   HISTOLOGIC CLASSIFICATION OF SOFT TISSUE TUMORS

Fibroblastic/myofibroblastic tumors
  Benign
    Nodular fasciitis (including intravascular/cranial)
    Proliferative fasciitis/myositis
    Organ-associated pseudosarcomatous myofibroblastic
      proliferations
    Ischemic fasciitis
    Fibroma of tendon sheath
    Pleomorphic fibroma of skin
    Nuchal-type fibroma/Gardner-associated fibroma
    Elastofibroma
    Nasopharyngeal angiofibroma
    Keloid
    Collagenous fibroma (desmoplastic fibroblastoma)
    Fibrous hamartoma of infancy
    Infantile digital fibromatosis
    Myofibroma/myofibromatosis
    Juvenile hyaline fibromatosis
    Gingival fibromatosis
    Fibromatosis colli
    Infantile fibromatosis
    Calcifying aponeurotic fibroma
    Calcifying fibrous pseudotumor
  Intermediate
    Adult-type fibromatosis
      Superficial (palmar, plantar, penile, knuckle pads)
      Deep (extra-abdominal, abdominal, intra-abdominal)
  Malignant
    Pleomorphic undifferentiated sarcoma/malignant fibrous
      histiocytoma
      Storiform-pleomorphic type
      Myxoid type
      Giant cell type
      Inflammatory type

Lipomatous tumors
  Benign
    Lipoma
    Angiolipoma
    Myolipoma
    Chondroid lipoma
    Spindle cell/pleomorphic lipoma
    Lipoblastoma/lipoblastomatosis
    Myelolipoma
    Hibernoma
    Lipomatosis
  Intermediate
    Atypical lipoma (superficial well-differentiated liposarcoma)
  Malignant
    Atypical lipomatous tumor/well-differentiated liposarcoma
      Lipoma-like
      Sclerosing
      Spindled
      Inflammatory
    Myxoid/round cell liposarcoma
    Pleomorphic liposarcoma
    Dedifferentiated liposarcoma

Smooth muscle tumors and related lesions
  Benign
    Leiomyoma
    Angiomyoma
    Intranodal palisaded myofibroblastoma
    Mammary myofibroblastoma
    Benign genital stromal tumors
      Angiomyofibroblastoma

Cellular angiofibroma/angiomyofibroblastoma of male genital
      tract
    Aggressive angiomyxoma
    Superficial cervicovaginal myofibroblastoma
    Intravenous leiomyomatosis
    Leiomyomatosis peritonealis disseminata
  Malignant
    Leiomyosarcoma

Extragastrointestinal stromal tumors
  Benign
  Malignant

Skeletal muscle tumors
  Benign
    Cardiac rhabdomyoma
    Adult rhabdomyoma
    Fetal rhabdomyoma
      Myxoid (classic)
      Intermediate (cellular, juvenile)
    Genital rhabdomyoma
  Malignant
    Embryonal rhabdomyosarcoma
      Usual type
      Botryoid type
      Spindle cell type
    Alveolar rhabdomyosarcoma
    Pleomorphic rhabdomyosarcoma
    Sclerosing rhabdomyosarcoma
    Other (rhabdoid features, anaplastic features)
    Rhabdomyosarcoma with ganglion cells (ectomesenchymoma)

Tumors of blood and lymph vessels
  Benign
    Papillary endothelial hyperplasia
    Hemangioma
      Capillary hemangioma
      Cavernous hemangioma
      Venous hemangioma
      Arteriovenous hemangioma
      Pyogenic granuloma
      Acquired tufted hemangioma
      Hobnail hemangioma
      Spindle cell hemangioma
    Lymphangioma
    Lymphiomyoma/lymphangiomyomatosis
    Angiomatosis
    Lymphangiomatosis
  Intermediate
    Epithelioid hemangioendothelioma
    Hobnail hemangioendothelioma (retiform, Dabska-type)
    Epithelioid sarcoma-like hemangioendothelioma
    Kaposiform hemangioendothelioma
    Polymorphous hemangioendothelioma
  Malignant
    Angiosarcoma
    Kaposi sarcoma

Perivascular tumors
  Benign
    Glomus tumor
      Usual type
      Glomangioma (glomuvenous malformation)
      Glomangiomyoma
      Glomangiomatosis
    Myopericytoma
    Hemangiopericytoma-like tumor of nasal passages

TABLE 1–2 Continued

Malignant
    Malignant glomus tumor

Synovial tumors
Benign
    Tenosynovial giant cell tumor
        Localized type
        Diffuse type
Malignant
    Malignant tenosynovial giant cell tumor

Mesothelial tumors
Benign
    Adenomatoid tumor
Intermediate
    Multicystic mesothelioma
    Well-differentiated papillary mesothelioma
Malignant
    Diffuse mesothelioma
        Epithelial type
        Sarcomatoid type
        Biphasic type

Peripheral nerve sheath tumors and related lesions
Benign
    Traumatic neuroma
    Mucosal neuroma
    Pacinian neuroma
    Palisaded encapsulated neuroma
    Morton's interdigital neuroma
    Nerve sheath ganglion
    Neuromuscular hamartoma
    Neurofibroma
        Usual type (localized)
        Diffuse
        Plexiform
        Epithelioid
        Pigmented
    Schwannoma
        Usual type
        Cellular
        Plexiform
        Degenerated (ancient)
        Epithelioid
        Neuroblastoma-like
    Melanotic schwannoma
    Perineurioma
        Intraneural
        Extraneural
    Granular cell tumor
    Neurothekeoma
        Myxoid type
        Cellular type
    Ectopic meningioma
    Glial heterotopia
Malignant
    Malignant peripheral nerve sheath tumor (MPNST)
        Usual type
        MPNST with rhabdomyoblastic differentiation (malignant
            Triton tumor)

Glandular MPNST
Epithelioid MPNST
Malignant granular cell tumor
Clear cell sarcoma of tendon and aponeurosis
Malignant melanotic schwannoma
Extraspinal ependymoma

Primitive neuroectodermal tumors and related lesions
Benign
    Ganglioneuroma
    Pigmented neuroectodermal tumor of infancy (retinal anlage
        tumor)
Malignant
    Neuroblastoma
    Ganglioneuroblastoma
    Ewing sarcoma/primitive neuroectodermal tumor
    Malignant pigmented neuroectodermal tumor of infancy

Paraganglionic tumors (paraganglioma)
Benign
Malignant

Extraskeletal osseous and cartilaginous tumors
Benign
    Myositis ossificans
    Fibro-osseous pseudotumor of digits
    Fibrodysplasia ossificans progressiva
    Extraskeletal chondroma/osteochondroma
    Extraskeletal osteoma
Malignant
    Extraskeletal chondrosarcoma
        Well-differentiated chondrosarcoma
        Myxoid chondrosarcoma
        Mesenchymal chondrosarcoma
    Extraskeletal osteosarcoma

Miscellaneous tumors
Benign
    Tumoral calcinosis
    Congenital granular cell tumor
    Myxoma
        Cutaneous
        Intramuscular
    Juxta-articular myxoma
    Ganglion
    Amyloid tumor
Intermediate
    Ossifying fibromyxoid tumor
    Inflammatory myxohyaline tumor
    Mixed tumor/myoepithelioma/parachordoma
    Pleomorphic hyalinizing angiectatic tumor
    Hemangiopericytoma/solitary fibrous tumor/giant cell
        angiofibroma
    Perivascular epithelioid cell family of tumors (PEComa)
Malignant
    Synovial sarcoma
    Alveolar soft part sarcoma
    Epithelioid sarcoma
    Desmoplastic small round cell tumor
    Malignant extrarenal rhabdoid tumor

a priori dictate a grade, and that the level of differentiation must be factored into the assignment of a grade. Over the ensuing decades following that publication, numerous studies reaffirmed the importance of grading and emphasized the primacy of necrosis and mitotic activity in assessing grade.[56–63] Some studies have further proposed the use of Ki-67 immunoreactivity or MIB-1 score/index[59,60,64–67] to accurately assess mitotic activity, and radiologists employ FDG-PET imaging not only for detection of but also for grading of sarcomas.[68]

The first large-scale effort to grade and stage sarcomas occurred in 1977 when Russell et al., using a database of 1000 cases and, employing the TNM staging system,[69] showed that incorporating a grade into the staging system achieved predictions of outcome.[70] Most importantly, in the absence of metastatic disease, grade essentially defined the clinical stage. This study is most often cited as providing the first reliable grading system in the United States, yet paradoxically it did not provide objective criteria for grading. Rather, grade was determined by a panel of experts based on their years of experience. The real contribution this paper provided to grading was the implied concept that certain histologic types of sarcomas were inherently low grade and others high grade, a premise of many grading systems.

Following that seminal publication, a number of grading systems were published internationally by Myrhe Jensen,[71,72] Costa,[58] Hashimoto,[73] van Unnik,[74] Gustafson,[75] and Markhede.[52] Although differing in emphasis, most relied on mitotic activity and necrosis in deriving a grade and some proposed that sarcoma-specific parameters should be employed. The number of grades varies among the staging systems ranging from two to four. Three-grade systems seem best suited for predicting patterns for survival and likely response to therapy.[76] Four-grade systems usually show little difference between the two lowermost grades; two-grade systems, which distinguish only between low-grade and high grade-sarcomas, are more readily related to the two

surgical therapies but make it difficult to deal with intermediate-grade sarcomas.

An early system proposed by Markhede et al.[52] outlined a four-tiered grading system based on cellularity, cellular pleomorphism, and mitotic activity. Grade correlated well with survival rates although patients with grade 1 and 2 tumors had a similar clinical course with no tumor-related deaths. The 5- and 10-year survival rates with grade 3 tumors were 68% and 55%, respectively, and with grade 4 tumors 47% and 26%, respectively. Myhre Jensen et al.[72] utilized a three-tiered system in evaluation of over 200 cases from Aarhus Musculoskeletal Tumour Centre and found 5-year survival rates of 97% for grade 1 tumors, 67% for grade 2 tumors, and 38% for grade 3 tumors. The respective 10-year survival rates were 93%, 57%, and 23% (Fig. 1–2). The authors concluded that mitotic activity was the main discriminating criterion but warned that delay in fixation, especially in the center of large tumors, may artificially reduce mitotic counts.

The system published by Costa et al.,[58] based on a review of 163 sarcomas from the National Cancer Institute (NCI), gained strongest hold in the United States. It used a combination of histologic diagnosis (Table 1–3), cellularity, cellular pleomorphism, and mitotic rate as criteria for grading; but it also included necrosis as an important determinant for predicting recurrence and survival rates. The authors employed a three-grade system and stressed that grade 2 and 3 tumors exhibiting moderate or marked necrosis (>15%) had a significantly poorer prognosis; thus, necrosis emerged as a major discriminating variable. The respective 5-year survival rates of patients with the three grades were 100%, 73%, and 46%.

The French system published by Trojani et al.[77] was developed by the French Federation of Cancer Centers Sarcoma Group (FNCLCC) based on an analysis of 155 adult patients with soft tissue sarcomas. On the basis of a multivariate analysis of the various histologic features, it selects a combination of cellular differentiation, mitotic rate, and tumor necrosis as parameters for this grading

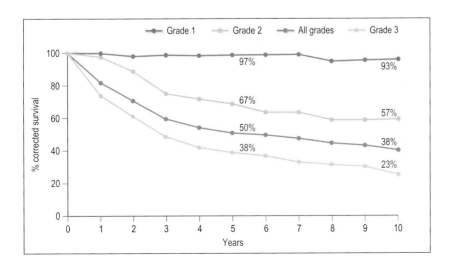

FIGURE 1–2 Grading system for soft tissue sarcomas based on three grades of malignancy. (From Myhre Jensen O, Kaae S, Madsen EH, et al. Histopathological grading in soft-tissue tumours: relation to survival in 261 surgically treated patients. Acta Pathol Microbiol Immunol Scand 1983; 91A:145.)

TABLE 1–3	ASSIGNED HISTOLOGIC GRADE ACCORDING TO HISTOLOGIC TYPE IN THE NCI SYSTEM			
Histologic type		**Grade 1**	**Grade 2**	**Grade 3**
Well-differentiated liposarcoma		+		
Myxoid liposarcoma		+		
Round cell liposarcoma			+	+
Pleomorphic liposarcoma				+
Fibrosarcoma			+	+
MFH, pleomorphic type			+	+
MFH, inflammatory type			+	+
MFH, myxoid type			+	
MFH, pleomorphic type			+	
DFSP		+		
Malignant granular cell tumor			+	+
Leiomyosarcoma		+	+	+
Malignant hemangiopericytoma		+	+	+
Rhabdomyosarcoma (all types)				+
Chondrosarcoma		+	+	+
Myxoid chondrosarcoma		+	+	
Mesenchymal chondrosarcoma				+
Osteosarcoma				+
Extraskeletal Ewing sarcoma				+
Synovial sarcoma				+
Epithelioid sarcoma			+	+
Clear cell sarcoma			+	+
Superficial MPNST			+	
Epithelioid MPNST			+	+
Malignant Triton tumor				+
Angiosarcoma			+	+
Alveolar soft part sarcoma				+
Kaposi sarcoma			+	+

Modified from Costa J, Wesley RA, Glatstein E, et al. The grading of soft tissue sarcomas: results of a clinicopathologic correlation in a series of 163 cases. Cancer 1984; 53:530. NCI, National Cancer Institute; MFH, malignant fibrous histiocytoma; DFSP, dermatofibrosarcoma protuberans; MPNST, malignant peripheral nerve sheath tumor. Tumor necrosis (microscopic) sarcoma for which the histologic typing is certain (e.g., alveolar soft part sarcoma).

TABLE 1–4	DEFINITIONS OF GRADING PARAMETERS FOR THE FNCLCC SYSTEM	
Parameter		**Criterion**
Tumor differentiation		
Score 1		Sarcoma closely resembling normal adult mesenchymal tissue (e.g., well-differentiated liposarcoma)
Score 2		Sarcomas for which histologic typing is certain (e.g., myxoid liposarcoma)
Score 3		Embryonal and undifferentiated sarcomas; sarcoma of uncertain type
Mitosis count		
Score 1		0–9/10 HPF
Score 2		10–19/10 HPF
Score 3		≥20/10 HPF
Tumor necrosis (microscopic)		
Score 0		No necrosis
Score 1		≤50% tumor necrosis
Score 2		>50% tumor necrosis
Histologic grade		
Grade 1		Total score 2, 3
Grade 2		Total score 4, 5
Grade 3		Total score 6, 7, 8

Modified from Coindre JM, Trojani M, Contesso G, et al. Reproducibility of a histopathologic grading system for adult soft tissue sarcomas. Cancer 1986; 58:306. FNCLCC, Fédération Nationale de Centres de Lutte Contre le Cancer; HPF, high-power field.

system. It assigns a score to each parameter and adds the scores together for a combined grade (Table 1–4). This study concluded that the histologic grade was the single most important factor for predicting survival rates; tumor depth (superficial versus deep) was another important prognostic parameter. The reproducibility of this system was tested by 15 pathologists; an agreement was reached in 81% of the cases for tumor necrosis, 74% for tumor differentiation, 73% for mitotic rate, and 75% for overall tumor grade, although the agreement as to histologic type was only 61%.

Both the FNLCC and NCI grading systems, the two most prevalent grading systems, have demonstrated prognostic value and share several features. Both emphasize the importance of recognizing histologic subtype (indirectly termed differentiation score in the French system) and both require an evaluation of the amount of necrosis. Both have undeniable shortcomings: the amount of necrosis emphasized by the NCI system is potentially affected by preferential sampling of necrotic and non-necrotic tissue and is not practical for evaluation of needle biopsy specimens. Moreover, retrospective analysis is complicated when an overall assessment of necrosis is not included in the gross description.

Although the French system relies on a more balanced evaluation of parameters (differentiation score, mitoses, necrosis), its principal weakness lies in the assignment of the differentiation score. Differentiation score is defined as the extent to which a tumor resembles adult mesenchymal tissue (score 1), the extent to which the histologic type is known (score 2), or the observation that the tumor is undifferentiated (score 3). Although a listing of the differentiation scores for the common tumors has been reported (Table 1–5), the rationale for some of these scores is not clear. For example, malignant fibrous histiocytoma is accorded a score of 2, whereas the inflammatory variant, an essentially identical lesion having inflammatory cells as its sole difference, is given a score of 3. There appears to be no scientific basis for this, but rather it seems to be a compensation factor to account for the worse prognosis of the retroperitoneal-based inflammatory malignant fibrous histiocytoma. Differentiation scores of 1, 2, or 3 may be given to fibrosarcoma, but the criteria for these distinctions are elusive. It must also be remembered that this system has been derived from resected specimens unmodified by treatment, a situation that is not analogous to our current practices, which are heavily weighted toward grading on biopsies or on resection specimens following irradiation or chemotherapy.

TABLE 1–5	TUMOR DIFFERENTIATION SCORE ACCORDING TO HISTOLOGIC TYPE IN THE UPDATED VERSION OF THE FNCLCC SYSTEM	
Histologic type		**Tumor differentiation score**
Well-differentiated liposarcoma		1
Myxoid liposarcoma		2
Round cell liposarcoma		3
Pleomorphic liposarcoma		3
Dedifferentiated liposarcoma		3
Well-differentiated fibrosarcoma		1
Conventional fibrosarcoma		2
Poorly differentiated fibrosarcoma		3
Well-differentiated MPNST		1
Conventional MPNST		2
Poorly differentiated MPNST		3
Epithelioid MPNST		3
Malignant triton tumor		3
Well-differentiated malignant hemangiopericytoma		2
Conventional malignant hemangiopericytoma		3
Myxoid MFH		2
Typical storiform/pleomorphic MFH		2
Giant-cell and inflammatory MFH		3
Well-differentiated leiomyosarcoma		1
Conventional leiomyosarcoma		2
Poorly differentiated/pleomorphic/epithelioid leiomyosarcoma		3
Biphasic/monophasic synovial sarcoma		3
Embryonal/alveolar/pleomorphic rhabdomyosarcoma		3
Well-differentiated chondrosarcoma		1
Myxoid chondrosarcoma		2
Mesenchymal chondrosarcoma		3
Conventional angiosarcoma		2
Poorly differentiated/epithelioid angiosarcoma		3
Extraskeletal osteosarcoma		3
Ewing sarcoma/PNET		3
Alveolar soft part sarcoma		3
Epithelioid sarcoma		3
Malignant rhabdoid tumor		3
Clear cell sarcoma		3
Undifferentiated sarcoma		3

Modified from Guillou L, Coindre J-M, Bonichon F, et al. Comparative study of the National Cancer Institute and French Federation of Cancer Centers Sarcoma Group grading systems in a population of 410 adult patients with soft tissue sarcoma. J Clin Oncol 1997; 15:350. PNET, primitive neuroectodermal tumor; see Tables 1–3 and 1–4 for other abbreviations.

Despite these issues and the fact that neither the NCI nor FNCLCC system has been formally endorsed either by the World Health Organization[51] or the Association of Directors of Anatomic and Surgical Pathology in the United States,[78] the French system is more universally used. In a recent study of soft tissue pathologists from 30 countries, more preferred the French system (37.3%) than the NCI (24%), Broders criteria (12%), Markhede system (1.3%) or other (15.3%)[79] systems, probably because it is more precisely defined and, therefore, reproducible. It also performs superiorly to the NCI system in a large dataset comparison. The two systems were compared by Guillou et al.[80] in adult patients with nonmeta-static soft tissue sarcomas. By univariate analysis, both systems were of prognostic value for predicting metastasis and overall survival. By multivariate analysis, a tumor size of 10 cm or more, a deep location, and a high tumor grade, irrespective of the system used, were found to be independent prognostic factors for the advent of metastases. Interestingly, there were grade discrepancies using these two grading systems in 34.6% of the cases. Use of the FNCLCC system resulted in an increased number of grade 3 tumors, a reduced number of grade 2 tumors, and a better correlation with overall and metastasis-free survival when compared with the NCI system.

LIMITATIONS OF GRADING

Despite the fact that there is widespread use of some form of grading system in the diagnosis and management of sarcomas, there is agreement among experts that no grading system performs well on every type of sarcoma. There are several reasons for this. In the most obvious situation, there are sarcomas in which the histologic subtype essentially defines behavior and, therefore, grade becomes redundant. This is best illustrated by well-differentiated liposarcoma (atypical lipomatous neoplasm), an inherently low-grade, nonmetastasizing lesion, and the majority of round cell sarcomas (e.g., alveolar rhabdomyosarcoma) which are inherently high grade.

A second problematic situation are the rare sarcomas that have been considered difficult, if not impossible, to grade. Epithelioid sarcoma, clear cell sarcoma, and alveolar soft part sarcoma are the most commonly cited examples of ungradable sarcomas, yet it is difficult to find a cogent explanation for this longstanding bias in the literature. It is possible that our grading systems fail to capture the correct histological information in grading these rare sarcomas or, perhaps, when compared to other sarcomas, nonhistological factors are far more influential in determining outcome than histological factors. What is clear, however, is that there is a substantial risk of distant metastasis in the long term, whereas in the short term (5 years), the interval for which traditional grading systems are most accurate, the risk may be low. Therefore, assignment of grade to these tumors does not guarantee biologic equivalency to other sarcomas of comparable grade.

In a number of sarcomas, clinical features play a larger role in determining prognosis. Cutaneous angiosarcomas are usually ungraded since multifocality and size are more predictive of outcome; paradoxically, angiosarcomas of deep soft tissue are probably amenable to grading. The difficulty of grading synovial sarcomas by histologic features has been noted in many studies,[81–83] leading Berghe et al.[84] to stratify synovial sarcoma into low and high risk groups using a combination of age, size, and presence or absence of poorly differentiated areas. Myxoid chondrosarcoma, long considered a low-grade lesion histologically, has late metastasis in approximately 40% of cases. By stratifying lesions by age, distal versus proximal location, and grade, Meis-Kindblom et al. were able to predict outcome.[85]

Leiomyosarcomas present another interesting paradigm. Various studies present conflicting views as to the predictive power of grading leiomyosarcomas, and there is emerging evidence that, as a group, myogenic tumors have a worse prognosis when matched for other variables.[86,87] Why this is true is not clear. However, a recent study, documenting the vascular origin of most somatic leiomyosarcomas, speculates that early hematogenous dissemination may account in part for this and proposes a risk model taking into account age, grade, and whether a tumor has been "disrupted" by prior surgical intervention.[88] Even among sarcomas that have traditionally been graded, we have begun to recognize the limitations of grading. For example, malignant peripheral nerve sheath tumors have customarily been graded, but the FNCLCC has recently indicated that assigned grade did not predict metastasis.

These models are not, strictly speaking, grading systems since they incorporate histologic, clinical, and demographic variables. Nonetheless, their use, most recently popularized with extragastrointestinal stromal tumors (see Chapter 19), gives some indication that we may gradually move in the direction of sarcoma-specific analyses which may be used in conjunction with or, in some cases, instead of grade. The advantage of such an approach is that it allows the most appropriate criteria to be employed for each sarcoma type to theoretically improve the ability to prognosticate. The disadvantage of this approach is that it presupposes an inordinate amount of clinical information for each sarcoma type, a challenge considering the rarity of these tumors of some of the subtypes. Moreover, the more specific these systems become, the more complicated they also become.

Another means of integrating clinical and pathologic data in a manner that accounts for sarcoma subtypes is the use of nomograms. This method collates multiple clinical and histologic parameters in a given patient and compares these data against a large population of patients with similar parameters whose outcome is known. A nomogram for 12-year sarcoma-specific mortality has been devised by Memorial Sloan Kettering Cancer Hospital (see Chapter 2).[89,90] Ultimately, nomograms could incorporate new molecular information with prognostic import.

In conclusion, despite the limitations noted above, grading remains one of the most powerful and inexpensive ways of assessing prognosis in a sarcoma and is currently regarded as a major independent predictor of metastasis in the major histologic types of adult soft tissue sarcomas.[91] Consequently, a grade should be provided by the pathologist, whenever possible. Putative

grade ranges for various sarcomas are shown in Figure 1–3. It should not be considered a substitute for an accurate histologic diagnosis, however. Grading, furthermore, plays no role in distinguishing benign and malignant lesions, and this distinction should always be made first, recognizing that some benign and reactive lesions may possess certain features (e.g., mitotic activity) that are also prevalent in sarcomas. Grading, like diagnosing soft tissue sarcomas, requires representative, well-fixed, well-stained histologic material which should be obtained prior to neoadjuvant therapy since this process alters many of the features necessary for accurate grading. Thick or heavily stained sections may be misleading since they may suggest less cellular differentiation than is actually present. Selection of the tissue sample and the length of fixation may also influence artificially the degree of necrosis and the mitotic index. Necrosis may be prominent in tumors that have been previously biopsied, irradiated, or embolized and, therefore, cannot be accurately assessed in these situations. Grading is usually based on the least differentiated area of a tumor unless it comprises a very minor component of the overall tumor.

STAGING SYSTEMS

Several staging systems have been developed for soft tissue sarcomas in an attempt to predict prognosis and to evaluate therapy by stratifying similar tumors according to prognostic factors such as histologic grade, tumor size, compartmentalization of the tumor, and the presence or absence of metastasis.[92] The two major staging systems used at present for adult soft tissue sarcomas were developed by The American Joint Committee on Cancer (AJCC)[69,70,93,94] and the Musculoskeletal Tumor Society as described by Enneking et al.[95-97] Each of these systems has advantages and disadvantages, as described below.

AJCC staging system

The original AJCC staging system was based on data obtained from a retrospective study of 702 sarcomas collected from 13 institutions. The study included only tumors that were diagnosed during the 15-year period 1954–1969, were histologically confirmed, had adequate follow-up information, and underwent primary treatment in the institution that contributed the specimen. Because the sample was too small to gain sufficient data on all well-defined soft tissue sarcomas, the staging system was limited to the eight most common types.[69,70] This system is based on the TNM staging system used for staging carcinomas, with the addition of histologic grade as a prognostic variable. Thus, the AJCC system, published in 1992,[93] is based on the size of the primary tumor (T), the involvement of lymph nodes (N), the presence of metastasis (M), and the type and grade of

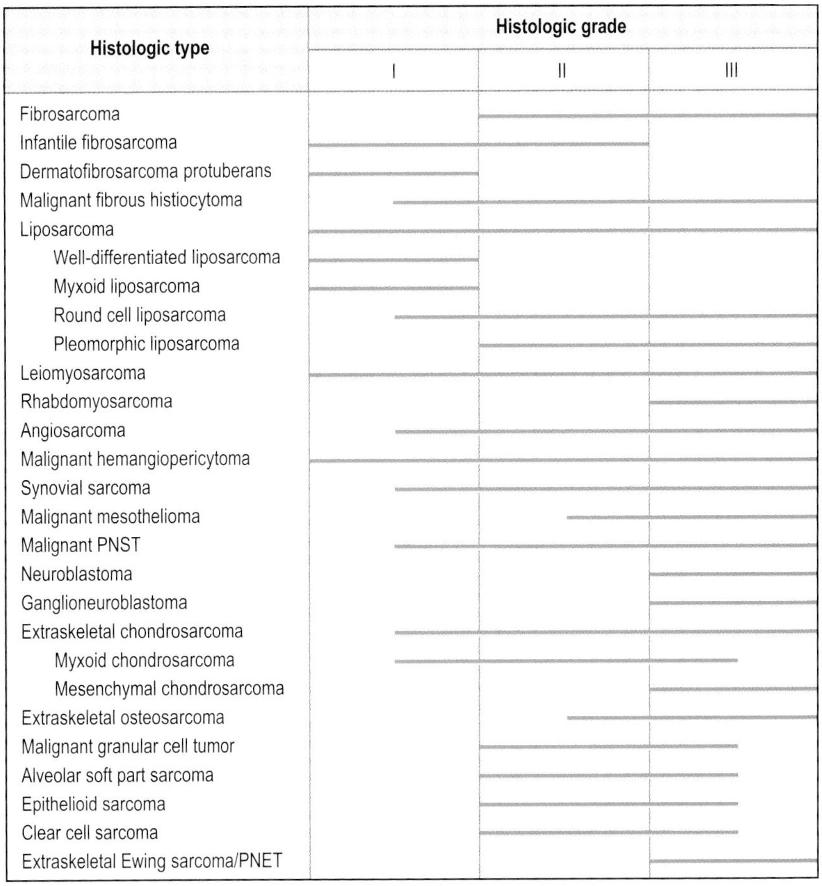

Histologic type	Histologic grade		
	I	II	III
Fibrosarcoma		——	——
Infantile fibrosarcoma	——	——	
Dermatofibrosarcoma protuberans	——		
Malignant fibrous histiocytoma	——	——	——
Liposarcoma	——	——	——
Well-differentiated liposarcoma	——		
Myxoid liposarcoma	——	——	
Round cell liposarcoma		——	——
Pleomorphic liposarcoma		——	——
Leiomyosarcoma	——	——	——
Rhabdomyosarcoma			——
Angiosarcoma	——	——	——
Malignant hemangiopericytoma	——	——	——
Synovial sarcoma	——	——	——
Malignant mesothelioma		——	——
Malignant PNST	——	——	——
Neuroblastoma			——
Ganglioneuroblastoma			——
Extraskeletal chondrosarcoma	——	——	——
Myxoid chondrosarcoma	——	——	——
Mesenchymal chondrosarcoma		——	——
Extraskeletal osteosarcoma		——	——
Malignant granular cell tumor	——	——	——
Alveolar soft part sarcoma	——	——	——
Epithelioid sarcoma	——	——	——
Clear cell sarcoma	——	——	——
Extraskeletal Ewing sarcoma/PNET			——

FIGURE 1–3 Soft tissue sarcomas. Estimated range of degree of malignancy based on histologic type and grade. Grade within the overall range depends on specific histologic features such as cellularity, cellular pleomorphism, mitotic activity, amount of stroma, infiltrative or expansive growth, and necrosis.

sarcoma (G). In 1997, several important modifications were made to the AJCC staging system.[94] Tumor depth, first shown to have prognostic significance in a large series of malignant fibrous histiocytomas by Weiss and Enzinger,[98,99] was subsequently incorporated into this staging system. In addition, grades 1 and 2 were grouped as low grade and grades 3 and 4 as high grade, whereas in a three-tiered grading system, grade 1 is considered "low grade" and grades 2 and 3 are "high grade." In the most recent AJCC staging system, the most significant change has been shifting of large, deep, low-grade lesions (G1T2bN0M0) from stage II to stage I (Table 1–6).[100]

Musculoskeletal Tumor Society staging system

The Enneking system, designed for sarcomas of both soft tissue and bone, distinguishes two anatomic settings: T1, intracompartmental tumors confined within the boundaries of well-defined anatomic structures, such as a functional muscle group, joint, and subcutis; and T2, extracompartmental neoplasms that arise within or involve secondarily extrafascial spaces or planes that have no natural anatomic barriers to extension. There are two grades (G1 and G2) and three stages. In this system, two grades are favored because they can be better related to the two surgical procedures (wide and radical excision) and because of the reported lack of any difference in the

metastatic rate between intermediate and high-grade tumors.[95–97] This staging system is summarized in Tables 1–7 and 1–8.

SIN system

Quite recently a new system, termed SIN, has been proposed, based on evaluation of three factors, size (S), vascular invasion (I), and necrosis (N) in 200 sarcomas derived from a large cohort of sarcoma patients treated in Sweden and France.[101] Each variable was analyzed in a dichotomous fashion (size $<$ or >8 cm; vascular invasion present/absent; necrosis present/absent). Outcome was strongly linked to the number of adverse factors and led to stratification into low- and high-risk groups. The low-risk group, defined as having 0–1 adverse factors, had an 81% 5-year survival compared to the high-risk group, having 2–3 adverse factors, with a 5-year survival of 32%. The authors suggest a binary or two-tiered system may offer an advantage over the AJCC system.

Advantages and disadvantages of staging systems

These two principal staging systems serve as a valuable guide to therapy and provide useful prognostic

TABLE 1–6 DEFINITIONS AND STAGING SYSTEM OF THE AMERICAN JOINT COMMITTEE ON CANCER

Primary tumor (T)
  TX Primary tumor cannot be assessed
  T0 No evidence of primary tumor
  T1 Tumor 5cm or less in greatest dimension
  T1a superficial tumor
  T1b deep tumor
Regional lymph nodes (N)
  NX Regional lymph nodes cannot be assessed
  N0 No regional lymph node metastasis
  N1 Regional lymph node metastasis

Distant metastasis (M)
  MX Distant metastasis cannot be assessed
  M0 No distant metastasis
  M1 Distant metastasis
Histopathologic grade
  GX Grade cannot be assessed
  G1 Well differentiated
  G2 Moderately differentiated
  G3 Poorly differentiated
  G4 Undifferentiated

Stage	Grade	Primary tumor	Regional lymph nodes	Distant metastasis
IA	G1 or G2	T1a or T1b	N0	M0
IB	G1 or G2	T2a	N0	M0
IIA	G1 or G2	T2b	N0	M0
IIB	G3 or G4	T1a or T1b	N0	M0
IIC	G3 or G4	T2a	N0	M0
III	G3 or G4	T2b	N0	M0
IV	Any G	Any T	N1	M0
	Any G	Any T	Any N	M1

From AJCC cancer staging handbook, 5th edn. Lippincott-Raven, Philadelphia, 1998 and Peabody TD, Gibbs CP, Simon MA. Evaluation and staging of musculoskeletal neoplasms. J Bone Joint Surg [Am] 1998; 86:1207.
Superficial tumor is located exclusively above the superficial fascia without invasion of the fascia; deep tumor is located either exclusively beneath the superficial fascia, or superficial to the fascia with invasion of or through the fascia, or superficial and beneath the fascia. Retroperitoneal, mediastinal, and pelvic sarcomas are classified as deep tumors.

TABLE 1–7 DEFINITIONS OF ANATOMIC EXTENT IN THE MUSCULOSKELETAL TUMOR SOCIETY STAGING SYSTEM

Intracompartmental (T1)		Extracompartmental (T2)
Intra-articular	→	Soft tissue extension
Superficial to deep fascia	→	Deep fascial extension
Paraosseous	→	Introsseous or extrafascial extension
Intrafascial compartment	→	Extrafascial compartment

Modified from Enneking WF, Spanier SS, Goodman MA. A system for the surgical staging of musculoskeletal sarcoma. Clin Orthop 1980; 153:106 and Peabody TD, Gibbs CP, Simon MA. Evaluation and staging of musculoskeletal neoplasms. J Bone Joint Surg [Am] 1998; 80:1204.

TABLE 1–8 MUSCULOSKELETAL TUMOR SOCIETY STAGING SYSTEM

Stage	Grade	Site	Metastasis
IA	G1	T1	M0
IB	G1	T2	M0
IIA	G2	T1	M0
IIB	G2	T2	M0
III	G1 or G2	T1 or T2	M1

Modified from Enneking WF, Spanier SS, Goodman MA. A system for the surgical staging of musculoskeletal sarcoma. Clin Orthop 1980; 153:106 and Peabody TD, Gibbs CP, Simon MA. Evaluation and staging of musculoskeletal neoplasms. J Bone Joint Surg [Am] 1998; 80:1204.

information. Although the AJCC system is applicable to soft tissue sarcomas at any site, the development of this system was based on studies that included lesions from a variety of anatomic locations, including the extremities, retroperitoneum, and head and neck. It is difficult to compare data from patients with tumors at these sites given the differences in the ability to eradicate tumors surgically in these anatomic locations. The AJCC system also uses 5 cm as an important dimension for determining prognosis, although the designation is somewhat arbitrary. The Musculoskeletal Tumor Society (Enneking) system, with its emphasis on compartmentalization, is most popular with surgeons and is best tailored for lesions in the extremities. It does not include the type, size, or depth of the tumor as separate parameters; and its two-tiered grading system may be too narrow for the wide biologic range of soft tissue sarcomas. Because of the need for adequately defining compartmentalization, the system does not lend itself to retrospective staging. Furthermore, this system was devised before the routine use of advanced imaging techniques such as magnetic resonance imaging and before the widespread use of adjuvant therapy.[92]

Obviously, staging soft tissue sarcomas requires a multidisciplinary approach with close cooperation among clinician, oncologist, and pathologist. In view of the relative rarity of these tumors, staging and grading are ideally carried out in large medical centers with special interest and experience in the diagnosis and management of soft tissue sarcomas. Moreover, prospective rather than retrospective studies are necessary to test the value of the various staging systems.

REFERENCES

Incidence

1. Jemal A, Siegel R, Ward E, et al. Cancer statistics, 2006. CA Cancer J Clin 2006; 56:106.
2. Ross JA, Severson RK, Davis S, et al. Trends in the incidence of soft tissue sarcomas in the United States from 1973 through 1987. Cancer 1993; 72:486.

Pathogenesis

3. Lavelle SM, Walton PW, Iomhair MM. Effect of irradiation, asbestos and chemical cocarcinogens on incidence of sarcoma on implants. Technol Health Care 2004; 12:217.
4. Aboulafia AJ, Brooks F, Piratzky J, et al. Osteosarcoma arising from heterotopic ossification after an electrical burn. A case report. J Bone Joint Surg [Am] 1999; 81:564.
5. Kirkpatrick CJ, Alves A, Kohler H, et al. Biomaterial-induced sarcoma: a novel model to study preneoplastic change. Am J Pathol 2000; 156:1455.
6. Wolf RF, Ng B, Weksler B, et al. Effect of growth hormone on tumor and host in an animal model. Ann Surg Oncol 1994; 1:314.
7. Madarnas P, Dube M, Rola-Pleszczynski M, et al. An animal model of Kaposi's sarcoma. II. Pathogenesis of dimethyl hydrazine induced angiosarcoma and colorectal cancer in three mouse strains. Anticancer Res 1992; 12:113.
8. Baas P, van 't Hullenaar N, Wagenaar J, et al. Occupational asbestos exposure: how to deal with suspected mesothelioma cases – the Dutch approach. Ann Oncol 2006; 17:848.
9. Price B, Ware A. Mesothelioma: risk apportionment among asbestos exposure sources. Risk Anal 2005; 25:937.
10. Fingerhut MA, Halperin WE, Marlow DA, et al. Cancer mortality in workers exposed to 2,3,7, 8-tetrachlorodibenzo-p-dioxin. N Engl J Med 1991; 324:212.
11. Kogevinas M, Becher H, Benn T, et al. Cancer mortality in workers exposed to phenoxy herbicides, chlorophenols, and dioxins. An expanded and updated international cohort study. Am J Epidemiol 1997; 145:1061.
12. Suruda AJ, Ward EM, Fingerhut MA. Identification of soft tissue sarcoma deaths in cohorts exposed to dioxin and to chlorinated naphthalenes. Epidemiology 1993; 4:14.
13. Costani G, Rabitti P, Mambrini A, et al. Soft tissue sarcomas in the general population living near a chemical plant in northern Italy. Tumori 2000; 86:381.
14. Tessari R, Canova C, Canal F, et al. Environmental pollution from dioxins and soft tissue sarcomas in the population of Venice and Mestre: an example of the use of current electronic information sources. Epidemiol Prev 2006; 30:191.
15. Eriksson M, Hardell L. Exposure to dioxins as a risk factor for soft tissue sarcoma: a population-based case-control study. J Natl Cancer Inst 1990; 82:486.
16. Hardell L, Eriksson M. The association between cancer mortality and dioxin exposure: a comment on the hazard of repetition of epidemiological misinterpretation. Am J Ind Med 1991; 19:547.
17. Hardell L, Eriksson M. Soft-tissue sarcoma and exposure to dioxins. Lancet 1986; 2:868.
18. Hardell L, Eriksson M, Axelson O. Agent Orange in war medicine: an aftermath myth. Int J Health Serv 1998; 28:715.
19. Hardell L, Eriksson M, Axelson O, et al. Increased risk of soft tissue sarcoma in persons exposed to dioxin. Lakartidningen 1991; 88:4005.
20. Bertazzi PA, Consonni D, Bachetti S, et al. Health effects of dioxin exposure: a 20-year mortality study. Am J Epidemiol 2001; 153:1031.
21. Balarajan R, Acheson ED. Soft tissue sarcomas in agriculture and forestry workers. J Epidemiol Community Health 1984; 38:113.
22. Smith AH, Patterson DG Jr, Warner ML, et al. Serum 2,3,7,8-tetrachlorodibenzo-p-dioxin levels of New Zealand pesticide applicators and their implication for cancer hypotheses. J Natl Cancer Inst 1992; 84:104.
23. Leiss JK, Savitz DA. Home pesticide use and childhood cancer: a case-control study. Am J Public Health 1995; 85:249.
24. Pahwa P, McDuffie HH, Dosman JA, et al. Hodgkin lymphoma, multiple myeloma, soft tissue sarcomas, insect repellents, and phenoxyherbicides. J Occup Environ Med 2006; 48:264.
25. Zahm SH, Ward MH. Pesticides and childhood cancer. Environ Health Perspect 1998; 106(Suppl 3):893.
26. Zahm SH, Fraumeni JF Jr. The epidemiology of soft tissue sarcoma. Semin Oncol 1997; 24:504.
27. Bertazzi PA, Zocchetti C, Guercilena S, et al. Dioxin exposure and cancer risk: A 15-year mortality study after the "Seveso accident." Epidemiology 1997; 8:646.
28. Kramarova E, Kogevinas M, Anh CT, et al. Exposure to Agent Orange and occurrence of soft-tissue sarcomas or non-Hodgkin lymphomas: an ongoing study in Vietnam. Environ Health Perspect 1998; 106(Suppl 2):671.
29. Clapp RW, Cupples LA, Colton T, et al. Cancer surveillance of veterans in Massachusetts, USA, 1982–1988. Int J Epidemiol 1991; 20:7.
30. Ward E, Boffetta P, Andersen A, et al. Update of the follow-up of mortality and cancer incidence among European workers employed in the vinyl chloride industry. Epidemiology 2001; 12:710.
31. Bosetti C, La Vecchia C, Lipworth L, et al. Occupational exposure to vinyl chloride and cancer risk: a review of the epidemiologic literature. Eur J Cancer Prev 2003; 12:427.
32. Rhomberg W. Exposure to polymeric materials in vascular soft-tissue sarcomas. Int Arch Occup Environ Health 1998; 71:343.
33. Mark RJ, Poen JC, Tran LM, et al. Angiosarcoma. A report of 67 patients and a review of the literature. Cancer 1996; 77:2400.
34. Billings SD, McKenney JK, Folpe AL, et al. Cutaneous angiosarcoma following breast-conserving surgery and radiation: an analysis of 27 cases. Am J Surg Pathol 2004; 28:781.
35. Arlen M, Higinbotham NL, Huvos AG, et al. Radiation-induced sarcoma of bone. Cancer 1971; 28:1087.
36. Patel SG, See AC, Williamson PA, et al. Radiation induced sarcoma of the head and neck. Head Neck 1999; 21:346.
37. Murray EM, Werner D, Greeff EA, et al. Postradiation sarcomas: 20 cases and a literature review. Int J Radiat Oncol Biol Phys 1999; 45:951.
38. Yap J, Chuba PJ, Thomas R, et al. Sarcoma as a second malignancy after treatment for breast cancer. Int J Radiat Oncol Biol Phys 2002; 52:1231.
39. Nakanishi H, Tomita Y, Myoui A, et al. Mutation of the p53 gene in postradiation sarcoma. Lab Invest 1998; 78:727.
40. Lipshutz GS, Brennan TV, Warren RS. Thorotrast-induced liver neoplasia: a collective review. J Am Coll Surg 2002; 195:713.
41. Ishikawa Y, Wada I, Fukumoto M. Alpha-particle carcinogenesis in Thorotrast patients: epidemiology, dosimetry, pathology, and molecular analysis. J Environ Pathol Toxicol Oncol 2001; 20:311.
42. Jenner RG, Boshoff C. The molecular pathology of Kaposi's sarcoma-associated herpesvirus. Biochim Biophys Acta 2002; 1602:1.
43. Schalling M, Ekman M, Kaaya EE, et al. A role for a new herpes virus (KSHV) in different forms of Kaposi's sarcoma. Nat Med 1995; 1:707.
44. Chang Y, Cesarman E, Pessin MS, et al. Identification of herpesvirus-like DNA sequences in AIDS-associated Kaposi's sarcoma. Science 1994; 266:1865.
45. Deyrup AT, Lee VK, Hill CE, et al. Epstein-Barr virus-associated smooth muscle tumors are distinctive mesenchymal tumors reflecting multiple infection events: a clinicopathologic and molecular analysis of 29 tumors from 19 patients. Am J Surg Pathol 2006; 30:75.
46. Cueni LN, Detmar M. New insights into the molecular control of the lymphatic vascular system and its role in disease. J Invest Dermatol 2006; 126:2167.
47. Roy P, Clark MA, Thomas JM. Stewart-Treves syndrome – treatment and outcome in six patients from a single centre. Eur J Surg Oncol 2004; 30:982.
48. Ruocco V, Schwartz RA, Ruocco E. Lymphedema: an immunologically vulnerable site for development of neoplasms. J Am Acad Dermatol 2002; 47:124.
49. Offori TW, Platt CC, Stephens M, et al. Angiosarcoma in congenital hereditary lymphoedema (Milroy's disease) – diagnostic beacons and a review of the literature. Clin Exp Dermatol 1993; 18:174.

Classification of soft tissue tumors

50. Fletcher CDM. The evolving classification of soft tissue tumours: an update based on the new WHO classification. Histopathology 2006; 48:3.
51. Fletcher CDM, Unni KK, Mertens FE. World Health Organization classification of tumours. pathology and genetics of tumours of soft tissue and bone. Lyon: IARC Press; 2002.
52. Markhede G, Angervall L, Stener B. A multivariate analysis of the prognosis after surgical treatment of malignant soft-tissue tumors. Cancer 1982; 49:1721.

Grading and staging soft tissue sarcomas

53. Kilpatrick SE. Histologic prognostication in soft tissue sarcomas: grading versus subtyping or both? A comprehensive review of the literature with proposed practical guidelines. Ann Diag Pathol 1999; 3:48.
54. Deyrup AT, Weiss SW. Grading of soft tissue sarcoma: the challenge of providing precise information in an imprecise world. Histopathology 2006; 48:42.

Grading systems

55. Broders AC, Hargrave R, Meyerding HW. Pathological features of soft tissue fibrosarcoma: with special reference to the grading of its malignancy. Surg Gynecol Obstet 1939; 69:267.
56. Coindre JM, Terrier P, Bui MB, et al. Prognostic factors in adult patients with locally controlled soft tissue sarcoma: a study of 546 patients from the French Federation of Cancer Centers Sarcoma Group. J Clin Oncol 1996; 14:869.
57. Coindre JM, Trojani M, Contesso G, et al. Reproducibility of a histopathologic grading system for adult soft tissue sarcoma. Cancer 1986; 58:306.
58. Costa J, Wesley RA, Glatstein E, et al. The grading of soft tissue sarcomas: results of a clinicohistopathologic correlation in a series of 163 cases. Cancer 1984; 53:530.
59. Jensen V, Hoyer M, Sorensen FB, et al. MIB-1 expression and iododeoxyuridine labelling in

soft tissue sarcomas: An immunohistochemical study including correlations with p53, bcl-2 and histological characteristics. Histopathology 1996; 28:437.

60. Jensen V, Sorensen FP, Bentzen SM, et al. Proliferative activity (MIB-1 index) is an independent prognostic parameter in patients with high-grade soft tissue sarcomas of subtypes other than malignant fibrous histiocytoma: A retrospective immunohistological study including 216 soft tissue sarcomas. Histopathology 1998; 32:536.

61. Parham DM, Webber BL, Jenkins JJ, et al. Non-rhabdomyosarcomatous soft tissue sarcomas of childhood: formulation of a simplified system for grading. Mod Pathol 1995; 8:705.

62. Rooser B, Attewell R, Berg MO, et al. Prognostication in soft tissue sarcoma: a model with four risk factors. Cancer 1988; 61:817.

63. Tsujimoto M, Aozasa K, Ueda T, et al. Multivariate analysis for histologic prognostic factors in soft tissue sarcomas. Cancer 1988; 62:994.

64. Hasegawa T, Yamamoto S, Yokoyama R, et al. Prognostic significance of grading and staging systems using MIB-1 score in adult patients with soft tissue sarcoma of the extremities and trunk. Cancer 2002; 95:843.

65. Hasegawa T, Yokoyama R, Lee YH, et al. Prognostic relevance of a histological grading system using MIB-1 for adult soft tissue sarcoma. Oncology 2000; 58:66.

66. Swanson SA, Brooks JJ. Proliferation markers Ki-67 and p105 in soft tissue lesions: correlation with DNA flow cytometric characteristics. Am J Pathol 1990; 137:1491.

67. Ueda T, Aozasa K, Tsujimoto M, et al. Prognostic significance of Ki-67 reactivity in soft tissue sarcomas. Cancer 1989; 63:1607.

68. Bastiannet E, Groen H, Jager PL, et al. The value of PDG-PET in the detection, grading and response to therapy of soft tissue and bone sarcoma: a systematic review of meta-analysis. Cancer Treat Rev 2004; 30:83.

69. Russell WO, Cohen J, Cutler S, et al. Staging system for soft tissue sarcoma. In: Task Force on Soft Tissue Sarcoma. American Joint Committee for Cancer staging and end results reporting. Chicago: American College of Surgeons; 1980.

70. Russell WO, Cohen J, Enzinger FM, et al. A clinical and pathological staging system for soft tissue sarcomas. Cancer 1977; 40:1562.

71. Myhre Jensen O, Hgh J, Stgaard SE, et al. Histopathological grading of soft tissue tumours: prognostic significance in a prospective study of 278 consecutive cases. J Pathol 1991; 163:19.

72. Myhre Jensen O, Kaae S, Madsen EH, et al. Histopathological grading in soft tissue tumours: relation to survival in 261 surgically treated patients. Acta Pathol Microbiol Immunol Scand 1983; 91A:145.

73. Hashimoto H, Daimaru Y, Takeshita S, et al. Prognostic significance of histologic parameters of soft tissue sarcomas. Cancer 1992; 70:2816.

74. Van Unnik JA, Coindre JM, Contesso C, et al. Grading of soft tissue sarcomas: experience of the EORTC soft tissue and bone sarcoma group. Eur J Cancer 1993; 29A:2089.

75. Gustafson P. Soft tissue sarcoma: epidemiology and prognosis in 508 patients. Acta Orthop Scand Suppl 1994; 259:1.

76. Kandel RA, Bell RS, Wunder JS, et al. Comparison between a 2- and 3-grade system in predicting metastatic-free survival in extremity soft-tissue sarcoma. J Surg Oncol 1999; 72:77.

77. Trojani M, Contesso G, Coindre JM, et al. Soft tissue sarcomas of adults: study of pathological and prognostic variables and definition of a histological grading system. Int J Cancer 1984; 33:37.

78. Association of Directors of Anatomic and Surgical Pathology. Recommendations for the reporting of soft tissue sarcomas. Hum Pathol 1999; 30:3.

79. Golouh R, Bracko M. What is the current practice in soft tissue sarcoma grading? Radiol Oncol 2001; 35:47.

80. Guillou L, Coindre J, Bonichon F, et al. Comparative study of the National Cancer Institute and French Federation of Cancer Centers Sarcoma Group grading systems in a population of 410 adult patients with soft tissue sarcoma. J Clin Oncol 1997; 15:350.

Limitations of grading

81. Wright PH, Sim FH, Soule EH, et al. Synovial sarcoma. J Bone Joint Surg [Am] 1982. 64:112.

82. Soule EH. Synovial sarcoma. Am J Surg Pathol 1986; 10:78.

83. Oda Y, Hashimoto H, Tsuneyoshi M, et al. Survival in synovial sarcoma: a multivariate study of prognostic factors with special emphasis on the comparison between early death and long term survival. Am J Surg Pathol 1993; 17:35.

84. Bergh P, Meis-Kindblom JM, Gherlinzoni F, et al. Synovial sarcoma: identification of low and high risk groups. Cancer 1999; 85:2596.

85. Meis-Kindblom JM, Bergh P, Gunterberg B, et al. Extraskeletal myxoid chondrosarcoma: a reappraisal of its morphologic spectrum and prognostic factors based on 117 cases. Am J Surg Pathol 1999; 23:636.

86. Deyrup AT, Haydon RC, Huo D, et al. Myoid differentiation and prognosis in adult pleomorphic sarcomas of the extremity: an analysis of 92 cases. Cancer 2003; 98:805.

87. Koea JB, Leung D, Lewis JJ, et al. Histopathologic type: an independent prognostic factor in primary soft tissue sarcoma of the extremity. Ann Surg Oncol 2003; 10:432.

88. Farshid G, Pradhan M, Goldblum J, et al. Leiomyosarcoma of somatic soft tissues: a tumor of vascular origin with multivariate analysis of outcome in 42 cases. Am J Surg Pathol 2002; 26:14.

89. Kattan MW, Leung DH, Brennan MF. Postoperative monogram for 12-year sarcoma-specific death. J Clin Oncol 2002; 20:791.

90. Eilber FC, Brennan MF, Eilber FR, et al. Validation of the postoperative nomogram for 12-year sarcoma-specific mortality. Cancer 2004; 101:2270.

91. Coindre JM, Terrier P, Guillou L, et al. Predictive value of grade for metastasis development in the main histologic types of adult soft tissue sarcomas. Cancer 2001; 91:1914.

Staging systems

92. Peabody TD, Gibbs CP, Simon MA. Evaluation and staging of musculoskeletal neoplasms. J Bone Joint Surg [Am] 1998; 80:1204.

93. Beahrs OH, Henson DE, Hutter RVP, et al. Manual for staging of cancer. 3rd edn. Philadelphia: Lippincott; 1992.

94. Fleming ID, Cooper JS, Henson GE, et al. AJCC cancer staging manual. 5th edn. Philadelphia: Lippincott-Raven; 1997.

95. Enneking WF. Musculoskeletal tumor surgery. New York: Churchill Livingstone; 1983.

96. Enneking WF, Spanier SS, Goodman MA. A system for the surgical staging of musculoskeletal sarcoma. Clin Orthop 1980; 153:106.

97. Enneking WF, Spanier SS, Malawar MM. The effect of the anatomic setting on the results of surgical procedures for soft part sarcoma of the thigh. Cancer 1981; 47:1005.

98. Weiss SW, Enzinger FM. Malignant fibrous histiocytoma: an analysis of 200 cases. Cancer 1978; 41:2250.

99. Weiss SW, Enzinger FM. Myxoid variant of malignant fibrous histiocytoma. Cancer 1977; 39:1672.

100. Greene FL, Page DL, Fleming ID, et al. AJCC cancer staging manual. 6th edn. New York: Springer-Verlag; 2002.

101. Gustafson P, Akerman M, Alvegard TA, et al. Prognostic information in soft tissue sarcoma using tumour size, vascular invasion and microscopic tumour necrosis – the SIN system. Eur J Cancer 2003; 39:1568.

CLINICAL EVALUATION AND TREATMENT OF SOFT TISSUE TUMORS

Peter W.T. Pisters

CHAPTER CONTENTS

INTRODUCTION

Although soft tissue sarcomas are a heterogeneous group of neoplasms, their clinical evaluation and treatment follow common principles. This chapter will focus on the clinical evaluation, determinants of prognosis and outcome, and treatment of patients with soft tissue sarcomas.

The frequency and anatomic distribution of 5781 consecutive patients with soft tissue sarcoma, referred to the University of Texas M.D. Anderson Cancer Center, are outlined in Figure 2–1. These data illustrate that the extremity is the most common anatomic site, accounting for approximately one-half of all cases. Other important anatomic sites include the retroperitoneum, head and neck, and body wall. The site-specific distribution of histologic subtypes is outlined in Figure 2.1. Of note, distribution of histologic subtypes is very dependent on anatomic site; for example, in the extremity, malignant fibrous histiocytoma (pleomorphic undifferentiated sarcoma), liposarcoma, and synovial sarcoma are common. In contrast, in the retroperitoneum, synovial sarcoma and malignant fibrous histiocytoma are relatively uncommon and other histologic subtypes, particularly leiomyosarcoma and liposarcoma, predominate. The reasons for this regional variation in histologic subtype are not understood.

CLINICAL EVALUATION

Clinical presentation and assessment

Most patients with suspected soft tissue neoplasms present with a painless mass, although pain is reported in one-third of cases.[1] Delay in diagnosis is common; the most common misdiagnoses include post-traumatic or spontaneous hematoma and "lipoma." Late diagnosis of patients with retroperitoneal sarcomas is very common because of the large size of the retroperitoneal space, generally slow growth rate, and the tendency of sarcomas to gradually displace rather than to invade and compromise adjacent viscera. Thus, retroperitoneal sarcomas can reach considerable size before diagnosis (Fig. 2–2).

Physical examination should include assessment of tumor size, relative mobility, and fixation. Patients with extremity soft tissue tumors should be evaluated for tumor-related neuropathy. Examination of regional lymph node basins should also be performed with the understanding that nodal metastases are relatively uncommon, occurring in less than 15% of patients with extremity soft tissue sarcomas.[2]

Pretreatment evaluation

The pretreatment evaluation of the patient with a suspected soft tissue malignancy includes biopsy diagnosis and radiologic staging to establish the extent of disease. Practical algorithms for evaluation of patients with extremity and retroperitoneal soft tissue masses are outlined in Figures 2–3 and 2–4.

Biopsy

Pretreatment biopsy of the primary tumor is essential for most patients presenting with soft tissue masses. In general, any soft tissue mass that is enlarging or is larger than 5 cm should be considered for biopsy. The preferred biopsy method is generally the least invasive technique that allows for definitive histologic assessment, including assessment of grade. Grade is particularly important to clinicians as it impacts treatment planning and treatment options.

Percutaneous core-needle biopsy (CNB) provides satisfactory diagnostic tissue for the diagnosis of most soft tissue neoplasms. CNB can be performed "blindly" in the clinic by clinicians without real-time radiologic control. However, many centers have moved to image-guided CNB performed by interventional radiologists.

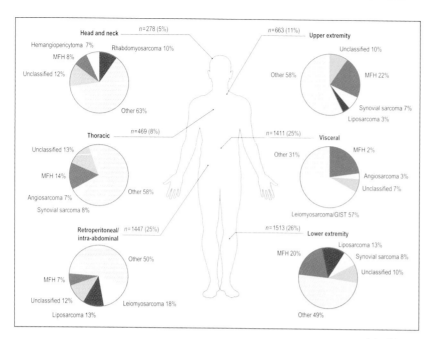

FIGURE 2–1 Anatomic distribution and site-specific histologic subtypes of 5781 consecutive soft tissue sarcomas seen at the University of Texas M.D. Anderson Cancer Center (MDACC Sarcoma Database, June 1996 to June 2006).

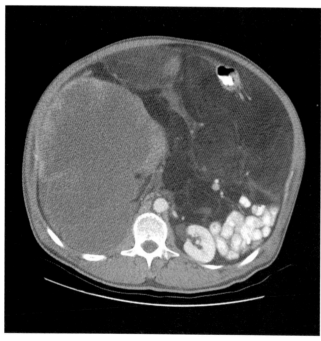

FIGURE 2–2 Contrast enhanced CT scan of a 52-year-old patient with retroperitoneal dedifferentiated liposarcoma. The CT findings illustrate both features of both well- and de-differentiated forms of liposarcoma which frequently coexist. The dedifferentiated component is the more solid-appearing, low-density mass situated in the right retroperitoneum while the well-differentiated component appears of disease has similar density to the subcutaneous (normal) fat and fills the retroperitoneum, displacing the contrast-filled small bowel to the anatomic left side and posteriorly.

Image-guided approaches allow for biopsy from the areas of the tumor felt to be most likely to harbor viable tumor (i.e., avoiding centrally necrotic areas). The use of real-time imaging also minimizes the risks for biopsy-related vascular or adjacent organ injury. In many centers, image-guided biopsy also allows for real-time pathology quality control by having a pathologist immediately available in the biopsy suite to evaluate the quality of tissue retrieved and its probable suitability for definitive diagnosis. Studies comparing CNB to traditional open surgical biopsy have demonstrated the safety, reliability, and cost-effectiveness of this approach.[3–5] Additional issues related to pathologic interpretation of CNB are discussed in Chapter 6.

Tumor recurrence in the needle track after percutaneous CNB is extremely rare. Indeed, there are only case reports in the literature. However, these rare cases have led some physicians to advocate tattooing the biopsy site for subsequent excision.[6] We have generally taken a practical approach to this issue and perform en-bloc resection of the needle track and percutaneous entry point when feasible but not if resection of the biopsy track requires a second incision or substantial modification of the surgical plan. The rare risks for needle track recurrence do not justify the added morbidity risk imposed by major alterations in the surgical plan.

Incisional biopsy is occasionally required to establish a definitive diagnosis for some soft tissue neoplasms. It has the advantage over CNB of providing more tissue for pathologic analysis and often additional tissue for tumor banking purposes. However, the morbidity of incisional biopsy can be considerable and includes the risks for anesthesia, bleeding, and wound healing problems. Given these risks and the greater financial costs of incisional biopsy, incisional biopsy is generally a secondary technique that may best be reserved for cases where a definitive diagnosis cannot be established by CNB.

Excisional biopsy may be appropriate for some patients who present with small superficial neoplasms located on the extremity or superficial body wall where the morbidity from this procedure is minimal. Although incisional biopsy may allow for a single diagnostic and therapeutic

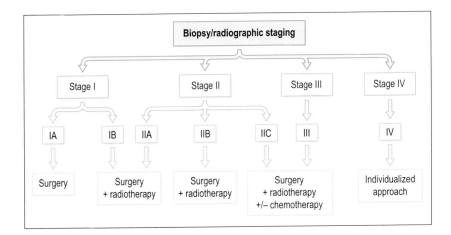

FIGURE 2–3 Pretreatment evaluation and staging algorithm for assessment of the patient presenting with an extremity soft tissue mass. AJCC, American Joint Commission on Cancer.[86] (From Pisters PWT, Ann Surg Oncol 1998; 5:464.

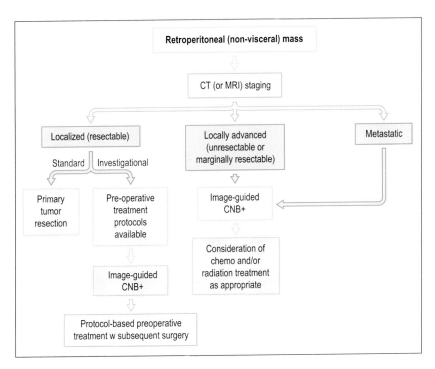

FIGURE 2–4 Pretreatment evaluation, staging, and treatment algorithm for assessment of the patient presenting with a retroperitoneal (non-visceral) mass. Patients should undergo pretreatment cross-sectional imaging by CT or MRI. Localized, radiologically resectable masses that are believed to be neoplastic can be treated by diagnostic and therapeutic primary tumor resection. In clinical settings, where preoperative treatment protocols are available, pretreatment image-guided core needle biopsy (CNB) should be used to establish the diagnosis of sarcoma for protocol eligibility. Patients with locally advanced (radiologically unresectable) or metastatic disease should undergo CNB for diagnosis followed by consideration of non-surgical treatments. In general, CNB is sufficient for diagnosis and surgery performed exclusively for diagnostic purposes (e.g., laparotomy for incisional biopsy) should be avoided whenever possible.

procedure in some clinical settings, its main disadvantage is that the malignant potential of the neoplasm is unknown at the time of biopsy and informed decisions on surgical margins are not possible. This leaves the operating surgeon with the choice of narrow or nonexistent surgical margins with generally lower risks for wound and functional morbidity or deliberately wide margins with generally greater risks for wound and functional morbidity. The oncologic appropriateness of the surgical margin cannot be assessed preoperatively and is difficult to assess with precision intraoperatively. This disadvantage makes excisional biopsy appropriate only for a small subset of patients who have small, superficial neoplasms and for whom re-excision is feasible should the final diagnosis indicate a malignant lesion with compromised margins.

Percutaneous fine needle aspiration (FNA) biopsy can also be used for cytologic assessment of some soft tissue neoplasms.[7,8] Accurate FNA diagnosis requires the avail-

ability of an expert cytopathologist experienced in the diagnosis of soft tissue sarcomas by cytology. From a practical standpoint, most centers (even academic centers) will not have a cytopathologist with sufficient experience to allow for use of FNA for routine diagnosis and classification of primary soft tissue neoplasms. Given the frequent difficulty in histopathologic diagnosis and classification of soft tissue sarcomas, the major utility of FNA cytology in most centers is for diagnosis of patients with suspected recurrent sarcoma. In such settings, there is already an established pathologic diagnosis such that only confirmation of a recurrence with similar features is required.

Staging

The relative rarity of soft tissue sarcomas, the anatomic heterogeneity of these lesions, and the presence of more than 50 recognized histologic subtypes of variable grades have made it difficult to establish a functional system that can accurately stage all forms of this disease. The staging system (6th edition) of the American Joint Committee on Cancer (AJCC) and the International Union Against Cancer (UICC) is the most widely employed staging system for soft-tissue sarcomas and is presented in Chapter 6.[9] The system is designed to optimally stage extremity tumors but is also applicable to torso, head and neck, and retroperitoneal lesions; it should not be used for sarcomas of the gastrointestinal tract or other parenchymal organs.

A major limitation of the present staging system is that it does not take into account the anatomic site of soft tissue sarcomas. Anatomic site, however, has been recognized as an important determinant of outcome.[10,11] Although site is not a specific component of any present staging system, outcome data should be reported on a site-specific basis.

PROGNOSTIC FACTORS

Clinicopathologic factors

Understanding the clinicopathologic factors that affect outcome is essential in formulating a treatment plan for the patient with soft tissue sarcoma. The three major clinicopathologic factors that establish the risk profile for a given patient are tumor size, anatomic depth relative to the investing fascia of the extremity or body wall musculature (superficial versus deep), and histologic grade.[12–14] Indeed these factors are all components of the AJCC staging system for soft tissue sarcoma.

In addition to the foregoing factors, anatomic site, histologic subtype, and margins status are also significant, but regrettably this information is not captured by the current staging system. Moreover, unlike other solid tumors, factors that predict local recurrence are different from those that predict distant metastasis and tumor-related death (Table 2–1).[12] In other words, patients with a constellation of adverse prognostic factors for local recurrence are not necessarily at increased risk for distant metastasis or tumor-related death and vice versa. Thus, clinicians and pathologists should be careful about using the terminology "high-risk disease" without qualification of which end point (local recurrence or overall survival) for which the patient is believed to be at increased risk.

Classification and prognostic significance of surgical margins

Surgeons should use the UICC resection (designated by the letter "R") classification system for integration of the operative findings and the final microscopic surgical margins. Under this classification system, an R0 resection is defined as macroscopically complete sarcoma resection with microscopically negative surgical margins; an R1 resection is macroscopically complete sarcoma resection with microscopically positive surgical margins, and an R2 resection is macroscopically incomplete (i.e., with gross residual disease) and microscopically positive surgical margins.

All therapeutic surgical procedures should be described in medical records using the R classification. To do so,

TABLE 2–1	**MULTIVARIATE ANALYSIS OF PROGNOSTIC FACTORS IN PATIENTS WITH EXTREMITY SOFT TISSUE SARCOMA**	
Endpoint	**Adverse prognostic factor**	**Relative risk**
Local recurrence	Fibrosarcoma	2.5
	Local recurrence at presentation	2.0
	Microscopically positive margin	1.8
	Malignant peripheral nerve sheath tumor	1.8
	Age >50 years	1.6
Distant recurrence	High grade	4.3
	Deep location	2.5
	Size 5.0–9.9 cm	1.9
	Leiomyosarcoma	1.7
	Nonliposarcoma histology	1.6
	Local recurrence at presentation	1.5
	Size ≥10.0 cm	1.5
Disease-specific survival	High grade	4.0
	Deep location	2.8
	Size ≥10.0 cm	2.1
	Malignant peripheral nerve sheath tumor	1.9
	Leiomyosarcoma	1.9
	Microscopically positive margin	1.7
	Lower extremity site	1.6
	Local recurrence at presentation	1.5

Adverse prognostic factors identified are independent by Cox regression analysis.[12] From Pisters et al. with permission from J Clin Oncol.

surgeons must await the final pathology report including margin assessment and then integrate the observed operative findings including the presence or absence of residual gross tumor with the final assessment of microscopic surgical margins. The operative report, discharge summary, and related medical records should describe the procedure using the R classification. As an example, a surgical procedure that involved wide local resection of a left anterior thigh soft tissue leiomyosarcoma with satisfactory gross tumor margins, no operatively defined residual gross tumor, and negative microscopic surgical margins would be described as "R0 resection of left anterior thigh leiomyosarcoma."

The type of microscopically positive surgical margins also appears important. For example, an R1 resection for a low-grade liposarcoma or an R1 after preoperative radiation treatment in which a microscopically positive margin is anticipated (and accepted) in order to preserve critical structures have a relatively low risk (<10%) for local recurrence.[15] In contrast, patients undergoing "unplanned" excision followed by a re-excision with positive margins (i.e., R1 re-resection) or patients with unanticipated positive margins after primary resection are at increased risk for local recurrence with local recurrence rates approaching 30%. Thus, the specific clinical setting needs to be considered when interpreting the relative risk for local recurrence after R1 resection.

Nomograms for assessment of individual patient prognosis

Kattan and colleagues from the Memorial Sloan-Kettering Cancer Center (MSKCC) have utilized a database of over 2000 prospectively followed adult patients with soft tissue sarcoma to predict the probability of sarcoma-specific death by 12 years.[10] The results have been used to construct and internally validate a nomogram to predict sarcoma-specific death (Fig. 2–5). This nomogram matches a patient's prognostic score against those of previously treated patients with comparable tumor and patient factors to estimate individual patient risk for sarcoma-related death. The MSKCC nomogram has been externally validated[16,17] and is considered to be an extremely valuable tool for individual patient counseling and determination of the frequency for individual patient follow-up. The nomogram is available for downloading to personal digital assistant devices at *www.nomograms.org*

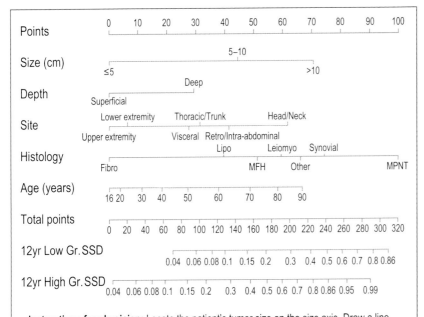

Instructions for physician: Locate the patient's tumor size on the size axis. Draw a line straight upwards to the points axis to determine how many points towards sarcoma-specific death the patient receives for his tumor size. Repeat this process for the other axis, each time drawing straight upward to the points axis. Sum the points achieved for each predictor and locate this sum on the Total Points axis. Draw a line straight down to either the Low Grade or High Grade axis to find the patient's probability of dying from sarcoma within 12 years assuming he or she does not die of another cause first.

Instruction to patient: "If we had 100 patients exactly like you, we would expect between <predicted percentage from nomogram –8%> and <predicted percentage + 8%> to die of sarcoma within 12 years if they did not die of another cause first, and death from sarcoma after 12 years is still possible."

FIGURE 2–5 Postoperative nomogram for 12-year sarcoma-specific deaths, in 2163 patients treated at Memorial Sloan-Kettering Cancer Center. Fibro, fibrosarcoma; Lipo, liposarcoma; Leiomyo, leiomyosarcoma; MFH, malignant fibrous histiocytoma; MPNT, malignant peripheral-nerve sheath tumor; GR, grade; SSD, sarcoma-specific death.[10] (From Kattan MW et al. J Clin Oncol 2002; 20:791, with permission.)

TREATMENT OF LOCALIZED PRIMARY EXTREMITY SARCOMAS

Surgery

Surgical resection remains the cornerstone of therapy for localized primary soft tissue sarcoma (STS). The discussion which follows focuses on soft tissue sarcomas in the limbs, the most common anatomic site of origin, but the principles of treatment are generally applicable for patients with sarcomas at other anatomic sites.

Historically, amputation was the primary treatment for patients with extremity STS. However, over the past 20 years, there has been a marked decline in the rate of amputation as the primary therapy for extremity STS. With the widespread application of multimodality treatment strategies, the vast majority of patients with localized soft tissue sarcoma of the extremities undergo limb-sparing treatment, and less than 10% of patients presently undergo amputation.[18,19]

Satisfactory local resection involves resection of the primary tumor with a margin of normal tissue around the lesion. Dissection along the tumor pseudocapsule (enucleation or "shelling out") is associated with local recurrence rates ranging between 33% and 63%.[20-22] In contrast, wide local excision with a margin of normal tissue around the lesion is associated with lower local recurrence rates in the range of 10–31%, as demonstrated in the surgery-alone control arms of randomized trials evaluating postoperative radiation therapy (RT) and in single-institution reports.[23-25]

The issue of what constitutes an acceptable gross surgical margin is complex, and there are limited prospective data specifically addressing surgical margins in STS surgery. Circumferential margin assessment in sarcomas is imprecise owing to the complex anatomy of each of these tumors and the tendency of soft tissue around the tumor to collapse and adopt its inherent shape when not under the continuous tension that is applied to the tissues as part of modern soft tissue surgery. This can result in significant discordance between the intraoperative perception and the pathologic evaluation of the gross surgical margin.

Unlike resections for cutaneous melanoma in which gross surgical margins can be measured with a ruler at the time of surgery, gross margins assessment for a soft tissue sarcoma cannot be measured so precisely. In addition, it is likely that not all soft tissues provide an equivalent barrier to tumor extension. For example, it is believed that a smaller gross margin that includes a fascial barrier is, in general, a more secure margin than a comparable gross margin that does not include fascia. For many of these reasons, margin assessment for sarcomas by both surgeons and pathologists will continue to have an unavoidable degree of imprecision that probably exceeds the inherent imprecision in the assessment of gross margins of other solid tumors.

Combined modality limb-sparing treatment

Currently, approximately 90% of patients with localized extremity sarcomas undergo limb-sparing treatment.[18,26] The use of limb-sparing multimodality treatment approaches for extremity sarcoma was based on an important phase III trial from the US National Cancer Institute (NCI) in which patients with extremity sarcomas amenable to limb-sparing surgery were randomly assigned to receive amputation or limb-sparing surgery with postoperative RT.[27,28] Both arms of this trial included postoperative chemotherapy with doxorubicin, cyclophosphamide, and methotrexate. With more than 9 years of follow-up information, this study established that for patients for whom limb-sparing surgery is an option, limb-sparing surgery combined with postoperative RT and chemotherapy yielded disease-related survival rates comparable to those for amputation and simultaneously preserved a functional extremity.[27,28] This trial established limb-sparing treatment as the standard treatment for patients with localized extremity soft tissue sarcoma. Amputation is used only in clinical settings in which local tumor anatomy precludes limb-sparing approaches most commonly as a result of tumor involvement of functionally significant neurovascular structures.

In the modern era, a discussion of limb-preserving approaches must be linked to discussion of the role of adjuvant therapies, most commonly radiation treatment. Several randomized, controlled trials have addressed issues surrounding the use of adjuvant therapy and collectively have established important milestones in the evolution of the local management of soft tissue sarcomas.

Yang et al. randomized 91 patients with high-grade extremity lesions following limb-sparing surgery to receive adjuvant chemotherapy alone or concurrent chemotherapy and RT.[24] An additional 50 patients with low-grade tumors were to receive adjuvant RT or no further treatment following limb-sparing surgery. The local control rate for those who received RT was 99% compared to 70% in the non-RT group ($p = 0.0001$).[24] The results were similar for high- and low-grade tumors (Table 2–2).

Adjuvant radiation using brachytherapy was also evaluated at the Memorial Sloan-Kettering Cancer Center (MSKCC) in a randomized trial of 126 cases treated between 1982 and 1987 (see Table 2–2).[23] Patients with localized extremity and superficial trunk sarcomas undergoing surgery were randomly assigned to be treated by surgery alone or a combination of surgery and brachytherapy. Brachytherapy (BRT) was administered postoperatively, via an iridium-192 implant which delivered

TABLE 2–2	**PHASE III TRIALS OF ADJUVANT RADIOTHERAPY FOR LOCALIZED EXTREMITY AND TRUNK SARCOMA STRATIFIED BY GRADE**						
Histologic grade	First author/institution	Treatment group	Radiation dose, Gy	No. patients	No. local failure (%)	LRFS %	OS %
High grade	Pisters/MSKCC[23]	Surgery + BRT	42–45	56	5 (9)	89	27
		Surgery	–	63	19 (30)	66	67
	Yang[27]	Surgery + XRT	45 + 18 (boost)	47	0 (0)	100	75
		Surgery	–	44	9 (20)	78	74
Low grade	Pisters[23]	Surgery + BRT	42–45	22	8 (36)	73	96
		Surgery	–	23	6 (26)	73	95
	Yang[27]	Surgery + BRT	45 + 18 (boost)	26	1 (4)	96	NR
		Surgery	–	24	8 (33)	63	NR

MSKCC, Memorial Sloan-Kettering Cancer Center; BRT, brachytherapy; LRFS, local recurrence-free survival; OS, overall survival; NCI, National Cancer Institute; XRT, external-beam radiotherapy; NR, not reported.

42–45 Gy over 4–6 days. At 5 years, the local control rate for high-grade tumors was 91% with BRT compared to 70% in surgery-alone controls ($p = 0.04$). Of note, no improvement in local control with BRT was evident for patients with the low-grade tumors (the local control rate was 74% with surgery alone and 64% with BRT). The full explanation for grade-specific differences in local control with BRT remains unresolved, although one suggestion implicates the relatively long cell cycle of low-grade tumors; low-grade tumor cells may not enter the radio-sensitive phases of the cell cycle during the relatively short BRT time.[23]

Taken together, the United States NCI and MSKCC randomized trials have provided the evidence to support surgery plus radiation as the standard approach for most patients with operable extremity and superficial trunk sarcomas. At this time, there are no controlled trials evaluating the use of radiation treatment for patients with sarcomas in non-extremity sites. However, most multidisciplinary groups have extrapolated from the foregoing data and have assumed that radiation improves local control for patients with non-extremity sarcomas as well.

Treatment by surgery alone – without radiotherapy

Radiation provides the unquestioned clinical benefit of decreasing local recurrence for the majority of patients with STS. However, the known secondary adverse effects of radiation, which include edema, fibrosis, and radiation-induced second malignancies, have also prompted clinicians to try to identify a subset of patients who could be treated by surgery alone without compromising local disease control. Careful patient selection for unimodality treatment by surgery alone is essential. Important criteria include an R0 resection in clinical settings in which the anatomic site clearly allows for adequate surgical margins. The importance of anatomic

site in considering treatment by surgery alone is illustrated by the hypothetical cases of two patients with 4 cm high-grade sarcomas – one in the anterior thigh and the second case with an identically sized tumor located in the wrist. Clearly, the first patient could undergo satisfactory treatment by surgery alone as the surgical margins can and should be satisfactory. This is not the case for the second patient since the wrist or other anatomically similar site is not amenable to wide margins without amputation and sacrifice of neurovascular structures. Table 2–2 summarizes recent reports of patients treated by surgery alone and demonstrates that very acceptable local control rates of 10% or less can be achieved in carefully selected patients treated by surgery alone.

Amputation

Although sparingly used, amputation is still appropriate treatment for a subset of patients who present with locally advanced primary tumors. Criteria for patient selection for amputation include:

- Radiologically defined major vascular, bony, or nerve involvement such that "limb sparing" primary tumor resection will result in critical loss of function or tissue viability;
- Localized non-metastatic disease. Amputation is usually not considered for patients with established metastatic disease.

For patients without limb sparing surgical options, amputation offers excellent local tumor control and the prospect of prompt rehabilitation and thus there remains a small but well-defined role for amputation in the management of patients with extremity STS.

Management of regional lymph nodes

There is no role for routine regional lymph node dissection in most patients with localized soft tissue sarcoma given the low (2–3%) incidence of lymph node metastasis in adults with sarcomas.[2,29] However, patients with angiosarcoma, embryonal/alveolar rhabdomyosarcoma, clear cell sarcoma, and epithelioid sarcoma are at increased risk for lymph node metastasis and should be carefully examined for lymphadenopathy. These patients should be considered for sentinel lymph node biopsy as part of definitive surgical treatment. Therapeutic lymph node dissection should be considered for patients with pathologically proven lymph node involvement who do not have radiologically defined metastatic disease. Therapeutic lymph node dissection may result in survival rates as high as 34%.[2]

The prognosis of patients with pathologically positive metastatic disease to lymph nodes has been generally regarded as similar to patients with visceral metastatic disease. However, a recent series of patients with isolated lymph node metastasis treated intensively with combined modality treatment showed somewhat better outcomes, approaching those of patients with localized, high-risk (stage III) disease. This report and the relative rarity of nodal involvement in patients with STS raise questions as to whether nodal involvement should be reconsidered in the future editions of the AJCC staging system.[30,31]

Radiotherapy

Rationale for combining radiotherapy with surgery

The use of RT in combination with surgery for soft tissue sarcomas is supported by two phase III clinical trials (see Table 2–2)[23,24] and is based on two premises: microscopic foci or residual disease can be destroyed by RT, and less radical surgery can be performed when surgery and RT are combined. Although the traditional belief was that soft tissue sarcomas were resistant to RT, radiosensitivity

assays performed on sarcoma cell lines grown in vitro have confirmed that the radiosensitivity of sarcomas is similar to that of other malignancies; this confirmation supports the first premise.[32,33] The second premise stresses the philosophy of preservation of form (including cosmesis where possible) and function as a goal for many patients with extremity, truncal, breast, and head and neck sarcomas.[34–36] Similar principles govern the frequent use of RT for sarcomas at anatomically challenging sites, such as the retroperitoneum, head and neck, or paravertebral regions.

Sequencing of radiotherapy and surgery

The optimal sequencing of surgery and radiation is a subject of considerable controversy and debate. Advantages of preoperative radiation include a generally lower radiation dose (50 Gy) and small field size with reduced risks for long-term treatment sequelae including edema and fibrosis. These advantages occur at the cost of increased risk for surgical wound complications resulting from radiation-related impairment in wound healing. Advantages of postoperative radiation treatment include the ability to treat pathologically diagnosed and staged patients with known margin status. However, postoperative radiation is usually administered to a higher dose (65 Gy) and is associated with greater risks for treatment-related, long-term complications including edema and fibrosis. Thus, treatment sequencing issues involve complicated trade-off issues that need to be individualized and carefully discussed with the patient.

The NCI of Canada/Canadian Sarcoma Group SR2 clinical trial (Fig. 2–6) is the only prospective, randomized comparison of preoperative versus postoperative RT.[37] Patients were randomly assigned to be treated by

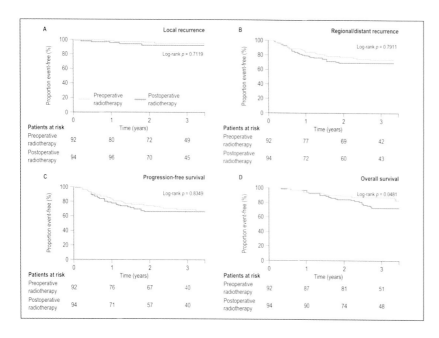

FIGURE 2–6 Kaplan–Meier plots for probability of local recurrence, metastasis (local and regional recurrence), progression-free survival, and overall survival in the Canadian Sarcoma Group randomized trial of the National Cancer Institute of Canada Clinical Trials Group comparing preoperative and postoperative radiotherapy.[37] Reproduced with permission of The Lancet Ltd. from O'Sullivan et al.

surgery with either pre- or postoperative radiation (with a radiation boost dose for patients with microscopically positive surgical margins). The primary end point of the trial was major wound complications. The SR2 trial demonstrated that wound complications were twice as common with preoperative RT as with postoperative RT (35% versus 17%), although the increased risk was almost exclusively confined to patients with sarcomas of the lower extremity. Of interest, a recent report from The University of Texas M.D. Anderson Cancer Center, using the same criteria for classifying wound complications as were used in the Canadian NCI trial, found almost identical results.[38]

The SR2 trial also provided important data on long-term treatment-related complications. Patients randomized to postoperative radiation had significantly greater rates of generally irreversible fibrosis and edema.[39] This observation is potentially important because patients with significant fibrosis, joint stiffness, or limb edema had significantly lower limb function scores at these later time points.[39] The analysis of late treatment effects demonstrated that radiation field size was associated with greater degrees of fibrosis and joint stiffness and also may be related to edema.[40]

The SR2 trial was neither designed nor statistically powered to compare traditional oncologic end points such as local control and overall survival (these were secondary end points in the trial). The 5-year results for preoperative versus postoperative respectively were, local control: 93% versus 92%; metastatic-relapse free: 67% versus 69%; recurrence-free survival: 58% versus 59%; overall survival: 73% versus 67% ($p = 0.48$); cause-specific survival: 78% versus 73% ($p = 0.64$).[41] Cox modeling showed only resection margins as significant for local control. Tumor size and grade were the only significant factors for metastatic relapse, overall survival, and cause-specific survival. Grade was the only consistent predictor of recurrence-free survival.[41]

For the present, decisions about preoperative versus postoperative RT should be individualized, taking into account tumor location, tumor size, RT field size, comorbidities, and risks. In general, preoperative RT provides some advantages over postoperative RT but exposes the patient to significantly increased risks of serious (generally reversible) postoperative wound complications. A summary of the relative indications that can be used to select patients for preoperative RT is provided in Table 2-3.

Radiation treatment techniques

Both external beam radiation treatment (EBRT) and brachytherapy (BRT) are used for patients with STS. There are no prospective trials which directly compare EBRT

TABLE 2-3 RELATIVE INDICATIONS FOR PREOPERATIVE RT, DESPITE CONCERNS RELATED TO WOUND COMPLICATIONS

Treatment context/sarcoma site	Issues of concern	Comments
Head and neck Paranasal sinus Skull base Cheek and face	Proximity to optic apparatus (eye, orbit, chiasma) Proximity to spinal cord, brainstem	Major visual functional deficit can be minimized Other "lesser" morbidities (dental, xerostomia) may also be less due to reduced doses and volumes
Split-thickness skin graft reconstruction (especially lower limb)	Skin graft breakdown and consequent infection	Many months to years of recreational and/or vocational disability may occur during healing (rare)
Large-volume GTV or CTV occupying coelomic cavities Retroperitoneum	Proximity to bowel, liver, kidney	Critical organs may be displaced by tumor or not fixed or adherent as is likely in postoperative setting Entire tumor treated prior to possible contamination of cavity
Some small bowel lesions	Proximity to critical anatomy, especially intestine with side wall adherence	Contamination of abdominal cavity renders postoperative RT unsuitable
Thoracic wall/pleura	Proximity to lung or cardiac structures	Lung may be displaced by chest wall or pleural tumor and can be avoided with preoperative RT, or permits GTV to be treated prior to operative contamination
Abdominal trunk walls, pelvic side wall	Proximity to kidney, bowel, liver, ovaries	Avoid CT encroachment on vulnerable anatomy GTV adjacent to dose-limiting critical anatomy
Thoracic inlet/upper chest	Proximity to brachial plexus	Dose limitation of critical anatomy lends itself to preoperative wall low neck RT. Additional volume considerations
Medial thigh (young male) Central limb tumor	Proximity to testes Proximity to other compartments	Permanent infertility may be avoided Permits partial circumferential sparing, which would not be feasible in postoperative setting

CT, clinical target volume; GTV, gross tumor volume; RT, radiotherapy.[34]
Reproduced with permission from Semin Radiat Oncol 1999; 9(4):328–348 by W.B. Saunders and Company.

and BRT, but each of these techniques has been compared with surgery alone.[23,24]

EBRT is the most commonly used radiation treatment technique for patients with STS. EBRT is widely available and can be administered by all radiation oncologists. It is also effective for patients with both high- and low-grade sarcomas. Treatment is usually administered on an outpatient basis in daily fractions of 1.8–2.0 Gy (Monday to Friday) to total doses of 50 Gy (pre-op dose; 5-week duration) or 60–66 Gy (post-op dose; 6.5 weeks).

In contrast, BRT for soft tissue sarcomas is only available in specific centers where there are trained radiation oncologists and appropriate radiation isotope storage and handling facilities, but does offer several advantages. Because of the shorter treatment time (4–6 days) compared to EBRT, it is usually administered on an inpatient basis during the same hospital stay and is more easily integrated into treatment protocols that include systemic chemotherapy. Since irradiated tissue volume is less, BRT may confer long-term functional advantages. Brachytherapy also costs US$1000 per patient less than external beam.[42] One specific limitation of BRT is that it should only be used for patients with high-grade sarcomas (and likely only for R0 cases) as the only randomized trial that evaluated this technique demonstrated that BRT does not appear effective for patients with low-grade sarcomas (see Table 2–2),[24,43,44] and retrospective data suggest that BRT may not provide optimal local control for R1 cases.[45]

Brachytherapy may also have an advantage in situations in which normal-tissue tolerance to conventional external beam radiation has been compromised such as: (1) a postoperative boost in patients who have received preoperative RT, or (2) radiation for local recurrence in a previously irradiated field.[46–49]

Intensity modulated radiation treatment (IMRT) is a radiation delivery technique which allows external beams designed with variable intensity to be delivered across their profiles in contrast to the uniform flat profile used in traditional external beam RT. These variable-intensity beams are not only shaped according to the needs of the target but also take into account the dose provided by the others. This allows the beams to closely conform to the target while avoiding other structures. It may be particularly valuable for tumors of complex shape such as sarcomas and has recently been used to treat large intra-abdominal targets including retroperitoneal sarcomas.[50] Clinical results are awaited from studies of these improvements in RT planning and delivery.

Chemotherapy

Chemotherapy is the mainstay of therapy for patients with metastatic (stage IV) soft tissue sarcomas. The use of chemotherapy in the adjuvant setting remains controversial. This section will review the use of chemotherapy in the adjuvant and metastatic settings. A brief discussion of chemotherapy combined with radiation therapy is also included in this section.

Chemotherapy following primary surgical resection

Although local or locoregional recurrence is a problem for a small subset of patients following primary therapy, the major risk to life in sarcoma patients is uncontrolled microscopic or macroscopic systemic disease. The availability of systemic therapy with proven, albeit often limited, ability to induce shrinkage of advanced sarcomas has raised the question of whether the early use of systemic treatment might affect microscopic metastatic disease and yield improvements in overall survival and disease-free survival.

Certainly for Ewing sarcoma/primitive neuroectodermal tumor (PNET), rhabdomyosarcoma, and osteogenic sarcoma adjuvant or neoadjuvant chemotherapy are an appropriate standard of care.[51–53] However, for more common soft tissue sarcomas such as leiomyosarcoma, liposarcoma, and high-grade malignant fibrous histiocytoma (MFH), also known as undifferentiated pleomorphic sarcoma, the benefit for chemotherapy, if there is one, is small.[54] Since adjuvant therapy is utilized by many practitioners for more common diseases where the benefit is a relatively small one, such as stage I breast cancer and stage II colon cancer, this small potential benefit is an issue that needs to be discussed on an individual basis. Certainly, the lack of available effective agents for metastatic sarcoma have impeded progress in this area, but the utility of imatinib in gastrointestinal stromal tumor (GIST) gives hope that new agents will contribute to the ultimate goal of any type of systemic therapy, specifically to increase the cure rate of new patients.

There have been over a dozen studies of anthracycline-based adjuvant chemotherapy for soft tissue sarcomas, which date back nearly as long as the initial development of doxorubicin.[55,56] These will not be reviewed here, since anthracycline/ifosfamide-based therapy constitutes a better standard of care in patients offered adjuvant chemotherapy, and only one of the studies completed by 1992 had used ifosfamide. The best summary of anthracycline-containing adjuvant-based chemotherapy for extremity sarcomas to date was the 1997 meta-analysis of 14 studies encompassing sarcomas of all anatomic sites.[57] In this study, 23 potential studies were considered, and 14 ultimately selected, constituting 1568 patients with soft tissue sarcomas of extremity and non-extremity sites with a median follow-up of 9.4 years. Pathology review was not centralized. The results of the meta-analysis, including the actuarial outcome probabilities and the hazard ratios, are summarized in Figure 2–7 and Table 2–4. Disease-free survival at 10 years was improved with chemotherapy from 45% to a highly statistically significant 55%, as was seen in several of the individual studies that comprised this population. Furthermore, local

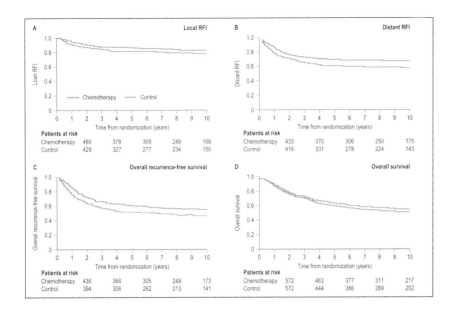

FIGURE 2–7 Actuarial curves from individual patient data meta-analysis. **(A)** Local recurrence-free interval (RFI). **(B)** Distant recurrence-free interval. **(C)** Overall recurrence-free survival. **(D)** Overall survival.[87] (Reproduced with permission of The Lancet Ltd. from Tierney JF, and The Sarcoma Meta-Analysis Collaboration.)

TABLE 2–4	HAZARD RATIOS FOR INDIVIDUAL PATIENT DATA META-ANALYSIS IN 1568 ADULTS FROM 14 TRIALS OF DOXORUBICIN-BASED CHEMOTHERAPY FOR SOFT TISSUE SARCOMA		
Hazard ratio	**Outcome**	**95% confidence intervals**	**p value**
Local RFI	0.73	0.56–0.94	0.016
Distant RFI	0.70	0.57–0.85	0.0003
Overall recurrence-free survival	0.75	0.64–0.87	0.0001
Overall survival	0.89	0.76–1.03	0.12

RFI, recurrent-free survival.
Data from the Sarcoma Data Base Meta-Analysis Collaboration.[58] Reproduced with permission from Verweij J and Seynaeve C, Semi Radiat Oncol, 1999; 9(4):352–359 by W.B. Saunders and Company.

disease-free survival was also improved at 10 years with chemotherapy, from 75% to 81% ($p = 0.016$). Most importantly, overall survival, also improved from 50% to 54% at 10 years, but was a favorable trend only, and not statistically significant ($p = 0.12$). The largest difference in overall survival was found in a post-hoc analysis of the 886 patients examined with extremity sarcomas. Overall survival was shown to improve by 7% in the group receiving chemotherapy ($p = 0.029$).

Many important interpretation issues have been summarized in a commentary on this meta-analysis.[58] As pointed out by Verweij and Seynaeve, these data have to be interpreted with caution, since (1) this was an unplanned subset analysis, (2) 18% of patients did not have histology available for review, (3) ineligibility rates were high, and (4) ≈6% of the patients from the largest contributing study to this meta-analysis did not have sarcoma after a repeat pathology review. Although the meta-analysis cannot replace a well-designed randomized study, it reinforces many of the findings from smaller

studies that local and distant recurrence-free survival is definitely improved, but not necessarily overall survival.

Adjuvant and neoadjuvant studies since the 1997 meta-analysis

The relevance of these older data to more modern practice may be limited because of improved imaging, widespread acceptance of limb-sparing surgery, and introduction of ifosfamide, more sophisticated pathological diagnosis, and better supportive care such as that offered by hematopoietic growth factors. Thus, the post-meta-analysis modern (i.e., modern chemotherapy drugs, dosing, and schedule) randomized trials may be the best group of studies to examine the question of the utility of adjuvant chemotherapy.

The largest modern-generation randomized trial was performed by the Italian Sarcoma Study Group (ISSG) in patients with primary or recurrent resected soft tissue sarcoma of the extremity or limb girdle treated or not treated with radiation.[59] One hundred and four patients with localized high-risk disease were randomized to receive no chemotherapy or to receive ifosfamide (1800 mg/m²/day for 5 consecutive days with mesna) and epirubicin (60 mg/m² on two consecutive days), with filgrastim support. Interim analysis in 1996 led to early conclusion of the trial when the study reached its primary end point of improved disease-free survival. Unfortunately, had this study commenced after the meta-analysis, it might have been constructed with a primary end point of overall survival. At a median follow-up of 36 months, overall survival in the chemotherapy arm was 72% compared to 55% for the control arm ($p = 0.002$). However, with longer-term follow-up, the overall survival difference is now no longer statistically significant on an intention-to-treat analysis.[59] This study was the strongest argument in the literature for the use of adjuvant chemotherapy. Nonetheless, interpretation of the study is made more difficult with the observation of equivalent distant ± local recurrence rates at 4 years. There are also subtle imbalances in the distribution of patients on the control and treatment arms of the study, which are difficult to evaluate given the heterogeneous nature of soft tissue sarcoma histology.

The data from this well-executed Italian study must also be taken into consideration with other data from two smaller studies. To examine the possible benefit of increased dose intensity in an adjuvant setting, an Austrian group studied 59 patients receiving no chemotherapy or doxorubicin 50 mg/m^2/cycle, dacarbazine 800 mg/m^2/cycle, and ifosfamide 6 g/m^2/cycle every 2 weeks with mesna and filgrastim support following surgical resection of the primary sarcoma. Overall survival and relapse-free survival did not differ significantly between the treatment arms at a mean follow-up of 41 months.[60] There were trends to improved recurrence-free survival, but the study was underpowered to detect a small difference in overall survival or disease-free survival. A randomized, phase II neoadjuvant study of doxorubicin 50 mg/m^2 and ifosfamide 5 g/m^2 by the EORTC and NCI-Canada also failed to show a survival advantage for the use of chemotherapy (estimated 5-year overall survival 64% for the control arm, 65% for the treatment arm).[61] Neoadjuvant chemotherapy is discussed in greater detail below. Finally, the EORTC have completed accrual in December, 2003, to an adjuvant trial (Study 62931) for high-grade soft tissue sarcomas for all sites, utilizing doxorubicin 75 mg/m^2 and ifosfamide 5000 mg/m^2 with filgrastim. Analysis will not be feasible until there has been sufficient follow-up.

Preoperative (neoadjuvant) chemotherapy

Preoperative chemotherapy has theoretical advantages over postoperative treatment. First, preoperative chemotherapy provides an in vivo test of chemotherapy sensitivity. Patients whose tumors show objective evidence of response are presumed to be the subset that may benefit most from further postoperative systemic treatment. In contrast, it is assumed that the population of non-responding patients will derive minimal or no benefit from further chemotherapy and can, therefore, be spared its toxicity. However, there are alternative ways to consider the subsets of patients identified by preoperative chemotherapy, i.e., the "responders" and the "non-responders." It is conceivable that patients who have tumors that respond well to preoperative chemotherapy simply have biologically less aggressive tumors that are destined to do well regardless of whether they receive chemotherapy (i.e., that response to chemotherapy simply selects out biologically favorable tumors). Using this perspective, one might also conclude that patients

who have tumors that appear resistant to chemotherapy have biologically more aggressive tumors not apparently impacted by conventional chemotherapy. This subset of patients is a group that could potentially benefit the most from the discovery of more effective systemic treatments.

A second potential advantage of preoperative chemotherapy is that it treats occult microscopic metastatic disease as soon as possible after the cancer diagnosis. This may theoretically prevent the development of chemotherapy resistance by isolated clones of metastatic cells or prevent the postoperative growth of microscopic metastases, but, given the nature of the growth of sarcomas, at most one or two doublings of the tumor would be affected, far fewer than the greater than 35 typically required in the development of a >1 cm tumor.

A third potential advantage of preoperative chemotherapy treatment is that chemotherapy-induced cytoreduction may permit a less radical and consequently less morbid surgical resection than would have been required initially. In patients with large soft tissue sarcomas of the extremities, chemotherapy-associated response may reduce the morbidity of limb-sparing surgical procedures and even allow patients who might otherwise have required an amputation to undergo limb-sparing surgery.

Investigators from the M.D. Anderson Cancer Center reported long-term results with doxorubicin-based preoperative chemotherapy for AJCC stages IIC and III (formerly AJCC stage IIIB) extremity soft tissue sarcomas.[62] In a series of 76 patients treated with doxorubicin-based preoperative chemotherapy, radiologic response rates were as follows: complete response, 9%; partial response, 19%; minor response, 13%; stable disease, 30%; and disease progression, 30%. The overall objective major response rate (complete plus partial responses) was 27%. At a median follow-up of 85 months, 5-year actuarial rates of local recurrence-free survival, distant metastasis-free survival, disease-free survival, and overall survival were 83%, 52%, 46%, and 59%, respectively. The event-free outcomes reported from the M.D. Anderson Cancer Center are similar to those observed with chemotherapy in the phase III postoperative chemotherapy trials. Furthermore, comparison of responding patients (complete and partial responses) and non-responding patients did not reveal any significant differences in event-free outcome.

In a prospective study from MSKCC, 29 patients with AJCC (4th edition) stage IIIB soft tissue sarcomas larger than 10 cm were treated with two cycles of a doxorubicin-based regimen prior to local therapy.[63] Subjective changes in the degree of primary tumor firmness and in imaging characteristics of the tumor (intratumoral necrosis and hemorrhage) were observed in many patients but were not quantifiable. Only one patient met the standard criteria for a partial response. Survival results in this population of high-risk patients were similar to those in historic controls treated with postoperative doxorubicin or patients treated with local therapy alone. The reasons for the apparent discrepancy in response rates between the reports from M.D. Anderson and MSKCC remain unclear. Possible explanations include the fact that the population treated at MSKCC appears to be a higher-risk population, with all patients having high-grade lesions larger than 10 cm, as is discussed below in studies examining retrospective data from both institutions. Moreover, the patients treated at MSKCC received a lower doxorubicin dose (60 mg/m^2) for fewer cycles (two). This may be important, given the known dose–response relationship with doxorubicin.[64]

Recently, ifosfamide-containing combinations have been used in the preoperative setting. Selected patients treated with aggressive ifosfamide-based regimens have had major responses, and preliminary results suggest that response rates may be higher than in historic controls treated with non-ifosfamide-containing regimens.[65] However, as noted above, the randomized phase II neoadjuvant study of doxorubicin and ifosfamide chemotherapy showed no benefit for the treatment arm, although the study was not specifically designed to determine a survival advantage.[61]

Combined preoperative chemotherapy and radiation therapy

With the advances made with combined-modality treatment of other solid tumors, there has been interest in combined-modality preoperative treatment (concurrent or sequential chemotherapy and RT) for patients with localized soft-tissue sarcomas. One putative advantage of preoperative chemo-radiation is the potential to shrink selected lesions resectable only by amputation sufficiently that they become amenable to a limb-sparing approach.

Concurrent chemotherapy and radiation has been employed extensively by Eilber and colleagues at UCLA and has been modified and examined by other groups.[66–68] The initial chemo-radiation treatment protocol typically involved intra-arterial doxorubicin with unusually high-dose per fraction RT (35 Gy of external beam radiation delivered in 10 daily fractions, which was reduced to 17.5 Gy in 5 daily fractions to minimize local toxicity). Although the intra-arterial route delivers chemotherapy more directly to the tumor, it is more complex, expensive, and prone to complications than intravenous chemotherapy.[69] Indeed, a prospective, randomized trial comparing preoperative intra-arterial doxorubicin to intravenous doxorubicin, both followed by 28 Gy of radiation delivered over 8 days and then surgical resection, showed no differences in local recurrence or survival.[70]

The largest study to date directly studying systemic chemotherapy combined with RT examined razoxane as the radiation-sensitizing agent was a randomized study of drug versus no drug in combination with radiation therapy for resectable or unresectable soft tissue sarcomas. Acute skin reactions were enhanced in the razoxane arm, but late toxicity was not greater than in the control arm. Although there are imbalances in the arms of the study for the 82 of 130 evaluable cases examined with gross disease RT (median dose 56–58 Gy) with razoxane (daily oral doses of 150 mg/m^2 throughout radiotherapy) showed an increased response rate (74% versus 49%), and improved local control rate (64 versus 30%; $p < 0.05$) compared to external beam radiation alone.[71]

Ifosfamide and cyclophosphamide have been routinely combined with radiation therapy as part of the definitive therapy for Ewing sarcoma and rhabdomyosarcoma in an attempt to continue systemic therapy at the same time as maximizing local control.[52,53] In general, toxicity does not appear to be greater than that of radiation alone. However, skin toxicity from the combination was greater in one study than that seen with radiation alone.[72]

An alternative sequential chemotherapy and radiation strategy in patients with localized, high-grade, large (>8 cm) extremity soft tissue sarcomas has been examined.[52,53] This treatment protocol involved three courses of doxorubicin, ifosfamide, mesna, and dacarbazine with two 22-Gy courses of radiation (11 fractions each) for a total preoperative radiation dose of 44 Gy. This was followed by surgical resection with careful microscopic assessment of surgical margins. An additional 16-Gy (8 fractions) boost dose was delivered for microscopically positive surgical margins. The outcomes of 48 patients treated with this regimen have been compared to those of matched historic controls and was superior to that of the historical control patients. The 5-year actuarial local control, freedom from distant metastasis, disease-free survival, and overall survival rate were 92% versus 86% ($p = 0.1155$), 75% versus 44% ($p = 0.0016$), 70% versus 42% ($p = 0.0002$), and 87% versus 58% ($p = 0.0003$) for the MAID and control patient groups, respectively. Febrile neutropenia was a complication in 25% of patients. Wound healing complications were substantial and occurred in 14 patients (29%) receiving the chemotherapy/radiation sequential therapy. One patient who received chemotherapy developed late fatal myelodysplasia. Given the favorable results of this study in comparison to historical controls, the Radiation Therapy Oncology Group is conducting a multi-institutional trial, modifying the chemotherapy in an attempt to address the local toxicity issue.

Although significant toxicity was observed, local control was improved in the prior study, raising the possibility that chemotherapy and radiation could be combined safely to decrease local control risk. Pisters and colleagues examined concurrent doxorubicin and irradiation in the neoadjuvant setting in 27 patients with extremity soft tissue sarcomas.[73] Preoperative external beam radiation was administered in 25 fractions of 2 Gy each. Doxorubicin was administered in escalating doses with a bolus followed by 4-day continuous infusion weekly. Radiographic restaging was performed 4–7 weeks after chemo-radiation. Patients with localized disease underwent surgical resection. The maximum tolerated dose of continuous-infusion doxorubicin combined with standard preoperative radiation was 17.5 mg/m^2/wk; 7/23 (30%) patients had grade 3 dermatologic toxicity at this dose level. Macroscopically complete resection (R0 or R1) was performed in all 26 patients who underwent surgery. For 22 patients who were treated with doxorubicin at the maximum tolerated dose and subsequent surgery, an encouraging 11 patients (50%) had 90% or greater tumor necrosis, including two patients who had complete pathologic responses. This approach is being further studied with other radiation-sensitizing agents, such as gemcitabine.[74]

Recent analyses of multicenter data regarding adjuvant therapy for STS

It is well recognized that different sarcoma subtypes have different chemosensitivity patterns. For example, malignant peripheral nerve sheath tumors are typically less sensitive to doxorubicin and leiomyosarcomas less sensitive to ifosfamide than other forms of sarcoma. Synovial sarcoma and myxoid/round cell liposarcoma appear to be more sensitive to chemotherapy in the metastatic setting than other subtypes of sarcoma and may well be two subtypes that respond to both anthracyclines and ifosfamide.[75] This argues that adjuvant chemotherapy should be examined on a subtype-specific basis. Combined non-randomized data from UCLA and MSKCC showed that adjuvant chemotherapy may, indeed, be useful for synovial sarcomas and myxoid/round cell liposarcoma, and argued for the use of chemotherapy in the neoadjuvant setting for all types of soft tissue sarcoma based on MSKCC and Dana-Farber institutional databases.[76–78] Interestingly, data of all patients treated or not treated with chemotherapy from M.D. Anderson and MSKCC indicated in the adjuvant or neoadjuvant setting that there was no statistical difference in overall survival in the group of patients who received chemotherapy versus those who did not.[79] However, these data are inherently biased in that it is likely that younger, healthier patients with larger high-grade tumors were those selected to receive chemotherapy. Even though there was no statistically significant difference in the group of patients who received chemotherapy and those who did not, there is still some shift toward patients with larger sarcomas and liposarcomas receiving chemotherapy, thereby possibly creating selection bias that allowed a group of patients with an inherently poorer outcome to do as well as those with a better outcome.

In summary, for AJCC stage III soft tissue sarcoma, if there is a benefit to chemotherapy in the adjuvant setting, it appears to be a small one. Therefore, dialogue with patients must include careful comparison of the small potential benefit and well-defined risks of systemic therapy. Above all, treatment must be individualized to the clinical setting. Younger patients with chemosensitive subtypes (e.g., myxoid/round cell liposarcoma, synovial sarcoma) may benefit most in this highly heterogeneous patient population.

TREATMENT OF LOCALLY ADVANCED DISEASE

Hyperthermic isolated limb perfusion

Hyperthermic isolated limb perfusion (HILP), an investigational technique in the United States (although recently approved by regulatory agencies in other parts of the world), has received considerable attention in the treatment of locally advanced, unresectable sarcomas of nonosseous tissues. HILP has been evaluated in two settings: (1) attempted limb preservation in cases of locally advanced extremity lesions surgically amenable only to amputation, and (2) functional extremity preservation for the short term in cases of locally advanced extremity lesions and synchronous pulmonary metastases (stage IV disease).

A multicenter phase II trial has evaluated a series of 55 patients with radiologically unresectable extremity soft tissue sarcomas using HILP with high-dose tumor necrosis factor-α, interferon-α, and melphalan.[80] A major tumor response was seen in 87% of patients: complete responses in 20 (36%) and partial responses in 28 (51%). Limb salvage was achieved in 84% of patients. Regional toxicity was limited, and systemic toxicity was minimal to moderate. There were no treatment-related deaths. This approach is being further evaluated in ongoing trials in Europe.

Radiation alone

Apart from patients with some very radiosensitive subtypes of sarcomas, most patients who undergo RT as the sole treatment modality for sarcoma have been deemed to have locally advanced unresectable disease. RT alone is a rare treatment choice that should be done only at centers skilled in the management of sarcomas; medically fit patients with grossly "unresectable" but non-metastatic disease should always be referred to a specialty center for multidisciplinary management, which may combine surgery, RT, and possibly chemotherapy. For example, proximal inguinal or axillary tumors that encircle major vascular structures in the proximal arm may be resected along with the involved vasculature and the

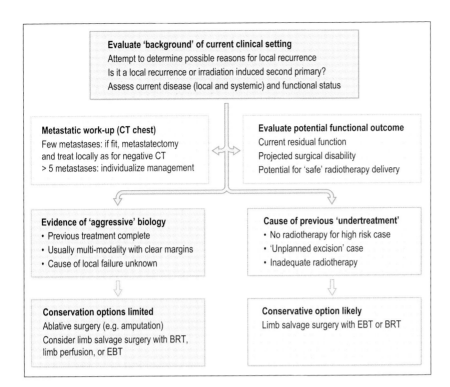

FIGURE 2–8 Schema for approaching the patient with local recurrence of soft-tissue sarcoma. The schema is oriented toward extremity lesions but is equally applicable to other anatomic sites (e.g., head and neck and retroperitoneum). BRT, brachytherapy; EBT, external-beam radiotherapy.[48] (Reproduced with permission from Catton CN et al. Seminars in Radiation Oncology 1999; 9(4):378.)

vessels reconstructed. Adjuvant RT is also generally used. Rarely, a patient with truly inoperable locally advanced disease may require RT alone, with either photon or particle (proton, neutron, or pion) beams.[81–85] No formal clinical trials have been performed to compare these strategies to each other, and they are generally administered in an adverse clinical setting. Local control has been reported in 40–70% of such cases treated with neutrons; treatment with photons produces local control in approximately 30% of cases.[82,83]

MANAGEMENT OF LOCAL RECURRENCE

If an isolated local recurrence is identified, the treatment goals are the same as for patients with primary tumors, namely, optimal local control while maintaining as much function and cosmesis as possible.[48] Early identification of local relapse may improve the chance of successful salvage therapy, and, like newly diagnosed patients, these patients are probably best managed in specialized multidisciplinary sarcoma centers. An approach to the evaluation and management of locally recurrent soft tissue sarcoma is summarized in Figure 2–8. The initial evaluation must include a full review of previous therapy because this will have a bearing on the therapeutic options available. Therefore, all prior surgery and pathology reports should be examined, as should reports on previous chemotherapy and previous RT, especially volume treated, dose, and energy of radiation.

Several distinct clinical settings are evident under the rubric of "locally recurrent" disease: (1) cases in which prior treatment did not include RT; (2) cases treated with RT in the past; (3) cases in which distant metastases are also present; and (4) cases in which it is difficult to distinguish between recurrence and secondary tumors induced by RT. Although the therapeutic options available are more limited in recurrent disease and the challenge posed by these cases that much more formidable, a proportion of these patients can be cured. Clinical experience is needed to determine which therapeutic options are appropriate in a given case of recurrent disease.

KEY POINTS

- Core needle biopsy is the preferred biopsy method for most patients with suspected sarcoma.

- Pretreatment staging should include an MRI (or CT) of the primary tumor site, chest X-ray, and chest CT (for patients with high-grade sarcomas)

- Surgery and pre- or postoperative external beam radiation treatment is the primary local treatment for most patients with localized disease. In many clinical settings, preoperative radiation should be considered because of the lower dose, smaller treatment volume, and lower risks for post-treatment edema and fibrosis.

- The role for routine administration of adjuvant chemotherapy treatment remains unclear.

- Patients with metastatic disease should be considered for chemotherapy treatment with carefully selected cases considered for metastasectomy.

REFERENCES

Clinical evaluation

1. Lawrence WJ, Donegan WL, Natarajan N, et al. Adult soft tissue sarcomas. A pattern of care survey of the American College of Surgeons. Ann Surg 1987; 205:349.
2. Fong Y, Coit DG, Woodruff JM, et al. Lymph node metastasis from soft tissue sarcoma in adults. Analysis of data from a prospective database of 1772 sarcoma patients. Ann Surg 1993; 217:72.
3. Ball AB, Fisher C, Pittam M, et al. Diagnosis of soft tissue tumours by Tru-Cut biopsy. Br J Surg 1990; 77:756.
4. Skrzynski MC, Biermann JS, Montag AG, et al. Diagnostic accuracy and charge-savings of outpatient core needle biopsy compared with open biopsy of musculoskeletal tumors. J Bone Joint Surg [A] 1996; 8:644.
5. Heslin MJ, Lewis JJ, Woodruff JM, et al. Core needle biopsy for diagnosis of extremity soft tissue sarcoma. Ann Surg Oncol 1997; 4:425.
6. Schwartz HS, Spengler DM. Needle tract recurrences after closed biopsy for sarcoma: three cases and review of the literature. Ann Surg Oncol 1997; 4:228.
7. Akerman M. Fine-needle aspiration cytology of soft tissue sarcoma: benefits and limitations. Sarcoma 1998; 2:155.
8. Kissin MW, Fisher C, Webb AJ, et al. Value of fine needle aspiration cytology in the diagnosis of soft tissue tumours: a preliminary study on the excised specimen. Br J Surg 1987; 74:479.
9. Soft tissue sarcoma. In: Greene F, Page D, Fleming ID, eds. American Joint Committee on Cancer (AJCC) staging manual. New York: Springer-Verlag; 2006:193.
10. Kattan MW, Leung DH, Brennan MF. Postoperative nomogram for 12-year sarcoma-specific death. J Clin Oncol 2002; 20:791.
11. Stojadinovic A, Yeh A, Brennan MF. Completely resected recurrent soft tissue sarcoma: primary anatomic site governs outcomes. J Am Coll Surg 2002; 194:436.

Prognostic factors

12. Pisters PWT, Leung DHY, Woodruff JM, et al. Analysis of prognostic factors in 1041 patients with localized soft tissue sarcomas of the extremities. J Clin Oncol 1996; 14:1679.
13. Coindre JM, Terrier P, Bui NB, et al. Prognostic factors in adult patients with locally controlled soft tissue sarcoma. A study of 546 patients from the French Federation of Cancer Centers Sarcoma Group. J Clin Oncol 1996; 14:869.
14. Gaynor JJ, Tan CC, Casper ES, et al. Refinement of clinicopathologic staging for localized soft tissue sarcoma of the extremity: A study of 423 adults. J Clin Oncol 1992; 10:1317.
15. Gerrand CH, Wunder JS, Kandel RA, et al. Classification of positive margins after resection of soft-tissue sarcoma of the limb predicts the risk of local recurrence. J Bone Joint Surg [Br] 2001; 83:1149.
16. Eilber FC, Brennan MF, Eilber FR, et al. Validation of the postoperative nomogram for 12-year sarcoma-specific mortality. Cancer 2004; 101:2270.
17. Mariani L, Miceli R, Kattan MW, et al. Validation and adaptation of a nomogram for predicting the survival of patients with extremity soft tissue sarcoma using a three-grade system. Cancer 2005; 103:402.

Treatment of localized primary extremity sarcomas

18. Williard WC, Collin CF, Casper ES, et al. The changing role of amputation for soft tissue sarcoma of the extremity in adults. Surg Gynecol Obstet 1992; 175:389.

19. Williard WC, Hajdu SI, Casper ES, et al. Comparison of amputation with limb-sparing operations for adult soft tissue sarcoma of the extremity. Ann Surg 1992; 215:269.
20. Bowden L, Booher RJ. The principles and techniques of resection of soft parts for sarcomas. Surgery 1958; 44:963.
21. Cantin J, McNeer GP, Chu FC, et al. The problem of local recurrence after treatment of soft tissue sarcoma. Ann Surg 1968;168:47.
22. Gerner RE, Moore GE, Pickren JW. Soft tissue sarcomas. Ann Surg 1975; 181:803.
23. Pisters PW, Harrison LB, Leung DH, et al. Long-term results of a prospective randomized trial of adjuvant brachytherapy in soft tissue sarcoma. J Clin Oncol 1996; 14:859.
24. Yang JC, Chang AE, Baker AR, et al. A randomized prospective study of the benefit of adjuvant radiation therapy in the treatment of soft tissue sarcomas of the extremity. J Clin Oncol 1998; 16:197.
25. Karakousis CP, Proimakis C, Walsh DL. Primary soft tissue sarcoma of the extremities in adults. Br J Surg 1995; 82:1208.
26. Brennan MF, Casper ES, Harrison LB, et al. The role of multimodality therapy in soft-tissue sarcoma. Ann Surg 1991; 214:328.
27. Yang JC, Rosenberg SA. Surgery for adult patients with soft tissue sarcomas. Semin Oncol 1989; 16:289.
28. Rosenberg SA, Tepper JE, Glatstein EJ, et al. The treatment of soft-tissue sarcomas of the extremities: prospective randomized evaluations of (1) limb-sparing surgery plus radiation therapy compared with amputation and (2) the role of adjuvant chemotherapy. Ann Surg 1982; 196:305.
29. Weingrad DN, Rosenberg SA. Early lymphatic spread of osteogenic and soft-tissue sarcomas. Surgery 1978; 84:231.
30. Behranwala KA, A'Hern R, Omar AM, et al. Prognosis of lymph node metastasis in soft tissue sarcoma. Ann Surg Oncol 2004; 11:714.
31. Riad S, Griffin AM, Liberman B, et al. Lymph node metastasis in soft tissue sarcoma in an extremity. Clin Orthop Rel Res 2004; 129.
32. Ruka W, Taghian A, Gioioso D, et al. Comparison between the in vitro intrinsic radiation sensitivity of human soft tissue sarcoma and breast cancer cell lines. J Surg Oncol 1996; 61:290.
33. Weichselbaum RR, Beckett MA, Simon MA, et al. In vitro radiobiological parameters of human sarcoma cell lines. Int J Radiat Oncol Biol Phys 1988; 15:937.
34. O'Sullivan B, Wylie J, Catton C, et al. The local management of soft tissue sarcoma. Semin Radiat Oncol 1999; 9:328.
35. Le Vay J, O'Sullivan B, Catton C, et al. An assessment of prognostic factors in soft-tissue sarcoma of the head and neck. Arch Otolaryngol Head Neck Surg 1994; 120:981.
36. McGowan TS, Cummings BJ, O'Sullivan B, et al. An analysis of 78 breast sarcoma patients without distant metastases at presentation. Int J Radiat Oncol Biol Phys 2000; 46:383.
37. O'Sullivan B, Davis AM, Turcotte R, et al. Preoperative versus postoperative radiotherapy in soft-tissue sarcoma of the limbs: a randomized trial. Lancet 2002; 359:2235.
38. Tseng JF, Ballo MT, Langstein H, et al. The effect of preoperative radiotherapy and reconstructive surgery on wound complications after resection of extremity soft-tissue sarcoma. Ann Surg Oncol 2006; In press.
39. Davis AM, O'Sullivan B, Turcotte R, et al. Late radiation morbidity following randomization to preoperative versus postoperative radiotherapy in extremity soft tissue sarcoma. Radiother Oncol 2005; 75:48.
40. O'Sullivan B, Davis A. A randomized phase III trial of preoperative compared to postoperative

radiotherapy in extremity soft tissue sarcoma. Proc ASTRO 2001; 51(3):151.
41. O'Sullivan B, Davis A, Turcotte R, et al. Five-year results of a randomized phase III trial of pre-operative vs post-operative radiotherapy in extremity soft tissue sarcoma. Proc Am Soc Clin Oncol 2004; 23:815.
42. Janjan NA, Yasko AW, Reece GP, et al. Comparison of charges related to radiotherapy for soft tissue sarcomas treated by preoperative external beam irradiation versus interstitial implantation. Ann Surg Oncol 1994; 1:415.
43. Suit HD, Mankin HJ, Wood WC, et al. Treatment of the patient with stage M0 soft tissue sarcoma. J Clin Oncol 1988; 6:854.
44. Pisters PWT, Harrison LB, Woodruff JM, et al. A prospective randomized trial of adjuvant brachytherapy in the management of low grade soft tissue sarcomas of the extremity and superficial trunk. J Clin Oncol 1994; 12:1150.
45. Alektiar KM, Velasco J, Zelefsky MJ, et al. Adjuvant radiotherapy for margin-positive high-grade soft tissue sarcoma of the extremity. Int J Radiat Oncol Biol Phys 2000; 48:1051.
46. Catton CN, Davis A, Bell RS, et al. Soft tissue sarcoma of the extremity. Limb salvage after failure of combined conservative therapy. Radiother Oncol 1996; 41:209.
47. Catton C, Swallow C, O'Sullivan B. A pilot study of external beam radiotherapy and pulsed dose rate brachytherapy for resectable retroperitoneal sarcomas. Radiother Oncol 1998; 47(Suppl 1):S30.
48. Catton CN, Swallow CJ, O'Sullivan B. Approaches to local salvage of soft tissue sarcoma after primary site failure. Semin Radiat Oncol 1999; 9:378.
49. Pearlstone D, Janjan NA, Feig BW, et al. Re-resection with brachytherapy for locally recurrent soft tissue sarcoma arising in a previously radiated field. Cancer J Sci Am 1999; 5:26.
50. Hong L, Alektiar K, Chui C, et al. IMRT of large fields: whole-abdomen irradiation. Int J Radiat Oncol Biol Phys 2002; 54:278.
51. Souhami RL, Craft AW, Van der Eijken JW, et al. Randomised trial of two regimens of chemotherapy in operable osteosarcoma: a study of the European Osteosarcoma Intergroup. Lancet 1997; 350:911.
52. Grier HE, Krailo MD, Tarbell NJ, et al. Addition of ifosfamide and etoposide to standard chemotherapy for Ewing's sarcoma and primitive neuroectodermal tumor of bone. N Engl J Med 2003; 348:694.
53. Crist WM, Anderson JR, Meza JL, et al. Intergroup rhabdomyosarcoma study – IV: results for patients with nonmetastatic disease. J Clin Oncol 2001; 19:3091.
54. Bramwell VH. Adjuvant chemotherapy for adult soft tissue sarcoma: is there a standard of care? J Clin Oncol 2001; 19:1235.
55. Wang JJ, Cortes E, Sinks LF, et al. Therapeutic effect and toxicity of adriamycin in patients with neoplastic disease. Cancer 1971; 28:837.
56. Benjamin RS, Wiernik PH, Bachur NR. Adriamycin chemotherapy – efficacy, safety, and pharmacologic basis of an intermittent single high-dosage schedule. Cancer 1974; 33:19.
57. Sarcoma Meta-analysis Collaboration. Adjuvant chemotherapy for localised resectable soft-tissue sarcoma of adults: meta-analysis of individual data. Lancet 1997; 350:1647.
58. Verweij J, Seynaeve C. The reason for confining the use of adjuvant chemotherapy in soft tissue sarcoma to the investigational setting. Semin Radiat Oncol 1999; 9:352.
59. Frustaci S, De Paoli A, Bidoli E, et al. Ifosfamide in the adjuvant therapy of soft tissue sarcomas. Oncology 2003; 65:80.

60. Brodowicz T, Schwameis E, Widder J, et al. Intensified adjuvant IFADIC chemotherapy for adult soft tissue sarcoma: a prospective randomized feasibility trial. Sarcoma 2000; 4:151.

61. Gortzak E, Azzarelli A, Buesa J, et al. A randomized phase II study on neo-adjuvant chemotherapy for 'high-risk' adult soft-tissue sarcoma. Eur J Cancer 2001; 37:1096.

62. Pisters PWT, Patel SR, Varma DGK, et al. Preoperative chemotherapy for stage IIIB extremity soft tissue sarcoma: long-term results from a single institution. J Clin Oncol 1997; 15:3481.

63. Casper ES, Gaynor JJ, Harrison LB, et al. Preoperative and postoperative adjuvant combination chemotherapy for adults with high grade soft tissue sarcoma. Cancer 1994; 73:1644.

64. O'Bryan RM, Baker LH, Gottlieb JE, et al. Dose response evaluation of adriamycin in human neoplasia. Cancer 1977; 39:1940.

65. Patel SR, Vadhan-Raj S, Papadopoulos NJ, et al. High-dose ifosfamide in bone and soft tissue sarcomas: results of phase II and pilot studies – dose–response and schedule dependence. J Clin Oncol 1997; 15:2378.

66. Eilber FR, Giuliano AE, Huth JH, et al. Neoadjuvant chemotherapy, radiation, and limited surgery for high grade soft tissue sarcoma of the extremity. In: Ryan JR, Baker LO, eds. Recent concepts in sarcoma treatment. Dordrecht, The Netherlands: Kluwer Academic Publishers; 1988:115–122.

67. Wanebo HJ, Temple WJ, Popp MB, et al. Preoperative regional therapy for extremity sarcoma. A tricenter update. Cancer 1995; 75:2299.

68. Levine EA, Trippon M, DasGupta TK. Preoperative multimodality treatment for soft tissue sarcomas. Cancer 1993; 71:3685.

69. Eilber FR, Eckardt J, Rosen G, et al. Preoperative therapy for soft tissue sarcoma. Hematol Oncol Clin North Am 1995; 9:817.

70. Eilber FR, Giuliano AE, Huth JF, et al. Intravenous (IV) vs. intraarterial (IA) adriamycin, 2800 Gy radiation and surgical excision for extremity soft tissue sarcomas: a randomized prospective trial. Proc Am Soc Clin Oncol 1990; 9:309.

71. Rhomberg W, Hassenstein EO, Gefeller D. Radiotherapy vs. radiotherapy and razoxane in the treatment of soft tissue sarcomas: final results of a randomized study. Int J Radiat Oncol Biol Phys 1996; 36:1077.

72. Cormier JN, Patel SR, Herzog CE, et al. Concurrent ifosfamide-based chemotherapy and irradiation. Cancer 2001; 92(6):1550.

73. Pisters PW, Ballo MT, Fenstermacher MJ, et al. Phase I trial of preoperative concurrent doxorubicin and radiation therapy, surgical resection, and intraoperative electron-beam radiation therapy for patients with localized retroperitoneal sarcoma. J Clin Oncol 2003; 21:3092.

74. Pisters PW, Ballo MT, Bekele N, et al. Phase I trial using toxicity severity weights for dose finding of gemcitabine combined with radiation therapy and subsequent surgery for patients with extremity and trunk soft tissue sarcomas. J Clin Oncol 2004; 22:9008.

75. Rosen G, Forscher C, Lowenbraun S, et al. Synovial sarcoma. Uniform response of metastases to high dose ifosfamide. Cancer 1994; 73:2506.

76. Eilber FC, Eilber FR, Eckardt JJ, et al. Impact of ifosfamide-based chemotherapy on survival in patients with primary extremity synovial sarcoma. J Clin Oncol 2004; 22:9017.

77. Eilber FC, Eilber FR, Eckardt J, et al. The impact of chemotherapy on the survival of patients with high-grade primary extremity liposarcoma. Ann Surg 2004; 240:686.

78. Grobmyer SR, Maki RG, Demetri GD, et al. Neo-adjuvant chemotherapy for primary high-grade extremity soft tissue sarcoma. Ann Oncol 2004; 15:1667.

79. Cormier JN, Huang X, Xing Y, et al. Cohort analysis of patients with localized, high-risk, extremity soft tissue sarcoma treated at two cancer centers: chemotherapy-associated outcomes. J Clin Oncol 2004; 22:4567.

Treatment of locally advanced disease

80. Eggermont AMM, Shraffordt Koops H, Lienard D, et al. Isolated limb perfusion with high-dose tumor necrosis factor-α in combination with interferon-v and melphalan for nonresectable extremity soft tissue sarcomas: a multicenter trial. J Clin Oncol 1996; 14:2653.

81. Isacsson U, Hagberg H, Johansson KA. Potential advantages of protons over conventional radiation beams for paraspinal tumours. Radiother Oncol 1997; 45:63.

82. Pickering DG, Stewart JS, Rampling R, et al. Fast neutron therapy for soft tissue sarcoma. Int J Radiat Oncol Biol Phys 1987; 13:1489.

83. Tepper JE, Suit HD. Radiation therapy alone for sarcoma of soft tissue. Cancer 1985; 56: 475.

84. Slater JD, McNeese MD, Peters LJ. Radiation therapy for unresectable soft tissue sarcomas. Int J Radiat Oncol Biol Phys 1986; 12:1729.

85. Greiner RH, Blattmann HJ, Thum P, et al. Dynamic pion irradiation of unresectable soft tissue sarcomas. Int J Radiat Oncol Biol Phys 1989; 17:1077.

86. Pisters PWT. Combined modality treatment of extremity soft tissue sarcomas. Ann Surg Oncol 1998; 5:464.

87. Tierney JF. Adjuvant chemotherapy for localised resectable soft-tissue sarcoma of adults: meta-analysis of individual data. Lancet 1997; 350:1647.

RADIOLOGIC EVALUATION OF SOFT TISSUE TUMORS

Mark D. Murphey and Mark J. Kransdorf

CHAPTER CONTENTS

The opinions or assertions contained herein are the private views of the authors and are not to be construed as official or as reflecting the views of the Departments of the Army, Navy or Defense.

INTRODUCTION

The radiologic evaluation of soft tissue tumors has evolved dramatically over the past 20 years because of the advent of computed tomography (CT) and subsequently magnetic resonance imaging (MRI). The goals of diagnostic imaging in evaluation of a soft tissue mass are: (1) identifying and characterizing the lesion; (2) distinguishing a neoplasm from a non-neoplastic process; (3) providing a specific diagnosis or reasonable differential diagnosis; (4) directing the biopsy to lesional tissue; and (5) staging. The radiologic literature suggests that a specific diagnosis can be obtained by imaging (CT or MRI) in 25% to 50% of cases.[1-8] However, we believe that this percentage will gradually increase and ultimately approach 75% to 90% (similar to bone tumors with radiography)[9] because more signs and characteristic MR findings of specific lesions are continually being described. These factors emphasize that the evaluation and treatment of soft tissue tumors requires a team approach, similar to bone tumors, and a close working relationship between the oncologic surgeon, musculoskeletal radiologist, and pathologist. The purpose of this chapter is to provide an overview of the radiologic evaluation of soft tissue tumors with particular emphasis on the implications for pathologists.

IMAGING EVALUATION AND OPTIONS

Advantages and disadvantages of various imaging modalities available for evaluation of soft tissue masses are listed in Tables 3-1 and 3-2.[10-12]

Radiographs

With the availability of high-technology imaging, the lowly radiograph is often forgotten in the evaluation of a soft tissue mass. Radiographs are frequently normal and unrewarding in evaluation of soft tissue masses. However, radiographs may detect subtle calcifications or underlying osseous abnormality critical for diagnosis that are more difficult to identify on cross-sectional imaging (ultrasonography [US], CT and MRI) (Figs 3-1, 3-2).[13-17] Because the value of radiographs cannot be determined in advance we believe this inexpensive modality should *always* be the initial imaging study for evaluation of a soft tissue mass.

Nuclear medicine

Nuclear medicine studies do not play a primary role in the evaluation of soft tissue masses. More recently, FDG (fluorine-18 fluro-2-deoxy-D-glucose) positron emission tomography (PET) has been used to assess soft tissue masses by measuring the avidity of glucose turnover (quantitated by use of the standardized uptake value [SUV]).[18-21] The role of FDG PET in distinguishing benign from malignant tumors (SUV greater than 2-3), evaluating the response of neoplasms to treatment (radiation and/or chemotherapy) and evaluating neoplasm recurrence following surgical resection[18-21] is currently under study. FDG PET images are also frequently matched to CT images (PET-CT fusion) to improve anatomic detail. As more experience with FDG PET is emerging, overlap between benign and malignant processes is becoming increasingly apparent (Fig. 3-3).

Ultrasound (US), CT and MRI

The use of cross-sectional imaging (US, CT and MR) markedly improves evaluation of soft tissue masses primarily because of superior contrast resolution.[1,2,4-8,13,22-34] However, MRI will be emphasized because the improved tissue characterization generally makes this modality optimal in the radiologic evaluation of soft tissue tumors.[1,2,4-6,8,13,26-35]

Varying the patient between prone and supine positions and placement of a marker over the soft tissue mass can be important with CT and MRI, particularly with

TABLE 3–1	NONCROSS-SECTIONAL IMAGING MODALITIES: ADVANTAGES AND DISADVANTAGES	
Modality	**Advantages**	**Disadvantages**
Radiographs	Low cost Availability Identifying and characterizing calcification can be pathognomonic (phleboliths in hemangioma; chondral bodies in synovial chondromatosis; peripheral rim in myositis ossificans) Identify underlying bone abnormality (osteochondroma, trauma deformity, periosteal reaction, cortical destruction, marrow invasion)	Usually non-specific Often do not identify masses when small Ionizing radiation
Nuclear medicine[a]	Intermediate cost Availability Gallium may help distinguish MPNST (uptake) from BPNST (no uptake)	Usually non-specific, mild uptake due to increased blood flow Often normal Ionizing radiation Lesions with calcification (myositis ossificans) more prominent uptake due to increased turnover calcium/phosphate)
Angiography	Availability Provides vascular road map for surgeon May embolize highly vascular tumors to lessen surgical blood loss or to definitively treat angiomatous lesions	Invasive Largely replaced by CT/MR angiography for vascular road map Ionizing radiation

[a]Bone scintigraphy unless otherwise specified.
MPNST, malignant peripheral nerve sheath tumor; BPNST, benign peripheral nerve sheath tumor.

TABLE 3–2	CROSS-SECTIONAL IMAGING MODALITIES: ADVANTAGES AND DISADVANTAGES	
Modality	**Advantages**	**Disadvantages**
Ultrasound (US)	Low cost Availability Cross-sectional multiplanar imaging Real-time (dynamic) scanning Lack of ionizing radiation Very good to evaluate superficial lesions Excellent to distinguish cystic lesions (ganglion, synovial cyst, bursa, abscess) from high water content solid masses (myxoid tumors) Identifying calcification Doppler for evaluation of vascularity	Very operator dependant Relatively high learning curve Some lesions not accessible to scan Underlying bone abnormalities not well evaluated Anatomy not as well defined for staging Limited ability to detect fat in lesions Often restricted field of view High physician time commitment Not good at characterizing calcification
Computed tomography (CT)	Availability Short scan times (limited motion artifact) Cross-sectional multiplanar imaging Optimal imaging to detect/characterize calcification (particularly if subtle or complex anatomy) Good for periscapular lesions Good for abdominal/chest wall lesions	Higher cost Ionizing radiation Not as good contrast resolution as US/MRI Need post-contrast images Potential allergic reaction May require imaging both sides for comparison
Magnetic resonance imaging (MRI)	No ionizing radiation Cross-sectional multiplanar imaging optimal method to characterize differing tissue components of lesion Optimal method to define anatomy for staging	Less availability High cost May need contrast (potential allergic reaction but much less than CT) Long scan times (motion artifact) Contraindications (claustrophobia, metallic foreign bodies, pacemakers) Metallic device artifact Not good at identifying/characterizing calcification

superficial lesions (e.g., subcutaneous lipoma) so that the tumor is not compressed (Fig. 3–4). The axial plane is almost invariably optimal for evaluation of a soft tissue mass. We believe both conventional T1-weighted (optimal for anatomic detail and staging of lesions) and T2-weighted images (optimal to detect abnormal tissue) should be obtained. The combination of signal intensity on these two pulse sequences provides information as to the potential type of tissue comprising the lesion (Table 3–3). A second orthogonal plane of imaging should also be performed either coronal (masses located medial or lateral in a compartment) or sagittal (masses located

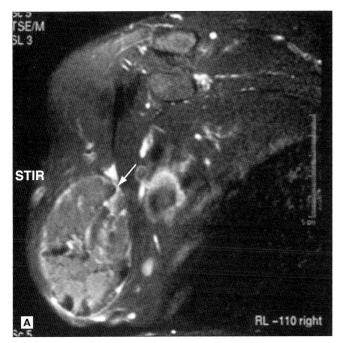

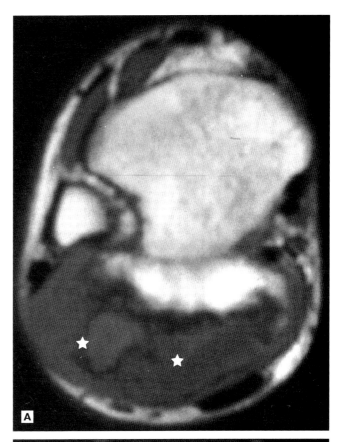

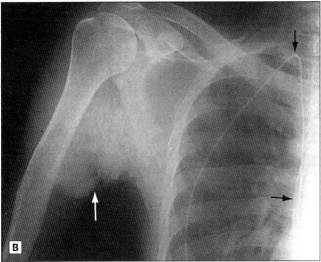

FIGURE 3–1 35-year-old man who was referred to a musculoskeletal radiologist for biopsy of a deep upper arm soft tissue mass by an orthopedic oncologist. **(A)** Coronal fat suppressed T2-weighted MR image shows a heterogeneous large, non-specific by intrinsic characteristics, soft tissue mass (arrow). **(B)** Radiograph reveals vague calcification (white arrow) throughout the lesion that cannot be recognized on MR and two large-bore catheters (black arrows) for hemodialysis in this chronic renal failure patient. Radiograph and clinical history are diagnostic of periarticular calcification related to renal failure (secondary tumoral calcinosis) and no biopsy was warranted. This case emphasizes the potential importance of both radiographs and clinical history in diagnosis of soft tissue masses.

FIGURE 3–2 Osteochondroma in a 12-year-old boy presenting as a palpable soft tissue mass. Axial **(A)** and sagittal STIR **(B)** MR images reveal the cartilaginous cap (white stars in A and arrow in B) causing the initial clinical presentation.

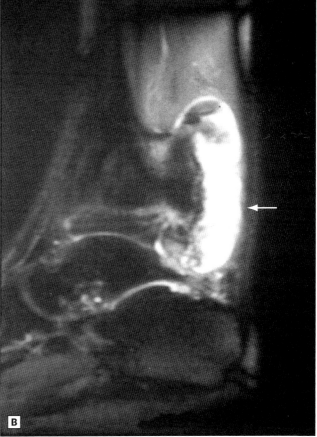

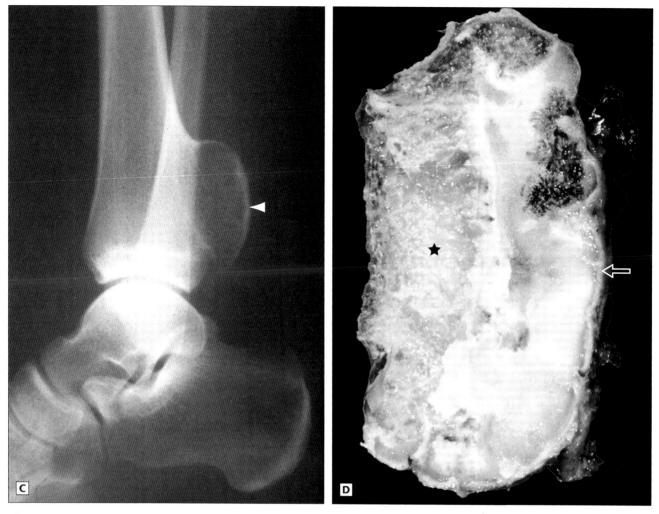

FIGURE 3–2 Continued. **(C)** Lateral radiograph reveals the obvious osteochondroma (arrowhead) with cortical and marrow continuity to the underlying tibia. **(D)** Photograph of sagittaly resected gross specimen demonstrated identical features with osteoid component (black star) and cartilage cap (open arrow) which was the cause of the palpable soft tissue mass on physical examination.

anterior or posterior in a compartment). Various sequences have been developed to subtract the fat signal (which makes it low signal intensity/black) which increases the conspicuity of abnormal tissue (Fig. 3–3b).[36–39] These include fat suppressed or fat saturated T2-weighted or short tau inversion recovery (STIR) MR sequences and these are often employed in the second plane in addition to T1-weighted images. A practical method to determining which pulse sequence you are viewing is to identify a normal water containing structure in the study (bladder, cerebrospinal fluid [CSF], joint fluid) and determine if it is low signal intensity (black and a T1-weighted sequence) or high signal intensity (white and a T2-weighted sequence) (Fig. 3–3b). Additional MR pulse sequences have been and continue to be developed that can be helpful in specific situations. Gradient-echo images are one example and may be used to identify hemosiderin (particularly helpful in hematoma and pigmented villonodular synovitis) and depict lesion–fat interfaces for neurovascular involvement.

CT or MRI following administration of intravenous contrast material improves contrast resolution in evaluation of soft tissue tumors.[40–51] In general, this is much more important for CT (several precontrast images should also be obtained for comparison) in differentiating soft tissue tumors from surrounding muscle due to its lower contrast resolution. Imaging following contrast is particularly important with masses that are high water content (cyst versus myxoid neoplasm) or are composed of prominent necrotic/hemorrhagic foci (nonenhancing areas) allowing identification and differentiation of these regions from enhancing solid cellular tissue (see later discussion) (Fig. 3–5).[52–54]

EVALUATION OF LESION

In addition to the age of the patient, the most important radiologic features in evaluation of soft tissue tumors are location and intrinsic imaging characteristics which include size, morphology, shape and extent.

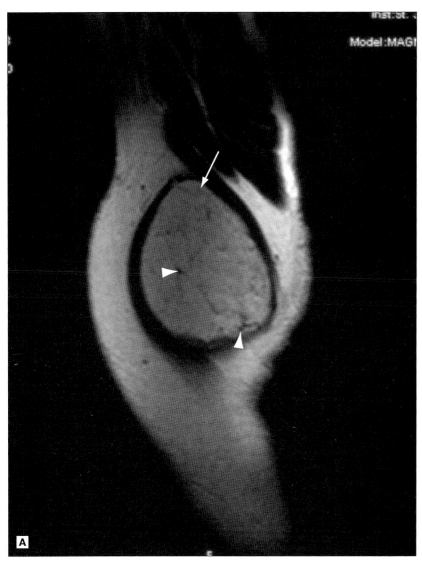

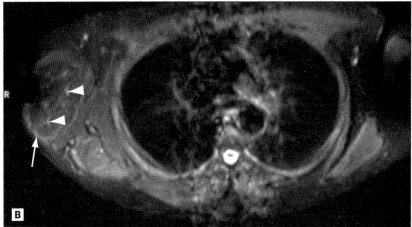

FIGURE 3–3 Hibernoma in a 63-year-old man with an upper arm soft tissue mass and PET imaging. **(A, B)** Sagittal T1-weighted (A) and axial fat suppressed T2-weighted (B) MR images show a soft tissue mass (arrow) nearly identical in intensity to subcutaneous fat. Curvilinear nonadipose components (small arrowheads) could be seen in a well-differentiated liposarcoma, although serpentine nature suggests these are vascular channels.

Location

Location is one of the most important clues to diagnosis.[13,55,56] Specific anatomic location (e.g., thigh) is available with cross-sectional imaging but is less informative than the compartment involved: subcutaneous, intermuscular, intramuscular, intra-articular/periarticular, and multiple lesions. Localization of soft tissue tumors to compartments is analogous to localization of bone tumors to epiphysis, metaphysis, or diaphysis and assists

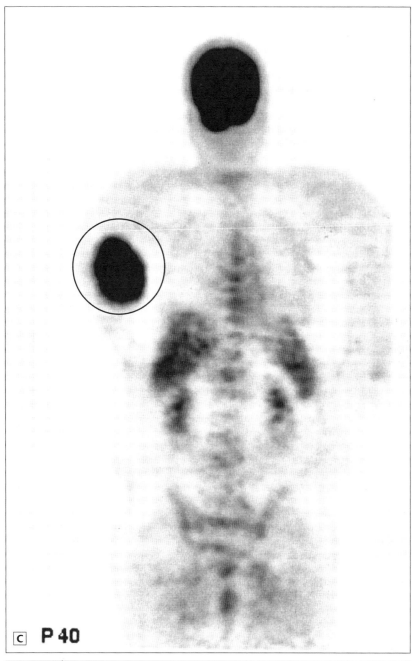

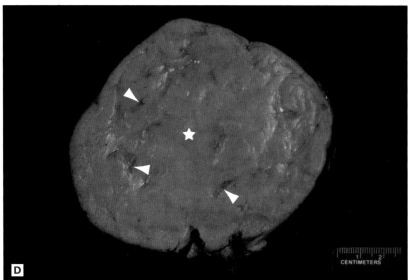

FIGURE 3–3 Continued. **(C)** PET imaging reveals marked increased uptake of radionuclide (circle). **(D)** Photograph of sectioned gross specimen demonstrated brown fat (star) and vascular channels (large arrowheads) corresponding to the imaging appearance. These vascular channels and degree of PET avidity would not be seen in well-differentiated liposarcoma and are pathognomonic for hibernoma. This case emphasizes that PET measures glucose turnover but not benignity versus malignancy, as this benign lesion (hibernoma) has more intense activity than the low-grade malignant tumor in the differential diagnosis (well-differentiated liposarcoma) in this instance.

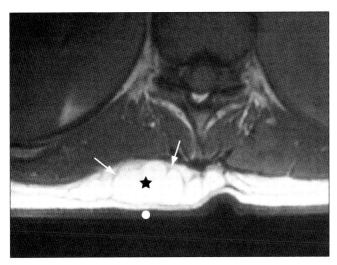

FIGURE 3–4 Small subcutaneous lipoma in the posterior subcutaneous tissues of the back. Axial T1-weighted MR image shows the subcutaneous lipoma (star) which could easily be compressed if the patient were imaged in a supine position. The small low-signal pseudocapsule (arrows) separates the lesion from the surrounding isointense subcutaneous fat. This distinction can be difficult (identifying a fatty tumor in a background of adipose tissue) and placement of a skin marker (white circle on posterior skin surface) is often helpful. Note that the lipoma is solely composed of fat with no nonadipose (thick septa or nodular foci) areas and represents a very typical imaging appearance.

TABLE 3–3	**MRI SIGNAL INTENSITY OF VARIOUS TISSUES**	
Tissue type	**T1ᵃ signal intensity**	**T2ᵇ signal intensity**
Fat	High	High
Bone marrow (yellow)	High	Intermediate
Bone marrow (red)	Intermediate	Intermediate
Tumorᶜ	Intermediate	High
Muscle	Intermediate	Intermediate to Low
Hyaline cartilage	Intermediate	High
Water	Very Low	Very High
Tendons/ligaments	Very Low	Very Low
Cortex	Very Low	Very Low
Fibrocartilage	Very Low	Very Low
Fibrous tissue	Low to Intermediate	Variableᵈ
Bloodᵉ	Variable	Variable

High, bright (white); Intermediate, gray; Low, dark (black).
ᵃT1-weighted images: Repetition time (TR) 500–1000 msec; echo times (TE) 10–30 msec.
ᵇT2-weighted images: > 1500 msec; TE > 90 msec.
ᶜTumor – majority of lesions.
ᵈHighly collagenized regions low signal, more cellular areas higher signal.
ᵉDependent on components of methemoglobin, hemosiderin, oxyhemoglobin, deoxyhemoglobin, frequently heterogeneous with areas of high signal on both T1 and T2 weighting except hemosiderin which is low signal on all pulse sequences.

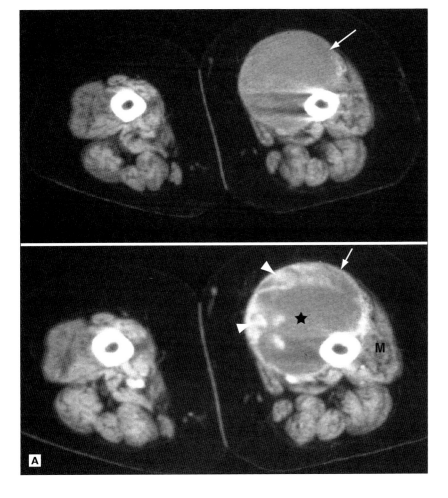

FIGURE 3–5 Malignant fibrous histiocytoma of the thigh with central necrosis in a 60-year-old woman. **(A)** Pre-(superior image) and post-contrast (image below) CT images show peripheral nodule enhancement (arrowheads) and nonenhancing necrotic region (star) of this large intramuscular thigh soft tissue mass (arrows in CT and MRI).

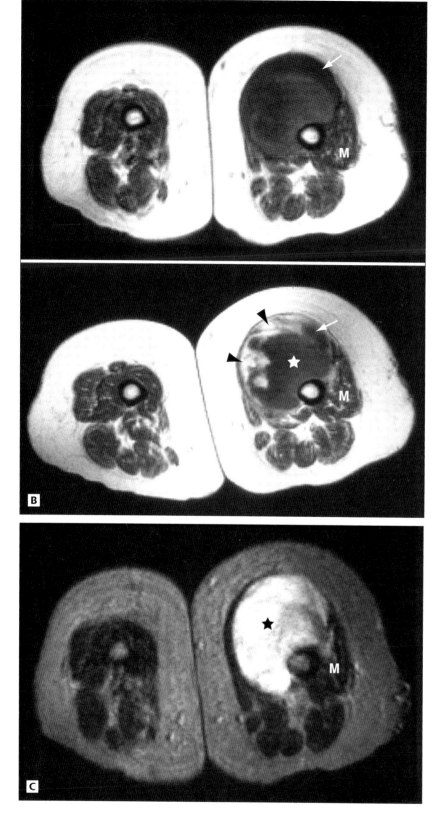

FIGURE 3–5 Continued. **(B)** Axial T1-weighted MR image before (superior image) and following contrast reveals identical peripheral nodular enhancement (arrowheads) and nonenhancing central necrosis (star). **(C)** Axial T2-weighted MR demonstrated diffuse high signal intensity in the soft tissue mass (star) not allowing distinction of the necrotic and non-necrotic regions.

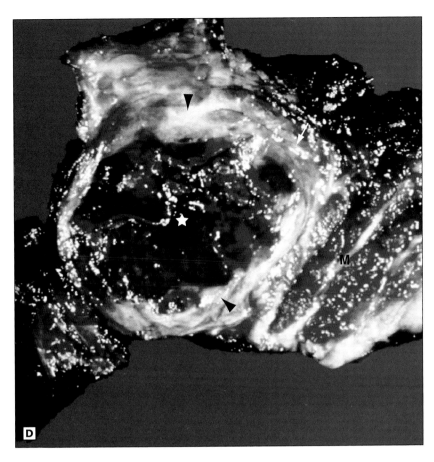

FIGURE 3–5 Continued. **(D)** Photograph of axially sectioned gross specimen shows identical features with central necrosis (star) and peripheral nodular viable neoplasm (arrowheads). This intramuscular mass replaces the normal muscle texture (M) on imaging (CT and MRI) and the gross specimen. Biopsy would need to be directed at solid peripheral areas and require imaging guidance (CT or sonography) to obtain diagnostic tissue.

TABLE 3–4 SOFT TISSUE MASS EVALUATION – LESION LOCATION

Subcutaneous	Angiomatous lesions	Intramuscular	Nodular fasciitis
	Benign fibrous histiocytoma		Angiomatous lesions
	Dermatofibrosarcoma protuberans (DFSP)		Lipoma
	Granuloma annulare		Malignant fibrous histiocytoma (MFH)
	Leiomyosarcoma		Fibrosarcoma
	Lipoma		Myxoma
	Lymphoma		Liposarcoma (well differentiated/ pleomorphic)
	Malignant fibrous histiocytoma (MFH)		Leiomyosarcoma/rhabdomyosarcoma
	Metastasis (particularly melanoma)		Soft tissue Ewing sarcoma/PNET
	Myxoma		Lipoma arborescens
	Nodular fasciitis	Intra-articular/juxta-articular	Pigmented villonodular synovitis
	Skin appendage tumors		Synovial chondromatosis
Intermuscular	Extraskeletal myxoid chondrosarcoma		Giant cell tumor of tendon sheath
	Fibromatosis		Synovial cyst, bursa, ganglion
	Ganglion, bursa and synovial cyst		Synovial hemangioma
	Leiomyosarcoma		Tumoral calcinosis
	Nodular fasciitis		Synovial sarcoma
	Neurogenic tumors		
	Synovial sarcoma		
	Lipoma and liposarcoma (myxoid)		

in differential diagnoses since some tumors are more likely to occur in certain compartments. Common benign and malignant lesions in these various compartments are listed in Table 3–4. There are exceptions to this concept such as a lesion deep to the scapular tip almost invariably represents elastofibroma (Fig. 3–6).[57–59]

Subcutaneous masses are extremely common clinically (Fig. 3–4). However, they are relatively infrequently evaluated by imaging owing to the "ease" of clinical evaluation. In contradistinction, deep-seated soft tissue masses (intermuscular, intramuscular, or intra-articular) are usually imaged because of inadequate clinical assessment.

Intermuscular soft tissue masses are usually adjacent to a rim of fat ("split-fat" sign) with the surrounding musculature draped around the lesion (Fig. 3–7). This is

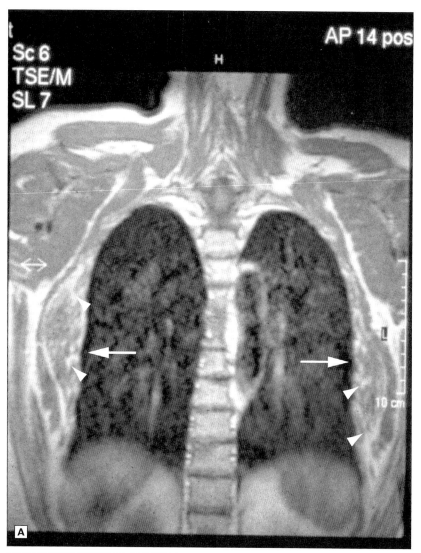

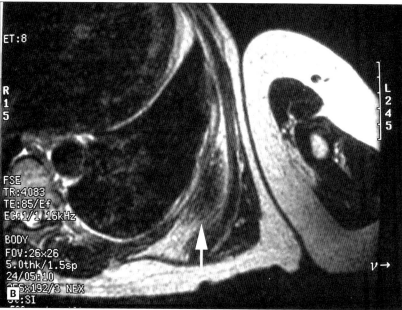

FIGURE 3–6 Elastofibroma in a 56-year-old woman deep to the scapular tip. **(A)** Coronal T1-weighted MR image shows bilateral soft tissue masses (arrows) deep to the scapular tips. There are small streaks of high signal intensity fat (arrowheads) within these masses. **(B)** T2-weighted MR image reveals nonadipose regions of low signal intensity (arrow) suggesting collagenized tissue. These features of location and appearance are pathognomonic of elastofibroma.

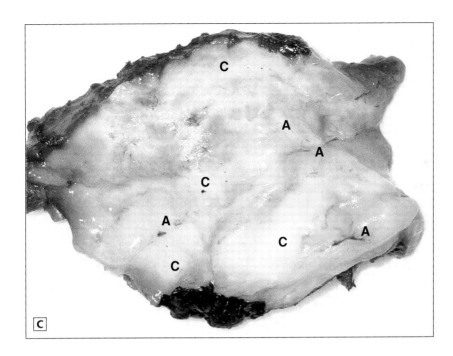

FIGURE 3–6 Continued. **(C)** Photograph of the gross specimen also reveals the intermixed collagenized elements (C) and adipose components (A) identical to imaging.

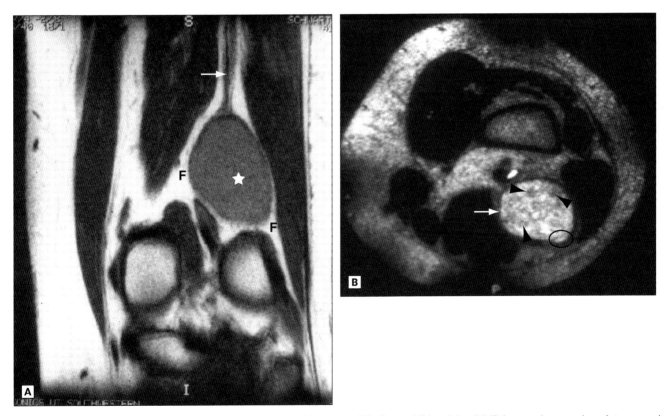

FIGURE 3–7 Schwannoma above the knee in a 49-year-old woman. **(A)** Coronal T1-weighted MR image shows a deep intermuscular mass (star) surrounded by fat (F – "split-fat" sign). Linear tubular extension superiorly represents the entering sciatic nerve (arrow) and creates a fusiform shaped mass. **(B)** Axial T2-weighted image also demonstrated the mass (large arrow) and reveals the "fascicular" sign with multiple small circular structures (arrowheads) and eccentric sciatic nerve (circle) distinguishing this lesion from a neurofibroma.

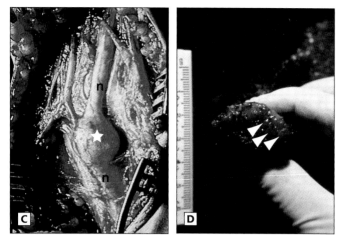

FIGURE 3–7 Continued. **(C)** Intraoperative photograph demonstrated the Schwannoma (star) as well as both the entering and exiting nerve (n). **(D)** Photograph of axially sectioned gross specimen reveals fascicular pattern (arrowheads) reflected on imaging.

best depicted by MRI but is also seen on US and CT. It occurs because the deep intermuscular tissue is primarily composed of fat and soft tissue masses arising in this location maintain a rim of adipose tissue as they enlarge. In large lesions the intermuscular location is often best determined by evaluating the superior and inferior aspect of the tumor.

Intramuscular masses replace the normal muscle texture signal intensity on MRI (Fig. 3–5). These lesions reveal surrounding muscle that typically lacks a fat rim unless they involve an entire compartment (Fig. 3–5).

Soft tissue masses that arise within or immediately adjacent to a joint have a relatively limited differential diagnosis and are usually benign. Synovial sarcoma is the most frequent malignancy, although it rarely originates in a joint (5–10% of cases).[13,55,56] Intra-articular lesions often diffusely involve the joint as seen with pigmented villonodular synovitis (Fig. 3–8), synovial chondromatosis, and lipoma arborescens.[15–17,60–63]

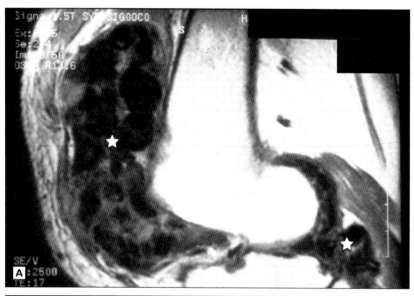

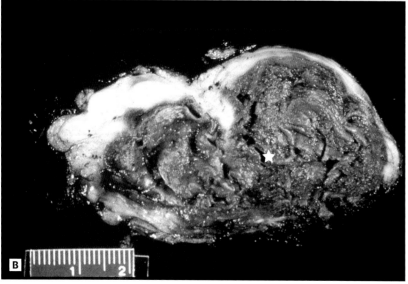

FIGURE 3–8 Pigmented villonodular synovitis (PVNS) in a 34-year-old woman involving the knee joint. **(A)** Sagittal proton density MR image shows massive involvement of the joint with tissue that demonstrates marked low signal (stars). **(B)** Photograph of gross specimen of a representative piece of the intra-articular tissue reveals marked brown color (*) related to extensive hemosiderin deposition causing the MR appearance characteristic of PVNS.

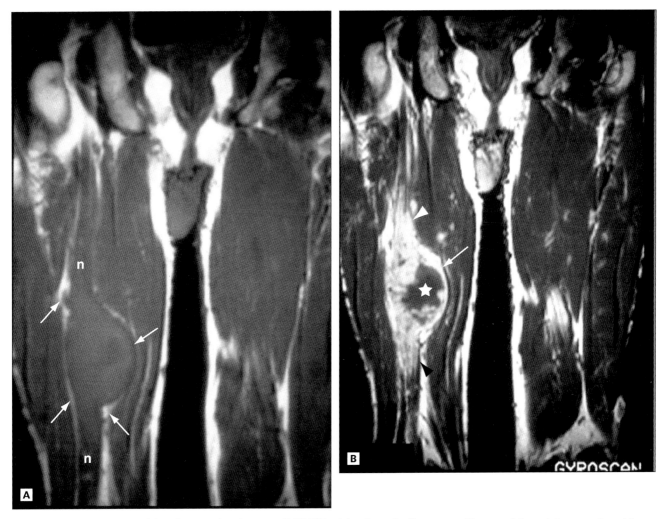

FIGURE 3–9 Malignant peripheral nerve sheath tumor (MPNST) arising in a plexiform neurofibroma of the sciatic nerve in a 42-year-old man with type I neurofibromatosis and recent rapidly enlarging thigh mass. **(A, B, C)** Coronal T1-weighted before (A) and after (B) intravenous contrast and fat suppressed T2-weighted (C) MR images show a fusiform shaped, intermuscular (split-fat sign – small arrows) soft tissue mass (large arrowheads) with marked thickening of the entering and exiting sciatic nerve (n) representing a plexiform neurofibroma. Note the large size of the MPNST (>5 cm), nonenhancing central necrosis (star), and growth along the exiting and entering nerves (large arrowheads) all indicative of sarcomatous degeneration. A second subcutaneous neurofibroma is seen superiorly (open arrow).

The detection of multiple soft tissue masses (or extensive/diffuse involvement) also markedly restricts the differential diagnosis and is generally associated with benign lesions, in contradistinction to other organ systems where this finding suggests malignancy. Lipomas are multiple in 5–15% of patients.[64-70] The fibromatoses and angiomatous lesions are multifocal in up to 20% of patients.[17,71-77] Patients with type 1 neurofibromatosis [NF 1] invariably reveal multiple neurogenic tumors and rapid enlargement of a lesion should be viewed as suggesting malignant degeneration to malignant peripheral nerve sheath tumor (Fig. 3–9).[78] Myxomas may be multiple in association with fibrous dysplasia (Mazabraud syndrome).[79,80] Finally, metastases may be multifocal, particularly to the subcutaneous tissue (e.g., melanoma, breast), or rarely to muscle (e.g., lung).

Intrinsic imaging characteristics

Whereas the compartmental location of a lesion provides a differential diagnosis, the intrinsic imaging characteristics often adds specificity. Those characteristics that frequently suggest the diagnosis include signal intensity, morphologic attributes and shape of the lesion. In addition, increasingly specific MRI findings are improving the confidence level of radiologic diagnosis. Detection of adipose tissue in a soft tissue mass limits the differential diagnosis to lipoma (Fig. 3–4), lipoblastoma, hibernoma (Fig. 3–3), hemangioma (with fat atrophy or overgrowth) (Fig. 3–10) and liposarcoma (Fig. 3–11).[66,68,70,81-95] Markedly low signal intensity on T2-weighted MRI may be related to rapidly flowing blood (arteriovenous hemangioma), calcification

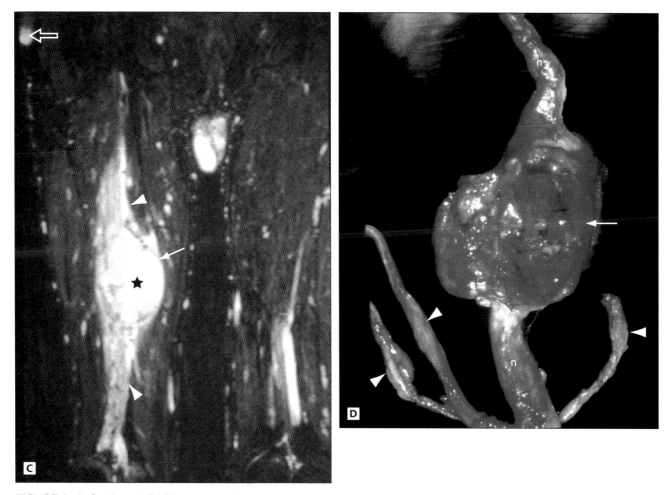

FIGURE 3–9 Continued. **(D)** Photograph of gross specimen reveals an identical appearance with the thickened plexiform neurofibroma diffusely involving the sciatic nerve (n) including its branches (small arrowheads) and the MPNST (arrow).

(extraskeletal osteosarcoma), hemosiderin (tenosynovial giant cell tumor, pigmented villonodular synovitis) (Fig. 3–8) or high collagen content (some cases of fibromatosis).[60–62,96–98]

Morphology and shape often reveal a characteristic imaging appearance of soft tissue masses that mirror the gross and histologic composition so that understanding the importance of this radiologic–pathologic correlation holds the key to continuous improvement in diagnostic acumen. Soft tissue tumors composed of serpentine channels and spaces invariably represent an angiomatous lesion (hemangioma or lymphangioma) (Fig. 3–10).[75] A tubular structure entering and exiting a fusiform mass suggests a nerve sheath tumor (Figs 3–7, 3–9).[99–108] Another characteristic sign

of a nerve sheath tumor is the "target" sign on T2-weighted MRI with a rim of high signal peripherally and low signal centrally. Linear extension along fascial planes or the skin ("fascial-tail" or "skin tail" sign) is common in the fibromatoses, nodular fasciitis, and dermatofibrosarcoma protuberans (Fig. 3–12).[13] Soft tissue neoplasms, both benign and malignant, usually have a relatively well-defined margin with little surrounding edema.[109,110] This is related to the pseudocapsule surrounding many soft tissue neoplasms and it is important to recognize that a well-defined margin does not imply a benign diagnosis. Prominent edema around a nontreated soft tissue mass may simulate a spiculated infiltrative and aggressive margin but should rather strongly suggest a reactive, traumatic, or inflammatory

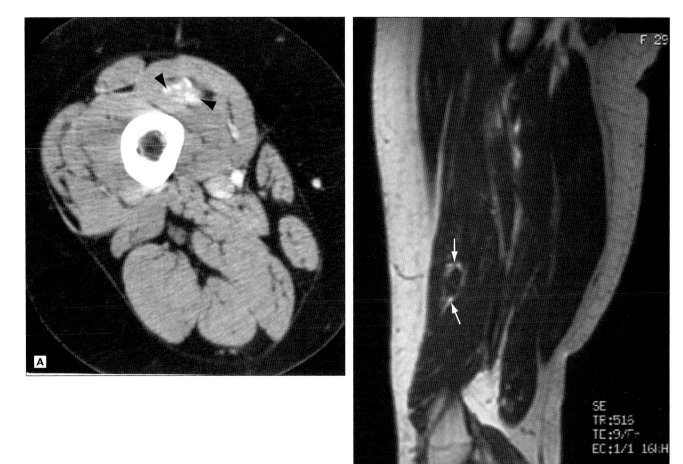

FIGURE 3–10 Intramuscular cavernous hemangioma of the thigh in a 29-year-old woman. **(A)** CT post-contrast shows the intramuscular soft tissue mass with multiple circular enhancing foci (black arrowheads). **(B)** Sagittal T1-weighted MR image reveals the intramuscular soft tissue mass with surrounding fat resulting from muscle atrophy (arrows).

process as opposed to neoplasm (Fig. 3–13). There are exceptions, however, and soft tissue metastases and myxoinflammatory fibroblastic sarcoma may show prominent surrounding edema.

Patient age must also be considered in determining the order of differential diagnoses of a soft tissue mass but is generally not as helpful as in bone tumors. For example, a deep soft tissue mass containing tissue with high water content (myxoid) and a small amount of fat in a patient over the age of 20 years almost certainly represents a myxoid liposarcoma.[90,92,111] In contrast, identical imaging features in a 2-year-old would invariably indicate a lipoblastoma (Fig. 3–14).[70,81,82] Additional relevant clinical history can also be an important factor in establishing an accurate diagnosis (Figs 3–1, 3–14). Table 3–5 shows differential diagnoses in order of decreasing frequency for three age groups: children, young adults, and older adults.

Lesion specificity by imaging

Imaging characteristics reportedly suggest a relatively specific diagnosis in 20–50% of soft tissue tumors.[1–8] We believe this percentage will gradually improve with recognition of increasingly specific MRI features, although probably not beyond 70–90%.[9] Imaging characteristics of soft tissue tumors and their relative specificity are listed in Tables 3–6 to 3–11.[112,113] Lesions with a

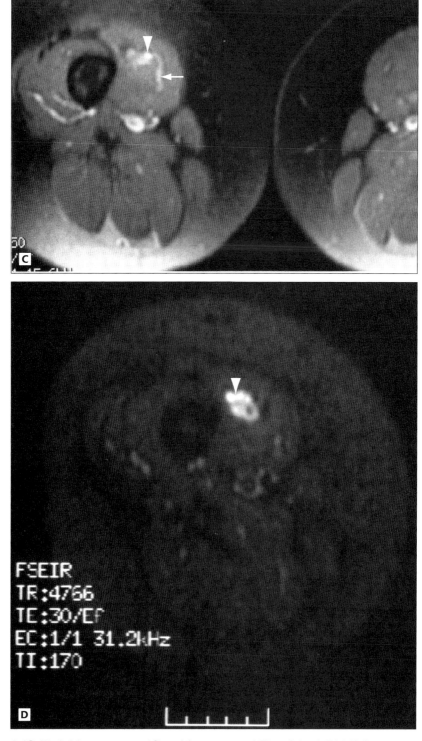

FIGURE 3–10 Continued. **(C, D)** Axial post-contrast (C) and fat suppressed T2-weighted (D) MR images demonstrate multiple high signal intensity circular vascular spaces (white arrowheads) and serpentine feeding vessel (arrow). These imaging features are pathognomonic of hemangioma.

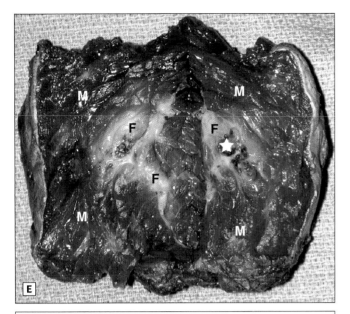

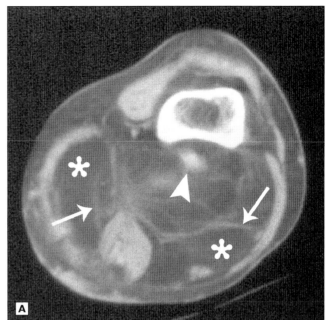

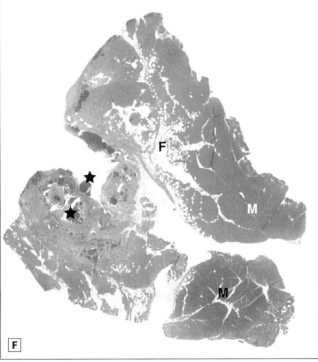

FIGURE 3–10 Continued. **(E, F)** Photograph of sectioned gross specimen (E) and photomicrograph (hematoxylin and eosin stain, ×10) shows identical features with blood filled spaces/channels (stars), fat atrophy of surrounding muscle (F) due to chronic ischemia and normal muscle (M).

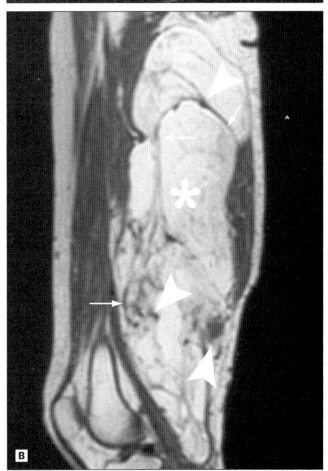

FIGURE 3–11 Well-differentiated liposarcoma of the thigh in a 65-year-old woman with a 3-year history of a slowly growing painless mass. **(A)** CT reveals the low attenuation fat (*) with numerous thick septa (>2 mm) (arrows) and encasement of the neurovascular bundle (arrowhead). **(B)** Sagittal T1-weighted MR image demonstrates a high signal intensity adipose lesion involving both intramuscular and intermuscular portions of the posterior thigh compartment (*) with thick septa (white arrows) and several areas of mild nodularity (arrowheads).

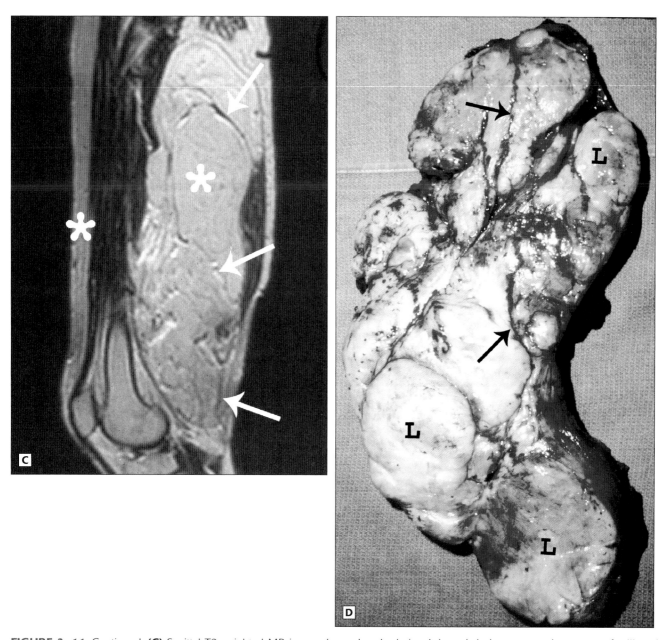

FIGURE 3–11 Continued. **(C)** Sagittal T2-weighted MR image shows that the lesional tissue is isointense to subcutaneous fat (*) and the thick septa reveal both high and low signal intensity (arrows). **(D)** Photograph of the sectioned gross specimen shows the yellow lipomatous tissue (L) and multiple septa (black arrows).

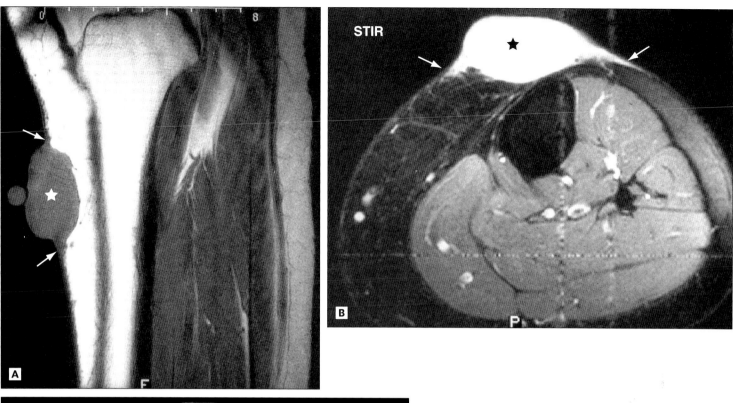

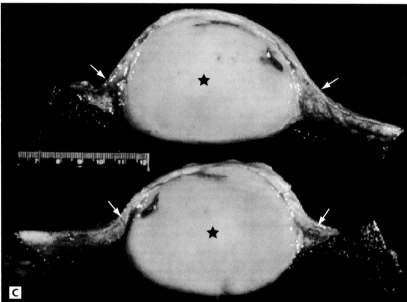

FIGURE 3–12 Dermatofibrosarcoma protuberans (DFSP) in a 38-year-old man with a slowly enlarging subcutaneous mass involving the skin. **(A)** Sagittal T1-weighted MR image shows a subcutaneous mass (star) protruding from and involving the skin. **(B)** Axial fat suppressed T2-weighted MR image reveals similar findings and high signal intensity in the mass (star). Linear extension along the skin ("skin-tail" sign) (arrows in A and B) are also seen on both images. **(C)** Photograph of sectioned gross specimen demonstrates manifestations identical to that seen on MR imaging with the mass (stars) and linear skin extension (arrows).

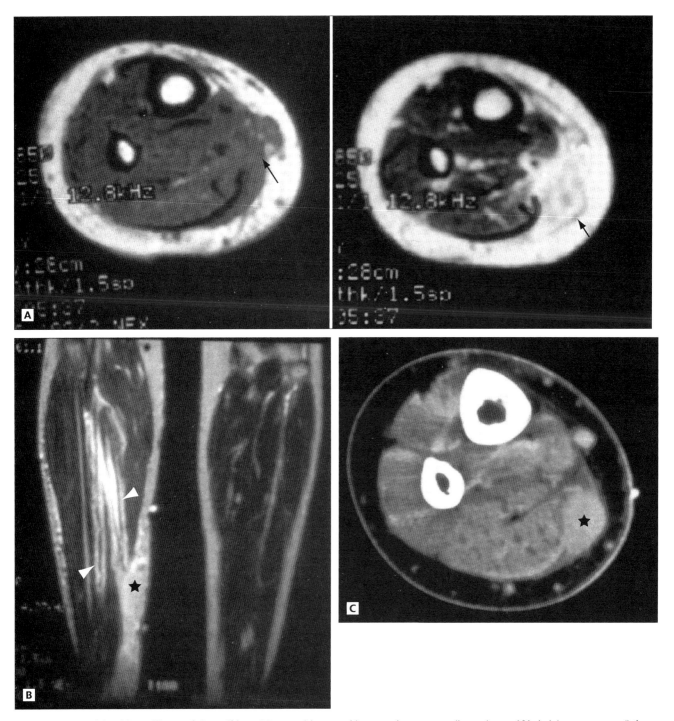

FIGURE 3–13 Myositis ossificans of the calf in a 39-year-old man with extensive surrounding edema. **(A)** Axial pre-contrast (left image) and post-contrast (right image) MR images show an enhancing ill-defined soft tissue mass (arrows). **(B)** Coronal T2-weighted MR reveals the soft tissue mass (star) and extensive edema (arrowheads) creating irregular margins and simulating aggressive growth. **(C)** CT at the time of the MR demonstrates the soft tissue mass (star) which is noncalcified.

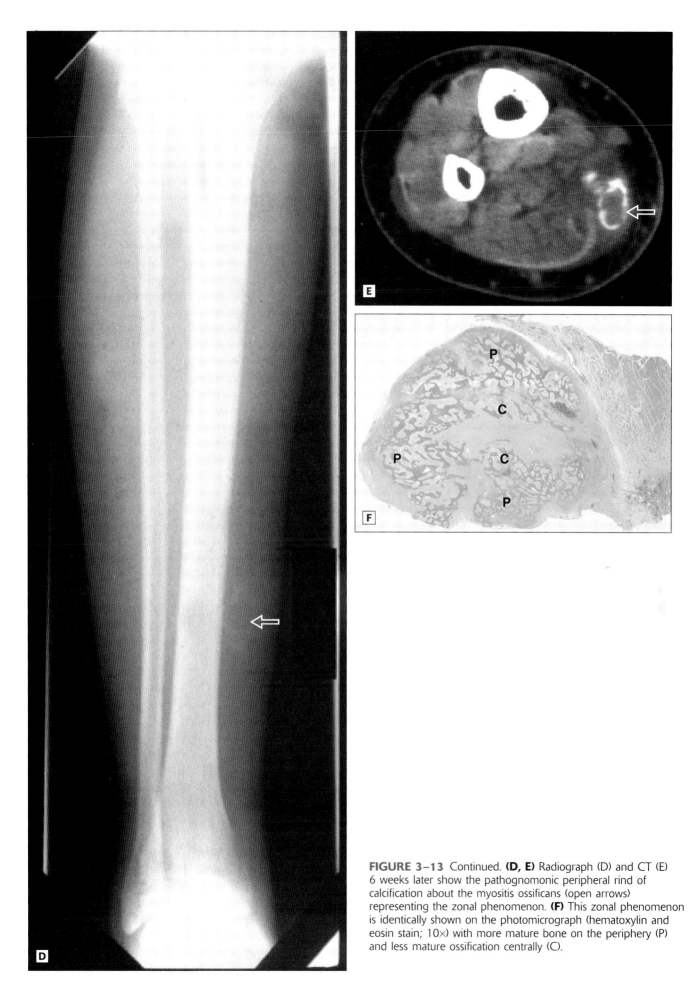

FIGURE 3–13 Continued. **(D, E)** Radiograph (D) and CT (E) 6 weeks later show the pathognomonic peripheral rind of calcification about the myositis ossificans (open arrows) representing the zonal phenomenon. **(F)** This zonal phenomenon is identically shown on the photomicrograph (hematoxylin and eosin stain; 10×) with more mature bone on the periphery (P) and less mature ossification centrally (C).

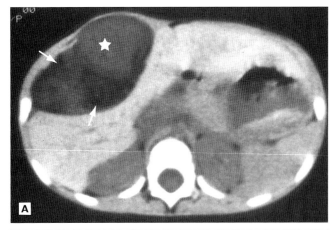

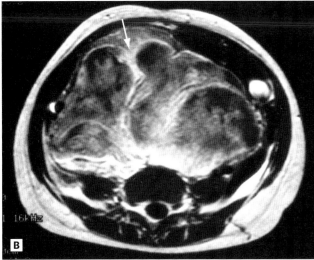

TABLE 3–5	SOFT TISSUE TUMOR DIFFERENTIAL DIAGNOSIS BY AGE

Child (<16 years)

Benign	Malignant
Hemangioma	Fibrosarcoma
Fibromatosis	Synovial sarcoma
Fibrous histiocytoma	Rhabdomyosarcoma
Granuloma annulare	

Young adult (16–45 years)

Benign	Malignant
Ganglion	MFH/Fibrosarcoma
Fibrous histiocytoma	Liposarcoma
Nodular fasciitis	Dermatofibrosarcoma
Neurogenic neoplasm (Schwannoma,	protuberans (DFSP)
neurofibroma)	Synovial sarcoma
Lipoma	MPNST
Hemangioma	

Older adult (46 years and up)

Benign	Malignant
Ganglion	MFH/Fibrosarcoma
Lipoma	Liposarcoma
Neurogenic neoplasm	Leiomyosarcoma
Fibrous histiocytoma	MPNST
Nodular fasciitis	DFSP
Myxoma	

From pathologic referral series AFIP, references 112 and 113, in order of decreasing frequency. MFH, malignant fibrous histiocytoma; MPNST, malignant peripheral nerve sheath tumor

FIGURE 3–14 Lipoblastoma of the abdominal wall in an infant simulating myxoid liposarcoma by intrinsic imaging characteristics. **(A)** CT shows a heterogeneous soft tissue mass with subtle fat peripherally (arrows) but more fluid attenuation in the remainder and majority of the lesion (star). **(B)** Axial gradient echo MR image reveals fat (arrow) only in the periphery with other predominant nonadipose regions. In an adult, this imaging appearance is diagnostic of myxoid liposarcoma. However, in an infant this diagnosis is untenable and the features are pathognomonic of lipoblastoma, emphasizing the importance of clinical information and patient age in some cases.

pathognomonic appearance (Table 3–12), typically benign lesions, on imaging may not require biopsy or excision, depending on the clinical situation. This emphasizes the need for a close working relationship between the oncologist/orthopedist and musculoskeletal radiologist and may change the types of soft tissue lesions the pathologist will evaluate in the future.

"Cystic" masses

Soft tissue masses demonstrating high water content on CT, MRI, or US suggesting a "cystic" lesion have differen-tial diagnostic possibilities restricted to those lesions listed in Table 3–13.[6,15,17,63,114–122] These lesions may all have similar appearances on noncontrast CT or MRI. CT demonstrates low attenuation and MRI shows low signal intensity on T1-weighting and very high signal on T2-weighting.[6,15,17,63,99] US reveals an anechoic lesion with posterior acoustic enhancement in truly cystic masses and, similar to other organ systems, is the most efficient and least expensive method to differentiate these lesions from cyst mimickers (myxoid neoplasms).[123]

Ganglion, synovial cyst, bursa, and lymphangioma are typically easily diagnosed by their characteristic location and intrinsic cystic imaging appearance (Fig. 3–15).[116–118,120,124] These lesions are frequently multiloculated with thin intervening septa. Ruptured synovial cysts, particularly popliteal, may dissect into the calf, simulating deep venous thrombosis clinically and creating a more complex appearance on imaging due to associated hemorrhage.[125] Imaging reveals this dissection as a long fusiform shape with frequent prominent surrounding edema resulting from tissue irritation allowing distinction from neoplasm (Fig. 3–16).

Perilabral/meniscal cysts adjacent to fibrocartilaginous structures have been referred to as ganglia and juxta-articular myxomas. However, it is now recognized that

TABLE 3–6 COMMON BENIGN SOFT TISSUE TUMORS: SPECIFIC IMAGING APPEARANCE

Diagnosis	Soft tissue tumor %[a]	Imaging appearance[b]	Estimated % with diagnostic imaging appearance
Lipoma and variants	16%	Extensive fat can be difficult to distinguish from well-differentiated liposarcoma	70–90% Often not requiring biopsy
Fibrous histiocytoma	13%	Non-specific, usually subcutaneous	0%
Nodular fasciitis	11%	Subcutaneous mass, particularly forearm, with linear extensions along fascia	Up to 50% Biopsy usually required
Hemangioma	8%	Serpentine channels/space with fat overgrowth	90–95% Biopsy not required
Fibromatosis (all types including infantile and fibroma)	8%	Mass along superficial fascia; low signal intensity bands; fascial tail sign, overall low signal intensity, location (foot, hand, shoulder)	50–70% Biopsy usually required, exception in superficial hand/foot lesions
Neurofibroma	5%	Intermuscular mass ("split-fat" sign) along major nerve, "entering/exiting tube" sign, "target" sign; "fascicular" sign, muscle atrophy, multiple lesions or plexiform morphology, <5 cm in size	70–90% Many not require biopsy
Schwannoma	5%	Same as above, may be able to distinguish from neurofibroma if nerve eccentric to mass	70–90% May not require biopsy
Giant cell tumor tendon sheath (GCTTS)	4%	Low signal intensity about tendon with blooming on gradient echo MRI due to hemosiderin	70–90% Often resected without biopsy
Myxoma	3%	High water content intramuscular mass with faint fat rim and edema; simulates a cyst on CT/MRI; sonography helpful, hypoechoic but solid mass	70–80% May not require biopsy if all pathognomonic findings present
Ganglion	0.9%, but much higher in nonreferral population	Cystic mass with septal or peripheral enhancement	>95% No biopsy required and often not resected
Myositis ossificans	0.7%, but much more common because most not resected	Diagnostic appearance on radiographs/CT with peripheral rim of ossification MRI can suggest a more aggressive lesion	>95% With development of ossificans rim (CT optimal). No biopsy needed

[a] From pathologic referral series AFIP, references 112 and 113.
[b] MRI appearance unless otherwise specified.

TABLE 3–7 UNCOMMON BENIGN SOFT TISSUE TUMORS: SPECIFIC IMAGING APPEARANCE

Diagnosis	Soft tissue tumor %[a]	Imaging appearance[b]	Estimated % with diagnostic imaging appearance
Leiomyoma	2%	May have extensive calcification (like in uterus) on radiographs; otherwise non-specific	0% Requires biopsy
Chondroma	2%	Ring and arc calcification on radiographs/CT; hand/foot/infrapatella location; high signal T2 and septal/peripheral enhancement	50–70% May not require biopsy
Fibroma of tendon sheath	2%	Similar to GCTTS but no hemosiderin	70–90% in differential with GCTTS often resected without biopsy
Hemangiopericytoma/solitary fibrous tumor	2%	Deep intermuscular mass with feeding vascular pedicle and intrinsic vessels	>50% in our experience but require biopsy and resection
Granular cell tumor	2%	Subcutaneous mass with prominent low signal intensity and may have mild surrounding edema	>50% in our experience but requires biopsy
Granuloma annulare/necrobiotic nodule	2%	Subcutaneous mass particularly pre-tibial in a child	>75%, may not require biopsy Lesions anterior to tibia
Proliferative fasciitis/myositis	1%	Non-specific appearance	0% Requires biopsy
Myofibromatosis	1%	Infant with associated bone lesions; may be multifocal	30–50% (only multifocal lesions) Biopsy for diagnosis
Glomus tumor	0.9%	Hand lesion related to nail bed, high signal T2	>90% Usually resected
Pigmented villonodular synovitis	0.9%	Diffuse intra-articular with low signal intensity and blooming on gradient sequences due to hemosiderin	>99% Usually resected without biopsy
Lymphangioma	0.9%	Cystic mass in neck in infant or young child <2 years of age	>95% Usually no biopsy required, may be resected or treated percutaneously with sclerosis

[a] From pathologic referral series AFIP, references 112 and 113.
[b] MRI appearance unless otherwise specified.

TABLE 3–8 RARE BENIGN SOFT TISSUE TUMORS: SPECIFIC IMAGING APPEARANCE

Diagnosis	Soft tissue tumor%[a]	Imaging appearance[b]	Estimated % with diagnostic imaging appearance
Lipoblastoma	0.6%	Fat in a mass without vascular structure in a patient less than 10 years of age	>95% No biopsy required
Fibrous hamartoma of infancy	0.5%	Heterogeneous lesion in axilla containing fat in an infant	50–75% in characteristic location but still requires biopsy
Neuroma	0.4% May be much more common (Morton neuroma)	Often characteristic appearance similar to neurogenic tumor and location/history	75–90% May not require biopsy
Paraganglioma	0.3%	Often characteristic by location (e.g., chemodectoma), vessels identified with salt/pepper appearance	>75% But usually requires resection
Tumoral calcinosis	0.3%	Para-articular calcification multiple sites; best on radiographs/CT	>95% Biopsy not usually required. Not typically resected
Elastofibroma	0.3%, but likely much more common (asymptomatic)	Characteristic periscapular location. Small mass with interspersed fat CT/MRI	>95% Biopsy not required nor is resection
Synovial chondromatosis	0.3%	Multiple calcifications (best on CT) and diffuse synovial abnormality	>95% Biopsy not required but often resected
Hibernoma	0.2%	Similar to fat but feeding vascular pedicle and internal vessels best on MRI. Marked uptake on PET unlike well-differentiated liposarcoma	>90% Biopsy or resection may not be required
Ganglioneuroma	0.2%	Location paraspinal, otherwise non-specific	0% Need biopsy/resection
Lipomatosis of nerve	0.1%	Fat about fascicles of enlarged nerve (usually median)	>99% No biopsy required

[a] From pathologic referral series AFIP, references 112 and 113.
[b] MRI appearance unless otherwise specified.

TABLE 3–9 COMMON MALIGNANT SOFT TISSUE TUMORS: SPECIFIC IMAGING APPEARANCE

Diagnosis	Soft tissue tumor %[a]	Imaging appearance[b]	Estimated % with diagnostic imaging appearance
MFH/Fibrosarcoma	49%	Non-specific intrinsically but intramuscular or deep subcutaneous mass in older patients	Suggestive appearance in majority >75% but not diagnostic. Biopsy/resection required
Well-differentiated liposarcoma	8%	Largely (>75%) fat with nodular or thick septa of nonadipose elements	>90% Often do not require biopsy and may not require resection
Leiomyosarcoma	8%	Non-specific appearance except when arise from vessel wall	<5% Requires biopsy and resection
MPNST	6%	Exiting/entering nerve with dominant mass; >5 cm and mildly irregular margins to distinguish from BPNST; often in association with NF	>70% Requires biopsy and resection
DFSP	6%	Subcutaneous mass with skin protuberance; also satellite lesions and extension along dermis ("skin tail" sign)	>70% Requires biopsy and resection
Synovial sarcoma	5%	Calcified (radiographs or CT) periarticular mass often very heterogeneous with hemorrhage; multilocular	>50% Requires biopsy and resection
Myxoid liposarcoma	4%	High water content mass with small amounts of fat (<5–10% of the lesions volume)	90–95% Requires biopsy and resection

[a] From pathologic referral series AFIP, references 112 and 113.
[b] MRI appearance unless otherwise specified.
MFH, malignant fibrous histiocytoma, currently referred to as undifferentiated high-grade pleomorphic sarcoma; includes all varieties and non-specific spindle cell sarcoma; MPNST, malignant peripheral nerve sheath tumor; BPNST, benign peripheral nerve sheath tumor; NF, neurofibromatosis type 1; DFSP, dermatofibrosarcoma protuberans (includes all variations and non-specific spindle cell sarcoma).

TABLE 3–10 UNCOMMON MALIGNANT SOFT TISSUE TUMORS: SPECIFIC IMAGING APPEARANCE

Diagnosis	Soft tissue tumor %[a]	Imaging appearance[b]	Estimated % with diagnostic imaging appearance
Extraskeletal chondrosarcoma	2%	Myxoid shows high water content; mesenchymal may show higher vascularity and enhancement; both chondroid calcification (CT or radiographs)	>50% because of calcification but requires biopsy and resection
Angiosarcoma	2%	Non-specific except in setting of chronic lymphedema with lobular, dominant skin mass	10% with lymphedema Requires biopsy and resection
Rhabdomyosarcoma	2%	Large often infiltrative intramuscular mass in child; alveolar types may have vascular structures and high signal on T2	40–50% Requires biopsy
Angiomatoid fibrous histiocytoma	2%	Multiloculated cystic appearance (fluid levels) with mild surrounding edema	>70% Biopsy and resection required
Pleomorphic liposarcoma	1%	Large mass with small amounts of fat (60–75%)	60–75% Requires biopsy and resection
Dedifferentiated liposarcoma	1%	Well-differentiated liposarcoma with nodular soft tissue component >1–2 cm in size	>95% Requires biopsy (both parts) and resection
Epithelioid sarcoma	1%	Subcutaneous/skin lesion of hand with non-specific features	0% Biopsy/resection required
Kaposi sarcoma	1%	Focal nodular skin mass in patient with AIDS	>50% Biopsy required
Malignant hemangiopericytoma	1%	Same as benign counterpart	>50% Biopsy/resection required
Extraskeletal Ewing/PNET/peripheral neuroepithelioma	1%	Non-specific but may see intrinsic high flow vessels	0% Biopsy required

[a]From pathologic referral series AFIP, references 112 and 113.
[b]MRI appearance unless otherwise specified.
PNET, primitive neuroectodermal tumor.

TABLE 3–11 RARE MALIGNANT SOFT TISSUE TUMORS: SPECIFIC IMAGING APPEARANCE

Diagnosis	Soft tissue tumor %[a]	Imaging appearance[b]	Estimated % with diagnostic imaging appearance
Clear cell sarcoma	1%	Growth in tendon/aponeurosis, may have mildly increased signal on T1 and low signal T2	60–70% Biopsy/resection required
Infantile fibrosarcoma	1%	Large mass in infant with high-flow vascular component	>90% Biopsy/resection required
Extraskeletal osteosarcoma	1%	Large mass in older patient with dense osteoid calcification (best on radiograph/CT)	>50% Biopsy/resection required
Alveolar soft part sarcoma	0.5%	Intramuscular mass with feeding vascular pedicle and very prominent high-flow vessels	>90% Biopsy/resection required
Neuroblastoma/ganglioneuroblastoma	0.5%	Non-specific in soft tissue; often paraspinal	0% Biopsy/resection required
Giant cell fibroblastoma	0.3%	Same as DFSP in an infant/child	>70% Requires biopsy/resection
Malignant granular cell tumor	0.2%	Same as benign granular cell tumor	>50% Requires biopsy/resection
Malignant giant cell tumor of tendon sheath (GCTTS)	0.1%	Same as benign GCTTS	70–90% Resection required
Malignant paraganglioma	0.1%	Same as benign paraganglioma	>75% Biopsy/resection required

[a]From pathologic referral series AFIP, references 112 and 113.
[b]MRI appearance unless otherwise specified.

these lesions result from traumatic tears with fluid extending through these injuries accumulating in an adjacent "cyst."[115,119,121] These lesions are likely to recur if the underlying cartilaginous damage is not repaired.

Liquefied hematoma and abscess formation may also cause "cystic" soft tissue masses.[13,126] Imaging typically reveals a much thicker and irregular wall about these lesions as compared to the pseudocapsule of high water content neoplasms. Hematomas may also reveal hemosiderin in thin or thick but smooth walls, in contrast to

neoplasms (Figs 3–5, 3–17). Abscess formation may also reveal linear extensions representing sinus tracts.

Myxomatous neoplasms that can simulate cystic masses on noncontrast CT and MRI because of their intrinsic high water content are listed in Table 3–13.[13,78–80,92,127–130] However, post-contrast peripheral nodular or mild diffuse enhancement distinguishes these lesions from a ganglion, synovial cyst, abscess, or hematoma, which demonstrates non-nodular, usually thin peripheral/septal enhancement. US is particularly useful for distinguishing these lesions because myxomatous lesions, while having a high water content, are still solid lesions and are hypoechoic but not anechoic as seen in cystic masses (Figs 3–15, 3–18).[116,123] Myxoid liposarcomas are particularly notorious for simulating a cyst (5–10% of cases) on imaging, although in our experience, 90–95% have a pathognomonic appearance because they contain small amounts of fat (5–10% or less of the tumor volume) on MRI, allowing accurate diagnosis (Fig. 3–18).[13,92,123]

Non-specific soft tissue masses

Soft tissue masses with a non-specific imaging appearance are becoming less common. Lesions that are small (<5 cm) with defined margins, homogeneity, and lack of neurovascular encasement are suggestive of a benign process.[51,109,110,131] In contrast, lesions that are large (>5 cm) with ill-defined margins, heterogeneity, and neurovascular or bone involvement are suggestive of an aggressive or malignant process. *However in our opinion,*

TABLE 3–12	SOFT TISSUE MASSES FREQUENTLY DIAGNOSED WITH IMAGING ALONE

Lipomatous lesions
Angiomatous lesions
Neurogenic tumors
Elastofibroma
Pigmented villonodular synovitis (PVNS)
Synovial chondromatosis
Myositis ossificans
Tumoral calcinosis
Ganglion
Synovial cyst
Giant cell tumor of tendon sheath
Fibromatosis (particularly superficial lesions hand/foot)
Nodular fasciitis
Myxoma
Abscess
Hematoma

TABLE 3–13	HIGH WATER CONTENT – "CYSTIC" MASSES	
Diagnosis	**Demographics**	**Imaging variation** [a]
Ganglion	Wrist (dorsal), foot, knee	May have thick but non-nodular wall and floating debris
Synovial cyst	Knee (popliteal-Baker cyst), iliopsoas, apophyseal	Neck connected to the joint; may have floating debris; ruptured cyst may have a more complex appearance
Bursa	Iliopsoas; about shoulder, knee and wrist	Characteristic locations; may have floating debris and surrounding edema if ruptured
Lymphangioma	Young patient (>90% less than age of 2 years) in neck	Usually multilocular; may have fluid levels if traumatized with hemorrhage
Perilabral/meniscal cyst	Knee, shoulder, hip related to fibrocartilaginous tear	Often complex appearance due to debris; MRI (modality of choice) to detect internal joint derangement
Hematoma	Thigh, retroperitoneal (clinical history helpful, patients often anticoagulated)	Complex thin/thick walled mass (non-nodular) with hemosiderin chronically. Surrounding edema often prominent initially
Abscess	History often helpful with inflammatory signs	Thick-walled mass usually not nodular. Prominent surrounding edema and sinus tract formation
Myxomatous neoplasm	Include myxoma, myxoid MFH/Fibrosarcoma, neurogenic neoplasm, myxoid liposarcoma and extraskeletal chondrosarcoma	Simulate cyst on noncontrast CT/MRI. Peripheral nodular or diffuse contrast enhancement, US hypoechoic but not truly cystic (anechoic)

[a] MRI appearance unless otherwise specified.
MFH, malignant fibrous histiocytoma currently referred to as undifferentiated high-grade pleomorphic sarcoma; includes all myxoid variations of fibrosarcoma.

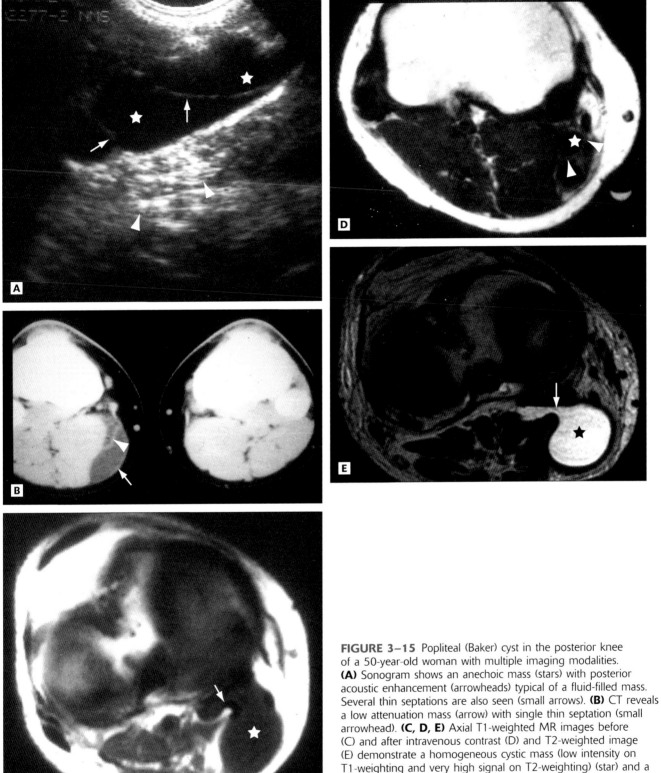

FIGURE 3–15 Popliteal (Baker) cyst in the posterior knee of a 50-year-old woman with multiple imaging modalities. **(A)** Sonogram shows an anechoic mass (stars) with posterior acoustic enhancement (arrowheads) typical of a fluid-filled mass. Several thin septations are also seen (small arrows). **(B)** CT reveals a low attenuation mass (arrow) with single thin septation (small arrowhead). **(C, D, E)** Axial T1-weighted MR images before (C) and after intravenous contrast (D) and T2-weighted image (E) demonstrate a homogeneous cystic mass (low intensity on T1-weighting and very high signal on T2-weighting) (star) and a neck extending back toward the joint (arrows). After contrast, thin peripheral and septal enhancement is seen (small arrowheads) confirming the cystic consistency of the lesion.

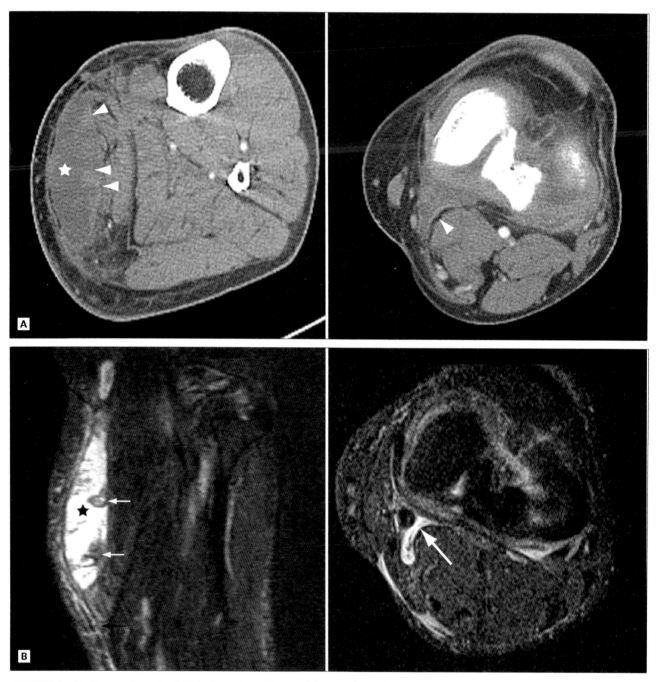

FIGURE 3–16 Ruptured popliteal (Baker) cyst in a 65-year-old man with calf pain. **(A)** CT at two levels shows a complex soft tissue mass (star) more inferiorly with nodular peripheral regions (small arrowheads, left image) and the neck of the synovial cyst connecting to the joint more superiorly (right image, large arrowhead). **(B)** Coronal (left image) and axial (right image) T2-weighted MR images reveal similar features of a long (15 cm) fusiform complex soft tissue mass (star) with solid components (small arrows). Surrounding edema (black arrows) is prominent and joint continuity through the neck is seen superiorly (large arrow).

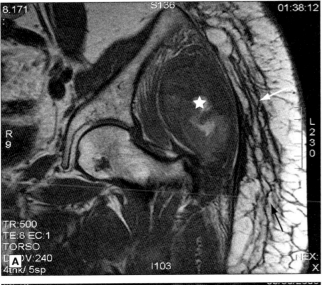

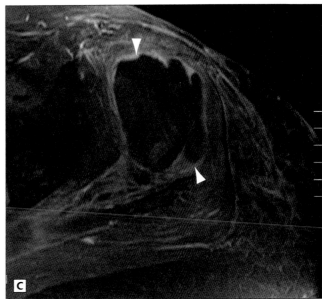

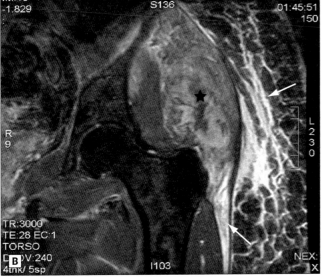

FIGURE 3–17 Hematoma, after a fall, involving the buttock of a 60-year-old woman on coumadin. **(A, B)** Coronal T1-weighted (A) and T2-weighted (B) MR images show a heterogeneous soft tissue mass (star) with extensive surrounding edema (arrows). **(C)** Axial post-contrast fat suppressed T1-weighted MR image reveals a thin rim of peripheral enhancement (arrowheads) about the hematoma without nodular foci.

MRI is not accurate enough to predict whether a soft tissue mass with non-specific intrinsic characteristics is benign or malignant. Therefore, such lesions require biopsy! Benign lesions that can demonstrate aggressive characteristics that simulate malignancy include hematoma (Fig. 3–17), fibromatosis, reactive lymph nodes, abscess, and myositis ossificans (Fig. 3–13). Malignant lesions that may reveal indolent features simulating benign disease include synovial sarcoma and myxoid liposarcoma.[13]

STAGING, BIOPSY AND TREATMENT FOLLOW-UP

There are numerous staging systems used in evaluation of soft tissue tumors discussed elsewhere in this text.[13,132–135] However, much of the information neces-

sary to stage soft tissue tumors can be obtained by imaging (particularly MRI). Important features to assess include: lesion extent (tumor crossing a major fascial plane to involve multiple compartments), size (lesion >5 cm) and involvement of adjacent bone, joint, or neurovascular structures.[124,136]

Biopsy of soft tissue masses is often performed percutaneously with imaging guidance (US or CT). Since limb salvage is the goal and treatment of choice in most soft sarcomas, nowhere is discussion between surgeon and radiologist more important so as not to violate tissues required in reconstruction.[137,138] In addition, it is essential that viable and representative tissue be obtained for pathologic evaluation and, for this reason, histologic analysis should be performed during the biopsy to ensure adequacy (Figs 3–18, 3–19).[13] Imaging can direct biopsy to non-necrotic and nonhemorrhagic foci of

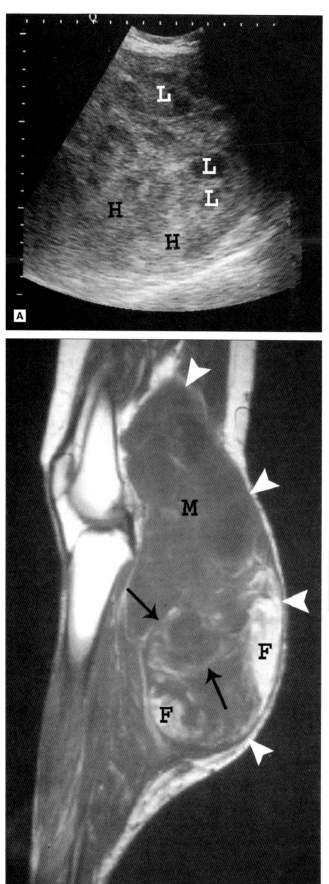

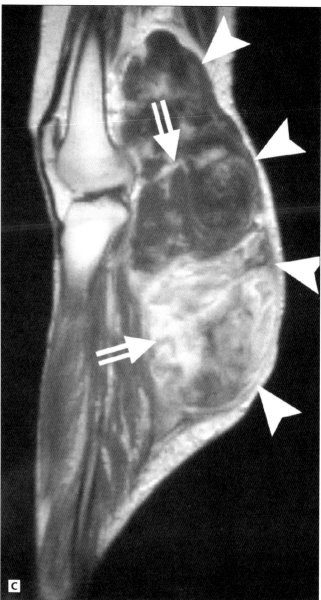

FIGURE 3–18 Myxoid liposarcoma of the popliteal region in a 60-year-old woman with a painless mass, which slowly increased in size over 6 years, clinically diagnosed as a popliteal cyst. **(A)** Sonogram reveals a heterogeneous mass with both low echogenicity areas (L) corresponding to myxoid tissue and regions of higher echogenicity (H). It is not possible to definitively identify fat, although the lesion is not cystic or in the expected location of a popliteal cyst and there is no neck of fluid extending toward the joint. **(B, C, D)** Sagittal T1-weighted MR images both before (B) and after (C) intravenous contrast and axial T2-weighted (D) MR image show a large heterogeneous intermuscular popliteal mass (arrowheads). The mass is deeper than expected for a Baker cyst and no neck of fluid extending to the joint is seen. The predominant signal intensity is that of a high water content mass (M) with low signal on T1-weighting and high signal on T2-weighting. However, focal areas in the septa (arrows) and several small nodular (F) regions (<10% of the tumor volume) are isointense to subcutaneous fat. Following contrast administration there is thick and nodular peripheral and septal enhancement most prominent inferiorly (open arrows).

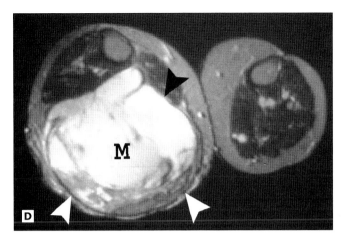

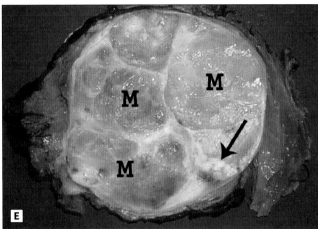

FIGURE 3–18 Continued. **(E)** Photograph of the axially sectioned gross specimen shows the high water content myxoid regions (M) and adipose areas (arrow) corresponding to the imaging appearance, that are diagnostic of myxoid liposarcoma. Biopsy of the more fat-containing regions as well as the myxoid areas may allow easier and more confident pathologic diagnosis in such a large mass.

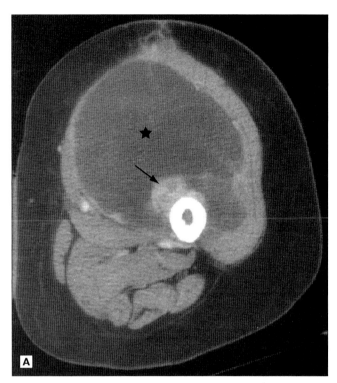

FIGURE 3–19 Malignant fibrous histiocytoma of the thigh presenting as a spontaneous hematoma in a 58-year-old man. **(A)** Axial post-contrast CT shows a large intramuscular anterior thigh soft tissue mass with large nonenhancing low attenuation component (star) representing hemorrhage and small solid neoplastic component with nodular enhancement (arrow).

tumor that harbor diagnostic tissue (Figs 3–5, 3–19). Lesions with areas of solid tissue differing in intrinsic imaging appearance (particularly on MRI) should have biopsy material from these varying regions as they likely contain different histological material (Fig. 3–20). This is particularly true in large masses and may dramatically alter diagnosis.

Response to chemotherapy and radiation can be assessed by imaging techniques and is most commonly judged by size and extent of necrosis.[139,140] Following therapy, perilesional edema is typically apparent on MRI. Following surgical resection, radiologic assessment (usually MRI) is directed at identifying local recurrence and distinguishing it from postoperative fibrosis (low signal intensity on all pulse sequences), lymphocele/ seroma (homogeneous very low signal intensity on T1-weighting and very high signal intensity on T2-weighting with thin rim and septal enhancement) (Fig. 3–21).[139,140] MRI following contrast is helpful in this assessment as most recurrent soft tissue neoplasms reveal diffuse enhancement. A focal soft tissue mass in a postsurgical site with any other intrinsic appearances than listed above for fibrosis or fluid collection likely represents recurrent neoplasm and should prompt biopsy (Fig. 3–21).

CONCLUSION

The role of imaging in evaluation of soft tissue tumors has dramatically progressed because of the advent of CT, US, and more recently MRI. The goals of imaging include:

1. Detection and characterization of the lesion;
2. Distinguishing neoplasm from non-neoplasm;
3. Constructing a differential diagnosis; and
4. Staging.

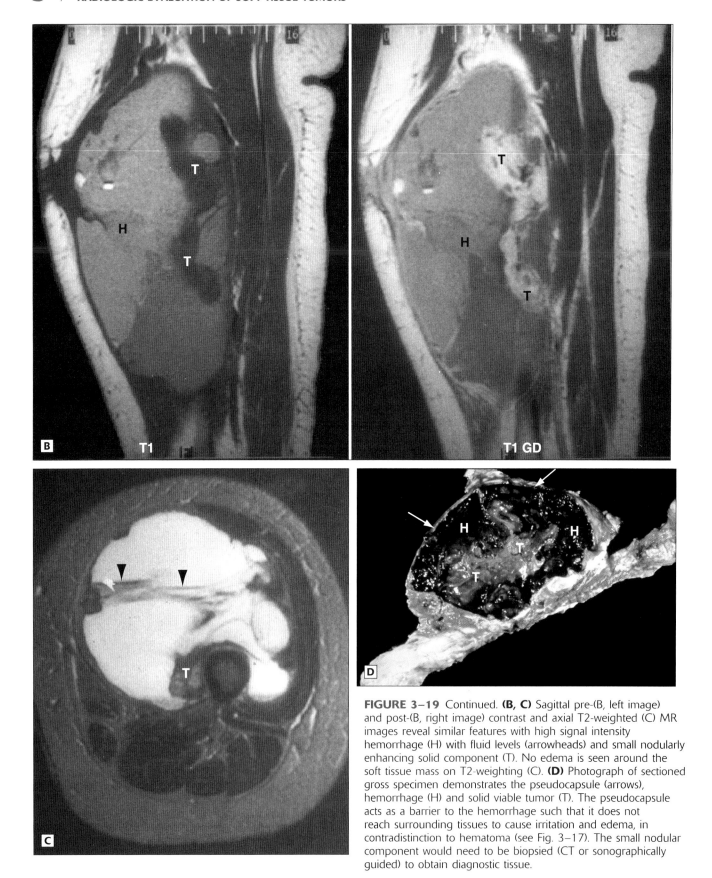

FIGURE 3–19 Continued. **(B, C)** Sagittal pre-(B, left image) and post-(B, right image) contrast and axial T2-weighted (C) MR images reveal similar features with high signal intensity hemorrhage (H) with fluid levels (arrowheads) and small nodularly enhancing solid component (T). No edema is seen around the soft tissue mass on T2-weighting (C). **(D)** Photograph of sectioned gross specimen demonstrates the pseudocapsule (arrows), hemorrhage (H) and solid viable tumor (T). The pseudocapsule acts as a barrier to the hemorrhage such that it does not reach surrounding tissues to cause irritation and edema, in contradistinction to hematoma (see Fig. 3–17). The small nodular component would need to be biopsied (CT or sonographically guided) to obtain diagnostic tissue.

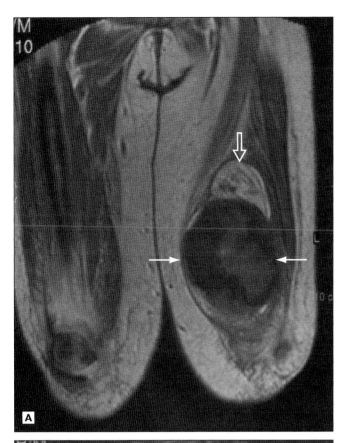

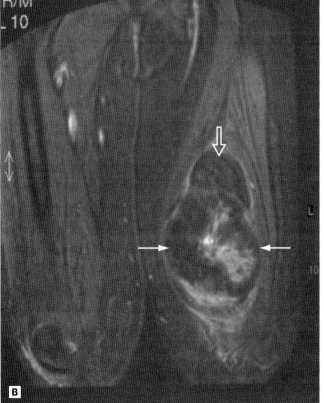

FIGURE 3–20 Dedifferentiated liposarcoma of the thigh in a 59-year-old woman with two differing solid components of tumor requiring biopsy. **(A, B)** Coronal T1-weighted (A) and fat suppressed T2-weighted (B) MR images show a large thigh soft tissue mass with two solid components. The superior component (open arrows) is comprised of adipose tissue with thick septa consistent with well-differentiated liposarcoma. The larger inferior component differs in signal intensity (arrows) representing the dedifferentiated region.

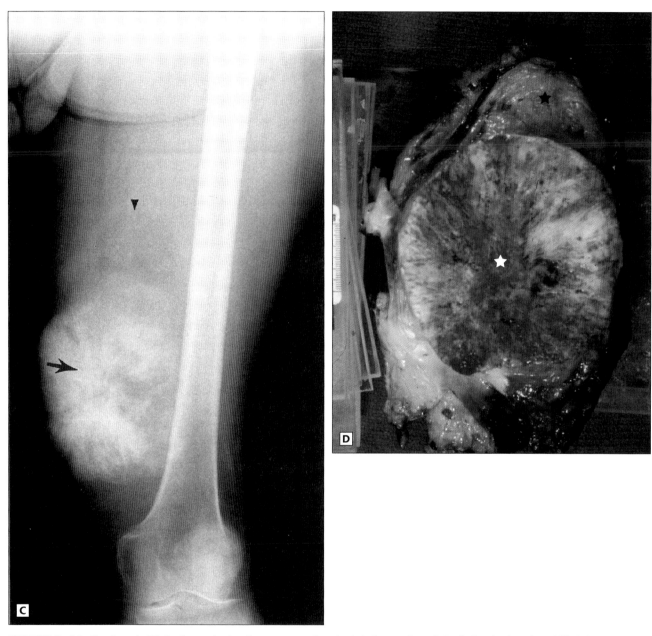

FIGURE 3–20 Continued. **(C)** Radiograph also demonstrates that the inferior portion of the lesion is densely calcified (small arrow) with faint radiolucency resulting from fat superiorly (arrowhead). **(D)** Photograph of the sectioned gross specimen reveals identical features, compared to imaging, with the well-differentiated liposarcomatous components superiorly (black star) and the high-grade osteosarcomatous component inferiorly (white star). Biopsy of only the superior component would have led to inappropriate initial treatment.

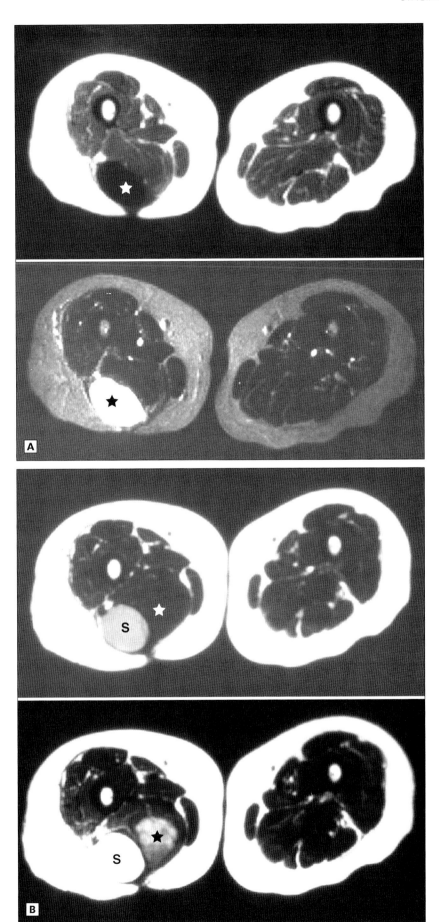

FIGURE 3–21 Postoperative seroma/ lymphocele and subsequent recurrent malignant fibrous histiocytoma (MFH) in the thigh of a 70-year-old woman. **(A)** Axial T1-weighted (upper image) and T2-weighted (lower image) MR images 1 year after surgery and adjuvant therapy for MFH shows a homogeneous low signal on T1-weighting and high signal on T2-weighting mass (star) in the postoperative site representing a lymphocele/ seroma. **(B)** Axial T1-weighted (upper image) and T2-weighted (lower image) MR images 18 months later reveal the continued lymphocele/seroma (S) but interval adjacent local recurrent MFH (star) with the appearance of solid tissue replacing the normal muscle texture seen previously in this region (normal muscle adjacent to lymphocele/seroma in A).

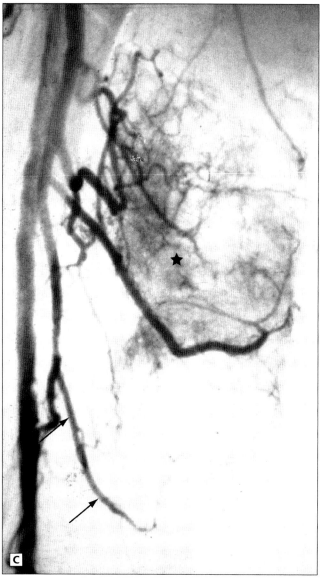

The most important radiologic features in evaluation of soft tissue tumors are the location of the lesion (subcutaneous, intermuscular, intramuscular, intra-articular/periarticular, and multiple lesions) and its intrinsic imaging characteristics (e.g., lesion morphology, shape, signal intensity and extent). In conjunction with the patient's age, these imaging morphology closely reflect the gross and histologic appearance of a soft tissue mass. In our opinion, recognizing and understanding the importance of this radiologic–pathologic correlation holds the key to the continued improvement in imaging diagnostic acumen. Soft tissue masses that frequently have pathognomonic imaging appearances include lipomatous lesions, angiomatous lesions, neurogenic tumors, "cystic" masses, elastofibroma, pigmented villonodular synovitis, synovial chondromatosis, and fibromatosis. Depending on the clinical situation, these lesions may not always require biopsy or resection. However, soft tissue tumors with a non-specific imaging appearance require biopsy to direct definitive treatment. Image-directed biopsy is essential to ensure that non-necrotic and nonhemorrhagic representative tissue is obtained for diagnosis. These factors emphasize that optimal pathologic evaluation of soft tissue tumors is similar to bone tumors in that the pathologic diagnosis should take into account the imaging findings whenever possible. This presupposes a team approach combining the skills of radiologists, pathologists, and oncologists with the ultimate goal of improving patient management and outcome.

FIGURE 3–21 Continued. **(C)** Arteriogram demonstrates tumor staining in the recurrent MFH (star) as opposed to draping of the vessels and lack of tumor staining about the fluid collection (arrows).

REFERENCES

Introduction

1. Berquist TH, Ehman RL, King BF, et al. Value of MR imaging in differentiating benign from malignant soft-tissue masses: study of 95 lesions. AJR Am J Roentgenol 1990; 155(6):1251.
2. Crim JR, Seeger LL, Yao L, et al. Diagnosis of soft-tissue masses with MR imaging: can benign masses be differentiated from malignant ones? Radiology 1992; 185(2):581.
3. Kransdorf MJ, Jelinek JS, Moser RP Jr, et al. Soft-tissue masses: diagnosis using MR imaging. AJR Am J Roentgenol 1989; 153(3):541.
4. Petasnick JP, Turner DA, Charters JR, et al. Soft-tissue masses of the locomotor system: comparison of MR imaging with CT. Radiology 1986; 160(1):125.

5. Totty WG, Murphy WA, Lee JK. Soft-tissue tumors: MR imaging. Radiology 1986; 160(1):135.
6. Sundaram M, McGuire MH, Herbold DR. Magnetic resonance imaging of soft tissue masses: an evaluation of fifty-three histologically proven tumors. Magn Reson Imaging 1988; 6(3):237.
7. Weekes RG, Berquist TH, McLeod RA, et al. Magnetic resonance imaging of soft-tissue tumors: comparison with computed tomography. Magn Reson Imaging 1985; 3(4):345.
8. Weekes RG, McLeod RA, Reiman HM, et al. CT of soft-tissue neoplasms. AJR Am J Roentgenol 1985; 144(2):355.
9. Murphey M, Nomikos G. Prospective diagnosis of soft tissue tumors. Radiology 2001; 221(p):473.

Imaging evaluation and options

10. Hammond JA, Driedger AA. Detection of malignant change in neurofibromatosis (von Recklinghausen's disease) by gallium-67 scanning. Can Med Assoc J 1978 2 6;119(4):352.
11. Kaplan IL, Swayne LC, Baydin JA. Uptake of Ga-67 citrate in a benign neurofibroma. Clin Nucl Med 1989; 14(3):224.
12. Levine E, Huntrakoon M, Wetzel LH. Malignant nerve-sheath neoplasms in neurofibromatosis: distinction from benign tumors by using imaging techniques. AJR Am J Roentgenol 1987; 149(5):1059.
13. Kransdorf MJ, Murphey M. Imaging of soft tissue tumors. 2nd edn. Philadelphia, PA: Lipponcott Williams & Wilkins; 2006.

14. Kransdorf MJ, Murphey MD. Radiologic evaluation of soft-tissue masses: a current perspective. AJR Am J Roentgenol 2000; 175(3):575.

15. Blandino A, Salvi L, Chirico G, et al. Synovial osteochondromatosis of the ankle: MR findings. Clin Imaging 1992; 16(1):34.

16. Kramer J, Recht M, Deely DM, et al. MR appearance of idiopathic synovial osteochondromatosis. J Comput Assist Tomogr 1993; 17(5):772.

17. Sundaram M, McGuire MH, Fletcher J, et al. Magnetic resonance imaging of lesions of synovial origin. Skeletal Radiol 1986; 5(2): 110.

18. Aoki J, Watanabe H, Shinozaki T, et al. FDG-PET for preoperative differential diagnosis between benign and malignant soft tissue masses. Skeletal Radiol 2003; 32(3):133.

19. Kapoor V, McCook BM, Torok FS. An introduction to PET-CT imaging. Radiographics 2004; 24(2):523.

20. Kostakoglu L, Hardoff R, Mirtcheva R, et al. PET-CT fusion imaging in differentiating physiologic from pathologic FDG uptake. Radiographics 2004; 24(5):1411.

21. Vernon CB, Eary JF, Rubin BP, et al. FDG PET imaging guided re-evaluation of histopathologic response in a patient with high-grade sarcoma. Skeletal Radiol 2003; 32(3):139.

22. Fornage BD, Tassin GB. Sonographic appearances of superficial soft tissue lipomas. J Clin Ultrasound 1991; 19(4):215.

23. Lin J, Fessell DP, Jacobson JA, et al. An illustrated tutorial of musculoskeletal sonography: part I, introduction and general principles. AJR Am J Roentgenol 2000; 175(3):637.

24. Lin J, Jacobson JA, Fessell DP,. An illustrated tutorial of musculoskeletal sonography: part 4, musculoskeletal masses, sonographically guided interventions, and miscellaneous topics. AJR Am J Roentgenol 2000; 175(6):1711.

25. Loyer EM, DuBrow RA, David CL, et al. Imaging of superficial soft-tissue infections: sonographic findings in cases of cellulitis and abscess. AJR Am J Roentgenol 1996; 166(1):149.

26. Aisen AM, Martel W, Braunstein EM, et al. MRI and CT evaluation of primary bone and soft-tissue tumors. AJR Am J Roentgenol 1986; 146(4):749.

27. Bloem JL, Taminiau AH, Eulderink F, et al. Radiologic staging of primary bone sarcoma: MR imaging, scintigraphy, angiography, and CT correlated with pathologic examination. Radiology 1988; 169(3):805.

28. Chang AE, Matory YL, Dwyer AJ, et al. Magnetic resonance imaging versus computed tomography in the evaluation of soft tissue tumors of the extremities. Ann Surg 1987; 205(4):340.

29. Dalinka MK, Zlatkin MB, Chao P, et al. The use of magnetic resonance imaging in the evaluation of bone and soft-tissue tumors. Radiol Clin North Am 1990; 28(2):461.

30. Demas BE, Heelan RT, Lane J, et al. Soft-tissue sarcomas of the extremities: comparison of MR and CT in determining the extent of disease. AJR Am J Roentgenol 1988; 150(3):615.

31. Panicek DM, Gatsonis C, Rosenthal DI, et al. CT and MR imaging in the local staging of primary malignant musculoskeletal neoplasms: report of the Radiology Diagnostic Oncology Group. Radiology 1997; 202(1):237.

32. Pettersson H, Gillespy T 3rd, Hamlin DJ, et al. Primary musculoskeletal tumors: examination with MR imaging compared with conventional modalities. Radiology 1987; 164(1):237.

33. Rubin DA, Kneeland JB. MR imaging of the musculoskeletal system: technical considerations for enhancing image quality and diagnostic yield. AJR Am J Roentgenol 1994; 163(5):1155.

34. Tehranzadeh J, Mnaymneh W, Ghavam C, et al. Comparison of CT and MR imaging in musculoskeletal neoplasms. J Comput Assist Tomogr 1989; 13(3):466.

35. Hudson TM, Hamlin DJ, Enneking WF, et al. Magnetic resonance imaging of bone and soft tissue tumors: early experience in 31 patients compared with computed tomography. Skeletal Radiol 1985; 13(2):134.

36. Dwyer AJ, Frank JA, Sank VJ, et al. Short-Ti inversion-recovery pulse sequence: analysis and initial experience in cancer imaging. Radiology 1988; 168(3):827.

37. Fujimoto H, Murakami K, Ichikawa T, et al. MRI of soft-tissue lesions: opposed-phase T2-weighted gradient-echo images. J Comput Assist Tomogr 1993; 17(3):418.

38. Shuman WP, Baron RL, Peters MJ, et al. Comparison of STIR and spin-echo MR imaging at 1.5 T in 90 lesions of the chest, liver, and pelvis. AJR Am J Roentgenol 1989; 152(4):853.

39. Mirowitz SA. Fast scanning and fat-suppression MR imaging of musculoskeletal disorders. AJR Am J Roentgenol 1993; 161(6):1147.

40. Benedikt RA, Jelinek JS, Kransdorf MJ, et al. MR imaging of soft-tissue masses: role of gadopentetate dimeglumine. J Magn Reson Imaging 1994; 4(3):485.

41. Harkens KL, Moore TE, Yuh WT, et al. Gadolinium-enhanced MRI of soft tissue masses. Australas Radiol 1993; 37(1):30.

42. Jordan RM, Mintz RD. Fatal reaction to gadopentetate dimeglumine. AJR Am J Roentgenol 1995; 164(3):743.

43. Omohundro JE, Elderbrook MK, Ringer TV. Laryngospasm after administration of gadopentetate dimeglumine. J Magn Reson Imaging 1992; 2(6):729.

44. Seeger LL, Widoff BE, Bassett LW, et al. Preoperative evaluation of osteosarcoma: value of gadopentetate dimeglumine-enhanced MR imaging. AJR Am J Roentgenol 1991; 157(2):347.

45. Shellock FG, Hahn HP, Mink JH, et al. Adverse reaction to intravenous gadoteridol. Radiology 1993; 189(1):151.

46. Takebayashi S, Sugiyama M, Nagase M, et al. Severe adverse reaction to iv gadopentetate dimeglumine. AJR Am J Roentgenol 1993; 160(3):659.

47. Tardy B, Guy C, Barral G, et al. Anaphylactic shock induced by intravenous gadopentetate dimeglumine. Lancet 1992; 339(8791):494.

48. Tishler S, Hoffman JC Jr. Anaphylactoid reactions to i.v. gadopentetate dimeglumine. AJNR Am J Neuroradiol 1990; 11(6):1167; discussion 8–9.

49. Verstraete KL, De Deene Y, Roels H, et al. Benign and malignant musculoskeletal lesions: dynamic contrast-enhanced MR imaging – parametric "first-pass" images depict tissue vascularization and perfusion. Radiology 1994; 192(3):835.

50. Beltran J, Chandnani V, McGhee RA Jr, et al. Gadopentetate dimeglumine-enhanced MR imaging of the musculoskeletal system. AJR Am J Roentgenol 1991; 156(3):457.

51. Mirowitz SA, Totty WG, Lee JK. Characterization of musculoskeletal masses using dynamic Gd-DTPA enhanced spin-echo MRI. J Comput Assist Tomogr 1992; 16(1):120.

52. Feydy A, Anract P, Tomeno B, et al. Assessment of vascular invasion by musculoskeletal tumors of the limbs: use of contrast-enhanced MR angiography. Radiology 2006; 238(2):611.

53. Kransdorf MJ, Murphey MD. The use of gadolinium in the MR evaluation of soft tissue tumors. Semin Ultrasound CT MR 1997; 18(4):251.

54. van der Woude HJ, Verstraete KL, Hogendoorn PC, et al. Musculoskeletal tumors: does fast dynamic contrast-enhanced subtraction MR imaging contribute to the characterization? Radiology 1998; 208(3):821.

Evaluation of lesion

55. Murphey M, Jelinek J, Kransdorf M, et al. Imaging of synovial sarcoma. Radiology 1998; 209(P):420.

56. Weiss S, Goldblum J. Malignant soft tissue tumors of uncertain type. In: Weiss S, Goldblum J, eds. Enzinger and Weiss's soft tissue tumors, 4th edn. St. Louis: Mosby; 2001:1483–1565.

57. Brandser EA, Goree JC, El-Khoury GY. Elastofibroma dorsi: prevalence in an elderly patient population as revealed by CT. AJR Am J Roentgenol 1998; 171(4):977.

58. Bui-Mansfield LT, Chew FS, Stanton CA. Elastofibroma dorsi of the chest wall. AJR Am J Roentgenol 2000; 175(1):244.

59. Kransdorf MJ, Meis JM, Montgomery E. Elastofibroma: MR and CT appearance with radiologic–pathologic correlation. AJR Am J Roentgenol 1992; 159(3):575.

60. Cotten A, Flipo RM, Chastanet P, et al. Pigmented villonodular synovitis of the hip: review of radiographic features in 58 patients. Skeletal Radiol 1995; 24(1):1.

61. Jelinek JS, Kransdorf MJ, Shmookler BM, et al. Giant cell tumor of the tendon sheath: MR findings in nine cases. AJR Am J Roentgenol 1994; 162(4):919.

62. Jelinek JS, Kransdorf MJ, Utz JA, et al. Imaging of pigmented villonodular synovitis with emphasis on MR imaging. AJR Am J Roentgenol 1989; 152(2):337.

63. Milgram JW. Synovial osteochondromatosis: a histopathological study of thirty cases. J Bone Joint Surg [Am] 1977; 59(6):792.

64. Barkhof F, Melkert P, Meyer S, et al. Derangement of adipose tissue: a case report of multicentric retroperitoneal liposarcomas, retroperitoneal lipomatosis and multiple subcutaneous lipomas. Eur J Surg Oncol 1991; 17(5):547.

65. Dolph JL, Demuth RJ, Miller SH. Familial multiple lipomatosis. Plast Reconstr Surg 1980; 66(4):620.

66. Dooms GC, Hricak H, Sollitto RA, et al. Lipomatous tumors and tumors with fatty component: MR imaging potential and comparison of MR and CT results. Radiology 1985; 157(2):479.

67. Hunter JC, Johnston WH, Genant HK. Computed tomography evaluation of fatty tumors of the somatic soft tissues: clinical utility and radiologic–pathologic correlation. Skeletal Radiol 1979 6; 4(2):79.

68. Kransdorf MJ, Moser RP Jr, Meis JM, et al. Fat-containing soft-tissue masses of the extremities. Radiographics 1991; 11(1):81.

69. Leffell DJ, Braverman IM. Familial multiple lipomatosis. Report of a case and a review of the literature. J Am Acad Dermatol 1986; 15(2 Pt 1):275.

70. Murphey MD, Carroll JF, Flemming DJ, et al. From the archives of the AFIP. Benign musculoskeletal lipomatous lesions. Radiographics 2004; 24(5):1433.

71. Buetow PC, Kransdorf MJ, Moser RP Jr, et al. Radiologic appearance of intramuscular hemangioma with emphasis on MR imaging. AJR Am J Roentgenol 1990; 154(3):563.

72. Derchi LE, Balconi G, De Flaviis L, et al. Sonographic appearances of hemangiomas of skeletal muscle. J Ultrasound Med 1989; 8(5):263.

73. Greenspan A, McGahan JP, Vogelsang P, et al. Imaging strategies in the evaluation of soft-tissue hemangiomas of the extremities: correlation of the findings of plain radiography, angiography, CT, MRI, and ultrasonography in 12 histologically proven cases. Skeletal Radiol 1992; 21(1):11.

74. McRae G, Murphey M, Temple H, et al. Imaging of soft tissue hemangioma with pathologic correlation (abstr). Radiology 1997; 205(P):449.

75. Murphey MD, Fairbairn KJ, Parman LM, et al. From the archives of the AFIP. Musculoskeletal angiomatous lesions: radiologic–pathologic correlation. Radiographics 1995; 15(4):893.

76. Nelson MC, Stull MA, Teitelbaum GP, et al. Magnetic resonance imaging of peripheral soft tissue hemangiomas. Skeletal Radiol 1990; 19(7):477.

77. Yuh WT, Kathol MH, Sein MA, et al. Hemangiomas of skeletal muscle: MR findings in five patients. AJR Am J Roentgenol 1987; 149(4):765.

78. Murphey MD, Smith WS, Smith SE, et al. From the archives of the AFIP. Imaging of musculoskeletal neurogenic tumors: radiologic–pathologic correlation. Radiographics 1999; 19(5):1253.

79. Sundaram M, McDonald DJ, Merenda G. Intramuscular myxoma: a rare but important association with fibrous dysplasia of bone. AJR Am J Roentgenol 1989; 153(1):107.

80. Wirth WA, Leavitt D, Enzinger FM. Multiple intramuscular myxomas. Another extraskeletal manifestation of fibrous dysplasia. Cancer 1971; 27(5):1167.

81. Chung EB, Enzinger FM. Benign lipoblastomatosis. An analysis of 35 cases. Cancer 1973; 32(2):482.

82. Jimenez JF. Lipoblastoma in infancy and childhood. J Surg Oncol 1986; 32(4):238.

83. Kransdorf MJ, Meis JM, Jelinek JS. Dedifferentiated liposarcoma of the extremities: imaging findings in four patients. AJR Am J Roentgenol 1993; 161(1):127.

84. Lateur L, Van Ongeval C, Samson I, et al. Case report 842. Benign hibernoma. Skeletal Radiol 1994; 23(4):306.

85. Leffert RD. Lipomas of the upper extremity. J Bone Joint Surg [Am] 1972; 54(6):1262.

86. London J, Kim EE, Wallace S, et al. MR imaging of liposarcomas: correlation of MR features and histology. J Comput Assist Tomogr 1989; 13(5):832.

87. Murphey M, Flemming D, Jelinek J, et al. Imaging of higher grade liposarcoma with pathologic correlation (abstr). Radiology 1997; 205(P):332.

88. Osment LS. Cutaneous lipomas and lipomatosis. Surg Gynecol Obstet 1968; 127(1):129.

89. Seynaeve P, Mortelmans L, Kockx M, et al. Case report 813: Hibernoma of the left thigh. Skeletal Radiol 1994; 23(2):137.

90. Jelinek JS, Kransdorf MJ, Shmookler BM, et al. Liposarcoma of the extremities: MR and CT findings in the histologic subtypes. Radiology 1993; 186(2):455.

91. Rydholm A, Berg NO. Size, site and clinical incidence of lipoma. Factors in the differential diagnosis of lipoma and sarcoma. Acta Orthop Scand 1983; 54(6):929.

92. Murphey MD, Arcara LK, Fanburg-Smith J. From the archives of the AFIP. Imaging of musculoskeletal liposarcoma with radiologic–pathologic correlation. Radiographics 2005; 25(5):1371.

93. Hosono M, Kobayashi H, Fujimoto R, et al. Septum-like structures in lipoma and liposarcoma: MR imaging and pathologic correlation. Skeletal Radiol 1997; 26(3):150.

94. Kransdorf MJ, Bancroft LW, Peterson JJ, et al. Imaging of fatty tumors: distinction of lipoma and well-differentiated liposarcoma. Radiology 2002; 224(1):99.

95. Ohguri T, Aoki T, Hisaoka M, et al. Differential diagnosis of benign peripheral lipoma from well-differentiated liposarcoma on MR imaging: is comparison of margins and internal characteristics useful? AJR Am J Roentgenol 2003; 180(6):1689.

96. Kransdorf MJ, Jelinek JS, Moser RP Jr, et al. Magnetic resonance appearance of fibromatosis. A report of 14 cases and review of the literature. Skeletal Radiol 1990; 19(7):495.

97. Quinn SF, Erickson SJ, Dee PM, et al. MR imaging in fibromatosis: results in 26 patients with pathologic correlation. AJR Am J Roentgenol 1991; 156(3):539.

98. Sundaram M, McGuire MH, Schajowicz F. Soft-tissue masses: histologic basis for decreased signal (short T2) on T2-weighted MR images. AJR Am J Roentgenol 1987; 148(6):1247.

99. Boutin RD, Pathria MN, Resnick D. Disorders in the stumps of amputee patients: MR imaging. AJR Am J Roentgenol 1998; 171(2):497.

100. Cerofolini E, Landi A, DeSantis G, et al. MR of benign peripheral nerve sheath tumors. J Comput Assist Tomogr 1991; 15(4):593.

101. Cohen EK, Kressel HY, Perosio T, et al. MR imaging of soft-tissue hemangiomas: correlation with pathologic findings. AJR Am J Roentgenol 1988; 150(5):1079.

102. Kumar AJ, Kuhajda FP, Martinez CR, et al. Computed tomography of extracranial nerve sheath tumors with pathological correlation. J Comput Assist Tomogr 1983; 7(5):857.

103. Redd RA, Peters VJ, Emery SF, et al. Morton neuroma: sonographic evaluation. Radiology 1989; 171(2):415.

104. Singson RD, Feldman F, Slipman CW, et al. Postamputation neuromas and other symptomatic stump abnormalities: detection with CT. Radiology 1987; 162(3):743.

105. Stull MA, Moser RP Jr, Kransdorf MJ, et al. Magnetic resonance appearance of peripheral nerve sheath tumors. Skeletal Radiol 1991; 20(1):9.

106. Suh JS, Abenoza P, Galloway HR, et al. Peripheral (extracranial) nerve tumors: correlation of MR imaging and histologic findings. Radiology 1992; 183(2):341.

107. Zanetti M, Ledermann T, Zollinger H, et al. Efficacy of MR imaging in patients suspected of having Morton's neuroma. AJR Am J Roentgenol 1997; 168(2):529.

108. Zanetti M, Strehle JK, Zollinger H, et al. Morton neuroma and fluid in the intermetatarsal bursae on MR images of 70 asymptomatic volunteers. Radiology 1997; 203(2):516.

109. Beltran J, Simon DC, Katz W, et al. Increased MR signal intensity in skeletal muscle adjacent to malignant tumors: pathologic correlation and clinical relevance. Radiology 1987; 162(1 Pt 1):251.

110. Hanna SL, Fletcher BD, Parham DM, et al. Muscle edema in musculoskeletal tumors: MR imaging characteristics and clinical significance. J Magn Reson Imaging 1991; 1(4):441.

111. Sundaram M, Baran G, Merenda G, et al. Myxoid liposarcoma: magnetic resonance imaging appearances with clinical and histological correlation. Skeletal Radiol 1990; 19(5):359.

112. Kransdorf MJ. Malignant soft-tissue tumors in a large referral population: distribution of diagnoses by age, sex, and location. AJR Am J Roentgenol 1995; 164(1):129.

113. Kransdorf MJ. Benign soft-tissue tumors in a large referral population: distribution of specific diagnoses by age, sex, and location. AJR Am J Roentgenol 1995; 164(2):395.

114. Rock MG, Pritchard DJ, Reiman HM, et al. Extra-abdominal desmoid tumors. J Bone Joint Surg [Am] 1984; 66(9):1369.

115. Burk DL Jr, Dalinka MK, Kanal E, et al. Meniscal and ganglion cysts of the knee: MR evaluation. AJR Am J Roentgenol 1988; 150(2):331.

116. De Flaviis L, Nessi R, Del Bo P, et al. High-resolution ultrasonography of wrist ganglia. J Clin Ultrasound 1987; 15(1):17.

117. Feldman F, Singson RD, Staron RB. Magnetic resonance imaging of para-articular and ectopic ganglia. Skeletal Radiol 1989; 18(5):353.

118. Haller J, Resnick D, Greenway G, et al. Juxtaacetabular ganglionic (or synovial) cysts: CT and MR features. J Comput Assist Tomogr 1989; 13(6):976.

119. Schuldt DR, Wolfe RD. Clinical and arthrographic findings in meniscal cysts. Radiology 1980; 134(1):49.

120. Schwimmer M, Edelstein G, Heiken JP, et al. Synovial cysts of the knee: CT evaluation. Radiology 1985; 154(1):175.

121. Tyson LL, Daughters TC Jr, Ryu RK, et al. MRI appearance of meniscal cysts. Skeletal Radiol 1995; 24(6):421.

122. Recht MP, Applegate G, Kaplan P, et al. The MR appearance of cruciate ganglion cysts: a report of 16 cases. Skeletal Radiol 1994; 23(8):597.

123. Ortega R, Fessell DP, Jacobson JA, et al. Sonography of ankle ganglia with pathologic correlation in 10 pediatric and adult patients. AJR Am J Roentgenol 2002; 178(6):1445.

124. Anderson MW, Temple HT, Dussault RG, et al. Compartmental anatomy: relevance to staging and biopsy of musculoskeletal tumors. AJR Am J Roentgenol 1999; 173(6):1663.

125. Ward EE, Jacobson JA, Fessell DP, et al. Sonographic detection of Baker's cysts: comparison with MR imaging. AJR Am J Roentgenol 2001; 176(2):373.

126. Liu PT, Leslie KO, Beauchamp CP, et al. Chronic expanding hematoma of the thigh simulating neoplasm on gadolinium-enhanced MRI. Skeletal Radiol 2006; 35(4):254.

127. Bancroft LW, Kransdorf MJ, Menke DM, et al. Intramuscular myxoma: characteristic MR imaging features. AJR Am J Roentgenol 2002; 178(5):1255.

128. Luna A, Martinez S, Bossen E. Magnetic resonance imaging of intramuscular myxoma with histological comparison and a review of the literature. Skeletal Radiol 2005; 34(1):19.

129. Murphey MD, Gross TM, Rosenthal HG. From the archives of the AFIP. Musculoskeletal malignant fibrous histiocytoma: radiologic–pathologic correlation. Radiographics 1994; 14(4):807; quiz 27.

130. Murphey MD, McRae GA, Fanburg-Smith JC, et al. Imaging of soft-tissue myxoma with emphasis on CT and MR and comparison of radiologic and pathologic findings. Radiology 2002; 225(1):215.

131. De Schepper AM, Ramon FA, Degryse HR. Statistical analysis of MRI parameters predicting malignancy in 141 soft tissue masses. Rofo 1992; 156(6):587.

Staging, biopsy and treatment follow-up

132. Enneking WF, Spanier SS, Goodman MA. A system for the surgical staging of musculoskeletal sarcoma. Clin Orthop Rel Res 1980 Nov-Dec(153):106.

133. Hajdu S. Pathology of soft tissue tumors. Philadelphia, PA: Lea & Febiger; 1979.

134. Mettlin C, Priore R, Rao U, et al. Results of the national soft-tissue sarcoma registry. J Surg Oncol 1982; 19(4):224.

135. Russell WO, Cohen J, Edmonson JH, et al. Staging system for soft tissue sarcoma. Semin Oncol 1981; 8(2):156.

136. Peabody TD, Simon MA. Principles of staging of soft-tissue sarcomas. Clin Orthop Rel Res 1993; Apr(289):19.

137. McDonald DJ. Limb-salvage surgery for treatment of sarcomas of the extremities. AJR Am J Roentgenol 1994; 163(3):509; discussion 14.

138. Rydholm A. Management of patients with soft-tissue tumors. Strategy developed at a regional oncology center. Acta Orthop Scand Suppl 1983; 203:13.

139. Choi H, Varma DG, Fornage BD, et al. Soft-tissue sarcoma: MR imaging vs sonography for detection of local recurrence after surgery. AJR Am J Roentgenol 1991; 157(2):353.

140. Kransdorf MJ, Murphey MD. Soft tissue tumors: post-treatment imaging. Radiol Clin North Am 2006; 44(3): 463.

CYTOGENETIC AND MOLECULAR GENETIC PATHOLOGY OF SOFT TISSUE TUMORS

Marc Ladanyi, Cristina R. Antonescu, and Paola Dal Cin

CHAPTER CONTENTS

INTRODUCTION

Previous editions of this text contained separate chapters for the cytogenetics and the molecular genetics of soft tissue tumors. Historically, this reflected the fact that, whereas much of our knowledge of the genetic pathology of this class of tumors was initially based on conventional karyotypic analysis, the molecular consequences of the cytogenetic alterations remained largely obscure. Chromosomal translocations, deletions, and amplifications provided novel diagnostic markers, even if their biology was not understood. Beginning in the early 1990s, as more and more of the genetic underpinnings were identified, namely the gene fusions resulting from the translocations, the tumor suppressor genes subject to deletion, and the oncogenes undergoing amplification, a more integrated understanding of the molecular genetic pathology of mesenchymal neoplasms began to emerge. In recent years, broad themes have become apparent at several levels, and these have been useful in organizing our thinking in this area. *At the cytogenetic level*, contrasting sarcomas with complex karyotypes and those with simple karyotypes has led to novel insights. *At the biological level*, oncogenic mechanisms have fallen into two broad categories, namely transcriptional deregulation and deregulated signaling. *At the practical level*, the rapid translation of tumor-type-specific genetic alterations into

molecular diagnostic markers stands in sharp contrast to the slow clinical adoption of less specific progression-related genetic alterations as prognostic markers. In this chapter, we provide a survey of the major cytogenetic and molecular genetic alterations in soft tissue tumors, focusing on those that are relevant to pathologic diagnosis and the development of more rational classification schemes, to clinical management and therapy selection, and to the understanding of the fundamental biology of these neoplasms.

GENERAL CONCEPTS IN CANCER GENETICS

In a landmark 2000 review, Hanahan and Weinberg distilled the pathobiology of cancer into six key features or "hallmarks," namely, self-sufficiency in growth signals, insensitivity to growth-inhibitory signals, evasion of programmed cell death (apoptosis), limitless replicative potential, sustained angiogenesis, and tissue invasion and metastasis.[1] The acquisition of these key features involves an essentially Darwinian process of random mutation followed by natural selection, the selection in this context being for autonomous proliferation. The pathways by which different cancers acquire the six hallmark capabilities clearly vary in terms of the specific genes involved. Whereas this six hallmark model also applies to sarcomas, the widely held notion of multistep carcinogenesis arising from the study of epithelial neoplasia, which encompasses a progression from preneoplastic lesions to invasive cancer, does not translate well to sarcomas, especially the so-called translocation sarcomas discussed in more detail below. In translocation sarcomas, no pre-neoplastic phase has been recognized and, in many cases, the translocation is the only identifiable genetic alteration, suggesting that the translocation may by itself provide several of the hallmarks of cancer. Furthermore, if one were to assume that differences among sarcoma types were as great if not greater than differences among epithelial cancers arising from different organs, issues of cell type specificity of oncogenic mechanisms take on a special importance.

The genetic alterations that allow a clone of cells to acquire the six hallmark properties of cancer affect three broad types of cancer genes: oncogenes, tumor suppressor genes, and caretaker genes.[2,3] These designations refer to how these genes contribute to cancer development and do not constitute specific gene families in terms of similarity of sequence or function. Oncogenes are cancer genes that achieve their oncogenic effect through increased or deregulated activity of one of the two copies of the gene in question.[2] This activation can occur by a mutation that alters the sequence of the protein in such a way that its function is aberrantly enhanced, by an increase in the number of gene copies (gene amplification), by a translocation that brings its expression under the control of the regulatory sequences (promoter) of another gene, or by a combination of the above. Examples relevant to mesenchymal tumors include *KIT* and *PDGFRA*, both activated by mutations, *MYCN* and *MDM2*, both activated by gene amplification, and *PLAG1* and *HMGA1*, activated by translocation-mediated promoter juxtaposition (see below for details). In addition, translocations that fuse the coding sequences of two genes to generate chimeric proteins are generally considered a special variety of oncogenes, known as fusion oncogenes, of which there are numerous examples in sarcomas.

Tumor suppressor genes, in contrast, typically exert their oncogenic effects through a loss of both functional gene copies.[2] This can be caused by one or more of the following mechanisms: mutations that result in a truncated or inactive protein, mutations that result in a dominant negative protein that interferes with the function of the normal protein produced by the remaining unmutated gene copy, large deletions affecting the gene, replacement of the remaining unmutated copy of the gene by the inactive copy (loss of heterozygosity by mitotic recombination), reduced expression due to hypermethylation of the gene's regulatory sequences, or interruption of the gene by a non-recurrent translocation. Key examples in sarcomas include the generic tumor suppressors *P53 (TP53)*, *RB1*, and *CDKN2A*, as well as sarcoma-specific suppressors such as *NF1* and *INI1 (SMARCB1)*. Classical tumor suppressor genes act through complete or near-complete loss of function of the protein in question within the cancer cell. However, for some non-classical tumor suppressors, haploinsufficiency, i.e., a loss of one copy resulting in 50% decreased protein function in the cell, may be pathogenetically significant,[4] but the extent of this type of mechanism in sarcomas requires further study.

The third major class of cancer genes are the so-called caretaker genes.[2] These genes contribute to oncogenesis through a loss of function mechanism but differ from conventional tumor suppressor genes in that this does not directly cause a malignant phenotype, i.e., it does not provide one of the six hallmark properties of cancer. Instead, the loss of function of caretaker genes increases the likelihood that oncogene activation or conventional tumor suppressor inactivation will occur. Caretaker genes are involved in the maintenance of genomic and chromosomal integrity and hence have also been referred to as stability genes. This class of cancer genes seems to have a more limited role in sarcomas than in lymphomas, leukemias, and carcinomas. Examples relevant to mesenchymal tumors include the occurrence of soft tissue sarcomas in Werner syndrome.[5]

In terms of functional classes, the vast majority of cancer genes belong to one of three groups: protein kinases, transcription factors, and DNA maintenance and repair proteins.[3] Whereas the last group correspond to the caretaker genes, the various protein kinases and transcription factors can function as either oncogenes or tumor suppressor genes.

GENERAL PRINCIPLES OF TRANSLOCATIONS

The importance of specific, recurrent chromosomal translocations to the biology and diagnosis of sarcomas warrants a more detailed discussion of this special class of genetic alterations. Specific intergenic rearrangements or gene fusions represent, in terms of numbers of different genes involved, the single most common type of somatic genetic alteration in human cancer. Over 75% of genes somatically altered in human tumors are translocated.[3] Biologically, these gene fusions operate either by promoter substitution or the formation of aberrant chimeric proteins. In the latter, the coding regions of two genes become fused and the new fusion gene encodes an abnormal, oncogenic protein with a novel combination of functional domains.

Chromosomal translocations constitute the majority of specific genetic alterations associated with sarcomas. In aggregate, fusion gene-related sarcomas may account for approximately a third of all sarcomas. These chromosomal translocations produce highly specific gene fusions. The specificity of these gene fusions and their prevalence in selected sarcomas are such that they have become a defining feature of many of these entities.[6-8] Two key concepts in translocation sarcomas are firstly, that these sarcomas contain their fusion gene from their earliest presentation and do not show a benign or premalignant phase; and secondly, the fusion gene is present in all tumor cells and is expressed throughout the clinical course. One of the key concepts relating to the structure of these translocations is that the genomic (DNA-level) breaks almost always occur within introns (not within exons) and that the exon sequences flanking the chimeric intron are then joined by transcription and splicing to form a chimeric mRNA (Fig. 4–1). As introns can be quite large and the genomic breaks can occur almost anywhere within them, this explains why tumor genomic DNA

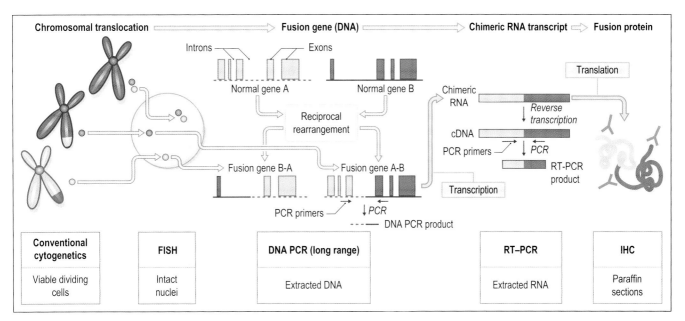

FIGURE 4–1 General principles of sarcoma translocation detection. The different approaches to the detection of a reciprocal translocation are schematized, ranging from conventional cytogenetics to the demonstration of the resulting fusion protein, along with the material needed for each assay. A break-apart FISH assay design is shown. Note that long-range DNA PCR and IHC detection are possible in only a minority of sarcoma translocations. IHC approaches usually use antibodies to one or both components of the fusion protein but are rarely specific for the fusion point.

rarely provides a usable starting point for detecting such translocations by polymeric chain reaction (PCR). In contrast, the consistent joining of the flanking exons by transcript splicing makes mRNA an extremely convenient target for PCR-based molecular detection (by reverse-transcriptase PCR [RT-PCR]) (Fig. 4.1).

Most of the major cytogenetically described translocations in sarcomas have by now been cloned. Table 4–1 lists the specific recurrent translocations reported in soft tissue neoplasms. Until a translocation is reported in more than one case of a given tumor, it is by definition non-recurrent. For many of the translocations in Table 4–1, rare non-recurrent variants have also been reported. Such unique fusions have been reported in alveolar rhabdomyosarcoma, angiomatoid fibrous histiocytoma, extraskeletal myxoid chondrosarcoma, Ewing sarcoma/ PNET, low-grade fibromyxoid sarcoma, inflammatory myofibroblastic tumor, and synovial sarcoma, and they are presented in the respective sections below. In addition, there have been unique gene fusions reported in some primitive undifferentiated sarcomas (sometimes called "Ewing sarcoma-like tumors") whose relationship to the canonical fusions remains unclear and whose conventional pathologic classification is uncertain.[9-13]

In sarcomas that have been extensively karyotyped, it is likely that only rare variant gene fusions remain to be identified. Novel fusions may remain to be discovered in sarcomas with only limited cytogenetic data, or if the translocations that generate them are difficult to detect in Giemsa-stained karyotypes or if they occur in a setting of highly complex karyotypes. As discussed below, the pathobiology of the oncogenic fusion proteins involves, in almost all instances, either transcriptional deregulation (most) or aberrant signaling (some).

Regarding the perennial question of how and why translocations arise,[14,15] a recent bioinformatic analysis of the sequence and structure of all genes involved in translocations has provided compelling new insights.[16] Comparing genes involved in translocations to control genes, striking differences emerge in overall gene size, average intron length, and length of the longest intron, all three of which are significantly greater in genes involved in translocations. However, so-called recombinogenic DNA sequence elements are not more frequent in translocated genes. This is notable because such DNA sequences had been previously proposed as explanations for the development of these translocations.[17,18] Contrary to these previous models, these data support the concept that the intronic breaks that lead to specific recurrent chromosomal translocations in cancer are largely random events (i.e., the risk of breaks is simply proportional to intron length) that become fixed through natural selection if they provide a growth advantage to the cell. Other factors that can be incorporated into this model include the increased "availability" of the genes for rearrangement that is created by the "open," less protected, chromatin conformation associated with gene transcription or replication,[19] and the unexpected proximity of some trans-

TABLE 4–1	RECURRENT CHROMOSOMAL TRANSLOCATIONS IN BENIGN AND MALIGNANT SOFT TISSUE TUMORS		
Soft tissue tumor	**Translocation**	**Gene fusion**	**Approximate prevalence[1]**
Alveolar rhabdomyosarcoma	t(2;13)(q35;q14)	PAX3-FKHR	65%
	t(1;13)(p36;q14)	PAX7-FKHR	15%
Angiomatoid fibrous histiocytoma	t(2;22)(q33;q12)	EWS-CREB1	*
	t(12;22)(q13;q12)	EWS-ATF1	*
	t(12;16)(q13;p11)	FUS-ATF1	*
Alveolar soft part sarcoma	t(X;17)(p11;q25)[2]	ASPL-TFE3	>95%
Clear cell sarcoma	t(12;22)(q13;q12)	EWS-ATF1	>90%
	t(2;22)(q33;q12)	EWS-CREB1	*
Dermatofibrosarcoma protuberans/giant cell fibroblastoma	t(17;22)(q21;q13)[3]	COL1A1-PDGFB	>90%
Desmoplastic fibroblastoma	t(2;11)(q31;q12)	Unknown	*
Desmoplastic small round cell tumor	t(11;22)(p13;q12)	EWS-WT1	>95%
Epithelioid hemangioendothelioma	t(1;3)(p36.3;q25)	Unknown	*
Extraskeletal myxoid chondrosarcoma	t(9;22)(q22-q3;q12)	EWS-NR4A3	75%
	t(9;17)(q22;q11)	TAF15-NR4A3	25%
Ewing sarcoma/PNET	t(11;22)(q24;q12)	EWS-FLI1	90%
	t(21;22)(q22;q12)	EWS-ERG	5%
	t(7;22)(p22;q12)	EWS-ETV1	<1%
	t(2;22)(q33;q12)	EWS-FEV	<1%
	t(17;22)(q12;q12)	EWS-E1AF	<1%
	t(16;21)(p11;q22)	FUS-ERG	<1%
Fibromyxoid sarcoma (low-grade)	t(7;16)(q33;p11.2)	FUS-CREB3L2	>95%
	t(11;16)(p13;p11.2)	FUS-CREB3L1	<5%
Giant cell tumor of tendon sheath	t(1;2)(p13;q37)	CSF1–COL6A3	*
Infantile fibrosarcoma	t(12;15)(p13;q26)	ETV6-NTRK3	>95%
Inflammatory myofibroblastic tumor	t with 2p23	ALK fusions	>50%
Lipoblastoma	t with 8q12	PLAG1 fusions	*
Lipoma, ordinary	t with 12q15	HMGA2 fusions	*
	t with 6p21	HMGA1 rearrangements[4]	*
Myxoid/round cell liposarcoma	t(12;16)(q13;p11)	FUS-CHOP	>95%
	t(12;22)(q13;q11)	EWS-CHOP	<5%
Pericytoma	t(7;12)(p2;q13)	ACTB-GLI	*
Synovial sarcoma	t(X;18)(p11.2;q11.2)	SYT-SSX1	65%
		SYT-SSX2	35%
		SYT-SSX4	<1%

[1] Insufficient data to estimate prevalence.
[2] Translocation usually present in unbalanced form as der(X) only (see text for details).
[3] Translocation usually present and amplified as ring chromosome (see text for details).
[4] HMGA1 rearrangements usually do not result in fusion transcripts (see text for details).

location partner genes due to the three dimensional arrangement of chromosomes in the nucleus. Evidence for the latter phenomenon has been presented in hematologic and thyroid cancers,[20,21] but not yet in sarcomas. In rare cases, sarcoma translocations may be related to radiotherapy-induced DNA damage.[22,23]

While the above discussion applies to recurrent reciprocal translocations, one should keep in mind that nonreciprocal or unbalanced translocations, even if recurrent, usually have different oncogenic consequences (exception: alveolar soft part sarcoma, see below), essentially representing a mechanism for gains or losses of genetic material. A notable recurrent unbalanced translocation in sarcomas is the der(16)t(1;16) seen in Ewing sarcoma,(24;25) and several other soft tissue sarcomas,[26–28] but the gene or genes whose gain or loss drives selection for this translocation remains unknown.

DIAGNOSTIC METHODS

Chromosome, fluorescence in situ hybridization, and gene nomenclature

According to standard chromosome nomenclature, chromosome regions are subdivided into bands and, at higher resolution, into sub-bands. For example, the designation 12q13 indicates chromosome 12, the long arm (q), region 1, band 3. On the ideogram, chromosome bands are numbered in an ascending fashion from centromere to telomere on each arm of the chromosome. Note that a limited number of bands is defined in each region, such that on a given chromosome band 13 may be followed by band 21, for example.

Due to the increase in the amount and variety of data on chromosome aberrations associated with neoplasia and the development and implementation of fluorescence in situ hybridization (FISH), a revised terminology was needed for describing acquired aberrations.[29] A fairly sophisticated set of rules now governs the description of chromosomal abnormalities. The convention is to specify first the total number of chromosomes followed by the sex chromosomes (e.g., the normal male karyotype is given as 46,XY). The autosomes are indicated only when an aberration or variant is present. In the description of a karyotype with chromosome abnormalities, sex chromosome aberrations are given first, followed by abnormalities of the autosomes listed in numerical order irrespective of the type of aberration. Aberrations are considered in two categories, numerical or structural. Numerical changes include either gain (+) or loss (−) of chromosomes (e.g., +7 indicates an extra copy of chromosome 7, or trisomy 7). The chromosome(s) involved in a structural change is specified in parentheses, directly following the symbol identifying the type of rearrangement [e.g., a translocation between chromosomes 12 and 16 as t(12;16)]. In all structural changes, the location of any given chromosome break is specified by the chromosome band in which that break has occurred (e.g., t(12;16)(q13;p11) describes a balanced translocation between the q13 band of chromosome 12 and the p11 band of chromosome 16). It is important to note that the chromosomes involved in a translocation are listed in numerical order and thus this nomenclature is not meant to provide information on the order of the genes involved in the oncogenic fusion product. Translocations involving the *EWS* (*EWSR1*) gene on chromosome 22 exemplify this situation. The most frequent structural changes in sarcomas include: translocation (t), in which chromatin is exchanged between two or more chromosomes; deletion (del), in which there is a net loss of chromatin; (add), in which there is additional material whose origin is uncertain by conventional G-banding; and derivative chromosome (der), in which one or more rearrangements within a single chromosome occurs. For instance, a derivative chromosome may be the result of a reciprocal translocation that is followed by loss of one of the two rearranged chromosomes (also known as unbalanced translocation).

A major advance in cancer cytogenetics has been the development of FISH analysis and related molecular cytogenetic techniques. FISH has been very effectively used to identify chromosomal regions, to reveal cryptic abnormalities, to describe complex chromosome rearrangements, and to detect chromosome rearrangements in interphase nuclei including those in paraffin-embedded, formalin-fixed tissues. The complementary use of conventional cytogenetic analysis and FISH has provided a remarkably powerful tool for cancer cytogenetics. Therefore, the current revised nomenclature also incorporates FISH data.[29] A type of probe commonly used in sarcomas is referred to as a break-apart probe. A break-apart probe set consists of a pair of probes that flank a gene locus of interest, is labeled in two different fluorochromes, and is especially useful for detecting chromosomal rearrangements of genes such as *EWS* for which the translocation partners may be variable.

Information of interest in interphase/nuclear in situ hybridization (nuc ish) includes the number of signals and their position relative to each other. For instance, a break-apart probe (e.g., *EWS*) is made of two DNA probes (*5'EWS* and *3'EWS*) from the same locus (22q12) that are labeled with different fluorophores to give, on normal chromosomes 22, either a single-color signal (e.g., yellow) or overlapping red and green signals (depending on the level of chromosome/DNA contraction in the individual interphase cells). When a chromosomal rearrangement such as a translocation causes a separation of the paired probes, two signals of different colors (e.g., orange and green) are seen, typically separated by at least the width of one signal. Therefore, abnormal cells will be described as nuc ish (*EWS*x2)(*5'EWS* sep *3'EWS* x1), meaning two *EWS* signals but one has separated into the 5' probe and the 3' probe presumably because of a translocation. An abbreviated list of symbols used to designate chromosome abnormalities as well as abbreviations utilized in describing results obtained by in situ hybridization in cancer cytogenetics is given in Table 4–2.

The nomenclature used to describe human genes in this chapter is either the official name as assigned by the Human Gene Nomenclature Committee (HUGO) (*www.gene.ucl.ac.uk/nomenclature*), or a more widely used common alias for the HUGO gene name (*www.gdb.org*). If the latter is used, the HUGO name is indicated in brackets the first time the gene is mentioned in the text, such as *CHOP (DDIT3)*, the former being the common name and the latter the HUGO name. Human genes and transcripts are written in uppercase italics, while the corresponding proteins are uppercase but not italicized.

Methodologic considerations

The application of long-term collagenase treatment for tissue disaggregation,[30] starting in the mid-1980s, greatly accelerated work in solid tumor cytogenetics. During the years in which these cytogenetic methodologies were being developed, adapted, and further refined for solid tumors, many differences arose among laboratories. However, today the protocols are more alike than they are dissimilar, despite the fact that there is a need to adapt them to the specific needs and conditions of each laboratory. There are several technical pitfalls that can affect cytogenetic analyses of clinical tumor samples:

1. Unpredictable growth of the neoplastic cells in tissue culture;
2. Overgrowth of neoplastic cells by reactive non-neoplastic cells;

TABLE 4–2	PARTIAL LIST OF SYMBOLS AND ABBREVIATED TERMS USED IN CANCER CYTOGENETICS
Symbol	**Definition**
Chromosome abnormalities	
add	Additional material of unknown origin
cp	Composite karyotype
del	Deletion
der	Derivative chromosome
dic	Dicentric chromosome
dmin	Double minute chromosome
dup	Duplication
hsr	Homogeneously staining region
i	Isochromosome
inc	Incomplete karyotype
ins	Insertion
inv	Inversion
mar	Marker chromosome
minus (–)	Loss
p	Short arm of a chromosome
plus (+)	Gain
q	Long arm of a chromosome
r	Ring chromosome
t	Translocation
In situ hybridization (ISH)	
amp	Amplified signal
con	Connected signals (signals are adjacent)
dim	Diminished signal intensity
FISH	Fluorescence in situ hybridization
double plus (++)	Duplication on a specific chromosome
ish	In situ hybridization on metaphases
minus (–)	Absent from a specific chromosome
multiplication sign (×)	Precedes the number of signal seen
nuc ish	Nuclear or interphase in situ hybridization
period (.)	Separates cytogenetics observation from results of ISH
plus (+)	Present on a specific chromosome
semicolon (;)	Separates probes on different derivative chromosomes
sep	Separated signals (signals are separated)
wcp	Whole chromosome paint

3. Contamination of tumor cultures by bacteria or fungi;
4. Predominance of nonviable tumor (necrotic sample).

A successful cytogenetic analysis is based on successful culture. The procedure for solid tumors begins in the operating room when the tumor is removed or biopsied. The tissue sample sent for cytogenetics must be sterile, must be representative of the tumor, and should be viable (i.e., not in a fixative solution). Optimally, the tumor biopsy is divided by the pathologist into sections to be used for pathological diagnosis, cytogenetics (culture), and molecular analyses (snap-frozen). At least 80% of all soft tissue tumors can be cultured successfully if the specimens are carefully selected by the pathologist to minimize necrotic and non-neoplastic components.

Solid tumor samples generally must be disaggregated by mechanical (mincing) and enzymatic (collagenase) methods before the cells are placed in tissue culture. To shorten the time in culture and avoid overgrowth of fibroblastic stroma, disaggregated cells are grown in chamber slides, which have the advantage of requiring only a small number of cells, and metaphases can be both harvested and stained using in situ techniques. Cell attachment, proliferation, and mitotic rate are monitored by daily examination of each culture through an inverted microscope. Selection of an appropriate point at which to harvest the cultures, as well as optimization of exposure to a mitotic spindle inhibitor that inhibits cell division at metaphase (e.g., colchicine) are also determined by daily monitoring. Harvesting and fixation of tumor cultures typically follow standard cytogenetic procedures for monolayer cultures with a very limited number of cells.

Most mesenchymal tumors can be karyotyped within 7 days after culture initiation and metaphases are best harvested after 1–3 days in culture, despite the fact that the yield of metaphases may be low at this point. This is because growth of some neoplastic populations can slow after 1–2 days in culture, or the neoplastic cells can be overgrown by fibroblasts or other non-neoplastic elements. Therefore, metaphase harvesting at multiple time points will improve the likelihood of a successful analysis. Overgrowth by reactive cells is the most common explanation for a normal diploid karyotype obtained after more than 10 days of culture.

The availability of fresh tumor, the differential diagnosis, and the need for rapid diagnostic cytogenetic results are factors in determining the order of performing molecular cytogenetic or molecular techniques (i.e., FISH and RT-PCR) or conventional cytogenetic analysis.

Molecular cytogenetics

The greater resolution afforded by molecular cytogenetics bridges the gap between classical cytogenetics and molecular genetics. Molecular cytogenetic techniques provide a critical role both in the diagnostic (e.g., detection of submicroscopic chromosomal aberrations) and research arenas (e.g., localization and mapping of chromosomal breakpoints and candidate disease genes).[31] FISH analysis is well suited to identify submicroscopic changes and define cryptic, and often complex, chromosome rearrangements. Moreover, FISH extends the application of diagnostic cytogenetics to all stages of the cell cycle, as dividing cells are no longer a prerequisite. As a result, with carefully designed probes, certain chromosome rearrangements (such as translocations) can be detected in non-dividing (interphase) nuclei without the need for cell culture. Thus, interphase cytogenetics using FISH provides cytogenetic information on specimens that are difficult or impossible to culture (e.g., fine needle aspirates, paraffin-embedded fixed tissues). FISH differs from conventional cytogenetics, however, in that effective application and interpretation of FISH relies upon an a priori knowledge of the targeted aberration and appropriate rational probe design. Validated FISH assays are assessed for reproducibility, specificity, and sensitivity, all of which must be established within each laboratory for every diagnostic probe. Such validation must also include testing of appropriate and relevant tissue samples.

A variety of different types of probes are used to detect chromosome abnormalities; however, the most frequently used probes in soft tissue neoplasms are alpha-satellite DNA probes (for pericentromeric repeat sequences specific for each chromosome) and unique locus-specific (or gene-specific) DNA sequences. Alpha-satellite probes to pericentromeric repeats allow the detection of monosomies, trisomies and other aneuploidies. These probes are also often used as a control for ploidy status when, for instance using a gene locus-specific probe to determine amplification. However, the ability to detect numerical abnormalities in a small neoplastic subpopulation

within a specimen (e.g., to assess minimal residual disease) is often hampered by hybridization inefficiencies, false background signals, and incomplete probe penetration in intact nuclei.

Probes that identify unique, locus-specific DNA sequences are typically genomic or cDNA clones, and vary in size from 1 to hundreds of kilobases. In most clinical cytogenetics laboratories, the detection of chromosome abnormalities is limited to probes that are commercially available, although some laboratories may develop "home-brew" probes for special studies or new sarcoma translocation genes. In sarcomas, the most frequently used method to detect a chromosome translocation is to employ DNA probes from one of the two loci involved. This type of probe design is referred to as a break-apart probe and has been described above (Fig. 4–2A). Another variation on FISH assays based on break-apart probes, frequently used in hematologic disorders, is the selection of two pairs of DNA probes that span

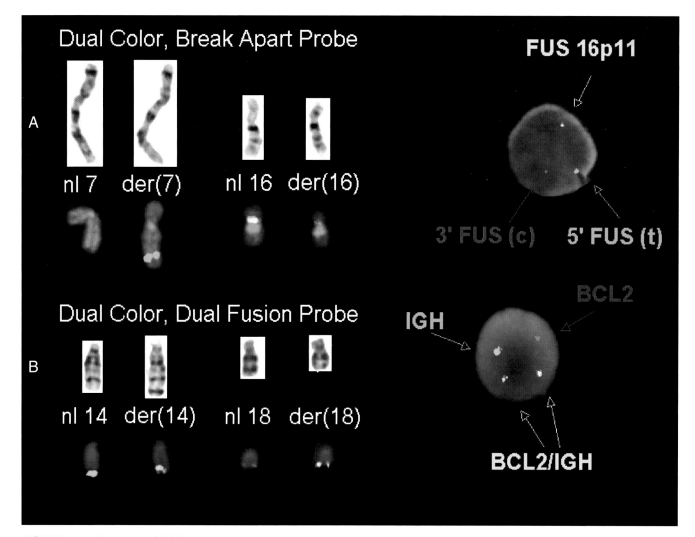

FIGURE 4–2 Two types of FISH assay designs for translocation detection (see text for details). nl, normal; c, centromeric; t, telomeric.

respectively both rearranged loci. A commonly used "dual-fusion" cocktail involves probes that span the *IGH* and *BCL2* loci, respectively, such that the hybridization pattern in a cell with a t(14;18)(q32;q21) shows not one but two yellow fusion signals [i.e., *IGH-BCL2* fusion on the der(14) and *BCL2-IGH* fusion on the der(18)], improving the specificity of the assay (Fig. 4–2B). Finally, FISH using differentially labeled probes allows simultaneous detection of multiple regions, which is particularly valuable when analyzing multiple abnormalities within a single cell.

As with any technique, it is necessary to understand the limitations of FISH; in certain instances, molecular analysis may be of greater sensitivity and utility.

In terms of sensitivity, break-apart probes are optimal for the detection of rearrangements consistently involving a single chromosomal region (e.g., *EWS*) in concert with several different chromosomal partners; however, by the same token, this design cannot identify the translocation partner and, therefore, will not distinguish between specific rearrangements, other than to confirm involvement of the common locus. In contrast, dual-fusion probes distinguish between different chromosomal partners in rearrangements, but require a separate assay for each combination [i.e., detection of *EWS* rearrangement in a t(11;22) or a t(21;22)].

Chromogenic in situ hybridization (CISH) is an alternative method in which the DNA probe is detected using a simple immunohistochemistry (IHC)-like peroxidase reaction. CISH is emerging as a practical, cost-effective, and valid alternative to FISH in testing for certain gene alterations.[32,33] CISH has some advantages over FISH: with CISH, a brightfield microscope is sufficient for scoring results; the methodology is less cumbersome and more economical; the signal intensity is not light-sensitive and therefore the signal does not fade over time; and, because pathologists are familiar with IHC signals and are able to correlate the CISH signals with histopathology, it permits particularly detailed histologic correlation in heterogeneous samples. On the other hand, with CISH the number of colors that can be distinguished by light microscopy is limited, and for this reason, most CISH applications have been directed towards the detection of numerical alterations (e.g., aneuploidy, amplification).

In terms of starting materials, interphase FISH/CISH can be performed using nuclei from touch or smear preparations, body fluid cell suspensions, or fresh tissue samples following enzymatic disaggregation, as well as from histologic sections of archival, formalin-fixed, paraffin-embedded tissue. With the latter, the thickness of tissue sections can affect hybridization quality and result interpretation. Specifically, the use of standard thickness histological sections (4 or 5 micrometers) in FISH/CISH assays can cause missed signals whenever sections cut through nuclei; analysis of many more cells is consequently necessary. This is a concern for the analysis of deletions or translocations, but is less problematic for the detection of amplifications. In contrast, the use of 50-micron-thick sections followed by isolation of intact nuclei allows the evaluation of intact nuclei and therefore circumvents the problems associated with sectioned nuclei.[34]

Recently developed multicolor FISH methods [e.g., spectral karyotyping (SKY), multicolor FISH (M-FISH), combined binary ratio (COBRA)-FISH] in which entire chromosomes are distinguished by different fluorescent labeling, can readily reveal complex inter-chromosomal rearrangements in a single hybridization experiment.[35] Their successful application depends upon the availability of a sufficient number of evaluable cells in metaphase. However, such techniques are not suitable for detecting intra-chromosomal rearrangements. Comparative genomic hybridization (CGH), as originally developed, involved labeling tumor DNA as a complex FISH probe and hybridizing it to normal metaphase chromosomes along with a reference DNA labeled with a different fluorophore, to define regions of gains or losses across all chromosomal regions.[36] Thus, this technique does not require viable or dividing tumor cells. Since this is a method in which bulk tumor DNA is extracted, normal DNA from admixed non-neoplastic cells can cause CGH to underestimate low-level copy number changes such as hemizygous loss or low amplification. More recently, conventional CGH has been made obsolete by the advent of array CGH, in which the tumor DNA is hybridized instead to high-density arrays of probes covering the entire genome.[37] Array CGH provides a much higher resolution genome-wide definition of genetic gains and losses. However, conventional and array-based CGH do not detect balanced chromosome translocations, a hallmark of many soft tissue tumors. Array-based CGH data in sarcomas are further discussed below.

Reverse-transcriptase-polymerase chain reaction

The second major diagnostic method for sarcoma translocations is reverse-transcriptase PCR (RT-PCR). The use of FISH to detect translocations has been described above. RT-PCR assays detect the specific fusion RNA transcribed from the fusion gene by using forward and reverse primers bracketing the fusion point in the RNA. In order to be used in the PCR reaction, the RNA has to be converted into a complementary DNA (cDNA) using the enzyme reverse-transcriptase. It should be noted that PCR using genomic DNA is usually not practical for the detection of most fusion genes because the genomic breakpoints are often scattered in large introns and only at the RNA level is there a highly consistent molecular structure. Thus, RT-PCR is the standard molecular approach for the detection of translocation-associated gene fusions. It is especially powerful because the splicing of the transcripts encoded by fusion genes typically results in very consistent fusion points that can be tightly bracketed by appropriate primers to generate relatively small RT-PCR products (e.g., 100–300 bp).

RT-PCR, as an RNA-based assay, is susceptible to failure due to poor RNA quality. As a PCR-based assay, it is also susceptible to false-positives due to PCR cross-contamination. It is critical to include two types of contamination controls: controls lacking only the template RNA (to detect contamination of the PCR reagents) and controls lacking only the reverse transcriptase (to detect contamination of the patient RNA sample).[6,38] Biologically, specific gene fusions are tumor-specific and appear necessary in the pathogenesis of specific cancers and therefore make near-perfect tumor markers. However, in practice, it is important to remember that technical limitations or errors in the detection of these translocations can lead to false-positives or false-negatives.[6,38]

Although RT-PCR is more sensitive and provides more detailed fusion information than FISH, it is less adaptable to paraffin material, and frozen tissue is generally preferred. Another important consideration for RT-PCR assays is that they require extensive knowledge of the specific exons involved by the gene fusions and of the variability in exon composition of some fusions. Recently, real-time RT-PCR, which employs highly sensitive fluorescent detection of PCR products as they are generated ("in real time"), has emerged as an improved strategy for RT-PCR detection of sarcoma fusion transcripts in archival pathology material,[39,40] with the added benefit of reducing cross-contamination risks by the closed tube detection of product and the avoidance of nested PCR.

RT-PCR and FISH are complementary methods for detecting sarcoma translocations. The use of one or the other as the first-line approach often reflects differences in local expertise. Most studies comparing both techniques in the sarcoma setting suggest that optimal diagnostic accuracy can be achieved when both are available.[41–44] The College of American Pathologists now offers regular proficiency testing for sarcoma translocation detection by FISH and RT-PCR.

The practical need for molecular testing in modern sarcoma diagnosis has recently been objectively evaluated in two clinical settings, namely the diagnosis of synovial sarcomas and Ewing sarcomas.[45,46] Based on these studies, after standard IHC panels are used, molecular confirmation of translocation status seems more often useful in diagnosing synovial sarcomas (useful in approximately 50%) than Ewing sarcomas (useful in approximately 10%). Some of the most common settings or indications for molecular diagnostic translocation testing in sarcomas include: (1) the differential diagnosis of undifferentiated small round cell sarcomas, Ewing/PNET versus desmoplastic small round cell tumor (DSCRT) versus poorly differentiated synovial sarcoma versus neuroblastoma; (2) the confirmation of alveolar subtype in rhabdomyosarcoma (as a prognostic factor);

(3) the distinction of monophasic synovial sarcoma from other spindle cell sarcomas; and (4) the confirmation of otherwise typical cases in older patients or in uncommon sites or in the setting of unusual histology or immunophenotype.

Immunohistochemical markers of genetic alterations

Many translocations can be "converted" into immunohistochemical assays based on the phenomenon of discordance in the expression levels of the amino- and carboxy-terminal ends of the product of gene B in tumors with A-B gene fusions, the markedly aberrant expression of the carboxy-terminal encoded by gene B in the context of these fusion proteins, or their expression in aberrant cell types or aberrant cellular compartments. This has been used as a basis for the immunohistochemical detection of oncogenic fusion proteins.[47] In sarcomas, this approach has been applied to the detection of the EWS-WT1 protein (Fig. 4–3A),[48,49] the ASPL-TFE3 protein (Fig. 4–3B),[50] the EWS-FLI1 protein,[51–53] and ALK fusion proteins.[54–56] Another strategy for converting molecular translocation detection into an immunohistochemical assay is provided by the rare gene fusions where a 5′ exon of gene B that is not normally translated becomes translated in the context of the fusion protein and therefore represents a novel peptide sequence that can be used to generate fusion protein-specific antibody. This approach has been elegantly demonstrated for FUS-CHOP and EWS-CHOP detection in myxoid liposarcomas.[57]

Although recurrent translocations are by far the most widely used markers, certain other genetic alterations are so closely associated with specific sarcomas that they can also form the basis for confirmatory immunohistochemical assays. This is the case with KIT (and PDGFRA) mutations in gastrointestinal stromal tumors.[58] However, KIT immunoreactivity in GIST is related to tumor cell lineage more than to the underlying mutation. Co-amplification of MDM2 and CDK4 in well-differentiated and dedifferentiated liposarcomas due to 12q amplification has emerged as a potentially useful marker in certain settings,[59,60] and this has been translated into a robust immunohistochemical assay.[61,62] Mutations involving the WNT pathway (in APC or in the β-catenin gene) are characteristic of (but not specific for) aggressive desmoid-type fibromatosis (see below). These mutations result in nuclear beta-catenin accumulation readily detected by immunohistochemistry.[63,64] Immunohistochemical analysis can be used to confirm the pathognomonic loss of INI1 in malignant rhabdoid tumors, and it appears fairly specific for this entity.[65]

Some immunohistochemical markers of genetic alterations are not restricted to any single sarcoma type but may be useful in other ways. Loss of PTEN staining,

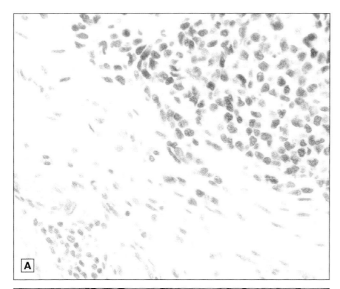

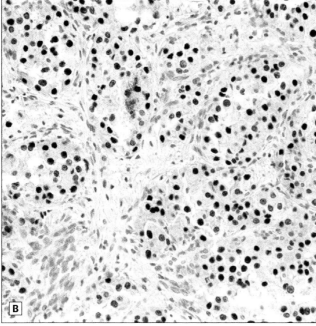

FIGURE 4–3 Two examples of IHC detection of translocation fusion proteins. **(A)** The detection of the EWS-WT1 protein using antibody to the WT1 carboxy-terminal. **(B)** The detection of the ASPL-TFE3 protein using antibody to a portion of TFE3 included in the fusion protein.

MAJOR PATHOGENETIC CLASSES OF SARCOMAS

For the discussion of genetic alterations in specific soft tissue tumors, we have chosen to group tumors into broad categories that integrate their cytogenetic features and their principal oncogenic mechanisms. These generally parallel each other insofar as sarcomas driven by transcriptional deregulation or deregulated signaling harbor specific translocations or point mutations and show relatively simple karyotypes with few changes. This is in contrast to sarcomas with highly complex karyotypes which are generally considered to have a different biology. The contrasting features of sarcomas with specific translocations ("translocation sarcomas") and those with complex karyotypes, presented in Table 4–3, were first highlighted in a 2003 conference report[71] and have become a widely used approach for discussing their biology.[8,72] However, these groupings should be considered as a conceptual framework that highlights the key shared features of different sarcomas, and not as an actual classification. For instance, the outcome of Ewing sarcomas[73] and myxoid liposarcomas[69,74] is dramatically worsened by p53/p14ARF pathway alterations; in contrast, most sarcomas lacking specific translocations show more frequent p53 alterations but these seem to have only a moderate clinical impact.[75] Another striking contrast emerges in telomere maintenance mechanisms, of which two main types have been described in human tumors: telomerase activation and the alternative lengthening of telomeres (ALT) mechanism. A predominance of telomerase activation in the absence of ALT appears to characterize sarcomas with specific chromosomal translocations, while a high prevalence of ALT is seen in sarcomas with non-specific complex karyotypes.[76–78] The reasons for this remain unclear. Other contrasting features are discussed in the following sections.

Sarcomas with chimeric transcription factors

The fusion genes produced by most sarcoma translocations encode chimeric transcription factors that cause transcriptional deregulation. Transcription factors have a modular structure consisting, at a minimum, of a transcription regulatory domain and a DNA binding domain. Transcription regulatory domains, because they do not show strong sequence conservation, are typically defined by functional assays and can either stimulate or repress gene transcription. DNA binding domains show strong sequence conservation which allows them to be grouped into families. One general rule of sarcomas with chimeric transcription factors is that all translocation variants associated with a specific sarcoma involve genes from the same transcription factor family as defined by the type of DNA binding domain. Translocations that lead to the

especially in conjunction with staining for phosphorylated AKT, may signal the presence of inactivating *PTEN* mutations.[66,67] Loss of staining for P16 or for its frequently co-deleted chromosomal neighbor, MTAP, can be used as a marker for *CDKN2A* homozygous deletion.[68,69] Finally, the association of P53 nuclear staining with *P53* missense mutations is well described, although its sensitivity and specificity can vary between tumor types and between studies.[70]

TABLE 4–3	SOME CONTRASTING ASPECTS OF SARCOMAS WITH SPECIFIC TRANSLOCATIONS AND SARCOMAS WITH COMPLEX KARYOTYPES	
	Sarcomas with specific translocations	**Sarcomas with non-specific genetic alterations**
Karyotypes	Usually simple	Usually complex
Translocations	Reciprocal & specific, producing fusion genes	Non-reciprocal & non-specific, causing gene copy number changes
Telomere maintenance mechanisms	Telomerase expression common, ALT[1] mechanism rare	ALT mechanism more common than telomerase
P53 pathway alterations	Relatively rare, but strong prognostic impact	More frequent, but limited or no prognostic impact
Incidence in bilateral retinoblastoma and Li-Fraumeni syndrome	Rare, if ever	Common
Similarity of gene expression profiles within each sarcoma type	Strong	Weak

[1] ALT, alternative lengthening of telomeres.

production of novel chimeric transcription factors generally either fuse two transcription factor genes or fuse one transcription factor gene with another gene encoding a domain which can function as a transcriptional activation domain. The modular structure of transcription factors allows their domains to be re-shuffled by these translocations, leading to new combinations of domains with aberrant properties.

Several features endow chimeric transcription factors with aberrant functional properties. Relative to the native translocation partners, there may be acquisition of new protein interactions (with coactivators, corepressors, chromatin binding proteins), acquisition of new target gene specificities (even if the primary structure of DNA-binding domain is not altered by the gene fusion),[79] and deregulation of expression relative to normal expression levels, cell type, developmental stage, or cell cycle timing. Transcription factors, as master regulators of the expression of multiple downstream "target genes", are themselves under tight control by other transcription factors that determine their expression by binding to the promoter region, located in the vicinity of their first exon. Within the context of fusion of genes A and B, the expression of the A-B fusion gene as a whole is largely driven by the promoter region of gene A, and this defines one aberrant aspect of chimeric transcription factors.

In broad terms, chimeric transcription factors are thought to deregulate the expression of specific repertoires of target genes, possibly orchestrating multiple oncogenic "hits". The identities of the specific target genes deregulated by each type of chimeric transcription factor are being gradually elucidated but a discussion of these studies is beyond the scope of this chapter. In general, the significance of individual target genes remains unclear and few if any have clear diagnostic or practical implications at present. The key role of these chimeric transcription factors in sarcoma pathogenesis is supported by their requirement for in vitro growth of corresponding sarcoma cell lines and the impact of relatively minor variability in

the structure of these chimeric proteins (due to variant cytogenetic or molecular breakpoints) on tumor phenotype and clinical behavior, as discussed in the specific sections below. Thus, the aberrant transcriptional protein is important for the maintenance of the malignant phenotype and seems to also determine the behavior of the sarcoma after initiation.

The specificity of chromosomal translocations in sarcomas is remarkable. The tumor-type specificity of sarcoma gene fusions may reflect a dynamic relationship with the cellular environment.[80] In this model, the gene fusion is oncogenic in a specific susceptible cell type at a particular developmental stage, and in turn, the gene fusion may then modify the phenotype of the susceptible cell. The need to target a specific mesenchymal cell type may account for the scarcity of transgenic mouse models for this class of sarcomas.[81,82] Aberrant transcription factors may be tolerated and transforming in only a very specific cell type. It has also become apparent that chimeric transcription factors may have a strong effect on cell lineage markers, in effect redirecting differentiation ("reprogramming"). Thus, the phenotype of the precursor cells may be difficult to infer from the phenotype of the translocation sarcoma, and, moreover, the precursor cells for a given type of translocation sarcoma may not be exactly identical from case to case. It has been found that introduction of the *EWS-FLI1* gene into neuroblastoma cells or embryonal rhabdomyosarcoma cells can shift their differentiation program to that of ES/PNET.[83,84] Likewise, *FUS-CHOP* can induce fibrosarcoma cells to display features of liposarcoma. This also raises the possibility that the precursor cells for different sarcomas may be similar. For instance, the introduction of *EWS-FLI1* or *FUS-CHOP* into primary mesenchymal progenitor cells leads to the formation of tumors with features of ES/PNET or liposarcoma, respectively.[85–87] Indeed, a recent study of Ewing sarcoma cell lines suggests that they originate from mesenchymal stem cells.[87a]

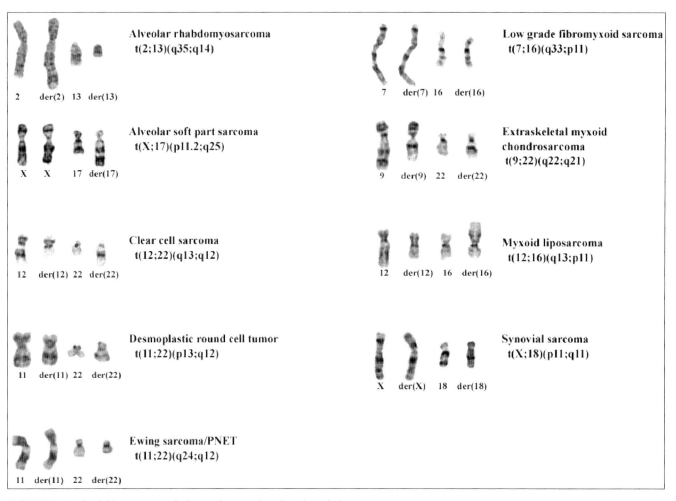

FIGURE 4-4 Partial karyotypes of nine major translocations in soft tissue sarcomas.

The following sections describe the genetic alterations in the major sarcomas driven by the transcriptional deregulation mediated by translocation-derived chimeric transcription factors. The major recurrent translocations are listed in Table 4–1. Partial karyotypes of nine major translocations in sarcomas are shown in Fig. 4–4.

1. Ewing sarcoma/peripheral neuroectodermal tumor

At the molecular level, Ewing sarcoma/peripheral neuroectodermal tumor (ES/PNET) is characterized by chromosomal translocations that fuse *EWS (EWSR1)*, located at 22q12, and a gene of the ETS family of transcription factors. In 90–95% of cases, the gene fusion is *EWS-FLI1*, consisting of the N-terminal portion of EWS and the C-terminal portion of FLI1 including the ETS DNA-binding domain. An *EWS-ERG* fusion, where the *ERG* gene from 21q22 substitutes for *FLI1*, is found in 5–10% of cases.[88,89] Very rare cases of ES/PNET show fusions of *EWS* to other *ETS* family genes [such as *ETV1, E1AF (ETV4)*, and *FEV*], or the *FUS-ERG* fusion.[90] These gene fusions are presumed to be the initiating oncogenic

event in ES/PNET, and appear to play a critical role in the proliferation and tumorigenesis of ES/PNET cells.[91,92]

The ETS family of transcription factors is defined by the ETS DNA-binding domain.[93] The EWS aminoterminal domain can function as a strong transactivation domain and its promoter is strongly and broadly activated, leading to relatively unrestricted high-level expression of the resulting fusion genes.[94,95] In contrast, expression of native FLI1 is tightly regulated and lineage-restricted.[96] Details of the biology of native EWS and FLI1, as well as the functional aspects of EWS-FLI1 and its possible non-transcriptional effects, are reviewed in detail elsewhere.[92]

EWS-FLI1 is structurally heterogeneous, with up to 18 possible types of in-frame *EWS-FLI1* chimeric transcripts, most of which have been observed in vivo.[88,95] The two main types, fusion of *EWS* exon 7 to *FLI1* exon 6 (type 1) and fusion of *EWS* exon 7 to *FLI1* exon 5 (type 2), account for about 85–90% of *EWS-FLI1* fusions.[88,97] In spite of this heterogeneity, each EWS-FLI1 fusion protein invariably contains the amino-terminal domain of EWS (exons 1 to 7), and the intact DNA-binding domain of

FLI1 (exon 9). The survival of patients whose tumor contains the type 1 *EWS-FLI1* fusion appears statistically better than those with other *EWS-FLI1* fusion types.[97–99] However, the clinical differences in these retrospective series have been moderate and the clinical utility of this observation remains uncertain. The variant *EWS-ERG* fusion has been found to be associated with clinical phenotypes indistinguishable from *EWS-FLI1*-positive ES/PNET.[100] The more immediate practical significance of *EWS-FLI1* structural variability is that not all forms of the *EWS-FLI1* fusion transcript may be detected in clinical material with a single RT-PCR primer pair, leading to a risk of false-negative results. Therefore, several RT-PCR assays with different primer pairs are typically needed to reliably exclude the presence of a *EWS-FLI1* fusion. The same concern applies to *EWS-ERG* detection, but to a lesser extent.

ES/PNET are also heterogeneous for the occurrence of genetic alterations involving certain critical regulators of cell cycle progression and apoptosis, in particular p16/p14ARF (encoded by *CDKN2A*) and p53.[101] Alterations in p53 or p16/p14ARF are found in about 25% of ES/PNET and define a subset with highly aggressive behavior and poor chemoresponse.[73]

2. Alveolar rhabdomyosarcoma

Alveolar rhabdomyosarcoma (ARMS) is associated with recurrent translocations fusing genes from the *PAX* family of transcription factors to *FKHR* (*FOXOA1*). Approximately 60–70% of histologically diagnosed ARMS involve a t(2;13)(q35;q14) leading to *PAX3-FKHR* gene fusion[102] and 10–20% have a t(1;13)(p36;q14) representing the variant *PAX7-FKHR* gene fusion.[103] However, 10–30% of histologic ARMS fail to exhibit any of these translocations.[104,105] Rare unique (so far non-recurrent) variant fusions have also been reported.[104,106] Morphologic evaluation alone is often insufficient to make the distinction between ARMS and embryonal rhabdomyosarcoma ERMS as some ARMS lack the alveolar architecture and ERMS can be cellular and poorly differentiated. Because this distinction is clinically critical in assigning patients to high-risk regimens, this is one of the most requested sarcoma translocation assays. Furthermore, *PAX3-FKHR*-positive appear significantly more aggressive tumors than those containing *PAX7-FKHR*.[105,107,108] *PAX3-FKHR* and *PAX7-FKHR*-expressing ARMS appear morphologically identical.

The PAX3-FKHR DNA-binding domain is contributed by the *PAX3* gene, containing the paired box domain and the adjacent homeodomain. PAX3-FKHR appears to be a stronger transactivator than native PAX3 and is also overexpressed at the RNA level relative to native PAX3 transcripts.[79] Interestingly, both PAX3 and PAX7 have well-studied roles in normal embryonic muscle development,[7] representing a rare instance in which the physiological role of one of the translocation partners in a sarcoma gene fusion can be linked to the phenotype of the associated sarcoma. An interesting special feature of ARMS with the *PAX7-FKHR* fusion is that the fusion gene is often duplicated or amplified.[109,110] Fusion-positive ARMS cases also show various other chromosomal gains and losses, some of which may function as secondary, cooperating genetic alterations.[111]

3. Desmoplastic small round cell tumor

The desmoplastic small round cell tumor (DSRCT) contains the characteristic *EWS-WT1* gene fusion in essentially all cases.[112,113] In the EWS-WT1 chimeric protein, the RNA-binding domain of EWS is replaced by a truncated but functional portion of the WT1 DNA-binding domain (3 of 4 zinc fingers). This altered WT1 DNA-binding domain is associated with altered binding affinity and specificity, resulting in only limited overlap between WT1 and EWS-WT1 transcriptional targets. At model promoters, the encoded chimeric EWS-WT1 protein functions as a strong transactivator.[114] Occasional *EWS-WT1* fusion structure variants have been reported.[115] The demonstration of the *EWS-WT1* fusion has been useful in establishing the diagnosis of DSRCT in extra-abdominal locations and other atypical settings.

4. Clear cell sarcoma

At least 90% of clear cell sarcomas (CCSs) are characterized cytogenetically by a recurrent chromosomal translocation, t(12;22), resulting in fusion of the *EWS* gene with the *ATF1* gene (activating transcription factor-1) on 12q13.[116–118] In the resulting chimeric protein the C-terminal of EWS is replaced by a functional basic DNA binding and leucine zipper dimerization (bZIP) DNA-binding domain of ATF1. ATF1 is a member of a subgroup of bZIP transcription factors that includes the cAMP-response-element-binding protein (CREB1). There is molecular heterogeneity among *EWS-ATF1* transcripts. Most cases show an in-frame transcript resulting from the fusion of *EWS* exon 8 to *ATF1* exon 4 ("type 1"). Some cases have a different *EWS-ATF1* fusion structure where the junction is between *EWS* exon 7 to *ATF1* exon 5 or between *EWS* exon 10 and *ATF1* exon 5.[117,118] In addition, some cases express two different fusion transcripts derived from the same fusion gene.[40]

A recurring theme in sarcoma translocations is that closely related gene family members can substitute for each other as translocation partners. Thus, it is not completely unexpected that *EWS-CREB1* has been identified as a variant fusion in CCS, generated by a t(2;22)(q33;q12) at the cytogenetic level.[119] Because this novel fusion was initially found in three CCS cases that arose in the gastrointestinal tract, it appears that this variant fusion may be preferentially associated with a gastrointestinal location, though some non-gastrointestinal CCS with *EWS-CREB1* may yet be identified as well.

Molecular approaches have provided seemingly conflicting data on the relationship of CCS to cutaneous melanoma. While most CCS share a melanocytic gene expression signature with melanomas,[120] the two are also clearly genetically distinct, as CCS lack the *BRAF* mutations commonly seen in melanomas,[121] whereas melanomas do not contain the *EWS-ATF1* fusion.[40,122,123]

5. Myxoid/round cell liposarcoma

The karyotypic hallmark of myxoid/round cell liposarcoma (MLS/RCLS) is the t(12;16)(q13;p11) present cytogenetically in more than 90% of cases.[124] The translocation leads to the fusion of the *CHOP* (*DDIT3*) and *FUS* genes at 12q13 and 16p11, respectively, and the resulting fusion gene encodes a FUS-CHOP chimeric protein.[125–127] The *FUS-CHOP* fusion is present in approximately 95% of cases. The remaining 5% of cases harbor a variant translocation, t(12;22)(q13;q12), in which *CHOP* fuses instead with *EWS*.[128] *FUS-CHOP* fusion transcripts occur as different recurrent structural variants based on the presence or absence of *FUS* exons 6 to 8 in the fusion product.[17,129] Thus, three major recurrent fusion transcript types have been reported: type 7-2 (type I), seen in about 20% of cases, type 5-2 (type II), seen in approximately two-thirds of cases, and type 8-2 (type III), seen in about 10%.[74,129,130]

Molecular detection of *FUS-CHOP* or *EWS-CHOP* has been used to establish the monoclonal origin of multifocal MLS/RCLS.[131] These two related fusions are highly specific for MLS, and are not found in morphologic mimics such as the predominantly myxoid well-differentiated liposarcomas of the retroperitoneum and myxofibrosarcomas.[132] Secondary *P53* alterations are sometimes observed and they are associated with a more aggressive course.[69,74]

6. Extraskeletal myxoid chondrosarcoma

Approximately 75–80% of extraskeletal myxoid chondrosarcoma (EMC) contain a characteristic t(9;22)(q22;q12) in which the *EWS* gene becomes fused to a gene located at 9q22 encoding an orphan nuclear receptor belonging to the steroid /thyroid receptor gene superfamily, *NR4A3* (formerly *CHN* or *TEC* or *NOR1*).[133–136] In another 15–20% of EMC, a gene at 17q11 highly related to *EWS*, *TAF15* (formerly *RBP56* or *TAF2N* or *hTAF$_{II}$68*), fuses with *NR4A3* instead.[136–138] In addition, two additional variant fusions involving *NR4A3* have been reported, each only in a single case.[139,140]

NR4A3 possesses structural features in common with other orphan receptors, including ligand-activated transcriptional regulators. As orphan receptors, the ligands which bind them have not been identified. NR4A3 contains a zinc finger DNA-binding domain similar to the DNA-binding domains of the retinoic acid gamma receptor and RXRβ. *EWS-NR4A3* show considerable variability in terms of exon composition, with the fusion joining *EWS* exon 12 to *NR4A3* exon 3 (type 1 fusion) in approximately two-thirds of cases and *EWS* exon 7 to *NR4A3* exon 2 (type 2 fusion) in another 20%.[136] The remaining 12% of *EWS-NR4A3* cases have other exon combinations.

The application of *EWS-NR4A3* detection has helped to further define EMC as an entity distinct from skeletal myxoid chondrosarcomas, which uniformly lack this specific fusion.[141,142]

7. Synovial sarcoma

Synovial sarcoma (SS) is characterized by the t(X;18)(p11.2;q11.2), which juxtaposes the *SYT* (*SS18*) gene on chromosome 18 to either the *SSX1* or the *SSX2* gene, both located at Xp11.2.[143–145] A rare but recurrent variant that also appears cytogenetically identical represents a *SYT-SSX4* fusion.[146,147] As well, there is another variant so far described in only a single case.[148] The term *SYT-SSX* is sometimes used to refer collectively to *SYT-SSX1* and *SYT-SSX2* (and *SYT-SSX4*). In spite of the fact that the SYT-SSX1 and SYT-SSX2 fusion proteins differ at only 13 amino acid positions,[149] the type of fusion is strongly correlated with epithelial differentiation (i.e., biphasic histology) in SS,[150] with the latter being observed in 35–50% of SS with the *SYT-SSX1* fusion but only in less than 10% of SS with *SYT-SSX2*. Thus, cases with *SYT-SSX1* are approximately five times as likely to show glandular epithelial differentiation. Fusion type is associated with moderate differences in clinical course (*SYT-SSX2* favorable) in some but not all studies.[150–153] These links between subtle differences in the SYT-SSX fusion protein and tumor differentiation patterns support the involvement of the fusion protein in key aspects of SS. The SYT-SSX chimeric transcriptional protein differs from most sarcoma translocation fusion proteins in that neither SYT nor the SSX proteins contain DNA-binding domains. Instead, they appear to be transcriptional regulators whose actions are mediated primarily through protein–protein interactions.[149,154]

The only secondary mutations described with any frequency in SS have been in genes encoding Wnt signaling pathway components. Mutations in several genes in this regulatory network have been reported in SS, specifically in the E-cadherin gene (13%), *APC* (8%), the β-catenin gene (8%), as well as in *PTEN* (8%).[155]

SYT-SSX translocation detection is frequently requested to help distinguish monophasic SS from other primitive spindle cell sarcomas, such as solitary fibrous tumor or malignant peripheral nerve sheath tumor (MPNSTs). It has also helped to establish the diagnosis of SS in many organ sites, most notably in the kidney.[156–160]

8. Alveolar soft part sarcoma

Alveolar soft part sarcoma (ASPS) is unusual in that its canonical translocation is usually unbalanced, specifically as a der(17)t(X;17)(p11;q25).[161,162] The der(17)t(X;17) has sometimes been described as an add(17)(q25) when the quality of the banding did not allow for positive identification of the additional material as the short arm of X. This translocation causes the fusion of the *TFE3* transcription factor gene (from Xp11.2) with a novel gene at 17q25, designated *ASPL* (*ASPSCR1*).[163] Both native TFE3 and native ASPL are normally expressed in almost all tissues. The TFE3 transcription factor contains a basic helix-loop-helix DNA binding domain and leucine zipper dimerization domain. The ASPL-TFE3 fusion replaces the amino-terminal portion of TFE3 by ASPL sequences, while retaining the TFE3 DNA-binding region, activation domain, and nuclear localization signal. The ASPL-TFE3 fusion protein localizes to the nucleus and can function as an aberrant transcription factor.[164] Although the presence of the *ASPL-TFE3* fusion is highly specific and sensitive for ASPS among sarcomas,[163] it should be noted that the same gene fusion is also found in a small but unique subset of renal adenocarcinomas.[165,166] Two forms of the *ASPL-TFE3* fusion transcript are known and differ in the inclusion of an additional *TFE3* exon in the less common fusion structure, designated type 2.[163] The application of immunohistochemistry to the detection of this fusion is described above.

9. Low-grade fibromyxoid sarcoma

Low-grade fibromyxoid sarcoma (LGFMS) contains a recurrent t(7;16)(q32-34;p11) that represents the formation of a *FUS-CREB3L2* fusion gene.[167] The detection of this fusion has emerged as a potentially useful marker for this still poorly defined tumor type.[168] CREB3L2 contains a basic DNA binding and leucine zipper dimerization (B-ZIP) motif, and belongs to the CREB transcription factor family, but is not closely related to ATF1 or CREB1. A peculiar feature of this gene fusion is that the molecular structure of the *FUS-CREB3L2* fusion transcript varies from case to case, as no simple recurrent exon-to-exon junctions are observed.[169] A rare variant involving the *CREB3L1* gene instead of *CREB3L2* was recently reported.[169]

10. Others

Recurrent transcription factor fusions have been described in several other poorly defined sarcomas. A novel class of pericytic spindle cell tumors with a t(7;12)(p21-22;q13-q15) contains a fusion of *ACTB* and *GLI (GLI1)*, leading to dysregulated *GLI* expression.[170] Tumors described as angiomatoid fibrous histiocytomas (AFH) are hemorrhagic, multicystic soft tissue tumors, associated with a distinctive histiocytoid morphology and frequent positivity for desmin, CD68, and EMA that occur typically in children and adolescents. Recent studies have shown that AFH contain the related *EWS-CREB1*, *EWS-ATF1*, and *FUS-ATF1* fusions in decreasing order of frequency.[171–173] This is notable because the former two are also seen in clear cell sarcoma and thus these fusions are found in two distinct sarcomas, and hence may be able to transform two different types of mesenchymal precursor cells, unlike other sarcoma-associated chimeric transcription factors. Finally, two recently reported cases of soft tissue sarcoma diagnosed as Ewing-like sarcoma, both with a t(4;19)(q35;q13), contained a novel *CIC-DUX4* fusion joining the *CIC* high mobility group box transcription factor gene to the double homeodomain gene *DUX4*.[11]

Sarcomas with genetic deregulation of kinase signaling

A second group of sarcomas is characterized by recurrent genetic alterations that directly result in a deregulation of kinase signaling pathways. Three types of such alterations have been observed: (1) translocations forming chimeric protein tyrosine kinases; (2) translocations encoding a chimeric autocrine growth factor; and (3) activating mutations in specific kinases. The fusion of the catalytic domain of a protein tyrosine kinase (PTK) with a ubiquitously expressed protein providing a dimerization domain produces a chimeric tyrosine kinase that is constitutively activated in a ligand-independent fashion. This type of mechanism is involved in the pathogenesis of inflammatory myofibroblastic tumor, as a result of *ALK* rearrangements (*TPM3-ALK*, etc.) and congenital fibrosarcoma, due to the *ETV6-NTRK3* fusion. A less common mechanism implicated in sarcomas with chromosomal translocations is the formation of a chimeric autocrine growth factor, exemplified by the *COL1A-PDGFB* fusion in dermatofibrosarcoma protuberans,[174] and more recently the *CSF1-COL6A3* fusion identified in giant cell tumor of tendon sheath.[175] Finally, gastrointestinal stromal tumor (GIST) is the example of a sarcoma with activating mutations in specific kinases. These different types of kinase-dependent sarcomas are discussed in the following sections.

1. Inflammatory myofibroblastic tumor

Inflammatory myofibroblastic tumor (IMT) is a mesenchymal neoplasm that affects mainly children and young adults, and is composed of a mixture of myofibroblastic cells, plasma cells, and lymphocytes in varying proportions. Genetic studies have shown chromosomal abnormalities of 2p23 and rearrangement of the *ALK* gene.[176]

Molecular studies have identified *ALK* fusions involving the genes for tropomyosins 3 and 4 (*TPM3* and *TPM4*),[177] the clathrin heavy chain (*CLTC*),[178] the cysteinyl-tRNA synthetase (*CARS*),[179] and the Ran-binding protein 2 (*RANBP2*),[180] and this list continues to grow. The common characteristic shared by these *ALK* fusion partners is the presence of an amino-terminal oligomerization motif which, once fused to a truncated tyrosine kinase (in this case, ALK), leads to activation of the kinase catalytic domain in a constitutive fashion.[181] Anti-ALK immunohistochemical studies show up-regulated ALK protein expression in about 60% of cases, although the percentage is lower in adult cases.[55] However, ALK positivity is not entirely specific for IMT and can be observed in some other mesenchymal neoplasms.[182]

2. Infantile or congenital variant of fibrosarcoma

This form of fibrosarcoma generally presents within the first 2 years of life and is associated with a much better prognosis than adult fibrosarcoma. Cytogenetically, it shows a recurrent t(12;15)(p13;q25), resulting in the *ETV6-NTRK3* fusion.[183,184] Trisomies for chromosomes 8, 11, 17, and 20 are nearly as characteristic as the *ETV6-NTRK3*, and appear to be acquired after the fusion gene.[185,186] NTRK3 is a transmembrane surface receptor for neurotrophin-3 and is primarily expressed in the central nervous system, where it is involved in growth and survival of neuronal cells.[187] ETV6 is a member of the ETS transcription factor gene family and is frequently targeted by chromosomal translocations in human cancer, especially in leukemias.[187] In leukemia translocations, ETV6 either contributes its ETS-type DNA domain or its dimerization domain. In congenital fibrosarcoma, the oligomerization domain of ETV6 is fused to the kinase domain of NTRK3, mediating ligand-independent dimerization and subsequent kinase activation. The *ETV6-NTRK3* fusion is absent in adult-type fibrosarcoma or in other pediatric cellular fibroblastic lesions such as infantile fibromatosis and myofibromatosis, and thus can be used as a molecular diagnostic test for infantile fibrosarcoma. However, *ETV6-NTRK3* is also present in the cellular and mixed variants of congenital mesoblastic nephroma (CMN),[184,186] suggesting a histogenetic relationship of this renal tumor with congenital fibrosarcoma.

It should be noted that the *ETV6-NTRK3* gene fusion is also present in secretory breast carcinoma and a rare subset of acute myeloid leukemias.[188,189] The occurrence of identical gene fusions in divergent tumor types seems to be common in sarcomas with chimeric PTK than in sarcomas with chimeric transcription factors. These findings suggest that oncogenic transformation in distinct cell types may be mediated by the activation of the same tyrosine kinase signaling pathway, independent of lineage constraints and without affecting differentiation programs. *ETV6-NTRK3* is the first translocation-associated

fusion identified in mesenchymal, epithelial, and hematopoietic malignancies. *ALK* fusions provide another example of a chimeric PTK observed in divergent cell lineages, given their presence in both IMT[177,178] and anaplastic large cell lymphoma.[190,191]

3. Dermatofibrosarcoma protuberans/giant cell fibroblastoma

The recurrent t(17;22)(q22;q13) resulting in *COL1A-PDGFB* fusion has been reported as a consistent finding in both dermatofibrosarcoma protuberans (DFSP) and giant cell fibroblastoma (GCF), supporting the concept of a common pathogenetic entity.[174,192] The t(17;22) is typically tandemly repeated and amplified within a supernumerary ring chromosome.[193] Such gains of *COL1A1-PDGFB* genomic copies may be associated with fibrosarcomatous transformation of DFSP.[194] The translocation fuses the strongly expressed collagen 1 alpha 1 (*COL1A1*) gene on chromosome 17 to the second exon of the platelet-derived growth factor-B (*PDGFB*) gene on chromosome 22. This distinctive translocation mechanism results in transcriptional up-regulation of the *PDGFB* gene in the context of the *COL1A1-PDGFB* fusion. The post-translationally processed form of the fusion protein gives rise to a fully functional and mature PDGF-B protein, which induces activation of its receptor, PDGFRB, through autocrine or paracrine routes.[195] A number of clinical studies have shown a high response rate to imatinib therapy in both locally advanced and metastatic DFSP.[196–198] As imatinib blocks PDGFRB signaling, these results support the concept that DFSP cells are dependent on aberrant activation of PDGFRB for cellular proliferation and survival.

4. Giant cell tumor of tendon sheath/pigmented villonodular synovitis

Giant cell tumor of tendon sheath (GCTTS) and the morphologically similar but more aggressive pigmented villonodular synovitis (PVNS) are composed of a mixture of giant cells, mononuclear cells, and inflammatory cells. Their neoplastic nature was long controversial, but this has now been resolved by the identification of a recurrent t(1;2)(p13;q37), resulting in a *CSF1-COL6A3* fusion, in a significant number of both GCTTS and PVNS.[175] This translocation results in overexpression of CSF1, which is detected in a minority of the intratumoral cells, whereas the majority of cells express CSF1R, as detected by in situ hybridization. Thus, only a minority of cells in GCTTS and PVNS appear neoplastic, while the remaining majority of cells are non-neoplastic and are recruited by the local overexpression of CSF1. This phenomenon, described as a "tumor landscaping" effect, indicates that aberrant CSF1 expression in the neoplastic cells leads to abnormal accumulation of CSF1R-positive non-neoplastic cells.

These findings are in keeping with the biology of CSF1, which mediates proliferation, differentiation, and activation of macrophages and their precursors.[199] In these tumors, the cells expressing CSF1 also express CD68, while lacking CD163, suggesting that the CSF1-expressing neoplastic cells may be derived from synovial lining cells.[175] Synovial lining cells in reactive synovitis express CSF1, providing additional support for this hypothesis. The evidence suggesting a central role for CSF1 in the pathogenesis of these tumors indicates that treatment with specific inhibitors of this pathway might be beneficial, especially in aggressive forms of PVNS that can recur and cause significant morbidity.

5. Gastrointestinal stromal tumors

Constitutive activation of either the KIT or PDGFRA receptor tyrosine kinases by oncogenic mutations plays a central pathogenetic role in gastrointestinal stromal tumors (GIST).[200] *KIT* was originally identified as the cellular homolog of the retroviral oncogene *v-kit* in the Hardy-Zuckerman 4-feline sarcoma virus.[201] In humans, the *KIT* gene maps to 4q12, in the vicinity of the genes encoding for *PDGFRA* and *FLK1* receptor tyrosine kinases. KIT belongs to the class III of receptor tyrosine kinases, together with macrophage colony stimulating factor (M-CSF) and PDGFRA, based on their sequence homology and similar conformational structure. The KIT receptor plays a critical role in the normal development and function of the interstitial cells of Cajal (ICC),[202–204] as well as in hematopoiesis, gametogenesis, and melanogenesis during embryonic development and in the postnatal organism. Activating *KIT* mutations have been implicated in the pathogenesis of several other human tumors including seminomas,[205] mastocytosis,[206] acute myelogenous leukemias,[207] and more recently in melanomas,[208] suggesting a broader role for KIT in oncogenesis.

In GIST, activating *KIT* mutations can involve either the extracellular or the cytoplasmic domains of the receptor. The majority of the mutations (70–75%) have been found in the juxtamembrane domain, in a hotspot region at the 5′ end of exon 11, involving codons 550–560.[209,210] By analogy with other receptor tyrosine kinases, the juxtamembrane domain may function as a negative regulator of the KIT kinase and disruption of the conformational integrity of this domain may impair its negative regulatory function. Thus, the oncogenic potential of juxtamembrane domain mutations is attributed to the loss of this inhibitory function. The types of mutations occurring in this hotspot are quite heterogeneous, including in-frame deletions of variable sizes, point mutations, or deletions preceded by substitutions. A second, less common, hotspot in the juxtamembrane domain is located at the 3′ end of exon 11, and these mutations are mainly internal tandem duplications (ITD).[209,211] Activating *KIT* mutations in the usual exon 11 hotspot do not

appear to be associated with a specific clinicopathologic phenotype, but the presence of deletions rather than substitutions predicts a more aggressive behavior.[212] Specifically, deletions affecting codons 557 and 558 predict a poor prognosis.[213,214] In contrast, GIST patients harboring the above-mentioned ITD 3′ end of exon 11 follow a more indolent clinical course and their tumors are preferentially located in the stomach.[209,211]

KIT exon 9 mutations occur in 10–15% of patients and define a distinct subset of GIST that are often located in the small bowel and show more aggressive behavior.[209,215] In contrast to the more common *KIT* mutations in exons 9 and 11, mutations have been rarely described in the kinase domain (exon 13 and 17).[216,217]

Approximately one-third of GIST lacking *KIT* mutations harbor a mutation in *PDGFRA*, within exons 12, 14, or 18.[218–220] *PDGFRA*-mutated GISTs show a preference for gastric location, epithelioid morphology, variable or absent KIT expression by IHC, and a more indolent clinical behavior.[220,221] In about 10% of patients, no detectable mutation is identified in either *KIT* or *PDGFRA*. In particular, GIST that occur in pediatric or neurofibromatosis type 1 patients are nearly always wild-type (i.e., not mutated) for both genes.[222–224] In the adult population, the wild-type GIST subset represents a heterogeneous group of patients with no particular association with anatomic location or clinical outcome. In contrast, pediatric GIST represent a distinct clinicopathologic and molecular subset, more common in females, with multifocal gastric tumors and epithelioid histology, indolent course, and absence of *KIT* or *PDGFRA* mutations.[224]

Although the pathologic diagnosis of GIST can be rendered on morphologic grounds in the majority of cases and supported by KIT (CD117) immunoreactivity, in approximately 4% of cases KIT is negative by IHC.[225] When compared with KIT-positive GIST, these KIT-negative cases are more likely to have epithelioid morphology, contain *PDGFRA* mutations, and arise outside the gastrointestinal tract. Since some GIST that are negative for KIT by IHC nonetheless contain imatinib-sensitive *KIT* or *PDGFRA* mutations, these patients should not be denied imatinib therapy based on the negative IHC result alone.

Most activating mutations in *KIT* or *PDGFRA* in GIST are sporadic and somatically acquired in the tumor cells. However, at least 11 families have been reported to carry a germline mutation in either *KIT* or *PDGFRA*.[226–228] Patients with this syndrome develop GIST which are usually multiple in number, smaller in size, and occur in a background of ICC hyperplasia, both adjacent to and remote from the neoplastic lesions. The consistent ICC hyperplasia suggests that constitutive activation of KIT (or PDGFRA) through oncogenic mutation is directly responsible for a polyclonal expansion of this subset of cells. While *KIT* mutation appears to be sufficient to result in the expansion of the myenteric plexus, additional somatic genetic alterations are presumably required to generate the neoplastic proliferations recognized as GIST. In addition, a significant number of familial GIST patients have cutaneous hyperpigmentation and, in rare cases, abnormalities of mast cells, such as urticaria pigmentosa or systemic mast cell disease. The observation that *KIT*-activating mutations may be inherited suggested that it might be possible to develop a murine model harboring a germline gain of function mutation, as a model for the studying of KIT oncogenic signaling mechanisms. Indeed, two such models have been created.[229,230]

Cytogenetically, GIST show rather simple karyotypes with common losses of chromosomes 14 and 22, in most cases present as early events, regardless of the tumor site, clinical outcome, or *KIT* genotype.[231,232] Additional chromosomal changes occur preferentially in high-risk and recurrent GIST, including loss of 9p and 1p, among others. GISTs have a very distinctive gene expression profile that distinguishes them as a group from other soft tissue sarcomas.[233,234] When comparing different pathologic or molecular subsets of GIST, there is some heterogeneity in gene expression patterns, correlated with tumor location and *KIT* genotype.[235,236]

Imatinib mesylate (STI571, Gleevec™, Novartis Pharmaceuticals, Basel, Switzerland) is a selective tyrosine kinase inhibitor whose targets include KIT and PDGFRA. Imatinib treatment achieves a partial response or stable disease in about 80% of patients with metastatic GIST.[237] Recent data suggest a correlation between imatinib response and the type of mutation, as tumors with an exon 9 mutation or wild-type *KIT* are less likely to respond to imatinib.[238,239] Although imatinib achieves a partial response or stable disease in the majority of GIST patients, complete and lasting responses are rare. About half of the patients who initially benefit from imatinib treatment eventually develop drug resistance. The most common mechanism of acquired resistance is through a second *KIT* mutation, usually located in the kinase domain, which disrupts imatinib binding by stabilizing the receptor in a constitutively active form.[240] Several second-generation tyrosine kinase inhibitors that show promising activity against imatinib-resistant GISTs are in the process of being tested in preclinical studies or clinical trials.

Sarcomas with complex karyotypes

It should be noted that the majority of malignant soft tissue tumors are not associated with specific chromosomal translocations or simple point mutations. In these remaining sarcomas, many complex cytogenetic aberrations leading to numerous genomic gains and losses have been described. Soft tissue sarcomas with complex unbalanced karyotypes lacking specific translocations include pleomorphic and dedifferentiated liposarcomas, angiosarcoma, leiomyosarcoma, neuroblastoma, mesothelioma, adult fibrosarcoma, and malignant fibrous histiocytoma (MFH), also known as pleomorphic sarcomas. Common cytogenetic findings in these sarcomas are listed in Table 4–4 and some are discussed in more detail below.

How do these sarcomas accumulate these complex karyotypic changes? The process is not simply age-related since some sarcomas in this group are pediatric (e.g., osteosarcoma). Two possible pathways of karyotypic complexity have been suggested by mouse models. Both have been associated with abrogation of p53 checkpoint function. In the first, progressive telomere erosion resulted

TABLE 4–4	COMMON CHROMOSOME CHANGES IN BENIGN AND MALIGNANT SOFT TISSUE TUMORS (OTHER THAN RECURRENT TRANSLOCATIONS)	
Soft tissue tumor	**Cytogenetic finding**	**Molecular event**
Atypical lipomatous tumor (atypical lipoma/ well-diff. liposarcoma)	+ring/long marker (amp12q15)	*MDM2, HMGA2*, and *CDK4* amplification
Desmoid type fibromatosis	Trisomy 8 and 20	?
	Deletion of 5q	*APC* loss
Epithelioid sarcoma, proximal type	t/del (22)(q11.2)	*INI1* loss
Gastrointestinal stromal tumor	Monosomy 14 and 22	?
	Deletion of 1p	?
Mesothelioma	Deletion 9p	*CDKN2A* loss
	Deletion 22q	*NF2* loss
Neuroblastoma	Hyperdiploidy, diploidy, near-diploidy, near-tetraploidy	?
	Deletion 1p36	?
	Deletion 11q23	?
	dmin, HSR	*NMYC* amplification
Perineurioma	Deletion 22q	*NF2* loss
Rhabdoid tumor (extrarenal)	t/del (22)(q11.2)	*INI1* loss
Spindle cell/pleomorphic lipoma	Deletion 13q or 16q	?
Schwannoma	Deletion of 22q	*NF2* loss

dmin, double minute chromosomes; HSR, homogeneously staining regions.

in associations between heterologous telomeres leading to chromosomal fusion-bridge-breakage cycles and non-reciprocal translocations,[241] as observed in some human sarcomas.[242,243] The unbalanced karyotype is then stabilized by the reactivation of telomerase or by the mechanism of alternative lengthening of telomeres, also described in human sarcomas.[244] In a second murine model of karyotypic complexity, impaired joining of nonhomologous ends promotes chromosomal translocations, amplifications, and deletions, due to an increase in unrepaired double-strand breaks. This mechanism has led to formation of soft tissue sarcomas in mice of the same histologic types as human sarcomas lacking specific translocations.[245]

Inactivation of the p53 pathway appears to be a key differentiating factor between sarcomas with simple genetic alterations and those with karyotypic complexity (Table 4–3). Among sarcomas with complex unbalanced karyotypes, p53 pathway alterations may be more prevalent but often have a weaker prognostic value than in translocation sarcomas, often requiring large numbers of patients to achieve statistical significance.[246,247] This may suggest that, in sarcomas with non-specific genetic alterations, p53 pathway inactivation may be a common early event, needed to overcome checkpoints triggered by senescence, telomere erosion, or double-strand breaks in the progression of these sarcomas. Its more widespread role in this class of sarcomas may account for its limited ability to define distinct clinical subsets in these tumors.

1. High-grade pleomorphic sarcomas

High-grade pleomorphic sarcomas, including many tumors formerly called MFH, generally have complex and nondistinctive karyotypes.[248] The only exception to this rule is dedifferentiated liposarcoma which, in addition to complex aberrations, retains the characteristic rings or giant markers derived from chromosome 12q, as seen in well-differentiated liposarcoma (see below).

2. Atypical lipomatous tumor/well-differentiated liposarcoma/dedifferentiated liposarcoma

Virtually all cases of atypical lipomatous tumor/well-differentiated liposarcoma (ALT/WDL) share the same cytogenetic features, namely supernumerary (extra) ring and/or giant marker chromosome(s) (Fig. 4–5). Such ring and/or giant marker chromosomes generally represent the sole chromosome abnormality in ALT/WDL coexist with a few other numerical/structural abnormalities and non-random telomeric associations. The tumor cells contain either a ring or a giant marker chromosome which can vary in size among the tumor cells in a given case because they are unstable during cell division.[249]

At the molecular level, these consist predominantly of amplicons involving the q13-q15 region of chromosome

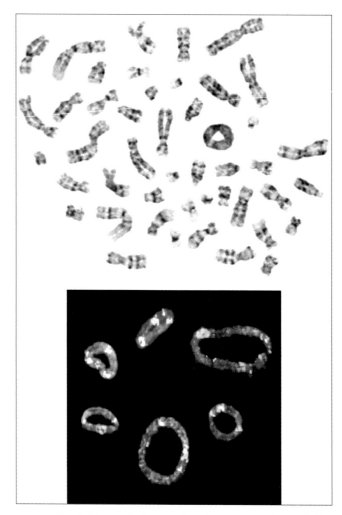

FIGURE 4–5 Ring and giant marker chromosomes in atypical lipoma (AL)/well-differentiated liposarcoma (WDLPS). Top panel shows Giemsa-stained metaphase chromosomes. Bottom panel shows ring chromosomes analyzed by spectral karyotyping (COBRA-FISH).

12. This region overlaps with the 12q14-15 region that is rearranged in a large number of lipomas and that contains numerous putative and established oncogenes. These include *MDM2*, *CDK4*, *HMGA2*, *GLI*, and *CHOP* among others. The potential roles of *MDM2*, *CDK4*, and *HMGA2* have been examined most extensively. However, the structure of these amplicons is complex and other genes may well also be significant. Similar rings and giant marker chromosomes are also seen in dedifferentiated liposarcoma, though a more complex karyotype is frequently observed. A recent study suggests that 1p32 amplification including the *JUN* gene may account for the impaired adipocytic differentiation in dedicated liposarcomas.[294a]

3. Neuroblastoma

Neuroblastoma is a genetically heterogeneous pediatric tumor with a remarkably variable clinical behavior.[250,251]

It has been a prototype for the use of genetic studies in guiding therapy selection. Low-risk disease is genetically characterized in most cases by a characteristic near-triploid karyotype (e.g., +7, +17, −3, −4, −11) and is mainly observed in children younger than 1 year. In contrast, high-risk, aggressive neuroblastomas tend to be diploid or tetraploid, but not triploid. Two high-risk groups have been defined by genetic data, both showing 17q gain in most cases. The first high-risk group shows *MYCN* amplification often accompanied by 1p36 deletion. The second high-risk group typically shows 11q deletion often accompanied by 3p deletion, without *MYCN* amplification or 1p deletion.[250,252] These groupings are not absolute and many of these genetic alterations have prognostic impacts that are independent of each other. For instance, 1p36 loss is associated with decreased progression-free survival even in the rare *MYCN* single copy cases in which it is detected.[253]

Because neuroblastoma cells generally fail to divide in culture, metaphases for conventional karyotyping are unavailable and, therefore, FISH is an essential adjunct method to detect *MYCN* amplification, 1p deletion, 11q23 deletion, 17q and ploidy status. Although a powerful *prognostic* marker, *MYCN* amplification is a moderately specific, relatively insensitive *diagnostic* marker for neuroblastoma. It is present in only about 22% of neuroblastomas, including about 30% of advanced-stage tumors. It has also been found occasionally in other sarcomas, especially in alveolar rhabdomyosarcoma, where it may also have a prognostic impact.[254] *MYCN* amplification is an early and stable event in neuroblastoma; it is present at diagnosis, stable over the course of the disease, and concordant at different sites.[255] Because it is prognostically significant and cannot be reliably predicted from histologic features, it remains an essential molecular marker in the management of neuroblastoma.

4. Leiomyosarcoma

Marked aneuploidy with complex chromosomal rearrangements is the karyotypic feature of the majority of soft tissue leiomyosarcomas (LMS), as well as those arising in of the uterus. No specific or recurrent change has been found in these tumors; however, some common gains or losses of genetic material have been detected by cytogenetic and CGH studies.[256] Among non-soft tissue LMS (mainly those of gastrointestinal and uterine origin), chromosome breaks at 1q21 are more frequent than those involving 1p13 or 10q22. While losses involving 1q and 3p are more frequent among soft tissue LMS, losses of chromosomes 14, 15, and 22q are more frequent in non-soft tissue LMS. These observations suggest that some aberrations may be more related to the site of origin than to the morphologic features of the tumors.[257]

5. Mesotheliomas

Though no specific chromosomal aberrations characterize malignant mesotheliomas, a number of recurrent abnormalities have been identified in karyotypes that are often extremely complex. Loss of 1p, 3p, 6q, 9p, and 22q are most frequently identified, suggesting that tumor suppressor genes mapping to these loci may play a role in mesothelioma tumorigenesis. The tumor suppressor gene *CDKN2A*, mapped to 9p21, encodes p16 and p14ARF, and has been found to be deleted in most mesothelioma cases with and without cytogenetic evidence of 9p deletion. At the molecular level, about 75–80% of cases show loss of both copies of *CDKN2A* and this proportion is even higher in cases with sarcomatous elements.[258,259] *CDKN2A* deletion can also function as a diagnostic marker for mesothelioma.[260] The small subset of cases without *CDKN2A* deletion shows longer overall survival.[261] *NF2* is a second important tumor suppressor gene in mesotheliomas and this subset of cases shows partial deletion 22q or monosomy 22.[262] No consistent genetic differences have been described between pleural and peritoneal mesotheliomas.

CHROMOSOME CHANGES IN BENIGN MESENCHYMAL TUMORS

It is interesting that many benign soft tissue tumors harbor specific genetic alterations that are quite distinct from those seen in sarcomas. This observation yet again highlights how seldom mesenchymal tumors progress from pre-neoplastic to benign to malignant, compared to epithelial cancers. Table 4–4 lists the major cytogenetic findings in benign soft tissue tumors and they are discussed in more detail below. Recurrent translocations in benign soft tissue tumors are included in Table 4–1.

Lipomas are the most common mesenchymal lesion studied cytogenetically and contain a recurrent t(3;12)(q28;q14).[263] Clonal chromosome abnormalities have been found in approximately 70% of these tumors, and the most frequently involved region is 12q13-q15. While the t(3;12)(q27-28;q13-q15) is found most often, virtually all chromosomes, except the Y, have been reported as partners in rearrangements involving 12q13-q15. 12q13-q15 involvement has been described in several other benign tumors, including uterine leiomyoma, endometrial polyps, pulmonary chondroid hamartoma, fibroadenoma, aggressive angiomyxoma, adenoma of the salivary glands, and soft tissue chondroma.

HMGA2 (formerly *HMGIC*), which maps to 12q15 (actually, 12q14.3), encodes a member of the high-mobility group A, small, non-histone, chromatin-associated proteins, HMGA2. It is consistently rearranged in all the mesenchymal tumors described above.[264] Though the 12q break appears at the cytogenetic level to be homogeneous, molecular studies have determined that the precise breakpoints are fairly heterogeneous. A variety of *HMGA2* rearrangements, some with an associated novel fusion transcript, have been demonstrated in these mesenchymal tumors. Most 12q rearrangements involve the large (140 kb) third intron of *HMGA2* and delete the 3′ portion of the gene, which encodes the protein binding domains.

The partner genes in the majority of *HMGA2* fusion transcripts are uncharacterized, novel DNA sequences. Most chimeric transcripts result in the addition of only a few amino acids (i.e., 1–10) to *HMGA2* exon 3. Consequently, one mechanistic possibility is that truncation of HMGA2 protein, rather than fusion to ectopic sequences, is the primary pathogenetic event.[265] It has therefore been suggested that the AT hook domain, encoded by exons 1–3, is the minimal region of HMGA2 required for full transforming activity.[266] A few *HMGA2* fusion transcripts have been further characterized in lipoma, including *HMGA2-LPP, HMGA2-LHFP, HMGA2-CMKOR1 (RDC1), HMGA2-NFIB,* and *HMGA2-EBF.*[267] Some specific *HMGA2* fusion genes (e.g., *HMGA2-LPP, HMGA2-NFIB*) have been found in different benign tumors, suggesting that they can transform a variety of cell types or that they occur in a pluripotent cell type.

In contrast to intragenic breaks, some benign tumors with 12q13-15 rearrangements show *HMGA2* breakpoints that fall outside the coding region, suggesting that disruption of regulatory sequences may lead to abnormal *HMGA2* expression. This has been demonstrated in uterine leiomyoma with t(12;14)(q15;q24),[268] and in aggressive angiomyxoma with a t(11;12)(q23;q15).[269]

A second group of lipomas are characterized by 6p21 rearrangement, to which another member of the HMG family, *HMGA1* (formerly *HMGIY*), maps. The majority of *HMGA1* breakpoints are located downstream of the coding region. It has been suggested that the dysregulation of *HMGA1* expression is mediated by replacement of negative regulatory sequences by enhancers from different translocation partners.[270] *HMGA1* rearrangements are also common in other benign tumors, including endometrial polyps and pulmonary chondroid hamartoma. In contrast to the range of fusion products involving HMGA2, only a single chimeric HMGA1 protein has been fully characterized.[271]

Furthermore, other benign adipose tissue tumors also show specific chromosome rearrangements. The characteristic cytogenetic abnormality in lipoblastoma, for example, involves 8q11-q13, to which *PLAG1* maps. Two different fusion genes have been reported: *HAS-PLAG1* and *COL1A2-PLAG1.*[272] The molecular consequence of these fusions is an activation of *PLAG1* transcription due to promoter substitution, as has been described

in pleomorphic adenoma of the salivary gland with a t(3;8)(p21;q12).

Hibernoma is characterized by involvement of 11q13, affecting not only the derivative 11, but also the apparently normal homolog. Heterozygous and homozygous deletions have been detected that are not limited to the 11q13.1 region surrounding *MEN1* but extend to 11q13.5.[273]

A specific t(11;16)(q13;p12-13) has been described in chondroid lipoma; however, the break in 11q13 appears to be at least 1 megabase proximal to the region rearranged in hibernoma.[274] Finally, monosomy or partial loss of either, or both, chromosomes 13 and 16 represents the most frequent aberration in spindle cell lipoma and pleomorphic lipoma.[275]

GENETICS OF FAMILIAL SARCOMAS AND THEIR SPORADIC COUNTERPARTS

Numerous familial sarcoma syndromes have been described.[276] The genetic basis of many of these has been elucidated. Some are associated with a broad spectrum of soft tissue sarcomas. For example, Li-Fraumeni syndrome is associated with germline *P53* mutation in most cases. Bone and soft tissue sarcomas are one of the classical syndromic tumors in Li-Fraumeni syndrome, along with breast carcinoma, brain cancers, and adrenocortical carcinoma.[277,278] The reported histologies of the soft tissue sarcomas have been rhabdomyosarcoma (usually embryonal), malignant fibrous histiocytoma, fibrosarcoma, and leiomyosarcoma.[277] It should be noted that patients with sarcoma but without a significant personal or family history are unlikely to harbor germline *P53* mutations;[279–281] however recent data suggest that certain DNA sequence polymorphisms (normal variants) that affect p53 pathway function may be associated with early-onset sporadic sarcomas from the complex karyotype group.[282,283]

Other familial sarcoma syndromes are associated with very specific sarcomas and the understanding of their genetic predisposition also illuminates understanding of their sporadic counterparts. Familial GIST has been described above. Three syndromes are briefly discussed here and other notable genetic syndromes associated with sarcomas, either as a primary or a rare manifestation, are listed in Table 4–5.

Neurofibromatosis type 1 and malignant peripheral nerve sheath tumor

Neurofibromatosis type 1 (NF1) is caused by germline inactivating mutations in the *NF1* gene and is defined by a variety of tumors, with neurofibromas and malignant peripheral nerve sheath tumors (MPNST) being

TABLE 4–5 | **GERMLINE GENETIC SYNDROMES WITH SOFT TISSUE TUMORS AS A COMMON OR RARE MANIFESTATION**

Disorder (OMIM number[1])	Inheritance[2]	Locus	Gene	Soft tissue tumors[3]
Bannayan-Riley-Ruvalcaba syndrome (153480)	AD	10q23	PTEN	Lipomas, hemangiomas
Beckwith-Wiedemann syndrome (130650)	Sporadic/AD	11p15	multiple	Embryonal rhabdomyosarcomas, myxomas, fibromas, hamartomas
Blue rubber bleb nevus syndrome (112200)	AD	?	?	Cavernous hemangiomas
Carney complex,[4] type I (160980)	AD	17q23-24	PRKAR1AK	Myxomas
Carney complex,[4] type II (605244)	AD	2p16	?	Myxomas
Costello syndrome (218040)	Sporadic	11p15	HRAS	Rhabdomyosarcomas, neuroblastomas
Familial adenomatous polyposis (175100), familial infiltrative fibromatosis (135290)	AD	5q21	APC	Desmoid tumors
Familial GIST syndrome (606764)	AD	4q12 4q12	KIT PDGFRA	GISTs
Familial hyperlipidemias, familial hypercholesterolemias	Multiple	Multiple	Multiple	Xanthoma tuberosum, tendinous xanthoma
Familial paragangliomas:	AD			Paragangliomas
type 1 (168000)		11q23	SDHD	
type 2 (601650)		11q13	?	
type 3 (605373)		1q21	SDHC	
type 4 (115310)		1p36	SDHB	
Familial paraganglioma and GIST[4] (606864)		?	?	Paragangliomas, GIST
Li-Fraumeni syndrome (151623)	AD AD	17p13 22q11	TP53 CHEK2	Rhabdomyosarcomas, other sarcomas
Lipomas, familial multiple (151900)	AD	12q14	HMGA2	Lipomas
Maffucci syndrome (166000)	Sporadic	3p22	PTHR1	Hemangiomas, angiosarcomas
Multiple endocrine neoplasia 2A and 2B				
Myofibromatosis (228550)	AR	?	?	Myofibromas
Nevoid basal cell carcinoma syndrome (Gorlin's) (109400)	AD	9q31	PTCH	Fetal rhabdomyomas, embryonal rhabdomyosarcomas, leiomyomas, leiomyosarcomas
Neurofibromatosis type 1 (162200)	AD	17q11	NF1	Neurofibromas, malignant peripheral nerve sheath tumors, paragangliomas
Neurofibromatosis type 2 (101000)	AD	22q12	NF2	Schwannomas
Nijmegen breakage syndrome (251260)	AR	8q21	NBS1	Perianal rhabdomyosarcomas
PTEN hamartoma-tumor syndromes:	AD	10q23	PTEN	
Cowden syndrome (158350)				Cutaneous sclerotic fibromas
Proteus syndrome (176920)				Lipomas
Bannayan syndrome (153480)				Lipomas, hemangiomas
Retinoblastoma (180200)	AD	13q14	RB1	Rhabdomyosarcomas, leiomyosarcomas
Rhabdoid predisposition syndrome (601607)	AD	22q11	SMARCB1	Malignant rhabdoid tumors
Rubinstein-Taybi syndrome (180849)	AD	16p13	CREBBP	Rhabdomyosarcomas, neuroblastomas
Tuberous sclerosis (191100)				Lymphangioleiomyomatosis, cutaneous angiofibroma, subungual fibromas
Tuberous sclerosis, type 1	AD	9q34	TSC1	
Tuberous sclerosis, type 2	AD	16p13	TSC2	
Venous malformations with glomus cells (138000)	AD	1p21-22		Glomus tumors
Von Hippel-Lindau (193300)	AD	3p25	VHL	Ocular hemangioblastomas
Werner syndrome (277700)	AR	8p11-12	WRN	MFH, leiomyosarcomas, fibrosarcomas

[1] Online Mendelian Inheritance in Man database (www.ncbi.nlm.nih.gov/entrez/query.fcgi?db=OMIM)
[2] AD, autosomal dominant; AR, autosomal recessive; Sporadic indicates that syndrome occurs as a new germline mutation with little or no data on transmission.
[3] For syndromes not primarily associated with sarcomas, data on types of sarcomas should be considered tentative because of the lack of histopathologic detail of many reports.
[4] Not to be confused with Carney's triad (gastric stromal sarcoma, paraganglioma, pulmonary chondroma), which is not familial.

most relevant to this section. In neurofibromas arising in NF1 patients, a double-hit model for *NF1* involving inactivation of the remaining functional copy of the *NF1* gene is well established.[284] This scenario has also been supported by mouse models of NF1.[285] In sporadic neurofibromas, acquired genetic alterations inactivating both copies of *NF1* have been documented.[286] MPNST are also associated with bi-allelic inactivation of *NF1*,[287] but their development additionally requires additional mutations in *CDKN2A* or *P53*, both in familial and sporadic cases,[287–290] as well as in animal models.[285]

Familial adenomatous polyposis and desmoids

Familial adenomatous polyposis (FAP) is caused by mutations in the adenomatous polyposis coli (*APC*) gene. Some cases are associated with extracolonic tumors (Gardner's syndrome), most notably deep (desmoid-type) fibromatoses, and this is correlated with the location of the mutation in the *APC* gene, specifically with mutations that result in truncation of the protein after codon 1444.[291,292] Notably, deep fibromatoses may be the first diagnostic clue to FAP,[293] or they may in rare cases be associated with only mild colonic disease.[294] The APC protein is involved in the regulation of β-catenin signaling. In the absence of functional APC, β-catenin moves to the nucleus and this forms the basis for the nuclear immunostaining for β-catenin that has been shown to be helpful in the diagnosis of familial and sporadic desmoid-type fibromatoses.[63,64] In contrast to FAP-associated desmoids, most sporadic desmoids show activating mutations in the β-catenin gene (*CTNNB1*) instead of inactivation of APC.[295]

Familial rhabdoid predisposition syndrome and malignant extrarenal rhabdoid tumors

Inactivation of the *INI1* tumor suppressor gene (*SMARCB1*), which resides on the long arm of chromosome 22, is the molecular hallmark of extrarenal (and renal) rhabdoid tumors.[296,297] Among sarcomas, *INI1* loss is seen in all cases of extrarenal rhabdoid tumors and has recently also been reported in a subset of epithelioid sarcomas.[298,299] Other cancers with discrete rhabdoid components do not show *INI1* loss, even in areas of rhabdoid morphology.[300]

The *INI1* gene encodes a protein involved in chromatin remodeling that is thought to regulate the access of certain transcription factors to their target genes. Its inactivation is thought to promote neoplasia by altering gene expression secondary to its effect upon chromatin structure.[296] The inactivation occurs by loss of both copies or an inactivating mutation in one copy with loss of the other copy (through monosomy or mitotic recombination with loss of heterozygosity).[301,302] *INI1* loss may require FISH and/or molecular techniques for detection

but immunohistochemistry for loss of nuclear staining is emerging as an attractive alternative.[65] A familial "rhabdoid predisposition syndrome" encompassing renal and extrarenal rhabdoid tumors has been described in which affected family members carry one copy of *INI1* with an inactivating mutation and then lose the remaining functional copy, leading to rhabdoid tumor development.[303]

CONTRIBUTIONS OF MICROARRAY STUDIES TO SARCOMA DIAGNOSIS AND CLASSIFICATION

High-density microarrays are used to measure, in a comprehensive manner ("profile"), gene expression patterns (when tumor RNA is tested) or gene copy number changes (when tumor genomic DNA is tested). Microarray-based studies are increasingly useful in addressing a wide variety of questions in sarcoma biology.[304–306] Here, we confine the discussion to their application as a source of diagnostic markers for sarcoma diagnosis and their role in clarifying sarcoma classification. It is likely that in the coming decade gene expression profiling will make significant contributions to the diagnosis and classification of sarcomas, just as translocation analysis has provided in the past decade.

A general observation of microarray-based expression profiling studies of sarcomas is that translocation-associated sarcomas are robustly clustered by expression profiling using cDNA microarrays, whereas so-called complex karyotype sarcomas tend to be less tightly clustered.[234,306,307] This is perhaps not unexpected because, firstly, the aberrant transcriptional proteins encoded by most translocation-derived fusion genes act primarily through changes in gene expression. Secondly, genomic copy number changes are associated with changes in the expression of the corresponding genes.[308,309] Thus, complex karyotype sarcomas that often show different gains and losses from case to case are also likely to show more variability in gene expression patterns, leading to less robust unsupervised clustering of the expression profiles. Of course, this by itself does not mean that complex karyotype sarcomas are less discrete entities than translocation-associated sarcomas, but may merely indicate that unsupervised clustering of expression data may not be the best approach to delineating them. Indeed, this tumor group may be more fruitfully studied by profiling of gene copy number changes using array-based CGH.[308,310,311] For instance, a number of studies have used profiling of gene copy number changes to propose relationships of subsets of tumors designated as malignant fibrous histiocytoma to leiomyosarcomas or liposarcomas.[312,313] Ultimately, integrated profiling of gene expression and genomic copy number changes may be the most efficient approach to understanding the biology and genetic heterogeneity of complex karyotype sarcomas, as exemplified by recent efforts in neuroblastoma.[314]

Although expression microarrays presently have no direct clinical application in sarcoma diagnosis, some of the data and insights these studies have provided are already having a practical impact because they are identifying differentially expressed genes that can be evaluated as new sarcoma-specific immunohistochemical markers. For instance, TLE1, a nuclear protein that functions as a transcriptional repressor of Wnt/β-catenin signaling, is one of the most consistent synovial sarcoma-associated genes in multiple expression microarray studies and its application as a robust immunohistochemical marker for this sarcoma has recently been demonstrated.[315] Likewise, several studies have used microarrays to identify genes differentially expressed between ARMS and ERMS.[106,316,317] The gene encoding transcription factor AP2-β (*TFAP2B*) has consistently stood out for its ARMS-associated expression and transcription factor AP2-β has now been validated as a useful marker for its distinction from ERMS.[318] Other new immunohistochemical markers emerging from microarray studies include ApoD as a novel marker for DFSP, among others.[319,320]

ACKNOWLEDGEMENTS

We thank Julia Bridge, Fred Barr, and William Gerald for critical reading. The FISH image in Figure 4–5 was provided by David Gisselsson. We apologize to colleagues whose papers could not be cited due to space considerations.

REFERENCES

General concepts in cancer genetics

1. Hanahan D, Weinberg RA. The hallmarks of cancer. Cell 2000; 100:57.
2. Vogelstein B, Kinzler KW. Cancer genes and the pathways they control. Nat Med 2004; 10:789.
3. Futreal PA, Coin L, Marshall M, et al. A census of human cancer genes. Nat Rev Cancer 2004; 4:177.
4. Santarosa M, Ashworth A. Haploinsufficiency for tumour suppressor genes: when you don't need to go all the way. Biochim Biophys Acta 2004; 1654:105.
5. Goto M, Miller RW, Ishikawa Y, et al. Excess of rare cancers in Werner syndrome (adult progeria). Cancer Epidemiol Biomarkers Prev 1996; 5:239.

General principles of translocations

6. Ladanyi M, Bridge JA. Contribution of molecular genetic data to the classification of sarcomas. Hum Pathol 2000; 31:532.
7. Xia SJ, Barr FG. Chromosome translocations in sarcomas and the emergence of oncogenic transcription factors. Eur J Cancer 2005; 41:2513.
8. Antonescu CR. The role of genetic testing in soft tissue sarcoma. Histopathology 2006; 48:13.
9. Mastrangelo T, Modena P, Tornielli S, et al. A novel zinc finger gene is fused to EWS in small round cell tumor. Oncogene 2000; 19:3799.
10. Yamaguchi S, Yamazaki Y, Ishikawa Y, et al. EWSR1 is fused to POU5F1 in a bone tumor with translocation t(6;22)(p21;q12). Genes Chromosomes Cancer 2005; 43:217.
11. Kawamura-Saito M, Yamazaki Y, Kaneko K, et al. Fusion between CIC and DUX4 up-regulates PEA3 family genes in Ewing-like sarcomas with t(4;19)(q35;q13) translocation. Hum Mol Genet 2006; 15:2125.
12. Mertens F, Wiebe T, Adlercreutz C, et al. Successful treatment of a child with t(15;19)-positive tumor. Pediatr Blood Cancer 2006 (in press).
13. Wang L, Bhargava R, Roulston D, et al. Undifferentiated small round cell sarcomas with rare EWS gene fusions. Identification of a novel EWS-SP3 fusion and of additional cases with the *EWS-ETV1* and *EWS-FEV* fusions. J Mol Diagn 2007 (in press).
14. Zucman-Rossi J, Legoix P, Victor JM, et al. Chromosome translocation based on illegitimate recombination in human tumors. Proc Natl Acad Sci USA 1998; 95:11786.
15. Aplan PD. Causes of oncogenic chromosomal translocation. Trends Genet 2006; 22:46.
16. Novo FJ, Vizmanos JL. Chromosome translocations in cancer: computational evidence for the random generation of double-strand breaks. Trends Genet 2006; 22:193.
17. Kanoe H, Nakayama T, Hosaka T, et al. Characteristics of genomic breakpoints in TLS-CHOP translocations in liposarcomas suggest the involvement of Translin and topoisomerase II in the process of translocation. Oncogene 1999; 18:721.
18. Hosaka T, Kanoe H, Nakayama T, et al. Translin binds to the sequences adjacent to the breakpoints of the TLS and CHOP genes in liposarcomas with translocation t(12;16). Oncogene 2000; 19:5821.
19. Chuang CH, Belmont AS. Close encounters between active genes in the nucleus. Genome Biol 2005; 6:237.
20. Roix JJ, McQueen PG, Munson PJ, et al. Spatial proximity of translocation-prone gene loci in human lymphomas. Nat Genet 2003; 34:287.
21. Nikiforova MN, Stringer JR, Blough R, et al. Proximity of chromosomal loci that participate in radiation-induced rearrangements in human cells. Science 2000; 290:138.
22. van de Rijn M, Barr FG, Xiong QB, et al. Radiation-associated synovial sarcoma. Hum Pathol 1997; 28:1325.
23. Egger JF, Coindre JM, Benhattar J, et al. Radiation-associated synovial sarcoma: clinicopathologic and molecular analysis of two cases. Mod Pathol 2002; 15:998.
24. Mugneret F, Lizard S, Aurias A, et al. Chromosomes in Ewing's sarcoma. ii. Nonrandom additional changes, trisomy 8 and der (16)t(1;16). Cancer Genet Cytogenet 1988; 32:239.
25. Hattinger CM, Rumpler S, Ambros IM, et al. Demonstration of the translocation der(16)t(1;16)(q12;q11.2) in interphase nuclei of Ewing tumors. Genes Chromosomes Cancer 1996; 17:141.
26. McManus AP, Min T, Swansbury GJ, et al. Der(16)t(1;16)(q21;q13) as a secondary change in alveolar rhabdomyosarcoma. A case report and review of the literature. Cancer Genet Cytogenet 1996; 87:179.
27. Day SJ, Nelson M, Rosenthal H, et al. Der(16)t(1;16)(q21;q13) as a secondary structural aberration in yet a third sarcoma, extraskeletal myxoid chondrosarcoma. Genes Chromosomes Cancer 1997; 20:425.
28. Mrozek K, Bloomfield CD. Der(16)t(1;16) is a secondary chromosome aberration in at least eighteen different types of human cancer. Genes Chromosomes Cancer 1998; 23:78.

Diagnostic methods

29. ISCN (2005). An international system for human cytogenetic nomenclature. Basel: Karger; 2005.
30. Limon J, Dal Cin P, Sandberg AA. Application of long-term collagenase disaggregation for the cytogenetic analysis of human solid tumors. Cancer Genet Cytogenet 1986; 23:305.
31. Ried T. Cytogenetics – in color and digitized. N Engl J Med 2004; 350:1597.
32. Bhargava R, Friedman O, Gerald WL, et al. Identification of MYCN gene amplification in neuroblastoma using chromogenic in situ hybridization (CISH): an alternative and practical method. Diag Mol Pathol 2005; 14:72.
33. Bhargava R, Lal P, Chen B. Chromogenic in situ hybridization for the detection of HER-2/neu gene amplification in breast cancer with an emphasis on tumors with borderline and low-level amplification: does it measure up to fluorescence in situ hybridization? Am J Clin Pathol 2005; 123:237.
34. Kuchinka BD, Kalousek DK, Lomax BL, et al. Interphase cytogenetic analysis of single cell suspensions prepared from previously formalin-fixed and paraffin-embedded tissues. Mod Pathol 1995; 8:183.
35. Speicher MR, Carter NP. The new cytogenetics: blurring the boundaries with molecular biology. Nat Rev Genet 2005; 6:782.
36. Kallioniemi A, Kallioniemi OP, Sudar D, et al. Comparative genomic hybridization for molecular cytogenetic analysis of solid tumors. Science 1992; 258:818.

37. Pinkel D, Albertson DG. Comparative genomic hybridization. Annu Rev Genomics Hum Genet 2005; 6:331.

38. Fletcher CDM, Fletcher JA, Dal Cin P, et al. Diagnostic gold standard for soft tissue tumours: morphology or molecular genetics? (letter). Histopathology 2001; 39:100.

39. Hostein I, Menard A, Bui BN, et al. Molecular detection of the synovial sarcoma translocation t(X;18) by real-time polymerase chain reaction in paraffin-embedded material. Diagn Mol Pathol 2002; 11:16.

40. Coindre JM, Hostein I, Terrier P, et al. Diagnosis of clear cell sarcoma by real-time reverse transcriptase-polymerase chain reaction analysis of paraffin embedded tissues: clinicopathologic and molecular analysis of 44 patients from the French Sarcoma Group. Cancer 2006; 107:1055.

41. Friedrichs N, Kriegl L, Poremba C, et al. Pitfalls in the detection of t(11;22) translocation by fluorescence in situ hybridization and RT-PCR. A single-blinded study. Diag Mol Pathol 2006; 15:83.

42. Qian X, Jin L, Shearer BM, et al. Molecular diagnosis of Ewing's sarcoma/primitive neuroectodermal tumor in formalin-fixed paraffin-embedded tissues by RT-PCR and fluorescence in situ hybridization. Diagn Mol Pathol 2005; 14:23.

43. Bridge RS, Rajaram V, Dehner LP, et al. Molecular diagnosis of Ewing sarcoma/primitive neuroectodermal tumor in routinely processed tissue: a comparison of two FISH strategies and RT-PCR in malignant round cell tumors. Mod Pathol 2006; 19:1.

44. Nishio J, Althof PA, Bailey JM, et al. Use of a novel FISH assay on paraffin-embedded tissues as an adjunct to diagnosis of alveolar rhabdomyosarcoma. Lab Invest 2006; 86:547.

45. Coindre JM, Pelmus M, Hostein I, et al. Should molecular testing be required for diagnosing synovial sarcoma? A prospective study of 204 cases. Cancer 2003; 98:2700.

46. Folpe AL, Goldblum JR, Rubin BP, et al. Morphologic and immunophenotypic diversity in Ewing family tumors: a study of 66 genetically confirmed cases. Am J Surg Pathol 2005; 29:1025.

47. Falini B, Mason DY. Proteins encoded by genes involved in chromosomal alterations in lymphoma and leukemia: clinical value of their detection by immunocytochemistry. Blood 2002; 99:409.

48. Gerald WL, Ladanyi M, de Alava E, et al. Clinical, pathologic, and molecular spectrum of tumors associated with t(11;22)(p13;q12): desmoplastic small round-cell tumor and its variants. J Clin Oncol 1998; 16:3028.

49. Barnoud R, Sabourin JC, Pasquier D, et al. Immunohistochemical expression of WT1 by desmoplastic small round cell tumor: a comparative study with other small round cell tumors. Am J Surg Pathol 2000; 24:830.

50. Argani P, Lal P, Hutchinson B, et al. Aberrant nuclear immunoreactivity for TFE3 in neoplasms with TFE3 gene fusions. A sensitive and specific immunohistochemical assay. Am J Surg Pathol 2003; 23:750.

51. Folpe AL, Hill CE, Parham DM, et al. Immunohistochemical detection of FLI-1 protein expression: a study of 132 round cell tumors with emphasis on CD99-positive mimics of Ewing's sarcoma/primitive neuroectodermal tumor. Am J Surg Pathol 2000; 24:1657.

52. Llombart-Bosch A, Navarro S. Immunohistochemical detection of EWS and FLI-1 proteins in Ewing sarcoma and primitive neuroectodermal tumors: comparative analysis with CD99 (MIC-2) expression. Appl Immunohistochem Mol Morphol 2001; 9:255.

53. Mhawech-Fauceglia P, Herrmann F, Bshara W, et al. FLI-1 expression in 4323 malignant and benign tumours: a multiple tumour tissue microarray analysis using polyclonal antibody. J Clin Pathol 2006; Epub ahead of print.

54. Coffin CM, Patel A, Perkins S, et al. ALK1 and p80 expression and chromosomal rearrangements involving 2p23 in inflammatory myofibroblastic tumor. Mod Pathol 2001; 14:569.

55. Cook JR, Dehner LP, Collins MH, et al. Anaplastic lymphoma kinase (ALK) expression in the inflammatory myofibroblastic tumor: a comparative immunohistochemical study. Am J Surg Pathol 2001; 25:1364.

56. Li XQ, Hisaoka M, Shi DR, et al. Expression of anaplastic lymphoma kinase in soft tissue tumors: an immunohistochemical and molecular study of 249 cases. Hum Pathol 2004; 35:711.

57. Oikawa K, Ishida T, Imamura T, et al. Generation of the novel monoclonal antibody against TLS/EWS-CHOP chimeric oncoproteins that is applicable to one of the most sensitive assays for myxoid and round cell liposarcomas. Am J Surg Pathol 2006; 30:351.

58. Corless CL, Fletcher JA, Heinrich MC. Biology of gastrointestinal stromal tumors. J Clin Oncol 2004; 22:3813.

59. Dei Tos AP, Doglioni C, Piccinin S, et al. Coordinated expression and amplification of the MDM2, CDK4, and HMGI-C genes in atypical lipomatous tumours. J Pathol 2000; 190:531.

60. Hostein I, Pelmus M, Aurias A, et al. Evaluation of MDM2 and CDK4 amplification by real-time PCR on paraffin wax-embedded material: a potential tool for the diagnosis of atypical lipomatous tumours/well-differentiated liposarcomas. J Pathol 2004; 202:95.

61. Binh MB, Sastre-Garau X, Guillou L, et al. MDM2 and CDK4 immunostainings are useful adjuncts in diagnosing well-differentiated and dedifferentiated liposarcoma subtypes: a comparative analysis of 559 soft tissue neoplasms with genetic data. Am J Surg Pathol 2005; 29:1340.

62. Binh MB, Garau XS, Guillou L, et al. Reproducibility of MDM2 and CDK4 staining in soft tissue tumors. Am J Clin Pathol 2006; 125:693.

63. Ng TL, Gown AM, Barry TS, et al. Nuclear beta-catenin in mesenchymal tumors. Mod Pathol 2005; 18:68.

64. Bhattacharya B, Dilworth HP, Iacobuzio-Donahue C, et al. Nuclear beta-catenin expression distinguishes deep fibromatosis from other benign and malignant fibroblastic and myofibroblastic lesions. Am J Surg Pathol 2005; 29:653.

65. Hoot AC, Russo P, Judkins AR, et al. Immunohistochemical analysis of hSNF5/INI1 distinguishes renal and extra-renal malignant rhabdoid tumors from other pediatric soft tissue tumors. Am J Surg Pathol 2004; 28:1485.

66. Thomas GV, Horvath S, Smith BL, et al. Antibody-based profiling of the phosphoinositide 3-kinase pathway in clinical prostate cancer. Clin Cancer Res 2004; 10:8351.

67. Kawaguchi K, Oda Y, Saito T, et al. Genetic and epigenetic alterations of the PTEN gene in soft tissue sarcomas. Hum Pathol 2005; 36:357.

68. Hustinx SR, Leoni LM, Yeo CJ, et al. Concordant loss of MTAP and p16/CDKN2A expression in pancreatic intraepithelial neoplasia: evidence of homozygous deletion in a noninvasive precursor lesion. Mod Pathol 2005; 18:959.

69. Oda Y, Yamamoto H, Takahira T, et al. Frequent alteration of p16(INK4a)/p14(ARF) and p53 pathways in the round cell component of myxoid/round cell liposarcoma: p53 gene alterations and reduced p14(ARF) expression both correlate with poor prognosis. J Pathol 2005; 207:410.

70. Hall PA, McCluggage WG. Assessing p53 in clinical contexts: unlearned lessons and new perspectives. J Pathol 2006; 208:1.

Major pathogenetic classes of sarcomas

71. Borden EC, Baker LH, Bell RS, et al. Soft tissue sarcomas of adults: state of the translational science. Clin Cancer Res 2003; 9:1941.

72. Helman LJ, Meltzer P. Mechanisms of sarcoma development. Nat Rev Cancer 2003; 3:685.

73. Huang HY, Illei PB, Zhao Z, et al. Ewing sarcomas with p53 mutations or p16/p14ARF homozygous deletions: a highly aggressive subset associated with poor chemoresponse. J Clin Oncol 2005; 23:548.

74. Antonescu CR, Tschernyavsky SJ, Decuseara R, et al. Prognostic impact of P53 status, TLS-CHOP fusion transcript structure, and histological grade in myxoid liposarcoma: a molecular and clinicopathologic study of 82 cases. Clin Cancer Res 2001; 7:3977.

75. Wurl P, Taubert H, Meye A, et al. Prognostic value of immunohistochemistry for p53 in primary soft-tissue sarcomas: a multivariate analysis of five antibodies. J Cancer Res Clin Oncol 1997; 123:502.

76. Ulaner GA, Hoffman AR, Otero J, et al. Divergent patterns of telomere maintenance mechanisms among human sarcomas: sharply contrasting prevalence of the alternative lengthening of telomeres mechanism in Ewing's sarcomas and osteosarcomas. Genes Chromosomes Cancer 2004; 41:155.

77. Montgomery E, Argani P, Hicks JL, et al. Telomere lengths of translocation-associated and nontranslocation-associated sarcomas differ dramatically. Am J Pathol 2004; 164:1523.

78. Henson JD, Hannay JA, McCarthy SW, et al. A robust assay for alternative lengthening of telomeres in tumors shows the significance of alternative lengthening of telomeres in sarcomas and astrocytomas. Clin Cancer Res 2005; 11:217.

79. Barr FG. Gene fusions involving PAX and FOX family members in alveolar rhabdomyosarcoma. Oncogene 2001; 20:5736.

80. Barr FG. Translocations, cancer and the puzzle of specificity. Nat Genet 1998; 19:121.

81. Perez-Losada J, Pintado B, Gutierrez-Adan A, et al. The chimeric FUS/TLS-CHOP fusion protein specifically induces liposarcomas in transgenic mice. Oncogene 2000; 19:2413.

82. Keller C, Arenkiel BR, Coffin CM, et al. Alveolar rhabdomyosarcomas in conditional Pax3:Fkhr mice: cooperativity of Ink4a/ARF and Trp53 loss of function. Genes Dev 2004; 18:2614.

83. Rorie CJ, Thomas VD, Chen P, et al. The Ews/Fli-1 fusion gene switches the differentiation program of neuroblastomas to Ewing sarcoma/peripheral primitive neuroectodermal tumors. Cancer Res 2004; 64:1266.

84. Hu-Lieskovan S, Zhang J, Wu L, et al. EWS-FLI1 fusion protein up-regulates critical genes in neural crest development and is responsible for the observed phenotype of Ewing's family of tumors. Cancer Res 2005; 65:4633.

85. Riggi N, Cironi L, Provero P, et al. Development of Ewing's sarcoma from primary bone marrow-derived mesenchymal progenitor cells. Cancer Res 2005; 65:11459.

86. Castillero-Trejo Y, Eliazer S, Xiang L, et al. Expression of the EWS/FLI-1 oncogene in murine primary bone-derived cells results in EWS/FLI-1-dependent, Ewing sarcoma-like tumors. Cancer Res 2005; 65:8698.

87. Riggi N, Cironi L, Provero P, et al. Expression of the FUS-CHOP fusion protein in primary mesenchymal progenitor cells gives rise to a model of myxoid liposarcoma. Cancer Res 2006; 66:7016.

87a. Tirode F, Laud-Duval K, Prieur A, et al. Mesenchymal stem cell features of Ewing tumors. Cancer Cell 2007; 11:421.

88. Zucman J, Melot T, Desmaze C, et al. Combinatorial generation of variable fusion proteins in the Ewing family of tumours. EMBO J 1993; 12:4481.

89. Sorensen PHB, Lessnick SL, Lopez-Terrada D, et al. A second Ewing's sarcoma translocation, t(21;22), fuses the EWS gene to another ETS-family transcription factor, ERG. Nature Genet 1994; 6:146.

90. Shing DC, McMullan DJ, Roberts P, et al. FUS/ERG gene fusions in Ewing's tumors. Cancer Res 2003; 63:4568.

91. Arvand A, Denny CT. Biology of EWS/ETS fusions in Ewing's family tumors. Oncogene 2001; 20:5747.

92. Ladanyi M. EWS-FLI1 and Ewing's sarcoma: recent molecular data and new insights. Cancer Biol Ther 2002; 1:330.

93. Sharrocks AD. The ETS-domain transcription factor family. Nat Rev Mol Cell Biol 2001; 2:827.

94. Aman P, Panagopoulos I, Lassen C, et al. Expression patterns of the human sarcoma-associated genes FUS and EWS and the genomic structure of FUS. Genomics 1996; 37:1.

95. Plougastel B, Zucman J, Peter M, et al. Genomic structure of the EWS gene and its relationship to EWSR1, a site of tumor-associated chromosome translocation. Genomics 1993; 18:609.

96. Truong AH, Ben David Y. The role of Fli-1 in normal cell function and malignant transformation. Oncogene 2000; 19:6482.

97. Zoubek A, Dockhorn-Dworniczak B, Delattre O, et al. Does expression of different EWS chimeric transcripts define clinically distinct risk groups of Ewing tumor patients? J Clin Oncol 1996; 14:1245.

98. de Alava E, Kawai A, Healey JH, et al. EWS-FLI1 fusion transcript structure is an independent determinant of prognosis in Ewing's sarcoma. J Clin Oncol 1998; 16:1248.

99. Aryee DN, Sommergruber W, Muehlbacher K, et al. Variability in gene expression patterns of Ewing tumor cell lines differing in EWS-FLI1 fusion type. Lab Invest 2000; 80:1833.

100. Ginsberg JP, de Alava E, Ladanyi M, et al. EWS-FLI1 and EWS-ERG gene fusions are associated with similar clinical phenotypes in Ewing's sarcoma. J Clin Oncol 1999; 17:1809.

101. Kovar H, Jug G, Aryee DNT, et al. Among genes involved in the RB dependent cell cycle regulatory cascade, the p16 tumor suppressor gene is frequently lost in the Ewing family of tumors. Oncogene 1997; 15:2225.

102. Galili N, Davis RJ, Fredericks WJ, et al. Fusion of a fork head domain gene to PAX3 in the solid tumour alveolar rhabdomyosarcoma. Nat Genet 1993; 5:230.

103. Davis RJ, D'Cruz CM, Lovell MA, et al. Fusion of PAX7 to FKHR by the variant t(1;13)(p36;q14) translocation in alveolar rhabdomyosarcoma. Cancer Res 1994; 54:2869.

104. Barr FG, Qualman SJ, Macris MH, et al. Genetic heterogeneity in the alveolar rhabdomyosarcoma subset without typical gene fusions. Cancer Res 2002; 62:4704.

105. Sorensen PH, Lynch JC, Qualman SJ, et al. PAX3-FKHR and PAX7-FKHR gene fusions are prognostic indicators in alveolar rhabdomyosarcoma: a report from the Children's Oncology Group. J Clin Oncol 2002; 20:2672.

106. Wachtel M, Dettling M, Koscielniak E, et al. Gene expression signatures identify rhabdomyosarcoma subtypes and detect a novel t(2;2)(q35;p23) translocation fusing PAX3 to NCOA1. Cancer Res 2004; 64:5539.

107. Kelly KM, Womer RB, Sorensen PHB, et al. Common and variant gene fusions predict distinct clinical phenotypes in rhabdomyosarcoma. J Clin Oncol 1997; 15:1831.

108. Anderson J, Gordon T, McManus A, et al. Detection of the PAX3-FKHR fusion gene in paediatric rhabdomyosarcoma: a reproducible predictor of outcome? Br J Cancer 2001; 85:831.

109. Barr FG, Nauta LE, Davis RJ, et al. In vivo amplification of the PAX3-FKHR and PAX7-FKHR fusion genes in alveolar rhabdomyosarcoma. Hum Mol Genet 1996; 5:15.

110. Weber-Hall S, McManus A, Anderson J, et al. Novel formation and amplification of the PAX7-FKHR fusion gene in a case of alveolar rhabdomyosarcoma. Genes Chromosomes Cancer 1996; 17:7.

111. Bridge JA, Liu J, Qualman SJ, et al. Genomic gains and losses are similar in genetic and histologic subsets of rhabdomyosarcoma, whereas amplification predominates in embryonal with anaplasia and alveolar subtypes. Genes Chromosomes Cancer 2002; 33:310.

112. Ladanyi M, Gerald W. Fusion of the EWS and WT1 genes in the desmoplastic small round cell tumor. Cancer Res 1994; 54:2837.

113. Gerald WL, Rosai J, Ladanyi M. Characterization of the genomic breakpoint and chimeric transcripts in the EWS-WT1 gene fusion of desmoplastic small round cell tumor. Proc Natl Acad Sci USA 1995; 92:1028.

114. Gerald WL, Haber DA. The EWS-WT1 gene fusion in desmoplastic small round cell tumor. Semin Cancer Biol 2005; 15:197.

115. Antonescu CR, Gerald WL, Magid MS, et al. Molecular variants of the EWS-WT1 gene fusion in desmoplastic small round cell tumor. Diagn Mol Pathol 1998; 7:24.

116. Zucman J, Delattre O, Desmaze C, et al. EWS and ATF-1 gene fusion induced by t(12;22) translocation in malignant melanoma of soft parts. Nat Genet 1993; 4:341.

117. Antonescu CR, Tschernyavsky SJ, Woodruff JM, et al. Molecular diagnosis of clear cell sarcoma: detection of EWS-ATF1 and MITF-M transcripts and histopathological and ultrastructural analysis of 12 cases. J Mol Diagn 2002; 4:44.

118. Panagopoulos I, Mertens F, Dbiec-Rychter M, et al. Molecular genetic characterization of the EWS/ATF1 fusion gene in clear cell sarcoma of tendons and aponeuroses. Int J Cancer 2002; 99:560.

119. Antonescu CR, Nafa K, Segal NH, et al. EWS-CREB1: a recurrent variant fusion in clear cell sarcoma. Association with gastrointestinal location and absence of melanocytic differentiation. Clin Cancer Res 2006; 12:5356.

120. Segal NH, Pavlidis P, Noble WS, et al. Classification of clear-cell sarcoma as a subtype of melanoma by genomic profiling. J Clin Oncol 2003; 21:1775.

121. Panagopoulos I, Mertens F, Isaksson M, et al. Absence of mutations of the BRAF gene in malignant melanoma of soft parts (clear cell sarcoma of tendons and aponeuroses). Cancer Genet Cytogenet 2005; 156:74.

122. Langezaal SM, Graadt van Roggen JF, Cleton-Jansen AM, et al. Malignant melanoma is genetically distinct from clear cell sarcoma of tendons and aponeurosis (malignant melanoma of soft parts). Br J Cancer 2001; 84:535.

123. Patel RM, Downs-Kelly E, Weiss SW, et al. Dual-color, break-apart fluorescence in situ hybridization for EWS gene rearrangement distinguishes clear cell sarcoma of soft tissue from malignant melanoma. Mod Pathol 2005; 18:1585.

124. Sreekantaiah C, Karakousis CP, Leong SP, et al. Cytogenetic findings in liposarcoma correlate with histopathologic subtypes. Cancer 1992; 69:2484.

125. Aman P, Ron D, Mandahl N, et al. Rearrangement of the transcription factor gene CHOP in myxoid liposarcomas with t(12;16)(q13;p11). Genes Chromosomes Cancer 1992; 5:278.

126. Crozat A, Aman P, Mandahl N, et al. Fusion of CHOP to a novel RNA-binding protein in human myxoid liposarcoma. Nature 1993; 363:640.

127. Rabbitts TH, Forster A, Larson R, et al. Fusion of the dominant negative transcription regulator CHOP with a novel gene FUS by translocation t(12;16) in malignant liposarcoma. Nat Genet 1993; 4:175.

128. Panagopoulos I, Hoglund M, Mertens F, et al. Fusion of the EWS and CHOP genes in myxoid liposarcoma. Oncogene 1996; 12:489.

129. Panagopoulos I, Mandahl N, Ron D, et al. Characterization of the CHOP breakpoints and fusion transcripts in myxoid liposarcomas with the 12;16 translocation. Cancer Res 1994; 54:6500.

130. Knight JC, Renwick PJ, Dal Cin P, et al. Translocation t(12;16)(q13;p11) in myxoid liposarcoma and round cell liposarcoma: molecular and cytogenetic analysis. Cancer Res 1995; 55:24.

131. Antonescu CR, Elahi A, Healey JH, et al. Monoclonality of multifocal myxoid liposarcoma. Confirmation by analysis of TLS-CHOP or EWS-CHOP rearrangements. Clin Cancer Res 2000; 6:2788.

132. Antonescu CR, Elahi A, Humphrey M, et al. Specificity of TLS-CHOP rearrangement for classic myxoid/round cell liposarcoma. Absence in predominantly myxoid well-differentiated liposarcomas. J Mol Diagnostics 2000; 2:132.

133. Labelle Y, Zucman J, Stenman G, et al. Oncogenic conversion of a novel orphan nuclear receptor by chromosome translocation. Hum Mol Genet 1995; 4:2219.

134. Clark J, Benjamin H, Gill S, et al. Fusion of EWS gene to CHN, a member of the steroid/thyroid receptor gene superfamily, in a human myxoid chondrosarcoma. Oncogene 1996; 12:229.

135. Brody RI, Ueda T, Hamelin A, et al. Molecular analysis of the fusion of EWS to an orphan nuclear receptor gene in extraskeletal myxoid chondrosarcoma. Am J Pathol 1997; 150:1049.

136. Panagopoulos I, Mertens F, Isaksson M, et al. Molecular genetic characterization of the EWS/CHN and RBP56/CHN fusion genes in extraskeletal myxoid chondrosarcoma. Genes Chromosomes Cancer 2002; 35:340.

137. Panagopoulos I, Mencinger M, Dietrich CU, et al. Fusion of the RBP56 and CHN genes in extraskeletal myxoid chondrosarcomas with translocation t(9;17)(q22;q11). Oncogene 1999; 18:7594.

138. Attwooll C, Tariq M, Harris M, et al. Identification of a novel fusion gene involving hTAF$_{II}$68 and CHN from a t(9;17)(q22;q11.2) translocation in an extraskeletal myxoid chondrosarcoma. Oncogene 1999; 18:7599.

139. Sjogren H, Wedell B, Meis-Kindblom JM, et al. Fusion of the NH2-terminal domain of the basic helix-loop-helix protein TCF12 to TEC in extraskeletal myxoid chondrosarcoma with translocation t(9;15)(q22;q21). Cancer Res 2000; 60:6832.

140. Hisaoka M, Ishida T, Imamura T, et al. TFG is a novel fusion partner of NOR1 in extraskeletal myxoid chondrosarcoma. Genes Chromosomes Cancer 2004; 40:325.

141. Antonescu CR, Argani P, Erlandson RA, et al. Skeletal and extraskeletal myxoid chondrosarcoma. A comparative clinicopathologic, ultrastructural and molecular study. Cancer 1998; 83:1504.

142. Okamoto S, Hisaoka M, Ishida T, et al. Extraskeletal myxoid chondrosarcoma: a clinicopathologic, immunohistochemical, and molecular analysis of 18 cases. Hum Pathol 2001; 32:1116.

143. Clark J, Rocques PJ, Crew AJ, et al. Identification of novel genes, SYT and SSX, involved in t(X;18)(p11.2;q11.2) translocation found in human synovial sarcoma. Nat Genet 1994; 7:502.

144. Crew AJ, Clark J, Fisher C, et al. Fusion of SYT to two genes, SSX1 and SSX2, encoding proteins with homology to the Kruppel-associated box in human synovial sarcoma. EMBO J 1995; 14:2333.

145. De Leeuw B, Balemans M, Olde Weghuis D, et al. Identification of two alternative fusion genes, SYT-SSX1 and SYT-SSX2, in t(X;18)(p11.2;q11.2)-positive synovial sarcomas. Hum Mol Genet 1995; 4:1097.

146. Skytting B, Nilsson G, Brodin B, et al. A novel fusion gene, SYT-SSX4, in synovial sarcoma. J Natl Cancer Inst 1999; 91:974.

147. Tamborini E, Papini D, Mezzelani A, et al. c-KIT and c-KIT ligand (SCF) in synovial sarcoma (SS): an mRNA expression analysis in 23 cases. Br J Cancer 2001; 85:405.

148. Storlazzi CT, Mertens F, Mandahl N, et al. A novel fusion gene, SS18L1/SSX1, in synovial sarcoma. Genes Chromosomes Cancer 2003; 37:195.

149. Ladanyi M. Fusions of the SYT and SSX Genes in synovial sarcoma. Oncogene 2001; 20:5755.

150. Kawai A, Woodruff J, Healey JH, et al. SYT-SSX gene fusion as a determinant of morphology and prognosis in synovial sarcoma. N Engl J Med 1998; 338:153.

151. Antonescu CR, Kawai A, Leung DH, et al. Strong association of SYT-SSX fusion type and morphologic epithelial differentiation in synovial sarcoma. Diagn Mol Pathol 2000; 9:1.

152. Ladanyi M, Antonescu CR, Leung DH, et al. Impact of SYT-SSX fusion type on the clinical behavior of synovial sarcoma. A multi-institutional retrospective study of 243 patients. Cancer Res 2002; 62:135.

153. Guillou L, Benhattar J, Bonichon F, et al. Histologic grade, but not SYT-SSX fusion type, is an important prognostic factor for patients with synovial sarcoma: a multicenter, retrospective analysis. J Clin Oncol 2004; 22:4040.

154. dos Santos NR, de Bruijn DR, Geurts van Kessel A. Molecular mechanisms underlying human synovial sarcoma development. Genes Chromosomes Cancer 2001; 30:1.

155. Saito T, Oda Y, Sakamoto A, et al. Prognostic value of the preserved expression of the E-cadherin and catenin families of adhesion molecules and of beta-catenin mutations in synovial sarcoma. J Pathol 2000; 192:342.

156. Argani P, Faria PA, Epstein JI, et al. Primary renal synovial sarcoma: molecular and morphologic delineation of an entity previously included among embryonal sarcomas of the kidney. Am J Surg Pathol 2000; 24:1087.

157. Saito T, Oda Y, Sugimachi K, et al. E-cadherin gene mutations frequently occur in synovial sarcoma as a determinant of histological features. Am J Pathol 2001; 159:2117.

158. Saito T, Oda Y, Sakamoto A, et al. APC mutations in synovial sarcoma. J Pathol 2002; 196:445.

159. Saito T, Oda Y, Kawaguchi K, et al. PTEN and other tumor suppressor gene mutations as secondary genetic alterations in synovial sarcoma. Oncol Rep 2004; 11:1011.

160. Saito T, Oda Y, Kawaguchi K, et al. E-cadherin mutation and snail overexpression as alternative mechanisms of E-cadherin inactivation in synovial sarcoma. Oncogene 2004; 23:8629.

161. Heimann P, Devalck C, Dubusscher C, et al. Alveolar soft-part sarcoma: further evidence by FISH for the involvement of chromosome band 17q25. Genes Chromosomes Cancer 1998; 23:194.

162. Joyama S, Ueda T, Shimizu K, et al. Chromosome rearrangement at 17q25 and Xp11.2 in alveolar soft-part sarcoma: a case report and review of the literature. Cancer 1999; 86:1246.

163. Ladanyi M, Lui MY, Antonescu CR, et al. The der(17)t(X;17)(p11;q25) of human alveolar soft part sarcoma fuses the TFE3 transcription factor gene to ASPL, a novel gene at 17q25. Oncogene 2001; 20:48.

164. Nagai M, Tsuda M, Saito T, et al. Functional properties of ASPL-TFE3 and identification of CYP17A and UPP1 as direct transcriptional targets. Proc Am Assoc Cancer Res 2005; 46:1067.

165. Argani P, Antonescu CR, Illei PB, et al. Primary renal neoplasms with the ASPL-TFE3 gene fusion of alveolar soft part sarcoma: a distinctive tumor entity previously included among renal cell carcinomas of children and adolescents. Am J Pathol 2001; 159:179.

166. Heimann P, El Housni H, Ogur G, et al. Fusion of a novel gene, RCC17, to the TFE3 gene in t(X;17)(p11.2;q25.3)-bearing papillary renal cell carcinomas. Cancer Res 2001; 61:4130.

167. Storlazzi CT, Mertens F, Nascimento A, et al. Fusion of the FUS and BBF2H7 genes in low-grade fibromyxoid sarcoma. Hum Mol Genet 2003; 12:2349.

168. Panagopoulos I, Storlazzi CT, Fletcher CD, et al. The chimeric FUS/CREB3l2 gene is specific for low-grade fibromyxoid sarcoma. Genes Chromosomes Cancer 2004; 40:218.

169. Mertens F, Fletcher CD, Antonescu CR, et al. Clinicopathologic and molecular genetic characterization of low-grade fibromyxoid sarcoma, and cloning of a novel FUS/CREB3L1 fusion gene. Lab Invest 2005; 85:408.

170. Dahlen A, Fletcher CD, Mertens F, et al. Activation of the GLI oncogene through fusion with the beta-actin gene (ACTB) in a group of distinctive pericytic neoplasms: pericytoma with t(7;12). Am J Pathol 2004; 164:1645.

171. Raddaoui E, Donner LR, Panagopoulos I. Fusion of the FUS and ATF1 genes in a large, deep-seated angiomatoid fibrous histiocytoma. Diagn Mol Pathol 2002; 11:157.

172. Hallor KH, Mertens F, Jin Y, et al. Fusion of the EWSR1 and ATF1 genes without expression of the MITF-M transcript in angiomatoid fibrous histiocytoma. Genes Chromosomes Cancer 2005; 44:97.

173. Antonescu CR, Dal Cin P, Nafa K, et al. EWS-CREB1 is the predominant gene fusion in so-called angiomatoid fibrous histiocytoma. (submitted) 2007.

174. Simon MP, Pedeutour F, Sirvent N, et al. Deregulation of the platelet-derived growth factor B-chain gene via fusion with collagen gene COL1A1 in dermatofibrosarcoma protuberans and giant-cell fibroblastoma. Nat Genet 1997; 15:95.

175. West RB, Rubin BP, Miller MA, et al. A landscape effect in tenosynovial giant-cell tumor from activation of CSF1 expression by a translocation in a minority of tumor cells. Proc Natl Acad Sci USA 2006; 103:690.

176. Griffin CA, Hawkins AL, Dvorak C, et al. Recurrent involvement of 2p23 in inflammatory myofibroblastic tumors. Cancer Res 1999; 59:2776.

177. Lawrence B, Perez-Atayde A, Hibbard MK, et al. TPM3-ALK and TPM4-ALK oncogenes in inflammatory myofibroblastic tumors. Am J Pathol 2000; 157:377.

178. Bridge JA, Kanamori M, Ma Z, et al. Fusion of the ALK gene to the clathrin heavy chain gene, CLTC, in inflammatory myofibroblastic tumor. Am J Pathol 2001; 159:411.

179. Cools J, Wlodarska I, Somers R, et al. Identification of novel fusion partners of ALK, the anaplastic lymphoma kinase, in anaplastic large-cell lymphoma and inflammatory myofibroblastic tumor. Genes Chromosomes Cancer 2002; 34:354.

180. Ma Z, Hill DA, Collins MH, et al. Fusion of ALK to the Ran-binding protein 2 (RANBP2) gene in inflammatory myofibroblastic tumor. Genes Chromosomes Cancer 2003; 37:98.

181. Schlessinger J. Cell signaling by receptor tyrosine kinases. Cell 2002; 103:211.

182. Cessna M. Expression of ALK1 and p80 in inflammatory myofibroblastic tumor and its mesenchymal mimics: a study of 135 cases. Mod Pathol 2002; 15:931.

183. Bourgeois JM, Knezevich SR, Mathers JA, et al. Molecular detection of the ETV6-NTRK3 gene fusion differentiates congenital fibrosarcoma from other childhood spindle cell tumors. Am J Surg Pathol 2000; 24:937.

184. Knezevich SR, McFadden DE, Tao W, et al. A novel ETV6-NTRK3 gene fusion in congenital fibrosarcoma. Nat Genet 1998; 18:184.

185. Schofield DE, Fletcher JA, Grier HE, et al. Fibrosarcoma in infants and children. Application of new techniques. Am J Surg Pathol 1994; 18:14.

186. Rubin BP, Chen CJ, Morgan TW, et al. Congenital mesoblastic nephroma t(12;15) is associated with ETV6-NTRK3 gene fusion. Cytogenetic and molecular relationship to congenital (infantile) fibrosarcoma. Am J Pathol 1998; 153:1451.

187. Lannon CL, Sorensen PH. ETV6-NTRK3: a chimeric protein tyrosine kinase with transformation activity in multiple cell lineages. Sem Cancer Biol 2005; 15:215.

188. Tognon C, Knezevich SR, Huntsman D, et al. Expression of the ETV6-NTRK3 gene fusion as a primary event in human secretory breast carcinoma. Cancer Cell 2002; 2:367.

189. Eguchi M, Eguchi-Ishimae M, Tojo A, et al. Fusion of ETV6 to neurotrophin-3 receptor TRKC in acute myeloid leukemia with t(12;15)(p13;q25). Blood 1999; 93:1355.

190. Lamant L, Dastugue N, Pulford K, et al. A new fusion gene TPM3-ALK in anaplastic large cell lymphoma created by a (1;2)(q25;p23) translocation. Blood 1999; 93:3088.

191. Touriol C, Greenland C, Lamant L, et al. Further demonstration of the diversity of chromosomal changes involving 2p23 in ALK-positive lymphoma: 2 cases expressing ALK kinase fused to CLTCL (clathrin chain polypeptide-like). Blood 2000; 95:3204.

192. Wang J, Hisaoka M, Shimajiri S, et al. Detection of COL1A1-PDGFB fusion transcripts in dermatofibrosarcoma protuberans by reverse transcription-

polymerase chain reaction using archival formalin-fixed, paraffin-embedded tissues. Diagn Mol Pathol 1999; 8:113.

193. Naeem R, Lux ML, Huang SF, et al. Ring chromosomes in dermatofibrosarcoma protuberans are composed of interspersed sequences from chromosomes 17 and 22. Am J Pathol 1995; 147:1553.

194. Abbott JJ, Erickson-Johnson M, Wang X, et al. Gains of COL1A1-PDGFB genomic copies occur in fibrosarcomatous transformation of dermatofibrosarcoma protuberans. Mod Pathol 2006; 19:1512.

195. Sjoblom T, Shimizu A, O'Brien KP, et al. Growth inhibition of dermatofibrosarcoma protuberans tumors by the platelet-derived growth factor receptor antagonist STI571 through induction of apoptosis. Cancer Res 2001; 61:5778.

196. Maki RG, Awan RA, Dixon RH, et al. Differential sensitivity to imatinib of 2 patients with metastatic sarcoma arising from dermatofibrosarcoma protuberans. Int J Cancer 2002; 100:623.

197. Sirvent N, Maire G, Pedeutour F. Genetics of dermatofibrosarcoma protuberans family of tumors: from ring chromosomes to tyrosine kinase inhibitor treatment. Genes Chromosomes Cancer 2003; 37:1.

198. McArthur GA, Demetri GD, Van Oosterom A, et al. Molecular and clinical analysis of locally advanced dermatofibrosarcoma protuberans treated with imatinib: Imatinib Target Exploration Consortium Study B2225. J Clin Oncol 2005; 23:866.

199. Barreda DR, Hanington PC, Belosevic M. Regulation of myeloid development and function by colony stimulating factors. Dev Comp Immunol 2004; 28:509.

200. Hirota S, Isozaki K, Moriyama Y, et al. Gain-of-function mutations of c-kit in human gastrointestinal stromal tumors. Science 1998; 279:577.

201. Besmer P, Murphy JE, George PC, et al. A new acute transforming feline retrovirus and relationship of its oncogene v-kit with the protein kinase gene family. Nature 1986; 320:415.

202. Huizinga JD, Thuneberg L, Kluppel M, et al. W/kit gene required for interstitial cells of Cajal and for intestinal pacemaker activity. Nature 1995; 373:347.

203. Maeda H, Yamagata A, Nishikawa S, et al. Requirement of c-kit for development of intestinal pacemaker system. Development 1992; 116:369.

204. Torihashi S, Ward SM, Nishikawa S, et al. c-kit-dependent development of interstitial cells and electrical activity in the murine gastrointestinal tract. Cell Tissue Res 1995; 280:97.

205. Tian Q, Frierson HF Jr, Krystal GW, et al. Activating c-kit gene mutations in human germ cell tumors. Am J Pathol 1999; 154:1643.

206. Nagata H, Worobec AS, Oh CK, et al. Identification of a point mutation in the catalytic domain of the protooncogene c-kit in peripheral blood mononuclear cells of patients who have mastocytosis with an associated hematologic disorder. Proc Natl Acad Sci USA 1995; 92:10560.

207. Gari M, Goodeve A, Wilson G, et al. c-kit proto-oncogene exon 8 in-frame deletion plus insertion mutations in acute myeloid leukaemia. Br J Haematol 1999; 105:894.

208. Willmore-Payne C, Holden JA, Tripp S, et al. Human malignant melanoma: detection of BRAF- and c-kit-activating mutations by high-resolution amplicon melting analysis. Hum Pathol 2005; 36:486.

209. Antonescu CR, Sommer G, Sarran L, et al. Association of KIT exon 9 mutations with nongastric primary site and aggressive behavior: KIT mutation analysis and clinical correlates of 120 gastrointestinal stromal tumors. Clin Cancer Res 2003; 9:3329.

210. Rubin BP, Singer S, Tsao C. KIT activation is a ubiquitous feature of gastrointestinal stromal tumors. Cancer Res 2001; 61:8118.

211. Lasota J, Dansonka-Mieszkowska A, Stachura T, et al. Gastrointestinal stromal tumors with internal tandem duplications in 3' end of KIT juxtamembrane domain occur predominantly in stomach and generally seem to have a favorable course. Mod Pathol 2003; 16:1257.

212. Andersson J, Bumming P, Meis-Kindblom JM, et al. Gastrointestinal stromal tumors with KIT exon 11 deletions are associated with poor prognosis. Gastroenterology 2006; 130:1573.

213. Martin J, Poveda A, Llombart-Bosch A, et al. Deletions affecting codons 557–558 of the c-KIT gene indicate a poor prognosis in patients with completely resected gastrointestinal stromal tumors: a study by the Spanish Group for Sarcoma Research (GEIS). J Clin Oncol 2005; 23:6190.

214. Wardelmann E, Losen I, Hans V, et al. Deletion of Trp-557 and Lys-558 in the juxtamembrane domain of the c-kit protooncogene is associated with metastatic behavior of gastrointestinal stromal tumors. Int J Cancer 2003; 106:887.

215. Lasota J, Kopczynski J, Sarlomo-Rikala M. KIT 1530ins6 mutation defines a subset of predominantly malignant gastrointestinal stromal tumors of intestinal origin. Hum Pathol 2003; 34:1306.

216. Lasota J, Wozniak A, Sarlomo-Rikala M. Mutations in exons 9 and 13 of KIT gene are rare events in gastrointestinal stromal tumors. A study of 200 cases. Am J Pathol 2000; 157:1091.

217. Lux ML, Rubin BP, Biase TL, et al. KIT extracellular and kinase domain mutations in gastrointestinal stromal tumors. Am J Pathol 2000; 156:791.

218. Heinrich MC. KIT mutational status predicts clinical response to STI571 in patients with metastatic gastrointestinal stromal tumors (GISTs). Proc ASCO 2002; 21:6.

219. Hirota S, Ohashi A, Nishida T, et al. Gain-of-function mutations of platelet-derived growth factor receptor alpha gene in gastrointestinal stromal tumors. Gastroenterology 2003; 125:660.

220. Lasota J, Dansonka-Mieszkowska A, Sobin LH, et al. A great majority of GISTs with PDGFRA mutations represent gastric tumors of low or no malignant potential. Lab Invest 2004; 84:874.

221. Wardelmann E, Hrychyk A, Merkelbach-Bruse S, et al. Association of platelet-derived growth factor receptor alpha mutations with gastric primary site and epithelioid or mixed cell morphology in gastrointestinal stromal tumors. J Mol Diagn 2004; 6:197.

222. Miettinen M, Lasota J, Sobin LH. Gastrointestinal stromal tumors of the stomach in children and young adults: a clinicopathologic, immunohistochemical, and molecular genetic study of 44 cases with long-term follow-up and review of the literature. Am J Surg Pathol 2005; 29:1373.

223. Miettinen M, Makhlouf H, Sobin LH, et al. Gastrointestinal stromal tumors of the jejunum and ileum: a clinicopathologic, immunohistochemical, and molecular genetic study of 906 cases before imatinib with long-term follow-up. Am J Surg Pathol 2006; 30:477.

224. Prakash S, Sarran L, Socci N, et al. Gastrointestinal stromal tumors in children and young adults: a clinicopathologic, molecular, and genomic study of 15 cases and review of the literature. J Pediatr Hematol Oncol 2005; 27:179.

225. Medeiros F, Corless CL, Duensing A, et al. KIT-negative gastrointestinal stromal tumors: proof of concept and therapeutic implications. Am J Surg Pathol 2004; 28:889.

226. Nishida T, Hirota S, Taniguchi M, et al. Familial gastrointestinal stromal tumours with germline mutation of the KIT gene. Nat Genet 1998; 19:323.

227. Robson ME, Glogowski E, Sommer G, et al. Pleomorphic characteristics of a germ-line KIT mutation in a large kindred with gastrointestinal stromal tumors, hyperpigmentation, and dysphagia. Clin Cancer Res 2004; 10:1250.

228. Isozaki K, Terris B, Belghiti J, et al. Germline-activating mutation in the kinase domain of KIT gene in familial gastrointestinal stromal tumors. Am J Pathol 2000; 157:1581.

229. Sommer G, Agosti V, Ehlers I, et al. Gastrointestinal stromal tumors in a mouse model by targeted mutation of the Kit receptor tyrosine kinase. Proc Natl Acad Sci USA 2003; 1 00:6706.

230. Rubin BP, Antonescu CR, Scott-Browne JP, et al. A knock-in mouse model of gastrointestinal stromal tumor harboring kit K641E. Cancer Res 2005; 65:6631.

231. Breiner JA, Meis-Kindblom J, Kindblom LG, et al. Loss of 14q and 22q in gastrointestinal stromal tumors (pacemaker cell tumors). Cancer Genet Cytogenet 2000; 120:111.

232. el-Rifai W, Sarlomo-Rikala M, Miettinen M, et al. DNA copy number losses in chromosome 14: an early change in gastrointestinal stromal tumors. Cancer Res 1996; 56:3230.

233. Allander SV, Nupponen NN, Ringner M, et al. Gastrointestinal stromal tumors with KIT mutations exhibit a remarkably homogeneous gene expression profile. Cancer Res 2001; 61:8624.

234. Segal NH, Pavlidis P, Antonescu CR, et al. Classification and subtype prediction of adult soft tissue sarcoma by functional genomics. Am J Pathol 2003; 163:691.

235. Antonescu CR, Viale A, Sarran L, et al. Gene expression in gastrointestinal stromal tumors is distinguished by KIT genotype and anatomic site. Clin Cancer Res 2004; 10:3282.

236. Subramanian S, West RB, Corless CL, et al. Gastrointestinal stromal tumors (GISTs) with KIT and PDGFRA mutations have distinct gene expression profiles. Oncogene 2004; 23:7780.

237. Demetri GD, von Mehren M, Blanke CD. Efficacy and safety of imatinib mesylate in advanced gastrointestinal stromal tumors. N Engl J Med 2002; 347:472.

238. Debiec-Rychter M, Dumez H, Judson I. Use of c-KIT/PDGFRA mutational analysis to predict the clinical response to imatinib in patients with advanced gastrointestinal stromal tumours entered on phase I and II studies of the EORTC Soft Tissue and Bone Sarcoma Group. Eur J Cancer 2004; 40:689.

239. Heinrich MC, Corless CL, Demetri GD, et al. Kinase mutations and imatinib response in patients with metastatic gastrointestinal stromal tumor. J Clin Oncol 2003; 21:4342.

240. Antonescu CR, Besmer P, Guo T, et al. Acquired resistance to imatinib in gastrointestinal stromal tumor occurs through secondary gene mutation. Clin Cancer Res 2005; 11:4182.

241. Artandi SE, Chang S, Lee SL, et al. Telomere dysfunction promotes non-reciprocal translocations and epithelial cancers in mice. Nature 2000; 406:641.

242. Gisselsson D, Jonson T, Petersen A, et al. Telomere dysfunction triggers extensive DNA fragmentation and evolution of complex chromosome abnormalities in human malignant tumors. Proc Natl Acad Sci USA 2001; 98:12683.

243. Gisselsson D, Pettersson L, Hoglund M, et al. Chromosomal breakage-fusion-bridge events cause genetic intratumor heterogeneity. Proc Natl Acad Sci USA 2000; 97:5357.

244. Scheel C, Schaefer KL, Jauch A, et al. Alternative lengthening of telomeres is associated with chromosomal instability in osteosarcomas. Oncogene 2001; 20:3835.

245. Sharpless NE, Ferguson DO, O'Hagan RC, et al. Impaired nonhomologous end-joining provokes soft tissue sarcomas harboring chromosomal translocations, amplifications, and deletions. Mol Cell 2001; 8:1187.

246. Drobnjak M, Latres E, Pollack D, et al. Prognostic implications of p53 nuclear overexpression and high proliferation index of Ki-67 in adult soft-tissue sarcomas. J Natl Cancer Inst 1994; 86:549.

247. Wurl P, Meye A, Lautenschlager C, et al. Clinical relevance of pRb and p53 co-overexpression in soft tissue sarcomas. Cancer Lett 1999; 139:159.

248. Mertens F, Fletcher CD, Dal Cin P, et al. Cytogenetic analysis of 46 pleomorphic soft tissue sarcomas and correlation with morphologic and clinical features: a report of the CHAMP Study Group. Chromosomes and Morphology. Genes Chromosomes Cancer 1998; 22:16.

249. Sandberg AA. Updates on the cytogenetics and molecular genetics of bone and soft tissue tumors: liposarcoma. Cancer Genet Cytogenet 2004; 155:1.

249a. Mariani O, Brennetot C, Coindre JM, et al. JUN oncogene amplification and overexpression block adipocytic differentiation in highly aggressive sarcomas. Cancer Cell 2007; 11:361.

250. Kushner BH, Cheung NK. Neuroblastoma – from genetic profiles to clinical challenge. N Engl J Med 2005; 353:2215.

251. Maris JM. The biologic basis for neuroblastoma heterogeneity and risk stratification. Curr Opin Pediatr 2005; 17:7.

252. Vandesompele J, Baudis M, De PK, et al. Unequivocal delineation of clinicogenetic subgroups and development of a new model for improved outcome prediction in neuroblastoma. J Clin Oncol 2005; 23:2280.

253. Attiyeh EF, London WB, Mosse YP, et al. Chromosome 1p and 11q deletions and outcome in neuroblastoma. N Engl J Med 2005; 353:2243.

254. Williamson D, Lu YJ, Gordon T, et al. Relationship between MYCN copy number and expression in rhabdomyosarcomas and correlation with adverse prognosis in the alveolar subtype. J Clin Oncol 2005; 23:880.

255. Brodeur GM, Hayes FA, Green AA, et al. Consistent N-myc copy number in simultaneous or consecutive neuroblastoma samples from sixty individual patients. Cancer Res 1987; 47:4248.

256. Sandberg AA. Updates on the cytogenetics and molecular genetics of bone and soft tissue tumors: leiomyosarcoma. Cancer Genet Cytogenet 2005; 161:1.

257. Mandahl N, Fletcher CD, Dal Cin P, et al. Comparative cytogenetic study of spindle cell and pleomorphic leiomyosarcomas of soft tissues: a report from the CHAMP Study Group. Cancer Genet Cytogenet 2000; 116:66.

258. Xiao S, Li D, Vijg J, et al. Codeletion of p15 and p16 in primary malignant mesothelioma. Oncogene 1995; 11:511.

259. Illei PB, Rusch VW, Zakowski MF, et al. Homozygous deletion of CDKN2A and co-deletion of the methylthioadenosine phosphorylase gene in the majority of pleural mesotheliomas. Clin Cancer Res 2003; 9:2108.

260. Illei PB, Ladanyi M, Rusch V, et al. CDKN2A deletion as a diagnostic marker for malignant mesothelioma in body cavity effusions. Cancer (Cancer Cytopathol) 2003; 99:51.

261. Lopez-Rios F, Chuai S, Flores R, et al. Global gene expression profiling of pleural mesotheliomas: overexpression of aurora kinases and P16/CDKN2A deletion as prognostic factors and critical evaluation of microarray-based prognostic prediction. Cancer Res 2006; 66:2970.

262. Sandberg AA, Bridge JA. Updates on the cytogenetics and molecular genetics of bone and soft tissue tumors. Mesothelioma. Cancer Genet Cytogenet 2001; 127:93.

Chromosome changes in benign mesenchymal tumors

263. Turc-Carel C, Dal Cin P, Rao U, et al. Cytogenetic studies of adipose tissue tumors. I. A benign lipoma with reciprocal translocation t(3;12)(q28;q14). Cancer Genet Cytogenet 1986; 23:283.

264. Hess JL. Chromosomal translocations in benign tumors: the HMGI proteins. Am J Clin Pathol 1998; 109:251.

265. Schoenmakers EF, Wanschura S, Mols R, et al. Recurrent rearrangements in the high mobility group protein gene, HMGI-C, in benign mesenchymal tumours. Nat Genet 1995; 10:436.

266. Rogalla P, Drechsler K, Frey G, et al. HMGI-C expression patterns in human tissues. Implications for the genesis of frequent mesenchymal tumors. Am J Pathol 1996; 149:775.

267. Nilsson M, Mertens F, Hoglund M, et al. Truncation and fusion of HMGA2 in lipomas with rearrangements of 5q32→q33 and 12q14→q15. Cytogenet Genome Res 2006; 112:60.

268. Quade BJ, Weremowicz S, Neskey DM, et al. Fusion transcripts involving HMGA2 are not a common molecular mechanism in uterine leiomyomata with rearrangements in 12q15. Cancer Res 2003; 63:1351.

269. Micci F, Panagopoulos I, Bjerkehagen B, et al. Deregulation of HMGA2 in an aggressive angiomyxoma with t(11;12)(q23;q15). Virchows Arch 2006; 448:838.

270. Kazmierczak B, Dal Cin P, Wanschura S, et al. HMGIY is the target of 6p21.3 rearrangements in various benign mesenchymal tumors. Genes Chromosomes Cancer 1998; 23:279.

271. Xiao S, Lux ML, Reeves R, et al. HMGI(Y) activation by chromosome 6p21 rearrangements in multilineage mesenchymal cells from pulmonary hamartoma. Am J Pathol 1997; 150:901.

272. Hibbard MK, Kozakewich HP, Dal Cin P, et al. PLAG1 fusion oncogenes in lipoblastoma. Cancer Res 2000; 60:4869.

273. Maire G, Forus A, Foa C, et al. 11q13 alterations in two cases of hibernoma: large heterozygous deletions and rearrangement breakpoints near GARP in 11q13.5. Genes Chromosomes Cancer 2003; 37:389.

274. Gisselsson D, Domanski HA, Hoglund M, et al. Unique cytological features and chromosome aberrations in chondroid lipoma: a case report based on fine-needle aspiration cytology, histopathology, electron microscopy, chromosome banding, and molecular cytogenetics. Am J Surg Pathol 1999; 23:1300.

275. Dal Cin P, Sciot R, Polito P, et al. Lesions of 13q may occur independently of deletion of 16q in spindle cell/pleomorphic lipomas. Histopathology 1997; 31:222.

Genetics of familial sarcomas and their sporadic counterparts

276. Lynch HT, Deters CA, Hogg D, et al. Familial sarcoma: challenging pedigrees. Cancer 2003; 98:1947.

277. Kleihues P, Schauble B, Zur HA, et al. Tumors associated with p53 germline mutations: a synopsis of 91 families. Am J Pathol 1997; 150:1.

278. Olivier M, Goldgar DE, Sodha N, et al. Li-Fraumeni and related syndromes: correlation between tumor type, family structure, and TP53 genotype. Cancer Res 2003; 63:6643.

279. Toguchida J, Yamaguchi T, Dayton SH, et al. Prevalence and spectrum of germline mutations of the p53 gene among patients with sarcoma. N Engl J Med 1992; 326:1301.

280. Moutou C, Le BC, Chompret A, et al. Genetic transmission of susceptibility to cancer in families of children with soft tissue sarcomas. Cancer 1996; 78:1483.

281. Hwang SJ, Lozano G, Amos CI, et al. Germline p53 mutations in a cohort with childhood sarcoma: sex differences in cancer risk. Am J Hum Genet 2003; 72:975.

282. Bond GL, Hu W, Bond EE, et al. A single nucleotide polymorphism in the MDM2 promoter attenuates the p53 tumor suppressor pathway and accelerates tumor formation in humans. Cell 2004; 119:591.

283. Bond GL, Hirshfield KM, Kirchhoff T, et al. MDM2 SNP309 accelerates tumor formation in a gender-specific and hormone-dependent manner. Cancer Res 2006; 66:5104.

284. Serra E, Puig S, Otero D, et al. Confirmation of a double-hit model for the NF1 gene in benign neurofibromas. Am J Hum Genet 1997; 61:512.

285. Cichowski K, Shih TS, Schmitt E, et al. Mouse models of tumor development in neurofibromatosis type 1. Science 1999; 286:2172.

286. Storlazzi CT, Von Steyern FV, Domanski HA, et al. Biallelic somatic inactivation of the NF1 gene through chromosomal translocations in a sporadic neurofibroma. Int J Cancer 2005; 117:1055.

287. Birindelli S, Perrone F, Oggionni M, et al. Rb and TP53 pathway alterations in sporadic and NF1-related malignant peripheral nerve sheath tumors. Lab Invest 2001; 81:833.

288. Legius E, Dierick H, Wu R, et al. TP53 mutations are frequent in malignant NF1 tumors. Genes Chromosomes Cancer 1994; 10:250.

289. Kourea HP, Orlow I, Scheithauer BW, et al. Deletions of the INK4A gene occur in malignant peripheral nerve sheath tumors but not in neurofibromas. Am J Pathol 1999; 155:1855.

290. Perrone F, Tabano S, Colombo F, et al. p15INK4b, p14ARF, and p16INK4a inactivation in sporadic and neurofibromatosis type 1-related malignant peripheral nerve sheath tumors. Clin Cancer Res 2003; 9:4132.

291. Caspari R, Olschwang S, Friedl W, et al. Familial adenomatous polyposis: desmoid tumours and lack of ophthalmic lesions (CHRPE) associated with APC mutations beyond codon 1444. Hum Mol Genet 1995; 4:337.

292. Bertario L, Russo A, Sala P, et al. Genotype and phenotype factors as determinants of desmoid tumors in patients with familial adenomatous polyposis. Int J Cancer 2001; 95:102.

293. Clark SK, Pack K, Pritchard J, et al. Familial adenomatous polyposis presenting

with childhood desmoids. Lancet 1997; 349:471.

294. Scott RJ, Froggatt NJ, Trembath RC, et al. Familial infiltrative fibromatosis (desmoid tumours) (MIM135290) caused by a recurrent 3' APC gene mutation. Hum Mol Genet 1996; 5:1921.

295. Tejpar S, Nollet F, Li C, et al. Predominance of beta-catenin mutations and beta-catenin dysregulation in sporadic aggressive fibromatosis (desmoid tumor). Oncogene 1999; 18:6615.

296. Versteege I, Sevenet N, Lange J, et al. Truncating mutations of hSNF5/INI1 in aggressive paediatric cancer. Nature 1998; 394:203.

297. Biegel JA, Zhou JY, Rorke LB, et al. Germ-line and acquired mutations of INI1 in atypical teratoid and rhabdoid tumors. Cancer Res 1999; 59:74.

298. Sevenet N, Lellouch-Tubiana A, Schofield D, et al. Spectrum of hSNF5/INI1 somatic mutations in human cancer and genotype-phenotype correlations. Hum Mol Genet 1999; 8:2359.

299. Modena P, Lualdi E, Facchinetti F, et al. SMARCB1/INI1 tumor suppressor gene is frequently inactivated in epithelioid sarcomas. Cancer Res 2005; 65:4012.

300. Fuller CE, Pfeifer J, Humphrey P, et al. Chromosome 22q dosage in composite extrarenal rhabdoid tumors: clonal evolution or a phenotypic mimic? Hum Pathol 2001; 32:1102.

301. Rousseau-Merck MF, Versteege I, Legrand I, et al. hSNF5/INI1 inactivation is mainly associated with homozygous deletions and mitotic recombinations in rhabdoid tumors. Cancer Res 1999; 59:3152.

302. Biegel JA, Tan L, Zhang F, et al. Alterations of the hSNF5/INI1 gene in central nervous system atypical teratoid/rhabdoid tumors and renal and extrarenal rhabdoid tumors. Clin Cancer Res 2002; 8:3461.

303. Sevenet N, Sheridan E, Amram D, et al. Constitutional mutations of the hSNF5/INI1 gene predispose to a variety of cancers. Am J Hum Genet 1999; 65:1342.

Contributions of microarray studies to sarcoma diagnosis and classification

304. Nielsen TO. Microarray analysis of sarcomas. Adv Anat Pathol 2006; 13:166.

305. West RB, van de RM. The role of microarray technologies in the study of soft tissue tumours. Histopathology 2006; 48:22.

306. Baird K, Davis S, Antonescu CR, et al. Gene expression profiling of human sarcomas: insights into sarcoma biology. Cancer Res 2005; 65:9226.

307. Nielsen TO, West RB, Linn SC, et al. Molecular characterisation of soft tissue tumours: a gene expression study. Lancet 2002; 359:1301.

308. Fritz B, Schubert F, Wrobel G, et al. Microarray-based copy number and expression profiling in dedifferentiated and pleomorphic liposarcoma. Cancer Res 2002; 62:2993.

309. Linn SC, West RB, Pollack JR, et al. Gene expression patterns and gene copy number changes in dermatofibrosarcoma protuberans. Am J Pathol 2003; 163:2383.

310. Ohguri T, Hisaoka M, Kawauchi S, et al. Cytogenetic analysis of myxoid liposarcoma and myxofibrosarcoma by array-based comparative genomic hybridisation. J Clin Pathol 2006; 59:978.

311. Heidenblad M, Hallor KH, Staaf J, et al. Genomic profiling of bone and soft tissue tumors with supernumerary ring chromosomes using tiling resolution bacterial artificial chromosome microarrays. Oncogene 2006; 25:7106.

312. Coindre JM, Hostein I, Maire G, et al. Inflammatory malignant fibrous histiocytomas and dedifferentiated liposarcomas: histological review, genomic profile, and MDM2 and CDK4 status favour a single entity. J Pathol 2004; 203:822.

313. Idbaih A, Coindre JM, Derre J, et al. Myxoid malignant fibrous histiocytoma and pleomorphic liposarcoma share very similar genomic imbalances. Lab Invest 2005; 85:176.

314. Wang Q, Diskin S, Rappaport E, et al. Integrative genomics identifies distinct molecular classes of neuroblastoma and shows that multiple genes are targeted by regional alterations in DNA copy number. Cancer Res 2006; 66:6050.

315. Terry J, Saito T, Subramanian S, et al. TLE1 as a diagnostic immunohistochemical marker for synovial sarcoma emerging from gene expression profiling studies. Am J Surg Pathol 2007; 31:240.

316. Davicioni E, Finckenstein FG, Shahbazian V, et al. Identification of a PAX-FKHR gene expression signature that defines molecular classes and determines the prognosis of alveolar rhabdomyosarcomas. Cancer Res 2006; 66:6936.

317. Laé M, Ahn EH, Mercado GE, et al. Global gene expression profiling of PAX-FKHR fusion-positive alveolar and PAX-FKHR fusion-negative embryonal rhabdomyosarcomas. J Pathol 2007; 212:143.

318. Wachtel M, Runge T, Leuschner I, et al. Subtype and prognostic classification of rhabdomyosarcoma by immunohistochemistry. J Clin Oncol 2006; 24:816.

319. West RB, Corless CL, Chen X, et al. The novel marker, DOG1, is expressed ubiquitously in gastrointestinal stromal tumors irrespective of KIT or PDGFRA mutation status. Am J Pathol 2004; 165:107.

320. West RB, Harvell J, Linn SC, et al. Apo D in soft tissue tumors: a novel marker for dermatofibrosarcoma protuberans. Am J Surg Pathol 2004; 28:1063.

FINE NEEDLE ASPIRATION BIOPSY OF SOFT TISSUE TUMORS

Kim R. Geisinger and Fadi W. Abdul-Karim

CHAPTER CONTENTS

INTRODUCTION

Fine needle aspiration biopsies (FNAB) are an established tool in the diagnostic armamentarium of many clinical practices. The initial diagnosis of mass lesions in both superficial (e.g., breast and thyroid) and deep (e.g., lung and pancreas) body sites is often readily assessed by FNAB. FNAB in the evaluation of primary soft tissue tumors, however, remains underutilized and, for some, is controversial.[1-18]

ADVANTAGES AND DISADVANTAGES

Several important challenges are inherent in the evaluation of soft tissue neoplasms. Many lesions, especially sarcomas, are rare so most practicing pathologists do not encounter these neoplasms on a routine basis and may not be familiar with their morphologic, clinical, and radiographic features. Soft tissue lesions also possess overlapping histopathologic and cytomorphologic attributes which are further compounded by the morphologic heterogeneity which may be present within some of these proliferations. For these reasons, some have advocated that the diagnoses and treatment of many soft tissue lesions, especially sarcomas, should occur within large, centralized medical facilities.[3,19,20]

FNAB of soft tissue masses possess a number of distinct advantages.[9,16,19-21] Compared to other techniques,

FNAB is a rapid outpatient procedure which permits on-site evaluation of specimen adequacy and which may provide an immediate diagnosis. This allows the orthopedic surgeon to discuss potential additional diagnostic procedures and therapeutic options during the initial visit. The aspiration procedure is well tolerated and local anesthesia is usually unnecessary. A major advantage of FNAB is that much greater sampling is possible. By altering the direction of the needle during a single puncture, multiple portions of the mass may be aspirated as compared to needle core biopsy. If necessary, multiple separate FNAB punctures may be performed during a single patient visit. Cellular material may be obtained during the same biopsy setting for electron microscopy, cytogenetics, molecular biologic analysis, and cell blocks. Cell blocks are preferable to direct smears for immunocytochemical studies.

FNAB also has a very low rate of significant clinical complications. Rarely, patients may suffer bleeding or develop edema and tenderness at the biopsy site. The procedure does not disrupt tissue planes or contaminate the subsequent surgical site. If not diagnostic, FNAB can be followed by another biopsy procedure. No instance of needle tracking of sarcomatous tumor cells by a fine needle has been documented. Finally, compared to all other biopsy techniques, FNAB is relatively inexpensive and viewed as very cost effective.

FNAB possess several distinct disadvantages, some of which are relatively specific to soft tissue lesions.[3,8,9,19,22,23] FNAB results in relatively small samples of a tumor. Inherent in the aspiration technique, there is dispersion of individual cells and loss of recognizable diagnostic tissue patterns. These limitations inevitably hinder the cytopathologist's ability to distinguish specific histologic type and subtype of tumors. There may be even more difficulty in distinguishing among benign cellular lesions and low-grade sarcomas. Accurate grading of many sarcomas may not be possible when utilizing current histopathologic classification schemes. In densely collagenized or sclerotic masses or highly vascular lesions, FNAB may provide only a sparse smear cellularity, making a benign versus malignant distinction impossible.

Although the exact role for FNAB in the clinical evaluation of soft tissue masses remains controversial, we believe that most published data and our own experiences strongly support its utility in accurately distinguishing between benign and malignant soft tissue tumors. Cytomorphologically, the most important feature in this decision process is the overall cellularity of the smears. Sarcomas usually yield moderately to highly cellular specimens, whereas benign mesenchymal lesions usually are more sparsely cellular. It is crucial to recognize, however, that there is overlap in this cellularity parameter. For example, aspirates of nodular fasciitis may yield numerous atypical-appearing spindle-shaped cells. Conversely, certain neoplasms, e.g., low-grade fibromyxoid sarcoma and richly collagenized malignancies, may not provide numerous neoplastic elements. This can be further complicated by poor sampling of the mass and extensive necrosis within the tumor. The classic cytologic attributes of malignancy also support the diagnosis of sarcoma. It is important to find diffuse and uniform hyperchromasia among essentially all of the aspirated tumor cells. The presence of moderate to marked pleomorphism, although certainly not specific, also leads to a diagnosis of malignancy. Irregularly contoured and variably thickened nuclear membranes are features of sarcoma. A word of caution concerning nucleoli is warranted in that they may be prominent in benign proliferations (e.g., granulation tissue) and inconspicuous in some malignancies (e.g., the myxoid sarcomas). The levels of reported diagnostic specificity and sensitivity are approximately 95% in establishing a diagnosis of sarcoma.[9,19] FNAB can also readily differentiate sarcomas from other malignancies which have spread to the soft tissues.

The diagnosis of a soft tissue tumor by aspiration biopsy necessitates the intimate cooperation of orthopedic surgeons, radiologists, and pathologists in order to optimize the integration of all clinically relevant information.[9,19] Whenever possible, an on-site evaluation by the pathologist is preferred as this expedites the opportunity for the pathologist to examine the patient, to review imaging studies, and to discuss the lesion with the surgeon. This also permits a timely assessment of specimen adequacy and possibly the rendering of an immediate interpretation.[24]

Another important reason for on-site evaluation is that it allows the pathologist to suggest further triage of the sample. Thus, additional needle punctures may be performed to obtain cellular material for cell blocks which may provide additional architectural data and a substrate for immunocytochemistry, cytogenetics, and a variety of molecular biologic assays.[25–30]

Generally, one can accurately subclassify soft tissue neoplasms on the basis of FNAB into clinically relevant categories that permit the initiation of therapy in many patients.[1,5,7,9,10,19,21,31,32] We classify soft tissue sarcomas in aspiration smears into six general categories on the basis of the predominant appearance of the specimen: myxoid, spindle cell, pleomorphic, polygonal cell, round cell, and miscellaneous.[9] We will expand upon this classification scheme in the following sections. In general, these categories correlate relatively well with the grade of the malignancy.

Histologic grade is one of the most significant and perhaps the most crucial single factor in predicting a patient's prognosis.[33] Within certain limitations, we believe that many soft tissue sarcomas can be accurately graded in smears in a clinically relevant manner.[9,16–20,32–36] However, not all authorities subscribe to this approach and some have discouraged this practice due to the limitations of FNAB.[22,33] The inability to assess mitotic figure counts, variability in cellularity from field to field, and the extent of tumor necrosis is prohibitive of accurate grading. The cytologist can only state that necrotic debris is absent or present in scant or large amounts. On the other hand, histologic subtype or degree of differentiation is somewhat different. In FNAB, a specific cell type can be identified in a large proportion of sarcomas.

Although many may not treat solely on the FNAB diagnosis, in some centers therapy is dictated by the FNAB interpretation. If tumors are considered low grade, surgery usually is the next step. However, if high grade, then preoperative chemotherapy may be administered to reduce the extent of surgery, e.g., limb-salvage therapy. Pleomorphic and round cell sarcomas are almost always high grade. Conversely, if identified accurately, well-differentiated liposarcomas are consistently low grade. Pure myxoid sarcomas are low grade. Polygonal cell and especially the spindle cell categories pose the greatest difficulties.[34,35]

Some authorities have provided data on the complementary nature of FNAB and needle core biopsies (NCB) in the outpatient setting for the primary diagnosis of soft tissue neoplasms.[1] More recently, several groups have compared these two diagnostic modalities in this exact clinical scenario. Yang and Damron evaluated 50 consecutive patients.[37] These authors averaged six needle core passes per patient (this number is high in our experience), followed by FNAB. The first procedure was performed by the surgeon, whereas the pathologist performed the aspiration. The authors concluded that NCB has a higher level of diagnostic accuracy in determining the nature of the neoplasm, establishing a histologic type and grade, and a specific diagnosis. Domanski et al. evaluated 130 consecutive patients in which both biopsy procedures were performed by the pathologist.[38] These authors concluded that the two techniques were complementary. It should be pointed out that both of these series included osseous as well as soft tissue lesions. Although more data can generally be acquired by NCB, the complementary nature is related to the many advantages of FNAB.

MYXOID SARCOMAS

The myxoid sarcomas include myxoid liposarcoma, myxoid malignant fibrous histiocytoma (high-grade myxofibrosarcoma) and extraskeletal myxoid chondrosarcoma. At low power, the most apparent feature of the smears is the voluminous extracellular matrix material (Fig. 5–1).[9,39,40] Often, the matrix fragments are irregularly shaped and moderately sized, with or without embedded tumor cells. With the Romanowsky stains, the matrix appears as homogeneous, fibrillar to structureless reddish purple material (Fig. 5–2). The matrix is typically metachromatic, especially in extracellular chondrosarcomas. With the Papanicolaou stain, the matrix is cyanophilic and often appears as a relatively watery pale-green substance (Fig. 5–1). The edges of the fragments may be sharply defined or blend irregularly with the background as delicate spicules which extend from the fragment. In the smear, the sarcoma cells are present in moderate to high numbers as individually dispersed elements, and in small aggregates, both embedded within the matrix and scattered in the background. Typically, the malignant cells are relatively small and have spindled, rounded, or stellate contours. Their precise shape is more apparent when they are unencumbered by the matrix. Most of the tumor cells are small to moderately sized, often with densely hyperchromatic solitary nuclei. Nucleoli are generally small and inconspicuous. A few multinucleated tumor giant cells may also be randomly distributed in the smears, especially with myxoid malignant fibrous histiocytoma (Fig. 5–3).

In aspirates from myxoid liposarcomas, the only cells of diagnostic value are lipoblasts.[9,38,39,41] Lipoblasts, however, may be sparse and require careful search. They

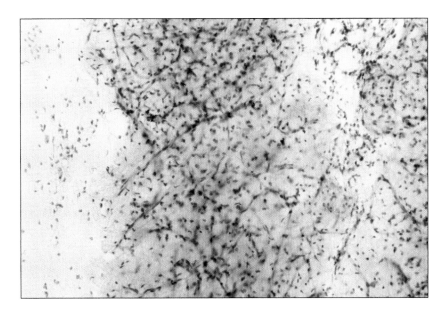

FIGURE 5–1 Myxoid liposarcoma. A moderate number of small uniform neoplastic cells with solitary hyperchromatic nuclei are set within abundant cyanophilic matrix, which also contains an obvious network of branched capillaries. Similar-appearing malignant cells are adjacent to the fragment of matrix. (Papanicolaou stain, ×40.)

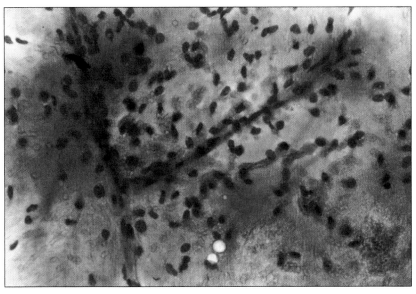

FIGURE 5–2 Myxoid liposarcoma. The small malignant cells are characterized by solitary darkly stained nuclei and high nucleocytoplasmic ratios. They appear to be fairly evenly scattered within the metachromatic matrix, which also contains a branched capillary. Two neoplastic cells have lipid vacuoles. (Diff-Quik stain, ×400.)

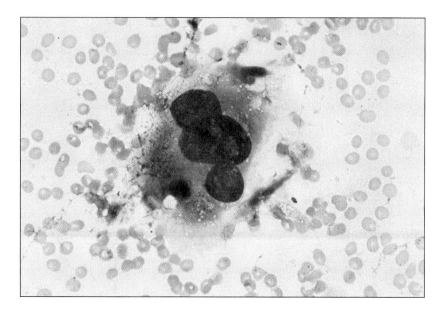

FIGURE 5–3 Myxoid malignant fibrous histiocytoma. Scattered bizarre-appearing tumor giant cells are characteristically present in small numbers. This cell is characterized by multiple variably sized nuclei with prominent nucleoli and abundant cytoplasm. The latter has indistinct edges which blend into the smear background. (Diff-Quik stain, ×400.)

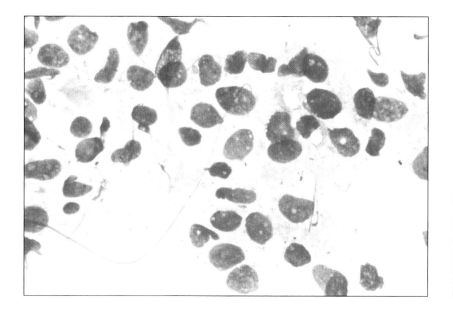

FIGURE 5–4 Round cell liposarcoma. The poorly differentiated variant of myxoid liposarcoma is composed of relatively small uniform malignant cells with round, large nuclei, scanty cytoplasm, and occasionally prominent nucleoli. Cytoplasmic lipid vacuoles may be seen within some of the cells. (Diff-Quik stain, ×400.)

are characterized by rounded contours and scant to moderate cytoplasm occupied by one or more sharply defined lipid vacuoles. The latter may be uniform in size or vary in diameter, but characteristically displace the nucleus eccentrically and indent or scallop its borders. Another highly distinctive feature of myxoid liposarcoma is the presence of branched delicate capillaries in the matrix material (Figs 5–1, 5–2). Larger round tumor cells with high nucleo-cytoplasmic ratios and occasional lipid vacuoles are seen in smears of poorly differentiated myxoid liposarcoma (Fig. 5–4). The finding of a low-grade component with malignant round cells in the same smear is a helpful clue to the correct classification. In smears, lipoblastoma may be indistinguishable from myxoid liposarcoma; thus, it is essential that patient age is integrated into the diagnosis.[42]

The most distinguishing feature of smears of myxoid malignant fibrous histiocytoma is the presence of moderate numbers of scattered bizarre tumor giant cells, generally multinucleated, with voluminous cytoplasm; these cells have indistinct edges that appear to blend into the smear background (Fig. 5–3).[9,39,40,43,44] Typically, the nuclei within a given cell vary in both size and outline.

The most distinctive attribute of extraskeletal myxoid chondrosarcomas is the extreme metachromasia and dense appearance of the matrix material,[39,40] features that contrast with the myxoid matrix of benign myxoid neoplasms.

The differential diagnosis of myxoid sarcomas includes benign myxoid soft tissue tumors, most commonly ganglion cysts and myxomas.[39,40,45,46] These masses may yield viscous aspiration fluid which is difficult to smear.[47] The smears are usually dominated by granular myxoid material in which are embedded paucicellular elements which resemble histiocytes. Although mitotic figures are sparse in aspirates of myxoid sarcomas, they are not present in samples of benign entities.

SPINDLE CELL SARCOMAS

This category includes fibrosarcoma, leiomyosarcoma, synovial sarcoma, malignant peripheral nerve sheath tumors, Kaposi sarcoma, low-grade fibromyxoid sarcoma, gastrointestinal stromal tumors (GIST), and some angiosarcomas.[9,12,13,30,34,35,43-66] This group poses the greatest diagnostic difficulties and has the greatest potential for false-negative diagnoses due to the difficulty in distinguishing benign proliferations from low-grade sarcomas.

Conversely, a variety of benign spindle cell proliferations may yield false-positive interpretations. In our experience, the two major attributes that allow an aspirate to be designated as sarcoma are moderate to high smear cellularity with some loss of cohesion and hyperchromatic nuclei. Based purely on the cytomorphology, it may be difficult or impossible to distinguish among the various spindle cell sarcomas and to grade them accurately. Neither nuclear configurations nor cytoplasmic features are of value in distinguishing among these neoplasms, especially the high-grade tumors.

In general, aspiration biopsies yield moderately to highly cellular smears (Fig. 5–5).[9] The major feature is a predominance of cells with elongated or spindled nuclei, paralleling the shape of the cell (Figs 5–6 to 5–8). The degree of intercellular cohesion may vary markedly from patient to patient and among the various spindle cell

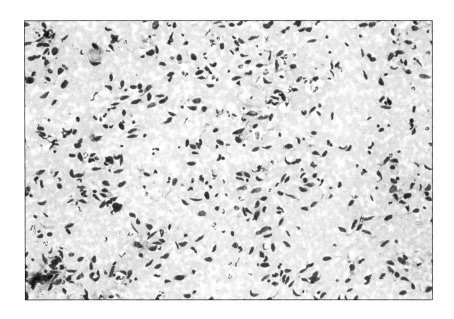

FIGURE 5–5 Malignant peripheral nerve sheath tumor. This extremely cellular aspirate is dominated by mildly pleomorphic and dissociated spindle-shaped malignant cells. There is almost no evidence of intercellular cohesion. The nucleo-cytoplasmic ratios appear high, although some possess elongated cytoplasmic tails. The spindle-shaped nuclei vary from smooth to buckled to wavy. (Diff-Quik stain, ×40.)

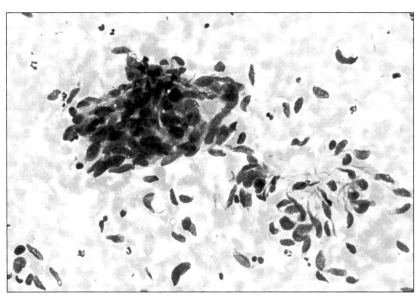

FIGURE 5–6 Synovial sarcoma. This highly cellular aspirate smear contains individual tumor cells, loose clusters, and a three-dimensional cohesive tumor fragment. The malignant cells are uniform, each possessing a single elongated nucleus and very high nucleo-cytoplasmic ratios. Nuclear contours vary from plump and ovoid to very elongated to comma-shaped. (Diff-Quik stain, ×250.)

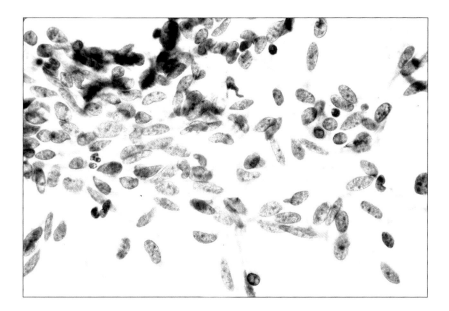

FIGURE 5–7 Malignant peripheral nerve sheath tumor. This cellular aspirate contains a loose aggregate of malignant cells. The edges of the aggregate appear irregular, resulting from individual cells falling away from its surface. Each cell has a solitary elongated nucleus with finely granulated, evenly distributed hyperchromatic chromatin and occasional minute nucleoli. No evidence of specific differentiation is seen. (Papanicolaou stain, ×400.)

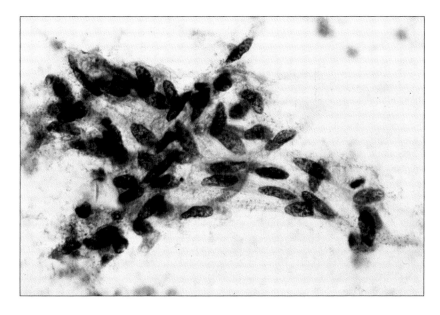

FIGURE 5–8 Leiomyosarcoma. The sarcomatous nuclei are large and hyperchromatic. Although the cells possess obvious dense cytoplasm, the cells are crowded due to higher nucleo-cytoplasmic ratios. (Papanicolaou stain, ×400.)

sarcomas. Some specimens are dominated by individually dispersed tumor cells and small loose aggregates, whereas in others, large tissue fragments predominate. In our experience, the latter situation is most characteristic of leiomyosarcomas. The edges of the neoplastic fragments are rendered indistinct by the detachment of cells from its surface. The neoplastic cells are usually mononuclear and monotonous. Their chromatin is finely to coarsely granular and may be either evenly or irregularly distributed. Generally, nucleoli are neither large nor prominent. The volume of cytoplasm varies from scant to moderate, and in some neoplasms, the tumor cells have long, tapering cytoplasmic tails. The application of ancillary diagnostic procedures such as immunocytochemistry, cytogenetics, and molecular assays of aspirated cellular material may assist in arriving at a specific diagnosis.

The most commonly aspirated benign spindle cell soft tissue lesions are nerve sheath neoplasms and nodular fasciitis. In most benign nerve sheath tumors, the cellularity of the smear is low to moderate.[67-70] The aspirated cells are consistently present in cohesive fragments having irregular contours and consisting of interlacing fascicles (Fig. 5–9). Most neoplastic cells have a solitary elongated nucleus with sharply pointed tips. Some of the nuclei may have a wavy outline. Although uncommon, hyperchromasia may be noted focally. Intranuclear vacuoles are present with some frequency. The cytoplasm of the tumor cells is generally inapparent and blends imperceptibly with the surrounding collagen in the fragments. Mitotic figures are not evident. A clinical clue to the diagnosis of a nerve sheath tumor is that aspiration incites pain that radiates along the involved nerve.

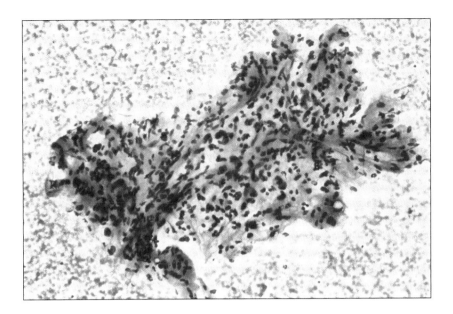

FIGURE 5–9 Schwannoma. This smear is characterized by a large cohesive fragment of tumor. Moderate numbers of neoplastic cells are situated within an abundant matrix. The pink-staining material represents both cytoplasm and collagen. Note the complete absence of individually dispersed tumor cells. (Diff-Quik stain, ×40.)

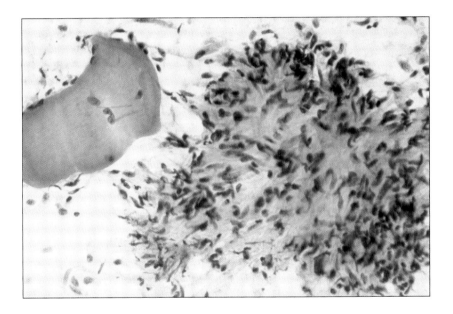

FIGURE 5–10 Nodular fasciitis. The classic loosely textured "tissue culture" appearance of nodular fasciitis is evident. Haphazardly positioned proliferating myofibroblasts are present within a pale stained, fibrillated myxoid matrix which also contains scattered lymphocytes. Although some of the nuclei of the proliferating cells are darkly stained, most are euchromatic. Adjacent to this fragment are individual myofibroblasts and skeletal muscle fibers. (Papanicolaou stain, ×40.)

In conjunction with the appropriate clinical presentation, the cytomorphology of aspirates of nodular fasciitis is often quite distinctive.[71–74] The smears are moderately to highly cellular and composed of singly dispersed cells, loose aggregates, and tissue fragments, all set in a metachromatic myxoid material. Within the fragments, the cells are loosely and haphazardly arranged, similar to the pattern of tissue cultures (Fig. 5–10). Although cellular shapes are variable, most are spindled with moderate volumes of faintly basophilic cytoplasm and one or two cytoplasmic tails. Most possess a solitary nucleus which is round with delicate, distinct membranes, vesicular chromatin, and distinct nucleoli which may be large and irregular in shape. Mitotic figures may also be present, at times numerous. The cytologic picture is completed by the presence of inflammatory cells.

FNAB of the fibromatoses notoriously may lead to false-negative (insufficient) specimens or false-positive diagnoses of sarcoma. The smears are variably cellular but tend to be less so than in sarcomas.[74] Presumably, this is related to the abundant collagen within the lesion. These cells are present both singly and in small, loose aggregates. Proliferating fibroblasts have solitary, uniform, elongated nuclei with delicate membranes, even fine chromatin, and inconspicuous nucleoli. One may find bipolar, tapering, long cytoplasmic tails. Mitotic figures are not expected.

PLEOMORPHIC SARCOMAS

The vast majority of the neoplasms in this category are pleomorphic malignant fibrous histiocytoma and pleomorphic liposarcomas.[8,9,44,59,75–78] However, other sarcomas may occasionally enter the differential diagnosis. In aspirate smears, pleomorphic sarcomas are almost always readily recognized as malignant and often as sarcomatous at low magnification. The direct smears are extremely cellular with little tendency for the malignant cells to aggregate.[9,41] An admixture of small round cells with high nucleo-cytoplasmic ratios, large spindled or polygonal cells with scant to moderate volumes of cytoplasm, and numerous bizarre tumor giant cells may be observed within a single field (Figs 5–11, 5–12). The giant cells contain hyperchromatic, multilobated nuclei, often with huge nucleoli. The giant cells typically have moderate to abundant cytoplasm with cell borders that blend imperceptibly into the background. The latter frequently contains necrotic debris. In general, it is impossible to distinguish among the different pleomorphic

sarcomas on smears. However, this limitation generally does not hinder subsequent clinical management of most patients.

The most common entities in the differential diagnosis are pleomorphic carcinomas of diverse sites. Notable examples are giant cell or sarcomatoid carcinomas of the lung, kidney, thyroid, and pancreas. On the basis of cytomorphology alone, some of these aspirates may be completely indistinguishable from those of sarcomas. In addition to clinical history, the smears should be carefully searched for the presence of residual epithelial differentiation in the form of cohesive aggregates of carcinoma cells with polygonal to columnar contours. Other malignancies which may fall into this morphologic pattern include melanoma and sarcomatoid mesothelioma. A few benign entities also need to be considered, including pleomorphic lipoma, ancient schwannoma,

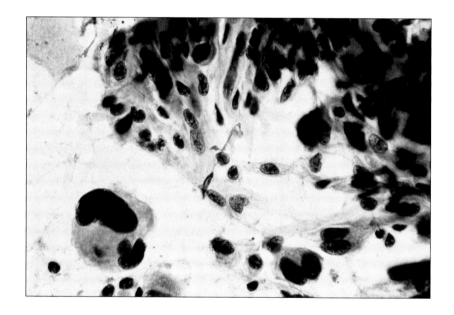

FIGURE 5–11 Malignant fibrous histiocytoma. Marked variability in the sizes and appearances of the malignant cells is apparent. Some tumor cells are relatively small with solitary hyperchromatic nuclei and inapparent cytoplasm. Others are larger with more polygonal or spindled shapes. Also present are several multinucleated tumor giant cells which have two or more extremely darkly stained nuclei and moderate to voluminous cytoplasm. Note that in several of the tumor giant cells, the nuclei form a characteristic acute angle with each other. (Papanicolaou stain, ×400.)

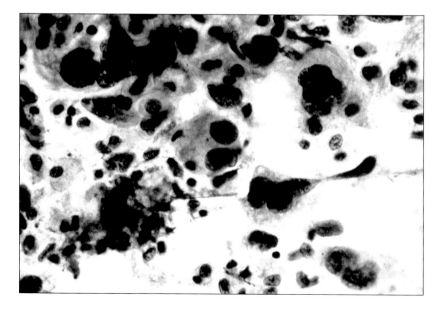

FIGURE 5–12 Malignant fibrous histiocytoma. Striking hyperchromasia and pleomorphism characterize the neoplastic nuclei and cells in this example. Multinucleated tumor giant cells, some with bizarre appearances, are evident in association with malignant cells having a more histiocytoid appearance. (Papanicolaou stain, ×400.)

and proliferative fasciitis/myositis (Fig. 5–13).[2,69,79] In most instances, when the clinical data are integrated with the aspiration cytomorphology, the correct interpretation can be rendered. Although less likely to be overdiagnosed as sarcoma, giant cell tumors of tendon sheath also need to be considered (Fig. 5–14).[80–83]

POLYGONAL CELL SARCOMAS

The least frequent of the FNAB categories of sarcomas is the polygonal or epithelial-like group. This includes epithelioid sarcoma, clear cell sarcoma, alveolar soft part sarcoma, malignant granular cell tumors, and the predominantly epithelioid types of other sarcomas (e.g., gastrointestinal stromal tumor and angiosarcoma).[49,50,84–92] Although smear cellularity is variable, it is usually moder-

ate to high, often with a largely dissociative pattern. The smears contain numerous individually dispersed malignant cells and small, generally flat aggregates (Figs 5–15, 5–16). The tumor cells have round or polygonal shapes, well-defined cellular borders, and at least a moderate volume of cytoplasm. Typically, they possess a solitary, often eccentrically positioned, round nucleus with a thick, distinct membrane, vesicular chromatin, and one or more large nucleoli. A small proportion of the neoplastic cells may be binucleated or even multinucleated. Alternatively, some cells have a spindled contour. In addition to subtle cytologic clues, an accurate clinical history and a judicious use of immunocytochemistry will allow distinction among these neoplasms.

The differential diagnosis is rather limited. It includes carcinoma or melanoma metastatic to soft tissue. In smears, a greater degree of intercellular cohesion, large

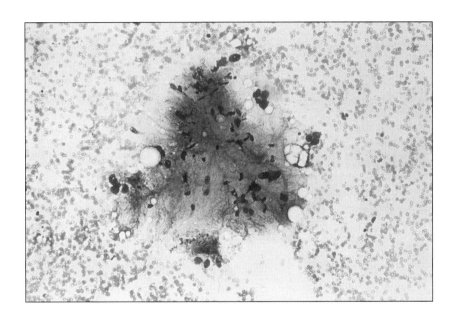

FIGURE 5–13 Pleomorphic lipoma. Scant cellularity characterizes this aspirate. Although most of the cells are small with solitary nuclei and apparently high nucleo-cytoplasmic ratios, others are larger. They vary from spindled to multinucleated tumor giant cells. A few neoplastic cells have prominent cytoplasmic lipid vacuoles. (Diff-Quik stain, ×40.)

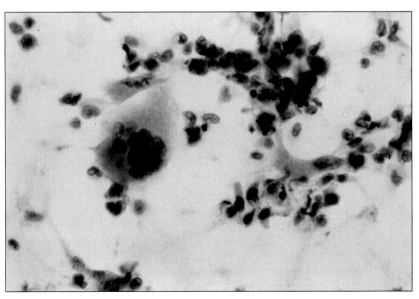

FIGURE 5–14 Giant cell tumor of tendon sheath. In contrast to the pleomorphic sarcomas, the nuclei within the giant cells are much smaller and more homogeneous. They have fine, even chromatin and small but distinct nucleoli. These giant cells have much more abundant cytoplasm and hence lower nucleo-cytoplasmic ratios. In the proper clinical setting, this should never be confused with a pleomorphic sarcoma. (Papanicolaou stain, ×100.)

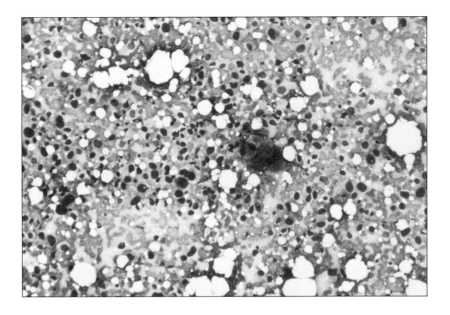

FIGURE 5–15 Clear cell sarcoma. Both high cellularity and a lack of cohesion characterize this aspirate. Most cells have large single nuclei with prominent nucleoli and scanty cytoplasm. A few larger and multinucleated neoplastic cells are also evident. (Diff-Quik stain, ×40.)

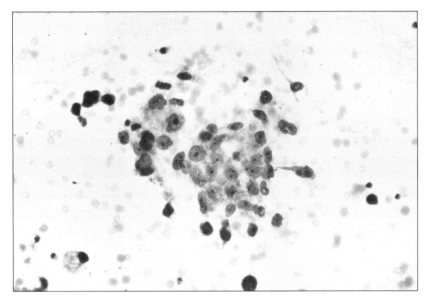

FIGURE 5–16 Epithelioid sarcoma. This cohesive aggregate has a distinct epithelioid appearance with the maintenance of cohesion, polygonal contours, and peripherally situated round nuclei. Nucleoli are also strikingly prominent. (Diff-Quik stain, ×250.)

cytoplasmic vacuoles, and three-dimensional aggregates favor metastatic carcinoma.

ROUND CELL SARCOMAS

Round cell sarcomas predominate in the pediatric population and young adults, and include rhabdomyosarcoma, extraskeletal Ewing sarcoma/primitive neuroectodermal tumor (ES/PNET), and intra-abdominal desmoplastic small round cell tumor (DSRCT).[8,9,93–101] Aspiration biopsies of these neoplasms typically yield highly cellular smears composed of relatively small, homogeneous malignant cells (Figs 5–17 to 5–20). The tumor cells have solitary nuclei with a high nucleo-cytoplasmic ratio. In embryonal rhabdomyosarcoma, however, the nuclei are hyperchromatic and a portion may have abundant cytoplasm and multiple nuclei (Fig. 5–19). Although nucleoli are usually inconspicuous in ES/PNET and DSRCT, they tend to be well developed in rhabdomyosarcoma (Fig. 5–20). Within a given specimen, uniformity of the cells is expected in the former two neoplasms, whereas pleomorphism is quite variable in the latter. This is the category in which ancillary diagnostic tests, performed on aspirated cellular material, is most helpful in determining an exact tumor type.

The major differential diagnosis is extranodal, primary non-Hodgkin B-cell lymphoma. These tumors almost never demonstrate any evidence of true intercellular cohesion. The cells tend to be homogeneous with round to irregular nuclear membranes and variably prominent nucleoli. Consistently, the nucleo-cytoplasmic ratio is very high. Lymphoglandular bodies are numerous in the background.[101]

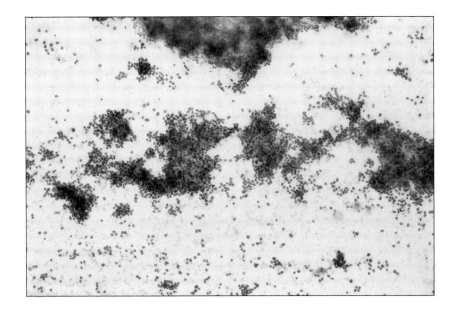

FIGURE 5–17 Alveolar rhabdomyosarcoma. On low power, high smear cellularity is apparent, with many of the tumor cells present in loosely cohesive fragments. This almost suggests a pseudoalveolar arrangement. In addition, individually dispersed neoplastic cells are evident. Even at this very low magnification, the striking uniformity of the cells is evident. Each cell possesses a solitary round nucleus which is surrounded by only a scanty rim of cytoplasm. (Diff-Quik stain, ×20.)

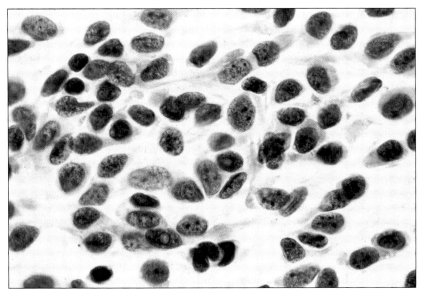

FIGURE 5–18 Embryonal rhabdomyosarcoma. Smear cellularity is high and cohesion is poorly preserved. The neoplastic cells are quite homogeneous in appearances. Each has a single ovoid nucleus with fine, even, hyperchromatic chromatin and minute nucleoli. Most cells possess scant cytoplasm in which the nucleus appears to be eccentrically positioned. A few tumor cells have long tapering cytoplasmic tails. (Hematoxylin and eosin, ×400.)

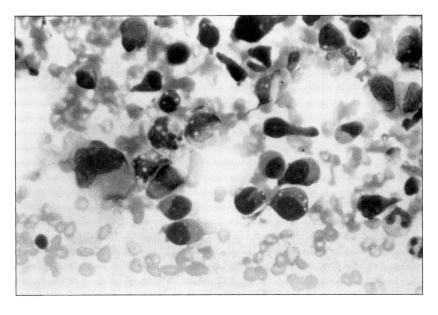

FIGURE 5–19 Embryonal rhabdomyosarcoma. A spectrum of cellular appearances is apparent. Most of the cells have solitary small round nuclei and rather high nucleocytoplasmic ratios. A tadpole cell is evident in the center of the field. Also note the presence of a large multinucleated tumor giant cell and the absence of intercellular cohesion. (Diff-Quik stain, ×400.)

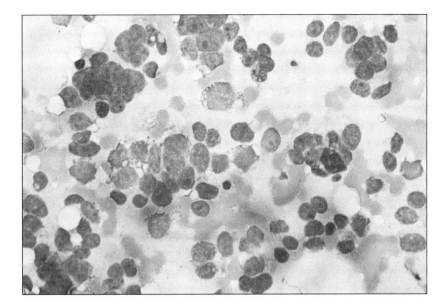

FIGURE 5–20 Primitive neuroectodermal tumor. Each malignant cell has a single round nucleus with very finely reticulated and evenly dispersed chromatin. For the most part, nucleoli are inconspicuous. In many cells, cytoplasm is barely visible, whereas others have small to large glycogen vacuoles. The presence of cohesion and the lack of lymphoglandular bodies helps to distinguish this from lymphoma. (Diff-Quik stain, ×400.)

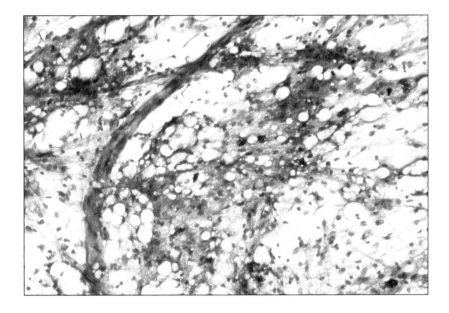

FIGURE 5–21 Well-differentiated liposarcoma. Unremarkable-appearing adipocytes are embedded within fibrous connective tissue. In addition, however, scattered cells have much larger nuclei. Some of these also appear to have cytoplasmic lipid vacuoles. In the proper clinical setting, this is diagnostic of liposarcoma. Vascularity is prominent. (Diff-Quik stain, ×40.)

MISCELLANEOUS SARCOMAS

A neoplasm that does not fit into any of the above categories is well-differentiated liposarcoma (atypical lipomatous neoplasm).[2,75,77,78] The aspiration cytomorphology of this neoplasm has only rarely been detailed. At best, smears are moderately cellular, and the sample may be mistaken for benign adipose tissue as it is composed mostly of fragments of mature-appearing fat cells (Fig. 5–21). The diagnosis of liposarcoma requires the finding of unequivocal lipoblasts with cytoplasmic lipid vacuoles that compress and distort the nucleus.

Other neoplasms which may fall into this category are gastrointestinal stromal tumor and angiosarcoma.[49,50,57] Paralleling their histologic appearances, these neoplasms may show a spectrum of cell contours, ranging from almost completely spindled to pure epithelioid cells. Many will contain a combination of the two cell types, as well as transitional forms.

ACCURACY

Only a few series with large numbers of patients have addressed the diagnostic accuracy of FNAB of soft tissue neoplasms.[1,3,5,7,10,14,17–19,21,103] There is a lack of standardization among these reports. Some studies have included patients with both benign and malignant neoplasms, whereas others have addressed only sarcomas. Some series are dedicated to the primary diagnosis of a mass, whereas others include patients with recurrent or metastatic sarcomas. Several investigations have included aspiration biopsies of both soft tissue and bone lesions, and it is not always clear how these statistical data are subdivided. Some authors have provided only the number of patients or specimens, whereas others have reported the levels of diagnostic sensitivity and specificity, rates of false-negative and false-positive diagnoses, or both.

Akerman and Willen have described the largest series.[19] Over a 20-year period, these investigators evaluated 517 patients with an aspirate for a primary diagnosis of a soft tissue neoplasm; of these, 315 were benign and 202 were sarcomas. The authors were able to distinguish benign from malignant in 94% of the patients. Their errors were equally divided between false-negative and false-positive diagnoses (14 each). As is the experience for many individuals, their area of greatest difficulty was spindle cell neoplasms followed by lipomatous tumors.

Brosjö et al. evaluated 342 patients with a relatively equal distribution between benign and malignant soft tissue tumors.[5] The cytologic diagnosis was conclusive in 300 patients (88%). There was a 5% false-negative rate among the 153 benign cytologic diagnoses and a 2% false-positive rate among the 147 malignant interpretations. Thus, a correct diagnosis was rendered in 97% of this population.

Oland et al. reported their experience with 196 patients who underwent FNAB of a soft tissue mass.[21] Patients who had a benign cytologic diagnosis (tumor or inflammation) were followed. Sixteen were diagnosed with metastatic carcinoma without subsequent surgery. A total of 48 patients underwent histologic examination of their masses following the aspiration biopsy, and all 25 cytologic diagnoses of frank sarcoma were confirmed; thus, there were no false-positive interpretations. Of the 17 benign soft tissue tumors diagnosed by cytology, one was a false-negative interpretation.

Liu et al. examined a series of 89 aspirates that included samples from 20 benign and 69 malignant masses, including 11 metastatic melanomas.[14] Each aspirate was independently evaluated by four pathologists who differed in their years of experience. Each evaluated these specimens in two settings: without and then later with the appropriate clinical history. In each of these two scenarios, each pathologist provided a precise cytopatho-logic diagnosis and classified the smears into one of four categories: benign, probably benign, probably malignant, or malignant. This data was then analyzed to create receiver operator characteristics (ROC) curves. Without the benefit of clinical history, the proportion of correct diagnosis ranged from 0.19 to 0.44. With the addition of clinical history, the proportion of accurate interpretations were improved to a range of 0.48 to 0.66. The proportion of correct diagnoses improved for all four pathologists. Difficulty was especially noted for benign spindle cell neoplasms.

CONCLUSION

Fine needle aspiration biopsy of soft tissue neoplasms has important limitations. Samples may be limited in cellularity to the point of being insufficient for a diagnosis, as soft tissue neoplasms have several attributes which may lead to poor cellularity on the smear. There are certain neoplasms in which a benign versus malignant designation cannot be made with certainty from FNAB. In addition, it may be impossible to predict the grade on the basis of the smear preparation; this is most commonly encountered with the spindle cell neoplasms. Based purely on cytomorphology, the exact cell type of many soft tissue neoplasms cannot be stated accurately; this is more likely with adult rather than childhood tumors. However, many of these problems are obviated by the use of ancillary diagnostic procedures on aspirated cellular material.

Still, FNAB of soft tissue neoplasms possesses a number of advantages that overall outweigh the disadvantages. Aspiration biopsy is easily performed in the outpatient setting and compared to other diagnostic procedures is relatively inexpensive. Aspiration biopsy provides a rapid, relatively nontraumatic procedure for sampling both superficial and deep-seated mass lesions. Soft tissue neoplasms can be recognized and accurately designated as benign or malignant in many instances. Multiple samples can also be obtained during a single clinical visit, thereby increasing the likelihood of specimen adequacy, including tissue for ancillary tests.

REFERENCES

Introduction

1. Bennert KW, Abdul-Karim FW. Fine needle aspiration cytology vs. needle core biopsy of soft tissue tumors – a comparison. Acta Cytol 1994; 38:381.
2. Akerman M, Rydholm A. Aspiration cytology of lipomatous tumors: a 10-year experience at an orthopedic oncology center. Diagn Cytolpathol 1987; 3:295.
3. Akerman M, Rydholm A, Persson BM. Aspiration cytology of soft tissue tumors: the 10-year experience of an orthopedic oncology center. Acta Orthop Scand 1985; 56:407.
4. Barth RJ, Merino MJ, Solomon D, et al. A prospective study of the value of core needle biopsy and fine needle aspiration in the diagnosis of soft tissue masses. Surgery 1992; 112:536.
5. Brosjö O, Bauer HCF, Kreisbergers A, et al. Fine needle aspiration biopsy of soft tissue tumors. Acta Orthop Scand 1994; 65(Suppl 256):108.
6. Cohen MB, Layfield LJ. Fine needle aspiration biopsy of soft tissue tumors. In: Schmidt WA, Miller TR, eds. Cytopathol annual 1994. Chicago: ASCP Press; 1994:101–132.
7. Costa MJ, Campman SC, Davis RL, et al. Fine-needle aspiration cytology of sarcoma: retrospective review of diagnostic utility and specificity. Diagn Cytopathol 1996; 15:23.
8. Gonzalez-Campora R, Munoz-Arias G, Otal-Salaverri C, et al. Fine needle aspiration cytology of primary soft tissue tumors: morphologic analysis of the most frequent types. Acta Cytol 1992; 36:905.
9. Kilpatrick SE, Geisinger KR. Soft tissue sarcomas: the utility and limitations of fine needle aspiration biopsy. Am J Clin Pathol 1998; 110:50.
10. Layfield LJ, Anders KH, Glasgow BJ, et al. Fine needle aspiration of primary soft tissue lesions. Arch Pathol Lab Med 1986; 110:420.
11. Layfield LJ, Liu K, Dodge RK. Logistic regression analysis of small round cell neoplasms: a cytologic study. Diagn Cytopathol 1999; 20:271.

12. Liu K, Dodge RK, Dodd LG, et al. Logistic regression analysis of low grade spindle cell lesions. A cytologic study. Acta Cytol 1999; 43:143.

13. Liu K, Dodge RK, Layfield LJ. Logistic regression analysis of high grade spindle cell neoplasms. A fine needle aspiration cytologic study. Acta Cytol 1999; 43:593.

14. Liu K, Layfield LJ, Coogan AC, et al. Diagnostic accuracy in fine-needle aspiration of soft tissue and bone lesions. Influence of clinical history and experience. Am J Clin Pathol 1999; 111:632.

15. Willén H, Akerman M, Carlén B. Fine needle aspiration (FNA) in the diagnosis of soft tissue tumours; a review of 22 years experience. Cytopathology 1995; 6:236.

16. Wakely PE Jr, Kineisl JS. Soft tissue aspiration cytopathology. Cancer Cytopathol 2000; 90(5):292.

17. Nagira K, Yamamoto T, Akisue T, et al. Reliability of fine-needle aspiration biopsy in the initial diagnosis of soft-tissue lesions. Diagn Cytopathol 2002; 27(6):354.

18. Dey P, Mallik MK, Gupta SK, et al. Role of fine needle aspiration cytology in the diagnosis of soft tissue tumours and tumour-like lesions. Cytopathology 2004; 15:32.

Advantages and disadvantages

19. Akerman M, Willen H. Critical review of the role of fine needle aspiration in soft tissue tumors. Pathol Case Rev 1998; 3:111.

20. Rydholm A. Centralization of soft tissue sarcoma. The southern Sweden experience. Acta Orthop Scand 1997; 68(Suppl 273):4.

21. Oland J, Rosen A, Reif R, et al. Cytodiagnosis of soft tissue tumors. J Surg Oncol 1986; 37:168.

22. Nguyen GK. What is the value of fine needle aspiration biopsy in the cytodiagnosis of soft tissue tumors? Diagn Cytopathol 1988; 4:352.

23. Shah MS, Garg V, Kapoor SK, et al. Fine-needle aspiration cytology, frozen section, and open biopsy: relative significance in diagnosis of musculoskeletal tumors. J Surg Orthop Adv 2003; 12(4):203.

24. Patel NP, Ward WG, Geisinger KR. Soft tissue fine needle aspiration biopsy (ST-FNAB) interpretation by house officers: analysis of preliminary vs final ST-FNAB diagnoses with tissue correlation. Modern Pathol 2006; 19:69A.

25. Rekhi B, Bhatnagar D, Bhatnagar A, et al. Cytomorphological study of soft tissue neoplasms: role of fluorescent immunocytochemistry in diagnosis. Cytopathology 2005; 16:219.

26. Kilpatrick SE, Bergman S, Pettenati MJ, et al. The usefulness of cytogenetic analysis in fine needle aspirates for the histologic subtyping of sarcomas. Modern Pathol 2006; 19:815.

27. Geisinger KR, Silverman JF, Cappellari JO, et al. Fine-needle aspiration cytology of malignant hemangiopericytomas with ultrastructural and flow cytometric analyses. Arch Pathol Lab Med 1990; 114:705.

28. Akhtar M, Ashraf AM, Sabbah R, et al. Small round cell tumor with divergent differentiation: cytologic, histologic and ultrastructural findings. Diagn Cytopathol 1994; 11:159.

29. Alkan S, Eltoum IA, Tabbara S, et al. Usefulness of molecular detection of human herpesvirus-8 in the diagnosis of Kaposi sarcoma by fine-needle aspiration. Am J Clin Pathol 1999; 111:91.

30. Akerman M, Ryd W, Skytting B. Fine-needle aspiration of synovial sarcoma. Criteria for diagnosis: retrospective reexamination of 37 cases, including ancillary diagnostics. A Scandinavian Sarcoma Group study. Diagn Cytopathol 2003; 28:232.

31. Kilpatrick SE, Ward WG, Cappellari JO, et al. Fine-needle aspiration biopsy of soft tissue sarcomas: a cytomorphologic analysis with emphasis on histologic subtyping, grading and therapeutic significance. Am J Clin Pathol 1999; 112:179.

32. Kilpatrick SE, Cappellari JO, Bos GD, et al. Is fine needle aspiration biopsy a practical alternative to open biopsy for the primary diagnosis of sarcoma? Experience with 140 patients. Am J Clin Pathol 2001; 115(1):59.

33. Guillou L, Coindre J-M. How should we grade soft tissue sarcomas and what are the limitations? Pathol Case Rev 1998; 3:105.

34. Weir MM, Rosenberg AE, Bell DA. Grading of spindle cell sarcomas in fine-needle aspiration biopsy specimens. Am J Clin Pathol 1999; 112:784.

35. Mathur S, Kapila K, Verma K. Accuracy of cytologic grading of spindle-cell sarcomas. Diagn Cytopathol 2003; 29(2):79.

36. Palmer HE, Mukunyadzi P, Culbreth W, et al. Subgrouping and grading of soft-tissue sarcomas by fine-needle aspiration cytology: a histopathologic correlation study. Diagn Cytopathol 2001; 24(5):307.

37. Yang YJ, Damron TA. Comparison of needle core biopsy and fine needle aspiration for diagnostic accuracy in musculoskeletal lesions. Arch Pathol Lab Med 2004; 128(7):759.

38. Domanski HA, Akerman M, Carlen B, et al. Core-needle biopsy performed by the cytopathologist: a technique to complement fine-needle aspiration of soft tissue and bone lesions. Cancer Cytopathol 2005; 105(4):229.

Myxoid sarcomas

39. Gonzalez-Campora R, Otal-Salaverri C, Helvia-Vazquez A, et al. Fine needle aspiration in myxoid tumors of the soft tissues. Acta Cytol 1990; 34:179.

40. Wakely PE Jr, Geisinger KR, Cappellari JO, et al. Fine-needle aspiration cytopathology of soft tissue: chromyxoid and myoid lesions. Diagn Cytopathol 1995; 12, 101.

41. Szadowska A, Lasota J. Fine needle aspiration cytology of myxoid liposarcoma: a study of 18 tumors. Cytopathology 1993; 4:99.

42. Kloboves-Prevodnik VV, Us-Krasovec M, Gale N, et al. Cytologic features of lipoblastoma: a report of three cases. Diagn Cytopathol 2005; 33(3):195.

43. Merck C, Hagmar B. Myxofibrosarcoma. A correlative cytologic and histologic study of 13 cases examined by fine needle aspiration cytology. Acta Cytol 1980; 24:137.

44. Klijanienko J, Cailland J-M, Lagace R, et al. Comparative fine-needle aspiration and pathologic study of malignant fibrous histiocytoma; cytodiagnosis of 95 tumors in 71 patients. Diagn Cytopathol 2003; 29:320.

45. Caraway NP, Staerkel GA, Fanning CV, et al. Diagnosing intramuscular myxoma by fine needle aspiration: a multidisciplinary approach. Diagn Cytopathol 1994; 11:255.

46. Wakely PE Jr, Bos GD, Mayerson I. The cytopathology of soft tissue myxomas: ganglia, juxta-articular myoid lesions, and intramuscular myxoma. Am J Clin Pathol 2005; 123:858.

Spindle cell sarcomas

47. Ferretti M, Gusella PM, Mancini AM, et al. Progressive approach to the cytologic diagnosis of retroperitoneal spindle cell tumors. Acta Cytol 1997; 41:450.

48. Powers CN, Berardo MD, Frable WJ. Fine needle aspiration biopsy: pitfalls in the diagnosis of spindle-cell lesions. Diagn Cytopathol 1994; 10:232.

49. Boucher LD, Swanson PE, Stanley MW, et al. Fine-needle aspiration of angiosarcoma. Acta Cytol 1998; 42:1289.

50. Klijanienko J, Calliwad JM, Lagace R, et al. Cytohistologic correlations in angiosarcoma including classic and epithelioid variants: Institut Curie's experience. Diagn Cytopathol 2003; 29(3):140.

51. Dahl I, Hagmar B, Agnervall L. Leiomyosarcoma of the soft tissue: a correlative cytological and histological study of 11 cases. Acta Pathol Microbiol Scand 1981; 89:285.

52. Tao LC, Davidson DD. Aspiration biopsy cytology of smooth muscle tumors: a cytologic approach to the differentiation between leiomyosarcoma and leiomyoma. Acta Cytol 1993; 37:300.

53. Barbazza R, Chiarelli S, Quintarelli GF, et al. Role of fine-needle aspiration cytology in the preoperative evolution of smooth muscle tumors. Diagn Cytopathol 1997; 16:326.

54. Jiménez-Heffernan JA, López-Ferrer P, Vicandi B, et al. Cytologic features of malignant peripheral nerve sheath tumor. Acta Cytol 1999; 43:175.

55. Gupta K, Dey P, Vasahist R. Fine-needle aspiration cytology of malignant peripheral nerve sheath tumors. Diagn Cytopathol 2004; 31(1):1.

56. Klijanienko J, Cailland J-M, Lagacé R, et al. Cytohistologic correlations of 24 malignant nerve sheath tumor (MPNST) in 17 patients: The Institut Curie experience. Diagn Cytopathol 2002; 27:103.

57. Elliott DD, Fanning CV, Caraway NP. The utility of fine-needle aspiration in the diagnosis of gastrointestinal stromal tumors. Cancer Cytopathol 2006; 108(1):49.

58. Hales M, Bottles K, Miller T, et al. Diagnosis of Kaposi's sarcoma by fine-needle aspiration biopsy. Am J Clin Pathol 1987; 88:20.

59. Berardo MD, Powers CN, Wakely P Jr, et al. Fine-needle aspiration cytopathology of malignant fibrous histiocytoma. Cancer Cytopathol 1997; 81:228.

60. Kilpatrick SE, Teot LA, Stanley MW, et al. Fine-needle aspiration biopsy of synovial sarcoma. A cytomorphologic analysis of primary recurrent, and metastatic tumors. Am J Clin Pathol 1996; 106:769.

61. Viguer JM, Jiménez-Heffernan JA, Vicandi B, et al. Cytologic features of synovial sarcoma with emphasis on the monophasic fibrous variant. A morphologic and immunocytological analysis of bcl-2 protein expression. Cancer Cytopathol 1998; 84:50.

62. Klijanienko J, Cailland J-M, Lagacé R, et al. Cytohistologic correlations in 56 synovial sarcomas in 36 patients: The Institut Curie experience. Diagn Cytopathol 2002; 27:96.

63. Ewing CA, Zakowski MF, Lin O. Monophasic synovial sarcoma: a cytologic spectrum. Diagn Cytopathol 2004; 30(1):19.

64. Lindberg GM, Maitra A, Gokaslan ST, et al. Low grade fibromyxoid sarcoma. Fine-needle aspiration cytology with histologic, cytogenetic, immunohistochemical, and ultrastructural correlation. Cancer Cytopathol 1999; 87:75.

65. Villaseñor EGE, Cedillo EAD, González LML. Fine needle aspiration cytology of low grade fibromyxoid sarcoma. Report of a case with histologic correlation. Acta Cytol 2004; 48:69.

66. Domanski HA. FNA diagnosis of dermatofibroma protuberans. Diagn Cytopathol 2005; 32:299.

67. Dahl I, Hagmar B, Idvall I. Benign solitary neurilemoma (schwannoma): A correlative cytological and histological study of 28 cases. Acta Pathol Microbiol Immunol Scan 1984; 92:91.

68. Resnick JM, Fanning CV, Caraway NP, et al. Percutaneous needle biopsy diagnosis of benign neurogenic neoplasms. Diagn Cytopathol 1997; 16:17.
69. Dodd LG, Marom EM, Dash RC, et al. Fine-needle aspiration cytology of "ancient" schwannoma. Diagn Cytopathol 1999; 20:307.
70. Henke AC, Salomão DR., Hughes JH. Cellular schwannoma mimics a sarcoma: an example of a potential pitfall in aspiration cytodiagnosis. Diagn Cytopathol 1999; 30:312.
71. Dahl I, Akerman M. Nodular fasciitis: a correlative cytologic and histologic study of 13 cases. Acta Cytol 1981; 25:215.
72. James LP. Cytopathology of mesenchymal repair. Diagn Cytopathol 1985; 1:91.
73. Kong CS, Cha I. Nodular fasciitis. Diagnosis by fine needle aspiration biopsy. Acta Cytol 2004; 48:473.
74. Raab SS, Silverman JF, McLeod DL, et al. Fine needle aspiration biopsy of fibromatoses. Acta Cytol 1993; 37:323.

Pleomorphic sarcomas

75. Walaas L, Kindblom LG. Lipomatous tumors: a correlative cytologic and histologic study of 27 tumors examined by fine needle aspiration cytology. Hum Pathol 1985; 16:6.
76. Walaas L, Angervall L, Hagmar B, et al. A correlative cytologic and histologic study of malignant fibrous histiocytoma: an analysis of 40 cases examined by fine needle aspiration cytology. Diagn Cytopathol 1986; 2:46.
77. Nemanqani D, Mourad WA. Cytomorphologic features of fine-needle aspiration of liposarcoma. Diagn Cytopathol 1999; 20:67.
78. Einarsdottir H, Skoog L, Soderlund V, et al. Accuracy of cytology for diagnosis of lipomatous tumors: comparison with magnetic resonance and computed tomography findings in 175 cases. Acta Radiol 2004; 45(8):840.
79. Rigby HS, Wilson V, Cawthorn S, et al. Fine needle aspiration of pleomorphic lipoma: a potential pitfall of cytodiagnosis. Cytopathology 1993; 4:55.
80. Wakely PE Jr, Frable WJ. Fine needle aspiration biopsy cytology of giant cell tumor of tendon sheath. Am J Clin Pathol 1994; 102:87.

81. Layfield LJ, Moffatt EJ, Dodd LG, et al. Cytologic findings in tenosynovial giant cell tumors investigated by fine-needle aspiration cytology. Diagn Cytopathol 1997; 16:317.
82. Iyer VK, Kapila K, Verma K. Fine-needle aspiration cytology of giant cell tumor of tendon sheath. Diagn Cytopathol 2003; 29(2):105.
83. Gupta K, Dey P, Goldsmith R, et al. Comparison of cytologic features of giant-cell tumor and giant-cell tumor of tendon sheath. Diagn Cytopathol 2004; 30:14.

Polygonal cell sarcomas

84. Caraway NP, Fanning CV, Wojeik EM, et al. Cytology of malignant melanoma of soft parts: fine needle aspirates and exfoliative specimens. Diagn Cytopathol 1993; 9:632.
85. Creager AJ, Pitman MB, Geisinger KR. Cytologic features of clear cell sarcoma (malignant melanoma) of soft parts. A study of fine-needle aspirates and exfoliative specimens. Am J Clin Pathol 2002; 117:217.
86. Lin O, Olgac S, Zakowski M. Cytological features of epithelioid mesenchymal neoplasms: a study of 21 cases. Diagn Cytopathol 2005; 32:5.
87. Kapila K, Chopra P, Verma K. Fine needle aspiration cytology of alveolar soft-part sarcoma. Acta Cytol 1985; 29:559.
88. Shabb N, Sneige N, Fanning CV, et al. Fine needle aspiration cytology of alveolar soft-part sarcoma. Diagn Cytopathol 1991; 7:293.
89. Lopez-Ferrer P, Jiménez-Hefferman JA, Vicandi B, et al. Cytologic features of alveolar soft part sarcoma: report of three cases. Diagn Cytopathol 2002; 27:115.
90. Pohar-Marinsek Z, Zidar A. Epithelioid sarcoma in FNAB smears. Diagn Cytopathol 1994; 11:367.
91. Geisinger KR, Kawamoto EH, Marshall RB, et al. Aspiration and exfoliative cytology, including ultrastructure, of a malignant granular cell tumor. Acta Cytol 1985; 29:593.
92. Dong Q, McKee G, Pitman M, et al. Epithelioid variant of gastrointestinal stromal tumor: diagnosis of fine-needle aspiration. Diagn Cytopathol 2003; 29(2):55.

Round cell sarcomas

93. Pettinato G, Swanson PE, Insabato L, et al. Undifferentiated small round-cell tumors of childhood: the immunocytochemical demonstration of myogenic differentiation in fine needle aspirates. Diagn Cytopathol 1989; 5:194.
94. Seidal T, Mark J, Hagmar B, et al. Alveolar rhabdomyosarcoma. A cytometric and correlated cytological and histological study. Acta Pathol Microbiol Scand (A) 1982; 90:345.
95. Seidal T, Walaas L, Kindblom LG, et al. Cytology of embryonal rhabdomyosarcoma. A cytologic, light microscopic, electron microscopic, and immunohistochemical study of seven cases. Diagn Cytopathol 1988; 4:292.
96. Akhtar M, Ali MA, Bakry M, et al. Fine needle aspiration biopsy of childhood rhabdomyosarcoma: cytologic, histologic, and ultrastructural correlations. Diagn Cytopathol 1992; 8:465.
97. Almeida M, Stastny JF, Wakely PE Jr, et al. Fine needle aspiration biopsy of childhood rhabdomyosarcoma: re-evaluation of the cytologic criteria for diagnosis. Diagn Cytopathol 1994; 11:231.
98. Berhant LE, Anderson LH, Taylor DA. Extraskeletal Ewing's sarcoma. Diagnosis of a case by fine needle aspiration cytology. Acta Cytol 1986; 30:683.
99. Renshaw AA, Pérez-Atayde AR, Fletcher JA, et al. Cytology of typical and atypical Ewing's sarcoma/PNET. Am J Clin Pathol 1996; 106:620.
100. Carraway NP, Fanning CV, Amato RJ, et al. Fine-needle aspiration of intra-abdominal desmoplastic small round cell tumor. Diagn Cytopathol 1993; 9:465.
101. Logrono R, Kurtycz DF, Sproat IA, et al. Diagnosis of recurrent desmoplastic small round cell tumor by fine needle aspiration. A case report. Acta Cytol 1997; 41:1402.
102. Meda BA, Buss DH, Woodruff RD, et al. Diagnosis and subclassification of primary and recurrent lymphoma. The usefulness and limitations of combined fine-needle aspiration cytomorphology and flow cytometry. Am J Clin Pathol 2000; 113:688.
103. Miralles TG, Gosalbez F, Menéndez P, et al. Fine needle aspiration cytology of soft-tissue lesions. Acta Cytol 1986; 30:671.

APPROACH TO THE DIAGNOSIS OF SOFT TISSUE TUMORS

CLINICAL INFORMATION

The diagnosis of a soft tissue lesion, as with other tumors, presupposes a modicum of clinical information and adequate, well-processed tissue. At a minimum, the pathologist should be apprised of the age of the patient, the location of the tumor, and its growth characteristics. In some cases the results of imaging studies, particularly magnetic resonance imaging (MRI), enhance one's understanding of the clinical extent of the lesion and its relationship to normal structures (see Chapter 3).

Although age rarely, if ever, suggests a particular diagnosis, the importance of this information is in knowing if the patient is a child. In general, there is little overlap between soft tissue tumors occurring in children and those seen in adults. Therefore, this critical piece of information essentially presents the pathologist with two groups of tumors from which a differential diagnosis can be constructed. For example, malignant fibrous histiocytoma (pleomorphic undifferentiated sarcoma) is essentially unheard of during childhood, so one should consider other diagnoses for a pleomorphic tumor in a child. On the other hand, neuroblastoma and angiomatoid fibrous histiocytoma rarely occur after childhood, and such diagnoses should always be made cautiously in adults.

Location, too, provides ancillary help in the differential diagnosis. Sarcomas, for the most part, develop as deeply located masses and infrequently present as superficial lesions. Exceptions do occur, however, and include lesions such as dermatofibrosarcoma protuberans, epithelioid sarcoma, and angiosarcoma (Table 6–1). It is also useful to recall that when carcinomas or melanomas metastasize to soft tissue, it is usually as small, superficial nodules rather than as large, deeply situated masses. In our experience, the most common carcinomas that present as soft tissue metastases are pulmonary and renal carcinomas, the former usually appearing as a subcutaneous mass on the chest wall and the latter as a soft tissue mass in nearly any location.

Unfortunately, there is a great deal of overlap between the manner of presentation of benign and malignant soft tissue masses, so this information may be least helpful to the pathologist. Most soft tissue sarcomas of the extremities are detected by the patient as a slowly growing mass that has been present for about 6 months at the time of diagnosis. The duration of benign lesions may be similar, although such lesions are generally described as static or slowly growing. An exception to the foregoing observation is the rapid development of some cases of nodular fasciitis. These superficial, reactive lesions may develop rapidly over a period of 1–3 weeks, and we have even encountered some that evolved in a few days, a pattern of growth that seldom if ever is encountered with a sarcoma. Thus, an astute general surgeon can sometimes suggest the diagnosis of fasciitis for a rapidly evolving superficial lesion of the extremity.

BIOPSY DIAGNOSIS

In the past the choice of biopsy technique for soft tissue masses was dictated by the size and location of the lesion (see Chapter 2). Incisional biopsy was considered the gold standard for large, deeply situated masses and provided ample material for diagnosis and ancillary studies. Its principal disadvantages included spillage of tumor into adjacent compartments due to poor hemostasis or faulty biopsy placement, complications of wound infection, and the usual requirement for hospitalization of the patient. Excisional biopsy, while more expedient and providing the entire lesion for examination, could only be performed on small, superficial lesions amenable to complete resection. The current reliance on minimally

TABLE 6–1	SUPERFICIAL SOFT TISSUE SARCOMAS

Dermatofibrosarcoma protuberans
Epithelioid sarcoma
Angiomatoid fibrous histiocytoma
Plexiform fibrohistiocytic tumor
Myxoid malignant fibrous histiocytoma (myxofibrosarcoma)
Angiosarcoma
Kaposi's sarcoma
Atypical fibroxanthoma

invasive techniques to procure tissue has changed the biopsy paradigm in the direction of the use of core needle biopsy. Based on the Memorial Sloan-Kettering Cancer Center experience, the incidence of core needle biopsies increased from less than 10% to nearly 80% during the early 1990s,[1] and in our hospital currently exceeds 90%. Consequently, the amount of material available to type and grade sarcomas has decreased and this trend is likely to continue unabated due to the emphasis on less costly outpatient care. Therefore, it is important to be aware of the limitations and pitfalls of core needle biopsy and to keep in mind a few basic principles.[2]

First, the pathologist should be aware of the expectation of the clinician. In some instances the goal of a core needle biopsy may be simply to establish that a soft tissue mass is a primary mesenchymal neoplasm as opposed to a lymphoma or metastatic lesion; a distinction usually easily made in a majority of cases with the use of adjuvant immunohistochemistry. If definitive surgery will be performed following the needle biopsy, then the most important priority is to determine if the lesion is a sarcoma or not. If, however, the intention is to provide preoperative (neoadjuvant) radio- or chemotherapy, every attempt should be made not only to make the diagnosis of sarcoma but also to classify and grade the lesion. It is not always possible to reliably grade a sarcoma on the basis of a core needle biopsy, however. In particular, it is difficult to discriminate a grade 2 from a grade 3 lesion. Pathologists may find that the best assessment they can give is the designation "low grade" or "high grade," recognizing that high grade will encompass both grade 2 and 3 lesions. Information is inevitably lost when collapsing a three-tiered system into a two-tiered one; however, a two-tiered system still performs reasonably well and is consistent with therapeutic considerations.[3]

In grading core needle biopsies, one can usually accept the presence of high-grade areas in several needle cores as diagnostic of a high-grade sarcoma due to the improbability that additional material will result in downgrading the lesion. At the same time one should also be unwilling to accept a lesion as low grade if the number of core biopsies is small, the lesion has not been sampled, or if imaging studies suggest features of a high-grade sarcoma (i.e., necrosis). Core needle biopsies containing necrosis usually imply a high-grade sarcoma, again because of the improbability that limited material captures a solitary or limited focus of necrosis. However, pathologists must be certain that necrosis is of the coagulative and not the hyaline type and is not reflective of prior therapy or surgical intervention. The corollary to the latter portion of this statement is that once radiation or chemotherapy has been administered, grading becomes unreliable due to alterations in nuclear features, mitotic activity, cellularity, and interstitial hyalinization. Therapy also induces necrosis, although it is not possible to discriminate spontaneous from therapy-induced necrosis. Most importantly, interpreting core needle biopsies implies a close dialogue with clinicians to resolve any inconsistencies between clinical and pathologic diagnoses.

FROZEN SECTION DIAGNOSIS

In the past, frozen section examinations were performed commonly with the expectation that definitive surgery would be accomplished during the same intraoperative procedure, but this trend is changing. Frozen sections are now obtained primarily to assure the surgeon that she or he has obtained representative, viable tissue that is adequate for a permanent section diagnosis or to evaluate margins. The former may be accomplished by freezing a portion of the biopsy material or sometimes, as in the case of a needle biopsy, performing a touch preparation. The presence of malignant cells in a non-necrotic background on a touch preparation ensures that the specimen is adequate. A background of reactive or necrotic cells suggests that a pseudocapsule has been biopsied or that the specimen is largely necrotic, requiring additional material depending on the clinical impression.

EVALUATION OF RESECTION SPECIMENS

Because there is a growing tendency to perform limb-sparing surgery for sarcomas of all types, the number of major amputation specimens received in the surgical pathology laboratory has markedly decreased compared to one to two decades ago. Most extremity sarcomas are removed with a wide local excision, usually combined with preoperative or postoperative radiotherapy. As with many other surgical specimens, the margins should be marked with permanent ink and blotted dry prior to the dissection of the specimen. Once incised, the gross characteristics of the tumor should be noted. If malignancy is suspected, careful assessment of the tumor as to its surroundings is mandatory. This includes the location of the lesion (e.g., subcutis, muscle) its size, its relation to vital structures (e.g., bone, neurovascular bundle), and the relative amount of necrosis present if it can be judged grossly. Size is important for providing an accurate T descriptor for the surgeon if the lesion is a sarcoma.

Lesions less than 5 cm are classified as T1, whereas those larger than 5 cm are classified as T2. Assessment of the degree of necrosis is important for untreated sarcomas, as this parameter is used in some grading systems. The extent of necrosis in lesions treated with preoperative irradiation or chemotherapy is also important, as it helps the clinical staff to assess the efficacy of preoperative irradiation or chemotherapy, although it does not carry the same implication as necrosis in an untreated lesion. Often, the gross appearance of the tumor is deceptive. Sarcomas may appear to be well circumscribed, for example, whereas some benign tumors suggest an infiltrative or invasive growth pattern. Also, the term *encapsulation* is often misleading and may invite inadequate excision by shelling out or enucleation of the tumor.

There are no dogmatic guidelines for sampling soft tissue tumors; to some extent, sampling is dictated by the specific case. In the case of a known benign lesion, a few representative sections suffice (or the entire lesion if it is small). With a sarcoma, the questions to be answered are different. For example, it may be less important to submit numerous sections for a high-grade sarcoma than for a low-grade lesion in which the sampling is being driven by the need to rule out the presence of high-grade areas. We have generally obtained one section for each centimeter of tumor diameter, with no more than about 10 sections if the lesion appeared more or less uniform. Representative sections of the margins or sections designed to show impingement of vital structures are also obtained. We select blocks for margins judiciously, depending on the gross appearance of the lesion. Lesions several centimeters away from a margin seldom have positive margins microscopically, so extensive margin sampling in these situations is less critical than with excisions containing grossly close margins. One exception is epithelioid sarcoma, a lesion that may be deceptive in its clinical extent grossly. Digital images can be useful for providing visual data as to the orientation of the specimen and sampling sites.

Most specimens are handled adequately as described above. However, in cases in which diagnostic difficulty is anticipated, it is useful to have frozen tissue in reserve in the event ancillary studies are important. It should be emphasized that there are certain tumors in which ancillary studies are essential. Notably, frozen tissue should be reserved for *N-myc* amplification studies of childhood neuroblastoma, and frozen tissue is highly recommended for use in national protocol studies for childhood rhabdomyosarcoma. Although we often perform cytogenetic studies on a wide variety of soft tissue lesions for research purposes, for the most part they do not contribute directly to the diagnosis or therapy; an exception is the differential diagnosis of round cell sarcoma in which the question of an extraskeletal Ewing's sarcoma has been raised but for which the histologic features do not permit an unequivocal diagnosis.

MICROSCOPIC EXAMINATION

The first and most important step in reaching a correct diagnosis is careful scrutiny of conventionally stained sections with light microscopy under low-power magnification. Useful microscopic features that can be identified at this point include the size and depth of the lesion, its relation to overlying skin and underlying fascia, and the nature of the borders (e.g., pushing, infiltrative).

Perhaps the most important question at this juncture is whether the lesion under study is a reactive process or a neoplasm. Reactive lesions may occur in superficial or deep soft tissue but tend to be more frequent in the former location (Table 6–2). A number of histologic features are suggestive of a reactive process. First, some reactive lesions display a distinct zonal quality. For example, in the case of fascial forms of nodular fasciitis and ischemic fasciitis, one encounters a cuff of proliferating fibroblasts that surround a central hypocellular zone of fibrinoid change. Myositis ossificans too displays a zonation that consists of centrifugal maturation of fibroblastic to osteoblastic mesenchyme. Cells comprising reactive lesions often have the appearance of tissue culture fibroblasts with large vesicular nuclei, prominent nucleoli, and striking cytoplasmic basophilia, reflecting the presence of abundant rough endoplasmic reticulum. Although mitotic figures may be numerous, important negative observations include no atypical mitotic figures or nuclear atypia, as one would expect in a sarcoma.

Once satisfied that a reactive lesion can be excluded, the pathologist is justified in proceeding with analysis of the neoplasm. At low power, one is usually struck with the architectural pattern, the appearance of the cells, and the characteristics of the stroma. These characteristics can lend themselves to the development of a number of differential diagnostic categories.

1. *Fasciculated spindle cell tumors.* These lesions comprise a large group of tumors (e.g., fibrosarcoma and synovial sarcoma) characterized by long fascicles (Table 6–3). Cellular schwannoma and fibromatosis must be distinguished from the others because they are nonmetastasizing tumors. Unlike the others, fibromatosis is typically a lesion of low cellularity and nuclear grade.

TABLE 6–2	**REACTIVE LESIONS SIMULATING A SARCOMA**

Nodular fasciitis
Intravascular and cranial fasciitis
Ischemic fasciitis (atypical decubital fibroplasia)
Organ-based fibromyxoid pseudotumors/postoperative spindle cell nodules
Proliferative fasciitis and myositis
Intravascular papillary endothelial hyperplasia
Myositis and panniculitis ossificans
Fibrodysplasia ossificans progressiva
Fibro-osseous pseudotumor of the digits

Cellular schwannoma, unlike the others, is characterized by diffuse, intense S-100 protein immunoreactivity.

2. *Myxoid lesions* (Table 6–4). Although nearly any soft tissue tumor may appear myxoid from time to time, a number of lesions display myxoid features consistently. In adults, the differential diagnosis of myxoid tumors includes myxoma, myxoid malignant fibrous histiocytoma (myxofibrosarcoma), myxoid liposarcoma, and myxoid chondrosarcoma. Analysis of the vascular pattern, degree of nuclear atypia, and occasionally the staining characteristics of the matrix aid in this distinction. For example, an intricate vasculature is a feature of both myxoid liposarcoma and myxoid malignant fibrous histiocytoma, but it is not a feature of myxoid chondrosarcoma or myxoma.

3. *Epithelioid tumors* (Table 6–5). For the differential diagnosis of epithelioid tumors, it is important to rule out metastatic carcinoma, melanoma, and even large-cell lymphomas before assuming that one is dealing with an epithelioid soft tissue tumor. Immunohistochemistry plays a decidedly pivotal role in this regard (discussed in greater detail in Chapter 7).

4. *Round cell tumors* (Table 6–6). Like epithelioid lesions, the differential diagnosis of round cell lesions can be broad; it presupposes excluding non-soft tissue lesions that may mimic a round cell sarcoma (e.g., lymphoma, carcinoma) and is greatly facilitated by the use of immunohistochemistry. It should also be borne in mind that the round cell tumor is not synonymous with round cell sarcoma, as benign lesions (e.g., glomus tumor, giant-cell poor forms of tenosynovial giant cell tumor) also enter the differential diagnosis. In general, the age of the patient helps narrow the possibilities. In children these lesions include neuroblastoma, rhabdomyosarcoma, Ewing's sarcoma/primitive neuroectodermal tumor (ES/PNET), and the rare desmoplastic small round cell tumor. Most of these diagnoses would not be considered in adults.

5. *Pleomorphic tumors* (Table 6–7). The differential diagnosis of pleomorphic sarcomas relies heavily on tumor sampling to identify areas of specific differentiation, sometimes in conjunction with immunohistochemistry. Pleomorphic undifferentiated sarcoma (malignant fibrous histiocytoma) is the most common pleomorphic sarcoma, but it should not be diagnosed in unusual situations unless carcinoma, melanoma, and lymphoma have been excluded.

TABLE 6–3 FASCICULATED SPINDLE CELL TUMORS
Fibromatosis (desmoid tumor)
Cellular schwannoma
Fibrosarcoma
Leiomyosarcoma
Spindle cell rhabdomyosarcoma
Synovial sarcoma
Malignant peripheral nerve sheath tumor

TABLE 6–4 MYXOID SOFT TISSUE LESIONS
Myxoma, cutaneous, intramuscular*
Aggressive angiomyxoma
Myxoid neurofibroma
Neurothekeoma
Myxoid chondroma
Myxoid lipoma (including myxoid spindle cell lipoma)
Lipoblastoma
Ossifying fibromyxoid tumor of soft parts
Myxoid liposarcoma*
Myxoid chondrosarcoma*
Myxoid dermatofibrosarcoma protuberans
Myxoid malignant fibrous histiocytoma (myxofibrosarcoma)*
Botryoid embryonal rhabdomyosarcoma
Myxoid leiomyosarcoma
*Most commonly encountered myxoid tumors.

TABLE 6–5 EPITHELIOID SOFT TISSUE TUMORS
Alveolar soft part sarcoma
Epithelioid sarcoma
Epithelioid angiosarcoma
Epithelioid hemangioendothelioma
Epithelioid hemangioma
Extragastrointestinal stromal tumor
Epithelioid variant of malignant peripheral nerve sheath tumor
Epithelioid schwannoma
Malignant rhabdoid tumor
Malignant mesothelioma
Synovial sarcoma (biphasic and predominantly monophasic epithelial)

TABLE 6–6 ROUND CELL SOFT TISSUE TUMORS
Alveolar rhabdomyosarcoma
Desmoplastic small cell round cell tumor of childhood
Embryonal rhabdomyosarcoma
Extraskeletal Ewing's sarcoma/primitive neuroectodermal tumor (ES/PNET)
Round cell liposarcoma
Cellular forms of extraskeletal myxoid chondrosarcoma
Mesenchymal chondrosarcoma
Small cell osteosarcoma
Malignant hemangiopericytoma
Glomus tumor
Tenosynovial giant cell tumor

TABLE 6–7 PLEOMORPHIC SARCOMAS
Pleomorphic undifferentiated sarcoma (malignant fibrous histiocytoma)
Pleomorphic liposarcoma
Pleomorphic rhabdomyosarcoma
Pleomorphic malignant peripheral nerve sheath tumor
Pleomorphic leiomyosarcoma

6. Hemorrhagic and vascular lesions (Table 6–8). Although sarcomas are generally highly vascularized, the number of soft tissue lesions that present as a hemorrhagic mass is limited and, interestingly, includes many nonvascular (i.e., nonendothelial) tumors. Conversely, many vascular tumors, such as intramuscular hemangiomas, do not have a hemorrhagic appearance. When evaluating vascular lesions, a good starting point is to ascertain whether the lesion is predominantly intravascular or extravascular (Table 6–9).[4] Intravascular lesions are nearly always benign and include primarily organizing thrombus/hematoma followed by the occasional angiocentric vascular tumor (Table 6–10). Extravascular lesions may be benign or malignant; features that favor benignancy include sharp circumscription, lobular arrangement of vessels, and the presence of both large (thick-walled) and small vessels. Angiosarcomas, on the other hand, have irregular margins, lack a lobular arrangement of vessels, and are composed of naked endothelial cells that dissect randomly through tissue planes. They usually occur in adults in the superficial soft tissues.

Further study of the sections can provide important information about the growth pattern, degree of cellularity, and amount and type of matrix formation. Growth patterns vary considerably, ranging from a fascicular, herringbone, or storiform (cartwheel, spiral nebula) pattern in fibroblastic, myofibroblastic, and fibrohistiocytic tumors to plexiform or endocrine patterns, palisading, and Homer-Wright and Flexner-Wintersteiner rosettes in various benign and malignant neural tumors. Biphasic cellular patterns with epithelial and spindle cell areas are characteristic of synovial sarcoma and mesothelioma. Although not all growth patterns permit a definitive diagnosis, they are of great help in narrowing the various differential diagnostic possibilities. Table 6–11 lists some of the most common architectural patterns in soft tissue pathology and relates them to the type of tumor in which they are found most frequently.

Other features, such as the amount and type of extracellular matrix, can be helpful in the differential diagnosis. Abundant myxoid material is produced by a variety of benign and malignant soft tissue tumors, ranging from myxoma and myxoid neurofibroma to myxoid liposarcoma and myxoid chondrosarcoma. It is usually an indication of a relatively slow-growing tumor, and it has been shown that the degree of myxoid change in some malignant tumors is inversely related to the metastatic rate (e.g., myxoid malignant fibrous histiocytoma, myxoid liposarcoma). Abundant collagen formation is also found more often in slowly growing tumors than in rapidly growing ones. However, this finding is not always significant and also may be a prominent feature of some highly malignant sarcomas, such as synovial sarcoma, malignant fibrous histiocytoma, and postirradiation sarcomas. Examination may also provide information as to the presence of calcification and metaplastic changes, especially metaplastic cartilage and bone formation. Table 6–12 summarizes these changes in a variety of soft tissue tumors.

The degree and type of cellular differentiation is best obtained under high-power examination. Lipoblasts, for example, are characterized by the presence of sharply

---

TABLE 6–8   HEMORRHAGIC LESIONS OF SOFT TISSUE

Organizing hemorrhage/hematoma
Aneurysmal fibrous histiocytoma
Angiomatoid fibrous histiocytoma
Angiosarcoma
High-grade sarcomas of various types (occasional)

TABLE 6–10   INTRAVASCULAR TUMORS AND PSEUDOTUMORS

Organizing thrombi and papillary endothelial hyperplasia
Intravascular fasciitis
Spindle cell hemangioma
Epithelioid hemangioendothelioma
Epithelioid hemangioma
Intimal sarcoma

TABLE 6–9   EVALUATION OF VASCULAR LESIONS

Parameter	Benign vascular lesion	Angiosarcoma
Age	All	Adults
Anatomic site	All	Superficial soft tissues usually
Predisposing factors		Lymphedema, radiation
Intravascular vs. extravascular	Either	Virtually always extravascular
Lobular growth	Often, particularly capillary hemangioma	No
Circumscription	Variable	No
Thick-walled vessels	Yes, particularly intramuscular hemangioma, angiomatosis	No

TABLE 6–11	CORRELATION OF GROWTH PATTERN AND TUMOR TYPE
Growth pattern	**Tumor type**
Alveolar	Alveolar soft part sarcoma; alveolar rhabdomyosarcoma
Acinar	Synovial sarcoma; mesothelioma
Biphasic	Synovial sarcoma; mesothelioma
Cording	Epithelioid hemangioendothelioma; myxoid chondrosarcoma; malignant peripheral nerve sheath tumor, epithelioid type; round cell liposarcoma (rare)
Fascicular	Fibromatosis (desmoid tumor); cellular schwannoma; fibrosarcoma; malignant peripheral nerve sheath tumor; synovial sarcoma
Endocrinoid (zellballen)	Paraganglioma; alveolar soft part sarcoma
Lobular, nodular, nest-like	Lipoblastoma; liposarcoma; epithelioid sarcoma; clear-cell sarcoma; fibrous hamartoma of infancy
Palisading	Schwannoma; malignant peripheral nerve sheath tumor; leiomyosarcoma; extragastrointestinal stromal tumor; synovial sarcoma (rare)
Plexiform	Neurofibroma; schwannoma (neurilemmoma); plexiform fibrohistiocytic tumor
Plexiform capillary	Myxoid liposarcoma; myxoid malignant fibrous histiocytoma (myxofibrosarcoma)
Pericytoma	Hemangiopericytoma; solitary fibrous tumor; synovial sarcoma; mesenchymal chondrosarcoma; malignant peripheral nerve sheath tumor; myofibromatosis; juxtaglomerular tumor; liposarcoma (rare)
Rosettes, pseudorosettes	Neuroblastoma; neuroepithelioma; malignant peripheral nerve sheath tumor (rare)
Storiform (cartwheel)	Dermatofibrosarcoma protuberans; fibrous histiocytoma; pleomorphic undifferentiated sarcoma (malignant fibrous histiocytoma); neurofibroma; perineurioma
Tubulopapillary	Mesothelioma

TABLE 6–12	CALCIFICATION, CHONDROID, AND OSSEOUS METAPLASIA IN SOFT TISSUE TUMORS		
Lesion	**Calcification**	**Chondriod**	**Osteoid**
Calcifying aponeurotic fibroma	+	+	–
Fibrodysplasia ossificans progressiva	+	+	+
Giant cell tumor	+	–	+
Hemangioma	+	–	+
Lipoma	+	+	+
Leiomyoma	+	–	–
Pleomorphic undifferentiated sarcoma (malignant fibrous histiocytoma)	–	–	+
Melanocytic schwannoma	+	–	–
Mesenchymal chondrosarcoma	–	+	+
Mesothelioma	–	+	–
Myofibromatosis	+	–	–
Myositis ossificans	–	+	+
Myxoid liposarcoma	–	+	–
Malignant mesenchymoma	–	+	+
Malignant peripheral nerve sheath tumor	–	+	–
Myxoid chondrosarcoma	–	+	–
Ossifying fibromyxoid tumor	–	+	+
Osteosarcoma	+	+	+
Panniculitis ossificans	–	–	+
Synovial sarcoma	+	+	+
Tumoral calcinosis	+	–	–

+, present (variable); –, usually absent.

defined intracellular droplets of lipid and one or more centrally or peripherally placed round or scalloped nuclei. Round and spindle-shaped rhabdomyoblasts can be usually identified in conventionally stained hematoxylineosin sections by their deeply eosinophilic cytoplasm with whorls of eosinophilic fibrillary material near the nucleus and cytoplasmic cross-striations. When interpreting these cells, however, caution is indicated because occasionally entrapped normal or atrophic fat or muscle tissue may closely resemble lipoblasts or rhabdomyoblasts, respectively. Differentiated smooth muscle cells are characterized by their elongated shape, eosinophilic longitudinal fibrils, and long, slender (cigar-shaped) nuclei, often with terminal juxtanuclear vacuoles. Other spindle cells are even more difficult to identify. Distinguishing fibroblasts, myofibroblasts, Schwann cells, and the spindle cells of synovial sarcoma and mesothelioma is more often based on the location and growth pattern

TABLE 6–13	BENIGN SOFT TISSUE TUMORS WITH NUCLEAR ATYPIA

Pleomorphic fibroma of the skin
Fibrous histiocytoma with bizarre cells
Pleomorphic lipoma
Pleomorphic leiomyoma
Ancient schwannoma
Symplastic glomus tumor

than on cytologic characteristics; positive identification of these cells frequently requires immunohistochemical studies or electron microscopic analysis. Cellular inclusions are rare in soft tissue pathology; alveolar soft part sarcoma can be identified by the characteristic intracellular periodic acid-Schiff (PAS)-positive crystalline material, and digital fibromatosis can be identified by eosinophilic inclusions consisting of actin-like microfilaments.

High-power examination is also essential for mitotic counts (e.g., the number of mitotic figures per 10 high-power fields [HPF]). Atypical mitotic figures are rare in benign soft tissue tumors and almost always indicate malignancy. Mitotic counts are useful for diagnosing benign and malignant nerve sheath tumors and tumors of smooth muscle tissue, but they are of little importance for the diagnosis of nodular fasciitis, localized and diffuse giant cell tumors, or malignant fibrous histiocytoma. Although nuclear atypia is more often associated with malignancy, it may occur as a degenerative feature in benign lesions (Table 6–13).

IMMUNOHISTOCHEMISTRY

Hematoxylin-eosin-stained sections represent the mainstay of diagnosis but occasionally must be supported by ancillary techniques. Formerly, histochemistry was commonly used for the diagnosis, but a burgeoning number of antibodies and refinement of the techniques have made immunohistochemistry the ancillary modality of choice for most diagnostic situations. Still, there are a few specific situations in which histochemistry provides information not easily obtained by immunohistochemistry. For example, identification of PAS-positive/diastase-resistant crystals is important for the diagnosis of alveolar soft part sarcoma; distinguishing epithelial mucin from mesenchymal mucin is best done by histochemistry. Although immunohistochemistry has improved the accuracy of diagnosis, one must be aware of the potential problems and limitations when interpreting these stains. Not only is it important to know the specificity of the antibody, one must also be aware of the artifacts that can occur in these preparations, such as non-specific staining of the edge of the tissue section (edge artifact) or necrotic zones,

diffusion or uptake of antigen into adjacent tissues or cells (e.g., myoglobin diffusion from necrotic muscle tissue into histiocytes), and the cross-reactivity of some antibodies (a phenomenon encountered more often with polyclonal than monoclonal antibodies).

To use immunostains in the most effective and cost-efficient way, it is useful to have an algorithmic approach in mind and to use these reagents in panels (see Chapter 7). For example, a panel of antibodies to differentiate carcinomas, melanomas, sarcomas, and lymphomas from one another would be selected before a series of B- and T-cell markers. In our experience, immunohistochemistry is an important if not obligate part of the work-up of certain soft tissue lesions, such as round cell sarcomas, epithelioid tumors, and pleomorphic tumors, particularly in the skin.

ELECTRON MICROSCOPY

Electron microscopy plays a far less prominent role in the diagnosis of soft tissue lesions than previously. This change is explained not only by the growing popularity of immunohistochemistry but also by the high cost and labor-intensive nature of electron microscopy, the relative inexperience of most pathologists in interpreting these studies, and the sampling issues inherent in this technique. Moreover, only a few ultrastructural markers lead to a specific histologic diagnosis, such as melanosomes in clear-cell sarcoma and malignant melanoma and Weibel-Palade bodies in vascular tumors. In most instances, the pathologist is called on to evaluate a constellation of less specific features and to decide, based on their frequency or prominence, the probability of a certain diagnosis, recognizing that a loss of differentiation by light microscopy is usually paralleled by a similar loss ultrastructurally.

Traditionally, electron microscopy has been most useful in the diagnosis of round cell sarcoma, but it should be pointed out that this is also the area in which immunohistochemistry and cytogenetics have made important strides. It is now rare that a diagnosis hinges on the results of electron microscopic analysis alone. Still, electron microscopy has yielded interesting information regarding the participation of myofibroblasts in many benign and malignant soft tissue lesions.

DIAGNOSTIC NOMENCLATURE

Even with complete sampling and ancillary studies, it may not be possible to classify all sarcomas accurately. In our consultation practice, approximately 10% of all sarcomas do not lend themselves to a definitive classification. Nonetheless, it is often possible for the pathologist to provide the clinician with sufficient information so therapy can proceed unencumbered. For example, when evaluating moderately differentiated spindle cell sarcomas, one cannot always distinguish a malignant peripheral nerve sheath tumor from a fibrosarcoma. Yet this distinction is not clinically important if the pathologist can assure the clinician that the lesion is malignant and can provide a histologic grade. Likewise, it is not worthwhile to labor exhaustively over classifying a pleomorphic sarcoma when the therapy does not differ. Thus, in these ambiguous diagnostic situations, there is no substitute for a constructive dialogue among the surgeon, pathologist, and oncologist to define the therapeutically relevant pathologic information. This has led to a managerial classification of soft tissue lesions (Table 6–14).[5] Such a system emphasizes the expected behavior rather than the histologic type. When the pathologist cannot be certain of the exact diagnosis, a managerial system can bridge the gap. For example, a low-grade myxoid sarcoma that does not seem to fall clearly into a specific diagnostic category could be labeled "low-grade myxoid sarcoma" with a comment that local recurrence rather than metastasis would be the expected behavior. The diagnosis "myxoid tumor with locally recurring potential" expresses the same information.

STANDARDIZED REPORTING OF SOFT TISSUE SARCOMAS

To convey the pathologic findings to clinicians unambiguously, we have found it useful to employ a checklist that can be translated into a standardized report (Table 6–15) using guidelines recently proposed by the Association of Directors of Anatomic and Surgical Pathology[6] and by the College of American Pathologists.[7] The three most important pieces of information the pathologist provides in a surgical pathology report, apart from the diagnosis of "sarcoma," are the grade, size, and depth of the lesion; each is an independent prognostic variable that figures prominently in the clinical stage (see Chapter 1).[8]

Grading system. The choice of a grading system is largely one of institutional, regional, or national preference, as all reported grading systems can be correlated with outcome (see Chapter 1).[9,10] The report should make clear the number of tiers in the grading system; for example, it is important to know whether a lesion is grade 2 of a four-tiered system or a three-tiered system. Alternatively, some prefer the simple labels "low grade" or "high grade," particularly when dealing with a core needle biopsy (see above).

TABLE 6–15	SARCOMA CASE CHECKLIST FOR STANDARD REPORTING OF RESECTION SPECIMENS

Tumor site
  Specimen type
    Intralesional, marginal, wide, radical, other
  Histologic type
  Grade
    System used (e.g., FNCLCC, NCI)
    Specify grade
  Size
    Three dimensions, if possible or greatest diameter (in centimeters)

Tumor depth
  Superficial (dermal; subcutaneous/suprafascial)
  Deep (fascial, subfascial, intramuscular, retroperitoneal, mediastinal, body cavity, head and neck)

Margins
  Positive/negative. Indicate distance for all margins <1.5 cm

Nodes
  Positive/negative

Necrosis
  Absent/present (microscopic)/present (macroscopic – approximate %)

Preresection treatment
  No therapy, chemotherapy, radiation, unknown

Ancillary studies
  State if tissue was sent for cytogenetics, molecular diagnostics, flow cytometry, or tissue banking

TNM code (see Chapter 1 for TNM parameters)

TABLE 6–14	MANAGERIAL DISEASE CATEGORIES			
Clinical status	**Behavior**	**Usual therapy**	**Examples**
Benign	Local excision usually curative; rare recurrence but not destructive; no metastasis	Local excision	Histologically benign tumors and pseudotumors
Borderline or intermediate	Local recurrence common and often destructive; metastases vary from none to few	Extended local to wide excision depending on circumstances	Fibromatosis (nonmetastasizing); dermatofibrosarcoma protuberans (rare metastasis)
Malignant	Local recurrence common; metastasis common; systemic disease sometimes present at onset	Wide excision; possible adjuvant therapy	Malignant fibrous histiocytoma

Modified from Kempson RL, Hendrickson MR. In: Weiss SW, Brooks JSJ, eds. An approach to the diagnosis of soft tissue tumors. In: Soft tissue tumors. Baltimore: Williams & Wilkins; 1996, with permission.

Tumor. The maximum dimensions of a tumor are given in metric units and in three dimensions if possible.

Location and depth. These tumor parameters are addressed by indicating whether it is superficial (above the fascia), deep (below the fascia or in muscle), or in a body cavity. For purposes of staging, deep lesions are defined as those in muscle, a body cavity, or the head and neck.[8]

Margins. It is believed that sarcomas excised with a less than 1.5–2.0-cm margin are prone to local recurrence[11] unless they are bordered by unbreached fascia or periosteum.[12] For this reason we comment on all positive margins (ink on the tumor) and the distance and location of all margins less than 1.5 cm. Positive margins imply a greater chance for distant metastasis with high-risk extremity sarcomas.[13]

Necrosis. Because necrosis is an integral part of some grading systems, it is useful to indicate whether necrosis is absent, microscopically present, or macroscopically present. If macroscopically present, we attempt to give some estimate of the amount. It should be kept in mind, however, that grading systems that rely on assessment of necrosis imply examination of surgical specimens that have not been altered by preoperative irradiation or chemotherapy. Once therapy is given, it is difficult to know to what extent necrosis is spontaneous versus therapy-induced. Nonetheless, if preoperative irradiation or chemotherapy has been undertaken, clinicians usually find that a statement as to the amount of viable tumor that remains is helpful.

Ancillary studies. It is useful if the report indicates what tissue has been archived for future use (tissue bank) or referred to other laboratories for additional tests or consultation.

Optional information. There are several other features on which pathologists may comment, including the mitotic rate, vascular invasion, nature of the margin (e.g., circumscribed, infiltrating), presence of an inflammatory infiltrate, and a preexisting benign lesion (e.g., sarcoma arising in a neurofibroma). None translates directly into patient management, and therefore they are considered optional in the report. In most instances, however, mitotic activity is assessed prior to arriving at a histologic grade.

REFERENCES

1. Heslin MJ, Lewis JJ, Woodruff JM. Core needle biopsy for diagnosis of extremity soft tissue sarcoma. Ann Surg Oncol 1997; 44:425.
2. Deyrup AT, Weiss SW. Grading of soft tissue sarcomas: the challenge of providing precise information in an imprecise world. Histopathol 2006; 48:42.
3. Kandel RA, Bell RS, Wunder JS, et al. Comparison between a 2 and 3 grade system in predicting metastatic-free survival in extremity soft tissue sarcoma. J Surg Oncol 1999; 72:77.
4. Weiss SW. The Vincent McGovern Memorial Lecture: Vascular tumors: a deductive approach to diagnosis. Surg Pathol 1989; 2:185.
5. Kempson RL, Hendrickson MR. In: Weiss SW, Brooks JSJ, eds. An approach to the diagnosis of soft tissue tumors. In: Soft tissue tumors. Baltimore: Williams & Wilkins; 1996.
6. Association of Directors of Anatomic and Surgical Pathology. Recommendations for the reporting of soft tissue sarcomas. Mod Pathol 1998; 11:1257.
7. Rubin BP, Fletcher CDM, Inwards CY, et al. CAP protocol for soft tissue and bone. Arch Pathol Lab Med 2006; 130(11):1616.
8. AJCC cancer staging handbook, 5th edn. Philadelphia: Lippincott Williams & Wilkins; 1998:139–146.
9. Coindre J-M, Terrier P, Bui NB, et al. Prognostic factors in adult patients with locally controlled soft tissue sarcomas: a study on 546 patients from the French Federation of Cancer Centers Sarcoma Group. J Clin Oncol 1996; 14:869.
10. Guillou L, Coindre J-M, Bonichon F, et al. Comparative study of the National Cancer Institute and French Federation of Cancer Centers Sarcoma Group grading systems in a population of 410 adult patients with soft tissue sarcomas. J Clin Oncol 1997; 15:350.
11. Pisters PWT, Leung DHY, Woodruff J, et al. Analysis of prognostic factors in 1,041 patients with localized soft tissue sarcomas of the extremities. J Clin Oncol 1996; 14:1679.
12. Rydholm A, Rooser B. Surgical margins for soft tissue sarcoma. J Bone Joint Surg [Am] 1987; 69:1074.
13. Heslin MJ, Woodruff JM, Brennan MF. Prognostic significance of a positive microscopic margin in high risk extremity soft tissue sarcoma: implications for management. J Clin Oncol 1996; 14:473.

IMMUNOHISTOCHEMISTRY FOR ANALYSIS OF SOFT TISSUE TUMORS

Andrew L. Folpe and Allen M. Gown

CHAPTER CONTENTS

Immunohistochemistry is the use of antibody-based reagents for localization of specific epitopes in tissue sections. In recent years, immunohistochemistry has become a powerful tool to assist the surgical pathologist in many clinically critical settings. It is important to recognize that immunohistochemistry has two components, each with its own strengths and weaknesses. These components may be thought of as the "hardware" (i.e., antibodies, detection systems) and the "software" (i.e., analytic processes). No matter how selective the antibodies or how powerful the detection system, the method fails if the analytic tools are inadequate. This chapter focuses on the antibody component of the hardware and the ways in which immunohistochemistry assists in the diagnosis of soft tissue neoplasms.

It cannot be overemphasized that immunohistochemistry is an adjunctive diagnostic technique to traditional morphologic methods in soft tissue pathology, as in any other area of surgical pathology. It is critical to recognize that the diagnosis of many soft tissue tumors does not require immunohistochemistry (e.g., adipocytic tumors), and that there are no markers or combinations of markers

that will distinguish benign from malignant tumors (e.g., the distinction of nodular fasciitis from leiomyosarcoma). Furthermore, reliable specific markers do not yet exist for certain mesenchymal cell types (e.g., osteoblasts, chondroblasts) and their tumors, and techniques other than immunohistochemistry, such as ultrastructural, cytogenetic, or molecular genetic study may prove more valuable in this setting. Lastly, it is important to acknowledge that a subset of soft tissue tumors defy classification, even with exhaustive immunohistochemistry, ultrastructural, and genetic study.

The expression of certain antigens, or clusters of antigens, is characteristic of some tumors. Whereas there are thousands of monoclonal and polyclonal antibodies available to assist in tumor diagnosis, only a small subset has proved to be of practical value in the diagnosis of soft tissue neoplasms. Tables 7–1 and 7–2 present an overview of the markers discussed in the sections below. The question marks highlight the gaps in our understanding of the cellular biology of many soft tissue tumors.

INTERMEDIATE FILAMENTS

The intermediate filaments comprise the major component of the cytoskeleton and consist of five major subgroups (vimentin, cytokeratins, desmin, neurofilaments, glial fibrillary acidic protein [GFAP]) and a small number of minor subgroups (e.g., nestin, peripherin).[1-3] Ultrastructurally, the intermediate filaments appear as wavy unbranched filaments that often occupy a perinuclear location in the cell. While it was originally thought that intermediate filament expression was restricted to specific cell types (e.g., cytokeratins in carcinomas, vimentin in sarcomas), this is now recognized as an oversimplification. The following sections on intermediate filaments concentrate not only on the normal pattern of expression of these proteins but also on the situations in which intermediate filaments show "anomalous expression."

Vimentin

Vimentin, a 57-kDa intermediate filament protein, is expressed in all mesenchymal cells. Vimentin is ubiqui-

TABLE 7–1	COMMON IMMUNOHISTOCHEMICAL MARKERS
Antibodies to	**Expressed by**
Cytokeratins	Carcinomas, epithelioid sarcoma, synovial sarcoma, some angiosarcomas and leiomyosarcomas, mesothelioma, extrarenal rhabdoid tumor
Vimentin	Sarcomas, melanoma, some carcinomas and lymphomas
Desmin	Benign and malignant smooth and skeletal muscle tumors
Glial fibrillary acidic protein	Gliomas, some schwannomas
Neurofilaments	Neuroblastic tumors
Pan-muscle actin	Benign and malignant smooth and skeletal muscle tumors, myofibroblastic tumors and pseudotumors
Smooth muscle actin	Benign and malignant smooth muscle tumors, myofibroblastic tumors and pseudotumors
Myogenic nuclear regulatory proteins (myogenin, MyoD1)	Rhabdomyosarcoma
S-100 protein	Melanoma, benign and malignant peripheral nerve sheath tumors, cartilaginous tumors, normal adipose tissue, Langerhans cells
Epithelial membrane antigen	Carcinomas, epithelioid sarcoma, synovial sarcoma, perineurioma, meningioma, anaplastic large cell lymphoma
CD31	Benign and malignant vascular tumors
von Willebrand factor (factor VIII-related protein)	Benign and malignant vascular tumors
CD34	Benign and malignant vascular tumors, solitary fibrous tumor, hemangiopericytoma, epithelioid sarcoma, dermatofibrosarcoma protuberans
CD99 (MIC2 gene product)	Ewing's sarcoma/primitive neuroectodermal tumor, some rhabdomyosarcomas, some synovial sarcomas, lymphoblastic lymphoma, mesenchymal chondrosarcoma, small cell osteosarcoma
CD45 (leukocyte common antigen)	Non-Hodgkin lymphoma
CD30 (Ki-1)	Anaplastic large cell lymphoma, embryonal carcinoma
CD68	Macrophages, fibrohistiocytic tumors, granular cell tumors, various sarcomas, melanomas, carcinomas
Melanosome-specific antigens (HMB-45, Melan-A, tyrosinase, microphthalmia transcription factor)	Melanoma, PEComa, clear cell sarcoma, melanotic schwannoma
MDM2/CDK4	Atypical lipomatous tumor and dedifferentiated liposarcoma
Claudin-1	Perineurioma, synovial sarcoma, epithelioid sarcoma, some Ewing's sarcoma/PNET
Glut-1	Perineurioma, infantile hemangioma
INI1	Expression lost in extrarenal rhabdoid tumor and epithelioid sarcoma
Protein kinase C θ	GIST
Bcl-2	Synovial sarcoma, solitary fibrous tumor, other spindle cell tumors

TABLE 7–2	SPECIFIC TUMOR TYPES, NORMAL COUNTERPARTS, AND USEFUL MARKERS

Tumor type	**Normal cell counterpart**	**Useful marker(s)**
Angiosarcoma	Endothelium	CD31, CD34, FLI-1, von Willebrand factor, ulex lectin
Leiomyosarcoma	Smooth muscle	Muscle (smooth) actins, desmin, caldesmon, myosin heavy chain
Rhabdomyosarcoma	Skeletal muscle	MyoD1, myogenin; muscle (sarcomeric) actins; desmin
Ewing's sarcoma/PNET	?	CD99 (p30/32-MIC2), FLI-1
Synovial sarcoma	?	Cytokeratin, EMA
Epithelioid sarcoma	?	Cytokeratin, CD34, INI1
Malignant peripheral nerve sheath tumor	Nerve sheath (e.g., Schwann cell, perineurial cell)	S-100, CD57, NGF receptor, EMA, claudin-1, Glut-1
Liposarcoma	Adipocyte	S-100 protein, MDM2, CDK4
Chondrosarcoma	Chondrocyte	S-100 protein
Osteogenic sarcoma	Osteocyte	Osteocalcin
Kaposi sarcoma	Endothelium	CD31, CD34, VEGFR3, LANA
Myofibroblastic lesions (e.g., nodular fasciitis)	Myofibroblast	Smooth muscle actins
Gastrointestinal stromal tumor	Interstitial cells of Cajal	CD117a (c-kit), CD34, protein kinase C θ
Hemangiopericytoma, solitary fibrous tumor	?	CD34, bcl-2
Glomus tumors	Glomus cell	Smooth muscle actins, type IV collagen
Angiomatoid (malignant) fibrous histiocytoma	?	Desmin, EMA, CD68
Alveolar soft part sarcoma	?	TFE3
Perivascular epithelioid cell neoplasms	?	Smooth muscle actins, melanocytic markers

tously expressed in all cells during early embryogenesis and is gradually replaced in many cells by type-specific intermediate filaments.[1,4] In some mesenchymal tissues vimentin is typically co-expressed along with the cell type-specific intermediate filaments (e.g., desmin and vimentin co-expression in muscle cells, vimentin and GFAP in some Schwann cells). Reversion to a pattern of vimentin expression is typically seen in cultured cells of many lineages.[5,6] Vimentin is also commonly expressed by sarcomatoid carcinomas at any site, an unfortunate fact that greatly limits its utility in the immunohisto-chemical distinction of carcinomas from sarcomas.[7-11] As a diagnostic reagent, antibodies to vimentin are of greatest utility in the diagnosis of carcinomas of uncertain primary site, where strong co-expression may be a clue to renal, endometrial, and thyroid carcinomas.[12] Vimentin immunoreactivity has been touted as a good marker of tissue preservation. However, vimentin expression, similar to that of all the intermediate filaments, is rather hardy and may remain present in tissues in which all other immunoreactivity has been lost.[13] The absence of vimentin expression may occasionally be a clue to the diagnosis of rare vimentin-negative mesenchymal tumors, such as alveolar soft part sarcoma and perivascular epithelioid cell neoplasms.[14,15]

Cytokeratins

Cytokeratins, the most complex members of the intermediate filament protein family, are a collection of more than 20 proteins. The cytokeratins may be grouped by their molecular weights (40–67 kDa) into acidic and basic subfamilies, or by their usual pattern of expression in simple or complex epithelium (Fig. 7–1). In practice, the cytokeratins are most commonly thought of in terms of low-molecular-weight cytokeratins (generally cytokeratins 8, 18, and 19) and high-molecular-weight cytokeratins (generally cytokeratins 1, 5, 10, and 14). Cytokeratins are highly sensitive markers for identifying carcinomas and are generally employed as markers distinguishing epithelial from nonepithelial tumors (i.e., lymphomas, sarcomas, melanomas) (Fig. 7–2). Over the past decade it has become abundantly clear that cytokeratin expression is not restricted to carcinomas.

Sarcomas with "true" epithelial differentiation: epithelioid sarcoma and synovial sarcoma

Among the sarcomas there are two patterns of cytokeratin expression. A small subset of sarcomas display true epithelial differentiation as defined by usual expression of cytokeratin and other epithelial proteins such as the desmoplakins and occludin (e.g., synovial sarcomas and epithelioid sarcomas).[16,17] Additionally, there is a larger group of tumors that occasionally display "anomalous" cytokeratin expression (i.e., cytokeratin expression by

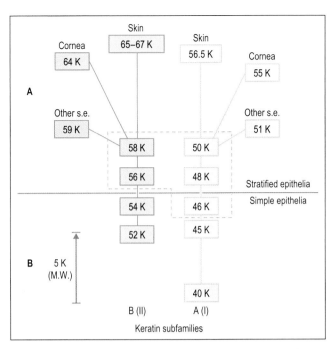

FIGURE 7–1 Subcategorization of acidic **(A)** and basic **(B)** cytokeratin subgroups within various tissues. (Modified from Cooper D, Schermer A, Sun TT. Classification of human epithelium and their neoplasms using monoclonal antibodies to keratins: strategies, applications, and limitations. Lab Invest 1985; 52:243, with permission.)

cells and tumors without true epithelial differentiation). Synovial sarcomas and epithelioid sarcomas are the best, if not the only, examples of sarcomas manifesting true epithelial differentiation (Fig. 7–3). Expression of both low and high-molecular-weight cytokeratin isoforms is seen in both synovial sarcoma and epithelioid sarcoma, confirming the presence of true epithelial differentiation.[18,19] Antibodies to specific cytokeratins, such as cytokeratins 7 and 19 for synovial sarcoma and cytokeratins 5/6 in epithelioid sarcoma, may also be diagnostically useful in selected cases.[19-21]

Anomalous cytokeratin expression

Anomalous cytokeratin expression is typically characterized by immunostaining (even under optimal technical conditions) in only a subset of the target cell population. In those cells, cytokeratin is present in only a portion of the cytoplasm, often yielding a "perinuclear" or "dot-like" pattern of immunostaining. This dot-like pattern is not always an indication of anomalous cytokeratin; however, as it is typically seen in some neuroendocrine carcinomas, including small cell carcinomas and Merkel cell tumors, and in extrarenal rhabdoid tumors (Fig. 7–4).[22-24] In addition, it is rare to find cytokeratins other than those corresponding to the Moll catalog 8 and 18 (corresponding to positivity with antibodies CAM5.2 or

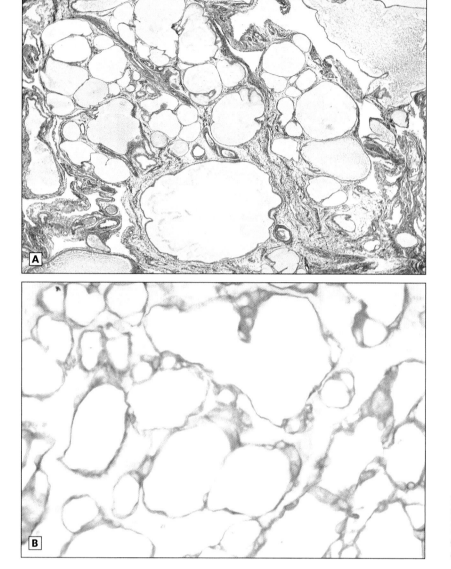

FIGURE 7–2 Cystic mesothelioma **(A)** immunostained for cytokeratin **(B)**. Demonstration of strong cytokeratin expression is useful for distinguishing this entity from cystic lymphangioma.

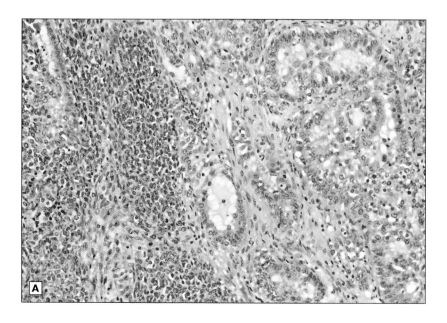

FIGURE 7–3 Biphasic synovial sarcoma with an evolving poorly differentiated cell population **(A)**. Poorly differentiated synovial sarcoma

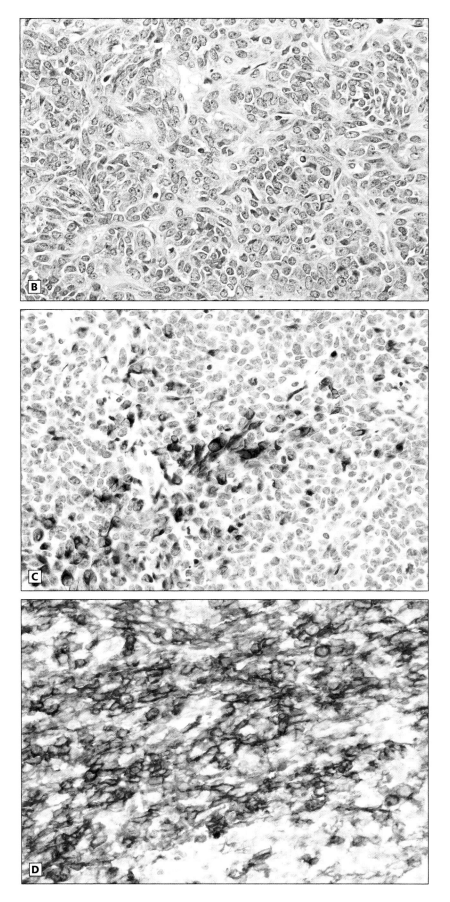

FIGURE 7–3 Continued. **(B)** demonstrating focal expression of high-molecular-weight cytokeratins. **(C)** Expression of cytokeratin in synovial sarcomas may be focal, and some express only high-molecular-weight isoforms. Many poorly differentiated synovial sarcomas also express CD99 **(D)**, and it is important not to mistake them for primitive neuroectodermal tumors.

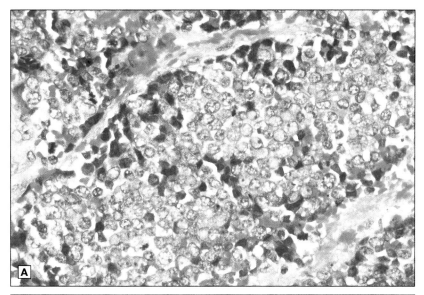

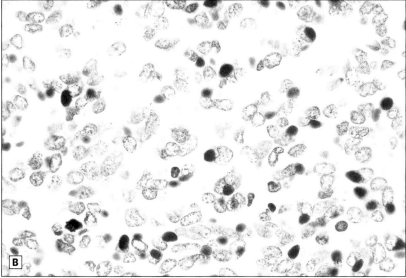

FIGURE 7–4 Merkel cell carcinoma **(A)** demonstrating characteristic expression of cytokeratin in a dot-like pattern **(B)**. Dot-like expression of cytokeratin and other intermediate filaments is not specific for neuroendocrine carcinomas and may be seen in any "small, blue round cell." Dot-like expression may also be a clue to anomalous intermediate filament expression.

35βH11) in tumors manifesting anomalous cytokeratin expression.[16]

Contrary to some earlier suggestions, anomalous cytokeratin expression is not a universal feature of sarcomas. It is, instead, a feature of a limited subset of nonepithelial tumors, particularly smooth muscle tumors, melanomas, and endothelial cell tumors; as such, it may serve as a clue to the diagnosis of these tumors. Interestingly, the normal cell counterparts of some of these tumors (i.e., smooth muscle cells and endothelial cells) have been found to express cytokeratins in nonmammalian species,[25] and in our experience are frequently cytokeratin-positive in routinely processed sections.

Smooth muscle cells and smooth muscle tumors

Frozen sections of the smooth muscle cell-rich myometrium of the uterus (along with myocardial cells) were first reported to "react with" various anti-cytokeratin antibodies. Brown et al.[26] and Norton et al.[27] verified these findings using slightly different techniques, although Norton et al. failed to find corroborative biochemical evidence of cytokeratin expression by these smooth muscle cells. Biochemical documentation of true "anomalous" cytokeratin expression of cytokeratins 8 and 18 was first presented by Gown and colleagues,[28] in which immunostaining was corroborated by Western blots; it was further documented by two-color immunofluorescence studies of myometrial smooth muscle cells grown in vitro. Subsequent studies have shown that at least 30% of leiomyosarcomas manifest cytokeratin.[29–31]

Melanomas

Despite the fact that many studies completed during the mid-1980s concluded that melanomas were vimentin-positive, cytokeratin-negative tumors,[32,33] Zarbo et al. first confirmed the cytokeratin positivity of many melanomas and demonstrated the positive immunostaining as a function of tissue preparation and fixation (with 21% of cases positive in frozen sections but far fewer in formalin-fixed, paraffin-embedded sections).[33] Zarbo et al. also performed one- and two-dimensional gel electrophoresis with immunoblotting, confirming that cytokeratin 8 was expressed by the tumor cell population.[33] Anomalous cytokeratin expression is generally a feature of metastatic, but not primary, melanomas.[34]

Angiosarcomas

Early reports suggested that vascular tumors manifesting epithelioid histologic features (e.g., epithelioid hemangioendothelioma and epithelioid angiosarcoma) express cytokeratin in most cases (Fig. 7–5).[35–39] The largest published series of angiosarcomas of deep soft tissue has documented cytokeratin expression in about one-third of cases.[40]

Small blue round cell tumors

A surprising number of tumors in the category of "small, blue round cell tumors" of childhood typically co-express cytokeratin in a pattern much like that of anomalous cytokeratin expression. These tumors include Ewing's sarcoma/primitive neuroectodermal tumor (PNET),[41–44] rhabdomyosarcoma,[45,46] Wilms' tumor,[47,48] and desmoplastic small round cell tumor of childhood.[49,50] Expression of low-molecular-weight cytokeratin isoforms may be seen in nearly 25% of Ewing's sarcoma/primitive neuroectodermal tumors, usually confined to less than 20% of the neoplastic cells;[41,42,44] expression of high-molecular-weight cytokeratins is far less common and is restricted to the rare "adamantinoma-like" variant of Ewing's sarcoma/primitive neuroectodermal tumor (Fig. 7–6).[44]

Cytokeratin expression in other sarcomas

The literature is replete with reports of cytokeratin expression in other sarcomas, including malignant fibrous histiocytoma,[51–54] chondrosarcoma,[55,56] osteosarcoma,[57,58] and malignant peripheral nerve sheath tumors.[21,59] Nonetheless, in our experience cytokeratin expression in these tumors is exceedingly rare.

It is important to remember that immunoreactivity and true antigen expression are not necessarily synonymous.[60] Several factors can theoretically account for positive cytokeratin immunostaining in tumors without true cytokeratin expression. This includes the use of antibodies at inappropriately high concentrations,[61,62] potentially altered specificities following the use of heat-induced epitope retrieval techniques ("antigen retrieval"),[61,62] and

the cross-reactivity of anti-cytokeratin antibodies with other proteins.[63] It is also important to distinguish reactive cytokeratin-positive cells, such as submesothelial fibroblasts, from the neoplastic cell population (Fig. 7–7). By employing an approach to immunohistochemistry that includes use of a panel of antibodies, the pathologist can generally avoid misinterpretation that might result from "misbehavior" of one antibody.

EPITHELIAL MEMBRANE ANTIGEN

Epithelial membrane antigen (EMA) is an incompletely characterized antigen that is present in a group of carbohydrate-rich, protein-poor, high-molecular-weight molecules present on the surface of many normal types of epithelium, including those in the pancreas, stomach, intestine, salivary gland, respiratory tract, urinary tract, and breast.[64,65] Among normal mesenchymal cells, EMA expression is limited to perineurial cells[66–69] and meningeal cells.[69,70] There are a limited number of uses for EMA in sarcoma diagnosis. EMA expression is a more sensitive, but less specific, marker of poorly differentiated synovial sarcomas; it may be helpful in cases with only focal (or absent) cytokeratin expression.[18] Perineuriomas and malignant peripheral nerve sheath tumors with perineurial differentiation are characterized by a sometimes subtle expression of EMA along cell processes, as well as by type IV collagen expression (Fig. 7–8).[71–75] Ectopic meningiomas, like their meningeal counterparts, are characterized by EMA and vimentin expression in the absence of cytokeratin expression.[69,70] Patchy expression of EMA (along with desmin and CD68) is seen in roughly 50% of angiomatoid fibrous histiocytomas.[76] More recently, however, with the widespread use of epitope retrieval techniques, it has been our experience that patchy EMA immunoreactivity may be seen in a somewhat broader range of mesenchymal tumors, emphasizing the need to employ antibodies to EMA as part of a panel of immunostains.

MARKERS OF MUSCLE DIFFERENTIATION

There are three types of muscle differentiation. The first is skeletal muscle differentiation, as recapitulated in rhabdomyoma and rhabdomyosarcoma. The second is "true" smooth muscle differentiation, reflected in leiomyoma and leiomyosarcoma. The third is "partial" smooth muscle differentiation, as seen in the myofibroblasts that constitute a significant population of cells in healing wounds and the stromal reaction to tumors. There is also a subset of soft tissue tumors (e.g., nodular fasciitis and myofibroblastoma), the phenotype of which bears great resemblance to myofibroblasts rather than true

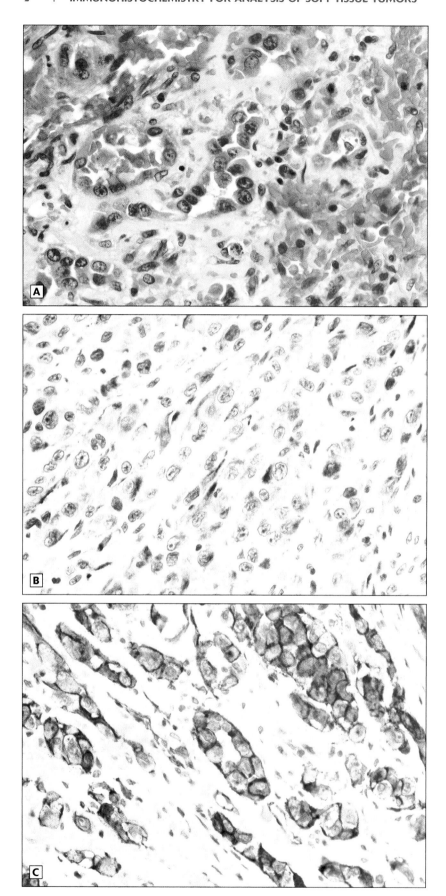

FIGURE 7–5 Epithelioid angiosarcoma **(A)** with strong expression of low-molecular-weight cytokeratin **(B)**. Vascular tumors, particularly epithelioid ones, commonly express low-molecular-weight cytokeratins and may be mistaken for carcinoma. Expression of CD31 **(C)**, a highly specific marker of endothelium, serves to distinguish keratin-positive angiosarcoma from carcinoma or epithelioid sarcoma.

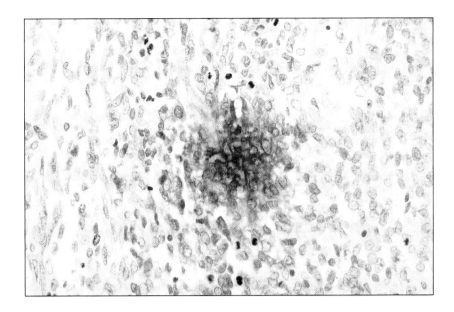

FIGURE 7–6 Overlay of dandruff on a slide, creating apparent focal cytokeratin expression.

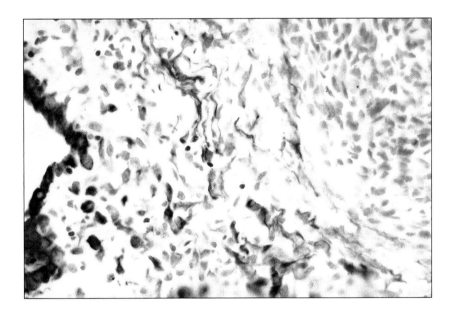

FIGURE 7–7 Low-molecular-weight cytokeratin expression in mesothelium (top) and in spindled submesothelial fibroblasts (middle). Expression of cytokeratin in these reactive submesothelial fibroblasts should be distinguished from cytokeratin expression in the adjacent infiltrating sarcoma (bottom).

smooth muscle cells. The principal markers of muscle differentiation are the intermediate filament desmin, the various actin isoforms, and the myogenic regulatory proteins.

Desmin

Desmin is the intermediate filament protein associated with both smooth and skeletal muscle differentiation; it is rarely expressed by myofibroblasts and their corresponding tumors. In skeletal muscle desmin is localized to the Z-zone between the myofibrils, where it presumably serves as binding material for the contractile apparatus.[77] In smooth muscle it is associated with cytoplasmic dense bodies and subplasmalemmal dense plaques.

Desmin may also be expressed by nonmuscle cells, including the fibroblastic reticulum cell of the lymph node,[78,79] the submesothelial fibroblast,[80] and endometrial stromal cells.[81] It is among the earliest muscle structural genes expressed in the myotome of embryos and has been regarded by some as the best single marker for the diagnosis of poorly differentiated rhabdomyosarcoma.[82,83] Although the early literature on desmin questioned its sensitivity in formalin-fixed, deparaffinized tissue sections,[84–86] more recent studies have borne out its excellent sensitivity. In our experience, with the use of heat-induced epitope retrieval techniques and modern antibodies such as D33, desmin is the most sensitive marker of skeletal and smooth muscle differentiation in terms of both the fraction of tumors so identified and the

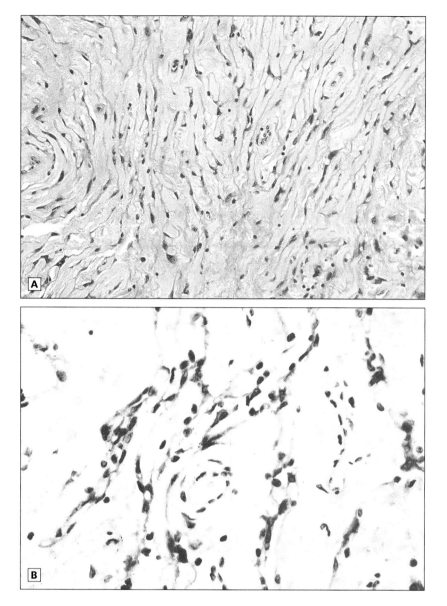

FIGURE 7–8 Malignant perineurioma **(A)** expressing epithelial membrane antigen **(B)**.

fraction of tumor cells in given tumors that are positive. Desmin expression is present in nearly 100% of rhabdomyosarcomas of all subtypes, including very poorly differentiated ones (Fig. 7–9).[73,86–93]

Desmin expression is apparently not as specific for muscle tumors as was originally thought, as it has also been described in Ewing's sarcoma/primitive neuroectodermal tumors,[44,94] desmoplastic small round cell tumors,[49,50,95] neuroblastoma,[96] mesothelial cells and tumors,[97] the blastemal component of Wilms' tumor,[98] giant cell tumors of the tendon sheath,[99] and ossifying fibromyxoid tumors of soft parts;[100] in none of these contexts is there thought to be true muscle differentiation (Fig. 7–10). Expression of desmin along with EMA and CD68, in the absence of other muscle markers, is highly characteristic of angiomatoid fibrous histiocytomas (Fig. 7–11).[76,101]

Actin

Actin, a ubiquitous protein, is expressed by all cell types; high concentrations of actins and unique isoforms, however, help make actin a marker of muscle differentiation. In general, actins can be grouped into muscle and nonmuscle isoforms, which differ by only a few amino acids in a protein with a molecular weight of 43000. It has, nevertheless, been possible to generate antibodies specific to muscle actins versus nonmuscle actins and to specific actin isotypes with respect to the various muscle types (e.g., smooth muscle versus skeletal muscle).[11,102–105] Although an early body of literature speaks to the "specificity" of anti-actin polyclonal antibodies for muscle cells, in most of these studies it is a quantitative rather than a qualitative phenomenon: that is, muscle cells have far more actin than many other cells, and demonstration

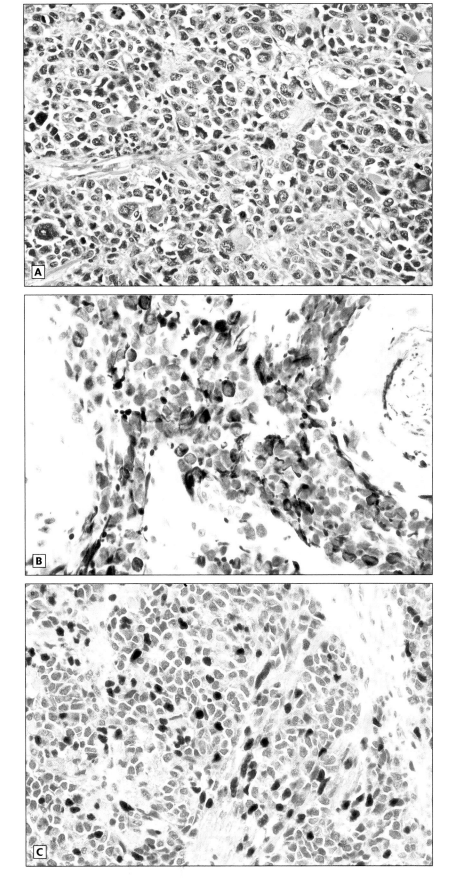

FIGURE 7–9 Alveolar rhabdomyosarcoma **(A)** demonstrating intense expression of desmin **(B)**. Although desmin is a highly sensitive marker of myogenous sarcomas, it may also be expressed in a variety of nonmyogenous tumors. The most specific markers of rhabdomyosarcoma are antibodies to myogenic nuclear regulatory proteins, such as MyoD1 **(C)** or myogenin. Only a nuclear pattern of expression of these proteins should be accepted.

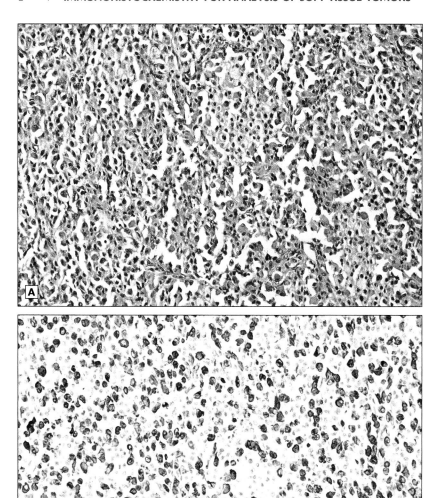

FIGURE 7–10 Diffuse-type tenosynovial giant cell tumor with a prominent population of large eosinophilic cells **(A)**. These eosinophilic cells may show intense positivity with antibodies to desmin **(B)** and may result in an erroneous diagnosis of rhabdomyosarcoma. Such desmin-positive cells are present in approximately 40% of tenosynovial giant cell tumors.

of positivity is determined on this basis alone. Whereas there are monoclonal antibodies that can identify all actin isoforms (i.e., the C4 clone[102]), given the sensitive immunohistochemical techniques available, this antibody cannot be used to distinguish muscle from nonmuscle actins. The antibody HHF35, which has been widely used to identify muscle cells and tumors, displays specificity for all muscle (versus nonmuscle) actins.[104,105] Antibody 1A4 is a monoclonal antibody which specifically identifies smooth muscle actin isoforms; it can thus distinguish smooth from skeletal muscle cells and tumors.[103] Smooth muscle actin isoforms are also expressed by myofibroblasts, and the characteristic pattern of actin expression in these cells may help distinguish them from true smooth muscle cells. In general, myofibroblasts show expression of smooth muscle actin only at the periphery of their cytoplasm ("tram-track" pattern);

this is in contrast to the uniform cytoplasmic expression in smooth muscle (Fig. 7–12). On occasion, this "tram-track" pattern is a clue that one is dealing with a myofibroblastic process (e.g., fasciitis) rather than a leiomyosarcoma. Antibody asr-1 is monoclonal and specifically identifies sarcomeric actins (skeletal, cardiac); it identifies rhabdomyosarcoma but not leiomyosarcoma.[11] One should be aware of the fact that some rhabdomyosarcomas, particularly the paratesticular spindle cell type, can express low levels of smooth muscle actins.[90]

Myogenic transcription factors

Myogenic regulatory proteins (i.e., transcription factors of the MyoD [myogenic determination] family) play a critical role in the commitment and differentiation of mesenchymal progenitor cells to the myogenic lineage

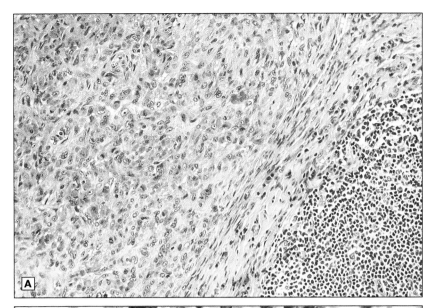

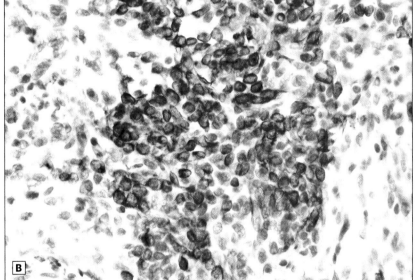

FIGURE 7–11 Angiomatoid fibrous histiocytoma **(A)** with strong expression of desmin **(B)**. These tumors characteristically co-express desmin and CD68 but are negative for all other muscle-related markers.

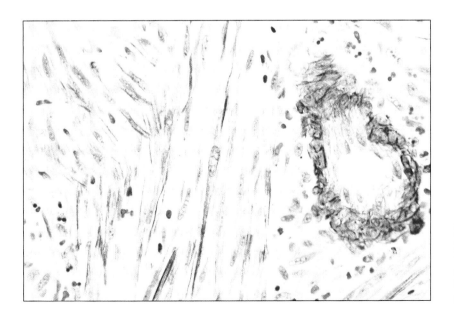

FIGURE 7–12 Immunostain for smooth muscle actin demonstrating the characteristic "tram-track" pattern of expression in myofibroblasts (left). This is in contrast to the uniform intracellular staining seen in true smooth muscle (right).

and subsequent maintenance of the skeletal muscle phenotype. MyoD1 and myogenin are members of the basic helix-loop-helix family of DNA binding myogenic nuclear regulatory proteins; the other members include Myf5 and MRF4.[106,107] These genes encode transcription factors, whose introduction into nonmuscle cells in culture can initiate muscle-specific gene expression and muscle differentiation.[107] In addition, such regulatory factors are expressed much earlier in the normal skeletal muscle differentiation program than structural proteins such as desmin, actin, and myosin; indeed, expression of these myogenic regulatory proteins leads to activation of the latter.[108,109] Antibodies to both MyoD1 and myogenin, but not the other myogenic nuclear regulatory proteins, have been studied in terms of diagnosing rhabdomyosarcoma. Both MyoD1 and myogenin are expressed in more than 90% of rhabdomyosarcomas of all subtypes.[87–89,110–118] Antibodies to both MyoD1 and myogenin show excellent specificity (Fig. 7–9). There is only a single report of nuclear immunoreactivity for MyoD1 in formalin-fixed, paraffin-embedded sections in a pleomorphic liposarcoma.[114,117,118] Four alveolar soft part sarcomas have been demonstrated to express MyoD1 by immunohistochemistry on frozen sections and by Western blot.[119] There have been no reports of myogenin immunoreactivity in nonrhabdomyosarcomas. Cytoplasmic immunoreactivity for MyoD1 has been reported in a small number of nonrhabdomyosarcomas, including primitive neuroectodermal tumor, Wilms' tumor, and undifferentiated sarcoma.[120] Only nuclear immunoreactivity for MyoD1 should be taken as evidence of skeletal muscle differentiation because the epitope recognized by the most commonly used antibody to MyoD1, 5.8A, includes amino acid sequences with close homology to the class 1 major histocompatibility antigen and transcription factors E2A and ITF-1,[110] suggesting that cytoplasmic immunoreactivity may represent a cross-reaction rather than true MyoD1 expression.

As noted above, both MyoD1 and myogenin are expressed by >95% of embryonal and alveolar rhabdomyosarcomas, including the well-differentiated spindle cell variant of ERMS and the solid variant of ARMS.[87–89,110–118] In general, ARMS express very high levels of myogenin and comparatively less MyoD1, whereas ERMS show the opposite pattern, or equal levels of expression.[115] The recently described sclerosing variant of RMS typically shows very strong expression of MyoD1, but only very focal myogenin expression.[87,88,116,121] Pleomorphic RMS are less frequently MyoD1 or myogenin positive, with a recent large series documenting expression in only 53% and 56% of cases, respectively.[89]

Although the available evidence appears to strongly support the view that MyoD1 and myogenin expression are highly specific for rhabdomyoblastic differentiation, it is important to realize that their expression does not obligate a diagnosis of rhabdomyosarcoma. In our expe-

rience and that of others, expression of MyoD1 and/or myogenin may be seen in a variety of rare tumors with rhabdomyoblastic differentiation including Wilms' tumors with myogenous differentiation, neuroendocrine carcinoma with rhabdomyoblastic differentiation, malignant glial tumors with myoblastic differentiation, malignant peripheral nerve sheath tumors with rhabdomyoblastic differentiation (malignant Triton tumor), and teratomas with rhabdomyoblastic differentiation.[117]

Myoglobin and other less commonly used markers

Antibodies to myoglobin, an oxygen-binding heme protein found in skeletal and cardiac muscle but not smooth muscle, were the first markers utilized in the immunohistochemical diagnosis of rhabdomyosarcoma.[77,122–126] Unfortunately, myoglobin is present in demonstrable amounts in fewer than 50% of rhabdomyosarcomas;[86,125] it may be identified in nonmyogenous tumor cells that are infiltrating skeletal muscle and phagocytosing myoglobin.[127] Commercially available myoglobin antibodies have a high level of non-specific, "background" staining, which may be difficult to distinguish from true myoglobin expression. This is in distinct contrast to desmin and the myogenic regulatory protein, which do not diffuse. We do not use antibodies to myoglobin in our routine practice. Other muscle markers that have been used for diagnosing rhabdomyosarcoma include antibodies to myosin,[125] creatine kinase subunit M,[124] and titin,[128] among others. In general, these alternative markers suffer from a lack of sensitivity and/or specificity, and their use cannot be recommended.

Recommendations for use of muscle markers

In summary, for identifying skeletal muscle differentiation, the myogenic regulatory proteins myogenin and MyoD1 are the most specific; antibodies to desmin and muscle actins (i.e., HHF35) are of high sensitivity but are not skeletal muscle-specific. For identification of smooth muscle differentiation (e.g., in leiomyosarcomas), antibodies to desmin and muscle actins (i.e., antibody HHF35) or smooth muscle α-actin (e.g., antibody 1A4) are the best markers of smooth muscle differentiation. For identifying myofibroblasts (e.g., the type of differentiation present in lesions such as nodular fasciitis), antibodies to desmin are useful only for distinguishing myofibroblasts from true smooth muscle cells, as the former (in contrast to the latter) generally do not express desmin.[129,130] Both cell types express smooth muscle actins, however, although myofibroblasts generally express the latter in a characteristic "wispy" or "tramtrack" pattern of immunostaining that, upon higher resolution, can be demonstrated to correspond to the peripheral bundles of actin filaments, which are the hallmark of this cell type. Myofibroblasts also lack expression of the smooth muscle and myoepithelial cell-associated proteins caldesmon and smooth muscle myosin heavy chain, and these markers may assist in the distinction of myofibroblastic and true smooth muscle proliferations.[131–133]

MARKERS OF NERVE SHEATH DIFFERENTIATION

S-100 protein

The S-100 protein is a 20-kDa acidic calcium-binding protein, so named for its solubility in 100% ammonium sulfate. The protein is composed of two subunits, α and β, which combine to form three isotypes. The α-α isotype is normally found in myocardium, skeletal muscle, and neurons; the α-β isotype is present in melanocytes, glia, chondrocytes, and skin adnexae; and the β-β isotype is seen in Langerhans cells and Schwann cells.[134]

Immunohistochemically, S-100 protein can be demonstrated in a large number of normal tissues, including some neurons and glia; Schwann cells; melanocytes; Langerhans cells; interdigitating reticulum cells of lymph nodes; chondrocytes; myoepithelial cells and ducts of sweat glands, salivary glands, and the breast; serous glands of the lung; fetal neuroblasts; and sustentacular cells of the adrenal medulla and paraganglia (Figs 7–13, 7–14).[135] In the immunohistochemical diagnosis of soft tissue neoplasms, S-100 protein is of most value as a marker of benign and malignant nerve sheath tumors and melanoma. S-100 protein is strongly and uniformly expressed in essentially all schwannomas.[135–137] The finding of uniform S-100 immunoreactivity may be a valuable clue to the diagnosis of cellular schwannoma,[138,139] as malignant peripheral nerve sheath tumors usually show only patchy, weak expression of S-100,[59,137,140,141] and fibrosarcomas would not be expected to be S-100-positive (Fig. 7–15). S-100 protein expression is much more variable in neurofibromas than in schwannomas.[137] S-100 protein expression is seen in 40–80% of malignant peripheral nerve sheath tumors.[59,137,140,141]

However, as may be inferred from the long list of normal tissues that express this protein, significant S-100 protein expression may be seen in a subset of non-neural tumors included in the differential diagnosis of malignant peripheral nerve sheath tumors: synovial sarcoma,[18,142,143] rhabdomyosarcoma,[46] leiomyosarcoma,[144] and myoepithelioma/parachordoma.[145–147] Other tumors that may express S-100 protein include adipocytic tumors, chondrocytic tumors, ossifying fibromyxoid tumor, and chordoma. Malignant melanomas of all types, including the desmoplastic and sarcomatoid variants, are almost always strongly positive for S-100 protein.[137,148,149] Uniform, strong S-100 protein expression may be a valuable clue that one is dealing with a melanoma rather than a malignant peripheral nerve sheath tumor of skin or soft tissue because, as noted above, S-100 protein expression in malignant peripheral nerve sheath tumors tends to be weaker and more patchy. It has been our experience that approximately 2–3% of melanomas are negative for S-100 protein; additional immunostaining for a melanosome-specific marker such as gp100 protein (identified by antibody HMB-45[150]) or Melan-A[151] is essential for arriving at the correct diagnoses in these cases.

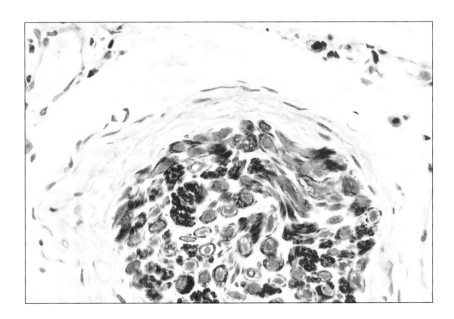

FIGURE 7–13 Nerve illustrating S-100 protein expression in Schwann cells. Note that the perineurial cells do not express S-100.

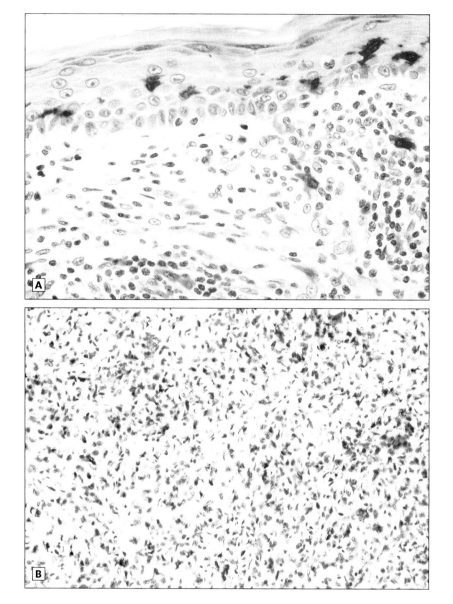

FIGURE 7–14 **(A)** Skin showing S-100 protein expression in both intraepidermal and dermal Langerhans cells. **(B)** Some dermal tumors, such as this benign fibrous histiocytoma, have a large number of infiltrating Langerhans cells. It is important to distinguish reactive from neoplastic subpopulations when interpreting immunostains of mesenchymal tumors.

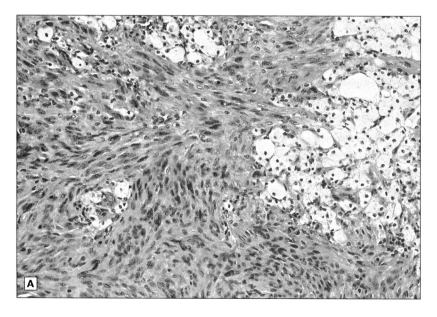

FIGURE 7–15 Cellular schwannoma **(A)** demonstrating uniform, intense S-100 protein expression **(B)**.

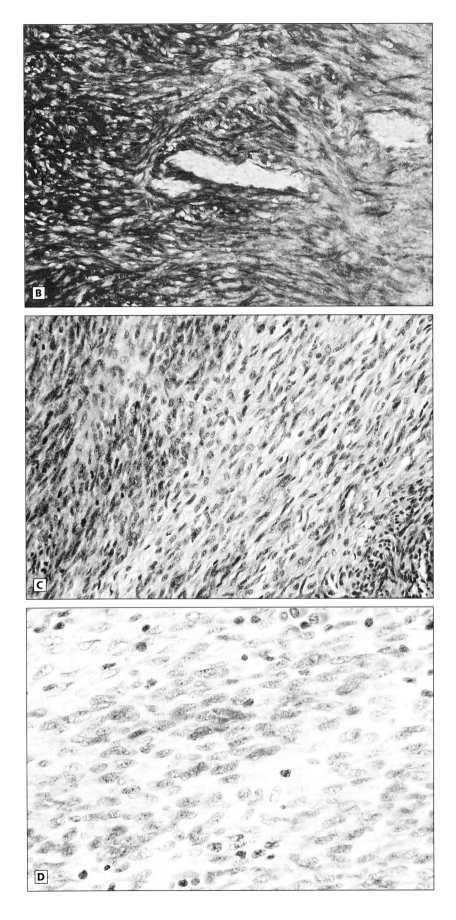

FIGURE 7–15 Continued. Such intense expression is characteristic of schwannomas and melanocytic tumors. In contrast, malignant peripheral nerve sheath tumors **(C)** typically show only patchy, weak S-100 expression **(D)**.

Claudin-1

The claudins are a family of approximately 20 homologous proteins that help determine tight junction structure and permeability, and that appear to be differentially expressed in tissues, with claudin-1 expression, for example, being relatively widespread among epithelia, and claudin-3 expression being confined to lung and liver epithelia.[152] They are integral transmembrane proteins that complex with other transmembrane proteins such as junctional adhesion molecule (JAM) and occludin, and interact with scaffolding proteins such as ZO-1, ZO-2 and ZO-3.[152] Among normal mesenchymal tissues, claudin-1 expression appears to be limited to perineurial cells.[153] In the appropriate histologic context, claudin-1 is a useful marker of perineuriomas, present in 20–90% of perineuriomas, but not in other tumors in this differential diagnosis, such as neurofibromas, schwannomas, low-grade fibromyxoid sarcoma, desmoplastic fibroblastoma, dermatofibrosarcoma protuberans, or fibromatosis (Fig. 7–16).[75,153] Aberrant, non-polarized expression of claudin-1 and other tight junction-related proteins is seen in a significant number of synovial sarcomas and Ewing's sarcoma/PNET.[17,154]

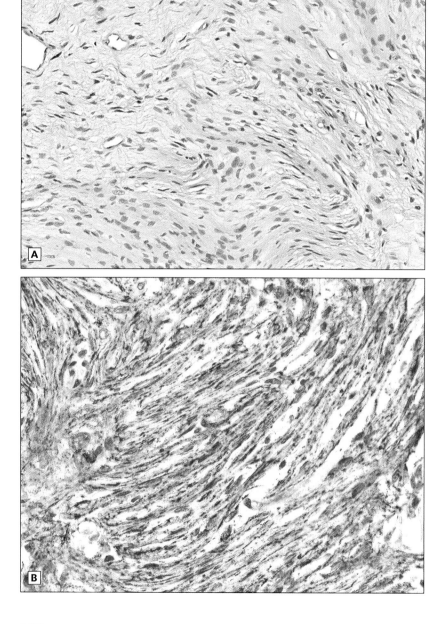

FIGURE 7–16 Perineurioma **(A)**, showing granular membrane immunoreactivity for claudin-1 **(B)**. Claudin-1 and/or Glut-1 may be useful additional markers of perineurial differentiation, particularly when EMA is weak or absent.

Glut-1

GLUT-1 is the erythrocyte-type glucose transporter protein, which plays a particular role in transporting glucose across epithelial and endothelial barrier tissues.[155] Expression of GLUT-1 protein has recently been demonstrated to be a consistent feature of normal perineurial cells and benign and malignant perineurial tumors.[156,157] However, GLUT-1 expression does not appear to have been systematically analyzed in other spindle cell and epithelioid tumors that may enter the differential diagnosis of perineurioma, and the specificity of GLUT-1 expression for perineurial tumors is unknown. GLUT-1 expression has been documented in a small number of epithelioid sarcomas.[158] Among vascular tumors, expression of GLUT-1 protein is seen in essentially all juvenile capillary hemangiomas, but not in other pediatric vascular tumors, including vascular malformations[159,160] and kaposiform hemangioendothelioma.[161] Its expression in vascular tumors appears unrelated to the proliferative activity of the lesions.

CD57

The 110-kDa protein CD57 is normally found on the surface of natural killer cells and T lymphocytes. Antibodies to this protein, including Leu7 and HNK-1, have been found to react with myelin-associated glycoprotein,[162] and both central nervous system oligodendroglia and peripheral Schwann cells may be CD57 positive.[163] Although CD57 immunoreactivity is present in most malignant peripheral nerve sheath tumors,[164,165] a significant percentage of other sarcomas, including synovial sarcoma[18,164] and leiomyosarcoma,[165] are also positive. This lack of specificity limits the utility of CD57 in the immunohistochemical diagnosis of sarcomas. There may be a very limited role for the use of antibodies to CD57 in concert with antibodies to the S-100 protein for confirmation of suspected malignant peripheral nerve sheath tumors.

p75NTR

The nerve growth factor receptor p75NTR, a low-affinity 75-kDa receptor, is normally expressed on neuronal axons, Schwann cells, perineurial cells, perivascular fibroblasts, outer follicular root sheath epithelium, and myoepithelium.[166,167] Expression of p75NTR has been reported in up to 80% of malignant peripheral nerve sheath tumors and nearly all schwannomas, granular cell tumors, and neurofibromas.[168] However, as with CD57, p75NTR expression is not limited to malignant peripheral nerve sheath tumors and may be seen in other sarcomas, including synovial sarcoma[18] and malignant melanoma.[167]

"NEUROECTODERMAL" MARKERS

CD99

The product of the pseudoautosomal MIC2 gene,[169] CD99 is a transmembrane glycoprotein of 30–32 kDa (p30/32).[170] Its exact function is unknown, although it appears to play a role in cellular adhesion and regulation of cellular proliferation.[171,172] The MIC2 gene is expressed, and the CD99 antigen is produced in nearly all human tissues, although the level of expression varies significantly. Normal tissues that commonly display strong CD99 expression include cortical thymocytes and Hassall's corpuscles, granulosa and Sertoli cells, endothelium, pancreatic islets, adenohypophysis, ependyma, and some epithelium, including urothelium, squamous epithelium, and columnar epithelium.[173,174]

The most important use of antibodies to CD99 is for immunohistochemical diagnosis of Ewing's sarcoma/primitive neuroectodermal tumor (ES/PNET). Many studies have shown that well over 90% of ES/PNETs express CD99, with a characteristic membranous pattern (Fig. 7–17).[173–179] Despite early claims that CD99 expression was also specific for ES/PNET, it has become increasingly obvious that this is not true.[173–179] It is particularly important to recognize that a significant subset of other small, blue, round cell tumors considered in the differential diagnosis of ES/PNET may express this antigen. CD99 expression is seen in more than 90% of lymphoblastic lymphomas,[180,181] 20–25% of primitive rhabdomyosarcomas,[174] more than 75% of poorly differentiated synovial sarcomas,[18,182,183] approximately 50% of mesenchymal chondrosarcomas,[184,185] and in rare cases of small cell osteosarcomas[186] and intra-abdominal desmoplastic round cell tumor.[50,187] CD99 expression has never been reported in neuroblastomas[173–179] and has been seen in only a single esthesioneuroblastoma.[188,189]

Immunohistochemical analysis of CD99 expression plays a limited role in the diagnosis of pleomorphic or spindle cell soft tissue neoplasms. As noted above, many synovial sarcomas express CD99, which may be helpful in discriminating them from malignant peripheral nerve sheath tumors and fibrosarcomas.[18,182,183] Expression of CD99 may also be seen in solitary fibrous tumors, mesotheliomas, leiomyosarcomas, and malignant fibrous histiocytomas.[174,190–192]

CD56 (neural cell adhesion molecule)

The 140-kDa isoform of the neural cell adhesion molecule, CD56, is an integral membrane glycoprotein that mediates calcium-independent homophilic cell–cell binding.[193,194] CD56 is expressed by many normal cells and tissues, including neurons, astrocytes, and glia of the cerebral cortex and cerebellum, adrenal cortex and medulla, renal proximal tubules, follicular epithelium of

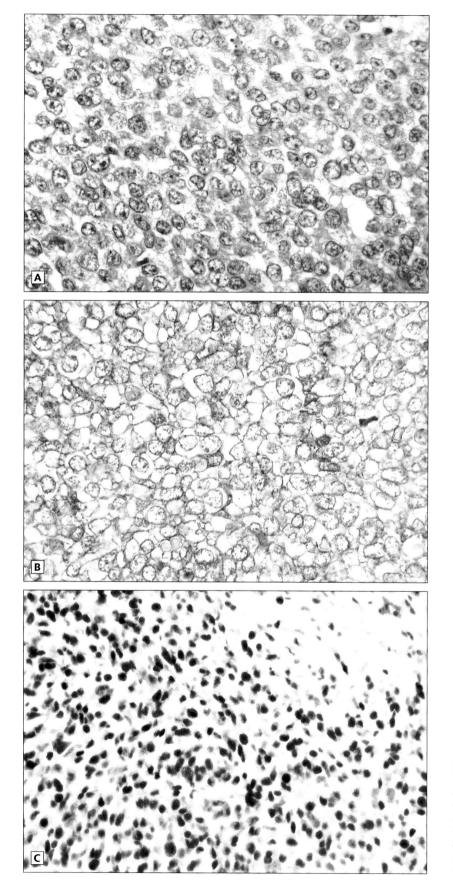

FIGURE 7–17 Ewing's sarcoma/primitive neuroectodermal tumor **(A)** with intense membranous expression of CD99 (MIC2) **(B)**. Although CD99 expression is highly characteristic of Ewing family tumors, it is not specific. Detection of nuclear expression of the carboxy-terminus of FLI-1 protein, expressed as a result of the Ewing's sarcoma-specific EWS/FLI-1 gene fusion, is a much more specific marker of these tumors **(C)**.

the thyroid; gastric parietal cells; cardiac muscle; regenerating and fetal skeletal muscle; pancreatic islet cells, and peripheral nerve.[195] CD56 is also ubiquitously expressed on human natural killer cells and on a subset of T lymphocytes.[196,197]

As might be expected from this long list of CD56-positive normal tissues, CD56 expression is widespread among sarcomas. Soft tissue tumors that often express CD56 include synovial sarcoma, malignant peripheral nerve sheath tumor, schwannoma, rhabdomyosarcoma, leiomyosarcoma, leiomyoma, chondrosarcoma, and osteosarcoma.[198–200] For this reason, examination of CD56 expression is not helpful when evaluating spindle cell soft tissue tumors. CD56 expression may, however, be useful for evaluating primitive "small, blue, round cell tumors," particularly in combination with CD99. CD56 expression is seen in only 10–25% of ES/PNET and in rare lymphoblastic lymphomas, compared with nearly 100% of neuroblastomas, poorly differentiated synovial sarcomas, alveolar and primitive embryonal rhabdomyosarcomas, small cell carcinomas, Wilms' tumors, and mesenchymal chondrosarcomas.[18,199,200] The absence of CD56 expression may be a clue to the diagnosis of ES/PNET in cases where results with more specific positive markers such as CD99, CD45, cytokeratin, and desmin are equivocal.

NB-84

Monoclonal antibody NB-84, raised against two neuroblastoma cell lines, recognizes an as yet uncharacterized 57-kDa molecule.[201] NB-84 is a highly sensitive marker of neuroblastoma, being positive in more than 95% of cases, including undifferentiated and poorly differentiated subtypes.[50,189,201–204] It is relatively specific for neuroblastoma, although 16–25% of ES/PNETs react with NB-84, as do a small number of rhabdomyosarcomas, esthesioneuroblastomas, Wilms' tumors, desmoplastic round cell tumors, and small cell osteosarcomas.[50,189,201–204] NB-84 antigen expression has not been examined in spindle cell soft tissue neoplasms.

MARKERS OF MELANOCYTIC DIFFERENTIATION

HMB-45

Monoclonal antibody HMB-45 identifies the Pmel 17 gene product gp100.[205] This gene product is a component of the premelanosomal/melanosomal melanogenic oxidoreductive enzymes and as such is melanosome-specific but not melanoma-specific.[206] HMB-45 is positive in the unusual myomelanocytic tumors that comprise the perivascular epithelioid cell family of tumors (angiomyolipoma, clear-cell tumor of lung, lymphangioleiomyoma-

tosis, soft tissue and bone PEComas),[14,207,208] but has not convincingly been shown to react with any tumor that does not contain melanosomes. Previous reports of HMB-45 positivity in carcinomas were based on the use of contaminated ascites fluid and have been retracted in the literature.[209] HMB-45 is generally negative in nevi and resting melanocytes but is expressed in approximately 85% of melanomas (Fig. 7–18).[205] Fewer than 10% of desmoplastic melanomas are HMB-45 positive.[210]

Melan-A

Melan-A, the product of the MART-1 gene (melanoma antigen recognized by T cells), is a 20–22-kDa component of the premelanosomal membrane.[151,211–214] Its function is unknown. Like HMB-45, Melan-A is a marker of melanosomes, not melanomas: it is also present in perivascular epithelioid cell tumors (PEComas) (Fig. 7–19).[14] Unlike HMB-45, Melan-A is positive in resting melanocytes and nevi. Melan-A is expressed by approximately 85% of epithelioid melanomas and has been reported to be present in upward of 50% of desmoplastic melanomas, although the true rate is almost certainly far lower and is probably the same as for HMB-45.[151,211–215] Melan-A is present in some HMB-45-negative melanomas and vice versa. One other interesting application of the most widely used antibody to Melan-A, A103, is for the diagnosis of adrenal cortical and other steroid-producing tumors. A103 has reproducible cross-reactivity with an unknown epitope present in these tumors, and it may be helpful for distinguishing adrenal cortical carcinomas from renal cell carcinoma.[213]

Microphthalmia transcription factor

Microphthalmia transcription factor (MiTF), the product of the microphthalmia (mi) gene located on chromosome 3p14.1, is a transcription factor critical for melanocyte development.[216–218] Mutations in mi were first described in mice in the 1940s and it was subsequently shown in humans that heterozygous mi deficiency results in Waardenburg's syndrome IIa, clinically defined by skin pigmentation abnormalities, bilateral hearing loss, and a white forelock.[219] Biochemical studies have shown that microphthalmia transcription factor, the protein encoded by mi, can transactivate several downstream gene promoters including genes ultimately responsible for melanin biosynthesis, namely tyrosinase and related pigmentation enzymes TRP-1 and TRP-2.[220] MiTF is expressed in essentially all resting melanocytes and nevi. Both melanocyte-specific and non-specific isoforms of this protein exist;[221] however, the commercially available antibodies to MiTF are not specific for the melanocytic isoforms, in our experience, despite claims to the contrary.

MiTF was initially described as highly sensitive and specific marker of melanoma, and is expressed in well

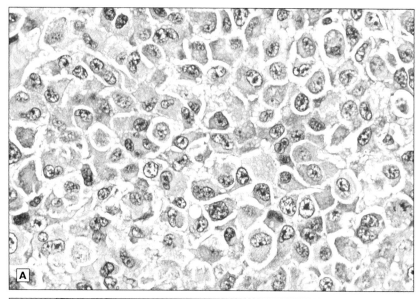

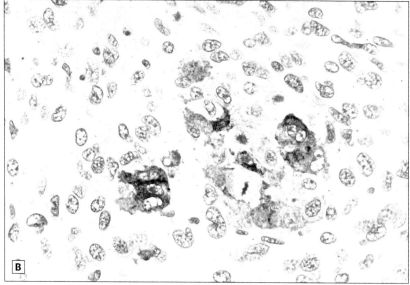

FIGURE 7–18 Malignant melanoma **(A)** immunostained with monoclonal antibody HMB-45 to gp100 protein **(B)**. HMB-45 is positive in approximately 85% of epithelioid melanomas but in only a small fraction of spindled melanomas.

over 90% of epithelioid melanomas.[222,223] Sarcomatoid melanomas are less often positive (40%) and true desmoplastic melanomas are very infrequently positive (<5%).[224,225] MiTF is also expressed in nearly all clear cell sarcomas (melanoma of soft parts) (Fig. 7–20).[224,226] MiTF expression may also be seen in PEComas of all types.[14,227] Because the commercially available antibodies are not specific for the melanocytic MiTF isoforms, MiTF expression is not limited to melanomas, and may be seen in leiomyosarcomas, atypical fibroxanthomas, atypical lipomatous neoplasms, and very rare carcinomas.[224,227] Thus, MiTF is best used for the confirmation of S-100 protein-positive, HMB-45/Melan-A/tyrosinase-negative tumors suspected of being melanomas. MiTF expression in the absence of S-100 protein expression is not diagnostic of melanoma.

Tyrosinase

Tyrosinase is an enzyme involved in the synthesis of melanin.[228] Antibodies to tyrosinase have recently been shown to have a sensitivity and specificity that is roughly equivalent to that of HMB-45 and Melan-A.[211,229] In general, we reserve the use of tyrosinase for cases strongly suspected of representing melanoma, which are negative with HMB-45 or A103.

MARKERS OF ENDOTHELIAL DIFFERENTIATION

A number of markers have been used to demonstrate endothelial differentiation, paralleling the progression in

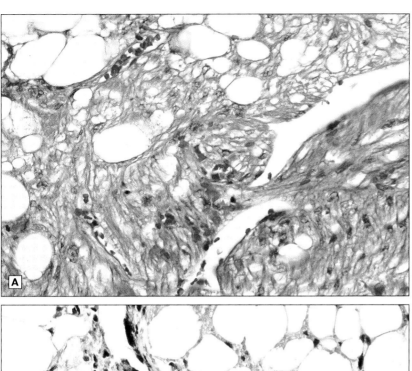

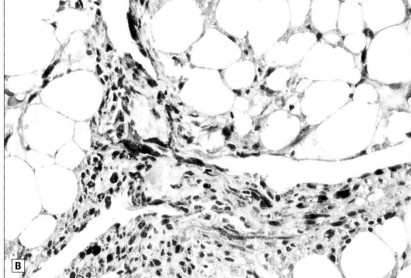

FIGURE 7–19 Angiomyolipoma **(A)**, showing Melan-A expression in epithelioid cells, spindled cells and in the cytoplasm of lipid-distended cells ("adipocytes") **(B)**. Co-expression of melanosome-related proteins, such as gp100 and Melan-A, with smooth muscle markers is characteristic of the perivascular epithelioid cell (PEComa) family of tumors.

our concept of spindle cell tumors manifesting endothelial differentiation. Endothelial markers include von Willebrand factor (factor VIII-associated protein, often erroneously referred to as factor VIII), CD34, CD31, and FLI-1. The pattern of expression of these markers in endothelial tumors is much like an overlapping Venn diagram, in which most tumors express all of these markers, but some express only a subset. Whereas early studies had suggested that markers such as von Willebrand factor (vWF) could differentially identify vascular versus lymphatic endothelium,[230-232] more recent studies have demonstrated that both vascular and lymphatic endothelium express all three markers; and novel markers such as podoplanin and vascular endothelial growth factor receptor-3 (positive on lymphatic endothelium and negative on vascular endothelium) are required to make this distinction.[233-235]

von Willebrand factor (factor VIII-related antigen)

The von Willebrand factor (vWF) was the first endothelium-specific marker employed in diagnostic immunohistochemical studies.[231] It was first used to identify the nature of the vinyl chloride-induced sarcomas of liver[236] and has subsequently been demonstrated to be a marker of vascular tumors of multiple sites, including but not limited to those of the central nervous system,[237] gastrointestinal tract,[238] and breast.[239] vWF is the least sensitive of the vascular markers and is positive in 50–75% of vascular tumors.[234] Although vWF expression is, in theory, absolutely specific for vascular tumors, technical problems limit its usefulness. vWF is not only produced by endothelial cells but circulates in the serum; and it therefore can be found often in zones of tumor necrosis and hemorrhage (Fig. 7–21).

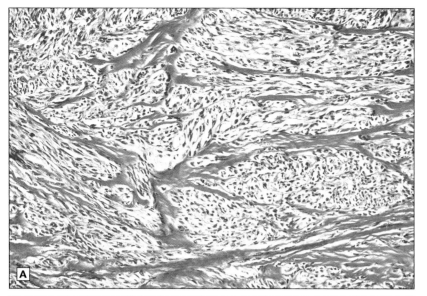

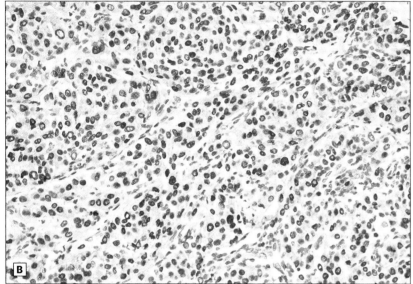

FIGURE 7–20 Clear cell sarcoma **(A)** with uniform nuclear expression of microphthalmia transcription factor **(B)**. Microphthalmia transcription factor is a highly sensitive marker of melanoma and of mesenchymal tumors with melanocytic differentiation.

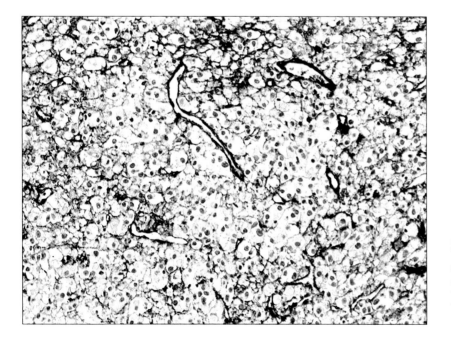

FIGURE 7–21 Immunostain for von Willebrand factor (factor VIII-related protein) showing spurious "membranous" positivity in a renal cell carcinoma. Staining of circulating vWF in the serum may be extremely difficult to distinguish from true membranous staining in an endothelial neoplasm.

CD34 (human hematopoietic progenitor cell antigen)

The function of CD34, a 110-kDa transmembrane glycoprotein, is unknown. It is expressed on hematopoietic stem cells, endothelium, the interstitial cells of Cajal, and a group of interesting dendritic cells present in the dermis, around blood vessels, and in the nerve sheath.[240] CD34 is expressed in more than 90% of vascular tumors[241] and is the most sensitive marker of Kaposi sarcoma.[234] As may be gathered from the above list of normal tissues, CD34 expression is not limited to vascular tumors. CD34 expression is well documented in dermatofibrosarcoma protuberans,[242] solitary fibrous tumors,[243] malignant peripheral nerve sheath tumors,[244] gastrointestinal stromal tumors,[245] and epithelioid sarcomas (Fig. 7–22).[19,20,246] CD34 is expressed by approximately 50–60% of epithelioid

sarcomas, compared with fewer than 2% of carcinomas. CD34 expression may be valuable for distinguishing cytokeratin-positive epithelioid angiosarcomas and epithelioid sarcomas from carcinoma.[19,20,246]

CD31 (platelet endothelial cell adhesion molecule-1)

The newest of the commonly used vascular markers, CD31 is the most sensitive and specific marker.[241,247] It is expressed in more than 90% of angiosarcomas, hemangioendotheliomas, hemangiomas, and Kaposi sarcoma and in fewer than 1% of carcinomas (probably much less than 1%) (Fig. 7–5). CD31 expression is not seen in any non-endothelial tissue or tumor, with the notable exception of macrophages and platelets (Fig. 7–23).[248] CD31

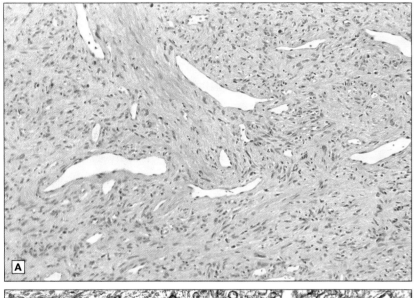

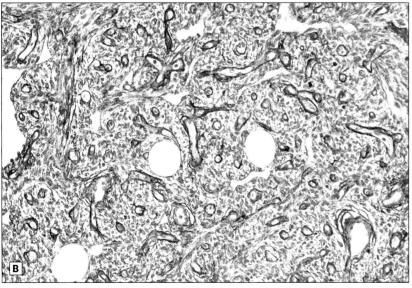

FIGURE 7–22 Solitary fibrous tumor **(A)** with uniform CD34 expression **(B)**.

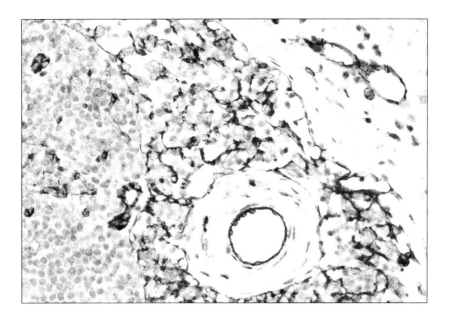

FIGURE 7–23 Granular, membranous CD31 expression in macrophages of the lymph node sinusoid. This granular expression in macrophages infiltrating a tumor may be mistaken for true expression by the tumor cells, leading to an erroneous diagnosis of angiosarcoma. CD31 expression in angiosarcomas is usually stronger and shows a linear, rather than granular, staining pattern (see also Fig. 7–5).

expression in intratumoral macrophages may result in the misdiagnosis of a nonvascular tumor as a vascular tumor, if one is not aware of this potential pitfall.[249] The CD31 expression seen in macrophages is distinctly granular, compared with the intense cytoplasmic and linear membranous staining of endothelium.

FLI-1

FLI-1 also is the only currently available nuclear marker of endothelial differentiation. FLI-1 is positive in >95% of endothelial neoplasms of all types and degrees of malignancy, including hemangiomas, hemangioendotheliomas, angiosarcomas, and Kaposi sarcoma.[250,251] FLI-1 is not expressed by epithelioid sarcomas, which is helpful in the distinction of these tumors from epithelioid forms of angiosarcoma.[250,251] Very rare melanomas, adenocarcinomas, and Merkel cell carcinomas have been reported to show focal FLI-1 positivity.[251] Merkel cell carcinomas may be strongly positive for FLI-1 in a subset of cases, although study of additional cases is necessary to determine the frequency of this occurrence. It is also very important not to mistake intratumoral FLI-1-positive endothelial cells and lymphocytes for positive tumor cells.

Ulex lectin

Ulex lectin was a popular alternative marker of endothelial cells and tumors.[252,253] Although it was initially praised for its great sensitivity for vascular tumors,[254,255] it was subsequently discovered that the sugar residue recognized by this lectin is also present on a wide range of epithelial tumors.[256–258] Ulex retains its high specificity for vascular tumors if its use is restricted to cytokeratin-negative tumors.

Vascular endothelial cell growth factor receptor-3 (VEGFR-3)

The platelet derived growth factor (PDGF) family, including vascular endothelial growth factor (VEGF), and the closely related molecules VEGF-B, VEGF-C and VEGF-D, play a significant role in angiogenesis and vascular permeability.[259] VEGF-C plays a critical role in lymphangiogenesis; in transgenic mice, VEGF-C has the ability to induce both lymphatic endothelial proliferation and lymphatic vessel formation.[260] In the adult, expression of the mRNA of the VEGF-C receptor, VEGFR-3 (FLT4) is limited almost exclusively to lymphatic endothelium, although it may be detected in other endothelia at earlier stages of development.[261] Early studies suggested that VEGFR-3 was a highly sensitive and specific marker of Kaposi sarcoma (KS), normal lymphatics, and lymphangiomas.[235] Two subsequent large studies confirmed its superb (>95%) sensitivity for KS, but also noted expression in close to 50% of angiosarcomas, some of which had features suggestive of lymphatic differentiation, occasional hemangiomas, and almost all cases of kaposiform hemangioendothelioma, Dabska tumor, and retiform hemangioendothelioma.[234,262] It is now generally conceded that VEGFR-3 expression is not specific for lymphatic differentiation in endothelial neoplasms. VEGFR-3 expression has not been documented in nonendothelial neoplasms.

Human herpesvirus 8 latency associated nuclear antigen (LANA)

An infectious etiology for Kaposi sarcoma has long been suspected, and epidemiological, serologic, and molecular genetic studies over the past 10–15 years have identified a novel herpesvirus, HHV-8, as the likely causative agent of KS.[263-267] HHV-8 is known to latently infect endothelial cells, as well as peripheral blood monocytes and B lymphocytes in patients with KS. LANA is one of the most highly expressed proteins during latent HHV-8 infection. The LANA protein is encoded by the open reading frame 73 (ORF73) of the HHV-8 genome, where it tethers viral DNA to host heterochromatin and is thereby required for persistence of viral DNA in dividing cells.[268] LANA also has an essential role in maintenance of the episomal DNA during latent infection and cell division, and also regulates gene expression in infected cells.[269,270] A relatively small number of studies have examined LANA expression by immunohistochemistry. Using a polyclonal antisera, Katano et al. found LANA expression in 100% of KS cases studied.[271] Three separate studies, all using the LNA53 monoclonal antibody, noted LANA expression in well over 90% of KS cases, as compared with 0% of non-KS controls.[272-274] Using the 13B10 clone, four very recent studies have noted LANA expression in very close to 100% of KS, as compared with 0% of non-KS potential mimics (Fig. 7–24).[275-278] LANA expression has not been reported in any non-KS tumor, with the notable exceptions of primary effusion lymphoma and Castleman disease.[272,273]

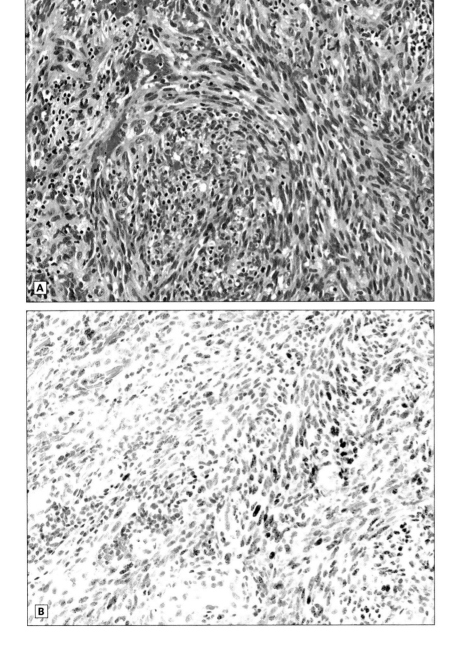

FIGURE 7–24 Kaposi sarcoma **(A)** showing strong nuclear expression of LANA protein **(B)**.

Type IV collagen

Type IV collagen, associated with basement membrane expression, is produced by smooth muscle, glomus cells, nerve sheath, and endothelial cells. In selected cases, demonstration of type IV collagen expression around clusters of cells, indicative of primitive vascular channel formation, may be a clue to the diagnosis of angiosarcoma.[279] Demonstration of uniform pericellular type IV collagen may also be a clue to the diagnosis of a glomus tumor (Fig. 7–25). In general, however, there are relatively few uses for collagen IV immunostains in the diagnosis of soft tissue neoplasms.

Recommendations for use of vascular markers

As a practical issue, it is best to employ a highly specific (e.g., antibodies to CD31) and a highly sensitive (e.g., antibodies to CD34) marker to assess the presence of endothelial differentiation in histologic and clinical settings in which the diagnosis of angiosarcoma is entertained. The endothelial markers are summarized in Table 7–3.

IMMUNOHISTOCHEMICAL DISTINCTION OF MESOTHELIOMA AND CARCINOMA

Few subjects have generated the remarkable proliferation of studies, papers, seminars, review articles, and courses as has the differential diagnosis of mesothelioma and carcinoma. In large part, this is probably due to the legal implications of the diagnosis of mesothelioma in the United States. Along with this proliferation of studies has come a sometimes bewildering number of new

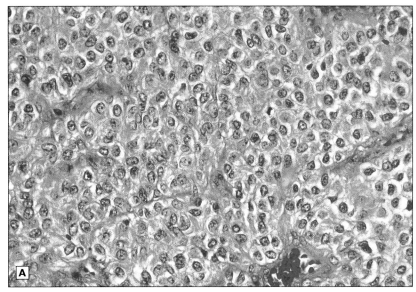

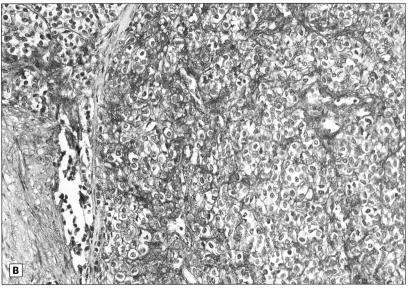

FIGURE 7–25 Malignant glomus tumor **(A)** with characteristic investment of individual cells by type IV collagen **(B)**. Pericellular type IV collagen is characteristic of tumors with glomus cell, endothelial, schwannian, perineurial, and smooth muscle differentiation.

TABLE 7–3	ENDOTHELIAL MARKERS			
Marker	Specificity	Sensitivity	Also identifies	
CD31	High	High	Macrophages	
CD34	Moderate	High	Epithelioid sarcoma, solitary fibrous tumor, DFSP, GIST	
vWF	High	Low	Megakaryocytes	
Ulex lectin	High*	Moderate	Many epithelia	
FLI-1	Moderate	High	Ewing's sarcoma/PNET, small lymphocytes	
Type IV collagen	Moderate*	Moderate	Glomus tumors, nerve sheath tumors, smooth muscle tumors	

vWF, von Willebrand factor.
*In the soft tissue (i.e., nonepithelial) tumor group.

TABLE 7–4	RECOMMENDED IMMUNOHISTOCHEMICAL PANEL FOR MESOTHELIOMA		
Antibodies to	Adenocarcinoma	Mesothelioma	Comments
Calretinin	5–5% positive	75–95% positive	High sensitivity in sarcomatoid mesothelioma
WT-1	Rarely positive (except ovarian serous carcinoma)	75–95% positive	Moderately high sensitivity in sarcomatoid mesothelioma (50–75%)
CK5/6	Rarely positive (positive in squamous cell carcinoma)	≈75% positive	Very low sensitivity in sarcomatoid mesothelioma (<25%)
Podoplanin (D2-40)	Negative	≈90% positive	Most sensitive marker for sarcomatoid mesothelioma
Tumor-associated glycoproteins (MOC-31, Bg8 or Ber-EP4)	Positive (sensitivity varies with tumor type)	Negative	Rarely positive

antibodies, each touted as more specific or sensitive than the last. Historically, the immunohistochemical diagnosis of mesothelioma was one of exclusion in that there were no positive markers of mesothelial differentiation. While traditionally, positive markers of adenocarcinoma/ negative markers of mesothelioma have included monoclonal antibodies to carcinoembryonic antigen (mCEA), monoclonal antibody LeuM1 to CD15, and monoclonal antibodies to the tumor-associated glycoproteins defined by antibodies B72.3 and Ber-EP4, more recently the antibodies MOC-31 and antibody Bg8 to the Lewis Y antigen have been demonstrated to have a higher sensitivity in a wider range of adenocarcinomas.[280] We have close to 20 years of experience in the use of these antibodies, and their range of reactivities in various carcinomas and mesotheliomas has been studied extensively. The combination of these four antibodies alone can distinguish more than 90% of pulmonary adenocarcinomas from mesothelioma.[281] It is therefore critical always to interpret the newer positive mesothelial markers, with which we have much less experience, in the context of the findings with negative markers. Recommendations for the immunodiagnosis of mesothelioma are given in Table 7–4.

Carcinoembryonic antigen and CD15 (LeuM1)

Carcinoembryonic antigen is expressed in approximately 85–90% of carcinomas of lung, gastric, and pancreaticobiliary origin but in only 15–30% of breast and ovarian carcinomas.[282–284] Rare mesotheliomas that are rich in hyaluronic acid may show false positivity for CEA.[285] However, unlike in adenocarcinomas, which are usually diffusely positive, this false positivity is seen only in scattered cells. The CD15 marker is expressed by a somewhat smaller number of carcinomas (60–75%) than is CEA.[286] As with CEA, rare hyaluronic acid-rich mesotheliomas show granular cytoplasmic positivity, and rare mesotheliomas have been reported to show strong CD15 expression.[287]

Tumor-associated glycoproteins (B72.3, Ber-EP4, Bg8, MOC-31)

The monoclonal antibodies B72.3 and Ber-EP4 are directed against different tumor-associated membrane glycoproteins, and have a higher sensitivity overall for adenocarcinomas compared with antibodies to CEA and CD15.[283,384,288] However, the adenocarcinoma markers with the greatest overall sensitivity and specificity are the glycoprotein identified by antibody MOC-31 and the Lewis Y antigen, identified by antibody Bg8.[288-292]

WT-1

A tumor-suppressor gene located on chromosome 11p13, WT-1, in contrast to other tumor-suppressor genes, is normally expressed only in certain tissues, including mesothelium. In paraffin sections 75–95% of mesotheliomas express this protein, compared with 25% of carcinomas metastatic to the pleura (Fig. 7–26).[288,290,293,294] The sensitivity and specificity of calretinin and WT-1 are roughly equivalent. WT-1 is routinely expressed by serous carcinomas of ovarian and extraovarian origin.

Other positive markers of mesothelioma (calretinin, cytokeratin 5/6, podoplanin)

The diagnosis of mesothelioma has been greatly assisted by the development of new positive markers expressed by mesotheliomas but not carcinomas. At the moment, the most promising markers include those to calretinin, mesothelin, the Wilms' tumor gene product WT-1, and cytokeratins 5/6. As noted above, it is critical to remember that these markers are not absolutely specific for mesothelioma, and as such the results of these markers should always be interpreted in the context of the well-established negative markers.

Calretinin, a calcium-binding protein originally identified in the retina, is probably the best studied of these new markers. Antibodies to calretinin recognize 75–95% of epithelial mesotheliomas and a smaller percentage of sarcomatoid mesotheliomas (about 50%) (Fig. 7–27).[294-296] A small percentage (5–15%) of carcinomas also express calretinin, including those of lung, colon, and ovarian origin.

Another useful positive mesothelioma marker is *cytokeratin 5/6*. Normal and neoplastic mesothelial cells express cytokeratins 4, 5, 6, 14, and 17, in addition to the cytokeratins (7, 8, 18, and 19) expressed by most glandular epithelium.[284] Cytokeratin 5/6 is expressed by 80–100% of mesotheliomas and only 15% of carcinomas, including those of lung and ovarian surface epithelial and endometrial origin.[297,298]

The most recent and perhaps most sensitive mesothelial-restricted marker is the monoclonal antibody D2–40-defined protein, *podoplanin*.[299,300] This marker, which also serves as a somewhat lymphatic endothelial restricted marker in other contexts,[301] also has a major advantage over other mesothelial markers in maintaining high sensitivity even in the context of sarcomatoid histology.

MARKERS OF GASTROINTESTINAL STROMAL TUMORS

CD117 (C-KIT)

The c-kit proto-oncogene product (CD117), a transmembrane receptor for stem cell factor, is normally expressed by mast cells, melanocytes, germ cells, various subsets of hematopoietic cells, and the interstitial cells of Cajal of the gastrointestinal tract.[245,302] CD117 is expressed by 85–95% of gastrointestinal stromal tumors.[245,303-306] In the gastrointestinal tract CD117 is a highly specific marker of gastrointestinal stromal tumors; it is not expressed by tumors typically in the differential diagnosis of a gastrointestinal mesenchymal tumor, such as leiomyomas, leiomyosarcomas, and nerve sheath tumors (Fig. 7–28).[245,303-303] CD117 is expressed by melanocytic tumors,

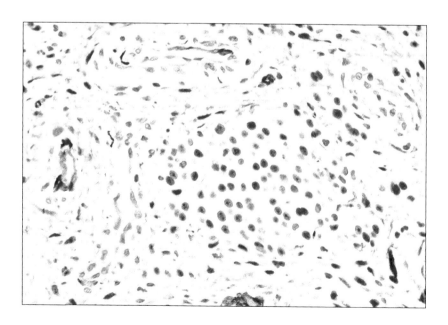

FIGURE 7–26 Nuclear WT-1 expression in an epithelioid mesothelioma. Note the typical cytoplasmic immunoreactivity of the endothelial cells. Only nuclear WT-1 expression should be accepted as positive.

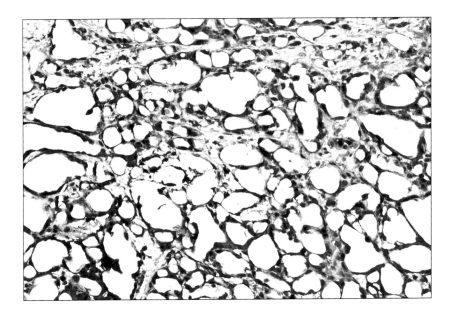

FIGURE 7–27 Intense nuclear and cytoplasmic calretinin expression in an adenomatoid tumor.

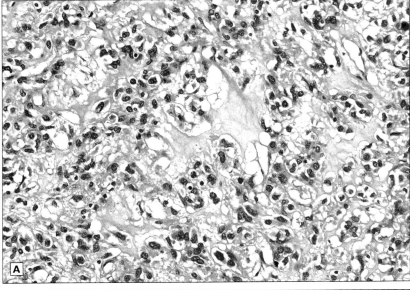

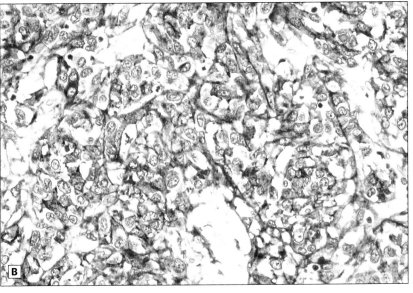

FIGURE 7–28 Gastrointestinal stromal tumor **(A)** with characteristic CD117 (c-kit) expression **(B)**. Such expression distinguishes stromal tumors from leiomyosarcomas and nerve sheath tumors.

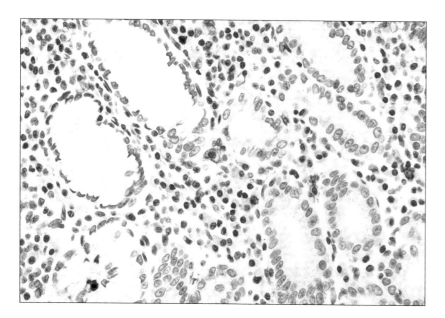

FIGURE 7–29 Mast cells in the lamina propria of the gut, demonstrating C117 (c-kit) expression. Failure to distinguish CD117 expression by mast cells infiltrating a nongastrointestinal stromal tumor from expression by tumor cells is a potential pitfall.

however, such as melanoma and clear cell sarcoma.[306] CD117 expression may also be seen in a minority of Ewing's sarcoma and PEComas.[14,44,307–310] In any type of tumor, care should be taken not to mistake mast cells in a tumor for scattered CD117-positive tumor cells (Fig. 7–29).

Protein kinase C θ

Protein kinase C θ is a recently described protein kinase involved in T-cell activation, skeletal muscle signal transduction and neuronal differentiation.[311–313] Overexpression of the protein kinase C θ gene in gastrointestinal stromal tumors (GIST) has been identified in two gene expression studies using DNA microarrays.[314,315] Most recently, two studies have shown expression of protein kinase C θ to be a highly sensitive and specific marker of GIST, including CD117-negative ones, with expression in 85–100% of routinely processed GIST, and in essentially no other mesenchymal or non-mesenchymal tumors, with the exception of <15% of schwannomas.[316,317]

USE OF IMMUNOHISTOCHEMISTRY AS A SURROGATE FOR THE PRESENCE OF TUMOR-SPECIFIC MOLECULAR ALTERATIONS

The immunohistochemical studies applied to sarcomas described to this point are employed to identify "cell type"-specific markers, i.e., to identify the "normal cell counterpart" to the mesenchymal tumor in question. There is an emerging class of soft tissue tumors, however, that does not appear to have a normal cell counterpart, and represents a set of tumors which are characterized, instead, by specific genetic alterations, usually chromosomal translocations. The latter can result in the abnormal juxtaposition of two genes, resulting in the neo-expression of one of the gene products, or a portion thereof. The latter can be identified by immunohistochemical studies, which thus serve as a surrogate for the presence of the chromosomal translocation. The following are five applications of this concept to soft tissue tumors.

FLI-1 as a marker of the t(11;22)(q24;q12) translocation of Ewing's sarcoma/primitive neuroectodermal tumor

The *FLI-1* gene and FLI-1 protein are best known for their critical role in the pathogenesis of Ewing's sarcoma/primitive neuroectodermal tumor. Over 85% of ES/PNET are characterized by the translocation t(11;22)(q24;q12) that results in the fusion of the *EWS* gene on chromosome 22 to the *FLI-1* gene on chromosome 11.[318–322] *FLI-1* is normally expressed in endothelial cells and in hematopoietic cells, including T lymphocytes.[323–325] The *FLI-1* gene has also recently been shown to play an important role in the embryological development of blood vessels and endothelial cells.[326]

FLI-1 is positive in 70–90% of genetically confirmed ES/PNET, reflecting the presence of the EWS-FLI-1 fusion protein.[44,251,324,325] Interestingly, FLI-1 may be positive in rare cases with known EWS-ERG fusions, probably reflecting protein homology between FLI-1 and ERG.[44] In contrast, FLI-1 is not positive in the great majority of other small blue round cell tumors, including RMS, mesenchymal chondrosarcoma, neuroblastoma, Wilms' tumor, and desmoplastic small round cell tumor.[251,325] Importantly, FLI-1 is uniformly expressed by lymphoblastic lymphomas, reflecting the normal presence of full-length FLI-1 protein in lymphocytes. As lymphoblastic lymphomas are also invariably positive for the Ewing's sarcoma-associated marker CD99, it is critical to consider this alternative diagnosis and to perform immunostains for other markers, such as CD43 and TDT, when indicated.

WT-1 as a marker of the t(11;22)(13;q24) translocation of desmoplastic small round cell tumor

Desmoplastic small round cell tumors (DSRCT) are characterized in almost all cases by a specific translocation, t(11;22)(p13;q24) which fuses the *EWS* and *WT1* genes and produces a fusion protein containing the carboxy-terminus of WT-1.[327-329] Antibodies directed against the carboxy-terminus of WT-1 have been shown to be highly sensitive (>90%) and relatively specific markers of desmoplastic round cell tumors, among small blue round cell tumors.[50,330-332] It is important to realize that many rhabdomyosarcomas express cytoplasmic wild-type WT-1, which will be identified by both amino- and carboxy-terminus antibodies, and which should be rigorously distinguished from the nuclear positivity seen in desmoplastic round cells tumors.[333] Wild-type WT-1 expression is also seen in Wilms' tumor, although this is seldom in the differential diagnosis of DRCT and is usually easily identified by routine microscopy.[331]

TFE3 as a marker of the der(17)t(X;17)(p11;q25) translocation of alveolar soft part sarcoma

Alveolar soft part sarcoma (ASPS) are characterized in almost all cases by a tumor-specific der(17)t(X;17)(p11;q25) that fuses the *TFE3* gene at Xp11 to the *ASPL* gene at 17q25, creating an ASPL-TFE3 fusion protein.[334] Recently, an antibody directed against the carboxy-terminus of the TFE3 transcription factor has been shown to be a highly sensitive and specific marker of ASPS (Fig. 7–30).[335] Although low levels of TFE3 expression is present in almost all normal tissues, strong nuclear expression of TFE3 is confined to tumors known to harbor TFE3 gene fusions, such as ASPS and rare pediatric renal carcinomas.[335] Only nuclear expression of TFE3 is of diagnostic value, as cytoplasmic staining (possibly nonspecific) is seen in a variety of tumors. Among other soft tissue tumors, TFE3 expression is confined to granular cell tumors[335] and to a small minority of PEComas.[14]

INI1 expression loss as a marker of monosomy or homozygous deletions of *hSNF5/INI-1/SMARCB1/BAF47* gene

The INI1 protein is the product of the *hSNF5/INI-1/SMARCB1/BAF47* gene, located on chromosome 22q11.2.[336-338] Loss of INI1, either in the form of monosomy 22 or as homozygous deletions in the gene itself have been strongly implicated in the pathogenesis of atypical teratoid/rhabdoid tumor of the central nervous system, as well as in extrarenal rhabdoid tumors.[339] The INI1 protein is felt to be a tumor suppressor, and as such is normally present within all normal tissues. By immunohistochemistry, loss of INI1 protein has been shown in all studied renal/extrarenal rhabdoid tumors and atypical teratoid/rhabdoid tumors and in four of six studied epithelioid sarcomas. In contrast, essentially all other carcinomas, sarcomas, and central nervous system neoplasms studied (with the exception of one medullary renal carcinoma) have been positive for INI1.[340-344] Although study of additional cases of extrarenal rhabdoid tumor and epithelioid sarcoma are clearly necessary, demonstration of loss of INI1 expression may prove to be a valuable adjunct in the diagnosis of these two entities.

Anaplastic lymphoma kinase

Anaplastic lymphoma kinase (ALK) is a transmembrane tyrosine kinase first identified as part of the characteristic t(2;5) (*NPM-ALK*) translocation seen in anaplastic large cell lymphomas[345] In normal tissues, expression of ALK protein is restricted to the central nervous system.[346] Inflammatory myofibroblastic tumors frequently contain chromosomal rearrangements that result in activation of the *ALK* gene, with subsequent overexpression of ALK protein in roughly 40% of cases.[347-351] However, overexpression of ALK may also be seen in a variety of other soft tissue tumors, including rhabdomyosarcoma, lipogenic tumors, Ewing's sarcoma, malignant fibrous histiocytoma, leiomyosarcoma, and others.[348,351] Thus, expression of ALK protein must be evaluated in the overall clinical and morphologic context, and as part of a panel of other immunostains.

OTHER MARKERS

CD68

The 110-kDa glycoprotein recognized by antibodies to CD68 (e.g., KP1, KI-M1P) is closely associated with, or a part of, lysosomes.[352] Although CD68 has been thought of as a marker of histiocytes (owing to the presence of large numbers of lysosomes in these cells), it is important to remember that CD68 is organelle-specific rather than lineage-specific. Although CD68 expression is commonly seen in "fibrohistiocytic" soft tissue tumors, such as benign and malignant fibrous histiocytoma, it may also be seen in a variety of other sarcomas, melanomas, and carcinomas.[353-356] For this reason, antibodies to CD68 play only a limited role in the diagnosis of soft tissue

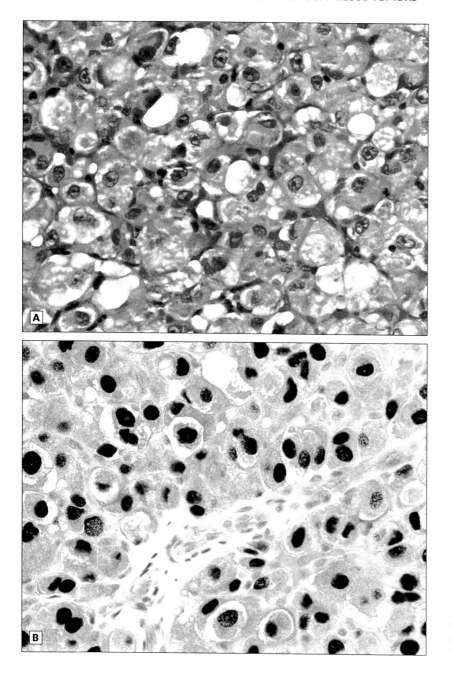

FIGURE 7–30 Alveolar soft part sarcoma **(A)**, showing nuclear positivity with anti-TFE3 antibody **(B)**, indicative of an ASPL-TFE3 fusion protein.

tumors. CD68 is expressed at high levels by lysosome-rich tumors such as granular cell tumors and may also be useful in bringing out the sometimes subtle round cell population of plexiform fibrohistiocytic tumors (Fig. 7–31).

β-catenin

β-catenin is a 92-kDa protein involved in both cadherin-mediated cellular cohesion, though binding to the cyto-plasmic tail of E-cadherin, and in intracellular signaling, as a component of the Wnt signaling pathway.[357] In normal cells, β-catenin expression is tightly regulated by the APC gene and by glycogen synthetase kinase 3-beta.[358–360] Loss of β-catenin regulation may be the result of either mutations in the APC genes, or in the β-catenin gene itself, resulting in accumulation of cytosolic β-catenin protein, and eventual translocation to the nucleus.

Essentially all familial fibromatoses contain mutation in the APC gene, whereas sporadic fibromatoses are more likely to contain β-catenin mutations.[361,362] As a consequence of these mutations, nuclear overexpression of β-catenin protein is seen in over 90% of fibromatoses.[363–367] Superficial fibromatoses lack β-catenin mutations, but also express nuclear β-catenin protein in approximately 90% of cases.[363] Nuclear β-catenin expression is relatively specific for fibromatoses, although it may also be seen in

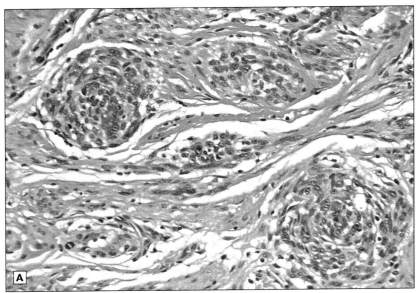

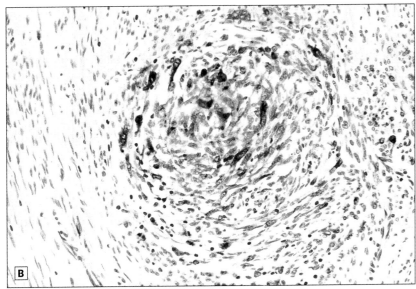

FIGURE 7–31 Plexiform fibrohistiocytic tumor **(A)** with strong CD68 expression in the histiocytoid nodules but not in the surrounding fibroblastic fascicles **(B)**.

a substantial minority of solitary fibrous tumors, synovial sarcomas, and endometrial stromal sarcomas, and in isolated cases of clear cell sarcoma, osteosarcoma, and liposarcoma.[367–370] Interestingly, desmoplastic fibromas of bone, which have been presumed to represent the bony counterpart of soft tissue fibromatoses, appear to lack β-catenin expression, suggesting a different pathogenesis for these morphologically identical lesions.[371]

MDM2

A nuclear phosphoprotein whose transcription is activated by the p53 gene, MDM2 binds the p53 gene and removes its block on the cell cycle at the G_1/S checkpoint.[372,373] The MDM2 marker has also been shown to exert an inhibitory effect through binding RB protein[374] and a stimulatory effect on the E2F family of transcrip-

tion factors.[375] Although overexpression of MDM2 has been previously documented in 33–37% of sarcomas, it does not appear to be of prognostic significance.[376–378] Most recently, MDM2 (and cdk4) expression has been shown to be highly characteristic of well-differentiated liposarcoma (atypical lipomatous tumor) and dedifferentiated liposarcoma, and detection of this protein may be useful in the distinction of these tumors from ordinary lipomas and other pleomorphic soft tissue sarcomas, respectively.[379–381]

Bcl-2

The bcl-2 protein is a mitochondrial and microsomal protein which plays a critical role in the prevention of cellular apoptosis.[382] Bcl-2 is normally expressed in a variety of normal cell types, including trophoblast, renal tubules and neurons.[383] Bcl-2 is perhaps best known for its role in the pathogenesis of follicular lymphomas, wherein the translocation t(14;18) results in fusion of the bcl-2 and immunoglobulin heavy chain genes, with subsequent overexpression of bcl-2 protein.[384] In soft tissue tumors, bcl-2 expression is relatively common in synovial sarcoma and solitary fibrous tumors, and some authors have suggested a role for this marker in the diagnosis of these entities.[191,192,385–388] However, careful reading of these same studies suggests that bcl-2 expression may actually be seen in most of the entities that enter into the differential diagnosis of monophasic synovial sarcoma and solitary fibrous tumor, and for this reason we do not advocate the use of bcl-2 immunostains in the diagnosis of soft tissue tumors.

PROGNOSTIC MARKERS

Ki-67

A 395-kDa nuclear antigen, Ki-67 is encoded by a single gene on chromosome 10, the expression of which is confined to late G_1, S, M, and G_2 growth phases.[389] It appears to be localized to the nucleolus and may be a component of nucleolar preribosomes.[390] In formalin-fixed tissue the most widely used antibody against this antigen is MIB-1. Several studies have documented a correlation between a high Ki-67 labeling index and poor prognostic features in soft tissue sarcomas.[391–394] Significant associations have been shown between a Ki-67 labeling index of more than 20% with high-grade, shortened overall survival and the development of metastatic disease.[395] In high-grade sarcomas of the extremities, a Ki-67 labeling index of more than 20% has been shown to be an independent predictor of distant metastases and tumor mortality.[396]

p53

The TP53 gene product, p53, is a nuclear phosphoprotein that appears to regulate transcription by arresting cells with damaged DNA in G_1 phase.[397–399] Mutations of the TP53 gene produce a mutant protein that loses its tumor-suppressing ability and has a longer half-life than wild-type p53;[397] this allows immunohistochemical detection of mutated p53. Overexpression of p53 has been examined in a variety of soft tissue sarcomas, with the incidence ranging from 9% to 41%.[378,396,400–404] Most studies of p53 expression in sarcomas have shown a correlation between p53 overexpression, high tumor grade, and worse outcome; however, p53 overexpression has not been shown to have prognostic significance independent of grade.[392,396,402–405]

p21^WAF1

A downstream effector of p53, p21^WAF1 is an inhibitor of the cyclin/cyclin-dependent kinase complexes.[406] Loss of normal p21^WAF1 expression has been documented in a subset of liposarcomas, including dedifferentiated, myxoid, and round cell liposarcomas, but has not yet been shown to be of prognostic significance.[372,373]

p16 AND p27^kip

The p16 and p27^kip markers are cyclin-dependent kinase inhibitors (CKIs) of the INK4 and KIP families, respectively.[406] These CKIs have been most extensively studied in malignant peripheral nerve sheath tumors. Loss of p16 expression, secondary to homozygous deletion of CDKN2A/p16, has been shown to be present in malignant peripheral nerve sheath tumors but not neurofibromas from patients with neurofibromatosis 1.[407] Loss of p27^kip constitutive expression has been implicated in the malignant transformation of neurofibromas.[408]

APPLICATION OF IMMUNOHISTOCHEMISTRY TO SARCOMA DIAGNOSIS: CLINICAL SCENARIOS

In general, it is advisable to have an initial panel of antibodies to analyze a sarcoma that is of uncertain differentiation histologically, including at least a representative of each of the antibody "groups" listed in Table 7–5. Of course, depending on the histologic setting of the tumor, it may or may not be necessary to include a member of each of the four groups.

Several common histologic scenarios of soft tissue tumors, in which immunohistochemistry can provide valuable clues to the correct diagnosis, are described below. These histologic settings include "the undifferentiated round cell tumor," "the monomorphic spindle cell tumor," and "the poorly differentiated epithelioid tumor."

TABLE 7–5	BASIC ANTIGEN GROUPS FOR SARCOMA IMMUNODIAGNOSIS	
Tumor group	**Markers**
Synovial sarcoma, epithelioid sarcoma	Cytokeratin, EMA
Nerve sheath group	S-100 protein, CD57, NGF receptor
Muscle group	Desmin, muscle actins, myogenic regulatory proteins
Endothelial group	CD31, CD34, FLI-1, vWF, ulex lectin

A basic principle in diagnostic immunohistochemistry that is illustrated in each of the four scenarios is the utilization of panels of antibodies, rather than single antibodies directed against markers of the suspected "correct" diagnosis. In general, such a panel should include not only antibodies that one would expect to be positive in a given tumor, but also antibodies that would be expected to be negative. This approach is essential for several reasons. First, many, if not most, antigens are expressed by more than one type of tumor. Second, for technical reasons, antibodies may show false-negative and, occasionally, false-positive results. Lastly, malignant cells may show unexpected or anomalous expression of antigens, and this may be very confusing if not interpreted within the context of other results.

The undifferentiated round cell tumor

The differential diagnosis of this case includes both sarcomas and non-sarcomas. As with all of our other diagnostic scenarios, the first task is to exclude a non-sarcoma. Non-sarcomatous neoplasms that might be legitimately included in this differential diagnosis include lymphoma, melanoma, and in an older patient, small cell carcinoma. Sarcomas that should be included in the differential diagnosis include Ewing's sarcoma/primitive neuroectodermal tumor (ES/PNET), rhabdomyosarcoma (RMS), poorly differentiated synovial sarcoma (PDSS), and desmoplastic round cell tumor (DRCT). Table 7–6 presents a screening panel of antibodies and the expected results for these tumors. The results of this panel dictate what additional studies are needed to confirm a specific diagnosis.

SMALL CELL CARCINOMA (poorly differentiated neuroendocrine carcinoma): Confirm with antibodies to chromogranin A or synaptophysin.

MELANOMA: Confirm with antibodies to melanosome-specific proteins (gp100, Melan-A, tyrosinase, microphthalmia transcription factor). As noted above, a small number of melanomas may be S-100 protein negative, and occasional melanomas express cytokeratin or desmin. Small cell melanomas of the sinonasal tract appear to be particularly likely to show the S-100 protein-negative/HMB-45-positive phenotype.

LYMPHOMA: Lymphoblastic lymphoma in children may be CD45 negative and CD99/FLI-1 positive, which can easily result in a misdiagnosis as ES/PNET. If the clinical or histologic features are suggestive of lymphoma, immunohistochemistry for terminal deoxyribonucleotide transferase (TDT) may be critically important in arriving at the correct diagnosis. In adults and children, anaplastic large cell lymphomas (which have a small cell variant) may also be CD45 negative. In this setting, antibodies to CD30 may be useful.

EWING'S SARCOMA/PRIMITIVE NEUROECTODERMAL TUMOR: As noted above, ES/PNET are unique among small blue round-cell tumors in that they do not usually express CD56. This negative finding may be useful in cases where CD99 is equivocal, or where there is anomalous expression of cytokeratin or desmin. Demonstration of FLI-1 protein expression may also be helpful.

RHABDOMYOSARCOMA: Confirm with myogenin or MyoD1.

POORLY DIFFERENTIATED SYNOVIAL SARCOMA: Cytokeratin expression is patchy or absent in some poorly differentiated synovial sarcomas. The addition of antibodies to EMA and high-molecular-weight cytokeratins may allow detection of scattered positive cells. Antibodies to type IV collagen also sometimes reveal nested growth, or "occult" glandular differentiation.

DESMOPLASTIC SMALL ROUND CELL TUMOR: Confirm with antibodies to carboxy-terminus WT-1 or FISH studies looking for presence of t(11;22)(p13;q12)

Monomorphic spindle cell tumors

The differential diagnosis of monomorphic spindle cell tumors often includes such entities as fibrosarcoma, monophasic fibrous synovial sarcoma, malignant peripheral nerve sheath tumor, and malignant solitary fibrous tumor. Table 7–7 presents a screening immunohistochemical panel and the expected result for each tumor.

The following comments should also be borne in mind when immunostaining monomorphic spindle cell tumors.

TABLE 7–6	SCREENING PANEL FOR UNDIFFERENTIATED ROUND CELL TUMOR						
Antibody to	Small cell carcinoma	Melanoma	Lymphoma	PNET	RMS	PDSS	DRCT
Pan-cytokeratin	Positive	Variable	Negative	Variable	Rare	Positive	Positive
S-100 protein	Negative	Positive	Negative	Variable	Rare	Variable	Negative
CD45	Negative	Negative	Positive #	Negative	Negative	Negative	Negative
Desmin	Negative	Variable	Negative	Rare	Positive	Negative	Positive
CD99	Negative	Negative	Variable	Positive	Variable	Positive	Rare

PNET, primitive neuroectodermal tumor; RMS, rhabdomyosarcoma; DRCT, desmoplastic round cell tumor; PDSS, poorly differentiated synovial sarcoma.
Lymphoblastic lymphomas may be CD45 negative. In children, screen with TdT and CD43 instead of CD45.

TABLE 7–7   SCREENING PANEL FOR MONOMORPHIC SPINDLE CELL TUMORS

Antibody to	Synovial sarcoma	MPNST	Fibrosarcoma	Leiomyosarcoma	Solitary fibrous tumor
Pan-cytokeratin	Positive	Negative	Negative	Rare	Rare
S-100 protein	Variable	Positive	Negative	Rare	Negative
CD34	Negative	Variable	Negative	Rare	Positive
Smooth muscle actin	Negative	Negative	Variable (myofibrosarcoma)	Positive	Negative

MPNST, malignant peripheral nerve sheath tumor.

TABLE 7–8   SCREENING PANEL FOR EPITHELIOID TUMORS IN SOFT TISSUE

Antibody to	Carcinoma	Melanoma	B- or T-cell lymphoma	Anaplastic large cell lymphoma	Epithelioid sarcoma	Epithelioid angiosarcoma
Cytokeratin	Positive	Variable	Negative	Negative	Positive	Variable
S-100 protein	Negative	Positive	Negative	Negative	Negative	Negative
CD45	Negative	Negative	Positive	Negative	Negative	Negative
CD30	Negative	Negative	Negative	Positive	Negative	Negative
CD31	Negative	Negative	Negative	Negative	Negative	Positive

TABLE 7–9   DISCRIMINATION OF CARCINOMA, EPITHELIOID SARCOMA, AND EPITHELIOID ANGIOSARCOMA

Antibody to	Carcinoma	Epithelioid sarcoma	Epithelioid angiosarcoma
High-molecular-weight cytokeratin	Variable	Variable	Negative
CD34	Negative	Variable	Positive
CD31	Negative	Negative	Positive
FLI-1	Negative	Negative	Positive
INI-1	Positive	Negative #	Positive

Normal tissues and most tumors express INI-1. Epithelioid sarcomas lose INI-1 expression.

SYNOVIAL SARCOMA: As noted above, cytokeratin and EMA expression may be focal in synovial sarcomas. Expression of CD34 is exceptionally rare in synovial sarcoma.

MALIGNANT PERIPHERAL NERVE SHEATH TUMOR: S-100 protein expression is often weak and focal. EMA, claudin-1 and Glut-1 expression may be seen in tumors with perineurial differentiation. Confirm with CD57 and p75NTR.

FIBROSARCOMA: It may show limited actin expression (myofibrosarcoma).

SOLITARY FIBROUS TUMOR: Occasional cases, particularly those with histologic features of malignancy, show anomalous cytokeratin expression. Strong CD34 expression is helpful in distinguishing such cases from monophasic synovial sarcoma.

Poorly differentiated epithelioid tumor

The differential diagnosis of poorly differentiated epithelioid tumors includes carcinoma, melanoma, lymphoma (including anaplastic large cell lymphoma), and epithelioid soft tissue tumors such as epithelioid sarcoma and angiosarcoma. The recommended panel of antibodies and their expected reactivities are presented in Table 7–8. This initial screening panel can make a specific diagnosis of melanoma, lymphoma, or anaplastic large cell lymphoma, but generally it is not able to discriminate carcinoma from epithelioid sarcoma or epithelioid angiosarcoma. These tumors can be reliably distinguished with the additional panel of antibodies listed in Table 7–9.

"Orphan sarcomas"

It should be noted, the above notwithstanding, that there remain "orphan sarcomas" without specific markers. This group includes tumors for which there is no known normal cell counterpart (e.g., malignant fibrous histiocytoma) and those for which there is a known cell counterpart (e.g., liposarcoma, osteogenic sarcoma, chondrosarcoma) but for which there are no reliable, useful specific markers at present. Whereas markers for osteosarcoma have been developed, such as osteocalcin and osteonectin, they have not proved to be more sensitive markers than is the histologic identification of tumor osteoid.[409]

CONCLUSION

Immunohistochemistry continues to be a rapidly evolving field, with a number of exciting new markers having already entered the armamentarium of the diagnostic pathologist, and more to come. In many respects, advances in the immunohistochemical diagnosis of soft tissue neoplasms serve as logical extensions of the ground-breaking cytogenetic and molecular genetic advances in our understanding of these tumors, with new markers such as FLI-1, WT-1, INI1, TFE3 and β-catenin serving as "surrogate" protein markers of underlying genetic events. It is anticipated that new markers will assist in the diagnosis of tumors with other, more recently described specific genetic events, such as the newly described translocation t(7;16)(q33;p11) seen in low-grade fibromyxoid sarcoma.[410,411]

REFERENCES

Intermediate filaments

1. Damjanov I. Antibodies to intermediate filaments and histogenesis. Lab Invest 1982; 47(3):215.
2. Denk H, Krepler R, Artlieb U, et al. Proteins of intermediate filaments. An immunohistochemical and biochemical approach to the classification of soft tissue tumors. Am J Pathol 1983; 110(2):193.
3. Osborn M, Weber K. Tumor diagnosis by intermediate filament typing: a novel tool for surgical pathology [Review]. Lab Invest 1983; 48(4):372.
4. Dahl D. The vimentin-GFA protein transition in rat neuroglia cytoskeleton occurs at the time of myelination. J Neurosci Res 1981; 6(6):741.
5. Connell ND, Rheinwald JG. Regulation of the cytoskeleton in mesothelial cells: reversible loss of keratin and increase in vimentin during rapid growth in culture. Cell 1983; 34(1):245.
6. Virtanen I, Lehto VP, Lehtonen E, et al. Expression of intermediate filaments in cultured cells. J Cell Sci 1981; 50:45.
7. Akhtar M, Tulbah A, Kardar AH, et al. Sarcomatoid renal cell carcinoma: the chromphobe connection. Am J Surgl Pathol 1997; 21(10):1188.
8. Eckert F, de Viragh PA, Schmid U. Coexpression of cytokeratin and vimentin intermediate filaments in benign and malignant sweat gland tumors. J Cutan Pathol 1994; 21(2):140.
9. Lopez-Beltran A, Escudero AL, Cavazzana AO, et al. Sarcomatoid transitional cell carcinoma of the renal pelvis. A report of five cases with clinical, pathological, immunohistochemical and DNA ploidy analysis. Pathol Res Pract 1996; 192(12):1218.
10. Meis JM, Ordonez NG, Gallager HS. Sarcomatoid carcinoma of the breast: an immunohistochemical study of six cases. Virchows Archiv A, Pathol Anat Histopathol 1987; 410(5):415.
11. Skalli O, Gabbiani G, Babai F, et al. Intermediate filament proteins and actin isoforms as markers for soft tissue tumor differentiation and origin. II. Rhabdomyosarcomas. Am J Pathol 1988; 130(3):515.
12. Azumi N, Battifora H. The distribution of vimentin and keratin in epithelial and nonepithelial neoplasms. A comprehensive immunohistochemical study on formalin- and alcohol-fixed tumors. Am J Clin Pathol 1987; 88(3):286.
13. Judkins AR, Montone KT, LiVolsi VA, et al. Sensitivity and specificity of antibodies on necrotic tumor tissue. Am J Clin Pathol 1998; 110(5):641.
14. Folpe AL, Mentzel T, Lehr HA, et al. Perivascular epithelioid cell neoplasms of soft tissue and gynecologic origin: a clinicopathologic study of 26 cases and review of the literature. Am J Surg Pathol 2005; 29(12):1558.
15. Fanburg-Smith JC, Miettinen M, Folpe AL, et al. Lingual alveolar soft part sarcoma; 14 cases: novel clinical and morphological observations. Histopathology 2004; 45(5):526.
16. Miettinen M. Keratin subsets in spindle cell sarcomas. Keratins are widespread but synovial sarcoma contains a distinctive keratin polypeptide pattern and desmoplakins. Am J Pathol 1991; 138(2):505.
17. Billings SD, Walsh SV, Fisher C, et al. Aberrant expression of tight junction-related proteins ZO-1, claudin-1 and occludin in synovial sarcoma: an immunohistochemical study with ultrastructural correlation. Mod Pathol 2004; 17(2):141.
18. Folpe AL, Schmidt RA, Chapman D, et al. Poorly differentiated synovial sarcoma: immunohistochemical distinction from primitive neuroectodermal tumors and high-grade malignant peripheral nerve sheath tumors. Am J Surg Pathol 1998; 22(6):673.
19. Miettinen M, Fanburg-Smith JC, Virolainen M, et al. Epithelioid sarcoma: an immunohistochemical analysis of 112 classical and variant cases and a discussion of the differential diagnosis. Hum Pathol 1999; 30(8):934.
20. Laskin WB, Miettinen M. Epithelioid sarcoma: new insights based on an extended immunohistochemical analysis. Arch Pathol Lab Med 2003; 127(9):1161.
21. Smith TA, Machen SK, Fisher C, et al. Usefulness of cytokeratin subsets for distinguishing monophasic synovial sarcoma from malignant peripheral nerve sheath tumor. Am J Clin Pathol 1999; 112(5):641.
22. Fanburg-Smith JC, Hengge M, Hengge UR, et al. Extrarenal rhabdoid tumors of soft tissue: a clinicopathologic and immunohistochemical study of 18 cases. Ann Diagn Pathol 1998; 2(6):351.
23. Hoefler H, Kerl H, Rauch HJ, et al. New immunocytochemical observations with diagnostic significance in cutaneous neuroendocrine carcinoma. Am J Dermatopathol 1984; 6(6):525.
24. Miettinen M, Lehto VP, Virtanen I, et al. Neuroendocrine carcinoma of the skin (Merkel cell carcinoma): ultrastructural and immunohistochemical demonstration of neurofilaments. Ultrastruct Pathol 1983; 4(2–3):219.
25. Jahn L, Fouquet B, Rohe K, et al. Cytokeratins in certain endothelial and smooth muscle cells of two taxonomically distant vertebrate species, *Xenopus laevis* and man. Differentiation 1987; 36(3):234.
26. Brown DC, Theaker JM, Banks PM, et al. Cytokeratin expression in smooth muscle and smooth muscle tumours. Histopathology 1987; 11(5):477.
27. Norton AJ, Thomas JA, Isaacson PG. Cytokeratin-specific monoclonal antibodies are reactive with tumours of smooth muscle derivation. An immunocytochemical and biochemical study using antibodies to intermediate filament cytoskeletal proteins. Histopathology 1987; 11(5):487.
28. Gown AM, Boyd HC, Chang Y, et al. Smooth muscle cells can express cytokeratins of "simple" epithelium. Immunocytochemical and biochemical studies in vitro and in vivo. Am J Pathol 1988; 132(2):223.
29. Miettinen M. Immunoreactivity for cytokeratin and epithelial membrane antigen in leiomyosarcoma. Arch Pathol Lab Med 1988; 112(6):637.
30. Ramaekers FC, Pruszczynski M, Smedts F. Cytokeratins in smooth muscle cells and smooth muscle tumours. Histopathology 1988; 12(5):558.
31. Tauchi K, Tsutsumi Y, Yoshimura S, et al. Immunohistochemical and immunoblotting detection of cytokeratin in smooth muscle tumors. Acta Pathol Japon 1990; 40(8):574.
32. Gown AM, Vogel AM. Monoclonal antibodies to human intermediate filament proteins. III. Analysis of tumors. Am J Clin Pathol 1985; 84(4):413.
33. Zarbo RJ, Gown AM, Nagle RB, et al. Anomalous cytokeratin expression in malignant melanoma: one- and two-dimensional Western blot analysis and immunohistochemical survey of 100 melanomas. Mod Pathol 1990; 3(4):494.
34. Ben-Izhak O, Stark P, Levy R, et al. Epithelial markers in malignant melanoma. A study of primary lesions and their metastases. Am J Dermatopathol 1994; 16(3):241.
35. Ben-Izhak O, Auslander L, Robinson S, et al. Epithelioid angiosarcoma of the adrenal gland with cytokeratin expression. Report of a case with accompanying mesenteric fibromatosis. Cancer 1992; 69(7):1808.
36. Gray MH, Rosenberg AE, Dickersin GR, et al. Cytokeratin expression in epithelioid vascular neoplasms. Hum Pathol 1990; 21(2):212.
37. O'Connell JX, Kattapuram SV, Mankin HJ, et al. Epithelioid hemangioma of bone. A tumor often mistaken for low-grade angiosarcoma or malignant hemangioendothelioma [see comments]. Am J Surg Pathol 1993; 17(6):610.
38. van Haelst UJ, Pruszczynski M, ten Cate LN, et al. Ultrastructural and immunohistochemical study of epithelioid hemangioendothelioma of bone: coexpression of epithelial and endothelial markers. Ultrastruct Pathol 1990; 14(2):141.
39. Wenig BM, Abbondanzo SL, Heffess CS. Epithelioid angiosarcoma of the adrenal glands. A clinicopathologic study of nine cases with a discussion of the implications of finding "epithelial-specific" markers. Am J Surg Pathol 1994; 18(1):62.
40. Meis-Kindblom JM, Kindblom LG. Angiosarcoma of soft tissue: a study of 80 cases. Am J Surg Pathol 1998; 22(6):683.

41. Collini P, Sampietro G, Bertulli R, et al. Cytokeratin immunoreactivity in 41 cases of ES/PNET confirmed by molecular diagnostic studies. Am J Surg Pathol 2001; 25(2):273.

42. Gu M, Antonescu CR, Guiter G, et al. Cytokeratin immunoreactivity in Ewing's sarcoma: prevalence in 50 cases confirmed by molecular diagnostic studies. Am J Surg Pathol 2000; 24(3):410.

43. Bridge JA, Fidler ME, Neff JR, et al. Adamantinoma-like Ewing's sarcoma: genomic confirmation, phenotypic drift. Am J Surg Pathol 1999; 23(2):159.

44. Folpe AL, Goldblum JR, Rubin BP, et al. Morphologic and immunophenotypic diversity in Ewing family tumors: a study of 66 genetically confirmed cases. Am J Surg Pathol 2005; 29(8):1025.

45. Miettinen M, Rapola J. Immunohistochemical spectrum of rhabdomyosarcoma and rhabdomyosarcoma-like tumors. Expression of cytokeratin and the 68-kD neurofilament protein. Am J Surg Pathol 1989; 13(2):120.

46. Coindre JM, de Mascarel A, Trojani M, et al. Immunohistochemical study of rhabdomyosarcoma. Unexpected staining with S100 protein and cytokeratin. J Pathol 1988; 155(2):127.

47. Droz D, Rousseau-Merck MF, Jaubert F, et al. Cell differentiation in Wilms' tumor (nephroblastoma): an immunohistochemical study. Hum Pathol 1990; 21(5):536.

48. Wick MR, Manivel C, O'Leary TP, et al. Nephroblastoma. A comparative immunocytochemical and lectin-histochemical study. Arch Pathol Lab Med 1986; 110(7):630.

49. Nikolaou I, Barbatis C, Laopodis V, et al. Intra-abdominal desmoplastic small-cell tumours with divergent differentiation. Report of two cases and review of the literature. Pathol Res Pract 1992; 188(8):981.

50. Ordonez NG. Desmoplastic small round cell tumor: II: an ultrastructural and immunohistochemical study with emphasis on new immunohistochemical markers. Am J Surg Pathol 1998; 22(11):1314.

51. Weiss SW, Bratthauer GL, Morris PA. Postirradiation malignant fibrous histiocytoma expressing cytokeratin. Implications for the immunodiagnosis of sarcomas [see comments]. Am J Surg Pathol 1988; 12(7):554.

52. Rosenberg AE, O'Connell JX, Dickersin GR, et al. Expression of epithelial markers in malignant fibrous histiocytoma of the musculoskeletal system: an immunohistochemical and electron microscopic study. Hum Pathol 1993; 24(3):284.

53. Litzky LA, Brooks JJ. Cytokeratin immunoreactivity in malignant fibrous histiocytoma and spindle cell tumors: comparison between frozen and paraffin-embedded tissues. Mod Pathol 1992; 5(1):30.

54. Miettinen M, Soini Y. Malignant fibrous histiocytoma. Heterogeneous patterns of intermediate filament proteins by immunohistochemistry. Arch Pathol Lab Med 1989; 13(12):1363.

55. Abramovici LC, Steiner GC, Bonar F. Myxoid chondrosarcoma of soft tissue and bone: a retrospective study of 11 cases. Hum Pathol 1995; 26(11):1215.

56. Hasegawa T, Seki K, Yang P, et al. Differentiation and proliferative activity in benign and malignant cartilage tumors of bone. Hum Pathol 1995; 26(8):838.

57. Dardick I, Schatz JE, Colgan TJ. Osteogenic sarcoma with epithelial differentiation. Ultrastruct Pathol 1992; 16(4):463.

58. Hasegawa T, Shibata T, Hirose T, et al. Osteosarcoma with epithelioid features. An immunohistochemical study. Arch Pathol Lab Med 1993; 117(3):295.

59. Hirose T, Hasegawa T, Kudo E, et al. Malignant peripheral nerve sheath tumors: an immunohistochemical study in relation to ultrastructural features. Hum Pathol 1992; 23(8):865.

60. Battifora H. Misuse of the term "expression" [letter; comment]. Am J Clin Pathol 1989; 92(5):708.

61. Swanson PE. HIERanarchy: the state of the art in immunohistochemistry [editorial]. Am J Clin Pathol 1997; 107(2):139.

62. Swanson PE. Heffalumps, jagulars, and cheshire cats. A commentary on cytokeratins and soft tissue sarcomas [see comments]. Am J Clin Pathol 1991; 95(4 Suppl 1):S2.

63. Bacchi CE, Zarbo RJ, Jiang JJ, et al. Do glioma cells express cytokeratin? Appl Immunohistochem 1995; 3(1):45.

Epithelial membrane antigen

64. Heyderman E, Steele K, Ormerod MG. A new antigen on the epithelial membrane: its immunoperoxidase localisation in normal and neoplastic tissue. Am J Clin Pathol 1979; 32(1):35.

65. Pinkus GS, Kurtin PJ. Epithelial membrane antigen – a diagnostic discriminant in surgical pathology: immunohistochemical profile in epithelial, mesenchymal, and hematopoietic neoplasms using paraffin sections and monoclonal antibodies. Hum Pathol 1985; 16(9):929.

66. Erlandson RA. The enigmatic perineurial cell and its participation in tumors and in tumorlike entities. Ultrastruct Pathol 1991; 15(4–5):335.

67. Theaker JM, Fletcher CD. Epithelial membrane antigen expression by the perineurial cell: further studies of peripheral nerve lesions. Histopathology 1989; 14(6):581.

68. Theaker JM, Gatter KC, Puddle J. Epithelial membrane antigen expression by the perineurium of peripheral nerve and in peripheral nerve tumours. Histopathology 1988; 13(2):171.

69. Theaker JM, Gillett MB, Fleming KA, et al. Epithelial membrane antigen expression by meningiomas, and the perineurium of peripheral nerve. Arch Pathol Lab Med 1987; 111(5):409.

70. Theaker JM, Gatter KC, Esiri MM, et al. Epithelial membrane antigen and cytokeratin expression by meningiomas: an immunohistological study. Am J Clin Pathol 1986; 39(4):435.

71. Ariza A, Bilbao JM, Rosai J. Immunohistochemical detection of epithelial membrane antigen in normal perineurial cells and perineurioma. Am J Surg Pathol 1988; 12(9):678.

72. Zamecnik M, Michal M. Malignant peripheral nerve sheath tumor with perineurial cell differentiation (malignant perineurioma). Pathol Internat 1999; 49(1):69.

73. Hirose T, Scheithauer BW, Sano T. Perineurial malignant peripheral nerve sheath tumor (MPNST): a clinicopathologic, immunohistochemical, and ultrastructural study of seven cases. Am J Surg Pathol 1998; 22(11):1368.

74. Perentes E, Nakagawa Y, Ross et al. Expression of epithelial membrane antigen in perineurial cells and their derivatives. An immunohistochemical study with multiple markers. Acta Neuropathol 1987; 75(2):160.

75. Hornick JL, Fletcher CD. Soft tissue perineurioma: clinicopathologic analysis of 81 cases including those with atypical histologic features. Am J Surg Pathol 2005; 29(7):845.

76. Fanburg-Smith JC, Miettinen M. Angiomatoid "malignant" fibrous histiocytoma: a

clinicopathologic study of 158 cases and further exploration of the nyoid phenotype. Hum Pathol 1999; 30(11):1336.

Markers of muscle differentiation

77. Kindblom LG, Seidal T, Karlsson K. Immunohistochemical localization of myoglobin in human muscle tissue and embryonal and alveolar rhabdomyosarcoma. Acta Pathol Microbiol Immunol Scand – Section A, Pathology 1982; 90(3):167.

78. Andriko JW, Kaldjian EP, Tsokos M, et al. Reticulum cell neoplasms of lymph nodes: a clinicopathologic study of 11 cases with recognition of a new subtype derived from fibroblastic reticular cells. Am J Surg Pathol 1998; 22(9):1048.

79. Cho J, Gong G, Choe G, et al. Extrafollicular reticulum cells in pathologic lymph nodes. J Korean Med Sci 1994; 9(1):9.

80. Van Muijen GN, Ruiter DJ, Warnaar SO. Coexpression of intermediate filament polypeptides in human fetal and adult tissues. Lab Invest 1987; 57(4):359.

81. Franquemont DW, Frierson HF Jr, Mills SE. An immunohistochemical study of normal endometrial stroma and endometrial stromal neoplasms. Evidence for smooth muscle differentiation. Am J Surg Pathol 1991; 15(9):861.

82. Altmannsberger M, Weber K, Droste R, et al. Desmin is a specific marker for rhabdomyosarcomas of human and rat origin. Am J Pathol 1985; 118(1):85.

83. Tsokos M. The role of immunocytochemistry in the diagnosis of rhabdomyosarcoma [editorial]. Arch Pathol Lab Med 1986; 110(9):776.

84. Azumi N, Ben-Ezra J, Battifora H. Immunophenotypic diagnosis of leiomyosarcomas and rhabdomyosarcomas with monoclonal antibodies to muscle-specific actin and desmin in formalin-fixed tissue. Mod Pathol 1988; 1(6):469.

85. Leader M, Collins M, Patel J, et al. Desmin: its value as a marker of muscle derived tumours using a commercial antibody. Virchows Archiv – A, Pathol Anat Histopathol 1987; 411(4):345.

86. Parham DM, Webber B, Holt H, et al. Immunohistochemical study of childhood rhabdomyosarcomas and related neoplasms. Results of an Intergroup Rhabdomyosarcoma Study Project. Cancer 1991; 67(12):3072.

87. Chiles MC, Parham DM, Qualman SJ, et al. Sclerosing rhabdomyosarcomas in children and adolescents: a clinicopathologic review of 13 cases from the Intergroup Rhabdomyosarcoma Study Group and Children's Oncology Group. Pediatr Dev Pathol 2004; 7(6):583.

88. Folpe AL, McKenney JK, Bridge JA, et al. Sclerosing rhabdomyosarcoma in adults: report of four cases of a hyalinizing, matrix-rich variant of rhabdomyosarcoma that may be confused with osteosarcoma, chondrosarcoma, or angiosarcoma. Am J Surg Pathol 2002; 26(9):1175.

89. Furlong MA, Mentzel T, Fanburg-Smith JC. Pleomorphic rhabdomyosarcoma in adults: a clinicopathologic study of 38 cases with emphasis on morphologic variants and recent skeletal muscle-specific markers. Mod Pathol 2001; 14(6):595.

90. Rubin BP, Hasserjian RP, Singer S, et al. Spindle cell rhabdomyosarcoma (so-called) in adults: report of two cases with emphasis on differential diagnosis. Am J Surg Pathol 1998; 22(4):459.

91. Coffin CM, Rulon J, Smith L, et al. Pathologic features of rhabdomyosarcoma before and after treatment: a clinicopathologic and immunohistochemical analysis. Mod Pathol 1997; 10(12):1175.

92. Rangdaeng S, Truong LD. Comparative immunohistochemical staining for desmin and muscle-specific actin. A study of 576 cases [see comments]. Am J Clin Pathol 1991; 96(1):32.

93. Truong LD, Rangdaeng S, Cagle P, et al. The diagnostic utility of desmin. A study of 584 cases and review of the literature [see comments]. Am J clin Pathol 1990; 93(3):305.

94. Parham DM, Dias P, Kelly DR, et al. Desmin positivity in primitive neuroectodermal tumors of childhood. Am J Surg Pathol 1992; 16(5):483.

95. Gerald WL, Miller HK, Battifora H, et al. Intra-abdominal desmoplastic small round-cell tumor. Report of 19 cases of a distinctive type of high-grade polyphenotypic malignancy affecting young individuals [see comments]. Am J Surg Pathol 1991; 15(6):499.

96. Sugimoto T, Ueyama H, Hosoi H, et al. Alpha-smooth-muscle actin and desmin expressions in human neuroblastoma cell lines. Int J Cancer 1991; 48(2):277.

97. Hurlimann J. Desmin and neural marker expression in mesothelial cells and mesotheliomas. HumaPathol 1994; 25(8):753.

98. Folpe AL, Patterson K, Gown AM. Antibodies to desmin identify the blastemal component of nephroblastoma. Mod Pathol 1997; 10(9):895.

99. Folpe AL, Weiss SW, Fletcher CDM, et al. Tenosynovial giant cell tumors: Evidence for a desmin-positive dendritic cell subpopulation. Mod Pathol 1998; 11(10):939.

100. Folpe AL, Weiss SW. Ossifying fibromyxoid tumor of soft parts: a clinicopathologic study of 70 cases with emphasis on atypical and malignant variants. Am J Surg Pathol 2003; 27(4):421.

101. Hasegawa T, Seki K, Ono K, et al. Angiomatoid (malignant) fibrous histiocytoma: a peculiar low-grade tumor showing immunophenotypic heterogeneity and ultrastructural variations. Pathol Int 2000; 50(9):731.

102. Lessard JL. Two monoclonal antibodies to actin: one muscle selective and one generally reactive. Cell Motil Cytoskel 1988; 10(3):349.

103. Skalli O, Ropraz P, Trzeciak A, et al. A monoclonal antibody against alpha-smooth muscle actin: a new probe for smooth muscle differentiation. J Cell Biol 1986; 103(6 Pt 2):2787.

104. Tsukada T, McNutt MA, Ross R, et al. HHF35, a muscle actin-specific monoclonal antibody. II. Reactivity in normal, reactive, and neoplastic human tissues. Am J Pathology 1987; 127(2):389.

105. Tsukada T, Tippens D, Gordon D, et al. HHF35, a muscle-actin-specific monoclonal antibody. I. Immunocytochemical and biochemical characterization. Am J Pathology 1987; 126(1):51.

106. Venuti JM, Morris JH, Vivian JL, et al. Myogenin is required for late but not early aspects of myogenesis during mouse development. J Cell Biol 1995; 128(4):563.

107. Weintraub H. The MyoD family and myogenesis: redundancy, networks, and thresholds. Cell 1993; 75(7):1241.

108. Dias P, Dilling M, Houghton P. The molecular basis of skeletal muscle differentiation. Semin Diagn Pathol 1994; 11(1):3.

109. Rudnicki MA, Jaenisch R. The MyoD family of transcription factors and skeletal myogenesis. Bioessays 1995; 17(3):203.

110. Dias P, Parham DM, Shapiro DN, et al. Monoclonal antibodies to the myogenic regulatory protein MyoD1: epitope mapping and diagnostic utility. Cancer Res 1992; 52(23):6431.

111. Wang NP, Marx J, McNutt MA, et al. Expression of myogenic regulatory proteins (myogenin and MyoD1) in small blue round cell tumors of childhood. Am J Pathol 1995; 147(6):1799.

112. Tonin PN, Scrable H, Shimada H, et al. Muscle-specific gene expression in rhabdomyosarcomas and stages of human fetal skeletal muscle development. Cancer Res 1991; 51(19):5100.

113. Kumar S, Perlman E, Harris CA, et al. Myogenin is a specific marker for rhabdomyosarcoma: an immunohistochemical study in paraffin-embedded tissues. Mod Pathol 2000; 13(9):988.

114. Cessna MH, Zhou H, Perkins SL, et al. Are myogenin and MyoD1 expression specific for rhabdomyosarcoma? A study of 150 cases, with emphasis on spindle cell mimics. Am J Surg Pathol 2001; 25(9):1150.

115. Dias P, Chen B, Dilday B, et al. Strong immunostaining for myogenin in rhabdomyosarcoma is significantly associated with tumors of the alveolar subclass. Am J Pathol 2000; 156(2):399.

116. Mentzel T, Katenkamp D. Sclerosing, pseudovascular rhabdomyosarcoma in adults. Clinicopathological and immunohistochemical analysis of three cases. Virchows Arch 2000; 436(4):305.

117. Folpe AL. MyoD1 and myogenin expression in human neoplasia: a review and update. Adv Anat Pathol 2002; 9(3):198.

118. Wesche WA, Fletcher CD, Dias P, et al. Immunohistochemistry of MyoD1 in adult pleomorphic soft tissue sarcomas. Am J Surg Pathol 1995; 19(3):261.

119. Rosai J, Dias P, Parham DM, et al. MyoD1 protein expression in alveolar soft part sarcoma as confirmatory evidence of its skeletal muscle nature. Am J Surg Pathol 1991; 15(10):974.

120. Dias P, Parham DM, Shapiro DN, et al. Myogenic regulatory protein (MyoD1) expression in childhood solid tumors: diagnostic utility in rhabdomyosarcoma. Am J Pathol 1990; 137(6):1283.

121. Croes R, Debiec-Rychter M, Cokelaere K, et al. Adult sclerosing rhabdomyosarcoma: cytogenetic link with embryonal rhabdomyosarcoma. Virchows Arch 2005; 446(1):64.

122. Mukai K, Rosai J, Hallaway BE. Localization of myoglobin in normal and neoplastic human skeletal muscle cells using an immunoperoxidase method. Am J Surg Pathol 1979; 3(4):373.

123. Brooks JJ. Immunohistochemistry of soft tissue tumors. Myoglobin as a tumor marker for rhabdomyosarcoma. Cancer 1982; 50(9):1757.

124. Tsokos M, Howard R, Costa J. Immunohistochemical study of alveolar and embryonal rhabdomyosarcoma. Lab Invest 1983; 48(2):148.

125. Jong AS, van Vark M, Albus-Lutter CE, et al. Myosin and myoglobin as tumor markers in the diagnosis of rhabdomyosarcoma. A comparative study. Am J Surg Pathol 1984; 8(7):521.

126. Seidal T, Kindblom LG, Angervall L. Myoglobin, desmin and vimentin in ultrastructurally proven rhabdomyomas and rhabdomyosarcomas. An immunohistochemical study utilizing a series of monoclonal and polyclonal antibodies. Appl Pathol 1987; 5(4):201.

127. Eusebi V, Bondi A, Rosai J. Immunohistochemical localization of myoglobin in nonmuscular cells. Am J Surg Pathol 1984; 8(1):51.

128. Osborn M, Hill C, Altmannsberger M, et al. Monoclonal antibodies to titin in conjunction with antibodies to desmin separate rhabdomyosarcomas from other tumor types. Lab Invest 1986; 55(1):101.

129. Iwasaki H, Isayama T, Ichiki T, et al. Intermediate filaments of myofibroblasts. Immunochemical and immunocytochemical analyses. Pathol Res Pract 1987; 182(2):248.

130. Kuhn C, McDonald JA. The roles of the myofibroblast in idiopathic pulmonary fibrosis. Ultrastructural and immunohistochemical features of sites of active extracellular matrix synthesis. Am J Pathol 1991; 138(5):1257.

131. Wang N-P, Wan BC, Skelly M, et al. Antibodies to novel myoepithelium-associated proteins distinguish benign lesions and carcinoma in situ from invasive carcinoma of the breast. Appl Immunohistochem 1997; 5(3):141.

132. Oliva E, Young RH, Amin MB, et l. An immunohistochemical analysis of endometrial stromal and smooth muscle tumors of the uterus: a study of 54 cases emphasizing the importance of using a panel because of overlap in immunoreactivity for individual antibodies. Am J Surg Pathol 2002; 26(4):403.

133. Nucci MR, O'Connell JT, Huettner PC, et al. h-Caldesmon expression effectively distinguishes endometrial stromal tumors from uterine smooth muscle tumors. Am J Surg Pathol 2001; 25(4):455.

Markers of nerve sheath differentiation

134. Taylor CR. Immunomicroscopy: a diagnostic tool for the surgical pathologist. Philadelphia: Saunders; 1986.

135. Kahn HJ, Marks A, Thom H, et al. Role of antibody to S100 protein in diagnostic pathology. Am J Clin Pathol 1983; 79(3):341.

136. Johnson MD, Glick AD, Davis BW. Immunohistochemical evaluation of Leu-7, myelin basic-protein, S100-protein, glial-fibrillary acidic-protein, and LN3 immunoreactivity in nerve sheath tumors and sarcomas. Arch Pathol Lab Med 1988; 112(2):155.

137. Weiss SW, Langloss JM, Enzinger FM. Value of S-100 protein in the diagnosis of soft tissue tumors with particular reference to benign and malignant Schwann cell tumors. Lab Invest 1983; 49(3):299.

138. White W, Shiu MH, Rosenblum MK, et al. Cellular schwannoma. A clinicopathologic study of 57 patients and 58 tumors. Cancer 1990; 66(6):1266.

139. Casadei GP, Scheithauer BW, Hirose T, et al. Cellular schwannoma. A clinicopathologic, DNA flow cytometric, and proliferation marker study of 70 patients. Cancer 1995; 75(5):1109.

140. Matsunou H, Shimoda T, Kakimoto S, et al. Histopathologic and immunohistochemical study of malignant tumors of peripheral nerve sheath (malignant schwannoma). Cancer 1985; 56(9):2269.

141. Meis JM, Enzinger FM, Martz KL, et al. Malignant peripheral nerve sheath tumors (malignant schwannomas) in children [see comments]. Am J Surg Pathol 1992; 16(7):694.

142. Fisher C, Schofield JB. S-100 protein positive synovial sarcoma. Histopathology 1991; 19(4):375.

143. Guillou L, Wadden C, Kraus MD, et al. S-100 protein reactivity in synovial sarcomas – A potentially frequent diagnostic pitfall. Immunohistochemical analysis of 100 cases. Appl Immunohistochem 1996; 4(3):167.

144. Kaddu S, Beham A, Cerroni L, et al. Cutaneous leiomyosarcoma. Am J Surg Pathol 1997; 1(9):979.

145. Kilpatrick SE, Hitchcock MG, Kraus MD, et al. Mixed tumors and myoepitheliomas of soft tissue: a clinicopathologic study of 19 cases with a unifying concept [see comments]. Am J Surg Pathol 1997; 21(1):13.

146. Fisher C. Parachordoma exists – but what is it? Adv Anat Pathol 2000; 7(3):141.

147. Michal M, Miettinen M. Myoepitheliomas of the skin and soft tissues. Report of 12 cases. Virchows Arch 1999; 434(5):393.

148. Nakajima T, Watanabe S, Sato Y, et al. Immunohistochemical demonstration of S100

protein in human malignant melanoma and pigmented nevi. Gann 1981; 72(2):335.

149. Nakajima T, Watanabe S, Sato Y, et al. Immunohistochemical demonstration of S100 protein in malignant melanoma and pigmented nevus, and its diagnostic application. Cancer 1982; 50(5):912.

150. Gown AM, Vogel AM, Hoak D, et al. Monoclonal antibodies specific for melanocytic tumors distinguish subpopulations of melanocytes. Am J Pathol 1986; 123(2):195.

151. Busam KJ, Chen YT, Old LJ, et al. Expression of melan-A (MART1) in benign melanocytic nevi and primary cutaneous malignant melanoma. Am J Surg Pathol 1998; 22(8):976.

152. Heiskala M, Peterson PA, Yang Y. The roles of claudin superfamily proteins in paracellular transport. Traffic 2001; 2(2):93.

153. Folpe AL, Billings SD, McKenney JK, et al. Expression of claudin-1, a recently described tight junction-associated protein, distinguishes soft tissue perineurioma from potential mimics. Am J Surg Pathol 2002; 26(12):1620.

154. Schuetz AN, Rubin BP, Goldblum JR, et al. Intercellular junctions in Ewing sarcoma/ primitive neuroectodermal tumor: additional evidence of epithelial differentiation. Mod Pathol 2005; 18(11):1403.

155. Mueckler M. Facilitative glucose transporters. Eur J Biochem 1994; 219(3):713.

156. Yamaguchi U, Hasegawa T, Hirose T, et al. Sclerosing perineurioma: a clinicopathological study of five cases and diagnostic utility of immunohistochemical staining for GLUT1. Virchows Arch 2003; 443(2):159.

157. Hirose T, Tani T, Shimada T, et al. Immunohistochemical demonstration of EMA/Glut1-positive perineurial cells and CD34-positive fibroblastic cells in peripheral nerve sheath tumors. Mod Pathol 2003; 16(4):293.

158. Smith ME, Awasthi R, O'Shaughnessy S, et al. Evaluation of perineurial differentiation in epithelioid sarcoma. Histopathology 2005; 47(6):575.

159. North PE, Waner M, Mizeracki A, et al. GLUT1: a newly discovered immunohistochemical marker for juvenile hemangiomas. Hum Pathol 2000; 31(1):11.

160. Leon-Villapalos J, Wolfe K, Kangesu L. GLUT-1: an extra diagnostic tool to differentiate between haemangiomas and vascular malformations. Br J Plast Surg 2005; 58(3):348.

161. Lyons LL, North PE, Mac-Moune Lai F, et al. Kaposiform hemangioendothelioma: a study of 33 cases emphasizing its pathologic, immunophenotypic, and biologic uniqueness from juvenile hemangioma. Am J Surg Pathol 2004; 28(5):559.

162. McGarry RC, Helfand SL, Quarles RH, et al. Recognition of myelin-associated glycoprotein by the monoclonal antibody HNK-1. Nature 1983; 306(5941):376.

163. Schuller-Petrovic S, Gebhart W, Lassmann H, et al. A shared antigenic determinant between natural killer cells and nervous tissue. Nature 1983; 306(5939):179.

164. Arber DA, Weiss LM. CD57 – A review. Appl Immunohistochem 1995; 3(3):137.

165. Swanson PE, Manivel JC, Wick MR. Immunoreactivity for Leu-7 in neurofibrosarcoma and other spindle cell sarcomas of soft tissue. Am J Pathol 1987; 126(3):546.

166. Thompson SJ, Schatteman GC, Gown AM, et al. A monoclonal antibody against nerve growth factor receptor. Immunohistochemical analysis of normal and neoplastic human tissue. Am J Clin Pathol 1989; 92(4):415.

167. Kanik AB, Yaar M, Bhawan J. P75 nerve growth factor receptor staining helps identify desmoplastic and neurotropic melanoma. J Cutan Pathol 1996;23(3):205.

168. Perosio PM, Brooks JJ. Expression of nerve growth factor receptor in paraffin-embedded soft tissue tumors. Am, J Pathol 1988; 132(1):152.

"Neuroectodermal" markers

169. Goodfellow PN, Pym B, Pritchard C, et al. MIC2: a human pseudoautosomal gene. Philos Trans R Soc Lond B Biol Sci 1988; 322(1208):145.

170. Fellinger EJ, Garin-Chesa P, Su SL, et al. Biochemical and genetic characterization of the HBA71 Ewing's sarcoma cell surface antigen. Cancer Res 1991; 51(1):336.

171. Gelin C, Aubrit F, Phalipon A, et al. The E2 antigen, a 32 kd glycoprotein involved in T-cell adhesion processes, is the MIC2 gene product. Embo J 1989; 8(11):3253.

172. Hamilton G, Mallinger R, Hofbauer S, et al. The monoclonal HBA-71 antibody modulates proliferation of thymocytes and Ewing's sarcoma cells by interfering with the action of insulin-like growth factor I. Thymus 1991; 18(1):33.

173. Fellinger EJ, Garin-Chesa P, Triche TJ, et al. Immunohistochemical analysis of Ewing's sarcoma cell surface antigen p30/32MIC2. Am J Pathol 1991; 139(2):317.

174. Stevenson A, Chatten J, Bertoni F, et al. CD99 (p30/32MIC2) neuroectodermal/Ewing's sarcoma antigen as an immunohistochemical marker. Review of more than 600 tumors and the literature experience. Appl Immunohistochem 1994; 2(4):231.

175. Ambros IM, Ambros PF, Strehl S, et al. MIC2 is a specific marker for Ewing's sarcoma and peripheral primitive neuroectodermal tumors. Evidence for a common histogenesis of Ewing's sarcoma and peripheral primitive neuroectodermal tumors from MIC2 expression and specific chromosome aberration. Cancer 1991; 67(7):1886.

176. Ramani P, Rampling D, Link M. Immunocytochemical study of 12E7 in small round-cell tumours of childhood: an assessment of its sensitivity and specificity. Histopathology 1993; 23(6):557.

177. Riopel M, Dickman PS, Link MP, et al. MIC2 analysis in pediatric lymphomas and leukemias. Hum Pathol 1994; 25(4):396.

178. Shanfeld RL, Edelman J, Willis JE, et al. Immunohistochemical analysis of neural markers in peripheral primitive neuroectodermal tumors (pPNET) without light microscopic evidence of neural differentiation. Appl Innmunohistochem 1997; 5(2):78.

179. Weidner N, Tjoe J. Immunohistochemical profile of monoclonal antibody O13: antibody that recognizes glycoprotein p30/32MIC2 and is useful in diagnosing Ewing's sarcoma and peripheral neuroepithelioma [see comments]. Am J Surg Pathol 1994; 18(5):486.

180. Vartanian RK, Sudilovsky D, Weidner N. Immunostaining of monoclonal antibody O13 (anti-MIC2 gene product [CD99]) in lymphomas. Impact of heat-induced epitope retrieval. Appl Immunohistochem 1996; 4(1):43.

181. Dorfman DM, Pinkus GS. CD99 (p30/ 32(MIC2)) immunoreactivity in the diagnosis of thymic neoplasms and mediastinal lymphoproliferative disorders. A study of paraffin sections using monoclonal antibody O13. Appl Immunohistochem 1996; 4(1):34.

182. Dei Tos AP, Wadden C, Calonje E, et al. Immunohistochemical demonstration of glycoprotein p30/32(MIC2) (CD99) in synovial sarcoma: a potential cause of diagnostic confusion. Appl Immunohistochem 1995; 3(3):168.

183. Pelmus M, Guillou L, Hostein I, et al. Monophasic fibrous and poorly differentiated synovial sarcoma: immunohistochemical reassessment of 60 t(X;18)(SYT-SSX)-positive cases. Am J Surg Pathol 2002; 26(11):1434.

184. Granter SR, Renshaw AA, Fletcher CD, et al. CD99 reactivity in mesenchymal chondrosarcoma. Hum Pathol 1996; 27(12):1273.

185. Devaney K, Abbondanzo SL, Shekitka KM, et al. MIC2 detection in tumors of bone and adjacent soft tissues. Clin Orthopaed Rel Res 1995; (310):176.

186. Devaney K, Vinh TN, Sweet DE. Small cell osteosarcoma of bone: an immunohistochemical study with differential diagnostic considerations [see comments]. Hum Pathol 1993; 24(11):1211.

187. Ordi J, de Alava E, Torne A, et al. Intraabdominal desmoplastic small round cell tumor with EWS/ERG fusion transcript. Am J Surg Pathol 1998; 22(8):1026.

188. Devaney K, Wenig BM, Abbondanzo SL. Olfactory neuroblastoma and other round cell lesions of the sinonasal region. Mod Pathol 1996; 9(6):658.

189. Folpe AL, Patterson K, Gown AM. Antineuroblastoma antibody NB-84 also identifies a significant subset of other small blue round cell tumors. Appl Immunohistochem 1997; 5(4):239.

190. Renshaw AA. O13 (CD99) in spindle cell tumors. Reactivity with hemangiopericytoma, solitary fibrous tumor, synovial sarcoma, and meningioma but rarely with sarcomatoid mesothelioma. Appl Immunohistochem 1995; 3(4):250.

191. Guillou L, Gebhard S, Coindre JM. Lipomatous hemangiopericytoma: a fat-containing variant of solitary fibrous tumor? Clinicopathologic, immunohistochemical, and ultrastructural analysis of a series in favor of a unifying concept. Hum Pathol 2000; 31(9):1108.

192. Guillou L, Gebhard S, Coindre JM. Orbital and extraorbital giant cell angiofibroma: a giant cell-rich variant of solitary fibrous tumor? Clinicopathologic and immunohistochemical analysis of a series in favor of a unifying concept. Am J Surg Pathol 2000; 24(7):971.

193. Cunningham BA, Hemperly JJ, Murray BA, et al. Neural cell adhesion molecule: structure, immunoglobulin-like domains, cell surface modulation, and alternative RNA splicing. Science 1987; 236(4803):799.

194. Edelman GM. Cell adhesion molecules in the regulation of animal form and tissue pattern. Annu Rev Cell Biol 1986; 2:81.

195. Shipley WR, Hammer RD, Lennington WJ, et al. Paraffin immunohistochemical detection of CD56, a useful marker for neural cell adhesion molecule (NCAM), in normal and neoplastic fixed tissues. Appl Immunohistochem 1997; 5(2):87.

196. Chan JK, Sin VC, Wong KF, et al. Nonnasal lymphoma expressing the natural killer cell marker CD56: a clinicopathologic study of 49 cases of an uncommon aggressive neoplasm. Blood 1997; 89(12):4501.

197. Lanier LL, Le AM, Civin CI, et al. The relationship of CD16 (Leu-11) and Leu-19 (NKH-1) antigen expression on human peripheral blood NK cells and cytotoxic T lymphocytes. J Immunol 1986; 136(12): 4480.

198. Mechtersheimer G, Staudter M, Moller P. Expression of the natural killer cell-associated antigens CD56 and CD57 in human neural and striated muscle cells and in their tumors. Cancer Res 1991; 51(4):1300.

199. Miettinen M, Cupo W. Neural cell adhesion molecule distribution in soft tissue tumors. Hum Pathol 1993; 24(1):62.

200. Garin-Chesa P, Fellinger EJ, Huvos AG, et al. Immunohistochemical analysis of neural cell adhesion molecules. Differential expression in

small round cell tumors of childhood and adolescence. Am J Pathol 1991; 139(2):275.

201. Thomas JO, Nijjar J, Turley H, et al. NB84: a new monoclonal antibody for the recognition of neuroblastoma in routinely processed material. J Pathol 1991; 163(1):69.

202. Miettinen M, Chatten J, Paetau A, et al. Monoclonal antibody NB84 in the differential diagnosis of neuroblastoma and other small round cell tumors. Am J Surg Pathol 1998; 22(3):327.

203. Bomken SN, Redfern K, Wood KM, et al. Limitations in the ability of NB84 to detect metastatic neuroblastoma cells in bone marrow. J Clin Pathol 2006; 59(9):927.

204. Sebire NJ, Gibson S, Rampling D. Immunohistochemical findings in embryonal small round cell tumors with molecular diagnostic confirmation. Appl Immunohistochem Mol Morphol 2005; 13(1):1.

Markers of melanocytic differentiation

205. Bacchi CE, Bonetti F, Pea M, et al. HMB-45. A review. Appl Immunohistochem 1996; 4(2):73.

206. Kapur RP, Bigler SA, Skelly M, et al. Anti-melanoma monoclonal antibody HMB45 identifies an oncofetal glycoconjugate associated with immature melanosomes. J Histochem Cytochem 1992; 40(2):207.

207. Pea M, Martignoni G, Zamboni G, et al. Perivascular epithelioid cell [letter; comment]. Am J Surg Pathol 1996; 20(9):1149.

208. Pea M, Martignoni G, Bonetti F, et al. Tumors characterized by the presence of HMB45-positive perivascular epithelioid cell (PEC) – A novel entity in surgical pathology. Electron J Pathol Histol 1997; 3(2):28.

209. Bonetti F, Pea M, Martignoni G, et al. False-positive immunostaining of normal epithelia and carcinomas with ascites fluid preparations of antimelanoma monoclonal antibody HMB45. Am J Clin Pathol 1991; 95(4):454.

210. Longacre TA, Egbert BM, Rouse RV. Desmoplastic and spindle-cell malignant melanoma. An immunohistochemical study. Am J Surg Pathol 1996; 20(12):1489.

211. Kaufmann O, Koch S, Burghardt J, et al. Tyrosinase, melan-A, and KBA62 as markers for the immunohistochemical identification of metastatic amelanotic melanomas on paraffin sections. Mod Pathol 1998; 11(8):740.

212. Busam KJ, Jungbluth AA. Melan-A, a new melanocytic differentiation marker. Adv Anat Pathol 1999; 6(1):12.

213. Busam KJ, Iversen K, Coplan KA, et al. Immunoreactivity for A103, an antibody to melan-A (Mart-1), in adrenocortical and other steroid tumors [see comments]. Am J Surg Pathol 1998; 22(1):57.

214. Jungbluth AA, Busam KJ, Gerald WL, et al. A103: An anti-melan-a monoclonal antibody for the detection of malignant melanoma in paraffin-embedded tissues [see comments]. Am J Surg Pathol 1998; 22(5):595.

215. Lim E, Browning J, Macgregor D, et al. Desmoplastic melanoma: comparison of expression of differentiation antigens and cancer testis antigens. Melanoma Res 2006; 16(4):347.

216. Hodgkinson CA, Moore KJ, Nakayama A, et al. Mutations at the mouse microphthalmia locus are associated with defects in a gene encoding a novel basic-helix-loop-helix-zipper protein. Cell 1993; 74(2):395.

217. Bentley NJ, Eisen T, Goding CR. Melanocyte-specific expression of the human tyrosinase promoter: activation by the microphthalmia gene product and role of the initiator. Molec Cell Biol 1994; 4(12):7996.

218. Hemesath TJ, Steingrimsson E, McGill G, et al. Microphthalmia, a critical factor in melanocyte development, defines a discrete transcription factor family. Genes Dev 1994; 8(22):2770.

219. Read AP, Newton VE. Waardenburg syndrome. J Med Genet 1997; 34(8):656.

220. Bertolotto C, Busca R, Abbe P, et al. Different cis-acting elements are involved in the regulation of TRP1 and TRP2 promoter activities by cyclic AMP: pivotal role of M boxes (GTCATGTGCT) and of microphthalmia. Mol Cell Biol 1998; 18(2):694.

221. Steingrimsson E, Copeland NG, Jenkins NA. Melanocytes and the microphthalmia transcription factor network. Annu Rev Genet 2004; 38:365.

222. King R, Weilbaecher KN, McGill G, et al. Microphthalmia transcription factor. A sensitive and specific melanocyte marker for melanoma diagnosis. Am J Pathol 1999; 155(3):731.

223. King R, Googe PB, Weilbaecher KN, et al. Microphthalmia transcription factor expression in cutaneous benign, malignant melanocytic, and nonmelanocytic tumors. Am J Surg Pathol 2001; 25(1):51.

224. Koch MB, Shih IM, Weiss SW, et al. Microphthalmia transcription factor and melanoma cell adhesion molecule expression distinguish desmoplastic/spindle cell melanoma from morphologic mimics. Am J Surg Pathol 2001; 25(1):58.

225. Granter SR, Weilbaecher KN, Quigley C, et al. Microphthalmia transcription factor: not a sensitive or specific marker for the diagnosis of desmoplastic melanoma and spindle cell (non-desmoplastic) melanoma. Am J Dermatopathol 2001; 23(3):185.

226. Granter SR, Weilbaecher KN, Quigley C, et al. Clear cell sarcoma shows immunoreactivity for microphthalmia transcription factor: further evidence for melanocytic differentiation. Mod Pathol 2001; 14(1):6.

227. Zavala-Pompa A, Folpe AL, Jimenez RE, et al. Immunohistochemical study of microphthalmia transcription factor and tyrosinase in angiomyolipoma of the kidney, renal cell carcinoma, and renal and retroperitoneal sarcomas: comparative evaluation with traditional diagnostic markers. Am J Surg Pathol 2001; 25(1):65.

228. Sanchez-Ferrer A, Rodriguez-Lopez JN, Garcia-Canovas F, et al. Tyrosinase: a comprehensive review of its mechanism. Biochimica et Biophysica Acta 1995; 1247(1):1.

229. Hofbauer GF, Kamarashev J, Geertsen R, et al. Tyrosinase immunoreactivity in formalin-fixed, paraffin-embedded primary and metastatic melanoma: frequency and distribution. J Cutan Pathol 1998; 25(4):204.

Markers of endothelial differentiation

230. Beckstead JH, Wood GS, Fletcher V. Evidence for the origin of Kaposi's sarcoma from lymphatic endothelium. Am J Pathol 1985; 119(2):294.

231. Burgdorf WH, Mukai K, Rosai J. Immunohistochemical identification of factor VIII-related antigen in endothelial cells of cutaneous lesions of alleged vascular nature. Am J Clin Pathol 1981; 75(2):167.

232. Hashimoto H, Muller H, Falk S, et al. Histogenesis of Kaposi's sarcoma associated with AIDS: a histologic, immunohistochemical and enzyme histochemical study. Pathol Res Pract 1987; 182(5):658.

233. Breiteneder-Geleff S, Matsui K, Soleiman A, et al. Podoplanin, novel 43-kd membrane protein of glomerular epithelial cells, is down-regulated in puromycin nephrosis. Am J Pathol 1997; 151(4):1141.

234. Folpe AL, Veikkola T, Valtola R, et al. Vascular endothelial growth factor receptor-3 (VEGFR-3): a marker of vascular tumors with presumed lymphatic differentiation, including Kaposi's sarcoma, kaposiform and Dabska-type hemangioendotheliomas, and a subset of angiosarcomas. Mod Pathol 2000; 13(2):180.

235. Jussila L, Valtola R, Partanen TA, et al. Lymphatic endothelium and Kaposi's sarcoma spindle cells detected by antibodies against the vascular endothelial growth factor receptor-3. Cancer Res 1998; 58(8):1599.

236. Fortwengler HP Jr, Jones D, Espinosa E, et al. Evidence for endothelial cell origin of vinyl chloride-induced hepatic angiosarcoma. Gastroenterology 1981; 80(6):1415.

237. Bohling T, Paetau A, Ekblom P, et al. Distribution of endothelial and basement membrane markers in angiogenic tumors of the nervous system. Acta Neuropathologica 1983; 62(1–2):67.

238. Ordonez NG, del Junco GW, et al. Angiosarcoma of the small intestine: an immunoperoxidase study. Am J Gastroenterol 1983; 78(4):218.

239. Merino MJ, Carter D, Berman M. Angiosarcoma of the breast. Am J Surg Pathol 1983; 7(1):53.

240. van de Rijn M, Rouse R. CD34: a review. Appl Immunohistochem 1994; 2(2):71.

241. Miettinen M, Lindenmayer AE, Chaubal A. Endothelial cell markers CD31, CD34, and BNH9 antibody to H- and Y-antigens – evaluation of their specificity and sensitivity in the diagnosis of vascular tumors and comparison with von Willebrand factor. Mod Pathol 1994; 7(1):82.

242. Kutzner H. Expression of the human progenitor cell antigen CD34 (HPCA-1) distinguishes dermatofibrosarcoma protuberans from fibrous histiocytoma in formalin-fixed, paraffin-embedded tissue [see comments]. J Am Acad Dermatol 1993; 28(4):613.

243. Westra WH, Gerald WL, Rosai J. Solitary fibrous tumor. Consistent CD34 immunoreactivity and occurrence in the orbit [see comments]. Am J Surg Pathol 1994; 18(10):992.

244. Weiss SW, Nickoloff BJ. CD-34 is expressed by a distinctive cell population in peripheral nerve, nerve sheath tumors, and related lesions [see comments]. Am J Surg Pathol 1993; 17(10):1039.

245. Kindblom LG, Remotti HE, Aldenborg F, et al. Gastrointestinal pacemaker cell tumor (GIPACT): gastrointestinal stromal tumors show phenotypic characteristics of the interstitial cells of Cajal. Am J Pathol 1998; 152(5):1259.

246. Sirgi KE, Wick MR, Swanson PE. B72.3 and CD34 immunoreactivity in malignant epithelioid soft tissue tumors. Adjuncts in the recognition of endothelial neoplasms. Am J Surg Pathol 1993; 17(2):179.

247. De Young BR, Frierson HF Jr, Ly MN, et al. CD31 immunoreactivity in carcinomas and mesotheliomas. Am J Clin Pathol 1998; 110(3):374.

248. Rizzo M, SivaSai KS, Smith MA, et al. Increased expression of inflammatory cytokines and adhesion molecules by alveolar macrophages of human lung allograft recipients with acute rejection: decline with resolution of rejection. J Heart Lung Transplant 2000; 19(9):858.

249. McKenney JK, Weiss SW, Folpe AL. CD31 expression in intratumoral macrophages: a potential diagnostic pitfall. Am J Surg Pathol 2001; 25(9):1167.

250. Folpe AL, Chand EM, Goldblum JR, et al. Expression of Fli-1, a nuclear transcription factor, distinguishes vascular neoplasms from potential mimics. Am J Surg Pathol 2001; 25(8):1061.

251. Rossi S, Orvieto E, Furlanetto A, et al. Utility of the immunohistochemical detection of FLI-1 expression in round cell and vascular neoplasm using a monoclonal antibody. Mod Pathol 2004; 17(5):547.

252. Miettinen M, Holthofer H, Lehto VP, et al. Ulex europaeus I lectin as a marker for tumors derived from endothelial cells. Am J Clin Pathol 1983; 79(1):32.

253. Walker RA. Ulex europeus I – peroxidase as a marker of vascular endothelium: its application in routine histopathology. J Pathology 1985; 146(2):123.

254. Alles JU, Bosslet K. Immunocytochemistry of angiosarcomas. A study of 19 cases with special emphasis on the applicability of endothelial cell specific markers to routinely prepared tissues. Am J Clin Pathol 1988; 89(4):463.

255. Schelper RL, Olson SP, Carroll TJ, et al. Studies of the endothelial origin of cells in systemic angioendotheliomatosis and other vascular lesions of the brain and meninges using ulex europaeus lectin stains. Clin Neuropathol 1986; 5(6):231.

256. Ching CK, Black R, Helliwell T, et al. Use of lectin histochemistry in pancreatic cancer. J Clin Pathol 1988; 41(3):324.

257. Khalifa MA, Sesterhenn IA. Tumor markers of epithelial ovarian neoplasms. Int J Gynecol Pathol 1990; 9(3):217.

258. Soderstrom KO. Lectin binding to prostatic adenocarcinoma. Cancer 1987; 60(8):1823.

259. Ferrara N, Davis-Smyth T. The biology of vascular endothelial growth factor. Endocr Rev 1997; 18(1):4.

260. Jeltsch M, Kaipainen A, Joukov V, et al. Hyperplasia of lymphatic vessels in VEGF-C transgenic mice [published erratum appears in Science 1997 Jul 25; 277(5325):463]. Science 1997; 276(5317):1423.

261. Kaipainen A, Korhonen J, Mustonen T, et al. Expression of the fms-like tyrosine kinase 4 gene becomes restricted to lymphatic endothelium during development. Proc Natl Acad Sci USA 1995; 92(8):3566.

262. Partanen TA, Alitalo K, Miettinen M. Lack of lymphatic vascular specificity of vascular endothelial growth factor receptor 3 in 185 vascular tumors. Cancer 1999; 86(11):2406.

263. Babal P, Pec J. Kaposi's sarcoma – still an enigma. J Eur Acad Dermatol Venereol 2003; 17(4):377.

264. Mbulaiteye SM, Parkin DM, Rabkin CS. Epidemiology of AIDS-related malignancies: an international perspective. Hematol Oncol Clin North Am 2003; 17(3):673, v.

265. Dukers NH, Rezza G. Human herpesvirus 8 epidemiology: what we do and do not know. Aids 2003; 17(12):1717.

266. Stebbing J, Portsmouth S, Bower M. Insights into the molecular biology and sero-epidemiology of Kaposi's sarcoma. Curr Opin Infect Dis 2003; 16(1):25.

267. Gandhi M, Greenblatt RM. Human herpesvirus 8, Kaposi's sarcoma, and associated conditions. Clin Lab Med 2002; 22(4):883.

268. Boshoff C, Schulz TF, Kennedy MM, et al. Kaposi's sarcoma-associated herpesvirus infects endothelial and spindle cells. Nat Med 1995; 1(12):1274.

269. Komatsu T, Ballestas ME, Barbera AJ, et al. The KSHV latency-associated nuclear antigen: a multifunctional protein. Front Biosci 2002; 7:d726.

270. Szekely L, Kiss C, Mattsson K, et al. Human herpesvirus-8-encoded LNA-1 accumulates in heterochromatin-associated nuclear bodies. J Gen Virol 1999; 80(Pt 11):2889.

271. Katano H, Sato Y, Kurata T, et al. High expression of HHV-8-encoded ORF73 protein in spindle-shaped cells of Kaposi's sarcoma. Am J Pathol 1999; 155(1):47.

272. Kellam P, Bourboulia D, Dupin N, et al. Characterization of monoclonal antibodies raised against the latent nuclear antigen of human herpesvirus 8. J Virol 1999; 73(6):5149.

273. Dupin N, Fisher C, Kellam P, et al. Distribution of human herpesvirus-8 latently infected cells in Kaposi's sarcoma, multicentric Castleman's disease, and primary effusion lymphoma. Proc Natl Acad Sci USA 1999; 96(8):4546.

274. Courville P, Simon F, Le Pessot F, et al. [Detection of HHV8 latent nuclear antigen by immunohistochemistry. A new tool for differentiating Kaposi's sarcoma from its mimics]. Ann Pathol 2002; 22(4):267.

275. Cheuk W, Wong KOY, Wong CSC, et al. Immunostaining for human herpesvirus 8 latent nuclear antigen-1 helps distinguish Kaposi sarcoma from its mimickers. Am J Clin Pathol 2004; 121:335.

276. Robin Y-M, Guillou L, Michels J-J, et al. Human herpesvirus 8 immunostaining. Am J Clin Pathol 2004; 121:330.

277. Patel RM, Goldblum JR, Hsi ED. Immunohistochemical detection of human herpes virus-8 latent nuclear antigen-1 is useful in the diagnosis of Kaposi sarcoma. Mod Pathol 2004; 17(4):456.

278. Hammock L, Reisenauer A, Wang W, et al. Latency-associated nuclear antigen expression and human herpesvirus-8 polymerase chain reaction in the evaluation of Kaposi sarcoma and other vascular tumors in HIV-positive patients. Mod Pathol 2005; 18(4):463.

279. Leong ASY, Vinyuvat S, Suthipintawong C, et al. Patterns of basal lamina immunostaining in soft-tissue and bony tumors. Appl Immunohistochem 1997; 5(1):1.

Immunohistochemical distinction of mesothelioma and carcinoma

280. Yaziji H, Battifora H, Barry TS. Evaluation of 12 antibodies for distinguishing epithelioid mesothelioma from adenocarcinoma: identification of a three-antibody immunohistochemical panel with maximal sensitivity and specificity. Mod Pathol 2006; 19(4):514.

281. Sheibani K, Esteban JM, Bailey A, et al. Immunopathologic and molecular studies as an aid to the diagnosis of malignant mesothelioma [see comments]. Hum Pathol 1992; 23(2):107.

282. Brown RW, Campagna LB, Dunn JK, et al. Immunohistochemical identification of tumor markers in metastatic adenocarcinoma. A diagnostic adjunct in the determination of primary site. Am J Clin Pathol 1997; 107(1):12.

283. Ordonez NG. Role of immunohistochemistry in differentiating epithelial mesothelioma from adenocarcinoma. Review and update. Am J Clin Pathol 1999; 112(1):75.

284. Ordonez NG. The immunohistochemical diagnosis of epithelial mesothelioma. Hum Pathol 1999; 30(3):313.

285. Robb JA. Mesothelioma versus adenocarcinoma: false-positive CEA and Leu-M1 staining due to hyaluronic acid [letter]. Hum Pathol 1989; 20(4):400.

286. Ordonez NG. Role of immunohistochemistry in distinguishing epithelial peritoneal mesotheliomas from peritoneal and ovarian serous carcinomas. Am J Surg Pathol 1998; 22(10):1203.

287. Wirth PR, Legier J, Wright GL Jr. Immunohistochemical evaluation of seven monoclonal antibodies for differentiation of pleural mesothelioma from lung adenocarcinoma. Cancer 1991; 67(3):655.

288. Ordonez NG. Value of the Ber-EP4 antibody in differentiating epithelial pleural mesothelioma from adenocarcinoma. The M.D. Anderson experience and a critical review of the literature. Am J Clin Pathol 1998; 109(1):85.

289. Oates J, Edwards C. HBME-1, MOC-31, WT1 and calretinin: an assessment of recently described markers for mesothelioma and adenocarcinoma. Histopathology 2000; 36(4):341.

290. Ordonez NG. Value of thyroid transcription factor-1, E-cadherin, BG8, WT1, and CD44S immunostaining in distinguishing epithelial pleural mesothelioma from pulmonary and nonpulmonary adenocarcinoma. Am J Surg Pathol 2000; 24(4):598.

291. Yaziji H, Battifora H, Barry TS, et al. Evaluation of 12 antibodies for distinguishing epithelioid mesothelioma from adenocarcinoma: identification of a three-antibody immunohistochemical panel with maximal sensitivity and specificity. Mod Pathol 2006; 19(4):514.

292. King JE, Thatcher N, Pickering CA, et al. Sensitivity and specificity of immunohistochemical markers used in the diagnosis of epithelioid mesothelioma: a detailed systematic analysis using published data. Histopathology 2006; 48(3):223.

293. Kumar-Singh S, Segers K, Rodeck U, et al. WT1 mutation in malignant mesothelioma and WT1 immunoreactivity in relation to p53 and growth factor receptor expression, cell-type transition, and prognosis. J Pathol 1997; 181(1):67.

294. Ordonez NG. The immunohistochemical diagnosis of mesothelioma: a comparative study of epithelioid mesothelioma and lung adenocarcinoma. Am J Surg Pathol 2003; 27(8):1031.

295. Ordonez NG. Value of calretinin immunostaining in differentiating epithelial mesothelioma from lung adenocarcinoma. Mod Pathol 1998; 11(10):929.

296. Doglioni C, Tos AP, Laurino L, et al. Calretinin: a novel immunocytochemical marker for mesothelioma. Am J Surg Pathol 1996; 20(9):1037.

297. Ordonez NG. Value of cytokeratin 5/6 immunostaining in distinguishing epithelial mesothelioma of the pleura from lung adenocarcinoma. Am J Surg Pathol 1998; 22(10):1215.

298. Clover J, Oates J, Edwards C. Anti-cytokeratin 5/6: a positive marker for epithelioid mesothelioma. Histopathology 1997; 31(2):140.

299. Ordonez NG. D2-40 and podoplanin are highly specific and sensitive immunohistochemical markers of epithelioid malignant mesothelioma. Hum Pathol 2005; 36(4):372.

300. Chu AY, Litzky LA, Pasha TL, et al. Utility of D2-40, a novel mesothelial marker, in the diagnosis of malignant mesothelioma. Mod Pathol 2005; 18(1):105.

301. Kahn HJ, Bailey D, Marks A. Monoclonal antibody D2-40, a new marker of lymphatic endothelium, reacts with Kaposi's sarcoma and a subset of angiosarcomas. Mod Pathol 2002; 15(4):434.

Markers of gastrointestinal stromal tumors

302. Hirota S, Isozaki K, Moriyama Y, et al. Gain-of-function mutations of c-kit in human gastrointestinal stromal tumors. Science 1998; 279(5350):577.

303. Hornick JL, Fletcher CD. Immunohistochemical staining for KIT (CD117) in soft tissue sarcomas is very limited in distribution. Am J Clin Pathol 2002; 117(2):188.

304. Fletcher CD, Berman JJ, Corless C, et al. Diagnosis of gastrointestinal stromal tumors: a consensus approach. Hum Pathol 2002; 33(5):459.

305. Reith JD, Goldblum JR, Lyles RH, et al. Extragastrointestinal (soft tissue) stromal tumors: an analysis of 48 cases with emphasis on histologic predictors of outcome. Mod Pathol 2000; 13(5):577.

306. Sarlomo-Rikala M, Kovatich AJ, Barusevicius A, et al. CD117: a sensitive marker for

gastrointestinal stromal tumors that is more specific than CD34. Mod Pathol 1998; 11(8):728.

307. Scotlandi K, Manara MC, Strammiello R, et al. C-kit receptor expression in Ewing's sarcoma: lack of prognostic value but therapeutic targeting opportunities in appropriate conditions. J Clin Oncol 2003; 21(10):1952.

308. Smithey BE, Pappo AS, Hill DA. C-kit expression in pediatric solid tumors: a comparative immunohistochemical study. Am J Surg Pathol 2002; 26(4):486.

309. Makhlouf HR, Remotti HE, Ishak KG. Expression of KIT (CD117) in angiomyolipoma. Am J Surg Pathol 2002; 26(4):493.

310. Hotfilder M, Lanvers C, Jurgens H, et al. c-KIT-expressing Ewing tumour cells are insensitive to imatinib mesylate (STI571). Cancer Chemother Pharmacol 2002; 50(2):167.

311. Altman A, Villalba M. Protein kinase C-theta (PKCtheta): it's all about location, location, location. Immunol Rev 2003; 192:53.

312. Altman A, Villalba M. Protein kinase C-theta (PKC theta): a key enzyme in T cell life and death. J Biochem (Tokyo) 2002; 132(6):841.

313. Villalba M, Altman A. Protein kinase C-theta (PKCtheta), a potential drug target for therapeutic intervention with human T cell leukemias. Curr Cancer Drug Targets 2002; 2(2):125.

314. Allander SV, Nupponen NN, Ringner M, et al. Gastrointestinal stromal tumors with KIT mutations exhibit a remarkably homogeneous gene expression profile. Cancer Res 2001; 61(24):8624.

315. Nielsen TO, West RB, Linn SC, et al. Molecular characterisation of soft tissue tumours: a gene expression study. Lancet 2002; 359(9314):1301.

316. Motegi A, Sakurai S, Nakayama H, et al. PKC theta, a novel immunohistochemical marker for gastrointestinal stromal tumors (GIST), especially useful for identifying KIT-negative tumors. Pathol Int 2005; 55(3):106.

317. Blay P, Astudillo A, Buesa JM, et al. Protein kinase C theta is highly expressed in gastrointestinal stromal tumors but not in other mesenchymal neoplasias. Clin Cancer Res 2004; 10(12 Pt 1):4089.

Use of immunohistochemistry as a surrogate for the presence of tumor-specific molecular alterations

318. Downing JR, Head DR, Parham DM, et al. Detection of the (11;22)(q24;q12) translocation of Ewing's sarcoma and peripheral neuroectodermal tumor by reverse transcriptase polymerase chain reaction. Am J Pathol 1993; 143(5):1294.

319. May WA, Gishizky ML, Lessnick SL, et al. Ewing sarcoma 11;22 translocation produces a chimeric transcription factor that requires the DNA-binding domain encoded by FLI1 for transformation. Proc Natl Acad Sci USA 1993; 90(12):5752.

320. May WA, Lessnick SL, Braun BS, et al. The Ewing's sarcoma EWS/FLI-1 fusion gene encodes a more potent transcriptional activator and is a more powerful transforming gene than FLI-1. Mol Cell Biol 1993; 13(12):7393.

321. Rao VN, Ohno T, Prasad DD, et al. Analysis of the DNA-binding and transcriptional activation functions of human Fli-1 protein. Oncogene 1993; 8(8):2167.

322. Giovannini M, Biegel JA, Serra M, et al. EWS-erg and EWS-Fli1 fusion transcripts in Ewing's sarcoma and primitive neuroectodermal tumors with variant translocations. J Clin Invest 1994; 94(2):489.

323. Deramaudt BM, Remy P, Abraham NG. Upregulation of human heme oxygenase gene expression by Ets-family proteins. J Cell Biochem 1999; 72(3):311.

324. Nilsson G, Wang M, Wejde J, et al. Detection of EWS/FLI-1 by immunostaining. An adjunctive tool in diagnosis of Ewing's sarcoma and primitive neuroectodermal tumor on cytological samples and paraffin-embedded archival material. Sarcoma 1999; 3:25.

325. Folpe AL, Hill CE, Parham DM, et al. Immunohistochemical detection of FLI-1 protein expression: a study of 132 round cell tumors with emphasis on CD99-positive mimics of Ewing's sarcoma/primitive neuroectodermal tumor. Am J Surg Pathol 2000; 24(12):1657.

326. Brown LA, Rodaway AR, Schilling TF, et al. Insights into early vasculogenesis revealed by expression of the ETS-domain transcription factor Fli-1 in wild-type and mutant zebrafish embryos. Mech Dev 2000; 90(2):237.

327. Ladanyi M, Gerald W. Fusion of the EWS and WT1 genes in the desmoplastic small round cell tumor. Cancer Res 1994; 54(11):2837.

328. de Alava E, Ladanyi M, Rosai J, et al. Detection of chimeric transcripts in desmoplastic small round cell tumor and related developmental tumors by reverse transcriptase polymerase chain reaction. A specific diagnostic assay. Am J Pathol 1995; 147(6):1584.

329. Gerald WL, Ladanyi M, de Alava E, et al. Clinical, pathologic, and molecular spectrum of tumors associated with t(11;22)(p13;q12): desmoplastic small round-cell tumor and its variants. J Clin Oncol 1998; 16(9):3028.

330. Charles AK, Moore IE, Berry PJ. Immunohistochemical detection of the Wilms' tumour gene WT1 in desmoplastic small round cell tumour. Histopathology 1997; 30(4):312.

331. Barnoud R, Sabourin JC, Pasquier D, et al. Immunohistochemical expression of WT1 by desmoplastic small round cell tumor: a comparative study with other small round cell tumors. Am J Surg Pathol 2000; 24(6):830.

332. Hill DA, Pfeifer JD, Marley EF, et al. WT1 staining reliably differentiates desmoplastic small round cell tumor from Ewing sarcoma/primitive neuroectodermal tumor. An immunohistochemical and molecular diagnostic study. Am J Clin Pathol 2000; 114(3):345.

333. Carpentieri DF, Nichols K, Chou PM, et al. The expression of WT1 in the differentiation of rhabdomyosarcoma from other pediatric small round blue cell tumors. Mod Pathol 2002; 15(10):1080.

334. Ladanyi M, Lui MY, Antonescu CR, et al. The der(17)t(X;17)(p11;q25) of human alveolar soft part sarcoma fuses the TFE3 transcription factor gene to ASPL, a novel gene at 17q25. Oncogene 2001; 20(1):48.

335. Argani P, Lal P, Hutchinson B, et al. Aberrant nuclear immunoreactivity for TFE3 in neoplasms with TFE3 gene fusions: a sensitive and specific immunohistochemical assay. Am J Surg Pathol 2003; 27(6):750.

336. Biegel JA. Molecular genetics of atypical teratoid/rhabdoid tumor. Neurosurg Focus 2006; 20(1):E11.

337. Biegel JA, Kalpana G, Knudsen ES, et al. The role of INI1 and the SWI/SNF complex in the development of rhabdoid tumors: meeting summary from the workshop on childhood atypical teratoid/rhabdoid tumors. Cancer Res 2002; 62(1):323.

338. Biegel JA, Zhou JY, Rorke LB, et al. Germ-line and acquired mutations of INI1 in atypical teratoid and rhabdoid tumors. Cancer Res 1999; 59(1):74.

339. Biegel JA, Tan L, Zhang F, et al. Alterations of the hSNF5/INI1 gene in central nervous system atypical teratoid/rhabdoid tumors and renal and extrarenal rhabdoid tumors. Clin Cancer Res 2002; 8(11):3461.

340. Hoot AC, Russo P, Judkins AR, et al. Immunohistochemical analysis of hSNF5/INI1 distinguishes renal and extra-renal malignant rhabdoid tumors from other pediatric soft tissue tumors. Am J Surg Pathol 2004; 28(11):1485.

341. Sigauke E, Rakheja D, Maddox DL, et al. Absence of expression of SMARCB1/INI1 in malignant rhabdoid tumors of the central nervous system, kidneys and soft tissue: an immunohistochemical study with implications for diagnosis. Mod Pathol 2006; 19(5):717.

342. Judkins AR, Burger PC, Hamilton RL, et al. INI1 protein expression distinguishes atypical teratoid/rhabdoid tumor from choroid plexus carcinoma. J Neuropathol Exp Neurol 2005; 64(5):391.

343. Perry A, Fuller CE, Judkins AR, et al. INI1 expression is retained in composite rhabdoid tumors, including rhabdoid meningiomas. Mod Pathol 2005; 18(7):951.

344. Judkins AR, Mauger J, Rorke LB, et al. Immunohistochemical analysis of hSNF5/INI1 in pediatric CNS neoplasms. Am J Surg Pathol 2004; 28(5):644.

345. Morris SW, Kirstein MN, Valentine MB, et al. Fusion of a kinase gene, ALK, to a nucleolar protein gene, NPM, in non-Hodgkin's lymphoma. Science 1994; 263(5151):1281.

346. Pulford K, Lamant L, Espinos E, et al. The emerging normal and disease-related roles of anaplastic lymphoma kinase. Cell Mol Life Sci 2004; 61(23):2939.

347. Griffin CA, Hawkins AL, Dvorak C, et al. Recurrent involvement of 2p23 in inflammatory myofibroblastic tumors. Cancer Res 1999; 59(12):2776.

348. Cessna MH, Zhou H, Sanger WG, et al. Expression of ALK1 and p80 in inflammatory myofibroblastic tumor and its mesenchymal mimics: a study of 135 cases. Mod Pathol 2002; 15(9):931.

349. Cook JR, Dehner LP, Collins MH, et al. Anaplastic lymphoma kinase (ALK) expression in the inflammatory myofibroblastic tumor: a comparative immunohistochemical study. Am J Surg Pathol 2001; 25(11):1364.

350. Coffin CM, Patel A, Perkins S, et al. ALK1 and p80 expression and chromosomal rearrangements involving 2p23 in inflammatory myofibroblastic tumor. Mod Pathol 2001; 14(6):569.

351. Li XQ, Hisaoka M, Shi DR, et al. Expression of anaplastic lymphoma kinase in soft tissue tumors: an immunohistochemical and molecular study of 249 cases. Hum Pathol 2004; 35(6):711.

Other markers

352. Holness CL, Simmons DL. Molecular cloning of CD68, a human macrophage marker related to lysosomal glycoproteins. Blood 1993; 81(6):1607.

353. Cassidy M, Loftus B, Whelan A, et al. KP-1: not a specific marker. Staining of 137 sarcomas, 48 lymphomas, 28 carcinomas, 7 malignant melanomas and 8 cystosarcoma phyllodes. Virchows Arch 1994; 424(6):635.

354. Smith ME, Costa MJ, Weiss SW. Evaluation of CD68 and other histiocytic antigens in angiomatoid malignant fibrous histiocytoma [see comments]. Am J Surg Pathol 1991; 15(8):757.

355. Dei Tos AP, Doglioni C, Laurino L, et al. KP1 (CD68) expression in benign neural tumours. Further evidence of its low specificity as a histiocytic/myeloid marker. Histopathology 1993; 23(2):185.

356. Gloghini A, Rizzo A, Zanette I, et al. KP1/CD68 expression in malignant neoplasms including lymphomas, sarcomas, and carcinomas. Am J Clin Pathol 1995; 103(4):425.

357. Taipale J, Beachy PA. The Hedgehog and Wnt signalling pathways in cancer. Nature 2001; 411(6835):349.

358. Barth AI, Nathke IS, Nelson WJ. Cadherins, catenins and APC protein: interplay between cytoskeletal complexes and signaling pathways. Curr Opin Cell Biol 1997; 9(5):683.

359. Rubinfeld B, Albert I, Porfiri E, et al. Binding of GSK3beta to the APC-beta-catenin complex and regulation of complex assembly. Science 1996; 272(5264):1023.

360. Hart MJ, de los Santos R, Albert IN, et al. Downregulation of beta-catenin by human Axin and its association with the APC tumor suppressor, beta-catenin and GSK3 beta. Curr Biol 1998; 8(10):573.

361. Alman BA, Li C, Pajerski ME, et al. Increased beta-catenin protein and somatic APC mutations in sporadic aggressive fibromatoses (desmoid tumors). Am J Pathol 1997; 151(2):329.

362. Miyoshi Y, Iwao K, Nawa G, et al. Frequent mutations in the beta-catenin gene in desmoid tumors from patients without familial adenomatous polyposis. Oncol Res 1998; 10(11–12):591.

363. Montgomery E, Lee JH, Abraham SC, et al. Superficial fibromatoses are genetically distinct from deep fibromatoses. Mod Pathol 2001; 14(7):695.

364. Abraham SC, Reynolds C, Lee JH, et al. Fibromatosis of the breast and mutations involving the APC/beta-catenin pathway. Hum Pathol 2002; 33(1):39.

365. Montgomery E, Torbenson MS, Kaushal M, et al. Beta-catenin immunohistochemistry separates mesenteric fibromatosis from gastrointestinal stromal tumor and sclerosing mesenteritis. Am J Surg Pathol 2002; 26(10):1296.

366. Bhattacharya B, Dilworth HP, Iacobuzio-Donahue C, et al. Nuclear beta-catenin expression distinguishes deep fibromatosis from other benign and malignant fibroblastic and myofibroblastic lesions. Am J Surg Pathol 2005; 29(5):653.

367. Ng TL, Gown AM, Barry TS, et al. Nuclear beta-catenin in mesenchymal tumors. Mod Pathol 2005; 18(1):68-.

368. Iwao K, Miyoshi Y, Nawa G, et al. Frequent beta-catenin abnormalities in bone and soft-tissue tumors. Jpn J Cancer Res 1999; 90(2):205.

369. Kuhnen C, Herter P, Muller O, et al. Beta-catenin in soft tissue sarcomas: expression is related to proliferative activity in high-grade sarcomas. Mod Pathol 2000; 13(9):1005.

370. Sato H, Hasegawa T, Kanai Y, et al. Expression of cadherins and their undercoat proteins (alpha-, beta-, and gamma-catenins and p120) and accumulation of beta-catenin with no gene mutations in synovial sarcoma. Virchows Arch 2001; 438(1):23.

371. Hauben EI, Jundt G, Cleton-Jansen AM, et al. Desmoplastic fibroma of bone: an immunohistochemical study including beta-catenin expression and mutational analysis for beta-catenin. Hum Pathol 2005; 36(9):1025.

372. Dei Tos AP, Doglioni C, Piccinin S, et al. Molecular abnormalities of the p53 pathway in dedifferentiated liposarcoma. J Pathol 1997; 181(1):8.

373. Dei Tos AP, Piccinin S, Doglioni C, et al. Molecular aberrations of the G1-S checkpoint in myxoid and round cell liposarcoma. Am J Pathol 1997; 151(6):1531.

374. Xiao ZX, Chen J, Levine AJ, et al. Interaction between the retinoblastoma protein and the oncoprotein MDM2. Nature 1995; 375(6533):694.

375. Martin K, Trouche D, Hagemeier C, et al. Stimulation of E2F1/DP1 transcriptional activity by MDM2 oncoprotein. Nature 1995; 375(6533):691.

376. Leach FS, Tokino T, Meltzer P, et al. p53 Mutation and MDM2 amplification in human soft tissue sarcomas. Cancer Res 1993; 53(10 Suppl):2231.

377. Oliner JD, Kinzler KW, Meltzer PS, et al. Amplification of a gene encoding a p53-associated protein in human sarcomas [see comments]. Nature 1992; 358(6381):80.

378. Cordon-Cardo C, Latres E, Drobnjak M, et al. Molecular abnormalities of mdm2 and p53 genes in adult soft tissue sarcomas. Cancer Res 1994; 54(3):794.

379. Binh MB, Sastre-Garau X, Guillou L, et al. MDM2 and CDK4 immunostainings are useful adjuncts in diagnosing well-differentiated and dedifferentiated liposarcoma subtypes: a comparative analysis of 559 soft tissue neoplasms with genetic data. Am J Surg Pathol 2005; 29(10):1340.

380. Coindre JM, Hostein I, Maire G, et al. Inflammatory malignant fibrous histiocytomas and dedifferentiated liposarcomas: histological review, genomic profile, and MDM2 and CDK4 status favour a single entity. J Pathol 2004; 203(3):822.

381. Coindre JM, Mariani O, Chibon F, et al. Most malignant fibrous histiocytomas developed in the retroperitoneum are dedifferentiated liposarcomas: a review of 25 cases initially diagnosed as malignant fibrous histiocytoma. Mod Pathol 2003; 16(3):256.

382. Hockenbery DM. bcl-2, a novel regulator of cell death. Bioessays 1995; 17(7):631.

383. LeBrun DP, Warnke RA, Cleary ML. Expression of bcl-2 in fetal tissues suggests a role in morphogenesis. Am J Pathol 1993; 142(3):743.

384. Weiss LM, Warnke RA, Sklar J, et al. Molecular analysis of the t(14;18) chromosomal translocation in malignant lymphomas. N Engl J Med 1987; 317(19):1185.

385. Nakanishi H, Ohsawa M, Naka N, et al. Immunohistochemical detection of bcl-2 and p53 proteins and apoptosis in soft tissue sarcoma: their correlations with prognosis. Oncology 1997; 54(3):238.

386. Suster S, Fisher C, Moran CA. Expression of bcl-2 oncoprotein in benign and malignant spindle cell tumors of soft tissue, skin, serosal surfaces, and gastrointestinal tract. Am J Surg Pathol 1998; 22(7):863.

387. Hasegawa T, Matsuno Y, Shimoda T, et al. Frequent expression of bcl-2 protein in solitary fibrous tumors. Jpn J Clin Oncol 1998; 28(2):86.

388. Chilosi M, Facchetti F, Dei Tos AP, et al. bcl-2 expression in pleural and extrapleural solitary fibrous tumours. J Pathol 1997; 181(4):362.

Prognostic markers

389. Gerdes J, Li L, Schlueter C, et al. Immunobiochemical and molecular biologic characterization of the cell proliferation-associated nuclear antigen that is defined by monoclonal antibody Ki-67. Am J Pathol 1991; 138(4):867.

390. Isola J, Helin H, Kallioniemi OP. Immunoelectron-microscopic localization of a proliferation-associated antigen Ki-67 in MCF-7 cells. Histochem J 1990; 22(9):498.

391. Choong PF, Akerman M, Willen H, et al. Prognostic value of Ki-67 expression in 182 soft tissue sarcomas. Proliferation – a marker of metastasis? APMIS 1994; 102(12):915.

392. Drobnjak M, Latres E, Pollack D, et al. Prognostic implications of p53 nuclear overexpression and high proliferation index of Ki-67 in adult soft-tissue sarcomas. J Natl Cancer Inst 1994; 86(7):549.

393. Levine EA, Holzmayer T, Bacus S, et al. Evaluation of newer prognostic markers for adult soft tissue sarcomas. J Clin Oncol 1997; 15(10):3249.

394. Ueda T, Aozasa K, Tsujimoto M, et al. Prognostic significance of Ki-67 reactivity in soft tissue sarcomas. Cancer 1989; 63(8):1607.

395. Rudolph P, Kellner U, Chassevent A, et al. Prognostic relevance of a novel proliferation marker, Ki-S11, for soft-tissue sarcoma. A multivariate study. Am J Pathol 1997; 150(6):1997.

396. Heslin MJ, Cordon-Cardo C, Lewis JJ, et al. Ki-67 detected by MIB-1 predicts distant metastasis and tumor mortality in primary, high grade extremity soft tissue sarcoma. Cancer 1998; 83(3):490.

397. Finlay CA, Hinds PW, Tan TH, et al. Activating mutations for transformation by p53 produce a gene product that forms an hsc70-p53 complex with an altered half-life. Mol Cell Biol 1988; 8(2):531.

398. Kastan MB, Onyekwere O, Sidransky D, et al. Participation of p53 protein in the cellular response to DNA damage. Cancer Res 1991; 51(23 Pt 1):6304.

399. Lane DP. Cancer. p53, guardian of the genome [news; comment] [see comments]. Nature 1992; 358(6381):15.

400. Castresana JS, Rubio MP, Gomez L, et al. Detection of TP53 gene mutations in human sarcomas. Eur J Cancer 1995; 5:735.

401. Golouh R, Bracko M, Novak J. Predictive value of proliferation-related markers, p53, and DNA ploidy for survival in patients with soft tissue spindle-cell sarcomas. Mod Pathol 1996; 9(9):919.

402. Kawai A, Noguchi M, Beppu Y, et al. Nuclear immunoreaction of p53 protein in soft tissue sarcomas. A possible prognostic factor. Cancer 1994; 73(10):2499.

403. Latres E, Drobnjak M, Pollack D, et al. Chromosome 17 abnormalities and TP53 mutations in adult soft tissue sarcomas. Am J Pathol 1994; 145(2):345.

404. Toffoli G, Doglioni C, Cernigoi C, et al. P53 overexpression in human soft tissue sarcomas: relation to biological aggressiveness. Ann Oncol 1994; 5(2):167.

405. Yang P, Hirose T, Hasegawa T, et al. Prognostic implication of the p53 protein and Ki-67 antigen immunohistochemistry in malignant fibrous histiocytoma. Cancer 1995; 76(4):618.

406. Sherr CJ. Cancer cell cycles. Science 1996; 274(5293):1672.

407. Nielsen GP, Stemmer-Rachamimov AO, Ino Y, et al. Malignant transformation of neurofibromas in neurofibromatosis 1 is associated with CDKN2A/p16 inactivation. Am J Pathol 1999; 155(6):1879.

408. Kourea HP, Orlow I, Scheithauer BW, et al. Deletions of the INK4A gene occur in malignant peripheral nerve sheath tumors but not in neurofibromas. Am J Pathol 1999; 155(6):1855.

Application of immunohistochemistry to sarcoma diagnosis: clinical scenarios

409. Fanburg JC, Rosenberg AE, Weaver DL, et al. Osteocalcin and osteonectin immunoreactivity in the diagnosis of osteosarcoma. Am J Clin Pathol 1997; 108(4):464.

410. Mertens F, Fletcher CD, Antonescu CR, et al. Clinicopathologic and molecular genetic characterization of low-grade fibromyxoid sarcoma, and cloning of a novel FUS/CREB3L1 fusion gene. Lab Invest 2005; 85(3):408.

411. Panagopoulos I, Storlazzi CT, Fletcher CD, et al. The chimeric FUS/CREB3l2 gene is specific for low-grade fibromyxoid sarcoma. Genes Chromosomes Cancer 2004; 40(3):218.

BENIGN FIBROBLASTIC/ MYOFIBROBLASTIC PROLIFERATIONS

Fibrous connective tissue consists principally of fibroblasts and an extracellular matrix containing fibrillary structures (collagen, elastin) and nonfibrillary extracellular matrix, or ground substance. Dense fibrous connective tissue, such as that found in tendons, aponeuroses, and ligaments, is composed predominantly of fibrillar collagen, whereas loose fibrous connective tissue contains a relative abundance of nonfibrillary ground substance.

Fibroblasts are the predominant cells in fibrous connective tissue. These cells are spindle-shaped with pale-staining, smoothly contoured oval nuclei, one or two minute nucleoli, and eosinophilic to basophilic cytoplasm, depending on the state of synthetic activity. The cytoplasmic borders are usually indistinct, although fibroblasts deposited in a rich myxoid stroma tend to assume a more stellate shape with multiple slender cytoplasmic extensions. Ultrastructurally, fibroblasts typically contain numerous, often dilated cisternae of rough endoplasmic reticulum, a large Golgi complex associated with small vesicles filled with granular or flocculent material, scattered mitochondria typically in a perinuclear location, many free ribosomes, occasional fat droplets, and slender microfilaments. Fibroblasts are responsible for

the intracellular assembly of various extracellular fibrillary and nonfibrillary products such as procollagen, protoelastin, and glycosaminoglycans, which form the ground substance of connective tissue.

Myofibroblasts share morphologic features with both fibroblasts and smooth muscle cells (Table 8–1).[1] Gabbiani et al. initially described these cells in granulation tissue[2] and later in Dupuytren's contracture.[3] Since this initial description, these cells have been described in such processes as responses to injury and repair phenomena, in quasineoplastic proliferative conditions, as part of the stromal response to neoplasia, and in a variety of benign and malignant neoplasms composed, at least in part, of myofibroblasts.[4–8] Ultrastructurally, myofibroblasts are characterized by indented nuclei with numerous, long cytoplasmic extensions. In the cytoplasm, bundles of microfilaments which are usually arranged parallel to the long axis of the cell are present with interspersed dense bodies. Subplasmalemmal plaques and pinocytotic vesicles are also numerous. The cells are partly enveloped by a basal lamina. The fibronexus, transmembrane complexes of intracellular microfilaments in continuity with the extracellular matrix, are also characteristic of this cell type.[9] Immunohistochemically, myofibroblasts may have a variable phenotype, including those that express (1) only vimentin (V type); (2) vimentin, smooth muscle α-actin, and desmin (VAD type); (3) vimentin and smooth muscle α-actin (VA type); and (4) vimentin and desmin (VD type) (Fig. 8–1).[10,11] These immunophenotypes differ depending on the type of myofibroblastic proliferation encountered.

Collagen is the main product of fibroblasts and the major constituent of the extracellular matrix. Up to 11 closely related but genetically distinct types of collagen are found in connective tissue, differing in the amino acid composition of their α chains.[12] Collagen chain polypeptides are synthesized on the ribosomes of the rough endoplasmic reticulum of fibroblasts and a variety of other cell types.[13] These precursor pro-α chains are then transported to the Golgi apparatus, where they coil into a triple helix, forming procollagens. After release from the Golgi apparatus, they are discharged into the pericellular matrix by exocytosis. Following enzymatic cleavage by procollagen peptidases, tropocollagen filaments

TABLE 8–1	ULTRASTRUCTURAL FEATURES OF MYOFIBROBLASTS COMPARED WITH FIBROBLASTS AND SMOOTH MUSCLE CELLS		
Feature	**Fibroblasts**	**Myofibroblasts**	**Smooth muscle cells**
Cell shape	Bipolar/tapered	Bipolar/stellate	Wider
Nucleus	Smooth	Deep marginations	Cigar-shaped
Golgi	+	+	Scanty
Rough endoplasmic reticulum	++	+	Scanty
Pinocytosis	–	+	
Attachment plaques	–	+	++
Dense bodies	–	+	++
External lamina	–	Interrupted	++
Cell–cell attachments	–	Gap, adherens	Continuous
Cell–stroma attachments (fibronexus)	–	++	Gap, adherens
			Attenuated

Modified from Fisher C. IAP presentation, Nice, France, October 1998.

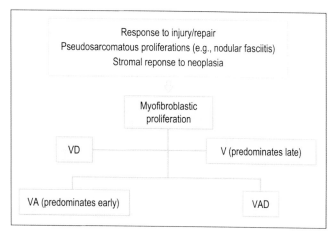

FIGURE 8–1 Immunophenotypes of myofibroblasts. V, vimentin; A, actin; D, desmin.

spontaneously aggregate in a staggered fashion, resulting in the formation of typical banded collagen fibrils with 64 nm periodicity. Long-spacing collagen with 240 nm periodicity is occasionally encountered in both normal and neoplastic tissues.

Type I collagen is ubiquitous and consists of parallel arrays of thick, closely packed banded fibrils. This type of collagen is found in the dermis, tendons, ligaments, bone, fascia, corneal tissue, and dentin. It is strongly birefringent and consists of two α_1 chains and one α_2 chain entwined in a helical configuration. *Type II collagen,* synthesized by chondroblasts, is found in the extracellular matrix of cartilage and in the notochord, nucleus pulposus, embryonic cornea, and vitreous body of the eye. *Type III collagen* is often associated with type I collagen, characteristically in loose connective tissue, including the dermis, blood vessel walls, and various glands and parenchymal organs. *Type IV collagen* is the major component of basal lamina. This collagen type is nonfibrillar and does not undergo any changes following secretion from the cell. *Type V collagen* is primarily found in

blood vessels and smooth muscle tissue. Other types of collagen (*types VII, VIII, IX*) are less common and less well defined. Reticular fibers form a delicate network of fibers that have the same cross-banding as collagen (67 nm) but differ from collagen fibers by their small size (approximately 50 nm in diameter) and their argyrophilia. They are composed mainly of type III collagen.[14] "Amianthoid" fibers are fused, abnormally thick collagen fibers with a typical periodicity but measuring up to 1000 nm in diameter.

Elastic fibers are usually closely associated with collagen fibers and are important components of the extracellular matrix of the dermis, large vessels, and internal organs such as the heart and the lung. Light microscopy reveals them to be slender, branching, highly refractile, weakly birefringent structures that stain with Weigert's resorcin-fuchsin, Verhoeff's, and aldehyde-fuchsin stains. Ultrastructurally, they have no cross-striations or banding. Elastic fibers are composed of two distinct components: *elastin,* a large amorphous homogeneous or finely granular structure of low electron density and peripherally located *microfibrils* which are 10–12 nm in length.[14] Elastin, the main component of elastic fibers, is synthesized and secreted as tropoelastin by fibroblasts; it typically contains large amounts of glycine, alanine, valine, and desmosine but little hydroxyproline. It is resistant to trypsin digestion but is hydrolyzed by elastase. Altered elastic fibers are found in a variety of heritable and acquired diseases and in the extracellular matrix of both benign and malignant neoplasms.[15,16]

The extracellular matrix is also composed in part of *glycoproteins,* including fibronectin and laminin. *Fibronectin* is a high-molecular-weight glycoprotein synthesized by fibroblasts and a variety of other cells. It affects cell-to-cell cohesion and the interaction between cells and the extracellular matrix, serving as a "molecular glue."[17] *Laminin* is a large glycoprotein distributed throughout the lamina lucida and lamina densa of the basement membrane.[18,19]

Glycosaminoglycans (*mucopolysaccharides*) form the ground substance of connective tissue. They are intimately associated with fibroblasts and collagen fibers, play an important role in salt and water distribution, and serve as a link in various cellular interactions. These substances are synthesized in fibroblasts or chondroblasts, where they are polymerized and sulfated in the Golgi complex. Chemically, they are linear polysaccharide chains of hexosamines (glycosamino-) and various sugars (-glycans) that are (with the exception of hyaluronic acid) bound to proteins. They have a high molecular weight, are negatively charged, and are capable of binding large amounts of fluids. These substances do not stain with hematoxylin and eosin but stain well with Alcian blue, colloidal iron, and toluidine blue.

One of the most important glycosaminoglycans is *hyaluronic acid,* a nonsulfated disaccharide chain composed of glucosamine and glucuronic acid. This substance is abundant in fibrous connective tissue and is the major component of synovial fluid. Histochemically, it is depolymerized and decolorized by hyaluronidase. *Chondroitin sulfates* (types 4 and 6) combine galactosamine and glucuronic acid, and these substances predominate in hyaline and elastic cartilage, nucleus pulposus, and intervertebral discs. Other glycosaminoglycans are *dermatan sulfate* and *heparin sulfate.* Dermatan sulfate is found predominantly in the dermis, tendons, and ligaments, whereas heparin sulfate is found in various structures rich in reticular fibers.[20]

BENIGN FIBROBLASTIC/ MYOFIBROBLASTIC PROLIFERATIONS

On the basis of distinct clinical and histologic features, there are four categories of fibroblastic/myofibroblastic lesions: (1) reactive lesions of which nodular fasciitis is the prototype; (2) fibromatoses, locally recurring but non-metastasizing lesions; (3) sarcomas with fibroblastic and/or myofibroblastic features that range in behavior from low to high grade; and (4) fibroblastic/myofibroblastic proliferations of infancy and childhood. The fourth category is included as a separate category because most fibroblastic/myofibroblastic lesions that occur during the first years of life have characteristic features that differ from those in older children and adults.

NODULAR FASCIITIS

Nodular fasciitis is a pseudosarcomatous, self-limiting reactive process composed of fibroblasts and myofibroblasts. Although first described by Kornwaler et al. in 1955 as "subcutaneous pseudosarcomatous fibromatosis," subsequent reports confirmed the benign nature of this proliferation.[21-23] Despite heightened awareness of this entity over the past 20 years and the topic of innumerable soft tissue seminars, nodular fasciitis is undoubtedly still the most common reactive or benign mesenchymal lesion that is misdiagnosed as a sarcoma given its characteristic rapid growth, rich cellularity, and mitotic activity. It is one of the most common soft tissue lesions and exceeds in frequency any other tumor or tumor-like lesion of fibrous tissue, which is attested to by the more than 1000 cases reviewed at the Armed Forces Institute of Pathology (AFIP) for a 20-year period and the large number of cases reported in the literature.

Although nodular fasciitis is clearly a benign process, the precise cause of this proliferation is unknown. Histologically, it bears a close resemblance to organizing granulation tissue, supporting a reactive proliferation that may be due to trauma, inconspicuous or otherwise. Morphologic variants of nodular fasciitis have been described, including intravascular, cranial, and ossifying fasciitis (described below), all of which have overlapping histologic features unified by a proliferation of cytologically bland fibroblasts and myofibroblasts. It is the differences in clinical, gross, and light microscopic features that warrant retention of these specific designations, although recognition as a reactive process is far more important than the ability to apply a precise name.

Clinical findings

Some patients provide a history of a rapidly growing mass or nodule that has been present for only 1–2 weeks. In about half of the cases there is associated soreness, tenderness, or slight pain. Numbness, paresthesia, or shooting pain is rare and develops only when the rapidly growing nodule exerts pressure on a peripheral nerve. Practically all lesions are solitary; among the AFIP cases there were only three in which two or more nodules were found at the same site. We have never encountered nodular fasciitis at multiple sites.

Although nodular fasciitis may occur in patients of any age, it is most common in adults 20–40 years of age (Fig. 8–2). In the series by Allen, only 14% of patients were less than 10 or more than 60 years of age.[24] Males and females are about equally affected. Most of the lesions grow rapidly and have a preoperative duration of 1 month or less. Although nodular fasciitis may occur virtually anywhere on the body, there is a distinct predilection for certain sites, the most common being the upper extremities, especially the volar aspect of the forearm, followed by the trunk, particularly the chest wall and back. Nodular fasciitis in the head and neck is next in frequency and is the most common site in infants and children.[25-27] It is less common in the lower extremities and infrequent in the hands and feet (Table 8–2). This lesion has also been reported in a variety of unusual locations, including the parotid gland (Fig. 8–3),[28] external ear,[29] oral cavity,[30] female genital tract,[31] ocular region,[32] and lymph node capsule (Fig. 8–4).

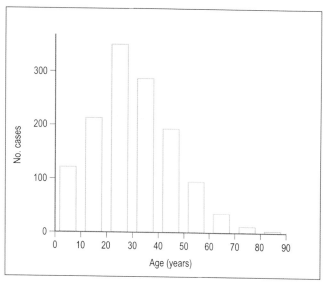

FIGURE 8–2 Age distribution for 1317 cases of nodular fasciitis.

Gross findings

The gross appearance of nodular fasciitis is highly dependent on the relative amounts of myxoid and fibrous stroma and the cellularity of the lesion. Most are relatively well circumscribed albeit nonencapsulated lesions, although some, particularly those centered about the deep fascia, are poorly circumscribed and appear to infiltrate the surrounding soft tissues. Most of the lesions are 2 cm or less in greatest dimension when they are excised.[33,34] Cases exceeding 3–5 cm in diameter should evoke concern about the diagnosis. Intramuscular lesions tend to be slightly larger than those found in the subcutaneous tissue.

The appearance of the cut surface depends on the relative amounts of myxoid and collagenous material. Those with a predominantly myxoid matrix are soft and gelatinous and grossly resemble other myxoid soft tissue lesions such as myxoma, ganglion, or benign peripheral nerve sheath tumors. Those with a pronounced collagenous stroma are firm and resemble other fibrous lesions such as fibromatosis or fibrosarcoma. Although extravasated erythrocytes are a frequent microscopic feature, these lesions are rarely grossly hemorrhagic.

Microscopic findings

Nodular fasciitis can be grouped into three subtypes based on their relation with the fascia. The *subcutaneous type*, the most common form of nodular fasciitis, is a well-circumscribed spherical nodule attached to the fascia but growing upward into the subcutis (Fig. 8–5). The *intramuscular type* is superficially attached to the fascia; it grows as an ovoid intramuscular mass and is often larger

TABLE 8–2	ANATOMIC DISTRIBUTION OF NODULAR FASCIITIS (1319 CASES)	
Anatomic location	**No. of patients**	**%**
Lower extremities	610	46
Head, neck	269	20
Trunk	235	18
Lower extremities	205	16
Total	1319	100

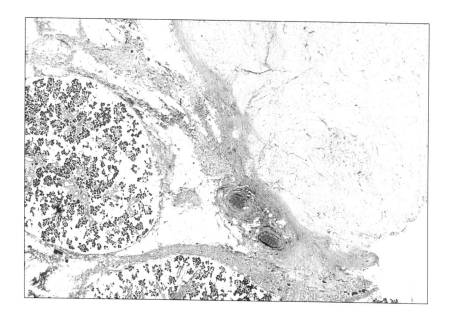

FIGURE 8–3 Nodular fasciitis involving the parotid gland. Note the circumscription and profuse myxoid change in the central portion of the lesion.

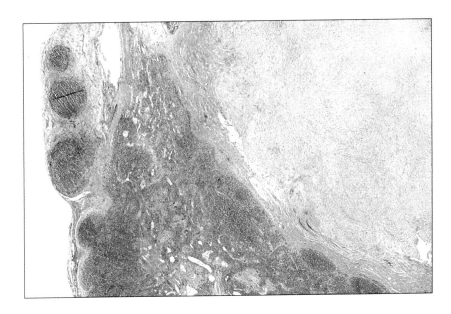

FIGURE 8–4 Rare example of nodular fasciitis involving the lymph node capsule.

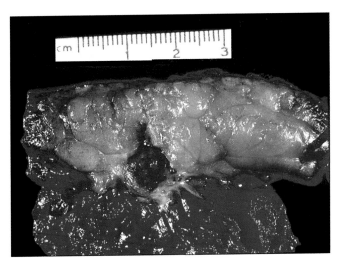

FIGURE 8–5 Gross appearance of the subcutaneous form of nodular fasciitis. The lesion is small and well circumscribed; it is superficially attached to the fascia.

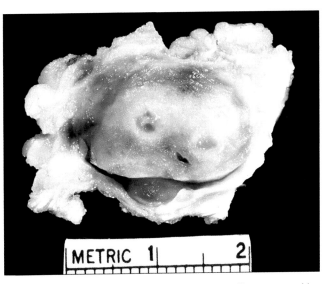

FIGURE 8–6 Nodular fasciitis with central cyst-like spaces, with accumulation of myxoid ground substance.

than the subcutaneous type. The *fascial type*, which is centered along the fascia, is less well circumscribed than the other forms, growing along the interlobular septa of the subcutaneous fat, resulting in a ray-like or stellate growth pattern. Rare examples of dermal nodular fasciitis have been reported.[35]

All cases of nodular fasciitis, regardless of whether they are predominantly fibrous or myxoid, are composed of plump, immature-appearing myofibroblasts that bear a close resemblance to the fibroblasts found in tissue culture or granulation tissue (Figs 8–6, 8–7). In general, the fibroblasts vary little in size and shape and have oval, pale-staining nuclei with prominent nucleoli. Mitotic

figures are fairly common, but atypical mitoses are virtually never seen (Fig. 8–8).

Characteristically, the fibroblasts are arranged in short, irregular bundles and fascicles and are accompanied by a dense reticulin meshwork and only small amounts of mature birefringent collagen. The intervening matrix is rich in mucopolysaccharides which stain readily with Alcian blue preparation and are depolymerized by hyaluronidase. The abundance of ground substance in most cases is responsible for the characteristic loosely textured, "feathery" pattern of nodular fasciitis; there are also cellular forms with only small amounts of interstitial myxoid material. Intermixed with the fibroblasts are

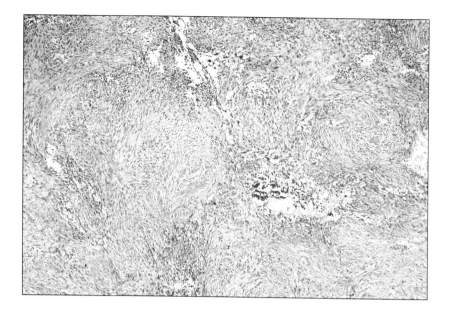

FIGURE 8–7 Nodular fasciitis showing varying cellularity with hypercellular spindle cell areas admixed with less cellular hyalinized zones.

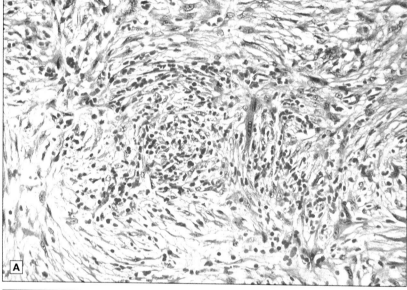

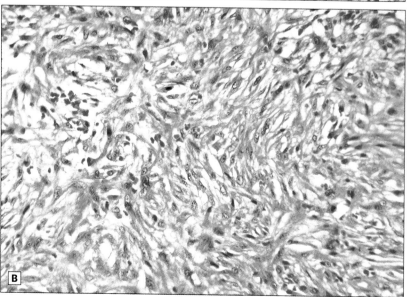

FIGURE 8–8 Nodular fasciitis. **(A)** Microhemorrhages between bundles of fibroblasts. **(B)** Bland cytologic features of cells in nodular fasciitis. There is an absence of nuclear hyperchromasia and variably sized nucleoli.

scattered lymphoid cells and erythrocytes and, in the more central portion of the lesion, a small number of lipid macrophages and multinucleated giant cells. Occasionally, there are associated areas of microhemorrhage, but siderophages are rare (Fig. 8–9).

There are minor variations in the histologic picture; sometimes the intramuscular form of nodular fasciitis contains residual atrophic muscle fibers and muscle giant cells; this feature, however, is much less pronounced in nodular fasciitis than in fibromatosis. The fascial type of nodular fasciitis may have cells arranged in a radial fashion around a central, poorly cellular, edematous area containing a mixture of mucoid material and fibrin. The myofibroblasts are closely associated with newly formed

vessels of narrow caliber; they have considerable mitotic activity, exceeding the average mitotic activity of the subcutaneous and intramuscular forms.

There is a close correlation between the microscopic picture and the preoperative duration of the lesion. Lesions of short duration tend to have a predominantly myxoid appearance (Fig. 8–10A,B), whereas those of longer duration are characterized by hyaline fibrosis (Fig. 8–10C,D), tissue shrinkage, and formation of minute fluid-filled spaces, or microcysts, a sequence closely paralleling the cicatrization of granulation tissue. In cases of long duration, the microcysts sometimes fuse and form a large centrally located cystic space (*cystic nodular fasciitis*).[36,37]

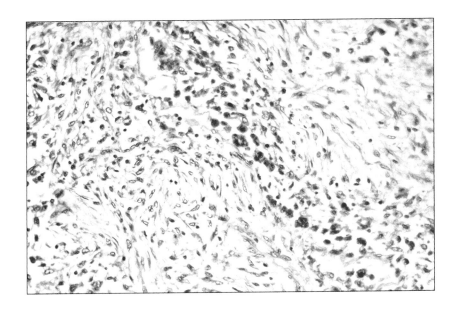

FIGURE 8–9 Nodular fasciitis with focal hemosiderin deposition, a feature rarely seen in this lesion.

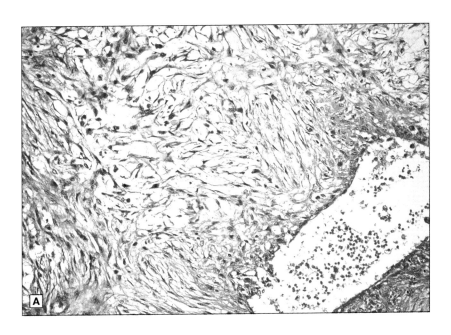

FIGURE 8–10 Nodular fasciitis. **(A)** Small area of myxoid breakdown imparting a loosely textured arrangement of fibroblasts.

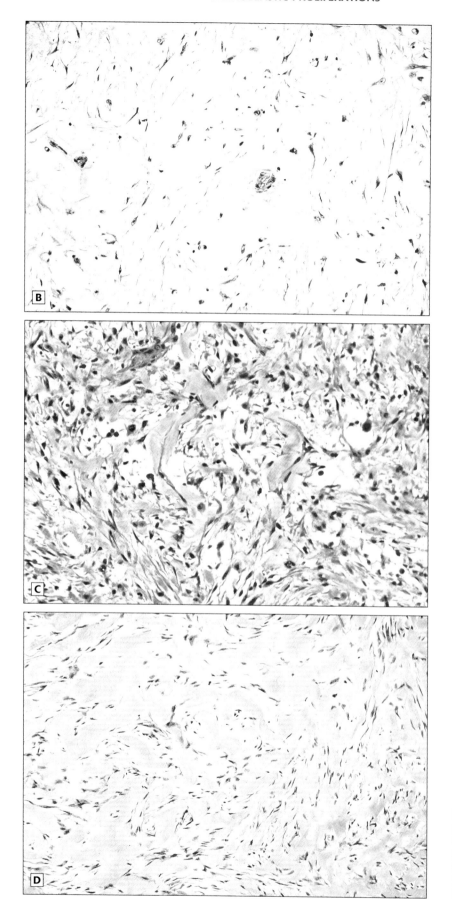

FIGURE 8–10 Continued. **(B)** More pronounced myxoid matrix with cells widely spaced by mucoid pools. **(C)** Nodular fasciitis showing hyaline fibrosis between fibroblasts. **(D)** Nodular fasciitis showing marked hyaline fibrosis, a feature usually encountered in lesions of long duration.

Ossifying fasciitis

On rare occasions a nodular fasciitis-like lesion has metaplastic bone, a condition described as *ossifying fasciitis*[38,39] or *fasciitis ossificans*[40,41] and, when arising from the periosteum, as *parosteal fasciitis* (Fig. 8–11).[42] Most of these lesions have features of both nodular fasciitis and myositis ossificans, but they are less well circumscribed than nodular fasciitis and lack the zonal maturation of myositis ossificans. Occasionally, small foci of metaplastic bone are also found in morphologically typical nodular fasciitis. *Panniculitis ossificans* and *fibro-osseous pseudotumor of the digits*[43,44] are closely related lesions that have a more irregular pattern and are somewhat akin to myositis ossificans. Rare cases of proliferative fasciitis, proliferative myositis, and cranial fasciitis may also contain foci of metaplastic bone.

Intravascular fasciitis

Intravascular fasciitis is a rare variant of nodular fasciitis characterized by involvement of small or medium-size veins or arteries.[45] It has been estimated to account for less than 3% of histologically proven cases of nodular fasciitis.[46] Males and females are equally affected, and most patients are young; very few patients are 30 years or older.[45,47] The typical presentation is that of a slowly growing, painless, solitary subcutaneous mass usually 2 cm or smaller. The upper extremity is the most common site, followed closely by the head and neck. Less common sites include the trunk and lower extremities.[46,48] Grossly, the lesions may be round or oval; or they may be elongated, multinodular, or plexiform, particularly those that grow as a predominantly intravascular mass (Fig. 8–12). Small to medium-size veins are most commonly affected,

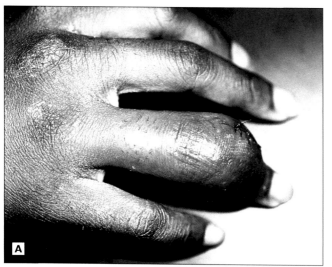

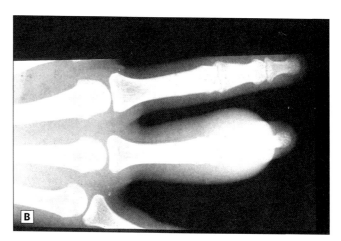

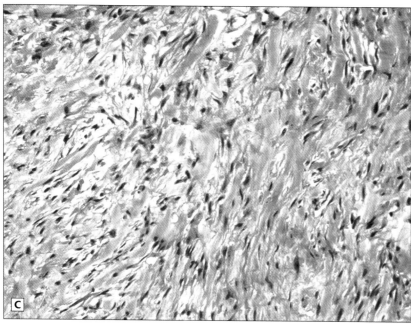

FIGURE 8–11 Parosteal fasciitis. **(A)** Gross appearance of parosteal fasciitis. **(B)** Accompanying radiograph of parosteal fasciitis. **(C)** Histologic appearance of parosteal fasciitis, which is identical to that seen in nodular fasciitis.

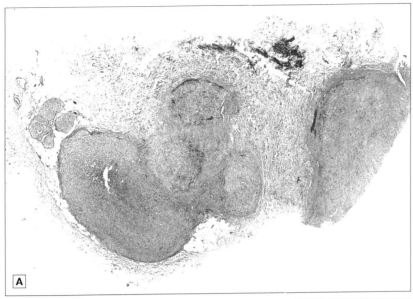

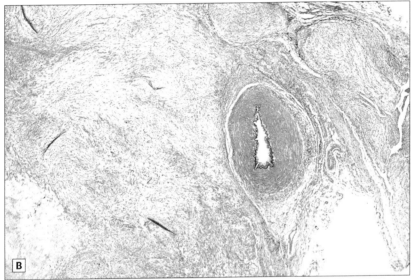

FIGURE 8–12 Intravascular fasciitis. **(A)** Low-power view showing multinodular growth in several markedly dilated veins. **(B)** Movat stain of intravascular fasciitis outlining intravascular growth of the spindle cell proliferation.

but some lesions involve arteries alone or are seen in conjunction with venous structures. In most cases there is involvement of the intima, media, adventitia, and perivascular soft tissue, frequently with a predominantly extravascular component, although some grow as an intraluminal polypoid mass (Fig. 8–13). The association with a vessel may be obscured by the proliferation such that special stains are required to highlight the involved vessel.

Histologically, the intravascular growth closely resembles nodular fasciitis, but it has a less prominent mucoid matrix and a conspicuous number of multinucleated giant cells resulting in a close resemblance to a benign fibrous histiocytoma or a giant cell tumor of soft parts (Figs 8–14, 8–15). Clefts are often present in areas where the proliferation has separated from the vessel wall. Because of the vessel involvement, this lesion may be confused with an organizing thrombus, intravascular capillary hemangioma, intravascular leiomyoma, or a sarcoma; 6 of 15 of the original lesions reported were initially confused with a sarcoma.[45] Despite the intravascular growth, there is no evidence of aggressive clinical behavior, recurrence, or metastasis.

Cranial fasciitis

Cranial fasciitis is a rapidly growing myofibroblastic proliferation which occurs chiefly, but not exclusively, in infants during the first year of life and involves the soft tissues of the scalp and the underlying skull.[49–52] It usually erodes the outer table of the cranium but not infrequently also penetrates the inner table, infiltrating the dura and sometimes even the leptomeninges. Radiographically, those that involve the underlying cranium create a lytic

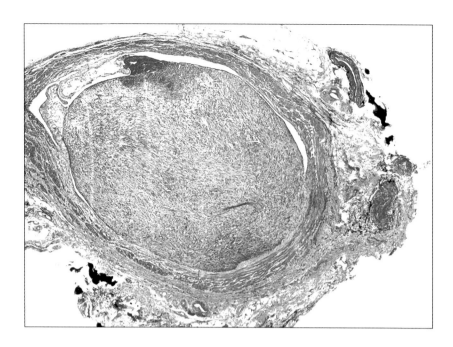

FIGURE 8–13 Movat stain of intravascular fasciitis highlighting the intravascular growth in a markedly dilated vein.

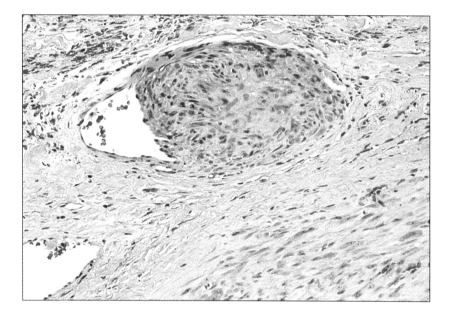

FIGURE 8–14 Small satellite nodule of intravascular fasciitis.

defect, often with a sclerotic rim (Fig. 8–16).[53] Histologically, cranial fasciitis exhibits the broad morphologic spectrum of nodular fasciitis; it is composed of a proliferation of fibroblasts and myofibroblasts deposited in a variably myxoid and hyalinized matrix, occasionally with foci of osseous metaplasia. The circumscription and the prominent myxoid matrix help distinguish the lesion from infantile fibromatosis or myofibromatosis.

Birth trauma may play a role in the development of the lesions; some affected children have been delivered by forceps.[49,54,55] Cranial fasciitis is a benign, probably reactive process that seems to arise from the galea aponeurotica or the epicranial aponeurosis; it infiltrates the incompletely formed cranial bone.

There is no relation between cranial fasciitis and the *"headbanger's tumor,"* a fibrosing lesion of the forehead with pigmentation of the overlying skin. Neither is there any association with an inherited fibrosing lesion of the scalp (*cutis verticis gyrata*) that occurs in adults and is associated with clubbing of the digits, enlargement of the distal extremities, and periosteal bone formation (pachydermoperiostosis).

Immunohistochemical findings

As one would expect in a lesion composed of myofibroblasts, most cells stain for smooth muscle actin and muscle-specific actin (Fig. 8–17).[34,56] Desmin is rarely

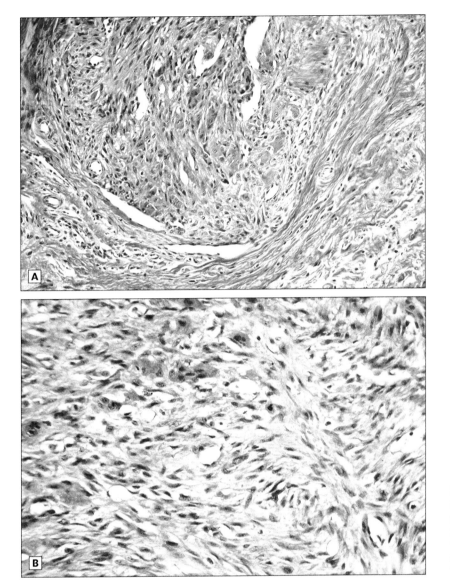

FIGURE 8–15 Intravascular fasciitis. **(A)** Intravascular proliferation of spindle-shaped cells with a conspicuous number of multinucleated giant cells. **(B)** Intravascular fasciitis composed of cytologically bland spindle cells similar to those found in nodular fasciitis.

expressed by the constituent cells; of the 53 cases stained by Montgomery and Meis, none expressed this antigen.[34] H-caldesmon has been purported to be a useful marker in distinguishing smooth muscle from myofibroblastic proliferations. Ceballos and colleagues and others found this marker to be consistently expressed by smooth muscle tumors but absent in nodular fasciitis.[57,57a] In small biopsy specimens, nodular fasciitis may be difficult to distinguish from a fibromatosis. β-catenin may be useful in this regard, since this antigen is consistently expressed by the nuclei in fibromatoses and is absent in the myofibroblasts of nodular fasciitis.[58] Immunostains for cytokeratin and S-100 protein are consistently negative.

Ultrastructural findings

Ultrastructurally, nodular fasciitis consists of elongated bipolar cells containing abundant rough endoplasmic reticulum, often filled with finely granular, electron-dense material. The nuclei have a smooth nuclear membrane and finely dispersed chromatin. In many of the cells there are also intracytoplasmic bundles of electron-dense microfilaments with focal condensation, pinocytotic vesicles, and occasional desmosomes.[59] Intracellular collagen fibers and fibronexus junctions are consistently identified, as one would expect in a predominantly myofibroblastic proliferation.[8,59]

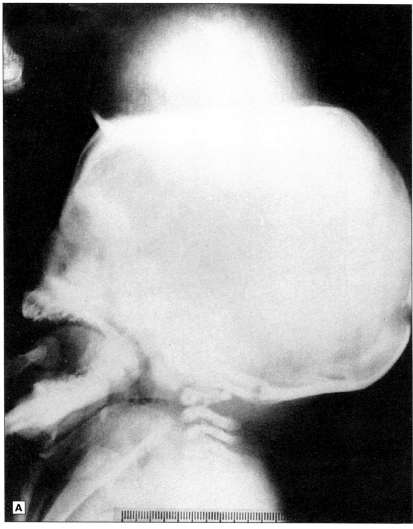

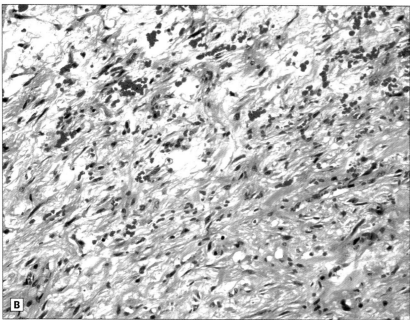

FIGURE 8–16 Cranial fasciitis.
(A) Radiograph of large soft tissue mass attached to the inner table of the skull in an infant. **(B)** Histologic picture of cranial fasciitis.

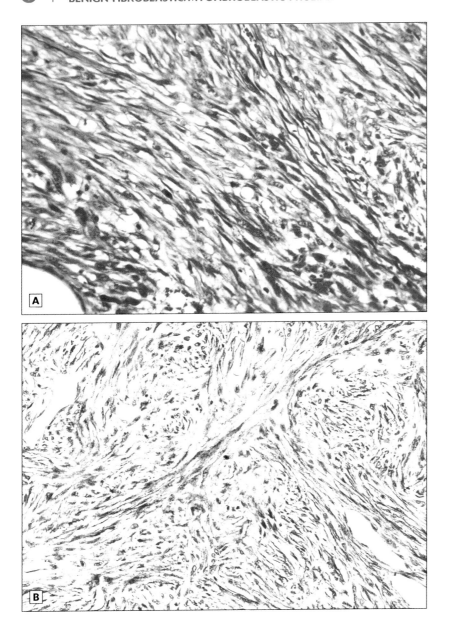

FIGURE 8–17 Nodular fasciitis. **(A)** Masson trichrome stain reveals fuchsinophilia of spindle cells. **(B)** Nodular fasciitis with diffuse smooth muscle actin immunoreactivity.

Ancillary findings

As suggested by the numerous mitotic figures that are typically present, nodular fasciitis has higher proliferative activity (as detected by antibodies to proliferating cell nuclear antigen) than other benign and malignant fibroblastic lesions.[60] However, the utility of these proliferative markers has not been established for distinguishing between these lesions for diagnostic purposes.

Few cases of nodular fasciitis have been evaluated cytogenetically. Rearrangements of 3q21 have been detected on several occasions,[61,62] confirming that karyotypic abnormalities may be found in reactive lesions. Another case of nodular fasciitis of the breast exhibited a 2;15 translocation, loss of chromosomes 2 and 13, and several

marker chromosomes.[63] A third report by Velagaleti et al. also documents a cytogenetic abnormality involving both homologues of chromosome 15, and the authors postulated a possible role for the *NTRK3* gene, a member of the neurotrophin transducing receptor family.[64] Contrary to these findings, using HUMARA-methylation-specific PCR, Koizumi and co-workers were unable to document clonality in 24 cases of nodular fasciitis from female patients.[65]

Differential diagnosis

Nodular fasciitis may be confused with numerous benign and malignant mesenchymal lesions, and the differential diagnosis depends on the relative amounts of myxoid and fibrous stroma and the cellularity of the lesion in question. As previously mentioned, nodular fasciitis remains the most common benign mesenchymal lesion misdiagnosed as a sarcoma. Hence, many cases of nodular fasciitis have been treated by unnecessary and overly radical surgery.

Although nodular fasciitis and *myxoma* may display a prominent myxoid matrix, the latter lesion is readily recognized by its paucity of cells and its poor vascularization. Myxomas also lack the zonal organization and regional heterogeneity of nodular fasciitis. Cellular nodular fasciitis may be confused with *fibrous histiocytoma*, and in a small number of cases distinction of these two lesions may be difficult if not somewhat arbitrary. The typical fibrous histiocytoma is dermis-based, less well circumscribed, and composed of a more polymorphous proliferation of spindle-shaped and round cells arranged in a more consistent storiform pattern. Secondary elements such as chronic inflammatory cells, xanthoma cells, siderophages, and Touton-type giant cells are also common. Peripherally located dense collagen fibers are typical; but similar-appearing fibers may occur in the central portion of nodular fasciitis, particularly in lesions of longer duration. Immunohistochemistry may play an ancillary role in distinguishing between these lesions, as most fibrous histiocytomas stain strongly for factor XIIIa,[66] in contrast to nodular fasciitis. Although smooth muscle actin can be focally present in some cases of fibrous histiocytoma,[67] most nodular fasciitis lesions stain diffusely for this antigen.[34] In general, however, the distinction between the two lesions is best made on histologic sections rather than on minor differences in immunophenotype.

Some cases of nodular fasciitis resemble *fibromatosis*. Grossly, fibromatosis is a large, poorly circumscribed lesion that typically infiltrates the surrounding soft tissue, in contrast to the circumscription of nodular fasciitis. Histologically, it is characterized by slender spindle-shaped fibroblasts arranged in long sweeping fascicles and separated by abundant collagen. Mitotic figures occur in both lesions, but they are much less frequent in musculoaponeurotic fibromatosis than in nodular fasciitis. Both lesions consistently express smooth muscle actin, but nuclear expression of β-catenin is characteristic of fibromatosis and absent in nodular fasciitis.[58]

Distinction from *fibrosarcoma* is primarily a matter of growth pattern and cellularity. The cells in fibrosarcoma are nearly always densely packed and are arranged in interweaving bundles, resulting in the characteristic "herringbone" pattern. Moreover, the individual cells are marked by a greater variation in size and shape, hyperchromatic nuclei, and a more pronounced mitotic rate, including atypical mitotic figures. The deep location, large size, and long duration of most fibrosarcomas also aid in the differential diagnosis.

Of the malignant myxoid lesions, *myxofibrosarcoma* (*myxoid malignant fibrous histiocytoma*) may closely resemble nodular fasciitis. This lesion occurs principally in patients older than 50 years and usually measures more than 3 cm when first excised. Microscopically, the cells show more nuclear pleomorphism, and there is typically a regular arborizing vasculature composed of coarse vessels, often invested with tumor cells. Atypical mitotic figures may be seen, as may areas of transition to a high-grade pleomorphic sarcoma.

Discussion

Although a well documented history of trauma is present in a small number of cases, nodular fasciitis is clearly a benign, reactive process that is likely triggered by local injury or in response to a localized inflammatory process. Regardless of the precise cause, histologic recognition of this reactive pattern is important to avoid misdiagnosing a sarcoma and unnecessary radical surgical treatment. The benign nature and excellent prognosis of nodular fasciitis has been well documented by numerous large clinicopathologic studies (Table 8–3). In the series of 895 cases reported by Allen,[24] only 9 (1%) reappeared after attempted complete surgical excision. Even those lesions that are incompletely excised rarely recur. Of the 18 cases of "recurrent nodular fasciitis" in the series by Bernstein and Lattes,[33] a review of the histology and clinical course led to revision of the original diagnosis in all 18 cases. In fact, these authors stated that recurrence of a lesion initially diagnosed as nodular fasciitis should lead to reappraisal of the original pathologic findings. Thompson and colleagues found a local recurrence rate of 9.3% in cases of nodular fasciitis of the external ear, a much higher rate of local recurrence when compared to nodular fasciitis at other sites.[29]

Several authors have reported the utility of fine-needle aspiration cytology for diagnosing nodular fasciitis.[68–70] However, this technique is limited by sampling error, and the aspirate must be interpreted in a clinical correlative fashion. In keeping with its benign nature, most cases of nodular fasciitis have been found to have a diploid DNA content.[71]

TABLE 8–3	RECURRENCE RATES IN LARGE SERIES OF NODULAR FASCIITIS	
Study	**Recurrence**	**%**
Bernstein and Lattes[33]	18/134*	13
Allen[24]	9/895	1

*Upon re-review, all recurrent lesions were reclassified as something other than nodular fasciitis.

PROLIFERATIVE FASCIITIS

Proliferative fasciitis, a term coined by Chung and Enzinger in 1975,[72] is the subcutaneous counterpart of proliferative myositis. Both of these lesions are pseudo-sarcomatous myofibroblastic proliferations characterized by the presence of unusual giant cells resembling ganglion cells. The microscopic appearance of the lesion is highly suggestive of a sarcoma, and many cases of this type have been misinterpreted in the past as embryonal rhabdomyosarcoma, ganglioneuroblastoma, or some other type of malignant neoplasm.

Clinical findings

Proliferative fasciitis is a lesion of adult life, with most patients being 40–70 years of age (mean 54 years).[72] Thus as a group, patients with proliferative fasciitis tend to be older than those with nodular fasciitis. It is uncommon for patients younger than 15 years of age to develop proliferative fasciitis.[73] There is no gender or race predilection, and most of the lesions occur in the subcutaneous tissues of the extremities, with the upper extremity (especially the forearm) affected more commonly than the lower extremity. The lesion also occurs with some frequency on the trunk and rarely on the head and neck.[74]

Clinically, most patients present with a firm, palpable subcutaneous nodule that is freely movable and unattached to the overlying skin, although about two-thirds of patients also have complaints of pain or tenderness. Most lesions measure less than 5 cm in greatest diameter, with a median size of 2.5 cm. Like nodular fasciitis, these lesions are typically rapidly growing, most being excised 2–6 weeks after their initial discovery. A history of trauma in the vicinity of the mass is elicited in about one-third of cases.[72]

Pathologic findings

Grossly, proliferative fasciitis is usually poorly circumscribed, forming an elongated or discoid-shaped mass that predominantly involves the subcutaneous tissue, although some involve the superficial fascia. Rare lesions also involve the superficial skeletal muscle, making it difficult to distinguish from proliferative myositis. The rare cases that arise during childhood tend to be more circumscribed and vaguely lobular, with only occasional extension along fascial planes.[73]

Microscopically, like nodular fasciitis, proliferative fasciitis is composed of tissue culture-like fibroblastic and myofibroblastic spindle cells that have bland cytologic features and are deposited in a variably myxoid and collagenous stroma. This proliferation extends along the interlobular septa of the subcutaneous tissue, with some extension along the superficial fascia (Fig. 8–18). The lesion is characterized by the presence of large, basophilic ganglion-like cells with one or two vesicular nuclei and prominent nucleoli. The cells have abundant basophilic, slightly granular cytoplasm but lack cross-striations typical of rhabdomyoblasts (Figs 8–19 to 8–21). Some cells have intracytoplasmic inclusions of collagen. These ganglion-like cells may be packed together or loosely arranged in aggregates. Multinucleated giant cells of the type seen in nodular fasciitis are rare in proliferative fasciitis. For unknown reasons, pediatric lesions tend to be more cellular (Fig. 8–22), have numerous mitoses, and have foci of acute inflammation and necrosis, features that are distinctly unusual in the typical adult form.[75] Childhood cases also tend to have less collagen and a less conspicuous myxoid matrix than their adult counterparts. Some lesions, particularly those that have been present for a long duration prior to excision, may have abundant hyalinized collagen that surrounds the ganglion-like cells, which could cause confusion with neoplastic osteoid and a misdiagnosis of osteosarcoma.

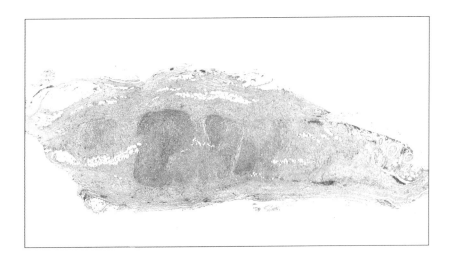

FIGURE 8–18 Proliferative fasciitis involving the subcutis.

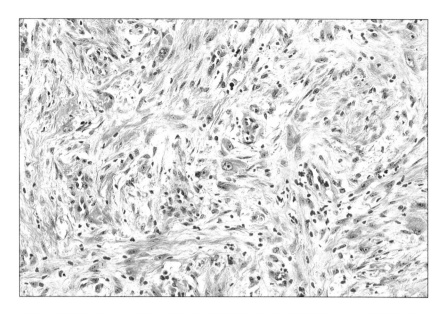

FIGURE 8–19 Proliferative fasciitis composed of a mixture of fibroblasts and giant cells with abundant basophilic cytoplasm bearing some resemblance to ganglion cells.

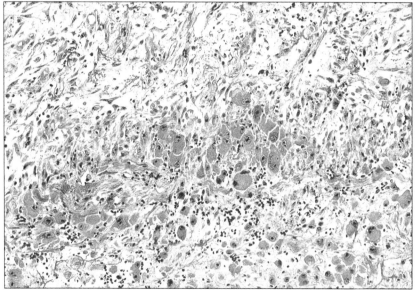

FIGURE 8–20 Peripheral portion of proliferative fasciitis with numerous ganglion-like giant cells.

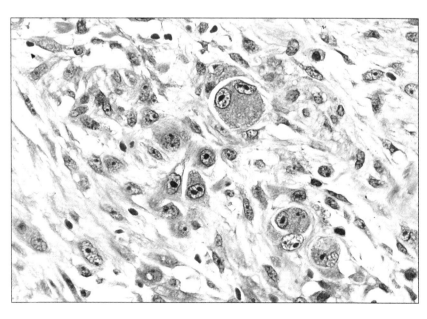

FIGURE 8–21 Proliferative fasciitis with large ganglion-like cells, some of which are multinucleated.

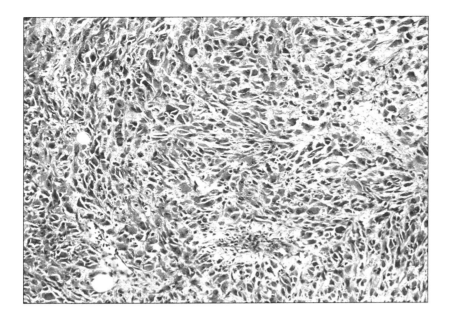

FIGURE 8–22 Proliferative fasciitis of childhood composed of round and polygonal cells with abundant cytoplasm and prominent nucleoli.

The immunohistochemical findings of proliferative fasciitis are similar to those of nodular fasciitis. The spindle and stellate-shaped cells stain for vimentin and both muscle-specific and smooth muscle actin. Some cells stain for CD68 (KP1); immunostains for cytokeratins, S-100 protein, and desmin are usually negative.[75,76] The ganglion-like cells may also stain for actin, although the staining is often focal and weak and may be membranous in distribution.[75]

Ultrastructurally, the spindle- and stellate-shaped cells have the typical features of fibroblasts and myofibroblasts.[77–79] The ganglion-like cells are characterized by abundant rough endoplasmic reticulum with dilated cisternae, some of which may contain short-spacing collagen fibrils.[80] Cell junctions and Z-line formations are not seen.

PROLIFERATIVE MYOSITIS

Proliferative myositis is the intramuscular counterpart of proliferative fasciitis. Although Kern is credited with the original description of proliferative myositis,[81] Ackerman probably reported the first cases in his study of "extraosseous non-neoplastic localized bone and cartilage formation."[82] Like proliferative fasciitis, it is a rapidly growing lesion that infiltrates muscle tissue in a diffuse manner and is characterized by bizarre giant cells bearing a close resemblance to ganglion cells.

Clinical findings

The symptoms are non-specific, and the diagnosis always rests on the histologic examination of tissue obtained by biopsy or excision. In most cases the lesion is first noted as a palpable, more or less discrete, solitary nodular mass that measures 1–6 cm in diameter. It rarely causes tenderness or pain, even though it may double in size within a period of a few days. The duration between onset and excision is usually less than 3 weeks.[83]

The patients tend to be older than those with nodular fasciitis, with a median age of 50 years.[83] Rare cases of proliferative myositis have been described in children.[75,84,85] There seems to be no predilection for either gender or any particular race. The lesion mainly affects the flat muscles of the trunk and shoulder girdle, especially the pectoralis, latissimus dorsi, or serratus anterior muscle. Occasionally, tumors are also found in the muscles of the thigh. Involvement of the head and neck is rare.[86,87]

Pathologic findings

Similar to proliferative fasciitis, proliferative myositis typically appears pale gray or scar-like, resulting in induration of the involved skeletal muscle (Fig. 8–23). When present in small or flat muscles, it often replaces most or all of the involved musculature. When involving large muscles, there is preferential involvement of the skeletal muscle immediately underneath the fascia with a progressive decrease in the central portion of the muscle in a wedge-like fashion.

The cellular components of proliferative myositis are identical to those found in proliferative fasciitis. There is a poorly demarcated proliferation of fibroblast-like cells that involve the epimysium, perimysium, and endomysium. Unlike the intramuscular form of nodular fasciitis and musculoaponeurotic fibromatosis, this cellular proliferation rarely completely replaces large areas of the involved muscle but, rather, is most striking in the subfascial region and interfascicular connective tissue septa.

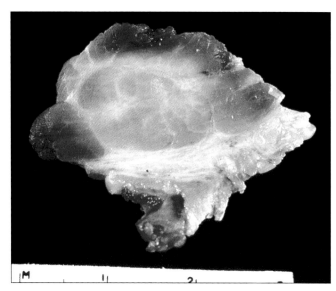

FIGURE 8–23 Proliferative myositis characterized by a poorly circumscribed scar-like fibrosing process involving muscle and muscle fascia.

The skeletal muscle fibers are relatively unaffected except for the presence of secondary atrophy, with neither sarcolemmal proliferation nor any evidence of skeletal muscle regeneration. This alternation of proliferating fibrous tissue with persistent atrophic skeletal muscle fibers results in a typical "checkerboard" pattern that is apparent at low magnification (Fig. 8–24). The other conspicuous histologic feature of proliferative myositis is the presence of large basophilic ganglion-like cells, identical to those found in proliferative fasciitis (Figs 8–25, 8–26). Mitotic figures are often easily identified in both the spindle and giant cells, although atypical mitoses are not seen. Rare lesions contain foci of metaplastic bone (Fig. 8–27).

The immunohistochemical and ultrastructural features of proliferative myositis are identical to those of proliferative fasciitis (Fig. 8–28).[88,89]

Trisomy 2 has been described in both proliferative fasciitis[90] and proliferative myositis.[91] McComb and colleagues reported a single case with a t(6;14)(q23;q32).[92] Flow cytometric DNA analysis of these lesions has revealed a uniformly diploid pattern.[76,93]

Differential diagnosis

Proliferative fasciitis and myositis may be mistaken for a variety of malignant neoplasms, most commonly *rhabdomyosarcoma* or *ganglioneuroblastoma*. In the series of 53 cases of proliferative fasciitis by Chung and Enzinger, 16 were originally diagnosed as a sarcoma.[72] Similarly, 14 of 33 cases of proliferative myositis reported by Enzinger and Dulcey were believed to be some type of

sarcoma.[83] Errors are most likely to occur with childhood cases where rhabdomyosarcoma is a strong diagnostic consideration. The history of a rapidly growing mass of short duration that typically attains a maximum size of less than 3 cm is more consistent with a reactive process than a sarcoma. Histologically, the ganglion-like cells lack cross-striations and show more cytoplasmic basophilia than is seen in rhabdomyoblasts. Although the immunohistochemical profiles may overlap, stains for desmin, myoglobin, and myogenin are negative in the ganglion-like cells, in contrast to the staining found in true rhabdomyoblasts. Although ganglioneuroblastoma is also a consideration, proliferative fasciitis and myositis lack a fibrillary background, and the ganglion-like cells may express actin, unlike true ganglion cells.

Discussion

Proliferative fasciitis and myositis, like nodular fasciitis, are self-limiting, benign, reactive processes that are probably preceded by some type of fascial or muscular injury resulting in a proliferation of myofibroblasts. However, only a small number of patients report a preceding injury in the exact location of the lesion, raising the possibility that causes other than mechanical trauma play a role in the development of proliferative fasciitis and myositis. Although some have reported the diagnosis of these lesions by fine-needle aspiration cytology, the unusual histologic features of these lesions warrant caution with this technique. Both proliferative fasciitis and myositis are adequately treated by local excision, and recurrence is exceedingly rare.

ORGAN-ASSOCIATED PSEUDOSARCOMATOUS MYOFIBROBLASTIC PROLIFERATIONS

Organ-associated pseudosarcomatous myofibroblastic proliferations, most of which arise in the genitourinary tract, have been described under an impressive variety of names, including *inflammatory pseudotumor, pseudosarcomatous myofibroblastic tumor, pseudosarcomatous myofibroblastic proliferation, pseudosarcomatous fibromyxoid tumor,* and even *nodular fasciitis.* Most commonly, those arising as a result of preceding trauma or surgical instrumentation have been referred to as *postoperative spindle cell nodule,*[94,95] whereas those arising spontaneously have often been referred to as inflammatory pseudotumor.[96–99] Certainly, the vast array of names used to describe these proliferations has contributed to some of the confusion. However, the major controversy has focused on whether these lesions are reactive or neoplastic, including whether these lesions are best designated as *inflammatory myofibroblastic tumor,* a term that implies a neoplastic process characterized by alterations of the *ALK* gene on

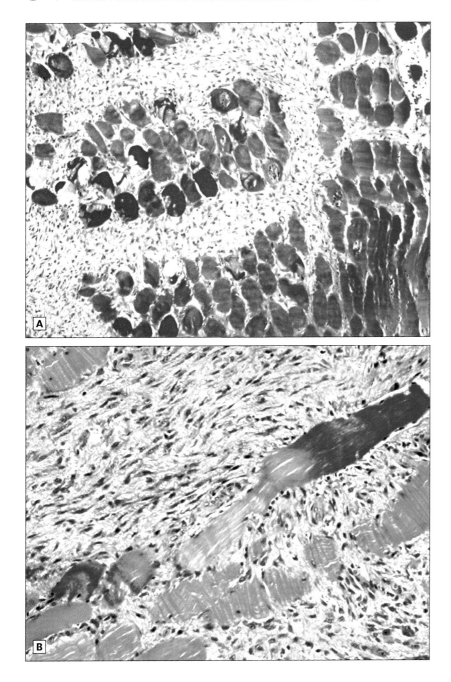

FIGURE 8–24 **(A)** Low-magnification view of proliferative myositis showing the characteristic "checkerboard" pattern. **(B)** Fasciitis-like area surrounding skeletal muscle fibers in a case of proliferative myositis.

2p23.[100–102] Two recent studies demonstrating *ALK* gene rearrangements, and immunostaining for the ALK protein suggest these lesions are neoplastic, although the two studies differ as to whether they believe the lesions are identical to inflammatory myofibroblastic tumor.[103,104] Harik et al. considers these lesions to be neoplastic but distinct from inflammatory myofibroblastic tumor and favors the term *pseudosarcomatous myofibroblastic proliferation*,[103] whereas the other group recommends calling them inflammatory myofibroblastic tumor.[104] What is clear, however, is that there is no histologic difference between lesions harboring *ALK* abnormalities and those that do not. Likewise, there are no significant histologic

differences between lesions that arise spontaneously and those that arise following instrumentation.

Clinical findings

Although these lesions can arise anywhere in the genitourinary tract including the prostate,[105–107] vagina,[100,108] urethra,[100,106,107] and ureter,[96] they are most common in the urinary bladder. For example, in the study by Hirsch and colleagues,[100] 21 of 27 pseudosarcomatous myofibroblastic proliferations of the genitourinary tract arose in the urinary bladder. Similarly, 42 of 46 "inflammatory myofibroblastic tumors" reported by Montgomery et al.

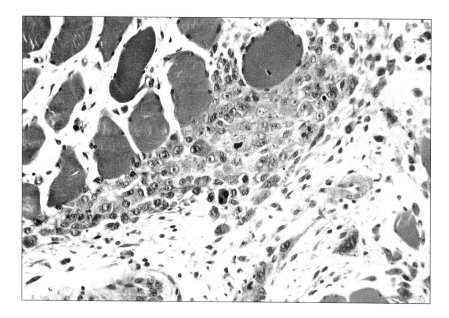

FIGURE 8–25 Proliferative myositis. Ganglion-like giant cells are seen immediately adjacent to and infiltrating skeletal muscle fibers.

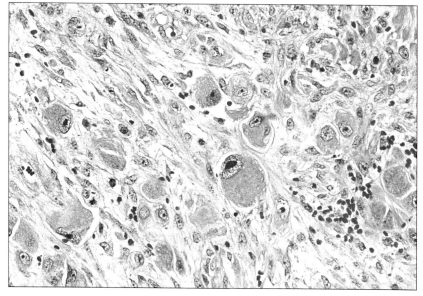

FIGURE 8–26 High-power view of ganglion-like giant cells in proliferative myositis.

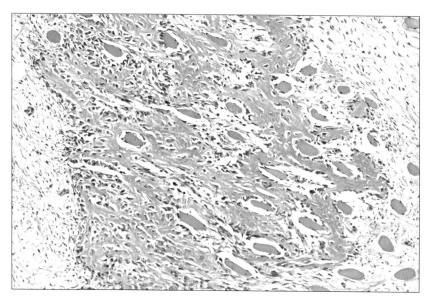

FIGURE 8–27 Unusual case of proliferative myositis with extensive metaplastic bone formation.

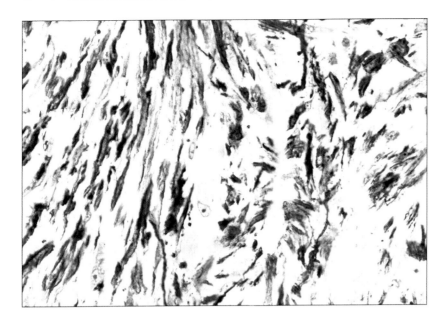

FIGURE 8–28 Proliferative myositis stained for smooth muscle actin. Most spindle cells stain for this antigen, but the ganglion-like cells in this case are negative.

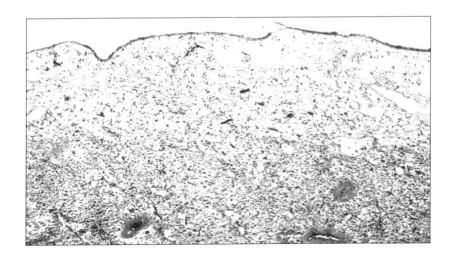

FIGURE 8–29 Inflammatory pseudotumor (pseudosarcomatous myofibroblastic proliferation) of the urinary bladder. Proliferation of spindle cells in a loose, edematous, myxoid stroma with mixed acute and chronic inflammatory cells.

arose in the urinary bladder.[104] Most commonly, patients present with hematuria, although some patients may present with dysuria, abdominal pain, or weight loss. Based upon the larger clinicopathologic studies, it is still unclear whether this lesion is more common in women or men. In the studies by Harik et al.[103] and Montgomery et al.,[104] males outnumbered females by a 2–3:1 ratio. However, Hirsch and colleagues found exactly the opposite, as women were affected three times as often as men.[100] Although the age range is broad, they most commonly arise in patients in their fourth to fifth decades of life. Approximately 20–25% of patients have a history of antecedent trauma or surgical instrumentation.[100,103,104] Those that arise secondary to surgical instrumentation usually become clinically apparent between 5 and 12 weeks following the surgical procedure.

Pathologic findings

Grossly, most lesions present as exophytic, nodular or polypoid intraluminal lesions that may extend deeply into the visceral organ from which they arise. They range in size from 1.5 cm to up to 12 cm, although most are between 3 and 5 cm at the time of excision. The lesion may be firm or soft, depending upon the relative amounts of fibrous and myxoid stroma present.

On microscopic examination, these lesions are characterized by a proliferation of spindle to stellate-shaped cells, often with a "tissue culture-like" appearance reminiscent of nodular fasciitis (Figs 8–29 to 8–31). The cells lack cytologic atypia or nuclear hyperchromasia and have bipolar or stellate-shaped cytoplasmic processes. Most commonly, the cells are widely separated and

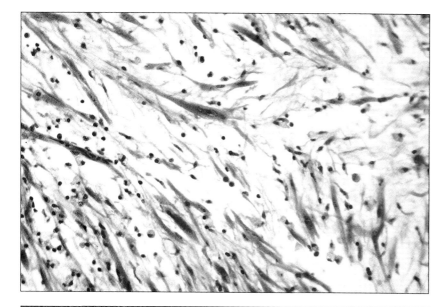

FIGURE 8–30 High-power view of inflammatory pseudotumor (pseudosarcomatous myofibroblastic proliferation) of the urinary bladder. Haphazard arrangement of spindle cells with bipolar or stellate-shaped cytoplasmic processes deposited in a myxoid stroma with scattered chronic inflammatory cells.

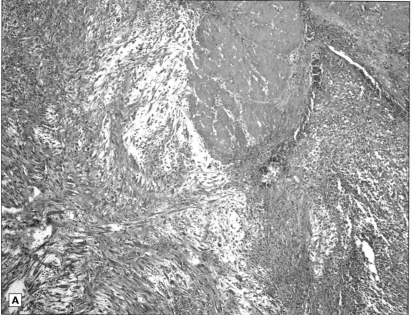

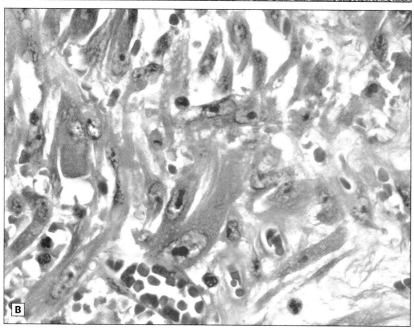

FIGURE 8–31 **(A)** Low-magnification view of a pseudosarcomatous myofibroblastic proliferation of the urinary bladder with infiltration of the muscularis propria. **(B)** High-magnification view of reactive-appearing spindled-shaped cells with prominent nucleoli.

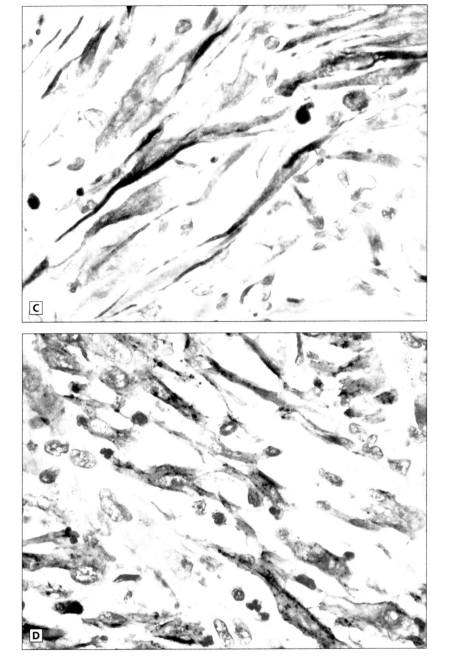

FIGURE 8–31 Continued. (C) Strong cytokeratin immunoreactivity in the constituent cells of a pseudosarcomatous myofibroblastic proliferation of the urinary bladder. (D) Strong ALK immunoreactivity in the same case is seen in Fig. 8–31C.

haphazardly distributed in a myxoid stroma composed predominantly of hyaluronic acid. Some cases are characterized by more cellular areas in which the cells are arranged in irregular fascicles with variable amounts of intercellular collagen. The cells have oval to spindle-shaped nuclei with open chromatin, variably sized nucleoli, and eosinophilic to amphophilic cytoplasm. Mitotic figures (MF) are present, usually with fewer than 1–2 MF/10 high-power fields (HPF), and they are not atypical. In the more myxoid zones, there is a prominent capillary network often associated with extravasated erythrocytes. A mixed inflammatory infiltrate composed of lymphocytes, plasma cells, eosinophils and occasional mast cells is usually conspicuous. When present, neutrophils are associated with areas of mucosal ulceration.

Some cases have histologic features that cause great concern for a malignancy. Rare examples have a brisk mitotic rate, with up to 20 MF/10 HPF. Invasion into the muscularis propria of the urinary bladder is a common finding, and some even infiltrate into the perivesicular adipose tissue. Although necrosis is usually focal and confined to the surface of the lesion and associated with mucosal ulceration, some cases show necrosis of the deeper tissue.

Immunohistochemical and ultrastructural findings

Immunohistochemically, the spindle cells stain strongly for vimentin and various muscle markers, including muscle-specific actin, smooth muscle actin, and desmin. In addition, many cases show focal or often diffuse staining for cytokeratins (Fig. 8–31C).[100,103,104] In the study by Harik and colleagues, 31 of 35 cases stained for cytokeratins.[103] Similarly, Montgomery and colleagues found 25 of 34 cases (73%) to stain for AE1/AE3, including 23 cases with strong, diffuse immunoreactivity.[104]

A significant percentage of these lesions also stain for ALK (Fig. 8–31D). However, there is an imperfect correlation between ALK immunoreactivity and detection of an *ALK* gene translocation by FISH (Table 8–4). In the study by Harik and co-workers, 12 of 26 (46%) cases stained for this antigen; analysis by FISH confirmed a translocation of the *ALK* gene in 4 of 6 (67%) ALK-positive tumors.[103] Montgomery and colleagues found 20 of 35 cases (57%) to stain for ALK, and 13 of 18 of these ALK-positive cases (72%) showed evidence of an *ALK* gene alteration by FISH.[104] In contrast, of the six ALK immunoreactive cases evaluated by Hirsch et al., none showed evidence of an *ALK* translocation by FISH.[100] More recently, Sukov et al. found *ALK* rearrangements in 14 of 21 cases (67%), with *ALK* staining in 13 of 21 cases

(62%).[104a] All cases with *ALK* expression harbored *ALK* rearrangements; one *ALK* negative case exhibited an *ALK* rearrangement. All of the other lesions studied (leiomyosarcomas, sarcomatoid carcinomas, embryonal rhabdomyosarcomas and lesions felt to be reactive were negative for *ALK* rearrangement and *ALK* staining.

Ultrastructurally, the cells show prominent myofibroblastic features with bipolar cytoplasmic processes containing abundant rough endoplasmic reticulum and peripheral bundles of thin filaments with focal densities and fibronexus junctions.[1]

Differential diagnosis

Although a pseudosarcomatous myofibroblastic proliferation should be suspected when one encounters a spindle cell lesion in the genitourinary tract, particularly in a patient who has undergone recent instrumentation at that site, numerous other benign and malignant spindle cell proliferations must be considered (Table 8–5). *Myxoid leiomyosarcoma* tends to occur in older patients and is quite rare before the age of 20 years. Microscopically, the lesion is composed of spindle cells with densely eosinophilic fibrillar cytoplasm, often with perinuclear vacuoles, deposited in a myxoid stroma. These lesions can also express cytokeratins, but they do not stain for ALK. Pseudosarcomatous myofibroblastic proliferations are characterized by a more prominent vasculature, more variable cellularity, and a more conspicuous inflammatory component. Moreover, these lesions characteristically have a "zonal" quality consisting of superficial (submucosal) myxoid zones juxtaposed to deep cellular zones associated with a prominent arcuate vascular pattern.

Botryoid-type rhabdomyosarcoma is also a diagnostic consideration; this lesion is characterized by the presence of a cambium layer under the epithelium composed of atypical, hyperchromatic cells, occasionally with overt rhabdomyoblastic differentiation. Immunohistochemical (myogenin) and ultrastructural analysis reveals evidence of skeletal muscle differentiation.

The immunohistochemical detection of epithelial differentiation in many pseudosarcomatous myofibroblastic proliferations often raises concern for a *sarcomatoid*

TABLE 8–4	FREQUENCY OF ALK IMMUNOREACTIVITY AND *ALK* GENE REARRANGEMENTS BY FISH IN PSEUDOSARCOMATOUS MYOFIBROBLASTIC PROLIFERATIONS/INFLAMMATORY MYOFIBROBLASTIC TUMORS OF THE URINARY BLADDER

Study	ALK staining	*ALK* gene rearrangements (FISH)
Tsuzuki et al.[101]	10/14	
Hirsch et al.[100]	10/21	0/6*
Harik et al.[103]	12/26	4/10**
Montgomery et al.[104]	20/35	13/18
Total	52/96 (54%)	17/34 (50%)

*All six cases tested stained for ALK.
**Includes four ALK-negative cases (0/4) and six ALK-positive cases (4/6).

TABLE 8–5	DIFFERENTIAL DIAGNOSTIC FEATURES OF GENITOURINARY PSEUDOSARCOMATOUS MYOFIBROBLASTIC PROLIFERATIONS

Feature	PMP	ML	B-RMS	SC
Cellularity	+	+/++	+/++	++
Growth pattern	Loose	Loose	Botryoid	Biphasic
Atypia	+	+/++	++	+++
Electron microscopy	Fibroblast/myofibroblast	Smooth muscle	Striated muscle	Epithelial
Cytokeratin	Frequent +	Rare	–	+
Desmin	±	+	+	±
SMA	+	+	–	±
ALK	50%	–	–	–

PMP, pseudosarcomatous myofibroblastic proliferation; ML, myxoid leiomyosarcoma; B-RMS, botryoid rhabdomyosarcoma; SC, sarcomatoid urothelial carcinoma.

urothelial carcinoma. The presence of marked cytologic atypia, atypical mitotic figures, non-myxoid zones with markedly increased cellularity, and the identification of an in-situ urothelial carcinoma are useful features in recognizing sarcomatoid urothelial carcinoma.[101,104] In addition, the expression of ALK in pseudosarcomatous myofibroblastic proliferations is a useful finding in this differential diagnosis.

Discussion

Whether these lesions should be considered true neoplasms or exuberant reactive proliferations is controversial, and as indicated above, there is some evidence to support both points of view. The history of prior surgical instrumentation in up to 25% of cases and the bland myofibroblastic appearance of the constituent cells, in association with a myxoinflammatory background, are hallmarks of many reactive soft tissue processes (most notably nodular fasciitis). However, most cases arise spontaneously without a history of prior surgical instrumentation. These lesions may show extensive mural growth with some infiltrating into the perivesicular adipose tissue. From an immunophenotypic standpoint, they are rather unique when compared to other pseudosarcomatous myofibroblastic proliferations, since most express cytokeratins, sometimes diffusely.

Although there are conflicting data, some of these lesions clearly harbor translocations of the *ALK* gene.[101-104] It is possible that some myofibroblastic proliferations of the genitourinary tract are reactive, whereas others are truly neoplastic and associated with *ALK* gene abnormalities. We and others believe there are some subtle differences which allow one to separate these lesions from the inflammatory myofibroblastic tumor in most instances. These lesions have a relative absence of plasma cells, a more prominent edematous stroma, and a lack of the peculiar ganglion-like cells of inflammatory myofibroblastic tumor.[100,103] It is also possible that pseudosarcomatous myofibroblastic proliferations and inflammatory myofibroblastic tumors represent various points within a single spectrum, as opposed to representing two distinct entities.

Regardless of whether one considers these reactive or neoplastic, the vast majority of these lesions arising in the genitourinary tract follow a benign course.[96,97,109-111] In the study by Harik and colleagues, follow-up information available in 28 patients with urinary bladder lesions revealed recurrences in only three patients, and none developed metastatic disease.[103] Hirsch and colleagues found 3 of 17 patients to develop non-destructive recurrences 3 months to 108 months following initial excision.[100] Montgomery et al. found a higher rate of local recurrence, as 10 of 32 patients with clinical follow-up developed local recurrence at a mean of 3 months following initial excision.[104] These authors found no association between the risk of local recurrence and histologic features or the presence or absence of ALK abnormalities. However, one of the cases in this study, a tumor involving the prostatic urethra and urinary bladder, showed features consistent with a "malignant inflammatory myofibroblastic tumor." This patient had a rapid recurrence of his tumor, and the patient died with intra-abdominal metastatic disease at 9 months, despite being treated aggressively with chemotherapy.

ISCHEMIC FASCIITIS (ATYPICAL DECUBITAL FIBROPLASIA)

Ischemic fasciitis and *atypical decubital fibroplasia* are synonyms for a pseudosarcomatous fibroblastic/myofibroblastic proliferation that predominantly involves soft tissues overlying bony prominences and occurs primarily in elderly and physically debilitated or immobilized patients.[112-116] Most of the patients are elderly, with a peak incidence during the eighth and ninth decades of life, although this lesion has rarely been described in adolescents (Table 8–6).[117] Females are affected slightly more commonly than males. Most patients present with a painless mass of short duration, usually less than 6 months; many but not all patients are debilitated or immobilized, bedridden, or wheelchair-bound. The soft tissues in the region of the shoulder are most commonly affected, followed by the soft tissues of the chest wall overlying the ribs, those overlying the sacrococcygeal region, or the greater trochanter.

Pathologic findings

Grossly, the lesion is poorly circumscribed and vaguely multinodular, often with a myxoid quality; it ranges from 1.0 to 8.5 cm in greatest diameter. It typically involves the subcutaneous tissue but may extend into the overlying dermis, with infrequent epidermal ulceration. In addition, the proliferation can involve the underlying skeletal muscles or adjacent periosteum.

TABLE 8–6	AGE DISTRIBUTION OF 34 PATIENTS WITH ISCHEMIC FASCIITIS REPORTED IN THE LITERATURE	
Age range (years)		**No. of patients**
0–10		0
11–20		1
21–30		2
31–40		1
41–50		0
51–60		1
61–70		3
71–80		13
81–90		11
91–100		2
Total		34

Microscopically, ischemic fasciitis has a zonal pattern, often with a central zone of liquefactive or focally coagulative necrosis surrounded by a fringe of proliferating vessels and fibroblasts (Figs 8–32, 8–33). The peripheral vessels are usually small, thin-walled, and ectatic; they are lined by prominent, occasionally atypical, endothelial cells (Fig. 8–34). In addition, a proliferation of plump fibroblasts form perivascular clusters or merge imperceptibly with the peripheral vessels. The fibroblasts may be cytologically atypical, with large, eccentric, often smudgy hyperchromatic nuclei, prominent nucleoli, and abundant basophilic cytoplasm. Some cells resemble the ganglion-like cells seen in proliferative fasciitis or myositis. The proliferation is usually paucicellular; although mitotic figures may be numerous, they are not atypical.

The peripheral vessels may contain fibrin thrombi and secondary acute inflammation with perivascular hyalinization. Multivacuolated muciphages can be seen in the myxoid zones and may mimic the lipoblasts of myxoid liposarcoma.

Immunohistochemically, the atypical fibroblast-like cells stain strongly and diffusely for vimentin but may also stain focally for both actin and CD68 (KP1),[116] suggesting focal myofibroblastic differentiation, a feature that has also been noted ultrastructurally.[118]

Differential diagnosis

In more than one-third of reported cases of ischemic fasciitis, a malignant diagnosis is seriously considered.[119,120]

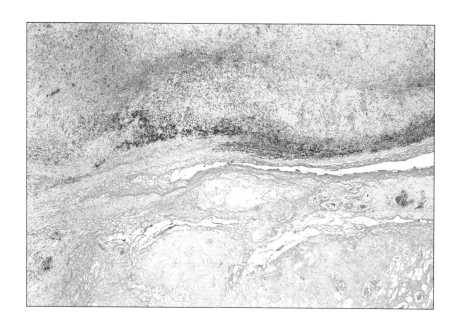

FIGURE 8–32 Low-power view of ischemic fasciitis showing a central zone of liquefactive necrosis with a proliferating fringe of fibroblasts and vessels. (Case courtesy of Dr. Elizabeth Montgomery, Johns Hopkins Hospital, Baltimore, Maryland.)

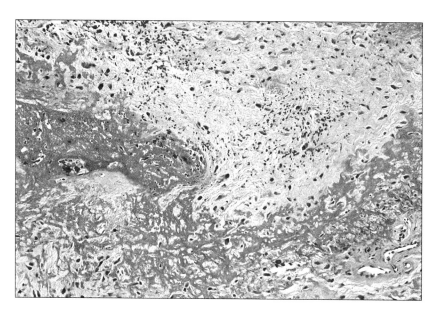

FIGURE 8–33 Interface between a liquefactive zone with fibrinous material and a reactive zone with atypical-appearing fibroblasts. (Case courtesy of Dr. Elizabeth Montgomery, Johns Hopkins Hospital, Baltimore, Maryland.)

Although the multinodular appearance with central necrosis is reminiscent of *epithelioid sarcoma*, the latter typically occurs on the distal extremity of young patients and is composed of cells with prominent cytoplasmic eosinophilia and cytokeratin immunoreactivity. *Myxoid liposarcoma* is also a consideration, but ischemic fasciitis lacks the organized plexiform vasculature typical of myxoid liposarcoma. Furthermore, although multivacuolated muciphages may be seen, true lipoblasts are not identified. *Myxofibrosarcoma* (*myxoid malignant fibrous histiocytoma*) lacks the zonation of ischemic fasciitis and the degenerative and reactive features, such as cells with smudgy chromatin, fat necrosis, hemosiderin deposition, and fibrin thrombi.

Discussion

Ischemic fasciitis is probably related to intermittent soft tissue ischemia with subsequent tissue breakdown and regenerative changes. Most lesions develop in areas where the subcutaneous tissue lies in close apposition to bone, often in patients with a clinical history of prolonged immobilization or trauma at that site. Histologically, the zonal quality is similar to that seen in other reactive fibroblastic and myofibroblastic proliferations. As suggested by Perosio and Weiss, the pathogenesis is probably similar to that of a decubitus ulcer, except that the ischemia may be less severe or of an intermittent nature, and it does not lead to breakdown of the overlying skin.[114]

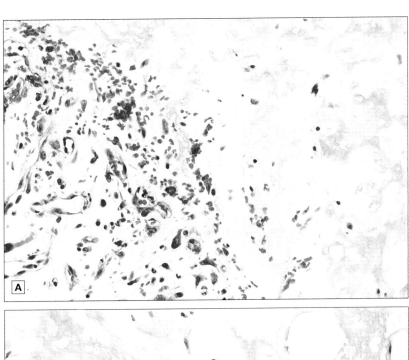

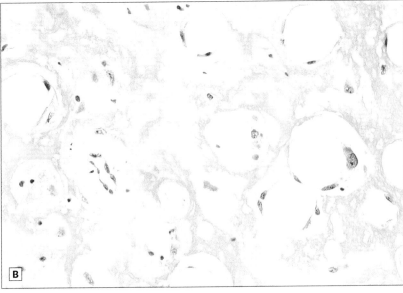

FIGURE 8–34 Ischemic fasciitis. **(A)** Interface between a zone of liquefactive necrosis and reactive fibroblastic and vascular proliferation. **(B)** High-power view of residual "ghosted" fat cells in a zone of coagulative necrosis.

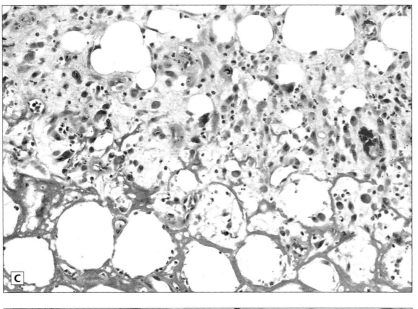

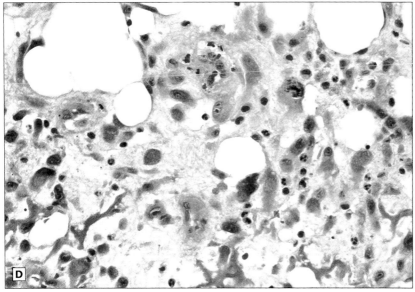

FIGURE 8–34 Continued. **(C)** Fibrinous material with an adjacent reactive fibroblastic zone. Some of the fibroblasts are round and similar to those seen in proliferative fasciitis. **(D)** High-power view of atypical fibroblasts in a reactive zone of ischemic fasciitis.

Although local recurrences have been described (presumably related to incomplete excision and regrowth due to the underlying ischemic process), most patients are cured by conservative excision, supporting its benign nature.[116] Awareness of this entity should allow the pathologist to avert a misdiagnosis of sarcoma and guide the clinical measures necessary to prevent subsequent recurrence or progression.

FIBROMA OF THE TENDON SHEATH

Fibroma of the tendon sheath is a slowly growing, dense, fibrous nodule that is firmly attached to the tendon sheath and is found most frequently in the hands and feet. Most cases evolve by way of a fasciitis-like proliferation which eventually hyalinizes, giving rise to a hypocellular nodule that characterizes the typical case. Its lobular configuration resembles that of a giant cell tumor of the tendon sheath, but it is much less cellular and lacks the polymorphic features of the latter lesion.

Fibroma of the tendon sheath is usually small (less than 2 cm) and typically has been present for some time and has increased slowly in size, often over many years. It is found most commonly in adults 20–50 years of age and is more than twice as common in men as in women.[121,122] Almost all of these tumors arise in the extremities; the upper extremity is more commonly affected than the lower extremity (Table 8–7). The most common sites of involvement in the upper extremity are the fingers (especially the thumb, index, and middle fingers), hand, and wrist, with only rare involvement of the forearm, elbow, or upper arm. Sites of involvement in the lower extremity are the knee, foot, ankle, and rarely the toe or leg.[123,124] As many as one-third of patients have slight tenderness, pain, or limited range of motion of the affected digit. A history of antecedent trauma has been reported in approximately 9% of cases.[122,125]

Pathologic findings

Most lesions are well circumscribed and have a lobular configuration, similar to that found with giant cell tumor of the tendon sheath. Attachment to a tendon or tendon sheath is visible in most but not all cases. On cut section, the lesions are usually uniform in appearance, with a gray or pearly white color. Occasionally, grossly myxoid and cystic areas are seen.

Microscopically, the lesion appears well circumscribed and lobulated or multilobulated and is composed of spindle-shaped cells resembling fibroblasts with elongated nuclei, fine chromatin, and small basophilic nucleoli. Most lesions lack cytologic atypia, although striking nuclear pleomorphism has been described (so-called pleomorphic fibroma of the tendon sheath).[126] In these unusual cases, the mitotic index is not commensurate with the degree of nuclear pleomorphism, suggesting a degenerative phenomenon. Stellate-shaped cells may also be present, particularly in myxoid zones. Most lesions are hypocellular, with widely spaced cytologically bland cells deposited in a densely eosinophilic hyalinized collagenous stroma. However, some have zones of increased cellularity in which the cells are arranged in either a storiform or fascicular growth pattern resembling nodular fasciitis (Figs 8–35, 8–36). These cellular areas always blend with less cellular collagenous areas. Not uncommonly, small myxoid zones are interspersed between the densely collagenized zones. A characteristic feature is the presence of elongated cleft-like spaces lined by flattened cells, particularly at the periphery of the lobules. These cells have been reported to stain for von Willebrand factor, suggesting that the spaces are truly vascular.[127] Some lesions contain multinucleated giant cells, but xanthoma cells and hemosiderin deposits are not present.

TABLE 8–7	ANATOMIC DISTRIBUTION OF 165 CASES OF FIBROMA OF THE TENDON SHEATH		
Site		**No.**	**%**
Upper extremities		145	88
Fingers		79	
Hands		41	
Wrist		17	
Forearm		4	
Elbow		3	
Upper arm		1	
Lower extremities		18	11
Knee		7	
Foot		5	
Ankle		3	
Toes		2	
Leg		1	
Trunk		2	1
Chest		1	
Back		1	

Data are from Chung and Enzinger[72] and Pulitzer et al.[125]

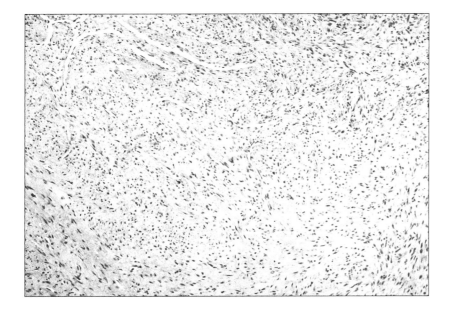

FIGURE 8–35 Cellular zone of a fibroma of the tendon sheath, including cleft-like spaces.

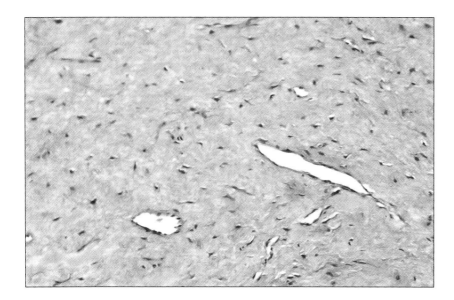

FIGURE 8–36 Fibroma of the tendon sheath composed of scattered spindle to stellate-shaped fibroblasts in a sparsely cellular and richly collagenous stroma.

Immunohistochemical and electron microscopic findings

The lesional cells co-express vimentin and muscle markers, including muscle-specific and smooth muscle actin, without staining for desmin.[128] In addition, stains for markers (albeit relatively non-specific) of monocytic-histiocytic differentiation, including CD68 (KP1) and HAM 56, may also be positive in some cases. Given the overlapping immunophenotype with giant cell tumor of the tendon sheath, some authors have proposed that fibroma and giant cell tumor of the tendon sheath represent histogenetically related lesions that are at the extremes in a spectrum of histiocytic-fibroblastic-myofibroblastic differentiation,[128,129] but this is doubtful given the fact that these tumors rarely contain areas resembling giant cell tumor.

Ultrastructurally, fibroma of the tendon sheath is composed of fibroblasts and myofibroblasts.[8,130] Cells with fibroblastic features (including abundant rough endoplasmic reticulum with dilated cisternae) predominate in the less cellular collagenized zones, whereas cells with myofibroblastic features (including actin-type intermediate filaments and dense bodies) predominate in the more cellular and myxoid zones.[131]

Differential diagnosis

The typical fibroma of the tendon sheath, composed of a hypocellular proliferation of bland spindle cells deposited in a densely collagenized stroma, is characteristic and unlikely to be confused with other entities; lesions that show more cellular zones may be confused with *fibrous histiocytoma* or *nodular fasciitis*. Pulitzer et al. reported that up to one-fourth of their cases had areas that were indistinguishable from nodular fasciitis,[125] and this has been

our experience as well. There are, however, minor differences in location and manner of presentation of the two lesions.

Although fibroma of the tendon sheath and *giant cell tumor of the tendon sheath* arise in similar locations and are grossly similar, giant cell tumor of the tendon sheath is composed of a proliferation of round cells (in contrast to spindle-shaped cells) and usually contains more multinucleated giant cells as well as xanthoma cells and hemosiderin deposits. Interestingly, translocations involving the long arm of chromosome 2 have been described in fibroma of tendon sheath [t(2;11)(q31-32;q12)][132] as well as giant cell tumor of tendon sheath,[133] but the breakpoints were found to be different (2q31-32 and 2q35-36, respectively). Sciot and co-workers also reported a case of fibroma of the tendon sheath with an 11q12 alteration.[134]

Rare fibromas of the tendon sheath show striking nuclear pleomorphism and may be confused with a pleomorphic sarcoma. However, the latter is characterized by greater cellularity and more mitotic activity, including atypical mitoses, as well as a more pronounced storiform growth pattern. Finally, simply based upon location, one could consider an *inflammatory myxohyaline tumor*, but this entity is characterized by an intimate admixture of inflammatory, myxoid, and hyalinized zones as well as bizarre cells resembling Reed-Sternberg cells or cytomegalovirus (CMV)-infected cells.

Discussion

Fibroma of the tendon sheath is a benign process that can recur but does not metastasize. In the series by Chung and Enzinger, 13 of 54 patients (24%) with follow-up information developed local recurrences, including three patients with two recurrences.[122] The lesions usually recurred 1–4 months after the initial surgery. Local excision and re-excision of recurrences is the treatment of choice.

The initial, transient cellular phase resembling nodular fasciitis strongly suggests that fibromas are reactive lesions. Friction inherent in the location of the lesion or vascular impairment may incite ongoing sclerosis. The possibility that a minority of fibromas arise secondary to hyalinization of benign mesenchymal tumors cannot be totally discounted and might account for the rare reports of clonality.

PLEOMORPHIC FIBROMA OF THE SKIN

Pleomorphic fibroma involving the skin is a relatively rare entity that shares histologic features with pleomorphic fibroma of the tendon sheath, particularly the presence of large pleomorphic, hyperchromatic cells deposited in a collagenized stroma. Clinically, most patients present with a slowly growing, asymptomatic, solitary lesion that appears as a flesh-colored, nonulcerated, dome-shaped papule. These lesions most commonly involve the papillary and reticular dermis of the extremities, followed by the trunk and the head and neck.[135,136] Some arise in a subungual location.[137,138] The tumor usually arises in adults, with a peak incidence during the fifth decade of life; women are affected slightly more commonly than men. The lesion is almost always 0.5–2.0 cm and clinically is often mistaken for a nevus, neurofibroma, or hemangioma.

Grossly, the mass is well circumscribed and involves the papillary and reticular dermis, resulting in a dome-shaped or polypoid lesion covered by a thin, nonulcerated epidermis, often associated with an epidermal collarette. Histologically, it is sparsely cellular and composed predominantly of thick, haphazardly arranged collagen. The characteristic feature is the presence of scattered spindle-shaped or stellate cells, including multinucleated giant cells with large pleomorphic, hyperchromatic nuclei and small nucleoli (Fig. 8–37). Mitotic figures are rare, but occasionally an atypical mitotic figure is seen.[135] The stroma may show focal or (rarely) diffuse myxoid change.[137,139] Adnexal structures are generally not found, and there may be a sparse intralesional lymphoplasmacytic infiltrate.

Immunohistochemically, the cells stain diffusely for vimentin, and variable numbers of cells also stain for muscle-specific actin, suggesting myofibroblastic differentiation.[136] The cells have also been reported to stain for CD34 and CD99.[140,141] Immunostains for S-100 protein, desmin, and cytokeratin are negative. Ultrastructurally, the fibroblast-like cells have complex nuclear contours and abundant rough endoplasmic reticulum.[142]

The differential diagnosis includes other cutaneous neoplasms characterized by the presence of pleomorphic cells. *Atypical fibroxanthoma* most commonly occurs as a rapidly growing lesion on sun-damaged skin of the face of elderly patients. It is characterized by much higher cellularity, cells with foamy cytoplasm, and a large number of typical and atypical mitotic figures. *Dermatofibroma with atypical cells*, also referred to as *dermatofibroma with monster cells*, *atypical cutaneous fibrous histiocytoma*, *pseudosarcomatous dermatofibroma*, and *atypical (pseudosarcomatous) cutaneous histiocytoma*, is a more densely cellular proliferation of pleomorphic cells, including cells with hemosiderin and foamy cytoplasm. In addition, most lesions have foci of typical fibrous histiocytoma. *Giant cell fibroblastoma* most commonly occurs as an infiltrative lesion on the trunk or extremities of patients less

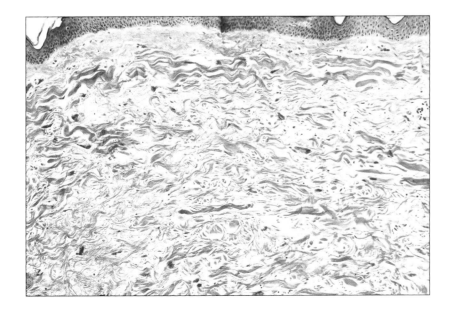

FIGURE 8–37 Pleomorphic fibroma of skin with scattered floret-like giant cells deposited in a densely collagenized dermis.

than 10 years of age. It is characterized by pseudovascular or angiectoid spaces lined by atypical spindle cells and floret-like giant cells. The absence of S-100 protein in pleomorphic fibroma of skin helps distinguish it from benign peripheral nerve sheath tumors with atypia (*ancient schwannoma* and *neurofibroma with atypia*).

Simple excision of this lesion is generally curative, as local recurrences are quite rare.

NUCHAL-TYPE FIBROMA AND GARDNER-ASSOCIATED FIBROMA

Nuchal fibroma is an uncommon fibrocollagenous proliferation that typically arises in the cervicodorsal region in adults. However, it is increasingly clear that this lesion is not restricted to a nuchal location, since it has been documented in a variety of other anatomic sites and as such is preferably referred to as nuchal-type fibroma.[143,144]

Patients typically present with a solitary unencapsulated subcutaneous mass in the cervicodorsal region. Extra-nuchal sites of involvement include the extremities,[144] buttock,[145] and lumbosacral area.[146,147] Regardless of anatomic site, nuchal-type fibroma is significantly more common in men, with a peak incidence during the third through fifth decades of life.[144] This process is strongly associated with diabetes mellitus, as up to 44% of patients with this lesion have diabetes.[144,148]

More recent reports clearly show a link to Gardner's syndrome, and such lesions have been referred to as Gardner-associated fibromas.[149–151a] This syndrome, caused by mutations in the adenomatous polyposis coli (*APC*) gene, is characterized by innumerable colonic polyps, osteomas and various soft tissue tumors. In 2001, Wehrli and colleagues reported 11 patients with solitary or multiple superficial and deep soft tissue fibromas histologically resembling nuchal fibromas.[152] Virtually all of these lesions arose in an extra-nuchal location, and in some cases represented the sentinel event leading to the detection of Gardner's syndrome. This lesion arises predominantly in infants, children, and adolescents, with no gender predilection. They may arise in the head and neck, extremities, chest wall, flank, back, and paraspinal region. A histologically similar lesion has been described in the mesentery as a possible "desmoid precursor lesion" in patients with familial adenomatous polyposis (FAP).[153] In fact, desmoid-type fibromatosis has been reported to arise in the sites of Gardner-associated fibromas following excision of the lesion.[154] Overall, about 45% of patients with this lesion subsequently develop a desmoid-type fibromatosis at some site.

Grossly, the lesions are unencapsulated and arise in the subcutaneous tissue, with minimal extension into the deep dermis, and occasionally the superficial skeletal muscle.[144] Most are 2.5–8.0 cm in greatest dimension at the time of excision, and the mass is usually present for several years prior to therapy. Lipoma is the most common preoperative diagnosis.

Microscopically, nuchal-type fibroma is quite bland; it is a hypocellular or almost completely acellular densely collagenized mass with scattered mature fibroblasts and islands of mature adipose tissue of varying size (Figs 8–38, 8–39). The mass is ill-defined, with some radiation of collagenous septa into the subcutaneous fat and deep dermis. Small nerves are frequently entrapped by this fibrous proliferation. Occasionally, altered elastic fibers similar to those seen in elastofibromas are identified. The spindle cells are positive for vimentin and CD34 and negative for smooth muscle actin and desmin. Some also stain for CD99. In the study by Coffin et al., 64% showed nuclear reactivity for β-catenin.[151a]

This lesion most commonly is mistaken for a *fibrolipoma*. Unlike nuchal-type fibroma, fibrolipoma is well circumscribed and encapsulated, has a greater proportion of the lesion composed of mature adipose tissue, and lacks entrapped nerves. The subcutaneous location and paucity of cells permit exclusion of *extra-abdominal fibromatosis*. The *nuchal fibrocartilaginous pseudotumor* arises in the posterior aspect of the base of the neck at the junction of the nuchal ligament and the deep cervical fascia and probably develops as a reaction to soft tissue injury.[155,156] Unlike the former lesion, nuchal-type fibroma lacks an association with ligaments, occurs superficial to the fascia, and lacks cartilaginous metaplasia. *Elastofibroma* typically occurs in the deep soft tissue in the vicinity of the inferomedial portion of the scapula. Given the observation of altered elastic fibers in nuchal-type fibroma, it is possible that these two lesions are closely related entities. Nuchal-type fibroma is benign but may recur if incompletely excised.[144]

ELASTOFIBROMA

Elastofibroma, an unusual fibroelastic pseudotumor, is most commonly encountered in elderly persons; it arises chiefly from the connective tissue between the inferomedial portion of the scapula and the chest wall. Originally described by Järvi and Saxén in 1961 as elastofibroma dorsi,[157] it has become increasingly apparent that identical lesions may be found in extra-scapular locations; thus the term elastofibroma is preferred.

Clinical findings

Most patients are elderly, with a peak incidence during the sixth and seventh decades of life;[158] only rare lesions have been described in children.[159] Women are affected more commonly than men. Most but not all patients have a history of intensive, often repetitive manual labor. Although thought to be rare, several autopsy studies have shown elastofibroma and pre-elastofibroma-like changes

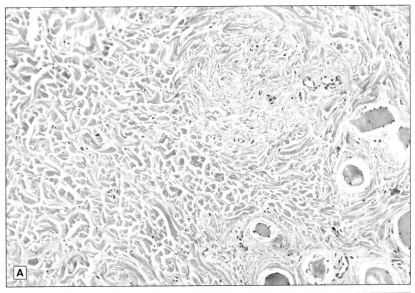

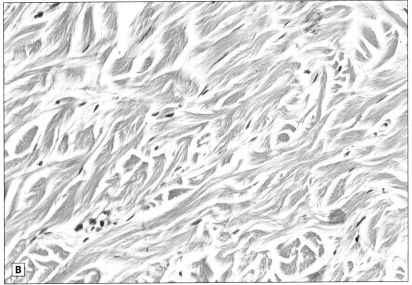

FIGURE 8–38 Nuchal fibroma. **(A)** Low-power view of nuchal fibroma, characterized by a hypocellular, densely collagenized mass with scattered fibroblasts among skeletal muscle fibers. **(B)** Scattered fibroblasts deposited in densely collagenized stroma.

in 13–17% of elderly individuals.[160,161] The most common presentation is that of a slowly growing, deep-seated mass that only rarely causes pain, tenderness, limitation of motion or scapular snapping.[162,163] Most arise from the connective tissue between the lower portion of the scapula and the chest wall, deep to the rhomboid major and latissimus dorsi muscles, with attachment to the periosteum and ligaments in the region of the sixth, seventh, and eighth ribs. Although usually unilateral, up to 10% of patients have bilateral lesions.[164,165] For example, Naylor et al. described the radiologic findings in 12 patients with elastofibroma; all patients in whom both sides of the chest wall were imaged had bilateral elastofibromas, suggesting subclinical bilateral involvement in many cases.[166] This lesion has been increasingly recognized by radio-logists on computed tomography (CT) and magnetic resonance imaging (MRI) as a poorly circumscribed, heterogeneous soft tissue mass with attenuation of signal intensity similar to that of skeletal muscle; it is interlaced with fat, allowing a presumptive diagnosis.[167,168] Numerous extra-scapular sites have been reported, including the oral cavity,[169] colon (resulting in a colonic polyp),[170] greater omentum,[171] deltoid region,[172] cornea,[173] stomach (in the region of a peptic ulcer),[174] and rectal submucosa.[175]

Pathologic findings

The mass is usually ill-defined, oblong or spherical, firm, and ranges 5–10 cm. The cut surface has a variegated

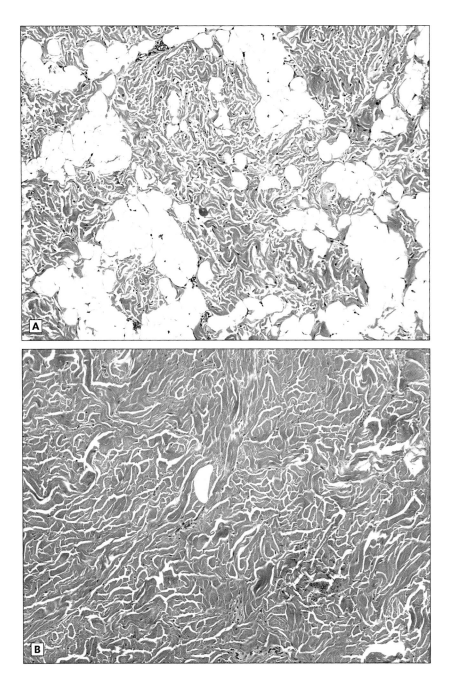

FIGURE 8-39 (A) Low-magnification view of a Gardner-associated fibroma showing interdigitation of mature fat and dense collagen. **(B)** Densely collagenous area of Gardner-associated fibroma.

appearance with small areas of adipose tissue interposed between gray-white fibrous areas, occasionally with cystic change (Fig. 8-40). Not infrequently, the surgeon is concerned about the possibility of a sarcoma, given the irregular margins and infiltration of skeletal muscle or periosteum.

On microscopic examination, the tumor-like mass consists of a mixture of intertwining swollen, eosinophilic collagen and elastic fibers in about equal proportions associated with occasional fibroblasts, small amounts of interstitial mucoid material, and variably

sized aggregates of mature fat cells. Typically, the elastic fibers have a degenerated, beaded appearance or are fragmented into small flower-like, serrated disks or globules (chenille bodies) with a distinct linear arrangement (Fig. 8-41).

Elastic stains (Verhoeff, Weigert, Gomori) reveal deeply staining, branched and unbranched fibers that have a central dense core and an irregular moth-eaten or serrated margin (Figs 8-42 to 8-44). The elastin-like material is removed by prior treatment of the sections with pancreatic or bacterial elastase and pepsin; collagenase or trypsin

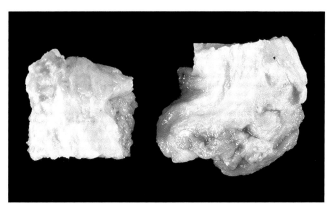

FIGURE 8–40 Elastofibroma. There is an intimate admixture of firm collagenous tissue with fat.

has no effect.[176,177] These altered elastic fibers can be recognized by specific antibodies to elastin,[178] and they exhibit a green fluorescence under ultraviolet light. The few spindle cells that are present express vimentin but are negative for smooth muscle actin, desmin, and S-100 protein.[56]

Ultrastructurally, the interspersed spindle cells have features of fibroblasts and myofibroblasts; some cells contain abundant dilated cisternae of rough endoplasmic reticulum, and others have cytoplasmic microfilaments and pinocytotic vesicles.[179] Non-membrane-bound dense granular bodies with an intensity similar to that of extracellular elastin and measuring 200–350 nm are present in the cytoplasm of fibroblasts, suggesting that these cells produce the abnormal extracellular elastic tissue.[180]

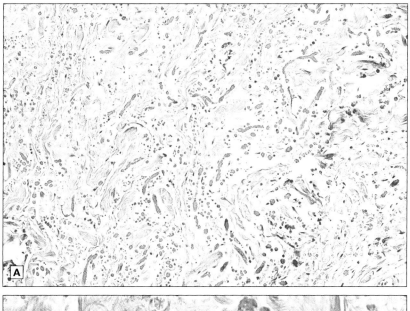

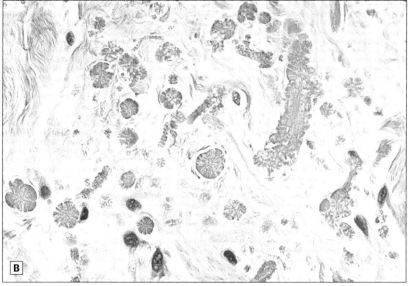

FIGURE 8–41 Elastofibroma. **(A)** Altered elastic fibers in a collagenous matrix. **(B)** Elastic fibers in cross-section showing a characteristic serrated edge (petaloid globules).

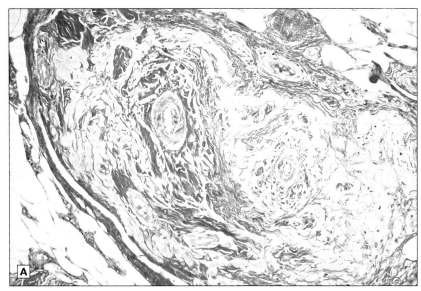

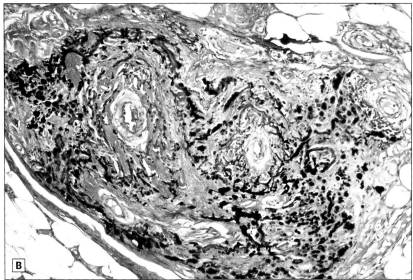

FIGURE 8–42 Elastofibroma. **(A)** Masson trichrome stain of elastofibroma outlining the collagen surrounding the abnormal elastic fibers. **(B)** Verhoeff elastin stain shows the mirror image, accentuating the abnormal elastic fibers.

Numerous electron-dense elongated and globular masses corresponding to the elastinophilic material seen on light microscopy are present in the collagenous stroma. A central core of more electron-lucent material resembling mature elastic tissue is surrounded by granular or fibrillary aggregations of electron-dense material resembling immature elastin or pre-elastin. The proximity of these aggregates to fibroblasts further supports a process of abnormal elastogenesis by these cells.[181] At high magnification, the outer zones are seen to consist of compactly and randomly arranged elastic microfibrils measuring approximately 12 nm in diameter.[182]

Differential diagnosis

The clinical and histologic features of elastofibroma are characteristic and are unlikely to be confused with those of other fibroblastic proliferations. De Nictolis et al.

described a case of an *elastofibrolipoma* arising in the mediastinum.[183] Unlike elastofibroma, the elastofibrolipoma is well circumscribed, is surrounded by a fibrous capsule, and has a more conspicuous adipose component in both the central and peripheral portions of the tumor. In a report of elastofibromatous change of the rectal submucosa,[175] the lesion closely mimicked amyloidosis, although elastic and Congo red stains allowed this distinction.

Discussion

The etiology of the abnormal elastic fibers has been debated since its initial description by Järvi and Saxén.[157] Whereas some have suggested that these fibers are derived from the elastotic degeneration of collagen fibers,[184] others believe they are derived from degeneration of preexisting elastic fibers or from disturbed elastic fibrillogenesis.[185] The preponderance of evidence suggests that

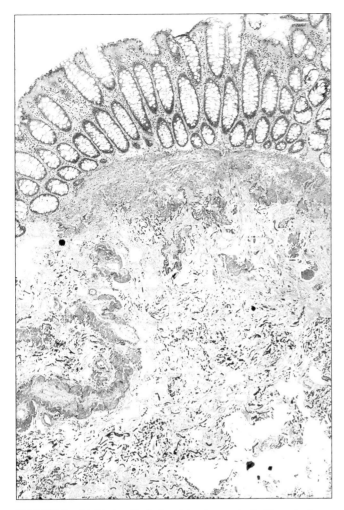

FIGURE 8–43 Verhoeff elastin stain shows elastic fibers in the submucosa of the rectum. This patient had a history of radiation therapy to this area.

elastofibroma is a degenerative pseudotumor that is the result of excessive formation of collagen and abnormal elastic fibers. Although friction between the inferior edge of the scapula and the underlying chest wall has been implicated as the cause of this abnormal elastogenesis, other factors such as radiation therapy may play a role,[175] particularly for lesions arising in extra-scapular sites. Interestingly, Nagamine et al. reported that about one-third of the patients with this lesion in Okinawa occurred in patients with a family history of elastofibroma, suggesting a genetic predisposition.[186] Others have found elastofibromas to arise in patients with other family members with this lesion.[187] Whether the central core of mature elastic tissue represents maturation of newly formed elastin fibers[188] or serves as a structural skeleton for newly formed elastin[179] is uncertain. Although most believe that fibroblasts and myofibroblasts serve as the source of the abnormal elastic fibers, some have proposed that elastofibromas arise from periosteum-derived

cells in response to repeated physical irritation in susceptible individuals.

Very few cases of elastofibroma have been evaluated cytogenetically, although alterations of the short arm of chromosome 1[189–191] and gains in the region of Xq[187] have been reported.

Elastofibroma is a benign lesion and best treated by conservative excision given that local recurrence is rare. This diagnosis can be made by fine needle aspiration cytology[192,193] or core biopsy[163] in the appropriate clinical and radiographic setting, thereby potentially avoiding additional unnecessary surgery. There are no reports of malignant transformation.

NASOPHARYNGEAL ANGIOFIBROMA

Nasopharyngeal angiofibroma is a relatively uncommon, histologically benign fibrovascular tumor which occurs virtually exclusively in the nasopharynx of adolescent boys. Although originally referred to as juvenile nasopharyngeal angiofibroma, some occur in adults, so this lesion is best referred to simply as nasopharyngeal angiofibroma.

Clinical findings

Most of these lesions occur in adolescent boys and young men 10–20 years of age, although it has also been reported in older patients.[194] Almost all of these tumors occur in males, with only a few having been reported in females.[195] As its name implies, virtually all of these cases arise in the nasopharynx, although tumors of identical morphology may arise at extra-nasopharyngeal sites, including the maxillary and ethmoid sinuses.[196] To this point, extra-nasopharyngeal angiofibromas have been restricted to the head and neck region and arise in patients who are slightly older and more likely to be female.[197]

Recently, a few patients with nasopharyngeal angiofibroma have also been found to have familial adenomatous polyposis (FAP).[198,199] Although mutations in the adenomatous polyposis coli (*APC*) gene on the long arm of chromosome 5 have not been detected in sporadic cases of nasopharyngeal angiofibroma,[200,201] most show evidence of a mutation in the β-catenin oncogene, resulting in strong and diffuse intranuclear accumulation of this protein.[202]

The common presenting symptoms are nasal obstruction, facial deformity, and repeated epistaxis. In some cases, excessive hemorrhage requires blood transfusions and hospitalization and on rare occasions is life-threatening. This tumor may even result in a consumptive coagulopathy, although this is an extremely rare complication.[203] Other symptoms include headache, sinusitis, otitis media, mastoiditis, and dacrocystitis.[204] Facial deformity of the orbital, temporal, and cheek region is not uncommon.[205]

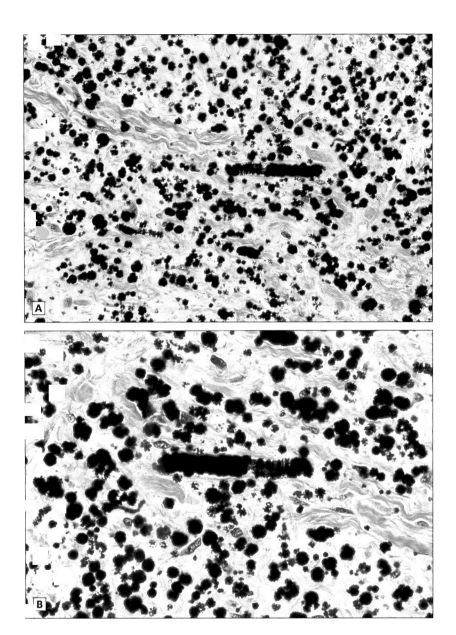

FIGURE 8–44 Elastofibroma. **(A)** Verhoeff elastin stain shows elongated and globoid elastic fibers. **(B)** High-power view of Verhoeff elastin stain showing elastic fibers with a dense core.

Physical examination typically reveals a variably sized, red or red-blue, lobulated or polypoid mass that can be easily seen through the nose or underneath the palate with a nasopharyngeal mirror. Most lesions originate from the superolateral nasopharyngeal area and, with growth, extend into the posterior aspect of the nasal cavity and superiorly into the sphenoid sinus. As the tumor enlarges, it extends through the pterygopalatine foramen and grows laterally into the pterygomaxillary and infratemporal fossae. It can extend into the soft tissues of the cheek and the orbit and often erodes bone with extension into the middle or anterior cranial fossae.

Radiologic techniques are useful for diagnostic and staging purposes. MRI and CT scans usually show a well-demarcated soft tissue mass in the nasopharynx with or without extension into the nasal cavity or paranasal sinuses, anterior bowing of the posterior wall of the maxillary sinus, and erosion of adjacent bony structures (Fig. 8–45). MRI appears to be superior to CT for demarcating the margin of the tumor from the surrounding soft tissue.[206] Angiography is useful for demonstrating the tumor's vascularity; transarterial embolization can be performed at the same time.[207] For cases in which the diagnosis remains in question following radiographic evaluation, a transnasal biopsy may be used to confirm the diagnosis. This procedure should be performed in an operating room, as significant hemorrhage requiring nasal packing or cautery may be encountered.[208]

Pathologic findings

The tumor is typically well circumscribed with a lobulated, smooth, glistening mucosal surface that may be focally ulcerated. The tissue is firm and rubbery; on cut section it has a spongy appearance owing to the presence of numerous vascular spaces characteristic of this lesion.

Nasopharyngeal angiofibroma has a very consistent histologic appearance, with little variation from case to case, with numerous vascular channels surrounded by dense paucicellular fibrous tissue (Fig. 8–46). The cells in the fibrous tissue are cytologically bland and may be spindle or stellate in shape with nuclei that lack hyperchromasia and have small nucleoli and little mitotic activity (Fig. 8–47). The dense fibrous stroma may show hyalinization or focal myxoid change, often with collagen fibers arranged in a parallel fashion. Mature fat entrapped within the lesion can occur, but is unusual.[209] The vascular channels are slit-like or dilated and vary in number, configuration, and thickness. Some vessels are surrounded by few if any smooth muscle cells, whereas others show focal pad-like thickenings.[210] Peripherally located vessels are often larger and of the arterial type with visible elastic laminae. However, the smaller vessels in the central portion of the tumor typically lack elastic laminae, which may explain the propensity for spontaneous or surgically induced hemorrhage.[210] The nature and organization of the vessels has suggested to some that this lesion could represent a vascular malformation as opposed to a neoplastic process.[204]

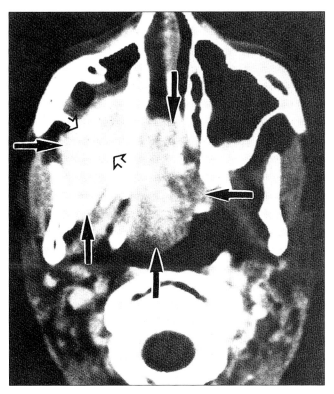

FIGURE 8–45 Nasopharyngeal angiofibroma involving the nasopharynx, nasal cavity, and right infratemporal fossa (arrows) and eroding through the posterior wall of the right maxillary antrum (small arrows). (From Chandler JR, Goulding R, Moskowitz L, et al. Nasopharyngeal angiofibromas: staging and management. Ann Otol Rhinol Laryngol 1984; 93:322.)

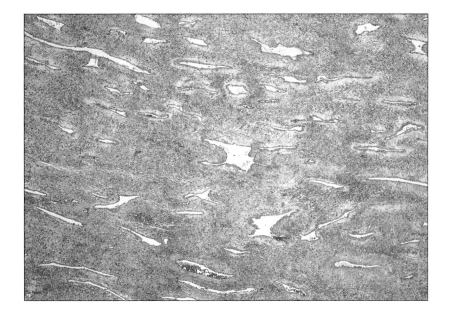

FIGURE 8–46 Nasopharyngeal angiofibroma consisting of dense fibrocollagenous tissue with interspersed vascular channels of varying caliber.

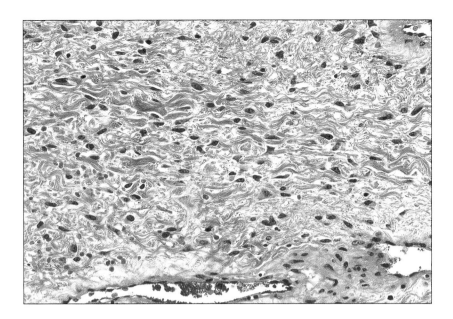

FIGURE 8–47 Nasopharyngeal angiofibroma composed of cytologically bland fibroblasts deposited in a dense collagenous stroma.

Immunohistochemical and electron microscopic findings

Immunohistochemically, the endothelial cells lining the slit-like or dilated vessels stain for endothelial markers, including von Willebrand factor, CD31, and CD34. The immediate perivascular cells show variable staining for smooth muscle actin, depending on the amount of perivascular smooth muscle.[210] The spindle and stellate-shaped cells deposited in the dense fibrous stroma stain for vimentin, although some also stain for smooth muscle actin. As one might expect in a tumor that occurs virtually exclusively in males, androgen receptors have been detected in the nuclei of endothelial and stromal cells using immunohistochemical techniques.[211,212] Strong and diffuse nuclear immunoreactivity for β-catenin is identified in the spindle cells in virtually all cases.[201,213] Zhang and colleagues have also found c-kit and nerve growth factor to be expressed in the majority of tumors.[213]

Ultrastructurally, the constituent cells reveal predominantly fibroblastic features.[214] Taxy suggested that at least some of these cells have myofibroblastic features, with bundles of intracellular filaments with focal densities, pinocytotic vesicles, and hemidesmosomes.[215] He also noted that many of these cells harbor electron-dense granular intranuclear inclusions, although the nature of these peculiar intranuclear granular inclusions remains unknown.

Discussion

Although nasopharyngeal angiofibroma is histologically benign, it may act in an aggressive fashion characterized by recurrences that can extend into and destroy adjacent bony structures. The likelihood of recurrence is most closely related to the adequacy of the initial surgical excision, which in turn depends on the tumor stage.[208] The type of surgical approach is dictated by the extent of the tumor, as determined by preoperative radiographic studies. For low-stage tumors, most propose a transnasal or intranasal endoscopic approach.[216–218] A transcranial approach may be more appropriate for tumors that have intracranial extension.[217,219] Preoperative transarterial embolization has been reported to result in decreased blood loss and a decreased rate of local recurrence.[220] Hormone therapy, including use of anti-androgenic agents, has generally been ineffective. Some authors advocate the use of radiation therapy, particularly for tumors with intracranial extension,[221,222] but radiation may cause osteonecrosis, and there have been reports of postradiation sarcomatous transformation into lesions that resemble fibrosarcoma[223] or malignant fibrous histiocytoma.[224]

GIANT CELL ANGIOFIBROMA

Giant cell angiofibroma is a distinctive tumor, originally described as arising in the orbit, but clearly having a much wider anatomic distribution than initially reported. This tumor shares morphologic features with solitary fibrous tumor and is currently considered "giant cell-rich variant of solitary fibrous tumor"[225] and is discussed in Chapter 36.

KELOID

Keloid is a benign dermal fibroproliferative process that occurs at sites of cutaneous injury and forms as a result of an abnormal wound healing process in genetically susceptible individuals.[226-228] It may be solitary or multiple and has a predilection for dark-skinned individuals.[229-231] Keloid (Greek: claw-like) was named for its multiple extensions, which bestow on the lesion an imaginary crab-like appearance. There are, in addition to its common cicatricial forms, "spontaneous" or "idiopathic" forms of the condition, but these too are likely the result of some minor infection or injury in areas with increased skin tension. *Hypertrophic scars*, lesions that remain confined to the original wound site, should be distinguished from keloids because of their substantially lower recurrence rate.

Clinical findings

Keloids usually manifest as well-circumscribed round, oval, or linear elevations of the skin and often extend with multiple processes into the surrounding areas. They may be asymptomatic but more often are described by the patient as being itchy, tender, or painful, possibly related to a small nerve fiber neuropathy secondary to the dense collagen.[232] In their earlier phase, keloids tend to be soft and erythematous; later they become increasingly indurated and turn white. They are found more commonly above than below the waist and have a predilection for the face, shoulders, forearms, and hands. About half of "spontaneous" keloids occur as a transverse band in the presternal region, probably the result of minor infection and increased skin tension in this region. In some patients keloids are limited to one portion of the body; thus they may develop after piercing the earlobes for earrings but are absent in an appendectomy scar (Figs 8–48, 8–49). Patients who develop keloids at multiple sites are generally younger and more likely to have a positive family history than those with solitary keloids.[229] In addition, women seem to be more likely than men to develop multiple keloids.

Keloids are induced by minor infections (especially acne and furuncles), smallpox and other vaccinations, tattooing and cautery, and laparotomies and various other surgical procedures.[233] Sometimes even minor injuries, such as needle marks or mosquito bites, produce small keloids of pinhead size. In some African countries, keloidal scarification is produced deliberately in a special design and is considered an adornment and mark of beauty. The condition occurs mainly during the late teens and early adult life. It is found rarely in infants, small children, or the aged. Although originally reported to be more common in women than men, more recent studies have found no significant difference in incidence between the genders.[234]

Keloids are more commonly encountered in dark-skinned persons, particularly those of African descent.[235] Of the various risk factors, a familial predisposition is clearly of paramount importance since up to 50% of affected individuals report another family member with a keloid.[229,231] Although an autosomal recessive pattern of inheritance was initially suggested, it is unclear whether the development of keloids is a complex oligogenic condition or inherited as a simple monogenic mendelian disorder.[226,236] Keloid formation has been reported in association with numerous dermatologic disorders, particularly acne vulgaris,[237] and some connective tissue diseases, including Ehlers-Danlos syndrome,[238] scleroderma,[239] and Rubinstein-Taybi syndrome.[240] An association of keloids with palmar, plantar, and penile fibromatosis has also been observed.[241]

Pathologic findings

Keloids are characterized by a fibrocollagenous proliferation of the dermis, with haphazardly arranged, thick, glassy, deeply acidophilic collagen fibers (Fig. 8–50). During the early phase, the lesions tend to be vascular, particularly at their periphery, accounting for the clinical

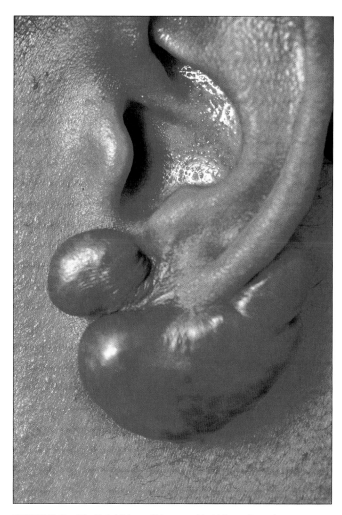

FIGURE 8–48 Keloid in a 25-year-old African-American woman. It appeared after the earlobes were pierced for earrings.

distributed than normal skin or even in hypertrophic scars.[244]

Differential diagnosis

Hypertrophic scars share the macroscopic features of keloids during the early phase of the lesion, but at later stages they flatten and have less mucoid matrix and few or no glassy collagen fibers. Unlike keloids, hypertrophic scars stay within the confines of the initial wound and increase in size by pushing out the margins of the scar, as opposed to invading the surrounding normal tissues.[226] The initial cellular phase is also marked by a larger proportion of myofibroblasts, which may play a role in the contraction and elevation of the lesion.[245] Features that are more commonly seen in keloids when compared to hypertrophic scars include a lack of flattening, minimal scarring of the papillary dermis, the absence of prominent vertically oriented blood vessels and the presence of a tongue-like advancing edge beneath a normal-appearing epidermis and papillary dermis.[246]

Collagenoma, a "connective tissue nevus," is an intradermal fibrocollagenous nodule that microscopically resembles a hypertrophic scar or keloid but there is no history of acne or dermal injury. The condition presents clinically as multiple discrete, asymptomatic, skin-colored, small nodules that affect mainly the regions of the trunk and the proximal portion of the upper extremities.[247] In general, they make their first appearance during the postpubertal period and are frequently found in two or more members of the same family. Their number is significantly increased during pregnancy.[248]

Circumscribed storiform collagenoma (*sclerotic fibroma*) and *fibrous papules of the face* are two other morphologically related lesions. The former presents as a solitary dermal nodule composed of glassy, thickened collagen fibers arranged in a storiform pattern, occasionally with bizarre multinucleated giant cells.[249] It is identical to the fibrous nodules that occur in the multiple hamartoma syndrome or Cowden's disease.[250] The term *fibrous papules of the face* has been applied to a small dome-shaped fibrous nodule of the nose and face with an "onionskin" periadnexal or perivascular collagen pattern. This lesion has also been described as perifollicular fibroma and melanocytic angiofibroma.[251]

Scleroderma (*morphea*) is characterized by thickening and altered staining characteristics of existing collagen fibers. There is no new fiber formation and consequently no elevation of the skin.

Keloidal dermatofibroma is a recently described variant of dermatofibroma that may also histologically resemble a keloid.[252] Clinically, these lesions appear similar to ordinary dermatofibromas but are characterized by the presence of keloid-like collagen admixed with elements typically present in the usual dermatofibroma, as well as strong factor XIIIa staining in the non-keloidal areas.

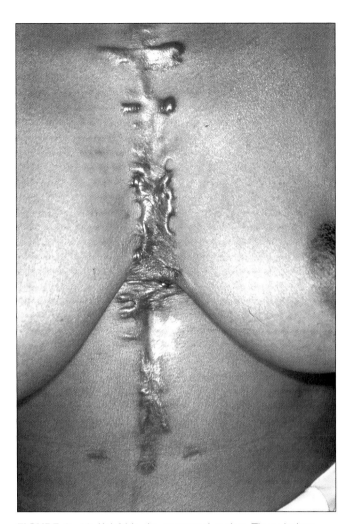

FIGURE 8–49 Keloid in the presternal region. These lesions may develop as the result of minor infection in an area of increased skin tension.

appearance of an erythematous lesion. Later lesions show decreased vascularity and more prominent hyalinization, which may undergo focal calcification or osseous metaplasia. Bland spindle-shaped cells are scattered throughout this hypocellular lesion. As the lesion grows, there is progressive displacement of the normal skin appendages, often with flattening or even atrophy of the overlying epidermis. Immunohistochemically, the spindle cells stain for vimentin. Although smooth muscle actin decorates the spindle cells of hypertrophic scars, the cells of keloids show minimal or no staining for this antigen.[242] Ultrastructurally, the constituent cells have the features of active fibroblasts, with abundant rough endoplasmic reticulum and prominent Golgi apparatus, although some cells are described as having myofibroblastic features.[243] Ultrastructural analysis also reveals collagen fibrils which are much larger and more irregularly

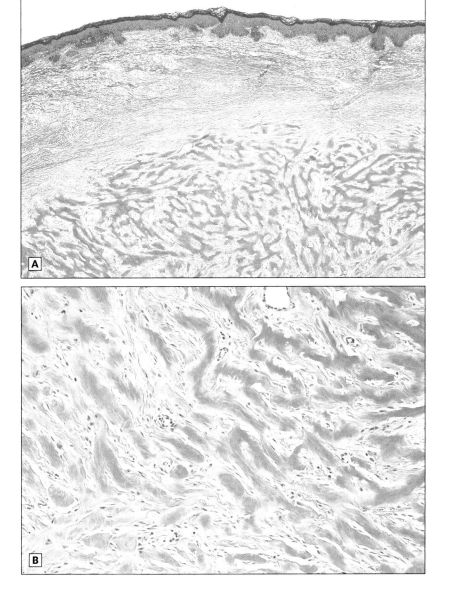

FIGURE 8–50 Keloid. **(A)** Low-power view. **(B)** Keloid displaying thick, glassy eosinophilic fibers in fibroblastic tissue.

Discussion

Numerous treatment modalities have been attempted to minimize local recurrence of keloids. The rate of local recurrence for surgical excision alone is high: 45–100%.[253,254] Surgery combined with topical injection of corticosteroids reduces the local recurrence rate to less than 50%.[246,255] Postoperative radiation therapy and high-dose-rate brachytherapy[256] have also been reported to have good results, with local recurrence rates of less than 10%. Numerous other therapeutic modalities, including laser therapy,[257] cryosurgery,[258] 5-fluorouracil,[259] and silicone gel or occlusive sheeting,[260,261] may also be effective. Patients who have a history of keloid formation should also avoid elective cosmetic procedures.

Unlike hypertrophic scars, keloids remain stationary or grow slowly and do not regress spontaneously. Although these lesions have a distinct tendency for local recurrence, the rate is highly dependent on the treatment. Immunohistochemical analyses of the proliferative activity of keloids using antibodies to Ki-67 or proliferating cell nuclear antigen have consistently found keloids to have a greater proliferative activity than is found in hypertrophic scars or normal skin, accounting for their tendency for continued growth.

Keloids are composed predominantly of type I collagen. Compared with normal skin, in which type I collagen constitutes approximately 75% of the collagen, this type of collagen comprises approximately 95% of the total collagen in keloids.[253] In addition, keloids have been reported to contain increased histamine,[262] fibronectin,[263] proline hydroxylase,[264] and elastin[265] compared to hypertrophic scars or normal skin. Numerous growth factors appear to be important in the pathogenesis of this lesion by inducing increased collagen synthesis by fibroblasts, including epidermal growth factor, platelet-derived growth factor receptors, and transforming growth factor-β1.[266-268] More recent studies have suggested that alterations in genes regulating apoptosis contribute to the fibroproliferative process;[269,270] fibroblasts in keloids have been shown to have a lower rate of apoptosis than normal fibroblasts, and alterations in p53, p63, and p73 have been implicated.[270-273]

DESMOPLASTIC FIBROBLASTOMA (COLLAGENOUS FIBROMA)

Desmoplastic fibroblastoma is a distinctive fibrous soft tissue tumor that typically occurs in the subcutaneous tissue or skeletal muscle of adults.[274-277] This tumor is rather nondescript in its morphologic appearance, and although first called desmoplastic fibroblastoma by Evans[274] in 1995, these lesions have been diagnosed as fibromas or some other benign mesenchymal lesion for many years. Most patients are in their fifth or sixth decade of life and present with a slowly growing, painless mass (Table 8-8). Few cases have been reported in children.[278,279] Men are affected three to four times more commonly than women.[280] The most common sites are the upper extremities, including the shoulder, upper arm, and forearm, followed by the lower extremity; rare lesions arise in the head and neck region.[281-283] Most are pre-dominantly subcutaneous, but some involve skeletal muscle exclusively. The vast majority of tumors are 4 cm or smaller at the time of excision.[280]

Pathologic findings

Grossly, desmoplastic fibroblastoma appears as a well-circumscribed, firm mass with a white to gray cut surface, without hemorrhage or necrosis. Microscopically, the tumor is more or less circumscribed but not infrequently infiltrates the surrounding soft tissues. The lesion is hypocellular and consists of widely spaced bland spindle to stellate-shaped cells embedded in a collagenous or myxo-collagenous stroma (Figs 8-51, 8-52). Mitotic figures are rare or absent, and necrosis is not present. Blood vessels are inconspicuous but may exhibit perivascular hyalinization.

TABLE 8-8	AGE DISTRIBUTION OF 63 PATIENTS WITH COLLAGENOUS FIBROMA	
Age range (years)		**Number of patients**
0–10		0
11–20		4
21–30		5
31–40		4
41–50		16
51–60		18
61–70		11
71–80		3
81–90		2

Modified from[280]: Miettinen M, Fetsch JF. Hum Pathol 1998; 29:676.

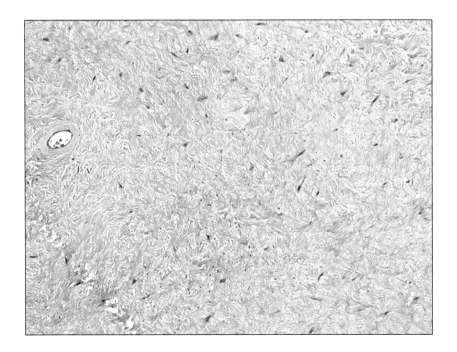

FIGURE 8–51 Desmoplastic fibroblastoma (collagenous fibroma). The lesion is hypocellular with widely spaced spindled and stellate-shaped cells embedded in a fibromyxoid stroma.

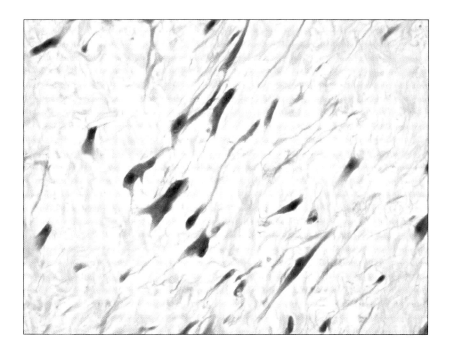

FIGURE 8–52 High-magnification view of bland spindled and stellate-shaped fibroblasts in a desmoplastic fibroblastoma (collagenous fibroma).

Immunohistochemically, the cells stain for vimentin, and most show focal staining for smooth muscle actin or muscle-specific actin.[284–286] In addition, rare cells may stain for cytokeratin.[280] Immunostains for desmin, CD34, and S-100 protein are typically negative. Ultrastructurally, the neoplastic cells have the features of fibroblasts and myofibroblasts, with dilated rough endoplasmic reticulum and few cells with pinocytotic vesicles and focal myofilaments with dense bodies.

Differential diagnosis

The differential diagnosis includes a variety of benign or low-grade, predominantly fibrous lesions. *Neurofibroma* is composed of cells with a wavy configuration deposited in a myxocollagenous stroma, often with "shredded carrot" bundles of collagen. Unlike desmoplastic fibroblastoma, S-100 protein is typically strongly positive in neurofibromas. *Fibromatosis*, even when hypocellular, is more cellular than desmoplastic fibroblastoma, more infiltrative, and the cells tend to be arranged in broad fascicles. *Calcifying fibrous pseudotumor*, which affects children and young adults, is characterized by psammomatous calcifications and a lymphoplasmacytic infiltrate. *Low-grade fibromyxoid sarcoma* is typically more cellular, with cells arranged in whorls and deposited in a variably fibromyxoid stroma. *Elastofibroma*, usually found in the subscapular area, is characterized by wavy elastic fibers that are not present in desmoplastic fibroblastoma. *Nodular fasciitis* of long duration can also resemble this lesion but usually has areas of increased cellularity and other features typical of nodular fasciitis, even if present focally.

Discussion

Most patients have been treated by conservative simple excision, and neither local recurrence nor metastasis has been reported. Because of the bland hypocellular appearance, it is not certain whether these lesions are the end-stage of a reactive process or a true neoplasm. Sciot et al.[134] reported two such tumors with aberrations of 11q12, similar to those described for fibroma of the tendon sheath, and an identical karyotype was reported in a single case by Bernal and colleagues.[287]

REFERENCES

1. Eyden B. The myofibroblast: a study of normal, reactive and neoplastic tissues, with an emphasis on ultrastructure. Part 2 – tumours and tumour-like lesions. J Submicrosc Cytol Pathol 2005; 37:231.
2. Gabbiani G, Ryan GB, Majne G. Presence of modified fibroblasts in granulation tissue and their possible role in wound contraction. Experientia 1971; 27:549.
3. Gabbiani G, Majno G. Dupuytren's contracture: Fibroblast contraction? An ultrastructural study. Am J Pathol 1972; 66:131.
4. Bhawan J. The myofibroblast. Am J Dermatopathol 1981; 3:73.
5. Gabbiani G. The myofibroblast in wound healing and fibrocontractive diseases. J Pathol 2003; 200:500.
6. Seemayer TA, Lagace R, Schurch W, et al. Myofibroblasts in the stroma of invasive and metastatic carcinoma: A possible host response to neoplasia. Am J Surg Pathol 1979; 3:525.
7. Eyden B. Fibroblast phenotype plasticity: relevance for understanding heterogeneity in "fibroblastic" tumors. Ultrastruct Pathol 2004; 28:307.
8. Eyden B. Electron microscopy in the study of myofibroblastic lesions. Semin Diagn Pathol 2003; 20:13.
9. Eyden B. The fibronexus in reactive and tumoral myofibroblasts: Further

characterisation by electron microscopy. Histol Histopathol 2001; 16:57.

10. Skalli O, Schurch W, Seemayer T, et al. Myofibroblasts from diverse pathologic settings are heterogeneous in their content of actin isoforms and intermediate filament proteins. Lab Invest 1989; 60:275.

11. Mentzel T, Katenkamp D. Myofibroblastic tumors. Brief review of clinical aspects, diagnosis and differential diagnosis. Pathologe 1998; 19:176.

12. Canty EG, Kadler KE. Procollagen trafficking, processing and fibrillogenesis. J Cell Sci 2005; 118:1341.

13. Leblond CP. Synthesis and secretion of collagen by cells of connective tissue, bone, and dentin. Anat Rec 1989; 224:123.

14. Ushiki T. Collagen fibers, reticular fibers and elastic fibers. A comprehensive understanding from a morphological viewpoint. Arch Histol Cytol 2002; 65:109.

15. Lewis KG, Bercovitch L, Dill SW, et al. Acquired disorders of elastic tissue: Part I. Increased elastic tissue and solar elastotic syndromes. J Am Acad Dermatol 2004; 51:1.

16. Lewis KG, Bercovitch L, Dill SW, et al. Acquired disorders of elastic tissue: Part II. Decreased elastic tissue. J Am Acad Dermatol 2004; 51:165.

17. Briggs SL. The role of fibronectin in fibroblast migration during tissue repair. J Wound Care 2005; 14:284.

18. Ekblom P, Lonai P, Talts JF. Expression and biological role of laminin-1. Matrix Biol 2003; 22:35.

19. Olsen D, Nagayoshi T, Fazio M, et al. Human laminin: cloning and sequence analysis of cDNAs encoding A, B1 and B2 chains, and expression of the corresponding genes in human skin and cultured cells. Lab Invest 1989; 60:772.

20. Gibbs RV. Cytokines and glycosaminoglycans (GAGs). Adv Exp Med Biol 2003; 535: 125.

Nodular fasciitis

21. Soule EH. Proliferative (nodular) fasciitis. Arch Pathol Lab Med 1962; 73:437.

22. Stout AP. Pseudosarcomatous fasciitis in children. Cancer 1961; 14:1216.

23. Meister P, Buckmann FW, Konrad E. Extent and level of fascial involvement in 100 cases with nodular fasciitis. Virchows Arch A Pathol Anat Histol 1978; 380:177.

24. Allen PW. Nodular fasciitis. Pathology 1972; 4:9.

25. Silva P, Bruce IA, Malik T, et al. Nodular fasciitis of the head and neck. J Laryngol Otol 2005; 119:8.

26. Handa Y, Asai T, Tomita Y. Nodular fasciitis of the forehead in a pediatric patient. Dermatol Surg 2003; 29:867.

27. Shin JH, Lee HK, Cho KJ, et al. Nodular fasciitis of the head and neck: Radiographic findings. Clin Imaging 2003; 27:31.

28. Abendroth CS, Frauenhoffer EE. Nodular fasciitis of the parotid gland. Report of a case with presentation in an unusual location and cytologic differential diagnosis. Acta Cytol 1995; 39:530.

29. Thompson LD, Fanburg-Smith JC, Wenig BM. Nodular fasciitis of the external ear region: a clinicopathologic study of 50 cases. Ann Diagn Pathol 2001; 5:191.

30. Dayan D, Nasrallah V, Vered M. Clinico-pathologic correlations of myofibroblastic tumors of the oral cavity: 1. Nodular fasciitis. J Oral Pathol Med 2005; 34:426.

31. Nielsen GP, Young RH. Mesenchymal tumors and tumor-like lesions of the female genital tract: a selective review with emphasis on recently described entities. Int J Gynecol Pathol 2001; 20:105.

32. Shields JA, Shields CL, Christian C, et al. Orbital nodular fasciitis simulating a dermoid cyst in an 8-month-old child. Case report and review of the literature. Ophthal Plast Reconstr Surg 2001; 17:144.

33. Bernstein KE, Lattes R. Nodular (pseudosarcomatous) fasciitis, a nonrecurrent lesion: clinicopathologic study of 134 cases. Cancer 1982; 49:1668.

34. Montgomery EA, Meis JM. Nodular fasciitis. Its morphologic spectrum and immunohistochemical profile. Am J Surg Pathol 1991; 15:942.

35. Kang SK, Kim HH, Ahn SJ, et al. Intradermal nodular fasciitis of the face. J Dermatol 2002; 29:310.

36. Dahl I, Angervall L, Magnusson S, et al. Classical and cystic nodular fasciitis. Pathol Eur 1972; 7:211.

37. Shimizu S, Hashimoto H, Enjoji M. Nodular fasciitis: An analysis of 250 patients. Pathology 1984; 16:161.

38. Daroca PJ Jr, Pulitzer DR, LoCicero J 3rd. Ossifying fasciitis. Arch Pathol Lab Med 1982; 106:682.

39. Innocenzi D, Giustini S, Barduagni F, et al. Ossifying fasciitis of the nose. J Am Acad Dermatol 1997; 37:357.

40. Kwittken J, Branche M. Fasciitis ossificans. Am J Clin Pathol 1969; 51:251.

41. Lui PC, Pang LM, Chu WC, et al. Pathologic quiz case: a solitary breast nodule in an elderly woman. Fasciitis ossificans of the breast. Arch Pathol Lab Med 2004; 128:e29.

42. Letts M, Pang E, Carpenter B, et al. Parosteal fasciitis in children. Am J Orthop 1995; 24:119.

43. de Silva MV, Reid R. Myositis ossificans and fibroosseous pseudotumor of digits: a clinicopathological review of 64 cases with emphasis on diagnostic pitfalls. Int J Surg Pathol 2003; 11:187.

44. Dupree WB, Enzinger FM. Fibro-osseous pseudotumor of the digits. Cancer 1986; 58:2103.

45. Patchefsky AS, Enzinger FM. Intravascular fasciitis: A report of 17 cases. Am J Surg Pathol 1981; 5:29.

46. Samaratunga H, Searle J, O'Loughlin B. Nodular fasciitis and related pseudosarcomatous lesions of soft tissues. Aust NZ J Surg 1996; 66:22.

47. Samaratunga H, Searle J, O'Loughlin B. Intravascular fasciitis: A case report and review of the literature. Pathology 1996; 28:8.

48. Sticha RS, Deacon JS, Wertheimer SJ, et al. Intravascular fasciitis in the foot. J Foot Ankle Surg 1997; 36:95.

49. Lauer DH, Enzinger FM. Cranial fasciitis of childhood. Cancer 1980; 45:401.

50. Cummings TJ, George TM, Fuchs HE, et al. The pathology of extracranial scalp and skull masses in young children. Clin Neuropathol 2004; 23:34.

51. Foureur N, Enjolras O, Boccon-Gibod L, et al. Cranial fasciitis of childhood. Ann Dermatol Venereol 2002; 129:732.

52. Keyserling HF, Castillo M, Smith JK. Cranial fasciitis of childhood. Am J Neuroradiol 2003; 24:1465.

53. Boddie DE, Distante S, Blaiklock CT. Cranial fasciitis of childhood: an incidental finding of a lytic skull lesion. Br J Neurosurg 1997; 11:445.

54. Hoya K, Usui M, Sugiyama Y, et al. Cranial fasciitis. Childs Nerv Syst 1996; 12:556.

55. Clapp CG, Dodson EE, Pickett BP, et al. Cranial fasciitis presenting as an external auditory canal mass. Arch Otolaryngol Head Neck Surg 1997; 123:223.

56. Kayaselcuk F, Demirhan B, Kayaselcuk U, et al. Vimentin, smooth muscle actin, desmin, S-100 protein, p53, and estrogen receptor expression in elastofibroma and nodular fasciitis. Ann Diagn Pathol 2002; 6:94.

57. Ceballos KM, Nielsen GP, Selig MK, et al. Is anti-h-caldesmon useful for distinguishing smooth muscle and myofibroblastic tumors? An immunohistochemical study. Am J Clin Pathol 2000; 114:746.

57a. Perez-Montiel MD, Plaza JA, Dominguez-Malagon H, et al. Differential expression of smooth muscle myosin, smooth muscle actin, H-caldesmon and calponin in the diagnosis of myofibroblastic and smooth muscle lesions of skin and soft tissue. Am J Dermatopathol 2006; 28:105.

58. Bhattacharya B, Dilworth HP, Iacobuzio-Donahue C, et al. Nuclear beta-catenin expression distinguishes deep fibromatosis from other benign and malignant fibroblastic and myofibroblastic lesions. Am J Surg Pathol 2005; 29:653.

59. Dominguez-Malagon H. Intracellular collagen and fibronexus in fibromatosis and other fibroblastic tumors. Ultrastruct Pathol 2004; 28:67.

60. Oshiro Y, Fukuda T, Tsuneyoshi M. Fibrosarcoma versus fibromatoses and cellular nodular fasciitis. A comparative study of their proliferative activity using proliferating cell nuclear antigen, DNA flow cytometry, and p53. Am J Surg Pathol 1994; 18:712.

61. Sawyer JR, Sammartino G, Baker GF, et al. Clonal chromosome aberrations in a case of nodular fasciitis. Cancer Genet Cytogenet 1994; 76:154.

62. Weibolt VM, Buresh CJ, Roberts CA, et al. Involvement of 3q21 in nodular fasciitis. Cancer Genet Cytogenet 1998; 106:177.

63. Birdsall SH, Shipley JM, Summersgill BM, et al. Cytogenetic findings in a case of nodular fasciitis of the breast. Cancer Genet Cytogenet 1995; 81:166.

64. Velagaleti GV, Tapper JK, Panova NE, et al. Cytogenetic findings in a case of nodular fasciitis of subclavicular region. Cancer Genet Cytogenet 2003; 141:160.

65. Koizumi H, Mikami M, Doi M, et al. Clonality analysis of nodular fasciitis by HUMARA-methylation-specific PCR. Histopathology 2005; 47:320.

66. Goldblum JR, Tuthill RJ. CD34 and factor-XIIIa immunoreactivity in dermatofibrosarcoma protuberans and dermatofibroma. Am J Dermatopathol 1997; 19:147.

67. Calonje E, Mentzel T, Fletcher CD. Cellular benign fibrous histiocytoma. clinicopathologic analysis of 74 cases of a distinctive variant of cutaneous fibrous histiocytoma with frequent recurrence. Am J Surg Pathol 1994; 18:668.

68. Kong CS, Cha I. Nodular fasciitis: diagnosis by fine needle aspiration biopsy. Acta Cytol 2004; 48:473.

69. Wong NL. Fine needle aspiration cytology of pseudosarcomatous reactive proliferative lesions of soft tissue. Acta Cytol 2002; 46:1049.

70. Aydin O, Oztuna V, Polat A. Three cases of nodular fasciitis: primary diagnoses by fine needle aspiration cytology. Cytopathology 2001; 12:346.

71. Ooe M, Ishiguro N, Kawashima M. Nuclear DNA content and distribution of Ki-67 positive cells in nodular fasciitis. J Dermatol 1993; 20:214.

Proliferative fasciitis

72. Chung EB, Enzinger FM. Proliferative fasciitis. Cancer 1975; 36:1450.

73. Kiryu H, Takeshita H, Hori Y. Proliferative fasciitis. Report of a case with histopathologic and immunohistochemical studies. Am J Dermatopathol 1997; 19:396.

74. Honda Y, Oh-i T, Koga M, et al. A case of proliferative fasciitis in the abdominal region. J Dermatol 2001; 28:753.

75. Meis JM, Enzinger FM. Proliferative fasciitis and myositis of childhood. Am J Surg Pathol 1992; 16:364.

76. Lundgren L, Kindblom LG, Willems J, et al. Proliferative myositis and fasciitis. A light and electron microscopic, cytologic, DNA-cytometric and immunohistochemical study. APMIS 1992; 100:437.

77. Diaz-Flores L, Martin Herrera AI, Garcia Montelongo R, et al. Proliferative fasciitis: ultrastructure and histogenesis. J Cutan Pathol 1989; 16:85.

78. Craver JL, McDivitt RW. Proliferative fasciitis: ultrastructural study of two cases. Arch Pathol Lab Med 1981; 105:542.

79. Ushigome S, Takakuwa T, Takagi M, et al. Proliferative myositis and fasciitis. Report of five cases with an ultrastructural and immunohistochemical study. Acta Pathol Jpn 1986; 36:963.

80. Ghadially FN, Thomas MJ, Jabi M, et al. Intracisternal collagen fibrils in proliferative fasciitis and myositis of childhood. Ultrastruct Pathol 1993; 17:161.

Proliferative myositis

81. Kern WH. Proliferative myositis; a pseudosarcomatous reaction to injury: a report of seven cases. Arch Pathol Lab Med 1960; 69:209.

82. Ackerman LV. Extra-osseous localized non-neoplastic bone and cartilage formation (so-called myositis ossificans): clinical and pathological confusion with malignant neoplasms. J Bone Joint Surg [Am] 1958; 40-A:279.

83. Enzinger FM, Dulcey F. Proliferative myositis. Report of thirty-three cases. Cancer 1967; 20:2213.

84. Pollock L, Fullilove S, Shaw DG, et al. Proliferative myositis in a child. A case report. J Bone Joint Surg [Am] 1995; 77:132.

85. Mulier S, Stas M, Delabie J, et al. Proliferative myositis in a child. Skeletal Radiol 1999; 28:703.

86. Dent CD, DeBoom GW, Hamlin ML. Proliferative myositis of the head and neck. Report of a case and review of the literature. Oral Surg Oral Med Oral Pathol 1994; 78:354.

87. Singh A, Philpott JM, Patel NN, et al. Proliferative myositis arising in the tongue. J Laryngol Otol 2000; 114:978.

88. Brooks JS. Immunohistochemistry of proliferative myositis. Arch Pathol Lab Med 1981; 105:682.

89. el-Jabbour JN, Bennett MH, Burke MM, et al. Proliferative myositis. An immunohistochemical and ultrastructural study. Am J Surg Pathol 1991; 15:654.

90. Dembinski A, Bridge JA, Neff JR, et al. Trisomy 2 in proliferative myositis. Cancer Genet Cytogenet 1992; 60:27.

91. Ohjimi Y, Iwasaki H, Ishiguro M, et al. Trisomy 2 found in proliferative myositis cultured cell. Cancer Genet Cytogenet 1994; 76:157.

92. McComb EN, Neff JR, Johansson SL, et al. Chromosomal anomalies in a case of proliferative myositis. Cancer Genet Cytogenet 199798:142.;

93. el-Jabbour JN, Wilson GD, Bennett MH, et al. Flow cytometric study of nodular fasciitis, proliferative fasciitis, and proliferative myositis. Hum Pathol 1991; 22:1146.

Organ-associated pseudosarcomatous myofibroblastic proliferations

94. Huang WL, Ro JY, Grignon DJ, et al. Postoperative spindle cell nodule of the prostate and bladder. J Urol 1990; 143:824.

95. Proppe KH, Scully RE, Rosai J. Postoperative spindle cell nodules of genitourinary tract resembling sarcomas. A report of eight cases. Am J Surg Pathol 1984; 8:101.

96. Horn LC, Reuter S, Biesold M. Inflammatory pseudotumor of the ureter and the urinary bladder. Pathol Res Pract 1997; 193:607.

97. Iczkowski KA, Shanks JH, Gadaleanu V, et al. Inflammatory pseudotumor and sarcoma of urinary bladder: differential diagnosis and outcome in thirty-eight spindle cell neoplasms. Mod Pathol 2001; 14:1043.

98. Jones EC, Clement PB, Young RH. Inflammatory pseudotumor of the urinary bladder. A clinicopathological, immunohistochemical, ultrastructural, and flow cytometric study of 13 cases. Am J Surg Pathol 1993; 17:264.

99. Nochomovitz LE, Orenstein JM. Inflammatory pseudotumor of the urinary bladder – possible relationship to nodular fasciitis. Two case reports, cytologic observations, and ultrastructural observations. Am J Surg Pathol 1985; 9:366.

100. Hirsch MS, Dal Cin P, Fletcher CD. ALK expression in pseudosarcomatous myofibroblastic proliferations of the genitourinary tract. Histopathology 2006; 48:569.

101. Tsuzuki T, Magi-Galluzzi C, Epstein JI. ALK-1 expression in inflammatory myofibroblastic tumor of the urinary bladder. Am J Surg Pathol 2004. 28:1609.

102. Freeman A, Geddes N, Munson P, et al. Anaplastic lymphoma kinase (ALK 1) staining and molecular analysis in inflammatory myofibroblastic tumours of the bladder: a preliminary clinicopathological study of nine cases and review of the literature. Mod Pathol 2004; 17:765.

103. Harik LR, Merino C, Coindre JM, et al. Pseudosarcomatous myofibroblastic proliferations of the bladder: a clinicopathologic study of 42 cases. Am J Surg Pathol 2006; 30:787.

104. Montgomery E, Shuster DD, Burkart A, et al. Inflammatory myofibroblastic tumors of the urinary tract: a clinicopathologic study of 46 cases, including a malignant example and a subset associated with high grade urothelial carcinoma. Am J Surg Pathol 2006; 30(12):1502.

104a. Sukov WR, Cheville JC, Carlson AW, et al. Utility of *ALK*-1 protein expression and *ALK* rearrangements in distinguishing inflammatory myofibroblastic tumor from malignant spindle cells lesions of the urinary bladder. Mod Pathol 2007; 20:592.

105. Young RH. Pseudoneoplastic lesions of the urinary bladder and urethra: a selective review with emphasis on recent information. Semin Diagn Pathol 1997; 14:133.

106. Young RH, Scully RE. Pseudosarcomatous lesions of the urinary bladder, prostate gland, and urethra. A report of three cases and review of the literature. Arch Pathol Lab Med 1987; 111:354.

107. Ro JY, el-Naggar AK, Amin MB, et al. Pseudosarcomatous fibromyxoid tumor of the urinary bladder and prostate: immunohistochemical, ultrastructural, and DNA flow cytometric analyses of nine cases. Hum Pathol 1993; 24:1203.

108. Guillou L, Costa J. Postoperative pseudosarcomas of the genitourinary tract. A diagnostic trap. Presentation of 4 cases of which 2 were studied immunohistochemically

and review of the literature. Ann Pathol 1989; 9:340.

109. Albores-Saavedra J, Manivel JC, Essenfeld H, et al. Pseudosarcomatous myofibroblastic proliferations in the urinary bladder of children. Cancer 1990; 66:1234.

110. Bulusu AD, Hopkins T. Inflammatory pseudotumor of the bladder. Urology 1998; 51:487.

111. Hojo H, Newton WA Jr, Hamoudi AB, et al. Pseudosarcomatous myofibroblastic tumor of the urinary bladder in children: a study of 11 cases with review of the literature. An intergroup rhabdomyosarcoma study. Am J Surg Pathol 1995; 19:1224.

Ischemic fasciitis (atypical decubital fibroplasia)

112. Washing D, Zaher A. Pathologic quiz case: a 76-year-old debilitated woman with a right thigh mass. Ischemic fasciitis (atypical decubital fibroplasia). Arch Pathol Lab Med 2004; 128: e139.

113. Baldassano MF, Rosenberg AE, Flotte TJ. Atypical decubital fibroplasia: a series of three cases. J Cutan Pathol 1998; 25:149.

114. Perosio PM, Weiss SW. Ischemic fasciitis: a juxta-skeletal fibroblastic proliferation with a predilection for elderly patients. Mod Pathol 1993; 6:69.

115. Zamecnik M, Michal M, Patrikova J. Atypical decubital fibroplasia (ischemic fasciitis) – a new pseudosarcomatous entity. Cesk Patol 1994; 30:130.

116. Montgomery EA, Meis JM, Mitchell MS, et al. Atypical decubital fibroplasia. A distinctive fibroblastic pseudotumor occurring in debilitated patients. Am J Surg Pathol 1992; 16:708.

117. Baranzelli MC, Lecomte-Houcke M, De Saint Maur P, et al. Atypical decubitus fibroplasia: a recent entity. Apropos of a case of an adolescent girl. Bull Cancer 1996; 83:81.

118. Fukunaga M. Atypical decubital fibroplasia with unusual histology. APMIS 2001; 109:631.

119. Scanlon R, Kelehan P, Flannelly G, et al. Ischemic fasciitis: an unusual vulvovaginal spindle cell lesion. Int J Gynecol Pathol 2004; 23:65.

120. Yamamoto M, Ishida T, Machinami R. Atypical decubital fibroplasia in a young patient with melorheostosis. Pathol Int 1998; 48:160.

Fibroma of the tendon sheath

121. Cooper PH. Fibroma of tendon sheath. J Am Acad Dermatol 1984; 11:625.

122. Chung EB, Enzinger FM. Fibroma of tendon sheath. Cancer 1979; 44:1945.

123. Hitora T, Yamamoto T, Akisue T, et al. Fibroma of tendon sheath originating from the knee joint capsule. Clin Imaging 2002; 26:280.

124. McGrory JE, Rock MG. Fibroma of tendon sheath involving the patellar tendon. Am J Orthop 2000; 29:465.

125. Pulitzer DR, Martin PC, Reed RJ. Fibroma of tendon sheath. A clinicopathologic study of 32 cases. Am J Surg Pathol 1989; 13:472.

126. Lamovec J, Bracko M, Voncina D. Pleomorphic fibroma of tendon sheath. Am J Surg Pathol 1991; 15:1202.

127. Jablokow VR, Kathuria S. Fibroma of tendon sheath. J Surg Oncol 1982; 19:90.

128. Maluf HM, DeYoung BR, Swanson PE, et al. Fibroma and giant cell tumor of tendon sheath: a comparative histological and immunohistological study. Mod Pathol 1995; 8:155.

129. Satti MB. Tendon sheath tumours: a pathological study of the relationship between

giant cell tumour and fibroma of tendon sheath. Histopathology 1992; 20:213.

130. Hashimoto H, Tsuneyoshi M, Daimaru Y, et al. Fibroma of tendon sheath: a tumor of myofibroblasts. A clinicopathologic study of 18 cases. Acta Pathol Jpn 1985; 35:1099.

131. Sarma DP, Weilbaecher TG, Rodriguez FH Jr. Fibroma of tendon sheath. J Surg Oncol 1986; 32:230.

132. Dal Cin P, Sciot R, De Smet L, et al. Translocation 2;11 in a fibroma of tendon sheath. Histopathology 1998; 32:433.

133. Dal Cin P, Sciot R, Samson I, et al. Cytogenetic characterization of tenosynovial giant cell tumors (nodular tenosynovitis). Cancer Res 1994; 54:3986.

134. Sciot R, Samson I, van den Berghe H, et al. Collagenous fibroma (desmoplastic fibroblastoma): genetic link with fibroma of tendon sheath? Mod Pathol 1999; 12:565.

Pleomorphic fibroma of skin

135. Kamino H, Lee JY, Berke A. Pleomorphic fibroma of the skin: a benign neoplasm with cytologic atypia. A clinicopathologic study of eight cases. Am J Surg Pathol 1989; 13:107.

136. Garcia-Doval I, Casas L, Toribio J. Pleomorphic fibroma of the skin, a form of sclerotic fibroma: an immunohistochemical study. Clin Exp Dermatol 1998; 23:22.

137. Hassanein A, Telang G, Benedetto E, et al. Subungual myxoid pleomorphic fibroma. Am J Dermatopathol 1998; 20:502.

138. Hsieh YJ, Lin YC, Wu YH, et al. Subungual pleomorphic fibroma. J Cutan Pathol 2003; 30:569.

139. Miliauskas JR. Myxoid cutaneous pleomorphic fibroma. Histopathology 1994; 24:179.

140. Mahmood MN, Salama ME, Chaffins M, et al. Solitary sclerotic fibroma of skin: a possible link with pleomorphic fibroma with immunophenotypic expression for O13 (CD99) and CD34. J Cutan Pathol 2003; 30:631.

141. Rudolph P, Schubert C, Zelger BG, et al. Differential expression of CD34 and ki-M1p in pleomorphic fibroma and dermatofibroma with monster cells. Am J Dermatopathol 1999; 21:414.

142. Ahn SK, Won JH, Lee SH, et al. Pleomorphic fibroma on the scalp. Dermatology 1995; 191:245.

Nuchal-type fibroma and Gardner-associated fibroma

143. Nielsen GP, O'Connell JX, Wehrli BM, et al. Collagen-rich tumors of soft tissues: An overview. Adv Anat Pathol 2003; 10:179.

144. Michal M, Fetsch JF, Hes O, et al. Nuchal-type fibroma: a clinicopathologic study of 52 cases. Cancer 1999; 85:156.

145. Shek TW, Chan AC, Ma L. Extranuchal nuchal fibroma. Am J Surg Pathol 1996; 20:902.

146. Balachandran K, Allen PW, MacCormac LB. Nuchal fibroma. A clinicopathological study of nine cases. Am J Surg Pathol 1995; 19:313.

147. Michal M. Non-nuchal-type fibroma associated with Gardner's syndrome. A hitherto unreported mesenchymal tumor different from fibromatosis and nuchal-type fibroma. Path Res Pract 2000; 196:857.

148. Banney LA, Weedon D, Muir JB. Nuchal fibroma associated with scleredema, diabetes mellitus and organic solvent exposure. Australas J Dermatol 2000; 41:39.

149. Dawes LC, La Hei ER, Tobias V, et al. Nuchal fibroma should be recognized as a new extracolonic manifestation of Gardner-variant familial adenomatous polyposis. Aust NZ J Surg 2000; 70:824.

150. Diwan AH, Graves ED, King JA, et al. Nuchal-type fibroma in two related patients with Gardner's syndrome. Am J Surg Pathol 2000; 24:1563.

151. Wehrli BM, Weiss SW, Yandow S, et al. Gardner-associated fibromas (GAF) in young patients: a distinct fibrous lesion that identifies unsuspected Gardner syndrome and risk for fibromatosis. Am J Surg Pathol 2001; 25:645.

151a. Coffin CM, Hornick JL, Zhou H, et al. Gardner fibroma: a clinicopathologic and immunohistochemical analysis of 45 patients with 57 fibromas. Am J Surg Pathol 2007; 31:410.

152. Wehrli BM, Weiss SW, Coffin CM. Gardner syndrome. Am J Surg Pathol 2001; 25:694.

153. Clark SK, Smith TG, Katz DE, et al. Identification and progression of a desmoid precursor lesion in patients with familial adenomatous polyposis. Br J Surg 1998; 85:970.

154. Allen PW. Nuchal-type fibroma appearance in a desmoid fibromatosis. Am J Surg Pathol 2001; 25:828.

155. Laskin WB, Fetsch JF, Miettinen M. Nuchal fibrocartilaginous pseudotumor: a clinicopathologic study of five cases and review of the literature. Mod Pathol 1999; 12:663.

156. O'Connell JX, Janzen DL, Hughes TR. Nuchal fibrocartilaginous pseudotumor: a distinctive soft-tissue lesion associated with prior neck injury. Am J Surg Pathol 1997; 21:836.

Elastofibroma

157. Järvi O, Saxén E. Elastofibroma dorsi. Acta Pathol Microbiol Scand 1961; 51:83.

158. Vastamaki M. Elastofibroma scapulae. Clin Orthop 2001; Nov(392):404.

159. Devaney D, Livesley P, Shaw D. Elastofibroma dorsi: MRI diagnosis in a young girl. Pediatr Radiol 1995; 25:282.

160. Giebel GD, Bierhoff E, Vogel J. Elastofibroma and pre-elastofibroma – a biopsy and autopsy study. Eur J Surg Oncol 1996; 22:93.

161. Järvi OH, Lansimies PH. Subclinical elastofibromas in the scapular region in an autopsy series. Acta Pathol Microbiol Scand [A] 1975; 83:87.

162. Majo J, Gracia I, Doncel A, et al. Elastofibroma dorsi as a cause of shoulder pain or snapping scapula. Clin Orthop 2001; Jul(388):200.

163. Hayes AJ, Alexander N, Clark MA, et al. Elastofibroma: a rare soft tissue tumour with a pathognomonic anatomical location and clinical symptom. Eur J Surg Oncol 2004; 30:450.

164. Heck S, Thomas G, Mader K, et al. Bilateral elastofibroma as an unusual cause of shoulder pain. Plast Reconstr Surg 2003; 112:1959.

165. Turna A, Yilmaz MA, Urer N, et al. Bilateral elastofibroma dorsi. Ann Thorac Surg 2002; 73:630.

166. Naylor MF, Nascimento AG, Sherrick AD, et al. Elastofibroma dorsi: radiologic findings in 12 patients. Am J Roentgenol 1996; 167:683.

167. Guha AR, Raja RC, Devadoss VG. Elastofibroma dorsi – a case report and review of literature. Int J Clin Pract 2004; 58:218.

168. Maldjian C, Adam RJ, Maldjian JA, et al. Elastofibroma of the neck. Skeletal Radiol 2000; 29:109.

169. Potter TJ, Summerlin DJ, Rodgers SF. Elastofibroma: the initial report in the oral mucosa. Oral Surg Oral Med Oral Pathol Oral Radiol Endod 2004; 97:64.

170. Hayashi K, Ohtsuki Y, Sonobe H, et al. Pre-elastofibroma-like colonic polyp: another cause of colonic polyp. Acta Med Okayama 1991; 45:49.

171. Tsutsumi A, Kawabata K, Taguchi K, et al. Elastofibroma of the greater omentum. Acta Pathol Jpn 1985; 35:233.

172. Mirra JM, Straub LR, Järvi OH. Elastofibroma of the deltoid. A case report. Cancer 1974; 33:234.

173. Hsu JK, Cavanagh HD, Green WR. An unusual case of elastofibroma oculi. Cornea 1997; 16:112.

174. Saint-Paul MC, Musso S, Cardot-Leccia N, et al. Elastofibroma of the stomach. Pathol Res Pract 2003; 199:637.

175. Goldblum JR, Beals T, Weiss SW. Elastofibromatous change of the rectum. A lesion mimicking amyloidosis. Am J Surg Pathol 1992; 16:793.

176. Madri JA, Dise CA, LiVolsi VA, et al. Elastofibroma dorsi: an immunochemical study of collagen content. Hum Pathol 1981; 12:186.

177. Nakamura Y, Okamoto K, Tanimura A, et al. Elastase digestion and biochemical analysis of the elastin from an elastofibroma. Cancer 1986; 58:1070.

178. Kumaratilake JS, Krishnan R, Lomax-Smith J, et al. Elastofibroma: disturbed elastic fibrillogenesis by periosteal-derived cells? An immunoelectron microscopic and in situ hybridization study. Hum Pathol 1991; 22:1017.

179. Kindblom LG, Spicer SS. Elastofibroma. A correlated light and electron microscopic study. Virchows Arch A Pathol Anat Histol 1982; 396:127.

180. Dixon AY, Lee SH. An ultrastructural study of elastofibromas. Hum Pathol 1980; 11:257.

181. Benisch B, Peison B, Marquet E, et al. Pre-elastofibroma and elastofibroma (the continuum of elastic-producing fibrous tumors). A light and ultrastructural study. Am J Clin Pathol 1983; 80:88.

182. Fukuda Y, Miyake H, Masuda Y, et al. Histogenesis of unique elastinophilic fibers of elastofibroma: ultrastructural and immunohistochemical studies. Hum Pathol 1987; 18:424.

183. De Nictolis M, Goteri G, Campanati G, et al. Elastofibrolipoma of the mediastinum. A previously undescribed benign tumor containing abnormal elastic fibers. Am J Surg Pathol 1995; 19:364.

184. Tighe JR, Clark AE, Turvey DJ. Elastofibroma dorsi. J Clin Pathol 1968; 21:463.

185. Kahn HJ, Hanna WM. "Aberrant elastic" in elastofibroma: an immunohistochemical and ultrastructural study. Ultrastruct Pathol 1995; 19:45.

186. Nagamine N, Nohara Y, Ito E. Elastofibroma in Okinawa. A clinicopathologic study of 170 cases. Cancer 1982; 50:1794.

187. Schepel JA, Wille J, Seldenrijk CA, et al. Elastofibroma: a familial occurrence. Eur J Surg 1998; 164:557.

188. Akhtar M, Miller RM. Ultrastructure of elastofibroma. Cancer 1977; 40:728.

189. Vanni R, Marras S, Faa G, et al. Chromosome instability in elastofibroma. Cancer Genet Cytogenet 1999; 111:182.

190. Batstone P, Forsyth L, Goodlad J. Clonal chromosome aberrations secondary to chromosome instability in an elastofibroma. Cancer Genet Cytogenet 2001; 128:46.

191. McComb EN, Feely MG, Neff JR, et al. Cytogenetic instability, predominantly involving chromosome 1, is characteristic of elastofibroma. Cancer Genet Cytogenet 2001; 126:68.

192. Harigopal M, Seshan SV, DeLellis RA, et al. Aspiration cytology of elastofibroma dorsi: case report with ultrastructural and immunohistochemical findings. Diagn Cytopathol 2002; 26:310.

FIBROMATOSES

Fibromatoses comprise a broad group of benign fibroblastic proliferations of similar microscopic appearance whose biologic behavior is intermediate between that of benign fibroblastic lesions and fibrosarcoma. Like fibrosarcoma, the fibromatoses are characterized by infiltrative growth and a tendency toward recurrence, but they never metastasize.

The various entities that constitute this group occur predominantly in adults and consist of highly differentiated fibroblasts and to a lesser degree myofibroblasts which form a firm, poorly circumscribed nodular mass which may be solitary or multiple and have a predilection for certain anatomic sites. The term *fibromatosis* should not be applied to non-specific reactive fibrous proliferations which are part of an inflammatory process or are secondary to injury or hemorrhage and have no tendency toward infiltrative growth or recurrence.

The fibromatoses can be divided into two major groups with several subdivisions (Table 9–1). *Superficial (fascial) fibromatoses* are small, slowly growing and of small size and arise from the fascia or aponeuroses and only rarely involve deep structures. The clinical course usually can be divided into an early, rather cellular proliferative phase and a late, richly collagenous regressive or contractile phase. *Deep (musculoaponeurotic) fibromatoses* are large, more rapidly growing tumors. Their biologic behavior is more aggressive than that of the superficial (fascial) fibromatoses; they have a high recurrence rate, and, as their name indicates, involve deep structures, particularly the musculature of the trunk and the extremities. The descriptive term *desmoid tumor*, coined by Mueller in 1838 to emphasize the band-like or tendon-like consistency of the lesions, is still widely used in the literature as a synonym for this type of fibromatosis. Other, less common synonyms such as *nonmetastasizing fibrosarcoma* and *grade 1 fibrosarcoma* should be discouraged, as both give the impression that fibromatosis is a sarcoma, and the latter implies metastatic potential.

Although all fascial and musculoaponeurotic fibromatoses are capable of recurrence after excision, the recurrence rate of the individual entities varies substantially. The risk of recurrence is governed less by the histologic picture than by the anatomic location of the lesion, the age of the patient, the size of the lesion and mode of therapy. In fact, histologic examination alone does not permit accurate prediction of the clinical course. Moreover, occasional fibromatoses do regress spontaneously, but the incidence and likelihood of regression, like that of recurrence, is unpredictable. These lesions do not undergo malignant transformation de novo, although there are rare reports of sarcomatous transformation after radiation therapy.[1]

PALMAR FIBROMATOSIS

Palmar fibromatosis, better known as *Dupuytren's disease* or *Dupuytren's contracture*, is by far the most common type of fibromatosis. Although it is named for Baron Guillaime Dupuytren, who reported this condition in 1831,[2] there are much earlier descriptions of this lesion. For example, Norse folklore from the twelfth century refers to the "MacCrimmons," a Scottish clan famed for its pipers, some of whom were unable to play because of digital contractures.[3,4] This form of superficial fibromatosis is characterized by a nodular fibroblastic proliferation which occurs in the volar surface of the hand and histologically closely resembles other forms of fibromatosis. The lesion appears to progress through a series of clinical and histologic stages and ultimately results in flexion contracture of the fingers, a complication that usually necessitates surgical therapy.

Clinical findings

Palmar fibromatosis is a relatively common condition that affects adults, with a rapid increase in incidence with advancing age. It has been estimated that almost 20% of

TABLE 9–1	CLASSIFICATION OF FIBROMATOSES

Superficial (fascial) fibromatoses
Palmar fibromatosis (Dupuytren's disease)
Plantar fibromatosis (Ledderhose's disease)
Penile fibromatosis (Peyronie's disease)
Knuckle pads
Deep (musculoaponeurotic) fibromatoses
Extra-abdominal fibromatosis (extra-abdominal desmoid)
Abdominal fibromatosis (abdominal desmoid)
Intra-abdominal fibromatosis (intra-abdominal desmoid)
Pelvic fibromatosis
Mesenteric fibromatosis
Mesenteric fibromatosis in Gardner syndrome

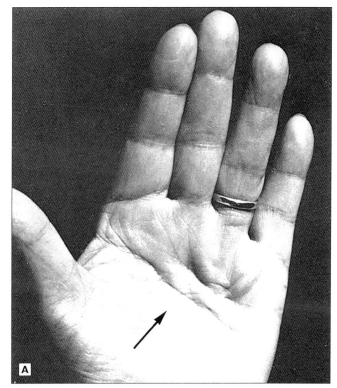

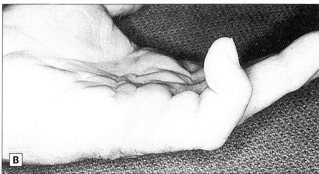

FIGURE 9–1 (A) Palmar fibromatosis with firm cord-like indurations and nodules causing puckering and dimpling (arrow) of the overlying skin. **(B)** Flexion contracture of the fifth finger (Dupuytren's contracture).

the general population is affected by 65 years of age. Patients younger than 30 years of age, particularly children, are seldom affected.[5,6] The condition is about three or four times more frequent in men than in women.[7] There is clearly a genetic susceptibility to this disease, as this form of fibromatosis is found virtually exclusively in Caucasians and is found only sporadically in those of Asian or African descent.[8] The highest prevalence of palmar fibromatosis is found in areas such as northern Scotland, Norway, Iceland, and Australia.[9]

The onset of the disease is slow and insidious, and the initial manifestation is typically an isolated, usually asymptomatic, firm nodule in the palmar surface of the hand. Because of the lack of symptoms at this stage, many patients ignore the presence of the nodule and do not seek medical therapy. There is a slight predilection for the right palmar surface, but almost 50% of cases are bilateral. Although clinical progression does not invariably occur, in many patients several months or years after the original appearance of the fibrous nodules, cord-like indurations or bands develop between nodules and adjacent fingers, often causing puckering and dimpling of the overlying skin (Fig. 9–1). These changes are usually most prominent on the ulnar side of the palm and are accompanied by flexion contractures that principally affect the fourth and fifth fingers of the hand. The thumb and index finger are least often affected. With increasing severity of the contractures, normal function of the hand becomes greatly impaired, and it is at this point that therapy is usually sought.

Concurrence of palmar fibromatosis with other diseases

Palmar fibromatosis has been linked with numerous other disease processes, including other forms of fibromatosis. Approximately 5–20% of cases of palmar fibromatosis are associated with plantar fibromatosis, and about 2–4% of patients also have penile fibromatosis (Peyronie's disease).[5,10] Knuckle pads (fibrous thickenings on the dorsal aspect of the proximal interphalangeal or metacarpophalangeal joints) have also been associated with palmar fibromatosis.[11] Rare patients have been described with polyfibromatosis syndrome, a condition characterized by the occurrence of several cutaneous fibroproliferative lesions, including Dupuytren's contracture and keloids.[12]

Palmar fibromatosis has been consistently linked with seemingly unrelated diseases. For example, approximately 20% of patients with diabetes mellitus have a palmar fibromatosis.[13] It is equally common in type 1 and type 2 diabetes mellitus, although it occurs at a younger age in patients with type 1.[14] Arkkila and co-workers found that the development of palmar fibromatosis in patients with diabetes mellitus was associated with increasing age and duration of the underlying disease.[15] Interestingly, there is a lower incidence of contractures when this lesion develops in diabetic patients. Although palmar fibromatosis is more common in men, in diabetic patients the gender ratio is almost equal.[15] Microvascular changes secondary to diabetes mellitus may result in local hypoxia, stimulating the fibroblastic proliferation.

The association between palmar fibromatosis and epilepsy was first noted by Lund in the 1940s in Denmark, with a prevalence of 50% among male patients and 25% among female patients.[16] Palmar fibromatosis occurs in all forms of epilepsy with equal frequency, and it is quite likely that it is closely related to the use of anticonvulsive drugs as opposed to the underlying disease itself.[17]

Alcoholics also have a high prevalence of Dupuytren's contracture.[18] The prevalence of palmar fibromatosis is far higher in alcoholics with liver disease than in those without liver disease, suggesting it is the effect of alcohol on the liver (rather than the direct effects of alcohol) that is the causative factor.[19] The effect of alcohol in the development of palmar fibromatosis may be exacerbated by cigarette smoking.[20]

Gross findings

The excised tissue consists of a single small nodule, usually measuring less than 1 cm in diameter, or an ill-defined conglomerate of several nodular masses intimately associated with a thickened palmar aponeurosis and subcutaneous fat. The tissue is firm and scar-like on palpation and on cut section reveals a gray-yellow to gray-white surface, although the color depends on the collagen content, which in turn depends on the age of the lesion. The gross specimen may also contain excised skin, and occasionally these nodular masses adhere to the overlying skin.

Microscopic findings

The microscopic findings depend on the age of the lesion. In general, plantar fibromatosis progresses from a proliferative nodular phase with relatively high cellularity, some mitotic activity and minimal collagen deposition to an involutional stage with increased myofibroblastic differentiation, decreased proliferative activity and increased collagen deposition to an end-stage that is less cellular and more collagenous.[5] The proliferative phase of the disease is characterized by a strikingly cellular proliferation of plump, immature-appearing spindle-shaped fibroblasts that form one or more nodules (Figs 9–2, 9–3). The fibroblasts are uniform in size and shape, with normochromatic nuclei and small, pinpoint nucleoli (Fig. 9–4). Mitotic figures may be identified but are usually not numerous. The cells are intimately associated with small to moderate amounts of collagen suspended in a mucopolysaccharide-rich matrix. Upon close examination, multinucleated giant cells are frequently seen.[5] Microhemorrhages with small deposits of hemosiderin and scattered chronic inflammatory cells may be present. The fibrous nodules originate within the palmar aponeurosis and extend into and replace the overlying subcutaneous fat.

Nodules that have been present a long time are less cellular and contain markedly increased amounts of dense birefringent collagen. The fibroblasts are smaller and more slender, and the fascial or aponeurotic cords between nodules are composed of dense fibrocollagen-

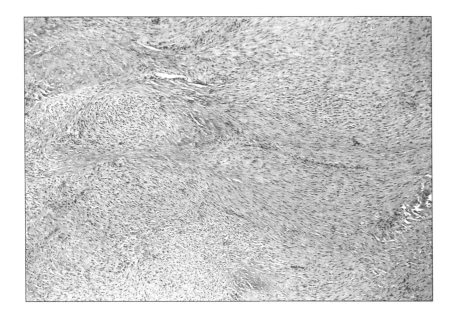

FIGURE 9–2 Palmar fibromatosis composed of parallel fascicles of slender fibroblasts separated by variable amounts of collagen.

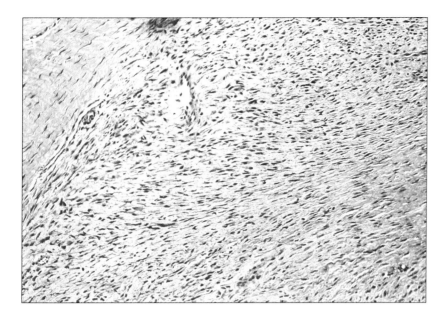

FIGURE 9–3 Uniform fibroblastic proliferation in palmar fibromatosis.

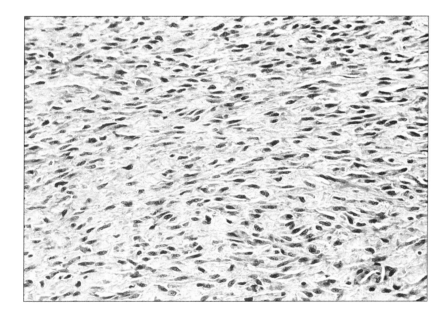

FIGURE 9–4 Early, rather cellular form of palmar fibromatosis showing uniform spindled cells separated by collagen.

ous tissue which resembles tendons. Osseous and cartilaginous metaplasia of the fibrous nodules may be seen, but is uncommon.

Electron microscopic and immunohistochemical findings

Gabbiani and Majno, the first to emphasize the presence of myofibroblasts in palmar fibromatosis, suggested that these cells played a role in the pathogenesis of the contraction observed clinically.[21] Since then, numerous reports have confirmed the role of myofibroblasts in this disease.[22] Ultrastructurally, the cells are characterized by deeply indented nuclei and cytoplasm with well-developed rough endoplasmic reticulum, longitudinally arranged microfilaments with interspersed dense bodies, subplasmalemmal plaques, partial envelopment by basal lamina, and the presence of fibronexus (Fig. 9–5). Ultrastructural studies have shown progression from a predominantly fibroblastic proliferative stage to an involutional stage composed predominantly of myofibroblasts, followed by a residual fibrocytic stage.[22] Throughout these stages there is a progressive decrease in cellularity with increased deposition of mature collagen, ultimately resulting in tendon-like structures.

Immunohistochemically, the spindle-shaped cells stain for vimentin and variably for smooth muscle actin and muscle-specific actin, depending on the stage and the

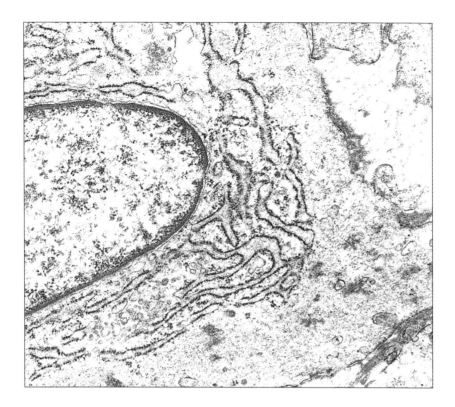

FIGURE 9–5 Electron microscopic picture of palmar fibromatosis showing a myofibroblast with well-developed rough endoplasmic reticulum, interspersed and focally condensed microfilaments, and partial basal lamina.

degree of myofibroblastic differentiation.[23] In addition, smooth muscle actin-positive cells are often numerous in apparently uninvolved dermis and provide a pool of progenitor cells from which new foci develop, accounting for the high rate of local recurrence.[24] Although the majority of palmar fibromatoses show nuclear β-catenin staining, the percentage of cells that stain is far less than that in deep fibromatoses.[25]

Other constituents of the extracellular matrix have also been identified by immunohistochemical means. Types III and VI collagen predominate during the early proliferative phase, whereas type I collagen increases during the involutional and residual phases.[26] Similarly, laminin and fibronectin appear to follow the distribution of myofibroblasts and decrease in quantity with increasing duration of the lesion.[27-29] Numerous growth factors, including transforming growth factor-β, platelet-derived growth factor, and basic fibroblast growth factor, have been implicated in the pathogenesis of this disease, as these growth factors are potent stimulators of collagen production.[30,31]

Cytogenetic findings

Standard karyotypic analysis of a large series of superficial fibromatoses has revealed clonal chromosomal aberrations in approximately 10% of cases.[32] The cytogenetic data pertaining specifically to palmar fibromatoses are sparse. DeWever and colleagues from the Chromosomes and Morphology Collaborative Group (CHAMP),

comprising cytogeneticists, pathologists and surgeons, carried out a systematic evaluation of 78 superficial and deep fibromatoses.[32] Of 28 superficial fibromatoses studied, only 3 cases showed cytogenetic aberrations, including 2 palmar fibromatoses with trisomy 8 and 1 plantar fibromatosis with trisomy 8 and loss of the X chromosome.

Differential diagnosis

In its most cellular phase, palmar fibromatosis may closely resemble *fibrosarcoma*. However, the cells of fibrosarcoma tend to be arranged in long fascicles or a herringbone pattern and show a greater degree of nuclear hyperchromasia, pleomorphism, and mitotic activity and occasionally necrosis. Furthermore, fibrosarcoma of the hand is rare, and, as stated by Fetsch and colleagues, "a healthy degree of skepticism is warranted whenever the diagnosis is suggested."[5] On those very rare occasions in which a fibrosarcoma does arise in this location, it is usually a deep-seated tumor that affects the aponeurosis and subcutaneous tissue only secondarily. In contrast, the cellular nodules in palmar fibromatosis arise within the aponeurosis and infiltrate the subcutaneous tissue.

The differential diagnosis also includes *cellular benign fibrous histiocytoma*. This is a dermal-based neoplasm that may secondarily involve the subcutaneous tissue. Although the central portion of the lesion may have a fascicular growth pattern reminiscent of palmar fibromatosis, the peripheral portion maintains a characteristic storiform growth pattern, and other features that are seen in the usual form of benign fibrous histiocytoma such as peripherally entrapped dense collagen bundles. *Calcifying (juvenile) aponeurotic fibroma* has a strong predilection for the palmar region of pediatric patients, but on rare occasions this lesion may be encountered in adults. Although fibromatosis-like areas are characteristically found, this lesion is also characterized by small foci of cords of epithelioid fibroblasts and distinctive chondroid nodules that frequently calcify. Finally, although *monophasic fibrous synovial sarcoma* can present as a mass in the hands or feet, it is composed of plumper spindled to epithelioid cells, frequently a hemangiopericytoma-like vascular pattern, stromal microcalcifications, immunoreactivity for cytokeratins and evidence of a t(X;18).

Treatment

Surgical extirpation remains the treatment of choice in patients with severe flexion contractures that impair normal hand function. Fasciotomy (subcutaneous division of the fibrous bands) leads to good immediate improvement of contractures of the metacarpophalangeal joints. This procedure has no effect on the progression of the disease, as it affects the proximal interphalangeal joint; thus long-term results are only marginal.[33] Furthermore, this procedure may result in injury to the digital arteries or nerves. More extensive surgical procedures, including wide or radical fasciectomy or dermofasciectomy, are usually advocated due to the lower risk of local recurrence.[34] The latter technique has been advocated for cases of recurrent Dupuytren's contracture requiring reoperation and as a primary procedure when there is significant skin involvement.[35] Potential nonsurgical therapies include the use of collagenase,[36] triamcinolone acetonide,[37] with variable success. Radiologic evaluation, particularly with magnetic resonance imaging (MRI), may be useful for determining the extent of the disease process, thereby facilitating the most appropriate surgical therapy.[38]

Discussion

The pathogenesis of palmar fibromatosis is multifactorial. It has been well established that there is a genetic component. Ling found that 68% of 50 index cases had a family history of the disease.[39] The presence of Dupuytren's contractures in identical twins has also been reported.[40] Lyall argued that an appropriate genetic background is inadequate by itself for the development of this disease; he reported two pairs of identical twins, in each of which only one twin had evidence of palmar fibromatosis.[40]

In addition to a genetic predisposition, other factors have been implicated, including trauma and microtrauma. Dupuytren himself suggested that repetitive minor trauma may be the major causative factor in this disease. Due to claims for compensation from patients with Dupuytren's contractures that the patients believed to be due to work injuries, Herzog undertook a review of the literature of over 1000 steelworkers, miners and clerks in 1951.[41] No significant difference was found in the prevalence of this disease between the different groups. Nevertheless, numerous case reports have implicated trauma as an etiologic factor. Furthermore, Liss and Stock reviewed 10 previously published studies and found good support for an association between hand vibration exposure and development of palmar fibromatosis.[42]

Kischer and Speer proposed that microvascular changes are a major etiologic factor in the development of palmar fibromatosis and other fibrosing lesions.[43] These authors observed microvascular occlusion in and around areas involved by the fibromatosis and proposed that hypoxia stimulates the excessive collagen production, possibly through generation of oxygen-free radicals. Such a hypothesis would be attractive for linking hyperlipidemia, diabetes mellitus, and cigarette smoking, all of which affect the microvasculature.

Finally, some have proposed an immunologic basis for this disease. Several studies have found circulating serum antibodies to collagen in some patients with palmar fibromatosis,[44] and others have found an increased prevalence of HLA-DR3,[45] a major histocompatibility complex class II antigen that is associated with autoimmune diseases. Although inflammation is usually not a conspicuous component of this disease, most of the inflammatory cells present are CD3+ lymphocytes and express HLA-DR antigen, suggesting a T cell-mediated autoimmune disorder.[46]

PLANTAR FIBROMATOSIS

Plantar fibromatosis, sometimes referred to as *Ledderhose's disease*, is characterized by a nodular fibrous proliferation arising within the plantar aponeurosis, usually in non-weight-bearing areas. Although Dupuytren recognized that a process similar to that occurring with palmar aponeurosis could involve plantar aponeurosis, it was Madelung who reported the first isolated case of plantar fibromatosis in 1875,[47] described in more detail by Ledderhose in 1897.[48] This condition appears to occur much less frequently than its palmar counterpart, but since it rarely produces a contracture and often has few if any symptoms, it is probably less frequently brought to the attention of physicians.[5,49]

Clinical findings

Like palmar fibromatosis, its incidence increases progressively with advancing age, although there is a much higher incidence in children and young persons. In the recent large study by Fetsch and colleagues, almost 44%

of 501 patients with plantar fibromatosis reviewed at the AFIP were 30 years of age or less.[5] In this same study of 56 cases of palmar or plantar fibromatosis in children and pre-adolescents, only 2 patients had palmar lesions. Overall, plantar fibromatosis affects males and females with similar frequency, but there is a striking female predilection in pediatric cases.[5] Approximately 30–35% of cases are bilateral, and in such cases, the lesions are usually metachronous with one lesion preceding the other by an interval of 2–7 years.[50]

Not infrequently, palmar and plantar fibromatoses affect the same patient, but the two lesions rarely occur at the same time; usually one precedes the other by 5–10 years. The association with penile fibromatosis (Peyronie's disease) is much less common. In a review of the literature by Pickren et al.,[51] only 1 of 104 patients with plantar fibromatosis had penile fibromatosis. Coexistence with dorsal knuckle pads has also been noted in up to 42% of cases.[52] Like palmar fibromatosis, this disease appears to be more common among epileptics, diabetics, alcoholics with liver disease and those with keloids. Fetsch and colleagues noted an apparent association with fifth finger clinodactyly, a finding in 3 of 23 (13%) patients with pediatric plantar fibromatosis.[5]

The lesion first appears as a single, firm subcutaneous thickening or nodule that adheres to the skin and is typically located in the medial plantar arch from the region of the navicular bone to the base of the first metatarsal.[5,53] It may be entirely asymptomatic but not infrequently causes mild pain after prolonged standing or walking.[54] Rarely, paresthesia of the distal portion of the sole of the foot and the undersurface of one or more toes may result when there is entrapment of the superficial plantar nerve.[55] Unlike its palmar counterpart, plantar fibromatosis only exceptionally results in contraction of the toes, presumably because the distal extensions of the plantar aponeurosis to the toes are much less well developed than in the hand. In patients with symptoms, plantar fibromatosis is often biopsied or excised at an earlier, more cellular stage than palmar fibromatosis and may cause serious diagnostic concern that a sarcoma is present, particularly fibrosarcoma.

Pathologic findings

Grossly and microscopically, the lesions are virtually indistinguishable from those found with palmar fibromatosis, although they are less often multinodular and only rarely contain the thick cords of fibrocollagenous tissue extending distally from the nodular growth (Fig. 9–6). Many of the lesions are highly cellular, but the cells lack nuclear hyperchromasia or pleomorphism and have small, pinpoint nucleoli (Figs 9–7, 9–8). Mitotic figures may also be identified but are few in number and are not atypical. Occasionally, one encounters mild perivascular chronic inflammation and deposits of hemosiderin; and in scattered lesions of long duration, focal chondroid or osseous metaplasia may be present.[56] Multinucleated giant cells are also a consistent but frequently overlooked feature.[5,57]

Immunohistochemically, as with palmar fibromatosis, this lesion is characterized by cells that stain for vimentin and in many cases for smooth muscle actin, indicating focal myofibroblastic differentiation. In addition, many of the growth factors identified in cases of palmar fibromatosis are also present in the plantar lesions and likely play an important role in stimulating collagen production by fibroblasts.[58,59]

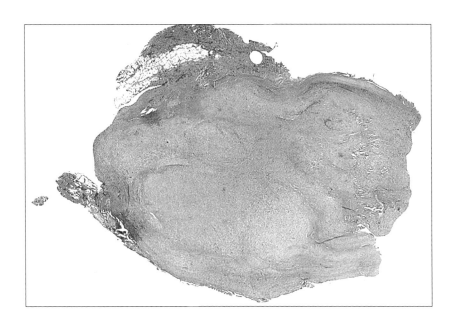

FIGURE 9–6 Plantar fibromatosis showing the characteristic nodular growth pattern.

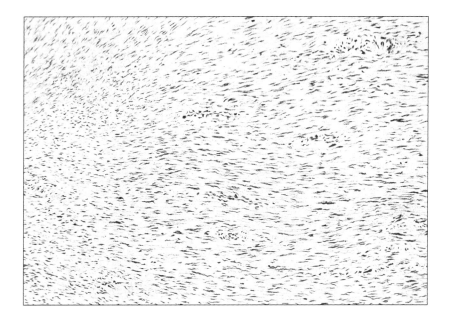

FIGURE 9–7 Plantar fibromatosis composed of uniform spindle-shaped cells arranged in long fascicles.

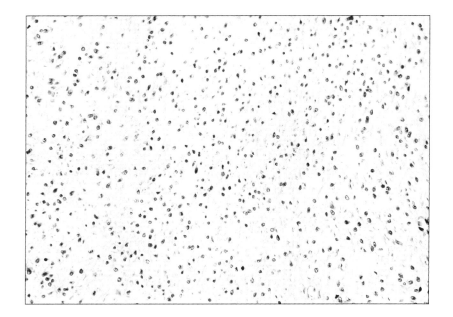

FIGURE 9–8 Plantar fibromatosis. Round-cell pattern caused by cross-section of spindle-shaped fibroblasts.

The differential diagnosis is similar to that described for palmar fibromatosis, but most commonly is restricted to *fibrosarcoma*. Although well-documented cases of fibrosarcoma in the foot have been reported, they are exceedingly rare and histologically are characterized by more hyperchromatic nuclei that show more nuclear pleomorphism and a higher degree of mitotic activity than that found with plantar fibromatosis.

Treatment

In most cases, surgical therapy is not required unless the nodules cause discomfort or disability. Although intra-lesional steroid injections have been effective in some cases,[60] surgical excision is the treatment of choice. Radiologic evaluation, particularly with MRI, may be useful for determining the extent of the disease process, thereby facilitating the most appropriate surgical therapy.[61,62] Simple excision of the lesion is associated with a high rate of local recurrence.[63] Complete fasciectomy, with or without skin grafting, is associated with a much lower rate of recurrence.[64] Most lesions recur less than 1 year after initial excision. There appears to be an increased risk of local recurrence in patients with multiple nodules, bilateral lesions, a positive family history, and those who develop a postoperative neuroma.[63,65]

Discussion

The etiology of plantar fibromatosis, like palmar fibromatosis, is probably multifactorial; and there seems to be a genetic predisposition. Like its palmar counterpart, cytogenetic aberrations have been reported in these lesions, including trisomies of chromosomes 8 and 14.[32,66] Trauma has frequently been considered an important factor in the pathogenesis of this disease. Certainly, the sole of the foot suffers a great variety of minor injuries over the years, and it is not surprising that a history of trauma can be elicited in many cases. There does not appear to be any occupational predilection, and most of these lesions arise in the medial portion of the plantar arch, an area least exposed to traumatic injury. The coexistence of the disease with epilepsy, diabetes, and alcohol-induced liver disease makes it likely that factors other than trauma are etiologically important.

PENILE FIBROMATOSIS (PEYRONIE'S DISEASE)

Although François de la Peyronie is generally credited with describing the disease that bears his name,[67] descriptions of this disease date back at least as far as the mid-sixteenth century.[68] It is considered a superficial form of fibromatosis that results in an ill-defined fibrous thickening or plaque-like mass in the shaft of the penis, frequently resulting in curvature of the erect penis. Despite numerous studies of the disease, its exact cause and pathogenesis are still unknown.

Clinical findings

Although once considered rare, this condition is clearly more common than previously believed. For example, in a study by Mulhall and colleagues, Peyronie's disease was found in 8.9% of men who were being screened for prostate cancer in the United States.[69] It is seen primarily in men 45–60 years of age; it rarely affects young adults, and there are no reports of cases in children. Most patients are white; the disease very rarely affects blacks or Orientals.[70,71]

The main complaint is a palpable plaque-like induration typically located on the dorsal or lateral aspect of the shaft of the penis causing the penis to curve toward the affected side. This curvature is the result of the relatively inelastic plaque-like scar tissue in the normally compliant tunica albuginea of the erectile body of the penis. It restricts expansion of the involved aspect of the penis during tumescence, limiting the extension of that segment of the penile shaft and causing the erection to be bent.[72] Associated symptoms include pain on erection and painful intercourse. Some patients who have penile curvature may have difficulty achieving an erection, presumably because the plaque-like induration impairs the veno-occlusive function of the tunica albuginea.

Penile fibromatosis is more common in patients with palmar and plantar fibromatosis than in the general population; its incidence varies from 2% to 4% in palmar fibromatosis and from 1% to 2% in plantar fibromatosis. There is also an increased incidence in epileptic and diabetic patients.[73] There have also been reports of an association between penile fibromatosis and Cogan syndrome (a vasculitis characterized by interstitial keratitis and vestibuloauditory symptoms[74]) Paget's disease of bone[75] and carcinoid syndrome.[76]

Gross findings

The fibrous mass chiefly involves fascial structures, corpus cavernosum, and rarely corpus spongiosum. It consists of dense, pearly white to gray-brown tissue that glistens on section; it averages 2 cm in greatest dimension.

Microscopic findings

There are relatively few descriptions of the pathologic features of Peyronie's disease. The most consistent histologic abnormality is the irregular orientation and character of the collagen within the tunica albuginea.[77] There is an increased number of cytologically bland fibroblasts associated with haphazardly arranged collagen bands, irregular collagen plates, or nodules (Fig. 9–9). There is also a marked reduction of elastic fibers in affected areas as demonstrated by elastic stains. Fibrin may or may not be present. Inflammatory cells, particularly lymphocytes and plasma cells, may be present in early lesions, predominantly in a perivascular location, both within and external to the tunica albuginea.[77] As the lesions persist, there tends to be a decrease in the amount of chronic inflammation with a progressive increase in the amount of fibrosis, often with focal calcification or ossification. Metaplastic cartilage has also been described.[78] It is important to be aware that penile epithelioid sarcoma may clinically mimic Peyronie's disease,[79] but the cells of epithelioid sarcoma are cytologically atypical and have densely eosinophilic cytoplasm.

Treatment

The optimal therapy for Peyronie's disease remains unresolved. Many nonsurgical therapies have been attempted, including vitamin E, potassium amino benzoate, colchicine, intralesional injections of corticosteroids, calcium channel blockers, shockwave therapy and collagenase, all with limited success.[80] Surgery appears to be the most effective treatment, although the best surgical technique is controversial.[81,82] Surgical candidates include patients who have erectile dysfunction and those whose penile curvature precludes intercourse. Straightening the penis

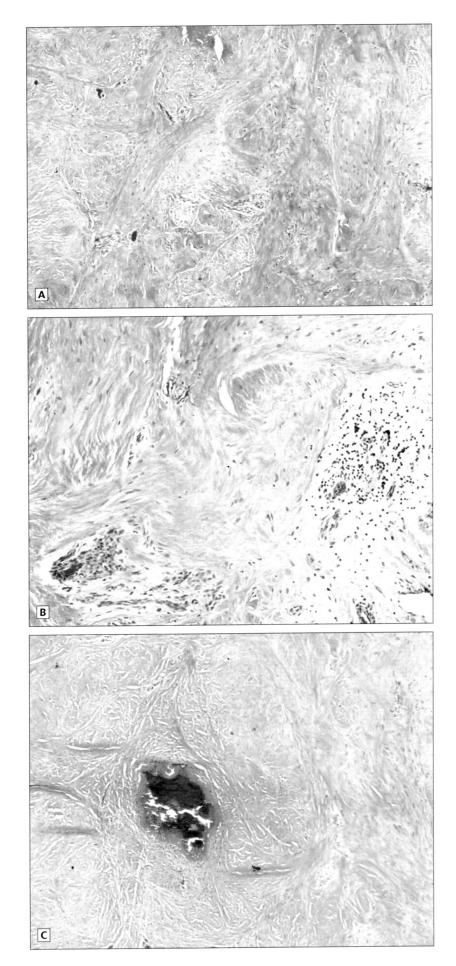

FIGURE 9–9 (A) Low magnification view of Peyronie's disease. The lesion is hypocellular and extensively hyalinized. **(B)** High-magnification view of hypocellular area of Peyronie's disease. A peripheral rim of lymphocytes is seen. **(C)** Focus of osseous metaplasia in Peyronie's disease.

usually requires at least partial excision of the plaque with surgery or laser therapy, coupled with some type of grafting procedure.[83,84] There is a significant rate of postoperative erectile dysfunction, so some patients also require placement of a penile prosthesis.[85] Given that about one-third of patients who remain untreated have spontaneous resolution of their symptoms, many urologists choose to observe these patients for a period of time before embarking on definitive therapy.

Discussion

The exact cause of Peyronie's disease is not clear. As with palmar and plantar fibromatoses, a genetic component has been suggested, perhaps requiring some environmental trigger. An inflammatory/infectious etiology was originally proposed, but more recent evidence makes an infectious etiology highly unlikely. There is evidence to support an autoimmune etiology, as this disease has been associated with several HLA tissue types, particularly HLA-DQ5.[86] Ralph and co-workers found that patients with early Peyronie's disease had immunoglobulin M (IgM) antibody deposition and a marked T-lymphocytic infiltrate with increased expression of HLA class II antigens.[87]

Trauma may also be an important etiologic factor. Devine et al. suggested that repetitive microvascular injury results in the deposition of fibrin followed by fibroblast activation and proliferation and subsequent collagen deposition.[88] Genes involved in collagen synthesis and myofibroblastic differentiation have also been found to be upregulated in this disease.[89] Interestingly, gene expression analysis has revealed a similar pattern of gene up- and down-regulation to that of palmar fibromatoses.[90]

Recently, an animal model for Peyronie's disease has been developed. Inducible nitric oxide synthetase (iNOS) has been shown to be up-regulated, while constitutive (endothelial) nitric oxide synthetase (eNOS) expression is down-regulated.[91] The exact role of nitric oxide synthetase in the pathophysiology of Peyronie's disease has yet to be fully elucidated, but it is likely to induce the production of reactive oxygen species and collagen deposition.[92,93] It is possible that Peyronie's disease does not represent a single distinct entity but a common morphologic appearance that occurs secondary to a variety of insults.

KNUCKLE PADS

Knuckle pads are flat or dome-shaped noninflammatory fibrous thickenings that occur on the dorsal aspect of the proximal interphalangeal or metacarpophalangeal joints and the paratenon of the extensor tendons (Fig. 9–10).[11] Most patients are asymptomatic, although some have mild tenderness or pain; the lesions rarely require surgical intervention. Knuckle pads comprise another fibrous proliferation not infrequently encountered in conjunction with palmar or plantar fibromatosis.[5,94] The knuckle pads may precede the onset of palmar or plantar fibromatosis and may disappear spontaneously after these lesions are excised. Like palmar and plantar fibromatoses, the knuckle pad chiefly affects patients during the fourth, fifth, and sixth decades of life and is observed more commonly in men than in women. *Pachydermodactyly* is a rare variant of this condition that occurs mainly in adolescent boys.[95] Microscopically, knuckle pads resemble palmar fibromatosis, but digital contractures do not occur. Grossly, knuckle pads may be confused with pad-like hyperkeratoses that occur secondary to occupational trauma (e.g., boxing) or self-manipulation.[96,97]

Bart-Pumphrey syndrome is an autosomal dominant disorder characterized by sensorineural hearing loss, palmoplantar keratoderma, leukonychia and knuckle pads, although there is considerable phenotypic variability.[98] Recently, this disorder has been associated with missense mutations in the *GJB2* gene, which encodes for a gap junction protein, connexin-26.[99] However, abnormalities of this gene have not been found in other superficial fibromatoses.

DEEP FIBROMATOSES

These lesions, whether they arise from the abdominal wall, mesentery or other extra-abdominal locations, share overlapping clinical, morphologic, immunohistochemical and molecular genetic features, although there are attributes which are unique to each. This discussion will focus on those features that are shared by the deep fibromatoses, as well as elaborate on those features which distinguish these entities from one another.

EXTRA-ABDOMINAL FIBROMATOSIS

Extra-abdominal fibromatosis arises principally from the connective tissue of muscle and the overlying fascia or aponeurosis (*musculoaponeurotic fibromatosis*); it chiefly affects the muscles of the shoulder, pelvic girdle and thigh of adolescents and young adults. Other terms used to describe this condition include *extra-abdominal desmoid, desmoid tumor, well-differentiated nonmetastasizing fibrosarcoma* or *grade 1 fibrosarcoma*. The term *aggressive fibromatosis* is often employed to emphasize its frequently aggressive behavior.

Extra-abdominal fibromatosis is one of the more common soft tissue lesions encountered by pathologists. Despite its relatively common occurrence, this tumor continues to present a problem in recognition and management, especially because of the striking discrepancy

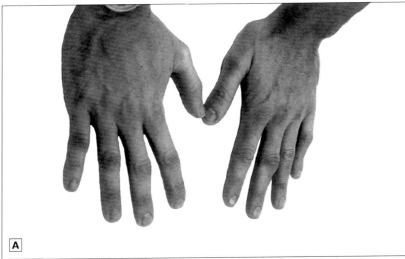

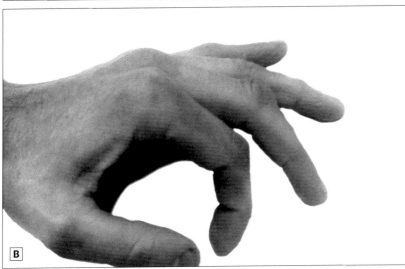

FIGURE 9-10 (A) Knuckle pads is a lesion marked by fibrous thickening over the extensor surfaces of the interphalangeal joints. It may be associated with both palmar and plantar fibromatosis. **(B)** Side view of knuckle pads.

between its deceptively bland microscopic appearance and its propensity to recur locally and infiltrate neighboring soft tissues.

Clinical findings

Extra-abdominal fibromatosis is most common in patients between puberty and 40 years of age, with a peak incidence between the ages of 25 and 35 years. Children are uncommonly affected; in the series by Rock et al., only 5% of the patients were 10 years of age or less, the youngest being 9 months old.[100] Women are more commonly affected than men.[101–103] In a study of 89 cases of "desmoid tumor" by Reitamo and colleagues, four major age groups were delineated where the site of the tumor, the gender of the patient, or both were nonrandomly distributed.[104] "Juvenile" tumors occurred predominantly in an extra-abdominal location, with a distinct predilection for girls younger than 15 years of age. "Fertile" tumors occurred nearly exclusively as abdominal tumors in fertile females. "Menopausal" tumors occurred predominantly in the

abdomen, with an approximately equal gender distribution. "Senescent" tumors were equally distributed between abdominal and extra-abdominal locations and showed no gender predilection.

Most patients present with a deeply situated, firm, poorly circumscribed mass that has grown insidiously and causes little or no pain. Decreased mobility of an adjacent joint may occur. Neurologic symptoms, including numbness, tingling, a "stabbing" or "shooting" pain, or motor weakness, may occur when the lesion compresses nearby nerves.

Radiographically, the lesion appears as a soft tissue mass that interrupts the adjacent intermuscular and soft tissue planes; it may encroach on adjacent bone, resulting in pressure erosion or superficial cortical defects. Up to 80% of affected patients have multiple minor bony anomalies of the mandible, chest, and long bones including cortical thickening, exostoses, and areas of cystic translucence or compact islands in the femur (or both).[105] As with other soft tissue tumors, computed tomography (CT) scans and MRI are helpful in the diagnosis and assessment of tumor extent prior to surgery. Pritchard et al. found a lower local recurrence rate after the introduction of these improved imaging techniques compared to the recurrence rate prior to their routine use.[102]

Anatomic location

The principal site of extra-abdominal fibromatosis is the musculature of the shoulder, followed by the chest wall and back, thigh, and head and neck (Table 9–2).

In the shoulder and neck region, the growth presents most often in the deltoid, scapular region, supraclavicular fossa, or posterior cervical triangle where it may extend into the anterior or posterior portion of the axilla and upper arm. Because of the numerous vital structures at this site, including nerves of the brachial plexus and large vessels, complete surgical excision of tumors in this location is often difficult if not impossible.

Fibromatoses in the region of the pelvic girdle primarily affect the gluteus muscle, whereas those in the region of the thigh affect the quadriceps muscle and muscles of the popliteal fossa. The hands and feet are rarely affected.[100]

The head and neck is not an unusual location for these lesions. As many as 23% of all extra-abdominal fibromatoses occur in this location.[106] In children, more than one-third of extra-abdominal fibromatoses are located in the head and neck.[107] The soft tissue of the neck is most commonly involved, followed by the face, oral cavity, scalp, paranasal sinuses, and orbit.[107] Clinically, fibromatoses arising in the head and neck are more aggressive than extra-abdominal fibromatoses arising elsewhere and are capable of massive destruction of adjacent bone and erosion of the base of the skull; they occasionally encroach on the trachea, sometimes with a fatal outcome.[107]

Fibromatosis of the breast may arise in the mammary gland or from extension of a lesion arising in the aponeu-rosis of the chest wall or shoulder girdle.[103,108,109] The differential diagnosis in this location includes metaplastic carcinoma, fibrosarcoma, and benign reactive processes such as nodular fasciitis and keloid.

Multicentric fibromatoses

Extra-abdominal fibromatoses are not infrequently multicentric.[110-113] Fong et al. found almost 5% of these lesions to be multicentric, typically involving one anatomic region of the body.[114] In most cases the second growth develops proximal to the primary lesion. Rarely, coexistence of abdominal and extra-abdominal fibromatoses has been observed in the same patient.[115]

Gross findings

The tumor is almost always confined to the musculature and the overlying aponeurosis or fascia. Large tumors may extend along the fascial plane or infiltrate the overlying subcutaneous tissue. Occasional lesions involve the periosteum and may lead to bone erosion, thereby closely resembling desmoplastic fibroma of bone.[116]

Most tumors measure 5–10 cm in greatest dimension, although lesions as large as 20 cm have been reported. The tumor is firm, cuts with a gritty sensation, and on cross-section reveals a glistening white, coarsely trabeculated surface resembling scar tissue (Figs 9–11, 9–12). Surgeons may have particular difficulty distinguishing recurrent fibromatosis from scar tissue related to prior excision.

Microscopic findings

Characteristically, the lesion is poorly circumscribed and infiltrates the surrounding tissue, usually striated musculature (Fig. 9–13). The proliferation consists of elongated,

TABLE 9–2	ANATOMIC DISTRIBUTION OF 367 CASES OF EXTRA-ABDOMINAL (DESMOID) FIBROMATOSIS	
Anatomic site	**No. of patients**	**%**
Head	7	1.9
Neck	28	7.6
Shoulder	81	22.1
Upper arm	21	5.7
Forearm	13	3.5
Hand	4	1.1
Chest wall; back	63	17.2
Mesentery	38	10.4
Buttock; hip	21	5.7
Thigh	46	12.5
Knee	27	7.4
Lower leg	17	4.6
Foot	1	0.3
Total	367	100.0

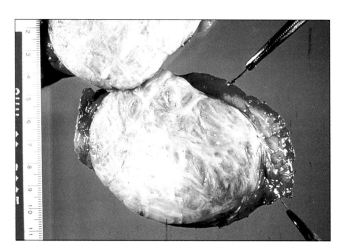

FIGURE 9–11 Extra-abdominal fibromatosis (desmoid tumor) involving the chest wall. The cut surface reveals a trabecular appearance reminiscent of that seen in uterine leiomyomas.

slender, spindle-shaped cells of uniform appearance surrounded and separated from one another by abundant collagen, with little or no cell-to-cell contact (Fig. 9–14). The cells lack nuclear hyperchromasia, but the cellularity varies from area to area. The constituent nuclei are small, pale-staining, and sharply defined, with one to three minute nucleoli (Figs 9–15, 9–16, 9–17). Clearly defined cellular boundaries can be discerned only in cases with a prominent myxoid matrix and relatively small amounts of collagen (Fig. 9–18).[117]

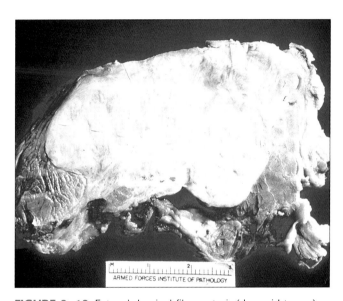

FIGURE 9–12 Extra-abdominal fibromatosis (desmoid tumor) involving the pectoralis muscle.

Cells and collagen fibers are usually arranged in sweeping bundles that are less well defined than those of fibrosarcoma. Glassy keloid-like collagen fibers or extensive hyalinization may be present and may obscure the basic pattern of the lesion (Fig. 9–19). At the periphery of the growth where the tumor has infiltrated muscle tissue, remnants of striated muscle fibers are frequently entrapped and undergo atrophy or form multinucleated giant cells that may be mistaken for malignancy (Fig. 9–20). Microhemorrhages and focal aggregates of lymphocytes are common. In rare instances there is calcification or chondroid or osseous metaplasia, but this is never a prominent feature of the tumor.

Immunohistochemical and ultrastructural findings

Immunohistochemically, the spindle cells stain with vimentin, smooth muscle actin and muscle-specific actin, consistent with fibroblastic/myofibroblastic differentiation. Rare cases also stain with antibodies to desmin. Inasmuch as virtually all deep fibromatoses have somatic β-catenin or adenomatous polyposis coli (*APC*) gene mutations leading to intranuclear accumulation of β-catenin, virtually all fibromatoses have diffuse β-catenin nuclear staining (Fig. 9–21).[118]

Ultrastructurally, musculoaponeurotic fibromatosis consists of a uniform population of elongated fibroblast-like cells often terminating in long, slender processes. Most nuclei are rounded or oval, but some cells show prominent nuclear indentations or clefts. There is a prominent rough endoplasmic reticulum that is partly dilated and contains granular or fibrillary material within

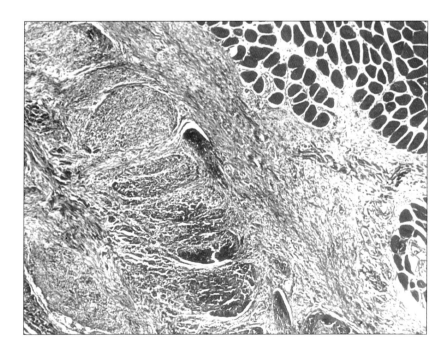

FIGURE 9–13 Extra-abdominal fibromatosis (extra-abdominal desmoid) invading striated muscle tissue.

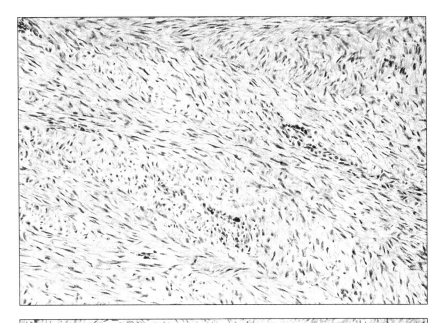

FIGURE 9–14 Interlacing bundles of fibroblasts separated by variable amounts of collagen in extra-abdominal fibromatosis.

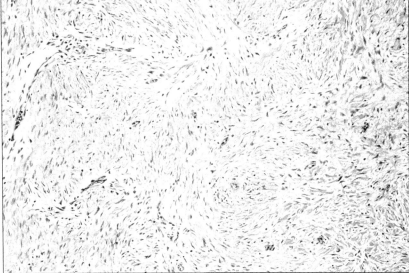

FIGURE 9–15 Extra-abdominal fibromatosis in which the cells are arranged in a focal storiform growth pattern.

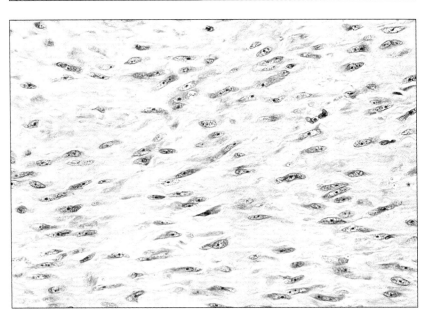

FIGURE 9–16 High-power view of extra-abdominal fibromatosis showing vesicular nuclei with minute nucleoli, rather indistinct cytoplasm, and interstitial collagen.

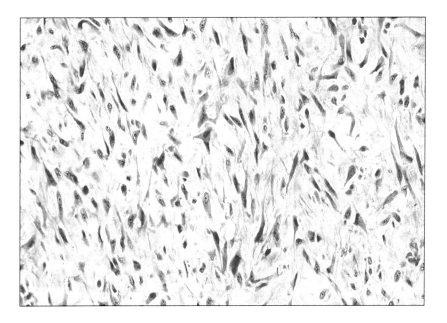

FIGURE 9–17 Stellate-shaped cells with uniform cytologic features in extra-abdominal fibromatosis.

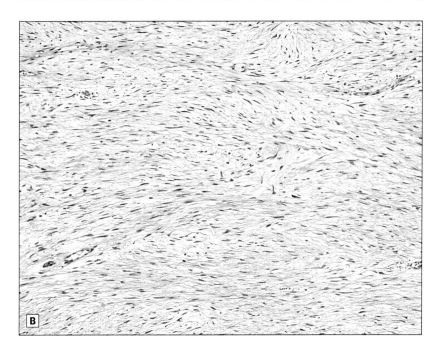

FIGURE 9–18 (A) Extra-abdominal fibromatosis with a partially myxoid matrix. Regularly distributed blood vessels are conspicuous. **(B)** High-magnification view of extra-abdominal fibromatosis with bland-appearing spindled cells arranged into short intersecting fascicles.

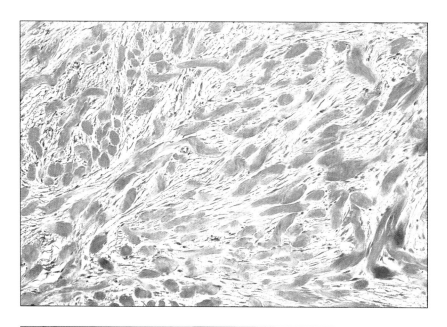

FIGURE 9–19 Fibromatosis with glassy hyalinized collagen fibers reminiscent of keloid, a rare feature of this tumor.

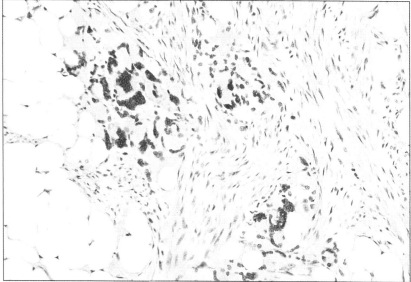

FIGURE 9–20 Peripheral portion of extra-abdominal fibromatosis with entrapped muscle giant cells.

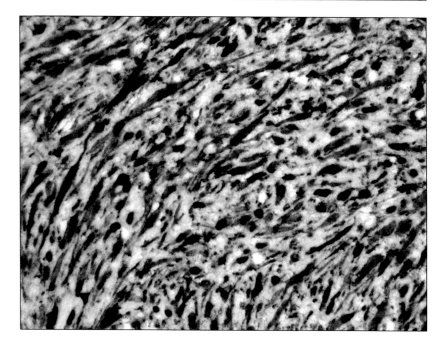

FIGURE 9–21 Nuclear beta-catenin immunoreactivity in an extra-abdominal fibromatosis.

the dilated spaces. The cytoplasm has a small number of mitochondria, a prominent Golgi apparatus, free ribosomes, and occasional pinocytotic vesicles and microtubules (Fig. 9–22). Some cells contain intracytoplasmic bundles of actin-type microfilaments measuring about 60 nm in diameter, often with areas of condensation (dense bodies).[119] Some cells contain incomplete or clumped basal lamina along the cell borders, all features characteristic of myofibroblasts. Intranuclear inclusions of collagen may be seen.[119] The stroma contains considerable amounts of collagen and ground substance.

Differential diagnosis

Fibromatosis most closely resembles fibrosarcoma on the one extreme and reactive fibrosis on the other. *Fibrosarcoma* is more uniformly cellular than fibromatosis, and the cells are arranged in a more consistent sweeping fascicular (herringbone) growth pattern. Unlike fibromatosis, the cells are often overlapping and separated by less collagen. The nuclei are more hyperchromatic and atypical and have more prominent nucleoli than those found in fibromatosis. Although it is important to remember that there can be considerable overlap in levels of mitotic activity between fibromatosis and well-differentiated fibrosarcoma, high mitotic counts (>1 per 10 high-power fields [HPF]) throughout a tumor should arouse suspicion of fibrosarcoma. A small biopsy specimen may lead

to a misdiagnosis, as some examples of fibrosarcoma have areas that are indistinguishable from fibromatosis and vice versa.

Fibromatosis can also be difficult to distinguish from *reactive fibroblastic/myofibroblastic proliferations* following injuries such as trauma, minor muscle tear, or intramuscular injection. Cytologically, these reactive proliferations are composed of cells indistinguishable from those found in fibromatosis. The low-magnification appearance is more useful for distinguishing these two entities since reactive processes have a more variable growth pattern and frequently have focal hemorrhage or hemosiderin deposition, often situated along vascular structures. In some cases iron stains are useful for highlighting hemosiderin that is difficult to identify on hematoxylin and eosin-stained sections. In addition, an infiltrative growth pattern is much more characteristic of fibromatosis.

Desmoplastic fibroma of bone is indistinguishable from fibromatosis, especially when it presents as a soft tissue mass after breaking through the thinned or expanded cortex of the involved bone.[120,121] This lesion predominates in the metaphyseal or diaphyseal portions of long bones (e.g., the femur) or in the jaw, and radiographic studies are essential for distinguishing between these histologically similar lesions.

Confusion with *myxoma* is possible, particularly if only a small amount of tissue (or needle biopsy) is available for examination. Myxoma is usually paucicellular, with

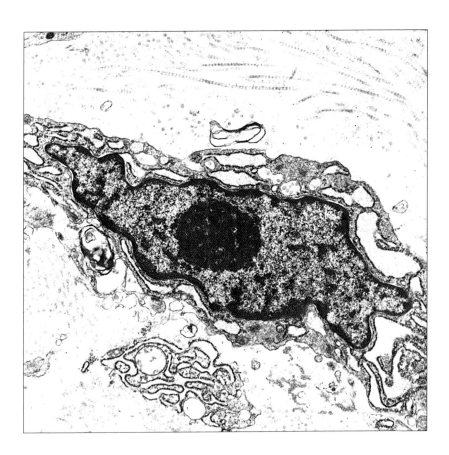

FIGURE 9–22 Fibroblast from typical extraabdominal fibromatosis. Note the prominent rough endoplasmic reticulum and mature collagen fibrils in the extracellular space. (From Taxy JB, Battifora H. The electron microscope in the study and diagnosis of soft tissue tumors. In: Trump BF, Jones RT, eds. Diagnostic electron microscopy. New York: Wiley; 1980.)

the cells separated from one another by abundant myxoid matrix. In contrast, fibromatosis always displays a greater degree of cellularity and more interstitial collagen than myxoma.

Fibrosarcomatous transformation of fibromatosis is exceedingly rare. Soule and Scanlon described and illustrated a case of typical fibromatosis of the inguinal region that evolved into a fibrosarcoma 10 years after initial excision and 9 years after radiotherapy.[1] Mooney et al. reported a case of metastasizing fibrosarcoma of the thigh that appeared 28 years after excision of a fibromatosis from the same region.[122] Following review of the slides from this reported case, Allen thought that the cells from the initial excision had too much nuclear hyperchromasia and atypia for fibromatosis and believed the lesion was a low-grade fibrosarcoma at the time of initial excision.[123] He went on to state that, "In my experience, all cases of metastasizing 'desmoid tumors' have proved to differ histologically from aggressive fibromatosis when the sections have been reviewed." Malignant transformation of fibromatosis may be erroneously suggested by occasional foci of increased cellularity and by exceptionally well-differentiated fibromatosis-like areas in some fibrosarcomas.

Clinical behavior

Despite its bland microscopic appearance, the tumor frequently behaves in an aggressive manner. Although incapable of metastasizing, extra-abdominal fibromatoses often recur; they can rarely cause death when they invade or compress a vital structure, such as occurs with tumors in the root of the neck and within the abdomen.[123] In most studies, the 5-year survival rate is better than 90%.[100,102]

The recurrence rate recorded in the literature is variable, ranging from as low as 19% to as high as 77%, with an average of approximately 40%.[101] In the study by Enzinger and Shiraki with a minimum 10 years of follow-up, 57% of tumors recurred.[117] In another large series of extra-abdominal desmoid tumors, Rock et al. found that 68% of patients experienced a recurrence an average 1.4 years after the initial treatment.[100] In a more recent study of 203 consecutive patients with extra-abdominal fibromatoses treated with surgery over a 35-year period at a single referral center, Gronchi and colleagues reported a local recurrence rate of 76% at 10 years.[124] Although tumor size was associated with risk of local recurrence, microscopically positive surgical margins did not predict recurrence risk, as one might anticipate. However, other studies have found the extent and adequacy of initial excision to be prognostically significant.[102,125,126]

Spontaneous regression of these tumors has been observed in sporadic cases, particularly in menarchal and menopausal patients. McDougall and McGarrity reported two cases of extra-abdominal fibromatoses that spontaneously regressed after menopause.[115] Enzinger and Shiraki reported a 36-year-old man with an extensive tumor involving the supraclavicular fossa, scalenus muscles, and brachial plexus that apparently resolved 9.5 years after the initial presentation.[117] A second patient, an elderly man with a large recurrent tumor of the axilla and chest wall, declined further treatment; 15 years later the tumor had substantially decreased in size and was no longer palpable.

Treatment

Because the microscopic picture does not reliably reflect the growth potential of the tumor, therapy is predicated on its extent and anatomic relations. Most authors recommend wide local excision unless there is a risk of significant compromise of function, as most studies have found a lower rate of recurrence when excision includes a wide margin of uninvolved structures around the grossly visible tumor. In view of the excellent prognosis for survival, amputation or other mutilating procedures should be done only for palliative purposes if the tumor recurs repeatedly and does not respond to adjuvant therapy or if the extent of the tumor or threat of complications leaves no other choice.

In situations where a wide local excision cannot be performed, postoperative radiation therapy seems to be indicated for primary tumors that are incompletely excised. Karakousis et al. reported local control in 96% of patients treated with surgical resection supplemented by postoperative radiation therapy.[127] Similarly, in an analysis of 54 patients who underwent surgery without prior radiation, compared to 35 patients who had postoperative radiation, Jelinek and co-workers found a 5-year local control rate of 81% for those who underwent radiation, compared to 53% for those treated with surgery alone.[128] Baliski and colleagues treated 13 patients with preoperative doxorubicin and radiotherapy, followed by resection 4 to 6 weeks later. Eleven of these patients remained free of disease for a median of 71 months following excision.[129] Very few other studies have evaluated neoadjuvant chemoradiotherapy.

As one might expect, imatinib mesylate (gleevec) therapy has been attempted in the salvage setting in patients with extra-abdominal fibromatoses.[130] In part, this is based upon some reports of KIT (CD117) immunoreactivity in some cases of fibromatosis.[131] However, we and others have found fibromatoses to be consistently negative for CD117, and these discrepancies likely are related to differences in antibodies and laboratory techniques.[132]

Cytotoxic and noncytotoxic drug therapy has also been attempted for the treatment of these tumors. Chemotherapeutic agents and nonsteroidal antiinflammatory prostaglandin-inhibiting drugs such as sudac and indometacin have been reported to cause stabilization or regression of both primary and recurrent tumors.[133] The efficacy of anti-estrogen therapy, including tamoxifen, progesterone, or the luteinizing hormone-releasing hormone analogue goserelin acetate is not fully established but appears to be promising.[134,135]

Discussion

Like other forms of fibromatosis, the etiology of extra-abdominal fibromatosis is probably multifactorial, as genetic, endocrine, and physical factors seem to play an important role in its pathogenesis. Features suggesting an underlying genetic basis are the occasional occurrence in siblings,[136] the presence of multiple bony abnormalities (in up to 80% of patients),[137] and the rare occurrence of extra-abdominal fibromatosis in patients with familial adenomatous polyposis (FAP),[138] described in greater detail below. In 1997, Lucas et al.[139] reported a uniform pattern of X chromosome inactivation, suggesting that this lesion is a true neoplasm. Subsequently, mutations of the APC/β-catenin pathway were identified in the majority of sporadic deep fibromatoses.[140-142]

Although clearly implicated in the development of abdominal fibromatosis (discussed below), endocrine factors may also play a role in the development and growth of extra-abdominal fibromatoses. Physical factors such as trauma or irradiation likely serve as a trigger mechanism, as examples of extra-abdominal fibromatosis have been reported in the chest wall following trauma[143] and reconstructive mammoplasty.[144] There have also been several reports of these lesions developing following radiation therapy for Hodgkin's disease.[145] Large studies of extra-abdominal fibromatosis have reported an antecedent history of trauma in 16–28% of cases.[102,105]

ABDOMINAL FIBROMATOSIS

Although abdominal fibromatosis is indistinguishable grossly and microscopically from extra-abdominal fibromatosis, it deserves separate consideration because of its characteristic location and its tendency to occur in women of childbearing age during or following pregnancy. The tumor arises from musculoaponeurotic structures of the abdominal wall, especially the rectus and internal oblique muscles and their fascial coverings.

Clinical findings

Abdominal fibromatosis occurs in young, gravid or parous women during gestation or, more frequently, during the first year following childbirth. Few cases have been reported in children of both genders (especially boys) and adult men. The relative frequency of abdominal and extra-abdominal desmoid tumors varies from one study to another. In a study carried out in Finland by Reitamo et al.,[104] abdominal fibromatoses (49%) outnumbered extra-abdominal (43%) and mesenteric (8%) fibromatoses. Most lesions are solitary, but patients with both abdominal and extra-abdominal fibromatoses have been described.[146]

Pathologic findings

The gross and microscopic appearances are virtually identical to those described for extra-abdominal fibromatosis, except that the average tumor is smaller and behaves less destructively than those in extra-abdominal locations. Most tumors measure 3–10 cm in greatest dimension, and when arising in the rectus muscle or its fascia, they usually remain at the site of origin and do not cross the abdominal midline.

Microscopically, these lesions are variably cellular and often predominantly hypocellular; they are composed of cells with normochromatic nuclei with small, pinpoint nucleoli. The cells lack nuclear pleomorphism, and only rare mitotic figures can be identified. Cells are arranged into ill-defined fascicles with dense collagen separating the individual tumor cells with infiltration of the surrounding muscle tissue.

Clinical behavior and therapy

As with all forms of fibromatosis, these lesions have a propensity to recur locally, although the rate of local recurrence (15–30%) is slightly lower than that of extra-abdominal fibromatosis (35–65%).[147,148] In most cases the lesions recur within the first 2 years after the initial excision or in connection with subsequent gestations or deliveries. Multiple recurrences are not uncommon. As with extra-abdominal fibromatosis, wide local excision with ample margins is the therapy of choice to limit the rate of local recurrence, and adjuvant radiation therapy may help achieve control of inoperable or recurrent tumors. There are relatively few data regarding the efficacy of cytotoxic and noncytotoxic agents.

Discussion

Like extra-abdominal fibromatosis, genetic, endocrine, and physical factors seem to play an important role in the development of these tumors. Some arise in the setting of FAP, often at the site of previous abdominal surgery.[149,150] Endocrine factors are clearly implicated by the frequent occurrence of this tumor during or after pregnancy, and there are reports of these tumors regressing with menopause.[151] Lipschutz and coworkers described the formation of desmoids in guinea pigs after prolonged estrogen administration and the prevention of these tumors by administration of testosterone, progesterone, and desoxycorticosterone.[152] The reported inhibitory effect of anti-estrogenic agents such as tamoxifen and raloxifene supports the role of hormonal factors in the development of this disease.[153]

Similar to extra-abdominal lesions, trauma may serve as a contributory cause, as some tumors have been reported to arise in the scars of radical nephrectomy sites,[154] the site of insertion of peritoneal dialysis catheters[155] and other abdominal operations (*cicatricial fibromatosis*). Because most patients with abdominal fibromatosis have no history of gross injury to this region, minor and undetected trauma such as minute muscle tears may conceivably serve as a contributing etiologic factor that triggers the fibrous growth in a hormonally or genetically predisposed individual.

INTRA-ABDOMINAL FIBROMATOSIS

The intra-abdominal fibromatoses are a group of closely related lesions (rather than a single entity) that pose similar problems for the histologic diagnosis but can be distinguished from one another by the clinical setting and location. This category includes pelvic fibromatoses and mesenteric fibromatoses, including those associated with FAP/Gardner syndrome.

Pelvic fibromatosis

Pelvic fibromatosis is a variant of abdominal fibromatosis, differing from the latter by its location in the iliac fossa and lower portion of the pelvis, where it manifests as a slowly growing palpable mass that is asymptomatic or causes only slight pain. Clinically, it is often mistaken for an ovarian neoplasm or a mesenteric cyst. Large tumors in this location may encroach on the urinary bladder, vagina, or rectum; or they may cause hydronephrosis or compress the iliac vessels.[156–158]

As with fibromatosis of the abdominal wall, the tumor arises from the aponeurosis or muscle tissue and occurs chiefly in young women 20–35 years of age; in most cases it is unrelated to gestation or childbirth. Grossly and microscopically, the tumor is indistinguishable from other forms of extra-abdominal or abdominal fibromatosis and requires similar modes of therapy.

Mesenteric fibromatosis

Fibromatosis is the most common primary tumor of the mesentery and accounts for approximately 8% of all fibromatoses. Although most cases are sporadic, some are associated with FAP/Gardner syndrome, trauma, or hyperestrogenic states. Most commonly, these tumors are located in the mesentery of the small bowel, but some originate from the ileocolic mesentery, gastrocolic ligament, omentum, or retroperitoneum. In the absence of a history of FAP, distinguishing this lesion from other fibrosing processes that occur in this location such as idiopathic retroperitoneal fibrosis or sclerosing mesenteritis, may be difficult, especially if the biopsy specimen is limited. Although several studies have focused on the distinction between mesenteric fibromatosis and gastrointestinal stromal tumor (GIST), the distinction is typically not difficult if one has some experience with both entities (see below).

As with pelvic fibromatosis, most patients present with an asymptomatic abdominal mass, although some have mild abdominal pain. Less commonly, patients present with gastrointestinal bleeding or an acute abdomen secondary to bowel perforation. Occasionally, the tumor is found incidentally at laparotomy performed for some other reason, including patients undergoing bowel resection for FAP.[159] Data on age and gender vary: in the largest series reported to date of 82 cases of mesenteric fibromatosis, Burke et al.[160] noted that the tumor was more commonly encountered in males and the mean age was 41 years.

Like many other neoplasms in the abdomen and retroperitoneum, most mesenteric fibromatoses are quite large at the time of excision, with the majority measuring 10 cm or more. Many have an initial phase of rapid growth; and complications may be caused by compression of the ureter, development of a ureteral fistula, or compression of the small or large intestines, sometimes complicated by intestinal perforation.[159–161] Grossly, most lesions are fairly well circumscribed, but like other forms of fibromatosis, there is microscopic infiltration into the surrounding soft tissues, including the bowel wall.

Microscopically, the lesions are composed of cytologically bland spindle-shaped or stellate cells evenly deposited in a densely collagenous stroma. Typically, there is variable cellularity, with some areas showing almost complete replacement by dense fibrous tissue. In others, the stroma shows marked myxoid change. Scattered keloid-type collagen fibers may be present, as are prominent dilated thin-walled veins and muscular hyperplasia of small arteries. Nodular lymphoid aggregates may be present at the advancing edge of the tumor.

The differential diagnosis includes *sclerosing (retractile) mesenteritis*, a lesion that appears to be related to *mesenteric panniculitis* and *mesenteric lipodystrophy*.[162] Like mesenteric fibromatosis, sclerosing mesenteritis typically involves the small bowel mesentery and presents as a solitary large mass, although multiple lesions or diffuse mesenteric thickening may also be seen. Histologically, sclerosing mesenteritis is composed of variable amounts of fibrosis, chronic inflammation and fat necrosis. Any of these three components may predominate in a given lesion. In difficult cases, immunohistochemical staining for β-catenin can be useful, since mesenteric fibromatosis consistently shows strong nuclear β-catenin staining, whereas sclerosing mesenteritis does not express this antigen (Table 9–3).[163]

TABLE 9–3	IMMUNOPHENOTYPIC FEATURES OF MESENTERIC FIBROMATOSIS COMPARED TO GASTROINTESTINAL STROMAL TUMOR AND SCLEROSING MESENTERITIS		
	GIST	Sclerosing mesenteritis	Mesenteric fibromatosis
CD117	+	−	−
β-catenin	−	−	+
CD34	+	−	−
SMA	±	+	±
Desmin	−	−	Rare
S-100 protein	−	−	−

GIST, gastrointestinal stromal tumor.

Inflammatory myofibroblastic tumor (also known as *inflammatory fibrosarcoma*) of the mesentery and retroperitoneum is also a diagnostic consideration, but this lesion is more cellular, has more pronounced cytologic atypia, and is less fibrotic and more inflamed than mesenteric fibromatosis.[164] Moreover, some, but not all, cases of inflammatory myofibroblastic tumor/inflammatory fibrosarcoma stain for ALK-1 protein, which is not found in mesenteric fibromatosis. *Idiopathic retroperitoneal fibrosis* (described in greater detail below) is usually more densely hyalinized and inflamed than fibromatosis.

Over the past several years, there have been several studies that have focused on distinguishing mesenteric fibromatosis from gastrointestinal stromal tumors (GIST) of the mesentery.[163,165,166] Distinguishing between these lesions is of clinical significance due to their vastly different therapeutic and prognostic implications. In a study of 25 cases of mesenteric fibromatosis, Rodriguez and colleagues found that GIST was by far the most common misdiagnosis, occurring in 52% of the cases.[165] Histologically, mesenteric fibromatosis is composed of a monotonous proliferation of cytologically bland spindled-shaped cells that are arranged into broad, sweeping fascicles and deposited in a finely collagenous stroma. Mitotic activity is typically low, and there is no evidence of necrosis. Keloidal-like collagen, an infiltrative growth pattern and prominent muscular arteries and dilated, thin-walled veins are also characteristic features. The histologic features of GIST are heterogeneous and can range from bland spindle cell tumors to highly cellular and overtly malignant epithelioid tumors. The confusion between these entities is compounded by reports of KIT (CD117) expression in mesenteric fibromatosis. For example, in the study by Yantiss and colleagues,[166] CD117 was expressed in 88% of the GIST, but was also found in 75% of fibromatoses. Similarly, 6 of 10 mesenteric fibromatoses reported by Montgomery et al. expressed CD117.[163] In both of these studies, CD34 was common in GIST but was not detected in mesenteric fibromatoses. It has been our experience that mesenteric fibromatoses are consistently negative for CD117. Nuclear β-catenin staining

characteristic of mesenteric fibromatosis (but absent in GIST) is also a useful finding.[163] Regardless of the immunophenotypic findings, mesenteric fibromatosis is sufficiently distinct from GIST on a morphologic basis such that immunohistochemistry does not necessarily have to be performed for diagnostic purposes in most cases (Table 9–4).

Like other forms of fibromatosis, tumors arising in this location have a propensity for local recurrence, although data on the recurrence rate differ greatly. In the study by Burke et al.[160] 23% of all tumors recurred, although there was a striking difference in recurrence rates between patients with (90%) and without (12%) FAP/Gardner syndrome. In fact, none of the patients with sporadic mesenteric fibromatosis had more than one recurrence, and none of these patients died as a direct result of their tumor. In contrast, most of the patients with FAP/Gardner syndrome had more than one recurrence, and four patients died of their tumor. Similar findings of aggressive behavior of mesenteric fibromatosis in this setting have been reported by others.[167,168]

Treatment is similar to that for extra-abdominal fibromatosis, but excision is often difficult because of the irregular growth pattern and intestinal attachment of the tumor. Other modes of therapy, including treatment with anti-estrogenic agents, cytotoxic chemotherapy and postoperative irradiation, have met with variable success.[169–171] Some have even attempted intestinal transplantation in those patients with tumors necessitating significant bowel resection.[172]

As with pelvic fibromatosis, the most likely cause appears to be tissue injury in a patient with a genetic predisposition to excessive fibrous growth. Of the patients without polyposis in the series by Burke et al.,[160] 12 (11%) had had abdominal surgery prior to detection of the fibromatosis. Rare cases of mesenteric fibromatosis have been reported following radiation therapy for Hodgkin's disease[173] or testicular seminoma.[93] Mesenteric fibromatosis may develop spontaneously in patients without polyposis or without prior surgical intervention. Although much less common than the association with abdominal fibromatosis, some mesenteric fibromatoses occur in patients with elevated serum estrogens. Of the 130 cases reported by Burke and co-workers, 6 were associated with hyperestrogenic states, including 4 patients in whom the tumor developed during pregnancy, 1 in whom the tumor developed 6 months postpartum, and 1 who was a male alcoholic with bilateral gynecomastia.[160]

Mesenteric fibromatosis in FAP/Gardner syndrome

Nichols was the first to recognize the association of desmoid tumors and FAP.[174] In 1951, Gardner reported the familial occurrence of intestinal polyposis, osteomas,

TABLE 9-4	**FEATURES USEFUL IN DISTINGUISHING BETWEEN MESENTERIC FIBROMATOSIS AND GASTROINTESTINAL STROMAL TUMOR**	
Feature	**Mesenteric fibromatosis**	**GIST**
Cell shape	Wavy, spindled	Spindled and/or epithelioid
Atypia	None	Variable
Growth pattern	Uniform, fascicular	Organoid, fascicles (variable)
Cellularity	Low to moderate	Moderate to high
Blood vessels	Regular, dilated and thin-walled	Hyalinized
Keloidal collagen	Frequent	Absent
Skeinoid fibers	Absent	May be present
Necrosis	Absent	May be present
Margins	Infiltrative	Often pushing
CD117	–	+
CD34	–	+
β-catenin	+ (nuclear)	–

GIST, gastrointestinal stromal tumor.
Modified from: Rodriguez JA, Guarda LA, Rosai J. Mesenteric fibromatosis with involvement of the gastrointestinal tract. Am J Clin Pathol 2004; 121:93.

fibromas, and epidermal or sebaceous cysts;[175] the term *Gardner syndrome* was coined by Smith in 1958.[176]

Gardner syndrome is inherited as an autosomal dominant trait that occurs in approximately half of the children of afflicted parents. It is more common in women than in men and is usually diagnosed in adults 25–35 years of age. Cutaneous cysts are present in 40–50% of patients, and osteomas can be detected in at least 35–50% of patients. Osteomas may occur anywhere in the skeleton but are usually found in the skull and facial bones, especially the maxilla, mandible, sphenoid, and frontal bone. Cortical thickening is more common in long bones.[177] As a rule, the cutaneous cysts and osteomas occur during childhood or the teenage years and precede the onset of polyposis and fibromatosis by 10–15 years.

Early cases tend to be asymptomatic or manifest with mild diarrhea and passage of small amounts of mucus or blood. At age 20–25 years, radiographic examination reveals numerous discrete filling defects in the colon characteristic of polyposis in about one-half of cases. The intestinal adenomatous polyps are indistinguishable from those seen with other forms of polyposis and are found throughout the intestinal tract; the colon and rectum are the two major sites, although adenomas may also occur in the ileum, duodenum, and stomach. Colorectal adenocarcinoma, often at multiple sites, usually occurs 10–15 years after the onset of polyposis, as most patients are diagnosed with carcinoma by 40 years of age, approximately 25 years earlier than the onset of colorectal carcinoma in the general population. Early detection of the disease permits proper surgical therapy before malignant transformation of the polyps takes place. Because the lesion usually does not manifest before the patient reaches reproductive age, genetic counseling and lifelong surveillance are important parts of therapy in patients with a positive family history. Many patients choose to undergo prophylactic colectomy, an operation

that has been made more palatable by the advent of the ileal pouch-anal anastomotic procedure (IPAA), which allows maintenance of fecal continence. Interestingly, although FAP/Gardner patients who have undergone an IPAA rarely develop pouchitis (as is frequently seen in patients with ulcerative colitis), we have certainly seen adenomas and even invasive adenocarcinomas develop in the pouch itself.

Mesenteric or retroperitoneal fibromatosis usually has its onset 1–2 years after excision of the diseased portion of the intestinal tract. Most large studies have found the incidence of fibromatosis in patients with polyposis to be in the vicinity of 10–15%,[160,178] and these lesions are the most common cause of death in polyposis patients after colectomy is performed.[179] Gurbuz et al. estimated the absolute risk of desmoids in polyposis patients to be 852 times that of the general population;[138] 68% of the patients had had abdominal surgery prior to discovery of the tumor. A similar-appearing tumor can also arise in the abdominal wall scar of the preceding laparotomy. Not all cases of fibromatosis develop as a result of surgical trauma; some have been noted prior to surgical intervention.

Clinically, the fibromatosis may be asymptomatic or may cause mild abdominal pain or intestinal obstruction as a result of infiltrative growth into the wall of the small or large bowel. Although most tumors grow slowly, Gold and Mucha reported mesenteric fibromatosis in a 40-year-old man that increased in size from 4 cm to 27 cm in greatest diameter over a period of 1 year.[180]

Histologically, the fibromatosis is virtually indistinguishable from those at other sites, and one cannot distinguish polyposis-related cases from sporadic cases by morphology. These tumors tend to have a prominent myxoid matrix. (Figs 9–23 to 9–26), and the cells may be arranged in a vague storiform pattern in addition to sweeping fascicles.

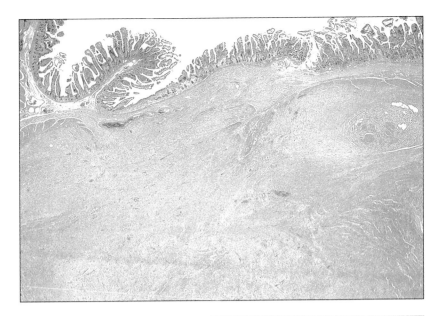

FIGURE 9–23 Low-power view of mesenteric fibromatosis in Gardner syndrome showing uniform fibrocollagenous growth infiltrating the wall of the small bowel.

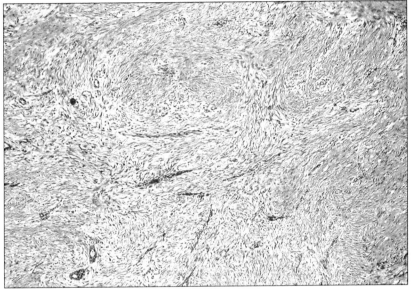

FIGURE 9–24 Orderly arrangement of uniform fibroblasts associated with moderate amounts of collagen and mucoid material in mesenteric fibromatosis.

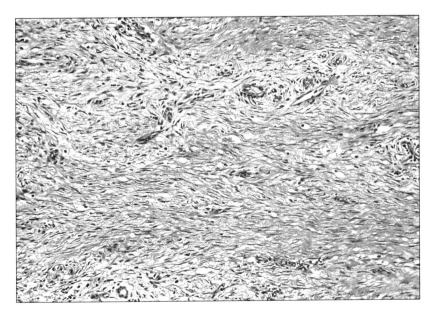

FIGURE 9–25 Uniform spindled proliferation in mesenteric fibromatosis.

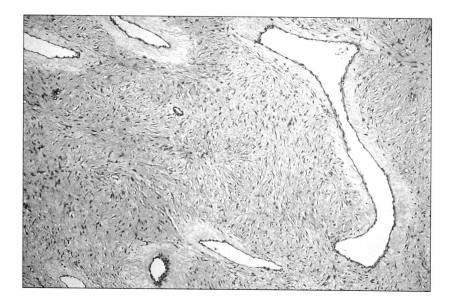

FIGURE 9–26 Prominent dilated blood vessels with perivascular hyalinization, a common feature of intra-abdominal fibromatosis.

As with mesenteric fibromatosis without polyposis, complete excision of the tumor is often difficult and necessitates removal of a sizable segment of the intestine together with the fibrous growth. For rapidly growing tumors, excision must be attempted to prevent complications caused by the presence of a massive, expanding intra-abdominal growth. Recurrence is common, and several studies have found a higher rate of recurrence and fatal complications in polyposis-related fibromatosis than in sporadic cases.[160] Endocrine therapy (tamoxifen and prednisolone), noncytotoxic drug therapy (sulindac and indometacin), and chemotherapy have been reported to be efficacious for treating recurrent or inoperable tumors.[169,170,181,182]

Discussion

Gardner syndrome is a genetically determined autosomal dominant disease caused by a germline abnormality of the adenomatous polyposis coli (*APC*) gene on the long arm of chromosome 5.[183] Cytogenetic and molecular genetic studies have reported abnormalities of this locus in mesenteric fibromatoses.[184,185] Studies suggest that mutations of the *APC* gene result in a protein product that loses the ability to degrade β-catenin, resulting in an elevated β-catenin protein level, which in turn promotes fibroblastic proliferation.[141,186] Other cytogenetic abnormalities include loss of the Y chromosome,[187] trisomy 8,[188,189] and trisomy 20.[188]

IDIOPATHIC RETROPERITONEAL FIBROSIS (ORMOND'S DISEASE)

Idiopathic retroperitoneal fibrosis is a rare fibrosing reactive process that may be confused with mesenteric fibromatosis and, as such, is discussed in this chapter. It is characterized by diffuse or localized fibroblastic proliferation and a chronic lymphoplasmacytic infiltrate in the retroperitoneum causing compression or obstruction of the ureters, aorta or other vascular structures. It is part of a spectrum of idiopathic fibroinflammatory reactions that may be grouped under the broader term of chronic periaortitis. Although described years earlier, it was not until the publication of two cases in the English literature by Ormond in 1948 that this disease became more widely recognized.[190,191]

The disease is quite uncommon, with an incidence estimated to be less than 1 per 10 000 patients.[192] It is two to three times more common in men, and most patients present during the fifth or sixth decade of life.[193] It is unusual before age 20 or over age 70, although there are reports of several cases arising in children.[194] Most patients present with vague, non-specific abdominal symptoms, including dull, poorly localized back or flank pain. Other common symptoms include weight loss, nausea or vomiting, malaise, anorexia, fever and hypertension.[195] The cause of the pain is probably related to ureteral obstruction or abnormal ureteral peristalsis.[196] Laboratory abnormalities include anemia, azotemia, elevated erythrocyte sedimentation rate, hypergammaglobulinemia and serum autoantibodies such as ANA.[195,197] Although most cases are idiopathic, some have been associated with the administration of certain drugs such as methysergide, an ergot derivative used to treat migraine headaches and pergolide, an anti-parkinsonian medication.[198] More recently, occupational asbestos exposure has also been associated with an increased risk.[199] Other cases of retroperitoneal fibrosis occur secondary to an exuberant desmoplastic response to a malignancy at this location. The tumors that are most frequently implicated include Hodgkin's disease and other types of lymphoma, retroperitoneal sarcomas, carcinoid tumors and a variety of carcinomas, including those from the breast, lung, stomach, colon, kidney, bladder, prostate and cervix.[200] Approximately 5–25% of abdominal aortic aneurysms are associated with perianeurysmal fibrosis, which likely represents an early or mild form of retroperitoneal fibrosis, as discussed below.

Pathologic findings

Grossly, the mass is dense, grayish-white, and plaque-like, usually arising at or just below the level of the aortic bifurcation. As it progresses, the plaque surrounds the aorta and inferior vena cava and spreads through the retroperitoneum in a perivascular distribution; it may extend into the pelvis to surround the iliac and gonadal vessels. In some cases, the plaque extends anteriorly along the celiac axis and superior mesenteric artery. Typically, one or both ureters, usually in the middle one-third, are encased by this fibrous proliferation, often resulting in hydronephrosis.

Microscopic examination reveals a fibrous proliferation, broad anastomosing bands of hyalinized collagen, and a lymphoplasmacytic infiltrate of variable density, with occasional germinal centers (Fig. 9–27). Macrophages and eosinophils may also be conspicuous, but neutrophils are generally absent. Several studies have found a progression from active inflammation to fibrosis through serial biopsies.[201] The aorta which is surrounded by the fibrous proliferation typically shows severe atherosclerosis with protrusion of atherosclerotic debris through the media into the adventitia with chronic inflammation within the aortic wall.[201]

Clinical behavior and therapy

Although spontaneous regression has been observed in some cases,[202] most patients require some form of treatment. Patients taking methysergide should stop the drug immediately, after which there is often relief of symptoms and regression of the fibrosis within a short time.[203,204] Surgical intervention is required in most patients. Multiple deep biopsies should be obtained to exclude the possibility of malignancy, as there may be a few malignant cells admixed within the fibrosis and inflammatory infiltrate. Ureterolysis (dissection of the ureters from the surrounding fibrosis) is often required to relieve the ureteral obstruction and restore normal renal function; some have reported success with laparoscopic ureterolysis and ureteral intraperitonealization.[205] Although ureterolysis successfully relieves ureteral obstruction in approximately 90% of cases, recurrent obstruction occurs in up to 22% of patients treated with ureterolysis alone, underlining the need for adjuvant medical therapy.[206] The antiinflammatory action of corticosteroids is effective for treating this disease, although there is less benefit if therapy is initiated during the later fibrotic stages.[207] A number of immunosuppressive agents including azathioprine, cyclophosphamide and methotrexate have been used in patients who did not respond to steroids, with variable success.[197,208,209] Antiestrogenic agents (tamoxifen) have also been tried in some patients, although their effectiveness is uncertain.[210] The prognosis for patients with malignant retroperitoneal fibrosis is exceedingly poor, but patients with the idiopathic form generally have a good prognosis with very few reports of death as a direct result of this disease.

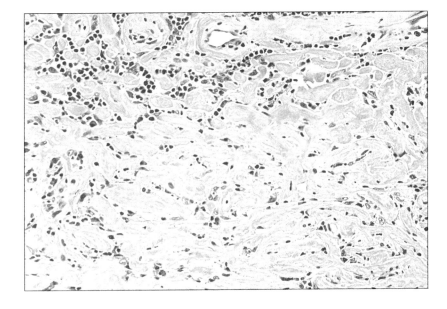

FIGURE 9–27 Anastomosing bands of hyalinized collagen admixed with a lymphoplasmacytic infiltrate in idiopathic retroperitoneal fibrosis.

Discussion

The exact cause of the idiopathic form of retroperitoneal fibrosis is unclear. The leading theory suggests that this fibrosing process is a local immune response to atherosclerotic plaque antigens such as oxidized low-density lipoproteins and ceroid.[201,211,212] There is morphologic evidence to support this view. Periaortic fibrosis is typically localized around that portion of the aorta with the most severe atherosclerotic disease. There is often inflammation of the aortic wall, not only in the areas of fibrosis but in portions of the aorta where there is no periaortic fibrosis, suggesting that the aortitis precedes the fibrosis.[213] IgG has been detected in close approximation to extracellular ceroid,[212] and serum antibodies to ceroid have been found to be more common in patients with chronic periaortitis than in control patients.[201] It has been speculated that rupture of an atherosclerotic plaque results in the release of ceroid, stimulating a chronic fibrosing inflammatory process.

Retroperitoneal fibrosis has been associated with a variety of other immune-mediated connective tissue diseases including systemic lupus erythematosus,[214] Wegener's granulomatosis,[215] and primary biliary cirrhosis.[216] Approximately 8–15% of patients have a histologically similar fibrosing process that occurs outside the retroperitoneum, including fibrosing mediastinitis, orbital fibrous pseudotumor, primary sclerosing cholangitis, and Reidel's thyroiditis.[217,218] Hughes and Buckley found that many of the spindle-shaped cells in this disease express the immunophenotype of a tissue macrophage, with expression of CD13, CD11c, CD68, HAM-56, and MAC 387.[219] Ranshaw and co-workers found increased levels of cytokine gene expression, including interleukins 1, 2, and 4, in aortic adventitial inflammatory cells associated with chronic periaortitis.[220] Given the ability of these cytokines to induce collagen production, their increased gene expression logically links periaortitis to idiopathic retroperitoneal fibrosis.

REFERENCES

Palmar fibromatosis

1. Soule EH, Scanlon PW. Fibrosarcoma arising in an extraabdominal desmoid tumor: Report of case. Mayo Clin Proc 1962; 37:443.
2. Dupuytren G. De la retraction des doigts par suite d'une affection de l'aponeurose palmaire: Description de la maladie, operation chirurgical qui convient dans de cas. J Univ Med Chir Prat Paris 1831; 5:348.
3. Hart MG, Hooper G. Clinical associations of Dupuytren's disease. Postgrad Med J 2005; 81:425.
4. Elliot D. The early history of Dupuytren's disease. Hand Clin 1999; 15:1.
5. Fetsch JF, Laskin WB, Miettinen M. Palmar-plantar fibromatosis in children and preadolescents: A clinicopathologic study of 56 cases with newly recognized demographics and extended follow-up information. Am J Surg Pathol 2005; 29:1095.
6. Rhomberg M, Rainer C, Gardetto A, et al. Dupuytren's disease in children – differential diagnosis. J Pediatr Surg 2002; 37:E7.
7. Mikkelsen OA. Dupuytren's disease – initial symptoms, age of onset and spontaneous course. Hand 1977; 9:11.
8. Saboeiro AP, Porkorny JJ, Shehadi SI, et al. Racial distribution of Dupuytren's disease in Department of Veterans Affairs patients. Plast Reconstr Surg 2000; 106:71.
9. Gudmundsson KG, Arngrimsson R, Sigfusson N, et al. Epidemiology of Dupuytren's disease: clinical, serological, and social assessment. The Reykjavik study. J Clin Epidemiol 2000; 53:291.
10. Burge P. Genetics of Dupuytren's disease. Hand Clin 1999; 15:63.
11. Mackey SL, Cobb MW. Knuckle pads. Cutis 1994; 54:159.
12. Lee YC, Chan HH, Black MM. Aggressive polyfibromatosis: A 10 year follow-up. Australas J Dermatol 1996; 37:205.
13. Ross DC. Epidemiology of Dupuytren's disease. Hand Clin 1999; 15:53.
14. Arkkila PE, Kantola IM, Viikari JS. Dupuytren's disease: association with chronic diabetic complications. J Rheumatol 1997; 24:153.
15. Arkkila PE, Kantola IM, Viikari JS, et al. Dupuytren's disease in type 1 diabetic patients: a five-year prospective study. Clin Exp Rheumatol 1996; 14:59.
16. Lund M. Dupuytren's contracture and epilepsy: Clinical connection between Dupuytren's contracture, fibroma plantae, periarthrosis humeri, helodermia, induratio penis plastica and epilepsy with attempt at pathogenetic evaluation. Acta Psychiatr Neurol 1941; 16:645.
17. Arafa M, Noble J, Royle SG, et al. Dupuytren's and epilepsy revisited. J Hand Surg 1992; 17:221.
18. Burge P, Hoy G, Regan P, et al. Smoking, alcohol and the risk of Dupuytren's contracture. J Bone Joint Surg [Br] 1997; 79:206.
19. Noble J, Arafa M, Royle SG, et al. The association between alcohol, hepatic pathology and Dupuytren's disease. J Hand Surg 1992; 17:71.
20. Gudmundsson KG, Arngrimsson R, Jonsson T. Dupuytren's disease, alcohol consumption and alcoholism. Scand J Prim Health Care 2001; 19:186.
21. Gabbiani G, Majno G. Dupuytren's contracture: Fibroblast contraction? An ultrastructural study. Am J Pathol 1972; 66:131.
22. Eyden B. Electron microscopy in the study of myofibroblastic lesions. Semin Diagn Pathol 2003; 20:13.
23. Tomasek J, Rayan GM. Correlation of alpha-smooth muscle actin expression and contraction in Dupuytren's disease fibroblasts. J Hand Surg 1995; 20:450.
24. McCann BG, Logan A, Belcher H, et al. The presence of myofibroblasts in the dermis of patients with Dupuytren's contracture. A possible source for recurrence. J Hand Surg [Br] 1993; 18:656.
25. Montgomery E, Lee JH, Abraham SC, et al. Superficial fibromatoses are genetically distinct from deep fibromatoses. Mod Pathol 2001; 14:695.
26. Magro G, Colombatti A, Lanzafame S. Immunohistochemical expression of type VI collagen in superficial fibromatoses. Pathol Res Pract 1995; 191:1023.
27. Kosmehl H, Berndt A, Katenkamp D, et al. Differential expression of fibronectin splice variants, oncofetal glycosylated fibronectin and laminin isoforms in nodular palmar fibromatosis. Pathol Res Pract 1995; 191:1105.
28. Magro G, Fraggetta F, Colombatti A, et al. Myofibroblasts and extracellular matrix glycoproteins in palmar fibromatosis. Gen Diagn Pathol 1997; 142:185.
29. Magro G, Fraggetta F, Travali S, et al. Immunohistochemical expression and distribution of alpha2beta1, alpha6beta1, alpha5beta1 integrins and their extracellular ligands, type IV collagen, laminin and fibronectin in palmar fibromatosis. Gen Diagn Pathol 1997; 143:203.
30. Alman BA, Greel DA, Ruby LK, et al. Regulation of proliferation and platelet-derived growth factor expression in palmar fibromatosis (Dupuytren contracture) by mechanical strain. J Orthop Res 1996; 14:722.
31. Magro G, Lanteri E, Micali G, et al. Myofibroblasts of palmar fibromatosis co-express transforming growth factor-alpha and epidermal growth factor receptor. J Pathol 1997; 181:213.
32. De Wever I, Dal Cin P, Fletcher CD, et al. Cytogenetic, clinical, and morphologic correlations in 78 cases of fibromatosis: A report from the CHAMP study group. Chromosomes and morphology. Mod Pathol 2000; 13:1080.
33. McCarthy DM. The long-term results of enzymic fasciotomy. J Hand Surg 1992; 17:356.
34. Armstrong JR, Hurren JS, Logan AM. Dermofasciectomy in the management of Dupuytren's disease. J Bone Joint Surg [Br] 2000; 82:90.
35. Brotherson TM, Balakrishnan C, Milner RH, et al. Long-term follow-up of dermofasciectomy for Dupuytren's contracture. Br J Plast Surg 1994; 47:440.
36. Badalamente MA, Hurst LC, Hentz VR. Collagen as a clinical target: nonoperative treatment of Dupuytren's disease. J Hand Surg 2002; 27:788.
37. Al-Qattan MM. The injection of nodules of Dupuytren's disease with triamcinalone acetonide. J Hand Surg [Am] 2001; 26:560.
38. Yacoe ME, Bergman AG, Ladd AL, et al. Dupuytren's contracture: MR imaging findings and correlation between MR signal intensity

and cellularity of lesions. AJR Am J Roentgenol 1993; 160:813.

39. Ling RS. The genetic factor. J Bone Joint Surg [Br] 1963; 45:709.

40. Lyall HA. Dupuytren's disease in identical twins. J Hand Surg 1993; 18:368.

41. Herzog EG. The aetiology of Dupuytren's contracture. Lancet 1951; 1:1305.

42. Liss GM, Stock SR. Can Dupuytren's contracture be work-related? Review of the evidence. Am J Ind Med 1996; 29:521.

43. Kischer CW, Speer DP. Microvascular changes in Dupuytren's contracture. J Hand Surg 1984; 9A:58.

44. Stollberger C, Finsterer J, Zlabinger GJ, et al. Antineutrophil cytoplasmic autoantibody-negative antiproteinase 3 syndrome presenting as vasculitis, endocarditis, polyneuropathy and Dupuytren's contracture. J Heart Valve Dis 2003; 12:530.

45. Neumuller J, Menzel J, Millesi H. Prevalence of HLA-DR3 and autoantibodies to connective tissue components in Dupuytren's contracture. Clin Immunol Immunopathol 1994; 71:142.

46. Baird KS, Alwan WH, Crossan JE, et al. T-cell-mediated response in Dupuytren's disease. Lancet 1993; 341:1622.

Plantar fibromatosis

47. Madelung OW. Die aetiologie und die operative behandlung der Dupuytren'schen fingerverkrumung. Berl Klin Wochenschr 1875; 12:191.

48. Ledderhose G. Pathologie der aponeurose des fusses und der hand. Arch Klin Chir 1897; 55:694.

49. Zgonis T, Jolly GP, Polyzois V, et al. Plantar fibromatosis. Clin Podiatr Med Surg 2005; 22:11.

50. Griffith JF, Wong TY, Wong SM, et al. Sonography of plantar fibromatosis. AJR Am J Roentgenol 2002; 179:1167.

51. Pickren JW, Smith AG, Stevenson TW, et al. Fibromatosis of the plantar fascia. Cancer 1951; 4:846.

52. Snyder M. Dupuytren's contracture and plantar fibromatosis: Is there more than a causal relationship? J Am Podiatr Assoc 1980; 70:410.

53. Aviles E, Arlen M, Miller T. Plantar fibromatosis. Surgery 1971; 69:117.

54. Landers PA, Yu GV, White JM, et al. Recurrent plantar fibromatosis. J Foot Ankle Surg 1993; 32:85.

55. Boc SF, Kushner S. Plantar fibromatosis causing entrapment syndrome of the medial plantar nerve. J Am Podiatr Med Assoc 1994; 84:420.

56. DeBrule MB, Mott RC, Funk C, et al. Osseous metaplasia in plantar fibromatosis: a case report. J Foot Ankle Surg 2004; 43:430.

57. Evans HL. Multinucleated giant cells in plantar fibromatosis. Am J Surg Pathol 2002; 26:244.

58. Alman BA, Naber SP, Terek RM, et al. Platelet-derived growth factor in fibrous musculoskeletal disorders: a study of pathologic tissue sections and in vitro primary cell cultures. J Orthop Res 1995; 13:67.

59. Zamora RL, Heights R, Kraemer BA, et al. Presence of growth factors in palmar and plantar fibromatoses. J Hand Surg 1994; 19:435.

60. Pentland AP, Anderson TF. Plantar fibromatosis responds to intralesional steroids. J Am Acad Dermatol 1985; 12:212.

61. Watson-Ramirez L, Rasmussen SE, Warschaw KE, et al. Plantar fibromatosis: use of magnetic resonance imaging in diagnosis. Cutis 2001; 68:219.

62. Recht MP, Donley BG. Magnetic resonance imaging of the foot and ankle. J Am Acad Orthop Surg 2001; 9:187.

63. Aluisio FV, Mair SD, Hall RL. Plantar fibromatosis: treatment of primary and recurrent lesions and factors associated with recurrence. Foot Ankle Int 1996; 17:672.

64. de Bree E, Zoetmulder FA, Keus RB, et al. Incidence and treatment of recurrent plantar fibromatosis by surgery and postoperative radiotherapy. Am J Surg 2004; 187:33.

65. Wapner KL, Ververeli PA, Moore JH Jr, et al. Plantar fibromatosis: a review of primary and recurrent surgical treatment. Foot Ankle Int 1995; 16:548.

66. Breiner JA, Nelson M, Bredthauer BD, et al. Trisomy 8 and trisomy 14 in plantar fibromatosis. Cancer Genet Cytogenet 1999; 108:176.

Penile fibromatosis (Peyronie's disease)

67. La Peyronie F. Sur quelques obstacles qui s'opposent a l'ejaculation naturelle de la semence. In: Mein De l'Academie Royale De Chir. Paris: 1743:425.

68. Dunsmuir WD, Kirby RS. François de la Peyronie (1678–1747): The man and the disease he described. Br J Urol 1996; 78:613.

69. Mulhall JP, Creech SD, Boorjian SA, et al. Subjective and objective analysis of the prevalence of Peyronie's disease in a population of men presenting for prostate cancer screening. J Urol 2004; 171:2350.

70. Hellstrom WJ. History, epidemiology, and clinical presentation of Peyronie's disease. Int J Impot Res 2003; 15:S91.

71. Briganti A, Salonia A, Deho F, et al. Peyronie's disease: A review. Curr Opin Urol 2003; 13:417.

72. Kadioglu A, Tefekli A, Erol B, et al. A retrospective review of 307 men with Peyronie's disease. J Urol 2002; 168:1075.

73. El-Sakka AI, Tayeb KA. Peyronie's disease in diabetic patients being screened for erectile dysfunction. J Urol 2005; 174:1026.

74. Ollivaud L, Godeau B, Lionnet F, et al. Cogan's syndrome and Peyronie's disease: a non-fortuitous association. Br J Rheumatol 1993; 32:1111.

75. Lyles KW, Gold DT, Newton RA, et al. Peyronie's disease is associated with Paget's disease of bone. J Bone Miner Res 1997; 12:929.

76. Bivens CH, Marecek RL, Feldman JM. Peyronie's disease – a presenting complaint of the carcinoid syndrome. N Engl J Med 1973; 289:844.

77. Davis CJ Jr. The microscopic pathology of Peyronie's disease. J Urol 1997; 157:282.

78. Anafarta K, Beduk Y, Uluoglu O, et al. The significance of histopathological changes of the normal tunica albuginea in Peyronie's disease. Int Urol Nephrol 1994; 26:71.

79. Hauck EW, Schmelz HU, Diemer T, et al. Epithelioid sarcoma of the penis – a rare differential diagnosis of Peyronie's disease. Int J Impot Res 2003; 15:378.

80. Levine LA. Review of current nonsurgical management of Peyronie's disease. Int J Impot Res 2003; 15:S113.

81. Hellstrom WJ, Usta MF. Surgical approaches for advanced Peyronie's disease patients. Int J Impot Res 2003; 15:S121.

82. Dean RC, Lue TF. Peyronie's disease: Advancements in recent surgical techniques. Curr Opin Urol 2004; 14:339.

83. Kalsi J, Minhas S, Christopher N, et al. The results of plaque incision and venous grafting (lue procedure) to correct the penile deformity of Peyronie's disease. Br J Urol Int 2005; 95:1029.

84. Austoni E, Colombo F, Romano AL, et al. Soft prosthesis implant and relaxing albuginea incision with saphenous grafting for surgical therapy of Peyronie's disease: a 5-year experience and long-term follow-up on 145 operated patients. Eur Urol 2005; 47:223.

85. Chaudhary M, Sheikh N, Asterling S, et al. Peyronie's disease with erectile dysfunction: penile modeling over inflatable penile prostheses. Urology 2005; 65:760.

86. Nachtsheim DA, Rearden A. Peyronie's disease is associated with an HLA class II antigen, HLA-DQ5, implying an autoimmune etiology. J Urol 1996; 156:1330.

87. Ralph DJ, Schwartz G, Moore W, et al. The genetic and bacteriological aspects of Peyronie's disease. J Urol 1997; 157:291.

88. Devine CJ Jr, Somers KD, Jordan SG, et al. Proposal: trauma as the cause of the Peyronie's lesion. J Urol 1997; 157:285.

89. Magee TR, Qian A, Rajfer J, et al. Gene expression profiles in the Peyronie's disease plaque. Urology 2002; 59:451.

90. Qian A, Meals RA, Rajfer J, et al. Comparison of gene expression profiles between Peyronie's disease and Dupuytren's contracture. Urology 2004; 64:399.

91. Bivalacqua TJ, Champion HC, Hellstrom WJ. Implications of nitric oxide synthase isoforms in the pathophysiology of Peyronie's disease. Int J Impot Res 2002; 14:345.

92. Mulhall JP. Expanding the paradigm for plaque development in Peyronie's disease. Int J Impot Res 2003; 15:S93.

93. Wegner HE, Fleige B, Dieckmann KP. Mesenteric desmoid tumor 19 years after radiation therapy for testicular seminoma. Urol Int 1994; 53:48.

Knuckle pads

94. Mikkelsen OA. Knuckle pads in Dupuytren's disease. Hand 1977; 9:301.

95. Chamberlain AJ, Venning VA, Wojnarowska F. Pachydermodactyly: A forme fruste of knuckle pads? Australas J Dermatol 2003; 44:140.

96. Dickens R, Adams BB, Mutasim DF. Sports-related pads. Int J Dermatol 2002; 41:291.

97. Kanerva L. Knuckle pads from boxing. Eur J Dermatol 1998; 8:359.

98. Allison JR Jr, Allison JR Sr. Knuckle pads. Arch Dermatol 1966; 93:311.

99. Richard G, Brown N, Ishida-Yamamoto A, et al. Expanding the phenotypic spectrum of Cx26 disorders: Bart-Pumphrey syndrome is caused by a novel missense mutation in GJB2. J Invest Dermatol 2004; 123:856.

Extra-abdominal fibromatosis

100. Rock MG, Pritchard DJ, Reiman HM, et al. Extra-abdominal desmoid tumors. J Bone Joint Surg [Am] 1984; 66:1369.

101. Pignatti G, Barbanti-Brodano G, Ferrari D, et al. Extraabdominal desmoid tumor. A study of 83 cases. Clin Orthop 2000; 375:207.

102. Pritchard DJ, Nascimento AG, Petersen IA. Local control of extra-abdominal desmoid tumors. J Bone Joint Surg [Am] 1996; 78:848.

103. Abbas AE, Deschamps C, Cassivi SD, et al. Chest-wall desmoid tumors: Results of surgical intervention. Ann Thorac Surg 2004; 78:1219.

104. Reitamo JJ, Hayry P, Nykyri E, et al. The desmoid tumor. I. Incidence, sex-, age- and anatomical distribution in the Finnish population. Am J Clin Pathol 1982; 77:665.

105. Hayry P, Reitamo JJ, Totterman S, et al. The desmoid tumor. II. Analysis of factors possibly contributing to the etiology and growth behavior. Am J Clin Pathol 1982; 77:674.

106. Abikhzer G, Bouganim N, Finesilver A. Aggressive fibromatosis of the head and neck: case report and review of the literature. J Otolaryngol 2005; 34:289.

107. Gnepp DR, Henley J, Weiss S, et al. Desmoid fibromatosis of the sinonasal tract and

nasopharynx. A clinicopathologic study of 25 cases. Cancer 1996; 78:2572.

108. Reis-Filho JS, Milanezi F, Pope LZ, et al. Primary fibromatosis of the breast in a patient with multiple desmoid tumors – report of a case with evaluation of estrogen and progesterone receptors. Pathol Res Pract 2001; 197:775.

109. Erguvan-Dogan B, Dempsey PJ, Ayyar G, et al. Primary desmoid tumor (extraabdominal fibromatosis) of the breast. AJR Am J Roentgenol 2005; 185:488.

110. Maurer F, Horst F, Pfannenberg C, et al. Multifocal extra-abdominal desmoid tumor – diagnostic and therapeutic problems. Arch Orthop Trauma Surg 1996; 115:359.

111. Weyl Ben Arush M, Meller I, Moses M, et al. Multifocal desmoid tumor in childhood: report of two cases and review of the literature. Pediatr Hematol Oncol 1998; 15:55.

112. Wagstaff MJ, Raurell A, Perks AG. Multicentric extra-abdominal desmoid tumours. Br J Plast Surg 2004; 57:362.

113. Rhys R, Davies AM, Mangham DC, et al. Sclerotome distribution of melorheostosis and multicentric fibromatosis. Skeletal Radiol 1998; 27:633.

114. Fong Y, Rosen PP, Brennan MF. Multifocal desmoids. Surgery 1993; 114:902.

115. McDougall A, McGarrity G. Extra-abdominal desmoid tumours. J Bone Joint Surg [Br] 1979; 61B:373.

116. Frick MA, Sundaram M, Unni KK, et al. Imaging findings in desmoplastic fibroma of bone: Distinctive T2 characteristics. AJR Am J Roentgenol 2005; 184:1762.

117. Enzinger FM, Shiraki M. Musculo-aponeurotic fibromatosis of the shoulder girdle (extra-abdominal desmoid). Analysis of thirty cases followed up for ten or more years. Cancer 1967; 20:1131.

118. Bhattacharya B, Dilworth HP, Iacobuzio-Donahue C, et al. Nuclear beta-catenin expression distinguishes deep fibromatosis from other benign and malignant fibroblastic and myofibroblastic lesions. Am J Surg Pathol 2005; 29:653.

119. Dominguez-Malagon H. Intracellular collagen and fibronexus in fibromatosis and other fibroblastic tumors. Ultrastruct Pathol 2004; 28:67.

120. Hauben EI, Jundt G, Cleton-Jansen AM, et al. Desmoplastic fibroma of bone: an immunohistochemical study including beta-catenin expression and mutational analysis for beta-catenin. Hum Pathol 2005; 36:1025.

121. Smith SE, Kransdorf MJ. Primary musculoskeletal tumors of fibrous origin. Semin Musculoskelet Radiol 2000; 4:73.

122. Mooney EE, Meagher P, Edwards GE, et al. Fibrosarcoma of the thigh 28 years after excision of fibromatosis. Histopathology 1993; 23:498.

123. Allen PW. The fibromatoses: A clinicopathologic classification based on 140 cases. Am J Surg Pathol 1977; 1:255.

124. Gronchi A, Casali PG, Mariani L, et al. Quality of surgery and outcome in extra-abdominal aggressive fibromatosis: a series of patients surgically treated at a single institution. J Clin Oncol 2003; 21:1390.

125. Easter DW, Halasz NA. Recent trends in the management of desmoid tumors. Summary of 19 cases and review of the literature. Ann Surg 1989; 210:765.

126. McKinnon JG, Neifeld JP, Kay S, et al. Management of desmoid tumors. Surg Gynecol Obstet. 1989; 169:104.

127. Karakousis CP, Mayordomo J, Zografos GC, et al. Desmoid tumors of the trunk and extremity. Cancer 1993; 72:1637.

128. Jelinek JA, Stelzer KJ, Conrad E, et al. The efficacy of radiotherapy as postoperative treatment for desmoid tumors. Int J Radiat Oncol Biol Phys 2001; 50:121.

129. Baliski CR, Temple WJ, Arthur K, et al. Desmoid tumors: A novel approach for local control. J Surg Oncol 2002; 80:96.

130. Mace J, Sybil Biermann J, Sondak V, et al. Response of extraabdominal desmoid tumors to therapy with imatinib mesylate. Cancer 2002; 95:2373.

131. Hornick JL, Fletcher CD. The significance of KIT (CD117) in gastrointestinal stromal tumors. Int J Surg Pathol 2004; 12:93.

132. Miettinen M. Are desmoid tumors kit positive? Am J Surg Pathol 2001; 25:549.

133. Leithner A, Schnack B, Katterschafka T, et al. Treatment of extra-abdominal desmoid tumors with interferon-alpha with or without tretinoin. J Surg Oncol 2000; 73:21.

134. Kinzbrunner B, Ritter S, Domingo J, et al. Remission of rapidly growing desmoid tumors after tamoxifen therapy. Cancer 1983; 52:2201.

135. Wilcken N, Tattersall MH. Endocrine therapy for desmoid tumors. Cancer 1991; 68:1384.

136. Ozuner G, Hull TL. Familial desmoids in association with adrenal and ovarian masses and leiomyomas: report of three cases. Dis Colon Rectum 1999; 42:529.

137. Reitamo JJ, Scheinin TM, Hayry P. The desmoid syndrome. New aspects in the cause, pathogenesis and treatment of the desmoid tumor. Am J Surg 1986; 151:230.

138. Gurbuz AK, Giardiello FM, Petersen GM, et al. Desmoid tumours in familial adenomatous polyposis. Gut 1994; 35:377.

139. Lucas DR, Shroyer KR, McCarthy PJ, et al. Desmoid tumor is a clonal cellular proliferation: PCR amplification of HUMARA for analysis of patterns of X-chromosome inactivation. Am J Surg Pathol 1997; 21:306.

140. Alman BA, Li C, Pajerski ME, et al. Increased beta-catenin protein and somatic APC mutations in sporadic aggressive fibromatoses (desmoid tumors). Am J Pathol 1997; 151:329.

141. Li C, Bapat B, Alman BA. Adenomatous polyposis coli gene mutation alters proliferation through its beta-catenin-regulatory function in aggressive fibromatosis (desmoid tumor). Am J Pathol 1998; 153:709.

142. Tejpar S, Nollet F, Li C, et al. Predominance of beta-catenin mutations and beta-catenin dysregulation in sporadic aggressive fibromatosis (desmoid tumor). Oncogene 1999; 18:6615.

143. Icard P, Le Rochais JP, Galateau F, et al. Desmoid fibromatosis of the shoulder and of the upper chest wall following a clavicular fracture. Eur J Cardiothorac Surg 1999; 15:723.

144. Aaron AD, O'Mara JW, Legendre KE, et al. Chest wall fibromatosis associated with silicone breast implants. Surg Oncol 1996; 5:93.

145. Gunther T, Buhtz P, Forgbert K, et al. Extra-abdominal aggressive fibromatosis after treatment of a morbus hodgkin. A case report. Gen Diagn Pathol 1995; 141:161.

Abdominal fibromatosis

146. Eccles DM, van der Luijt R, Breukel C, et al. Hereditary desmoid disease due to a frameshift mutation at codon 1924 of the APC gene. Am J Hum Genet 1996; 59:1193.

147. Sorensen A, Keller J, Nielsen OS, et al. Treatment of aggressive fibromatosis: A retrospective study of 72 patients followed for 1–27 years. Acta Orthop Scand 2002; 73:213.

148. Stojadinovic A, Hoos A, Karpoff HM, et al. Soft tissue tumors of the abdominal wall: analysis of disease patterns and treatment. Arch Surg 2001; 136:70.

149. Marone U, Amore A, Pezzullo L, et al. Giant desmoid tumor of the abdominal wall associated with familial adenomatous polyposis. Tumori 2003; 89:331.

150. Bandipalliam P, Balmana J, Syngal S. Comprehensive genetic and endoscopic evaluation may be necessary to distinguish sporadic versus familial adenomatous polyposis-associated abdominal desmoid tumors. Surgery 2004; 135:683.

151. Durkin AJ, Korkolis DP, Al-Saif O, et al. Full-term gestation and transvaginal delivery after wide resection of an abdominal desmoid tumor during pregnancy. J Surg Oncol 2005; 89:86.

152. Lipshutz H. Painful knuckle pads. Plast Reconstr Surg 1961; 28:420.

153. Picariello L, Tonelli F, Brandi ML. Selective oestrogen receptor modulators in desmoid tumours. Expert Opin Investig Drugs 2004; 13:1457.

154. Fujita K, Sugao H, Tsujikawa K, et al. Desmoid tumor in a scar from radical nephrectomy for renal cancer. Int J Urol 2003; 10:274.

155. Mall JW, Philipp AW, Zimmerling M, et al. Desmoid tumours following long-term Tenckhoff peritoneal dialysis catheters. Nephrol Dial Transplant 2002; 17:945.

Intra-abdominal fibromatosis

156. Huang GS, Lee HS, Lee CH, et al. Pelvic fibromatosis with massive ossification. AJR Am J Roentgenol 2005; 184:1029.

157. Mariani A, Nascimento AG, Webb MJ, et al. Surgical management of desmoid tumors of the female pelvis. J Am Coll Surg 2000; 191:175.

158. Chao AS, Lai CH, Hsueh S, et al. Successful treatment of recurrent pelvic desmoid tumour with tamoxifen: Case report. Hum Reprod 2000; 15:311.

159. Hartley JE, Church JM, Gupta S, et al. Significance of incidental desmoids identified during surgery for familial adenomatous polyposis. Dis Colon Rectum 2004; 47:334.

160. Burke AP, Sobin LH, Shekitka KM. Mesenteric fibromatosis. A follow-up study. Arch Pathol Lab Med 1990; 114:832.

161. Richard HM 3rd, Thall EH, Mitty H, et al. Desmoid tumor-ureteral fistula in Gardner's syndrome. Urology 1997; 49:135.

162. Emory TS, Monihan JM, Carr NJ, et al. Sclerosing mesenteritis, mesenteric panniculitis and mesenteric lipodystrophy: a single entity? Am J Surg Pathol 1997; 21:392.

163. Montgomery E, Torbenson MS, Kaushal M, et al. Beta-catenin immunohistochemistry separates mesenteric fibromatosis from gastrointestinal stromal tumor and sclerosing mesenteritis. Am J Surg Pathol 2002; 26:1296.

164. Meis JM, Enzinger FM. Inflammatory fibrosarcoma of the mesentery and retroperitoneum. A tumor closely simulating inflammatory pseudotumor. Am J Surg Pathol 1991; 15:1146.

165. Rodriguez JA, Guarda LA, Rosai J. Mesenteric fibromatosis with involvement of the gastrointestinal tract. A GIST simulator: a study of 25 cases. Am J Clin Pathol 2004; 121:93.

166. Yantiss RK, Spiro IJ, Compton CC, et al. Gastrointestinal stromal tumor versus intra-abdominal fibromatosis of the bowel wall: A clinically important differential diagnosis. Am J Surg Pathol 2000; 24:947.

167. Sturt NJ, Gallagher MC, Bassett P, et al. Evidence for genetic predisposition to desmoid tumours in familial adenomatous polyposis independent of the germline APC mutation. Gut 2004; 53:1832.

168. Soravia C, Berk T, McLeod RS, et al. Desmoid disease in patients with familial adenomatous polyposis. Dis Colon Rectum 2000; 43:363.

169. Tonelli F, Ficari F, Valanzano R, et al. Treatment of desmoids and mesenteric fibromatosis in familial adenomatous polyposis with raloxifene. Tumori 2003; 89:391.

170. Hansmann A, Adolph C, Vogel T, et al. High-dose tamoxifen and sulindac as first-line

treatment for desmoid tumors. Cancer 2004; 100:612.

171. Okuno SH, Edmonson JH. Combination chemotherapy for desmoid tumors. Cancer 2003; 97:1134.

172. Tzakis AG, Tryphonopoulos P, De Faria W, et al. Partial abdominal evisceration, ex vivo resection, and intestinal autotransplantation for the treatment of pathologic lesions of the root of the mesentery. J Am Coll Surg 2003; 197:770.

173. Bar-Maor JA, Shabshin U. Mesenteric fibromatosis. J Pediatr Surg 1993; 28:1618.

174. Nichols RW. Desmoid tumors: A report of 31 cases. Arch Surg 71923; :227.

175. Gardner EJ. A genetic and clinical study of intestinal polyposis, a predisposing factor for carcinoma of the colon and rectum. Am J Hum Genet 1951; 3:167.

176. Smith WG. Multiple polyposis, Gardner's syndrome and desmoid tumors. Dis Colon Rectum 1958; 1:323.

177. Gorlin RJ, Chaudhary AP. Multiple osteomatosis, fibromas, lipomas and fibrosarcomas of the skin and mesentery, epidermoid inclusion cysts of the skin, leiomyomas and multiple intestinal polyposis: a heritable disorder of connective tissue. N Engl J Med 1960; 263:1151.

178. Clark SK, Smith TG, Katz DE, et al. Identification and progression of a desmoid precursor lesion in patients with familial adenomatous polyposis. Br J Surg 1998; 85:970.

179. Parc Y, Piquard A, Dozois RR, et al. Long-term outcome of familial adenomatous polyposis patients after restorative coloproctectomy. Ann Surg 2004; 239:378.

180. Gold RS, Mucha SJ. Unique case of mesenteric fibrosis in multiple polyposis. Am J Surg 1975; 130:366.

181. Tulchinsky H, Keidar A, Goldman G, et al. Surgical treatment and long-term outcome of patients with familial adenomatous polyposis: 16 years experience at the Tel Aviv Sourasky Medical Center. Isr Med Assoc J 2005; 7:82.

182. Tulchinsky H, Keidar A, Strul H, et al. Extracolonic manifestations of familial adenomatous polyposis after proctocolectomy. Arch Surg 2005; 140:159.

183. Kinzler KW, Nilbert MC, Su LK, et al. Identification of FAP locus genes from chromosome 5q21. Science 1991; 253:661.

184. Miyaki M, Konishi M, Kikuchi-Yanoshita R, et al. Coexistence of somatic and germ-line mutations of APC gene in desmoid tumors from patients with familial adenomatous polyposis. Cancer Res 1993; 53:5079.

185. Okamoto M, Sato C, Kohno Y, et al. Molecular nature of chromosome 5q loss in colorectal tumors and desmoids from patients with familial adenomatous polyposis. Hum Genet 1990; 85:595.

186. Rubinfeld B, Albert I, Porfiri E, et al. Loss of beta-catenin regulation by the APC tumor suppressor protein correlates with loss of structure due to common somatic mutations of the gene. Cancer Res 1997; 57:4624.

187. Bridge JA, Sreekantaiah C, Mouron B, et al. Clonal chromosomal abnormalities in desmoid tumors. Implications for histopathogenesis. Cancer 1992; 69:430.

188. Dal Cin P, Sciot R, Van Damme B, et al. Trisomy 20 characterizes a second group of desmoid tumors. Cancer Genet Cytogenet 1995; 79:189.

189. Fletcher JA, Naeem R, Xiao S, et al. Chromosome aberrations in desmoid tumors. Trisomy 8 may be a predictor of recurrence. Cancer Genet Cytogenet 1995; 79:139.

Idiopathic retroperitoneal fibrosis
(Ormond's disease)

190. Ormond JK. Bilateral ureteral obstruction due to envelopment and compression by an inflammatory retroperitoneal process. J Urol 1948; 59:1072.

191. Ormond JK. Idiopathic retroperitoneal fibrosis: An established clinical entity. JAMA 1960; 174:1561.

192. Gilkeson GS, Allen NB. Retroperitoneal fibrosis. A true connective tissue disease. Rheum Dis Clin North Am 1996; 22:23.

193. Loffeld RJ, van Weel TF. Tamoxifen for retroperitoneal fibrosis. Lancet 1993; 341:382.

194. Sherman C, Winchester P, Brill PW, et al. Childhood retroperitoneal fibrosis. Pediatr Radiol 1988; 18:245.

195. Vaglio A, Corradi D, Manenti L, et al. Evidence of autoimmunity in chronic periaortitis: a prospective study. Am J Med 2003; 114:454.

196. Baker LR, Mallinson WJ, Gregory MC, et al. Idiopathic retroperitoneal fibrosis. A retrospective analysis of 60 cases. Br J Urol 1987; 60:497.

197. Marcolongo R, Tavolini IM, Laveder F, et al. Immunosuppressive therapy for idiopathic retroperitoneal fibrosis: a retrospective analysis of 26 cases. Am J Med 2004; 116:194.

198. Agarwal P, Fahn S, Frucht SJ. Diagnosis and management of pergolide-induced fibrosis. Mov Disord 2004; 19:699.

199. Uibu T, Oksa P, Auvinen A, et al. Asbestos exposure as a risk factor for retroperitoneal fibrosis. Lancet 2004; 363:1422.

200. Kottra JJ, Dunnick NR. Retroperitoneal fibrosis. Radiol Clin North Am 1996; 34:1259.

201. Parums DV, Brown DL, Mitchinson MJ. Serum antibodies to oxidized low-density lipoprotein and ceroid in chronic periaortitis. Arch Pathol Lab Med 1990; 114:383.

202. Tiptaft RC, Costello AJ, Paris AM, et al. The long-term follow-up of idiopathic retroperitoneal fibrosis. Br J Urol 1982; 54:620.

203. Lees AJ. Fibrosis due to ergot derivatives: Exposure to risk should be weighed up. Prescrire Int 2002; 11:186.

204. Cai FZ, Tesar P, Klestov A. Methysergide-induced retroperitoneal fibrosis and pericardial effusion. Intern Med J 2004; 34:297.

205. Wen CC, Wang DS. Laparoscopic ureterolysis for benign and malignant conditions. J Endourol 2005; 19:710.

206. Vaglio A, Buzio C. Chronic periaortitis: A spectrum of diseases. Curr Opin Rheumatol 2005; 17:34.

207. Kardar AH, Kattan S, Lindstedt E, et al. Steroid therapy for idiopathic retroperitoneall fibrosis: dose and duration. J Urol 2002; 168:550.

208. Harreby M, Bilde T, Helin P, et al. Retroperitoneal fibrosis treated with methylprednisolone pulse and disease-modifying antirheumatic drugs. Scand J Urol Nephrol 1994; 28:237.

209. Grotz W, von Zedtwitz I, Andre M, et al. Treatment of retroperitoneal fibrosis by mycophenolate mofetil and corticosteroids. Lancet 1998; 352:1195.

210. Tan MO, Uygur MC, Diker Y, et al. Remission of idiopathic retroperitoneal fibrosis after sequential therapy with corticosteroids and tamoxifen. Urol Int 2003; 71:426.

211. Mitchinson MJ. Aortic disease in idiopathic retroperitoneal and mediastinal fibrosis. J Clin Pathol 1972; 25:287.

212. Parums DV, Chadwick DR, Mitchinson MJ. The localisation of immunoglobulin in chronic periaortitis. Atherosclerosis 1986; 61:117.

213. Mitchinson MJ. Chronic periaortitis and periarteritis. Histopathology 1984; 8:589.

214. Okada H, Takahira S, Sugahara S, et al. Retroperitoneal fibrosis and systemic lupus erythematosus. Nephrol Dial Transplant 1999; 14:1300.

215. de Roux-Serratrice C, Serratrice J, Granel B, et al. Periaortitis heralding Wegener's granulomatosis. J Rheumatol 2002; 29:392.

216. Tang KH, Schofield JB, Powell-Jackson PR. Primary biliary cirrhosis and idiopathic retroperitoneal fibrosis: A rare association. Eur J Gastroenterol Hepatol 2002; 14:783.

217. Dehner LP, Coffin CM. Idiopathic fibrosclerotic disorders and other inflammatory pseudotumors. Semin Diagn Pathol 1998; 15:161.

218. Szarf G, Bluemke DA. Case 83: multifocal fibrosclerosis with mediastinal-retroperitoneal involvement. Radiology 2005; 235:829.

219. Hughes D, Buckley PJ. Idiopathic retroperitoneal fibrosis is a macrophage-rich process. Implications for its pathogenesis and treatment. Am J Surg Pathol 1993; 17:482.

220. Ramshaw AL, Roskell DE, Parums DV. Cytokine gene expression in aortic adventitial inflammation associated with advanced atherosclerosis (chronic periaortitis). J Clin Pathol 1994; 47:721.

FIBROUS TUMORS OF INFANCY AND CHILDHOOD

CHAPTER CONTENTS

Fibrous tumors of infancy and childhood can be divided into two large groups. The first group consists of lesions that correspond to similar lesions in adults in terms of clinical setting, microscopic picture, and behavior. Typical examples of such lesions are nodular fasciitis, palmar or plantar fibromatosis, and abdominal or extra-abdominal fibromatosis. The second group consists of fibrous lesions that are peculiar to infancy and childhood and generally have no clinical or morphologic counterpart in adult life. The latter are less common; because of their unusual microscopic features, they pose a special problem in diagnosis. In fact, the microscopic picture often fails to accurately reflect the biologic behavior, and features such as cellularity and rapid growth may be mistaken for evidence of malignancy, sometimes leading to unnecessary and excessive therapy. Accurate interpretation and diagnosis of these lesions are therefore of utmost importance for predicting clinical behavior and for selecting the proper forms of therapy (Table 10–1).

FIBROUS HAMARTOMA OF INFANCY

Fibrous hamartoma of infancy is a distinctive, benign, fibrous growth that most frequently occurs during the first 2 years of life. This lesion was first reported by Reye in 1956 as *subdermal fibromatous tumor of infancy*.[1] In 1965, Enzinger reviewed a series of 30 cases from the files of the AFIP and suggested the term *fibrous hamartoma of infancy* to emphasize its organoid microscopic appearance and its frequent occurrence at birth and during the immediate postnatal period.[2]

Clinical findings

The lesion virtually always develops during the first 2 years of life (median age 10 months) as a small, rapidly growing mass in the subcutis or reticular dermis. Rare lesions have been reported in older infants and children. About 15–25% of cases are present at birth.[2,3] Like other fibrous tumors in children, it is more common in boys than in girls, with boys affected two to three times more often.[3] The mass is often freely movable; occasionally it is fixed to the underlying fascia but only rarely involves the superficial portion of the musculature. These lesions grow rapidly from the outset up to the age of about 5 years. The growth of the lesion then slows but does not cease or regress spontaneously.[4]

Most occur above the waist, with the most common location being the anterior or posterior axillary fold, followed in frequency by the upper arm, thigh, inguinal and pubic region, shoulder, back, and forearm. This lesion has also been described in unusual locations, including the scrotum,[5] labium majus,[6] scalp,[7] and gluteal region.[8] Few cases have been described in the feet or hands,[9] a feature that helps distinguish this lesion from infantile digital fibromatosis and calcifying aponeurotic fibroma. Virtually all cases are solitary, with only rare reports of multiple lesions in the same patient.[2] There is no evidence of increased familial incidence or of associated malformations or other neoplasms. Antecedent trauma is occasionally reported at the time of presentation, but is likely unrelated to its pathogenesis.[10]

Gross findings

The excised lesion tends to be poorly circumscribed and consists of an intimate mixture of firm gray-white tissue

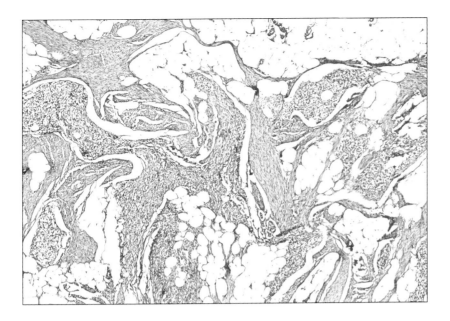

FIGURE 10–1 Fibrous hamartoma of infancy showing a characteristic organoid pattern composed of interlacing fibrous trabeculae, islands of loosely arranged spindle-shaped cells, and mature adipose tissue.

TABLE 10–1   **CLINICOPATHOLOGIC CHARACTERISTICS OF FIBROUS TUMORS OF INFANCY AND CHILDHOOD**

Histologic diagnosis	Age (years)	Location	Solitary	Multiple	Regression
Fibrous hamartoma	B-2	Axilla, inguinal area	+	–	–
Digital fibromatosis	B-2	Fingers, toes	+	+	+
Myofibromatosis	B-A	Soft tissue, bone, viscera	+	+	+
Hyaline fibromatosis	2-A	Dermis, subcutis	–	+	–
Gingival fibromatosis	B-A	Gingiva, hard palate	+	+	+
Fibromatosis colli	B-2	Sternocleidomastoid muscle	+	Bilateral	+
Infantile fibromatosis	B-4	Musculature	+	–	–
Congenital/infantile fibrosarcoma	B-2	Musculature	+	–	–
Calcifying aponeurotic fibroma	2-A	Hands, feet	+	–	+

A, adult life; B, birth.

and fat. In some cases the fatty component is inconspicuous, whereas in others it occupies a large portion of the tumor, thereby resembling a fibrolipoma. Most measure 3–5 cm in greatest diameter, but tumors as large as 15 cm have been reported.

Microscopic findings

Fibrous hamartoma of infancy is characterized by three distinct components forming a vague, irregular, "organoid" pattern (Figs 10–1, 10–2): (1) well-defined intersecting trabeculae of fibrous tissue of varying size and shape and composed of well-oriented spindle-shaped cells (predominantly myofibroblasts) separated by varying amounts of collagen (Figs 10–3, 10–4); (2) loosely textured areas consisting chiefly of immature small, round, or stellate cells in a matrix of Alcian blue-positive hyaluronidase sensitive material (Figs 10–5 to 10–7); and (3) varying amounts of interspersed mature fat, which may be present only at the periphery of the lesion or may be the major component. Despite the lack of clear boundaries between the fat in the tumor and that in the surrounding subcutis, there is little doubt that the fat is an integral part of the lesion. In fact, in many cases its total amount exceeds many times the amount of fat normally present in the surrounding subcutis. In some cases the immature small round cells in the myxoid foci are oriented around small veins.[11]

Some tumors show an additional tissue component, a peculiar fibrosing process that has a superficial resemblance to a neurofibroma.[2] It consists of thick collagen fibers and scattered fibroblasts that replace the fat in the loosely textured mesenchymal areas; sometimes it is the principal component of the tumor.

Immunohistochemical and ultrastructural findings

Immunohistochemically, staining for vimentin is positive in both the trabecular and loosely cellular areas.

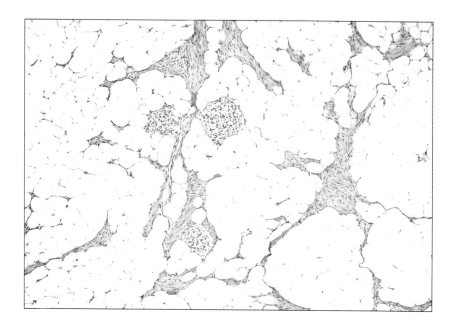

FIGURE 10–2 Fibrous hamartoma of infancy with an organoid pattern but composed predominantly of mature adipose tissue.

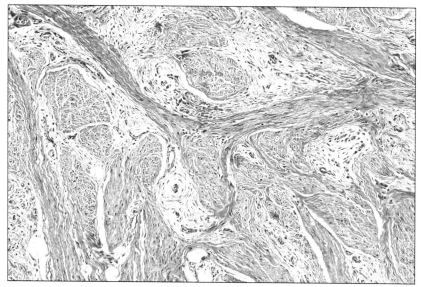

FIGURE 10–3 Fibrous hamartoma of infancy with interlacing fibrous trabeculae and interspersed myxoid zones.

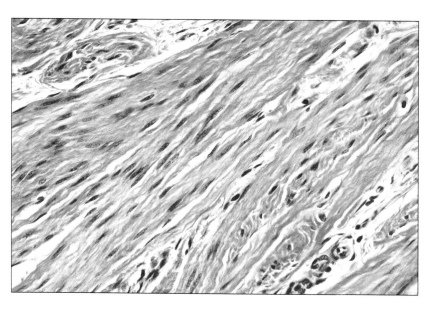

FIGURE 10–4 High-power view of spindle-shaped cells in fibrous trabeculae of a fibrous hamartoma of infancy.

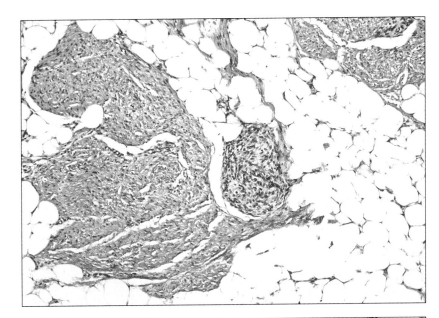

FIGURE 10–5 Fibrous hamartoma of infancy showing an admixture of mature adipose tissue, fibrous trabeculae, and a nodule of spindle-shaped cells.

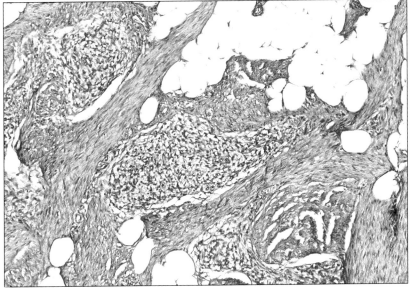

FIGURE 10–6 Organoid pattern with a characteristic arrangement of the three distinct components typical of fibrous hamartoma of infancy.

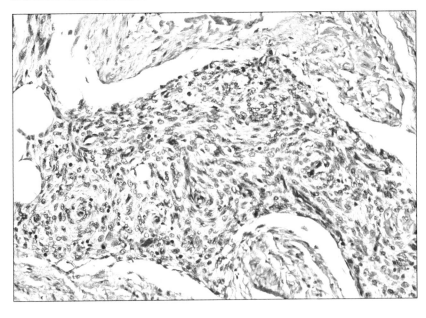

FIGURE 10–7 High-power view of cytologically bland spindle-shaped cells deposited in a myxoid stroma in a fibrous hamartoma of infancy.

Actin immunoreactivity is present only in the trabecular component,[12] and desmin is rarely expressed. In some cases, the spindle cell component stains for CD34.

Ultrastructurally, the lesional cells have both fibroblastic and myofibroblastic features, with some cells showing partial envelopment by basal lamina, pinocytotic vesicles, myofilaments with focal dense bodies, and occasional subplasmalemmal densities.[12] The immature-appearing cells resemble immature mesenchymal cells with few intracytoplasmic organelles.

Differential diagnosis

In most cases the "organoid" pattern characteristic of fibrous hamartoma of infancy is readily recognized, so the lesion is not difficult to distinguish from other entities. On occasion, when the myofibroblastic areas predominate, the lesion may be difficult to distinguish from infantile fibromatosis, diffuse myofibromatosis, and calcifying aponeurotic fibroma. *Infantile fibromatosis* may encroach on the subcutis in a similar trabecular manner, but this tumor arises primarily in muscle rather than in the subcutis and lacks the "organoid" pattern of fibrous hamartoma. *Diffuse myofibromatosis*, typically nodular or multinodular, is characterized by light-staining nodules separated by or associated with hemangiopericytoma-like vascular areas. *Calcifying aponeurotic fibroma* may grow in the same trabecular manner, especially during its earliest phase, when there is still little or no calcification. However, the older age of the children and the location of the tumor in the palm of the hand permit an unequivocal diagnosis.

Awareness of the characteristic "organoid" pattern also facilitates distinction from *infantile fibrosarcoma* and *embryonal rhabdomyosarcoma*. Because some fibrous hamartomas of infancy occur in the scrotal region, the *spindle cell form of embryonal rhabdomyosarcoma* enters the differential diagnosis, but this lesion generally occurs in older children and is composed of cells with more cytologic atypia.

Discussion

It is important to recognize and distinguish fibrous hamartoma of infancy from other forms of fibromatosis because it is a benign lesion that, despite its focal cellularity, is usually cured by local excision. As many as 16% locally recur,[2,3] but recurrences are nondestructive and are generally cured by local re-excision.

The true nature of fibrous hamartoma of infancy remains obscure. Although Reye suggested that it might be a reparative process,[1] there are no histologic features that suggest the lesion is a response to local injury. As its name implies, most have advocated the hamartomatous nature of this lesion, but it is not possible to exclude the possibility that it is a benign neoplasm. A single case of fibrous hamartoma of infancy with a t(2;3)(q31;q21) has been reported.[13]

INFANTILE DIGITAL FIBROMATOSIS

Infantile digital fibromatosis is a distinctive fibrous tumor of infancy characterized by its occurrence in the fingers and toes, a marked tendency for local recurrence, and the presence of characteristic inclusion bodies in the cytoplasm of the neoplastic fibroblasts. In 1957, Jensen et al. reported seven patients whose presentations were consistent with this entity but referred to these lesions as *digital neurofibrosarcoma in infancy*.[14] Enzinger subsequently reported seven cases in 1965 as *infantile dermal fibromatosis*.[15]

Clinical findings

Most patients present with a firm, broad-based, hemispheric or dome-shaped, nontender nodule with a smooth, glistening surface that is skin-colored or pale red. They are usually small, rarely exceeding 2 cm in greatest diameter. Almost all of these lesions are noted within the first 3 years of life, with most recognized by 1 year of age. Up to one-third of cases are already present at birth.[16,17] Rare examples have been described in older children, adolescents, and even in adults.[18–20] Unlike most other forms of fibromatosis, the condition seems to be slightly more common in girls than in boys, but there is no evidence of any familial tendency. Recently, this lesion has been identified in patients with terminal osseous dysplasia and pigmentary defects, possibly inherited in an X-lined dominant fashion.[21,22]

The nodules are more often found in the fingers than the toes and in most instances are located on the sides or dorsum of the distal or middle phalangeal joints, especially of the third, fourth, and fifth digits. Although the thumb is rarely affected, none involving the great toe has been reported. The lesions may be single or multiple and often affect more than one digit of the same hand or foot. Occasionally they involve both the fingers and toes of the same patient. Very few cases have been described as occurring outside the hands and feet. Purdy and Colby reported a case with typical eosinophilic perinuclear inclusions that occurred in the upper arm of a 2½-year-old child near an old injection site.[23] Pettinato et al. described two cases of "extradigital inclusion body fibromatosis" in the breasts of 24- and 53-year-old women.[24]

Although pain and tenderness are not typical symptoms, associated functional impairment or joint deformities may be present, such as lateral deviation or flexion deformities of the adjacent joints. These deformities typically remain unchanged following surgical removal of the lesions.

Pathologic findings

The excised lesions are small, firm masses that are covered on one side by intact skin and have a solid white cut surface (Fig. 10–8). They show little variation in their microscopic appearance; like the desmoid form of infantile fibromatosis, they consist of a uniform proliferation of fibroblasts surrounded by a dense collagenous stroma (Fig. 10–9). They are poorly circumscribed and extend from the epidermis into the deeper portions of the dermis and subcutis, typically surrounding the dermal appendages. The overlying epidermis is usually minimally altered, with slight hyperkeratosis or acanthosis.

The most striking feature of the tumor is the presence of small, round inclusions in the cytoplasm of the fibroblasts. The number of inclusions varies from case to case. In some they are numerous and easily detected, whereas in others they are scarce and difficult to find with hematoxylin and eosin-stained slides. Typically, these inclusions are situated close to the nucleus from which a narrow clear zone (Fig. 10–10) often separates them. They are eosinophilic and resemble erythrocytes except for their more variable size (3–15 μm), intracytoplasmic location, and lack of refringence. Numerous histochemical preparations can be used to highlight these inclusions; they stain a deep red with Masson trichrome stain (Fig. 10–11), but do not stain with periodic acid-Schiff (PAS), Alcian blue, or colloidal iron stains.

Immunohistochemical and ultrastructural findings

Immunohistochemically, the spindled cells stain consistently for actin, but variable results have been obtained

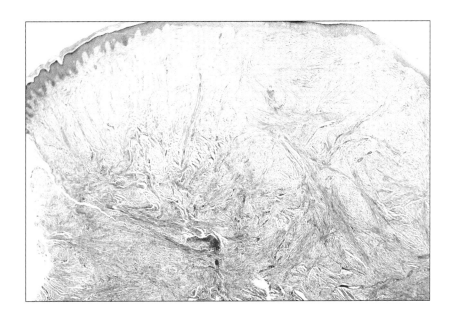

FIGURE 10–8 Low-power view of a broad-based hemispheric dermal nodule composed of spindle-shaped cells, characteristic of infantile digital fibromatosis.

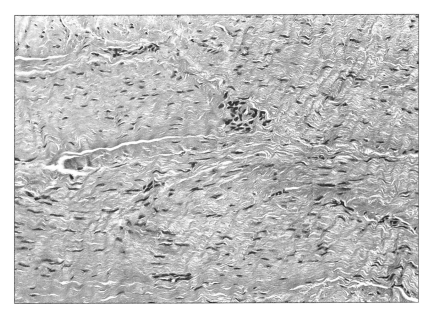

FIGURE 10–9 Infantile digital fibromatosis, composed of a uniform proliferation of fibroblasts surrounded by a dense collagenous stroma.

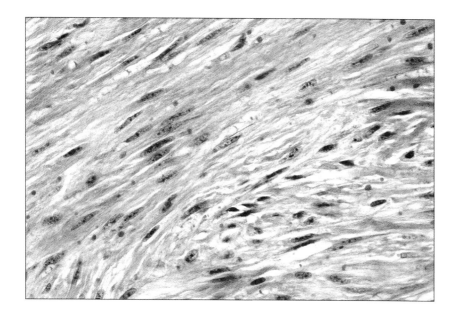

FIGURE 10–10 Infantile digital fibromatosis. Fibroblasts with characteristic intracytoplasmic inclusions separated by a narrow clear zone.

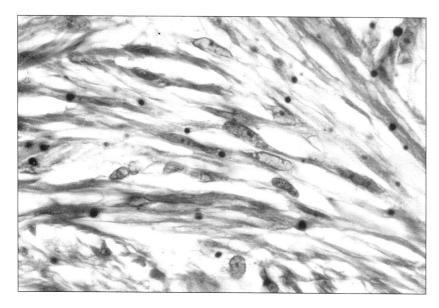

FIGURE 10–11 Masson trichrome stain demonstrating intracytoplasmic inclusions characteristic of infantile digital fibromatosis.

with respect to actin immunoreactivity of the inclusion bodies themselves. Most of the earlier studies using formalin-fixed tissues were unable to demonstrate actin staining of the inclusion bodies.[25] However, actin staining of the inclusion bodies has been demonstrated using alcohol-fixed tissue as well as KOH and trypsin-pretreated formalin-fixed tissue.[26]

Bhawan et al. were the first to emphasize the myofibroblastic nature of many of the cells in infantile digital fibromatosis and proposed the alternate term *infantile digital myofibroblastoma*.[27] The myofibroblasts contain narrow intracellular bundles of 5–7 nm microfilaments with interspersed dense bodies and occasional patches of basal lamina.[28] These strap-like bundles of filaments are continuous with the juxtanuclear inclusion bodies, which also consist of fibrillary and granular material that has no limiting membrane and seems to originate in the endo-

plasmic reticulum (Fig. 10–12). Small membrane-bound vesicles may also be found in the inclusion bodies and are probably derived from entrapped cell organelles.[29]

Prognosis and therapy

Although 60% of these lesions recur locally, the ultimate prognosis is excellent. Recurrences usually appear at the same site within a few weeks or months after the initial excision.[30] Although there is an initial period of growth, if watched for a long enough period of time many lesions regress spontaneously.[31] Most authors advocate conservative treatment,[32] since there is no evidence of aggressive behavior or malignant transformation. Some advocate a "watch and wait" approach following a diagnosis, given the high rate of spontaneous regression, but surgical excision is usually undertaken. Mohs' micrographic

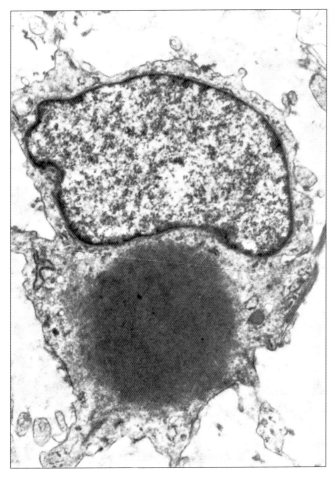

FIGURE 10–12 Infantile digital fibromatosis. Electron microscopy shows an inclusion within the fibroblast. (From Taxy JB, Battifora H. The electron microscope in the study and diagnosis of soft tissue tumors. In: Trump BF, Jones RT, ed. Diagnostic Electron Microscopy. New York: Wiley; 1980, with permission.)

surgery may be effective in minimizing the risk of local recurrence.[33] Deformities and contractures develop in some cases, regardless of whether the lesions are removed surgically, and surgical correction of contractures and functional changes is sometimes necessary.

Discussion

The exact nature of the inclusions is not clear. Because of the resemblance of these inclusions to the viroplasm of fibroblasts infected with SHOPE fibroma virus, Battifora and Hines proposed a possible viral etiology.[34] The immunohistochemical and ultrastructural findings strongly suggest that the inclusions are related to the intracellular bundles of microfilaments and represent densely packed masses of actin microfilaments.[25] The occurrence of extradigital post-traumatic lesions that are histologically indistinguishable from those on the digits[35] and antecedent trauma related to digital lesions[36] suggests that trauma may stimulate development of the lesion. Inclusion bodies identical to those found in infantile digital fibromatosis have also been described in a variety of tumors including a fibrous tumor of the tongue,[37] a dermal fibrous lesion in the toxic oil epidermic syndrome,[38] an endocervical polyp,[39] a vulvar angioleiomyoma,[40] and fibroepithelial proliferations of the breast, including phyllodes tumor.[41]

MYOFIBROMA AND MYOFIBROMATOSIS

Myofibromatosis was initially described in 1951 by Williams and Schrum, who designated the lesions *congenital fibrosarcoma*.[42] Three years later, Stout renamed the entity *congenital generalized fibromatosis*,[43] and he described two male infants who died soon after birth with multiple fibrous nodules in soft tissues and internal organs. In 1965 Kauffman and Stout grouped their cases of "congenital fibromatosis" into two categories: (1) a multiple form, with lesions restricted to skin, subcutaneous tissue, skeletal muscle, and bone and characterized by a good prognosis; and (2) a generalized form, with visceral lesions and a poor prognosis.[44] Following recognition of the myofibroblastic nature of the constituent cells, Chung and Enzinger reported 61 cases of this entity and renamed it *infantile myofibromatosis*.[45] We prefer the terms *myofibroma* and *myofibromatosis* for solitary and multiple lesions, respectively, not only because these lesions occur in infants, children, and adults and have a prominent myofibroblastic component but also because their behavior distinguishes them from other, more aggressive types of fibromatosis.

Clinical findings

Myofibroma manifests as a single swelling or mass most commonly in the dermis and subcutis. It measures a few millimeters to several centimeters in diameter. The more superficially located nodules are freely movable, and when skin is involved, the lesion can manifest as a purplish macule giving the impression of a hemangioma. Some lesions are more deeply seated and appear to be fixed. Although Chung and Enzinger found solitary lesions to be almost three times as common as the multicentric form,[45] in a review of the literature of 170 cases by Wiswell et al. solitary lesions were half as common as the multicentric form.[46] The condition is almost twice as common in males as in females, and both the solitary and multicentric forms occur not only in infants and children but also in adults.[47–49]

Solitary nodules are found most commonly in the general region of the head and neck, including the scalp, forehead, orbit, parotid region, and oral cavity.[50,51] The trunk is the second most commonly affected site, followed by the lower and upper extremities. There have

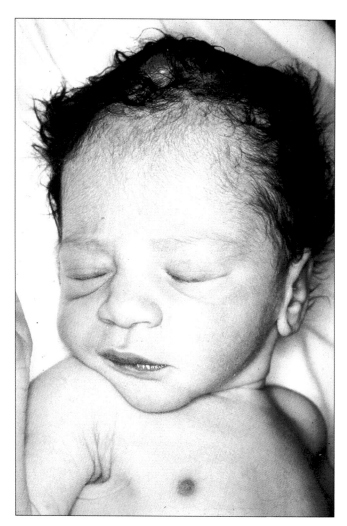

FIGURE 10–13 Newborn infant with myofibromatosis, with numerous dermal and subcutaneous nodules of the head and neck region.

also been several reports of solitary intraosseous myofibromas,[52,53] most of which have involved the craniofacial bones. Solitary lesions involving the viscera are rare.[54–56]

In patients with multiple lesions (*myofibromatosis*), the individual nodules have essentially the same appearance as the solitary nodules; they occur not only in dermis and subcutis but also in muscle, the internal organs, and the skeleton. Up to 40% of patients have visceral lesions that are invariably present at birth (Fig. 10–13). The nodules may be numerous, especially when they are in the subcutis, lung, or skeleton; in several patients more than 50 nodules were counted. Schaffzin et al. reported a newborn girl who had 59 subcutaneous nodules noted at birth.[57] Heiple et al. also described an infant who had more than 100 lesions in the skeleton that involved both flat and long bones.[58] In the latter case, the nodules were recognized only after the infant suffered a fracture in a minor fall and underwent a radiographic examination of the injured leg.

Apart from the soft tissues and the skeleton, the most common sites of organ involvement are the lung, heart, gastrointestinal tract, and pancreas and rarely the central nervous system.[46] Internal lesions often cause symptoms such as severe respiratory distress, vomiting, or diarrhea, which often fail to respond to therapy and prove fatal within a few days or weeks after birth. Others cause few symptoms, making it likely that some internal lesions remain unrecognized. The nodules grow principally during the immediate perinatal period. Lesional growth is not restricted to this period, and continued enlargement or formation of new nodules may be observed during infancy or even later in life.[59]

Radiographically, the bone lesions are circumscribed lytic areas with marginal sclerosis and without penetration of the cortex in most cases.[60] Occasionally, however, a soft tissue lesion may extend into the underlying bone. Extraosseous lesions may show weak radiodensity as a result of focal calcification (Figs 10–14, 10–15).[61] Magnetic resonance imaging (MRI) is useful in planning the extent of surgery.[62]

Pathologic findings

As a rule, the nodules in the dermis and subcutis are better delineated than those in the muscle, bone, or viscera (Fig. 10–16). They are rubbery or firm and scarlike in consistency and typically have a white-gray or pink surface; they vary greatly in size, averaging 0.5–1.5 cm in greatest diameter. Large lesions may ulcerate the overlying epidermis.

Microscopically, *myofibroma* and *myofibromatosis* have similar features. At low magnification, there is typically a nodular or multinodular growth pattern that appears biphasic owing to the alternation of light- and dark-staining areas. The light-staining areas consist mainly of plump myoid spindle cells with eosinophilic cytoplasm arranged in nodules, short fascicles, or whorls (Fig. 10–17). The nuclei are elongated and tapering or cigar-shaped and lack nuclear atypia. Some foci have extensive hyalinization. These areas are usually located more peripherally, although in some cases they are distributed haphazardly throughout the lesion. Immunohistochemically, the cells are immunoreactive for vimentin and actin but do not stain for desmin or S-100 protein, consistent with myofibroblastic differentiation.[63,64]

The dark-staining areas of the lesion, usually centrally located, are composed of round or polygonal cells with slightly pleomorphic hyperchromatic nuclei or small spindle cells arranged around a distinct hemangiopericytoma-like vascular pattern (Figs 10–18, 10–19). These primitive cells have vesicular nuclei, small amounts of eosinophilic cytoplasm, indistinct cell margins and a low mitotic index. In some cases focal hemorrhage, cystic degeneration, or coagulative necrosis is present, often with foci of calcification. Peripherally

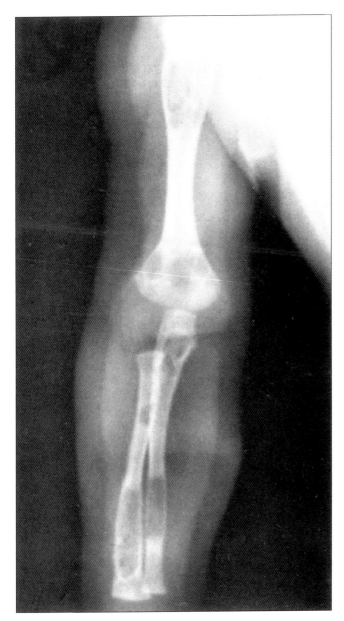

FIGURE 10–14 Infantile myofibromatosis, multicentric type, with extensive bone involvement of the right arm. (From Brill PW, Yandow DR, Langer LO, et al. Congenital generalized fibromatosis: case report and literature review. Pediatr Radiol 1982; 12:269, with permission.)

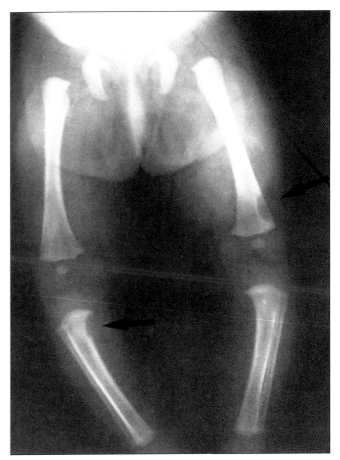

FIGURE 10–15 Infantile myofibromatosis, multicentric type, with multiple bone involvement (arrows). These osseous lesions tend to regress spontaneously and usually are no longer demonstrable after a few years.

located chronic inflammatory cells, including lymphocytes and plasma cells, may be present. Because of these cellular and richly vascular areas and the extensive necrosis, these lesions can be mistaken for a sarcoma. In addition, the presence of intravascular growth, a feature that is present in up to one-fifth of cases, may also be worrisome but does not seem to have any prognostic significance. Some cases are composed almost exclusively of these cellular areas (so-called monophasic cellular variant of infantile myofibromatosis), which may represent the earliest stage of the disease.[65]

Recently, Coffin and colleagues analyzed 59 IMTs with histologic atypia and/or clinical aggressiveness.[235a] The majority of these lesions occurred in the abdomen or pelvis (64%). Thirty-three patients had local recurrences including 6 patients with both local recurrences and distant metastases. Lesions located in an abdominopelvic location were more likely to recur. Interestingly, absence *ALK* expression was associated with older age, distant metastases and death from disease.

Immunohistochemical and ultrastructural findings

Immunohistochemically, the primitive-appearing cells stain focally and weakly for actin. Fletcher et al. thought these cells had smooth muscle differentiation based on the immunohistochemical expression of desmin.[66] However, a study by the same authors several years later found an absence of desmin staining in these primitive cells, and they suggested that the discrepant results were obtained because of the use of an outdated polyclonal anti-chicken antibody.[67] Ultrastructurally, there is general

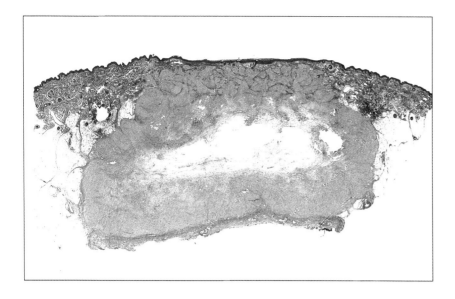

FIGURE 10–16 Low-power view of a solitary myofibroma involving the dermis and subcutis.

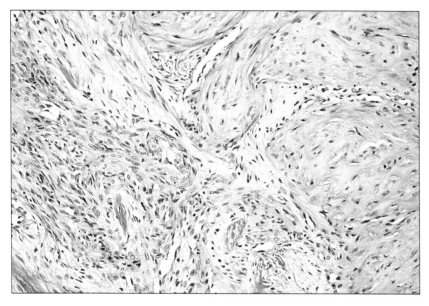

FIGURE 10–17 Infantile myofibromatosis, solitary type, consisting of broad bundles of plump myoid spindle cells with eosinophilic cytoplasm.

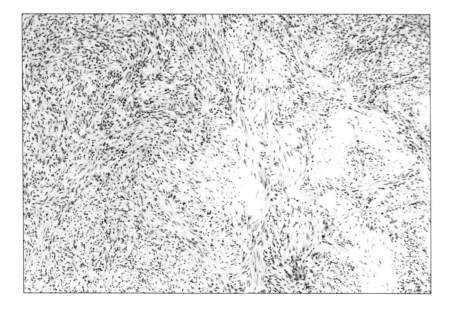

FIGURE 10–18 Infantile myofibromatosis, solitary type, composed predominantly of darkly staining spindle-shaped cells with intermixed plumper myoid-like cells.

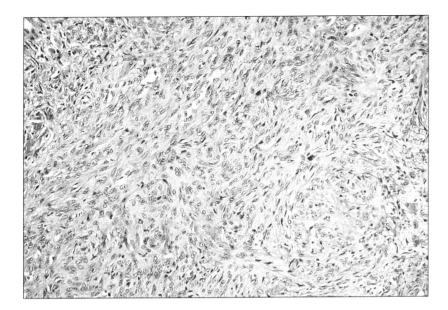

FIGURE 10–19 Infantile myofibromatosis with cellular proliferation of ovoid cells without cytologic atypia.

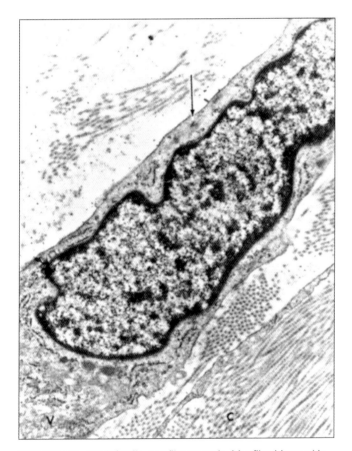

FIGURE 10–20 Infantile myofibromatosis. Myofibroblasts with condensed filamentous material (arrow). (From Benjamin SP, Mercer RD, Hawk W. Myofibroblastic contraction in spontaneous regression of multiple congenital mesenchymal hamartomas. Cancer 1977; 40:2343, with permission.)

agreement that the predominant cells are fibroblasts and myofibroblasts, with prominent endoplasmic reticulum, intracytoplasmic microfilaments, dense bodies, focal basal lamina, and occasional fibronexus junctions (Fig. 10–20).[63,68]

Differential diagnosis

The differential diagnosis of this lesion depends in part on whether the eosinophilic myofibroblasts or more primitive small cells predominate in a given lesion. The peripheral areas of myofibroma can resemble nodular fasciitis, fibrous histiocytoma, neurofibroma, or infantile fibromatosis. *Nodular fasciitis* is a rare lesion in newborns and infants but certainly should be considered in the differential diagnosis in adults. Nodular fasciitis arises from the fascia, has a more prominent myxoid matrix, and usually contains scattered chronic inflammatory cells and occasional erythrocytes. The hemangiopericytoma-like pattern characteristic of myofibroma is absent in nodular fasciitis. The peripheral areas may also resemble *neurofibroma*, but the myofibroblastic cells lack S-100 protein. Clinically, myofibromatosis should not be confused with *type 1 neurofibromatosis (NF-1)*, as myofibromatosis manifests with multiple nodules at birth or within the first few weeks of life, whereas neurofibromatosis affects older children with evidence of multiple café au lait spots and other stigmata of NF-1. Interestingly, there is one report of solitary myofibroma arising in a patient with well-documented NF-1.[69] *Fibrous histiocytoma* is composed of a polymorphous proliferation of cells arranged in a more pronounced storiform pattern. Although smooth muscle actin may be found in fibrous histiocytoma, the staining is usually focal. Furthermore, the cells of fibrous histiocytoma usually express factor XIIIa. Solitary forms of the disease may be mistaken for *infantile fibromatosis*. The latter tends to be less well circumscribed, arise in muscle, and show a more uniform spindle cell pattern. In addition, infantile fibromatosis shows neither central necrosis nor a central hemangiopericytoma-like vascular pattern.

Myofibromatosis has a number of clinical and morphologic similarities with *infantile hemangiopericytoma*.[70] As in myofibromatosis, most infantile hemangiopericytomas are present at birth or occur early in life, with a predilection for boys. Although most are solitary subcutaneous lesions, both multicentricity and visceral involvement have been described. In addition, the main affected sites are similar between these lesions. Histologically, the central immature-appearing areas of myofibromatosis are indistinguishable from those of infantile hemangiopericytoma. Upon review of 11 cases originally diagnosed as infantile hemangiopericytoma, Mentzel et al. found focal mature-appearing, actin-positive, spindle-shaped cells similar to those seen in myofibromatosis in all cases.[70] These authors proposed that infantile hemangiopericytoma and myofibromatosis represent different stages of maturation of a single entity, a contention supported by others.[71,72]

Finally, biopsy specimens obtained from the central portion of this lesion may have features that resemble various types of sarcoma, particularly those composed of small round cells arranged around a hemangiopericytoma-like vasculature. Such lesions include peripheral primitive neuroectodermal tumor, mesenchymal chondrosarcoma, malignant hemangiopericytoma, and poorly differentiated synovial sarcoma. A battery of immunostains, including those for cytokeratins, S-100 protein, and CD99, can assist in the differential diagnosis. Although not always present, identifying peripheral myoid-appearing cells is the most useful feature for recognizing myofibromatosis.

Discussion

The clinical course seems to be largely determined by the extent of the disease. Solitary and multiple lesions confined to soft tissues and bone (with no evidence of visceral involvement) carry an excellent prognosis; they tend to regress spontaneously and rarely require more than a diagnostic biopsy.[45,73] In the review by Wiswell et al., only 5 of 54 (9%) solitary lesions recurred locally following excision, even after incomplete excision.[46] In addition, 11 of 18 patients with multicentric lesions without visceral involvement and follow-up of more than 1 year had spontaneous regression of the lesions. Chung and Enzinger found that only 3 of 28 solitary lesions (11%) locally recurred, and several of the multicentric lesions without visceral involvement showed spontaneous regression.[45] Fukasawa and colleagues documented massive apoptosis in two cases of infantile myofibromatosis and proposed that this mechanism may account for the high rate of spontaneous regression of these lesions.[74]

The prognosis is much less favorable in newborns and infants with multiple visceral lesions, and as many as 75% of them die with signs of respiratory distress or diarrhea soon after birth.[45,46] There are exceptions, however. Hatzidaki et al. reported one case of a child with multicentric visceral involvement with apparent spontaneous regression of the lesions.[75] Similarly, Zeller et al. reported an unusual case of an 8-month-old boy with numerous osteolytic lesions throughout the skeleton that resulted in a softened thoracic wall and respiratory failure.[76] Supportive therapy was given, and many of the lesions subsequently regressed. More recently, low-dose chemotherapy has been shown to be efficacious in some patients with multicentric visceral involvement.[77-79]

Myofibroma and myofibromatosis are clearly expressions of a benign, self-limiting, localized or generalized process that consists to a large degree of cells with the characteristics of myofibroblasts. Several studies have documented a familial occurrence, including the presence of this lesion in siblings, suggesting an autosomal recessive pattern of inheritance.[80,81] Others have described multiple generations of families with an autosomal dominant pattern.[82] Very few cases have been studied cytogenetically. Stenman and co-workers reported a case of solitary myofibroma with a del(6)(q12;q15).[83] Monosomy 9q and trisomy 16q have also been reported.[84]

JUVENILE HYALINE FIBROMATOSIS

Juvenile hyaline fibromatosis is another rare hereditary disease that bears a superficial resemblance to myofibromatosis but differs by its cutaneous distribution of the tumor nodules, the histologic picture, and associated clinical features. The condition was first described by Murray in 1873 as *molluscum fibrosum in children*, and was thought to represent an unusual variant of neurofibromatosis.[85] Whitfield and Robinson offered a follow-up report of these three cases in 1903.[86] Amazingly, no further reports occurred until 1962, when Puretic et al. reported a case under the name *mesenchymal dysplasia*.[87] A variety of terms were used in subsequent reports, including systemic hyalinosis[88] and disseminated painful fibromatosis.[89] Kitano coined the term "juvenile hyaline fibromatosis," which has become the preferred term.[90] This entity appears to be rare, as fewer than 70 cases have been recorded in the world literature.[91]

Clinical findings

Clinical onset is usually noted from 2 months to 5 years of age, but they may be congenital.[92] Some patients are initially diagnosed much later in life (fourth or fifth decade).[91,93] Boys are affected slightly more commonly than girls.[94] The condition is characterized by multiple cutaneous papules, nodules, or masses, gingival hypertro-

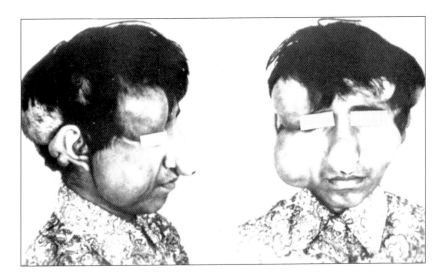

FIGURE 10–21 Juvenile hyaline fibromatosis. Multiple masses involve the scalp and face. (Courtesy of Prof. Dr. Eduardo Carceres, Director, Instituto Nacional de Enfermades Neoplasicas, Lima, Peru.)

phy, joint contractures, and osteolytic defects. The skin lesions have been grouped into three types: (1) small, pearly papules on the face and neck; (2) small nodules and large plaques with a translucent appearance and a gelatinous consistency developing on fingers and ears and around the nose; and (3) firm, large, subcutaneous tumors with a predilection for the scalp, trunk, and limbs (Fig. 10–21).[95] The lesions vary in size from 1 mm to as large as 10 cm; they are slow-growing and painless and have a tendency to recur following excision. The number of cutaneous lesions varies from case to case, but some patients have been found to have more than 100 tumors in various parts of the body.[96] Occasional patients also have perianal papillomatous lesions.[97] Most patients have extracutaneous findings. Gingival hypertrophy and painful flexion contractures of the major joints are present in most patients, and these findings may precede the development of skin lesions.[98] More than 60% of patients reveal multiple osteolytic defects on radiographic examination.[94] Histologic examination of tissue obtained from these bony defects reveals infiltration of hyaline material similar to that seen in the skin and muscle.[99] Most patients report painful, debilitating flexion contractures of large joints, often resulting in marked deformity and generalized stiffness.[100] Other unusual associations include coexisting squamous cell carcinoma of the oral cavity[101] and bullous pemphigoid.[102]

Pathologic findings

The tumors are poorly circumscribed and consist of cords of spindle-shaped cells embedded in a homogeneous eosinophilic matrix (Figs 10–22 to 10–24). They are often found in the dermis, subcutis, and gingiva, although the bone and joints may also be involved. Deposition of this amorphous eosinophilic matrix is widespread in some patients; Kitano et al. reported one patient with autopsy-proven deposition of this substance in the tongue, esophagus, stomach, intestine, thymus, spleen and lymph nodes.[103] Early lesions show increased cellularity and less prominent stroma, whereas the large, older lesions are less cellular and contain more ground substance. The matrix stains positively with PAS and Alcian blue but does not stain with toluidine blue or Congo red. Elastic tissue is completely absent. Occasional nodules reveal marked calcification, including calcospherites.[104] Multinucleated giant cells may occasionally be seen.[105]

Electron microscopic examination reveals scattered fibroblast-like cells with enlarged rough endoplasmic reticulum and a prominent Golgi apparatus containing cystic vesicles filled with a fibrillar and granular material as well as aggregates of microfilaments or fibril-filled balls of varying size.[106,107] Large amounts of microfibrillary material are present in the interstices, with occasional alignment of the fibrils to mature, normal, and long-spaced collagen fibers. Immunohistochemically, the spindled cells are negative for actins.[108] However, there is a conspicuous population of CD68-positive macrophages found between the spindled cells.[105]

Differential diagnosis

Multicentric infantile myofibromatosis is composed of multiple nodules that are almost always present at birth or appear during the first year of life. In general, the nodules are better circumscribed and are found not only in the subcutis but also in muscle, bone, and viscera. Microscopically, they consist of broad, interlacing bundles of plump myofibroblasts, often with a central hemangiopericytoma-like area composed of primitive-appearing cells. The gums or joints are never involved. *Neurofibromatosis* tends to make its first appearance in slightly older children and is associated with café au lait spots; the tumors are composed of hyperchromatic serpentine nuclei in a fibrillary eosinophilic matrix and are positive

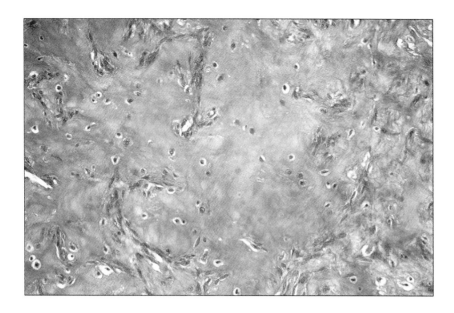

FIGURE 10–22 Hypocellular zone of a juvenile hyaline fibromatosis. Scattered cells with bland nuclei are deposited in a densely hyalinized stroma.

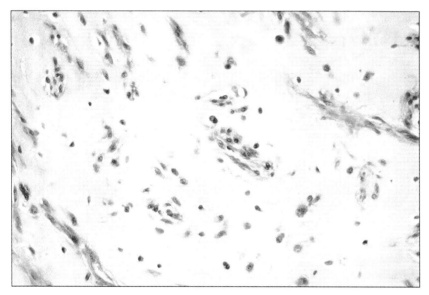

FIGURE 10–23 Juvenile hyaline fibromatosis. High-power view of cytologically bland cells deposited in a densely hyalinized stroma.

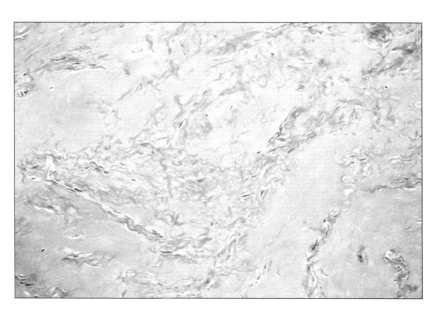

FIGURE 10–24 Juvenile hyaline fibromatosis. This lesion of long duration is almost completely acellular.

for S-100 protein. *Gingival fibromatosis*, a lesion with a similar hereditary pattern, is limited to the gums of the upper and lower jaws and consists of dense, scar-like connective tissue rich in collagen. *Cylindromas*, or turban tumors, are confined to the head.

Winchester syndrome, a rare autosomal hereditary disease, is characterized by densely cellular, poorly demarcated fibrous proliferations in the dermis, subcutis, and joints without deposition of a hyaline matrix; periarticular thickening and limited motion in the limbs and the spine, corneal opacities and radiographic changes of bones and joints are also part of this disorder.[109] The precise relation between juvenile hyaline fibromatosis, Winchester syndrome, and *infantile systemic hyalinosis* is unclear, and some believe that these conditions represent different expressions of the same disorder.[91,110]

Discussion

Although most lesions in this condition are formed during childhood, new lesions may continue to appear into adult life. The nodules continue to grow slowly and may ulcerate the overlying skin. Although local recurrence does occur, Woyke et al. reported a patient who underwent successful surgical removal of more than 100 tumors over a period of 19 years with good cosmetic results.[96] Hence, these authors advocate surgical excision of all newly discovered tumors and hypertrophic gingival tissue. On the other hand, Quintal and Jackson reported a patient who had numerous surgical excisions over a period of 34 years and found that the therapy was as mutilating as the disease.[111] The tumors do not appear to respond to radiotherapy.[111] Most patients with long-term follow-up are severely physically handicapped by joint contractures.[112] Some patients may even develop upper airway obstruction due to the profound gingival hypertrophy that may occur.[113,114] Other patients die in early infancy from overwhelming infection.[100]

The condition is inherited as an autosomal recessive trait. It usually affects more than one sibling of the same family. Although we are not aware that it has ever been observed in more than one generation, consanguinity of the parents of the afflicted children has been reported.[115] In 2002, Rahman and co-workers performed a genome-wide linkage search in two families with this disease and identified a region of homozygosity on chromosome 4q21.[116] Subsequently, Dowling et al. identified disease-causing mutations in the capillary morphogenesis factor-2 (*CMG2*) gene on 4q21 in both juvenile hyaline fibromatosis and infantile systemic hyalinosis, further supporting the link between these conditions.[117] Other workers confirmed the central role of *CMG2* in the pathogenesis of this disease.[118] Defects in this gene likely cause aberrant synthesis of glycosaminoglycans by fibroblasts, which in turn alter the macromolecular organization of collagen.[119]

GINGIVAL FIBROMATOSIS

Gingival fibromatosis is a rare benign fibroproliferative disorder that has been described under various names, including *idiopathic* or *hereditary gingival fibromatosis*,[120,121] *hereditary gingival hyperplasia*,[122] *congenital macrogingivae*,[123] *generalized hypertrophy of the gums*,[124] and *gingival elephantiasis*.[125] It is a clinically distinct entity that chiefly affects young persons of both genders and has a tendency for recurrent local growth. Lesions may be idiopathic or familial, and some are associated with a heterogeneous group of hereditary syndromes. Takagi et al.[126] classified gingival fibromatosis into six categories: (1) isolated familial gingival fibromatosis; (2) isolated idiopathic gingival fibromatosis; (3) gingival fibromatosis associated with hypertrichosis; (4) gingival fibromatosis associated with hypertrichosis and mental retardation or epilepsy (or both); (5) gingival fibromatosis with mental retardation, epilepsy, or both; and (6) gingival fibromatosis associated with hereditary syndromes.

Clinical findings

The principal complaint is of a slowly growing, ill-defined enlargement or swelling of the gingivae, causing little pain but considerable difficulty in speaking and eating. The gingival overgrowth may be to such a degree that the teeth are completely covered and the lips are prevented from closing.[127] The lesions may also extend over the hard palate, resulting in a deformity of the contour of the palate.[126] Some patients also have marked swelling of the jaw bone. In some cases the gingival swelling is minimal and limited to a small portion of the gum (*localized type*), but in most cases it is extensive and bilateral, involving the gingival tissues of both the upper and lower jaws and the hard palate (*generalized type*). Idiopathic cases are slightly more common than familial cases. Among the idiopathic cases, the generalized type outnumbers the localized type by almost 2 to 1.[126] Most familial cases are generalized, as relatively few localized familial cases have been documented.[128] The condition occurs at any age, but most present at the time of eruption of the deciduous or permanent teeth. In fact, it has been postulated that the erupting teeth trigger the fibrous growth, as evidenced by effective treatment with tooth extraction alone in some cases. Patients with the familial form of the disease tend to be younger than those with the idiopathic form. Up to 8% of cases are found at birth or immediately after delivery.[126]

Hypertrichosis is found in almost 10% of patients with this condition. Some patients also have mental retardation or epilepsy (or both), although the latter features can also be present in the absence of hypertrichosis. The gingival fibromatosis associated with these conditions generally occurs at a younger age than in the idiopathic form and is more common in females.

This condition may also be associated with a variety of syndromes. *Zimmerman-Laband syndrome* is a rare autosomal dominant disorder characterized by gingival fibromatosis, various skeletal anomalies including dysplasia of the distal phalanges of thumbs and halluces, vertebral defects and hepatosplenomegaly.[129-131] Stefanova and colleagues reported a t(3;8)(p21.2;q24.3) in a patient with this syndrome,[132] although this observation has yet to be reproduced by others. Gingival fibromatosis has also been found to be associated with cherubism (*Ramon syndrome*),[133,134] hearing loss and supernumerary teeth,[135,136] *Klippel-Trenaunay-Weber syndrome*,[137] prune-belly syndrome,[138] and growth hormone deficiency.[139]

Pathologic findings

Grossly, the growth consists of dense scar-like tissue that cuts with difficulty and has a gray-white glistening surface. On microscopic examination, the lesions (which vary little in appearance) consist of poorly cellular, richly collagenous fibrous connective tissue underneath a normal or acanthotic squamous epithelium. Mild perivascular chronic inflammation and small foci of dystrophic calcification may be present.[140] The histologic features of the familial and idiopathic forms are indistinguishable. Ultrastructurally, the lesion is composed mainly of fusiform fibroblast-like cells surrounded by an extracellular matrix with abundant collagen fibrils and flocculent material.[141]

Differential diagnosis

There is a striking resemblance between gingival fibromatosis and hypertrophy of the gums following prolonged therapy with diphenylhydantoin sodium (Dilantin, phenytoin sodium).[142] In epileptic patients treated with this drug, it is difficult if not impossible to determine the cause of the gingival overgrowth. However, patients with gingival fibromatosis and epilepsy were described prior to the use of phenytoin, indicating that the changes are not entirely drug-induced. Other drugs including immunosuppressive agents (ciclosporin A) and calcium channel blockers (nifedipine) can induce the same changes.[143] Lesions of similar appearance may also be found during pregnancy and as the result of chronic gingivitis. In most of these cases, a detailed clinical and family history permits the correct diagnosis. *Juvenile hyaline fibromatosis*, a hereditary lesion that may involve the gingiva in a similar manner, can be distinguished by its association with multiple cutaneous tumors and the characteristic microscopic appearance, especially the prominent PAS-positive hyaline matrix.

Discussion

Surgical excision of the hyperplastic tissue is frequently followed by local recurrence. However, the overgrowth may recede or disappear with tooth extraction. Many authors recommend excision of the excess tissue and removal of all teeth in severe cases.[121]

Approximately 35% of cases of gingival fibromatosis are familial; however, there is clearly genetic heterogeneity. While some cases appear to be inherited in an autosomal recessive manner, most have an autosomal dominant pattern of inheritance. Several genes have been associated with gingival fibromatosis, including mutations at 2p21-p22, possibly involving the *SOS-1* gene,[144-146] as well as alterations at 5q13-q22.[147] The fibroblasts in this condition have a higher proliferative rate than normal gingival fibroblasts,[148] possibly mediated by autocrine stimulation by TGF-β1.[149]

FIBROMATOSIS COLLI

Fibromatosis colli has long been recognized as a peculiar benign fibrous growth of the sternocleidomastoid muscle that usually appears during the first weeks of life and is often associated with muscular torticollis, or wryneck. It bears a close resemblance to other forms of infantile fibromatosis but is sufficiently different in its microscopic appearance and behavior to warrant separation as a distinct entity. This lesion occurs in approximately 0.4% of live births.[150] The finding of torticollis is not synonymous with the presence of fibromatosis colli, as nearly 80 entities have been reported to cause torticollis (acquired torticollis).[151] In a retrospective study of 58 patients with infantile torticollis using MRI, Parikh and colleagues found evidence of fibromatosis colli in 7 patients.[152]

Clinical findings

Characteristically, the lesion manifests between the second and fourth weeks of life as a mass lying in or replacing the mid to lower portion of the sternocleidomastoid muscle, especially its sternal or clavicular portion. The lesion is movable only in a horizontal plane and never affects the overlying skin. Rare cases also simultaneously involve the trapezius muscle.[153] Most commonly, a 1–3 cm long, hard mass or "bulb" is palpable at the base of the sternocleidomastoid muscle 2–4 weeks after birth. Almost all cases are unilateral, with a slight predilection for the right side of the neck; rare cases of bilateral fibromatosis colli have been described.[154] Most authors have found a slight predilection for this lesion to occur in boys.[155]

Initially, the mass grows rapidly, but after a few weeks or months the growth slows and becomes stationary. In many cases, spontaneous regression occurs by the age of 1–2 years, and the lesion may no longer be palpable. During the initial growth period, torticollis (rotation and tilting of the head to the affected side) occurs in only about one-fourth to one-third of cases and usually is mild and transient. In addition, the face and skull on the affected side may begin to appear smaller, resulting in facial asymmetry and plagiocephaly; there is flattening of the affected side of the face with posterior displacement of the ipsilateral ear.[155] A number of patients with this lesion present with torticollis later in life, as the affected sternocleidomastoid muscle is incapable of keeping pace with the growth and elongation of the sternocleidomastoid muscle on the opposite side, causing functional imbalance and torticollis.

Fibromatosis colli is associated with a high incidence of difficult deliveries, including breech[156] (reported in up to 60% of patients) and forceps deliveries.[153] Several reports have noted an association with other congenital anomalies, including rib cage anomalies[156] and ipsilateral congenital dysplasia of the hip.[157]

Rare cases of fibromatosis colli appear to be familial. A hereditary component to this disease was first proposed by Joachimsthal in 1905,[158] and since that time there have been numerous reports of familial muscular torticollis.[159] Isigkeit reported that 11.2% of 1388 patients with fibromatosis colli had a positive family history and concluded that this condition is a hereditary disease that is influenced by environmental factors.[160]

Pathologic findings

When the growth is excised at an early stage, the specimen consists of a small mass of firm tissue averaging 1–2 cm in diameter. The cut surface is gray-white and glistening and blends imperceptibly with the surrounding skeletal muscle. Microscopic examination discloses partial replacement of the sternocleidomastoid muscle by a diffuse fibroblastic proliferation of varying cellularity (Figs 10–25, 10–26). The constituent cells lack significant nuclear hyperchromasia, pleomorphism, and mitotic

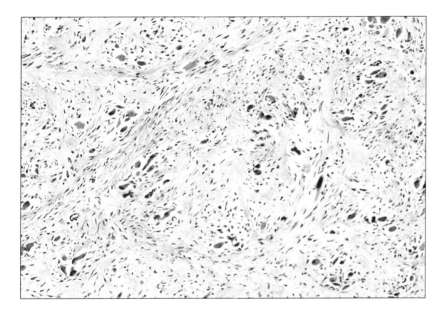

FIGURE 10–25 Fibromatosis colli in a 4-month-old boy. Note the intimate mixture of fibrous tissue and entrapped and partly atrophic muscle fibers.

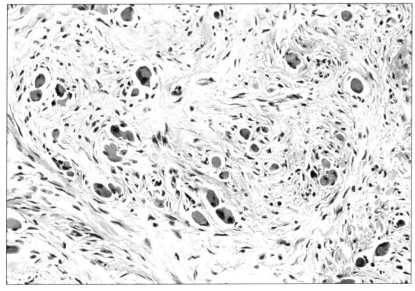

FIGURE 10–26 Fibromatosis colli. Separation of atrophic muscle fibers by dense fibrous tissue.

activity. Scattered throughout the lesion are residual muscle fibers that have undergone atrophy or degeneration with swelling, loss of cross-striations, and proliferation of sarcolemmal nuclei. This intimate mixture of proliferated fibroblasts and residual atrophic skeletal muscle fibers is fully diagnostic of the lesion and should not be confused with the infiltrative growth of a malignant neoplasm. Lesions of longer duration typically show less cellularity and more stromal collagen, but there does not appear to be a correlation between the histologic picture and the age of the patient. Although hemosiderin deposits are present in some cases, they are never a prominent feature. Unlike *fibrosing myositis*, there is no inflammatory infiltrate; unlike *fibrodysplasia ossificans progressiva*, there are no associated malformations of the hands or feet. Fine-needle aspiration cytology is a useful diagnostic modality and may obviate the need for further surgery.[161–163] As one might expect, the aspirate is characterized by bland spindle-shaped fibroblasts of low cellularity admixed with degenerating skeletal muscle fibers.

Prognosis and treatment

After a stationary period of several months, the growth slowly subsides and spontaneously resolves in up to 70% of cases by 1 year of age without surgical treatment.[157] It does not recur, nor is there aggressive growth into the surrounding tissues, although some patients develop a compensatory thoracic scoliosis, persistent head tilt, or obvious cosmetic deformity.[156] Recommendations as to the best type of therapy differ. Most advocate a conservative approach for patients younger than 1 year of age, often with implementation of an exercise program.[153] Surgery is a more effective mode of therapy for patients more than 1 year of age.[156,164] Ferkel et al.[165] reported better surgical results with release of the sternal and clavicular heads of the sternocleidomastoid muscle, but most have not found that one surgical approach is better than another.

Discussion

The cause of the growth has been the subject of considerable debate in the literature. In view of the unusually high incidence of breech and forceps deliveries, birth injury may play a role in the pathogenesis.[166] As far back as 1838, Stromeyer proposed that rupture of the sternocleidomastoid muscle during birth results in formation of a hematoma with subsequent fibrous replacement of the sternocleidomastoid muscle.[167] However, microscopic examination reveals little evidence of an organizing hematoma, and few cases exhibit deposition of hemosiderin. The fact that coexistent facial deformities are often present at birth and the development of these lesions in patients following cesarean section[168] cast doubt on this hypothesis. Others have postulated

that abnormal intrauterine positioning results in occlusion of the sternocleidomastoid branch of the superior thyroid artery, resulting in ischemic necrosis of the sternocleidomastoid muscle.[169] Certainly, contributing genetic factors are suggested by the reports of familial fibromatosis colli and association of the growth with congenital malformations.

INFANTILE FIBROMATOSIS (LIPOFIBROMATOSIS)

Fibromatoses occurring in infancy and early childhood consist of two morphologically distinct types. One type is essentially identical to adult-type fibromatoses. This discussion will focus on the other type, which is unique to childhood and has also been termed *lipofibromatosis*. It mainly affects children from birth to 8 years of age and is slightly more common in boys than girls. There are considerable variations in its morphologic appearance, depending on the stage of differentiation of the constituent fibroblasts.

Stout was the first to identify and describe the childhood form of fibromatosis as a distinct entity,[43] but relatively few cases have been added to the literature since then.

Clinical findings

Most patients present with a solitary firm mass that is poorly circumscribed and deep-seated and that usually has grown rapidly during the preceding weeks or months. In almost all cases, the mass is noted during the first 8 years of life, most commonly before age 2. Although most patients are asymptomatic, some report pain or tenderness of the involved site.[170] The mass typically originates in skeletal muscle, especially the muscles of the head and neck, shoulder and upper arm, and thigh.[171–173] The preferred sites in the head and neck region are the tongue, mandible, maxilla, and mastoid process.[174] Unusual sites in the head and neck region include the nose and paranasal sinuses[175] and parotid gland.[176] Intracranial extension may occur, but is not common.[177] As the lesion progresses, it may infiltrate adjacent muscles and grow around vessels and nerves, with resultant tenderness, pain, or functional disturbances. Involvement of the joint capsule can lead to contracture and restriction of movement.

Radiographic examination shows a soft tissue mass sometimes associated with bowing or deformation of bone, especially in cases in which the onset was during the first 2–3 years of life and has been present for several months or years.[178,179] Lesions in the regions of the mandible, maxilla, or mastoid frequently involve bone; it may be difficult to determine whether the mass arose in the soft tissues, periosteum, or bone,[180] thereby making

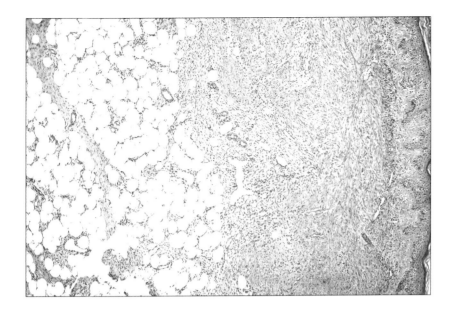

FIGURE 10–27 Infantile fibromatosis. Replacement of muscle tissue by fibrous tissue and mature fat bearing a superficial resemblance to a lipomatous tumor. The lesion was excised from the right arm of a 2-year-old girl.

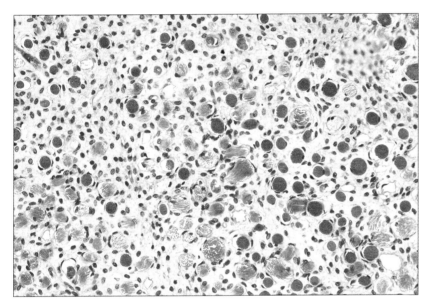

FIGURE 10–28 Infantile fibromatosis, diffuse type, removed from the trapezius muscle of a 5½-month-old girl. The absence of digital malformations helps distinguish it from an early nonossifying stage of fibrodysplasia ossificans progressiva.

distinction from desmoplastic fibroma of bone difficult in some cases.

Pathologic findings

Grossly, the tumor is a firm, ill-defined scar-like mass of gray-white tissue measuring 1–10 cm in greatest dimension. The tumor is not encapsulated and usually is excised together with portions of the involved muscle and subcutaneous fat.

Microscopically, infantile fibromatosis has a wide morphologic spectrum reflecting progressive stages in the differentiation of the fibroblasts. The more common form of infantile fibromatosis is the *diffuse* (*mesenchymal*) type. This form, found chiefly in infants during the first few months of life, is characterized by small, haphazardly arranged, round or oval cells deposited in a myxoid background (Figs 10–27 to 10–33). The cells are intermediate in appearance between primitive mesenchymal cells and fibroblasts, and they are often intimately associated with residual muscle fibers and lipocytes. The interspersed lipocytes are probably the result of ex vacuo fatty proliferation secondary to muscular atrophy of the infiltrated and immobilized muscle tissue. Some cases have extensive lipocytic elements, a condition referred to as *lipofibromatosis*. In a study of 45 cases of pediatric lipofibromatosis, Fetsch and colleagues found significant overlap with infantile fibromatosis and suggested that this lesion comprised part of the spectrum of infantile fibromatosis.[181] Peripherally located lymphocytic inflammation is often present. These areas blend with a more cellular proliferation composed chiefly of plump and spindle-shaped fibroblasts arranged in distinct bundles and fascicles. It may be highly cellular and mitotically

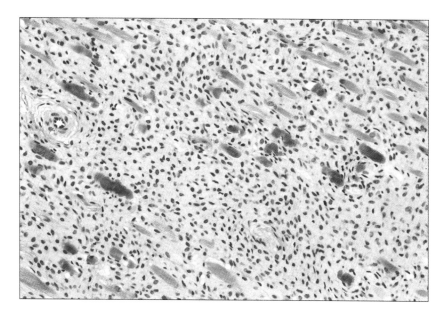

FIGURE 10–29 Infantile fibromatosis, diffuse type. Note the separation of striated muscle fibers by primitive fibroblasts with little variation in size and shape.

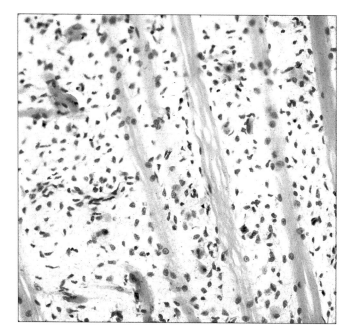

FIGURE 10–30 Higher-magnification view of a diffuse-type infantile fibromatosis. Primitive fibroblasts are seen separating striated muscle fibers.

active, making distinction from infantile fibrosarcoma exceedingly difficult in some cases.

The less common form of infantile fibromatosis (*desmoid type*) is virtually indistinguishable from the adult form of fibromatosis (desmoid tumor). This type usually occurs in children older than 5 years of age, and its behavior appears to be similar to that of the adult form of fibromatosis.[182] Although the morphology is similar to adult lesions, calcification and/or ossification is a feature peculiar to pediatric cases.[172,183]

Like other forms of fibromatosis, infantile fibromatosis is composed of a mixture of fibroblasts and myofi-

broblasts with prominent, often dilated endoplasmic reticulum and bundles of peripherally located microfilaments in some cells.[184] Immunohistochemically, the more primitive-appearing cells characteristic of the diffuse type and the plump spindle-shaped cells of both types stain for vimentin, with variable staining for muscle markers including muscle-specific actin, smooth muscle actin, and desmin.[185]

Differential diagnosis

The differential diagnosis depends on the type of infantile fibromatosis encountered. The diffuse (mesenchymal) type frequently causes diagnostic problems, as it may be confused with a wide variety of myxoid or lipomatous lesions because of the prominent myxoid stroma and the partial replacement of the infiltrated muscle by lipocytes. *Myxoid liposarcoma* is virtually unheard of in children younger than 5 years of age and is characterized by the presence of a uniform plexiform capillary pattern and variable numbers of typical lipoblasts. *Lipoblastomatosis*, the infantile counterpart of lipoma, can be distinguished by its distinctly lobular pattern and the uniform appearance of the constituent lipoblasts. There may be some resemblance to *botryoid rhabdomyosarcoma*, which has a similar age incidence; but this lesion is uncommon in the musculature and nearly always occurs in the wall of mucosa-lined cavities such as the urinary bladder or vagina. *Fibrodysplasia ossificans progressiva* bears some resemblance to the diffuse form of infantile fibromatosis, but patients with this disorder have bilateral malformations and shortening of fingers and toes (microdactylia). Confusion may also occur with the early stages of *calcifying aponeurotic fibroma*, although this lesion is characterized by its location in the palmar and plantar regions as

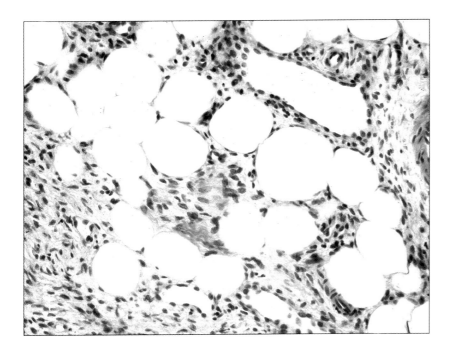

FIGURE 10–31 Infantile fibromatosis, diffuse type. Immature fibroblasts are seen infiltrating between adipocytes.

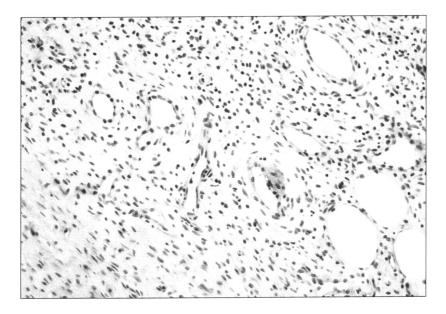

FIGURE 10–32 Infantile fibromatosis, diffuse type. Immature fibroblasts are deposited in a myxoid background.

well as foci of linear calcifications and chondroid metaplasia.

The most difficult problem in the differential diagnosis is distinguishing the more cellular variants of infantile fibromatosis from *congenital/infantile fibrosarcoma* (Table 10–2). The latter tumor resembles the adult form of fibrosarcoma, with characteristic high cellularity, arrangement in a uniform herringbone pattern, and a high mitotic rate. In addition, zones of hemorrhage and necrosis are not uncommon. In our experience, distinction between infantile fibromatosis and congenital/infantile fibrosarcoma is usually feasible if one pays attention to the infiltrative growth pattern of fibromatosis and its variation in the degree of cellularity, often with alternating cellular

and more collagenous areas, resembling the desmoid form. Yet in some cases reliable distinction between these entities is difficult if not impossible. Cytogenetic and molecular genetic analyses are highly reliable in this distinction. By traditional cytogenetics, congenital/infantile fibrosarcoma is characterized by gains of chromosomes 8, 11, 17, and 20.[186,187] These alterations are not found in infantile fibromatosis, although gains in chromosome 17 gave been reported in some cases.[188] As described in greater detail elsewhere in this chapter, congenital/infantile fibrosarcoma is characterized by a t(12;15)(p13;q25), resulting in the fusion of the *ETV* gene (chromosome 12) with the *NTRK3* gene (chromosome 15), which can be reliably detected by a variety of molecular techniques.[189]

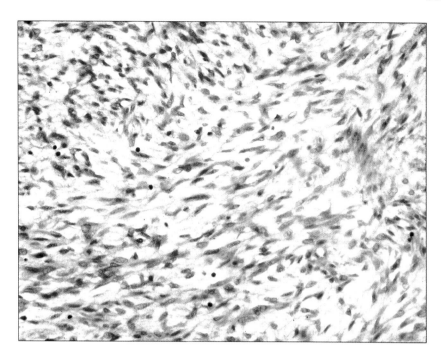

FIGURE 10–33 Infantile fibromatosis closely resembling the adult form of fibromatosis.

TABLE 10–2	SUMMARY OF FEATURES DISTINGUISHING INFANTILE FIBROMATOSIS AND INFANTILE FIBROSARCOMA	
Feature	**Infantile fibromatosis**	**Congenital/infantile fibrosarcoma**
Cellularity	Variable	Moderate to high
Herringbone pattern	Absent	Usually present
Mitotic figures	Rare	Few to many
Hemorrhage	Absent	Often present
Necrosis	Absent	Often present
t(12;15)(p13;q25)	Absent	Present

Discussion

Although infantile fibromatosis does not metastasize, it may reach a large size and, like other forms of fibromatosis, tends to recur locally when inadequately excised. In the series by Faulkner et al.,[171] none of the patients developed metastatic disease or died as a direct result of their tumor, but 41 of 63 patients (65%) developed local recurrences, with 51% recurring less than 1 year after initial excision, and 90% recurring within 3 years. The status of the resection margins was the only significant prognostic factor, as those patients who had undergone a wide local excision with tumor-free margins were significantly less likely to develop local recurrence. Histologic features do not allow accurate prediction of the clinical course,[171,173] although some have found a correlation between a large number of slit-like blood vessels and increased numbers of undifferentiated mesenchymal cells and risk of recurrence.[185] In rare cases, encroachment on critical structures, particularly those of the head and neck, may result in the patient's death.[190]

Complete excision with ample margins is the treatment of choice, although it is difficult in some anatomic locations and may be impossible without disfigurement or dysfunction. There is relatively little information as to the efficacy of adjuvant chemotherapy or radiotherapy, but some have found these modalities to be of therapeutic benefit.[191]

The cause of infantile fibromatosis is not clear. As with other forms of fibromatosis, trauma has been implicated as an inciting factor. In the series by Faulkner et al., 17% of patients had a history of antecedent trauma in the vicinity of the lesion.[171] Coffin and Dehner reported two cases that arose at sites of previous surgery.[173] Unlike many other fibrous lesions, increased familial incidence has not been observed with this type of fibromatosis.

CONGENITAL/INFANTILE FIBROSARCOMA

Fibrosarcoma in newborns, infants, and small children bears some resemblance to adult fibrosarcoma, but it must be considered a separate entity because of its markedly different clinical behavior as well as its distinctive molecular alterations. On one hand, it must be distinguished from richly cellular forms of infantile fibro-matosis, a lesion that lacks metastatic capability; on the other hand, it must be separated from more aggressive childhood sarcomas (e.g., embryonal rhabdomyosar-coma), which are prone to metastasize and require more radical therapy. Fibrosarcomas in older children behave similarly to those seen in adults.

Congenital/infantile fibrosarcoma is relatively rare. The first detailed clinicopathologic study of this entity was reported by Stout in 1962.[192] He reviewed 31 cases from the literature and added 23 cases of "juvenile fibro-sarcoma," 11 of which developed during the first 5 years of life and 4 of which were present at birth. He suggested that fibrosarcomas arising in this group of patients were more indolent than their adult counterparts. Although several subsequent smaller series of congenital/infantile fibrosarcoma were reported, it was not until Chung and Enzinger's series of 53 cases (reported in 1976) did con-clusive evidence support this tumor as a distinct entity.[193] Similar conclusions were reached by Soule and Pritchard in their report of 110 cases, including 70 previously published cases and 40 new cases from the files of the Mayo Clinic.[194]

Clinical findings

The principal manifestation of the disease is a nontender, painless swelling or mass that ranges from 1 to 20 cm. Up to one-third of the tumors are present at birth; in most cases the mass becomes evident during the first year of life. In the series by Chung and Enzinger, 20 of 53 tumors (38%) were present at birth, and 27 (51%) were noted before 3 months of life.[193] Similarly, 40 (36%) of the 110 cases reported by Soule and Pritchard were con-genital.[194] Males are affected slightly more commonly than females. The principal sites of involvement are the extremities, especially the regions of the foot, ankle, and lower leg and the hand, wrist, and forearm. The next most common sites of involvement are the trunk and head and neck regions, although these tumors have also been reported in locations such as the retroperitoneum,[195] mesentery,[196] ovary,[197] and bowel.[198]

Radiographic examination may show, in addition to a soft tissue mass, cortical thickening, bending deformities, and rarely extensive destruction of the underlying bone (Fig. 10–34).[193] Both MRI and ultrasound are useful in the evaluation of these tumors, including the detection of congenital tumors in utero.[199]

Gross findings

The tumors vary considerably in size. Some are only a few centimeters when first detected, whereas others are extremely large and may replace the entire distal portion of the involved limb. Some patients present with a large exophytic mass that ulcerates the overlying skin. Most are

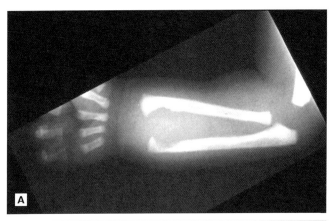
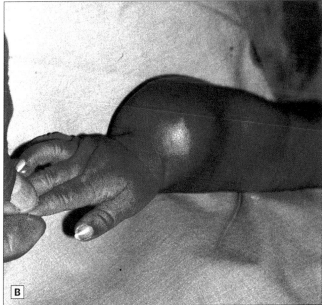

FIGURE 10–34 Radiograph **(A)** and gross photomicrograph **(B)** of a congenital fibrosarcoma in a 1-day-old infant.

poorly circumscribed, fusiform or disk-shaped, and have a gray-white or pale pink cut surface. Large tumors may be markedly distorted by central necrosis or hemorrhage (Fig. 10–35), whereas others show extensive myxoid or cystic change.

Microscopic findings

Most of these tumors closely resemble their adult coun-terparts and are composed of sheets of solidly packed, spindle-shaped cells that are relatively uniform in appear-ance and arranged in bundles or fascicles, imparting a herringbone appearance. The cells show little nuclear pleomorphism and are mitotically active, but their numbers vary from area to area in the same tumor. Tumors with abundant collagen tend to be more fascicu-lated and often approach the appearance of an adult fibrosarcoma (sometimes referred to as the "desmoplas-

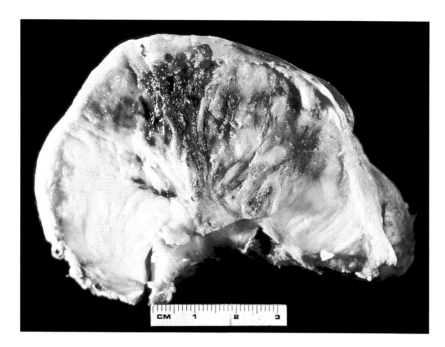

FIGURE 10–35 Infantile fibrosarcoma of the right shoulder in a 1-month-old boy, showing marked interstitial hemorrhage.

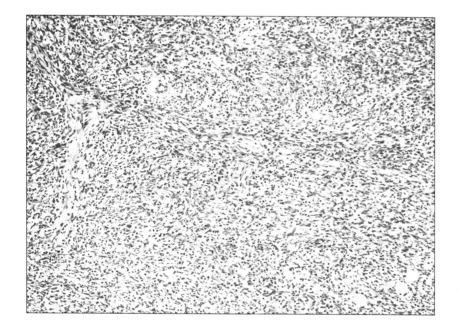

FIGURE 10–36 Infantile fibrosarcoma composed of uniform, well-oriented fibroblasts arranged in a fascicular growth pattern.

tic" type). Tumors with minimal amounts of collagen, on the other hand, show a lesser degree of cellular polarity and consist of small, more rounded, immature-appearing cells with only focal evidence of fibroblastic differentiation ("medullary" type) (Figs 10–36 to 10–38).[200]

As in the adult fibrosarcoma, bizarre cells and multinucleated giant cells are rare. Scattered chronic inflammatory cells, particularly lymphocytes, are another common, sometimes striking feature that helps distinguish infantile from adult fibrosarcoma. A hemangiopericytoma-like vascular pattern may be prominent (Fig. 10–39) and can cause confusion with infantile hemangiopericytoma.

Immunohistochemical and ultrastructural findings

Immunohistochemically, the spindle cells of congenital/infantile fibrosarcoma stain for vimentin and variably for muscle markers including muscle-specific and smooth muscle actin.[173] The more primitive-appearing ovoid cells tend not to express these muscle markers. Ultrastructural examination reveals fibroblast-like cells with large irregular nuclei, one or two nucleoli, free ribosomes, a well-developed Golgi apparatus, and a prominent, often dilated rough endoplasmic reticulum, sometimes

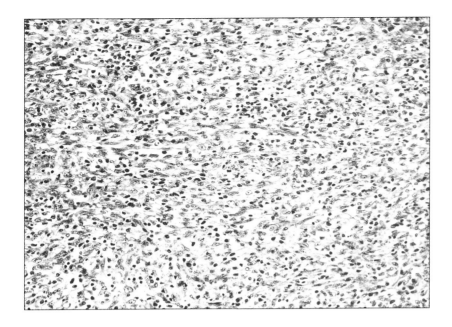

FIGURE 10–37 Characteristic microscopic view of an infantile fibrosarcoma with immature-appearing fibroblasts associated with small round cells, probably lymphocytes.

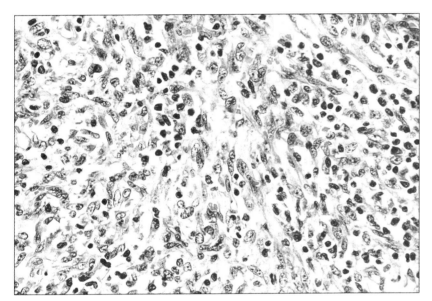

FIGURE 10–38 High-power view of immature-appearing fibroblasts with a prominent lymphocytic infiltrate, characteristic of infantile fibrosarcoma.

containing amorphous material.[68,201] Bundles of thin filaments and fibronexus junctions characteristic of myofibroblastic differentiation may be present.[68,202]

Cytogenic and molecular genetic findings

Numerous studies have noted a nonrandom gain of chromosomes 11, 20, 17, and 8 (in descending order of frequency) in congenital/infantile fibrosarcomas.[186,187,203] Using FISH techniques, Schofield et al. found gains of these chromosomes (in various combinations) in 11 of 12 infantile fibrosarcomas in patients less than 2 years of age.[186] In contrast, alterations of these chromosomes were not found in four fibrosarcomas in patients 6–17 years of age. Interestingly, one of three cases of "cellular fibromatosis" also showed the above cytogenetic abnor-

malities, suggesting that "these two entities are on a spectrum and that their distinction may not be clear-cut."[186]

Most congenital/infantile fibrosarcomas and cellular mesoblastic nephromas have the same diagnostic chromosomal translocation: t(12;15)(p13; q25).[189,204] This translocation results in fusion of the *ETV6* gene (also known as *TEL*) on chromosome 12 with the neurotrophin-3 receptor *NTRK3* (also known as *TRKC*) gene on chromosome 15. Although this translocation is difficult to detect by conventional cytogenetic means, it can be readily demonstrated by RT-PCR or FISH using frozen or paraffin-embedded tissue.[205–208] Given the similar histologic and cytogenetic findings in congenital/infantile fibrosarcoma and cellular mesoblastic nephroma, it has been suggested that these two lesions are histogenetically related entities arising in soft tissue

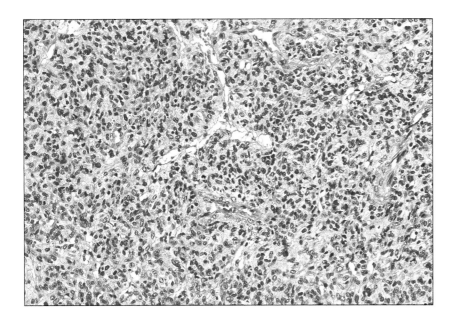

FIGURE 10–39 Infantile fibrosarcoma composed of immature-appearing fibroblasts arranged around a prominent hemangiopericytoma-like vascular pattern.

and renal locations, respectively.[204,209] Interestingly, secretory breast carcinoma has also been found to harbor this translocation.[210]

Differential diagnosis

The microscopic picture may be confused with that of other mesenchymal neoplasms, but in most cases the uniformity of the spindle-shaped tumor cells, the solid growth pattern, the fascicular arrangement, and the lack of any other form of cellular differentiation seen by electron microscopy and immunohistochemistry permit a reliable diagnosis.

Spindle cell rhabdomyosarcoma is a subtype of embryonal rhabdomyosarcoma that may be difficult to distinguish from congenital/infantile fibrosarcoma. This tumor is most often encountered in the paratesticular region and the head and neck, but it may also be present at other sites, including the extremities. Histologically, this variant of rhabdomyosarcoma is composed of uniform spindle cells with eosinophilic fibrillar cytoplasm and elongated hyperchromatic nuclei separated by abundant, partly hyalinized collagen. Immunohistochemically, this tumor characteristically expresses desmin and myogenin, which are usually absent in congenital/infantile fibrosarcoma.

In 1993, Lundgren et al. described three cases of *infantile rhabdomyofibrosarcoma*, each of which was initially diagnosed as congenital/infantile fibrosarcoma.[211] This tumor, which was observed in children 3 months to 3 years of age, has features that overlap spindle cell rhabdomyosarcoma and desmoplastic portions of congenital/infantile fibrosarcoma. Immunohistochemically, the cells express vimentin, smooth muscle actin, and desmin but not myoglobin (not tested for MyoD1 or myogenin); they have the ultrastructural features of rhabdomyoblasts, fibroblasts, and myofibroblasts. By cytogenetics, 2 of the

3 cases reported by Lundgren et al. showed monosomy of chromosome 19 and 22, among other abnormalities;[211] a case reported by Miki et al. showed der (2) t(2;11)(q37;q13).[212] Two of the patients developed metastases and died within 2 years of the primary operation; the third patient was alive with a local recurrence. The exact nature of this tumor is still not clear. It may represent an intermediate form between a congenital/infantile fibrosarcoma and a spindle cell rhabdomyosarcoma. The authors also raised the possibility that some tumors reported as congenital/infantile fibrosarcoma that have metastasized and followed a fatal course may actually be examples of this entity.

Congenital/infantile fibrosarcoma with a marked degree of vascularity may be difficult to distinguish from *infantile hemangiopericytoma*. The latter is marked by a distinct lobulated arrangement and more regularly distributed dilated vascular channels that form a branching, or "staghorn," pattern. In some cases, clear distinction is difficult and mandates examination of multiple sections from different portions of the tumor. Some authors have reported tumors with overlapping histologic features and have proposed that these two entities represent a histologic continuum.[71]

Perhaps the most difficult lesion to distinguish from congenital/infantile fibrosarcoma is the cellular form of *infantile fibromatosis* (Table 10–2). Some authors have reported cases in which the primary tumor had the appearance and growth pattern of infantile fibromatosis, whereas the recurrent tumor showed more cellularity and was virtually indistinguishable from fibrosarcoma.[193] On the other hand, we have also observed tumors with a fibrosarcoma-like appearance in the primary neoplasm and a fibromatosis-like appearance in the recurrence. Detection of the t(12;15) by cytogenetic or molecular techniques allows for distinction between these lesions.

Discussion

Compared with adult fibrosarcoma, the clinical course of congenital/infantile fibrosarcoma is a favorable one. Of the 48 patients with follow-up in the study by Chung and Enzinger, only 8 (17%) developed one or more local recurrences 6 weeks to 10 years after the initial excision.[193] Only 4 (8%) of the 48 patients died of metastatic disease, and one patient was living 6.5 years after lobectomy for metastatic tumor. The 5-year survival rate in this series was 84%. The recurrent and nonrecurrent groups showed no demonstrable differences in regard to tumor site, age at onset, or size of the tumor. However, the initial therapy was more radical for the tumors that neither recurred nor metastasized. Most studies have found that neither cellularity, mitotic counts, or the extent of tumor necrosis correlate well with clinical behavior.[193,213] Blocker et al. found that tumors located in the axial skeleton behaved more aggressively than those found peripherally.[214] There are reports of incompletely excised infantile fibrosarcomas that have not recurred or metastasized after several years,[215] as well as sporadic reports of spontaneous regression.[216]

Despite rapid growth and a high degree of cellularity, most congenital/infantile fibrosarcomas are cured by wide local excision. A number of reports have indicated that preoperative chemotherapy is useful for decreasing tumor bulk, enabling a more conservative surgical approach.[217-219] There are also reports of success with postoperative chemotherapy[220] and with chemotherapy alone as a mode of treatment for inoperable tumors.[221] The value of radiotherapy is difficult to assess, as it has been used only in selected cases.[202] In view of the generally favorable clinical course, it appears that adjuvant radiotherapy and chemotherapy should be reserved for congenital/infantile fibrosarcomas that are unresectable or have recurred or metastasized.

INFLAMMATORY MYOFIBROBLASTIC TUMOR

Inflammatory myofibroblastic tumor is a histologically distinctive lesion that occurs primarily in the viscera and soft tissue of children and young adults and usually pursues a benign clinical course. Although original descriptions of this lesion focused on its occurrence in the lung,[222] inflammatory myofibroblastic tumor has been described in virtually every anatomic location and under many appellations including plasma cell granuloma,[223] plasma cell pseudotumor,[224] inflammatory myofibrohistiocytic proliferation,[225] omental-mesenteric myxoid hamartoma[226] and, most commonly, inflammatory pseudotumor.[227] The term inflammatory myofibroblastic tumor is preferred, as "inflammatory pseudotumor" has been applied to diverse entities,[228] including pseudo-sarcomatous myofibroblastic proliferations of the lower genitourinary tract (see Chapter 8), infectious lesions (including those secondary to *Mycobacterium avium intracellulare*),[229] Epstein-Barr virus-associated follicular dendritic cell tumors usually found in the liver or spleen,[230] and reactive "inflammatory pseudotumors" of lymph nodes (Fig. 10–40).[231] This discussion focuses on extrapulmonary inflammatory myofibroblastic tumors.

Clinical findings

Inflammatory myofibroblastic tumors have been reported in virtually every anatomic site. Table 10–3 provides a partial list of sites of inflammatory myofibroblastic tumor that have been reported in just the last 5 years. The most common sites of extrapulmonary inflammatory myofibroblastic tumor are the mesentery and omentum.[232] In a seminal study by Coffin et al.,[232] 36 of 84 extrapulmonary lesions (43%) arose at these sites. Although the age range is broad, extrapulmonary inflammatory myofibroblastic tumors show a predilection for children, with a mean age of approximately 10 years. Females are affected slightly more commonly than males.

Presenting symptoms depend on the site of primary tumor involvement. Patients with intra-abdominal tumors most commonly complain of abdominal pain or an abdominal mass with increased girth, occasionally with signs and symptoms of gastrointestinal obstruction. Some patients have prominent systemic manifestations, including fever, night sweats, weight loss and malaise. Laboratory abnormalities are present in a small number of patients and include an elevated erythrocyte sedimentation rate, anemia, thrombocytosis, and hypergammaglobulinemia, which often resolve when the lesion is excised.[232,233]

Gross findings

Grossly, most lesions are lobular, multinodular, or bosselated with a hard or rubbery cut surface that appears white, gray, tan-yellow, or red (Fig. 10–41). Some cut with a gritty sensation due to the presence of calcifications. Although most are solitary tumors, multiple nodules generally restricted to the same anatomic location are found in almost one-third of cases.[232,234] The tumors range in size from 2 to 20 cm, but most are 5–10 cm.

Microscopic findings

A variety of histologic patterns may be seen, and different patterns may be found in the same tumor. Some tumors are composed predominantly of cytologically bland spindle- or stellate-shaped cells loosely arranged in a myxoid or hyaline stroma with scattered inflammatory cells, somewhat resembling nodular fasciitis. Others

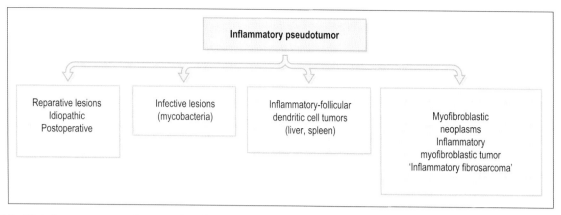

FIGURE 10–40 Inflammatory pseudotumor. A variety of lesions of differing etiologies have been referred to as inflammatory pseudotumor. (Modified from Chan JKC. Inflammatory pseudotumor: a family of lesions of diverse nature and etiologies. Adv Anat Pathol 1996; 3:156.)

TABLE 10–3	**EXTRAPULMONARY ANATOMIC SITES OF INFLAMMATORY MYOFIBROBLASTIC TUMOR REPORTED SINCE 2001**	
Anatomic site	**First Author (year)**	**Reference**
Bone	Gasparotti et al. (2003)	258
Breast	Ilvan et al. (2005)	259
CNS	Jeon et al. (2005)	260
GI tract	SantaCruz et al. (2002)	261
Heart	Li et al. (2002)	262
Hepatobiliary	Dasgupta et al. (2004)	263
Kidney	Kapusta et al. (2003)	264
Larynx	Rodrigues et al. (2005)	265
Mediastinum	Makimoto et al. (2005)	266
Mesentery	Corapcioglu et al. (2005)	267
Omentum	Hagenstad et al. (2003)	253
Oral cavity	Fang and Dym (2004)	268
Orbit/ocular region	O'Malley et al. (2004)	269
Pancreas	Pungpapong et al. (2004)	270
Paratesticular region	Kapur et al. (2004)	271
Parotid gland	Van Weert et al. (2005)	272
Sinus	Karakok et al. (2002)	273
Spinal column	Lacoste-Collin et al. (2003)	274
Spleen	Mosunjac et al. (2001)	275
Trachea	Browne et al. (2004)	276
Urachus	Nascimento et al. (2004)	277
Uterus	Rabban et al. (2005)	278

are composed of a compact proliferation of spindle-shaped cells arranged in a storiform or fascicular growth pattern (Figs 10–42 to 10–45). In these foci, the nuclei tend to be elongated but lack significant hyperchromasia or cytologic atypia. Mitotic figures are variable but not atypical. These foci are usually associated with a prominent lymphoplasmacytic infiltrate, occasionally with formation of germinal centers. Other foci may be sparsely cellular, with cytologically bland cells deposited in a sclerotic stroma resembling a scar. Lymphocytes and plasma cells are often seen in these foci, and small punctate areas of calcification or metaplastic bone may be observed.

In some lesions there is pronounced cytologic atypia, with cells containing large nuclei and distinct nucleoli. Some tumors have large histiocytoid cells resembling ganglion cells or Reed-Sternberg cells.[235,235a]

Immunohistochemical and ultrastructural findings

The tumor cells stain strongly for vimentin and variably with myoid markers including smooth muscle actin, muscle-specific actin, and desmin. In the study by Meis and Enzinger,[234] smooth muscle actin and muscle-specific actin marked 90% and 83% of cases, respectively. On the

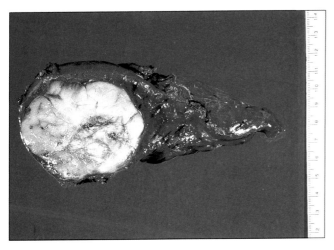

FIGURE 10–41 Gross appearance of an inflammatory myofibroblastic tumor in the left upper lobe of the lung of a 21-year-old woman.

other hand, there was equivocal desmin staining in only 1 of 11 (9%) cases. Coffin and colleagues found staining for smooth muscle actin, muscle-specific actin, and desmin in 92%, 89%, and 69% of cases, respectively.[232] Focal cytokeratin immunoreactivity was noted in 36% of the cases in the study by Coffin et al.[232] and 77% of the cases in the study by Meis and Enzinger,[234] predominantly in portions of the tumor that were in a submesothelial location. CD68 staining is found in up to 25% of cases. As discussed below, some but not all inflammatory myofibroblastic tumors stain for ALK.

Ultrastructurally, most of the constituent cells have fibroblastic features with a well-developed Golgi apparatus, abundant rough endoplasmic reticulum and extracellular collagen. However, some cells show unequivocal evidence of myofibroblastic differentiation with intracytoplasmic thin filaments, dense bodies, and fibronexus junctions.[68,201]

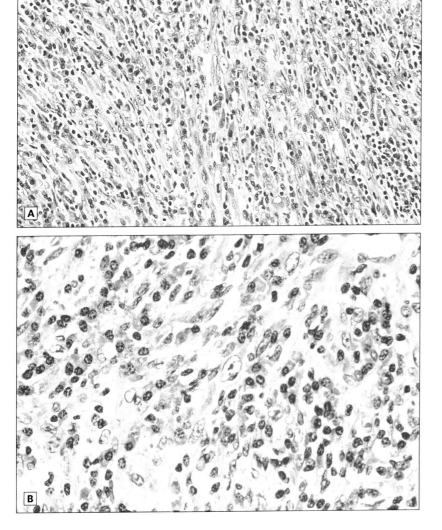

FIGURE 10–42 Inflammatory myofibroblastic tumor. **(A)** Low-power view showing an admixture of spindle-shaped and ovoid cells with a prominent inflammatory infiltrate. **(B)** High-power view of an inflammatory myofibroblastic tumor. Note the conspicuous admixture of lymphocytes and plasma cells.

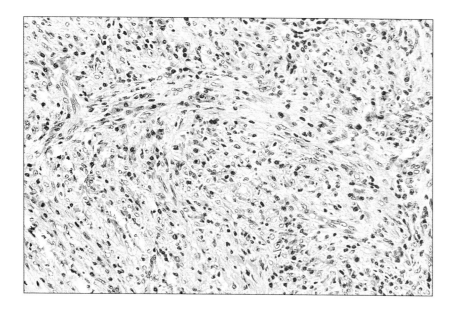

FIGURE 10–43 Inflammatory myofibroblastic tumor. Cytologically bland spindle-shaped cells are intimately admixed with a predominantly plasmacytic infiltrate.

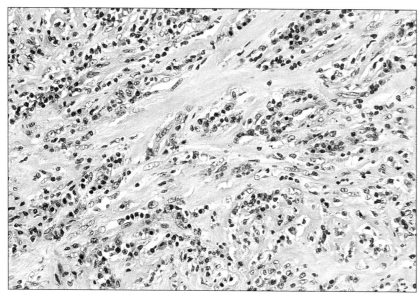

FIGURE 10–44 Less cellular inflammatory myofibroblastic tumor than that depicted in Figures 10–42 and 10–43. Plate-like collagen is present.

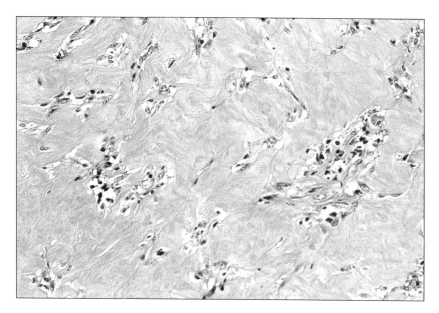

FIGURE 10–45 Hypocellular inflammatory myofibroblastic tumor composed predominantly of sclerotic fibrous tissue with scattered spindle-shaped and inflammatory cells.

Cytogenetic findings

A number of inflammatory myofibroblastic tumors have been studied cytogenetically and have been found to harbor clonal cytogenetic aberrations, especially at 2p22–24.[236-240] The anaplastic lymphoma kinase (*ALK*) gene, located on 2p23, has been implicated in the pathogenesis of this lesion. This gene codes for a tyrosine kinase receptor that is a member of the insulin growth factor receptor superfamily. *ALK* rearrangements result in constitutive expression and activation of this gene with abnormal phosphorylation of cellular substrates. Fusion partners that appear to be important in the oncogenesis of at least some of these tumors include tropomyosin 3 (*TPM3-ALK*) and tropomyosin 4 (*TPM4-ALK*).[241] Other less common fusion partners for *ALK* have been reported including the clathrin heavy-chain gene (*CLTC*),[242] the cysteinyl-tRNA synthetase gene (*CARS*),[243] the *ATIC* gene,[244] and the *RANBP-2* gene.[245] There is evidence to suggest that different fusion partners result in different patterns of ALK immunoreactivity, including diffuse cytoplasmic, granular cytoplasmic, membranous, and nuclear patterns of staining.[241,246-248] Overall, between 36% and 60% of inflammatory myofibroblastic tumors stain for ALK.

Differential diagnosis

The differential diagnosis of this lesion depends on the clinicopathologic setting, including the patient's age, gender, tumor location, and number of lesions. *Inflammatory malignant fibrous histiocytoma* is characterized by bizarre pleomorphic cells that may be obscured by numerous xanthomatous and inflammatory cells. For tumors composed of elongated spindle cells with eosinophilic cytoplasm arranged in a focal fascicular growth pattern, differentiation from *inflammatory leiomyosarcoma* may pose a problem. However, the nuclei in leiomyosarcoma are cigar-shaped and arranged in a more regular fascicular growth pattern. Rare inflammatory myofibroblastic tumors have a conspicuous population of large multinucleated tumor cells with prominent nucleoli bearing a resemblance to the Reed-Sternberg cells of *Hodgkin's disease*. The immunohistochemical reactivity of the spindle and ganglion-like cells for actins and ALK and negativity for CD15 and CD30 assist in distinguishing these two entities. Inflammatory myofibroblastic tumor can occasionally arise in the gastrointestinal tract and can be confused with an *inflammatory fibroid polyp*.[249] The latter is a benign lesion that most often occurs in the stomach and ileum as a solitary submucosal polyp. Histologically, this lesion is dominated by stellate-shaped cells deposited in a myxoid stroma with reactive blood vessels and mixed inflammatory cells, particularly eosinophils. *Gastrointestinal stromal tumors* (GIST) may occasionally closely resemble an inflammatory myofibroblastic tumor, but GIST consistently stain for CD117 and CD34, and are ALK negative. Although they share some histologic similarities, inflammatory myofibroblastic tumor can be distinguished from the group of inflammatory fibrosclerosing lesions, including *sclerosing mediastinitis*, *idiopathic retroperitoneal fibrosis*, and *Riedel's thyroiditis*, by paying close attention to the clinical setting and gross and microscopic findings. These lesions tend to occur in older patients and, although mass-forming, are usually ill-defined, entrapping the normal tissues in the vicinity. They tend to have more prominent sclerosis and phlebitis than the typical inflammatory myofibroblastic tumor. Other fibroinflammatory processes that occur in this location, including *xanthogranulomatous inflammation secondary to Erdheim-Chester disease* and *pseudotumor resulting from atypical mycobacterial infection*, also may be in the differential diagnosis and can be distinguished by virtue of their distinct clinicopathologic setting.

Finally, the question as to whether inflammatory myofibroblastic tumor and *inflammatory fibrosarcoma* are the same tumor, distinct entities, or represent a spectrum has been debated.[234,250,251] Certainly, these two entities share clinical and pathologic features; as stated by Coffin et al., the distinction of inflammatory fibrosarcoma "from inflammatory myofibroblastic tumor may be more semantic than real."[232] We, however, believe the two lesions are the same and, therefore, that these terms are completely synonymous, although we prefer the term inflammatory myofibroblastic tumor because of its more universal usage.

Discussion

There have been a number of controversial issues with respect to these lesions over the years, such as whether the lesions are a homogeneous entity, if they are neoplastic, and, if neoplastic, their level of malignancy. It seems reasonably certain that the lesions reported under the various terms noted above indeed refer to the same process, although the features of any given lesion may vary somewhat depending on the degree of inflammation, sclerosis, and cellularity. In our opinion, it is not possible to make histologic distinctions between lesions reported by some authors as inflammatory fibrosarcoma and by others as inflammatory myofibroblastic tumor. In support of this statement is the fact that there is overlap in case material reported in the two largest studies under the two preceding terms.[232,234] There is also compelling evidence that these lesions are true neoplasms rather than pseudotumors. Many have been associated with aggressive local behavior that has resulted in some deaths. In addition, as previously mentioned, some (but not all) tumors show aberrations of the *ALK-1* gene, supportive evidence of a neoplastic process.

Based on the two largest studies of abdominal and retroperitoneal lesions, it is clear that tumors in this location have a propensity for more aggressive behavior than their extra-abdominal counterparts, with recurrence rates of 23–37%.[232,234] The major question seems to be whether these lesions have metastatic potential or whether multiple lesions in a single patient represent multifocal disease. Coffin et al.,[232] in a series of 53 cases with follow-up, reported no instances of metastasis, whereas 3 of 27 patients reported by Meis and Enzinger[234] developed metastasis to lung and brain. The reasons for this discrepancy are not clear. In at least one case reported by Meis and Enzinger (case 26), the simultaneous presentation of histologically bland mediastinal and cerebral lesions with no evidence of disease nearly 4 years after surgery raises the possibility that these lesions may be multifocal. However, there are other reports which clearly indicate that some examples of this tumor metastasize and can result in patient death.[235a,252,253] Debelenko and colleagues reported a primary lesion and metastasis with identical fusions of the *ALK* gene and cysteinyl-tRNA (*CARS*) gene, supporting a metastasis as opposed to multifocal disease.[243] Finally, there are rare reports of inflammatory myofibroblastic tumors merging into frankly malignant-appearing neoplasms.[232,235a,254,255]

The mainstay of therapy is surgical resection with re-excision of recurrent tumors. Some have advocated chemotherapy and radiation therapy in recurrent or metastatic cases.[254,256] Cellularity, mitotic counts, and extent of inflammation do not appear to be prognostic markers; in contrast, cytologic atypia, ganglion-like cells, *p53* expression, and DNA aneuploidy may be useful for identifying tumors that are more likely to pursue an aggressive clinical course.[257]

CALCIFYING APONEUROTIC FIBROMA

Originally described as *juvenile aponeurotic fibroma* by Keasbey in 1953,[279] fewer than 150 cases of calcifying aponeurotic fibroma have been recorded in the literature. Although initially reported in children and adolescents between birth and 16 years of age, it has subsequently become apparent that this lesion affects a much wider age range than other forms of juvenile fibromatosis and may occur in young adults and rarely in older adults.[280] Keasbey described its characteristic histologic picture, its predilection for the palm and fingers of the hand, and its propensity to locally recur after excision. In view of the wide age range of patients, the term juvenile aponeurotic fibroma was changed to aponeurotic fibroma[281] and *calcifying aponeurotic fibroma*.[282]

Clinical findings

Most patients present with a slowly growing, painless mass in the hands or feet of several months' or even years' duration. In most cases the mass is poorly circumscribed and causes neither discomfort nor limitation of movement, although some patients do have complaints of mild tenderness.[283] Grossly, lesions that have been present for several years are often more sharply circumscribed and distinctly nodular than those of shorter duration.

Most lesions occur in children, with a peak incidence of 8–14 years. Although most small series have not reported a distinct gender predilection, 70% of the patients in the series by Allen and Enzinger were male.[283] There is no record of increased familial incidence. The two principal sites of growth are the hands and the feet. In the hand, the most common sites are the palm and fingers. The dorsum of the hand is rarely involved.[284] Fewer lesions occur on the plantar surface of the foot or ankle region and rarely the toes. Isolated tumors have been observed at other sites, including the neck, forearm, thigh, popliteal fossa, knee, and soft tissues of the lumbosacral region.[283,285-287] They may be found in the subcutaneous tissue or attached to the aponeurosis, tendons, or fascia. Preoperative radiographic examination reveals a faint mass, frequently with calcific stippling, especially in the more heavily calcified tumors. MRI is more precise at outlining the anatomic extent of the process and is useful in planning the surgical excision.[288]

Gross findings

Most lesions are ill-defined, firm or rubbery, and graywhite, usually less than 3 cm in greatest diameter. Older lesions are more grossly well circumscribed, although there is typically microscopic infiltration of the surrounding soft tissues even in these cases. Portions of the surrounding fat, skeletal muscle, and fibrous tissue frequently merge with the tumor. In some cases, calcifications are evident as small white flecks (Fig. 10–46), but in heavily calcified cases they may be more grossly apparent. On sectioning, the lesion often has a gritty sensation due to these calcifications.

Microscopic findings

The histologic picture varies little from case to case. It reveals a fibrous growth that extends with multiple processes into the surrounding tissue with more centrally located foci of calcification and cartilage formation. The cellularity of the lesion varies from region to region and is composed of plump fibroblasts with round or ovoid nuclei and indistinctly outlined cytoplasm separated by a densely collagenous stroma (Figs 10–47 to 10–51). Despite the focal cellularity of the lesion, mitotic figures are scarce. Not infrequently, the fibrous growth is attached to a tendon or aponeurosis and encircles blood vessels and nerves. Unlike other forms of fibromatosis, there

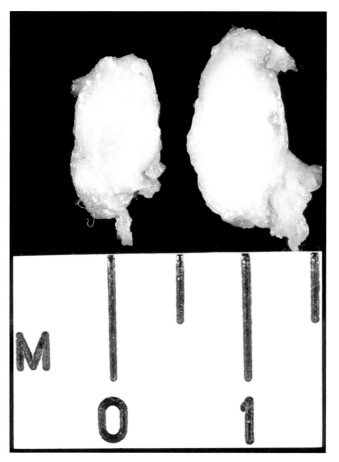

FIGURE 10–46 Calcifying aponeurotic fibroma in the palm of a 4-year-old-boy. Note the small white flecks, indicative of calcification.

tends to be orientation of the stromal cells. There may be a vague cartwheel or whorled pattern, or the nuclei may line up in columns, occasionally resulting in marked nuclear palisading.

Focal calcification is invariably present except in lesions in infants or small children. Calcification and cartilage formation are much more pronounced in lesions removed from older children and young adults. The calcifications are usually small and vary from fine granules or string-like deposits to large amorphous masses. In many cases these calcified foci are surrounded by radiating columns of cells that resemble chondrocytes, with rounded nuclei lying in lacunae (Fig. 10–49). These cartilage-like cells are often aligned in linear columns that radiate from the center of the calcified areas, although there may be a circumferential arrangement as well. Occasionally, multinucleated giant cells resembling osteoclasts are present adjacent to the calcific foci (Fig. 10–52), but they may also be seen adjacent to noncalcified fibrocartilage-like tissue. Ossification occurs but is rare.

Differential diagnosis

The differential diagnosis differs from case to case, depending on the age of the patient at the time the lesion is excised. In infants and small children, when there is still little or no calcification, this lesion may be difficult to distinguish from *infantile fibromatosis*. However, infantile fibromatosis most commonly presents as a soft tissue mass in the head and neck and the proximal extremities; involvement of the distal extremities is rare. Moreover, the fibroblasts of infantile fibromatosis are more elongated and are often deposited in a myxoid background, and foci of calcification and ossification are uncommon. Giant cells, a common feature of calcifying aponeurotic fibroma, are not typical of fibromatosis. *Palmar* and *plantar fibromatoses* may occur in children but are not common, especially palmar lesions. They are more nodular in appearance, and lack calcification or chondroid differentiation. Malignant spindle cell tumors, such as *monophasic fibrous-type synovial sarcoma*, may rarely be mistaken for calcifying aponeurotic fibroma with a prominent spindle cell pattern. Immunoreactivity for epithelial markers and analysis for *SYT* gene aberrations allow for recognition of synovial sarcoma.

In older patients, distinction of the growth from a *soft part chondroma* may cause considerable difficulty, especially since both lesions are most common in the hands. However, soft part chondromas more frequently affect older adults and have a lower rate of local recurrence than aponeurotic fibromas. Histologically, soft part chondromas are well-circumscribed, lobulated masses that are sharply demarcated from the surrounding soft tissues. Furthermore, the extent of chondroid differentiation is far better developed in soft tissue chondromas than aponeurotic fibromas.

Ultrastructural findings

Calcifying aponeurotic fibromas have a biphasic pattern consisting of fibroblasts and occasional myofibroblasts and cartilage cells, with a well-developed granular endoplasmic reticulum, a prominent Golgi complex, and multiple microvilli.[289] These cells are surrounded by an intercellular matrix containing fine fibrils and spherical granules.

Discussion

Because of its infiltrative nature, the calcifying aponeurotic fibroma is characterized by a high rate of local recurrence. In the series by Allen and Enzinger, 10 of 19 lesions recurred 1 month to 11 years after the initial excision.[283] The authors did not identify any histologic features that predicted recurrence but did note that young patients, particularly those under 5 years of age, had a higher risk of recurrence. Very few cases of malignant transformation

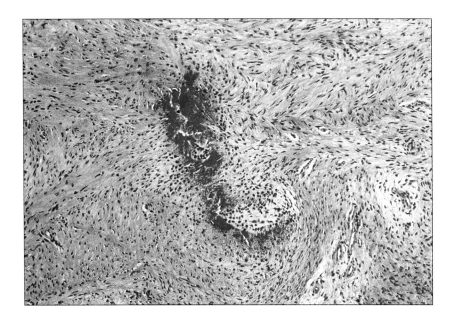

FIGURE 10–47 Calcifying aponeurotic fibroma with early focal calcification.

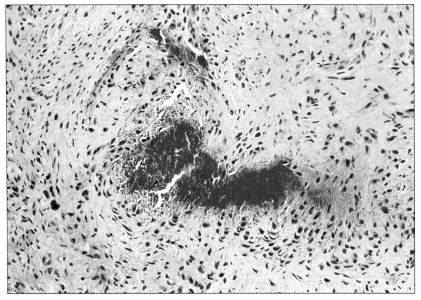

FIGURE 10–48 Calcifying aponeurotic fibroma showing hyalinization of the fibrous tissue in the vicinity of heavily calcified areas.

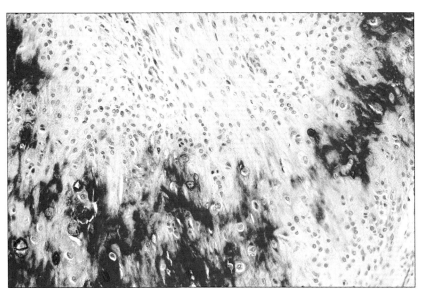

FIGURE 10–49 Calcifying aponeurotic fibroma with small round cells radiating from the calcified areas and arranged in linear arrays.

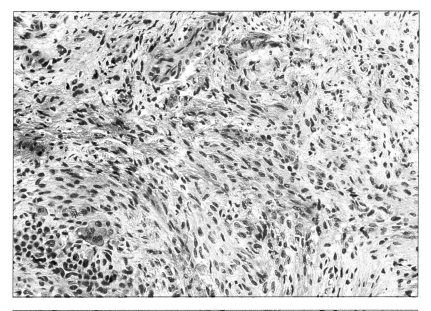

FIGURE 10–50 High-power view of the cellular portion of a calcifying aponeurotic fibroma.

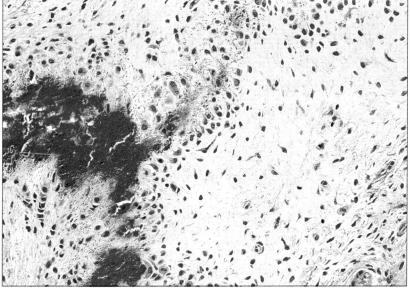

FIGURE 10–51 Calcifying aponeurotic fibroma with focal cartilaginous metaplasia in an area of calcification.

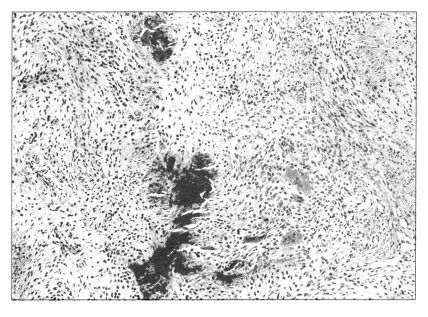

FIGURE 10–52 Calcifying aponeurotic fibroma with multinucleated giant cells adjacent to an area of calcification.

have been reported.[290] Lafferty et al. reported a calcifying aponeurotic fibroma of the palm in a 3-year-old girl that metastasized as a metastatic fibrosarcoma to the lungs and bones 5 years after a second local excision.[291] One of us (S.W.W.) has also reviewed a single case of malignant transformation of a calcifying aponeurotic fibroma.

Surgical management should be conservative for all tumors with the typical appearance of a calcifying aponeurotic fibroma. In fact, excision and re-excision, if necessary, are preferable to radical or mutilating surgical procedures to maintain function of the extremity.

There seem to be two phases in the development of this tumor: (1) an initial phase, which is more common in infants and small children, in which the tumor grows diffusely, often lacks calcification, and bears a resemblance to infantile fibromatosis; and (2) a late phase, in which the tumor is more compact and nodular and shows a more prominent degree of calcification and cartilage formation. In some of the latter cases, calcification and cartilage formation are so prominent it may be difficult to distinguish this lesion from a calcifying soft part chondroma.

CONGENITAL AND ACQUIRED MUSCULAR FIBROSIS

Muscular fibrosis was first defined as an entity by Hnevkovsky in 1961 as *progressive fibrosis of vastus intermedius muscle in children*.[292] Since 1961, numerous examples of this condition have been reported in the literature; most affected the quadriceps muscle,[293] although a few have been reported in the gluteus,[294] deltoid,[295] triceps,[296] and gastrocnemius muscles.[297] Both congenital and acquired lesions of this type have been described.

Clinical findings

Although the onset of the lesion usually dates back to the first year of life, the mass develops slowly and often does not become apparent before the second or third year of life. Clinically, most patients present with a progressive, painless mass or cord-like induration of the involved muscle. Lesions are generally poorly circumscribed and may occur on one or both sides. Progressive fibrosis results in shortening and contracture of the involved muscle, which leads to various functional disturbances depending on the extent of the fibrosis and the muscle involved. Concomitant dimpling or depressions of the overlying skin are observed occasionally; they are most likely a result of fatty atrophy and extension of the fibrosing process into the adjacent fascia and subcutaneous fat.

The fibrosing process is most commonly encountered in the quadriceps muscle, where it usually affects the distal portion of the vastus intermedius and vastus lateralis. It severely limits the range of active and passive flexion of the knee joint and causes difficulty squatting and sitting straight as well as an abnormal gait. In some cases the patella dislocates laterally every time the knee is flexed. Involvement of the gluteus muscle may lead to external rotation and abduction contracture of the hip in a seated position and a waddling gait. Napiontek and Ruszkowski reported a case of gluteal fibrosis following intramuscular injection that resulted in paralytic foot-drop secondary to sciatic nerve injury and external rotation contracture of the hip.[298] Involvement of the deltoid muscle may cause abduction contracture of the shoulder and lateral elevation of the arms.[299]

Pathologic findings

Grossly, the involved muscle shows patchy, firm, scar-like, gray or gray-yellow areas that consist microscopically of a conglomerate of collagenous fibrous tissue, residual partly degenerated atrophic muscle fibers, and replacement of atrophic muscle by mature fat. Not infrequently, the fibrosis extends into the muscle fascia or aponeurosis and even into the subcutaneous fat. There is no evidence of foreign body reaction or significant inflammation.

Discussion

Various concepts have been suggested as to the most likely cause of the fibrosing process. Lloyd-Roberts and Thomas[300] and Gunn[301] were the first to recognize the association of this lesion with multiple intramuscular injections. In many cases the patients have a history of severe illness during infancy and treatment with multiple intramuscular injections of antibiotics or other medications. No single drug has been incriminated as the cause of the fibrosis, although antibiotics appear to be the most frequently injected medication. It has been proposed that the intramuscular injection results in chemical myositis or pressure ischemia with subsequent fibrosis.[299] Given the fact that only a small number of infants who undergo this type of therapy develop intramuscular fibrosis, other predisposing factors have been suggested. There are reports of muscle fibrosis in children who have had the lesions since birth, with no history of intramuscular injections. There is no clear hereditary pattern, but the condition has been observed in four pairs of siblings[302] and several pairs of identical twins.[303,304]

To regain a normal range of function, tenotomy (rather than physical therapy or other conservative measures) is the treatment of choice. Most patients regain full range of motion, although a subset of patients continue to have functional impairment of the involved extremity.[293]

CEREBRIFORM FIBROUS PROLIFERATION (PROTEUS SYNDROME)

Proteus syndrome, a rare entity, is included here because the cerebriform or gyriform fibrous proliferation characteristically found on the volar surfaces may be mistaken for fibromatosis. Although isolated or localized cerebriform fibrous proliferations have been described,[305] they occur more commonly in conjunction with a complex group of lesions involving the skin, soft tissue, and skeleton. Proteus syndrome was first described by Cohen and Hayden in 1979[306] and named by Wiedemann in 1983[307] after the Greek ocean deity, Proteus (the polymorphous), because of the broad range of its features. Although "the elephant man," Joseph Merrick, was originally believed to have neurofibromatosis, evidence indicates that he suffered from Proteus syndrome.[308]

Patients with the Proteus syndrome exhibit a constellation of congenital and developmental defects that cannot be classified into previously defined disorders, and these patients demonstrate wide morphologic variability.[309,310] Manifestations include gigantism of the hands or feet (macrodactyly), asymmetry, skeletal abnormalities including hemihypertrophy and exostoses (particularly cranial exostoses),[311] and a variety of cutaneous abnormalities including epidermal nevi and lipomatous and hemangiomatous tumors. The lipomatous proliferations may be present in the subcutis but may also affect the abdomen, pelvis, and mesentery.[312,313] The cerebriform fibrous changes affect the plantar surfaces and to a lesser degree the palmar surfaces, and they are associated with unilateral or bilateral macrodactyly or hypertrophy of long bones (partial gigantism). Grossly, there is marked thickening of the skin in the volar areas resulting in a coarse cerebriform or gyriform pattern (Fig. 10–53).

Microscopically, the plantar and palmar lesions consist of dense fibrosis involving both the dermis and subcutis, with hyperkeratosis of the overlying skin (Figs 10–54 to 10–56).[314] Uitto et al. showed that these lesions consist almost exclusively of type I collagen and suggested an underlying defect in the production of collagenase.[315]

The cause of the Proteus syndrome is unknown. There is no gender predilection, and all reported cases appear to be sporadic.[313] Mutations in the *PTEN* tumor suppressor gene have been reported in some patients.[316,317] Mutations in this gene have not been found in many patients with Proteus syndrome, suggesting that mutations in other genes are involved or that current clinical diagnostic criteria are overly inclusive.

CALCIFYING FIBROUS PSEUDOTUMOR

Originally reported as *childhood fibrous tumor with psammoma bodies*,[318] calcifying fibrous pseudotumor is a rare entity; it is a hypocellular, fibrous lesion that most often

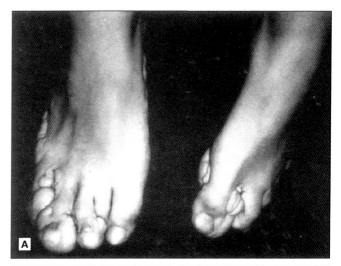

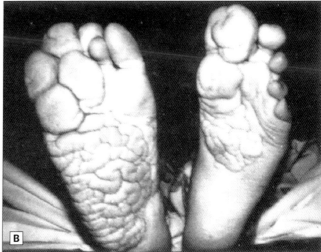

FIGURE 10–53 Bilateral cerebriform (gyriform) fibrous proliferation of toes **(A)** and plantar surfaces **(B)**. This process may occur alone or in conjunction with lipomatous and hemangiomatous tumors and various skeletal changes, including scoliosis, multiple exostoses, and craniofacial asymmetry (Proteus syndrome).

affects patients during the second or third decade of life.[319,320] Females are affected slightly more commonly than males. Most patients present with a slowly growing, painless mass in the subcutaneous or deep soft tissues which may be associated with systemic symptoms. The lesions most commonly arise in the extremities, followed by the trunk, inguinal and scrotal regions, and head and neck. Rare lesions have also been described in the omentum/mesentery,[321] mediastinum,[322,323] pleura,[324,325] and peritoneum.[326] Most are 3–5 cm at the time of excision, but the lesions can be as large as 15 cm.

On gross examination, the mass is well circumscribed, somewhat lobulated, and solid or firm; it has a uniform gray-white fibrous appearance on cross-section. It often cuts with a gritty sensation due to the extensive calcifica-

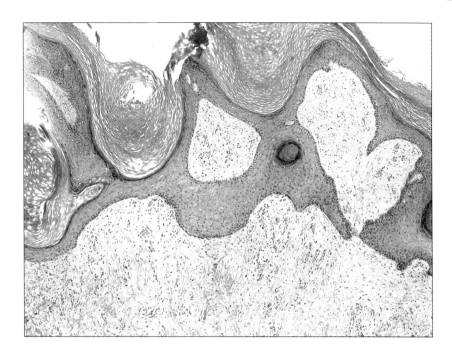

FIGURE 10–54 Proteus syndrome. The lesion shows evidence of acanthosis and hyperkeratosis of the overlying epithelium associated with dermal fibrosis and mild chronic inflammation.

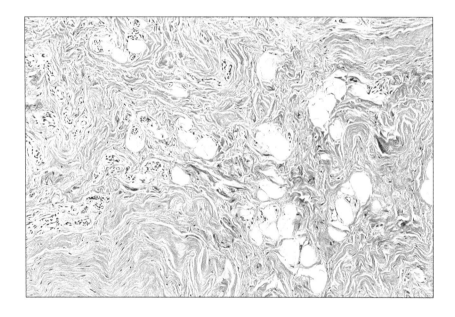

FIGURE 10–55 Proteus syndrome. Hypocellular dense collagen with admixed adipocytes.

tions which are typically present. Histologically, the mass is well circumscribed, nonencapsulated, and composed chiefly of hyalinized birefringent fibrosclerotic tissue with a variable inflammatory infiltrate composed of lymphocytes and plasma cells, with the formation of occasional germinal centers. The lesions are hypocellular, with scattered cytologically bland, fibroblastic or myofibroblastic spindle cells.[319,320] A characteristic feature is the presence of dystrophic, frequently psammomatous calcifications that may be focally present or comprise most of the tumor (Fig. 10–57). Immunohistochemically, these cells stain diffusely for vimentin. Variable immunoreactivity for muscle-specific actin, smooth muscle actin, and

desmin has been reported.[320] In our experience, scattered cells express these markers, but they are never diffusely positive. Many of the lesional cells express CD34 and/or factor XIIIa.[320,327] However, stains for ALK, a marker found in many (but not all) inflammatory myofibroblastic tumors, is consistently negative in calcifying fibrous pseudotumor.[320,328]

The differential diagnosis includes inflammatory myofibroblastic tumor, reactive nodular fibrous pseudotumor, fibromatosis, nodular fasciitis, fibroma of the tendon sheath, calcifying aponeurotic fibroma, and amyloidoma. *Inflammatory myofibroblastic tumor* is generally more cellular, less hyalinized, and typically lacks

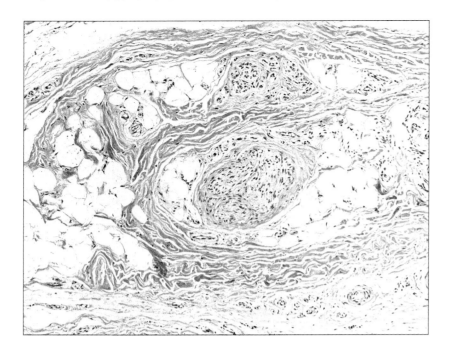

FIGURE 10–56 Benign lipomatous lesion with entrapped nerves in a patient with Proteus syndrome.

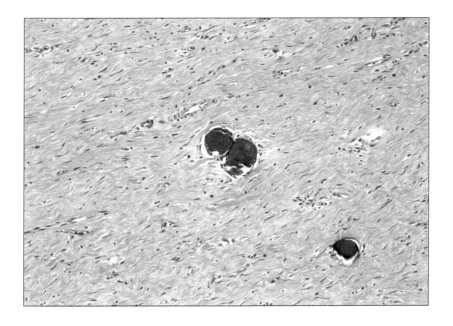

FIGURE 10–57 Calcifying fibrous pseudotumor chiefly composed of a uniform dense collagenous matrix with psammomatous calcifications and scattered spindle-shaped and inflammatory cells.

calcifications. However, clearly there is histologic overlap of these lesions, and it has been proposed that calcifying fibrous pseudotumor represents a late sclerosing phase of inflammatory myofibroblastic tumor.[319,329,330] Van Dorpe et al. described an intra-abdominal tumor, which arose in a 17-year-old female, with features overlapping those seen in these two entities, as well as transitional stages between calcifying fibrous pseudotumor and inflammatory myofibroblastic tumor.[329] However, calcifying fibrous pseudotumor is consistently negative for ALK, and there is no evidence to suggest that alterations of the *ALK* gene are involved in its pathogenesis.

Yantiss and colleagues described a fibroinflammatory lesion which typically arises in the mesentery and coined the term *"reactive nodular fibrous pseudotumor."*[331] Although there are some similarities to calcifying fibrous pseudotumor, the authors argued that this entity is distinct based upon histologic and immunohistochemical grounds. In contrast to reactive nodular fibrous pseudotumor, calcifying fibrous pseudotumor is usually more cellular, the infiltrate contains lymphocytes, plasma cells and granulocytes, and calcifications are characteristic. The lesional cells of reactive nodular fibrous pseudotumor express actins, desmin, and CD117, and are negative for CD34.

Fibromatosis is less well circumscribed, and histologically the spindle cells typically infiltrate the surrounding soft tissues. In addition, fibromatosis is characterized by greater cellularity with arrangement in a prominent fascicular growth pattern. Microcalcifications are extremely uncommon in fibromatosis. *Nodular fasciitis* is composed of tissue culture-like spindle cells deposited in a myxoid stroma that lacks microcalcifications. Unlike calcifying fibrous pseudotumor, *fibroma of the tendon sheath* typically arises in the distal extremities. It is composed chiefly of densely sclerotic collagen, but there are frequently areas of increased cellularity, some of which resemble nodular fasciitis. In addition, elongated slit-like spaces are typical, and calcifications are not present. *Calcifying aponeurotic fibroma* usually arises in the hands or feet, is less well circumscribed than calcifying fibrous pseudotumor, and is characterized by band-like calcifications frequently surrounded by cartilaginous metaplasia and multinucleated giant cells. Unlike amyloid tumor (*amyloidoma*), calcifying fibrous pseudotumor is devoid of giant cells or demonstrable amyloid, as Congo red stains are negative.

Although metastases have not been reported, some lesions locally recur.[319,332] In the study by Nascimento and colleagues, 3 of the 10 cases with clinical follow-up recurred, including 2 cases that recurred more than once.[320] Nevertheless, this lesion is clearly benign, and conservative excision seems reasonable.

REFERENCES

Fibrous hamartoma of infancy

1. Reye RD. A consideration of certain subdermal fibromatous tumours of infancy. J Pathol Bacteriol 1956; 72:149.
2. Enzinger FM. Fibrous hamartoma of infancy. Cancer 1965; 18:241.
3. Dickey GE, Sotelo-Avila C. Fibrous hamartoma of infancy: current review. Pediatr Dev Pathol 1999; 2:236.
4. Efem SE, Ekpo MD. Clinicopathological features of untreated fibrous hamartoma of infancy. J Clin Pathol 1993; 46:522.
5. Thami GP, Jaswal R, Kanwar AJ. Fibrous hamartoma of infancy in the scrotum. Pediatr Dermatol 1998; 15:326.
6. Stock JA, Niku SD, Packer MG, et al. Fibrous hamartoma of infancy: a report of two cases in the genital region. Urology 1995; 45:130.
7. Eppley BL, Harruff R, Shah M, et al. Fibrous hamartomas of the scalp in infancy. Plast Reconstr Surg 1994; 94:195.
8. Imaji R, Goto T, Takahashi Y, et al. A case of recurrent and synchronous fibrous hamartoma of infancy. Pediatr Surg Int 2005; 21:119.
9. Ashwood N, Witt JD, Hall-Craggs MA. Fibrous hamartoma of infancy at the wrist and the use of MRI in preoperative planning. Pediatr Radiol 2001; 31:450.
10. German DS, Paletta CE, Gabriel K. Fibrous hamartoma of infancy. Orthopedics 1996; 19:258.
11. Fletcher CD, Powell G, van Noorden S, et al. Fibrous hamartoma of infancy: a histochemical and immunohistochemical study. Histopathology 1988; 12:65.
12. Groisman G, Lichtig C. Fibrous hamartoma of infancy: an immunohistochemical and ultrastructural study. Hum Pathol 1991; 22:914.
13. Lakshminarayanan R, Konia T, Welborn J. Fibrous hamartoma of infancy: a case report with associated cytogenetic findings. Arch Pathol Lab Med 2005; 129:520.

Infantile digital fibromatosis

14. Jensen AR, Martin LW, Longino LA. Digital neurofibrosarcoma in infancy. J Pediatr 1957; 51:566.
15. Enzinger FM. Dermal fibromatosis. In: Tumors of bone and soft tissue. Chicago: Year Book; 1965:375.
16. Kang SK, Chang SE, Choi JH, et al. A case of congenital infantile digital fibromatosis. Pediatr Dermatol 2002; 19:462.

17. Kanwar AJ, Kaur S, Thami GP, et al. Congenital infantile digital fibromatosis. Pediatr Dermatol 2002; 19:370.
18. Sungur N, Kilinc H, Ozdemir R, et al. Infantile digital fibromatosis: an unusual localization. J Pediatr Surg 2001; 36:1587.
19. Plusje LG, Bastiaens M, Chang A, et al. Infantile-type digital fibromatosis tumour in an adult. Br J Dermatol 2000; 143:1107.
20. Rimareix F, Bardot J, Andrac L, et al. Infantile digital fibroma – report on eleven cases. Eur J Pediatr Surg 1997; 7:345.
21. Drut R, Pedemonte L, Rositto A. Noninclusion-body infantile digital fibromatosis: a lesion heralding terminal osseous dysplasia and pigmentary defects syndrome. Int J Surg Pathol 2005; 13:181.
22. Bacino CA, Stockton DW, Sierra RA, et al. Terminal osseous dysplasia and pigmentary defects: clinical characterization of a novel male lethal X-linked syndrome. Am J Med Genet 2000; 94:102.
23. Purdy LJ, Colby TV. Infantile digital fibromatosis occurring outside the digit. Am J Surg Pathol 1984; 8:787.
24. Pettinato G, Manivel JC, Gould EW, et al. Inclusion body fibromatosis of the breast. Two cases with immunohistochemical and ultrastructural findings. Am J Clin Pathol 1994; 101:714.
25. Mukai M, Torikata C, Iri H, et al. Immunohistochemical identification of aggregated actin filaments in formalin-fixed, paraffin-embedded sections. I. A study of infantile digital fibromatosis by a new pretreatment. Am J Surg Pathol 1992; 16:110.
26. Choi KC, Hashimoto K, Setoyama M, et al. Infantile digital fibromatosis. Immunohistochemical and immunoelectron microscopic studies. J Cutan Pathol 1990; 17:225.
27. Bhawan J, Bacchetta C, Joris I, et al. A myofibroblastic tumor. Infantile digital fibroma (recurrent digital fibrous tumor of childhood). Am J Pathol 1979; 94:19.
28. Mukai M, Torikata C, Iri H, et al. Infantile digital fibromatosis. An electron microscopic and immunohistochemical study. Acta Pathol Jpn 1986; 36:1605.
29. Hayashi T, Tsuda N, Chowdhury PR, et al. Infantile digital fibromatosis: a study of the development and regression of cytoplasmic inclusion bodies. Mod Pathol 1995; 8:548.
30. Khan N, Alam K, Maheshwari V, et al. Recurrent infantile digital fibromatosis – a rare entity. Indian J Pathol Microbiol 2001; 44:135.

31. Kawaguchi M, Mitsuhashi Y, Hozumi Y, et al. A case of infantile digital fibromatosis with spontaneous regression. J Dermatol 1998; 25:523.
32. Falco NA, Upton J. Infantile digital fibromas. J Hand Surg [Am] 1995; 20:1014.
33. Albertini JG, Welsch MJ, Conger LA, et al. Infantile digital fibroma treated with Mohs' micrographic surgery. Dermatol Surg 2002; 28:959.
34. Battifora H, Hines JR. Recurrent digital fibromas of childhood. An electron microscope study. Cancer 1971; 27:1530.
35. Miyamoto T, Mihara M, Hagari Y, et al. Posttraumatic occurrence of infantile digital fibromatosis. A histologic and electron microscopic study. Arch Dermatol 1986; 122:915.
36. Kawabata H, Masada K, Aoki Y, et al. Infantile digital fibromatosis after web construction in syndactyly. J Hand Surg [Am] 1986; 11:741.
37. Canioni D, Richard S, Rambaud C, et al. Lingual localization of an inclusion body fibromatosis (Reye's tumor). Pathol Res Pract 1991; 187:886.
38. Navas-Palacios JJ, Conde-Zurita JM. Inclusion body myofibroblasts other than those seen in recurring digital fibroma of childhood. Ultrastruct Pathol 1984; 7:109.
39. Yusoff KL, Spagnolo DV, Digwood KI. Atypical cervical polyp with intracytoplasmic inclusions. Pathology 1998; 30:215.
40. Terada S, Suzuki N, Uchide K, et al. Vulvar angioleiomyoma. Arch Gynecol Obstet 1993; 253:51.
41. Ortega E, Aranda FI, Chulia MT, et al. Phyllodes tumor of the breast with actin inclusions in stromal cells: diagnosis by fine-needle aspiration cytology. Diagn Cytopathol 2001; 25:115.

Myofibroma and myofibromatosis

42. Williams JO, Schrum D. Congenital fibrosarcoma: report of a case in a newborn infant. AMA Arch Pathol 1951; 51:548.
43. Stout AP. Juvenile fibromatosis. Cancer 1954; 7:953.
44. Kauffman SL, Stout AP. Congenital mesenchymal tumors. Cancer 1965; 18:460.
45. Chung EB, Enzinger FM. Infantile myofibromatosis. Cancer 1981; 48:1807.
46. Wiswell TE, Davis J, Cunningham BE, et al. Infantile myofibromatosis: the most common fibrous tumor of infancy. J Pediatr Surg 1988; 23:315.

47. Swierkowski P, Seex K. Soft tissue solitary adult myofibroma in an intervertebral foramen. A NZ J Surg 2004; 74:1028.
48. Oliver RJ, Coulthard P, Carre C, et al. Solitary adult myofibroma of the mandible simulating an odontogenic cyst. Oral Oncol 2003; 39:626.
49. Granter SR, Badizadegan K, Fletcher CD. Myofibromatosis in adults, glomangiopericytoma, and myopericytoma: a spectrum of tumors showing perivascular myoid differentiation. Am J Surg Pathol 1998; 22:513.
50. Liu CJ, Chang KW. "Infantile" myofibroma of the oral cavity: Report of case. J Oral Maxillofac Surg 2001; 59:471.
51. Foss RD, Ellis GL. Myofibromas and myofibromatosis of the oral region: a clinicopathologic analysis of 79 cases. Oral Surg Oral Med Oral Pathol Oral Radiol Endod 2000; 89:57.
52. Tsuji M, Inagaki T, Kasai H, et al. Solitary myofibromatosis of the skull: a case report and review of literature. Childs Nerv Syst 2004; 20:366.
53. Sedghizadeh PP, Allen CM, Kalmar JR, et al. Solitary central myofibroma presenting in the gnathic region. Ann Diagn Pathol 2004; 8:284.
54. Ng WT, Book KS, Ng WF. Infantile myofibromatosis of the ovary presenting with ascites. Eur J Pediatr Surg 2001; 11:415.
55. Ozturk A, Gunes T, Cetin N, et al. Congenital multiple myofibromatosis: is it really due to underestrogenic stimulation?. Pediatr Int 2004; 46:91.
56. Kaplan SS, Ojemann JG, Grange DK, et al. Intracranial infantile myofibromatosis with intraparenchymal involvement. Pediatr Neurosurg 2002; 36:214.
57. Schaffzin EA, Chung SM, Kaye R. Congenital generalized fibromatosis with complete spontaneous regression. A case report. J Bone Joint Surg [Am] 1972; 54:657.
58. Heiple KG, Perrin E, Aikawa M. Congenital generalized fibromatosis: a case limited to osseous lesions. J Bone Joint Surg [Am] 1972; 54:663.
59. Hogan SF, Salassa JR. Recurrent adult myofibromatosis. A case report. Am J Clin Pathol 1992; 97:810.
60. Hasegawa T, Hirose T, Seki K, et al. Solitary infantile myofibromatosis of bone. An immunohistochemical and ultrastructural study. Am J Surg Pathol 1993; 17:308.
61. Chateil JF, Brun M, Lebail B, et al. Infantile myofibromatosis. Skeletal Radiol 1995; 24:629.
62. Koujok K, Ruiz RE, Hernandez RJ. Myofibromatosis: imaging characteristics. Pediatr Radiol 2005; 35:374.
63. Hicks J, Mierau G. The spectrum of pediatric fibroblastic and myofibroblastic tumors. Ultrastruct Pathol 2004; 28:265.
64. Jurcic V, Perkovic T, Pohar-Marinsek Z, et al. Infantile myofibroma in a prematurely born twin: a case report. Pediatr Dermatol 2003; 20:345.
65. Zelger BW, Calonje E, Sepp N, et al. Monophasic cellular variant of infantile myofibromatosis. An unusual histopathologic pattern in two siblings. Am J Dermatopathol 1995; 17:131.
66. Fletcher CD, Achu P, Van Noorden S, et al. Infantile myofibromatosis: a light microscopic, histochemical and immunohistochemical study suggesting true smooth muscle differentiation. Histopathology 1987; 11:245.
67. Beham A, Badve S, Suster S, et al. Solitary myofibroma in adults: clinicopathological analysis of a series. Histopathology 1993; 22:335.

68. Eyden B. Electron microscopy in the study of myofibroblastic lesions. Semin Diagn Pathol 2003; 20:13.
69. De Schepper S, Janssens S, Messiaen L, et al. Multiple myofibromas and an epidermal verrucous nevus in a child with neurofibromatosis type 1. Dermatology 2004; 209:223.
70. Mentzel T, Calonje E, Nascimento AG, et al. Infantile hemangiopericytoma versus infantile myofibromatosis. Study of a series suggesting a continuous spectrum of infantile myofibroblastic lesions. Am J Surg Pathol 1994; 18:922.
71. Variend S, Bax NM, van Gorp J. Are infantile myofibromatosis, congenital fibrosarcoma and congenital haemangiopericytoma histogenetically related? Histopathology 1995; 26:57.
72. Dictor M, Elner A, Andersson T, et al. Myofibromatosis-like hemangiopericytoma metastasizing as differentiated vascular smooth-muscle and myosarcoma. Myopericytes as a subset of "myofibroblasts." Am J Surg Pathol 1992; 16:1239.
73. Tokano H, Ishikawa N, Kitamura K, et al. Solitary infantile myofibromatosis in the lateral orbit floor showing spontaneous regression. J Laryngol Otol 2001; 115:419.
74. Fukasawa Y, Ishikura H, Takada A, et al. Massive apoptosis in infantile myofibromatosis. A putative mechanism of tumor regression. Am J Pathol 1994; 144:480.
75. Hatzidaki E, Korakaki E, Voloudaki A, et al. Infantile myofibromatosis with visceral involvement and complete spontaneous regression. J Dermatol 2001; 28:379.
76. Zeller B, Storm-Mathisen I, Smevik B, et al. Cure of infantile myofibromatosis with severe respiratory complications without antitumour therapy. Eur J Pediatr 1997; 156:841.
77. Gandhi MM, Nathan PC, Weitzman S, et al. Successful treatment of life-threatening generalized infantile myofibromatosis using low-dose chemotherapy. J Pediatr Hematol Oncol 2003; 25:750.
78. Day M, Edwards AO, Weinberg A, et al. Brief report: successful therapy of a patient with infantile generalized myofibromatosis. Med Pediatr Oncol 2002; 38:371.
79. Williams W, Craver RD, Correa H, et al. Use of 2-chlorodeoxyadenosine to treat infantile myofibromatosis. J Pediatr Hematol Oncol 2002; 24:59.
80. Bracko M, Cindro L, Golouh R. Familial occurrence of infantile myofibromatosis [25 refs]. Cancer 1992; 69:1294.
81. Narchi H. Four half-siblings with infantile myofibromatosis: a case for autosomal-recessive inheritance. Clin Genet 2001; 59:134.
82. Zand DJ, Huff D, Everman D, et al. Autosomal dominant inheritance of infantile myofibromatosis. Am J Med Genet 2004; 126:261.
83. Stenman G, Nadal N, Persson S, et al. Del(6)(q12q15) as the sole cytogenetic anomaly in a case of solitary infantile myofibromatosis. Oncol Rep 1999; 6:1101.
84. Sirvent N, Perrin C, Lacour JP, et al. Monosomy 9q and trisomy 16q in a case of congenital solitary infantile myofibromatosis. Virchows Arch 2004; 445:537.

Juvenile hyaline fibromatosis

85. Murray J. On three peculiar cases of molluscum fibrosum in children. Med Chir Trans 1873; 38:235.
86. Whitfield A, Robinson AH. A further report of a remarkable series of cases of molluscum

fibrosum in children. Med Chir Trans 1903; 86:293.
87. Puretic S, Puretic B, Fiser-Herman M. A unique form of mesenchymal dysplasia. Br J Dermatol 1962; 74:8.
88. Alfi OS, Heuser ET, Landing BH, et al. A syndrome of systemic hyalinosis, short-limb dwarfism and possible thymic dysplasia. Birth Defects Orig Artic Ser 1975; 11:57.
89. Nezelof C, Letourneux-Toromanoff B, Griscelli C, et al. Painful disseminated fibromatosis (systemic hyalinis): a new hereditary collagen dysplasia. Arch Fr Pediatr 1978; 35:1063.
90. Kitano Y. Juvenile hyalin fibromatosis. Arch Dermatol 1976; 112:86.
91. Allen PW. Selected case from the Arkadi M. Rywlin International Pathology Slide Seminar: Hyaline fibromatosis. Adv Anat Pathol 2001; 8:173.
92. Fayad MN, Yacoub A, Salman S, et al. Juvenile hyaline fibromatosis: two new patients and review of the literature. Am J Med Genet 1987; 26:123.
93. Fetisovova Z, Adamicova K, Pec M, et al. Dermatological findings in an adult patient with juvenile hyaline fibromatosis. J Eur Acad Dermatol Venereol 2003; 17:473.
94. Gilaberte Y, Gonzalez-Mediero I, Lopez Barrantes V, et al. Juvenile hyaline fibromatosis with skull-encephalic anomalies: a case report and review of the literature. Dermatology 1993; 187:144.
95. Finlay AY, Ferguson SD, Holt PJ. Juvenile hyaline fibromatosis. Br J Dermatol 1983; 108:609.
96. Woyke S, Domagala W, Markiewicz C. A 19-year follow-up of multiple juvenile hyaline fibromatosis. J Pediatr Surg 1984; 19:302.
97. Kan AE, Rogers M. Juvenile hyaline fibromatosis: an expanded clinicopathologic spectrum. Pediatr Dermatol 1989; 6:68.
98. O'Neill DB, Kasser JR. Juvenile hyaline fibromatosis. A case report and review of musculoskeletal manifestations. J Bone Joint Surg [Am] 1989; 71:941.
99. Bas NS, Guzey FK, Emel E, et al. A solitary calvarial lytic lesion with typical histopathological findings of juvenile hyaline fibromatosis. J Neurosurg 2005; 103:285.
100. Bedford CD, Sills JA, Sommelet-Olive D, et al. Juvenile hyaline fibromatosis: a report of two severe cases. J Pediatr 1991; 119:404.
101. Kawasaki G, Yanamoto S, Mizuno A, et al. Juvenile hyaline fibromatosis complicated with oral squamous cell carcinoma: A case report. Oral Surg Oral Med Oral Pathol Oral Radiol Endod 2001; 91:200.
102. Shimizu K, Ogawa F, Hamasaki Y, et al. A case of bullous pemphigoid arising in juvenile hyaline fibromatosis with oral squamous cell carcinoma. J Dermatol 2005; 32:650.
103. Kitano Y, Horiki M, Aoki T, et al. Two cases of juvenile hyalin fibromatosis. Some histological, electron microscopic, and tissue culture observations. Arch Dermatol 1972; 106:877.
104. Ko CJ, Barr RJ. Calcospherules associated with juvenile hyaline fibromatosis. Am J Dermatopathol 2003; 25:53.
105. Haleem A, Al-Hindi HN, Juboury MA, et al. Juvenile hyaline fibromatosis: morphologic, immunohistochemical, and ultrastructural study of three siblings. Am J Dermatopathol 2002; 24:218.
106. Remberger K, Krieg T, Kunze D, et al. Fibromatosis hyalinica multiplex (juvenile hyalin fibromatosis). Light microscopic, electron microscopic, immunohistochemical, and biochemical findings. Cancer 1985; 56:614.

107. Winik BC, Boente MC, Asial R. Juvenile hyaline fibromatosis: ultrastructural study. Am J Dermatopathol 1998; 20:373.

108. Ugras S, Akpolat N, Metin A. Juvenile hyaline fibromatosis in one Turkish child. Turk J Pediatr 2000; 42:264.

109. Prapanpoch S, Jorgenson RJ, Langlais RP, et al. Winchester syndrome. A case report and literature review. Oral Surg Oral Med Oral Pathol 1992; 74:671.

110. Urbina F, Sazunic I, Murray G. Infantile systemic hyalinosis or juvenile hyaline fibromatosis? Pediatr Dermatol 2004; 21:154.

111. Quintal D, Jackson R. Juvenile hyaline fibromatosis. A 15-year follow-up. Arch Dermatol 1985; 121:1062.

112. Schaller M, Stengel-Rutkowski S, Sollberg S, et al. Juvenile hyaline fibromatosis. Hautarzt 1997; 48:253.

113. Karabulut AB, Ozden BC, Onel D, et al. Management of airway obstruction in a severe case of juvenile hyaline fibromatosis. Ann Plast Surg 2005; 54:328.

114. Seefelder C, Ko JH, Padwa BL. Fibreoptic intubation for massive gingival hyperplasia in juvenile hyaline fibromatosis. Paediatr Anaesth 2000; 10:682.

115. Senzaki H, Kiyozuka Y, Uemura Y, et al. Juvenile hyaline fibromatosis: a report of two unrelated adult sibling cases and a literature review. Pathol Int 1998; 48:230.

116. Rahman N, Dunstan M, Teare MD, et al. The gene for juvenile hyaline fibromatosis maps to chromosome 4q21. Am J Hum Genet 2002; 71:975.

117. Dowling O, Difeo A, Ramirez MC, et al. Mutations in capillary morphogenesis gene-2 result in the allelic disorders juvenile hyaline fibromatosis and infantile systemic hyalinosis. Am J Hum Genet 2003; 73:957.

118. Hanks S, Adams S, Douglas J, et al. Mutations in the gene encoding capillary morphogenesis protein 2 cause juvenile hyaline fibromatosis and infantile systemic hyalinosis. Am J Hum Genet 2003; 73:791.

119. Katagiri K, Takasaki S, Fujiwara S, et al. Purification and structural analysis of extracellular matrix of a skin tumor from a patient with juvenile hyaline fibromatosis. J Dermatol Sci 1996; 13:37.

Gingival fibromatosis

120. Bakaeen G, Scully C. Hereditary gingival fibromatosis in a family with the Zimmermann-Laband syndrome. J Oral Pathol Med 1991; 20:457.

121. Cuestas-Carnero R, Bornancini CA. Hereditary generalized gingival fibromatosis associated with hypertrichosis: report of five cases in one family. J Oral Maxillofac Surg 1988; 46:415.

122. Emerson TG. Hereditary gingival hyperplasia: a familial pedigree of four generations. Oral Surg Oral Med Oral Pathol 1965; 19:1.

123. Byers LT, Jurkiewicz N. Congenital macrogingivae and hypertrichosis with subsequent giant fibroadenoma of the breasts. J Plast Reconstr Surg 1961; 27:608.

124. Heath C. Two cases of hypertrophy of the gums and alveoli treated by operation. Trans Odont Soc Great Britain 1989; 11:18.

125. Weski H. Elephantiasis gingivae hereditaria. Dtsch Monatsschur Zahnh 1920; 38:557.

126. Takagi M, Yamamoto H, Mega H, et al. Heterogeneity in the gingival fibromatoses. Cancer 1991; 68:2202.

127. Bittencourt LP, Campos V, Moliterno LF, et al. Hereditary gingival fibromatosis: review of the literature and a case report. Quintessence Int 2000; 31:415.

128. Redman RS, Ward CC, Patterson RH. Focus of epithelial dysplasia arising in hereditary gingival fibromatosis. J Periodontol 1985; 56:158.

129. Holzhausen M, Goncalves D, Correa F de O, et al. A case of Zimmermann-Laband syndrome with supernumerary teeth. J Periodontol 2003; 74:1225.

130. Holzhausen M, Ribeiro FS, Goncalves D, et al. Treatment of gingival fibromatosis associated with Zimmermann-Laband syndrome. J Periodontol 2005; 76:1559.

131. Shah N, Gupta YK, Ghose S. Zimmermann-Laband syndrome with bilateral developmental cataract – a new association?. Int J Paediatr Dent 2004; 14:78.

132. Stefanova M, Atanassov D, Krastev T, et al. Zimmermann-Laband syndrome associated with a balanced reciprocal translocation t(3;8)(p21.2;q24.3) in mother and daughter: molecular cytogenetic characterization of the breakpoint regions. Am J Med Genet A 2003; 117:289.

133. Pina-Neto JM, Moreno AF, Silva LR, et al. Cherubism, gingival fibromatosis, epilepsy, and mental deficiency (Ramon syndrome) with juvenile rheumatoid arthritis. Am J Med Genet 1986; 25:433.

134. Ramon Y, Berman W, Bubis JJ. Gingival fibromatosis combined with cherubism. Oral Surg Oral Med Oral Pathol 1967; 24:435.

135. Wynne SE, Aldred MJ, Bartold PM. Hereditary gingival fibromatosis associated with hearing loss and supernumerary teeth – a new syndrome. J Periodontol 1995; 66:75.

136. Kasaboglu O, Tumer C, Balci S. Hereditary gingival fibromatosis and sensorineural hearing loss in a 42-year-old man with Jones syndrome. Genet Couns 2004; 15:213.

137. Hallett KB, Bankier A, Chow CW, et al. Gingival fibromatosis and Klippel-Trenaunay-Weber syndrome. Case report. Oral Surg Oral Med Oral Pathol Oral Radiol Endod 1995; 79:578.

138. Harrison M, Odell EW, Agrawal M, et al. Gingival fibromatosis with prune-belly syndrome. Oral Surg Oral Med Oral Pathol Oral Radiol Endod 1998; 86:304.

139. Radhakrishnan S, Rajan P. Gingival fibromatosis and growth hormone deficiency syndrome – report of a rare case and review of literature. Indian J Dent Res 2003; 14:170.

140. Sakamoto R, Nitta T, Kamikawa Y, et al. Histochemical, immunohistochemical, and ultrastructural studies of gingival fibromatosis: a case report. Med Electron Microsc 2002; 35:248.

141. Barros SP, Merzel J, de Araujo VC, et al. Ultrastructural aspects of connective tissue in hereditary gingival fibromatosis. Oral Surg Oral Med Oral Pathol Oral Radiol Endod 2001; 92:78.

142. Kataoka M, Kido J, Shinohara Y, et al. Drug-induced gingival overgrowth – a review. Biol Pharm Bull 2005; 28:1817.

143. Sano M, Ohuchi N, Inoue T, et al. Proliferative response to phenytoin and nifedipine in gingival fibroblasts cultured from humans with gingival fibromatosis. Fundam Clin Pharmacol 2004; 18:465.

144. Ye X, Shi L, Cheng Y, et al. A novel locus for autosomal dominant hereditary gingival fibromatosis, GINGF3, maps to chromosome 2p22.3-p23.3. Clin Genet 2005; 68:239.

145. Zhang Y, Gorry MC, Hart PS, et al. Localization, genomic organization, and alternative transcription of a novel human SAM-dependent methyltransferase gene on chromosome 2p22-p21. Cytogenet Cell Genet 2001; 95:146.

146. Hart TC, Pallos D, Bowden DW, et al. Genetic linkage of hereditary gingival fibromatosis to chromosome 2p21. Am J Hum Genet 1998; 62:876.

147. Xiao S, Bu L, Zhu L, et al. A new locus for hereditary gingival fibromatosis (GINGF2) maps to 5q13-q22. Genomics 2001; 74:180.

148. Almeida JP, Coletta RD, Silva SD, et al. Proliferation of fibroblasts cultured from normal gingiva and hereditary gingival fibromatosis is dependent on fatty acid synthase activity. J Periodontol 2005; 76:272.

149. Martelli-Junior H, Cotrim P, Graner E, et al. Effect of transforming growth factor-beta1, interleukin-6, and interferon-gamma on the expression of type I collagen, heat shock protein 47, matrix metalloproteinase (MMP)-1 and MMP-2 by fibroblasts from normal gingiva and hereditary gingival fibromatosis. J Periodontol 2003; 74:296.

Fibromatosis colli

150. Coventry MB, Harris LE, Bianco AJ Jr, et al. Congenital muscular torticollis (wryneck). Postgrad Med 1960; 28:383.

151. Kiwak KJ. Establishing an etiology for torticollis. Postgrad Med 1984; 75:126.

152. Parikh SN, Crawford AH, Choudhury S. Magnetic resonance imaging in the evaluation of infantile torticollis. Orthopedics 2004; 27:509.

153. Lawrence WT, Azizkhan RG. Congenital muscular torticollis: a spectrum of pathology. Ann Plast Surg 1989; 23:523.

154. Kumar V, Prabhu BV, Chattopadhayay A, et al. Bilateral sternocleidomastoid tumor of infancy. Int J Pediatr Otorhinolaryngol 2003; 67:673.

155. Blythe WR, Logan TC, Holmes DK, et al. Fibromatosis colli: a common cause of neonatal torticollis. Am Fam Physician 1996; 54:1965.

156. Canale ST, Griffin DW, Hubbard CN. Congenital muscular torticollis. A long-term follow-up. J Bone Joint Surg [Am] 1982; 64:810.

157. Binder H, Eng GD, Gaiser JF, et al. Congenital muscular torticollis: results of conservative management with long-term follow-up in 85 cases. Arch Phys Med Rehabil 1987; 68:222.

158. Joachimsthal G. Handbuch der orthopadischen chirurgie, vol 1, sect 2. In: Jena: Gustav Fischer; 1905:234.

159. Thompson F, McManus S, Colville J. Familial congenital muscular torticollis: case report and review of the literature. Clin Orthop 1986; 202:193.

160. Isigkeit E. Untersuchungen uber die hereditat orthopadischer leiden. Arch Orthop Unfallchir 1931; 30:459.

161. Sharma S, Mishra K, Khanna G. Fibromatosis colli in infants. A cytologic study of eight cases. Acta Cytol 2003; 47:359.

162. Kurtycz DF, Logrono R, Hoerl HD, et al. Diagnosis of fibromatosis colli by fine-needle aspiration. Diagn Cytopathol 2000; 23:338.

163. Pereira S, Tani E, Skoog L. Diagnosis of fibromatosis colli by fine needle aspiration (FNA) cytology. Cytopathology 1999; 10:25.

164. Ling CM, Low YS. Sternomastoid tumor and muscular torticollis. Clin Orthop 1972; 86:144.

165. Ferkel RD, Westin GW, Dawson EG, et al. Muscular torticollis. A modified surgical approach. J Bone Joint Surg [Am] 1983; 65:894.

166. Suzuki S, Yamamuro T, Fujita A. The aetiological relationship between congenital torticollis and obstetrical paralysis. Int Orthop 1984; 8:175.

167. Stromeyer GF. Beitrage zur operativen orthopadik oder erfahrungen uber die subcutane durchschneidung berkurzter muskeln und deren schnen. Hannover: Helwing; 1838.

168. Kiesewetter WB, Nelson PK, Palladino VSea. Neonatal torticollis. JAMA 1955; 157:1281.

169. Nove-Josserand G, Viannay C. Pathogenie du torticolis congenital. Rev Orthop 1906; 7:397.

Infantile fibromatosis (lipofibromatosis)

170. Rao BN, Horowitz ME, Parham DM, et al. Challenges in the treatment of childhood fibromatosis. Arch Surg 1987; 122:1296.

171. Faulkner LB, Hajdu SI, Kher U, et al. Pediatric desmoid tumor: retrospective analysis of 63 cases. J Clin Oncol 1995; 13:2813.

172. Dehner LP, Askin FB. Tumors of fibrous tissue origin in childhood. A clinicopathologic study of cutaneous and soft tissue neoplasms in 66 children. Cancer 1976; 38:888.

173. Coffin CM, Dehner LP. Fibroblastic-myofibroblastic tumors in children and adolescents: a clinicopathologic study of 108 examples in 103 patients. Pediatr Pathol 1991; 11:569.

174. Thompson DH, Khan A, Gonzalez C, et al. Juvenile aggressive fibromatosis: report of three cases and review of the literature. Ear Nose Throat J 1991; 70:462.

175. Mannan AA, Ray R, Sharma SC, et al. Infantile fibromatosis of the nose and paranasal sinuses: report of a rare case and brief review of the literature. Ear Nose Throat J 2004; 83:481.

176. Ramanathan RC, Thomas JM. Infantile (desmoid-type) fibromatosis of the parotid gland. J Laryngol Otol 1997; 111:669.

177. Flacke S, Pauleit D, Keller E, et al. Infantile fibromatosis of the neck with intracranial involvement: MR and CT findings. AJNR Am J Neuroradiol 1999; 20:923.

178. Robbin MR, Murphey MD, Temple HT, et al. Imaging of musculoskeletal fibromatosis. Radiographics 2001; 21:585.

179. Ahn JM, Yoon HK, Suh YL, et al. Infantile fibromatosis in childhood: findings on MR imaging and pathologic correlation. Clin Radiol 2000; 55:19.

180. Wilkins SA Jr, Waldron CA, Mathews WH, et al. Aggressive fibromatosis of the head and neck. Am J Surg 1975; 130:412.

181. Fetsch JF, Miettinen M, Laskin WB, et al. A clinicopathologic study of 45 pediatric soft tissue tumors with an admixture of adipose tissue and fibroblastic elements, and a proposal for classification as lipofibromatosis. Am J Surg Pathol 2000; 24:1491.

182. Scougall P, Staheli LT, Chew DE, et al. Desmoid tumors in childhood. Orthop Rev 1987; 16:481.

183. Fromowitz FB, Hurst LC, Nathan J, et al. Infantile (desmoid type) fibromatosis with extensive ossification. Am J Surg Pathol 1987; 11:66.

184. Rodu B, Weathers DR, Campbell WG Jr. Aggressive fibromatosis involving the paramandibular soft tissues. A study with the aid of electron microscopy. Oral Surg Oral Med Oral Pathol 1981; 52:395.

185. Schmidt D, Klinge P, Leuschner I, et al. Infantile desmoid-type fibromatosis. Morphological features correlate with biological behaviour. J Pathol 1991; 164:315.

186. Schofield DE, Fletcher JA, Grier HE, et al. Fibrosarcoma in infants and children. Application of new techniques. Am J Surg Pathol 1994; 18:14.

187. Mandahl N, Heim S, Rydholm A, et al. Nonrandom numerical chromosome aberrations (+8, +11, +17, +20) in infantile fibrosarcoma. Cancer Genet Cytogenet 1989; 40:137.

188. Flores-Stadler EM, Chou PM, Barquin N, et al. Fibrous tumors in children – a morphologic and interphase cytogenetic analysis of problematic cases. Int J Oncol 2000; 17:433.

189. Knezevich SR, McFadden DE, Tao W, et al. A novel ETV6-NTRK3 gene fusion in congenital fibrosarcoma. Nat Genet 1998; 18:184.

190. Ayala AG, Ro JY, Goepfert H, et al. Desmoid fibromatosis: a clinicopathologic study of 25 children. Semin Diagn Pathol 1986; 3:138.

191. Raney B, Evans A, Granowetter L, et al. Nonsurgical management of children with recurrent or unresectable fibromatosis. Pediatrics 1987; 79:394.

Congenital/infantile fibrosarcoma

192. Stout AP. Fibrosarcoma in infants and children. Cancer 1962; 15:1028.

193. Chung EB, Enzinger FM. Infantile fibrosarcoma. Cancer 1976; 38:729.

194. Soule EH, Pritchard DJ. Fibrosarcoma in infants and children: a review of 110 cases. Cancer 1977; 40:1711.

195. Ramphal R, Manson D, Viero S, et al. Retroperitoneal infantile fibrosarcoma: clinical, molecular, and therapeutic aspects of an unusual tumor. Pediatr Hematol Oncol 2003; 20:635.

196. Coffin CM, Jaszcz W, O'Shea PA, et al. So-called congenital-infantile fibrosarcoma: does it exist and what is it? Pediatr Pathol 1994; 14:133.

197. Iiboshi Y, Azuma T, Kitayama Y, et al. Successful excision of a congenital, prenatally diagnosed fibrosarcoma involving the entire right ovary. Pediatr Surg Int 2003; 19:683.

198. Shima Y, Ikegami E, Takechi N, et al. Congenital fibrosarcoma of the jejunum in a premature infant with meconium peritonitis. Eur J Pediatr Surg 2003; 13:134.

199. Huang SY, Wang CW, Wang CJ, et al. Combined prenatal ultrasound and magnetic resonance imaging in an extensive congenital fibrosarcoma: a case report and review of the literature. Fetal Diagn Ther 2005; 20:266.

200. Dahl I, Save-Soderbergh J, Angervall L. Fibrosarcoma in early infancy. Pathol Eur 1973; 8:193.

201. Fisher C. Myofibroblastic malignancies. Adv Anat Pathol 2004; 11:190.

202. Kodet R, Stejskal J, Pilat D, et al. Congenital-infantile fibrosarcoma: a clinicopathological study of five patients entered on the Prague Children's Tumor Registry. Pathol Res Pract 1996; 192:845.

203. Bernstein R, Zeltzer PM, Lin F, et al. Trisomy 11 and other nonrandom trisomies in congenital fibrosarcoma. Cancer Genet Cytogenet 1994; 78:82.

204. Rubin BP, Chen CJ, Morgan TW, et al. Congenital mesoblastic nephroma t(12;15) is associated with ETV6-NTRK3 gene fusion: cytogenetic and molecular relationship to congenital (infantile) fibrosarcoma. Am J Pathol 1998; 153:1451.

205. Adem C, Gisselsson D, Dal Cin P, et al. ETV6 rearrangements in patients with infantile fibrosarcomas and congenital mesoblastic nephromas by fluorescence in situ hybridization. Mod Pathol 2001; 14:1246.

206. Sheng WQ, Hisaoka M, Okamoto S, et al. Congenital-infantile fibrosarcoma. A clinicopathologic study of 10 cases and molecular detection of the ETV6-NTRK3 fusion transcripts using paraffin-embedded tissues. Am J Clin Pathol 2001; 115:348.

207. Bourgeois JM, Knezevich SR, Mathers JA, et al. Molecular detection of the ETV6-NTRK3 gene fusion differentiates congenital fibrosarcoma from other childhood spindle cell tumors. Am J Surg Pathol 2000; 24:937.

208. Argani P, Fritsch MK, Shuster AE, et al. Reduced sensitivity of paraffin-based RT-PCR assays for ETV6-NTRK3 fusion transcripts in morphologically defined infantile

fibrosarcoma. Am J Surg Pathol 2001; 25:1461.

209. Argani P, Fritsch M, Kadkol SS, et al. Detection of the ETV6-NTRK3 chimeric RNA of infantile fibrosarcoma/cellular congenital mesoblastic nephroma in paraffin-embedded tissue: application to challenging pediatric renal stromal tumors. Mod Pathol 2000; 13:29.

210. Makretsov N, He M, Hayes M, et al. A fluorescence in situ hybridization study of ETV6-NTRK3 fusion gene in secretory breast carcinoma. Genes Chromosomes Cancer 2004; 40:152.

211. Lundgren L, Angervall L, Stenman G, et al. Infantile rhabdomyofibrosarcoma: a high-grade sarcoma distinguishable from infantile fibrosarcoma and rhabdomyosarcoma. Hum Pathol 1993; 24:785.

212. Miki H, Kobayashi S, Kushida Y, et al. A case of infantile rhabdomyofibrosarcoma with immunohistochemical, electronmicroscopical, and genetic analyses. Hum Pathol 1999; 30:1519.

213. Cecchetto G, Carli M, Alaggio R, et al. Fibrosarcoma in pediatric patients: results of the Italian Cooperative Group studies (1979–1995). J Surg Oncol 2001; 78:225.

214. Blocker S, Koenig J, Ternberg J. Congenital fibrosarcoma. J Pediatr Surg 1987; 22:665.

215. Wilson MB, Stanley W, Sens D, et al. Infantile fibrosarcoma – a misnomer? Pediatr Pathol 1990; 10:901.

216. Spicer RD. Re: "chemotherapy for infantile fibrosarcoma." Med Pediatr Oncol 1993; 21:80.

217. Grohn ML, Borzi P, Mackay A, et al. Management of extensive congenital fibrosarcoma with preoperative chemotherapy. A NZ J Surg 2004; 74:919.

218. Loh ML, Ahn P, Perez-Atayde AR, et al. Treatment of infantile fibrosarcoma with chemotherapy and surgery: results from the Dana-Farber Cancer Institute and Children's Hospital, Boston. J Pediatr Hematol Oncol 2002; 24:722.

219. Kurkchubasche AG, Halvorson EG, Forman EN, et al. The role of preoperative chemotherapy in the treatment of infantile fibrosarcoma. J Pediatr Surg 2000; 35:880.

220. Surico G, Muggeo P, Daniele RM, et al. Chemotherapy alone for the treatment of congenital fibrosarcoma. Is surgery always needed? Med Pediatr Oncol 2003; 40:268.

221. McCahon E, Sorensen PH, Davis JH, et al. Non-resectable congenital tumors with the ETV6-NTRK3 gene fusion are highly responsive to chemotherapy. Med Pediatr Oncol 2003; 40:288.

Inflammatory myofibroblastic tumor

222. Spencer H. The pulmonary plasma cell/histiocytoma complex. Histopathology 1984; 8:903.

223. Warter A, Satge D, Roeslin N. Angioinvasive plasma cell granulomas of the lung. Cancer 1987; 59:435.

224. Pisciotto PT, Gray GF Jr, Miller DR. Abdominal plasma cell pseudotumor. J Pediatr 1978; 93:628.

225. Tang TT, Segura AD, Oechler HW, et al. Inflammatory myofibrohistiocytic proliferation simulating sarcoma in children. Cancer 1990; 65:1626.

226. Gonzalez-Crussi F, deMello DE, Sotelo-Avila C. Omental-mesenteric myxoid hamartomas. Infantile lesions simulating malignant tumors. Am J Surg Pathol 1983; 7:567.

227. Ramachandra S, Hollowood K, Bisceglia M, et al. Inflammatory pseudotumour of soft tissues: a clinicopathological and

immunohistochemical analysis of 18 cases. Histopathology 1995; 27:313.

228. Chan JKC. Inflammatory pseudotumor: a family of lesions of diverse nature and etiologies. Adv Anat Pathol 1996; 3:156.

229. Umlas J, Federman M, Crawford C, et al. Spindle cell pseudotumor due to *Mycobacterium avium-intracellulare* in patients with acquired immunodeficiency syndrome (AIDS). Positive staining of mycobacteria for cytoskeleton filaments. Am J Surg Pathol 1991; 15:1181.

230. Shek TW, Ho FC, Ng IO, et al. Follicular dendritic cell tumor of the liver. Evidence for an Epstein-Barr virus-related clonal proliferation of follicular dendritic cells. Am J Surg Pathol 1996; 20:313.

231. Davis RE, Warnke RA, Dorfman RF. Inflammatory pseudotumor of lymph nodes. Additional observations and evidence for an inflammatory etiology. Am J Surg Pathol 1991; 15:744.

232. Coffin CM, Watterson J, Priest JR, et al. Extrapulmonary inflammatory myofibroblastic tumor (inflammatory pseudotumor). A clinicopathologic and immunohistochemical study of 84 cases. Am J Surg Pathol 1995; 19:859.

233. Souid AK, Ziemba MC, Dubansky AS, et al. Inflammatory myofibroblastic tumor in children. Cancer 1993; 72:2042.

234. Meis JM, Enzinger FM. Inflammatory fibrosarcoma of the mesentery and retroperitoneum. A tumor closely simulating inflammatory pseudotumor. Am J Surg Pathol 1991; 15:1146.

235. Mirra M, Falconieri G, Zanconati F, et al. Inflammatory fibrosarcoma: another imitator of Hodgkin's disease? Pathol Res Pract 1996; 192:474.

235a. Coffin CM, Hornick JL, Fletcher CDM. Inflammatory myofibroblastic tumor: comparison of clinicopathologic, histologic and immunohistochemical features including *ALK* expression in atypical and aggressive cases. Am J Surg Pathol 2007; 31:510.

236. Griffin CA, Hawkins AL, Dvorak C, et al. Recurrent involvement of 2p23 in inflammatory myofibroblastic tumors. Cancer Res 1999; 59:2776.

237. Su LD, Atayde-Perez A, Sheldon S, et al. Inflammatory myofibroblastic tumor: cytogenetic evidence supporting clonal origin. Mod Pathol 1998; 11:364.

238. Snyder CS, Dell'Aquila M, Haghighi P, et al. Clonal changes in inflammatory pseudotumor of the lung: A case report. Cancer 1995; 76:1545.

239. Treissman SP, Gillis DA, Lee CL, et al. Omental-mesenteric inflammatory pseudotumor. Cytogenetic demonstration of genetic changes and monoclonality in one tumor. Cancer 1994; 73:1433.

240. Yousem SA, Shaw H, Cieply K. Involvement of 2p23 in pulmonary inflammatory pseudotumors. Hum Pathol 2001; 32:428.

241. Lawrence B, Perez-Atayde A, Hibbard MK, et al. TPM3-ALK and TPM4-ALK oncogenes in inflammatory myofibroblastic tumors. Am J Pathol 2000; 157:377.

242. Bridge JA, Kanamori M, Ma Z, et al. Fusion of the ALK gene to the clathrin heavy chain gene, CLTC, in inflammatory myofibroblastic tumor. Am J Pathol 2001; 159:411.

243. Debelenko LV, Arthur DC, Pack SD, et al. Identification of CARS-ALK fusion in primary and metastatic lesions of an inflammatory myofibroblastic tumor. Lab Invest 2003; 83:1255.

244. Debiec-Rychter M, Marynen P, Hagemeijer A, et al. ALK-ATIC fusion in urinary bladder inflammatory myofibroblastic tumor. Genes Chromosomes Cancer 2003; 38:187.

245. Ma Z, Hill DA, Collins MH, et al. Fusion of ALK to the ran-binding protein 2 (RANBP2) gene in inflammatory myofibroblastic tumor. Genes Chromosomes Cancer 2003; 37:98.

246. Cessna MH, Zhou H, Sanger WG, et al. Expression of ALK1 and p80 in inflammatory myofibroblastic tumor and its mesenchymal mimics: a study of 135 cases. Mod Pathol 2002; 15:931.

247. Cook JR, Dehner LP, Collins MH, et al. Anaplastic lymphoma kinase (ALK) expression in the inflammatory myofibroblastic tumor: a comparative immunohistochemical study. Am J Surg Pathol 2001; 25:1364.

248. Chan JK, Cheuk W, Shimizu M. Anaplastic lymphoma kinase expression in inflammatory pseudotumors. Am J Surg Pathol 2001; 25:761.

249. Makhlouf HR, Sobin LH. Inflammatory myofibroblastic tumors (inflammatory pseudotumors) of the gastrointestinal tract: how closely are they related to inflammatory fibroid polyps? Hum Pathol 2002; 33:307.

250. Coffin CM, Dehner LP, Meis-Kindblom JM. Inflammatory myofibroblastic tumor, inflammatory fibrosarcoma, and related lesions: an historical review with differential diagnostic considerations. Semin Diagn Pathol 1998; 15:102.

251. Coffin CM, Humphrey PA, Dehner LP. Extrapulmonary inflammatory myofibroblastic tumor: a clinical and pathological survey. Semin Diagn Pathol 1998; 15:85.

252. Morotti RA, Legman MD, Kerkar N, et al. Pediatric inflammatory myofibroblastic tumor with late metastasis to the lung: case report and review of the literature. Pediatr Dev Pathol 2005; 8:224.

253. Hagenstad CT, Kilpatrick SE, Pettenati MJ, et al. Inflammatory myofibroblastic tumor with bone marrow involvement. A case report and review of the literature. Arch Pathol Lab Med 2003; 127:865.

254. Dishop MK, Warner BW, Dehner LP, et al. Successful treatment of inflammatory myofibroblastic tumor with malignant transformation by surgical resection and chemotherapy. J Pediatr Hematol Oncol 2003; 25:153.

255. Donner LR, Trompler RA, White RR 4th. Progression of inflammatory myofibroblastic tumor (inflammatory pseudotumor) of soft tissue into sarcoma after several recurrences. Hum Pathol 1996; 27:1095.

256. Chun YS, Wang L, Nascimento AG, et al. Pediatric inflammatory myofibroblastic tumor: anaplastic lymphoma kinase (ALK) expression and prognosis. Pediatr Blood Cancer 2005; 45:796.

257. Hussong JW, Brown M, Perkins SL, et al. Comparison of DNA ploidy, histologic, and immunohistochemical findings with clinical outcome in inflammatory myofibroblastic tumors. Mod Pathol 1999; 12:279.

258. Gasparotti R, Zanetti D, Bolzoni A, et al. Inflammatory myofibroblastic tumor of the temporal bone. AJNR Am J Neuroradiol 2003; 24:2092.

259. Ilvan S, Celik V, Paksoy M, et al. Inflammatory myofibroblastic tumor (inflammatory pseudotumor) of the breast. APMIS 2005; 113:66.

260. Jeon YK, Chang KH, Suh YL, et al. Inflammatory myofibroblastic tumor of the central nervous system: clinicopathologic analysis of 10 cases. J Neuropathol Exp Neurol 2005; 64:254.

261. SantaCruz KS, McKinley ET, Powell RD Jr, et al. Inflammatory myofibroblastic tumor of the gastroesophageal junction in childhood. Pediatr Pathol Mol Med 2002; 21:49.

262. Li L, Cerilli LA, Wick MR. Inflammatory pseudotumor (myofibroblastic tumor) of the heart. Ann Diagn Pathol 2002; 6:116.

263. Dasgupta D, Guthrie A, McClean P, et al. Liver transplantation for a hilar inflammatory myofibroblastic tumor. Pediatr Transplant 2004; 8:517.

264. Kapusta LR, Weiss MA, Ramsay J, et al. Inflammatory myofibroblastic tumors of the kidney: a clinicopathologic and immunohistochemical study of 12 cases. Am J Surg Pathol 2003; 27:658.

265. Rodrigues M, Taylor RJ, Sun CC, et al. Inflammatory myofibroblastic tumor of the larynx in a 2-year-old male. ORL J Otorhinolaryngol Relat Spec 2005; 67:101.

266. Makimoto Y, Nabeshima K, Iwasaki H, et al. Inflammatory myofibroblastic tumor of the posterior mediastinum: an older adult case with anaplastic lymphoma kinase abnormalities determined using immunohistochemistry and fluorescence in situ hybridization. Virchows Arch 2005; 446:451.

267. Corapcioglu F, Kargi A, Olgun N, et al. Inflammatory myofibroblastic tumor of the ileocecal mesentery mimicking abdominal lymphoma in childhood: report of two cases. Surg Today 2005; 35:687.

268. Fang JC, Dym H. Myofibroblastic tumor of the oral cavity. A rare clinical entity. NY State Dent J 2004; 70:28.

269. O'Malley DP, Poulos C, Czader M, et al. Intraocular inflammatory myofibroblastic tumor with ALK overexpression. Arch Pathol Lab Med 2004; 128:e5.

270. Pungpapong S, Geiger XJ, Raimondo M. Inflammatory myofibroblastic tumor presenting as a pancreatic mass: a case report and review of the literature. J Pathol 2004; 5:360.

271. Kapur P, Treat K, Chuang AT, et al. Pathologic quiz case: paratesticular mass in a young man. Inflammatory myofibroblastic tumor of the paratestis. Arch Pathol Lab Med 2004; 128:589.

272. Van Weert S, Manni JJ, Driessen A. Inflammatory myofibroblastic tumor of the parotid gland: case report and review of the literature. Acta Otolaryngol (Stockh) 2005; 125:433.

273. Karakok M, Ozer E, Sari I, et al. Inflammatory myofibroblastic tumor (inflammatory pseudotumor) of the maxillary sinus mimicking malignancy: a case report of an unusual location (is that a true neoplasm?). Auris Nasus Larynx 2002; 29:383.

274. Lacoste-Collin L, Roux FE, Gomez-Brouchet A, et al. Inflammatory myofibroblastic tumor: a spinal case with aggressive clinical course and ALK overexpression. Case report. J Neurosurg 2003; 98:218.

275. Mosunjac MB, Feliciano DV, Majmudar B. Pathologic quiz case: a mass of the spleen. Inflammatory myofibroblastic tumor of the spleen. Arch Pathol Lab Med 2001; 125:1607.

276. Browne M, Abramson LP, Chou PM, et al. Inflammatory myofibroblastic tumor (inflammatory pseudotumor) of the neck infiltrating the trachea. J Pediatr Surg 2004; 39:e1.

277. Nascimento AF, Dal Cin P, Cilento BG, et al. Urachal inflammatory myofibroblastic tumor with ALK gene rearrangement: a study of urachal remnants. Urology 2004; 64:140.

278. Rabban JT, Zaloudek CJ, Shekitka KM, et al. Inflammatory myofibroblastic tumor of the uterus: a clinicopathologic study of 6 cases emphasizing distinction from aggressive mesenchymal tumors. Am J Surg Pathol 2005; 29:1348.

Calcifying aponeurotic fibroma

279. Keasbey LE. Juvenile aponeurotic fibroma (calcifying fibroma): a distinctive tumor

arising in the palms and soles of young children. Cancer 1953; 6:338.

280. Sferopoulos NK, Kotakidou R. Calcifying aponeurotic fibroma: a report of three cases. Acta Orthop Belg 2001; 67:412.

281. Keasbey LE, Fanselau HA. The aponeurotic fibroma. Clin Orthop 1961; 19:115.

282. Iwasaki H, Enjoji M. Calcifying aponeurotic fibroma. Fukuoka Acta Med 1973; 64:52.

283. Allen PW, Enzinger FM. Juvenile aponeurotic fibroma. Cancer 1970; 26:857.

284. Adeyemi-Doro HO, Olude O. Juvenile aponeurotic fibroma. J Hand Surg [Br] 1985; 10:127.

285. Fetsch JF, Miettinen M. Calcifying aponeurotic fibroma: a clinicopathologic study of 22 cases arising in uncommon sites. Hum Pathol 1998; 29:1504.

286. Murphy BA, Kilpatrick SE, Panella MJ, et al. Extra-acral calcifying aponeurotic fibroma: a distinctive case with 23-year follow-up. J Cutan Pathol 1996; 23:369.

287. Sharma R, Punia RS, Sharma A, et al. Juvenile (calcifying) aponeurotic fibroma of the neck. Pediatr Surg Int 1998; 13:295.

288. Kwak HS, Lee SY, Kim JR, et al. MR imaging of calcifying aponeurotic fibroma of the thigh. Pediatr Radiol 2004; 34:438.

289. Iwasaki H, Kikuchi M, Eimoto T, et al. Juvenile aponeurotic fibroma: An ultrastructural study. Ultrastruct Pathol 4:75, 1983.

290. Amaravati R. Rare malignant transformation of a calcifying aponeurotic fibroma. J Bone Joint Surg [Am] 2002; 84:1889.

291. Lafferty KA, Nelson EL, Demuth RJ, et al. Juvenile aponeurotic fibroma with disseminated fibrosarcoma. J Hand Surg [Am] 1986; 11:737.

Congenital and acquired muscular fibrosis

292. Hnevkovsky O. Progressive fibrosis of the vastus intermedius muscle in children. J Bone Joint Surg [Br] 1961; 43:318.

293. Mukherjee PK, Das AK. Injection fibrosis in the quadriceps femoris muscle in children. J Bone Joint Surg [Am] 1980; 62:453.

294. Peiro A, Fernandez CI, Gomar F. Gluteal fibrosis. J Bone Joint Surg [Am] 1975; 57:987.

295. Goodfellow JW, Nade S. Flexion contracture of the shoulder joint from fibrosis of the anterior part of the deltoid muscle. J Bone Joint Surg [Br] 1969; 51:356.

296. Varma BP, Chandra U. Bilateral ankylosis of the elbows in extension due to contracture of the triceps. A case report. Int Surg 1969; 52:337.

297. Matsusue Y, Yamamuro T, Ohta H, et al. Fibrotic contracture of the gastrocnemius muscle. A case report. J Bone Joint Surg [Am] 1994; 76:739.

298. Napiontek M, Ruszkowski K. Paralytic drop foot and gluteal fibrosis after intramuscular injections. J Bone Joint Surg [Br] 1993; 75:83.

299. Groves RJ, Goldner JL. Contracture of the deltoid muscle in the adult after intramuscular injections. J Bone Joint Surg [Am] 1974; 56:817.

300. Lloyd-Roberts GC, Thomas TG. The etiology of quadriceps contracture in children. J Bone Joint Surg [Br] 1964; 46:498.

301. Gunn DR. Contracture of the quadriceps muscle: a discussion on the etiology and relationship to recurrent dislocation of the patella. J Bone Joint Surg [Br] 1964; 46:492.

302. Shen YS. Abduction contracture of the hip in children. J Bone Joint Surg [Br] 1975; 57:463.

303. Chiu SS, Furuya K, Arai T, et al. Congenital contracture of the quadriceps muscle. Four case reports in identical twins. J Bone Joint Surg [Am] 1974; 56:1054.

304. Fairbank TJ, Barrett AM. Vastus intermedius contracture in early childhood: case report in identical twins. J Bone Joint Surg [Br] 1961; 43:326.

Cerebriform fibrous proliferation (Proteus syndrome)

305. Smeets E, Fryns JP, Cohen MM Jr. Regional Proteus syndrome and somatic mosaicism. Am J Med Genet 1994; 51:29.

306. Cohen MM Jr, Hayden PW. A newly recognized hamartomatous syndrome. Birth Defects Orig Artic Ser 1979; 15:291.

307. Wiedemann HR, Burgio GR, Aldenhoff P, et al. The Proteus syndrome. Partial gigantism of the hands and/or feet, nevi, hemihypertrophy, subcutaneous tumors, macrocephaly or other skull anomalies and possible accelerated growth and visceral affections. Eur J Pediatr 1983; 140:5.

308. Tibbles JA, Cohen MM Jr. The Proteus syndrome: the elephant man diagnosed. Br Med J (Clin Res Ed) 1986; 293:683.

309. Turner JT, Cohen MM Jr, Biesecker LG. Reassessment of the Proteus syndrome literature: application of diagnostic criteria to published cases. Am J Med Genet A 2004; 130:111.

310. Biesecker LG, Happle R, Mulliken JB, et al. Proteus syndrome: diagnostic criteria, differential diagnosis, and patient evaluation. Am J Med Genet 1999; 84:389.

311. Adolphs N, Tinschert S, Bier J, et al. Craniofacial hyperostoses in Proteus syndrome – a case report. J Craniomaxillofac Surg 2004; 32:391.

312. White NJ, Cochrane DD, Beauchamp R. Paraparesis caused by an angiolipomatous hamartoma in an adolescent with Proteus syndrome and scoliosis. J Neurosurg 2005; 103:282.

313. Cohen MM Jr. Proteus syndrome: an update. Am J Med Genet C Semin Med Genet 2005; 137:38.

314. Nguyen D, Turner JT, Olsen C, et al. Cutaneous manifestations of Proteus syndrome: correlations with general clinical severity. Arch Dermatol 2004; 140:947.

315. Uitto J, Bauer EA, Santa Cruz DJ, et al. Decreased collagenase production by regional fibroblasts cultured from skin of a patient with connective tissue nevi of the collagen type. J Invest Dermatol 1982; 78:136.

316. Loffeld A, McLellan NJ, Cole T, et al. Epidermal naevus in Proteus syndrome showing loss of heterozygosity for an inherited PTEN mutation. Br J Dermatol 2006; 154:1194.

317. Smith JM, Kirk EP, Theodosopoulos G, et al. Germline mutation of the tumour suppressor PTEN in Proteus syndrome. J Med Genet 2002; 39:937.

Calcifying fibrous pseudotumor

318. Rosenthal NS, Abdul-Karim FW. Childhood fibrous tumor with psammoma bodies. Clinicopathologic features in two cases. Arch Pathol Lab Med 1988; 112:798.

319. Fetsch JF, Montgomery EA, Meis JM. Calcifying fibrous pseudotumor. Am J Surg Pathol 1993; 17:502.

320. Nascimento AF, Ruiz R, Hornick JL, et al. Calcifying fibrous 'pseudotumor': clinicopathologic study of 15 cases and analysis of its relationship to inflammatory myofibroblastic tumor. Int J Surg Pathol 2002; 10:189.

321. Ben-Izhak O, Itin L, Feuchtwanger Z, et al. Calcifying fibrous pseudotumor of mesentery presenting with acute peritonitis: case report with immunohistochemical study and review of literature. Int J Surg Pathol 2001; 9:249.

322. Dumont P, de Muret A, Skrobala D, et al. Calcifying fibrous pseudotumor of the mediastinum. Ann Thorac Surg 1997; 63:543.

323. Chon SH, Lee CB, Oh YH. Calcifying fibrous pseudotumor causing thoracic outlet syndrome. Eur J Cardiothorac Surg 2005; 27:353.

324. Jang KS, Oh YH, Han HX, et al. Calcifying fibrous pseudotumor of the pleura. Ann Thorac Surg 2004; 78:e87.

325. Ammar A, El Hammami S, Horchani H, et al. Calcifying fibrous pseudotumor of the pleura: a rare location. Ann Thorac Surg 2003; 76:2081.

326. Konstantakos AK, Shuck JM. Calcifying fibrous pseudotumor of the anterior parietal peritoneum: treatment by laparoscopic resection. Surgery 2005; 137:257.

327. Hill KA, Gonzalez-Crussi F, Omeroglu A, et al. Calcifying fibrous pseudotumor involving the neck of a five-week-old infant. Presence of factor XIIIa in the lesional cells. Pathol Res Pract 2000; 196:527.

328. Sigel JE, Smith TA, Reith JD, et al. Immunohistochemical analysis of anaplastic lymphoma kinase expression in deep soft tissue calcifying fibrous pseudotumor: evidence of a late sclerosing stage of inflammatory myofibroblastic tumor? Ann Diagn Pathol 2001; 5:10.

329. Van Dorpe J, Ectors N, Geboes K, et al. Is calcifying fibrous pseudotumor a late sclerosing stage of inflammatory myofibroblastic tumor? Am J Surg Pathol 1999; 23:329.

330. Jimenez-Heffernan JA, Urbano J, Tobio R, et al. Calcifying fibrous pseudotumor: a rare entity related to inflammatory pseudotumor. Acta Cytol 2000; 44:932.

331. Yantiss RK, Nielsen GP, Lauwers GY, et al. Reactive nodular fibrous pseudotumor of the gastrointestinal tract and mesentery: a clinicopathologic study of five cases. Am J Surg Pathol 2003; 27:532.

332. Maeda T, Hirose T, Furuya K, et al. Calcifying fibrous pseudotumor: an ultrastructural study. Ultrastruct Pathol 1999; 23:189.

FIBROSARCOMA

Definitionally, the cells of fibrosarcoma recapitulate the appearance of the normal fibroblast. This admittedly broad definition has resulted in a great deal of subjectivity as to which spindle cell, collagen-forming tumors were appropriately termed fibrosarcoma and which were better classified as another form of sarcoma. Depending on the era and the criteria in vogue at that time, the incidence and behavior of this neoplasm have varied greatly. This trend is well illustrated by a series of studies from the Mayo Clinic over a period of 50 years. In 1936 Meyerding et al.[1] reported that 65% of soft tissue sarcomas were fibrosarcoma, a figure revised to 12% in 1974 by Pritchard et al.[2] and to even less by Scott et al. in 1989.[3]

On closer scrutiny, several factors are probably responsible for the apparent decline in the incidence of fibrosarcoma. The categorization by many pathologists of high-grade, pleomorphic spindle cell tumors with fibroblastic and myofibroblastic differentiation as "malignant fibrous histiocytoma," as opposed to fibrosarcoma, certainly has contributed to this trend. Second, refinement of histologic criteria resulted in the segregation of fibromatosis (desmoid tumors) as a unique group of tumors distinct from fibrosarcoma. Lastly, with the advent of immunohistochemistry, cytogenetics and, more recently, molecular genetic techniques, it became possible to more reproducibly recognize monophasic fibrous synovial sar-

comas and malignant peripheral nerve sheath tumors, which were probably frequently misclassified as fibrosarcomas. Despite significant progress in this area, the differential diagnosis of spindle cell tumors remains a difficult, challenging, and sometimes unsolvable problem, especially when only a small biopsy specimen is available for microscopic examination.

As a result of the foregoing trends, a number of general statements can be made concerning the diagnosis of fibrosarcoma:

1. Fibrosarcoma has become, in large part, a diagnosis of exclusion. It presupposes that diagnoses such as monophasic fibrous synovial sarcoma and malignant peripheral nerve sheath tumor have been excluded by the appropriate immunohistochemical, ultrastructural, or cytogenetic/molecular genetic studies.
2. Fibrosarcomas, like other fibroblastic tumors (e.g., fibromatosis), may have a variable component of neoplastic cells with features of myofibroblasts. Therefore, the finding of various actin isoforms within these tumors does not mitigate against the diagnosis of fibrosarcoma. On the other hand, there are some spindle cell sarcomas that are composed predominantly of cells with myofibroblastic differentiation, and the entity of "myofibrosarcoma" has become increasingly accepted.
3. Collagen-forming, spindle cell tumors of high nuclear grade showing fibroblastic differentiation are, by convention, classified as pleomorphic undifferentiated sarcomas (malignant fibrous histiocytoma; see Chapter 14). Consequently, lesions diagnosed as fibrosarcoma, for the most part, occupy the low-grade end (grades 1 and 2) of a spectrum that includes pleomorphic undifferentiated sarcoma/malignant fibrous histiocytoma at the high-grade end. However, there are rare examples of high-grade fibrosarcoma that have histologic features distinct from pleomorphic undifferentiated sarcoma.

Despite the fact that the incidence of fibrosarcoma has markedly decreased in recent years, there have been renewed efforts to identify unique subsets or variants within this group of lesions. Although it is still not clear

TABLE 11-1	CLASSIFICATION OF FIBROSARCOMA

Adult-type fibrosarcoma
  Classic type
  Myxoid type (myxofibrosarcoma; low-grade myxoid MFH)
  Fibromyxoid type (low-grade fibromyxoid sarcoma/hyalinizing
    spindle cell tumor with giant rosettes)
  Sclerosing epithelioid type

Juvenile/infantile fibrosarcoma

TABLE 11-2	ANATOMIC LOCATIONS OF FIBROSARCOMA		
Anatomic location		**No. patients**	**%**
Lower extremities		313	45
Upper extremities		195	28
Trunk		118	17
Head, neck		69	10
Total		695	100

Data are from the Armed Forces Institute of Pathology.

to what extent these variants are biologically different from one another, they certainly have distinct histologic features that allow their identification in a more or less consistent fashion. These variants include myxoid fibrosarcoma (myxofibrosarcoma), low-grade fibromyxoid sarcoma/hyalinizing spindle cell tumor with giant rosettes, and sclerosing epithelioid fibrosarcoma, all of which are discussed in this chapter (Table 11–1). Congenital/infantile-type fibrosarcoma and inflammatory myofibroblastic tumor ("inflammatory fibrosarcoma") are discussed in Chapter 10, given their distinctive clinical and genetic features. This chapter will also include a discussion of those sarcomas that are composed predominantly of myofibroblasts (myofibrosarcoma), an entity that has only begun to gain acceptance over the past 5 years.

CLINICAL FINDINGS

Like most other sarcomas, fibrosarcoma causes no characteristic symptoms and is difficult to diagnose clinically. Most patients present with a solitary palpable mass ranging from 3 to 8 cm in greatest dimension. It is slowly growing and usually painless; pain is encountered more commonly with synovial sarcoma and malignant peripheral nerve sheath tumor than with fibrosarcoma.

The skin overlying the tumor is generally intact, although more superficially located neoplasms that grow rapidly or have been traumatized may result in ulceration of the skin. Such tumors, particularly when clinically neglected, may form large fungating masses in the areas of ulceration. The preoperative duration of symptoms varies greatly and ranges from as little as a few weeks to as long as 20 years, although the average preoperative duration is 3 years. Fibrosarcoma may occur at any age but is most common in the third through fifth decades of life. Most studies have reported a slightly higher incidence of the tumor in men than in women. For instance, Scott and co-workers noted that 61% of the 132 patients with fibrosarcoma were men.[3]

The tumor may occur in any soft tissue site but is most common in the deep soft tissues of the lower extremities, particularly the thigh and knee, followed by the upper extremities and trunk (Table 11–2). There are numerous reports of fibrosarcoma in the head and neck, including the nasal cavity, paranasal sinuses, and nasopharynx.[4–8]

Rare examples of this tumor have been reported in virtually every anatomic site including the breast,[9] thyroid,[10] heart,[11] liver,[12] and central nervous system.[13]

Fibrosarcoma predominantly involves deep structures, where it tends to originate from the intramuscular and intermuscular fibrous tissue, fascial envelopes, aponeuroses, and tendons. Deeply situated tumors may even encircle bone and cause radiographically demonstrable periosteal and cortical thickening; in such cases distinction from parosteal osteosarcoma may be difficult. Other radiographic findings, in addition to a soft tissue mass, include occasional foci of calcification and ossification, although this feature is much more common with synovial sarcoma than fibrosarcoma. Fibrosarcomas arising from the subcutis, excluding those that arise in dermatofibrosarcoma protuberans, are rare and tend to originate in tissues damaged by radiation, heat, or scarring (described later in this chapter).

Most patients lack systemic manifestations except weight loss in those with tumors of large size and long duration and in cases where tumors have metastasized widely. Hypoglycemia, presumably due to the production of insulin-like substances secreted from the tumor, has been reported.[14,15]

GROSS FINDINGS

Generally, the excised tumor consists of a solitary, soft to firm, fleshy, rounded or lobulated mass that is gray-white to tan-yellow and measures 3–8 cm in greatest dimension. Small tumors tend to be well circumscribed and frequently are partly or completely encapsulated. Large tumors are less well defined; they often extend with multiple processes into the surrounding tissues or grow in a diffusely invasive or destructive manner. The frequent circumscription of small fibrosarcomas can be misleading and may result in an erroneous diagnosis of a benign tumor and inadequate surgical therapy.

MICROSCOPIC FINDINGS

Although there are minor variations in the histologic picture, most fibrosarcomas have in common a rather uniform fasciculated growth pattern consisting of fusiform or spindle-shaped cells that vary little in size and shape, have scanty cytoplasm with indistinct cell borders, and are separated by interwoven collagen fibers arranged in a parallel fashion. Mitotic activity varies, but caution should be exercised when diagnosing fibrosarcoma in the absence of mitotic figures. Multinucleated giant cells or giant cells of bizarre size and shape are rarely a feature of this tumor.

Histologic grading of fibrosarcomas is based on the cellularity and differentiation, mitotic activity, and necrosis. *Low-grade fibrosarcomas* are characterized by a uniform, orderly appearance of the spindle cells associated with abundant collagen (Figs 11–1 to 11–4). In some cases the cells are oriented in curving or interlacing fascicles, forming a classic herringbone pattern. In others, the cells are separated by thick, wire-like collagen fibers. Secondary features are common. Low-grade fibrosarcomas may show focal chondro-osseous differentiation. Some tumors have areas that are less cellular or extensively myxoid (Fig. 11–5) and closely mimic portions of fibromatosis, thereby making distinction of these two lesions difficult in some cases, particularly when only a small sample is available for evaluation.

High-grade fibrosarcomas are characterized by closely packed, less well-oriented tumor cells that are small, ovoid or rounded, and associated with less collagen (Fig. 11–6). The fascicular or herringbone growth pattern is less distinct, the nuclei are more pleomorphic, mitotic figures are more numerous, and there are areas of necrosis and/or hemorrhage.

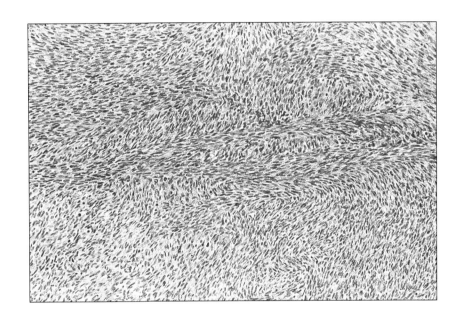

FIGURE 11–1 Low-power view of a fibrosarcoma exhibiting a distinct fascicular (herringbone) pattern.

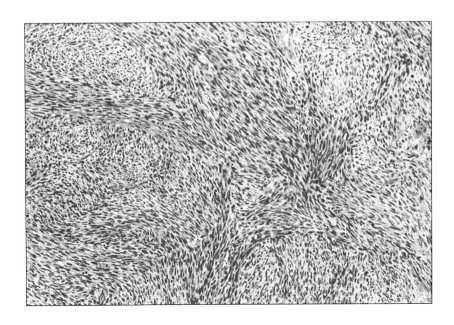

FIGURE 11–2 Fibrosarcoma consisting of uniform spindle cells showing little variation in size and shape and a distinct fascicular pattern.

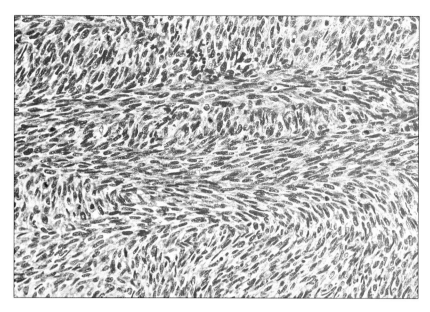

FIGURE 11-3 Fibrosarcoma showing arrangement of the fibroblasts in distinct intersecting fascicles (herringbone pattern).

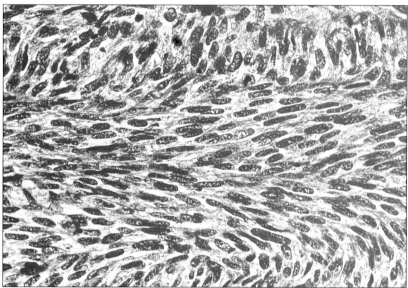

FIGURE 11-4 High-power view of fibrosarcoma showing uniformity of the tumor cells and the characteristic fascicular pattern.

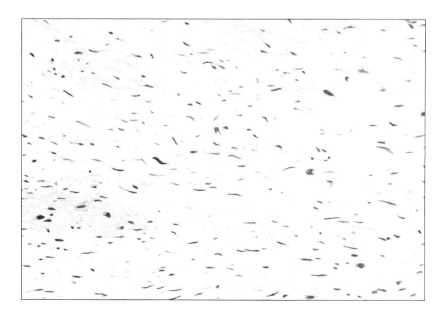

FIGURE 11-5 Fibrosarcoma with extensive myxoid change. The fibroblasts are widely separated by abundant myxoid stroma, making the fascicular pattern less conspicuous.

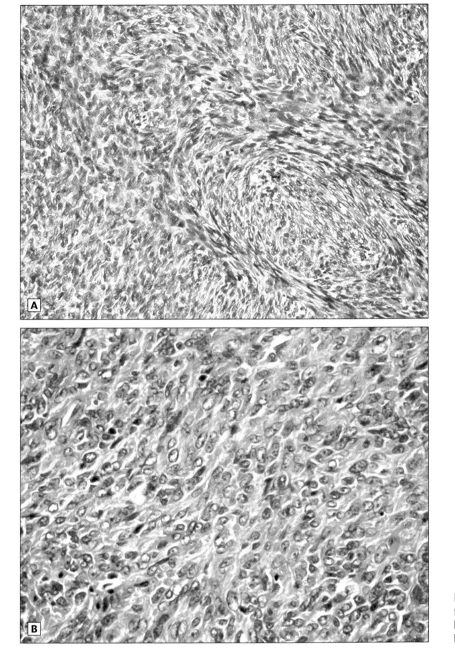

FIGURE 11–6 (A,B) High-grade fibrosarcoma characterized by closely packed, less well-oriented, rounded tumor cells with high-grade nuclear features.

IMMUNOHISTOCHEMICAL AND ULTRASTRUCTURAL FINDINGS

Fibrosarcomas express vimentin, but they do not exhibit any other lineage-specific markers such as keratin or S-100 protein. The lack of cytokeratin immunoreactivity aids in distinction from monophasic fibrous synovial sarcoma. Negative immunostaining for S-100 protein distinguishes fibrosarcoma from spindle cell or desmoplastic malignant melanomas but not necessarily from malignant peripheral nerve sheath tumors, as only 50–60% of the latter stain focally for this antigen. In some fibrosarcomas, scattered cells stain for smooth muscle or muscle-specific actin, reflecting focal myofibroblastic differentiation.

As might be anticipated from the light microscopic features, the tumors are largely composed of elongated fibroblastic cells with irregularly outlined or indented nuclei, infrequent nucleoli, and prominent rough endoplasmic reticulum that is often dilated and contains granular or amorphous material. Some cells contain, in addition, intracytoplasmic bundles of microfilaments measuring up to 60 nm in diameter, focal condensations or dense bodies, and sometimes basal lamina material, features characteristic of myofibroblasts.[16] Suh et al. studied the ultrastructural features of 60 fibrosarcomas and found myofibroblastic differentiation in scattered cells in 33 of the tumors.[17]

DIFFERENTIAL DIAGNOSIS

It is often difficult to distinguish fibrosarcoma from other spindle cell tumors, and in many instances only careful examination of multiple sections and ancillary studies permit a correct diagnosis. *Benign processes* likely to be mistaken for fibrosarcoma range from nodular fasciitis to cellular benign fibrous histiocytoma and fibromatosis. *Malignant neoplasms* considered in the differential diagnosis are much more numerous and include most commonly malignant peripheral nerve sheath tumor, malignant fibrous histiocytoma, and monophasic fibrous synovial sarcoma. Other tumors that tend to simulate fibrosarcoma include sarcomatoid mesothelioma, clear cell sarcoma, epithelioid sarcoma, dermatofibrosarcoma protuberans, desmoplastic leiomyosarcoma, spindle cell forms of rhabdomyosarcoma, malignant melanoma, and spindle cell carcinoma. Because the differential diagnosis of most of these tumors is discussed elsewhere, the following comments are limited to lesions most frequently confused with fibrosarcoma.

Nodular fasciitis, a pseudosarcomatous reactive myofibroblastic proliferation that grows rapidly and is marked by its cellularity and immature cellular appearance, differs from fibrosarcoma by its smaller size and microscopically by its more irregular growth pattern; characteristically, its cells are arranged in short bundles – never in long, sweeping fascicles or a herringbone pattern as in fibrosarcoma. The cells lack nuclear hyperchromasia, and there is usually a prominent myxoid matrix and scattered chronic inflammatory cells.

Cellular benign fibrous histiocytoma may be difficult to distinguish from fibrosarcoma since this lesion is characteristically cellular and often forms fascicles. However, the fascicles are usually not as regular or sweeping as those seen in fibrosarcoma. Areas of more conventional benign fibrous histiocytoma may be present and are extremely useful in this distinction. In most cases, cellular benign fibrous histiocytoma is situated in the dermis or subcutis; unlike fibrosarcoma, it is rarely found in deep soft tissue structures. Mitotic figures are present in cellular benign fibrous histiocytoma, but the presence of atypical mitotic figures lends strong support to a diagnosis of malignancy. The cells also characteristically express factor XIIIa antigen.

Musculoaponeurotic fibromatosis (desmoid tumor) has a growth pattern similar to that of fibrosarcoma but is less cellular and contains more collagen. The cells are uniformly spindled, with delicate chromatin and one or two minute nucleoli. In general, the cells do not touch one another but, rather, are separated by collagen, whereas the cells of fibrosarcoma frequently overlap with closely spaced hyperchromatic nuclei. Low levels of mitotic activity may be present in fibromatosis such that considerable overlap in mitotic activity between fibromatosis and fibrosarcoma may be encountered (Table 11–3). Thus, mitotic activity is not a reliable discriminant between fibromatosis and fibrosarcoma when dealing with low levels of mitotic activity (<50/50 high-power fields [HPF]) but might become useful when higher levels of mitotic activity (>50/50 HPF) are present. Because fibromatosis-like areas may be present in low-grade fibrosarcoma, careful sampling of the tumor is mandatory. Clinical considerations are of little help for distinguishing these tumors because they may occur at the same location and in patients of similar age.

Pleomorphic undifferentiated sarcoma (malignant fibrous histiocytoma) has been included in many of the earlier reports of poorly differentiated or pleomorphic fibrosarcomas. Clinically, these tumors principally arise in elderly persons, with a peak during the seventh decade; microscopically, they are characterized by a storiform to haphazard growth pattern and the presence of multinucleated bizarre giant cells, often with eosinophilic cytoplasm and containing delicate droplets of lipid material. Siderophages and xanthoma cells are also common features that assist in the diagnosis. Transitions between fibrosarcoma and pleomorphic undifferentiated sarcoma do occur, suggesting a form of tumor progression in some cases. Admittedly, where one draws the line between a high-grade fibrosarcoma and a pleomorphic undifferentiated sarcoma is, at times, quite subjective.

TABLE 11–3	COMPARISON OF HISTOLOGIC FEATURES OF LOW-GRADE FIBROSARCOMA AND FIBROMATOSIS	
Parameter	**Low-grade fibrosarcoma**	**Fibromatosis**
Cellularity	Low to moderate	Low to moderate
Nuclear overlap	Present	Usually absent
Nuclear hyperchromasia	Present	Absent
Nucleoli	More prominent	Inconspicuous
Mitotic figures	1+ to 3+	1+
Necrosis	Rare	Absent
Vessel wall infiltration	Rare	Absent

Malignant peripheral nerve sheath tumor (MPNST) may display areas that are virtually indistinguishable from fibrosarcoma. However, by definition, some evidence of nerve sheath differentiation must be evident to support the diagnosis of MPNST. For example, cells showing neural differentiation often have a wavy or buckled appearance, rather than the finely tapered fibroblasts of fibrosarcoma. Although the cells can be arranged into an irregular fascicular growth pattern, the long, sweeping fascicles characteristic of fibrosarcoma are usually not present. Moreover, the cells of MPNST tend to show perivascular cuffing and may be arranged in distinct whorls or palisades. At low magnification, MPNST often shows a "marbled" appearance with alternating myxoid and cellular zones. In addition, MPNST may show transitions between malignant and benign neurofibroma-like areas. The finding of S-100 protein in scattered tumor cells supports a diagnosis of MPNST, although up to 50% of cases do not stain for this antigen, and S-100 protein staining is not specific for MPNST.

Monophasic fibrous synovial sarcoma may also closely simulate a fibrosarcoma, although it is generally composed of more ovoid-appearing cells arranged in an irregular fascicular growth pattern. Moreover, many of these sarcomas have areas in which the cells contain more eosinophilic cytoplasm with a suggestion of cellular cohesion, even if well-formed glands are not present. Immunohistochemically, almost all cases of synovial sarcoma express at least one epithelial marker, a feature not found in fibrosarcoma. The identification of t(X;18) by fluorescence in situ hybridization (FISH) or reverse transcriptase-polymerase chain reaction (RT-PCR) is a highly sensitive and specific method for identifying a tumor as a synovial sarcoma. In essence, fibrosarcoma is a diagnosis of exclusion.

CLINICAL BEHAVIOR

It is difficult to compare the results of published studies, as many of the tumors included in older series probably represent entities other than fibrosarcoma. Few studies have utilized immunohistochemistry and/or molecular genetics to exclude other lesions in the differential diagnosis. As such, the rate of local recurrence varies significantly among studies. For example, Mackenzie noted a recurrence in 93 (49%) of 190 cases[18] and Pritchard et al. in 113 (57%) of 199 cases.[2] In the study by Scott and co-workers, the overall rate of recurrence was 42% at 5 years.[3] In that study, although neither tumor grade nor tumor stage was associated with an increased risk of local recurrence, the status of the surgical margins was strongly predictive; the 5-year cumulative probability of local recurrence was 79% in tumors with inadequate surgical margins and 18% in tumors treated by wide or radical excision.

Metastasis of fibrosarcoma occurs almost exclusively by way of the bloodstream. The lung is the principal metastatic site, followed by the skeleton, especially the vertebrae and skull. Most metastases are noted within the first 2 years after diagnosis, although some patients, particularly those with low-grade fibrosarcomas, develop metastasis late in their course. Lymph node metastasis is rare, occurring in less than 8% of cases;[2] the relative incidence is, of course, influenced by the number of autopsy cases in the reported material because lymph nodes tend to be involved in the terminal phase of the disease. As such, regional lymph node excision is not a necessary part of the initial therapeutic regimen.

The rate of metastasis varies widely among studies. Scott et al. found 1-, 2-, and 5-year metastasis rates to be 34%, 52%, and 63%, respectively.[3] Using a four-grade classification scheme, these authors noted an increased risk of metastasis with increasing tumor grade. Patients with grade 1 or 2 tumors had a 5-year metastasis rate of 43% compared to 82% for those patients with grade 4 tumors.

Survival rates also vary considerably, especially in earlier descriptions of the tumor. More recent reports suggest a 5-year survival rate near 40%.[3] These data differ considerably from those of Castro et al.,[19] who reported a 5-year survival rate of 70% and a 10-year rate of 60%. In the latter series, however, it is not clear whether fibromatoses were included as grade 1 fibrosarcomas.

Most studies have found a significant relation between tumor grade and survival. This point was clearly established as early as 1939 by Broders et al.,[20] who demonstrated close parallels between prognosis and histologic features. Mackenzie, employing a three-grade classification, reported 5-year survival rates of 82.2% for grade 1, 55.0% for grade 2, and 35.5% for grade 3 tumors.[18] Scott et al., using a four-grade classification, noted 58% survival for grades 1 or 2, 34% for grade 3, and 21% for grade 4.[3] It is evident from these data that prognosis is least favorable with tumors that are richly cellular, have more than two mitotic figures per high-power field, contain little collagen, and show evidence of necrosis.

A second and equally important factor when determining prognosis is the adequacy of the initial excision. Bizer reported a 5-year survival rate of 30% for patients treated by local excision and 78% for those treated by radical excision.[21] Likewise, Scott et al. found a 29% 5-year survival rate for the group treated with inadequate margins and a 40% rate for those treated with adequate margins.[3] In the latter series the incidence of recurrence was even more closely related to the extent of surgery, as those with positive margins were more than four times as likely to develop a recurrence than those treated with wide margins. There was no clear relation between the extent of surgery and metastasis.

DISCUSSION

Little is known about the cytogenetic and molecular genetic alterations in fibrosarcoma. In contrast to congenital/infantile fibrosarcoma, adult fibrosarcoma does not appear to have a characteristic cytogenetic abnormality, although multiple complex chromosomal rearrangements have been reported.[22,23] Limon et al. reported a nonrandom chromosomal change involving t(2;19) with involvement of 2q21-qter.[23]

Considering the prominent role of fibroblasts in post-traumatic repair, it is not surprising that trauma has been implicated repeatedly as a possible and even likely causative factor.[24] Stout, for example, reported 36 cases of fibrosarcoma arising in scar tissue (*cicatricial fibrosarcoma*) or at the site of a former injury.[25] One patient had suffered an injury at age 9 years and developed a fibrosarcoma in the scar at age 35. Ivins et al.[26] noted a history of preceding trauma in 19 of 78 cases of fibrosarcoma but concluded that "only in one an etiologic significance was remotely possible." Fibrosarcoma has also been reported to arise in a draining sinus of long duration.[27] Evaluation of the significance of these cases is difficult. In some of them trauma may be a contributing factor, whereas in others trauma may merely serve to alert the patient or the physician to the presence of the disease and may be an incidental finding rather than a tumor-provoking factor.

Factors other than trauma have also been implicated to induce or contribute to the development of fibrosarcoma. Burns et al. reported a tumor arising in a 31-year-old man 10 years after a plastic Teflon-Dacron prosthetic vascular graft was placed for a lacerated femoral artery;[28] a similar case was described by O'Connell et al.[29] Eckstein et al.[30] reported a fibrosarcoma that arose in the vicinity of a total knee joint prosthesis.

FIBROSARCOMA VARIANTS

Fibrosarcoma, sclerosing epithelioid type

Sclerosing epithelioid fibrosarcoma is an unusual but distinctive variant of fibrosarcoma composed of epithelioid cells arranged in nests and cords and deposited in a densely hyalinized collagenous matrix. Since the initial description of this tumor by Meis-Kindblom and colleagues in 1995,[31] relatively few reports of this neoplasm have appeared in the literature.

Clinical findings

Most patients present with a deep-seated mass that is painful in up to one-third of cases. The age range is wide, with a median age of approximately 45 years; there does not seem to be any striking gender predilection.[31,32] The most common location is the deep soft tissues of the lower extremity or limb girdle followed by the trunk, upper extremities and limb girdle, and head and neck region.[31–33] Other unusual locations include the ovary,[34] retroperitoneum,[35] pelvis,[36] neuraxis,[37] and bone.[38,39]

Pathologic findings

Grossly, the tumor is usually well circumscribed and lobulated, bosselated, or multinodular; most are 5–10 cm in greatest diameter. Occasional tumors show cystic or myxoid change, and some have a gritty sensation upon sectioning due to focal calcifications. Most arise within the skeletal muscles of the extremities, deep fascia, or periosteum; some invade adjacent bone or the deep subcutaneous tissue.

Although grossly well circumscribed, there is characteristically infiltration of the surrounding soft tissues. At low magnification, the tumor is hypocellular with extensive areas of densely hyalinized stroma (Fig. 11–7). The neoplastic cells are predominantly epithelioid in appearance and are arranged in a variety of patterns, including nests, cords, strands, and occasionally acini or alveoli. The cells have oval to round angulated nuclei with finely stippled or vesicular chromatin, small basophilic nucleoli, and scanty cleared-out or faintly eosinophilic cytoplasm. Mitotic figures (MFs) are generally inconspicuous, but occasional tumors are characterized by a high mitotic rate (>5 MF/10 HPF). Necrosis may be seen in up to one-third of cases. The stroma is composed predominantly of deeply acidophilic collagen, which in some foci nearly completely obliterates the neoplastic cells, resulting in hypocellular occasionally calcified zones. Myxoid and chondro-osseous areas may be present. Branching vessels that are frequently hyalinized and organized in a hemangiopericytoma-like pattern may also be present. Peripherally located cleft-like spaces filled with tumor, suggesting true angiolymphatic invasion, may be seen. In almost all cases the tumor shows foci of spindle-shaped sarcoma similar to conventional fibrosarcoma. Occasionally, there are areas which closely resemble low-grade fibromyxoid sarcoma/hyalinizing spindle cell tumor with giant rosettes.[34,40]

Immunohistochemical and ultrastructural findings

Virtually all tumors stain strongly and diffusely for vimentin, but importantly, up to 50% have a membranous pattern of immunoreactivity to epithelial membrane antigen (EMA), contributing to confusion with carcinoma, epithelioid sarcoma, and synovial sarcoma.[41,42] However, cytokeratins are typically not expressed by the neoplastic cells. Neural markers including S-100 protein and neuron-specific enolase are positive in a small number of cases. Stains for desmin, smooth muscle actin, HMB-45, CD68, leukocyte common antigen, and CD34 are typically negative.

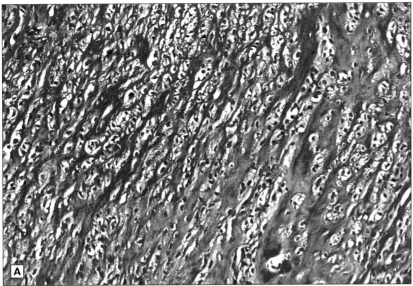

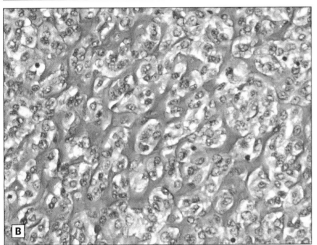

FIGURE 11–7 (A) Sclerosing epithelioid fibrosarcoma characterized by abundant hyalinized collagen between small, rounded tumor cells with clear cytoplasm. **(B)** High-magnification view of malignant epithelioid cells in sclerosing epithelioid fibrosarcoma. (Photograph courtesy of Dr. Cristina Antonescu, Memorial Sloan Kettering Cancer Center, New York, NY.)

Ultrastructurally, the neoplastic cells have the features of fibroblasts and sometimes myofibroblasts, with a large Golgi apparatus and abundant rough endoplasmic reticulum, usually arranged in parallel arrays, and often dilated and filled with granular or fibrillar material.[43,44] Intermediate filaments, sometimes arranged in perinuclear whorls, are present. Intracytoplasmic collagen may be seen, and most cells contain particulate glycogen. The tumor cells are intimately associated with dense bundles or irregular whorls of stromal collagen. Hanson and colleagues described one case with features suggesting perineurial differentiation.[45]

Cytogenetic findings

Very few cases of sclerosing epithelioid fibrosarcoma have been studied cytogenetically. Gisselsson et al. reported a case arising in a 14-year-old boy with a complex karyotype with amplification of 12q13 and 12q15 (including the *HMGIC* gene) as well as 9q13 rearrangement.[46]

Donner and colleagues described a tumor arising in the calf of a 55-year-old man with involvement of 6q15, 22q13 and Xq13.[41] Another case was found to have a dert(10;17)(p11;q11).

Differential diagnosis

The differential diagnosis includes a wide range of both benign and malignant lesions composed, at least in part, of epithelioid cells. In the series by Meis-Kindblom et al.,[31] many of the cases were submitted in consultation with a diagnosis of a benign lesion, including nodular fasciitis, fibrous histiocytoma, myositis ossificans, hyalinized leiomyoma, or desmoid tumor, perhaps accounting for the large number of cases treated with inadequate surgical excision in that series.

The most difficult differential diagnostic considerations are other malignant epithelioid neoplasms, particularly *infiltrating lobular carcinoma* and *infiltrating signet ring adenocarcinoma*. This distinction is made more difficult by the immunohistochemical expression of EMA in up to one-half of cases of sclerosing epithelioid fibrosarcoma. Identification of conventional areas of fibrosarcoma and ultrastructural features indicative of fibroblastic or myofibroblastic differentiation allow this distinction. The absence of leukocyte common antigen is helpful for distinguishing this tumor from a *sclerosing lymphoma*. *Clear cell sarcoma* is characterized by a more uniform pattern of nested cells with vesicular nuclei and macronucleoli. Although S-100 protein is present in a few cases of sclerosing epithelioid fibrosarcoma, the absence of HMB-45 helps distinguish between these lesions. The more nested and cord-like areas of sclerosing epithelioid fibrosarcoma may resemble *ossifying fibromyxoid tumor of soft parts*, but the latter entity is characterized by a peripherally located incomplete shell of lamellar bone in most cases and is composed of cells of lower nuclear grade. *Synovial sarcoma*, particularly those with poorly differentiated areas, may be composed of round cells often arranged around a hemangiopericytoma-like vascular pattern, with the immunohistochemical expression of epithelial markers. All of these features are similar to those of sclerosing epithelioid fibrosarcoma, and thus the recognition of lower-grade biphasic or monophasic synovial sarcoma is useful for this distinction. Cytogenetic or molecular genetic identification of the t(X;18) characteristic of synovial sarcoma is extremely helpful. Distinction from *malignant peripheral nerve sheath tumor* may be difficult, particularly because both tumors may express S-100 protein and neuron-specific enolase. Recognizing that the tumor originated from a nerve or a surrounding benign peripheral nerve sheath tumor is useful in this regard. In equivocal cases, ultrastructural analysis may be the best way to arrive at a definitive diagnosis. Finally, the recently described *sclerosing rhabdomyosarcoma* may closely resemble sclerosing epithelioid fibrosarcoma.[47] The former may show overt rhabdomyoblastic differentiation in the form of strap cells, and the cells typically express desmin, often in a peculiar dot-like pattern. MyoD1 is strongly expressed by the neoplastic cells, but myogenin staining is less impressive.

Discussion

Comparing the clinical behavior of this variant of fibrosarcoma to conventional fibrosarcoma is difficult, particularly because fibrosarcoma has essentially become a diagnosis of exclusion. In the study by Meis-Kindblom et al.,[31] 8 of 15 (53%) patients in whom follow-up information was available developed local recurrence a median 4.8 years after diagnosis. Metastases, most commonly to the lungs, followed by the pleura/chest wall, bones, and brain, were detected in 43% of patients. Of the six patients with metastatic disease, four died and two were alive with pulmonary metastases 14 years after the initial diagnosis. Patients with tumors on the trunk, those with large

tumors, and those of male gender may have a worse prognosis. In the study by Antonescu and colleagues,[40] of 14 patients with more than 1 year of follow-up, 12 (86%) developed distant metastases, and eight patients (57%) died as a direct result of their tumor. Wide surgical excision is the mainstay of therapy, and long-term follow-up is indicated as some patients develop local recurrence or metastatic disease late in their course.

Fibrosarcoma, myxoid type (myxofibrosarcoma or low-grade myxoid malignant fibrous histiocytoma)

The term *myxofibrosarcoma* was originally proposed by Angervall et al. to describe a group of fibroblastic lesions that show a spectrum of cellularity, nuclear pleomorphism, and mitotic activity ranging from a hypocellular lesion with minimal cytologic atypia to a more cellular lesion with features bordering on those of pleomorphic-storiform malignant fibrous histiocytoma (MFH).[48] These tumors have been subdivided into three[48,49] or four[49] grades based on the degree of cellularity, nuclear pleomorphism, and mitotic activity. There is a continuum between low- and high-grade variants, as indicated by the presence of low-grade areas in high-grade lesions and a histologic progression of low-grade to high-grade tumors in recurrences.[48–50] Comparing data among these studies is somewhat difficult, as the proportion of myxoid areas in the tumor required for inclusion has varied. For example, all of the tumors reported by Merck et al.[51] and Angervall et al.[48] were "wholly, or almost wholly, myxomatous in appearance," whereas Mentzel and co-workers[49] required only 10% of the tumor to show prominent myxoid change to be included in their study. In their initial description of the *myxoid variant of MFH*, Weiss and Enzinger required at least 50% of the tumor to be composed of myxoid areas.[52] In our opinion, the term *myxofibrosarcoma* should be used only for tumors that are predominantly (>50%) myxoid and of low nuclear grade. Failure to adhere to these guidelines results in a heterogeneous group of lesions of variable biologic course that overlap considerably with myxoid MFH and even other high-grade pleomorphic sarcomas. The following discussion focuses on the low-grade tumors in the myxofibrosarcoma spectrum. The entity of myxoid MFH is discussed in Chapter 14.

Clinical findings

The tumor most commonly arises as a slowly enlarging, painless mass in the extremities of elderly patients. Although the age range is broad, most patients are in their fifth to seventh decades of life, and men are affected slightly more often than women. The most common site is the extremities, with a predilection for the lower extremities. The tumor is found less commonly on the upper extremities, trunk, and head and neck region. Rare examples have also been described in the skin,[53] genitourinary tract,[54] gastrointestinal tract,[55] and breast.[56] This tumor is very uncommon in the abdominal cavity and retroperitoneum, and in fact extensive sampling and/or molecular genetic analysis usually reveals the myxofibrosarcoma to be a component of a dedifferentiated liposarcoma.[57-59]

Pathologic findings

Myxofibrosarcoma is usually centered in the subcutaneous tissue and is composed of multiple gelatinous nodules that have a tendency to spread in a longitudinal manner. In almost one-third of cases the tumor involves underlying skeletal muscle. Deep-seated lesions tend to be less nodular, demonstrate a more infiltrative growth pattern, and are usually larger than their superficial counterparts.

Histologically, low magnification reveals a multinodular tumor of low cellularity (Fig. 11–8). The constituent cells are generally spindle or stellate shaped and are deposited in a myxoid matrix composed predominantly of hyaluronic acid. The cells have slightly eosinophilic cytoplasm and indistinct cell borders; the nuclei are hyperchromatic, are mildly pleomorphic, and have only rare mitotic figures (Fig. 11–9). Occasional tumor cells show cytoplasmic vacuolation, but true lipoblasts are not seen. Most tumors have elongated, curvilinear capillaries; there is a tendency for the tumor cells to align themselves along the vessel periphery. Recently, Nascimento and colleagues described an epithelioid variant of myxofibrosarcoma, which accounted for only 3% of all myxofibrosarcomas seen in their consultation material.[59a]

Immunohistochemically, the cells stain strongly and diffusely for vimentin, although focal staining for muscle-specific actin and smooth muscle actin may be seen, indicative of myofibroblastic differentiation.[49,50] Electron microscopically, the cells are seen to have prominent, sometimes dilated, rough endoplasmic reticulum, a well-developed Golgi apparatus, and moderate numbers of mitochondria.[32] A minority of cells show features suggesting myofibroblastic differentiation.

Cytogenetic findings

Fewer than 70 cases of myxofibrosarcoma (or myxoid MFH) have been studied cytogenetically. Most cases with cytogenetic aberrations have shown a highly complex karyotype, often with triploid or tetraploid alterations. As one might expect from a low-grade sarcoma, ring chromosomes have been reported in some cases.[60] Study of several cases by comparative genomic hybridization has revealed genomic imbalances, including losses of 6p and gains of 9q and 12q.[61] Sawyer and colleagues reported a reciprocal t(10;17)(p11.2;q23) in a single case of myxofibrosarcoma,[62] whereas another case was found to have a t(2;15)(p23;q21.2) and an interstitial deletion of 7q.[63]

Recently, Willems and colleagues evaluated the karyotype and clinicopathologic features of 32 cases of myxofibrosarcoma.[64] Most cases showed complex cytogenetic anomalies, and such alterations were found in tumors of all grades. However, no tumor-specific chromosomal abnormalities were identified. Interestingly, those cases that locally recurred showed more complex cytogenetic aberrations than those which did not. The authors proposed the concept of progression of myxofibrosarcoma

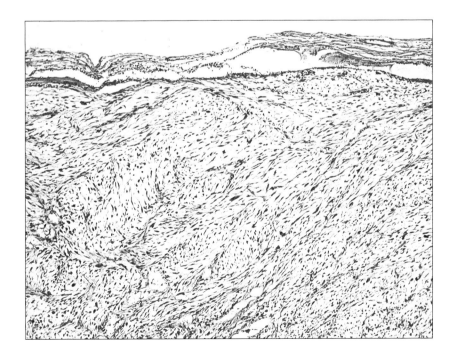

FIGURE 11–8 Myxofibrosarcoma. The spindle cells are minimally pleomorphic and separated by copious amounts of myxoid stroma.

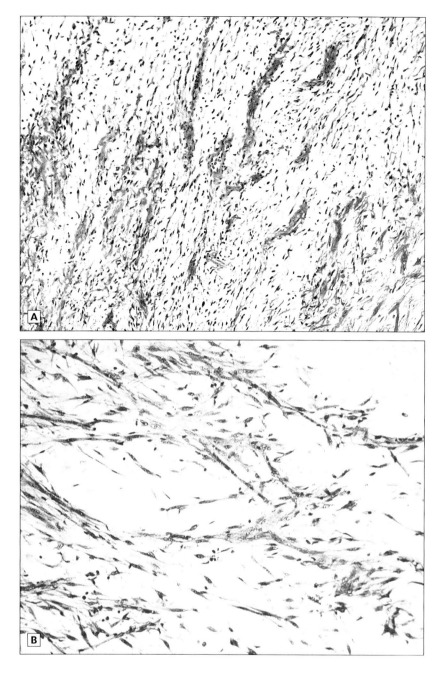

FIGURE 11–9 (A) Characteristic curvilinear vascular pattern seen in myxofibrosarcoma. **(B)** Myxoid zone of low-grade fibromyxoid sarcoma. The lesion is of low cellularity and composed of bland spindle-shaped cells.

as a multistep genetic process governed by genetic instability.

Differential diagnosis

The differential diagnosis includes a wide array benign and malignant myxoid soft tissue neoplasms. Tumors that are uniformly low grade and lack a transition to a higher-grade lesion may be easily mistaken for a benign lesion. *Nodular fasciitis* is characterized by a proliferation of fibroblasts and myofibroblasts that lack nuclear hyperchromasia, although mitotic figures are often easily seen. Other features, such as the presence of slit-like spaces, extravasated erythrocytes, and keloid-like collagen, help

distinguish nodular fasciitis from myxofibrosarcoma. *Myxoma* typically presents as a large, painless, fluctuant intramuscular mass composed of oval-shaped cells deposited in an abundant hyaluronic acid-rich myxoid matrix. The cellularity of a myxoma may overlap with that of myxofibrosarcoma, but the cells show less atypia and mitotic activity. Furthermore, myxoma is hypovascular and lacks the curvilinear vessels characteristically found in myxofibrosarcoma. *Spindle cell lipoma* is a benign lipomatous tumor typically found in the subcutaneous tissue of the posterior neck, shoulder, or back region of elderly people, mostly men. The spindle cells lack cytologic atypia and mitotic activity, and they stain for CD34. Mature lipocytes and ropey collagen fibers are also characteristic of this lesion. *Nerve sheath myxoma* or *myxoid neurothekeoma* is typically a small, solitary, intradermal or subcutaneous multinodular tumor often located on the fingers. Although some show nuclear pleomorphism, most are composed of cells with less atypia than those found in myxofibrosarcoma; this tumor also lacks the curvilinear vessels found in the latter lesion. In addition, the cells typically stain strongly for S-100 protein.

Myxofibrosarcoma must also be distinguished from other myxoid sarcomas that tend to be more clinically aggressive. *Myxoid liposarcoma* has less cytologic atypia, a fine plexiform vascular pattern without perivascular tumor cell condensation, and scattered lipoblasts. Clinically, myxoid liposarcoma is almost always deep-seated and occurs predominantly in the thigh or popliteal fossa of middle-aged adults. *Extraskeletal myxoid chondrosarcoma* is a multinodular neoplasm composed of rounded cells arranged in strands and cords deposited in a chondroitin sulfate-rich myxoid stroma. These lesions tend to show prominent hemorrhage and lack the curvilinear vessels of myxofibrosarcoma. We have found analysis by FISH for evidence of a *FUS* or *EWS* translocation to be useful in this differential diagnosis, as these aberrations can be detected in myxoid liposarcoma and extraskeletal myxoid chondrosarcoma, respectively.

Perhaps the most difficult distinction is from *low-grade fibromyxoid sarcoma* (Table 11–4), which is also discussed in this chapter. Clinically, this tumor occurs in young patients and has a tendency for multiple recurrences, with a risk of metastasis, if the lesion is incompletely excised. Histologically, it is composed of cytologically bland spindle cells arranged in a whorled pattern in a variably myxoid and fibrous stroma. In contrast, myxofibrosarcoma is always predominantly myxoid, and the cells show more cytologic atypia than those found in low-grade fibromyxoid sarcoma. Detection of a *FUS* translocation is a strong confirmatory finding for low-grade fibromyxoid sarcoma.

Discussion

The clinical behavior of myxofibrosarcoma appears to be closely related to the tumor grade. For example, Merck and colleagues found the risk of local recurrence to be 38%, 48%, 51%, and 61% for grade 1, 2, 3, and 4 tumors, respectively.[51] In contrast, in the study by Mentzel et al.,[49] the rate of local recurrence was independent of histologic grade, as 6 of 12 (50%) low-grade lesions recurred; one patient developed eight recurrences (Table 11–5). Two subcutaneous low-grade lesions recurred as higher-grade lesions with increased cellularity, nuclear pleomorphism, and mitotic activity. Adequate initial surgical therapy is necessary to limit the rate of local recurrence and the subsequent risk of histologic progression. The risk of metastasis is minimal for pure low-grade tumors. In the study by Merck et al.,[51] although 35% of patients developed metastases, none of the eight patients with grade 1 tumors did so. Similarly, Angervall and co-workers found that no patient with a grade 1 tumor developed metastatic disease, although two of seven patients with grade 2 tumors eventually did so (Tables 11–6, 11–7).[48]

Huang and co-workers evaluated 49 myxofibrosarcomas treated and followed up at a single institution.[65] With a median follow-up period of 55 months, local

TABLE 11–4	DISTINCTION OF LOW-GRADE FIBROMYXOID SARCOMA FROM MYXOFIBROSARCOMA	
Feature	**LGFMS**	**Myxofibrosarcoma**
Peak age	Young to middle age	Elderly
Depth	Skeletal muscle	Subcutaneous tissue
Stroma	Alternating myxoid and fibrous	Usually uniformly myxoid
Atypia	Absent to minimal	More prominent
Metastasis	Up to 50% of cases	Rare

LGFMS, low-grade fibromyxoid sarcoma.

TABLE 11–5	RELATION BETWEEN HISTOLOGIC GRADE AND RATE OF LOCAL RECURRENCE FOR MYXOFIBROSARCOMA			
	Local recurrence			
Study	**Grade 1**	**Grade 2**	**Grade 3**	**Grade 4**
Mentzel et al.[49]*	6/12 (50%)	9/13 (69%)	18/33 (55%)	
Angervall et al.[48]	0/2	2/7 (29%)	6/10 (60%)	7/11 (64%)
Merck et al.[51]	3/8 (38%)	13/27 (48%)	21/41 (51%)	17/28 (61%)

*Used only a three-grade scale.

TABLE 11–6	RELATION BETWEEN HISTOLOGIC GRADE AND RATE OF METASTASIS FOR MYXOFIBROSARCOMA			
	Metastasis			
Study	**Grade 1**	**Grade 2**	**Grade 3**	**Grade 4**
Mentzel et al.[49]*	0/12	5/13 (38%)	10/34 (29%)	
Angervall et al.[48]	0/2	2/7 (29%)	2/11 (18%)	3/11 (27%)
Merck et al.[51]	0/8	6/28 (21%)	21/45 (47%)	11/29 (38%)

*Used only a three-grade scale.

TABLE 11–7	RATES OF LOCAL RECURRENCE AND METASTASIS FOR GRADE 1 (LOW-GRADE) MYXOFIBROSARCOMA	
Study	**Recurrence**	**Metastasis**
Mentzel et al.[49]	6/12 (50%)	0/12
Angervall et al.[48]*	0/2	0/2
Merck et al.[51]*	3/8 (38%)	0/8

*Used a four-grade scale; data include only tumors designated grade 1.

recurrence and distant metastases were detected in 28 (57%) and 7 (14%) patients, respectively. Only one patient developed metastasis without having had a prior local recurrence. The 5-year recurrence-free survival, metastasis-free survival and disease-specific mortality rates were 41%, 90%, and 4.4%, respectively. Tumor size larger than 5 cm, tumor necrosis, and <75% of myxoid areas were significantly associated with disease-specific mortality, the former two factors being the most predictive of metastasis.

Fibrosarcoma, fibromyxoid type (low-grade fibromyxoid sarcoma/hyalinizing spindle cell tumor with giant rosettes)

The low-grade fibromyxoid sarcoma was first recognized by Evans in 1987, when he reported bland fibromyxoid neoplasms arising in the deep soft tissue of two young women.[66] Although initially diagnosed as benign, both tumors eventually metastasized; subsequent reports have verified the metastatic potential of this histologically deceptive neoplasm. Although there was a great deal of skepticism as to whether this tumor was a specific entity, subsequent clinicopathologic, cytogenetic, and molecular genetic studies have confirmed this lesion as a distinct variant of fibrosarcoma. This sarcoma is probably more common than the literature would lead one to believe, as some have undoubtedly been diagnosed as myxofibrosarcoma, low-grade myxoid sarcoma, not otherwise specified, or a variety of other benign or malignant fibrous or myxoid neoplasms.

Hyalinizing spindle cell tumor with giant rosettes is an unusual fibrous tumor of deep soft tissues first delineated in 1997 by Lane et al.[67] in a series of 19 cases. Virtually all reported cases have behaved in an indolent fashion, although rare examples exhibit aggressive clinical behavior, including both early and late metastases. There is significant histologic and molecular genetic overlap with low-grade fibromyxoid sarcoma, and there is sufficient evidence to support the contention that this tumor represents a variant of the latter.[68–71]

Clinical findings

Most patients with low-grade fibromyxoid sarcoma are young to middle-aged adults, but this tumor may arise in patients as young as 3 years and as old as 78 years.[71] Males are affected more commonly than females. The usual presentation is that of a slowly growing, painless, deep soft tissue mass that ranges from 1 to 18 cm in greatest diameter, although most are 8–10 cm. The tumor most commonly arises in the deep soft tissue of the lower extremities, particularly the thigh, followed, in decreasing order of frequency, by the chest wall/axilla, shoulder region, inguinal region, buttock, and neck. Rare cases have also been described in unusual sites including the retroperitoneum,[72] small bowel mesentery,[73] mediastinum,[74] and paravertebral region.[75]

Most patients with hyalinizing spindle cell tumor with giant rosettes are in their third or fourth decade of life, and men are affected twice as often as women. The most common presenting symptom is a painless, deep-seated, slowly enlarging mass that may be present months to years prior to presentation. The tumor is most common in the extremities, particularly the thigh. Other sites of involvement are the chest wall, axilla, buttock, head and neck, omentum, pelvis, and mediastinum.[76–78] The overlapping clinical features and anatomic sites of involvement with low-grade fibromyxoid sarcoma are further evidence that these neoplasms are related.

Gross findings

Most examples of low-grade fibromyxoid sarcoma/hyalinizing spindle cell tumor with giant rosettes arise in the skeletal muscle, although some appear to be centered in the subcutaneous tissue, with minimal or no muscle involvement. Recently, Billings and colleagues described a sizable group of these tumors that involve the dermis as well.[79] Although typically grossly well circumscribed, there is often extensive microscopic infiltration into the surrounding soft tissues. On cut section, the tumor often has a yellow-white appearance with focal areas with a glistening appearance secondary to the accumulation of myxoid ground substance. Some exhibit cystic degeneration, but neither necrosis nor hemorrhage is present.

Microscopic findings

Characteristically, low-grade fibromyxoid sarcoma is of low or moderate cellularity composed of bland spindle-shaped cells with small hyperchromatic oval nuclei, finely clumped chromatin, and one to several small nucleoli.

The cells have indistinct pale eosinophilic cytoplasm and show only mild nuclear pleomorphism with little mitotic activity. The cells are deposited in a fibrous and myxoid stroma that tends to vary in different areas of the tumor (Figs 11–10 to 11–12). In general, the lesions appear more fibrous than myxoid. The myxoid zones may abut abruptly with the fibrous zones, or there may be a gradual transition between these areas. Cells with a stellate configuration are often present in the myxoid zones, and they are generally arranged in a whorled or random fashion (Figs 11–13, 11–14). There is often a prominent network of curvilinear and branching capillary-sized blood vessels in the myxoid zones, somewhat reminiscent (although thicker walled) of that seen in myxoid liposarcoma (Fig. 11–15),[71] sometimes with perivascular hypercellularity. The stroma stains with Alcian blue which is completely

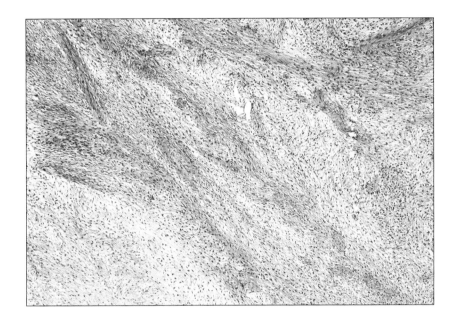

FIGURE 11–10 Low-grade fibromyxoid sarcoma. At low power, alternating areas with a fibrous and myxoid stroma are apparent.

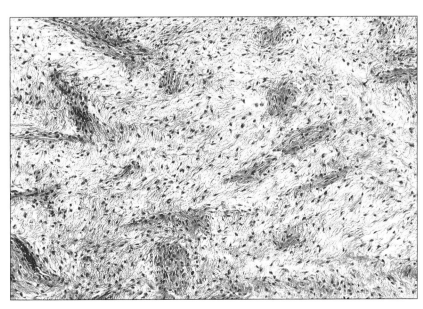

FIGURE 11–11 Low-grade fibromyxoid sarcoma with alternating fibrous and myxoid areas. The cells commonly show a whorled pattern of growth.

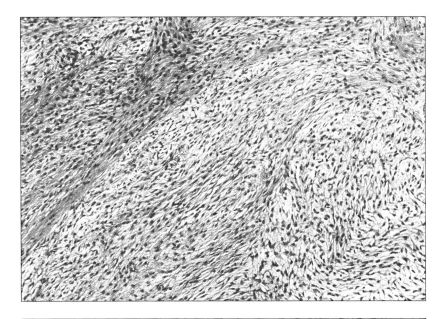

FIGURE 11–12 Junction between fibrous and myxoid zones in low-grade fibromyxoid sarcoma.

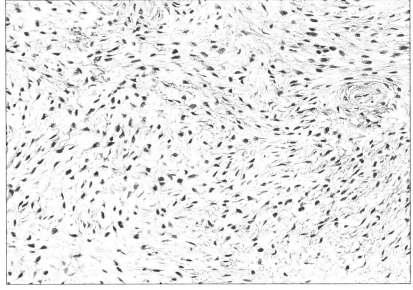

FIGURE 11–13 Myxoid zone of low-grade fibromyxoid sarcoma. The lesion is of low cellularity and composed of bland spindle-shaped cells.

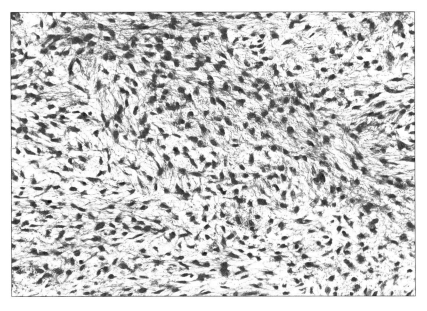

FIGURE 11–14 More cellular area of a low-grade fibromyxoid sarcoma. The cells have a stellate appearance and are evenly distributed within a fibromyxoid stroma.

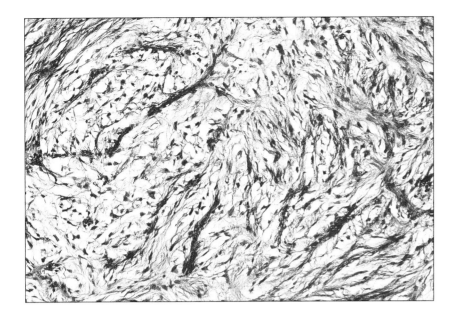

FIGURE 11–15 Low-grade fibromyxoid sarcoma showing a prominent network of branching capillary-sized blood vessels reminiscent of myxoid liposarcoma.

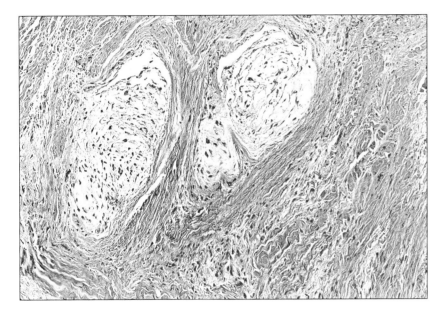

FIGURE 11–16 Although grossly well circumscribed, low-grade fibromyxoid sarcoma often shows microscopic infiltration of the surrounding soft tissues by small myxoid nodules.

removed by pretreatment with hyaluronidase.[80,81] Epithelioid cells may also be present focally, and there are areas of intermediate-grade fibrosarcoma in about 15–20% of cases.[71]

Although this neoplasm is characterized by a deceptively bland appearance, recurrences may show areas of increased cellularity and mitotic activity, sometimes with the formation of hypercellular nodules (Figs 11–16, 11–17).[72,82] Evans reported one case that progressed to a neoplasm composed of sheets of anaplastic round cells 30 years after the initial excision.[73] We have reviewed rare cases that show areas of transition to a high-grade pleomorphic spindle cell sarcoma. In most cases, recurrences and metastases resemble the primary lesions, although we have seen a case in which the metastasis had a predominantly primitive round cell appearance.

Hyalinizing spindle cell tumor with giant rosettes is characterized by spindle-shaped cells arranged into a variety of patterns and deposited in a densely hyalinized stroma punctuated by large collagen rosettes (Figs 11–18 to 11–20). Cellularity varies from case to case and in different areas of the same tumor. In most areas, the cells are arranged in irregular crisscrossing fascicles separated by moderate amounts of collagen (Fig. 11–21), often with a "cracking" artifact around the elongated fibroblastic cells. In some areas there is extensive stromal hyalinization with a paucity of neoplastic cells, whereas in others the cells are deposited in a myxoid stroma that may have a delicate arborizing vasculature (Figs 11–22, 11–23). The tumor cells have irregular or wavy nuclei with a mild degree of nuclear atypia. Mitotic figures are difficult to find, usually with fewer than one MF/50 HPF. Like

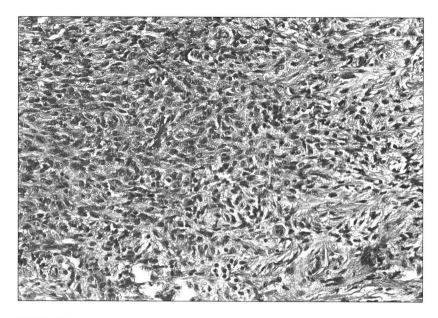

FIGURE 11–17 Recurrent low-grade fibromyxoid sarcoma showing an area of increased cellularity and nuclear pleomorphism.

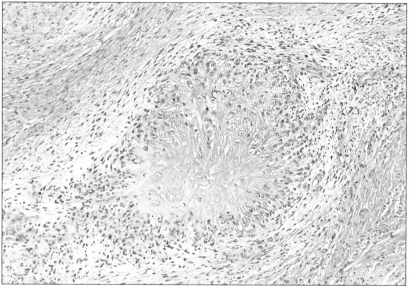

FIGURE 11–18 Hyalinizing spindle cell tumor with giant rosettes. The most characteristic feature is the presence of large collagen rosettes.

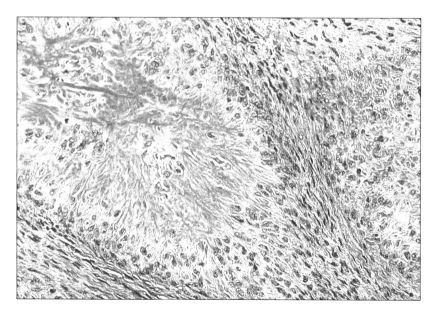

FIGURE 11–19 Trichrome stain of collagen rosette in a case of hyalinizing spindle cell tumor demonstrating that the central eosinophilic portion of the rosette is composed of collagen.

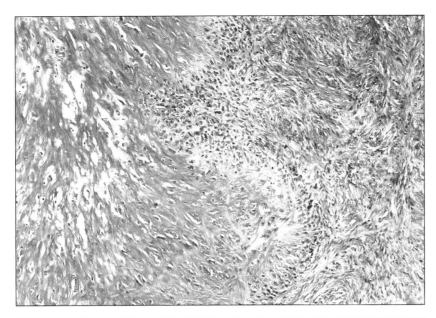

FIGURE 11–20 Hyalinizing spindle cell tumor with giant rosettes showing transition between a collagen rosette and a more cellular fibrosarcoma-like area.

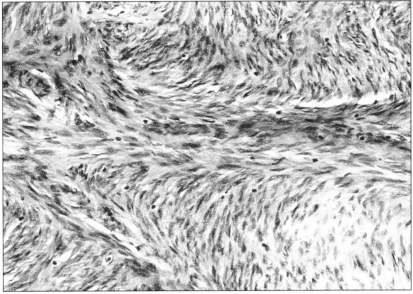

FIGURE 11–21 Fibrosarcoma-like area in a case of hyalinizing spindle cell tumor with giant rosettes. The cells are arranged into irregular crisscrossing fascicles.

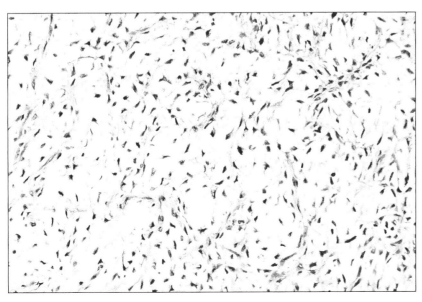

FIGURE 11–22 Myxoid zone of hyalinizing spindle cell tumor with giant rosettes. The neoplastic cells are widely separated by myxoid stroma, and a plexiform vasculature is apparent.

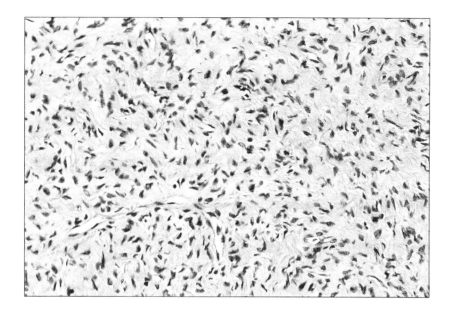

FIGURE 11–23 Hyalinizing spindle cell tumor with giant rosettes. Spindled stroma shows greater cellularity than in Figure 11–22. Cells have an irregular wavy shape somewhat reminiscent of cells in neurofibroma.

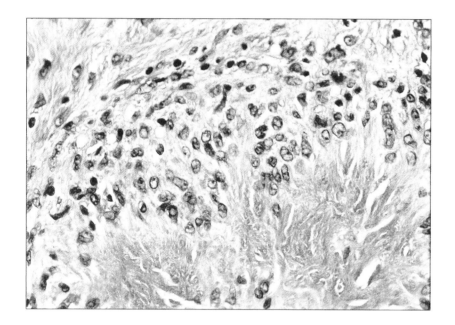

FIGURE 11–24 Rounded cells comprising the periphery of a rosette in a case of hyalinizing spindle cell tumor with giant rosettes. A few of the cells have intranuclear cytoplasmic inclusions.

ordinary fibromyxoid sarcoma, areas of an intermediate-grade fibrosarcoma may be present. The most characteristic feature is the presence of a variable number of large rosette-like structures that merge abruptly or imperceptibly with the surrounding hyalinized or spindled stroma. The rosettes, which tend to cluster together, are composed of a central core of brightly eosinophilic birefringent collagen arranged centrifugally from the center surrounded by rounded to ovoid cells that have clear to eosinophilic cytoplasm and little to no nuclear atypia or mitotic activity. Occasional cells show intranuclear cytoplasmic inclusions (Fig. 11–24). Other features include the presence of hemosiderin deposition, cystic degeneration, calcification, osseous and chondroid metaplasia, and peripheral chronic inflammation.[83,84]

Immunohistochemical and ultrastructural findings

Immunohistochemically, the neoplastic cells in low-grade fibromyxoid sarcoma stain strongly and diffusely for vimentin. Focal immunoreactivity for muscle markers including smooth muscle actin and muscle-specific actin may be present, suggesting myofibroblastic differentiation in at least some of the cells. Rare cases show focal staining for desmin, CD34, and cytokeratins. The cells do not stain for β-catenin, a useful finding when deep fibromatosis is a diagnostic consideration.

The immunophenotype of hyalinizing spindle cell tumor with giant rosettes is quite similar to that seen in low-grade fibromyxoid sarcoma. Both the spindle-shaped and ovoid cells comprising the rosettes stain strongly for vimentin. S-100 protein, Leu-7, and neuron-specific enolase are frequently present in the rounded cells but are less often identified in the spindled cells.[67,77]

Ultrastructurally, the neoplastic cells of low-grade fibromyxoid sarcoma are slender spindle-shaped cells with limited amount of cytoplasm and long, nonbranching, delicate cell processes.[32] Most of the cells have a moderate number of cytoplasmic organelles, including mildly well-developed rough endoplasmic reticulum cisternae. Abundant arrays of vimentin intermediate filaments are also present. Long, narrow cell processes with numerous pinocytotic vesicles are also a characteristic feature, and somewhat reminiscent of the ultrastructural features seen in perineurioma.[32,81,85] Although Nielsen et al.[84] noted that the cells surrounding the collagen rosettes exhibited ultrastructural features similar to those of the spindle-shaped cells, de Pinieux et al.[86] found that the rounded cells surrounding the collagen rosettes had schwannian features. Focal myofibroblastic differentiation may also be seen.[87]

Cytogenetic findings

Cytogenetically, early studies of low-grade fibromyxoid sarcoma revealed evidence of a supernumerary ring chromosome containing material from chromosomes 7 and 16, as detected by comparative genomic hybridization.[88] Subsequently, several studies confirmed the presence of a characteristic translocation involving the *FUS* gene on chromosome 7 and the *CREB3L2* gene on chromosome 16.[89,90] This same translocation was identified in cases of hyalinizing spindle cell tumor with giant rosettes, supporting the identity of these two tumors.[91] Mertens and colleagues reported the presence of a *FUS/CREB3L2* fusion in 22 of 23 (96%) cases of low-grade fibromyxoid sarcoma;[92] none of the other fibrous or myxoid neoplasms tested showed evidence of this fusion transcript, supporting the sensitivity and specificity of this translocation. In a recent study, Matsuyama et al. found evidence of a FUS/*CREB3L2* fusion transcript in 14 of 16 (88%) cases of low grade fibromyxoid sarcoma using RT-PCR on formalin-fixed, paraffin-embedded tissue.[92a] Currently, we utilize fixed, paraffin-embedded tissue using a breakapart probe for the *FUS* gene to support this diagnosis, which can be extremely difficult to make on morphologic and immunohistochemical grounds, particularly in a small biopsy specimen.

Differential diagnosis

The differential diagnosis of low-grade fibromyxoid sarcoma includes numerous benign and malignant soft tissue lesions characterized by a variably fibrous and myxoid stroma. *Myxoid neurofibroma* is composed of cells with more slender and wavy nuclei that consistently express S-100 protein. *Perineurioma* may resemble the fibrous whorled areas seen in low-grade fibromyxoid

sarcoma, but the immunohistochemical detection of epithelial membrane antigen allows its distinction. Some areas of low-grade fibromyxoid sarcoma may resemble *nodular fasciitis*, but the latter lesion is characterized by cells that resemble tissue culture fibroblasts. Other features of fasciitis, such as cleft-like spaces, extravasation of erythrocytes, and the presence of multinucleated giant cells, are not found in low-grade fibromyxoid sarcoma. *Cellular myxoma* occasionally can resemble low-grade fibromyxoid sarcoma. However, the lesion lacks the abrupt transition between fibrous and myxoid zones and lacks evidence of a *FUS* translocation.[93] *Desmoid fibromatoses* are composed of nuclei that tend to be plumper and more vesicular and are arranged in a fascicular growth pattern. The cells consistently show nuclear β-catenin staining. The *myxoid variant of dermatofibrosarcoma protuberans* (DFSP) may resemble the myxoid zones of low-grade fibromyxoid sarcoma. Given that low-grade fibromyxoid sarcoma can arise in a superficial location, the distinction between these tumors can be challenging. However, the cells of DFSP are arranged in a monotonous storiform pattern and consistently stain for CD34.

Malignant peripheral nerve sheath tumors may contain myxoid foci, but the cells are more elongated or wavy, are typically arranged in an irregular fascicular growth pattern, and stain for S-100 protein in up to 60% of cases. In addition, ultrastructural analysis reveals evidence of schwannian differentiation. *Spindle cell liposarcoma* usually arises in the subcutaneous tissue of adults and always contains an atypical lipomatous component that includes the presence of lipoblasts. The myxoid zones of low-grade fibromyxoid sarcoma may also resemble *myxoid liposarcoma*, particularly the cases with a well-developed plexiform vascular pattern. However, low-grade fibromyxoid sarcoma lacks lipoblasts, and adequate sampling always reveals fibrous areas. Cytogenetically, myxoid liposarcoma is characterized by t(12;16)(q13; p11). Like low-grade fibromyxoid sarcoma, aberrations of the *FUS* gene on 16p11 are characteristic. Thus, one must correlate the results of FISH analysis with the morphologic features of the tumor in question.

The lesion with which low-grade fibromyxoid sarcoma is most easily confused is *myxofibrosarcoma*, a neoplasm at the lower end of the spectrum that overlaps with myxoid malignant fibrous histiocytoma.[94] Unlike low-grade fibromyxoid sarcoma, which typically arises in the skeletal muscle of young patients, myxofibrosarcoma commonly arises in the subcutaneous tissues of the extremities of elderly patients. Histologically, myxofibrosarcoma is uniformly myxoid, lacks alternating fibrous zones, and always has a greater degree of nuclear pleomorphism and hyperchromasia. Antonescu and coworkers found subtle ultrastructural differences between these two lesions, with a more inactive or primitive form of fibroblastic differentiation in low-grade fibromyxoid sarcoma.[32]

Hyalinizing spindle cell tumor with giant rosettes may be confused with other tumors with giant collagen-containing rosettes, including *neuroblastoma-like neurilemmoma*, in which the rosettes are made up of a core of collagen flanked by small, rounded, differentiated Schwann cells.[95] Rare cases of *osteosarcoma* have been reported to contain similar rosettes, but in these cases the central core is composed of an osteoid-like material, often with central calcification, and surrounded by cells with more nuclear pleomorphism than those encountered in the hyalinizing spindle cell tumor.[96] The spindle-shaped areas may also resemble *fibromatosis*, but the latter lesion is characterized by more uniform cellularity with arrangement into a distinct fascicular growth pattern and an absence of rosette-like structures.

Discussion

Although originally considered distinctive entities, low-grade fibromyxoid sarcoma and hyalinizing spindle cell tumor with giant rosettes are now regarded as part of a histologic spectrum. The reasons for believing them to be the same are as follows: similarity in age and location, virtual identity of the spindled stroma (Fig. 11–25) including the occasional presence of intermediate-grade fibrosarcoma and the presence of the same characteristic translocation [t(7;16)].[91,97]

Despite its deceptively bland histologic appearance, low-grade fibromyxoid sarcoma was originally thought to have a high rate of local, often repeated recurrence as well as pulmonary metastases in a significant percentage of cases. Prior to 2000, approximately 65% of cases reported in the literature had locally recurred 6 months to 50 years after initial excision, with many patients developing multiple recurrences. In fact, Evans reported one case in which the patient developed 17 recurrences over a 29-year period.[73] Metastases were reported to be present at the time of initial excision or developed late in the clinical course. Evans described one case that metastasized 45 years after the initial presentation.[73] The lung has been involved in virtually all cases with metastatic disease.

In the original report of hyalinizing spindle cell tumor with giant rosettes by Lane et al.,[67] follow-up information available for 12 of the 19 patients showed only one instance of local recurrence and no evidence of metastatic disease. Woodruff et al., however, reported a tumor that arose in the arm of a 28-year-old woman that had the typical features of hyalinizing spindle cell tumor with giant rosettes; it ultimately metastasized to the lung 4 years after presentation.[70] Farinha and colleagues reported a patient with prolonged survival following detection of pulmonary metastases from an 11 cm thigh mass.[98] We, too, have reviewed a case in consultation that produced metastasis 8 years after the initial resection, and Chang et al. reported a case that metastasized 11 years after initial detection.[68]

In 2000, Folpe and colleagues reported the clinicopathologic features of 73 cases of low-grade fibromyxoid sarcoma, some of which had overlapping features with hyalinizing spindle cell tumor with giant rosettes.[71] Follow-up information was obtained in 54 cases, with a median follow-up period of 24 months. Of this group, five patients developed local recurrences, three developed metastatic disease, and only one patient died as a direct result of the tumor. Importantly, the diagnosis of low-grade fibromyxoid sarcoma/hyalinizing spindle cell tumor with giant rosettes was made prospectively in 51 patients, and none of these patients developed metastatic disease. Thus, the significantly better prognosis in this study compared with prior studies was felt to reflect the fact that all were initially diagnosed as sarcomas and treated with aggressive surgery. This is in stark contrast to

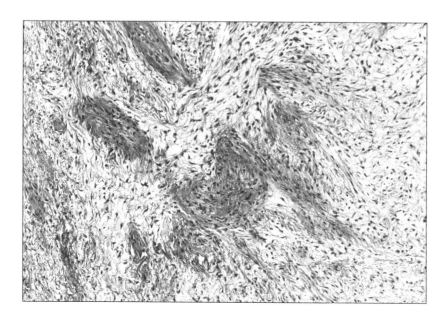

FIGURE 11–25 Alternating fibrous and myxoid zones in a hyalinizing spindle cell tumor with giant rosettes. Such zones are reminiscent of low-grade fibromyxoid sarcoma.

patients reported in the earlier studies, most of whom were originally diagnosed with and treated for a benign neoplasm. Although the presence of small areas of higher-grade fibrosarcoma has not been shown to be an adverse prognostic indicator, the significance of larger high-grade areas has yet to be determined. Low-grade fibromyxoid sarcoma/hyalinizing spindle cell tumor is best considered a low-grade sarcoma, and wide surgical excision with indefinite follow-up is the treatment of choice.

FIBROSARCOMATOUS CHANGE ARISING IN DERMATOFIBROSARCOMA PROTUBERANS

Up to 10% of cases of dermatofibrosarcoma protuberans have fascicular areas of increased cellularity, nuclear pleomorphism, and mitotic activity, and resemble conventional soft tissue fibrosarcoma. The significance of fibrosarcomatous change in dermatofibrosarcoma protuberans is discussed in greater detail in Chapter 13.

POSTRADIATION FIBROSARCOMA

Although high-grade pleomorphic sarcomas are by far the most common postradiation sarcoma, there is clearly a higher incidence of fibrosarcoma in patients who have been exposed to radiation than in the general population. There are numerous reports in which a fibrosarcoma originated at the site of therapeutic irradiation for various benign and malignant neoplasms[99-101] and for non-neoplastic disorders such as psoriasis and hypertrichosis.[25]

The latency period between irradiation and tumor development is of significance when evaluating these cases. The tumor usually develops 4–15 years following irradiation, although periods as short as 15 months have been reported.[102] Tumors appearing less than 2 years following irradiation are unlikely to be radiation-induced. Opinions vary as to the significance of the radiation dose for tumor development, and both small and large doses have been implicated as being more likely to produce radiation-related neoplasms. In general, the prognosis for patients developing postradiation fibrosarcoma is poor, as most patients die within 2 years of the development of the tumor. Rearrangements of the *RET* oncogene have been implicated in the development of postradiation fibrosarcoma.[103]

FIBROSARCOMA ARISING IN BURN SCARS

Although less common than postradiation fibrosarcoma, there are rare cases of fibrosarcoma arising in scars formed at sites of thermal injury. Nearly all of the affected patients have suffered extensive burns as children and developed tumors after an interval of 30 years or more.[104] For example, Pack and Ariel described a 53-year-old man who developed a fibrosarcoma arising in a burn scar suffered at age 6.[15] Carcinomas are more common than sarcomas as a late sequence of thermal injury (Marjolin's ulcer) and usually develop after a 30- to 40-year latent period.[105] Immunohistochemical analysis with cytokeratins, including high-molecular-weight cytokeratins, is useful for excluding the possibility of a desmoplastic or spindle cell carcinoma before rendering a diagnosis of fibrosarcoma arising in a burn scar.

MYOFIBROSARCOMA (MYOFIBROBLASTIC SARCOMA)

As mentioned earlier in this chapter, scattered cells in typical cases of fibrosarcoma may stain for smooth muscle or muscle-specific actin, and ultrastructural data support the presence of cells with myofibroblastic differentiation in otherwise typical fibrosarcoma. The issue as to whether there are sarcomas composed predominantly or exclusively of myofibroblasts remains a contentious one, primarily because the diagnostic criteria for recognizing such tumors remain obscure. Schürch and colleagues stated that benign and malignant neoplasms composed of myofibroblasts reported in the literature lack specific myofibroblastic features.[106,107] According to these authors, myofibroblasts can only be recognized by the ultrastructural identification of stress fibers, well-developed microtendons (fibronexus) and intercellular intermediate-type end-gap junctions.[106] Because of the heterogeneous immunophenotype of myofibroblasts with regard to intermediate filaments and actin isoforms, these authors argued that categorizing a cell as a myofibroblast by its immunohistochemical staining pattern alone is imprecise.[107] Others have argued that myofibroblastic sarcomas are recognizable even in the absence of the aforementioned ultrastructural features.[108-110] In our opinion, myofibroblastic sarcomas do exist but are uncommon. Although one may suspect a myofibrosarcoma on the basis of routine morphology, we believe that confirmation of myofibroblastic differentiation requires at least supportive immunohistochemical analysis and, ideally, ultrastructural evaluation, although the minimal ultrastructural criteria required for recognizing such cells are yet to be well defined. Since high-grade myofibroblastic sarcomas likely get grouped with other high-grade pleomorphic sarcomas or so-called malignant fibrous histiocytoma,[111,112] this discussion will focus on low-grade myofibrosarcomas.

Clinical findings

Low-grade myofibrosarcoma can arise in patients of virtually any age, but most patients are in their fourth decade of life, and there is a predilection for males. In the study by Mentzel and colleagues describing 18 such tumors (5 of which had supportive ultrastructural findings), these tumors occurred in 10 men and 7 women between 19 and 72 years.[108] In the study of 15 case of myofibrosarcoma reported by Montgomery and co-workers, the tumors arose in 11 men and 4 women aged 33 to 73 years, with a median age of 54 years.[112] Most patients present with a slowly enlarging, painless mass with tumor size ranging from 1.5 cm to 12 cm. The most common site of involvement is the head and neck region (especially the oral cavity and tongue), followed by the extremities and trunk.[108,112] Rare cases involving the adrenal gland,[113] breast,[114,115] and bone[111] have also been described.

Pathologic findings

Grossly, most tumors are firm and have a pale fibrous-appearing cut surface with ill-defined margins, although some are well circumscribed and have pushing margins.

Histologically, this tumor is characterized by a proliferation of spindled to stellate-shaped cells arranged into intersecting fascicles, sheets, or storiform whorls, with variable collagenous or myxoid stroma and scanty inflammation. Some tumors closely resemble nodular fasciitis (Figs 11–26 to 11–28). The cells have ill-defined pale eosinophilic cytoplasm. The nuclei are usually fusiform in shape, and most have an evenly dispersed chromatin pattern, although at least focal nuclear hyperchromasia is seen. Mitotic activity is typically low, and necrosis is absent in low-grade lesions. The cells typically infiltrate the surrounding soft tissue structures, an important feature that helps to distinguish this lesion from a reactive process.

Immunohistochemical and ultrastructural findings

The cells usually show a delicate "tram track" pattern of actin staining, especially with smooth muscle actin (Table 11–8). Fewer than 50% of cases express desmin, usually in a small percentage of cells.[108,112] These antigens can be expressed together or separately, but more commonly low-grade myofibrosarcoma reveals a smooth muscle actin-positive/desmin-negative immunophenotype. In addition, calponin is usually diffusely positive, whereas h-caldesmon shows only focal expression in occasional cases.[109] These immunophenotypic findings, which are quite similar to those of nodular fasciitis, are potentially useful in distinguishing low-grade myofibrosarcoma from leiomyosarcoma, which usually expresses both calponin and h-caldesmon. Some low-grade myofibrosarcomas also express fibronectin, but not collagen IV or laminin. The neoplastic cells are typically negative for S-100 protein, CD34, CD99, ALK, epithelial markers, and myogenin.

Ultrastructurally, the neoplastic cells contain indented or clefted nuclei, numerous rough endoplasmic reticulum, randomly oriented intermediate filaments, and thin filaments with focal dense bodies and focal subplasmalemmal attachment plaques, a discontinuous basal lamina, and micropinocytotic vesicles.[109,110,116] In some cases, fibronectin fibrils and fibronexus junctions can be demonstrated.

Cytogenetic findings

Given the difficulty in recognizing this tumor and the lack of uniformly accepted criteria, it is not surprising that very

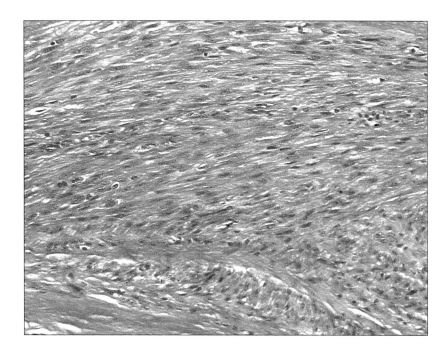

FIGURE 11–26 Myofibrosarcoma composed of intersecting fascicles of spindled cells with palely eosinophilic cytoplasm. (Case courtesy of Dr. Cyril Fisher, Royal Marsden Hospital, London, England.)

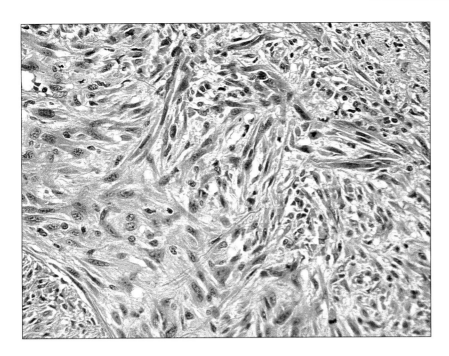

FIGURE 11–27 Myofibrosarcoma composed of spindled to stellate-shaped cells resembling nodular fasciitis. (Case courtesy of Dr. Cyril Fisher, Royal Marsden Hospital, London, England.)

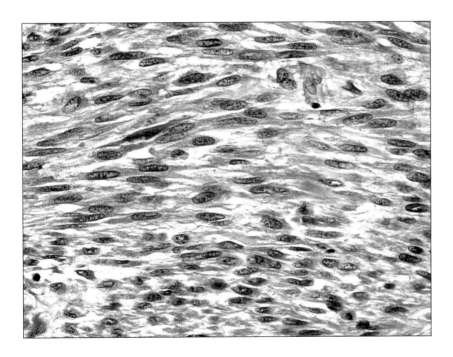

FIGURE 11–28 Myofibrosarcoma composed of uniform plump spindled cells with palely eosinophilic cytoplasm somewhat resembling leiomyosarcoma. (Case courtesy of Dr. Cyril Fisher, Royal Marsden Hospital, London, England.)

TABLE 11–8	IMMUNOPHENOTYPIC FEATURES OF MYOFIBROSARCOMA COMPARED TO FIBROSARCOMA AND LEIOIMYOSARCOMA		
	Myofibrosarcoma	**Fibrosarcoma**	**Leiomyosarcoma**
Desmin	±	–	+
SMA	+	±	+
MSA	±	–	+
Calponin	+	–	+
h-caldesmon	–	–	+

Modified from: Fisher C. Myofibrosarcoma. Virch Arch 2004; 445:215.

few examples of this tumor have been studied by cytogenetics. The few cases that have been studied have shown a moderate number of non-characteristic chromosomal aberrations and show a far simpler karyotype than that typically seen in high-grade pleomorphic sarcomas.[117]

Differential diagnosis

Low-grade myofibrosarcoma can resemble reactive processes or benign myofibroblastic neoplasms on the one hand and spindle cell sarcomas on the other. Some cases very closely resemble *nodular fasciitis*, a reactive pseudosarcomatous proliferation that typically appears suddenly and grows rapidly. Nodular fasciitis rarely exceeds 5 cm and is most often located in the subcutis. Regional heterogeneity with zonation is a characteristic feature, and the constituent cells lack nuclear hyperchromasia. Invariably, low-grade myofibrosarcoma shows at least scattered hyperchromatic nuclei, which are not seen in nodular fasciitis. Any case of recurrent nodular fasciitis should engender reconsideration of that diagnosis, and such cases are sometimes better classified as low-grade myofibrosarcoma.

Leiomyosarcoma is also frequently a diagnostic consideration. However, leiomyosarcoma typically has alternating fascicles of cells that are less tapered and have blunt-ended nuclei with perinuclear vacuoles. The cells also typically have more densely eosinophilic fibrillar cytoplasm. Although the immunophenotype overlaps with that seen in low-grade myofibrosarcoma, leiomyosarcoma typically coexpresses calponin and h-caldesmon, whereas low-grade myofibrosarcoma does not express h-caldesmon. *Fibrosarcoma* is composed of more uniformly hyperchromatic and atypical cells arranged into longer sweeping fascicles with the characteristic herringbone growth pattern. At most, fibrosarcoma shows only focal myoid differentiation by immunohistochemistry.

Discussion

Low-grade myofibrosarcoma is usually an indolent tumor, although there is a propensity for local recurrence if the lesion is incompletely excised. Occasionally, the tumor can progress to a higher-grade sarcoma in a recurrence. Overall, approximately 33% of these tumors locally recur, and fewer than 10% have been reported to metastasize. In the study by Montgomery and colleagues, four of nine grade 1 tumors recurred, as did three of four grade 2 tumors.[112] However, many of these tumors were initially incompletely excised, and prospective studies of well-characterized tumors that have been appropriately treated have not been reported. In this same study, although none of the grade 1 tumors metastasized, one of four grade 2 tumors metastasized to the lungs. Others have confirmed the capacity of this tumor to metastasize.[118] Increased proliferative activity and necrosis may portend a more aggressive clinical behavior.[112] Surgery is the mainstay of therapy.[119] For those rare examples that are more superficially located, Mohs' micrographic surgery seems to minimize the risk of local recurrence.[120]

REFERENCES

1. Meyerding HW, Broders AC, Hargrave RL. Clinical aspects of fibrosarcoma of the soft tissues of the extremities. Surg Gynecol Obstet 1936; 62:1010.
2. Pritchard DJ, Soule EH, Taylor WF, et al. Fibrosarcoma – a clinicopathologic and statistical study of 199 tumors of the soft tissues of the extremities and trunk. Cancer 1974; 33:888.
3. Scott SM, Reiman HM, Pritchard DJ, et al. Soft tissue fibrosarcoma. A clinicopathologic study of 132 cases. Cancer 1989; 64:925.

Clinical findings

4. Conley J, Stout AP, Healey WV. Clinicopathologic analysis of eighty-four patients with an original diagnosis of fibrosarcoma of the head and neck. Am J Surg 1967; 114:564.
5. Fu YS, Perzin KH. Nonepithelial tumors of the nasal cavity, paranasal sinuses, and nasopharynx. A clinicopathologic study. VI. Fibrous tissue tumors (fibroma, fibromatosis, fibrosarcoma). Cancer 1976; 37:2912.
6. Greager JA, Reichard K, Campana JP, et al. Fibrosarcoma of the head and neck. Am J Surg 1994; 167:437.
7. Heffner DK, Gnepp DR. Sinonasal fibrosarcomas, malignant schwannomas, and "triton" tumors. A clinicopathologic study of 67 cases. Cancer 1992; 70:1089.

8. Mark RJ, Sercarz JA, Tran L, et al. Fibrosarcoma of the head and neck. The UCLA experience. Arch Otolaryngol Head Neck Surg 1991; 117:396.
9. Ingle A, Bindu R, Hayatnagarkar N, et al. Fibrosarcoma of breast. Indian J Pathol Microbiol 2004; 47:228.
10. Gatta G, Capocaccia R, Stiller C, et al. Childhood cancer survival trends in Europe: a EUROCARE working group study. J Clin Oncol 2005; 23:3742.
11. Odim J, Reehal V, Laks H, et al. Surgical pathology of cardiac tumors. Two decades at an urban institution. Cardiovasc Pathol 2003; 12:267.
12. Kelle S, Paetsch I, Neuss M, et al. Primary fibrosarcoma of the liver infiltrating the right atrium of the heart. Int J Cardiovasc Imaging 2005; 21:655.
13. Cai N, Kahn LB. A report of primary brain fibrosarcoma with literature review. J Neurooncol 2004; 68:161.
14. Lengle SJ, Hecht ST, Link DP, et al. Palliative embolization of fibrosarcoma for control of tumor-induced hypoglycemia. Cardiovasc Intervent Radiol 1995; 18:255.
15. Pack GT, Ariel IM. Fibrosarcoma of the soft somatic tissues; a clinical and pathologic study. Surgery 1952; 31:443.

Immunohistochemical and ultrastructural findings

16. Eyden B. Fibroblast phenotype plasticity: relevance for understanding heterogeneity in

"fibroblastic" tumors. Ultrastruct Pathol 2004; 28:307.
17. Suh CH, Ordonez NG, Mackay B. Fibrosarcoma: observations on the ultrastructure. Ultrastruct Pathol 1993; 17:221.

Clinical behavior

18. MacKenzie DH. Fibroma: a dangerous diagnosis. A review of 205 cases of fibrosarcoma of soft tissues. Br J Surg 1964; 51:607.
19. Castro EB, Hajdu SI, Fortner JG. Surgical therapy of fibrosarcoma of extremities: a reappraisal. Arch Surg 1973; 107:284.
20. Broders AC, Hargrave R, Meyerding HW. Pathological features of soft tissue fibrosarcoma: with special reference to the grading of its malignancy. Surg Gynecol Obstet 1939; 69:267.
21. Bizer LS. Fibrosarcoma. Report of sixty-four cases. Am J Surg 1971; 121:586.

Discussion

22. Dal Cin P, Pauwels P, Sciot R, et al. Multiple chromosome rearrangements in a fibrosarcoma. Cancer Genet Cytogenet 1996; 87:176.
23. Limon J, Szadowska A, Iliszko M, et al. Recurrent chromosome changes in two adult fibrosarcomas. Genes Chromosomes Cancer 1998; 21:119.
24. Delpla PA, Rouge D, Durroux R, et al. Soft tissue tumors following traumatic injury: two observations of interest for the medicolegal

causality. Am J Forensic Med Pathol 1998; 19:152.

25. Stout AP. Fibrosarcoma: the malignant tumor of fibroblasts. Cancer 1948; 1:30.

26. Ivins JC, Dockerty MB, Ghormley RK. Fibrosarcoma of the soft tissues of the extremities; a review of 78 cases. Surgery 1950; 28:495.

27. Denham RH, Dingley F. Fibrosarcoma occurring in a draining sinus. J Bone Joint Surg 1963; 45:384.

28. Burns WA, Kanhouwa S, Tillman L, et al. Fibrosarcoma occurring at the site of a plastic vascular graft. Cancer 1972; 29:66.

29. O'Connell TX, Fee HJ, Golding A. Sarcoma associated with Dacron prosthetic material: case report and review of the literature. J Thorac Cardiovasc Surg 1976; 72:94.

30. Eckstein FS, Vogel U, Mohr W. Fibrosarcoma in association with a total knee joint prosthesis. Virchows Arch A Pathol Anat Histopathol 1992; 421:175.

Fibrosarcoma variants

31. Meis-Kindblom JM, Kindblom LG, Enzinger FM. Sclerosing epithelioid fibrosarcoma: a variant of fibrosarcoma simulating carcinoma. Am J Surg Pathol 1995; 19:979.

32. Antonescu CR, Baren A. Spectrum of low-grade fibrosarcomas: a comparative ultrastructural analysis of low-grade myxofibrosarcoma and fibromyxoid sarcoma. Ultrastruct Pathol 2004; 28:321.

33. Battiata AP, Casler J. Sclerosing epithelioid fibrosarcoma: a case report. Ann Otol Rhinol Laryngol 2005; 114:87.

34. Watanabe K, Suzuki T. Epithelioid fibrosarcoma of the ovary. Virchows Arch 2004; 445:410.

35. Jiao YF, Nakamura S, Sugai T, et al. Overexpression of MDM2 in a sclerosing epithelioid fibrosarcoma: genetic, immunohistochemical and ultrastructural study of a case. Pathol Int 2002; 52:135.

36. Arya M, Garcia-Montes F, Patel HR, et al. A rare tumour in the pelvis presenting with lower urinary symptoms: "sclerosing epithelioid fibrosarcoma". Eur J Surg Oncol 2001; 27:121.

37. Bilsky MH, Schefler AC, Sandberg DI, et al. Sclerosing epithelioid fibrosarcomas involving the neuraxis: report of three cases. Neurosurgery 2000; 47:956.

38. Chow LT, Lui YH, Kumta SM, et al. Primary sclerosing epithelioid fibrosarcoma of the sacrum: a case report and review of the literature. J Clin Pathol 2004; 57:90.

39. Abdulkader I, Cameselle-Teijeiro J, Fraga M, et al. Sclerosing epithelioid fibrosarcoma primary of the bone. Int J Surg Pathol 2002; 10:227.

40. Antonescu CR, Rosenblum MK, Pereira P, et al. Sclerosing epithelioid fibrosarcoma: a study of 16 cases and confirmation of a clinicopathologically distinct tumor. Am J Surg Pathol 2001; 25:699.

41. Donner LR, Clawson K, Dobin SM. Sclerosing epithelioid fibrosarcoma: a cytogenetic, immunohistochemical, and ultrastructural study of an unusual histological variant. Cancer Genet Cytogenet 2000; 119:127.

42. Hindermann W, Katenkamp D. Sclerosing epithelioid fibrosarcoma. Pathologe 2003; 24:103.

43. Eyden BP, Manson C, Banerjee SS, et al. Sclerosing epithelioid fibrosarcoma: a study of five cases emphasizing diagnostic criteria. Histopathology 1998; 33:354.

44. Reid R, Barrett A, Hamblen DL. Sclerosing epithelioid fibrosarcoma. Histopathology 1996; 28:451.

45. Hanson IM, Pearson JM, Eyden BP, et al. Evidence of nerve sheath differentiation and high grade morphology in sclerosing epithelioid fibrosarcoma. J Clin Pathol 2001; 54:721.

46. Gisselsson D, Andreasson P, Meis-Kindblom JM, et al. Amplification of 12q13 and 12q15 sequences in a sclerosing epithelioid fibrosarcoma. Cancer Genet Cytogenet 1998; 107:102.

47. Folpe AL, McKenney JK, Bridge JA, et al. Sclerosing rhabdomyosarcoma in adults: report of four cases of a hyalinizing, matrix-rich variant of rhabdomyosarcoma that may be confused with osteosarcoma, chondrosarcoma, or angiosarcoma. Am J Surg Pathol 2002; 26:1175.

48. Angervall L, Kindblom LG, Merck C. Myxofibrosarcoma. A study of 30 cases. Acta Pathol Microbiol Scand [A] 1977; 85A:127.

49. Mentzel T, Calonje E, Wadden C, et al. Myxofibrosarcoma. clinicopathologic analysis of 75 cases with emphasis on the low-grade variant. Am J Surg Pathol 1996; 20:391.

50. Fukunaga M, Fukunaga N. Low-grade myxofibrosarcoma: progression in recurrence. Pathol Int 1997; 47:161.

51. Merck C, Angervall L, Kindblom LG, et al. Myxofibrosarcoma. A malignant soft tissue tumor of fibroblastic-histiocytic origin. A clinicopathologic and prognostic study of 110 cases using multivariate analysis. Acta Pathol Microbiol Immunol Scand Suppl 1983; 282:1.

52. Weiss SW, Enzinger FM. Myxoid variant of malignant fibrous histiocytoma. Cancer 1977; 39:1672.

53. Fujimura T, Okuyama R, Terui T, et al. Myxofibrosarcoma (myxoid malignant fibrous histiocytoma) showing cutaneous presentation: report of two cases. J Cutan Pathol 2005; 32:512.

54. Denschlag D, Kontny U, Tempfer C, et al. Low-grade myxofibrosarcoma of the vulva in a 15-year-old adolescent: a case report. Int J Surg Pathol 2005; 13:117.

55. Song HK, Miller JI. Primary myxofibrosarcoma of the esophagus. J Thorac Cardiovasc Surg 2002; 124:196.

56. Orosz Z, Rohonyi B, Luksander A, et al. Pleomorphic liposarcoma of a young woman following radiotherapy for epithelioid sarcoma. Pathol Oncol Res 2000; 6:287.

57. Huang HY, Brennan MF, Singer S, et al. Distant metastasis in retroperitoneal dedifferentiated liposarcoma is rare and rapidly fatal: a clinicopathological study with emphasis on the low-grade myxofibrosarcoma-like pattern as an early sign of dedifferentiation. Mod Pathol 2005; 18:976.

58. Hisaoka M, Morimitsu Y, Hashimoto H, et al. Retroperitoneal liposarcoma with combined well-differentiated and myxoid malignant fibrous histiocytoma-like myxoid areas. Am J Surg Pathol 1999; 23:1480.

59. Hasegawa T, Seki K, Hasegawa F, et al. Dedifferentiated liposarcoma of retroperitoneum and mesentery: varied growth patterns and histological grades – a clinicopathologic study of 32 cases. Hum Pathol 2000; 31:717.

59a. Nascimento A, Bertoni F, Fletcher CDM. Epithelioid variant of myxofibrosarcoma: expanding the clinicopathologic spectrum of myxofibrosarcoma in a series of 17 cases. Am J Surg Pathol 2007; 31:99.

60. Meloni-Ehrig AM, Chen Z, Guan XY, et al. Identification of a ring chromosome in a myxoid malignant fibrous histiocytoma with chromosome microdissection and fluorescence in situ hybridization. Cancer Genet Cytogenet 1999; 109:81.

61. Simons A, Schepens M, Jeuken J, et al. Frequent loss of 9p21 (p16(INK4A)) and other genomic imbalances in human malignant fibrous histiocytoma. Cancer Genet Cytogenet 2000; 118:89.

62. Sawyer JR, Binz RL, Gilliland JC, et al. A novel reciprocal (10;17)(p11.2;q23) in myxoid

fibrosarcoma. Cancer Genet Cytogenet 2001; 124:144.

63. Clawson K, Donner LR, Dobin SM. Translocation (2;15)(p23;q21.2) and interstitial deletion of 7q in a case of low-grade myxofibrosarcoma. Cancer Genet Cytogenet 2001; 127:140.

64. Willems SM, Debiec-Rychter M, Szuhai K, et al. Local recurrence of myxofibrosarcoma is associated with increase in tumour grade and cytogenetic aberrations, suggesting a multistep tumour progression model. Mod Pathol 2006; 19:407.

65. Huang HY, Lal P, Qin J, et al. Low-grade myxofibrosarcoma: a clinicopathologic analysis of 49 cases treated at a single institution with simultaneous assessment of the efficacy of 3-tier and 4-tier grading systems. Hum Pathol 2004; 35:612.

66. Evans HL. Low-grade fibromyxoid sarcoma. A report of two metastasizing neoplasms having a deceptively benign appearance. Am J Clin Pathol 1987; 88:615.

67. Lane KL, Shannon RJ, Weiss SW. Hyalinizing spindle cell tumor with giant rosettes: a distinctive tumor closely resembling low-grade fibromyxoid sarcoma. Am J Surg Pathol 1997; 21:1481.

68. Chang E, Lee A, Lee E, et al. Hyalinizing spindle cell tumor with giant rosettes with pulmonary metastasis after a long hiatus: a case report. J Korean Med Sci 2004; 19:619.

69. O'Sullivan MJ, Sirgi KE, Dehner LP. Low-grade fibrosarcoma (hyalinizing spindle cell tumor with giant rosettes) with pulmonary metastases at presentation: case report and review of the literature. Int J Surg Pathol 2002; 10:211.

70. Woodruff JM, Antonescu CR, Erlandson RA, et al. Low-grade fibrosarcoma with palisaded granulomalike bodies (giant rosettes): report of a case that metastasized. Am J Surg Pathol 1999; 23:1423.

71. Folpe AL, Lane KL, Paull G, et al. Low-grade fibromyxoid sarcoma and hyalinizing spindle cell tumor with giant rosettes: a clinicopathologic study of 73 cases supporting their identity and assessing the impact of high-grade areas. Am J Surg Pathol 2000; 24:1353.

72. Goodlad JR, Mentzel T, Fletcher CD. Low-grade fibromyxoid sarcoma: clinicopathological analysis of eleven new cases in support of a distinct entity. Histopathology 1995; 26:229.

73. Evans HL. Low-grade fibromyxoid sarcoma. A report of 12 cases. Am J Surg Pathol 1993; 17:595.

74. Takanami I, Takeuchi K, Naruke M. Low-grade fibromyxoid sarcoma arising in the mediastinum. J Thorac Cardiovasc Surg 1999; 118:970.

75. Rando G, Buonuomo V, D'Urzo C, et al. Fibromyxoid sarcoma in a 4-year-old boy: case report and review of the literature. Pediatr Surg Int 2005; 21:311.

76. Galetta D, Cesario A, Margaritora S, et al. Primary mediastinal hyalinizing spindle cell tumor with giant rosettes. Ann Thorac Surg 2004; 77:2206.

77. Fras AP, Frkovic-Grazio S. Hyalinizing spindle cell tumor with giant rosettes of the broad ligament. Gynecol Oncol 2001; 83:405.

78. Koishi A, Gomibuchi H, Inoue J, et al. Hyalinizing spindle cell tumor with giant rosettes of the omentum. J Obstet Gynaecol Res 2003; 29:388.

79. Billings SD, Giblen G, Fanburg-Smith JC. Superficial low-grade fibromyxoid sarcoma (Evans tumor): a clinicopathologic analysis of 19 cases with a unique observation in the pediatric population. Am J Surg Pathol 2005; 29:204.

80. Shidham VB, Ayala GE, Lahaniatis JE, et al. Low-grade fibromyxoid sarcoma: clinicopathologic case report with review of the literature. Am J Clin Oncol 1999; 22:150.

81. Zamecnik M, Michal M. Low-grade fibromyxoid sarcoma: a report of eight cases with histologic, immunohistochemical, and ultrastructural study. Ann Diagn Pathol 2000; 4:207.

82. Dvornik G, Barbareschi M, Gallotta P, et al. Low grade fibromyxoid sarcoma. Histopathology 1997; 30:274.

83. Scolyer RA, McCarthy SW, Wills EJ, et al. Hyalinizing spindle cell tumour with giant rosettes: report of a case with unusual features including original histological and ultrastructural observations. Pathology 2001; 33:101.

84. Nielsen GP, Selig MK, O'Connell JX, et al. Hyalinizing spindle cell tumor with giant rosettes: a report of three cases with ultrastructural analysis. Am J Surg Pathol 1999; 23:1227.

85. Franchi A, Massi D, Santucci M. Hyalinizing spindle cell tumor with giant rosettes and low-grade fibromyxoid sarcoma: an immunohistochemical and ultrastructural comparative investigation. Ultrastruct Pathol 2003; 27:349.

86. de Pinieux G, Anract P, le Charpentier M, et al. A case of hyalinizing spindle cell tumor with giant rosettes in the presacral region. Immunohistochemical and ultrastructural study. Ann Pathol 1998; 18:488.

87. Dobashi Y, Noguchi T, Nasuno S, et al. Hyalinizing spindle cell tumor with giant rosettes: report of a case showing remarkable myofibroblastic differentiation. Pathol Res Pract 2001; 197:691.

88. Mezzelani A, Sozzi G, Nessling M, et al. Low-grade fibromyxoid sarcoma. A further low-grade soft tissue malignancy characterized by a ring chromosome. Cancer Genet Cytogenet 2000; 122:144.

89. Storlazzi CT, Mertens F, Nascimento A, et al. Fusion of the FUS and BBF2H7 genes in low grade fibromyxoid sarcoma. Hum Mol Genet 2003; 12:2349.

90. Panagopoulos I, Storlazzi CT, Fletcher CD, et al. The chimeric FUS/CREB3l2 gene is specific for low-grade fibromyxoid sarcoma. Genes Chromosomes Cancer 2004; 40:218.

91. Reid R, de Silva MV, Paterson L, et al. Low-grade fibromyxoid sarcoma and hyalinizing spindle cell tumor with giant rosettes share a common t(7;16)(q34;p11) translocation. Am J Surg Pathol 2003; 27:1229.

92. Mertens F, Fletcher CD, Antonescu CR, et al. Clinicopathologic and molecular genetic characterization of low-grade fibromyxoid sarcoma, and cloning of a novel FUS/CREB3L1 fusion gene. Lab Invest 2005; 85:408.

92a. Matsuyama A, Hisaoka M, Shimajiri S, et al. Molecular detection of FUS-CREB3L2 fusion transcripts in low-grade fibromyxoid sarcoma using formalin-fixed, paraffin-embedded tissue specimens. Am J Surg Pathol 2006; 30:1077.

93. Nielsen GP, O'Connell JX, Rosenberg AE. Intramuscular myxoma: a clinicopathologic study of 51 cases with emphasis on hypercellular and hypervascular variants. Am J Surg Pathol 1998; 22:1222.

94. Oda Y, Takahira T, Kawaguchi K, et al. Low-grade fibromyxoid sarcoma versus low-grade myxofibrosarcoma in the extremities and trunk. A comparison of clinicopathological and immunohistochemical features. Histopathology 2004; 45:29.

95. Goldblum JR, Beals TF, Weiss SW. Neuroblastoma-like neurilemoma. Am J Surg Pathol 1994; 18:266.

96. Kim H, Park C, Lee YB, et al. Case report 643: osteosarcoma of ribs with giant rosettoid structures. Skeletal Radiol 1990; 19:609.

97. Bejarano PA, Padhya TA, Smith R, et al. Hyalinizing spindle cell tumor with giant rosettes – a soft tissue tumor with mesenchymal and neuroendocrine features. An immunohistochemical, ultrastructural, and cytogenetic analysis. Arch Pathol Lab Med 2000; 124:1179.

98. Farinha P, Oliveira P, Soares J. Metastasizing hyalinizing spindle cell tumour with giant rosettes: report of a case with long survival. Histopathology 2000; 36:92.

Postradiation fibrosarcoma

99. Gnanalingham KK, Chakraborty A, Galloway M, et al. Osteosarcoma and fibrosarcoma caused by postoperative radiotherapy for a pituitary adenoma. Case report. J Neurosurg 2002; 96:960.

100. Kirova YM, Vilcoq JR, Asselain B, et al. Radiation-induced sarcomas after radiotherapy for breast carcinoma: a large-scale single-institution review. Cancer 2005; 104:856.

101. Thijssens KM, van Ginkel RJ, Suurmeijer AJ, et al. Radiation-induced sarcoma: a challenge for the surgeon. Ann Surg Oncol 2005; 12:237.

102. Aydin F, Ghatak NR, Leshner RT. Possible radiation-induced dural fibrosarcoma with an unusually short latent period: case report. Neurosurgery 1995; 36:591.

103. Ito T, Seyama T, Iwamoto KS, et al. In vitro irradiation is able to cause RET oncogene rearrangement. Cancer Res 1993; 53:2940.

Fibrosarcoma arising in burn scars

104. Ozyazgan I, Kontas O. Burn scar sarcoma. Burns 1999; 25:455.

105. Giblin T, Pickrell K, Pitts Wea. Malignant degeneration in burn scars: Marjolin's ulcer. Ann Surg 1965; 162:291.

Myofibrosarcoma (myofibroblastic sarcoma)

106. Schürch W, Seemayer TA, Gabbiani G. The myofibroblast: a quarter century after its discovery. Am J Surg Pathol 1998; 22:141.

107. Lagace R, Seemayer TA, Gabbiani G, et al. Myofibroblastic sarcoma. Am J Surg Pathol 1999; 23:1432.

108. Mentzel T, Dry S, Katenkamp D, et al. Low-grade myofibroblastic sarcoma: analysis of 18 cases in the spectrum of myofibroblastic tumors. Am J Surg Pathol 1998; 22:1228.

109. Fisher C. Myofibrosarcoma. Virchows Arch 2004; 445:215.

110. Fisher C. Myofibroblastic malignancies. Adv Anat Pathol 2004; 11:190.

111. Watanabe K, Ogura G. Fibronexus in "malignant fibrous histiocytoma" of the bone: a case report of pleomorphic myofibrosarcoma. Ultrastruct Pathol 2002; 26:47.

112. Montgomery E, Goldblum JR, Fisher C. Myofibrosarcoma: a clinicopathologic study. Am J Surg Pathol 2001; 25:219.

113. McLaughlin SA, Schmitt TM, Huguet KL, et al. Myofibrosarcoma of the adrenal gland. Am Surg 2005; 71:191.

114. Gocht A, Bosmuller HC, Bassler R, et al. Breast tumors with myofibroblastic differentiation: clinico-pathological observations in myofibroblastoma and myofibrosarcoma. Pathol Res Pract 1999; 195:1.

115. Taccagni G, Rovere E, Masullo M, et al. Myofibrosarcoma of the breast: review of the literature on myofibroblastic tumors and criteria for defining myofibroblastic differentiation. Am J Surg Pathol 1997; 21:489.

116. Eyden B. The myofibroblast: a study of normal, reactive and neoplastic tissues, with an emphasis on ultrastructure. Part 2—Tumours and tumour-like lesions. J Submicrosc Cytol Pathol 2005; 37:231.

117. Fletcher CD, Dal Cin P, de Wever I, et al. Correlation between clinicopathological features and karyotype in spindle cell sarcomas. A report of 130 cases from the CHAMP study group. Am J Pathol 1999; 154:1841.

118. Watanabe K, Ogura G, Tajino T, et al. Myofibrosarcoma of the bone: a clinicopathologic study. Am J Surg Pathol 2001; 25:1501.

119. Keller C, Gibbs CN, Kelly SM, et al. Low-grade myofibrosarcoma of the head and neck: importance of surgical therapy. J Pediatr Hematol Oncol 2004; 26:119.

120. Chiller K, Parker D, Washington C. Myofibrosarcoma treated with Mohs micrographic surgery. Dermatol Surg 2004; 30:1565.

BENIGN FIBROHISTIOCYTIC TUMORS

CHAPTER CONTENTS

The concept of fibrohistiocytic neoplasms has been challenged largely because the malignant forms (i.e., malignant fibrous histiocytoma) consistently lack histiocytic features and because some, but not all, when carefully studied, show a subtle degree of differentiation. Nonetheless, many benign fibrohistiocytic lesions are, in fact, truly derived from histiocytes (e.g., juvenile xanthogranuloma, xanthoma), and, for this reason, there remains some merit in retaining this category. This has been recently endorsed by the World Health Organization[1] recognizing that use of the term "fibrohistiocytic" is descriptive and merely denotes a lesion composed of cells that resemble normal histiocytes and fibroblasts.

Benign fibrohistiocytic tumors, however, are a pathogenetically diverse group of lesions. Xanthoma is a "pseudotumor" which usually arises in response to a disturbance in serum lipids. The preponderance of evidence suggests fibrous histiocytoma is a true neoplasm with a definite growth potential but a limited capacity for aggressive behavior. Between these extremes are lesions of an indeterminate nature, exemplified by juvenile xanthogranuloma. Although juvenile xanthogranuloma resembles a tumor morphologically, it usually regresses with time, thereby raising the question of its proper position in the spectrum between hyperplasia and neoplasia. The present classification represents a practical, rather than a conceptual, approach aimed at defining differences among several histologically similar lesions (Table 12–1).

TABLE 12–1	CLASSIFICATION OF HISTIOCYTIC SYNDROMES IN CHILDREN

Class I: Langerhans cell histiocytosis
Forms of histiocytosis X (including eosinophilic granuloma and Hand-Schüller-Christian disease, among others)

Class II: mononuclear phagocytes other than Langerhans cells
Hemophagocytic lymphohistiocytosis
Infection-associated hemophagocytic syndrome
Sinus histiocytosis with massive lymphadenopathy
Juvenile xanthogranuloma
Reticulohistiocytoma

Class III: malignant histiocytic disorders
Acute monocytic leukemia
Malignant histiocytosis
True histiocytic lymphomas

Data are from the Writing Group of the Histiocyte Society.[87]

FIBROUS HISTIOCYTOMA

Fibrous histiocytoma is a neoplastic or quasi-neoplastic lesion composed of a mixture of fibroblastic and histiocytic cells that are arranged in sheets or short fascicles and that are accompanied by varying numbers of inflammatory cells, foam cells, and siderophages. Most commonly this tumor occurs in the dermis and superficial subcutis, and rarely in deep soft tissues. When located in the skin, fibrous histiocytoma is also referred to as dermatofibroma.[2,3] In this chapter we use the all-inclusive term "fibrous histiocytoma" to refer to lesions of the dermis and soft tissue. The terms histiocytoma cutis, nodular subepidermal fibrosis, and sclerosing hemangiomas, once used as synonyms for fibrous histiocytomas, are now archaic.

Clinical findings

Cutaneous fibrous histiocytoma is a solitary, slowly growing nodule that usually makes its appearance during early or mid-adult life. A subset occurs following minor trauma or insect bites. Although any part of the skin surface may be affected, it is most common on the extremities.[4] Roughly one-third of these tumors are multiple and present metachronously. Synchronous development can occur in the setting of immunosuppression, particularly systemic lupus erythematosus[5] but is not associated with human herpesvirus 8 (HHV8),[6] as has been demonstrated for other multifocal tumors such as Kaposi's sarcoma. Cutaneous fibrous histiocytomas are elevated or pedunculated lesions measuring from a few millimeters to a few centimeters in diameter (Figs 12–1 to 12–3). Rarely, they result in a depressed area in the skin ("atrophic dermatofibroma").[7] They impart a red to red-brown to blue-black color to the overlying skin. Although usually ascribed to the presence of hemosi-

derin, epidermal hyperpigmentation has recently been attributed to lesional expression of stem cell factor and an increase in tyrosinase-positive melanocytes.[8] Such lesions may be confused clinically with malignant melanoma. The presence of a central dimple on lateral compression is regarded as a useful clinical sign for distinguishing it from melanoma.[9] Deeply situated fibrous histiocytomas are less common than cutaneous ones. The relative incidence is difficult to determine because the latter are less likely to be subjected to biopsy or excised than the former. In a study by Fletcher,[10] only three cases of fibrous histiocytoma involving skeletal muscle were culled from more than 1000 fibrohistiocytic tumors. Like their cutaneous counterparts, they present as painless

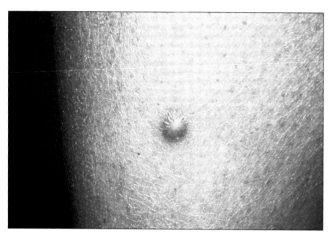

FIGURE 12–1 Red nodular appearance of a benign fibrous histiocytoma. (Case courtesy of Dr. John T. Headington.)

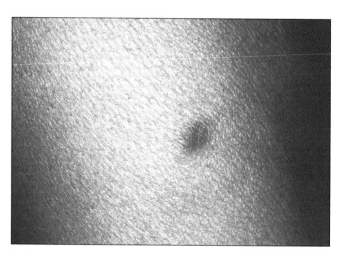

FIGURE 12–2 Benign fibrous histiocytoma with a pigmented appearance. (Case courtesy of Dr. John T. Headington.)

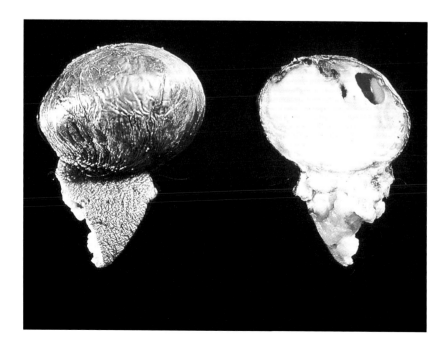

FIGURE 12–3 Gross appearance of a pedunculated cutaneous fibrous histiocytoma. The light color of the lesion is a result of the presence of large amounts of lipid. Focal cyst formation is also present.

masses, usually on an extremity. Although they develop at any age, most occur between the ages of 20 and 40 years. They tend to be larger than the cutaneous tumors. Nearly half of these tumors are 5 cm or more when excised, in contrast to most cutaneous fibrous histiocytomas, which are less than 3 cm, in our experience. Grossly, they are circumscribed, yellow or white masses that may have focal areas of hemorrhage.

Microscopic findings

The cutaneous fibrous histiocytoma consists of a nodular cellular proliferation involving dermis and occasionally subcutis (Fig. 12–4). The tumor is not sharply defined (Fig. 12–5) laterally and typically interdigitates with dermal collagen ("collagen trapping"). The overlying epidermis frequently shows some degree of hyperplasia including acanthosis or elongation and widening of the rete pegs (Fig. 12–6). The presence of a rim of normal dermis between epidermis and tumor is variable. At the deep margin, the tumor extends small tentacles for short distances into the subcutis (Fig. 12–7) or, less commonly, has a smoothly contoured margin (Fig. 12–8). Both types contrast with the deeply penetrating border of dermatofibrosarcoma protuberans. Most cutaneous fibrous histiocytomas consist of short, intersecting fascicles of fibroblastic cells (Figs 12–9 to 12–15). The fascicles usually form a loose crisscross pattern or a vague storiform pattern (Fig. 12–9). Occasional rounded "histiocytic" cells accompany the spindle cells, but they rarely

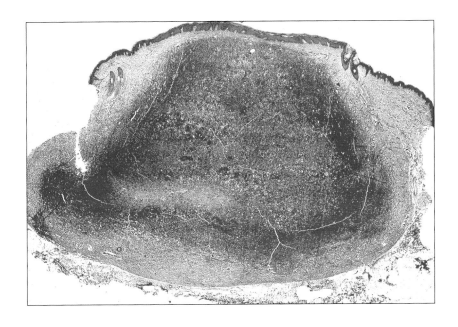

FIGURE 12–4 Low-power view of a cutaneous fibrous histiocytoma. The lesion is confined to the dermis and has a smooth, bulging deep margin.

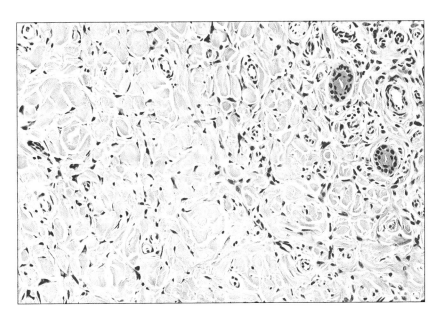

FIGURE 12–5 Lateral border of a fibrous histiocytoma illustrating entrapment of collagen.

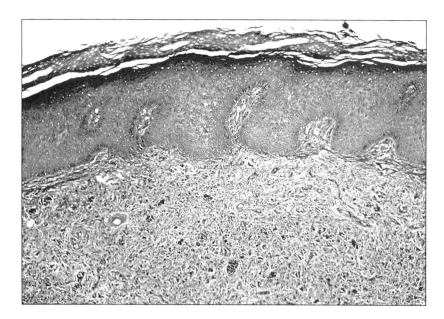

FIGURE 12–6 Epithelial hyperplasia overlying a fibrous histiocytoma.

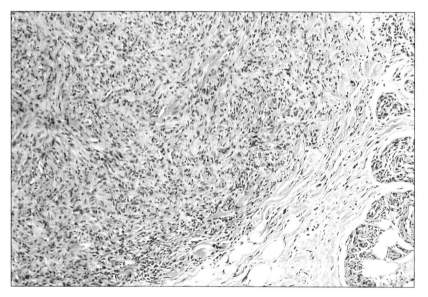

FIGURE 12–7 Smoothly contoured deep border of a fibrous histiocytoma.

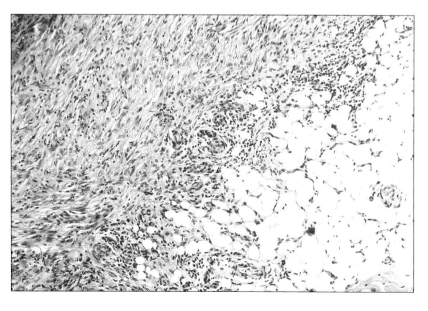

FIGURE 12–8 Minimal irregular penetration of the subcutis at the deep border of a fibrous histiocytoma contrasts with the more infiltrative border of dermatofibrosarcoma protuberans.

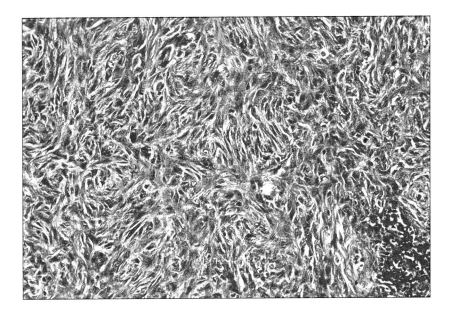

FIGURE 12–9 Fibrous histiocytoma with a predominantly spindled appearance.

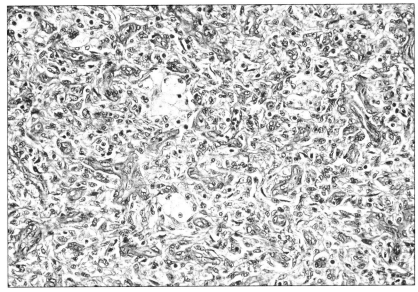

FIGURE 12–10 Fibrous histiocytoma with a mixture of spindled and xanthomatous cells.

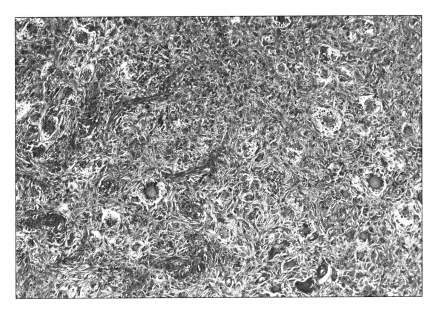

FIGURE 12–11 Fibrous histiocytoma with numerous Touton giant cells.

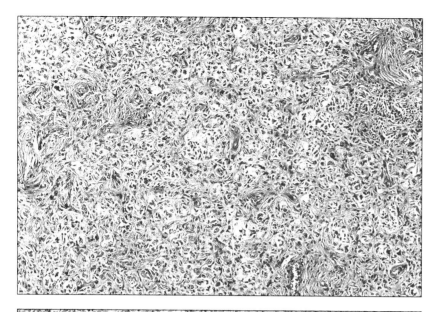

FIGURE 12–12 Fibrous histiocytoma with a lipidized appearance and some nuclear atypia.

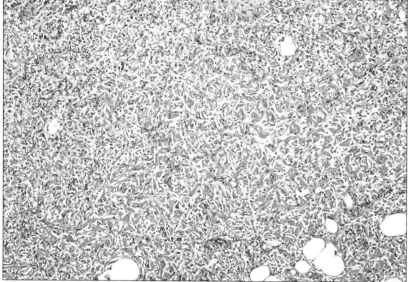

FIGURE 12–13 Fibrous histiocytoma with interstitial and perivascular hyalinization.

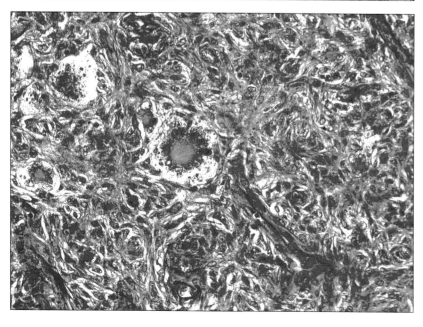

FIGURE 12–14 Touton giant cells containing lipid and hemosiderin.

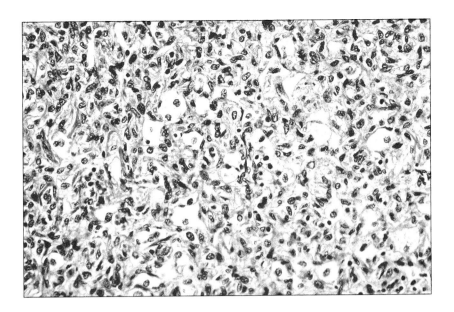

FIGURE 12–15 Xanthoma cells within fibrous histiocytoma.

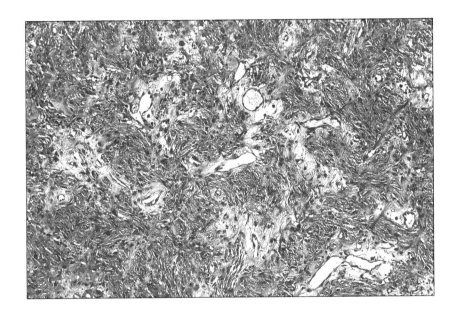

FIGURE 12–16 Fibrous histiocytoma of soft tissue. In contrast to cutaneous fibrous histiocytomas, these lesions have a more distinct storiform pattern but lack the variety of secondary elements such as xanthoma cells and siderophages.

predominate. Multinucleated giant cells of the foreign body or Touton type are a typical feature of this form of fibrous histiocytoma and often contain phagocytosed lipid and hemosiderin (Fig. 12–14). Inflammatory cells, particularly lymphocytes and xanthoma cells, are scattered randomly throughout the tumors but vary greatly in number. The stroma consists of a delicate collagen network surrounding individual cells. In a small number of cases, the vessels and stroma exhibit striking hyalinization (Figs 12–12, 12–13). Cystic areas of hemorrhage are common (see Figs 12–30 to 12–32) and, when prominent, result in large accumulations of hemosiderin in the tumor cells. When this feature is striking, some have employed the term "aneurysmal"[11–13] fibrous histiocytoma (see below). A number of other unusual features is

seen in these lesions, including clear-cell change, granular cell change, nuclear palisading, extensive hyalinization, and lipidization (see below). Recently, it was pointed out that fibrous histiocytomas occasionally evoke an unusual mesenchymal response around them, usually in the form of proliferation of mature smooth muscle.[14]

Deep fibrous histiocytomas are similar to their cutaneous counterparts, but they usually have a more prominent storiform pattern and fewer secondary elements such as xanthoma cells (Figs 12–16 to 12–18). The stroma often undergoes myxoid change (Fig. 12–17) or hyalinization. In unusual cases, dense bundles of collagen (amianthoid fibers) and even metaplastic osteoid are detected. Not infrequently, deep fibrous histiocytomas blend with areas indistinguishable from a benign hemangiopericy-

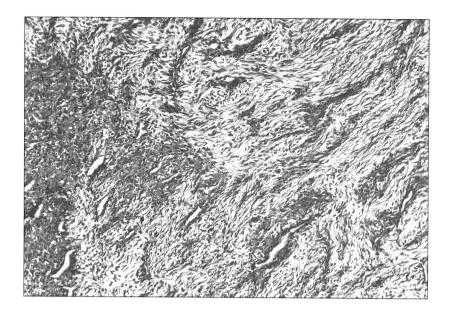

FIGURE 12-17 Fibrous histiocytoma of soft tissue with myxoid areas.

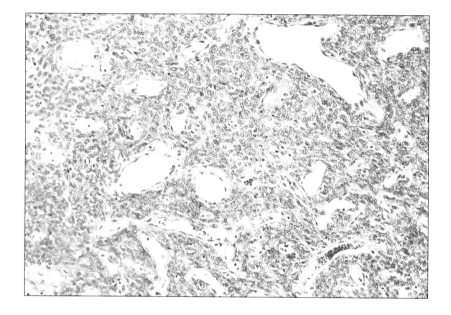

FIGURE 12-18 Hemangiopericytoma-like area within a fibrous histiocytoma of soft tissue.

toma (Fig. 12–18). This combination of hemangiopericytic and fibrohistiocytic areas is particularly characteristic of fibrous histiocytomas of the orbit.

The benign nature of fibrous histiocytoma is usually apparent histologically. The cells are well differentiated and exhibit little pleomorphism and usually little or no mitotic activity (Fig. 12–19). The occasional pleomorphic cells with hyperchromatic nuclei and clear to eosinophilic cytoplasm (Fig. 12–20), referred to by some as "monster cells,"[15] within an otherwise typical fibrous histiocytoma seem to be a degenerative phenomenon and do not affect the prognosis adversely.[15,16] However, the presence of both pleomorphism and mitotic activity suggests a more aggressive lesion, either atypical fibrous histiocytoma (see below) or superficial malignant fibrous

histiocytoma. A small subset of fibrous histiocytomas known as "cellular fibrous histiocytomas" is characterized by somewhat longer, cellular fascicles of spindle cells bereft of other cellular elements. Although benign, these lesions have a high local recurrence rate and are discussed below.

Immunohistochemical findings

The majority of fibrous histiocytomas displays immunostaining for factor XIIIa in a significant population of cells, leading some to conclude that these tumors arise from dermal dendrocytes[17] (Fig. 12–21). Whether factor XIIIa stains tumor elements or reactive dermal dendrocytes that populate benign fibrous histiocytomas is a

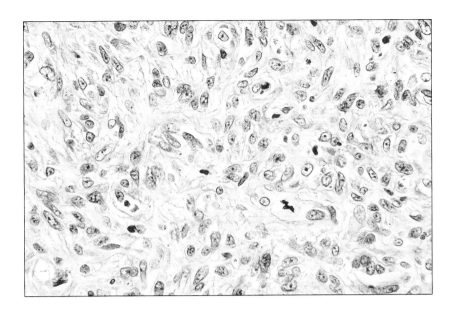

FIGURE 12–19 Plump spindle cells with benign fibrous histiocytoma displaying an occasional mitotic figure.

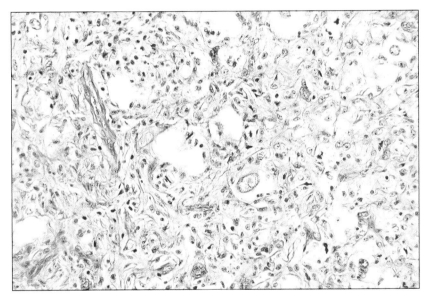

FIGURE 12–20 Pleomorphic (monster) cell within an otherwise benign fibrous histiocytoma of the skin.

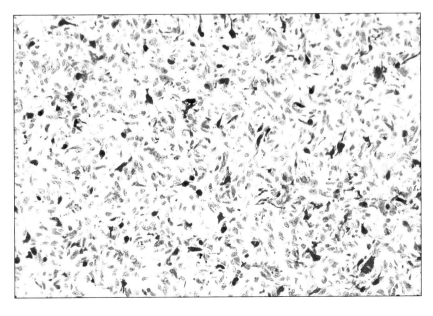

FIGURE 12–21 Factor XIIIa immunostain of a fibrous histiocytoma showing numerous positively staining dendritic cells.

matter of debate.[18] However, since factor XIIIa is present in many mesenchymal lesions, its presence per se is not diagnostic of fibrous histiocytomas and must be interpreted in the context of the case. The combination of factor XIIIa and CD34 is commonly used to distinguish benign fibrous histiocytoma from dermatofibrosarcoma protuberans, however (see Differential diagnosis). Myoid markers (e.g., desmin, smooth muscle myosin[19]) are occasionally present in fibrous histiocytomas and are significant only to call attention to the fact that their sporadic presence should not be construed as evidence of a smooth muscle neoplasm.

Electron microscopic studies have shown a spectrum of cell types in these tumors. Cells resembling fibroblasts represent one end of this spectrum. They contain organized lamellae of rough endoplasmic reticulum but few or no lipid droplets and no phagolysosomes.[20] Depending on the functional state of these cells, they may acquire features of myofibroblasts. The other end of the spectrum is represented by rounded cells resembling histiocytes with numerous cell processes, mitochondria, and phagolysosomes.

Differential diagnosis

Fibrous histiocytomas are most frequently confused with other benign lesions, notably nodular fasciitis, neurofibroma, and leiomyoma. Although *nodular fasciitis* may display a storiform pattern, it is distinguished from fibrous histiocytoma by its loosely arranged bundles of fibroblasts. Cellular areas containing proliferating fibroblasts alternate with loose myxoid zones containing extravasated red blood cells and inflammatory cells. The vasculature in fasciitis is seldom as orderly or as uniform as that of fibrous histiocytoma. Finally, because most cases of fasciitis are excised during the period of active growth, they usually manifest much more mitotic activity than a fibrous histiocytoma of comparable cellularity. In our experience it is difficult, if not impossible, to distinguish the early (cellular) phase of nodular fasciitis from a benign fibrous histiocytoma. Fortunately, from a practical point of view, this diagnostic imprecision has little adverse effect on patient care. The distinction between a fibrous histiocytoma and a *neurofibroma* is usually not difficult. Neurofibromas contain a population of Schwann cells expressing S-100 protein and having serpentine nuclei. Additional features of neural differentiation may include organoid structures reminiscent of sensory receptors or vague nuclear palisading. The usual lack of any storiform pattern or significant inflammation in the neurofibroma further underscores the difference between the two tumors. Sclerotic forms of *leiomyoma* may resemble a fibrous histiocytoma. However, smooth muscle tumors have a more distinct fascicular growth pattern. Their blunt-ended nuclei are plumper, and the cytoplasm typically has longitudinal striations corre-

sponding to the presence of myofilamentous material, which can be accentuated with Masson trichrome stain. They strongly express smooth muscle actin and muscle-specific actin in a diffuse pattern, unlike the focal immunoreactivity noted in benign fibrous histiocytomas reflective of myofibroblastic differentiation.

Most importantly, fibrous histiocytoma must be distinguished from dermatofibrosarcoma protuberans. Like fibrous histiocytoma, *dermatofibrosarcoma protuberans* occurs in the dermis and subcutis but typically displays extensive subcutaneous involvement in the form of long, penetrating tentacles of tumor. It is also characterized by a more uniform cellular population and lacks giant cells, inflammatory cells, and xanthomatous elements. Its fascicles, composed of slender attenuated cells, are longer and arranged in a distinct storiform pattern, unlike the short curlicue fascicles of fibrous histiocytoma. Its margins are infiltrative, in contrast to the better defined margins of fibrous histiocytoma. Immunostaining reveals distinct differences in the cellular composition of these tumors as well. Fibrous histiocytomas contain a significant population of factor XIIIa-positive cells. Usually CD34 is absent within lesional cells, although CD34-positive dendritic cells are sometimes observed at the periphery of a fibrous histiocytoma and presumably represent collections of normal dermal elements. Dermatofibrosarcoma protuberans, on the other hand, contains only scattered factor XIIIa-positive cells but, in striking contrast to benign fibrous histiocytoma, expresses CD34 in a significant portion of neoplastic cells (Fig. 12–22). The combination of these two stains, in our experience, has proved to be reasonably reliable for distinguishing these two lesions, which often cause diagnostic problems, particularly when only a superficial biopsy specimen is available for review. Recently, it has been suggested that immunostaining for HMGA1 and HMGA2, which are positive in fibrous histiocytomas and negative in dermatofibrosarcomas, provides discriminatory power equivalent to factor XIIIa and CD34.[21]

The difference between benign and frankly *malignant fibrous histiocytomas* is usually obvious because the latter is a pleomorphic, deeply situated tumor with numerous typical and atypical mitotic figures and prominent areas of hemorrhage and necrosis. Less obvious is the difference between this tumor and the *angiomatoid form of fibrous histiocytoma*. The latter is a tumor of childhood characterized by sheets of histiocytic cells interrupted by cystic areas of hemorrhage. They are surrounded by a dense cuff of lymphocytes and plasma cells but almost never have giant cells or xanthoma cells as does the fibrous histiocytoma.

Discussion

Whether benign fibrous histiocytomas are reactive or neoplastic is still debated. The most frequently cited argu-

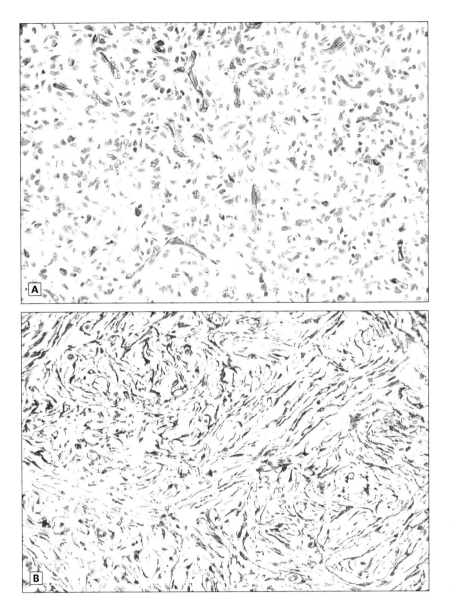

FIGURE 12–22 CD34 immunostains of benign fibrous histiocytoma and dermatofibrosarcoma protuberans. **(A)** CD34 immunostain of fibrous histiocytoma decorates normal vessels. **(B)** CD34 immunostain of a dermatofibrosarcoma protuberans in which the majority of tumor cells is decorated.

ments in favor of a reactive condition include the frequency with which minor trauma antedates the lesions, the accompanying inflammatory component, and the evolutionary stages of this disease. On the other hand, there is growing and reasonably compelling evidence that a least a subset are neoplastic. In general, benign fibrous histiocytomas do not involute and, in fact, are associated with a definable rate of local recurrence, and in exceptional instances, metastases. Clonality, furthermore, has been documented in 30–100% of cases examined.[22–25] There seems to be some preliminary evidence suggesting a correlation between clonality and the appearance of the fibrous histiocytoma. For example, in the study by Vanni et al.,[23] clonality was slightly more common in cellular as opposed to conventional fibrous histiocytomas and Hui et al. noted that histiocytic-appearing lesions were more often clonal.[25] The fact that the incidence of clonality varies from study to study and perhaps even amongst

the various types of fibrous histiocytoma lends credence to the idea that fibrous histiocytomas may be a heterogeneous group of lesions, only some of which are neoplastic.

Regardless of the above debate, generalizations can be made concerning behavior. Fewer than 5% of cutaneous fibrous histiocytomas recur following local excision.[3,18] In our unpublished experience, the overall recurrence rate of cutaneous and soft tissue fibrous histiocytomas is approximately 10% following conservative therapy. Those located in deep soft tissue have a recurrence rate that is somewhat higher and is reflective of the larger size and incompleteness of the surgical excision. In this regard, Franquemont et al.[26] reported a recurrence rate of nearly 50% for fibrous histiocytomas (eight cases) that extended into the subcutis or grew in a multinodular fashion (or both); and Font and Kidayat[27] noted that 57% of orbital fibrous histiocytomas with infiltrative margins or hypercellular zones (or both) recurred compared with 31% of those without these features. Mentzel et al. likewise have commented on the fact that facial fibrous histiocytomas, which frequently invade subcutis and muscle, have a high rate of recurrence.[28]

Nearly every histologic feature used to assess malignancy of tumors in general has been recorded in clinically benign fibrous histiocytomas as an isolated finding (i.e., increased cellularity,[29] necrosis,[10] vascular invasion,[3,10] mitotic activity, atypia[15,16]) and sometimes even in company with one another without adverse consequences. Therefore, it is important to recognize the underlying nature of the lesion to know what significance to place on many of these features. A useful guideline is that benign fibrous histiocytomas may show enhanced cellularity and some level of mitotic activity (e.g., cellular fibrous histiocytoma) and still be considered benign. Likewise, benign fibrous histiocytomas may display nuclear atypia on a degenerative basis in the form of large "monster cells" set amidst the typical backdrop of banal neoplastic cells. Such lesions also are clinically benign. The presence of both mitotic activity and atypia (especially atypical mitotic figures) in the same lesion should be a cause for concern and raise the question of the so-called "atypical fibrous histiocytomas" (see below) or more ominous lesions such as atypical fibroxanthoma or superficial malignant fibrous histiocytoma. Having said this, there are anecdotal examples of histologically benign fibrous histiocytomas that have produced metastases. Two cases were reported by Colome-Grimmer and Evans.[30] Both were small (2 cm) cutaneous lesions that recurred, producing regional lymph node (and ultimately pulmonary) metastasis. The metastases appeared similar to the primary lesions, and both patients were alive 4 and 8 years after resection of the pulmonary deposits. Guillou et al.[31] described three patients with fibrous histiocytomas of the aneurysmal, cellular, or atypical type who developed regional lymph node metastases but who had a protracted course and favorable outcome.[31] We, too, have seen an instance of pulmonary metastasis from a benign cutaneous fibrous histiocytoma in which the metastasis also appeared benign (Fig. 12–23). Fortunately, such cases are rare and should not alter the approach to patients with these tumors.

VARIANTS OF BENIGN FIBROUS HISTIOCYTOMA

There are a number of histologic variants of benign fibrous histiocytoma. With the exception of the cellular and epithelioid forms, these designations are of minor importance. Cellular fibrous histiocytoma appears to have a higher risk of local recurrence and often poses a diagnostic challenge to distinguish it from more aggressive lesions such as fibrosarcoma, whereas the epithelioid fibrous histiocytoma can be confused with tumors of melanocytic lineage.

Cellular fibrous histiocytoma

Cellular fibrous histiocytoma is a designation used for lesions characterized by increased cellularity and a more fascicular (and less storiform) growth pattern. Some cases of "dermatofibroma with subcutaneous extension"[32,33] and "dermatofibroma with potential for local recurrence"[26] are examples of this variant. Occurring in an age range and anatomic location similar to those for ordinary benign fibrous histiocytoma, these lesions are composed of a relatively monomorphic population of plump spindle cells arranged in longer fascicles with fewer inflammatory cells and giant cells (Figs 12–24, 12–25). In addition,

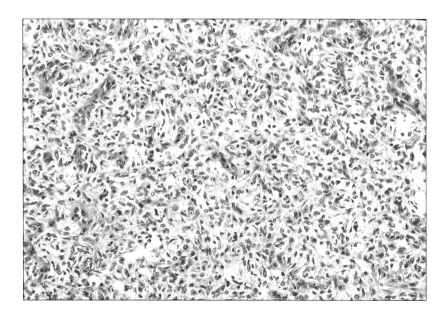

FIGURE 12–23 Benign fibrous histiocytoma that produced pulmonary metastasis.

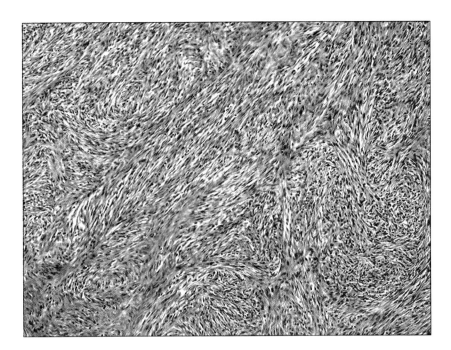

FIGURE 12–24 Cellular fibrous histiocytoma illustrating monomorphic spindle cells arranged in short and long fascicles.

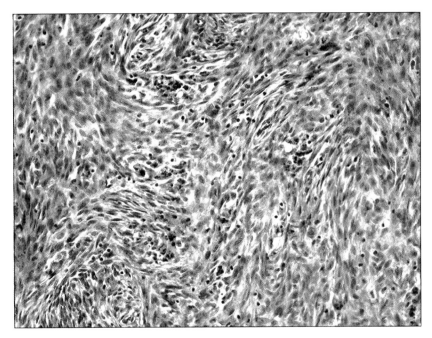

FIGURE 12–25 Cellular fibrous histiocytoma.

mitotic activity is usually somewhat higher (mean 3 mitoses/10 high-power fields [HPF]), and subcutaneous extension more common (30%), than in the usual fibrous histiocytoma. About 10% undergo spontaneous central necrosis. Although the local recurrence rate of 25% for this form of fibrous histiocytoma seemingly contrasts with that of the ordinary form, it has not been demonstrated that cellularity is an independent predictor of recurrence. The high incidence of extension into the subcutis by this form of fibrous histiocytoma suggests that this feature might be equally significant. Nonetheless, we believe it is still useful to recognize the cellular form of fibrous histiocytoma as a distinct variant, but we think it

is also important to comment on extensive subcutaneous extension when present in fibrous histiocytomas of the usual type as a possible predictor of recurrence. Recently, a distinct chromosomal translocation has been identified in this form of fibrous histiocytoma,[23] but it is not clear whether it uniquely identifies this variant or is a feature of all fibrous histiocytomas.

Epithelioid fibrous histiocytoma

Epithelioid fibrous histiocytoma is defined as a fibrous histiocytoma in which one-half or more of the cells assume a rounded epithelioid shape.[34-36] It presents as a solitary, red cutaneous nodule with an epidermal collarette similar to that of a pyogenic granuloma. The cells, large and polygonal with abundant eosinophilic cytoplasm, resemble those of a reticulohistiocytoma. Transitions to areas of conventional fibrous histiocytoma are frequent (Figs 12–26 to 12–28). Epithelioid fibrous histiocytoma contains a variable population of CD34-positive dermal fibroblasts and factor XIIIa-positive dendritic histiocytes which supports the idea that these tumors arise from the dermal microvascular unit.[37] The unusual appearance of this variant of fibrous histiocytoma often raises the possibility of a number of other lesions, Spitz nevus being a prime consideration. Epithelioid fibrous histiocytomas are S-100 protein negative, however.

Aneurysmal fibrous histiocytoma

Approximately 1–2% of benign fibrous histiocytomas undergo extensive cystic hemorrhage. Dubbed "aneurysmal fibrous histiocytomas," their significance resides in the fact that they can evolve rapidly as a result of spontaneous intralesional hemorrhage.[11–13,38] Their blue to black color suggests the clinical diagnosis of a vascular or melanocytic tumor. At low power, these lesions are seen to contain large blood-filled spaces lined by discohesive fragments of tumor rather than endothelium (Figs 12–29 to 12–32). Hemosiderin may be abundant, and mitotic activity is often noted in the immediate vicinity of the hemorrhage. A 20% recurrence rate has been reported for

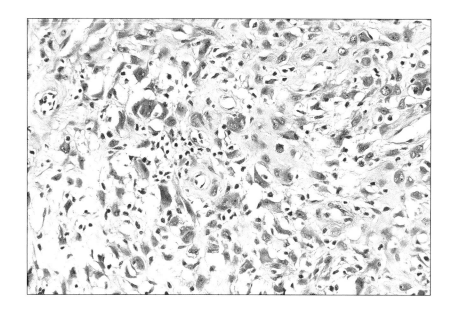

FIGURE 12–26 Epithelioid fibrous histiocytoma.

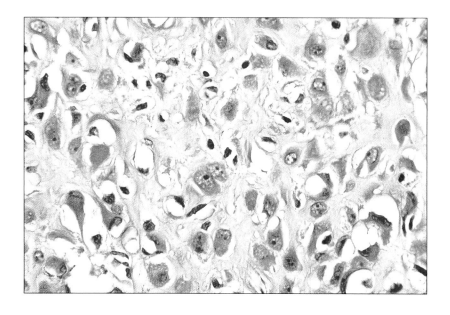

FIGURE 12–27 High-power view of an epithelioid fibrous histiocytoma.

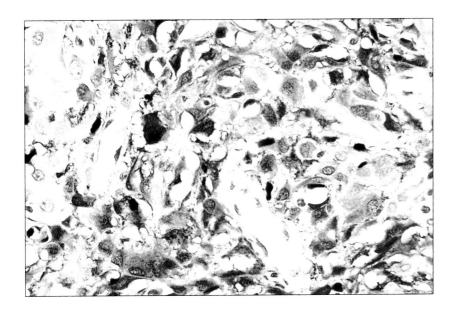

FIGURE 12–28 Factor XIIIa immunostain decorates cells of an epithelioid fibrous histiocytoma.

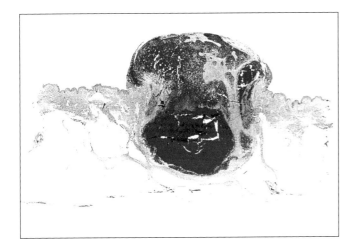

FIGURE 12–29 Aneurysmal fibrous histiocytoma.

these tumors, but there are too few cases to know if this is meaningful. Despite the similarity of names, the aneurysmal fibrous histiocytoma should be clearly distinguished from the angiomatoid (malignant) fibrous histiocytoma of childhood, a subcutaneous lesion often associated with systemic symptoms (see Chapter 13).

Minor histologic variants

There are a number of rare and minor variants of benign fibrous histiocytoma.[15,28,39–41] They are principally important in that they evoke a somewhat different list of diagnostic considerations. Zelger et al. described a *"clear cell dermatofibroma"* in which most of the cells underwent a translucent clear-cell change (Fig. 12–33).[42] This lesion must be distinguished from clear-cell carcinomas or melanocytic tumors involving the skin. The cells are positive for factor XIIIa but not for melanocytic antigens.

Lipidized (ankle-type) fibrous histiocytoma, typically a lesion of the lower leg, particularly ankle, is usually larger than the usual fibrous histiocytomas and is characterized by foamy histiocytes situated within a hyalinized collagenous or osteoid-like stromal backdrop (Fig. 12–34).[43] Fortuitous palisading of nuclei ("palisaded fibrous histiocytoma"[40]), extensive myxoid change ("myxoid dermatofibroma"[41]) and granular cell change have also been noted in fibrous histiocytomas.

ATYPICAL FIBROUS HISTIOCYTOMA

A very small number of fibrous histiocytomas have borderline histologic features that include significantly more atypia and mitotic activity than are encountered in the usual type. Kaddu et al. have recently coined the term "atypical fibrous histiocytomas" for these lesions.[44] They differ from atypical fibroxanthoma/superficial malignant fibrous histiocytomas in their predilection for younger individuals (mean 38 years) and in a distribution that favors the extremities as opposed to the sun-exposed surfaces of the face and neck. The average size is less than 2 cm. The majority are restricted to the dermis with superficial subcutaneous involvement in one-third of cases. In our opinion, the diagnosis of atypical fibrous histiocytoma needs to be made judiciously and should be applied *only to those cases in which there is a clear-cut background of classic fibrous histiocytoma* but which display areas of more generalized atypia than the occasional "monster cell" described above and increased mitotic activity, including atypical forms (Figs 12–35, 12–36). Follow-up information in 21 patients[44] followed for approximately 4 years disclosed local recurrences in three patients and distant metastases in two, one of whom died.

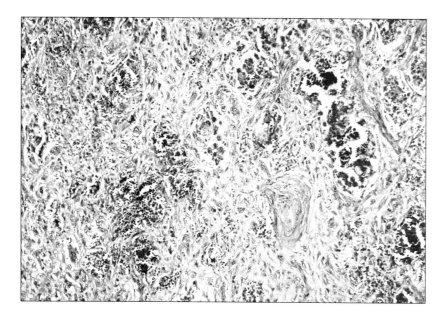

FIGURE 12-30 Cystic hemorrhage in an aneurysmal fibrous histiocytoma.

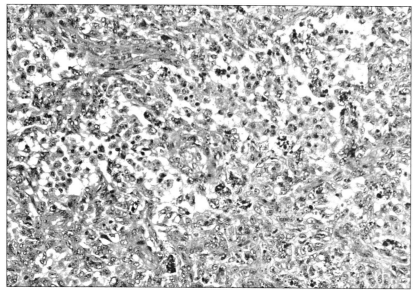

FIGURE 12-31 Hemosiderin deposits in an aneurysmal fibrous histiocytoma.

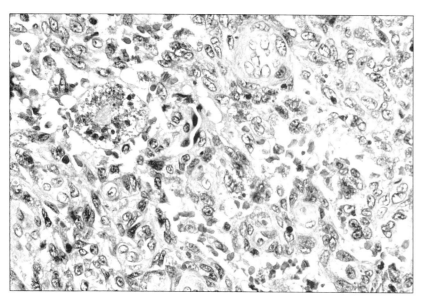

FIGURE 12-32 Hemosiderin deposits and cystic hemorrhage in an aneurysmal fibrous histiocytoma.

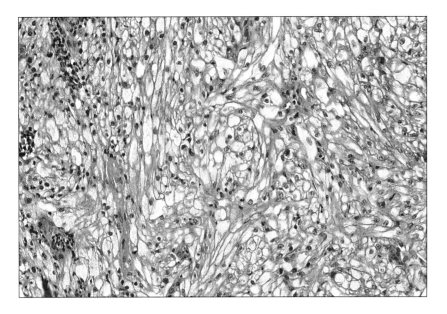

FIGURE 12–33 Clear-cell fibrous histiocytoma (dermatofibroma).

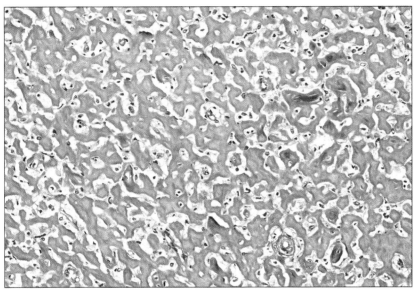

FIGURE 12–34 Lipidized fibrous histiocytoma.

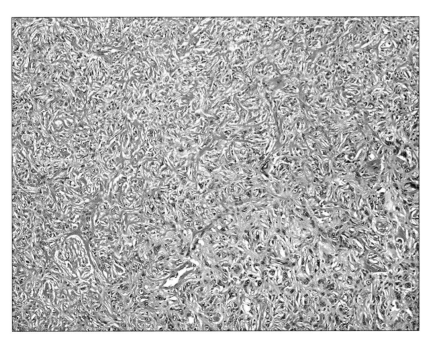

FIGURE 12–35 Atypical fibrous histiocytoma showing interface between classic benign fibrous histiocytoma (upper left) and more atypical areas (lower right).

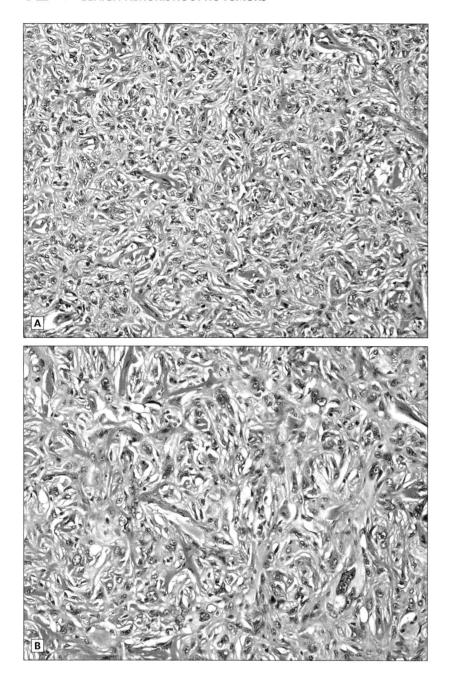

FIGURE 12–36 Atypical fibrous histiocytoma showing areas of classic benign fibrous histiocytoma **(A)** and more atypical areas **(B)**. Same case as Figure 13–35.

JUVENILE XANTHOGRANULOMA

Juvenile xanthogranuloma is a stable or regressing histiocytic lesion that usually occurs during childhood.[45-55] It has recently been reclassified from a non-X form of histiocytosis to a dendritic cell-related histiocytic proliferation. This nosological change places it conceptually closer to Langerhans cell histiocytosis and distinct from the macrophage-related histiocytic proliferations which include Rosai-Dorfman disease. The lesion(s) usually develop during infancy and is (are) characterized by one or more cutaneous nodules and less often by additional lesions in deep soft tissue or organs.[45,46] As a rule, those

that develop after the age of 2 years or in adults are usually solitary.[48] Tahan et al.[48] suggested that juvenile xanthogranuloma be reduced to xanthogranuloma because 15–30% of these lesions occur in individuals older than 20 years of age. Use of this term alone, we believe, could be problematic, as xanthogranuloma has been used for a variety of tumorous and reactive conditions whose pathogenesis varies.

Clinical findings and gross appearance

This disease may occur exclusively as a cutaneous lesion or a disease affecting deep soft tissue or parenchymal organs. In the more common cutaneous form, one or more nodules develop shortly after birth, although approximately one-third of patients have lesions at birth.[46] Two-thirds of patients develop the lesions by the age of 6 months. Depending on the series, 10–40% of patients develop the lesion after the age of 20 years. There is no underlying lipid abnormality, and no well-established familial incidence, although rare reports have documented the disease in parent and offspring.

About half of the lesions develop on the head and neck, followed by the trunk and extremities. They measure a few millimeters to a few centimeters in diameter. The early lesions are red papules (Fig. 12–37), and the older lesions are brown or yellow. Following a limited period of growth, most nodules regress spontaneously, leaving a depressed, sometimes hyperpigmented area of skin. In patients with numerous skin nodules, the tumors may appear in crops. Older lesions begin to regress as new ones emerge, so lesions of various ages may be present simultaneously. Although most lesions subside by ado-

lescence, those that develop after age 20 may persist in a stable form.

In the less common form of the disease, cutaneous lesions may be accompanied by similar lesions in other sites, such as the eye, lung, epicardium, oral cavity, and testis. Less than 5% of cases occur in deep soft tissue (usually skeletal muscle) or parenchymal organs.[45,46] In such patients, the presenting symptoms are often referable to the extracutaneous tumor, and the skin lesions may be overlooked or appear later. The eye is the most common extracutaneous site, and patients may present with anterior chamber hemorrhage and glaucoma.

Microscopic findings

Juvenile xanthogranulomas are similar whether they occur in children or adults.[47] There is a tendency, however, for deep lesions to appear more monomorphic and less lipidized (Figs 12–38, 12–39).[51] Lesions consist of sheets of histiocytes involving the dermis and extending to, but not invading, the flattened epidermis (Fig. 12–8). The infiltrate closely apposes adnexal structures and extends into the subcutis. Deeply situated juvenile xanthogranulomas appear circumscribed but blend with or infiltrate skeletal muscle at their periphery (Fig. 12–39). In both forms of the disease the histiocytes are well differentiated and exhibit little pleomorphism and only rare mitoses. The appearance of the lesions varies in a more or less time-dependent fashion and with the amount of lipid present. "Early" lesions have little lipid; hence the cells have a homogeneous amphophilic or eosinophilic cytoplasm (Fig. 12–40). In the older, more "classic" lesions, the cells have a finely vacuolated or even xanthomatous cytoplasm (Figs 12–41, 12–42). Giant cells, including Touton giant cells, are typical of this lesion (Figs 12–43, 12–44) but may vary considerably in number from one area to another or from lesion to lesion. Usually, a modest number of inflammatory cells is present, consisting of both acute and chronic inflammatory cells, especially eosinophils. Longstanding or regressive lesions eventually develop interstitial fibrosis and even a vague storiform pattern (Fig. 12–45), so they may resemble the more conventional fibrous histiocytoma seen in adults.

Electron microscopic studies show that the cells have characteristics of histiocytes.[51,52] They have numerous pseudopodia, lipid droplets, and lysosomes. Lipid, however, is not present to any extent within vessel walls, in contrast to certain types of eruptive xanthoma. Langerhans granules, tubular organelles associated with forms of histiocytosis X, have not been demonstrated. The cells express CD68, α_1-antitrypsin, α_1-antichymotrypsin, lysozyme,[47,50] CD31, and factor XIIIa.[46,53] They are consistently negative for CD1a and usually negative for S-100 protein,[46] both of which can be used to distinguish this lesion from Langerhans cell histiocytosis (see below).

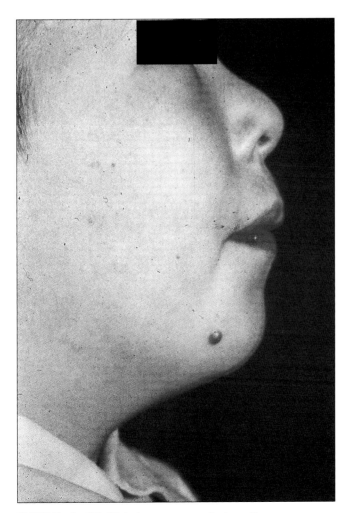

FIGURE 12–37 Clinical appearance of a juvenile xanthogranuloma. (Case courtesy of Dr. Elson Helwig.)

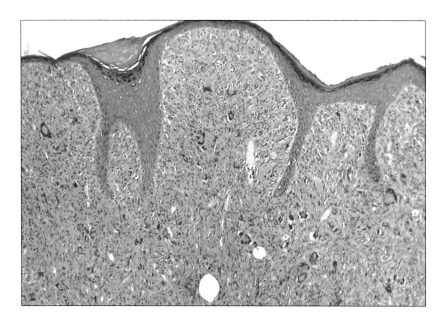

FIGURE 12–38 Juvenile xanthogranuloma.

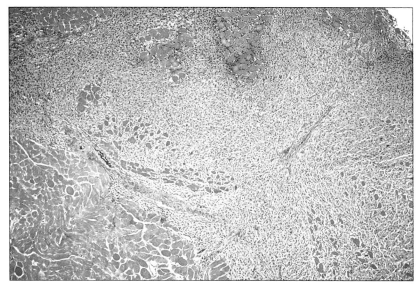

FIGURE 12–39 Deep juvenile xanthogranuloma infiltrating muscle.

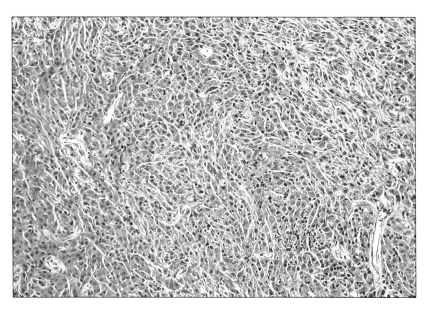

FIGURE 12–40 Early juvenile xanthogranuloma composed of nonlipidized histiocytes.

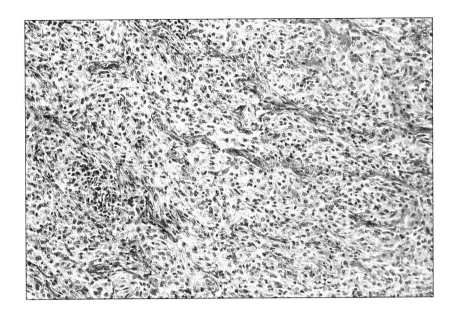

FIGURE 12–41 Lipidized juvenile xanthogranuloma.

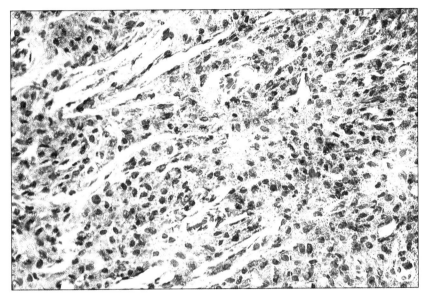

FIGURE 12–42 Fat stain showing extensive lipid within a juvenile xanthogranuloma.

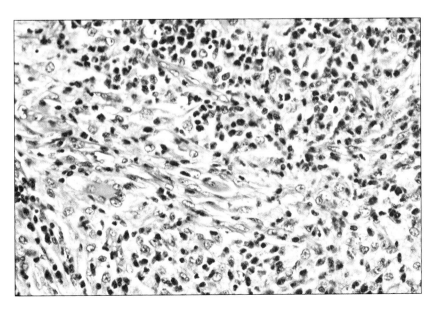

FIGURE 12–43 Juvenile xanthogranuloma with an eosinophilic infiltrate.

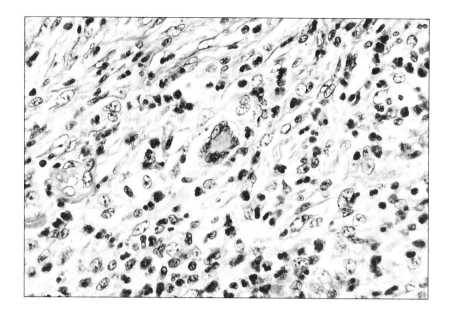

FIGURE 12–44 Juvenile xanthogranuloma with eosinophils and Touton giant cells.

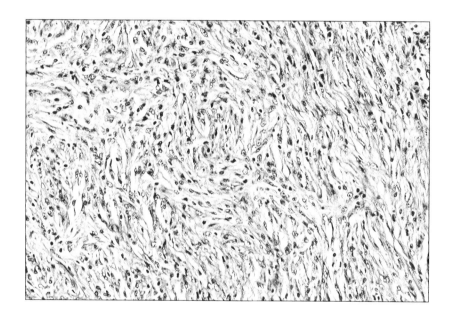

FIGURE 12–45 Late juvenile xanthogranuloma with fibrosis.

Differential diagnosis

Even though juvenile xanthogranuloma and Langerhans cell histiocytosis are both considered dendritic cell-related histiocytic proliferations, there are still compelling biological reasons to distinguish between these two disorders. In contrast to Langerhans cell histiocytosis involving the skin, juvenile xanthogranuloma does not generally invade the epidermis and shows greater cellular cohesion and fewer eosinophils. Touton giant cells, a feature of juvenile xanthogranuloma, are typically absent in Langerhans cell histiocytosis; when these cells are scarce, distinction of the two diseases may be difficult. In these situations, ultrastructural studies documenting the presence or absence of Langerhans' gran-ules and immunostaining for S-100 protein may be required. The latter is strongly positive in Langerhans cell histiocytosis but is negative or present in scattered cells in juvenile xanthogranuloma. Usually, juvenile xanthogranuloma can be easily distinguished from *xanthomas* histologically because the latter contain a more uniform population of foamy cells and lack Touton giant cells and acute inflammation. Moreover, xanthomas associated with hypercholesterolemia often have large extracellular cholesterol deposits. The greater uniformity of juvenile xanthogranuloma, the usual lack of a storiform pattern, and the distinctive clinical setting distinguish it from *solitary fibrous histiocytoma of adults*.

Clinical behavior

The prognosis for patients with this disease is excellent. The skin lesions usually regress or at least stabilize with time, and even large, deeply located tumors pursue a favorable course. In the recent experience reported from the Kiel Registry, 83% of patients were cured following excision, 10% experienced recurrence, and 7% developed additional lesion(s) in the same general vicinity as the original tumor.[46] Death from disease may occur in systemic cases. Dehner documented two deaths among eight patients with systemic disease.[53] Surgical excision is the mainstay of treatment for patients with solitary or limited disease, whereas multimodal chemotherapy is the treatment of choice for the rare patient with systemic disease.[46]

SOLITARY RETICULOHISTIOCYTOMA

Reticulohistiocytoma is a distinctive but rare lesion of adult life. It consists of nodules of eosinophilic histiocytes, often exhibiting multinucleation. It has been suggested that the solitary forms of reticulohistiocytoma are similar to adult xanthogranulomas, the distinction being largely based on whether there is a predominance of multinucleated eosinophilic histiocytes. On the other hand, solitary reticulohistiocytoma appears to be a fundamentally different disease from multicentric reticulohistiocytomas, both clinically and immunophenotypically.[56]

Solitary reticulohistiocytoma is a nodular dermatosis (reticulohistiocytoma, reticulohistiocytic granuloma)[56,57] that develops at any body site. Most patients are adult men, and fewer than one-fifth have multiple tumors.[56] The lesions are yellow-brown papules composed of dense circumscribed dermal nodules of deeply eosinophilic histiocytes (Figs 12–46 to 12–48). Multinucleated forms, often 20–30 times larger than their mononuclear counterparts, with abundant nuclei are common. The so-called oncocytic histiocytes may display some degree of nuclear atypia, and occasionally mitotic figures are noted. In some areas there is a subtle degree of spindling of the histiocytes, although frankly spindled areas and Touton giant cells such as are seen in fibrous histiocytomas are absent. Occasional lymphocytes are present. Immunohistochemically, the lesions express several markers associated with the non-X forms of histiocytosis. They consistently express CD68, variably α_1-antitrypsin, and lysozyme; but they lack S-100 protein.[58] They also express muscle-specific actin, an antigen that has been identified in the mononuclear cells of giant cell tumors of bone and soft tissue giant cell tumors of low malignant potential (see Chapter 13).

Isolated cutaneous lesions with some degree of pleomorphism must be distinguished from *superficial forms of malignant fibrous histiocytoma* (malignant giant cell tumor of soft parts), *carcinoma*, and *melanoma*. In contrast to superficial forms of malignant fibrous histiocytoma, these tumors are smaller and have fewer mitotic figures, less prominent spindling, and no necrosis. Unlike melanoma, there is no junctional activity, more interstitial collagen, and a less distinct organoid growth pattern. The frequent accompaniment of acute inflammatory cells and numerous multinucleated cells also aids in this distinction.

The lesions pursue a benign or self-limiting course. In one study[56] most patients with follow-up information were cured by simple excision; two patients developed a recurrence, and three had a nodule elsewhere. Several patients with multiple nodules noted spontaneous regression of a lesion.

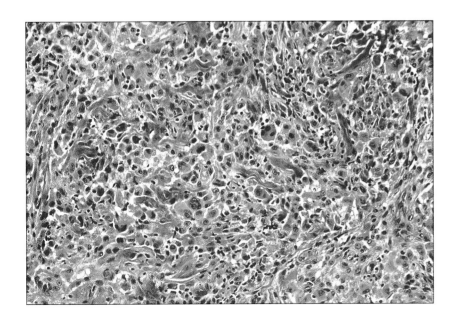

FIGURE 12–46 Reticulohistiocytoma.

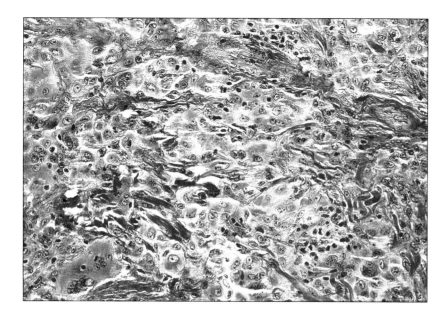

FIGURE 12–47 Reticulohistiocytoma.

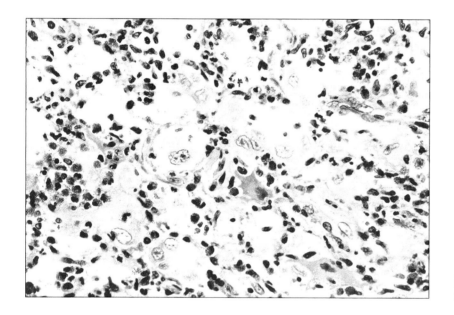

FIGURE 12–48 High-power view of a reticulohistiocytoma.

MULTICENTRIC RETICULOHISTIOCYTOSIS

In contrast to the cutaneous disease, multicentric reticulohistiocytosis is a systemic, occasionally paraneoplastic disease characterized by myriad symptoms including progressive symmetric, erosive arthritis, episodes of pyrexia, and weight loss.[59-65] Multiple cutaneous and mucosal nodules follow the arthritis within a period of months to years, although occasionally the skin lesions initiate the disease. The disease may be associated with a number of other conditions including tuberculosis, diabetes, Sjögren syndrome, hypothyroidism, Wegener's granulomatosis, polyarteritis,[60,66,67] celiac disease, and systemic lupus erythematosus.[58] In addition, malignancies of various types (e.g., carcinoma of the colon, breast, lung, ovary, and cervix; sarcoma; lymphoma) develop in about 30% of patients.[59,68] In one dramatic case, the constitutional symptoms regressed when the underlying neoplasm was treated.[57] Despite the fact that the various lipid materials accumulate within lesional cells, no consistent or specific serum lipid abnormality has been identified. The disease is usually marked by a waxing and waning course over a period of several years, eventually leaving most patients with a disfiguring, crippling arthritis that most severely affects the distal interphalangeal joint and bears some similarity to rheumatoid arthritis (Fig. 12–49).

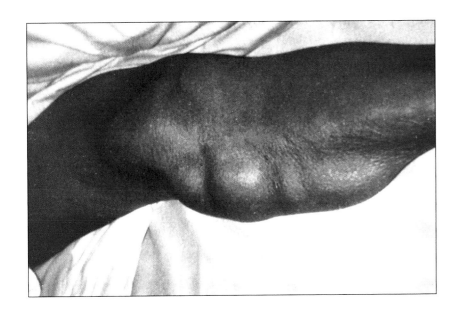

FIGURE 12–49 Deforming arthritis of the elbow in a patient with multicentric reticulohistiocytosis.

Pathologic findings

The cutaneous lesions consist of circumscribed collections of histiocytes confined to the dermis or extending to the epidermis and subcutis. Delicate reticulin fibers are present around individual cells, and occasionally acute and chronic inflammatory cells are present. Although multinucleated eosinophilic histiocytes characterize both this disease and the solitary reticulohistiocytoma, these histiocytes tend to be smaller, are less eosinophilic, and show only a minor degree of multinucleation. Similar deposits may be seen in other involved organs such as synovium, bone, and lymph nodes. In most cases they stain strongly with Sudan black B fat stain, oil red O, and periodic acid-Schiff (PAS) after diastase digestion and are believed to contain a mixture of phospholipid, mucoprotein or glycoprotein, and neutral fat.[59] Immunohistochemically, these cells contrast slightly with those of solitary reticulohistiocytoma in that they lack muscle-specific actin and factor XIIIa; but they express CD68, α_1-antitrypsin, and lysozyme. Electron microscopy shows that the histiocytes have numerous lipid droplets and a dilated rough endoplasmic reticulum filled with granular material.[63] Langerhans granules, tubular structures present in certain normal and neoplastic histiocytes, are usually not identified in multicentric reticulohistiocytosis,[69,70] although there have been some reports to the contrary.[71,72]

Discussion

Usually, this disease poses few diagnostic problems for the pathologist because evaluation of the skin lesions is aided immeasurably by the clinical history and in some cases by a confirmatory biopsy of synovium or other tissue. The etiology of this condition remains obscure, however. Because a disproportionately large number of patients with multicentric reticulohistiocytosis have associated malignancies or other systemic disease, some have suggested that the disease is a reflection of an altered immune state. It furthermore appears that the histiocytes in these lesions have the ability to secrete a wide variety of substances that may be responsible for many of the manifestations of the disease.[70,73,74] β-Interleukin-1β and platelet-derived growth factor-β, both of which promote synovial proliferation, can be identified immunohistochemically in the histiocytes.[73] Urokinase is elevated in synovial tissue and could, by activation of collagenase, account for the destruction of articular tissue. Although in the past there was little or no therapy for the disease, a number of reports have attested to alleviation of the condition with the use of chemotherapeutic agents, including alkylating agents.[75-77]

XANTHOMA

Xanthoma is a localized collection of tissue histiocytes containing lipid.[78-82] It is not a true tumor but, rather, a reactive histiocytic proliferation that occurs in response to alterations in serum lipids. Xanthomas develop in most primary and some secondary (e.g., primary biliary cirrhosis, diabetes mellitus) hyperlipoproteinemias and occasionally in the normolipemic state. A brief synopsis of the various primary hyperlipidemias and their associated defects is provided in Table 12–2. Usually, xanthomas occur in the skin and subcutis,[83-86] but occasionally they involve deep soft tissue such as tendons (xanthoma of the tendon sheath)[84,87-89] or synovium.[90]

TABLE 12–2	PLASMA LIPOPROTEIN PHENOTYPES					
Disorder	**I**	**IIa**	**IIb**	**III**	**IV**	**V**
Lipoprotein elevation	Chylomicrons	LDL	LDL, VLDL	Chylomicrons, VLDL remnants	VLDL	Chylomicrons, VLDL
Xanthoma	Eruptive	Tendon, tuberous	None	Palmar, tuberous, eruptive	None	Eruptive
Molecular defect	Lipoprotein lipase, apoC-II	LDL receptor, apoB-100	Unknown	ApoE	Unknown	Unknown

*Modified from Rader DJ. Disorders of lipid metabolism. In: Kelley WN, ed. Textbook of internal medicine, 3rd edn. Philadelphia: Lippincott-Raven; 1997.
LDL, low density lipoproteins; VLDL, very low density lipoproteins; apo/Apo, apolipoprotein.

TABLE 12–3	COMPARISON OF CLINICAL TYPES OF XANTHOMA		
Type of xanthoma	**Association with lipoprotein phenotype**	**Location**	**Histologic appearance**
Eruptive	I, III, V	Predilection for buttocks	Foamy and nonfoamy histiocytes
Tuberous	IIa, III	Elbows, buttocks, knees, fingers	Foamy histiocytes, extracellular cholesterol deposits, fibrosis, inflammation
Tendinous	IIa, cerebrotendinous xanthomatosis	Tendons of hands and feet, Achilles tendon	Similar to tuberous xanthoma
Xanthelasma	IIa, III	Eyelids	Foamy histiocytes
Plane	Primary biliary cirrhosis III, normolipemic states	Skin creases of palms	Foamy histiocytes

Clinical findings and gross appearance

Cutaneous xanthomas are designated according to their gross appearance and clinical presentation (Table 12–3). Eruptive xanthomas are small, yellow papules with a predilection for the gluteal surfaces. They develop in individuals with hyperlipoproteinemia types I, III, and V. Tuberous xanthomas, large plaque-like lesions of the subcutis, are usually located on the buttocks, elbows, knees, and fingers and are seen with type IIa or III hyperlipoproteinemia. Plane xanthomas occur in skinfolds, such as the palmar creases, and are characteristic of type III hyperlipoproteinemia; they may also be associated with primary biliary cirrhosis. Occasionally, they occur in normolipemic persons, and in this setting they have a high association with reticuloendothelial malignancies.[85,91] Xanthelasmas are xanthomas of the eyelid and usually are observed in normolipemic persons, although they also occur in those with type IIa or III hyperlipoproteinemia. These last three types of xanthoma contain large amounts of cholesterol and its esters, which may be demonstrated under polarized light in fresh tissue as birefringent crystals.

Deep xanthomas occur most frequently in tendon or synovium, and rarely bone. Most tendinous xanthomas occur in the setting of hypercholesterolemia associated with type IIa hyperlipoproteinemia (Fig. 12–50). Usually, the severity of the xanthoma is roughly proportional to the severity and duration of the increased cholesterol levels. A rare inherited disease known as cerebrotendinous xanthomatosis is now also recognized as a cause of

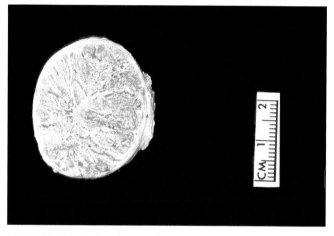

FIGURE 12–50 Xanthoma of the Achilles tendon cut in cross-section. White bands correspond to residual tendinous tissue that has been spread apart by xanthomatous infiltration.

bilateral xanthomas occurring exclusively in the Achilles tendon.[92–94] This disease is an autosomal recessive disorder caused by mutations in the gene for sterol 27-hydroxylase, an enzyme important for hepatic bile acid synthesis. As a result, bile acids are synthesized to the end product cholestanol, which accumulates systemically, producing multiple signs and symptoms including dementia, ataxia, cataracts, and tendinous xanthomas. Recognition of this disease is important, as early treatment with chenodeoxycholic acid can prevent progression of clinical symptoms.

Most tendinous xanthomas present as painless, slowly growing masses that produce few symptoms unless joint function is compromised. The lesions may be solitary or multiple, and they occur in sites subjected to minor trauma such as the finger, wrist, and ankle. They are usually a few centimeters in diameter, although large lesions in excess of 20 cm have been reported in the Achilles tendon (Fig. 12–50). Xanthomas may be circumscribed or diffuse and are firmly attached to tendon but not to overlying skin. On cut section they have a variegated color ranging from yellow to brown to white, depending on the amount of lipid, hemorrhage, and fibrosis present from area to area. Like tuberous and plane xanthomas, they also have a high cholesterol content.

Microscopic findings

The various types of xanthoma differ in histologic appearance. Eruptive xanthoma, which represents an acute, evanescent lesion, contains a large proportion of nonfoamy histiocytes in addition to occasional foam cells and inflammatory cells. Tuberous and tendinous xanthomas are essentially identical (Figs 12–51 to 12–53). Although in their early stages they may contain some nonfoamy histiocytes, the typical appearance is that of sheets of foamy histiocytes interspersed with occasional inflammatory cells. The histiocytes are bland with small pyknotic nuclei. Some cells contain fine granules of hemosiderin. Collections of extracellular cholesterol (cholesterol clefts) flanked by giant cells are conspicuous. Varying amounts

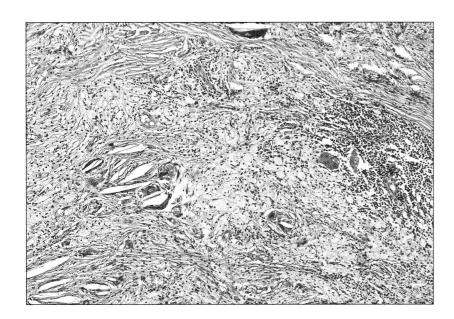

FIGURE 12–51 Tuberous xanthoma of the leg consisting of xanthoma cells admixed with inflammatory cells and giant cells surrounding cholesterol-containing clefts.

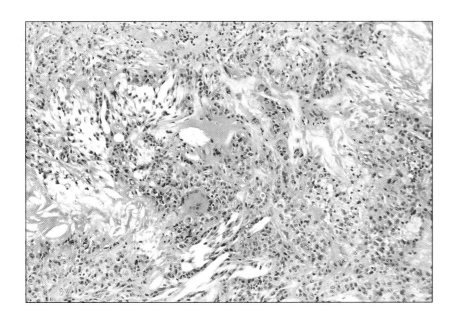

FIGURE 12–52 Tuberous xanthoma with xanthoma cells but without fibrosis or inflammation.

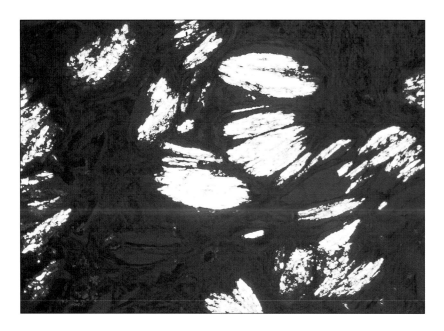

FIGURE 12–53 Frozen section of a xanthoma viewed under polarized light to illustrate numerous birefringent cholesterol crystals.

of fibrosis may be present but are most marked in long-standing lesions. Plane xanthoma and xanthelasma are characterized by sheets of xanthoma cells, but they rarely exhibit the degree of fibrosis present in the foregoing two lesions. Ultrastructurally, xanthoma cells of all of these lesions are similar and contain numerous clear vacuoles, presumably representing cholesterol or its esters. Eruptive xanthomas, in addition, have fat in the vessel walls and tissue macrophages.

Discussion

Cutaneous xanthomas usually present few problems in diagnosis or management. The superficial location, gross appearance, and associated clinical findings leave little doubt as to the diagnosis. Xanthomas of the tendon sheath may be more problematic. The deep location and slow, persistent growth occasionally raise the question of sarcoma. When a biopsy is done, such lesions should be adequately sampled because giant cell tumors of the tendon sheath, diffuse villonodular synovitis, or sarcomas with xanthomatous change may focally resemble this lesion. The diagnosis of xanthoma of the tendon sheath should always be considered in a patient with hypercholesterolemia, especially if the lesions are multiple.

Because of the nonneoplastic nature of these lesions, conservative therapy is generally recommended. In fact, xanthelasmas and tuberous xanthomas have regressed on medical therapy alone,[86,95] although months or years may be required before tangible benefits are appreciated. Soft tissue radiographs may be helpful for serial assessment of tendinous xanthomas under treatment.[96] Surgery, includ-

ing excision with tendon reconstruction, has been reserved for large or symptomatic xanthomas. Surgically treated xanthomas may slowly recur, although generally reoperation is not necessary.[87] Irradiation has also been employed as therapy for these lesions, but there are few data to support its efficacy. Long-term treatment of cerebrotendinous xanthomatosis with chenodeoxycholic acid has resulted in alleviation of some of the neurologic symptoms but has not affected the tendinous xanthomas.[97]

Although xanthomas were formerly considered neoplastic, their association with hyperlipidemic states leaves little doubt that they are reactive lesions. Current evidence suggests that the lipid in them is derived from blood.[98–100] It has been demonstrated experimentally that serum lipoproteins leave the vascular compartment, traverse small vessels, and enter the macrophages of soft tissue.[99] This series of events can be confirmed ultrastructurally by the sequential finding of lipoprotein between endothelium and basement membrane and finally in the pericytes. Once ingested by macrophages, the lipoprotein is degraded to lipid, and the lipid is released to the extracellular space. The fibrosis characteristic of mature or long-standing xanthomas is believed to be related to the fibrogenic properties of extracellular cholesterol.[58] Although xanthomas can potentially occur at any soft tissue site, the localization stimulus seems directly related to the vascular permeability, as agents that increase permeability (e.g., histamine) can accelerate xanthoma formation at a given site.[99] Likewise, minor trauma or injury that results in histamine release also accelerates xanthoma formation.[101] This observation provides an explanation for the common occurrence of such lesions in the tendons of the hands and feet.

MISCELLANEOUS HISTIOCYTIC REACTIONS RESEMBLING A NEOPLASM

Histiocytic reactions may be difficult to distinguish from neoplasms when they are localized lesions with few inflammatory cells. In these cases it is necessary to obtain detailed clinical data, perform special staining procedures for microorganisms, and examine the specimen under polarized light for foreign material before rendering a diagnosis. Even under the best circumstances, the etiology of some histiocytic proliferations remains enigmatic. The more distinctive histiocytic reactions with known etiologies are discussed below.

Infectious disease

Gram-positive and Gram-negative bacteria can induce inflammatory changes similar to those of xanthogranuloma. The lesions are composed of sheets of foamy histiocytes set against a mixed background of inflammatory cells. They differ from a neoplastic xanthogranuloma by the presence of focal abscesses and numerous microorganisms in the histiocytes. We have seen several cases of chronic staphylococcal infection with this appearance, and we are aware of a similar lesion of the retroperitoneum secondary to *Arizona hinshawii*, a Gram-negative bacillus.[102]

Histoid leprosy, a rare form of lepromatous leprosy described by Wade[103,104] in 1963, grossly and microscopically resembles fibrous histiocytoma (Figs 12–54 to 12–56). Unlike the usual type of lepromatous leprosy, which spreads in an infiltrative manner, this disease develops as an expansile nodule of the subcutis and dermis. The cells resemble fibroblasts rather than histiocytes and are often arranged in a storiform pattern.

Although the similarity of this disease to a true fibrous histiocytoma is striking, numerous intracellular acid-fast bacilli can be demonstrated with special stains (e.g., Fite-Feraco) (Fig. 12–56). Because this form of leprosy occurs in patients with longstanding lepromatous leprosy treated with sulfones, it has been suggested that these lesions are the result of emergence of sulfone-resistant bacilli.

Mycobacterial pseudotumors, first recognized by Wood et al. in an immunosuppressed patient, have been reported most recently in AIDS patients in a variety of sites, most commonly lymph nodes but also skin/subcutis.[105,106] The lesions are analogous to those of histoid leprosy in that they consist of a tumorous proliferation of spindled and epithelioid histiocytes arranged in vague fascicles and associated with occasional chronic inflammatory cells (Figs 12–57, 12–58). The cells are laden with numerous acid-fast bacilli easily demonstrable with appropriate stains (Fig. 12–59). The lesional cells are CD68 and S-100 protein positive, confirming their histiocytic lineage. In some cases desmin has been demonstrated but has been attributed to immunoreactivity of the bacilli.[107]

Malacoplakia

Malacoplakia is a rare inflammatory disease believed to represent an unusual host response to infection with a variety of organisms, including *Escherichia coli*, *Klebsiella*, and acid-fast bacilli. The reaction results in the formation of yellow plaque-like lesions on the mucosal surface of the affected organs.[108] The disease typically develops in the genitourinary tract, particularly the bladder, although it may affect the soft tissues of the retroperitoneum as well. It is characterized by sheets of pale, slightly granular, or vacuolated histiocytes (von Hansemann's cells) containing PAS-positive, diastase-resistant inclusions in the

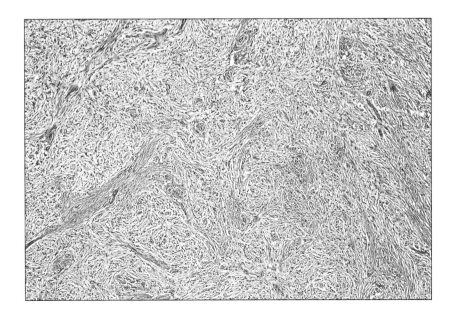

FIGURE 12–54 Histoid leprosy with a pattern similar to that of a fibrous histiocytoma.

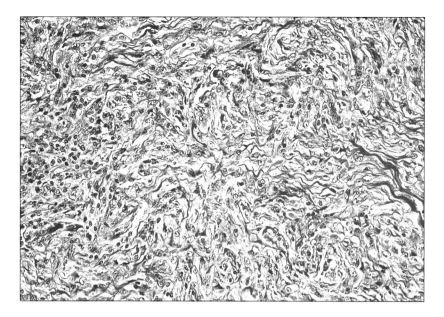

FIGURE 12–55 Medium-power view of histoid leprosy.

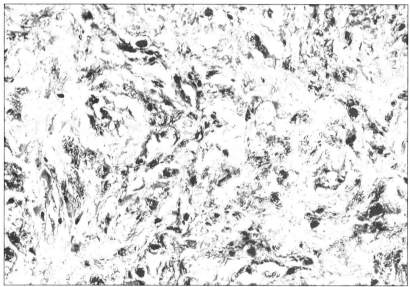

FIGURE 12–56 Fite-Feraco stain demonstrates numerous intracellular acid-fast bacilli in histoid leprosy.

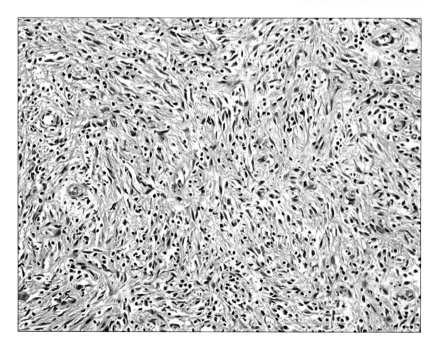

FIGURE 12–57 Atypical mycobacterial pseudotumor.

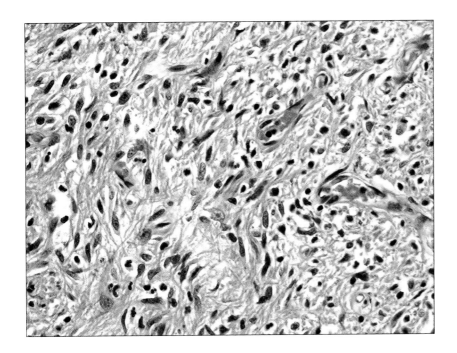

FIGURE 12–58 Atypical mycobacterial pseudotumor.

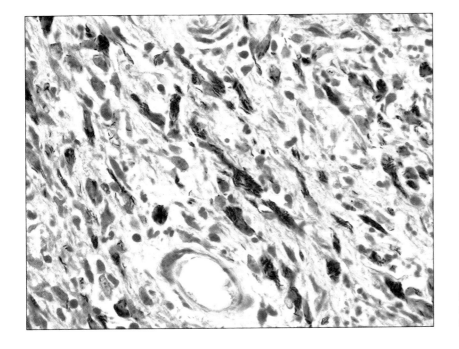

FIGURE 12–59 Acid-fast stain in atypical mycobacterial pseudotumor demonstrating organisms in spindled histiocytes.

cytoplasm (Fig. 12–60). Lymphocytes, plasma cells, and neutrophils are typically abundant. The distinctive Michaelis-Gutmann bodies, small calcospherites that consist of a mixture of organic and inorganic materials including calcium and phosphate, can be identified within the histiocytes and extracellularly (Fig. 12–61). Electron microscopic studies show that the von Hansemann histiocytes contain numerous phagolysosomes, occasional bacterial forms, and lamellated crystalline bodies representing the early stage of Michaelis-Gutmann bodies.[109]

Extranodal (soft tissue) Rosai-Dorfman disease

Rosai-Dorfman disease is a polyclonal histiocytic disorder of uncertain etiology, which, although originally described as a lymph node disease,[110] occurs in sundry locations including soft tissue. Although the nature of the proliferating histiocyte is still unknown, its appearance and immunophenotype most closely approximate an activated macrophage.[111] Approximately 10% of all cases of Rosai-Dorfman disease are associated with soft tissue involvement, and in some cases it is the sole manifestation of the

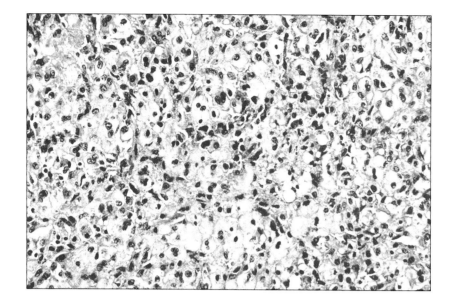

FIGURE 12–60 Malacoplakia of the retroperitoneum with solid sheets of histiocytes admixed with inflammatory cells.

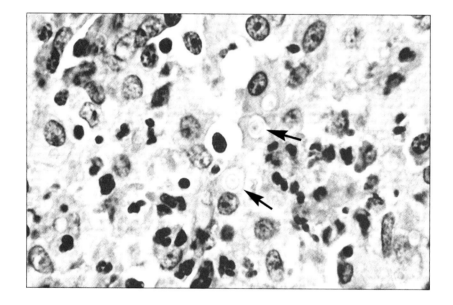

FIGURE 12–61 High-power view of malacoplakia showing Michaelis-Gutmann bodies (arrows) in occasional cells.

disorder.[112,113] However, the actual incidence of associated lymphadenopathy in patients with soft tissue lesions depends greatly on the bias of the study. In the study by Foucar et al.[112] most had lymphadenopathy, whereas in the study by Montgomery et al.[113] only a few did (4 of 23). The former study was based on a referral of all cases to the National Sinus Histiocytosis with Massive Lymphadenopathy (SHML) Registry at Yale University, whereas the latter represented referral cases to the Soft Tissue Registry of the Armed Forces Institute of Pathology (AFIP). Patients with soft tissue Rosai-Dorfman disease tend to be older than those with lymph node-based disease.

Microscopically, the lesions consist of sheets or syncytia of large, pale histiocytes with large, round, vesicular nuclei with some degree of atypia (Figs 12–62, 12–63). Mitotic figures are usually difficult to detect or are absent altogether. The cytoplasm of the histiocytes may contain lymphocytes (emperipolesis), although this is seldom as striking as in the lesions of lymph nodes. Microabscesses, when present, suggest the possibility of an infectious process. The feature that tends to complicate the diagnosis of these unusual lesions is the presence of fibrosis, which distorts the sheet-like growth pattern, creating instead a storiform pattern. Predictably, the latter pattern, in association with atypical histiocytes, is often construed as evidence that one is dealing with a fibrohistiocytic tumor. The histiocytes of Rosai-Dorfman disease consistently and strongly express S-100 protein and occasionally other histiocytic antigens[114] including CD1a. They do not contain Birbeck granules, however.

The presence of S-100 protein is useful for discriminating these lesions from malignant fibrous histiocytomas

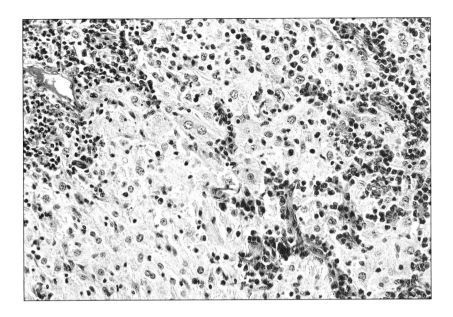

FIGURE 12–62 Extranodal Rosai-Dorfman disease characterized by sheets of pale histiocytes with voluminous cytoplasm.

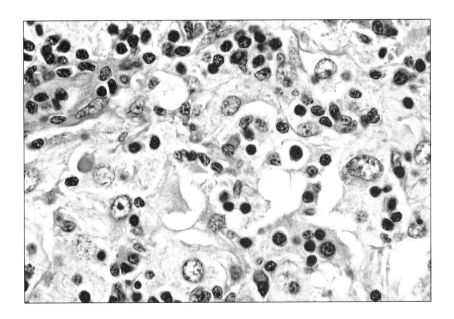

FIGURE 12–63 High-power view of Rosai-Dorfman disease illustrating mild nuclear atypia and emperipolesis.

and histiocytic proliferations of infectious etiology. Obviously, this antigen does not discriminate examples of soft tissue Rosai-Dorfman disease from Langerhans cell histiocytosis, although usually the cytologic differences between the proliferating histiocytes in the two conditions and the differences in the inflammatory cells accompanying them readily permit this distinction. The data, at present, suggest that the prognosis of soft tissue Rosai-Dorfman disease is excellent. Most patients with isolated soft tissue masses appeared well following surgery, although some developed recurrent disease. A significant number of patients with isolated cutaneous disease resolve.[115]

Histiocytic reactions to endogenous and exogenous material

Silica reaction

Although the usual response to silica in soft tissue is a localized foreign body reaction, exuberant reactions to the material simulate a fibrohistiocytic neoplasm (Figs 12–64, 12–65). In our experience, the latter form of soft tissue silicosis is probably related to the presence of large amounts of silica. It seems principally to be an iatrogenic disease secondary to the now obsolete injection therapy for hernias.[116] Clinically, these lesions present as slowly enlarging tumorous masses, usually in the inguinal region

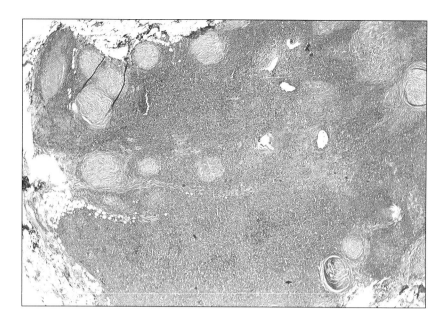

FIGURE 12–64 Silica reaction in the inguinal region. Lesion is composed of sheets of well-differentiated histiocytes interlaced with fibrous bands.

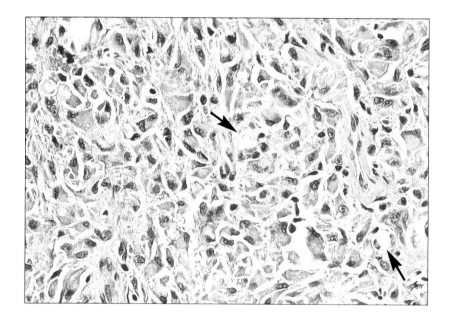

FIGURE 12–65 Silica reaction in the inguinal region showing well-differentiated histiocytes. Spicules of foreign material can be seen in the cytoplasm of some histiocytes, but full elucidation requires polarization.

or abdominal wall. Typically, they occur many years after the injection of silica, so the causal relation of the injection is minimized or overlooked. Grossly, the lesions are ill-defined, gray-yellow masses with a gritty consistency on cutting. They consist of sheets of histiocytes with a clear or amphophilic cytoplasm. Although usually well differentiated, the histiocytes occasionally display moderate pleomorphism. Mitotic figures are rare. PAS-positive, diastase-resistant bodies may be present in the histiocytes and probably represent large phagolysosomes, organelles involved in the intracellular storage of silica. Numerous silica crystals can be identified under polarized light. A striking feature of the lesion is the large amount of fibrosis. The collagen varies from delicate interstitial or perivascular fibers in the early stages to broad bands and finally

mats or large nodules. The presence of silica, extensive fibrosis, scarcity of mitotic figures, and poorly developed vasculature all serve to distinguish these lesions from benign or malignant fibrous histiocytomas.

Polyvinylpyrrolidone granuloma

Polyvinylpyrrolidone (PVP) is a polymer of vinylpyrrolidone, which was used notably as a plasma expander during wartime and until recently was utilized in various intravenous preparations in Asia. It has been marketed under various names, including Plasgen, Periston, Plasmagel, Biseko, Blutogen, and Subplasm. Because of its hydroscopic properties it has also been used as a retardant in various injectable medicines (hormones, antihypertensives, local anesthetics), as a clarifier in fruit juices, and as a resin in hair sprays.[117] The molecular weight of PVP varies depending on its chain length (MW 10 000–200 000 daltons). Low molecular-weight PVP is filtered by the glomerulus and cleared by the kidney, whereas high molecular-weight PVP (MW 50 000 daltons or more) is retained indefinitely by the body and is stored throughout the reticuloendothelial system. The common appearance of PVP disease following intravenous injection of the substance is that of blue-gray histiocytes lining the sinusoids of the liver, spleen, and lymph nodes. A second form of PVP disease presumably occurs following inhalation of the substance from hair spray.[118] The alveolar walls are thickened, and macrophages fill the alveolar spaces. An uncommon form of PVP disease is a localized pseudotumor,[119–121] presumably caused by local injection

of the material. Cases reported in the literature have documented PVP pseudotumors secondary to the anesthetic Depot-Impletol[122] and vasopressin.[121]

Histologically, these lesions are composed of numerous histiocytes massively engorged with PVP (Figs 12–66 to 12–68). The material appears glassy blue or blue-gray in sections stained with hematoxylin-eosin. The histiocytes form sheets or small clusters in a matrix containing copious amounts of foreign material. Giant cells are occasionally present and may be helpful in suggesting the diagnosis of a foreign body reaction. Another feature suggesting a reactive process is the manner in which the histiocytes "percolate" around the adnexal structures, nerves, and vessels. Typically there are few if any inflammatory cells and no necrosis. The tinctoral properties of PVP have been well documented and serve to distinguish

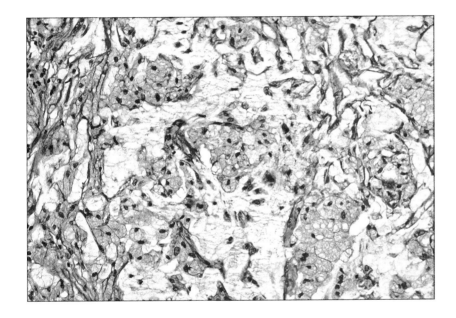

FIGURE 12–66 Polyvinylpyrrolidone (PVP) granuloma. Clusters of bubbly histiocytes are suspended in pools of basophilic-appearing PVP.

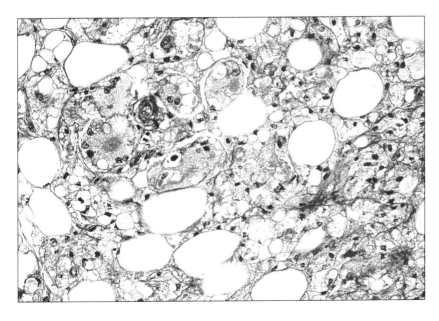

FIGURE 12–67 Multinucleated histiocytes filled with PVP.

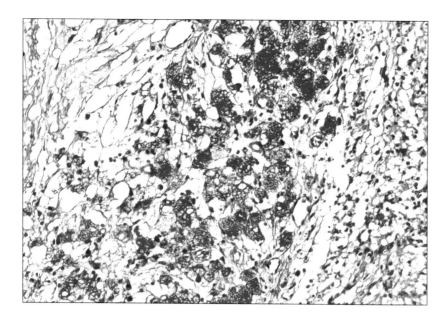

FIGURE 12–68 Congo red staining of PVP.

TABLE 12–4	STAINING REACTIONS OF POLYVINYLPYRROLIDONE

Positive
Congo red
Sirius red
Mucicarmine
Colloidal iron

Negative
Periodic acid-Schiff (PAS)
Alcian blue

this lesion from other myxoid lesions (Table 12–4).[123] PVP characteristically does not stain with Alcian blue and therefore stains differently from all myxoid tumors of soft tissue, such as liposarcoma, chondrosarcoma, and chordoma. It does not stain blue with Giemsa stain and should therefore not be confused with the syndrome of sea-blue histiocytes. PVP is carminophilic, and this fact should be kept in mind, as occasional cases of PVP granuloma have been mistaken for infiltrating carcinomas of the signet-ring type.[123] The best stains for demonstrating the cytoplasmic material are Congo red or Sirius red. Ultrastructurally, the material is contained in large membrane-limited vacuoles believed to be distended lysosomes. Dense bodies, probably composed of ferritin, are condensed at the periphery of the vacuoles.

Granular cell reaction

Collections of histiocytes with granular eosinophilic cytoplasm occasionally accumulate at the site of surgical trauma.[124] These peculiar histiocytic reactions bear a close similarity to granular cell tumor (Figs 12–69 to 12–71) but can usually be differentiated from the foregoing by the fact that the nuclei in these reactions are rather small and inconspicuous and the granules are large and coarsely textured (Fig. 12–71). Furthermore, the cells often surround nodules of granuloamorphous debris similar to the cytoplasmic granular material (Figs 12–69, 12–70). Sobel et al.[124] pointed out that the staining reactions serve to distinguish the two lesions. The ceroid-lipofuscin substance in these histiocyte reactions is usually acid fast and autofluorescent compared with that of the granular cell tumor.

Crystal-storing histiocytosis resembling rhabdomyoma

Crystal-storing histiocytosis is a rare condition in which tumorous deposits of histiocytes containing crystalline immunoglobulin occur in soft tissue.[125,126] A small number of cases have been reported, all of which were associated with a lymphoplasmacytic neoplasm and monoclonal immunoglobulin production. It appears that the immunoglobulin is crystallized locally and phagocytosed by histiocytes, which become massively distorted by the material. The histiocytes are large, rounded to angular cells that occasionally appear multinucleated (Figs 12–72, 12–73). The crystalline material varies in size, but the largest deposits can be visualized easily by light microscopy. The histiocytic cells can be few in number or so abundant that the underlying lymphoplasmatic neoplasm is overlooked, resulting in an erroneous diagnosis of rhabdomyoma.[126] However, the cells can be clearly identified as histiocytic by strong immunostaining for CD68. Ultrastructurally, the crystalline material displays a lattice pattern with a periodicity of 45–60 Angstroms consistent with immunoglobulin (Fig. 12–74).

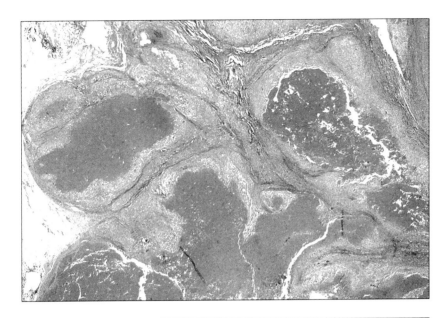

FIGURE 12–69 Granular cell reaction showing a fringe of histiocytes surrounding the core of the granuloamorphous material.

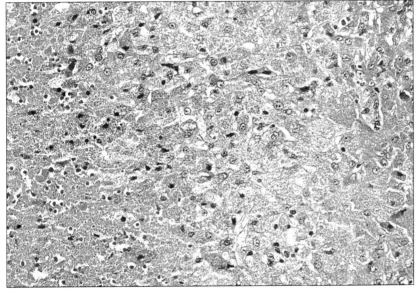

FIGURE 12–70 Histiocytic reaction with "granular cell" features at the site of previous surgery.

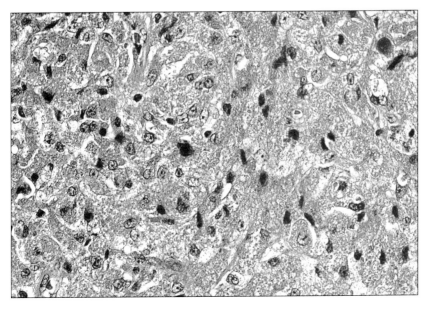

FIGURE 12–71 High-power view of granular-appearing histiocytes in granular cell reactions.

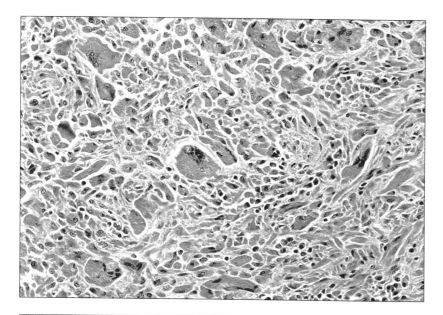

FIGURE 12–72 Crystalline storing histiocytosis in a patient with lymphoplasmatic lymphoma.

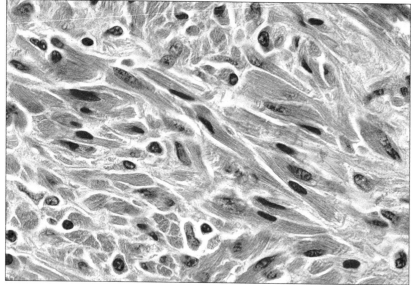

FIGURE 12–73 High-power view of crystal-containing histiocytes from Figure 12–67 showing massive distortion and spindling as a result of intracytoplasmic crystalline immunoglobulin.

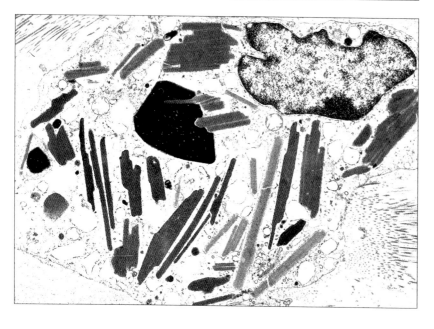

FIGURE 12–74 Electron micrograph of crystalline immunoglobulin from Figure 12–68 showing periodicity.

REFERENCES

General

1. Fletcher CD, Unni KK, Mertens F. World Health Organization Classification of Tumours. Pathology and Genetics of Tumors of Soft Tissue and Bone. Lyon: IARC Press; 2002:109–124.
2. Katenkamp D, Stiller D. Cellular composition of the so-called dermatofibroma (histiocytoma cutis). Virchows Arch [Pathol Anat] 1975; 367:325.
3. Niemi KM. The benign fibrohistiocytic tumours of the skin. Acta Dermatol Venereol 1970; 50(Suppl 63):1.
4. Gonzalez S, Duarte I. Benign fibrous histiocytoma of the skin: a morphologic study of 290 cases. Pathol Res Pract 1982; 174:379.
5. Newman DM, Walter JB. Multiple dermatofibromas in patients with systemic lupus erythematosus on immunosuppressive therapy. N Engl J Med 1973; 289:842.
6. Foreman K, Bonish BMS, Nickoloff B. Absence of human herpesvirus 8 DNA sequences in patients with immunosuppression-associated dermatofibroma. Arch Dermatol 1997; 133:108.
7. Beer M, Eckert F, Schmoeckel C. The atrophic dermatofibroma. J Am Acad Dermatol 1991; 25:1081.
8. Shishido E, Kadono S, Manaka I, et al. The mechanism of epidermal hyperpigmentation in dermatofibromas is associated with stem cell factor and hepatocyte growth factor expression. J Invest Dermatol 2001; 117:627.
9. Fitzpatrick TB, Gilchrest BA. Dimple sign to differentiate benign from malignant pigmented cutaneous lesions. N Engl J Med 1977; 296:1518.
10. Fletcher CD. Benign fibrous histiocytoma of subcutaneous and deep soft tissue: a clinicopathologic analysis of 21 cases. Am J Surg Pathol 1990; 14:801.
11. Calonje E, Fletcher CDM. Aneurysmal benign fibrous histiocytoma: clincopathological analysis of 40 cases of a tumor frequently misdiagnosed as a vascular neoplasm. Histopathology 1995; 26:323.
12. McKenna DB, Kavanagh GM, McLaren KM, et al. Aneurysmal fibrous histiocytoma: an unusual variant of cutaneous fibrous histiocytoma. J Eur Acad Dermatol Venereol 1999; 12:238.
13. Santa Cruz DJ, Kyriakos M. Aneurysmal ("angiomatoid") fibrous histiocytoma of the skin. Cancer 1981; 47:2053.
14. LeBoit PE, Barr RJ. Smooth muscle proliferation in dermatofibromas. Am J Dermatopathol 1994; 16:155.
15. Tamada S, Ackerman AB. Dermatofibroma with monster cells. Am J Dermatopathol 1987; 9:380.
16. Beham A, Fletcher CD. Atypical "pseudosarcomatous" variant of cutaneous benign fibrous histiocytoma: report of eight cases. Histopathology 1990; 17:167.
17. Cerio R, Spaull J, Wilson Jones E. Histiocytoma cutis: a tumour of dermal dendrocytes (dermal dendrocytoma). Br J Dermatol 1989; 120:197.
18. Calonje E, Fletcher CDM. Cutaneous fibrohistiocytic tumors: an update. Adv Anat Pathol 1994; 1:2.
19. Bruecks AK, Trotter MJ. Expression of desmin and smooth muscle myosin heavy chain in dermatofibromas. Arch Path Lab Med 2002; 126:1179.
20. Mihatsch-Konz B, Schaumburg-Lever G, Lever WR. Ultrastructure of dermatofibroma. Arch Derm Forsch 1973; 246:181.
21. Li N, McNiff J, Hui P, et al. Differential expression of HMGA1 and HMGA2 in dermatofibroma and dermatofibrosarcoma protuberans: potential diagnostic applications, and comparison with histologic findings, CD34, and factor XIIIa immunoreactivity. Am J Dermatopathol 2004; 26:267.
22. Chen TC, Kuo T, Chan HL. Dermatofibroma is a clonal proliferative process. J Cut Path 2000; 27:36.
23. Vanni R, Marras S, Faa G, et al. Cellular fibrous histiocytoma of the skin: evidence of a clonal process with different karyotype from dermatofibrosarcoma. Genes Chromosomes Cancer 1997; 18:314.
24. Vanni R, Fletcher CD, Sciot R, et al. Cytogenetic evidence of clonality in cutaneous benign fibrous histiocytomas: a report of the CHAMP study groups. Histopathology 2000; 37:212.
25. Hui P, Glusac EJ, Sinard JH, et al. Clonal analysis of cutaneous fibrous histiocytomas (dermatofibroma). J Cut Path 2002; 29:385.
26. Franquemont DW, Cooper PH, Shmookler BM, et al. Benign fibrous histiocytoma of the skin with potential for local recurrence: a tumor to be distinguished from dermatofibroma. Mod Pathol 1990; 3:58.
27. Font RL, Kidayat AA. Fibrous histiocytoma of the orbit: a clinicopathologic study of 150 cases. Hum Pathol 1982; 13:199.
28. Mentzel T, Calonje E, Fletcher CDM. Dermatomyofibroma: additional observations on a distinctive cutaneous myofibroblastic tumour with emphasis on differential diagnosis. Br J Dermatol 1993; 129:69.
29. Calonje E, Mentzel T, Fletcher CDM. Cellular benign fibrous histiocytoma: clinicopathologic analysis of 74 cases of a distinctive variant of cutaneous fibrous histiocytoma with frequent recurrence. Am J Surg Pathol 1994; 18:668.
30. Colome-Grimmer MI, Evans HL. Metastasizing cellular dermatofibroma: a report of two cases. Am J Surg Pathol 1996; 20:1361.
31. Guillou L, Gebhard S, Slameron M, et al. Metastasizing fibrous histiocytoma of the skin: a clinicopathologic and immunohistochemical analysis of three cases. Mod Pathol 2000; 13:654.
32. Kamino H, Jacobson M. Dermatofibroma extending into the subcutaneous tissue: differential diagnosis from dermatofibrosarcoma protuberans. Am J Surg Pathol 1990; 14:1156.
33. Zelger B, Sidoroff A, Stanzl U, et al. Deep penetrating dermatofibroma versus dermatofibrosarcoma protuberans: a clinicopathologic comparison. Am J Surg Pathol 1994; 18:677.
34. Glusac EJ, Barr RJ, Everett MA, et al. Epithelioid cell histiocytoma: a report of 10 cases including a new cellular variant. Am J Surg Pathol 1994; 18:583.
35. Singh GAC, Calonje E, Fletcher CDM. Epithelioid benign fibrous histiocytoma of skin: clinicopathological analysis of 20 cases of a poorly known variant. Histopathology 1994; 24:123.
36. Wilson Jones E, Cerio R, Smith NP. Epithelioid cell histiocytoma: a new entity. Br J Dermatol 1989; 120:185.
37. Silverman JS, Glusac EJ. Epithelioid cell histiocytoma – histogenetic and kinetics analysis of dermal microvascular unit dendritic cell subpopulations. J Cut Path 2003; 30:415.
38. Zelger BW, Zelger BG, Steiner H, et al. Aneurysmal and hemangiopericytoma-like fibrous histiocytoma. J Clin Pathol 1996; 49:313.
39. Kamino H, Reddy VB, Gero M, et al. Dermatomyofibroma: a benign cutaneous plaque-like proliferation of fibroblasts in young adults. J Cutan Pathol 1992; 19:85.
40. Schwob VS, Santa Cruz DJ. Palisading cutaneous fibrous histiocytoma. J Cutan Pathol 1986; 13:403.
41. Zelger BG, Calonje E, Zelger B. Myxoid dermatofibroma. Histopathology 1999; 34:357.
42. Zelger B, Steiner H, Kutzner H. Clear cell dermatofibroma. Am J Surg Pathol 1996; 20:483.
43. Iwata J, Fletcher CD. Lipidized fibrous histiocytoma: clinicopathologic analysis of 22 cases. Am J Dermatopathol 2000; 22:126.
44. Kaddu S, McMenamin ME, Fletcher CD. Atypical fibrous histiocytoma of the skin: clinicopathologic analysis of 59 cases with evidence of infrequent metastasis. Am J Surg Pathol 2002; 26:35.

Juvenile xanthogranuloma

45. Helwig EB, Hackney VC. Juvenile xanthogranuloma (nevoxantho-endothelioma). Am J Pathol 1954; 30:625.
46. Janssen D, Harms D. Juvenile xanthogranuloma in childhood and adolescence: a clinicopathologic study of 129 patients from the Kiel Pediatric Tumor Registry. Am J Surg Pathol 2005; 29:21.
47. Zelger B, Cerio R, Orchard G, et al. Juvenile and adult xanthogranuloma: a histological and immunohistochemical comparison. Am J Surg Pathol 1994; 18:126.
48. Tahan SR, Pastel-Levy C, Bhan AK, et al. Juvenile xanthogranuloma: clinical and pathologic characterization. Arch Pathol Lab Med 1989; 113:1057.
49. Cohen BA, Hood A. Xanthogranuloma: report on clinical and histologic findings in 64 patients. Pediatr Dermatol 1989; 6:262.
50. Nascimento AG. A clinicopathologic and immunohistochemical comparative study of cutaneous and intramuscular forms of juvenile xanthogranuloma. Am J Surg Pathol 1997; 21:645.
51. Esterly NB, Sahihi T, Medenica M. Juvenile xanthogranuloma: an atypical case with a study of ultrastructure. Arch Dermatol 1972; 105:99.
52. Gonzalez-Crussi F, Campbell RJ. Juvenile xanthogranuloma: ultrastructural study. Arch Pathol 1970; 89:65.
53. Dehner LP. Juvenile xanthogranulomas in the first two decades of life: a clinicopathologic study of 174 cases with cutaneous and extracutaneous manifestations. Am J Surg Pathol 2003; 27:579.
54. Kraus MD, Haley JC, Ruiz R, et al. "Juvenile" xanthogranuloma: an immunophenotypic study with a reappraisal of histogenesis. Am J Dermatopathol 2001; 23:104.
55. Zelger BW, Cerio R. Xanthogranuloma is the archetype of non-Langerhans cell histiocytoses. Br J Dermatol 2001; 145:369.

Reticulohistiocytoma

56. Purvis WE, Helwig EB. Reticulohistiocytic granuloma ("reticulohistiocytoma") of the skin. Am J Clin Pathol 1954; 24:1005.
57. Montgomery H, Polley HF, Pugh DG. Reticulohistiocytoma (reticulohistiocytic granuloma). Arch Dermatol 1958; 77:61.
58. Zelger B, Cerio R, Soyer HP, et al. Reticulohistiocytoma and multicentric reticulocytosis: histopathologic and immunophenotypic distinct entities. Am J Dermatopathol 1994; 16:577.
59. Barrow MV, Holubar K. Multicentric reticulohistiocytosis. Medicine 1969; 48:287.
60. Conaghan P, Miller M, Dowling JP, et al. A unique presentation of multicentric reticulohistiocytosis in pregnancy. Arthritis Rheum 2003; 36:269.
61. Davies BT, Wood SR. The so-called reticulohistiocytoma of the skin: a comparison of two distinct types. Br J Dermatol 1955; 67:205.
62. Davies NEJ, Roenigk HH, Hawk WA, et al. Multicentric reticulohistiocytosis: report of a case with histochemical studies. Arch Dermatol 1968; 97:543.

63. Flam M, Ryan SC, Mah-Poy GL, et al. Multicentric reticulohistiocytosis: report of a case with atypical features and electron microscopic study of skin lesions. Am J Med 1972; 52:841.

64. Orkin M, Goltz RW, Good RA, et al. A study of multicentric reticulohistiocytosis. Arch Dermatol 1964; 89:640.

65. Taylor DR. Multicentric reticulohistiocytosis. Arch Dermatol 1977; 113:330.

66. Oliver GF, Umbert I, Winkelmann RK, et al. Reticulohistiocytoma cutis: review of 15 cases and an association with systemic vasculitis in two cases. Clin Exp Dermatol 1990; 15:1.

67. Shiokawa S, Shingu M, Nishimura M, et al. Multicentric reticulohistiocytosis associated with subclinical Sjögren's syndrome. Clin Rheumatol 1991; 10:201.

68. Kuramoto Y, Iizawa O, Matsunaga J. Development of Ki-1 lymphoma in a child suffering from multicentric reticulohistiocytosis. Acta Dermatol Venereol 1991; 71:448.

69. Kuwabara H, Uda H, Tanaka S. Multicentric reticulohistiocytosis: report of a case with electron microscopic studies. Acta Pathol Jpn 1992; 42:130.

70. Lotti T, Santucci M, Casigliani R, et al. Multicentric reticulohistiocytosis: report of three cases with evaluation of tissue proteinase activity. Am J Dermatopathol 1988; 10:497.

71. Ehrlich GE, Young I, Nosheny SZ, et al. Multicentric reticulohistiocytosis (lipoid dermatoarthritis). Am J Med 1972; 52:830.

72. Hashimoto K, Pritzker MS. Electron microscopic study of reticulohistiocytoma. Arch Dermatol 1973; 107:263.

73. Nakajima Y, Sato K, Morita H, et al. Severe progressive erosive arthritis in multicentric reticulohistiocytosis: possible involvement of cytokines in synovial proliferation. J Rheumatol 1992; 19:1643.

74. Zagala A, Guyot A, Bensa JC, et al. Multicentric reticulohistiocytomas: a case with enhanced interleukin-1, prostaglandin E_2, and interleukin-2 secretion. J Rheumatol 1988; 15:136.

75. Ginsburg WW, O'Duffy JD, Morris JL, et al. Multicentric reticulohistiocytosis: response to alkylating agents in six patients. Ann Intern Med 1989; 11:384.

76. Kenik JG, Fok F, Huerter CJ, et al. Multicentric reticulohistiocytosis in a patient with malignant melanoma: a response to cyclophosphamide and a unique cutaneous feature. Arthritis Rheum 1990; 33:1047.

77. Lambert CM, Nuki G. Multicentric reticulohistiocytosis with arthritis and cardiac infiltration: regression following treatment for underlying malignancy. Ann Rheum Dis 1992; 51:815.

Xanthoma

78. Crocker AC. Skin xanthomas in childhood. Pediatrics 1951; 8:573.

79. Fredrickson DS, Lees RS. A system for phenotyping hyperlipoproteinemia. Circulation 1965; 31:321.

80. Marcoval J, Moreno A, Bordas X, et al. Diffuse plane xanthoma: clinicopathologic study of 8 cases. J Am Acad Dermatol 1998; 39:439.

81. Wilkes LL. Tendon xanthoma in type IV hyperlipoproteinemia. South Med J 1977; 70:254.

82. Wilson DE, Flowers CM, Hershgold EJ, et al. Multiple myeloma, cryoglobulinemia, and xanthomatosis: distinct clinical and biochemical syndromes in two patients. Am J Med 1975; 59:721.

83. Beerman H. Lipid diseases as manifested in the skin. Med Clin North Am 1951; 35:433.

84. Cristol DS, Gill AB. Xanthoma of tendon sheath. JAMA 1943; 122:1013.

85. Montgomery H. Cutaneous xanthomatosis. Ann Intern Med 1939; 13:671.

86. Montgomery H, Osterberg AE. Xanthomatosis: correlation of clinical histopathologic and chemical studies of cutaneous xanthoma. Arch Dermatol Syph 1938; 37:373.

87. Fahey JJ, Stark HH, Donovan WF, et al. Xanthoma of the Achilles tendon: seven cases with familial hyperbetalipoproteinemia. J Bone Joint Surg [Am] 1973; 55:1197.

88. Friedman MS. Xanthoma of the Achilles tendon. J Bone Joint Surg 1947; 29:760.

89. McWhorter JE, Weeks C. Multiple xanthoma of the tendons. Surg Gynecol Obstet 1925; 40:199.

90. DeSanto DA, Wilson PD. Xanthomatous tumors of joints. J Bone Joint Surg 1939; 21:531.

91. Lynch PJ, Winkelmann RK. Generalized plane xanthoma and systemic disease. Arch Dermatol 1966; 93:639.

92. Hughes JD, Meriwether TW. Familial pseudohypertrophy of tendoachillis with multisystem disease. South Med J 1971; 64:311.

93. Kearns WP, Wood WS. Cerebrotendinous xanthomatosis. Arch Ophthalmol 1976; 94:148.

94. Sloan HR, Frederickson DS. Rare familial diseases with neutral lipid storage: Wolman's disease, cholesterol ester storage disease, and cerebrotendinous xanthomatosis. In: Stanbury JB, Wyngaarden JB, Frederickson DS, eds. Metabolic basis of inherited disease, 3rd edn. New York: McGraw-Hill; 1972.

95. Buxtorf JC, Beaumont V, Jactot B, et al. Regression de xanthomes et medicaments hypolipidemiants. Atherosclorosis 1974; 19:1.

96. Gattereau A, Davignon J, Levesque HP. Roentgenological evaluation of Achilles tendon xanthomatosis. Lancet 1971; 2:705.

97. Berginer VM, Salen G, Shefer S. Long-term treatment of cerebrotendinous xanthomatosis with chenodeoxycholic acid. N Engl J Med 1984; 311:1649.

98. Parker F, Odland GF. Electron microscopic similarities between experimental xanthoma and human eruptive xanthomas. J Invest Dermatol 1969; 52:136.

99. Parker F, Odland GF. Experimental xanthoma: a correlative biochemical, histologic, histochemical, and electron microscopic study. Am J Pathol 1968; 53:537.

100. Walton KW, Thomas C, Dunkerley DJ. The pathogenesis of xanthomata. J Pathol 1973; 109:271.

101. Scott PJ, Winterbourn CC. Low density lipoprotein accumulation in actively growing xanthomas. J Atheroscler Res 1967; 7:207.

Miscellaneous histiocytic reactions resembling tumor

102. Keren DF, Rawlings W, Murray HW, et al. *Arizona hinshawii* osteomyelitis with antecedent enteric fever and sepsis: a case report and review of the literature. Ann J Med 1976; 60:577.

103. Mansfield RE. Histoid leprosy. Arch Pathol 1969; 87:580.

104. Wade HW. Histoid variety of lepromatous leprosy. Int J Leprosy 1963; 31:129.

105. Logani S, Lucas DR, Cheng J, et al. Spindle cell tumors associated with mycobacteria in lymph nodes of HIV-positive patients: "Kaposi sarcoma with mycobacteria" and "mycobacterial pseudotumor." Am J Surg Pathol 1999; 23:656.

106. Wood C, Nickoloff BJ, Todes-Taylor NR. Pseudotumor resulting from atypical mycobacterial infection: a "histoid" variety of *Mycobacterium avium-intracelluare* complex infection. Am J Clin Pathol 1985; 83:524.

107. Umlas J, Federman M, Crawford C, et al. Spindle cell pseudotumor due to *Mycobacterium avium-intracellulare* in patients with acquired immunodeficiency syndrome (AIDS). Positive staining of mycobacteria for cytoskeleton filaments. Am J Surg Pathol 1991; 15:1181.

108. Damjanov I, Katz SM. Malakoplakia. Pathol Annu 1981; 16:103.

109. Font RL, Bersani TA, Eagle RC. Malakoplakia of the eyelid: clinical, histopathologic and ultrastructural characteristics. Ophthalmology 1988; 95:61.

110. Rosai J, Dorfman RF. Sinus histiocytosis with massive lymphadenopathy: a pseudolymphomatous benign disorder: analysis of 34 cases. Cancer 1972; 30:1174.

111. Favara BE, Feller AC, Pauli M, et al: Contemporary classification of histiocytic disorders. Med Pediatr Oncol 1997; 29:157.

112. Foucar E, Rosai J, Dorfman RF. Sinus histiocytosis with massive lymphadenopathy (Rosai-Dorfman disease): review of the entity. Semin Diagn Pathol 1990; 7:19.

113. Montgomery EA, Meis JM, Frizzera G. Rosai-Dorfman disease of soft tissue. Am J Surg Pathol 1992; 16:122.

114. Eisen RN, Buckley PJ, Rosai J. Immunophenotypic characterization of sinus histiocytomas with massive lymphadenopathy (Rosai-Dorfman disease). Semin Diagn Pathol 1990; 7:74.

115. Brenn T, Calonje E, Grantner SR, et al. Cutaneous Rosai-Dorfman disease is a distinct clinical entity. Am J Dermatopathol 2002; 24:385.

116. Weiss SW, Enzinger FM, Johnson FB. Silica reaction simulating fibrous histiocytoma. Cancer 1978; 42:2738.

117. Wessel W, Schoog M, Winkler E. Polyvinylpyrrolidone (PVP): its diagnostic, therapeutic, and technical application and consequences thereof. Arzneim Forsch 1971; 21:1468.

118. Bergman M, Flance IJ, Cruz PT, et al. Thesaurosis due to inhalation of hair spray: report of twelve new cases including three autopsies. N Engl J Med 1962; 266:750.

119. Bubis JJ, Cohen S, Dinbar J, et al. Storage of polyvinylpyrrolidone mimicking a congenital mucolipid storage disease in a patient with Munchausen's syndrome. Isr J Med Sci 1975; 11:999.

120. Hizawa K, Inaba H, Nakanishi S, et al. Subcutaneous pseudosarcomatous polyvinylpyrrolidone granuloma. Am J Surg Pathol 1984; 8:393.

121. Reske-Nielsen E, Bojsen-Moller M, Vetner M, et al. Polyvinylpyrrolidone-storage disease: light and microscopical, ultrastructural, and chemical verification. Acta Pathol Microbiol Scand 1976; 84A:397.

122. Gille J, Brandau H. Fremdkorpergranulation in der Brusdruse nach Injektion eines polyvinylpyrrolidonhaltigen Praparats: eine Fallbeobactung. Geburtsch Frauenheilkd 1975; 35:799.

123. Kuo TT, Hsueh S. Mucicarminophilic histiocytosis: a polyvinylpyrrolidone (PVP) storage disease simulating signet ring carcinoma. Am J Surg Pathol 1984; 8:419.

124. Sobel H, Arvin E, Marquet E, et al. Reactive granular cells in sites of trauma: a cytochemical and ultrastructural study. Am J Clin Pathol 1974; 61:223.

125. Harada M, Shimada M, Fuhayama M, et al. Crystal-storing histiocytosis associated with lymphoplasmacytic lymphoma mimicking Weber-Christian disease: immunohistochemical, ultrastructural and gene-rearrangement studies. Hum Pathol 1996; 27:84.

126. Kapadia SB, Enzinger FM, Heffner DK, et al. Crystal-storing histiocytosis associated with lymphoplasmacytic neoplasm: report of three cases mimicking adult rhabdomyoma. Am J Surg Pathol 1993; 17:461.

FIBROHISTIOCYTIC TUMORS OF INTERMEDIATE MALIGNANCY

CHAPTER CONTENTS

Fibrohistiocytic tumors of intermediate malignancy originally included only dermatofibrosarcoma protuberans and the closely related giant cell fibroblastoma. This category now embraces a number of other lesions such as the plexiform fibrohistiocytic tumor and angiomatoid fibrous histiocytoma. All are characterized by a significant risk of local recurrence but a limited risk of regional and distant metastasis. They differ from the malignant fibrous histiocytoma in this important respect. They also occur in a decidedly younger population; indeed, some seem to occur almost exclusively in children. As with malignant fibrous histiocytoma, there seems to be a general consensus that most of these lesions do not display true histiocytic differentiation. Their present classification, therefore, is considered a tentative one pending a general consensus on reclassification. On the one hand, the dermatofibrosarcoma and its juvenile counterpart, giant cell fibroblastoma, seem to be most closely related to a fibroblast; and indeed the discovery of CD34 immunoreactivity in these two lesions provides a linkage to the CD34+ dendritic cells that populate the dermis. On the other hand, the plexiform fibrohistiocytic tumor seems to most closely approach the spirit of the term "fibrohistiocytic." It has a bimodal population of cells, one of which has the histologic and immunophenotypic properties of a histiocyte and the other resembling a myofibroblast. The cells of many angiomatoid fibrous histiocytomas have a striking "histiocytic" appearance, contain phagocytosed particles of hemosiderin, and occasionally express the histiocytic marker CD68 but more frequently express various myoid markers.

DERMATOFIBROSARCOMA PROTUBERANS

Dermatofibrosarcoma protuberans, first described in 1924 by Darier and Ferrand[1] as "progressive and recurring dermatofibroma," is a nodular cutaneous tumor characterized by a prominent storiform pattern. Over the years it has been considered a fibroblastic, histiocytic, and neural tumor. It bears some histologic similarity to benign fibrous histiocytoma; on this basis it, along with its pigmented counterpart (Bednar tumor), was classified with the fibrohistiocytic neoplasms. In contrast to fibrous histiocytoma, dermatofibrosarcoma protuberans grows in a more infiltrative fashion and has a greater capacity for local recurrence. Moreover, in unusual instances it metastasizes, although distant metastasis is usually a late event.

Clinical findings

Dermatofibrosarcoma protuberans typically presents during early or middle adult life as a nodular cutaneous mass. Although early studies reflected its rarity in children,[2-5] there is an increasing number of reports of its appearing in the pediatric age group. In fact, given the indolent growth and long preclinical duration, it is likely that many begin during childhood and become apparent only during young adulthood.[3] Males are affected more frequently than females. Although these tumors occur at almost any site, they are seen most frequently on the trunk and proximal extremities (Table 13–1). Unusual sites for this tumor are the vulva and parotid. Antecedent trauma, reported in about 10–20% of cases, is probably coincidental.[4-6]

In most cases this tumor is characterized by slow but persistent growth over a long period, often several years. The clinical and gross appearances, then, are determined to a great extent by the stage of the disease. The initial manifestation is usually the development of a firm, plaque-like lesion of the skin, often with surrounding red to blue discoloration.[5] These lesions have been compared with the morphea of scleroderma or morphea-like basal

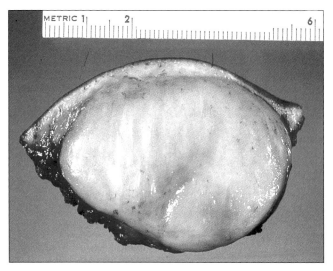

FIGURE 13–1 Typical dermatofibrosarcoma protuberans involving the dermis and subcutis in a nodular fashion.

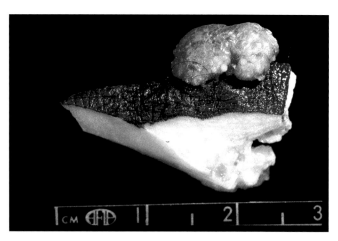

FIGURE 13–2 Small dermatofibrosarcoma displaying protuberant growth.

TABLE 13-1	ANATOMIC DISTRIBUTION OF DERMATOFIBROSARCOMA PROTUBERANS (1960–1979)		
Anatomic location		**No. of cases**	**%**
Head and neck		124	14.5
Upper extremity		155	18.2
Trunk		404	47.4
Lower extremity		170	19.9
Total		853	100

Data are from the Armed Forces Institute of Pathology (AFIP).

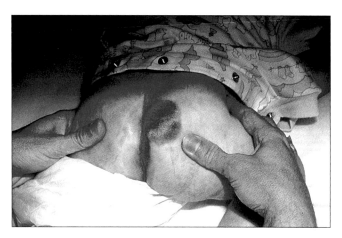

FIGURE 13–3 Dermatofibrosarcoma protuberans from the buttock of young child. It has the red color that some of these lesions exhibit.

cell carcinoma. Rarely, the lesions appear as an area of atrophy. Less often, multiple small subcutaneous nodules appear initially rather than a plaque. The plaque may grow slowly or remain stationary for a variable period, eventually entering a more rapid growth phase and giving rise to one or more nodules. Thus, only in the fully developed lesion is the typical "protuberant" appearance manifested. Neglected tumors may achieve enormous proportions and have multiple satellite nodules. Despite the large size of many of these tumors, though, the patients appear surprisingly well and lack the signs of cachexia associated with malignancies.

Gross findings

Most of these tumors are biopsied during the nodular stage; therefore the specimen consists of a solitary, protuberant, gray-white mass involving subcutis and skin (Figs 13–1 to 13–3). The average size at surgery is approximately 5 cm.[5] Multiple discrete masses are usually not seen in the original tumor but are more characteristic of recurrent lesions (Fig. 13–4).[5] The skin overlying these tumors is taut or even ulcerated. Skeletal muscle exten-

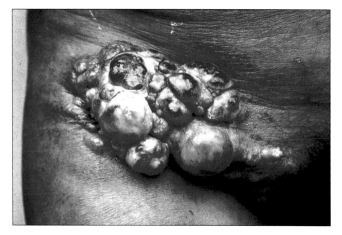

FIGURE 13–4 Gross appearance of an advanced case of dermatofibrosarcoma protuberans with multiple tumor nodules.

sion is uncommon except in large or recurrent lesions. Rarely this tumor is confined to the subcutis and lacks dermal involvement altogether. Occasionally, areas of the tumor have a translucent or gelatinous appearance corresponding microscopically to myxoid change. Hemorrhage and cystic change are sometimes seen in the tumors, but necrosis, a common feature of malignant fibrous histiocytoma, is rare.

Microscopic findings

Despite the apparent gross circumscription of these lesions, the tumor diffusely infiltrates the dermis and subcutis (Fig. 13–5). The tumor may reach the epidermis or leave an uninvolved zone of dermis just underneath the epidermis. In either event, the overlying epidermis does not usually display the hyperplasia that characterizes some cutaneous fibrous histiocytomas (dermatofibromas).[5] The peripheral portions of the tumor have a deceptively bland appearance due in part to the marked attenuation of the cells at their advancing edge. This is especially true in superficial areas, where the spread of slender cells between preexisting collagen is easily mistaken for cutaneous fibrous histiocytoma (dermatofibroma) (Fig. 13–6A). In deep regions, the tumor spreads along connective tissue septa and between adnexae (Fig. 13–7), or it intricately interdigitates with lobules of subcutaneous fat, creating a lace-like or honeycomb effect (Fig. 13–6B).

The central or main portion of the tumor is composed of a uniform population of slender fibroblasts arranged in a distinct, often monotonous, storiform pattern around an inconspicuous vasculature (Figs 13–8, 13–9). There is usually little nuclear pleomorphism and only low to moderate mitotic activity. Secondary elements such as giant cells, xanthoma cells, and inflammatory elements are few in number or absent altogether. In this respect, dermatofibrosarcoma protuberans displays remarkable uniformity compared with other fibrohistiocytic neoplasms. Although most tumors are characterized by these highly ordered cellular areas, occasional tumors contain myxoid areas (Fig. 13–10). These myxoid areas occur in both primary and recurrent lesions and are characterized by the interstitial accumulation of ground substance material. As myxoid change of the stroma becomes more pronounced, the storiform pattern becomes less distinct and the vascular pattern more apparent. By virtue of these features, such tumors can resemble myxoid liposarcoma (Fig. 13–10B).

Giant cells, similar to those in giant cell fibroblastoma, can be identified in a small percentage of otherwise typical dermatofibrosarcomas. An unusual feature of dermatofibrosarcoma protuberans is the myoid nodule (Fig. 13–11). Originally construed as evidence of myofibroblastic differentiation,[7] these structures seem to be centered in some cases around blood vessels,[8,9] and likely represent an unusual nonneoplastic vascular response to the tumor. Infrequently, dermatofibrosarcoma protuberans contains areas that are indistinguishable from fibrosarcoma (Figs 13–12 to 13–14). Characterized by long fascicles of spindle cells with more nuclear atypia and mitotic activity, these areas usually sharply abut conventional low-grade areas. Mitotic activity usually averages more than 5 mitotic figures/10 high-power fields (HPF), in contrast to areas of conventional dermatofibrosarcoma protuberans, which usually have fewer than 5 mitotic figures/10 HPF. In exceptional instances, dermatofibrosarcoma protuberans contains areas resembling malignant fibrous histiocytoma (Figs 13–15, 13–16).[10,11] Fibrosarcomatous areas were originally believed to be more common in recurrent lesions, but recent studies have documented that the contrary is true.[10] The biologic

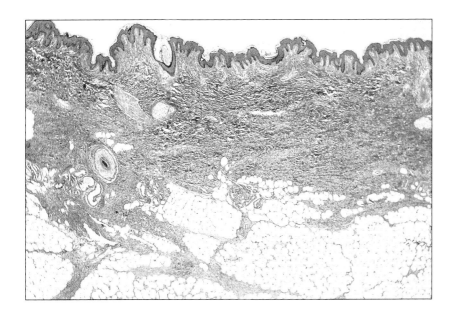

FIGURE 13–5 Plaque form of dermatofibrosarcoma protuberans illustrating the expansion of the interface between dermis and subcutis and the extension into subcutaneous fat.

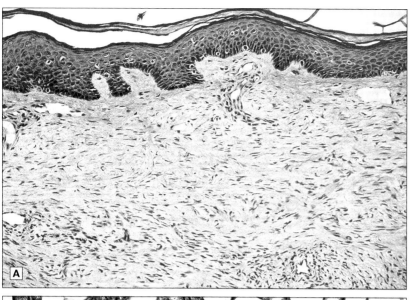

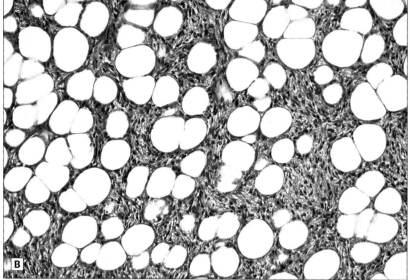

FIGURE 13–6 Superficial **(A)** and deep **(B)** extensions of dermatofibrosarcoma protuberans. Spread of the tumor between preexisting collagen of the dermis may simulate the appearance of a cutaneous fibrous histiocytoma **(A)**. At the deep margin the tumor intricately interdigitates with normal fat **(B)**.

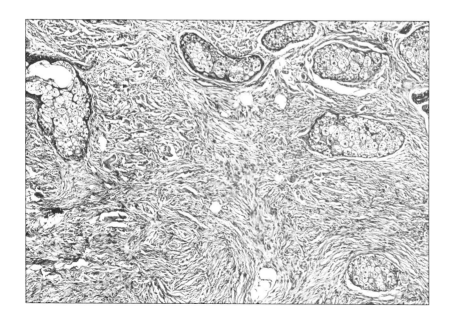

FIGURE 13–7 Dermatofibrosarcoma protuberans infiltrating between adnexal structures.

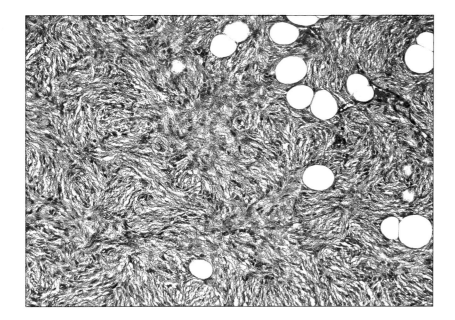

FIGURE 13–8 Slender spindle cells arranged in a distinct storiform pattern characterize most of these tumors.

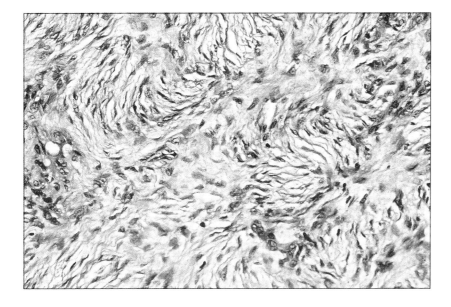

FIGURE 13–9 Dermatofibrosarcoma protuberans showing greater interstitial collagenization.

significance of sarcomatous areas in dermatofibrosarcoma protuberans is discussed below. Metastatic deposits from this tumor occur most commonly in the lung and secondly in regional lymph nodes, where they may resemble the parent tumor or may appear more pleomorphic, like a fibrosarcoma (Fig. 13–17).

Immunohistochemical and ultrastructural findings

Dermatofibrosarcoma protuberans is characterized by the nearly consistent presence of CD34 (Fig. 13–18), the human progenitor cell antigen, in a significant proportion of its cells.[10,12,13] Although this antigen has been identified in a growing number of soft tissue tumors, its presence in dermatofibrosarcoma protuberans suggests a

close linkage to the normal CD34[+] dendritic cells of the dermis, including those that ensheath the adnexae, nerves, and vessels.[13] The nearly consistent expression of this antigen has also proved useful for distinguishing dermatofibrosarcoma protuberans from benign fibrous histiocytoma, especially when dealing with small biopsies. Only occasional benign fibrous histiocytomas express this antigen.[10] Caution should be used when interpreting CD34 immunostains in spindle cell tumors of the skin, being certain that positively staining cells are neoplastic, not entrapped normal dermal dendritic cells. Apolipoprotein D has been identified immunohistochemically within a significant percentage of dermatofibrosarcomas and seems to discriminate them well from benign fibrous histiocytomas.[14] Because of the sensitivity of CD34 in the diagnosis of dermatofibrosarcoma protuberans, there has

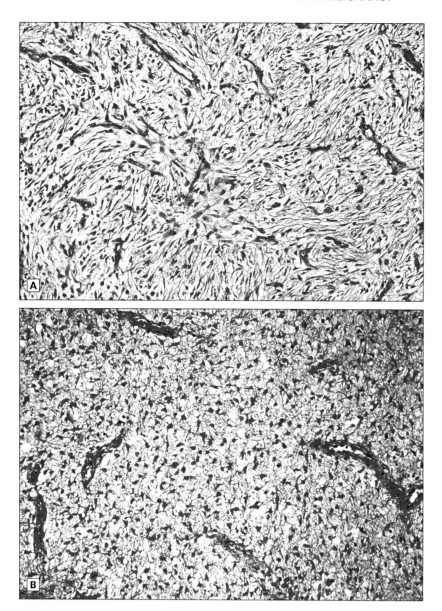

FIGURE 13–10 (A) Myxoid change in dermatofibrosarcoma protuberans. **(B)** When the myxoid change is prominent, the storiform pattern may be lacking altogether, and the tumor may resemble a myxoid liposarcoma.

been little recent interest in studying these lesions ultrastructurally. Earlier studies indicated that the cells resemble fibroblasts,[15] although some have noted certain modifications that suggest perineural differentiation.[16,17] These features included convoluted nuclei, elaborate cell processes, moderate numbers of desmosomes, and incomplete basal lamina (Fig. 13–19).

Cytogenetic analysis

Both dermatofibrosarcoma and giant cell fibroblastoma are characterized by either the presence of a supernumerary ring chromosome[18] consisting of low-level amplification of sequences from chromosomes 17 and 22,[19,20] and uncommonly 8[21] or alternatively linear translocation derivatives. The presence of a ring versus a linear translocation may be related to age.[18,21] Specifically, adult cases typically possess the ring chromosome, whereas pediatric

cases have the linear translocation derivative.[18] Either event fuses exon 2 of the platelet-derived growth factor β-chain (PDGFβ) gene to various exons of the collagen type 1 α1 gene (COL1A1) resulting in a fusion transcript that places PDGFβ under the control of the COL1A1 promotor.[22,23] The fusion protein is processed to an end product that is indistinguishable from normal PDGFβ.[23] Overproduction of PDGFβ by dermatofibrosarcoma results in autocrine stimulation and cell proliferation, a sequence of events that can be interrupted by specific tyrosine kinase inhibitors (see below).

Differential diagnosis

The most common problem in the differential diagnosis is distinguishing this tumor from other fibrohistiocytic neoplasms. Dermatofibrosarcoma protuberans has a more uniform appearance, more distinct storiform

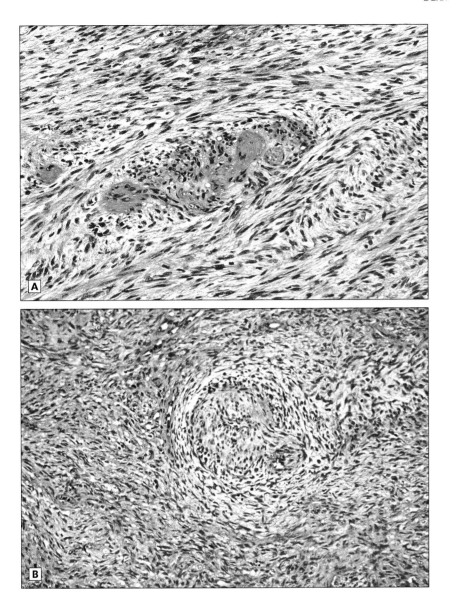

FIGURE 13–11 **(A)** Myoid balls within dermatofibrosarcoma protuberans. **(B)** Myoid ball centered around a small vessel.

pattern, and fewer secondary elements (i.e., giant cells, inflammatory cells) than either a benign or malignant fibrous histiocytoma. The distinction between *benign fibrous histiocytoma* and dermatofibrosarcoma occasionally proves difficult when only the superficial portion of the dermatofibrosarcoma is present in a biopsy specimen, because these areas appear so well differentiated (Table 13–2). Under these circumstances, knowledge of the size and configuration of the lesion in question suggests the diagnosis, and biopsy of a deeper portion confirms it. In addition, because CD34 is almost always expressed by dermatofibrosarcoma and far less so by benign fibrous histiocytoma, CD34 is an extremely useful antigen for solving this problem.[12,13] The recent observation that benign fibrous histiocytomas express HMGA1 and HMGA2 but dermatofibrosarcomas do not suggests that these may in time become useful markers.[24] *Malignant fibrous histiocytoma* (pleomorphic undifferentiated

sarcoma) is not often confused with this tumor because it is characterized by far greater pleomorphism, mitotic activity, and necrosis. Moreover, its typical deep location in muscle and more rapid growth are at variance with the indolent course of this tumor. Rarely, one encounters dermatofibrosarcoma protuberans with areas of malignant fibrous histiocytoma (Figs 13–15, 13–16). As indicated earlier, when such areas represent more than just a microscopic focus, they should be diagnosed as "sarcoma arising in dermatofibrosarcoma protuberans."

A second common problem is the confusion of this tumor with benign neural tumors, specifically a diffuse form of *neurofibroma*. This is most likely to occur when dermatofibrosarcoma is in the plaque stage or when a biopsy is done on only the periphery of the tumor. However, neurofibroma usually contains tactoid structures or other features of neural differentiation, and it lacks the highly cellular areas with mitotic figures that

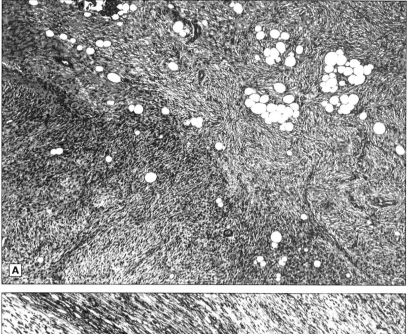

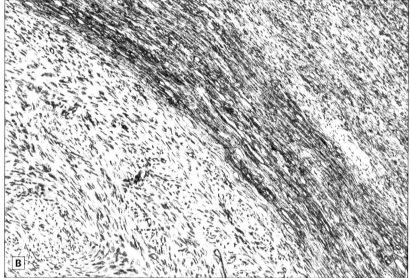

FIGURE 13–12 **(A)** Dermatofibrosarcoma protuberans showing the transition to fibrosarcoma (lower left corner). **(B)** CD34 immunostain in a dermatofibrosarcoma (upper right) with fibrosarcomatous areas. Note the marked diminution of CD34 immunostain in the fibrosarcomatous portion of the tumor (lower left).

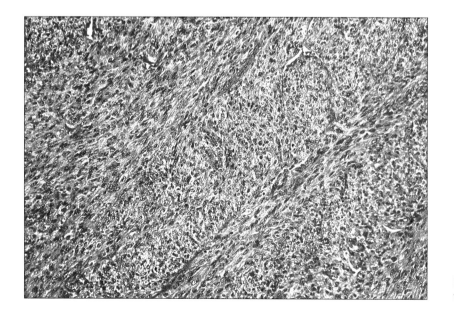

FIGURE 13–13 Fibrosarcomatous areas within dermatofibrosarcoma protuberans.

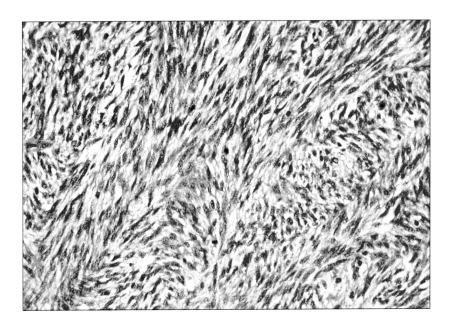

FIGURE 13–14 Fibrosarcomatous areas showing increased cellularity and mitotic activity.

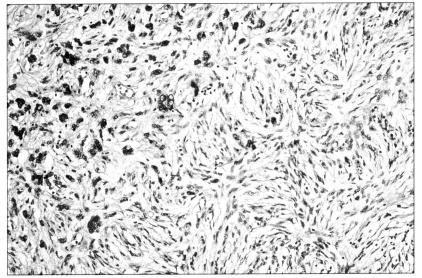

FIGURE 13–15 Dermatofibrosarcoma protuberans with transformation to malignant fibrous histiocytoma.

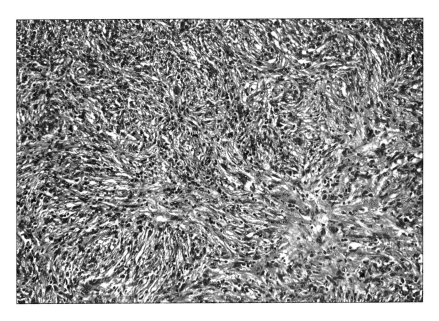

FIGURE 13–16 Malignant fibrous histiocytoma-like areas in dermatofibrosarcoma protuberans.

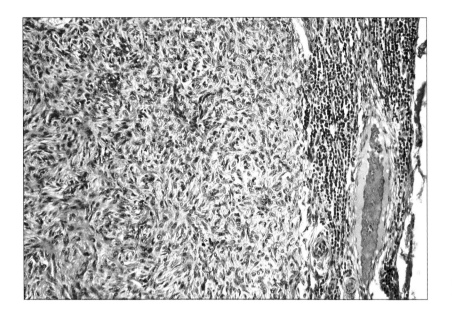

FIGURE 13–17 Lymph node metastasis from dermatofibrosarcoma protuberans.

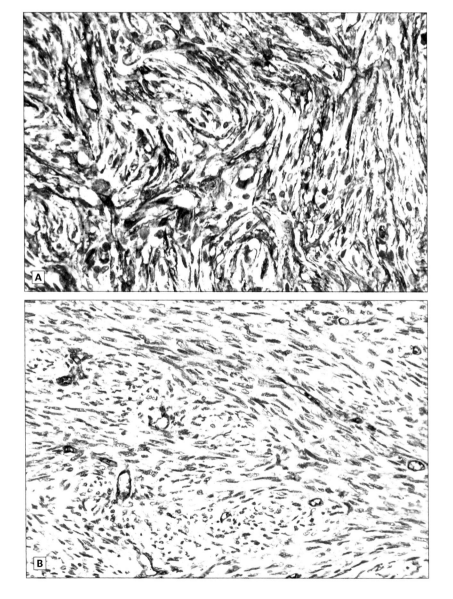

FIGURE 13–18 CD34 immunoreactivity within a conventional dermatofibrosarcoma **(A)** compared to markedly reduced immunoreactivity within a fibrosarcomatous area of dermatofibrosarcoma protuberans **(B)**.

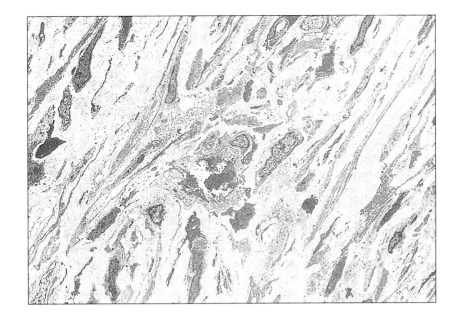

FIGURE 13–19 Electron micrograph of dermatofibrosarcoma protuberans showing the center of a storiform area occupied by a small vessel. Fibroblast-like cells spin out from the vessel and have numerous slender processes that may join each other by means of specialized cell contacts. (From Taxy JB, Battifora H. The electron microscope in the study and diagnosis of soft tissue tumors. In: Trump BF, Jones RT, eds. Diagnostic Electron Microscopy. New York: Wiley; 1980.)

TABLE 13–2	COMPARISON OF FIBROUS HISTIOCYTOMA AND DERMATOFIBROSARCOMA PROTUBERANS	
Parameter	**Benign fibrous histiocytoma**	**Dermatofibrosarcoma**
Common locations	Extremities	Trunk; groin
Size	Usually small	Small to large
Growth pattern	Short fascicles, haphazard	Monotonous storiform
Cell population	Plump spindle cells often admixed with inflammatory cells, siderophages, giant cells	Slender spindle cells with few if any secondary elements
Hemorrhage	Occasional	No
Subcutaneous extension	Occasional and limited	Consistent and extensive
CD34	Focal staining in occasional cases	Diffuse and extensive staining in most cases
Local recurrence	5–10%	20–50%
Metastasis	Anecdotal cases only	Rare in conventional form; potentially higher if fibrosarcoma present with inadequate local control
Malignant transformation	Anecdotal cases only	Fibrosarcoma in occasional cases

characterize the central portion of a dermatofibrosarcoma. The presence of S-100 protein in virtually all neurofibromas and its absence in dermatofibrosarcoma is an additional point of contrast.

Finally, highly myxoid forms of dermatofibrosarcoma may resemble *myxoid liposarcoma* by virtue of the prominent vasculature and bland stellate or fusiform cells. However, the superficial location, gross configuration, CD34 immunoreactivity, and complete absence of lipoblasts should raise serious questions concerning the diagnosis of liposarcoma. In such cases, additional sampling of the tumor or review of the original material in a recurrent lesion may reveal the diagnostic cellular areas.

Discussion

Unlike the benign fibrous histiocytoma it resembles, dermatofibrosarcoma protuberans is a locally aggressive neoplasm that recurs in up to one-half of patients.[5,25,26] The high recurrence rate in part reflects the extensive infiltration of the tumor compared with fibrous histiocytoma and failure to appreciate this phenomenon at the time of surgery. It is clear that prompt wide local excision (2–3 cm), the standard of practice for this lesion, can markedly alter the recurrence rate. Recurrence rates reported in the literature for patients treated by wide local excision average range from 10–20% compared to 43%

when the excision was undefined or conservative.[27] In addition, recurrence rates in cases treated primarily at large referral centers are low (1.75–33%),[4,6,28] again suggesting that adequate initial surgery is essential for minimizing recurrences. The risk of local recurrence, furthermore, correlates well with the extent of the wide excision. If the excision margin is 3 cm or more, the recurrence rate is 20%, compared with 41% if the margin is 2 cm or less.[29] If local recurrence develops, it is usually within 3 years of the initial surgery,[25] although about one-third of patients will develop recurrences after 5 years, attesting to the need for long-term follow-up. In patients who develop multiple recurrences, progressively shorter intervals between successive recurrences have been noted.[5]

Mohs' micrographic surgery has been met with growing enthusiasm for treatment of this disease.[30–34] Those who advocate this approach point out that dermatofibrosarcoma protuberans occasionally grows in an asymmetric fashion from its epicenter such that a traditional wide local excision fails to remove all tumor in a subset of cases.[35] Mohs' surgery offers the potential to achieve clear margins with minimum removal of normal tissue, an advantage particularly attractive for sites such as the head and neck. Local recurrence rates following Mohs' surgery are less than 10% and in some studies approach 0%.[26,32,33]

Despite its locally aggressive behavior, this tumor infrequently metastasizes and therefore should be clearly distinguished from conventional sarcomas. The incidence of metastasis is difficult to assess because of the bias introduced when selectively reporting metastasizing tumors, the inability to determine if sarcomatous areas were noted in a subset of reported cases, and the lack of uniform treatment. In general, however, for the ordinary dermatofibrosarcoma protuberans uncomplicated by areas of fibrosarcoma, metastasis appears to be an uncommon event. In one large study of 115 patients, no metastases were observed,[5] whereas, in two other studies, 5 of 86 patients[25] and 4 of 96 patients[4] developed metastases. In the latter study the follow-up period was 15 years. Thus, long-term follow-up may reveal higher metastatic rates than previously reported. Of the 471 patients reported in the literature, 16 (3.4%) developed metastatic disease.[4] About three-fourths of patients with metastases have hematogenous spread to the lungs, and one-fourth have lymphatic spread to regional lymph nodes. Metastases to other sites, such as the brain, bones, and heart, have also been documented. Although some metastasizing cases have clearly originated from tumors with areas of "sarcoma" (see below), some have not.[36]

Metastasizing lesions share some common clinical features. They are almost always recurrent lesions, and there is usually an interval of several years between diagnosis and metastasis. The low incidence of regional lymph node metastasis and the negative findings in a small series of blind lymph node dissections do not warrant routine node dissection. Resection of isolated pulmonary metastases has been advocated because of the overall low-grade behavior of the tumor. Radiotherapy has been recommended for large, unresectable tumors or postoperatively for margin-positive tumors.[37] Molecular targeting of dermatofibrosarcoma protuberans with imatanib mesylate has recently been employed in patients with advanced or metastatic disease with significant reductions in tumor burden.[38–40]

SARCOMA ARISING IN DERMATOFIBROSARCOMA PROTUBERANS (FIBROSARCOMATOUS VARIANT OF DERMATOFIBROSARCOMA PROTUBERANS)

There has been increasing awareness that a small subset of dermatofibrosarcomas contain areas indistinguishable from conventional fibrosarcoma (and rarely malignant fibrous histiocytoma).[8,10,11,41,42] This has led to the use of the term "fibrosarcomatous variant of dermatofibrosarcoma" and the suggestion that these lesions pursue a more aggressive course, although the risk of distant metastasis is debated. These tumors share the same general clinical properties as ordinary dermatofibrosarcoma protuberans, and in most cases the sarcomatous foci are noted in the original tumor.

To diagnose sarcoma arising in dermatofibrosarcoma protuberans we have generally used a constellation of features: the "sarcomatous" foci should constitute at least 5–10% of the tumor, in contrast to simply a rare to occasional microscopic focus. These zones are characterized by a fascicular (rather than storiform) architectural pattern and are composed of plump spindle cells of high nuclear grade. Mitotic activity is increased in these areas, whereas CD34 immunoreactivity is often diminished (Fig. 13–19B), compared to the surrounding dermatofibrosarcoma. In addition, fibrosarcomatous areas are also characterized by a higher MIB-1 labeling index and increased p53 immunostaining than the classic areas. Although we have never required an absolute level of mitotic activity to diagnose sarcomatous change, mitotic activity within these sarcomatous areas averages 7–15/10 HPF[10,41] compared to 1–3/10 HPF in dermatofibrosarcoma.

The significance of sarcomatous forms of dermatofibrosarcoma protuberans has been the subject of a number of studies. Although it seems logical that high-grade areas within a low-grade lesion would affect behavior adversely, early studies failed to confirm this hypothesis in a statistically meaningful fashion.[43] Ding and Enjoji suggested that fibrosarcomatous areas within dermatofibrosarcoma protuberans are associated with a higher local recurrence rate and thus a more aggressive course, but the status and adequacy of surgical excisions in these cases was not

TABLE 13–3	SARCOMA ARISING IN DERMATOFIBROSARCOMA PROTUBERANS		
Study	No. of patients*	Recurrence rate (%)	Metastatic rate (%)
Mentzel et al.[41]	34	58	14.7
Pizarro et al.[45]	19	42	33.0
Goldblum et al.[10]	18	22	0

*Patients with follow-up information.

TABLE 13–4	SARCOMAS ARISING IN DERMATOFIBROSARCOMA PROTUBERANS TREATED WITH WIDE LOCAL EXCISION, WITH FOLLOW-UP INFORMATION	
Study	No. of patients	Metastasis
Goldblum et al.[10]	18	0/18
Mentzel et al.[41]	6	0/6
Diaz-Cascajo et al.[92]	3	1/3
O'Connell et al.[93]	2	0/2
Total	29	1/29

made clear.[43] Connelly and Evans[44] reported no difference in the local recurrence rate or in time to recurrence compared with conventional dermatofibrosarcoma protuberans but noted that two of their six patients with fibrosarcomatous areas developed metastatic disease. Two large studies by Mentzel et al.[41] and Pizarro et al.,[45] on the other hand, revealed higher local recurrence rates (58% and 42%, respectively) and metastatic rates (13.7% and 33.0%, respectively) (Table 13–3). In neither study, however, did it appear that wide local excision with clear margins was achieved in most cases. A more recent study of 41 patients has documented a 10% incidence of metastasis in fibrosarcomatous dermatofibrosarcoma protuberans but again patients in that study appear not to have received optimal surgical therapy.[46] All received local excisions that often left positive margins and three of four patients with metastasis also experienced local recurrences, again suggesting inadequate primary surgery. Because the ability to eradicate tumor locally arguably affects the risk of subsequent dissemination, none of these studies addressed the behavior of this neoplasm in the context of the current standard of practice. In our experience with 18 patients treated by wide local excision and clear margins and with a minimum follow-up of 5 years, local recurrence rates are essentially identical to those of ordinary dermatofibrosarcoma protuberans; and we noted no instance of metastasis.[10] Similarly, culling cases from the literature of sarcomatous dermatofibrosarcoma in which wide local excisions were performed, only one instance of metastasis was noted (Table 13–4). To clearly resolve the issue of metastasis in fibrosarcomatous dermatofibrosarcoma protuberans, follow-up of a larger cohort of patients treated with adequate surgery and who achieve negative margins is needed.

In summary, although dermatofibrosarcoma protuberans containing fibrosarcoma may well be an inherently more aggressive neoplasm, this behavior can be favorably influenced by wide local excision to the extent that there may be little increased risk of distant metastasis over that of conventional dermatofibrosarcoma protuberans. Thus, wide local excision should be even more forcefully encouraged than for conventional dermatofibrosarcoma protuberans.

BEDNAR TUMOR (PIGMENTED DERMATOFIBROSARCOMA PROTUBERANS, STORIFORM NEUROFIBROMA)

In 1957, Bednar[47] described a group of nine cutaneous tumors characterized by indolent growth and a prominent storiform pattern and in four cases by the presence of melanin pigment. He regarded these tumors as variants of neurofibroma (*storiform neurofibroma*) and cited as evidence the presence of similar areas within neural nevi[48] and the presence of melanin. We reserve the term *Bednar tumor* for tumors that resemble dermatofibrosarcoma protuberans but that, in addition, have melanin pigment. These tumors are uncommon,[43,47,49–52] as evidenced by the fact that Bednar gleaned only four cases from among 100 000 biopsy specimens; in our experience these tumors account for fewer than 5% of all cases of dermatofibrosarcoma protuberans. Although, as suggested by Bednar, these tumors may represent neural lesions, their nonpigmented portions are virtually identical to dermatofibrosarcoma protuberans. Moreover, their clinical and gross features are similar. Most are slowly growing cutaneous masses that extend to the epidermis and advance into the deep subcutis. The number of melanin-bearing cells varies widely within these tumors. In some, large numbers of melanin-containing cells cause black discoloration of the tumor (Fig. 13–20), whereas in others melanin is so sparse it can be appreciated only microscopically. These cells are scattered irregularly throughout the tumor (Fig. 13–21A). Their tentacle-like processes emanating from a central nucleus-containing zone give them a characteristic bipolar or multipolar shape, depending on the plane of the section (Fig. 13–21B). They stain with conventional

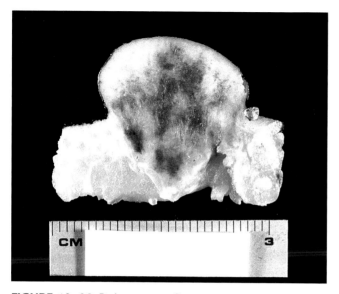

FIGURE 13–20 Bednar tumor. Gross appearance of the tumor is identical to conventional dermatofibrosarcoma protuberans, but the substance of the tumor is flecked with melanin pigment.

melanin stains and ultrastructurally contain mature membrane-bound melanosomes. Electron microscopic studies reveal that most areas of Bednar tumors are composed of slender fibroblastic cells arranged in a delicate collagen matrix (Fig. 13–22), although other areas have cells more suggestive of Schwann cell differentiation (Fig. 13–23). The cells have numerous interlocking processes elaborately invested with basal laminae. Mature and immature melanosomes can be identified within the tumor cells. We have suggested that this finding indicates that the tumor synthesizes rather than phagocytoses melanin (Fig. 13–24), whereas others have suggested that the tumor is simply colonized by melanin-bearing cells.[52] On the other hand, we have not been able to identify S-100 protein,[50] which is present in many neural tumors, in Bednar tumors or their nonpigmented counterparts.

Because of the rarity of this tumor, there are few collective data in the literature concerning its behavior, although overall it appears to be similar to dermatofibro-

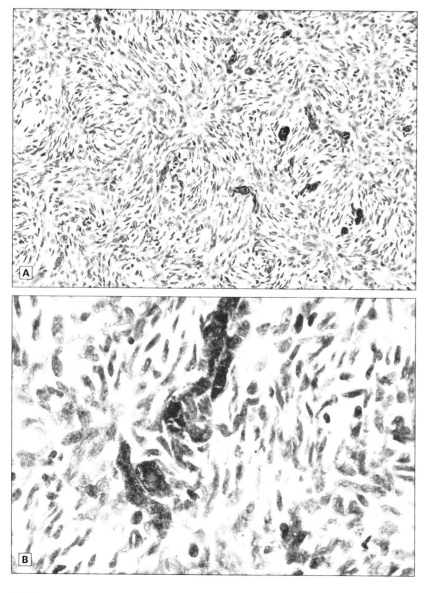

FIGURE 13–21 Pigmented dermatofibrosarcoma protuberans (Bednar tumor) **(A)** showing dendritic pigmented cells **(B)**.

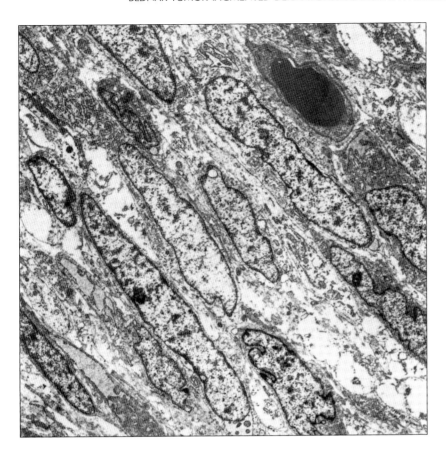

FIGURE 13–22 The predominant cells in a Bednar tumor have features of fibroblasts (×5700). (From Dupree SB, Langloss JM, Weiss SW. Pigmented dermatofibrosarcoma protuberans (Bednar tumor): a pathologic, ultrastructural, and immunohistochemical study. Am J Surg Pathol 1985; 9:630, with permission.)

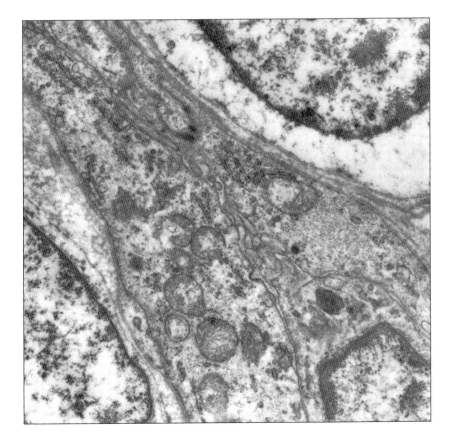

FIGURE 13–23 Schwann cell-like areas of a Bednar tumor where cells have interlacing processes, junctions, and basal lamina (×24800). (From Dupree WB, Langloss JM, Weiss SW. Pigmented dermatofibrosarcoma protuberans (Bednar tumor): a pathologic, ultrastructural, and immunohistochemical study. Am J Surg Pathol 1985; 9:630, with permission.)

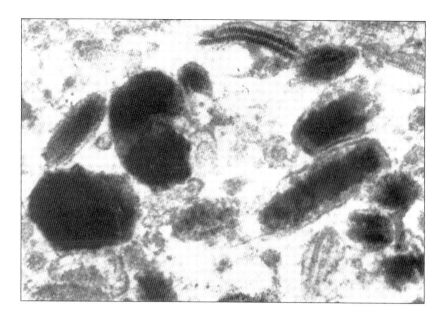

FIGURE 13-24 Mature and immature melanosomes in a Bednar tumor (×93 900). (From Dupree WB, Langloss JM, Weiss SW. Pigmented dermatofibrosarcoma protuberans (Bednar tumor): a pathologic, ultrastructural, and immunohistochemical study. Am J Surg Pathol 1985; 9:630, with permission.)

sarcoma protuberans. In addition, these tumors may display fibrosarcomatous areas.[53] There are also rare examples of metastasis, some with areas of fibrosarcoma,[53,54] including one report in the literature of a Bednar tumor with pulmonary metastasis.[55]

GIANT CELL FIBROBLASTOMA

Giant cell fibroblastoma was first described in 1982 by Shmookler and Enzinger, who suggested that it represents a juvenile form of dermatofibrosarcoma protuberans, a view reinforced in their seminal publication in 1989.[56] Subsequent reports reaffirmed it as an entity[57-64] and embraced this notion for describing tumors with hybrid features or lesions that evolved from one pattern to the other.[57,59,60,65-69]

Finally, the two lesions have been shown to have the same cytogenetic abnormality (supernumerary ring chromosome derived from chromosomes 17 and 22),[70] although there is some evidence that the ring chromosome occurs in cases of dermatofibrosarcoma, whereas the linear derivative chromosome occurs in giant cell fibroblastoma.[18] Both, however, result in the same molecular event (see above).

Clinical findings

Giant cell fibroblastoma develops as a painless nodule or mass in the dermis or subcutis, with a predilection for the back of the thigh, inguinal region, and chest wall. It affects predominantly infants and children, being encountered only infrequently in adults.[58,71] In our experience, about two-thirds of the children were younger than 5 years of age when brought to medical attention, and the median age was 3 years. About two-thirds of patients are male.

Pathologic findings

Grossly, the lesions consist of gray to yellow mucoid masses that are poorly circumscribed and measure 1–8 cm. They are composed of loosely arranged, wavy spindle cells with a moderate degree of nuclear pleomorphism that infiltrate the deep dermis and subcutis and encircle adnexal structures in a fashion similar to dermatofibrosarcoma protuberans (Figs 13–25 to 13–32). The tumors vary in cellularity from those approximating the cellularity of dermatofibrosarcoma protuberans (Figs 13–27, 13–31) to those that are hypocellular with a myxoid or hyaline stroma (Figs 13–28 to 13–30). The characteristic feature of the tumor is the peculiar pseudovascular spaces which seem to reflect a loss of cellular cohesion. Large and irregular in shape, the pseudovascular spaces are lined by a discontinuous row of multinucleated cells that represent variants of the basic proliferating tumor cell (Figs 13–26, 13–32). Although these cells appear to contain multiple overlapping nuclei, as seen by light microscopy, they actually represent multiple sausage-like lobations of a single nucleus when studied ultrastructurally (Fig. 13–33).[56] Immunohistochemical studies indicate that these tumors express vimentin but lack S-100 protein and vascular markers.[71] Most giant cell fibroblastomas express CD34, a feature they share with dermatofibrosarcoma protuberans.

Differential diagnosis

In our early experience about 40% of giant cell fibroblastomas were misdiagnosed as *sarcoma*. Because of the

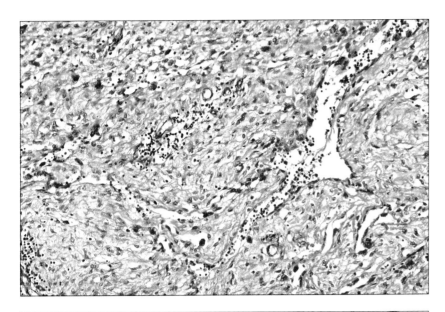

FIGURE 13–25 Classic appearance of a giant cell fibroblastoma showing pseudovascular spaces lined by giant cells.

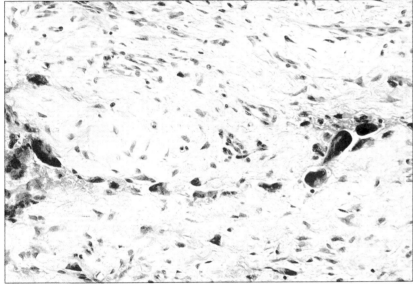

FIGURE 13–26 Hyperchromatic giant cells lining pseudovascular spaces in a giant cell fibroblastoma.

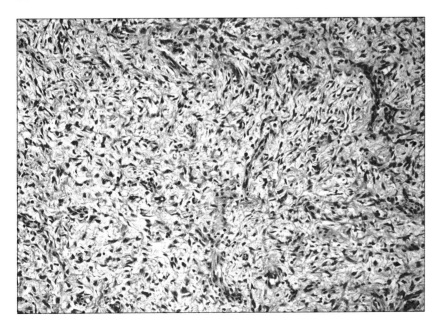

FIGURE 13–27 Cellular areas in a giant cell fibroblastoma (×160).

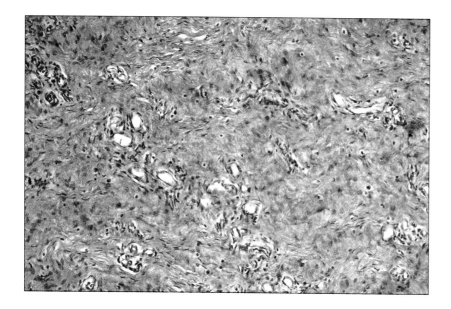

FIGURE 13–28 Hypocellular hyalinized zones in a giant cell fibroblastoma (×160).

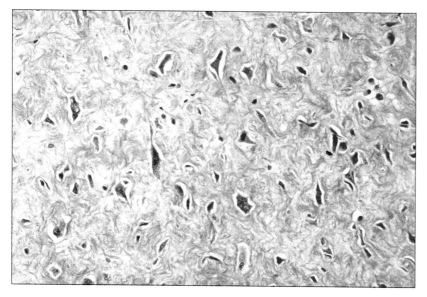

FIGURE 13–29 Markedly hyalinized area in a giant cell fibroblastoma.

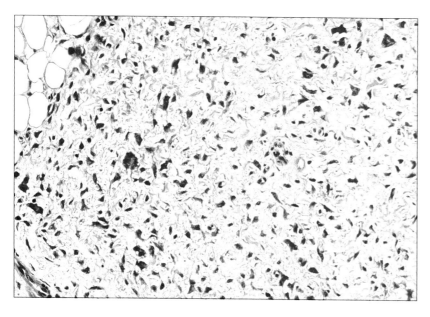

FIGURE 13–30 Hypocellular area in a giant cell fibroblastoma with giant cells not associated with pseudovascular spaces.

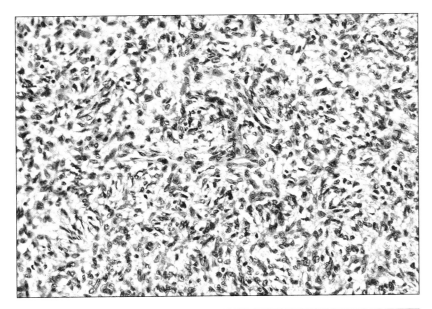

FIGURE 13–31 Dermatofibrosarcoma protuberans-like area in a giant cell fibroblastoma.

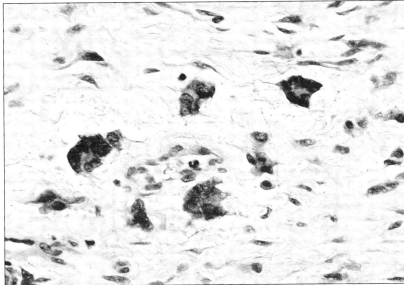

FIGURE 13–32 Giant cells in a giant cell fibroblastoma.

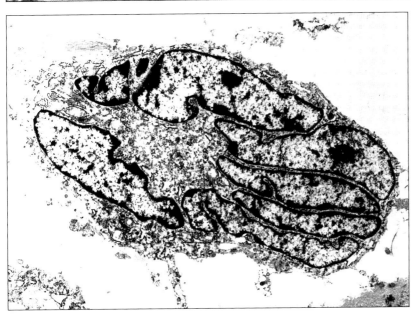

FIGURE 13–33 Electron micrograph of giant cells illustrating a hypersegmented nucleus. (Courtesy of Dr. Barry Schmookler.)

myxoid areas and hyperchromatic giant cells, there is a tendency to assume they represent examples of myxoid liposarcoma or myxoid malignant fibrous histiocytoma occurring in an unusually young individual. Important clues to the diagnosis include the superficial location, lack of an intricate vasculature, and the presence of hyperchromatic cells lying preferentially along the pseudovascular spaces.

Discussion

There have been fewer reports of giant cell fibroblastoma than dermatofibrosarcoma protuberans in the literature. Recurrences have developed in about one-half of cases, but metastases have not been reported. Treatment of these tumors ideally is wide local excision. If limited therapy is contemplated, conscientious follow-up is advisable to document and treat recurrences.

It is well accepted that giant cell fibroblastoma and dermatofibrosarcoma are slightly different expressions of the same neoplasm. Like dermatofibrosarcoma protuberans, giant cell fibroblastoma occurs in superficial soft tissues, with a strong predilection for the abdominal wall, back, and groin. Even more compelling is the observation that hybrid tumors occur. For example, occasional dermatofibrosarcomas of adults contain giant cells or foci similar to those of giant cell fibroblastoma.[67] Less frequently, otherwise typical giant cell fibroblastomas of childhood contain areas of dermatofibrosarcoma protuberans. There have also been a number of recorded instances in which either dermatofibrosarcoma protuberans or giant cell fibroblastoma has recurred and recapitulated the pattern of the other tumor in the recurrence.[63,66,68] Finally, the giant cell fibroblastoma displays a cytogenetic abnormality identical to that of dermatofibrosarcoma protuberans (see above).

ANGIOMATOID FIBROUS HISTIOCYTOMA

Previously termed *angiomatoid malignant fibrous histiocytoma*,[72] this distinctive tumor of children and young adults has been renamed *angiomatoid fibrous histiocytoma*, a designation that reflects the relative rarity of metastasis and the overall excellent clinical course.

Clinical findings

Angiomatoid fibrous histiocytoma, a tumor that occurs primarily in children and young adults, is rarely encountered in adults over age 40. It develops as a slowly growing nodular, multinodular, or cystic mass of the hypodermis or subcutis. It most often occurs on the extremities. Local symptoms such as pain and tenderness are uncommon, but systemic symptoms such as anemia, pyrexia, and

weight loss are occasionally encountered and suggest the production of cytokines by the neoplasm.

Gross and microscopic findings

The tumors are firm, circumscribed lesions that usually measure a few centimeters in diameter and vary in color from gray-tan to red-brown, depending on the amount of hemosiderin present. One of the most characteristic features is the presence of irregular blood-filled cystic spaces best appreciated on cross section (Fig. 13–34). This feature may be so striking as to give the impression of a hematoma, hemangioma, or a thrombosed vessel.

These lesions are characterized by three features: irregular solid masses of histiocyte-like cells, cystic areas of hemorrhage, and chronic inflammation. In general, the solid masses of histiocyte-like cells interspersed with areas of hemorrhage occupy the central portion of the tumor, and the inflammatory cells form a dense peripheral cuff that blends with the surrounding pseudocapsule (Figs 13–35 to 13–43).

The histiocyte-like cells are usually quite uniform; they have a round or oval nucleus and a faintly staining eosinophilic cytoplasm often containing finely particulate hemosiderin. In most instances the cells are bland, such that some may be confused with the histiocytes of granulomas (Figs 13–41, 13–42). In about one-fifth of cases, significant nuclear atypia or hyperchromatic giant cells are present (Fig. 13–43), a feature that does not correlate with aggressive behavior.[73] In a small number of cases, myxoid change may develop in the tumor. Lipid and especially hemosiderin are present in the cells, but xanthoma cells are usually absent. Multifocal hemorrhage is a striking feature in all cases and results in the formation of irregular cystic spaces (Figs 13–37, 13–38). Although these spaces resemble vascular spaces, they are not lined

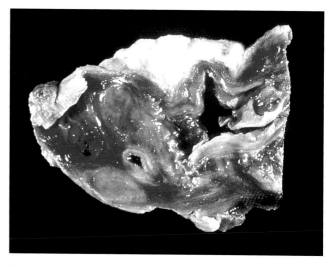

FIGURE 13–34 Gross specimen of an angiomatoid fibrous histiocytoma illustrating cystic change and a hemosiderin-stained tumor. Normal fat is present at the periphery.

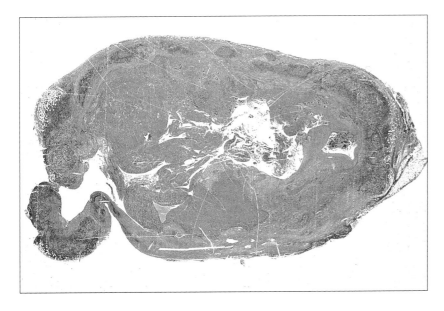

FIGURE 13–35 Angiomatoid fibrous histiocytoma shows a partially cystic tumor mass surrounded by a dense fibrous pseudocapsule and prominent lymphoid cuff.

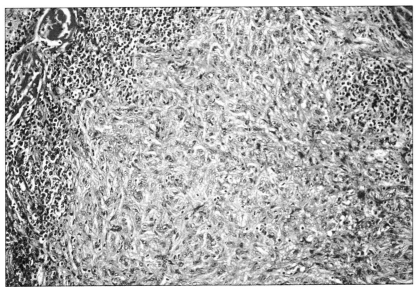

FIGURE 13–36 Angiomatoid fibrous histiocytoma. Histiocyte-like cells are arranged in solid sheets. Lymphoid infiltrate surrounds the tumor nodule.

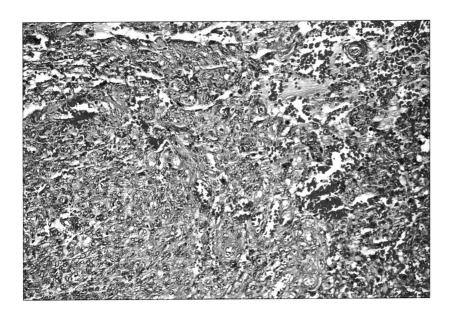

FIGURE 13–37 Areas of microscopic hemorrhage and cystic change in an angiomatoid fibrous histiocytoma.

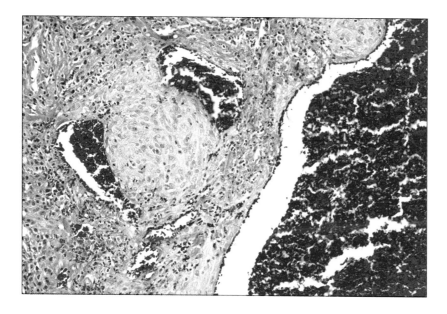

FIGURE 13–38 Cystic hemorrhage in an angiomatoid fibrous histiocytoma.

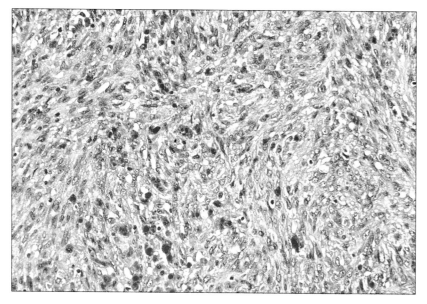

FIGURE 13–39 Spindle cell area in an angiomatoid fibrous histiocytoma.

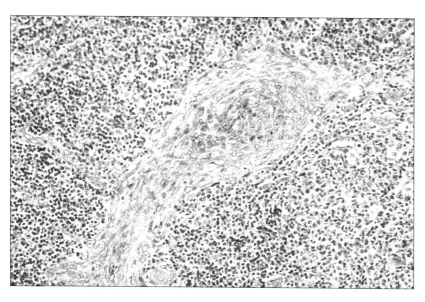

FIGURE 13–40 Tentacle-like extension of tumor in an angiomatoid fibrous histiocytoma surrounded by a chronic inflammatory response.

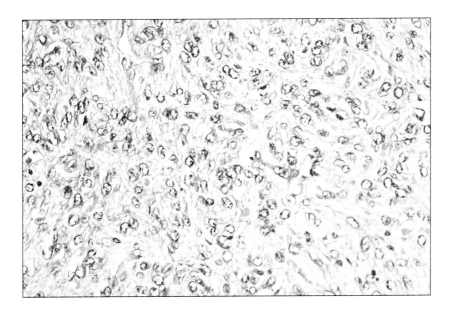

FIGURE 13–41 Histiocyte-like cells in an angiomatoid fibrous histiocytoma.

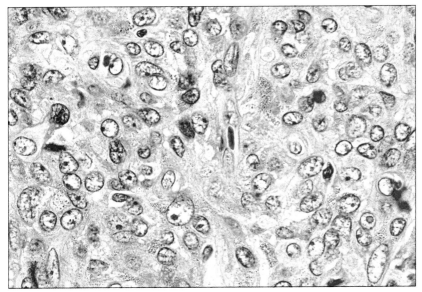

FIGURE 13–42 Histiocyte-like cells in an angiomatoid fibrous histiocytoma.

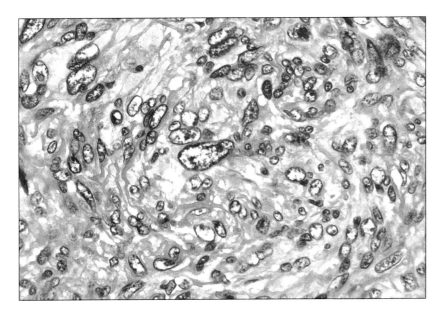

FIGURE 13–43 Cellular atypia in angiomatoid fibrous histiocytoma.

by endothelium but, rather, by flattened tumor cells. Small vessels may be present at the periphery of the nodules, but they do not seem to be the major components of these tumors. Inflammatory cells consist of a mixture of lymphocytes and plasma cells. Germinal center formation is occasionally observed, a feature suggesting lymph node metastasis, especially if the tumor represents a recurrence. The resemblance to a lymph node is further heightened by the thick pseudocapsule, a structure often interpreted as a lymph node capsule. However, unlike a true lymph node, there are no subcapsular or medullary sinuses, and germinal center formation occurs randomly around the tumor, without a predilection for the subcapsular zone. Differentiation of these tumors from hemorrhagic fibrous histiocytomas is discussed in Chapter 12.

Discussion

Angiomatoid fibrous histiocytoma was originally believed to be a reasonably aggressive neoplasm based on follow-up of a small number of cases ascertained retrospectively.[72] In the most recent large study of 86 patients, only one patient developed a regional lymph node metastasis and one, a local recurrence.[74] A number of factors can be correlated with the risk of local recurrence, including infiltrating margins, location on the head and neck, and involvement of skeletal muscle rather than the subcutis.[75] Complete surgical excision without adjuvant therapy is the appropriate treatment for these low-grade tumors.

Since the original description of this tumor in 1979, a number of views have been espoused concerning the line of differentiation. Although the lesions have a decidedly histiocytic appearance and show ample evidence of phagocytosis of hemosiderin, immunohistochemical analysis of histiocytic antigens has been disappointing.[75] The tumors do not express muramidase or L-1. About half express CD68 (KP-1),[75] probably because of acquisition of this antigen by cells that are phagocytic and have a high density of phagolysosomes. An intriguing observation is the finding of desmin within half of these cases[74,76,77] and other muscle markers within a smaller percentage (muscle-specific actin, heavy-caldesmon, smooth muscle actin, and calponin).[76] CD99 is also present in about one-half of cases.[74] The close association of these tumors with lymphoid tissue as well as this myoid phenotype has led to the postulate that these cells may be related to the desmin-positive stromal cells of lymph node.[74] Recently, it has been shown that this tumor possesses a fusion gene which incorporates either *EWSR1* or *FUS* genes with the *ATF-1* gene. The *EWSR1-ATF1* fusion is molecularly similar to that of clear cell sarcoma yet paradoxically results in a histologically dissimilar lesion without expression of the MITF-M transcript as occurs in clear cell sarcoma.[78,79]

PLEXIFORM FIBROHISTIOCYTIC TUMOR

Clinical findings

Plexiform fibrohistiocytic tumor, like giant cell fibroblastoma and angiomatoid fibrous histiocytoma, occurs almost exclusively in children and young adults and is rarely encountered after the age of 30 years.[80] It typically presents as a slowly growing mass of the deep dermis and subcutaneous tissues. In our experience, the most common location is the upper extremity (63%) followed by the lower extremity (14%).

Gross and microscopic findings

The lesions are relatively small (1–3 cm), ill-defined masses with a gray-white trabecular appearance. In its most typical form (about 40% of cases) the lesion contains a mixture of two components: a differentiated fibroblastic component and a round cell histiocytic component containing multinucleated giant cells. At low-power microscopy one is impressed by the numerous tiny cellular nodules that occupy the dermis and subcutaneous tissue (Figs 13–44, 13–45). These nodules are composed of nests of histiocytic cells that often contain multinucleated, osteoclast-like giant cells and occasionally undergo focal hemorrhage (Figs 13–46 to 13–50). The cells in these nodules are well differentiated and do not display atypia or significant levels of mitotic activity. The nodules, in turn, are circumscribed by short fascicles of fibroblastic cells (Figs 13–47 to 13–49) that intersect slightly or ramify in the soft tissue, creating a plexiform growth pattern. The fascicles of spindle cells to some extent resemble fibromatosis, except that the cells are usually plumper and the fascicles shorter than those of fibromatosis. In the less typical case, the two components described above may not be equally represented. For example, in a few cases the nodules of giant cells are rare or absent, and only short intersecting fascicles of plump spindle cells are seen. In other cases there may be a blending of the nodules and fascicles; and the cells in these two zones may appear to be in an intermediate stage between fibroblasts and histiocytes.

Ancillary studies

Immunohistochemically, the multinucleated giant cells and many of the mononuclear cells express CD68, suggesting true histiocytic differentiation, whereas the spindle cells express smooth muscle actin, as one would expect of myofibroblasts (Fig. 13–51). The cells do not contain other histiocytic markers such as HLA-DR, lysozyme, or L-2; nor are S-100 protein, keratin, desmin, and Factor XIIIa present.

Ultrastructural studies have identified cells with features of histiocytes and myofibroblasts.[81] In a large series

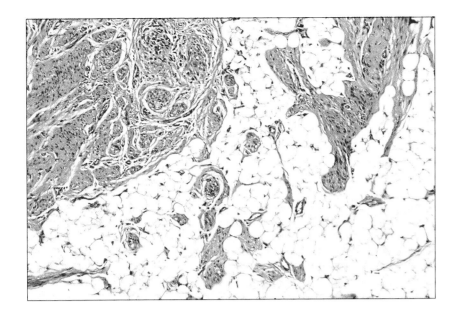

FIGURE 13–44 Plexiform fibrohistiocytic tumor showing ramifying fascicles of tumor in the subcutis.

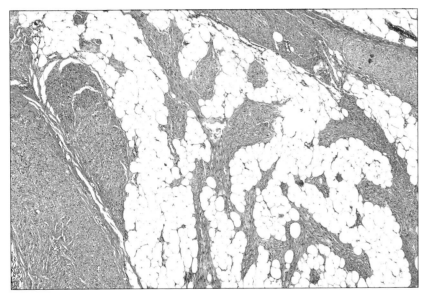

FIGURE 13–45 Plexiform fibrohistiocytic tumor showing relatively acellular ramifying fascicles in the subcutis.

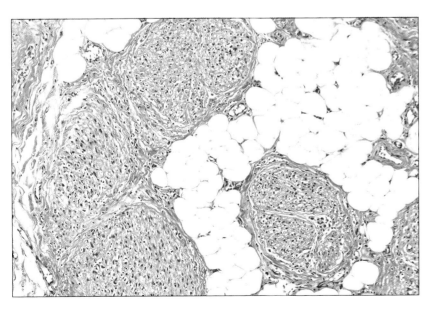

FIGURE 13–46 Irregular fascicles and nodules of a plexiform fibrohistiocytic tumor.

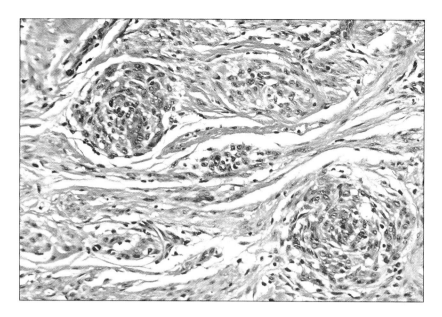

FIGURE 13–47 Typical "biphasic" appearance of a plexiform fibrohistiocytic tumor. Histiocyte-like nodules circumscribed by fibromatosis-like areas.

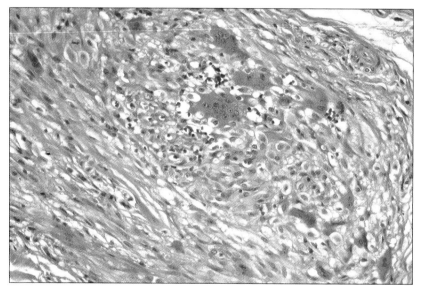

FIGURE 13–48 Nodules of histiocyte-like cells in a plexiform fibrohistiocytic tumor.

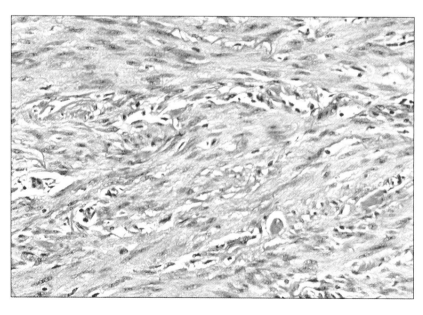

FIGURE 13–49 Plexiform fibrohistiocytic tumor with areas of short, ramifying fascicles of fibroblasts without histiocytes.

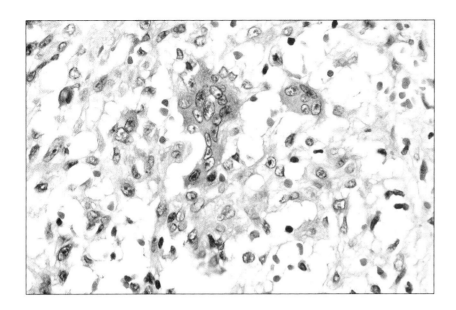

FIGURE 13–50 Plexiform fibrohistiocytic tumor with a high-power view of histiocyte-like cells comprising tumor nodules.

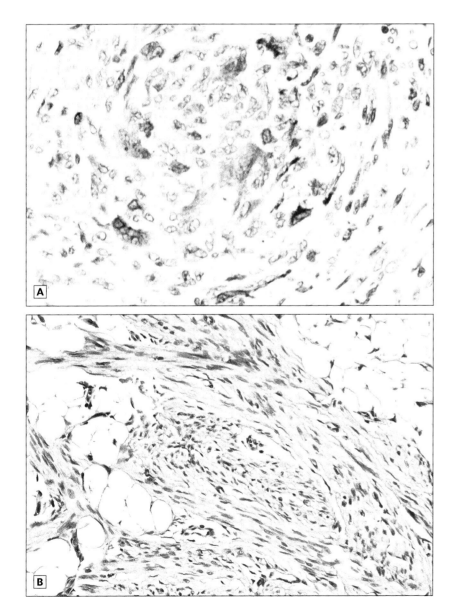

FIGURE 13–51 CD68 immunostain of a plexiform fibrohistiocytic tumor showing positivity of histiocytic giant cell nodules **(A)** and no positivity of fibroblastic areas **(B)**.

reported by Remstein et al., all cases were diploid with an S-phase fraction of 0.93–7.22%.[82] Cytogenetic analysis has been carried out in a few cases. One patient had a complex karyotype with numerous deletions, whereas the other had a t(4;15)(q21;q15).[83,84]

Differential diagnosis

A variety of benign diagnoses that includes granuloma, fibrous hamartoma, fibrous histiocytoma, giant cell tumor, and fibromatosis is entertained in these cases. The most important distinctions are those that materially affect the management of the patient. It is essential to distinguish the lesion from an infectious granulomatous process. In the typical case the presence of associated fibroblastic cuffing of the histiocytic nodules is usually sufficient to suggest an alternative diagnosis. In tumors that are predominantly histiocytic, the important observations include the fact that these tumors do not have a surrounding inflammatory infiltrate, nor do the histiocytic nodules undergo central necrosis. Predominantly fibroblastic forms of plexiform fibrohistiocytic tumor may resemble fibromatosis, but in fibromatosis the fascicles are wider, longer, and composed of more slender fibroblastic cells.

Discussion

Based on three series, these tumors appear to be low-grade neoplasms that frequently recur (12.5–40%) within 1–2 years of the original diagnosis.[83,85,86] Lymph node metastases have been observed in only two cases,[83,85] and only three patients in the literature have had histologically proven pulmonary metastases, one of whom died of the disease. It should be noted that there may be pulmonary metastases at the time of presentation, emphasizing the need for careful initial evaluation. Unfortunately, no histologic parameters (e.g., mitotic activity, vascular invasion) have been correlated with aggressive behavior. Ideally, these lesions are completely, if not widely, excised. It does not seem appropriate to commit the patient to adjuvant therapy based on the limited risk of regional or distant disease.

SOFT TISSUE GIANT CELL TUMOR OF LOW MALIGNANT POTENTIAL

In 1999, the term "soft tissue giant cell tumors of low malignant potential" was proposed for a group of lesions that represents the benign end of the spectrum of malignant giant cell tumor of soft parts (malignant fibrous histiocytoma, giant cell type) and that seem to be the soft tissue analogue of giant cell tumor of bone.[87] These lesions were first described in two nearly simultaneous publications during the 1970s.[88,89] Salm and Sissons

reported a group of 10 giant cell tumors of soft parts that they likened to giant cell tumors of bone,[89] and Guccion and Enzinger noted a subset of malignant giant cell tumors of soft parts characterized by "less atypia and mitotic activity" and that did not give rise to metastatic disease.[88] Two additional studies were subsequently published.[90,91]

Although seemingly a new entity, these lesions were probably grouped with a number of other lesions in the past, such as tenosynovial giant cell tumor, malignant giant cell tumor of soft parts, plexiform fibrohistiocytic tumor, and even epithelioid sarcoma. Although to date there has not been an instance of metastasis from any of these lesions, logically one might expect to encounter rare instances of metastasis similar to those seen with giant cell tumor of bone.

Clinical and pathologic features

These lesions tend to occur in all age groups and may develop in superficial or deep soft tissue, most commonly on the arm or hand. They consist of multiple tumor nodules that diffusely infiltrate soft tissue. The nodules are composed of bland mononuclear cells, short spindle cells, and osteoclasts (Figs 13–52 to 13–54). By definition, the mononuclear and giant cells in these lesions lack the striking atypia that is the hallmark of giant cell forms of malignant fibrous histiocytoma (Fig. 13–53). Despite the lack of nuclear atypia, they often have brisk mitotic activity; about one-half display vascular invasion (as may be seen with giant cell tumor of bone), although necrosis is not seen. Metaplastic bone and angiectatic spaces reminiscent of the changes of aneurysmal bone cysts can be seen (Figs 13–55, 13–56). Soft tissue giant cell tumors have an immunophenotypic profile similar to that of giant cell tumor of bone in that they express CD68 and smooth muscle actin, and the osteoclastic giant cells express the osteoclast-specific marker tartrate-resistant acid phosphatase (TRAP). However, they lack CD45, S-100 protein, desmin, and lysozyme.

Differential diagnosis

In our experience these tumors are most often confused with tenosynovial giant cell tumor or malignant giant cell tumor of soft parts (malignant fibrous histiocytoma, giant cell type). Apart from the rather significant difference in location, *tenosynovial giant cell tumor* usually has prominent stromal hyalinization and a more heterogeneous population of cells, including xanthoma cells, siderophages, and lymphocytes. Giant cell forms of malignant fibrous histiocytoma, by definition, contain mononuclear and giant cells with significant levels of atypia. In addition, necrosis and atypical mitotic figures are often present. Areas of *plexiform fibrohistiocytic tumor* bear a startling resemblance to these tumors. Clearly, identification

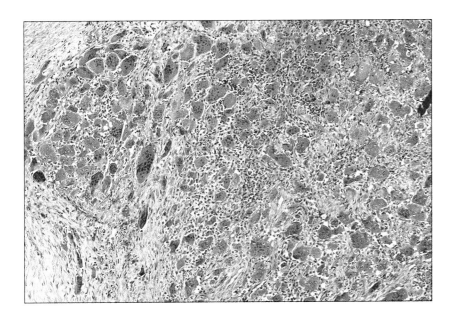

FIGURE 13–52 Giant cell tumor of low malignant potential with coarse nodular architecture.

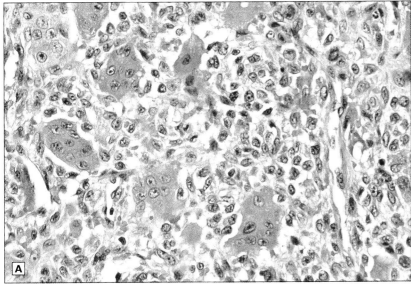

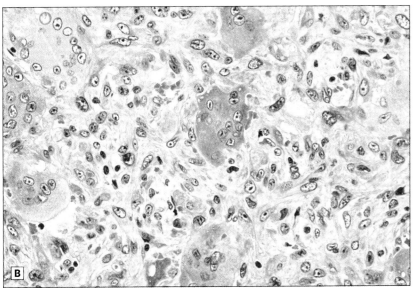

FIGURE 13–53 Giant cell tumor of low malignant potential with mild **(A)** and moderate **(B)** atypia of the mononuclear tumor cells. This contrasts with the marked atypia of classic malignant fibrous histiocytoma, giant cell type.

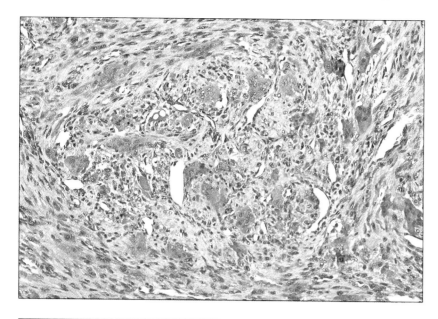

FIGURE 13–54 Giant cell tumor of low malignant potential showing spindling of cells.

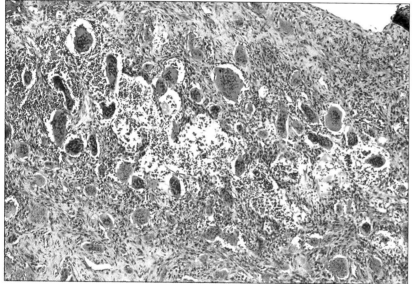

FIGURE 13–55 Aneurysmal bone cyst-like changes in a giant cell tumor of low malignant potential.

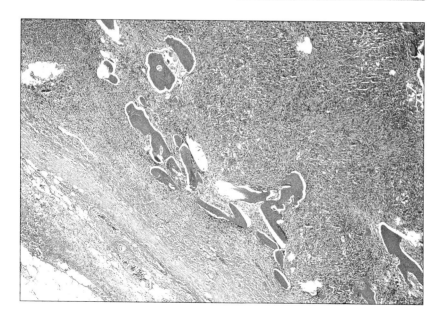

FIGURE 13–56 Metaplastic bone formation in a giant cell tumor of low malignant potential.

of the bimodal population of cells and the dermal/subcutaneous location aid in the distinction. Lastly, *epithelioid sarcomas* and *nodular fasciitis with giant cells* should always be excluded before diagnosing a soft tissue giant cell tumor of low malignant potential. Keratin, present in epithelioid sarcoma, is absent in these tumors.

Clinical behavior

The clinical behavior of this group of tumors is considerably better than that reported for malignant giant cell tumor of soft parts. Of our 17 patients, four developed recurrences but none had metastasis.[87]

REFERENCES

Dermatofibrosarcoma protuberans and bednar tumor

1. Darier J, Ferrand M. Dermatofibromas progressifs et recidivants ou fibrosarcomes de la peau. Ann Dermatol Syph 1924; 5:545.
2. Degos R, Mouly R, Civatte J, et al. Dermatofibro-sarcome de Darier-Ferrand, datant de 70 ans, opere au stade ultime de tumeur monstrueuse. Bull Soc Fr Derm Syph 1967; 74:190.
3. McKee PH, Fletcher CD. Dermatofibrosarcoma protuberans presenting in infancy and childhood. J Cutan Pathol 1991; 18:241.
4. Petoin DS, Verola O, Banzet P, et al. Dermatofibrosarcome de Darier et Ferrand: etude de 96 cas sur 15 ans. Chirurgie 1985; 111:132.
5. Taylor HB, Helwig EB. Dermatofibrosarcoma protuberans: a study of 115 cases. Cancer 1962; 15:717.
6. Pack GT, Tabah EJ. Dermatofibrosarcoma protuberans. Arch Surg 1951; 62:391.
7. Calonje E, Fletcher CDM. Myoid differentiation in dermatofibrosarcoma protuberans and its fibrosarcomatous variant: clinicopathologic analysis of 5 cases. J Cutan Pathol 1996; 23:30.
8. Morimitsu Y, Hisaoka M, Okamoto S, et al. Dermtofibrosarcoma protuberans and its fibrosarcomatous variant with areas of myoid differentiation: a report of three cases. Histopathology 1998; 32:547.
9. Sanz-Trelles A, Ayala-Carbonero A, Rodrigo-Fernandex I, et al. Leiomyomatous nodules and bundles of vascular origin in the fibrosarcomatous variant of dermatofibrosarcoma protuberans. J Cutan Pathol 1998; 25:44.
10. Goldblum JR, Reith JD, Weiss SW. Sarcomas arising in dermatofibrosarcoma protuberans: a reappraisal of biologic behavior in eighteen cases treated by wide local excision with extended clinical follow up. Am J Surg Pathol 2000; 24:1125.
11. O'Dowd J, Laidler P. Progression of dermatofibrosarcoma protuberans to malignant fibrous histiocytoma: report of a case with implications for tumour histogenesis. Hum Pathol 1988; 19:368.
12. Goldblum JR, Tuthill RJ. CD34 and factor XIIIa immunoreactivity in dermatofibrosarcoma protuberans and dermatofibroma. Am J Dermatopathol 1997; 19:147.
13. Weiss SW, Nickoloff BJ. CD34 is expressed by a distinctive cell population in peripheral nerve, nerve sheath tumors, and related lesions. Am J Surg Pathol 1993; 17:1039.
14. West RB, Harvell J, Linn SC, et al. ApoD in soft tissue tumors: a novel marker for dermatofibrosarcoma protuberans. Am J Surg Pathol 2004; 28:1063.
15. Gutierrez G, Ospina JE, de Baez NE, et al. Dermatofibrosarcoma protuberans. Int J Dermatol 1984; 23:396.
16. Alguacil-Garcia A, Unni KK, Goellner JR. Histogenesis of dermatofibrosarcoma protuberans: an ultrastructural study. Am J Clin Pathol 1978; 69:427.

17. Hashimoto K, Brownstein MH, Jakobiec FA. Dermatofibrosarcoma protuberans. Arch Dermatol 1974; 110:874.
18. Sirvant N, Maire G, Pedeutour F. Genetics of dermatofibrosarcoma protuberans family of tumors: from ring chromosomes to tyrosine kinase inhibitor treatment. Genes Chromosomes Cancer 2003; 37:1.
19. Mandahl N, Heim S, Willen H, et al. Supernumerary ring chromosome as the sole cytogenetic abnormality in a dermatofibrosarcoma protuberans. Cancer Genet Cytogenet 1990; 49:273.
20. Simon M-P, Pedeutour F, Sirbent N, et al. Deregulation of the platelet-derived growth factor β-chain gene via fusion with collagen gene COL1A1 in dermatofibrosarcoma protuberans and giant cell fibroblastoma. Nat Genet 1997; 15:95.
21. Nishio J, Iwasaki H, Ohjimi Y, et al. Supernumerary ring chromosomes in dermatofibrosarcoma protuberans may contain sequences from 8q11.2-qter and 17q21-qter: a combined cytogenetic and comparative genomic hybridization study. Cancer Genet Cytogenet 2001; 129:102.
22. O'Brien KP, Seroussi E, Dal Cin P, et al. Various regions within the alpha-helical domain of the COL1A1 gene are fused to the second exon of the PDGFB gene in dermatofibrosarcomas and giant-cell fibroblastoma. Genes Chromosomes Cancer 1998; 23:187.
23. Shimizu A, O'Brien KP, Sjoblom T, et al. The dermatofibrosarcoma protuberans associated collagen type I/platelet derived growth factor (PDGF) β chain fusion gene generates a transforming protein that is processed to functional PDGF-ββ. Cancer Res 1999; 59:3719.
24. Li N, McNiff J, Hui P, et al. Differential expression of HMGA1 and HMGA2 in dermatofibroma and dermatofibrosarcoma protuberans: potential diagnostic applications and comparison with histologic findings, CD34, and Factor XIIIa immunoreactivity. Am J Dermatopathol 2004; 26:267.
25. McPeak CJ, Cruz T, Nicastri AD. Dermatofibrosarcoma protuberans: an analysis of 86 cases – five with metastasis. Ann Surg 1967; 166(Suppl 12):803.
26. Fiore M, Miceli R, Mussi C, et al. Dermatofibrosarcoma protuberans treated at a single institution: a surgical disease with a high cure rate. J Clin Oncol 2005; 23:7669.
27. Gloster HM, Harris KR, Roenigk RK. A comparison between Mohs' micrographic surgery and wide surgical excision for the treatment of dermatofibrosarcoma protuberans. J Am Acad Dermatol 1996; 35:82.
28. Burkhardt BR, Soule EH, Winkelmann RK. Dermatofibrosarcoma protuberans: study of 56 cases. Am J Surg 1966; 111:638.
29. Roses DF, Valensi Q, Latrenta G, et al. Surgical treatment of dermatofibrosarcoma protuberans. Surg Gynecol Obstet 1986; 162:44.
30. Robinson JK. Dermatofibrosarcoma protuberans resected by Mohs' surgery (chemosurgery): a 5-year prospective study. J Am Acad Dermatol 1985; 12:1093.

31. Nouri K, Lodha R, Jimenez G, et al. Mohs' micrographic surgery for dermatofibrosarcoma protuberans: University of Miami and NYU experience. Dermatolog Surg 2002; 28:1060.
32. Wacker J, Khan-Durani B, Hartschuh W. Modified Mohs' micrographic surgery in the treatment of dermatofibrosarcoma protuberans: analysis of 22 patients. Ann Surg Oncol 2004; 11:438.
33. Snow SN, Gordon EM, Larson PO, et al. Dermatofibrosarcoma protuberans: a report on 29 patients treated with Mohs' micrographic surgery with long term follow up and review of the literature. Cancer 2004; 101:28.
34. Ah-Weng A, Marsden JR, Sanders DS, et al. Dermatofibrosarcoma protuberans treated by micrographic surgery. Br J Cancer 2002; 87:1386.
35. Ratner D, Thomas CO, Johnson TM, et al. Mohs' micrographic surgery for the treatment of dermatofibrosarcoma protuberans. J Am Acad Dermatol 1997; 37:600.
36. Kahn LB, Saxe N, Gordon W. Dermatofibrosarcoma protuberans with lymph node and pulmonary metastases. Arch Dermatol 1978; 114:599.
37. Suit H, Sprior I, Mankin HJ, et al. Radiation in management of patients with dermatofibrosarcoma protuberans. J Clin Oncol 1996; 145:2365.
38. Rubin BP, Schuetze SM, Eary JF, et al. Molecular targeting of platelet-derived growth factor β by imatanib mesylate in a patient with metastatic dermatofibrosarcoma protuberans. J Clin Oncol 2002; 20:3586.
39. McArthur GA, Demetri GD, van Oosterom A, et al. Molecular and clinical analysis of locally advanced dermatofibrosarcoma protuberans treated with imatinib: Imatinib Target Exploration Consortium Study. J Clin Oncol 2005; 23:866.
40. Labropoulos SV, Fletcher JA, Olivera AM, et al. Sustained complete remission of metastatic dermatofibrosarcoma protuberans with imatinib mesylate. AntiCancer Drugs 2005; 16:461.

Sarcoma arising in dermatofibrosarcoma protuberans

41. Mentzel T, Beham A, Katemkamp D, et al. Fibrosarcomatous ("high grade") dermatofibrosarcoma protuberans: clinicopathologic and immunohistochemical study of a series of 41 cases with emphasis on prognostic significance. Am J Surg Pathol 1998; 22:576.
42. Wrotnowski U, Cooper PH, Shmookler BM. Fibrosarcomatous change in dermatofibrosarcoma protuberans. Am J Surg Pathol 1988; 12:287.
43. Ding JA, Enjoji M. Dermatofibrosarcoma protuberans with fibrosarcomatous areas: a clinicopathologic study of nine cases and a comparison with allied tumors. Cancer 1989; 64:7212.
44. Connelly JH, Evans HL. Dermatofibrosarcoma protuberans: a clinicopathologic review with emphasis on fibrosarcomatous areas. Am J Surg Pathol 1992; 16:921.

45. Pizarro GB, Fanburg JC, Miettinen M. Dermatofibrosarcoma protuberans (DFSP) with fibrosarcomatous transformation: re-explored. Mod Pathol 1997; 10:13A.
46. Abbott JJ, Oliveira AM, Nascimento AG. The prognostic significance of fibrosarcomatous transformation in dermatofibrosarcoma protuberans. Am J Surg Pathol 2006; 30:436.

Bednar tumor

47. Bednar B. Storiform neurofibromas of the skin, pigmented and nonpigmented. Cancer 1957; 10:368.
48. Bednar B. Storiform neurofibroma in core of naevocellular naevi. J Pathol 1970; 101:199.
49. Ding JA, Hashimoto H, Sugimoto T, et al. Bednar tumor (pigmented dermatofibrosarcoma protuberans): an analysis of six cases. Acta Pathol Jpn 1990; 40:744.
50. Dupree WB, Langloss JM, Weiss SW. Pigmented dermatofibrosarcoma protuberans (Bednar tumor): a pathologic, ultrastructural, and immunohistochemical study. Am J Surg Pathol 1985; 9:630.
51. Fletcher CD, Theaker JM, Flanagan A, et al. Pigmented dermatofibrosarcoma protuberans (Bednar tumour): melanocytic colonization or neuroectodermal differentiation? A clinicopathological and immunohistochemical study. Histopathology 1988; 13:631.
52. Tsuneyoshi M, Enjoji M. Bednar tumor (pigmented dermatofibrosarcoma protuberans): an analysis of six cases. Acta Pathol Jpn 1990; 40:744.
53. Bisceglia M, Vairo M, Calonje E, et al. Pigmented fibrosarcomatous dermatofibrosarcoma protuberans (Bednar tumor): 3 case reports, analogy with conventional type and review of the literature. Pathologica 1997; 89:264.
54. Onoda N, Tsutsumi Y, Kakudo K, et al. Pigmented dermatofibrosarcoma protuberans (Bednar tumor): an autopsy case with systemic metastasis. Acta Pathol Jpn 1990; 40:935.
55. Ozawa A, Niizuma K, Onkido M, et al. Pigmented dermatofibrosarcoma protuberans: an analysis of six cases. Acta Pathol Jpn 1990; 40:935.

Giant cell fibroblastoma

56. Shmookler BM, Enzinger FM, Weiss SW. Giant cell fibroblastoma: a juvenile form of dermatofibrosarcoma protuberans. Cancer 1989; 15:2154.
57. Abdul-Karim FW, Evans HL, Silva EG. Giant cell fibroblastoma: a report of three cases. Am J Clin Pathol 1985; 83:165.
58. Barr RJ, Young EM, Liao SY. Giant cell fibroblastoma: an immunohistochemical study. J Cutan Pathol 1986; 13:301.
59. Chou P, Gonzalez-Crussi F, Mangkornkanok M. Giant cell fibroblastoma. Cancer 1989; 63:756.
60. Dymock RB, Allen PW, Stirling JW, et al. Giant cell fibroblastoma: a distinctive recurrent tumor of childhood. Am J Surg Pathol 1987; 11:263.
61. Kanai Y, Mukai M, Sugiura H, et al. Giant cell fibroblastoma: a case report and immunohistochemical comparison with ten cases of dermatofibrosarcoma protuberans. Acta Pathol Jpn 1991; 41:552.

62. Michal M, Zamecnik M. Giant cell fibroblastoma with a dermatofibrosarcoma protuberans component. Am J Dermatopathol 1992; 14:549.
63. Nair R, Kane SV, Borges A, et al. Giant cell fibroblastoma. J Surg Oncol 1993; 53:136.
64. Rosen LB, Amazon K, Weitzner J, et al. Giant cell fibroblastoma: a report of a case and review of the literature. Am J Dermatopathol 1989; 11:242.
65. Alguacil-Garcia A. Giant cell fibroblastoma recurring as a dermatofibrosarcoma protuberans. Am J Surg Pathol 1991; 15:798.
66. Allen PW, Zwi J. Giant cell fibroblastoma transforming into dermatofibrosarcoma protuberans [letter]. Am J Surg Pathol 1992; 15:1127.
67. Beham A, Fletcher CD. Dermatofibrosarcoma protuberans with areas resembling giant cell fibroblastoma: report of two cases. Histopathology 1990; 17:165.
68. Coyne J, Kaftan SM, Craig RD. Dermatofibrosarcoma protuberans recurring as a giant cell fibroblastoma. Histopathology 1992; 21:184.
69. Maeda T, Hirose T, Furuya K, et al. Giant cell fibroblastoma associated with dermatofibrosarcoma protuberans: a case report. Mod Pathol 1998; 11:491.
70. Dal Cin PD, Sciot R, De Wever I, et al. Cytogenetic and immunohistochemical evidence that giant cell fibroblastoma is related to dermatofibrosarcoma protuberans. Genes Chromosomes Cancer 1996; 15:73.
71. Fletcher CD. Giant cell fibroblastoma of soft tissue: a clinicopathologic and immunohistochemical study. Histopathology 1988; 13:499.

Angiomatoid fibrous histiocytoma

72. Enzinger FM. Angiomatoid malignant fibrous histiocytoma: a distinct fibrohistiocytic tumor of children and young adults simulating a vascular neoplasm. Cancer 1979; 44:2147.
73. Costa MJ, Weiss SW. Angiomatoid malignant fibrous histiocytoma: a follow-up study of 108 cases with evaluation of possible histologic predictors of outcome. Am J Surg Pathol 1990; 14:1126.
74. Fanburg-Smith JC, Miettinen M. Angiomatoid "malignant" fibrous histiocytoma: a clinicopathologic study of 158 cases and further exploration of the myoid phenotype. Hum Path 1999; 30:1336.
75. Pettinato G, Manivel JC, De Rosa G, et al. Angiomatoid malignant fibrous histiocytoma: cytologic, immunohistochemical, ultrastructural, and flow cytometric study of 20 cases. Mod Pathol 1990; 3:479.
76. El-Naggar AK, Ro JY, Ayala AG, et al. Angiomatoid malignant fibrous histiocytoma: flow cytometric DNA analysis of six cases. Surg Oncol 1989; 40:201.
77. Fletcher CD. Angiomatoid "malignant fibrous histiocytoma": an immunohistochemical study indicative of myoid differentiation. Hum Pathol 1991; 22:563.
78. Waters BL, Panagopoulos I, Allen EE. Genetic characterization of angiomatoid fibrous histiocytoma identifies fusion of the FUS and ATF-1 genes induced by a chromosomal

translocation involving bands 12q13 and 16p11.
79. Hallor KH, Mertens F, Ji Y, et al. Fusion of the EWSR1 and ATF1 genes without expression of the MITF-M transcript in angiomatoid fibrous histiocytoma. Genes Chromosomes Cancer 2005; 44:97.

Plexiform fibrohistiocytic tumor

80. Enzinger FM, Zhang RY. Plexiform fibrohistiocytic tumor presenting in children and young adults: an analysis of 65 cases. Am J Surg Pathol 1988; 12:818.
81. Hollowood K, Holley MP, Fletcher CD. Plexiform fibrohistiocytic tumour: clinicopathological, immunohistochemical and ultrastructural analysis in favour of a myofibroblastic lesion. Histopathology 1991; 19:503.
82. Remstein E, Arndt CA, Nascimento AG. Plexiform fibrohistiocytic tumor: clinicopathologic analysis of 22 cases. Am J Surg Pathol 1999; 23:662.
83. Redlich GC, Montgomery KD, Allgood GA, et al. Plexiform fibrohistiocytic tumor with a clonal cytogenetic anomaly. Cancer Genet Cytogenet 1999; 108:141.
84. Smith S, Fletcher CD, Smith MA, et al. Cytogenetic analysis of a plexiform fibrohistiocytic tumor. Cancer Genet Cytogenet 1990; 48:31.
85. Angervall L, Kindsblom LG, Lindholm K, et al. Plexiform fibrohistiocytic tumor: report of a case involving preoperative aspiration cytology and immunohistochemical and ultrastructural analysis of surgical specimens. Pathol Res Pract 1992; 188:350.
86. Giard F, Bonneau R, Raymond GP. Plexiform fibrohistiocytic tumor. Dermatologica 1991; 183:290.

Soft tissue giant cell tumor of low malignant potential

87. Folpe AL, Morris RJ, Weiss SW. Soft tissue giant cell tumor of low malignant potential: a proposal for the reclassification of malignant giant cell tumor of soft parts. Mod Pathol 1999; 12:894.
88. Guccion JG, Enzinger FM. Malignant giant cell tumor of soft parts: an analysis of 32 cases. Cancer 1972; 29:1518.
89. Salm R, Sissons HA. Giant cell tumors or soft tissues. J Pathol 1972; 107:27.
90. O'Connell JX, Wehrli BM, Nielsen GP, et al. Giant cell tumors of soft tissue: a clinicopathologic study of 18 benign and malignant tumors. Am J Surg Pathol 2000; 24:386.
91. Oliviera AM, Dei Tos AP, Fletcher CDM, et al. Primary giant cell tumor of soft tissues: a study of 22 cases. Am J Surg Pathol 2000; 24:248.
92. Diaz-Cascajo C, Weyers W, Borrego L, et al. Dermatofibrosarcoma protuberans with fibrosarcomatous areas; a clinicopathologic and immunohistochemical study in four cases. Am J Dermatopathol 1997; 19:562.
93. O'Connell JX, Trotter MJ. Fibrosarcomatous dermatofibrosarcoma protuberans; a variant. Mod Pathol 1996; 9:273.

MALIGNANT FIBROUS HISTIOCYTOMA (PLEOMORPHIC UNDIFFERENTIATED SARCOMA)

CHAPTER CONTENTS

The concept of malignant fibrous histiocytoma has undergone significant change over the past four decades. The term was first introduced in 1963 to refer to a group of soft tissue tumors, characterized by a storiform, or cartwheel-like, growth pattern, that were believed to be derived from histiocytes[1,2] on the basis of early tissue culture studies demonstrating ameboid movement and phagocytosis of explanted tumor cells. Ultrastructural studies both endorsed and refuted the histiocytic origin of these tumors, however. With the advent of immunohistochemistry and the accessibility of numerous monoclonal antibodies directed against various structural proteins of specific cell types, the phenotype of this tumor was shown to be more closely aligned with a fibroblast than a histiocyte.[3–6] Furthermore, many, but not all, lesions labeled as "malignant fibrous histiocytoma" could, upon close scrutiny, be subclassified as lineage-specific sarcomas, an observation that led some to conclude that the entity of malignant fibrous histiocytoma did not exist at all.[7] The extent to which malignant fibrous histiocytomas can be subclassified as sarcomas of alternative type is, in large part, dependent on definitional criteria and the number of ancillary studies a pathologist is willing to bring to bear on the evaluation of a pleomorphic sarcoma. There is still no general agreement as to what percentage of pleomorphic sarcomas, when subjected to rigorous evaluation, remain unclassified.[8] Recent studies report percentages from 20 to 70%.[8–11] The largest study to date, published by the Swedish Sarcoma Group, indicates that of the approximately 300 cases referred centrally with a diagnosis of malignant fibrous histiocytoma, the diagnosis was confirmed in 70% after re-evaluation and additional immunohistochemistry.[10] These discrepancies, nonetheless, underscore the fact that the criteria by which a pleomorphic tumor is provisionally labeled as a malignant fibrous histiocytoma as well as the criteria by which some are reclassified differ from institution to institution.

Whatever the true incidence of malignant fibrous histiocytoma there is a general agreement that the term "malignant fibrous histiocytoma" should be used synonymously with pleomorphic sarcoma which, by a combination of sampling and immunohistochemistry, shows no definable line of differentiation[8] and by electron microscopy manifests fibroblastic/myofibroblastic features.[9,12,13] As increasingly more advanced technologies are brought to bear on the evaluation of pleomorphic sarcomas, this definition may well change. In this regard, it has been shown with comparative genomic hybridization studies that some retroperitoneal malignant fibrous histiocytomas of the storiform and inflammatory type are dedifferentiated liposarcomas,[14] and with gene expression profiling some leiomyosarcomas and malignant fibrous histiocytomas are closely linked by hierarchical clustering.[15–17]

During this transitional era it is judicious to employ both terms in diagnostic reports so as to avert any misunderstanding with clinicians who continue to be familiar with the term malignant fibrous histiocytoma and would be confused if suddenly this term were to be dropped in favor of pleomorphic undifferentiated sarcoma. The term atypical fibroxanthoma continues to be in use for pleomorphic undifferentiated sarcomas of the skin which appear to be the superficial counterpart of malignant fibrous histiocytoma.

ATYPICAL FIBROXANTHOMA (PLEOMORPHIC UNDIFFERENTIATED SARCOMA OF SKIN)

Atypical fibroxanthoma is a cutaneous pleomorphic undifferentiated sarcoma (malignant fibrous histiocytoma) which typically occurs on sun-damaged, actinic skin of the elderly.[18–20] Its superficial location has generally been credited with its excellent clinical outcome. In any event, the diagnosis of atypical fibroxanthoma needs to be strictly defined so that it does not include other pleomorphic tumors of the skin (e.g., melanoma) or deeply invasive sarcomas that are well known to have metastatic potential.

Clinical findings

Atypical fibroxanthomas typically occur on the exposed surface of the head and neck, particularly the nose, cheek, and ear of elderly individuals. Those rare atypical fibroxanthomas thought to occur on the extremities of young individuals are now thought to be examples of atypical fibrous histiocytomas (see Chapter 13). Solar and therapeutic radiation are strong predisposing factors in the pathogenesis of this disease. This belief is supported by the common occurrence of the tumor on sun-damaged skin, its frequent association with other actinic lesions (e.g., basal cell carcinoma, squamous carcinoma), and the identification of both ultraviolet related mutations and photoproducts within these lesions.[21,22] The incidence of previous irradiation varies from less than 5% in some series[20] to more than 50% in others.[23] In most instances the latent period between the previous radiation exposure and the appearance of the atypical fibroxanthoma is more than 10 years and thus well in keeping with the accepted interval for a radiation-induced tumor.

Gross and microscopic findings

Grossly, the lesions are solitary nodules or ulcers usually measuring less than 2 cm in diameter (Figs 14–1, 14–2). Their appearance is not distinctive, and for this reason, a variety of preoperative diagnoses is considered, including basal cell carcinoma, squamous carcinoma, pyogenic granuloma, and sebaceous cyst.

These tumors are expansile dermal nodules that abut the epidermis, causing pressure atrophy or ulceration (Fig. 14–3). Alternatively, a *grenz* zone of uninvolved dermis is present. The tumor compresses the skin appendages laterally and extends into the subcutis. By definition, the tumor does not extensively involve the subcutis, nor invades deeper structures such as fascia or muscle. Areas adjacent to these lesions may display solar elastosis, vascular dilatation, and capillary proliferation.

Histologically, these tumors resemble pleomorphic forms of malignant fibrous histiocytoma, although some can have a more monomorphic fascicular appearance resembling a fibrosarcoma. Most are characterized by bizarre cells arranged in a haphazard or vaguely fascicular pattern (Fig. 14–4). Rarely, a storiform pattern is evident. The cells are spindle-shaped or round, and they exhibit multinucleation, pleomorphism, and numerous typical and atypical mitotic figures. The cells occasionally have small droplets of neutral fat and periodic acid-Schiff (PAS)-positive, diastase-resistant material, two features that probably reflect, in part, degenerative changes. Hemorrhage is occasionally prominent within atypical fibroxanthoma and may lead to extensive hemosiderin deposits which should be distinguished from melanin. Occasional inflammatory cells are present; and rarely osteoclastic giant cells[24] or osteoid[25] are seen. Clear cell[26,27]

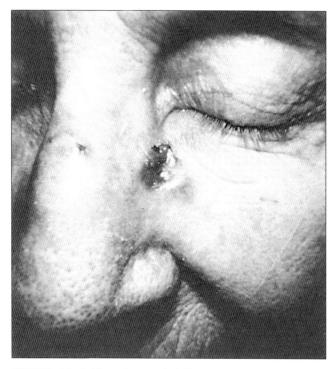

FIGURE 14–1 Ulcerating atypical fibroxanthoma from the nose of an 80-year-old woman. Grossly, the tumor resembled a basal cell carcinoma. (From Fretzin DF, Helwig EB. Atypical fibroxanthoma of the skin. Cancer 1973; 31:1541.)

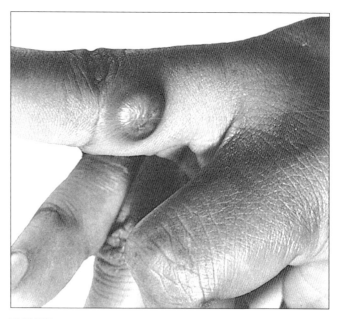

FIGURE 14–2 Nodular atypical fibroxanthoma from the finger of a 36-year-old woman. Atypical fibroxanthomas in young patients typically occur on the extremities, in contrast to those in elderly patients, which are located on sun-exposed or actinic-damaged surfaces. (From Fretzin DF, Helwig EB. Atypical fibroxanthoma of the skin. Cancer 1973; 31:1541.)

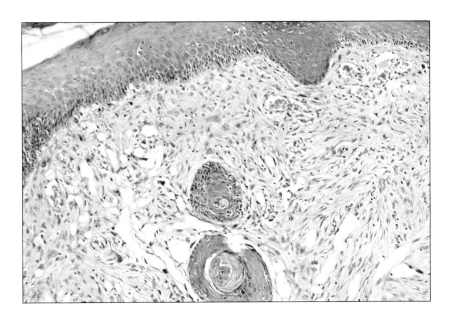

FIGURE 14–3 Atypical fibroxanthoma abutting epidermis. Dilated capillaries are commonly seen adjacent to and in the tumor.

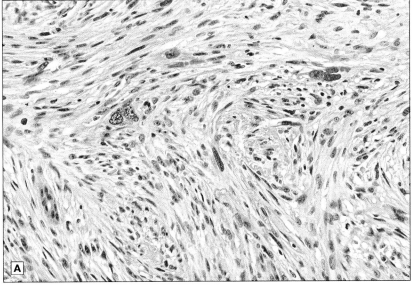

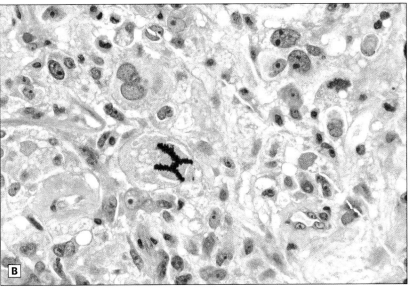

FIGURE 14–4 Bizarre cells comprising atypical fibroxanthoma vary from plump spindled cells to large round cells. **(A)** Pleomorphism is marked; and mitotic figures, including atypical forms, are common **(B)**.

and granular cell variants[28] of atypical fibroxanthoma have been described but are rare. The former, containing large foamy CD68-positive cells, raises a different set of differential considerations including balloon cell melanoma, sebaceous carcinoma, and pleomorphic liposarcoma.

Atypical fibroxanthomas are typically negative for S-100 protein, cytokeratin, and various melanin-related markers, but may express actin and calponin due to focal myofibroblastic differentiation. The ultrastructural features of this tumor are similar to those of malignant fibrous histiocytoma and include cells with fibroblastic/myofibroblastic features.

Differential diagnosis

Since the diagnosis of atypical fibroxanthoma implies a biologically innocuous lesion, it is important that it be carefully distinguished from superficial forms of malignant fibrous histiocytoma which have some capacity for distant metastasis. In our opinion, if a tumor is large (>2 cm), extensively involves the subcutis, penetrates fascia and muscle, or displays necrosis or vascular invasion, it should be diagnosed as a malignant fibrous histiocytoma, as such tumors run a definite risk of recurrence and metastasis. In our opinion, most cases of so-called metastasizing atypical fibroxanthoma are likely lesions improperly diagnosed as superficial malignant fibrous histiocytoma.

In assessing a pleomorphic tumor of the skin, immunostains are important to rule out a carcinoma, melanoma, angiosarcoma, and pleomorphic form of leiomyosarcoma. The usual primary immunohistochemical panel includes pancytokeratin and S-100 protein whereas a secondary panel might include actin, desmin, CD31 (a vascular marker), and melanin-specific markers, depending on the appearance of the lesion and the results of the first panel. One should be reminded that S-100 protein-positive histiocytes and CD31-positive histiocytes (see Chapter 7) may be encountered in atypical fibroxanthomas and should be carefully distinguished from the lesional cells.

Discussion

Although this tumor is histologically indistinguishable from some forms of malignant fibrous histiocytoma, it deserves a special designation because of its almost uniformly excellent prognosis following conservative therapy. In one of the largest series in the literature, only nine of 140 patients had a recurrence, and none developed metastasis;[20] a slightly smaller series documented no recurrences or metastasis among 86 patients.[29] Recently, the lack of H-ras and K-ras mutations in atypical fibroxanthoma compared to malignant fibrous histiocytoma has been suggested as another difference, apart from superficial location, which may explain the difference in outcome.[30]

MALIGNANT FIBROUS HISTIOCYTOMA (PLEOMORPHIC UNDIFFERENTIATED SARCOMA)

Depending on definitional criteria, malignant fibrous histiocytoma still accounts for a significant proportion of, sarcomas occurring in late adult life.[10,31] It manifests a broad range of histologic appearances and for that reason is divided into several subtypes: storiform-pleomorphic, myxoid (myxofibrosarcoma), giant cell (malignant giant cell tumor of soft parts), and inflammatory (xanthosarcoma, malignant xanthogranuloma), some of which have prognostic significance.

The most common form of malignant fibrous histiocytomas, consisting of a mixture of storiform and pleomorphic areas, is descriptively termed *storiform-pleomorphic type*. Depending on the relative proportions of these areas, the tumor may appear well differentiated and resemble dermatofibrosarcoma protuberans, or it may appear highly anaplastic. This subtype serves as the prototype for much of our thinking concerning the behavior of this group of neoplasms. The *myxoid type*, which accounts for roughly one-fourth of malignant fibrous histiocytomas, is the second most common variety.[32] It is characterized by prominent myxoid change of the stroma and contains cellular areas indistinguishable from the foregoing type. It is distinguished from the storiform-pleomorphic type not only because of its distinctive appearance but also because of its better prognosis. The last two types are less common. The *giant cell type* (malignant giant cell tumor of soft parts)[33] contains numerous osteoclast-type giant cells, and the *inflammatory type* is characterized by a predominance of xanthoma cells and acute inflammatory cells.

Clinical findings

The clinical features of the various subtypes are similar and are considered together. Malignant fibrous histiocytoma is characteristically a tumor of late adult life, with most cases occurring in persons between the ages of 50 and 70 years.[31] Tumors in children with the same histologic features as the adult forms of malignant fibrous histiocytoma are rare, and this diagnosis should always be made with caution in patients under 20 years of age. Approximately two-thirds of malignant fibrous histiocytomas occur in men, and whites are affected more often than blacks or Asians. The tumor occurs most frequently on the lower extremity (Figs 14–5, 14–6), especially the thigh, followed by the upper extremity and retroperitoneum (Fig. 14–7). A notable exception is inflammatory malignant fibrous histiocytoma, which is most often

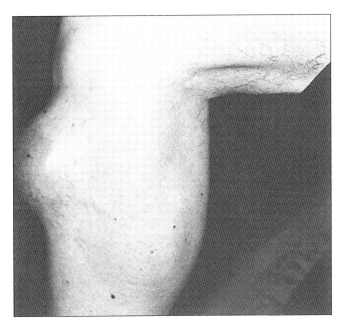

FIGURE 14-5 Malignant fibrous histiocytoma of the lower leg of a 62-year-old man. (From Guccion JG, Enzinger FM. Malignant giant cell tumor of soft parts: an analysis of 32 cases. Cancer 1972; 29:1518.)

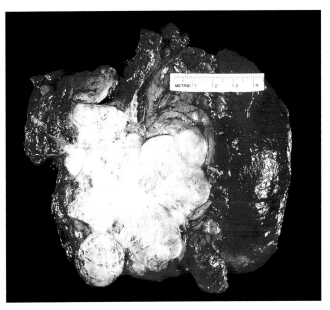

FIGURE 14-7 Gross appearance of a malignant fibrous histiocytoma of the retroperitoneum. The tumor is a multinodular white mass arising adjacent to the kidney.

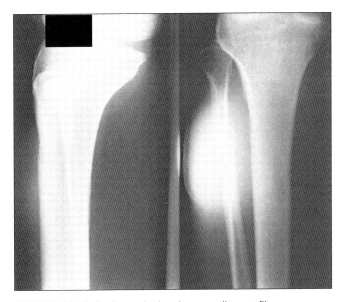

FIGURE 14-6 Radiograph showing a malignant fibrous histiocytoma of the lower leg (same case as in Figure 14-5). Ill-defined soft tissue mass has eroded a portion of the tibial cortex.

located in the retroperitoneum; relatively few are found in the extremities.

When on an extremity, the tumor presents as a painless, enlarging mass usually of several months' duration but occasionally much longer, depending on the rate of growth. Rapid acceleration of the growth rate prompts the patient to seek medical attention quickly. As with other sarcomas, growth rate acceleration has been observed during pregnancy.[31] In contrast to patients with lesions of the extremity, patients with retroperitoneal tumors develop constitutional symptoms including anorexia, malaise, weight loss, and signs of increasing abdominal pressure.

Occasionally, fever and leukocytosis with neutrophilia or eosinophilia dominate the clinical presentation of this disease. This unusual constellation of symptoms has been documented for the inflammatory type of malignant fibrous histiocytoma,[34] although rarely it occurs with the other subtypes.[35] These paraneoplastic signs and symptoms appear to be the result of tumor-related production of cytokines,[36] which have included interleukins (IL-6, IL-8)[35] and tumor necrosis factor. The symptoms usually remit following removal of the tumor. Rarely, hypoglycemia occurs in association with this disease,[31,34] and has recently been shown to be due to big insulin-like growth factor II.[37] Malignant fibrous histiocytoma rarely presents as a metastatic tumor without a clinically evident primary lesion, although a small percentage of patients present with synchronous primary and metastatic disease.[38] A number of cytogenetic abnormalities has been identified in malignant fibrous histiocytomas.[39-45] Emerging evidence suggests that certain chromosomes appear to be structurally rearranged more consistently than others in this disease.

Etiologic factors

Like atypical fibroxanthomas, there is excellent circumstantial evidence that some of these tumors are radiation

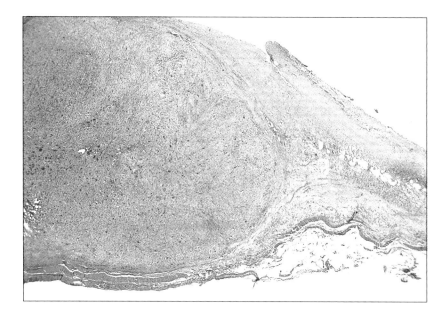

FIGURE 14–8 Malignant fibrous histiocytoma arising in and extending along superficial fascia.

induced and may occur following radiation for tumors of various types after an interval of several years. Aside from these sporadic iatrogenic tumors, there are few data on etiologic factors for this disease. About 10% of patients with malignant fibrous histiocytoma have had or subsequently develop a second neoplasm. This does not seem statistically meaningful in view of the generally older age of these patients and the accepted risk of a second neoplasm complicating the course of a first. Several malignant fibrous histiocytomas have occurred in patients exposed to phenoxy acids, although a direct causal relation has not been established.[46] The tumor has also been reported in a patient with Lynch II syndrome.[47] Intraosseous malignant fibrous histiocytomas have occurred in preexisting bone infarcts and at the site of shrapnel injury.[48]

Gross findings

Typically, the lesions are solitary, multilobulated, fleshy masses 5–10 cm in diameter when first detected (Fig. 14–7), although retroperitoneal lesions are much larger than lesions in the extremities.[49] About two-thirds of these tumors are located in skeletal muscle, and fewer than 10% are confined to the subcutis. Tumors located adjacent to bone may induce mild degrees of periosteal reaction or cortical erosion, which can be detected radiographically. Although malignant fibrous histiocytoma has a circumscribed appearance grossly, it often spreads for a considerable distance along fascial planes (Fig. 14–8) or between muscle fibers microscopically, which accounts for its high rate of local recurrence.

On cut section, most tumors are gray to white (Fig. 14–9), but this pattern may be modified by an abundance of one or more elements. For example, the inflammatory form of malignant fibrous histiocytoma (*malignant*

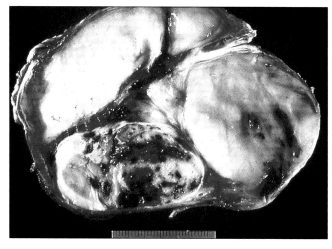

FIGURE 14–9 Typical gross appearance of a malignant fibrous histiocytoma showing a multinodular white mass with areas of hemorrhage and necrosis.

xanthogranuloma, xanthosarcoma) may have a yellow hue because of the predominance of xanthoma cells (see Fig. 14–33, below), whereas hemorrhagic tumors appear brown. Myxoid malignant fibrous histiocytoma typically has a translucent mucoid appearance (see Fig. 14–20, below) and in this respect cannot be distinguished grossly from other myxoid sarcomas, such as myxoid liposarcoma. In contrast to less aggressive fibrohistiocytic tumors, hemorrhage and necrosis are common features of this tumor. In fact, about 5% of malignant fibrous histiocytomas undergo such extensive hemorrhage that they present clinically as fluctuant masses and are diagnosed as cystic hematomas.[31] Nonetheless, residual tumor cells can be identified microscopically in the wall of such "cysts," leaving no doubt as to the correct diagnosis.

Malignant fibrous histiocytoma: storiform-pleomorphic type

Microscopically, the storiform-pleomorphic form of malignant fibrous histiocytoma has a highly variable morphologic pattern and shows frequent transitions from storiform to pleomorphic areas (Figs 14–10 to 14–17), although the emphasis in most tumors is on haphazardly arranged pleomorphic zones. Storiform areas consist of plump spindle cells arranged in short fascicles in a cartwheel, or storiform, pattern around slit-like vessels. The spindle cells are well differentiated and resemble fibroblasts. Although such tumors resemble dermatofibrosarcoma protuberans, they differ by a less distinctive storiform pattern and by the presence of occasional plump histiocytic cells, numerous typical and atypical mitotic figures,

and secondary elements including xanthoma cells and chronic inflammatory cells. Although this pattern of malignant fibrous histiocytoma is easily recognized, it is seldom seen throughout the entire tumor. Instead, most tumors have a combination of storiform and pleomorphic areas, with a preponderance on the latter. Least often, tumors have a fascicular growth pattern and resemble fibrosarcomas, except for scattered giant cells. In contrast to the storiform areas, pleomorphic areas contain plumper fibroblastic cells and more rounded histiocytic cells arranged haphazardly with no particular orientation to vessels. Pleomorphism and mitotic activity are usually more prominent. A characteristic feature of these areas is the presence of large numbers of giant cells with multiple hyperchromatic irregular nuclei. The intense eosinophilia of these giant cells often suggests cells with myoblastic

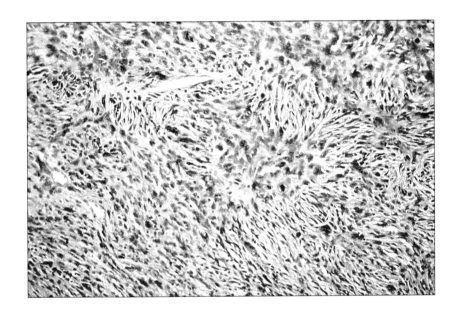

FIGURE 14–10 Malignant fibrous histiocytoma, storiform-pleomorphic type, with a predominantly storiform pattern. Tumors may resemble dermatofibrosarcoma at low power but are distinguished from them by the greater degree of nuclear atypia and mitotic activity.

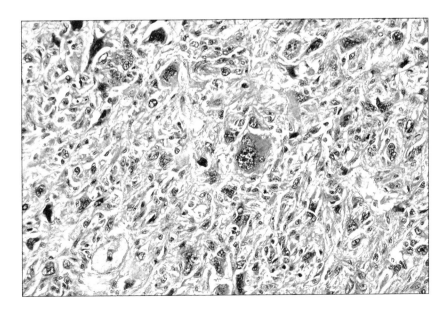

FIGURE 14–11 Malignant fibrous histiocytoma, storiform-pleomorphic type, with a pleomorphic pattern. Anaplastic tumor cells are arranged haphazardly in sheets.

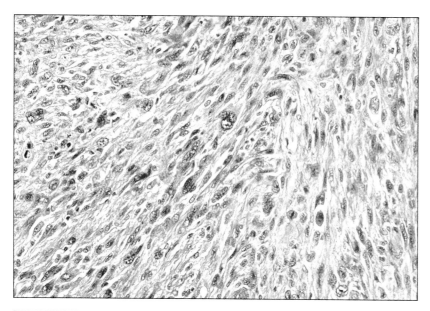

FIGURE 14–12 Malignant fibrous histiocytoma, storiform-pleomorphic type, with a predominantly fascicular pattern. Tumors of this type are classified by some as pleomorphic (high-grade) fibrosarcomas.

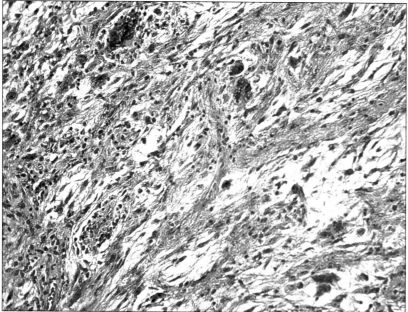

FIGURE 14–13 Malignant fibrous histiocytoma, storiform-pleomorphic type, with focal (microscopic) areas of myxoid change. Myxoid forms of malignant fibrous histiocytoma, in contrast, should have a predominantly (>50%) myxoid pattern.

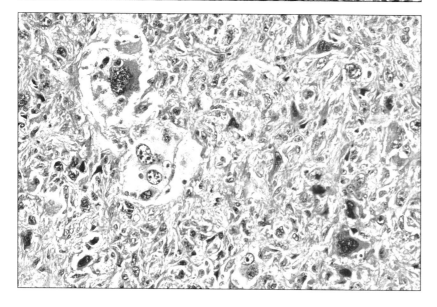

FIGURE 14–14 Cells in a malignant fibrous histiocytoma are characterized by an extreme degree of pleomorphism and occasional multinucleation. Bizarre cells may vary from deeply eosinophilic to xanthomatous. In the past, pleomorphic eosinophilic cells in these tumors were confused with rhabdomyoblasts, and the lesions were regarded as pleomorphic rhabdomyosarcomas.

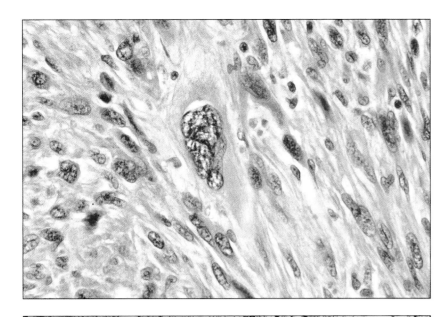

FIGURE 14–15 Bizarre spindled cells in a malignant fibrous histiocytoma.

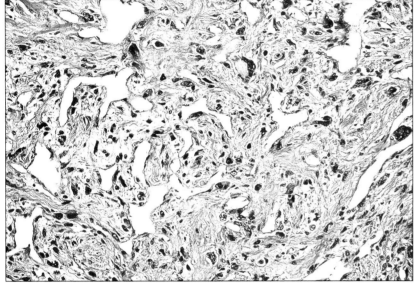

FIGURE 14–16 Hemangiopericytoma-like vascular pattern in a malignant fibrous histiocytoma.

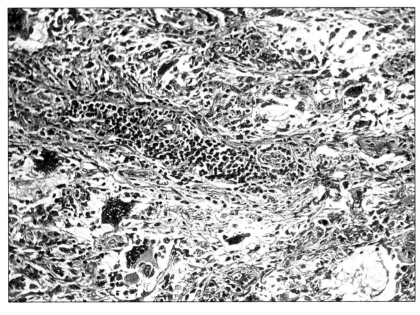

FIGURE 14–17 Malignant fibrous histiocytoma with a focally dense lymphocytic infiltrate. Chronic inflammation is a common feature in many malignant fibrous histiocytomas.

differentiation (Fig. 14–14). Although small droplets of neutral fat and PAS-positive, diastase-resistant droplets may be seen in mononuclear cells in this tumor, they are especially prominent in the giant cells and probably reflect degenerative changes.

The stroma and secondary elements vary considerably in the storiform and pleomorphic areas. Usually, the stroma consists of delicate collagen fibrils encircling individual cells but occasionally collagen deposition is extensive and widely separates cells. Focal myxoid change is also a common phenomenon and consists of localized collections of hyaluronidase-sensitive acid mucopolysaccharide (Fig. 14–13). When this change becomes especially prominent, the tumors are classified as myxoid variants of malignant fibrous histiocytoma. Rarely, the stroma contains metaplastic osteoid or chondroid. If, however, bone or cartilage is extensive and/or appears immature, the tumor should be classified as an osteo- or chondrosarcoma. The vasculature, although elaborate, is seldom appreciated unless it becomes dilated and resembles that of a hemangiopericytoma (Fig. 14–16). Modest numbers of lymphocytes or plasma cells characterize most of these tumors, although in about one-fifth of cases can be quite numerous and include an intense neutrophilic infiltrate (Fig. 14–17). Intermingling of the neoplastic cells and lymphocytes at the periphery may simulate lymphoma, particularly Hodgkin's disease.

Metastatic deposits from malignant fibrous histiocytoma involve organs in a nodular fashion. In rare instances, metastatic lesions to lymph nodes are diffuse and consist of nests of cells scattered throughout a lymph node, thereby resembling lymphoma. However, adjacent nodes can usually be found with the more typical solid pattern of involvement. Metastatic lesions in general resemble the original tumor.

Immunohistochemical findings

The role of immunohistochemistry in the diagnosis of malignant fibrous histiocytoma has traditionally been an ancillary one, primarily serving as a means to exclude other pleomorphic tumors such as anaplastic carcinoma and sarcoma, which may bear a resemblance to malignant fibrous histiocytoma. Thus, the diagnosis of malignant fibrous histiocytoma continues to presuppose excellent sampling and evaluation of hematoxylin-eosin-stained sections. Despite the limited diagnostic applications of immunohistochemistry, they have provided ample evidence that these tumors do not display features of monocytes or macrophages[50,51] but, rather, fibroblasts. Reliable histiocytic markers such as Leu-3, Leu-M3, and CD68 have not been identified in these tumors,[51] while fibroblast-associated antigens can be identified on the surface of the cells.[5,51]

Tumors that qualify by light microscopy as malignant fibrous histiocytomas may focally express a number of

intermediate filaments such as keratin, desmin, and neurofilament protein.[3,4,52–56] Although initially dismissed as a technical artifact or cross-reactivity, true expression of these proteins occurs,[23,57] and the incidence increases as the sensitivity of the detection method is enhanced.[54] The issue then becomes whether a minor degree of immunoreactivity of certain antigens in a pleomorphic undifferentiated sarcoma should be considered sufficient evidence of specific differentiation and, accordingly, alter the diagnosis. Although a controversial question, we have adopted the approach that focal immunoreactivity for intermediate filaments such as keratin or desmin in an otherwise undifferentiated pleomorphic sarcoma (malignant fibrous histiocytoma) alone is not sufficient to alter the diagnosis. On the other hand, diffuse immunoreactivity is more likely reflective of specific differentiation (see below).

Ultrastructural findings

With widespread use of immunohistochemistry, electron microscopic studies have assumed a diminished role in the diagnosis of malignant fibrous histiocytoma. Since there are no ultrastructural features that are specific for malignant fibrous histiocytoma, electron microscopy is best used for ruling out the presence of organelles indicating a higher order of differentiation. Within malignant fibrous histiocytomas one can identify several cell types. These include a small number of primitive mesenchymal cells with a narrow rim of cytoplasm largely devoid of organelles except for a few free ribosomes,[58] spindled fibroblastic cells with an elongated nucleus, prominent nucleoli, and abundant lamellae of rough endoplasmic reticulum (Fig. 14–18),[9,13,58] and myofibroblasts with

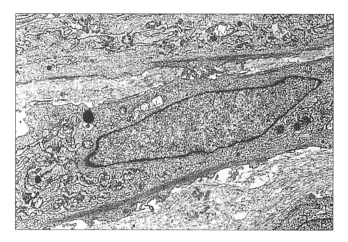

FIGURE 14–18 Electron micrograph showing fibroblast-like cells comprising a malignant fibrous histiocytoma. Cells are elongated with numerous profiles of rough endoplasmic reticulum. Actin-like filaments are often clustered underneath the cytoplasmic membrane (×17 000). (Courtesy of Dr. Bruce Mackay, M.D. Anderson Cancer Hospital.)

nuclear clefts, peripheral myofilament bundles with dense bodies, pinocytotic vesicles and fragments of external lamina.[9] About one-third of malignant fibrous histiocytomas display myofibroblastic features (so-called pleomorphic myofibroblastomas). This subset does not differ in any meaningful way from those that do not, although they have a greater tendency to express myogenic markers by immunohistochemistry.[9]

Differential diagnosis

The most common problem in the differential diagnosis is separating malignant fibrous histiocytoma from other malignant tumors that display a comparable degree of cellular pleomorphism, such as anaplastic carcinoma and pleomorphic forms of liposarcoma, leiomyosarcoma, and rhabdomyosarcoma. Careful sampling in conjunction with a targeted panel of immunostains is the mainstay of diagnosis. Pleomorphic liposarcoma, in particular, may have areas that closely simulate malignant fibrous histiocytomas but ultimately is diagnosed by the presence of pleomorphic lipoblasts. Dedifferentiated liposarcomas are identified by virtue of areas of well-differentiated or low-grade liposarcoma. It is especially important that retroperitoneal lesions be well sampled since a recent study suggests that many malignant fibrous histiocytomas in this location, when carefully sampled and analyzed for amplification of 12q13-15, prove to be dedifferentiated liposarcomas.[59] The distinction between pleomorphic leiomyosarcomas and malignant fibrous histiocytoma is probably the most problematic and controversial area in differential diagnosis. Unless there are light microscopic areas that are diagnostic of smooth muscle differentiation, one is usually forced to decide the extent to which immunoreactivity for various myogenic markers is reflective of smooth muscle differentiation. We have generally required either significant amounts of actin immunoreactivity or, alternatively, some degree of both actin and desmin for the diagnosis of pleomorphic leiomyosarcomas. In evaluating actin immunoreactivity it is important to distinguish the peripheral actin immunoreactivity of myofibroblasts occurring in malignant fibrous histiocytoma from the diffuse actin immunoreactivity of smooth muscle cells in leiomyosarcomas. The diagnosis of pleomorphic rhabdomyosarcomas is often suggested by intense cytoplasmic eosinophilia,

cell-to-cell molding, and presence of strap cells. Since they also express the nuclear regulatory proteins specific for skeletal muscle differentiation, myoD1 and myogenin, their diagnosis can be definitively made by immunohistochemistry.

Depending on the clinical situation, the differential diagnosis of malignant fibrous histiocytoma should also include an anaplastic carcinoma. This is especially true for lesions in the retroperitoneum, those based in or around epithelial organs, or those occurring in patients known to have a previous carcinoma. Immunostains for pancytokeratin are invaluable in this distinction, although, as noted above, keratin is expressed focally in a small percentage of malignant fibrous histiocytomas. Electron microscopy may also aid in the distinction by detecting minor degrees of epithelial differentiation not readily apparent by light microscopy, such as numerous large intercellular junctions or tonofibrils.

Discussion

The vast majority of malignant fibrous histiocytomas are high-grade lesions having a local recurrence rate ranging 19–31%, a metastatic rate of 31–35%, and a 5-year survival of 65–70% (Table 14–1).[10,50–63] Both local recurrence and distant metastases develop within 12–24 months of diagnosis. Only a minority of patients develops metastases after 5 years,[10] with the common metastatic sites being lung (90%), bone (8%), and liver (1%). Regional lymph node metastases are decidedly uncommon and develop in 4–17% of patients.[64–66]

The factors that correlate consistently with metastasis, survival, or both are depth, tumor size, grade, histologic subtype, necrosis, and local recurrence, although they are not necessarily independent variables. For example, size and depth appear to co-vary[61] because large tumors tend to be deep tumors, and highly myxoid forms of malignant fibrous histiocytoma tend to be smaller and more superficial than nonmyxoid forms (Tables 14–2, 14–3). Recently, it has been pointed out that the impact of prognostic factors for metastases in malignant fibrous histiocytoma is not constant but rather time-dependent.[10] Necrosis and local recurrence are significant predictors of metastasis within the first two years of diagnosis and throughout a longitudinal follow-up period, whereas only tumor depth and local recurrence were significant

TABLE 14–1	BEHAVIOR OF MALIGNANT FIBROUS HISTIOCYTOMA			
Author	**No. of patients**	**Local recurrence (%)**	**Metastasis (%)**	**5-year survival (%)**
Salo et al.[61]	239	19	35	65
Le Doussal et al.[60]	216	31	33	70
Zagars et al.[63]	271	21	31	68
Engellau[10]	338	29	33	

predictors beyond 2 years. Conceptually, this suggests that there may be considerable biologic heterogeneity within traditionally defined risk groups.

There has been recent interest in correlating various cytogenetic abnormalities in malignant fibrous histiocytoma with clinical parameters.[40-43,67-69] More than 80% of malignant fibrous histiocytomas show gains affecting 1p31, 1q21-22, 17q23qter, 20q 9q31, 5p14-pter, and 7q32 by comparative genomic hybridization and about 50% display losses of 9p21, 10q, 11q23qter, and 13q10-q31. Gains at 7q32 in one study were a predictor of a worse metastasis-free and overall survival in a multivariate analysis with tumor size and grade. Because this chromosomal region is seldom amplified in other cancers, the authors have suggested that it represents a unique prognostic marker of malignant fibrous histiocytoma. Frequent deletions at the p16(INK4A) and RB1 loci provide support that loss of these tumor suppressor genes is also important in tumorigenesis.[70]

Malignant fibrous histiocytoma: myxoid type (high-grade myxofibrosarcoma)

The myxoid type of malignant fibrous histiocytoma is characterized by myxoid areas in association with cellular areas indistinguishable from ordinary malignant fibrous histiocytoma (Figs 14–19 to 14–23).[32] Although the proportion of myxoid and cellular areas can vary in these tumors, at least half of the tumor should appear myxoid before it is designated a "myxoid variant."

The myxoid areas appear either as small foci blending with the adjacent cellular areas or as large areas abutting cellular areas with little transition (Fig. 14–21). In the extreme case, an entire nodule of a tumor may appear myxoid and an adjacent nodule cellular. Qualitatively, the myxoid zones are similar to the cellular zones; they differ principally in their interstitial accumulation of hyaluronidase-sensitive acid mucopolysaccharide. As a result, the storiform pattern becomes less evident and the vasculature more prominent (Fig. 14–22A, B). The vessels typically form arcs along which tumor cells and inflammatory cells condense. Less often, the vessels are extremely delicate and assume an intricate plexiform pattern similar to that of myxoid liposarcoma.

As in the cellular areas, the cells in the myxoid zones show a spectrum of differentiation, ranging from well-differentiated fibroblasts to cells showing pleomorphism, mitotic activity, and multinucleation. Highly myxoid tumors with a predominance of the former cells are easily confused with myxoma or nodular fasciitis (Fig. 14–22C, D). Occasionally, cells in the myxoid zones resemble

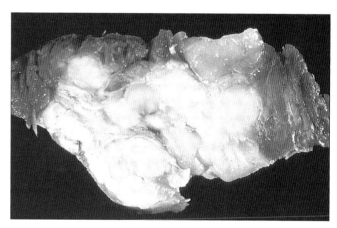

FIGURE 14–19 Gross specimen of myxoid malignant fibrous histiocytoma depicting the gelatinous appearance of several of the tumor nodules.

TABLE 14–2	INDEPENDENT FAVORABLE PROGNOSTIC FACTORS WITH RESPECT TO DISEASE-SPECIFIC SURVIVAL IN MALIGNANT FIBROUS HISTIOCYTOMA

UICC/AJCC stage I or II
Freedom from gross disease following initial treatment
Superficial location
Myxoid subtype
Age <50 years

Modified from Le Doussal V, Coindre J-M, Leroux A, et al. Prognostic factors for patients with localized primary malignant fibrous histiocytoma. Cancer 1996; 77:1823.

TABLE 14–3	DISEASE-SPECIFIC SURVIVAL FOR MALIGNANT FIBROUS HISTIOCYTOMA BY STAGE		
		Disease-specific survival (%)	
Stage	**No. of patients**	**5 years**	**10 years**
Stage I			
Low grade (<5 cm)	17	100	100
Stage II			
Low grade (>5 cm deep)	100	83	79
Stage III			
High grade (5–10 cm deep)	55	59	48
High grade (>10 cm deep)	59	34	31

Modified from AJCC Stage of 239 Patients with Extremity Malignant Fibrous Histiocytoma.

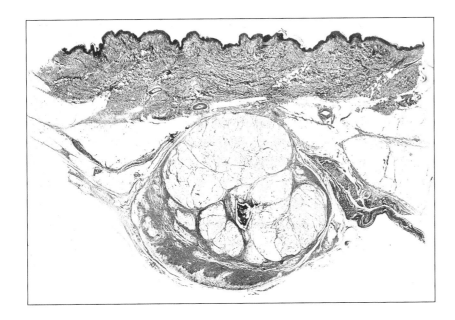

FIGURE 14–20 Low-power view of a superficial (subcutaneous) myxoid malignant fibrous histiocytoma. Most of the tumor is myxoid, but at the deep border there is a rim of typical (nonmyxoid) malignant fibrous histiocytoma.

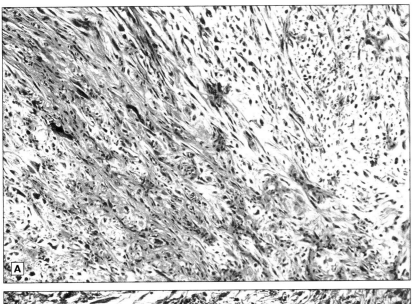

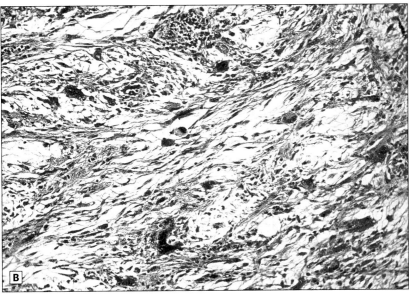

FIGURE 14–21 Broad myxoid zones may sharply abut cellular areas **(A)** or may be scattered in small microscopic foci throughout the myxoid malignant fibrous histiocytoma **(B)**.

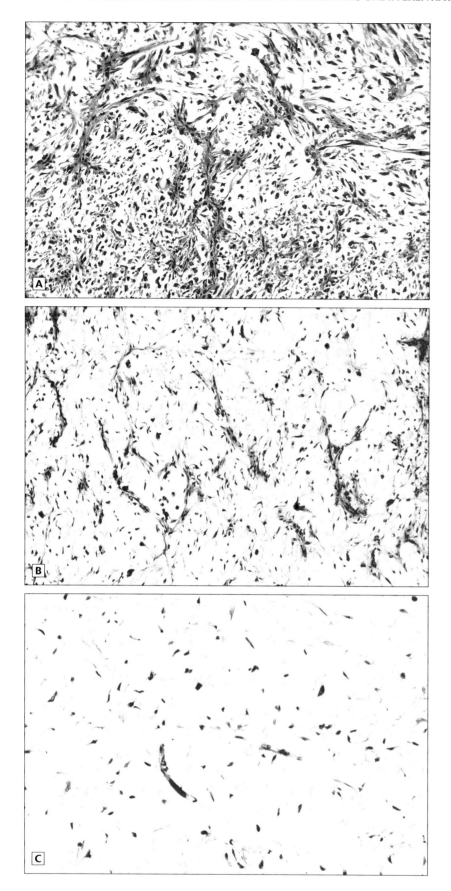

FIGURE 14–22 Range of cellularity that may be encountered in myxoid malignant fibrous histiocytoma/myxofibrosarcoma spectrum of lesions from most cellular **(A)** to least cellular **(D)**. **(A, B)** Easily recognized pleomorphic lesions fall in the spectrum of malignant fibrous histiocytomas. **(C, D)** Different areas in the same tumor have less cellularity and atypia and might be classified as "low-grade myxofibrosarcoma."

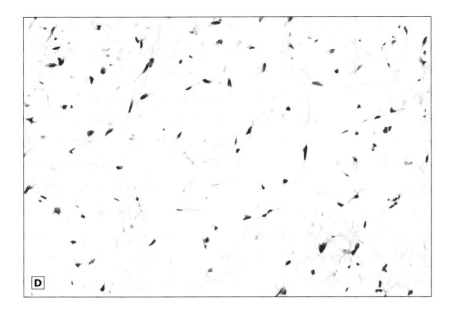

FIGURE 14–22 Continued. **(D)** Note the lack of vascularity. It superficially resembles a myxoma except for the greater degree of nuclear atypia.

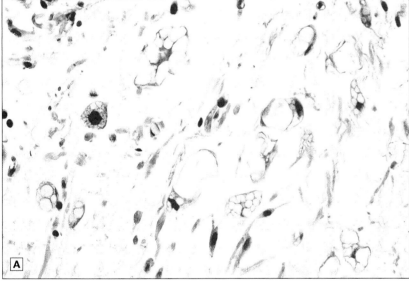

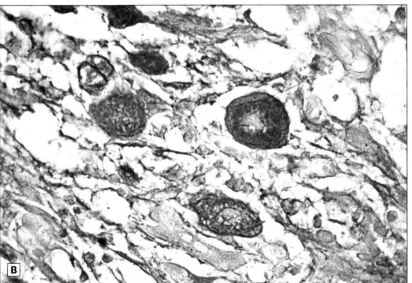

FIGURE 14–23 Pseudolipoblasts in a myxoid malignant fibrous histiocytoma. Tumor cells become distended with hyaluronic acid and resemble lipoblasts. Note, however, that the vacuoles are ill-defined and do not cause the sharp indentation of the nucleus seen in true lipoblasts **(A)**. Vacuoles stain positively for hyaluronic acid with Alcian blue **(B)**.

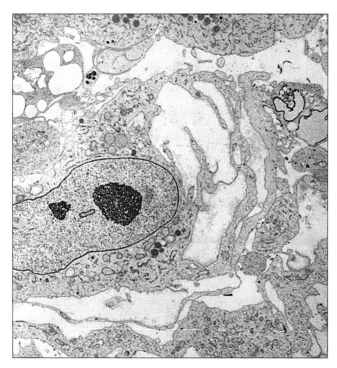

FIGURE 14-24 Electron micrograph of a myxoid malignant fibrous histiocytoma. Cells are surrounded by abundant ground substance. Vacuolation of cells is caused by numerous invaginations of the cytoplasmic membrane, trapping ground substance around the nucleus, and by dilatation of the endoplasmic reticulum. (Courtesy of Dr. Bruce Mackay.)

lipoblasts because of their coarse cytoplasmic vacuoles (Fig. 14–23), but unlike lipoblasts, the vacuoles contain acid mucin rather than neutral fat. Like classic malignant fibrous histiocytoma, the cells within the myxoid variant have features of fibroblasts (Fig. 14–24). The vacuolation seems to be the result of dilatation of the endoplasmic reticulum and formation of "pseudocanaliculi" by delicate cytoplasmic processes.

Differential diagnosis

The most important aspect of the differential diagnosis is the clear distinction of this lesion from benign myxoid lesions, such as nodular fasciitis and myxoma. Although nodular fasciitis may have focal myxoid change, it lacks the extensive orderly vasculature, bizarre cells, and atypical mitotic figures seen in myxoid malignant fibrous histiocytoma. Myxomas also lack the extensive vasculature of the malignant fibrous histiocytoma and usually have small cells with minimal atypia and few if any mitotic figures.

The sarcoma most nearly resembling this tumor is liposarcoma. Although myxoid liposarcoma resembles this tumor grossly, it consists of a more uniform population of small spindle cells embedded in a clear matrix with a delicate plexiform vasculature. Bizarre cells are

absent, and mitotic figures are infrequent. Lipoblasts are usually present. Pleomorphic liposarcoma, on the other hand, does have bizarre cells similar to myxoid malignant fibrous histiocytoma, but it has a cellular rather than a myxoid background, is more uniform in appearance, and contains lipoblasts.

Discussion

Identification of a myxoid variant of malignant fibrous histiocytoma was proposed not only because of its distinctive appearance but also because of its better prognosis compared with the storiform-pleomorphic type.[33,71] By definition, this tumor is composed of cells that qualitatively resemble those of an ordinary malignant fibrous histiocytoma, implying that the cells have a moderate or marked degree of nuclear atypia. In addition, at least one-half of the tumor should be characterized by an abundant myxoid background. Defined in this fashion, the lesions can be shown to have a better prognosis than the ordinary forms of malignant fibrous histiocytoma.

This tumor recurs in almost two-thirds of cases but metastasizes in only about one-fourth. The indolent course of the tumor is, furthermore, underscored by the longer interval between the time of diagnosis and metastasis. Although the better prognosis is due in part to the fact that such lesions tend to segregate more often to the superficial soft tissues and to be smaller, it has been shown by multivariate analysis that the myxoid subtype is an independent prognostic factor.

The terms myxofibrosarcoma and myxoid malignant fibrous histiocytoma are often used synonymously with the following qualifications. Myxofibrosarcoma was originally coined in the 1970s for low-grade myxoid fibrosarcomas that tended to segregate to the superficial soft tissues.[72] More recently, the term has been applied to a spectrum of myxoid fibroblastic/myofibroblastic tumors that range from low- to high-grade lesions and which can very greatly in the degree of myxoid change.[73,74] Use of this term in the latter unqualified manner is of dubious clinical value, as it can refer to lesions that vary from grade I to grade III and which can be predominantly myxoid or cellular. Because all data derived from large studies indicating the improved outcome of myxoid forms of malignant fibrous histiocytoma use stringent criteria for diagnosis (a tumor >50% myxoid), acceptance of loose diagnostic criteria inevitably erodes the prognostic importance of this subtype and leads to general confusion regarding its behavior. If the term myxofibrosarcoma is used, it should be clearly stipulated whether the lesion is considered low or high grade. On the other hand, the term myxoid malignant fibrous histiocytoma generally implies at least an intermediate-grade tumor. For these reasons we have adopted the approach shown in Figure 14–25. Highly myxoid fibroblastic/myofibroblastic sarcomas (>50% myxoid) can be

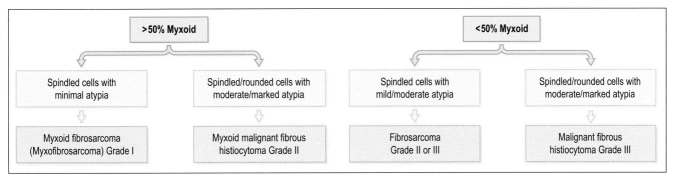

```
┌─────────────────────────────────────────────────────────────────────────────────────────────┐
│              [>50% Myxoid]                                      [<50% Myxoid]                   │
│                                                                                                │
│   ┌──────────────────┐  ┌──────────────────┐      ┌──────────────────┐  ┌──────────────────┐  │
│   │ Spindled cells with│  │ Spindled/rounded cells│      │ Spindled cells with│  │ Spindled/rounded cells│  │
│   │  minimal atypia   │  │ with moderate/marked  │      │ mild/moderate atypia│  │ with moderate/marked  │  │
│   │                   │  │      atypia       │      │                   │  │      atypia       │  │
│   └──────────────────┘  └──────────────────┘      └──────────────────┘  └──────────────────┘  │
│                                                                                                │
│   ┌──────────────────┐  ┌──────────────────┐      ┌──────────────────┐  ┌──────────────────┐  │
│   │ Myxoid fibrosarcoma│  │ Myxoid malignant fibrous│     │   Fibrosarcoma    │  │ Malignant fibrous │  │
│   │(Myxofibrosarcoma) │  │ histiocytoma Grade II │      │  Grade II or III  │  │ histiocytoma Grade III│  │
│   │     Grade I       │  │                   │      │                   │  │                   │  │
│   └──────────────────┘  └──────────────────┘      └──────────────────┘  └──────────────────┘  │
└─────────────────────────────────────────────────────────────────────────────────────────────┘
```

FIGURE 14–25 Proposed nomenclature for myxoid fibroblastic and fibrohistiocytic neoplasms.

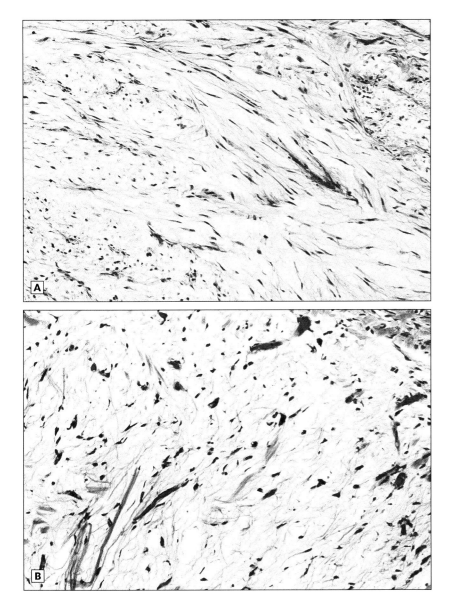

FIGURE 14–26 Comparison of a classic "low-grade myxofibrosarcoma" or fibrosarcoma, myxoid type, grade I **(A)** with a myxoid malignant fibrous histiocytoma, grade II **(B)**. Although both are predominantly myxoid, myxofibrosarcomas are composed of differentiated spindled cells arranged in fascicles, whereas myxoid fibrous histiocytomas are composed of stellate, spindled, and pleomorphic cells arranged haphazardly.

divided into two groups depending on the level of atypia. We refer to those with minimal atypia as low grade (grade 1) "myxofibrosarcoma" (Fig. 14–26A), whereas those with significant atypia are designated myxoid malignant fibrous histiocytoma, grade 2 (Figs 14–22A,

B, 14–26B). Predominantly nonmyxoid lesions (<50% myxoid) are designated fibrosarcoma or malignant fibrous histiocytoma, depending on the level of atypia, and are graded accordingly. These lesions may be grade 2 or 3.

Malignant fibrous histiocytoma: giant cell type (pleomorphic undifferentiated sarcoma with giant cells)

The giant cell type of malignant fibrous histiocytoma, also termed malignant giant cell tumor of soft parts,[34,75] is a multinodular tumor composed of a mixture of spindled, rounded, and osteoclast-type giant cells. Dense, fibrous bands containing vessels encircle the nodules of tumor, and secondary hemorrhage and necrosis are commonly present in them (Fig. 14–27). As in other malignant fibrous histiocytomas the relative amounts of the three cell types vary. Most tumors contain all three cell types arranged randomly, with some tendency for the fibroblasts to aggregate at the periphery of a nodule (Figs 14–28 to 14–31). The cells display pleomorphism and mitotic activity and often contain ingested material such as lipid and hemosiderin. The hallmark of this tumor is the giant cell. Although these cells resemble normal osteoclasts, they are usually not found in association with osteoid, and their nuclei tend to be of high nuclear grade. Hemorrhage tends to be common in these lesions (Fig. 14–31) and occasionally forms large cystic hemorrhagic spaces.

Focal osteoid or mature bone is present (Fig. 14–28) in approximately half of the cases. This material is usually located at the periphery of a tumor nodule and appears to be produced by neoplastic cells. In view of this feature,

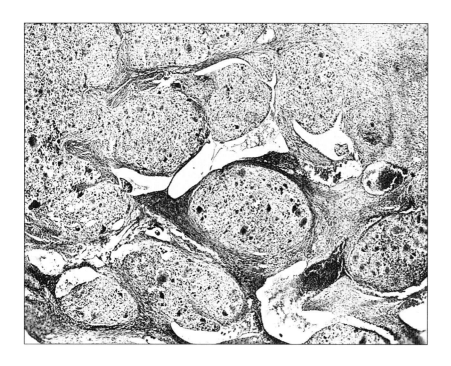

FIGURE 14–27 Characteristic multinodular pattern of the giant cell type of malignant fibrous histiocytoma (×38). (From Guccion JG, Enzinger FM. Malignant giant cell tumor of soft parts: an analysis of 32 cases. Cancer 1972; 29:1518.)

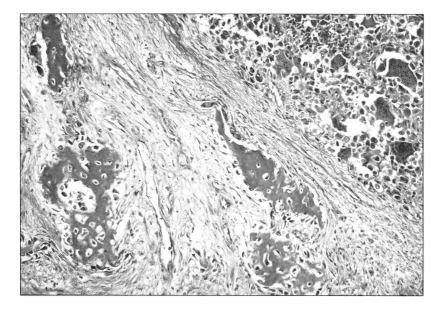

FIGURE 14–28 Giant cell form of malignant fibrous histiocytoma showing a shell of woven bone at the periphery.

the question can legitimately be raised as to whether this tumor is one of bone-forming mesenchyme. Ultrastructural studies have presented divergent views on this point.[19,76]

A subset of giant cell tumors of soft parts is composed of cells lacking significant nuclear atypia but with mitotic activity and vascular invasion. These lesions, resembling giant cell tumors of bone, are considered giant cell tumors of low malignant potential because they produce metastasis infrequently (see Chapter 13).

Differential diagnosis

The distinctive appearance of this neoplasm usually causes few problems with the diagnosis. Deeply situated tumors may raise the question of a giant cell tumor of bone involving soft tissue. This tumor, however, has a degree of multinodularity not generally encountered in giant cell tumors of bone and does not create major osseous defects as would be expected in a bone tumor.

Discussion

Although there are considerably fewer data concerning this form of malignant fibrous histiocytoma compared with data for the foregoing types, the original study of 32 cases[34] indicates the same general tendencies as discussed previously. Superficial tumors involving the subcutis or fascia have a much better prognosis than deeply situated tumors. Two-thirds of superficial tumors recur, but only about one-sixth metastasize. On the other hand, about 40% of deep tumors recur, and about half metastasize, a proportion roughly comparable to the ordinary forms of malignant fibrous histiocytoma.

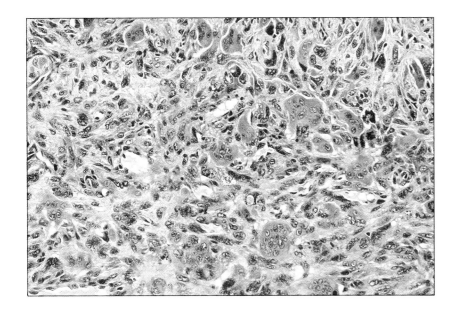

FIGURE 14–29 Giant cell form of malignant fibrous histiocytoma.

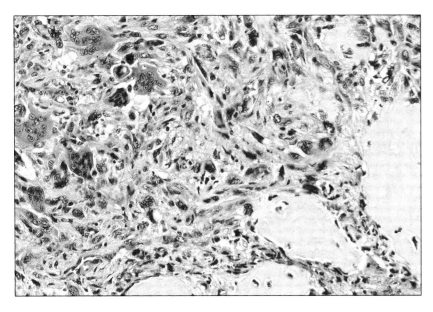

FIGURE 14–30 Giant cell form of malignant fibrous histiocytoma containing less mature bone in the tumor.

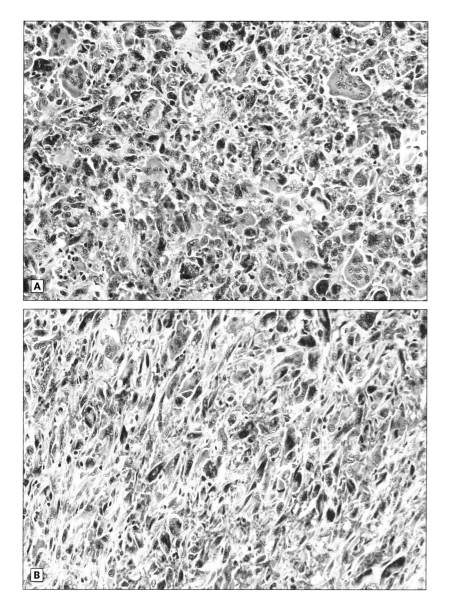

FIGURE 14–31 Hemorrhagic areas in a giant cell form of malignant fibrous histiocytoma that vary from having a predominantly round cell population with numerous osteoclast-like giant cells with high-grade nuclear atypia **(A)** to a spindled population **(B)**.

Malignant fibrous histiocytoma: inflammatory type (pleomorphic undifferentiated sarcoma with prominent inflammation)

The inflammatory form of malignant fibrous histiocytoma is a rare tumor found almost exclusively in the retroperitoneum and is characterized by both a prominent xanthomatous and neutrophilic infiltrate, the former imparting to the tumor its almost invariable yellow color (Fig. 14–32A). Analysis of tumor extracts has documented eosinophilic and neutrophilic chemotactic activity along with myelopoietic activity, suggesting that production of specific cytokines by the tumor could explain all of the unusual associated blood manifestations.[37,77]

Histologically, the tumor is composed of benign- and malignant-appearing xanthoma cells, the latter often

assuming a gigantic size with bizarre nuclei. Typically, these neoplastic cells display phagocytosis of neutrophils, a feature that helps distinguish them from anaplastic lymphoma in which inflammatory cells typically are not internalized by the neoplastic lymphoid cells (Figs 14–33 to 14–37). The neoplastic cells in malignant fibrous histiocytomas express vimentin but not various leukocyte lineage markers (CD15, CD20, CD45), although they may contain CD68 as a reflection of their phagocytic activity. The inflammatory component is characteristically prominent and usually consists of a mixture of acute and chronic inflammatory cells with marked prominence on the former. A delicate vasculature is sometimes appreciated throughout the tumor, creating a superficial resemblance to granulation tissue. There are frequent transitions to spindled areas with a fascicular or even a storiform

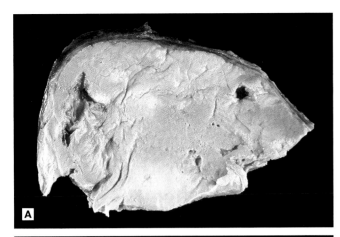

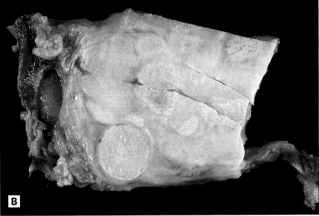

FIGURE 14–32 Gross appearance of a malignant fibrous histiocytoma with a tawny yellow color **(A)**. In some portions of the tumor there were areas of conventional malignant fibrous histiocytoma. **(B)** Interface of conventional malignant fibrous histiocytoma (white areas) with the inflammatory areas.

growth pattern (Fig. 15–32B). These areas resemble the more typical malignant fibrous histiocytomas and are therefore of great help in establishing a diagnosis. Metastases from this tumor usually resemble the parent lesion; when the metastases are different, they usually appear to be less xanthomatous and more fibroblastic.

Differential diagnosis

The differential diagnosis consists primarily of distinguishing this tumor from non-neoplastic xanthomatous processes. Although xanthogranulomatous pyelonephritis may involve the retroperitoneal soft tissue, it first and foremost affects the kidneys and is accompanied by the usual constellation of symptoms of urinary tract infection. Xanthogranulomatous inflammatory processes may also be seen in other settings, some of which are related to infectious agents. Thus, culture of these lesions and bacterial stains are mandatory. Ultimately, the distinction of this tumor from xanthogranulomatous inflammation rests on the documentation of atypia or mitotic activity in the xanthoma cells or fibroblastic areas resembling the usual form of malignant fibrous histiocytoma. Therefore, careful sampling of large xanthomatous lesions, especially in the retroperitoneum, is of the utmost importance.

The malignant tumor most often confused with inflammatory malignant fibrous histiocytoma is lymphoma. Small biopsy specimens or peripheral sampling of large tumors may result in close intermingling of rounded histiocyte-like cells with inflammatory cells, simulating the pattern of lymphoma. Although the clinical

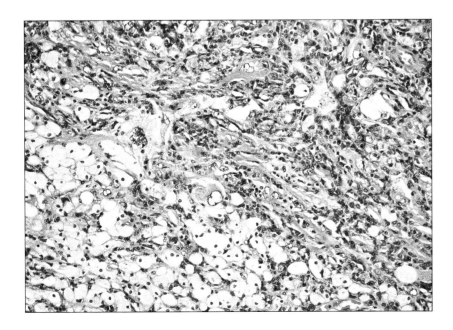

FIGURE 14–33 Inflammatory malignant fibrous histiocytoma showing transition to a conventional malignant fibrous histiocytoma (top right).

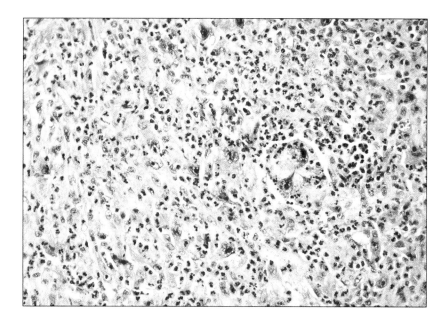

FIGURE 14-34 Inflammatory malignant fibrous histiocytoma with a predominance of neutrophils, some in tumor cells.

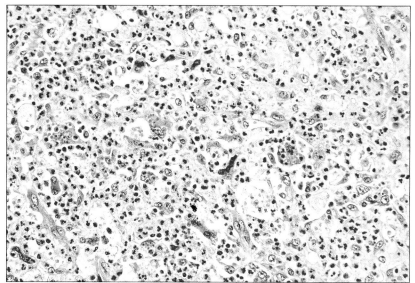

FIGURE 14-35 Inflammatory malignant fibrous histiocytoma.

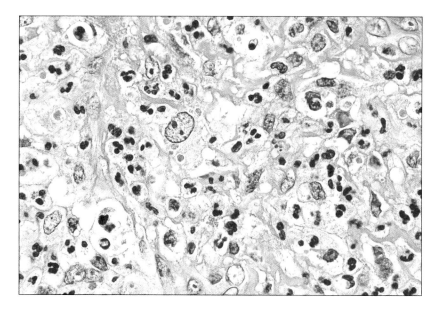

FIGURE 14-36 High-power view of cells in an inflammatory malignant fibrous histiocytoma. The round neoplastic cells sometimes resemble the cells in anaplastic large cell lymphomas or Hodgkin's disease.

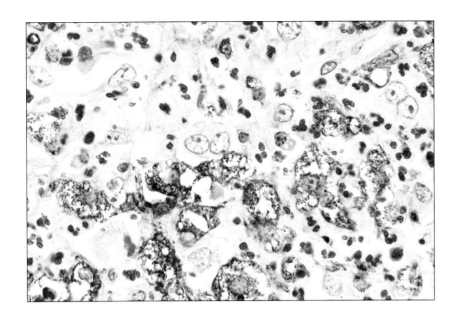

FIGURE 14–37 CD68 stain of an inflammatory malignant fibrous histiocytoma with staining of benign xanthoma cells. Some phagocytic tumor cells also stain. Other leukocyte lineage markers are not present in the neoplastic cells in the tumor.

symptoms of fever and leukemoid reaction, which occasionally characterize inflammatory malignant fibrous histiocytoma, are rare with lymphoma, it is often necessary to perform a number of immunostaining procedures to establish the diagnosis. Negative immunostaining for leukocyte common antigen, Leu-M1, and other leukocyte lineage markers are helpful for distinguishing the two lesions, particularly when only a small needle biopsy is available. In our experience, leukocyte lineage markers are not identified in the neoplastic cells of inflammatory malignant fibrous histiocytoma, although CD68 may be identified in neoplastic cells that have evidence of phagocytosis (Fig. 14–37).[77]

Discussion

In the past it has been difficult to characterize the behavior of these tumors because of the uncertainty of the diagnosis in some cases and the limited follow-up information in others. In a review of 29 acceptable cases from the literature[78] approximately half of the patients had persistent or recurrent disease, and about one-third developed distant metastases in such sites as the liver, lung, and lymph nodes. The aggressive nature of the tumor is corroborated by another report of seven cases[34] in which virtually all patients suffered severe effects of local disease, and four eventually developed metastases. Although it is obvious that these lesions are malignant, it is not clear to what extent they should be regarded as comparable to the other forms of malignant fibrous histiocytoma. The deep location of most of these tumors, the surgical inaccessibility, and the therapeutic delays resulting from diagnostic errors adversely affect the prognosis of these cases.

Although it is sometimes claimed that inflammatory forms of malignant fibrous histiocytoma are, in effect, lymphomas that are misdiagnosed, this is clearly an overstatement. It is true that failure to exclude other tumors that legitimately enter the differential diagnosis can lead to overdiagnosis, but application of immunohistochemistry to this problem area helps considerably. When evaluating small needle biopsy specimens with a presumptive diagnosis of inflammatory malignant fibrous histiocytoma, immunostains for leukocyte lineage markers and for cytokeratin serve to rule out retroperitoneum-based carcinomas and lymphomas (including Hodgkin's disease), which occasionally have a striking inflammatory infiltrate. Likewise, a recent study suggests that some inflammatory forms of malignant fibrous histiocytoma represent dedifferentiated liposarcomas,[14] again reinforcing the need to carefully sample any lesion presumed to represent a malignant fibrous histiocytoma.

REFERENCES

1. Ozzello L, Stout AP, Murray MR. Cultural characteristics of malignant histiocytomas and fibrous xanthomas. Cancer 1963; 16:331.
2. O'Brien JE, Stout AP. Malignant fibrous xanthomas. Cancer 1964; 17:1445.
3. Roholl PJ, Kleyne J, Elbers J, et al. Characterization of tumour cells in malignant fibrous histiocytomas and other soft tissue tumours in comparison with malignant histiocytes. I. Immunohistochemical study on paraffin sections. J Pathol 1985; 147:87.
4. Roholl PJM, Kleyne J, Van Unnik JAM. Characterization of tumour cells in malignant fibrous histiocytomas and other soft tissue tumors, in comparison with malignant histiocytes. II. Immunoperoxidase study on cryostat sections. Am J Pathol 1985; 121:269.
5. Iwasaki H, Isayama T, Johzaki H, et al. Malignant fibrous histiocytoma: evidence of perivascular mesenchymal cell origin immunocytochemical studies with monoclonal anti-MFH antibodies. Am J Pathol 1987; 128:528.
6. Iwasaki H, Isayama T, Ohjimi Y, et al. Malignant fibrous histiocytoma: a tumor of facultative histiocytes showing mesenchymal differentiation in cultured cell lines. Cancer 1992; 69:437.
7. Fletcher CD. Pleomorphic malignant fibrous histiocytoma: fact or fiction? A critical reappraisal based on 159 tumors diagnosed as

pleomorphic sarcoma. Am J Surg Pathol 1992; 16:213.

8. Fletcher CDM, Unni KK, eds. Pathology and genetics: tumors of soft tissues and bone. World Health Organization Classification of Tumours. Lyon: IARC Press; 2002:102–103; 120–126.

9. Montgomery E, Fisher C. Myofibroblastic differentiation in malignant fibrous histiocytoma (pleomorphic myxofibrosarcoma): a clinicopathologic study. Histopathology 2001; 38:499.

10. Engellau J, Anderson H, Rydholm A, et al. Time dependence of prognostic factors for patients with soft tissue sarcomas: a Scandinavian Group Study of 338 malignant fibrous histiocytomas. Cancer 2004; 100:2233.

11. Fletcher CDM, Gustafson P, Rydlholm A, et al. Clinicopathologic re-evaluation of 100 malignant fibrous histiocytomas: prognostic relevance of subclassification. J Clin Oncol 2001; 19:3045.

12. Kindblom LG, Widehn S, Meis-Kindblom JM. The role of electron microscopy in the diagnosis of pleomorphic sarcomas of soft tissue. Semin Diagn Pathol 2003; 20:72.

13. Suh CH, Orgonez NG, Mackay B. Malignant fibrous histiocytoma: an ultrastructural perspective. Ultrastruct Pathol 2000; 24:243.

14. Coindre JM, Hostein I, Maire G, et al. Inflammatory malignant fibrous histiocytomas and dedifferentiated liposarcomas: histological review, genomic profile, and MDM2 and CDK4 status favour a single entity. J Pathol 2004; 203:822.

15. Nielsen TO, Wes RB, Linn SC, et al. Molecular characterization of soft tissue tumours: a gene expression study. Lancet 2002; 359:1301.

16. Derrre J, Lagace R, Nicolas A, et al. Leiomyosarcomas and most malignant fibrous histiocytomas share very similar comparative genomic hybridization imbalances: an analysis of a series of 27 leiomyosarcomas. Lab Invest 2001; 81:211.

17. Sabah JA, Cummins R, Leader M, et al. Leiomyosarcoma and malignant fibrous histiocytoma share similar allelic imbalance pattern at 9p. Virchows Arch 2005; 446:251.

Atypical fibroxanthoma

18. Alguacil-Garcia A, Unni KK, Goellner JR, et al. Atypical fibroxanthoma of the skin. Cancer 1977; 40:1471.

19. Dahl L. Atypical fibroxanthoma of the skin: a clinicopathological study of 57 cases. Acta Pathol Microbiol Scand 1976; 84:183.

20. Fretzin DF, Helwig EB. Atypical fibroxanthoma of the skin. Cancer 1973; 31:1541.

21. Dei Tos AP, Maestro R, Doglioni C, et al. Ultraviolet induced p53 mutations in atypical fibroxanthoma. Am J Pathol 1994; 145:11.

22. Sakamoto A, Oda Y, Itakura E, et al. Immunoexpression of ultraviolet photoproducts and p53 mutation analysis in atypical fibroxanthoma and superficial malignant fibrous histiocytoma. Mod Pathol 2001; 14:581.

23. Hudson AW, Winkelmann RK. Atypical fibroxanthoma of the skin: a reappraisal of 19 cases in which the original diagnosis was spindle-cell squamous carcinoma. Cancer 1972; 29:413.

24. Khan ZM, Cockerell CJ. Atypical fibroxanthoma with osteoclast-like multinucleated giant cells. Am J Dermatopathol 1997; 19:174.

25. Chen KTK. Atypical fibroxanthoma of the skin with osteoid production. Arch Dermatol 1980; 116:113.

26. Requena L, Sanguezca OP, Sanchez YE, et al. Clear cell atypical fibroxanthoma. J Cutan Pathol 1997; 24:176.

27. Crowson AN, Carlson-Sweet K, Macinnis C, et al. Clear cell atypical fibroxanthoma: a clinicopathologic study. J Cutan Pathol 2002; 29:374.

28. Orosz Z. Atypical fibroxanthoma with granular cells. Histopathology 1998; 33:88.

29. Mirza B, Weedon D. Atypical fibroxanthoma: a clinicopathologic study of 89 cases. Australasian J Dermtol 2005; 46:235.

30. Sakamoto A, Oda Y, Itakura E, et al. H-K- and N ras gene mutation in atypical fibroxanthoma and malignant fibrous histiocytoma. Human Pathol 2001; 32:1225.

Malignant fibrous histiocytoma

31. Weiss SW, Enzinger FM. Malignant fibrous histiocytoma: an analysis of 200 cases. Cancer 1978; 41:2250.

32. Weiss SW, Enzinger FM. Myxoid variant of malignant fibrous histiocytoma. Cancer 1977; 39:1672.

33. Guccion JG, Enzinger FM. Malignant giant cell tumor of soft parts: an analysis of 32 cases. Cancer 1972; 29:1518.

34. Kyriakos M, Kempson RL. Inflammatory fibrous histiocytoma: an aggressive and lethal lesion. Cancer 1976; 37:1584.

35. Hamada T, Komiya S, Hiraoka K, et al. IL-6 in a pleomorphic type of malignant fibrous histiocytoma presenting high fever. Hum Pathol 1998; 29:758.

36. Isoda M, Yasumoto S. Eosinophil chemotactic factor derived from a malignant fibrous histiocytoma. Clin Exp Dermatol 1986; 11:253.

37. Kageyama K, Moriyama T, Hizuka N, et al. Hypoglycemia associated with big insulin-like growth factor II produced during development of malignant fibrous histiocytoma. Endocrine J 2003; 50:753.

38. Rooser B, Willen H, Gustafson P, et al. Malignant fibrous histiocytoma of soft tissue: a population-based epidemiologic and prognostic study of 137 patients. Cancer 1991; 67:499.

39. Bridge JA, Sanger WG, Shaffer B, et al. Cytogenetic findings in malignant fibrous histiocytoma. Cancer Genet Cytogenet 1987; 29:97.

40. Choong PF, Mandahl N, Mertens F, et al. 19p⁺ marker chromosome correlates with relapse in malignant fibrous histiocytoma. Genes Chromosomes Cancer 1996; 16:88.

41. Lararamendy ML, Tarkkanen M, Blomqvist C, et al. Comparative genomic hybridization of malignant fibrous histiocytoma reveals a novel prognostic marker. Am J Pathol 1997; 151:1153.

42. Mairal A, Terrier P, Chibon F, et al. Loss of chromosome 13 is the most frequent genomic imbalance in malignant fibrous histiocytoma: a comparative genomic hybridization analysis of a series of 30 cases. Cancer Genet Cytogenet 1999; 111:134.

43. Meloni-Ehrig AM, Chen Z, Guan XY, et al. Identification of a ring chromosome in a myxoid malignant fibrous histiocytoma with chromosome microdissection and fluorescence in situ hybridization. Cancer Genet Cytogenet 1999; 109:81.

44. Orndal C, Mandahl N, Carlen B, et al. Near-haploid clones in a malignant fibrous histiocytoma. Cancer Genet Cytogenet 1992; 60:147.

45. Rydholm A, Mandahl N, Heim S, et al. Malignant fibrous histiocytomas with a 19p+ marker chromosome have increased relapse rate. Genes Chromosomes Cancer 1990; 2:296.

46. Eriksson M, Hardell L, Berg NO, et al. Soft tissue sarcomas and exposure to chemical substances: a case referent study. Br J Ind Med 1981; 38:27.

47. Buckley C, Thomas V, Cros J, et al. Cancer family syndrome associated with multiple malignant melanomas and a malignant fibrous histiocytoma. Br J Dermatol 1992; 126:83.

48. Lindeman G, McKay MJ, Taubman KL, et al. Malignant fibrous histiocytoma developing in bone 44 years after shrapnel trauma. Cancer 1990; 66:2229.

49. Pezzi CM, Rawlings MS Jr, Esgro JJ, et al. Prognostic factors in 227 patients with malignant fibrous histiocytoma. Cancer 1992; 69:2098.

50. Brecher ME, Franklin WA. Absence of mononuclear phagocyte antigens in malignant fibrous histiocytoma. Am J Clin Pathol 1986; 86:344.

51. Wood GS, Beckstead JH, Turner RR, et al. Malignant fibrous histiocytoma tumor cells resemble fibroblasts. Am J Surg Pathol 1986; 10:323.

52. Hirose T, Sano T, Hizawa K. Ultrastructural study of the myxoid area of malignant fibrous histiocytomas. Ultrastruct Pathol 1988; 12:621.

53. Lawson CW, Fisher C, Garter KC. An immunohistochemical study of differentiation in malignant fibrous histiocytoma. Histopathology 1987; 11:375.

54. Litzky LA, Brooks JJ. Cytokeratin immunoreactivity in malignant fibrous histiocytoma and spindle cell tumors: comparison between frozen and paraffin-embedded tissues. Mod Pathol 1992; 5:30.

55. Miettinen M, Soini Y. Malignant fibrous histiocytoma: heterogeneous patterns of intermediate filament proteins by immunohistochemistry. Arch Pathol Lab Med 1989; 113:1363.

56. Weiss SW, Bratthauer GL, Morris PA. Postirradiation malignant fibrous histiocytoma expressing cytokeratin: implications for the immunodiagnosis of sarcomas. Am J Surg Pathol 1988; 12:554.

57. Evans HL, Smith JL. Spindle cell squamous carcinoma and sarcoma-like tumors of the skin: a comparative study of 38 cases. Cancer 1980; 45:2687.

58. Fu Y-S, Gabbiani G, Kaye GI, et al. Malignant soft tissue tumors of probable histiocytic origin (malignant fibrous histiocytoma): general considerations and electron microscopic and tissue culture studies. Cancer 1975; 35:176.

59. Coindre JM, Mariani O, Chibon F, et al. Most malignant fibrous histiocytomas developed in the retroperitoneum are dedifferentiated liposarcomas: a review of 25 cases initially diagnosed as malignant fibrous histiocytoma. Mod Pathol 2003; 16:256.

60. Le Doussal V, Coindre J-M, Leroux A, et al. Prognostic factors for patients with localized primary malignant fibrous histiocytoma. Cancer 1996; 77:1823.

61. Salo JC, Lewis JJ, Woodruff JM, et al. Malignant fibrous histiocytoma of the extremity. Cancer 1999; 85:1765.

62. Gibbs JF, Huang PP, Lee RJ. Malignant fibrous histiocytoma: an institutional review. Cancer Investigation 2001; 19:23.

63. Zagars GK, Mullen JR, Pollack A. Malignant fibrous histiocytoma: outcome and prognostic factors following conservation surgery and radiotherapy. Int J Oncol Biol Phys 1996; 34:983.

64. Bertoni F, Capanna R, Biagini R, et al. Malignant fibrous histiocytoma of soft tissue: an analysis of 78 cases located and deeply seated in the extremities. Cancer 1985; 56:356.

65. Kearney MM, Soule EH, Ivins JC. Malignant fibrous histiocytoma: a retrospective study of 167 cases. Cancer 1980; 45:167.

66. Belaal A, Kandil A, Allam A, et al. Malignant fibrous histiocytoma: a retrospective study of 109 cases. Am J Clin Oncol 2002; 25:16.

67. Mandahl N, Heim S, Willen H, et al. Characteristic karyotypic anomalies identify

subtypes of malignant fibrous histiocytoma. Genes Chromosomes Cancer 1989; 1:9.

68. Mertens F, Fletcher CDM, Dal Cin P, et al. Cytogenetic analysis of 46 pleomorphic sarcomas and correlation with morphological and clinical features: a report of the CHAMP Study Group. Genes Chromosomes Cancer 1998; 22:16.

69. Simons R, Hofstra R, Hollema H, et al. Inclusion of malignant fibrous histiocytoma in the tumour spectrum associated with hereditary nonpolyposis colorectal cancer. Genes Chromosomes Cancer 2000; 29:353.

70. Chibon F, Mairal A, Freneaux P, et al. The Rb1 gene is the target of chromosome 13 deletions in malignant fibrous histiocytoma. Cancer Res 2000; 60:6339.

71. Kindblom LG, Merck C, Svendsen P. Myxofibrosarcoma: a pathological-anatomical, microangiopathic and angiographic correlative study of eight cases. Br J Radiol 1977; 50:876.

72. Mentzel T, Calonje E, Wadden C, et al. Myxofibrosarcoma: clinicopathologic analysis of 75 cases with emphasis on the low-grade variant. Am J Surg Pathol 1996; 20:391.

73. Michael RH, Dorfman HD. Malignant fibrous histiocytoma associated with bone infarcts. Clin Orthop 1976; 118:180.

74. Alguacil-Garcia A, Unni KK, Goellner JR. Malignant giant cell tumor of soft parts: ultrastructural study of four cases. Cancer 1977; 40:244.

75. Van Haelst UJGM, de Haas van Dorsser AH. Giant cell tumor of soft parts: an ultrastructural study. Virchows Arch [Pathol Anat] 1976; 371:199.

76. Takahashi K, Kimura Y, Naito M, et al. Inflammatory fibrous histiocytoma presenting leukemoid reaction. Pathol Res Pract 1989; 184:498.

77. Khalidi H, Singleton T, Weiss SW. Inflammatory malignant fibrous histiocytoma: distinction from Hodgkin's disease and non-Hodgkin's lymphoma by a panel of leukocyte markers. Mod Pathol 1997; 10:438.

78. Kahn LB. Retroperitoneal xanthogranuloma and xanthosarcoma (malignant fibrous xanthoma). Cancer 1973; 31:411.

BENIGN LIPOMATOUS TUMORS

CHAPTER CONTENTS

The significance and multiple functions of fat are not always fully appreciated. Fat serves not only as one of the principal and most readily available sources of energy in the body; it functions as a barrier for the conservation of heat and as mechanical protection of the underlying tissues against physical injury. Two basic forms of adipose tissue can be distinguished, *white fat* and *brown fat*.

WHITE FAT

White fat makes its first appearance at a relatively late stage of development; it is rarely encountered before the third or fourth month of intrauterine life. In its earliest stages, after 10–14 weeks' gestation, it consists of aggregates of mesenchymal cells that are condensed around proliferating primitive blood vessels.[1-4] Following this stage, the stellate-shaped preadipocytes are organized into lobules that contain a rich network of proliferating capillaries. At later stages (14–24 weeks' gestation), small oil red O-positive and sudanophilic lipid droplets appear in these cells, gradually converting them to rounded or spherical, multivacuolated lipoblasts. Intracellular glycogen is usually present at this stage of development. The multiple lipid droplets then fuse to form a single vacuole and displace the nucleus marginally, forming the mature fat cell, or lipocyte. Small aggregates of lipocytes form lobules that make their first appearance in the regions of the face, neck, breast, and abdominal wall followed by the back and shoulders. The lobules multiply and enlarge, and by the end of the fifth month a continuous subcutaneous layer of fat is formed in the extremities.[3]

Postnatally, white fat cells enlarge significantly during the first 6 months of life without a significant increase in cell number.[3] This phase is followed by a progressive increase in adipocyte number, although the cell size remains fairly constant. At puberty there is a marked increase in both adipocyte size and number. After puberty, new adipocytes continue to form throughout adult life, although at a much slower rate.[5]

Fat serves several functions, including thermal insulation and mechanical protection. Its main role is the uptake, synthesis, and storage of lipid and the release of free fatty acids in response to hormonal and neural stimuli. This function is mediated by lipoprotein lipase, an enzyme synthesized by adipocytes and transferred to the luminal surface of endothelial cells.

Histologically, differentiated white fat consists of spherical or polygonal cells in which most of the cytoplasm has been replaced by a single large lipid droplet, leaving only a narrow rim of cytoplasm at the periphery. The eccentrically placed nucleus is flattened and is crescent-shaped on cross-section; not infrequently it contains one small lipid invagination (Lochkern). The white fat cells (lipocytes) measure up to 120 μm in diameter. Like any metabolically active tissue, white fat is highly vascularized, a feature that is more evident in atrophic fat than in normal fat. In the subcutis and to a lesser extent in deeper tissues, the fat cells are arranged in distinct lobules separated by a thin membrane of fibrous connective tissue. The lobular architecture of white fat is most prominent in areas subjected to pressure and probably has a cushioning effect.

According to Napolitano's classic description, the ultrastructure of adipose tissue cells during the earliest stage of development closely resembles that of fibroblasts.[6,7] The cells are spindle-shaped, have slender cytoplasmic extensions, and contain small spherical mitochondria and abundant highly organized endoplasmic reticulum. At later stages of development the endoplasmic reticulum becomes less conspicuous, and one or more inclusions of non-membrane-bound lipid make their appearance in the cytoplasm, usually adjacent to the nucleus. There are also irregular, smooth-surfaced, membrane-limited vesicles, a rather poorly developed Golgi apparatus, and glycogen granules (in close association with the lipid inclusions). An amorphous basal lamina sets the cells apart from the surrounding collagen and occasional nonmyelinated nerves; the basal lamina is present at all stages of cellular differentiation and helps distinguish preadipocytes from fibroblasts.

Continued accumulation of cytoplasm and increasing amounts of intracellular lipid lead to more-rounded cells, which are characterized by a large, centrally located lipid droplet, a thin rim of cytoplasm, and a peripherally placed, flattened, or crescent-shaped nucleus. There is a membrane separating the central lipid inclusion from the surrounding cytoplasm. This "signet ring" stage of cellular development represents the lipocyte of mature adipose tissue.

BROWN FAT

The precursors of brown fat are spindle-shaped cells that are closely related to a network of capillaries.[8] Subsequently, there is proliferation of capillaries and brown adipocytes, with organization into lobules by fibrous connective tissue septa. As the cells accumulate lipid, they are initially unilocular; but with further lipid accumulation, multiple cytoplasmic lipid vacuoles appear. Brown fat is found mainly in infants and children and gradually disappears from most sites with increasing age. In children, brown fat deposits are most conspicuous in the interscapular region, around the blood vessels and muscles of the neck, around the structures of the mediastinum, adjacent to the lung hila, on the anterior abdominal wall, and surrounding intra-abdominal and retroperitoneal structures including the kidneys, pancreas, and spleen. During adulthood, deposits of brown fat persist around the kidneys, adrenal glands, and aorta and within the mediastinum and neck.

The principal function of brown fat is heat production, a process principally controlled by the release of nore-pinephrine from sympathetic nerves. Brown fat may also play a role in weight regulation in adults.[9] Santos et al. found an increased amount of periadrenal fat in malnourished people at autopsy, suggesting a compensatory increase in nonshivering thermogenesis to maintain body temperature in those with diminished subcutaneous fat.[10]

The term brown fat refers to its gross appearance, which results from its abundant vascularity and numerous mitochondria. Compared to white fat, brown fat tends to have a more prominent lobulated growth pattern. Its cells are smaller (25–40 μm in diameter), are round or polygonal, and contain a large amount of cytoplasm that stains deeply eosinophilic with hematoxylin-eosin. The cells are mostly multivacuolated, with distinctly granular cytoplasm between the individual lipid droplets. Intermixed with these cells are nonvacuolated, purely granular cells and cells with a single large lipid vacuole, resembling lipocytes. The nuclei are rounded and situated in a central position, although the nucleus may be displaced to the periphery in cells with large lipid vacuoles as in white fat. The cells are arranged in distinct lobular aggregates and are intimately associated with a prominent vascular network and numerous nerves.

There are apparent transitions between brown and white fat in both humans and animals, but brown fat can be clearly identified by electron microscopy. The brown fat cell is smaller and can be recognized by small lipid inclusions with mitochondria that are both numerous and more complex in structure. There are also scattered ribosomes, variable amounts of glycogen, and a poorly developed endoplasmic reticulum.

MOLECULAR BIOLOGY

The *CHOP* gene, located on the long arm of chromosome 12, appears to be involved in adipocytic differentiation.[11] This gene encodes a member of the CCAAT/enhancer binding protein family (C/EBP), which may be an inhibitor of other C/EBP transcription factors known to be important in cell proliferation. Members of the C/EBP group are highly expressed in fat and are involved in the growth arrest of terminally differentiated adipocytes.[12]

IMMUNOHISTOCHEMISTRY

Adipocytes and benign and malignant fatty tumors stain positively for vimentin and S-100 protein.[13,14] More recently, an antibody to the adipocyte lipid-binding protein p422 (also known as aP2), a protein expressed exclusively in preadipocytes late in adipogenesis, has been found to stain only lipoblasts and brown fat cells, as well as liposarcomas.[2] The diagnostic utility of this antibody has yet to be proven.

CLASSIFICATION OF BENIGN LIPOMATOUS TUMORS

It is widely assumed that benign lipomatous tumors represent a common group of neoplasms that cause few complaints or complications and present little diagnostic difficulty. This may be largely true for the ordinary subcutaneous lipoma, but it does not take into account the enormous variety of benign tumors and tumor-like lesions of adipose tissue that are well defined but often have received little attention in the medical literature. In fact, it is our personal experience that benign lipomatous tumors are among the most frequently received in our consultation practice.

The bulk of lipomatous tumors may be grouped into four categories including:

1. *Superficial lipoma*, a tumor composed of mature fat and arising in the superficial (subcutaneous) soft tissues, represents by far the most common mesenchymal neoplasm.
2. *Deep lipomas* arise from or are intimately associated with tissues deep to the subcutis or with specific anatomic sites. The main subdivisions of this group are angiomyolipoma, intramuscular and intermuscular lipoma, lipoma of the tendon sheath, neural fibrolipoma with and without macrodactyly (fibrolipomatous hamartoma), and lumbosacral lipoma.
3. *Infiltrating* or *diffuse neoplastic* or *non-neoplastic proliferations of mature fat* may cause compression of vital structures or may be confused with atypical lipomatous neoplasm/well-differentiated liposarcoma. This group is composed of six entities: diffuse lipomatosis, pelvic lipomatosis, symmetric lipomatosis (Madelung's disease), adiposis dolorosa (Dercum's disease), steroid lipomatosis, and nevus lipomatosus.
4. *Variants of lipoma* are much less common and differ from ordinary lipoma by a characteristic microscopic picture and specific clinical setting. These include angiolipoma, myolipoma, angiomyolipoma, myelolipoma, chondroid lipoma, spindle cell/pleomorphic lipoma, hibernoma and lipoblastoma/lipoblastomatosis.

When describing these entities, we have made no attempt to distinguish between true neoplasms, hamartomatous processes, and localized overgrowth of fat, as it would be largely speculative and of little practical consequence. In the past 10 years, cytogenetic data have contributed significantly to our understanding of the

TABLE 15–1	PRINCIPAL CHROMOSOMAL ABERRATIONS OF BENIGN LIPOMATOUS TUMORS	
Tumor	**Chromosomal aberration**
Lipoma (ordinary)	Translocations involving 12q13–15
	Interstitial deletions of 13q
	Rearrangements involving 6p21–23
Angiolipoma	None
Spindle cell/pleomorphic lipoma	Loss of 16q13
	Unbalanced 13q alterations
Lipoblastoma/lipoblastomatosis	Translocations involving 8q11–13
Hibernoma	Translocations involving 11q13
	Translocations involving 10q22

pathogenesis of both benign and malignant lipomatous tumors. Although cytogenetic analysis is of limited diagnostic utility in this group of benign lipomatous tumors, the knowledge gained by such analyses has allowed a better understanding of how these lipomatous tumors are related to one another (Table 15–1).

LIPOMA

Solitary lipomas, consisting entirely of mature fat, have been largely ignored in the literature, because they grow insidiously and cause few problems other than those of a localized mass. Many lipomas remain unrecorded or are brought to the attention of a physician only if they reach a large size or cause cosmetic problems or complications because of their anatomic site. As a consequence, the reported incidence of lipoma is certainly much lower than the actual incidence. Even if we consider only the recorded data, however, lipomas outnumber other benign or malignant soft tissue tumors by a considerable margin and undoubtedly represent the most common soft tissue tumor. This is true for the solitary subcutaneous lipoma and for lipomas in general, regardless of histologic type.

Age and gender incidence

Lipoma is rare during the first two decades of life and usually makes its appearance when fat begins to accumulate in inactive individuals. Most become apparent in patients 40–60 years of age. When not excised, they persist for the remainder of life, although they hardly increase in size after the initial growth period. Statistics as to gender incidence vary, but most report a higher incidence in men.[15] There seems to be no difference in regard to race; and in the United States, whites and African-Americans are affected in proportion to their distribution in the general population.

Localization

Two types of solitary lipoma can be distinguished. *Subcutaneous (superficial) lipomas* are most common in the regions of the upper back and neck, shoulder, and abdomen, followed in frequency by the proximal portions of the extremities, chiefly the upper arms, buttocks, and upper thigh. They are seldom encountered in the face, hands, lower legs or feet.

Deep lipomas are rare in comparison. They are often detected at a relatively late stage of development and consequently tend to be larger than more superficial lipomas. Numerous sites may be involved. When in the extremities, they often arise from the subfascial tissues of the hands and feet, where they may be mistaken for ganglion cysts.[16] They may also arise from juxta-articular regions or the periosteum (*parosteal lipoma*), sometimes causing nerve compression, erosion of bone, or focal cortical hyperostosis.[17] Deep lipomas in the region of the head occur chiefly in the forehead and scalp;[18] those in the trunk are found principally in the thorax and mediastinum, chest wall and pleura, pelvis and paratesticular region.[19]

In the gastrointestinal tract, lipomas are mainly seen in the submucosa and subserosa of the small and large intestines, often as an incidental finding at endoscopy.[20,21] They are solitary or multiple and present as a sessile or pedunculated mass; sometimes, they are associated with ulceration and bleeding or intussusception.

Deep or subfascial lipomas tend to be less well circumscribed than superficial ones, and their contours are usually determined by the space they occupy. Intrathoracic lipomas, for instance, may extend from the upper mediastinum, neck, or subpleural region (*cervicomediastinal lipoma*) into the subcutis of the chest wall, sometimes assuming an hourglass configuration (*transmural lipoma*). Deep-seated lipomas of the hand or wrist form irregular masses with multiple processes underneath fascia or aponeuroses; they may attain a large size and, on rare occasions, extend from the palm to the dorsal surface of the hand. These tumors must be distinguished from lipomas growing in the tendon sheath (*endovaginal lipomas*) and those involving major nerves in the regions of the hand and wrist (*neural fibrolipomas*), which usually occur in young patients.

There are also rare lipoma-like fatty proliferations in the region of the umbilicus and inguinal ring (*hernial lipoma*) that may be associated with direct or indirect hernias or merely simulate a hernia clinically. A similar overgrowth of fat arising from surgical scars has been termed *incisional lipoma*.

Clinical findings

The usual clinical history of lipoma is that of an asymptomatic, slowly growing, round or discoid mass with a soft or doughy consistency. There is usually good mobility, with dimpling of the skin on movement. Pain is rare with ordinary lipomas; when it occurs it is a late symptom generally confined to large angiolipomas or lipomas that compress peripheral nerves. Although this may seem intuitive, lipomas are more common in obese persons and often increase in size during a period of rapid weight gain. In contrast, severe weight loss in cachectic patients or during periods of prolonged starvation rarely affects the size of a lipoma, suggesting that the fatty tissue of lipomas (or liposarcomas) is largely unavailable for general metabolism.

Deep or subfascial lipomas may cause a variety of symptoms, depending on their site and size. The symptoms range from a feeling of fullness and discomfort on motion and, rarely, restriction of movement with lipomas of the hand to dyspnea or palpitation with mediastinal tumors. Although some benign lipomatous tumors have been described in the retroperitoneum, most reported in the early literature probably represent well-differentiated liposarcomas rather than lipomas.

Imaging studies are extremely helpful for diagnosis; lipomas present as globular radiolucent masses clearly outlined by the greater density of the surrounding tissue. Computed tomography (CT) scans reveal a mass having the appearance of subcutaneous fat and, like fat, having a much more uniform density than liposarcomas. On magnetic resonance imaging (MRI) both benign and malignant lipomatous tumors exhibit a high signal intensity on T1-weighted images.[22]

Gross findings

Subcutaneous lipoma usually manifests as a soft, well-circumscribed, thinly encapsulated, rounded mass varying in size from a few millimeters to 5 cm or more (median: 3 cm); lipomas larger than 10 cm are uncommon. On cross-section, the lipoma is pale yellow to orange and has a uniform greasy surface and an irregular lobular pattern (Fig. 15–1A). Lipomas of deeper structures vary much more in shape, but they also tend to be well delineated from the surrounding tissues by a thin capsule. Focal discoloration caused by hemorrhage or fat necrosis occurs, but it is much less common than in liposarcomas.

Microscopic findings

Lipomas differ little in microscopic appearance from the surrounding fat as they are composed of mature fat cells, but the cells vary slightly in size and shape and are somewhat larger, measuring up to 200 μm in diameter (Fig. 15–1B). The nuclei are fairly uniform and, importantly, there is an absence of nuclear hyperchromasia. Subcutaneous lipomas are usually thinly encapsulated and have a distinct lobular pattern. Deep-seated lipomas have a more irregular configuration, largely depending on the

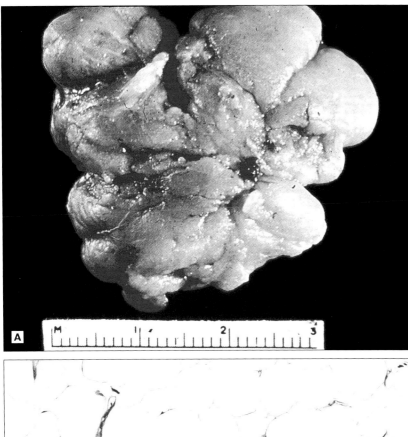

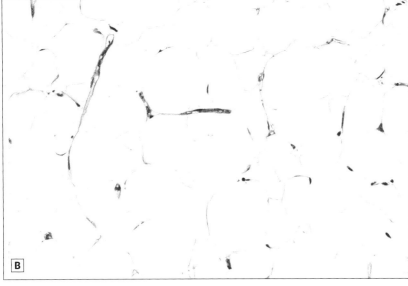

FIGURE 15–1 (A) Lipoma showing a distinct multilobular pattern and uniform yellow color. **(B)** Lipoma consisting throughout of mature fat cells has only a slight variation in cellular size and shape.

site of origin. All are well vascularized, but under normal conditions the vascular network is compressed by the distended lipocytes and is not clearly discernible. The rich vascularity of these tumors becomes apparent in atrophic lipomas in which the markedly reduced volume of the lipocytes reveals the intricate vascular network in the interstitial space.

Lipomas are occasionally altered by an admixture of other mesenchymal elements that comprise an intrinsic part of the tumor. The most common of these elements is fibrous connective tissue, which is often hyalinized and may or may not be associated with the capsule or the fibrous septa (*fibrolipomas*). *Sclerotic lipomas* have a predi-

lection to occur on the scalp or hands of young men and are composed predominantly of sclerotic fibrous tissue with only focal lipocytic areas.[23] *Myxolipomas* are benign lipomatous tumors that are replaced by mucoid substances that stain well with Alcian blue and are removed or depolymerized by prior treatment of the sections with testicular hyaluronidase (Fig. 15–2).[24] Some of these lesions have an abundance of thin- and thick-walled blood vessels and have been termed *vascular myxolipoma* or *angiomyxolipoma*.[25,26] Distinction of these tumors from *myxomas* and *myxoid liposarcomas* may on occasion be difficult. In general, however, the presence of transitional zones between fat and myxoid areas helps rule out

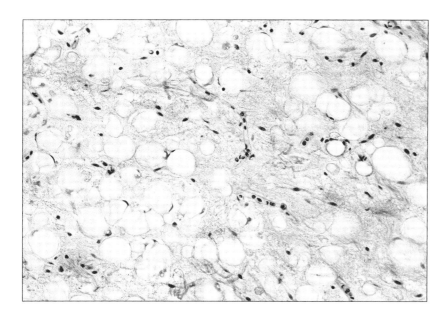

FIGURE 15–2 Lipoma with myxoid change.

myxoma, and the absence of lipoblasts and a diffuse plexiform capillary pattern militates against myxoid liposarcoma. Vacuolated cells containing mucoid material are occasionally seen in myxolipomas and angiomyxolipomas; but unlike neoplastic lipoblasts, these cells lack hyperchromatic nuclei and distinctly outlined lipid droplets within the cytoplasm. Like normal fat cells, the cytoplasmic rim of the fat cells of lipoma is immunoreactive for S-100 protein.

Cartilaginous or osseous metaplasia (*chondrolipoma, osteolipoma*) is rare and is mainly encountered in lipomas of large size and long duration.[27–29] *Myolipoma*, which has a distinct smooth muscle component, and *chondroid lipoma*, a tumor displaying features of both chondrolipoma and hibernoma, are discussed below as separate entities.

Secondary changes occur occasionally as the result of impaired blood supply or traumatic injury. Prolonged ischemia may lead to infarction, hemorrhage, and calcification and may result in cyst-like changes. Similarly, infection or trauma may cause fat necrosis and local liquefaction of fat, a process marked by phagocytic activity and formation of lipid cysts. Characteristically, nests of foamy macrophages are found in the intercellular spaces or around lipocytes that have ruptured or been traumatized (Fig. 15–3). This process is sometimes accompanied by multinucleated giant cells and scattered inflammatory elements, chiefly lymphocytes or plasma cells. As for lipogranuloma, hyaline fibrosis and calcification may become prominent features during the late stages of this process. Rarely, there is a nodular pattern caused by encapsulation of the necrotic lobules of fat. In some cases cystic spaces are lined by an eosinophilic, hyaline membrane with pseudopapillary luminal projections (membranous fat necrosis).[30]

Ultrastructure

Like normal white fat, lipomas are composed of mature lipocytes with a single centrally positioned large lipid vacuole and peripherally placed cytoplasm and nucleus. The cytoplasm consists of smooth membrane-bound vesicles, ribosomes, and round or oval mitochondria, together with small amounts of glycogen, rough endoplasmic reticulum, and an inconspicuous Golgi apparatus. The nuclei display peripheral condensation of chromatin and prominent nucleoli. There are also numerous pinocytotic vesicles and a well-developed basal lamina.[31] Small spindle cells with occasional lipid vacuoles are often situated along the interstitial capillaries and are probably potential precursors of adipocytes (preadipocytes).[32]

Cytogenetic findings

Approximately 55-75% of lipomas have chromosomal aberrations.[33–35] Of these, approximately 75% show a balanced karyotype, and most have 46 chromosomes. Cytogenetic aberrations seem to increase in prevalence with increasing patient age.[33,34] There are essentially three major subgroups of cytogenetic aberrations. Approximately two-thirds of tumors with an abnormal karyotype have 12q13-15 aberrations. Although 12q13-15 can combine with many different bands in virtually all chromosomes, the most common is a t(3;12)(q27-28;q13-15), found in approximately 20% of cases with an aberration of 12q13-15. Less than 10% of cases with 12q13-15 aberrations involve 1p36, 1p32-34, 2p22-24, 2q35-37, 5q33, 11q13 and 12p11-12, among others.

Approximately one-third of lipomas with an abnormal karyotype do not harbor aberrations of 12q13-15.

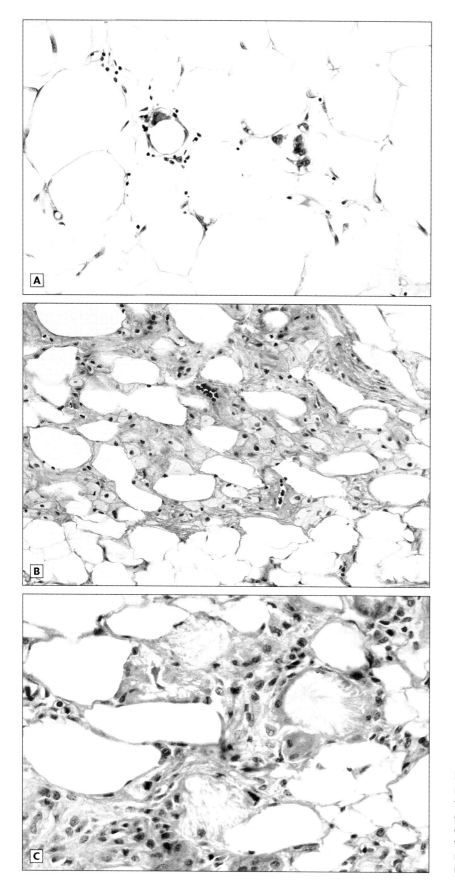

FIGURE 15–3 (A) Lipoma with focal fat necrosis with rare macrophage nuclei and vacuolated cytoplasm between mature fat cells. **(B)** Lipoma with a more extensive area of fat necrosis. Numerous macrophage nuclei with granular cytoplasm are seen between mature adipocytes. **(C)** Rare example of fat necrosis in a newborn infant.

Of these, the most commonly involved loci include 6p21-23, 13q11-12, and 12q22-24. The only recurrent translocation involving 6p21-23 is a t(3;6)(q27-28;p21-23). Various combinations can occur in the same tumor, including simultaneous 13q11-12 and 6p21-23 rearrangements or 13q11-12 and 12q13-15 rearrangements, but aberrations of 6p and 12q rarely occur together.

At the molecular level, the *HMGIC* (*HMGA2*) gene, which encodes for a member of the high mobility group of proteins and is located on 12q15, seems to be affected in some cases with 12q13-15 rearrangements.[36,37] The t(3;12) results in a fusion of the *HMGIC* gene on 12q15 with the *LPP* gene on 3q27-28.[38] This fusion gene has also been detected in some parosteal lipomas and pulmonary chondroid hamartomas.[39,40] Aberrations of 6p21-23 may involve the *HMGIY* gene (*HMGA1B*).[41,42] Tallini and colleagues developed monoclonal antibodies to *HMGIC* and *HMGIY* and immunoreactivity with these antibodies was found to correlate very well with cytogenetic alterations.[42]

Behavior and treatment

Lipomas are completely benign, but they may recur locally (fewer than 5%). Malignant change is virtually unheard of, and only a few cases have been reported in the literature. It is likely, however, that some of them are pleomorphic lipomas, and others are atypical lipomatous tumors (well-differentiated liposarcomas) in which the malignant characteristics were absent or missed when the tumor was first examined. Deep lipomas have a greater tendency to recur, presumably because of the difficulty with complete surgical removal.

Discussion

Aside from the relatively small number of patients in whom an increased familial incidence of lipomas can be demonstrated, little is known about the pathogenesis of these tumors. Certainly, lipomas are more common in obese than in slender persons and perhaps as a consequence are more frequently encountered in patients older than 45 years. An increased incidence of lipomas is also claimed for diabetic patients and those with elevated serum cholesterol. It is doubtful, however, whether the stated association of lipoma with rheumatoid arthritis or with a family history of cancer is more than a mere coincidence.

Trauma or irradiation may lead to overgrowth of fat indistinguishable from a lipoma. In particular, such lesions, often exceeding 10 cm in diameter, have been observed to develop secondary to blunt, bruising injuries, often preceded by a large hematoma.[43]

MULTIPLE LIPOMAS

Approximately 5–8% of all patients with lipomas have multiple tumors that are indistinguishable grossly and microscopically from solitary lipomas. The term "lipomatosis" has been used to describe this lesion, but we prefer to use this name for a diffuse overgrowth of mature adipose tissue (described later in this chapter).

Multiple lipomas vary in number from a few to several hundred lesions, and they occur predominantly in the upper half of the body, with a predilection for the back, shoulder, and upper arms. Not infrequently the lipomas are arranged in a symmetric distribution, with a slight predilection for the extensor surfaces of the extremities. They are about three times as common in men as in women. Most have their onset during the fifth and sixth decades, although occasional lesions appear as early as puberty. Local excision and suction lipectomy have been recommended as the treatments of choice.[44]

There is a definite hereditary trait in about one-third of patients with this condition (*familial multiple lipomas*).[45,46] For instance, in one of our cases, multiple lipomas were observed in members of the same family during three successive generations. Most cases seem to be inherited in an autosomal dominant manner.[47] Mutation in the tRNA gene of mitochondrial DNA has been implicated in this syndrome.[48]

There is no evidence of any chemical differences in the composition of solitary and multiple lipomas. Associated hypercholesterolemia, however, has been noted repeatedly.[49] An increased incidence of multiple lipomas has also been reported in diabetic patients at the site of insulin injections,[50] and during pregnancy.[51]

The question of a relationship between multiple lipomas and neurofibromatosis has been raised repeatedly in the literature, but to our knowledge there is no convincing proof of this association.[52] In fact, given the frequency of lipomas and the relative frequency of neurofibromatosis, these entities probably occur together fortuitously.

There are several syndromes with multiple lipomatous lesions: *Bannayan-Zonana syndrome* is characterized by the congenital association of multiple lipomas (including lipomatosis of the thoracic and abdominal cavity in some cases), hemangiomas, and macrocephaly.[53-55] *Cowden syndrome* consists of multiple lipomas and hemangiomas associated with goiter and lichenoid, papular, and papillomatous lesions of the skin and mucosae. Mutations in the *PTEN* gene have been identified in both of these inherited hamartoma syndromes.[56,57] *Frohlich syndrome*, also known as prune-belly syndrome, is defined by multiple lipomas, obesity and sexual infantilism.[58] *Proteus syndrome* is marked by multiple lipomatous lesions, including pelvic lipomatosis, fibroplasia of the feet and hands, skeletal hypertrophy, exostoses and scoliosis, and various pigmented lesions of the skin.[59]

ANGIOLIPOMA

Angiolipoma occurs chiefly as a subcutaneous nodule in young adults, often making its first appearance when the patient is in the late teens or early twenties; it is rare in children and, unlike solitary or multiple subcutaneous lipomas, in patients older than 50 years. It also seems to be more common in males. About 5% of cases are familial.[60] The forearm is by far the most common site; almost two-thirds of all angiolipomas are found in this location. Next in frequency are the trunk and upper arm. Like all lipomas, it seldom occurs in the face, scalp, hands, and feet. Spinal angiolipoma is a specific entity that should be distinguished from cutaneous angiolipoma.[61] In addition, intramuscular hemangiomas, sometimes referred to as "infiltrating angiolipoma," is distinct from cutaneous angiolipoma.

Multiple angiolipomas are much more common than solitary ones and account for about two-thirds of all angiolipomas.[62,63] Characteristically, angiolipomas are tender to painful (often only on touch or palpation) particularly during the initial growth period; frequently, pain becomes less severe or ceases entirely when the tumor reaches its final size, which is rarely more than 2 cm. There seems to be no correlation between the degree of vascularity and the occurrence or intensity of pain,[64] nor is the pain intensified by heat, cold, or venous occlusion.

At operation, angiolipomas are always located in the subcutis, where they present as encapsulated yellow nodules with a more or less pronounced reddish tinge (Fig. 15–4). Microscopy reveals these nodules to consist of mature fat cells separated by a branching network of small vessels (Fig. 15–5); the proportion of fatty tissue and vascular channels varies, but usually the vascularity is slightly more prominent in the subcapsular areas (Fig. 15–6). Late forms of this tumor frequently undergo perivascular and interstitial fibrosis. Characteristically, the vascular channels contain fibrin thrombi (Fig. 15–7), a feature that is absent in ordinary lipomas.[64] Dixon and colleagues demonstrated fluorescein-labeled antihuman fibrinogen in the thrombi and, to a lesser degree, in the surrounding endothelial cells.[64] Mast cells are often conspicuous in angiolipomas, another feature that distinguishes this tumor from the usual lipoma. Some tumors are highly cellular and composed almost entirely of vascular channels (cellular angiolipoma) (Fig. 15–8).[65–67]

Ultrastructurally, the angiolipoma consists of adipocytes and interspersed vascular structures lined by elongated endothelial cells with irregular finger-like extensions, basal lamina, and long, tight junctions, and surrounded by pericytes. Compared with normal endothelium, Weibel-Palade bodies are scarce. The fibrin thrombi are associated with disrupted endothelial cells.

Unlike ordinary lipomas, which usually have karyotypic abnormalities involving 12q, 6p, and 13q (described previously), all karyotyped angiolipomas, except one, have been reported to show a normal karyotype.[35,68] The only exception was a single case reported by Mandahl et al., which showed a t(X;2) as the sole anomaly.[35] Sciot and co-workers argued that the normal karyotype characteristic of this tumor is more in keeping with a nonneoplastic lesion, possibly a hamartoma.[68] Furthermore, because hemangiomas also usually have a normal

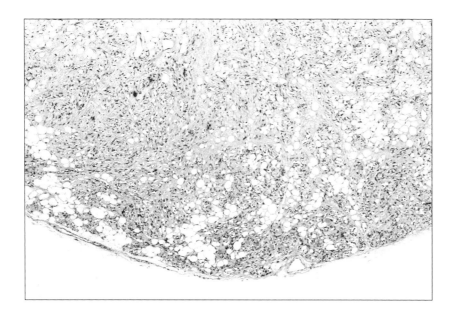

FIGURE 15–4 Angiolipoma showing sharp circumscription and proliferation of numerous vascular channels between mature fat cells.

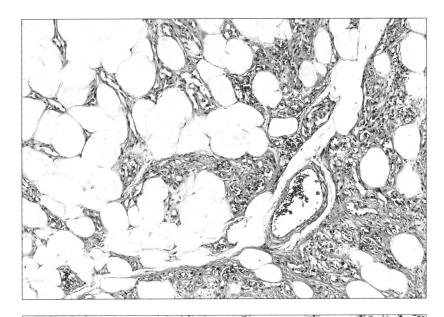

FIGURE 15–5 Angiolipoma consisting of a mixture of fat cells and narrow vascular channels. The vascularity is more prominent in the subcapsular areas.

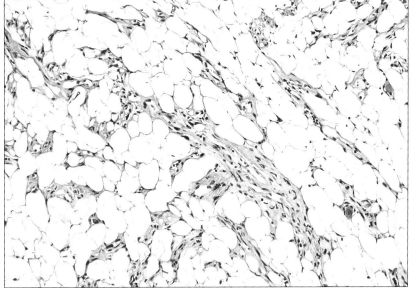

FIGURE 15–6 Angiolipoma with small vessels with an infiltrative-like appearance between mature fat cells.

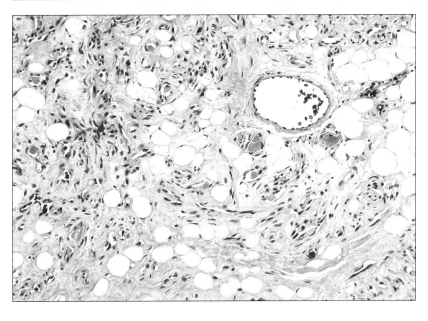

FIGURE 15–7 Angiolipoma with fibrin thrombi, a characteristic feature of this tumor.

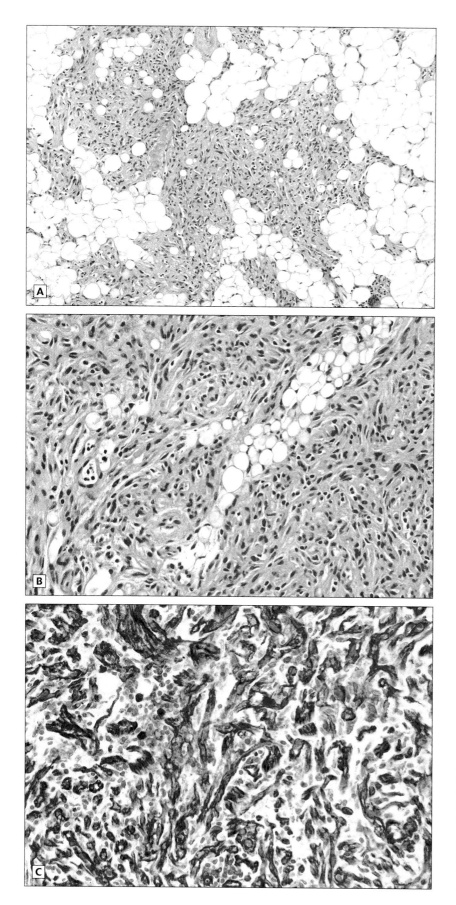

FIGURE 15-8 (A) Low-power appearance
of an angiolipoma with increased cellularity.
(B) High-power view of a cellular area of the
angiolipoma, with virtually complete
replacement by proliferating small vessels.
Lesions of this type have been mistaken for
Kaposi sarcoma or spindle cell angiosarcoma.
(C) Cellular angiolipoma stained for CD31,
indicating that virtually all of the spindle cells
are endothelial cells.

karyotype, it raises the possibility that a vascular proliferation is the primary component of this tumor.

The differential diagnosis of this lesion in part depends on the density of vessels. The hypovascular lesions may be difficult to distinguish from *ordinary lipomas*, although the identification of microthrombi allows this distinction. *Intramuscular hemangioma*, at one time referred to as *cellular* or *infiltrating angiolipoma*, should not be difficult to distinguish from the more superficially located angiolipoma; despite similarities in name, the latter can be correctly diagnosed if attention is paid to the encapsulation of the lesion, the presence of microthrombi, and the small size, multiplicity, and subcutaneous location of the lesion. The cellular angiolipoma may be difficult to distinguish from *Kaposi sarcoma*. Like cellular angiolipoma, Kaposi sarcoma can be found as multiple subcutaneous nodules in young men. However, Kaposi sarcoma has slit-like vascular spaces and periodic acid-Schiff (PAS)-positive globules in the cytoplasm of some of the cells, and it lacks microthrombi. Moreover, this lesion is characterized by immunoreactivity for human herpesvirus (HHV)-8.

Angiolipomas are benign. There is no evidence that these lesions ever undergo malignant transformation.

MYOLIPOMA

Myolipoma is a rare variant of lipoma marked by the proliferation of mature fat and mature smooth muscle tissue. The alternate term *extrauterine lipoleiomyoma* may also be used, but we prefer myolipoma, since the former implies some relationship to uterine smooth muscle tumors. The tumor occurs in adults, most commonly during the fifth and sixth decades of life, with a predilection for women. Myolipoma is most often found in the retroperitoneum, abdomen, pelvis, inguinal region, or abdominal wall.[69-74] The extremities may also be involved, usually as a subcutaneous mass that can also involve the superficial muscular fascia.[71] Most patients present with a painless mass, but in some cases the tumor is found incidentally because of its propensity to arise in deep locations. Deep-seated tumors tend to be large, obtaining an average size of 15 cm. Subcutaneous lesions tend to be much smaller.

Grossly, the tumors are completely or partially encapsulated with a glistening, yellow-white cut surface; tumors with a prominent smooth muscle component have large areas of white or gray firm tissue with a whorled appearance. Histologically, myolipoma consists of a variable admixture of mature adipose tissue and bundles or sheets of well-differentiated smooth muscle, both of which lack nuclear atypia, although one case of myolipoma with "bizarre," presumably degenerative, nuclei has been described. Generally, the smooth muscle component is regularly interspersed with the adipose tissue, imparting a sieve-like appearance at low magnification (Fig. 15–9). The smooth muscle bundles are typically arranged in short interweaving fascicles and are characterized by cytologically bland oval nuclei with longitudinally oriented deeply eosinophilic fibrillar cytoplasm. The adipose tissue component is entirely mature, and lacks floret-like giant cells or lipoblasts.[69,71] Some lesions have prominent stromal sclerosis and chronic inflammation. Medium-caliber arteries with thick muscular walls, characteristic of angiomyolipoma, are absent.

The smooth muscle element stains well with Masson trichrome preparation, and the cells are immunoreactive for smooth muscle actin and desmin (Fig. 15–10). Estrogen receptor positivity has also been noted, but very

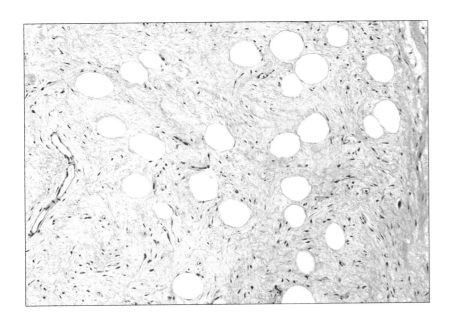

FIGURE 15–9 Myolipoma with a mixture of elongated eosinophilic smooth muscle cells and adipocytes.

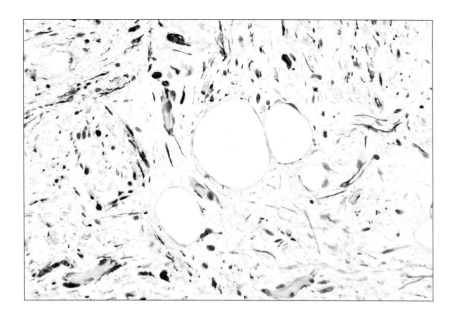

FIGURE 15–10 Myolipoma stained for desmin, showing that virtually all of the spindle cells are smooth muscle cells.

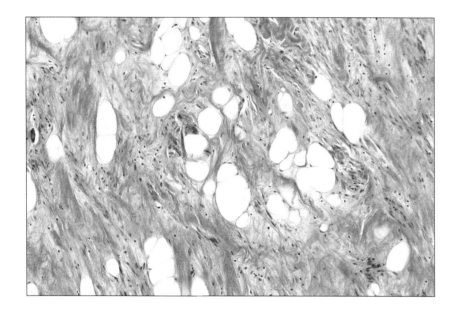

FIGURE 15–11 Uterine leiomyoma with fatty degeneration. This lesion is composed predominantly of mature smooth muscle cells, with only focal areas of mature fat cells. Fatty degeneration of smooth muscle tumors of soft tissue is rare.

few cases have been evaluated for the expression of this antigen.[75] Electron microscopy confirms the coexistence of mature smooth muscle and adipocytic differentiation.

The differential diagnosis includes spindle cell lipoma, angiolipoma, angiomyolipoma, leiomyoma with fatty degeneration, and dedifferentiated liposarcoma. *Spindle cell lipoma* is composed of cytologically bland spindle-shaped cells that do not have smooth muscle differentiation. The spindle cells stain for CD34 but not for smooth muscle markers. Furthermore, spindle cell lipoma is rare in the retroperitoneum, abdomen, and pelvis. *Angiomyolipoma* often presents as a large retroperitoneal mass, as does myolipoma. It differs from myolipoma by the presence of medium-sized arteries with thick muscular walls,

as well as HMB-45 immunoreactive epithelioid smooth muscle cells. Unlike angiomyolipoma, myolipoma is not associated with tuberous sclerosis. *Leiomyoma with fatty degeneration* lacks the regular distribution of fat that is present in myolipoma (Fig. 15–11). Furthermore, fatty degeneration of smooth muscle tumors of soft tissue is rare. Finally, *dedifferentiated liposarcoma* can be distinguished from myolipoma by the presence of atypical hyperchromatic cells in the adipocytic component and cytologic atypia with mitotic activity in the dedifferentiated component.

Myolipoma, despite its frequently large size and occurrence in deep soft tissue locations, is a benign neoplasm, with no reported recurrence or metastasis.

CHONDROID LIPOMA

The chondroid lipoma is a rare, benign fatty tumor found in the subcutaneous tissue or in deeper soft tissues predominantly in the limbs and limb girdles of adult women. Although it is clinically benign, it is another example of a pseudosarcoma in that it may be mistaken for a myxoid liposarcoma or chondrosarcoma. Although first recognized as a distinct entity in 1993 by Meis and Enzinger,[76] it was probably first described by Chan and colleagues as an "extraskeletal chondroma with lipoblast-like cells."[77]

Clinical findings

Although the age range is broad, most patients are in the third or fourth decade of life, and there is a striking predilection for this tumor to occur in women. In the largest series to date from the Armed Forces Institute of Pathology (AFIP) (20 cases), there were 16 females and 4 males ranging in age from 14 to 70 years, with a median age of 35 years.[76] Most patients present with a slowly growing painless mass that is often present for several years prior to excision. This lesion most commonly arises in the proximal extremity or limb girdle. Less common sites include the distal extremities, trunk, and the head and neck region, especially the oral cavity.[78-80] Radiologic studies show a heterogeneous soft tissue mass that has features different than typical lipoma, but not distinctive enough to be diagnostic.[81,82] The diagnosis can be suggested by fine needle aspiration in the hands of a skilled cytopathologist with some experience with this rare tumor.[83,84]

Pathologic findings

Grossly, the tumor is well demarcated and often encapsulated with a yellow, white, or pink-tan cut surface. It ranges in size from 1 to 11 cm (mean: 4 cm). Some lesions are located entirely within the subcutaneous tissue, whereas others involve the superficial fascia or skeletal muscle, and some are entirely intramuscular.

Microscopically, chondroid lipoma has a lobular pattern and consists of strands and nests of round cells deposited in a myxochondroid or hyalinized fibrous background. Some cells have eosinophilic, granular cytoplasm, whereas others have lipid vacuoles indicative of lipoblastic differentiation (Figs 15–12, 15–13). Most commonly, these multivacuolated cells predominate, although in some cases they may be less conspicuous. The cells are not pleomorphic, nor do they show significant mitotic activity. They stain positively with oil red O and PAS stains, consistent with the presence of intracytoplasmic neutral fat and glycogen. A mature adipose tissue component may be present only focally, or it may be the predominant component of the tumor. The extracellular matrix is often extensively myxoid and may be intermingled with zones of hyalinization and fibrin deposition reminiscent of serous atrophy of fat. The matrix is stained with Alcian blue or colloidal iron stains and is usually partially or completely resistant to hyaluronidase digestion. Most lesions are vascular, with thick-walled blood vessels and cavernous thin-walled vascular spaces. Other changes include the presence of hemorrhage, hemosiderin deposition, focal calcification, and hyalinized zones.

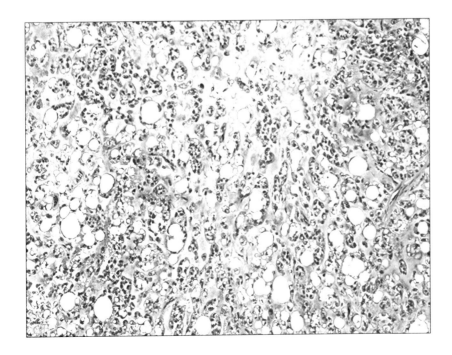

FIGURE 15–12 Chondroid lipoma showing nests of vacuolated cells deposited in a chondroid-like matrix associated with mature fat cells.

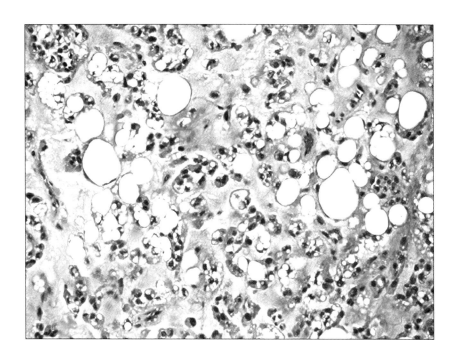

FIGURE 15–13 High-power view of a chondroid lipoma showing vacuolated cells associated with mature fat cells. Some of the vacuolated cells closely simulate lipoblasts.

TABLE 15–2	ULTRASTRUCTURAL FEATURES OF CHONDROID LIPOMA AND COMPARISON WITH EARLY LIPOBLASTS/PREADIPOCYTES AND CHONDROBLASTS/EARLY CHRONDROCYTES		
Feature	**Chondroid lipoma**	**Early lipoblasts/ preadipocytes**	**Chrondroblasts/ early chondrocytes**
Nuclear shape	Irregular clefts	Smooth-scalloped	Multilobulated
Nucleoli	Small to medium size; central or peripheral	Small and central	Small and central
Rough endoplasmic reticulum	Sparse to abundant	Decreasing with maturation	Abundant
Mitochondria	Moderate	Moderate	Abundant
Intermediate filaments	Sparse	Bundles	Diffuse network
Lipid droplets	Many small, few large or single	Many small to few large	Few and small
Glycogen	Sparse to abundant	Little or none	Abundant
External lamina	None	Present	None
Pinocytotic vesicles	None to sparse	Prominent	None to few
Cell membrane	Smooth	Smooth	Spike-like projections
"Protruding bodies"	Prominent	None	None
Matrix	Abundant, cartilaginous	Myxoid early	Abundant, cartilaginous

Modified from Kindblom L-G, Meis-Kindblom JM. Chondroid lipoma: an ultrastructural and immunohistochemical analysis with further observations regarding its differentiation. Hum Pathol 1995; 26:706.

By immunohistochemistry, the tumor cells stain positively for vimentin and S-100 protein, with focal staining for CD68 in the vacuolated tumor cells. Some lesions also show focal cytokeratin immunoreactivity, although immunostains for epithelial membrane antigen are negative.[76] Ultrastructurally, the cells have abundant intra-cytoplasmic lipid and glycogen, as well as numerous pinocytotic vesicles, characteristic of white adipocytes.[85] Nielson and colleagues found no evidence of true cartilaginous differentiation.[85] On the other hand, Kindblom and Mies-Kindblom found a spectrum of differentiation, ranging from primitive cells sharing features of chondroblasts and prelipoblasts, to lipoblasts, preadipocytes, and mature adipocytes.[86] These authors also described rather distinctive knob-like protrusions of the cell membrane containing amorphous, granular material that appeared to be extruded into the adjacent matrix. The myxohyaline matrix itself had ultrastructural features of cartilage (Table 15–2).

Cytogenetic findings

Several examples of chondroid lipoma have been found to harbor a balanced translocation t(11;16)(q13;p12-

13),[87–89] which seems to be characteristic of this lesion, although very few cases have been studied.

Differential diagnosis

The differential diagnosis of chondroid lipoma is broad and includes myxoid liposarcoma, extraskeletal myxoid chondrosarcoma, soft tissue chondroma, and myoepithelial tumors. *Myxoid liposarcoma* may have hibernoma-like cells deposited in a myxoid matrix that on occasion shows chondroid metaplasia.[90] However, unlike chondroid lipoma, this tumor is composed predominantly of mildly atypical spindled cells deposited around a delicate, plexiform vascular pattern. *Extraskeletal myxoid chondrosarcoma* typically has fibrous septa that impart a distinct lobulated appearance. The cells of extraskeletal myxoid chondrosarcoma are more uniformly round or oval, have eosinophilic cytoplasm and few if any intracytoplasmic vacuoles. *Soft tissue chondroma* occurs in the hands and feet and often contains multinucleated giant cells and true hyaline cartilage. *Myoepithelial tumors*, including mixed tumor, tend to be more superficially located and typically display epithelial areas. The myoepithelial cells may have cytoplasmic vacuoles, but they are usually not multivacuolated. Immunohistochemically, myoepithelial cells stain more uniformly for cytokeratins and are marked by antibodies to epithelial membrane antigen and actins.

Discussion

Chondroid lipoma, despite its worrisome histologic appearance, is clearly benign; the lesion does not recur, nor does it metastasize. All available evidence supports a neoplastic, not a reactive, origin.

SPINDLE CELL/PLEOMORPHIC LIPOMA

Although spindle cell lipoma and pleomorphic lipoma were described as separate but related entities in the last edition of this textbook, given the clear-cut overlapping clinical, histologic, immunohistochemical, and cytogenetic features, these lesions are best considered as one entity, although there may be considerable histologic variation within this family of tumors. Some cases may be pure spindle cell or pleomorphic lipomas, but many show overlapping features of spindle cell and pleomorphic lipoma within the same tumor.

Spindle cell lipoma was originally described as a distinct entity by Enzinger and Harvey in 1975.[91] Several years later (1981), Shmookler and Enzinger described a series of 48 cases of pleomorphic lipoma.[92] Although spindle cell and pleomorphic lipomas at one time were grouped under the term "atypical lipoma" by some authors,[93,94] it is clear this family of tumors is sufficiently

characteristic to justify consideration as an entity distinct from atypical lipoma/atypical lipomatous tumor/well-differentiated liposarcoma.

Clinical findings

Spindle cell/pleomorphic lipoma occurs in a characteristic clinical setting, arising mainly in men 45–60 years of age in the subcutaneous tissue of the posterior neck, shoulder, and back (Fig. 15–14).[91,92,95,95a] Approximately 80% of these tumors arise in this characteristic location, but 20% arise in unusual locations, thereby making these cases more difficult to diagnose (Table 15–3). For example, a significant number of cases arising outside of the usual location occur in the oral cavity.[96–98] Other unusual locations include the parapharynx,[99] hypopharynx,[100] parotid gland,[101] spermatic cord,[102] and female genital tract.[103] Similarly, pleomorphic lipoma has also been described in a myriad of unusual locations (tonsillar fossa,[104] orbit,[105] tongue,[106] vulva).[107] In general, spindle cell/pleomorphic lipoma is not encountered in adolescents or children. There is a striking predilection for men. For example, 91% of patients with spindle cell lipoma in the study from the AFIP were men,[91] and 30 of 48 patients with pleomorphic lipoma were men.[92] Like ordinary lipomas, spindle cell/pleomorphic lipoma manifests as a slowly growing, typically solitary, circumscribed or encapsulated, painless, firm nodule, usually centered in the subcutaneous tissue. It is often present for years prior to excision. Very rarely, these lesions can arise in multiple sites, either as synchronous or metachronous lesions.[108,109] Fanburg-Smith et al. reported 18 patients with multiple spindle cell lipomas, including 7 familial cases.[110] Most of these patients presented with their initial tumors on the posterior neck or upper back, with subsequent lesions developing bilaterally on the upper neck, shoulders, arms, chest, and then axillae; spread is in a predominantly caudal direction. Some cases involve the dermis or have predominantly dermal involvement.[107,111] Interestingly, Reis-Filho and colleagues found these dermal lesions to arise more frequently in women, and they tended to be less circumscribed than their subcutaneous counterparts. Moreover, there seemed to be a wider anatomic distribution.[107] Other examples involve the superficial skeletal muscle or are located exclusively in an intramuscular location.[112,113]

Pathologic findings

Grossly, spindle cell/pleomorphic lipoma resembles the usual type of lipoma, except for gray-white gelatinous foci, representing the areas of increased cellularity (Fig. 15–15). Some tumors show extensive myxoid change, whereas others are predominantly lipomatous. Although some tumors are quite large (up to 14 cm), most are between 3 and 5 cm. The tumor is usually well

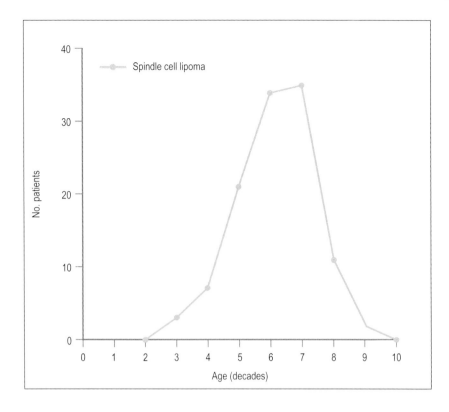

TABLE 15–3	**ANATOMIC DISTRIBUTION OF PLEOMORPHIC LIPOMA**	
Anatomic location	**No. of patients**	**%**
Neck	27	48
Shoulder	7	13
Back	6	11
Head	5	9
Upper extremity	4	7
Lower extremity	3	5
Chest wall / axilla	3	5
Buttock	1	2
Total	56	100

Data from Azzopardi JG, Iocco J, Salm R. Pleomorphic lipoma: a tumour simulating liposarcoma. Histopathology 1983; 7:511,[95a] and Shmookler BM, Enzinger FM. Pleomorphic lipoma: a benign tumor simulating liposarcoma: a clinicopathologic analysis of 48 cases. Cancer 1981; 47:126.

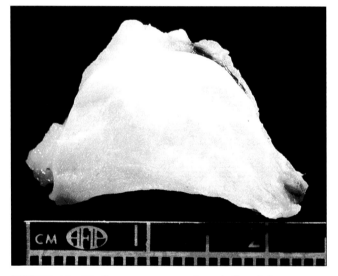

FIGURE 15–15 Gross appearance of a spindle cell lipoma showing a well-circumscribed mass with gray-white foci between areas that resemble the usual type of lipoma.

circumscribed and easily distinguished from the surrounding subcutaneous tissue (Fig. 15–16). Rare examples have a plexiform architecture and are composed of multiple small nodules separated by collagen.[114]

Microscopically, spindle cell/pleomorphic lipoma can vary widely in its appearance. Some tumors are predominantly composed of mature adipose tissue with only scattered spindle cell or pleomorphic elements (described further below). Other tumors are predominantly solid and lack any significant lipomatous component. Very rarely, one encounters a spindle cell/pleomorphic lipoma nearly devoid of fat, and such cases are obviously quite

challenging since the lipomatous nature of the neoplasm is not obvious. Finally, although some examples are purely spindled or purely pleomorphic, many show overlapping features, and either cell type can predominate.

The classic spindle cell lipoma consists of a relative equal mixture of mature fat and spindle cells. The spindle cells are uniform with a single elongated nucleus and narrow, bipolar cytoplasmic processes (Fig. 15–17). Nucleoli are inconspicuous, as are mitotic figures. The

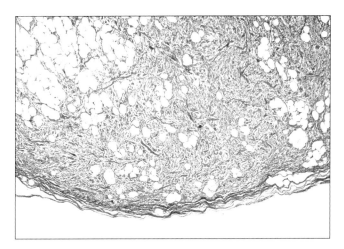

FIGURE 15–16 Spindle cell lipoma. Note the circumscription of the lesion and irregular distribution of the spindle cell areas between mature fat cells.

cells may be haphazardly distributed but tend to be arranged in short, parallel bundles, often with striking nuclear palisading reminiscent of a neural tumor. The cells are deposited in a mucoid matrix composed of hyaluronic acid and mixed with a varying number of characteristic birefringent collagen fibers (Fig. 15–18). In some cases, the tumors are highly myxoid and hypocellular with haphazardly arranged spindled cells; such cases may be easily confused with a myxoma. The vascular pattern is usually inconspicuous and consists of a few small or intermediate-sized, thick-walled vessels, although some examples have a prominent plexiform vascular pattern reminiscent of myxoid liposarcoma (Fig. 15–19), while others show a predominantly hemangiopericytoma-like vascular pattern.[115,116] A pseudoangiomatous variant, characterized by irregular branching spaces with well-formed connective tissue projections,

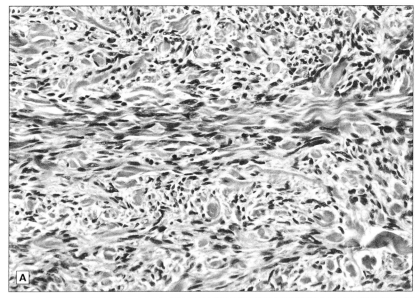

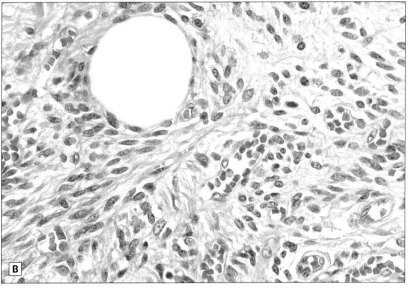

FIGURE 15–17 (A) Cellular area of a spindle cell lipoma showing spindle cells arranged in short bundles and separated by dense collagen. **(B)** High-power view of cytologically bland spindle cells in a spindle cell lipoma. The cells are uniform, with an elongated nucleus and bipolar cytoplasmic processes.

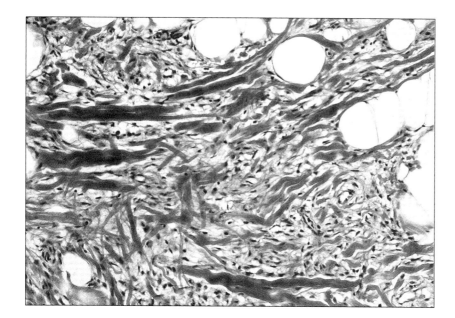

FIGURE 15–18 Spindle cell lipoma with characteristic ropey collagen bundles between bland spindle cells.

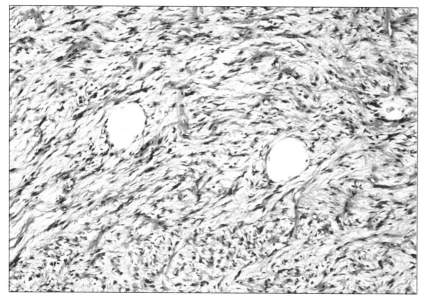

FIGURE 15–19 Spindle cell lipoma with extensive myxoid change. Such areas may resemble myxoid liposarcoma.

has also been described (Figs 15–20, 15–21).[117,118] Mast cells are a conspicuous feature in almost all cases. Rare tumors show small foci of osseous or cartilaginous metaplasia.[115]

The classic pleomorphic lipoma is characterized by the presence of scattered, bizarre giant cells that frequently have a concentric floret-like arrangement of multiple hyperchromatic nuclei about a deeply eosinophilic cytoplasm (Figs 15–22 to 15–24). Ropey collagen bundles identical to those found in spindle cell lipoma are also characteristic. Some tumors also have extensive myxoid change, and mast cells are usually prominent. A pseudo-angiomatous variant of pleomorphic lipoma has also been described.[119]

Immunohistochemical and ultrastructural findings

Immunohistochemically, the cells in spindle cell/pleomorphic lipoma stain strongly for CD34 (Figs 15–25, 15–26),[120,121] but they are not immunoreactive for actin or desmin. Although S-100 protein stains the nuclei of mature lipocytes, neither the spindled cells nor the atypical or floret-like giant cells stain for this antigen.[122] BCL-2 is also frequently positive in spindle cell/pleomorphic lipoma, but we have not found this marker to be particularly helpful in distinguishing this lesion from other lesions in the differential diagnosis, since many of those lesions also stain for this antigen.[123]

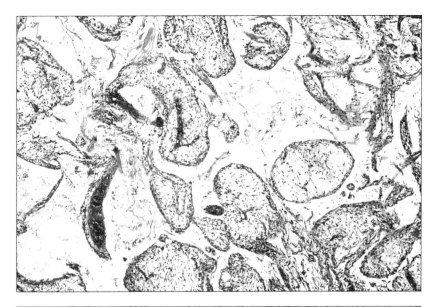

FIGURE 15-20 Spindle cell lipoma with pseudoangiomatous features characterized by irregular branching spaces with well-formed connective tissue projections.

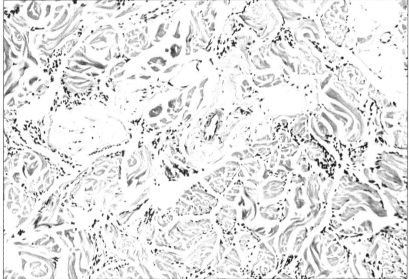

FIGURE 15-21 Pseudoangiomatous variant of a spindle cell lipoma closely resembling angiosarcoma. Short bundles of cytologically bland spindle cells are separated by dense connective tissue projections, simulating the dissecting pattern of angiosarcoma.

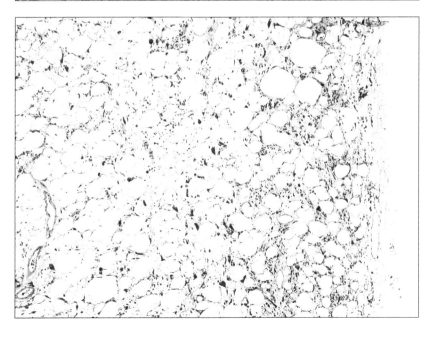

FIGURE 15-22 Pleomorphic lipoma. The lesion is typically well circumscribed and separated from the surrounding subcutaneous tissue.

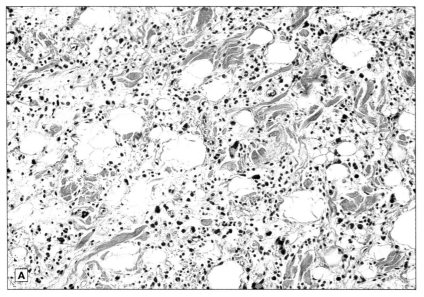

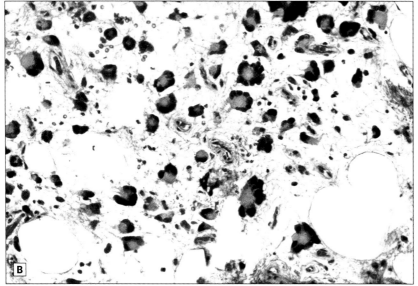

FIGURE 15–23 **(A)** Pleomorphic lipoma, characterized by a mixture of mature fat cells, multinucleated giant cells, and ropey collagen bundles similar to those found in spindle cell lipoma. **(B)** Pleomorphic lipoma with numerous multinucleated floret-like giant cells deposited in a myxoid stroma.

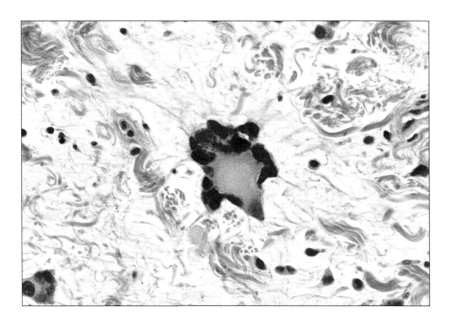

FIGURE 15–24 High-power view of a typical multinucleated floret-like giant cell as seen in pleomorphic lipomas. There is a wreath-like arrangement of hyperchromatic nuclei about a deeply eosinophilic cytoplasm.

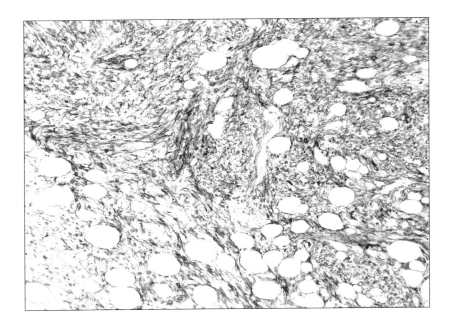

FIGURE 15–25 Diffuse CD34 immunoreactivity in a spindle cell lipoma.

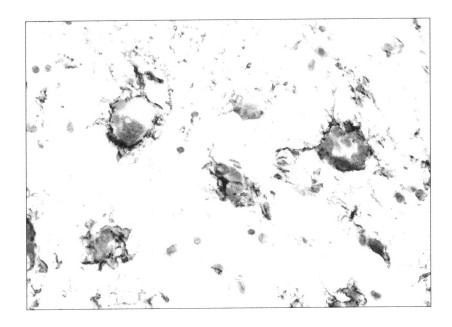

FIGURE 15–26 CD34 immunoreactivity in the multinucleated giant cells of a pleomorphic lipoma.

Ultrastructurally, the cells have abundant rough endoplasmic reticulum, a well-formed Golgi apparatus, and nonmembrane-bound lipoid vacuoles (Fig. 15–27).[124,125] An interrupted basal lamina is also present.

Cytogenetic findings

Aside from the overlapping clinical, morphologic, and immunohistochemical findings that link spindle cell and pleomorphic lipoma, these lesions also share the same cytogenetic aberrations – that is, most show loss of 16q material and less frequently material from 13q.[35,115,126,127] These unique cytogenetic abnormalities, coupled with

the usual absence of giant marker and ring chromosomes that are typically seen in atypical lipomatous tumor/well-differentiated liposarcoma, support the relation between spindle cell and pleomorphic lipoma as well as their distinction from atypical lipomatous tumor/well-differentiated liposarcoma.[128–132]

Differential diagnosis

The differential diagnosis of spindle cell/pleomorphic lipoma depends upon which elements predominate. Classic spindle cell lipoma can be confused with *dermatofibrosarcoma protuberans* (DFSP). However, DFSP

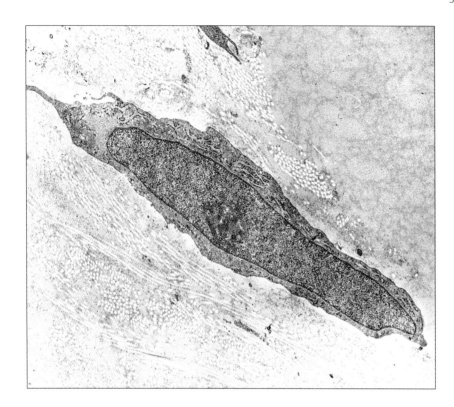

FIGURE 15–27 Electron micrograph of a spindle cell lipoma. Note the close resemblance to a fibroblast and the presence of collagen fibrils in the extracellular space.

typically arises in the dermis and is composed of a proliferation of plump CD34-positive spindled cells arranged in a monotonous storiform pattern with infiltration into the underlying subcutaneous tissue. DFSP tends to arise in younger patients and lacks the characteristic ropey collagen of spindle cell/pleomorphic lipoma. *Nodular fasciitis* has a more variable appearance, with tissue culture fibroblast-like cells characterized by smooth muscle actin positivity and an absence of CD34 staining. Spindle cell lipoma has histologic features that overlap with those seen in *angiomyofibroblastoma*, a superficially located vulvar tumor, which on occasion can also arise in the male genital tract. Both lesions may contain variable amounts of mature adipose tissue, and both are characteristically CD34 positive. Histologically, angiomyofibroblastoma tends to have a more prominent vascular pattern consisting of uniformly distributed thick-walled blood vessels as well as a predominance of epithelioid (as opposed to spindled) cells. At this point, the precise relationship between spindle cell lipoma and angiomyofibroblastoma is not clear. Given the striking nuclear palisading present in some spindle cell lipomas as well as the conspicuous mast cell infiltrate, *schwannoma* and *neurofibroma* are sometimes diagnostic considerations. The cells of these benign peripheral nerve sheath tumors tend to be more wavy or buckled in appearance, and although the cells may express CD34, they invariably express S-100 protein, a marker that is negative in spindle cell lipoma.

Perhaps the lesions that are most easily confused with classic spindle cell lipoma are *myofibroblastoma* (*mammary or mammary-type*), *solitary fibrous tumor*, and *hemangiopericytoma*. These lesions all share overlapping morphologic features, although each has distinctive features that account for the original belief that each was distinct from one another. However, as we have encountered lesions with features that overlap these entities, we believe it is possible or perhaps even likely that all of these lesions are histogenetically related. It is possible these tumors are derived from a CD34-positive perivascular stem cell with the capacity for lipocytic and fibroblastic/myofibroblastic differentiation, but this theory has yet to be proven. The differential diagnostic considerations for each of these entities will be discussed in their respective chapters.

Spindle cell lipoma may also be mistaken for several sarcomas, including *myxoid liposarcoma* or *spindle cell liposarcoma*. Some examples of spindle cell lipoma are diffusely myxoid and have a prominent plexiform vascular pattern reminiscent of that seen in myxoid liposarcoma. However, spindle cell lipoma is more circumscribed and superficially located than myxoid liposarcoma, lacks lipoblasts, and is characterized by ropey collagen bundles. Although some CD34 immunoreactivity may be seen in myxoid liposarcoma, it is not the diffuse, strong CD34 staining that one sees in spindle cell lipoma. In difficult cases, fluorescence in situ hybridization (FISH) analysis for aberrations of *DDIT3* and/or *FUS* genes can be helpful. Similarly, spindle cell liposarcoma, a rare variant of

TABLE 15–4	COMPARISON OF PLEOMORPHIC LIPOMA, WELL-DIFFERENTIATED LIPOSARCOMA, AND PLEOMORPHIC LIPOSARCOMA		
Feature	**Pleomorphic lipoma**	**ALT/WDL**	**Pleomorphic liposarcoma**
Favored site(s)	Subcutis of posterior neck, back, and shoulders	Deep soft tissue of extremities, retroperitoneum	Extremities
Peak age (years)	45–60	50–70	50–70
Floret-like cells	Characteristic	Present	Rare
Pleomorphic lipoblasts	Absent	Present	Characteristic
Cytogenetics	Loss of 16q, 13q	Giant marker and ring chromosomes	Varied complex abnormalities
Metastasis	None	Extremely rare, except in dedifferentiated cases	Common

ALT/WDL, atypical lipomatous tumor/well-differentiated liposarcoma.

liposarcoma, is characterized by relatively bland spindle cells, mature fat, scattered lipoblasts, and only rare cells that may stain for CD34.

Classic pleomorphic lipoma may be difficult to distinguish from the *sclerosing type of atypical lipomatous tumor/ well-differentiated liposarcoma*. This distinction can usually be accomplished on the basis of the typical setting of pleomorphic lipoma on the shoulder or head and neck region, its location in subcutaneous tissue, and its circumscription. Although multinucleated floret-like giant cells are characteristic of pleomorphic lipoma, they are not pathognomonic, as such cells are occasionally also seen in atypical lipomatous tumor/well-differentiated liposarcoma (as well as a variety of other nonlipogenic neoplasms) (Table 15–4). The ropey collagen bundles characteristic of pleomorphic lipoma are an extremely useful distinguishing feature, since this collagen pattern is not seen in atypical lipomatous tumor/well-differentiated liposarcoma. Finally, as previously mentioned, detection of the characteristic cytogenetic aberrations present in each of these lipomatous neoplasms can be extremely helpful in difficult cases. FISH analysis for *MDM2* amplification can be utilized on paraffin-embedded tissues, although this test is not yet routinely used.

Discussion

Spindle cell/pleomorphic lipoma is a completely benign lesion. Even if incompletely excised, the tumor only very exceptionally recurs, and neither dedifferentiation nor metastasis has been reported. Even those cases of pleomorphic lipoma with lipoblasts and atypical mitotic figures have behaved in a clinically benign fashion. The exact nature of the spindled and pleomorphic cells is uncertain, as it is difficult to distinguish early fibroblasts from prelipoblasts by electron microscopy.[91] Based on the finding of CD34 immunoreactivity in spindle cell lipomas, Suster and Fisher suggested that this lesion is a dendritic interstitial cell neoplasm located in fat rather than a true lipogenic neoplasm.[120]

BENIGN LIPOBLASTOMA AND LIPOBLASTOMATOSIS

Benign lipoblastoma and lipoblastomatosis refer, respectively, to the circumscribed and diffuse forms of the same tumor. This tumor is a peculiar variant of lipoma and lipomatosis occurring almost exclusively during infancy and early childhood. The lesions differ from lipoma and lipomatosis by their cellular immaturity and their close resemblance to fetal adipose tissue.

Lipoblastomatosis was named in 1958 by Vellios et al., who reported an infiltrating lipoblastoma in the region of the anterior chest wall, axilla, and supraclavicular region of an 8-month-old girl.[133] The tumor had not recurred after 30 months. Earlier, Van Meurs reported a similar tumor as "embryonic lipoma." He demonstrated its transformation (or maturation) to a common lipoma with repeated biopsies.[134]

Clinical findings

Lipoblastoma is a tumor of infancy. It is usually noted during the first 3 years of life and occasionally at birth.[135–138] Sporadic examples have also been described in older children and very uncommonly in adults (Table 15–5).[139,140] Most studies have found a predilection for this tumor to occur in boys. It is found most commonly in the upper and lower extremities as a painless nodule or mass. Less common sites of involvement include the head and neck area,[141] trunk,[142] mediastinum,[143] mesentery,[144] omentum,[145] scrotum,[146] and retroperitoneum[147] (Table 15–6). Two types of lipoblastoma have been described; circumscribed (*benign lipoblastoma*) and diffuse (*diffuse lipoblastomatosis*). The more common circumscribed form, located in the superficial soft tissues, clinically simulates a lipoma. The diffuse type tends to infiltrate not only the subcutis but also the underlying muscle tissue, has an infiltrative growth pattern, and a greater tendency to recur.[148–150] Most patients present with a slowly growing soft tissue mass, although some

TABLE 15–5	AGE DISTRIBUTION OF LIPOBLASTOMA/ LIPOBLASTOMATOSIS PATIENTS AT THE TIME OF OPERATION	
Age (months)	**No. of patients**	**%**
0–11	26	36
12–23	19	26
24–35	10	14
36–47	4	5
48–59	5	7
60–70	3	4
71–83	2	3
≥84	4	5
Total	73	100

Data are from references 135, 137, 138.

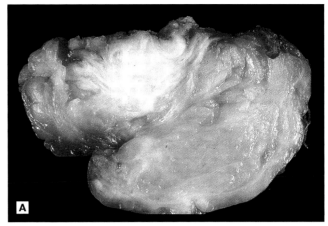

TABLE 15–6	ANATOMIC DISTRIBUTION OF LIPOBLASTOMA/LIPOBLASTOMATOSIS	
Anatomic site	**No. of patients**	**%**
Head and neck	**10**	14
Mediastinum	**1**	2
Upper extremity	**19**	26
Hand	8	
Elbow	1	
Upper arm	2	
Shoulder	3	
Axilla	4	
Forearm	1	
Lower extremity	**29**	40
Buttock	8	
Groin	4	
Thigh	11	
Lower leg	6	
Trunk	**10**	14
Back	5	
Labia	2	
Chest wall	3	
Retroperitoneum	**3**	4
Total	72	100

Data are from references 135, 137, 138.

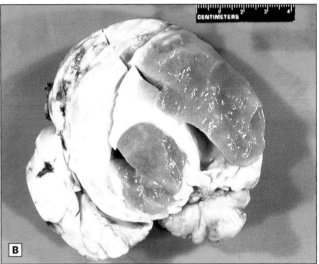

FIGURE 15–28 (A) Gross appearance of a lipoblastoma. This lesion is well circumscribed and has a predominantly fatty appearance, although focal cartilaginous metaplasia (white to gray area) is present. **(B)** Lipoblastoma with multinodular appearance and foci with extensive myxoid change.

report tumors with a rapid period of growth.[151] Depending on the tumor size and location, the mass may compress adjacent structures and interfere with function. For example, tumors arising in the head and neck may cause airway obstruction and respiratory insufficiency.[152] Tumors can also involve the spinal canal, resulting in hemiparesis or even quadriparesis.[153,154] Radiologic studies typically show a well-delineated soft tissue mass with the density of adipose tissue, although neither CT nor MRI reliably distinguishes this lesion from lipoma or liposarcoma.[82]

Pathologic findings

On sectioning, lipoblastoma is paler than the ordinary lipoma, and its cut surfaces are distinctly myxoid or gelat-inous (Fig. 15–28). Most tumors are 3–5 cm in diameter, although some are much larger, and occasionally weigh as much as 1 kg.[155,156]

Histologically, this tumor is composed of irregular small lobules of immature fat cells separated by connective tissue septa of varying thickness and mesenchymal areas with a loose myxoid appearance (Fig. 15–29). The individual lobules are composed of lipoblasts in different stages of development, ranging from primitive, stellate, and spindle-shaped mesenchymal cells (preadipocytes) to lipoblasts approaching the univacu-olar "signet ring" picture of a mature fat cell. The degree of cellular differentiation may be the same throughout the tumor, or it may vary in different tumor lobules. There are occasional examples in which the cells are more rounded and finely vacuolated with intracellular eosinophilic granules, resembling the cells of brown

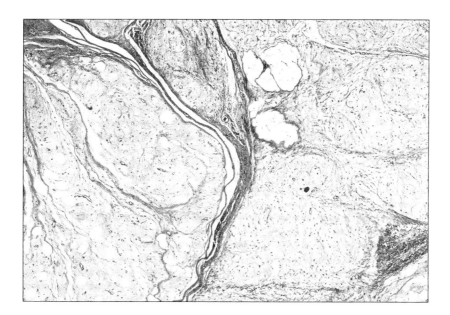

FIGURE 15–29 Lipoblastoma with the characteristic multilobular pattern. Many of the nodules show extensive myxoid change.

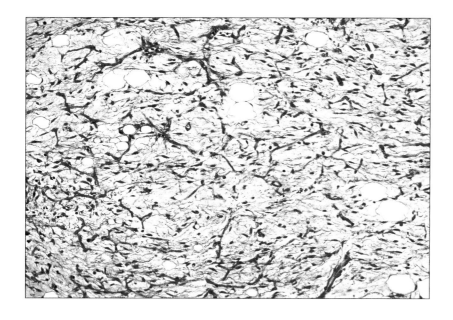

FIGURE 15–30 Lipoblastoma of a 1-year-old child composed of lipoblasts and a prominent mucoid matrix. A plexiform vasculature reminiscent of myxoid liposarcoma is also apparent.

fat.[135] Characteristically, the lipoblasts are surrounded by mucinous material rich in hyaluronic acid, the amount of which is inversely proportional to the degree of cellular differentiation.

Some examples with prominent myxoid change show a plexiform vascular pattern quite reminiscent of myxoid liposarcoma (Fig. 15–30). We have seen examples of lipoblastoma which, at least in areas, are indistinguishable from myxoid liposarcoma. The cellular composition is the same regardless of whether the tumor is circumscribed or diffuse. Diffuse tumors (*diffuse lipoblastomatosis*), however, have a less pronounced lobular pattern and usually contain an admixture of residual muscle fibers similar to intramuscular lipoma. Cases with sheets of primitive mesenchymal cells or broad fibrous septa may be mistaken for infantile fibromatosis. Cellular maturation of lipoblastoma has been observed in multiple follow-up biopsies (Fig. 15–31).[137,157]

Ultrastructural studies disclose a variable picture. As in normal developing fat, the cells display a wide morphologic spectrum ranging from immature mesenchymal cells and preadipocytes to multivacuolar lipoblasts and univacuolar lipocytes. The lipoblasts contain numerous vesicles, round to oval mitochondria, and well-developed Golgi membranes.[150,158] Pinocytotic vesicles are abundant along the plasma membrane. Stellate mesenchymal cells with prominent rough endoplasmic reticulum may be present in the peripheral portions of the lobules.[159]

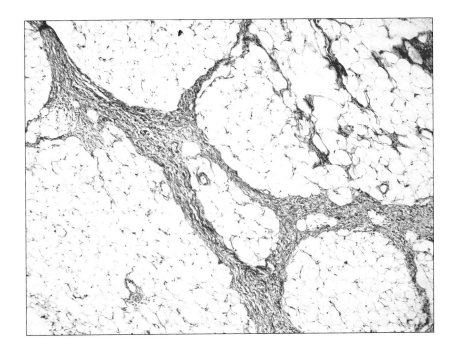

FIGURE 15–31 Recurrent lipoblastoma composed of multiple lobules of mature-appearing fat cells separated by fibrous septa. Some examples of lipoblastoma show maturation in recurrent lesions.

Cytogenetic findings

The most characteristic cytogenetic alteration is rearrangement of 8q11-13.[160] In the study by Gisselsson and colleagues, 11 of 16 cases had rearrangement of 8q12 involving the *PLAG1* gene.[161] Fusion genes have been identified resulting from *PLAG1* rearrangements including *HAS2/PLAG1* and *COL1A2/PLAG1*.[162,163] The *HAS2* gene is located on 8q24 and the *COL1A2* gene is on 7q22. Interestingly, *PLAG1* alterations have been detected by FISH in all cell types within lipoblastoma, including primitive mesenchymal cells, suggesting neoplastic origin in a primitive mesenchymal precursor cell.[161] Polysomy of chromosome 8 might represent an alterative oncogenic mechanism, since this was found in 3 of 16 cases of lipoblastoma without a *PLAG1* rearrangement.[161]

Differential diagnosis

The principal differential diagnostic consideration is *myxoid liposarcoma*. Unlike lipoblastoma, which is a tumor of infancy and early childhood predominantly occurring in patients less than 5 years of age, myxoid liposarcoma has a peak incidence during the third through sixth decades of life. Occasional myxoid liposarcomas have been reported during adolescence, but such cases are exceedingly rare under the age of 10 years. Histologically, both lesions may be lobulated, contain lipoblasts, and spindle cells deposited in a myxoid stroma with a prominent plexiform capillary network. However, lipoblastoma is more lobulated than most myxoid liposarcomas. Although myxoid liposarcoma lacks marked nuclear atypia or hyperchromasia, such features are usually present focally, whereas lipoblastoma lacks nuclear atypia altogether. Foci of hypercellularity may be found in myxoid liposarcoma but are not found in extraseptal loci in lipoblastoma. Microcystic spaces may be present in lipoblastoma but are more often found and are more pronounced in myxoid liposarcoma. Finally, as previously mentioned, lipoblastoma is characterized cytogenetically by deletions of 8q11-13 and lacks the characteristic t(12;16) translocation in myxoid liposarcoma. We have evaluated several highly myxoid lipoblastomas by FISH to document the absence of *DDIT3* and *FUS* alterations.

Lipoblastoma may also be confused with other benign adipose tissue tumors, including *ordinary lipoma* and *hibernoma*. Ordinary lipoma is less cellular than lipoblastoma and lacks lipoblasts, whereas hibernoma consists at least in part of brown fat cells with mitochondria-rich, eosinophilic, granular cytoplasm. The latter two entities have cytogenetic abnormalities distinct from those found in lipoblastoma.

Discussion

The prognosis is excellent. The reported rate of local recurrence ranges from 9%[137] to 22% in the series reported by Mentzel et al.[135] Recurrence is not related to any morphologic features such as lobulation, myxoid change, or degree of adipocytic differentiation. Recurrences for the most part develop in patients with diffuse rather than circumscribed lipoblastomas, particularly those whose tumors are incompletely excised. Therefore, wide local excision of the diffuse or infiltrating type of lipoblastomatosis is well advised.

ANGIOMYOLIPOMA

Angiomyolipoma is a member of an ever-expanding family of neoplasms with perivascular epithelioid cell differentiation (PEComas). Other members of this family of tumors include clear cell "sugar" tumor of the lung, lymphangioleiomyomatosis, clear cell myomelanocytic tumor of the falciform ligament/ligamentum teres, and clear cell tumors of the pancreas, uterus, and other soft tissue sites. Rather than discuss angiomyolipoma in this chapter, it is more appropriately described in the chapter on PEComas (Chapter 36).

MYELOLIPOMA

Although myelolipoma, a tumor-like growth of mature fat and bone marrow elements, is most common in the adrenal glands, it also rarely occurs in extra-adrenal sites including the thoracic,[164] retroperitoneum and presacral region,[165] mediastinum,[166] liver,[167] spleen,[168] testis,[169] and lung.[170] It must be distinguished from *extramedullary hematopoietic tumors*, which are more often multiple than solitary, are frequently associated with splenomegaly and hepatomegaly, and are secondary to severe anemia (thalassemia, hereditary spherocytosis), various myeloproliferative diseases, myelosclerosis, and skeletal disorders.[171]

Myelolipomas are quite rare in young patients,[172] and most are encountered in persons older than 40 years. Small tumors tend to be asymptomatic and often are detected as incidental findings during radiologic studies or surgery for some unrelated disease or at autopsy.[173] Some of these tumors can grow to enormous sizes, and there are innumerable case reports of "giant" myelolipomas, including one tumor weighing 6000 grams.[174] These large tumors tend to cause symptoms including abdominal pain, constipation, or nausea.[175] Very uncommonly, these tumors can even spontaneously rupture and cause massive retroperitoneal hemorrhage.[176]

Radiologically, myelolipoma presents as a well-circumscribed radiolucent mass, usually in the adrenal gland, where it causes inferior renal displacement which can be seen on intravenous urography. A confident diagnosis can often be made using CT and MRI scans,[177] but endoscopic ultrasound or CT-guided needle biopsy of the lesion may be required for a definitive diagnosis.[178]

Grossly, myelolipoma has the features of a lipoma; but when the myeloid elements prevail, the tumor assumes a more grayish or grayish-red appearance. Most are between 3 and 7 cm, but as previously mentioned, some can become enormous. Microscopically, the lesion is composed of a mixture of bone marrow elements and lipocytes in varying proportions (Fig. 15–32). Some exhibit extensive myxoid change.[179]

The histogenesis of this lesion is not clear. Many of the reported tumors have been associated with hormonally active neoplasms, including adrenocortical adenomas,[180] adrenocortical carcinomas,[181] and pheochromocytomas.[182] Others have been described in association with adrenocortical hyperplasia,[183] 17- or 21-hydroxylase deficiency,[184,185] and Conn syndrome.[186] It has been proposed that these lesions arise by hormonally driven metaplasia of undifferentiated adrenal stromal cells or, in the case of extra-adrenal myelolipomas, from choristomatous hematopoietic stem cell rests.[187] Only one case of myelolipoma has been studied by cytogenetics, revealing a t(3;21) (q25;p11), suggesting a neoplastic process. More recently, Bishop et al. found the majority of myelolipomas to have nonrandom X-chromosome inactivation, further supporting a clonal origin.[188]

INTRAMUSCULAR AND INTERMUSCULAR LIPOMAS

Intramuscular and intermuscular lipomas are relatively common. They concern both clinicians and pathologists because of their large size, deep location, and infiltrating growth. Intramuscular lipomas outnumber intermuscular lipomas by a considerable margin, but many lesions involve both muscular and intermuscular tissues.[19,189] The condition has also been described in the literature as an *infiltrating lipoma*.[190]

The tumor arises at all ages, but most occur in adults 30–60 years of age. Occasionally, it is encountered in children.[191] In such cases, distinction from diffuse lipomatosis and lipoblastomatosis may be difficult, if not impossible. There is general agreement that men are more often afflicted than women. The most common sites of involvement are the large muscles of the extremities, especially those of the thigh, shoulder, and upper arm. Unusual cases have also been described in the paraspinal muscles,[192] chest wall,[193] muscles of the head and neck (temporalis, sternocleidomastoid),[194,195] and distal extremities.[196] Most are slowly growing, painless masses that often become apparent only during muscle contraction when the tumor is converted to a firm spherical mass. On occasion, movement causes aching or pain,[197] but the pain is rarely severe. Their size ranges from minute lesions to tumors 20 cm or more in diameter. Occasional tumors are found on routine radiologic examination because intramuscular lipomas, like other forms of lipoma, are radiolucent and are readily demonstrated radiographically (Fig. 15–33).[198]

Grossly, cross-sections of the intramuscular lipoma reveal gradual replacement of the muscle tissue by fat that may extend beyond the muscle fascia into the intermuscular connective tissue spaces. On longitudinal section it often assumes a striated appearance owing to the proliferation of fat cells between muscle fibers (Fig. 15–34).

Microscopic examination reveals lipocytes that infiltrate muscle in a diffuse manner. The entrapped muscle

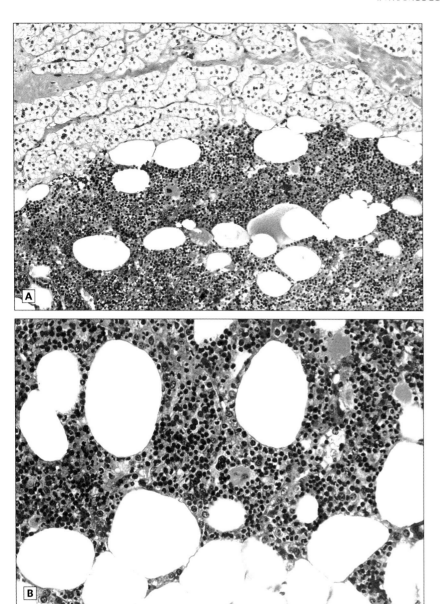

FIGURE 15–32 (A) Low-power view of a myelolipoma with an admixture of adrenal cortical cells, mature fat cells, and myeloid elements. **(B)** High-power view of a myelolipoma with a mixture of mature fat cells and bone marrow elements, including megakaryocytes.

fibers usually show few changes other than various degrees of muscular atrophy (Fig. 15–35). Characteristically, the lipocytes are mature; there are no lipoblasts or cells with atypical nuclei as in *atypical lipomatous tumor* (*well-differentiated liposarcoma*). Nonetheless, careful sampling of these tumors is mandatory because portions of an intramuscular atypical lipomatous tumor may be indistinguishable from those of intramuscular lipoma. We generally recommend submitting at least one section per centimeter of tumor for histologic evaluation. *Diffuse lipoblastomatosis and lipomatosis*, lesions that occur mostly in infants and children, affect the subcutis *and* muscle, and generally more than one muscle is involved. Furthermore, these lesions tend to be more distinctly lobulated than intramuscular lipoma, with connective tissue septa of varying thickness and lobules composed of lipoblasts

in different stages of development. On occasion, however, we believe these lesions can be indistinguishable. In some *intramuscular hemangiomas*, "ex vacuo" growth of fat may simulate the picture of an intramuscular lipoma; such cases have been misinterpreted as "angiolipoma." It can be quite easy to mistake an intramuscular hemangioma with fat for an intramuscular lipoma with a few blood vessels.

Very few cases of intramuscular lipoma have been studied by cytogenetics. Heim and colleagues reported a t(3;12)(q27;q13),[199] whereas Bao and Miles reported a case with a t(1;4;12)(q25,q27;q15).[191] It is possible that FISH analysis for *MDM2* and 12q amplification could be helpful in distinguishing intramuscular lipoma from atypical lipomatous tumor, since these alterations are frequently detected in the latter and not in the former.[200]

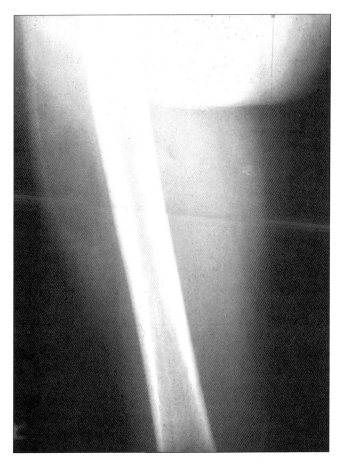

FIGURE 15–33 Radiograph of an intramuscular lipoma involving the muscles of the thigh. Note the sharply circumscribed radiolucent mass surrounded by a rim of muscle tissue.

The prospect of cure is excellent if the tumor is completely removed. In the AFIP series, 85% of patients remained well following the initial excision; the tumor recurred in the other 15%.[201] Overall, the recurrence rate reported in the literature has varied from as little as 3.0%[189] to as much as 62.5%,[190] undoubtedly depending on the completeness of the excision and on the criteria employed for diagnosis and distinction from an intramuscular atypical lipomatous tumor.

LIPOMAS OF TENDON SHEATHS AND JOINTS

Lipomas of the tendon sheaths and joints are rare. There are two types: (1) solid fatty masses that extend along tendons for varying distances; and (2) *lipoma-like* lesions that consist chiefly of hypertrophic synovial villi distended by fat, most commonly seen in the region of the knee joint (*lipoma arborescens*). When they occur in tendon sheaths, these lesions have been described as *endovaginal* tumors, in contrast to *epivaginal* tumors (e.g., deep lipomas arising outside the tendon sheath).

Lipoma of the tendon sheath occurs with about equal frequency in both genders and chiefly in young persons (15–35 years);[202] it affects the wrist and hand and less commonly the ankle and foot. About half are bilateral and show a symmetric distribution. Occasionally, they involve both the hands and feet of the same individual. By the time the patient seeks treatment most of the lesions have been present for several years. Symptoms include

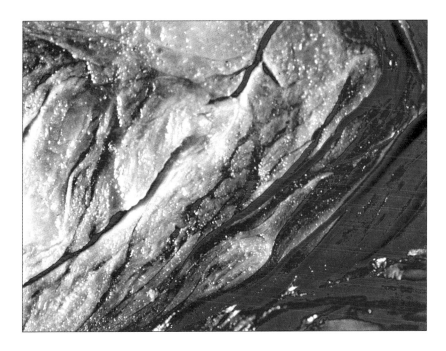

FIGURE 15–34 Partial replacement of muscle tissue by fat in an intramuscular lipoma.

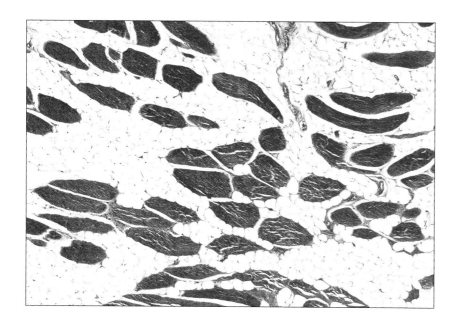

FIGURE 15-35 Intramuscular lipoma with entrapped striated muscle fibers in cross-section. There is some atrophy of the fat cells but no lipoblasts or cells with hyperchromatic nuclei as in well-differentiated liposarcoma.

severe pain, trigger finger,[203] or symptoms of carpal tunnel syndrome.[204] Rupture of a tendon secondary to lipoma of the tendon sheath has been reported. As with other types of lipoma, radiologic examination shows a mass of less density than the surrounding tissue, which may be helpful for the diagnosis.[205]

Lipoma in joints (*lipoma arborescens*) is far more common than lipoma of the tendon sheath. The condition most commonly affects the knee joint, particularly the suprapatellar pouch;[206,207] rare cases occur in the shoulder,[208] hip,[209] and elbow.[210] Most patients are adults, although there are some reports of this lesion in children.[211] Men are affected more commonly than women. The typical presentation is insidious swelling of the knee with intermittent effusions followed by progressive pain and debilitation.[206] Although most patients have only one joint affected (usually the knee), this process can occasionally be bilateral[212-214] or even affect multiple joints.[215,216] Arthrography reveals irregular, non-specific filling defects, most commonly in the posteromedial aspect of the suprapatellar pouch. CT, MRI and high-resolution ultrasonography are extremely useful in making a diagnosis.[217,218] Using MRI, Vilanova and colleagues found this lesion to be associated with some other type of chronic pathology of the joint in virtually all cases, including joint effusion (100%), degenerative changes (87%), meniscal tear (72%), synovial cysts (38%), bone erosions (25%), and synovial chondromatosis (13%).[218] Grossly and microscopically, the lesion consists of fibrofatty tissue or thickened, grape-like or finger-like villi infiltrated by fat and lined by synovium. Some cases are associated with osseous or chondroid metaplasia.[219] Arthroscopy with synovectomy is adequate therapy in most cases.[220]

Lipoma arborescens is probably a reactive process, given its close association with other types of chronic joint pathology. Hallel et al. proposed the term "villous lipomatous proliferation of the synovial membrane" to avoid confusion with a neoplastic process.[221] It is likely some of the symmetric lipoma arborescens-like lesions of the tendon sheath are also reactive hyperplastic lesions associated with various forms of chronic tenosynovitis.

LUMBOSACRAL LIPOMA

Lumbosacral lipoma is another curious type of lipomatous growth that deserves recognition because of its close relation to the spinal cord and its coverings. It is characterized by a diffuse proliferation of mature fat overlying the lower portion of the spine in the lumbosacral region. The lesion is always associated with spina bifida or a similar laminar defect (lipomyeloschisis), and there is a stalk-like connection (tethered cord) between the fatty growth and a portion of the spinal cord that often also harbors an intradural or extradural lipoma. The stalk may cause traction and ischemia. Lipomas extending from the middle to one side are more likely to contain a meningocele or a myelocele. According to Rickwood et al., its overall incidence is slightly less than 1 in 10 000 live births.[222]

Clinically, lumbosacral lipoma is asymptomatic initially and is noted only because of the presence of a large soft tissue mass or because of a sinus, skin tag, hemangioma, or excessive hair associated with a soft swelling in the lumbosacral region. Later, in about two-thirds of cases, progressive myelopathy or radiculopathy causes motor or sensory disturbances in the lower legs, bladder, or bowel.[223,224]

The lesion affects females almost twice as often as males and is encountered mainly in infants or children between birth and 10 years of age.[225,226] Occasional cases in adults have been reported;[227] Loeser and Lewin described a case in a 34-year-old man who complained of weakness of 4–5 years' duration in both legs, associated with a spina bifida at L4–5 and an intradural filling defect.[228] In the series of Lassman and James, all 19 patients had evidence of spina bifida, and 9 had evidence of progressive neuropathy.[229] The authors also found 26 cases of lumbosacral lipoma among 100 cases of occult spina bifida.

Sonography, CT scans, or MRI are essential for diagnosis and for planning therapy; these procedures show not only the exact position of the cord and its relation to the lipoma but also the association of the mass with spina bifida or some degree of sacral dysgenesis.[230,231] Some cases can even be diagnosed antenatally.[232]

At operation, the lipomatous growth is usually unencapsulated and consists of lobulated adipose tissue microscopically indistinguishable from lipoma. In some cases, vascular proliferation and smooth muscle tissue are present in addition to the adipocytes. Unusual elements may rarely be found within the adipose tissue including islets of neuroglia, ependyma-lined tubular structures, primitive neural tissue, teratomatous elements, and even a neuromuscular choristoma.[233-235]

Surgical exploration – laminectomy and division of the stalk and fibrous bands that have formed at the upper margin of the spinal defect – should be performed as early as possible, preferably prior to the onset of neurologic symptoms.[236,237] Early treatment, however, does not prevent the development of neurologic defects in the long term, as a significant percentage of patients ultimately develop urinary bladder dysfunction and other signs of neurologic deterioration.[238,239]

NEURAL FIBROLIPOMA (LIPOFIBROMATOUS HAMARTOMA OF NERVES)

Neural fibrolipoma is a tumor-like lipomatous process that involves principally the volar aspects of the hands, wrists, and forearms of young persons. It usually manifests as a soft, slowly growing mass consisting of proliferating fibrofatty tissue surrounding and infiltrating major nerves and their branches. Other terms applied to this condition include *lipofibromatous hamartoma of nerves*,[240] *neural lipofibromatous hamartoma*,[240a] *and neurolipomatosis*.[241] About one-third of neural fibrolipomas are associated with overgrowth of bone and macrodactyly of the digits innervated by the affected nerve. In the series of 26 cases reported from the AFIP, seven were associated with macrodactyly.[242] Lesions of this type have also been described as *macrodystrophia lipomatosa*,[243] but we prefer the term *neural fibrolipoma with macrodactyly*.

The lesion is almost always seen during the first three decades of life, usually because of increasing pain, tenderness, diminished sensation, or paresthesias associated with a gradually enlarging mass causing compression neuropathy. There may also be some loss of strength. Growth is usually slow and in most patients has been noted for many years. Lesions present at birth or infancy far outnumber those recognized later in childhood or adult life. Females predominate when the lesion is associated with macrodactyly, but males are affected more commonly when macrodactyly is absent. The left hand is more often involved than the right. There may be a genetic predisposition, but there is no history of any hereditary disorders. Carpal tunnel syndrome is a late complication of some lesions. Findings on MRI are virtually pathognomonic and reveal a fusiform enlargement of the affected nerve secondary to fatty infiltration.[244,245]

At operation, neural fibrolipoma presents as a soft, gray-yellow, fusiform, sausage-shaped mass that has diffusely infiltrated and replaced portions of a large nerve and its branches (Figs 15–36, 15–37). The median nerve and its digital branches are affected in most cases, but other nerves including the ulnar, radial, peroneal, and cranial nerves may be involved. The lesion consists of fibrofatty tissue that grows along epi- and perineurium and surrounds and infiltrates the nerve trunk (Fig. 15–38). Prolonged duration and compression of nerves by the fatty tissue result in neural degeneration and atrophy, which accounts for the usual late appearance of symptoms. Rare cases show foci of metaplastic bone.[246] Masses of fibrofatty tissue may also be found outside the involved nerves, unattached to either the overlying skin or neighboring tendons and indistinguishable from a deep-seated lipoma. There is also marked, often concentric thickening

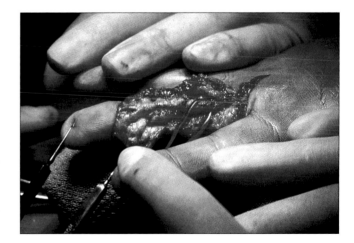

FIGURE 15–36 Neural fibrolipoma with a fusiform, sausage-shaped mass caused by diffuse infiltration of a digital nerve.

of the perineurium and the perivascular fibrous tissue. Sometimes the affected nerve may show a pseudo-onion bulb formation, thereby mimicking an intraneural perineurioma. The diffuse infiltrative character of the lesion distinguishes it from localized and circumscribed lipomas of nerves occurring elsewhere in the body, including lipomas originating in the spinal canal. Unlike *neuromas* and *neurofibromas*, there is atrophy rather than proliferation of neural elements. Clear distinction from *diffuse lipomatosis with overgrowth of bone* is not always possible, but diffuse lipomatosis is primarily a lesion of the subcutis and muscle and only secondarily affects nerves.

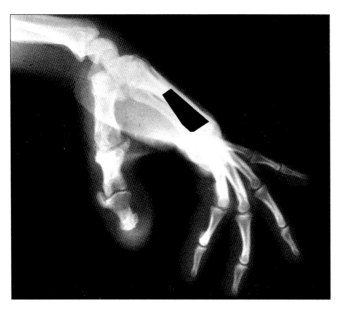

FIGURE 15–37 Radiograph displaying macrodactyly in a patient with an associated neural fibrolipoma.

There is no effective therapy for neural fibrolipoma. Complete excision of the fibrofatty growth is contraindicated because it may cause severe sensory or motor disturbances. If necessary, biopsy of a small cutaneous nerve can establish the diagnosis.[247] Pain and sensory loss may be partially or completely relieved by dividing the transverse carpal ligament and decompressing the median nerve.[248]

DIFFUSE LIPOMATOSIS

Diffuse lipomatosis may be defined as a rare, diffuse overgrowth of mature adipose tissue that usually affects large portions of an extremity or the trunk. Although it simulates liposarcoma by its size and aggressive growth, it is indistinguishable from lipoma microscopically. Like lipoma, it consists entirely of mature fat; and despite its frequently rapid enlargement, there are no lipoblasts or cellular pleomorphism.

The condition is not limited to the panniculus, and in nearly all cases subcutis and muscle are diffusely involved. Many lesions are associated with osseous hypertrophy, leading to macrodactyly or giantism of a digit or limb (Fig. 15–39).[249] Unlike neural fibrolipoma, there is no involvement of nerves, and the process is not limited to the extremities. Association with lipomas or angiomas in other portions of the body is by no means rare. In addition to the extremities and trunk, the lesion occurs in the head and neck, intestinal tract, and abdominal cavity.[250-254] Most cases have their onset during the first 2 years of life, but we and others have also observed typical examples of this tumor in adolescents and adults (Fig. 15–40).[255] Kindblom and colleagues reported an unusual case of diffuse lipomatosis of the leg that occurred

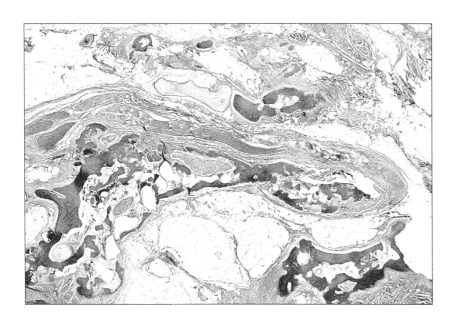

FIGURE 15–38 Low-power view of a neural fibrolipoma with extensive osseous metaplasia.

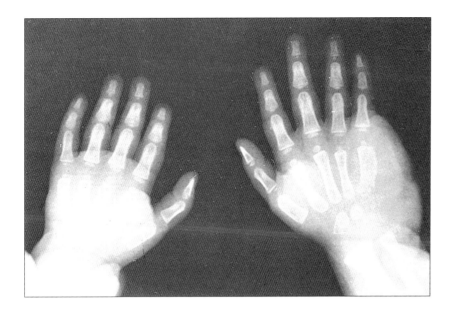

FIGURE 15–39 Diffuse lipomatosis of the right hand with slight overgrowth of phalangeal bones.

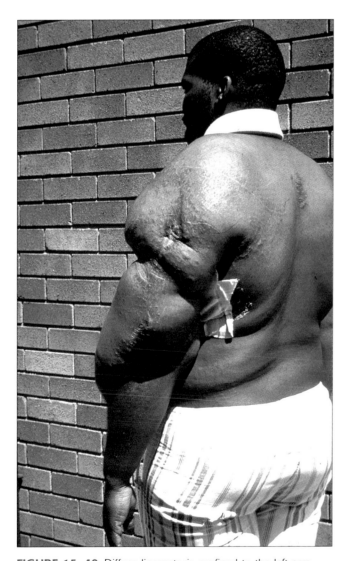

FIGURE 15–40 Diffuse lipomatosis confined to the left arm.

following poliomyelitis.[256] This lesion has been associated with tuberous sclerosis in several reports.[257,258]

The differential diagnosis may be difficult. *Intramuscular lipomas* exhibit a similar microscopic picture, but these tumors are always confined to muscle or intermuscular tissue spaces and usually contain a larger number of entrapped muscle fibers. *Diffuse angiomatosis* may be accompanied by considerable fatty and osseous overgrowth, but it is always recognizable by its more pronounced vascular pattern. *Atypical lipomatous tumor (well-differentiated liposarcoma)* is usually less of a problem if the tumor is carefully sampled for evidence of enlarged hyperchromatic nuclei. Distinction is also facilitated by the age of the patient. Liposarcomas are exceedingly rare during infancy, and virtually all lipoblastic tumors seen during this period are examples of lipoblastoma or lipoblastomatosis.

Diffuse lipomatosis tends to recur, often repeatedly over many years. It may reach a large size and in rare instances causes severely impaired function, necessitating drastic surgery.

SYMMETRIC LIPOMATOSIS

Symmetric lipomatosis is a rare, fascinating disease that has also been described under the eponyms *Madelung's disease*[259] and *Launois-Bensaude syndrome*.[260] Originally described by Brodie in 1846,[261] the disease was not well described until Madelung reported a series of cases with "horse collar" cervical involvement by adipose tissue.[259] It was further described in 1889 by Launois and Bensaude in a report of 65 cases.[260] Patients with this condition suffer from massive symmetric deposition of mature fat in the region of the neck, so the head appears to be pushed forward by a hump that has been likened to a horse collar or doughnut-shaped ring (*lipoma annulare colli*) (Fig. 15–41).

The disease affects middle-aged men almost exclusively, particularly those of Mediterranean origin.[262,263] Excessive alcohol intake or liver disease has been reported in 60–90% of patients in various series, although the precise role of these factors in the development of the lipomatosis is unclear.[264-266] The fatty deposits grow insidiously, frequently over many years; and in contrast to Dercum's disease (adiposis dolorosa), they are non-tender and painless. They are chiefly located bilaterally in the region of the neck but also may involve the cheeks, breast, upper arm, and axilla. The distal portions of the forearm and leg remain unaffected. Up to 86% of patients have a predominantly axonal sensorimotor neuropa-thy,[267-270] and up to 50% have central nervous system involvement, including hearing loss, atrophy of the optic nerve, and cerebellar ataxia.[271] Most cases are sporadic, but a few are familial, possibly in an autosomal dominant mode of inheritance.[47,272] It has also been suggested that occult malignancy is found with increased frequency in patients with symmetric lipomatosis.[273]

The fatty deposits are poorly circumscribed and affect both the subcutis and deep soft tissue spaces, frequently extending in tongue-like projections between the cervical and thoracic muscles. Massive deposits in the deep portion of the neck, larynx, and mediastinum may cause dysphagia, stridor, and respiratory embarrassment[274,275] or progressive vena caval compression.[276] As a rule, patients with this condition are not particularly obese, a fact that adds to the striking appearance of the fatty deposits in the neck. Both CT and MRI are useful for determining the extent of fat accumulation, particularly in deep soft tissue sites.[277] Grossly and microscopically, the accumulated fat is indistinguishable from mature fat, except for varying degrees of fibrosis and, rarely, calcification and ossification.

The exact cause of the condition remains obscure. A variety of metabolic disturbances such as hyperuricemia and gout, hyperlipidemia,[278] and diabetes[279] have been associated with symmetric lipomatosis, but these findings are inconsistent. It has been suggested that the increased synthesis of fat is the result of a defect in catecholamine-stimulated lipolysis.[280] Others have proposed that functional sympathetic denervation results in the hypertrophy of embryologic brown fat.[281] Zancanaro et al. found that the adipose tissue in symmetric lipomatosis ultrastructurally resembles brown fat.[282] More recently, a mitochondrial cytopathy, with point mutations at the MERRF (myoclonus epilepsy and ragged-red fibers syndrome) locus of the human mitochondrial genes, has been implicated in the pathogenesis.[283,284]

Although conservative surgery and liposuction have been used effectively to treat the disease,[265,285-287] it may not be necessary, as in some cases the deposited fat recedes with abstinence from alcohol and correction of nutritional deficiencies.[288] In a study of 31 patients with follow-up, eight (25.8%) patients died during this period including three with sudden death.[289] All three of these patients had severe autonomic neuropathy and none had coronary artery disease.

Symmetric lipomatosis must be distinguished from *adiposis dolorosa* (*Dercum's disease*). The latter condition is marked by tender or painful, diffuse or nodular accumulation of subcutaneous fat. It occurs predominantly in postmenopausal women and primarily affects the regions of the pelvic girdle and the thigh. The lesion is associated with marked asthenia (e.g., loss of strength and fatigue with the least amount of effort), depression, and psychic disturbances.

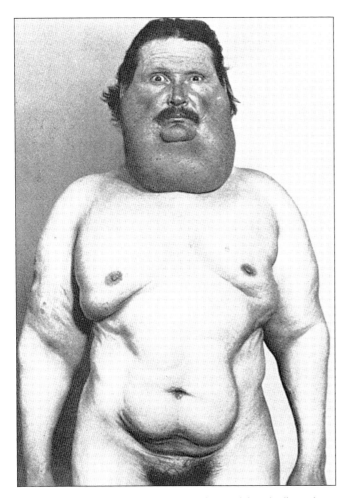

FIGURE 15–41 Symmetric lipomatosis (Madelung's disease). (From Saalfeld E, Saalfeld U. Klinic der gutartigen Tumoren; Handbuch der Haut und Geschlechtskrankheiten, Geschwuelst der Haut. Berlin: Julius Springer; 1932, with permission.)

PELVIC LIPOMATOSIS

Pelvic lipomatosis, first described by Engels in 1959,[290] is characterized by an overgrowth of fat in the perirectal and perivesical regions, causing compression of the lower urinary tract and rectosigmoid colon. The lesion is probably more common than is implied by the relatively small number of cases so far described.[291–293]

The condition chiefly affects black men during the third and fourth decades of life. Women are rarely affected.[294] In a review of the literature, Heyns found a male/female ratio of 18:1.[295] In this same review, 67% of patients were black and 78% were 20–60 years old. The only clinical complaints during the early stages of the disease are mild perineal pain and increased urinary frequency. At later stages, patients often complain of hematuria, constipation, nausea, lower abdominal pain, or backache of increasing severity and sometimes edema of the lower extremities.[296] Rarely, pelvic lipomatosis causes venous obstruction resulting in recurrent deep venous thrombosis.[297] Hypertension is present in about one-third of patients, and some can even develop uremia secondary to renal failure.[298] Pelvic lipomatosis also has an unusual association with cystitis cystica or cystitis glandularis in up to 75% of cases,[299,300] and rare cases have been associated with adenocarcinoma of the urinary bladder.[301–305]

Radiographically (excretory urography and CT scan), the typical findings include a pear- or gourd-shaped urinary bladder with an elevated base, a high-lying prostate gland, and straightening and tubular narrowing of the rectosigmoid as the result of extrinsic pressure by a radiolucent mass (Fig. 15–42). The mass may cause dilatation and medial displacement of one or both ureters and occasionally unilateral or bilateral hydronephrosis. CT and MRI reveal a homogeneous perivesical mass with linear densities, reflecting fibrous bands within the proliferated fatty tissue.[306]

Pelvic lipomatosis is the result of massive overgrowth of fat in the perivesical and perirectal portions of the pelvic retroperitoneum. The fatty growth is diffuse rather than nodular and consists entirely of mature fat indistinguishable grossly and microscopically from fatty tissue elsewhere in the body. Increased vascularity, fibrosis, and inflammatory changes may be present but are rare.

The cause of this overgrowth is unknown, but it appears that it is a hyperplastic rather than a neoplastic process that almost always is limited to the pelvic region. Cases with associated multiple lipomas and manifestations of Proteus syndrome have been reported, however.[307,308] *Lipomatosis of the ileocecal region* (submucosal, polypoid fatty infiltration of the ileocecal valve) and *renal replacement lipomatosis* (secondary to long-standing inflammation and calculi with severe atrophy and destruction of the renal parenchyma) should not be confused with this lesion. The symmetric diffuse growth and absence of atypical nuclei help rule out liposarcoma. However, this distinction becomes even more difficult if fat necrosis is prominent.[309]

Prediction of the clinical course is difficult in the individual case. Frequently, pelvic lipomatosis is a slowly progressive process that may cause vesicoureteric obstruction, hydronephrosis, and uremia requiring surgical intervention, mainly urinary diversion and attempts to excise the accumulated fat.[310]

STEROID LIPOMATOSIS

The term *steroid lipomatosis* is used here to describe a benign, diffuse fatty overgrowth caused by prolonged stimulation by adrenocortical hormones. The condition may be endogenous, as in Cushing's disease and adrenal

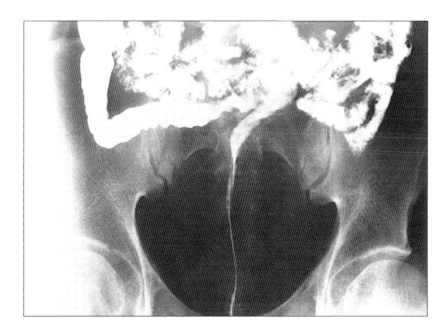

FIGURE 15–42 Radiograph of pelvic lipomatosis with marked compression of the rectum by the accumulated radiolucent fat.

cortical hyperplasia, or the result of prolonged corticosteroid therapy or steroid immunosuppression in transplant patients. As with Cushing's disease, the newly formed fat is unevenly distributed and tends to be concentrated in certain portions of the body. In some cases the accumulation of fat is found mainly in the face (moon face), episternal region (dewlap), or interscapular region (buffalo hump); in others it is limited to the mediastinum,[311] pericardium,[312] paraspinal region,[313] mesentery,[314] retroperitoneum,[315] or epidural space.[316] Symptoms vary depending on the location of the fatty deposition but are usually the result of compression of vital structures in a confined space, such as compression of the trachea in the mediastinum or the spinal cord in the spinal canal. CT scans or MRI and demonstration of increased serum and urine cortisol levels are essential for diagnosis. Steroid lipomatosis tends to resolve when the steroid concentration is lowered. In HIV patients, the use

of protease inhibitors is associated with abdominal obesity, buffalo hump, decreased facial and subcutaneous fat, hyperlipidemia, and type 2 diabetes mellitus (so-called HAART-associated dysmetabolic syndrome or HIV-associated lipodystrophy).[317-319]

NEVUS LIPOMATOSUS CUTANEOUS SUPERFICIALIS

First described by Hoffman and Zurhelle in 1921,[320] nevus lipomatosus cutaneous superficialis is a relatively rare lesion characterized by groups of ectopic fat cells in the papillary or reticular dermis. Two clinical forms have been identified. The multiple form (classic type) is characterized by multiple soft nontender skin-colored or yellow papules, nodules, or plaques that usually develop shortly after birth or during the first two decades of life (Figs 15–43, 15–44).[321-323] The distribution of these

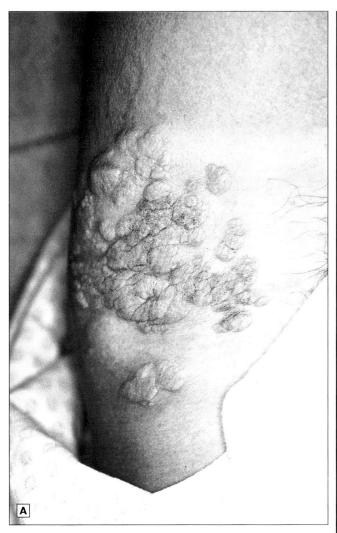
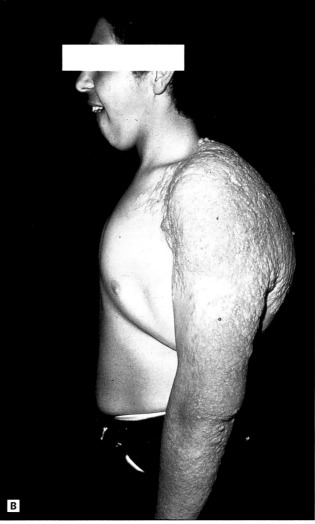

FIGURE 15–43 (A) Classic type of nevus lipomatosus cutaneous superficialis, characterized by multiple skin-colored papules, nodules, and plaques. **(B)** Unusual form of nevus lipomatosus cutaneous superficialis, with numerous lesions localized to the middle to upper back and proximal portion of the left arm.

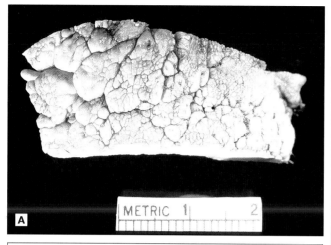

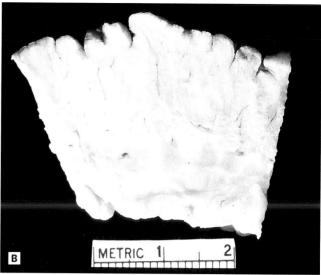

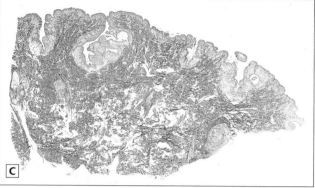

FIGURE 15–44 (A) Nevus lipomatosus cutaneous superficialis showing cerebriform wrinkled skin. **(B)** Cross-section of a nevus lipomatosus cutaneous superficialis showing the characteristic dermal accumulation of fat. **(C)** Low-power view of nevus lipomatosus cutaneous superficialis with characteristic infoldings of epidermis and accumulation of mature fat in the dermis.

lesions is usually linear or along the lines of the skinfolds with a predilection for the pelvic girdle, most commonly the buttock, sacrococcygeal region, and upper portion of the posterior thigh.[324] Rare cases of this form have also been described in the scalp,[325] shoulder,[326] abdomen,[324] thorax,[327] and back.[328] Less commonly, these lesions arise as solitary nodules that usually develop after the age of 20 years. There is no site predilection for the solitary form; and the lesions have been reported to occur on the scalp,[329] forehead,[330] back,[331] extremities,[327] and face.[332,333] There is no gender prevalence, and patients are otherwise in good health.

Microscopically, the nodules are composed of aggregates of mature fat cells in the mid and upper dermis, sometimes with keratotic plugs, increased vascularity, and scattered lymphocytes, mast cells, and histiocytes (Fig. 15–45).

Like other connective tissue nevi, this lesion should be considered a developmental anomaly or hamartomatous growth. Several electron microscopic studies have suggested that the adipose tissue is derived from precursor cells arising from or in close proximity to dermal blood vessels.[324] Treatment is not necessary other than for cosmetic reasons, and the lesion does not generally recur following simple excision.

Another peculiar variant of this condition is marked by excessive symmetric, circumferential folds of skin with underlying nevus lipomatosus that affects the neck, forearms, and lower legs and resolves spontaneously during childhood; it has been aptly described as the *Michelin tire baby syndrome*. The syndrome is inherited as an autosomal dominant trait and is characterized by deletion of chromosome 11. Association with smooth muscle hamartomas and multiple anomalies has been described.

HIBERNOMA

The term *hibernoma* was coined by Gery in 1914,[334] and should be retained even though not all hibernomas occur at the few sites in which brown fat is encountered in humans. Such terms as *lipoma of immature adipose tissue*, *lipoma of embryonic fat*, and *fetal lipoma* have also been proposed by some authors because brown fat bears a close resemblance to early stages in the development of white fat.

Clinical findings

Hibernomas occur chiefly in adults, with a peak incidence during the third decade of life; patients with

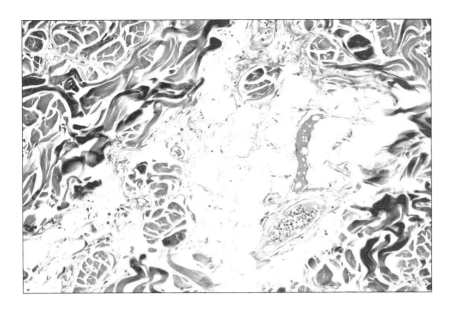

FIGURE 15–45 Nevus lipomatosus cutaneous superficialis with separation of dermal collagen by mature fat.

hibernomas are on average considerably younger than those with lipoma. In the largest series published to date (170 cases derived from the files of the AFIP), there were 99 men and 71 women, whose ages ranged from 2 to 75 years (mean: 38 years).[335] Nine of these patients were in the pediatric age range. There are several other reports of hibernomas arising in infants, but it is possible these are examples of lipoblastoma, perhaps with rare cells resembling brown fat.[336,337] Although traditionally believed to arise most commonly from the scapular and interscapular regions, in the AFIP series, the most common site was the soft tissues of the thigh, followed by the shoulder, back, neck, chest, arm, and abdominal cavity/retroperitoneum, in descending order of frequency. There are several reports of this tumor arising in the mediastinum,[338,339] breast,[340] and even within the adrenal gland.[341] Clinically, hibernomas are slowly growing painless tumors that typically arise in the subcutis, although about 10% of cases are intramuscular. They are often noted several years before they are excised.[335,342]

Pathologic findings

Hibernomas are usually well-defined, soft, and mobile and are 5–15 cm (mean: 9.3 cm) in diameter, although tumors as large as 24 cm have been reported.[335] Their color varies from tan to a deep red-brown (Fig. 15–46). CT scans and MRI reveal a lipomatous tumor but are unreliable for distinguishing hibernoma from liposarcoma.[29,82,343,344] However, the morphologic findings in fine needle aspiration specimens are quite reproducible and are helpful in excluding a preoperative diagnosis of liposarcoma.[345,346]

Microscopically, Furlong and colleagues described four morphologic variants of hibernoma.[335] The most

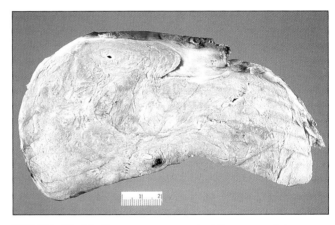

FIGURE 15–46 Gross appearance of a hibernoma of the retroperitoneum.

common (typical, accounting for 140 of 170 cases), displays a distinct lobular pattern and is composed of cells that show varying degrees of differentiation, ranging from uniform, round to ovoid, granular eosinophilic cells with a distinct cellular membrane to multivacuolated cells with multiple, small, oil red O-positive lipid droplets and centrally placed nuclei (Figs 15–47 to 15–50). There are also intermixed univacuolar cells with one or more large lipid droplets and peripherally placed nuclei resembling lipocytes. Fourteen of 170 cases in the AFIP series showed prominent myxoid change (myxoid variant) (Fig. 15–51). The lipoma-like variant (12 of 170 cases) is composed predominantly of univacuolated lipocytes with only occasional cells showing hibernomatous features. Very rarely, the cells take on a spindle cell morphology (spindle cell variant, accounting for four of 170 cases). The latter group tend to occur on the neck and scalp and

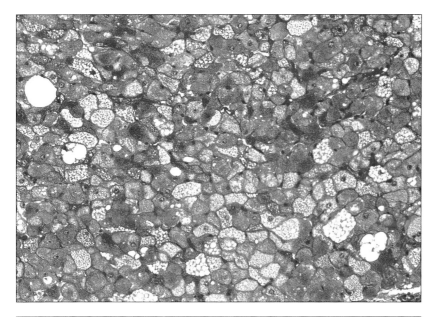

FIGURE 15–47 Hibernoma composed predominantly of vacuolated granular eosinophilic cells.

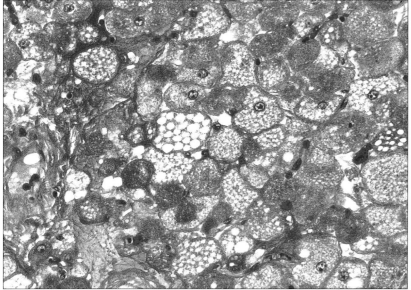

FIGURE 15–48 High-power view of granular and multivacuolated cells in a hibernoma.

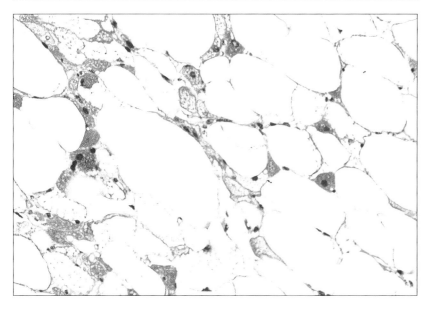

FIGURE 15–49 Hibernoma showing gradual transition between brown and white fat cells.

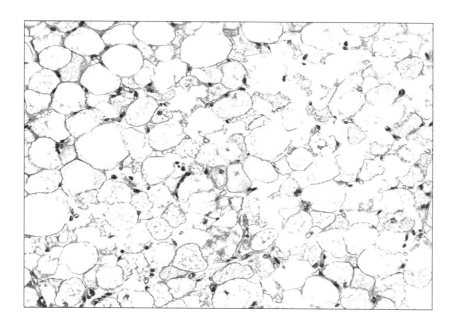

FIGURE 15–50 Hibernoma composed predominantly of fat cells with multiple cytoplasmic vacuoles.

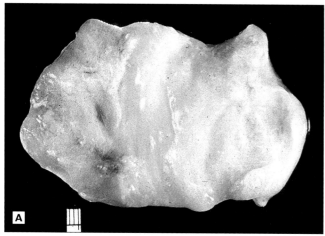

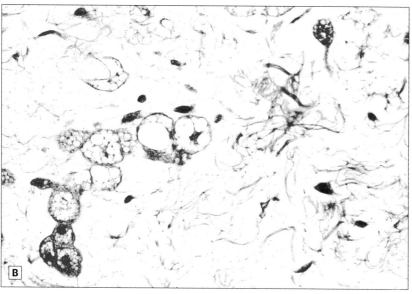

FIGURE 15–51 (A) Gross appearance of a hibernoma with extensive myxoid change. **(B)** Hibernoma with extensive myxoid change, with multivacuolated fat cells deposited in a mucoid matrix.

can be easily confused with a spindle cell lipoma. For all subtypes, the vascular supply is considerably more prominent in hibernomas than in lipomas. In fact, the distinct brown color of hibernoma is due to the prominent vascularity and abundant mitochondria in the tumor.

Immunohistochemical and ultrastructural findings

Although immunohistochemistry is usually not necessary, these lesions usually stain strongly for S-100 protein.[335] Rarely, the cells stain for CD34, although this seems limited to the spindle cell variant. Ultrastructural studies reveal multivacuolated and univacuolated cells packed with round to tubular mitochondria with parallel transverse cristae, a varying number of well-defined lipid droplets, and occasional lysosomes with a well-formed limiting membrane.[347] In addition, there are pinocytotic vesicles and a well-defined basal lamina. The nucleus contains uniformly distributed chromatin condensed under a well-defined nuclear membrane. The scarcity of rough endoplasmic reticulum and a prominent Golgi apparatus distinguish the cells from the preadipocytes of white fat.

Cytogenetic findings

Lake other benign lipomatous tumors, hibernomas have a characteristic cytogenetic aberration. Structural rearrangements of 11q13-21 are most common, but there does not appear to be a consistent translocation partner.[348–351] These chromosomal rearrangements are more complex than can be detected by chromosome banding analysis, but they can be demonstrated by metaphase FISH analysis.[352] The precise gene involved in this aberration is not yet known, but recent studies implicate involvement of the *GARP* gene on 11q13.5.[353]

Differential diagnosis

The likelihood of confusion with other tumors is minimal. *Adult rhabdomyoma* is composed of similar eosinophilic cells, but its cells are larger and contain considerable amounts of glycogen and, on careful search, crystals and cross-striations. *Granular cell tumors* bear a superficial resemblance to hibernoma but are readily distinguished by the complete absence of intracellular oil red O-positive lipid vacuoles. S-100 protein staining is not helpful since both tumors are typically positive. We are uncertain as to the existence of malignant hibernoma. We have encountered possible cases but have interpreted them microscopically as variants of round cell liposarcoma with multivacuolar eosinophilic lipoblasts; some of these cases have been confirmed by cytogenetic or molecular analysis.

Discussion

Hibernoma is a benign tumor. In the study by Furlong and colleagues, follow-up in 66 patients (mean follow-up period: 7.7 years) revealed no local recurrences or evidence of aggressive behavior, even though many of these tumors were incompletely excised.[335]

REFERENCES

White fat

1. Poissonnet CM, LaVelle M, Burdi AR. Growth and development of adipose tissue. J Pediatr 1988; 113:1.
2. Joyner CJ, Triffitt J, Puddle B, et al. Development of a monoclonal antibody to the aP2 protein to identify adipocyte precursors in tumors of adipose differentiation. Pathol Res Pract 1999; 195:461.
3. Poissonnet CM, Burdi AR, Garn SM. The chronology of adipose tissue appearance and distribution in the human fetus. Early Hum Dev 1984; 10:1.
4. Poissonnet CM, Burdi AR, Bookstein FL. Growth and development of human adipose tissue during early gestation. Early Hum Dev 1983; 8:1.
5. Ailhaud G, Massiera F, Weill P, et al. Temporal changes in dietary fats: role of n-6 polyunsaturated fatty acids in excessive adipose tissue development and relationship to obesity. Prog Lipid Res 2006; 45:203.
6. Napolitano I.M. Observations on the fine structure of adipose cells. Ann NY Acad Sci 1965; 131:34.

7. Napolitano L. The differentiation of white adipose cells. An electron microscope study. J Cell Biol 1963; 18:663.

Brown fat

8. Nnodim JO. Development of adipose tissues. Anat Rec 1987; 219:331.
9. Brooks JJ, Perosio PM. Adipose tissue. In: Histology for pathologists. 2nd edn. Philadelphia: Lippincott-Raven; 1997:167.
10. Santos GC, Araujo MR, Silveira TC, et al. Accumulation of brown adipose tissue and nutritional status. A prospective study of 366 consecutive autopsies. Arch Pathol Lab Med 1992; 116:1152.

Molecular biology

11. Ladanyi M. The emerging molecular genetics of sarcoma translocations. Diagn Mol Pathol 1995; 4:162.
12. Adelmant G, Gilbert JD, Freytag SO. Human translocation liposarcoma-CCAAT/enhancer binding protein (C/EBP) homologous protein (TLS-CHOP) oncoprotein prevents adipocyte differentiation by directly interfering with C/EBPbeta function. J Biol Chem 1998; 273:15574.

Immunohistochemistry

13. Haimoto H, Kato K, Suzuki F, et al. The ultrastructural changes of S-100 protein localization during lipolysis in adipocytes. An immunoelectron-microscopic study. Am J Pathol 1985; 121:185.
14. Weiss SW, Langloss JM, Enzinger FM. Value of S-100 protein in the diagnosis of soft tissue tumors with particular reference to benign and malignant Schwann cell tumors. Lab Invest 1983; 49:299.

Lipoma

15. Rydholm A, Berg NO. Size, site and clinical incidence of lipoma. Factors in the differential diagnosis of lipoma and sarcoma. Acta Orthop Scand 1983; 54:929.
16. Oster LH, Blair WF, Steyers CM. Large lipomas in the deep palmar space. J Hand Surg [Am] 1989; 14:700.
17. Seki N, Okada K, Miyakoshi N, et al. Common peroneal nerve palsy caused by parosteal lipoma of the fibula. J Orthop Sci 2006; 11:88.
18. El-Monem MH, Gaafar AH, Magdy EA. Lipomas of the head and neck: presentation variability and diagnostic work-up. J Laryngol Otol 2006; 120:47.

19. Fletcher CD, Martin-Bates E. Intramuscular and intermuscular lipoma: neglected diagnoses. Histopathology 1988; 12:275.

20. Wiech T, Walch A, Werner M. Histopathological classification of nonneoplastic and neoplastic gastrointestinal submucosal lesions. Endoscopy 2005; 37:630.

21. Thompson WM. Imaging and findings of lipomas of the gastrointestinal tract. AJR Am J Roentgenol 2005; 184:1163.

22. Munk PL, Lee MJ, Janzen DL, et al. Lipoma and liposarcoma: evaluation using CT and MR imaging. AJR Am J Roentgenol 1997; 169:589.

23. Zelger BG, Zelger B, Steiner H, et al. Sclerotic lipoma: lipomas simulating sclerotic fibroma. Histopathology 1997; 31:174.

24. Chitnis M, Steyn T, Koeppen P, et al. Differentiation of a benign myxolipoma from a myxoid liposarcoma by tumour karyotyping – a diagnosis missed. Pediatr Surg Int 2002; 18:83.

25. Lee HW, Lee DK, Lee MW, et al. Two cases of angiomyxolipoma (vascular myxolipoma) of subcutaneous tissue. J Cutan Pathol 2005; 32:379.

26. Tardio JC, Martin-Fragueiro LM. Angiomyxolipoma (vascular myxolipoma) of subcutaneous tissue. Am J Dermatopathol 2004; 26:222.

27. Kruger S, Kisse B, Stahlenbrecher A, et al. Chondrolipoma of the hand: a case report. Acta Orthop Belg 2004; 70:495.

28. Castilho RM, Squarize CH, Nunes FD, et al. Osteolipoma: a rare lesion in the oral cavity. Br J Oral Maxillofac Surg 2004; 42:363.

29. Gaskin CM, Helms CA. Lipomas, lipoma variants, and well-differentiated liposarcomas (atypical lipomas): results of MRI evaluations of 126 consecutive fatty masses. AJR Am J Roentgenol 2004; 182:733.

30. Ramdial PK, Madaree A, Singh B. Membranous fat necrosis in lipomas. Am J Surg Pathol 1997; 21:841.

31. Kim YH, Reiner L. Ultrastructure of lipoma. Cancer 1982; 50:102.

32. Solvonuk PF, Taylor GP, Hancock R, et al. Correlation of morphologic and biochemical observations in human lipomas. Lab Invest 1984; 51:469.

33. Sreekantaiah C, Leong SP, Karakousis CP, et al. Cytogenetic profile of 109 lipomas. Cancer Res 1991; 51:422.

34. Willen H, Akerman M, Dal Cin P, et al. Comparison of chromosomal patterns with clinical features in 165 lipomas: a report of the CHAMP study group. Cancer Genet Cytogenet 1998; 102:46.

35. Mandahl N, Hoglund M, Mertens F, et al. Cytogenetic aberrations in 188 benign and borderline adipose tissue tumors. Genes Chromosomes Cancer 1994; 9:207.

36. Ashar HR, Tkachenko A, Shah P, et al. HMGA2 is expressed in an allele-specific manner in human lipomas. Cancer Genet Cytogenet 2003; 143:160.

37. Schoenmakers EF, Wanschura S, Mols R, et al. Recurrent rearrangements in the high mobility group protein gene, HMGI-C, in benign mesenchymal tumours. Nat Genet 1995; 10:436.

38. Petit MM, Mols R, Schoenmakers EF, et al. LPP, the preferred fusion partner gene of HMGIC in lipomas, is a novel member of the LIM protein gene family. Genomics 1996; 36:118.

39. Petit MM, Swarts S, Bridge JA, et al. Expression of reciprocal fusion transcripts of the HMGIC and LPP genes in parosteal lipoma. Cancer Genet Cytogenet 1998; 106:18.

40. von Ahsen I, Rogalla P, Bullerdiek J. Expression patterns of the LPP-HMGA2 fusion transcript in pulmonary chondroid hamartomas with t(3;12)(q27 approximately 28;q14 approximately 15). Cancer Genet Cytogenet 2005; 163:68.

41. Kazmierczak B, Dal Cin P, Wanschura S, et al. HMGIY is the target of 6p21.3 rearrangements in various benign mesenchymal tumors. Genes Chromosomes Cancer 1998; 23:279.

42. Tallini G, Vanni R, Manfioletti G, et al. HMGI-C and HMGI(Y) immunoreactivity correlates with cytogenetic abnormalities in lipomas, pulmonary chondroid hamartomas, endometrial polyps, and uterine leiomyomas and is compatible with rearrangement of the HMGI-C and HMGI(Y) genes. Lab Invest 2000; 80:359.

43. Theumann N, Abdelmoumene A, Wintermark M, et al. Posttraumatic pseudolipoma: MRI appearances. Eur Radiol 2005; 15:1876.

Multiple lipomas

44. Constantinidis J, Steinhart H, Zenk J, et al. Combined surgical lipectomy and liposuction in the treatment of benign symmetrical lipomatosis of the head and neck. Scand J Plast Reconstr Surg Hand Surg 2003; 37:90.

45. Keskin D, Ezirmik N, Celik H. Familial multiple lipomatosis. Isr Med Assoc J 2002; 4:1121.

46. Toy BR. Familial multiple lipomatosis. Dermatol Online J 2003; 9:9.

47. Stoll C, Alembik Y, Truttmann M. Multiple familial lipomatosis with polyneuropathy, an inherited dominant condition. Ann Genet 1996; 39:193.

48. Gamez J, Playan A, Andreu AL, et al. Familial multiple symmetric lipomatosis associated with the A8344G mutation of mitochondrial DNA. Neurology 1998; 51:258.

49. Moi L, Canu C, Pirari P, et al. Dercum's disease: a case report. Ann Ital Med Int 2005; 20:187.

50. Tranquada RE. Subcutaneous lipomas at sites of insulin injection. Report of a case. Diabetes 1966; 15:807.

51. Benny PS, MacVicar J. Multiple lipomas in pregnancy. Br Med J 1979; 1:1679.

52. Oktenli C, Gul D, Deveci MS, et al. Unusual features in a patient with neurofibromatosis type 1: multiple subcutaneous lipomas, a juvenile polyp in ascending colon, congenital intrahepatic portosystemic venous shunt, and horseshoe kidney. Am J Med Genet A 2004; 127:298.

53. Wanner M, Celebi JT, Peacocke M. Identification of a PTEN mutation in a family with Cowden syndrome and Bannayan-Zonana syndrome. J Am Acad Dermatol 2001; 44:183.

54. Celebi JT, Tsou HC, Chen FF, et al. Phenotypic findings of Cowden syndrome and Bannayan-Zonana syndrome in a family associated with a single germline mutation in PTEN. J Med Genet 1999; 36:360.

55. Celebi JT, Chen FF, Zhang H, et al. Identification of PTEN mutations in five families with Bannayan-Zonana syndrome. Exp Dermatol 1999; 8:134.

56. Woodhouse JB, Delahunt B, English SF, et al. Testicular lipomatosis in Cowden's syndrome. Mod Pathol 2005; 18:1151.

57. Celebi JT, Ping XL, Zhang H, et al. Germline PTEN mutations in three families with Cowden syndrome. Exp Dermatol 2000; 9:152.

58. Angerpointner TA. Prune-belly syndrome with anorectal malformation. J Pediatr Surg 2005; 40:894.

59. Cohen MM Jr. Proteus syndrome: an update. Am J Med Genet C Semin Med Genet 2005; 137:38.

Angiolipoma

60. Cina SJ, Radentz SS, Smialek JE. A case of familial angiolipomatosis with Lisch nodules. Arch Pathol Lab Med 1999; 123:946.

61. Konya D, Ozgen S, Kurtkaya O, et al. Lumbar spinal angiolipoma: case report and review of the literature. Eur Spine J 2006; 15(6):1025.

62. Levitt J, Lutfi Ali SA, Sapadin A. Multiple subcutaneous angiolipomas associated with new-onset diabetes mellitus. Int J Dermatol 2002; 41:783.

63. Chung JY, Ramos-Caro FA, Beers B, et al. Multiple lipomas, angiolipomas, and parathyroid adenomas in a patient with Birt-Hogg-Dube syndrome. Int J Dermatol 1996; 35:365.

64. Dixon AY, McGregor DH, Lee SH. Angiolipomas: an ultrastructural and clinicopathological study. Hum Pathol 1981; 12:739.

65. Kazakov DV, Hes O, Hora M, et al. Primary intranodal cellular angiolipoma. Int J Surg Pathol 2005; 13:99.

66. Kahng HC, Chin NW, Opitz LM, et al. Cellular angiolipoma of the breast: immunohistochemical study and review of the literature. Breast J 2002; 8:47.

67. Kanik AB, Oh CH, Bhawan J. Cellular angiolipoma. Am J Dermatopathol 1995; 17:312.

68. Sciot R, Akerman M, Dal Cin P, et al. Cytogenetic analysis of subcutaneous angiolipoma: further evidence supporting its difference from ordinary pure lipomas: A report of the CHAMP study group. Am J Surg Pathol 1997; 21:441.

Myolipoma

69. Michal M. Retroperitoneal myolipoma. A tumour mimicking retroperitoneal angiomyolipoma and liposarcoma with myosarcomatous differentiation. Histopathology 1994; 25:86.

70. Brown PG, Shaver EG. Myolipoma in a tethered cord. Case report and review of the literature. J Neurosurg 2000; 92:214.

71. Meis JM, Enzinger FM. Myolipoma of soft tissue. Am J Surg Pathol 1991; 15:121.

72. Oh MH, Cho IC, Kang YI, et al. A case of retroperitoneal lipoleiomyoma. J Korean Med Sci 2001; 16:250.

73. Sonobe H, Ohtsuki Y, Iwata J, et al. Myolipoma of the round ligament: report of a case with a review of the English literature. Virchows Arch 1995; 427:455.

74. Takahashi Y, Imamura T, Irie H, et al. Myolipoma of the retroperitoneum. Pathol Int 2004; 54:460.

75. Ben-Izhak O, Elmalach I, Kerner H, et al. Pericardial myolipoma: a tumour presenting as a mediastinal mass and containing oestrogen receptors. Histopathology 1996; 29:184.

Chondroid lipoma

76. Meis JM, Enzinger FM. Chondroid lipoma. A unique tumor simulating liposarcoma and myxoid chondrosarcoma. Am J Surg Pathol 1993; 17:1103.

77. Chan JK, Lee KC, Saw D. Extraskeletal chondroma with lipoblast-like cells. Hum Pathol 1986; 17:1285.

78. Darling MR, Daley TD. Intraoral chondroid lipoma: a case report and immunohistochemical investigation. Oral Surg Oral Med Oral Pathol Oral Radiol Endod 2005. 99:331.

79. Furlong MA, Fanburg-Smith JC, Childers EL. Lipoma of the oral and maxillofacial region: site and subclassification of 125 cases. Oral Surg Oral Med Oral Pathol Oral Radiol Endod 2004; 98:441.

80. Gomez-Ortega JM, Rodilla IG, Basco Lopez de Lerma JM. Chondroid lipoma. A newly described lesion that may be mistaken for

malignancy. Oral Surg Oral Med Oral Pathol Oral Radiol Endod 1996; 81:586.

81. Logan PM, Janzen DL, O'Connell JX, et al. Chondroid lipoma: MRI appearances with clinical and histologic correlation. Skeletal Radiol 1996; 25:592.

82. Murphey MD, Carroll JF, Flemming DJ, et al. From the archives of the AFIP: benign musculoskeletal lipomatous lesions. Radiographics 2004; 24:1433.

83. Jimenez-Heffernan JA, Gonzalez-Peramato P, Perna C. Diagnosis of chondroid lipoma by fine-needle aspiration biopsy. Arch Pathol Lab Med 2002; 126:773.

84. Yang YJ, Damron TA, Ambrose JL. Diagnosis of chondroid lipoma by fine-needle aspiration biopsy. Arch Pathol Lab Med 2001; 125:1224.

85. Nielsen GP, O'Connell JX, Dickersin GR, et al. Chondroid lipoma, a tumor of white fat cells. A brief report of two cases with ultrastructural analysis. Am J Surg Pathol 1995; 19:1272.

86. Kindblom LG, Meis-Kindblom JM. Chondroid lipoma: an ultrastructural and immunohistochemical analysis with further observations regarding its differentiation. Hum Pathol 1995; 26:706.

87. Ballaux F, Debiec-Rychter M, De Wever I, et al. Chondroid lipoma is characterized by t(11;16)(q13;p12-13). Virchows Arch 2004; 444:208.

88. Gisselsson D, Domanski HA, Hoglund M, et al. Unique cytological features and chromosome aberrations in chondroid lipoma: a case report based on fine-needle aspiration cytology, histopathology, electron microscopy, chromosome banding, and molecular cytogenetics. Am J Surg Pathol 1999; 23:1300.

89. Thomson TA, Horsman D, Bainbridge TC. Cytogenetic and cytologic features of chondroid lipoma of soft tissue. Mod Pathol 1999; 12:88.

90. Siebert JD, Williams RP, Pulitzer DR. Myxoid liposarcoma with cartilaginous differentiation. Mod Pathol 1996; 9:249.

Spindle cell/pleomorphic lipoma

91. Enzinger FM, Harvey DA. Spindle cell lipoma. Cancer 1975; 36:1852.

92. Shmookler BM, Enzinger FM. Pleomorphic lipoma: a benign tumor simulating liposarcoma. A clinicopathologic analysis of 48 cases. Cancer 1981; 47:126.

93. Azumi N, Curtis J, Kempson RL, et al. Atypical and malignant neoplasms showing lipomatous differentiation. A study of 111 cases. Am J Surg Pathol 1987; 11:161.

94. Evans HL, Soule EH, Winkelmann RK. Atypical lipoma, atypical intramuscular lipoma, and well differentiated retroperitoneal liposarcoma: a reappraisal of 30 cases formerly classified as well differentiated liposarcoma. Cancer 1979; 43:574.

95. Angervall L, Dahl I, Kindblom LG, et al. Spindle cell lipoma. Acta Pathol Microbiol Scand [A] 1976; 84:477.

95a. Azzopardi JG, Iocco J, Salm R. Pleomorphic lipoma: a tumor stimulating liposarcoma. Histopathology 1983; 7:511.

96. Clark S, Greenwood M, Fullarton M, et al. An unusual case of floor of mouth swelling: case report, differential diagnosis and a review of the literature. Dent Update 2005; 32:617.

97. Agoff SN, Folpe AL, Grieco VS, et al. Spindle cell lipoma of the oral cavity. Report of a rare intramuscular case with fine needle aspiration findings. Acta Cytol 2001; 45:93.

98. Piattelli A, Fioroni M, Rubini C. Spindle cell lipoma of the oral cavity: Report of a case. J Oral Maxillofac Surg 1999; 57:624.

99. Baumann I, Dammann F, Horny HP, et al. Spindle cell lipoma of the parapharyngeal

space: first report of a case. Ear Nose Throat J 2001; 80:244.

100. Cantarella G, Neglia CB, Civelli E, et al. Spindle cell lipoma of the hypopharynx. Dysphagia 2001; 16:224.

101. Fasig JH, Robinson RA, McCulloch TM, et al. Spindle cell lipoma of the parotid: fine-needle aspiration and histologic findings. Arch Pathol Lab Med 2001; 125:820.

102. Al Rashid M, Soundra Pandyan GV. Spindle cell lipoma of the spermatic cord. Saudi Med J 2004; 25:667.

103. Zahn CM, Kendall BS, Liang CY. Spindle cell lipoma of the female genital tract. A report of two cases. J Reprod Med 2001; 46:769.

104. Singh N, Dabral C, Singh PA, et al. Pleomorphic lipoma of the tonsillar fossa – a case report. Indian J Pathol Microbiol 2003; 46:476.

105. Daniel CS, Beaconsfield M, Rose GE, et al. Pleomorphic lipoma of the orbit: a case series and review of literature. Ophthalmology 2003; 110:101.

106. Atik E, Usta U, Aydin NE. Pleomorphic lipoma of the tongue. Otolaryngol Head Neck Surg 2002; 126:430.

107. Reis-Filho JS, Milanezi F, Soares MF, et al. Intradermal spindle cell/pleomorphic lipoma of the vulva: case report and review of the literature. J Cutan Pathol 2002; 29:59.

108. Kaku N, Kashima K, Daa T, et al. Multiple spindle cell lipomas of the tongue: report of a case. APMIS 2003; 111:581.

109. Harvell JD. Multiple spindle cell lipomas and dermatofibrosarcoma protuberans within a single patient: evidence for a common neoplastic process of interstitial dendritic cells? J Am Acad Dermatol 2003; 48:82.

110. Fanburg-Smith JC, Devaney KO, Miettinen M, et al. Multiple spindle cell lipomas: a report of 7 familial and 11 nonfamilial cases. Am J Surg Pathol 1998; 22:40.

111. Matsushima N, Maeda M, Takeda K. Dermal spindle cell lipoma of the posterior neck: CT and MR findings. Eur Radiol 2003; 13:241.

112. Usta U, Turkmen E, Mizrak B, et al. Spindle cell lipoma in an intramuscular location. Pathol Int 2004; 54:734.

113. Horiuchi K, Yabe H, Nishimoto K, et al. Intramuscular spindle cell lipoma: case report and review of the literature. Pathol Int 2001; 51:301.

114. Zelger BW, Zelger BG, Plorer A, et al. Dermal spindle cell lipoma: plexiform and nodular variants. Histopathology 1995; 27:533.

115. Fletcher CD, Martin-Bates E. Spindle cell lipoma: a clinicopathological study with some original observations. Histopathology 1987; 11:803.

116. Warkel RL, Rehme CG, Thompson WH. Vascular spindle cell lipoma. J Cutan Pathol 1982; 9:113.

117. Hawley IC, Krausz T, Evans DJ, et al. Spindle cell lipoma – a pseudoangiomatous variant. Histopathology 1994; 24:565.

118. Richmond I, Banerjee SS. Spindle cell lipoma – a pseudoangiomatous variant. Histopathology 1995; 27:201.

119. Diaz-Cascajo C, Borghi S, Weyers W. Pleomorphic lipoma with pseudopapillary structures: a pleomorphic counterpart of pseudoangiomatous spindle cell lipoma. Histopathology 2000; 36:475.

120. Suster S, Fisher C. Immunoreactivity for the human hematopoietic progenitor cell antigen (CD34) in lipomatous tumors. Am J Surg Pathol 1997; 21:195.

121. Templeton SF, Solomon AR Jr. Spindle cell lipoma is strongly CD34 positive. An immunohistochemical study. J Cutan Pathol 1996; 23:546.

122. Beham A, Schmid C, Hodl S, et al. Spindle cell and pleomorphic lipoma: an

immunohistochemical study and histogenetic analysis. J Pathol 1989; 158:219.

123. Suster S, Fisher C, Moran CA. Expression of bcl-2 oncoprotein in benign and malignant spindle cell tumors of soft tissue, skin, serosal surfaces, and gastrointestinal tract. Am J Surg Pathol 1998; 22:863.

124. Bolen JW, Thorning D. Spindle-cell lipoma. A clinical, light- and electron-microscopical study. Am J Surg Pathol 1981; 5:435.

125. Pitt MA, Roberts IS, Curry A. Spindle cell and pleomorphic lipoma: an ultrastructural study. Ultrastruct Pathol 1995; 19:475.

126. Dal Cin P, Sciot R, Polito P, et al. Lesions of 13q may occur independently of deletion of 16q in spindle cell/pleomorphic lipomas. Histopathology 1997; 31:222.

127. Mandahl N, Mertens F, Willen H, et al. A new cytogenetic subgroup in lipomas: loss of chromosome 16 material in spindle cell and pleomorphic lipomas. J Cancer Res Clin Oncol 1994; 120:707.

128. Meis-Kindblom JM, Sjogren H, Kindblom LG, et al. Cytogenetic and molecular genetic analyses of liposarcoma and its soft tissue simulators: recognition of new variants and differential diagnosis. Virchows Arch 2001; 439:141.

129. Mentzel T. Lipomatous tumors of the skin and soft tissue. New entities and concepts. Pathologe 2000; 21:441.

130. Rosai J, Akerman M, Dal Cin P, et al. Combined morphologic and karyotypic study of 59 atypical lipomatous tumors. Evaluation of their relationship and differential diagnosis with other adipose tissue tumors (a report of the CHAMP study group). Am J Surg Pathol 1996; 20:1182.

131. Rubin BP, Dal Cin P. The genetics of lipomatous tumors. Semin Diagn Pathol 2001; 18:286.

132. Rubin BP, Fletcher CD. The cytogenetics of lipomatous tumours. Histopathology 1997; 30:507.

Benign lipoblastoma and lipoblastomatosis

133. Vellios F, Baez J, Shumacker HB. Lipoblastomatosis: a tumor of fetal fat different from hibernoma; report of a case, with observations on the embryogenesis of human adipose tissue. Am J Pathol 1958; 34:1149.

134. Van Meurs DP. The transformation of an embryonic lipoma to a common lipoma. Br J Surg 1947; 34:282.

135. Mentzel T, Calonje E, Fletcher CD. Lipoblastoma and lipoblastomatosis: a clinicopathological study of 14 cases. Histopathology 1993; 23:527.

136. Singh V, Raju R, Singh M, et al. Congenital lipoblastoma of the scalp. Am J Perinatol 2004; 21:377.

137. Collins MH, Chatten J. Lipoblastoma/ lipoblastomatosis: a clinicopathologic study of 25 tumors. Am J Surg Pathol 1997; 21:1131.

138. Chung EB, Enzinger FM. Benign lipoblastomatosis. An analysis of 35 cases. Cancer 1973; 32:482.

139. Sciot R, De Wever I, Debiec-Rychter M. Lipoblastoma in a 23-year-old male: Distinction from atypical lipomatous tumor using cytogenetic and fluorescence in-situ hybridization analysis. Virchows Arch 2003; 442:468.

140. Lae ME, Pereira PF, Keeney GL, et al. Lipoblastoma-like tumour of the vulva: report of three cases of a distinctive mesenchymal neoplasm of adipocytic differentiation. Histopathology 2002; 40:505.

141. Rosen A, Jedynak AR, Respler D. Lipoblastoma of the neck mimicking cystic hygroma. Otolaryngol Head Neck Surg 2005; 132:511.

142. Adnani A, Chellaoui M, Chat L, et al. Unusual appearance of axillary lipoblastoma of infancy. J Radiol 2005; 86:1043.

143. Raman Sharma R, Mahapatra AK, Pawar SJ, et al. An unusual posterior mediastinal lipoblastoma with spinal epidural extension presenting as a painful suprascapular swelling: case report and a brief review of the literature. J Clin Neurosci 2002; 9:204.

144. Al-Salem AH, Al-Nazer M. Mesenteric lipoblastoma in a 2-year-old child. Pediatr Surg Int 2003; 19:115.

145. Soin S, Andronikou S, Lisle R, et al. Omental lipoblastoma in a child: diagnosis based on CT density measurements. J Pediatr Hematol Oncol 2006; 28:57.

146. Somers GR, Teshima I, Nasr A, et al. Intrascrotal lipoblastoma with a complex karyotype: a case report and review of the literature. Arch Pathol Lab Med 2004; 128:797.

147. Dokucu AI, Ozturk H, Yildiz FR, et al. Retroperitoneal lipoblastoma involving the right common iliac artery and vein. Eur J Pediatr Surg 2003; 13:268.

148. Coffin CM. Lipoblastoma: an embryonal tumor of soft tissue related to organogenesis. Semin Diagn Pathol 1994; 11:98.

149. Jung SM, Chang PY, Luo CC, et al. Lipoblastoma/lipoblastomatosis: a clinicopathologic study of 16 cases in Taiwan. Pediatr Surg Int 2005; 21:809.

150. Hicks J, Dilley A, Patel D, et al. Lipoblastoma and lipoblastomatosis in infancy and childhood: histopathologic, ultrastructural, and cytogenetic features. Ultrastruct Pathol 2001; 25:321.

151. al-Qattan MM, Weinberg M, Clarke HM. Two rapidly growing fatty tumors of the upper limb in children: lipoblastoma and infiltrating lipoma. J Hand Surg [Am] 1995; 20:20.

152. Lorenzen JC, Godballe C, Kerndrup GB. Lipoblastoma of the neck: a rare cause of respiratory problems in children. Auris Nasus Larynx 2005; 32:169.

153. O'Brien D, Aquilina K, Farrell M, et al. Cervical lipoblastomatosis producing quadriparesis: case report of surgery with chemotherapy and 10-year follow-up. Childs Nerv Syst 2005; 21:165.

154. Sun JJ, Rasgon BM, Hilsinger RL Jr. Lipoblastomatosis of the neck causing hemiparesis: a case report and review of the literature. Head Neck 2003; 25:337.

155. Nmadu PT. Giant lipoblastoma: a case report. Ann Trop Paediatr 1992; 12:417.

156. Pollono DG, Tomarchio S, Drut R, et al. Retroperitoneal and deep-seated lipoblastoma: diagnosis by CT scan and fine-needle aspiration biopsy. Diagn Cytopathol 1999; 20:295.

157. Harrer J, Hammon G, Wagner T, et al. Lipoblastoma and lipoblastomatosis: a report of two cases and review of the literature. Eur J Pediatr Surg 2001; 11:342.

158. Gaffney EF, Vellios F, Hargreaves HK. Lipoblastomatosis: ultrastructure of two cases and relationship to human fetal white adipose tissue. Pediatr Pathol 1986; 5:207.

159. Bolen JW, Thorning D. Benign lipoblastoma and myxoid liposarcoma: a comparative light- and electron-microscopic study. Am J Surg Pathol 1980; 4:163.

160. Chen Z, Coffin CM, Scott S, et al. Evidence by spectral karyotyping that 8q11.2 is nonrandomly involved in lipoblastoma. J Mol Diagn 2000; 2:73.

161. Gisselsson D, Hibbard MK, Dal Cin P, et al. PLAG1 alterations in lipoblastoma: involvement in varied mesenchymal cell types and evidence for alternative oncogenic mechanisms. Am J Pathol 2001; 159:955.

162. Hibbard MK, Kozakewich HP, Dal Cin P, et al. PLAG1 fusion oncogenes in lipoblastoma. Cancer Res 2000; 60:4869.

163. Morerio C, Rapella A, Rosanda C, et al. PLAG1-HAS2 fusion in lipoblastoma with masked 8q intrachromosomal rearrangement. Cancer Genet Cytogenet 2005; 156:183.

Myelolipoma

164. Franiel T, Fleischer B, Raab BW, et al. Bilateral thoracic extraadrenal myelolipoma. Eur J Cardiothorac Surg 2004; 26:1220.

165. Mariappan MR, Fadare O, Ocal IT. Pathologic quiz case: a 74-year-old man with an incidental retroperitoneal tumor found at autopsy. Presacral myelolipoma. Arch Pathol Lab Med 2004; 128:591.

166. Gao B, Sugimura H, Sugimura S, et al. Mediastinal myelolipoma. Asian Cardiovasc Thorac Ann 2002; 10:189.

167. Savoye-Collet C, Goria O, Scotte M, et al. MR imaging of hepatic myelolipoma. AJR Am J Roentgenol 2000; 174:574.

168. Cina SJ, Gordon BM, Curry NS. Ectopic adrenal myelolipoma presenting as a splenic mass. Arch Pathol Lab Med 1995; 119:561.

169. Adesokan A, Adegboyega PA, Cowan DF, et al. Testicular "tumor" of the adrenogenital syndrome: a case report of an unusual association with myelolipoma and seminoma in cryptorchidism. Cancer 1997; 80:2120.

170. Lu X, Xiao L. Myelolipoma of the lung: a case report. Chin Med J 2003; 116:951.

171. Remstein ED, Kurtin PJ, Nascimento AG. Sclerosing extramedullary hematopoietic tumor in chronic myeloproliferative disorders. Am J Surg Pathol 2000; 24:51.

172. Cobanoglu U, Yaris N, Cay A. Adrenal myelolipoma in a child. Pediatr Surg Int 2005; 21:500.

173. Meyer A, Behrend M. Presentation and therapy of myelolipoma. Int J Urol 2005; 12:239.

174. Akamatsu H, Koseki M, Nakaba H, et al. Giant adrenal myelolipoma: report of a case. Surg Today 2004; 34:283.

175. Sharma MC, Kashyap S, Sharma R, et al. Symptomatic adrenal myelolipoma. Clinicopathological analysis of 7 cases and brief review of the literature. Urol Int 1997; 59:119.

176. Nakajo M, Onohara S, Shinmura K, et al. Embolization for spontaneous retroperitoneal hemorrhage from adrenal myelolipoma. Radiat Med 2003; 21:214.

177. Pereira JM, Sirlin CB, Pinto PS, et al. CT and MR imaging of extrahepatic fatty masses of the abdomen and pelvis: techniques, diagnosis, differential diagnosis, and pitfalls. Radiographics 2005; 25:69.

178. Jhala NC, Jhala D, Eloubeidi MA, et al. Endoscopic ultrasound-guided fine-needle aspiration biopsy of the adrenal glands: analysis of 24 patients. Cancer 2004; 102:308.

179. Shapiro JL, Goldblum JR, Dobrow DA, et al. Giant bilateral extra-adrenal myelolipoma. Arch Pathol Lab Med 1995; 119:283.

180. Matsuda T, Abe H, Takase M, et al. Case of combined adrenal cortical adenoma and myelolipoma. Pathol Int 2004; 54:725.

181. Sun X, Ayala A, Castro CY. Adrenocortical carcinoma with concomitant myelolipoma in a patient with hyperaldosteronism. Arch Pathol Lab Med 2005; 129:e144.

182. Ukimura O, Inui E, Ochiai A, et al. Combined adrenal myelolipoma and pheochromocytoma. J Urol 1995; 154:1470.

183. Courcoutsakis NA, Patronas NJ, Cassarino D, et al. Hypodense nodularity on computed tomography: novel imaging and pathology of micronodular adrenocortical hyperplasia associated with myelolipomatous changes. J Clin Endocrinol Metab 2004; 89:3737.

184. Nagai T, Imamura M, Honma M, et al. 17 alpha-hydroxylase deficiency accompanied by adrenal myelolipoma. Intern Med 2001; 40:920.

185. Oliva A, Duarte B, Hammadeh R, et al. Myelolipoma and endocrine dysfunction. Surgery 1988; 103:711.

186. Whaley D, Becker S, Presbrey T, et al. Adrenal myelolipoma associated with Conn syndrome: CT evaluation. J Comput Assist Tomogr 1985; 9:959.

187. Fowler MR, Williams RB, Alba JM, et al. Extra-adrenal myelolipomas compared with extramedullary hematopoietic tumors: a case of presacral myelolipoma. Am J Surg Pathol 1982; 6:363.

188. Bishop E, Eble JN, Cheng L, et al. Adrenal myelolipomas show nonrandom X-chromosome inactivation in hematopoietic elements and fat: support for a clonal origin of myelolipomas. Am J Surg Pathol 2006; 30:838.

Intramuscular and intermuscular lipomas

189. Kindblom LG, Angervall L, Stener B, et al. Intra- and intermuscular lipoma. Nord Med 1971; 86:1455.

190. Dionne GP, Seemayer TA. Infiltrating lipomas and angiolipomas revisted. Cancer 1974; 33:732.

191. Bao L, Miles L. Translocation (1;4;12)(q25;q27;q15) in a childhood intramuscular lipoma. Cancer Genet Cytogenet 2005; 158:95.

192. Dattolo RA, Nesbit GM, Kelly KE, et al. Infiltrating intramuscular lipoma of the paraspinal muscles. Ann Otol Rhinol Laryngol 1995; 104:582.

193. Pant R, Poh AC, Hwang SG. An unusual case of an intramuscular lipoma of the pectoralis major muscle simulating a malignant breast mass. Ann Acad Med Singapore 2005; 34:275.

194. Uemura T, Suse T, Yokoyama T, et al. Intramuscular benign lipoma of the temporalis muscle. Scand J Plast Reconstr Surg Hand Surg 2002; 36:231.

195. Moumoulidis I, Durvasula P, Jani P. Well-circumscribed intramuscular lipoma of the sternocleidomastoid muscle. Auris Nasus Larynx 2004; 31:283.

196. Zamora MA, Zamora CA, Samayoa EA, et al. High-resolution ultrasonography in an aggressive thenar intramuscular lipoma. J Ultrasound Med 2005; 24:1151.

197. Warner JJ, Madsen N, Gerber C. Intramuscular lipoma of the deltoid causing shoulder pain. Report of two cases. Clin Orthop 1990; 253:110.

198. Matsumoto K, Hukuda S, Ishizawa M, et al. MRI findings in intramuscular lipomas. Skeletal Radiol 1999; 28:145.

199. Heim S, Mandahl N, Kristoffersson U, et al. Reciprocal translocation t(3;12)(q27;q13) in lipoma. Cancer Genet Cytogenet 1986; 23:301.

200. Scolozzi P, Lombardi T, Maire G, et al. Infiltrating intramuscular lipoma of the temporal muscle. A case report with molecular cytogenetic analysis. Oral Oncol 2003; 39:316.

201. Enzinger FM. Benign lipomatous tumors simulating a sarcoma. In: Management of primary bone and soft tissue tumors. Chicago: Year Book; 1977.

Lipomas of tendon sheaths and joints

202. Bryan RS, Dahlin DC, Sullivan CR. Lipoma of the tendon sheath. J Bone Joint Surg [Am] 1956; 38:1275.

203. Pampliega T, Arenas AJ. An unusual trigger finger. Acta Orthop Belg 1997; 63:132.
204. Kremchek TE, Kremchek EJ. Carpal tunnel syndrome caused by flexor tendon sheath lipoma. Orthop Rev 1988; 17:1083.
205. Sheldon PJ, Forrester DM, Learch TJ. Imaging of intraarticular masses. Radiographics 2005; 25:105.
206. Davies AP, Blewitt N. Lipoma arborescens of the knee. Knee 2005; 12:394.
207. Kim RS, Song JS, Park SW, et al. Lipoma arborescens of the knee. Arthroscopy 2004; 20:e95.
208. Nisolle JF, Blouard E, Baudrez V, et al. Subacromial-subdeltoid lipoma arborescens associated with a rotator cuff tear. Skeletal Radiol 1999; 28:283.
209. Wolf RS, Zoys GN, Saldivar VA, et al. Lipoma arborescens of the hip. Am J Orthop 2002; 31:276.
210. Doyle AJ, Miller MV, French JG. Lipoma arborescens in the bicipital bursa of the elbow: MRI findings in two cases. Skeletal Radiol 2002; 31:656.
211. Haasbeek JF, Alvillar RE. Childhood lipoma arborescens presenting as bilateral suprapatellar masses. J Rheumatol 1999; 26:683.
212. Al-Ismail K, Torreggiani WC, Al-Sheikh F, et al. Bilateral lipoma arborescens associated with early osteoarthritis. Eur Radiol 2002; 12:2799.
213. Dinauer P, Bojescul JA, Kaplan KJ, et al. Bilateral lipoma arborescens of the bicipitoradial bursa. Skeletal Radiol 2002; 31:661.
214. Cil A, Atay OA, Aydingoz U, et al. Bilateral lipoma arborescens of the knee in a child: a case report. Knee Surg Sports Traumatol Arthrosc 2005; 13:463.
215. Bejia I, Younes M, Moussa A, et al. Lipoma arborescens affecting multiple joints. Skeletal Radiol 2005; 34:536.
216. Siva C, Brasington R, Totty W, et al. Synovial lipomatosis (lipoma arborescens) affecting multiple joints in a patient with congenital short bowel syndrome. J Rheumatol 2002; 29:1088.
217. Learch TJ, Braaton M. Lipoma arborescens: high-resolution ultrasonographic findings. J Ultrasound Med 2000; 19:385.
218. Vilanova JC, Barcelo J, Villalon M, et al. MR imaging of lipoma arborescens and the associated lesions. Skeletal Radiol 2003; 32:504.
219. Kurihashi A, Yamaguchi T, Tamal K, et al. Lipoma arborescens with osteochondral metaplasia – a case mimicking synovial osteochondromatosis in a lateral knee bursa. Acta Orthop Scand 1997; 68:304.
220. Ozalay M, Tandogan RN, Akpinar S, et al. Arthroscopic treatment of solitary benign intra-articular lesions of the knee that cause mechanical symptoms. Arthroscopy 2005; 21:12.
221. Hallel T, Lew S, Bansal M. Villous lipomatous proliferation of the synovial membrane (lipoma arborescens). J Bone Joint Surg [Am] 1988; 70:264.

Lumbosacral lipoma

222. Rickwood AMK, Hemalatha V, Zachary RB. Lipoma of the cauda equina (lumbosarcal lipoma): a study of 74 cases operated in childhood. Z Kinderchir 1979; 27:159.
223. Rawashdeh YF, Jorgensen TM, Olsen LH, et al. The outcome of detrusor myotomy in children with neurogenic bladder dysfunction. J Urol 2004; 171:2654.
224. Fujimura M, Kusaka Y, Shirane R. Spinal lipoma associated with terminal syringohydromyelia and a spinal arachnoid cyst in a patient with cloacal exostrophy. Childs Nerv Syst 2003; 19:254.
225. Dorward NL, Scatliff JH, Hayward RD. Congenital lumbosacral lipomas: pitfalls in analysing the results of prophylactic surgery. Childs Nerv Syst 2002; 18:326.
226. Cornette L, Verpoorten C, Lagae L, et al. Closed spinal dysraphism: a review on diagnosis and treatment in infancy. Eur J Paediatr Neurol 1998; 2:179.
227. Wang TC, Yu CL, Hsu JC, et al. F wave monitoring during surgery for adult tethered cord syndrome – a case report. Acta Anaesthesiol Sin 2000; 38:167.
228. Loeser JD, Lewin RJ. Lumbosacral lipoma in the adult: case report. J Neurosurg 1968; 29:405.
229. Lassman LP, James CC. Lumbosacral lipomas: critical survey of 26 cases submitted to laminectomy. J Neurol Neurosurg Psychiatry 1967; 30:174.
230. Hashiguchi K, Morioka T, Fukui K, et al. Usefulness of constructive interference in steady-state magnetic resonance imaging in the presurgical examination for lumbosacral lipoma. J Neurosurg 2005; 103:537.
231. Kawamura T, Morioka T, Nishio S, et al. Cerebral abnormalities in lumbosacral neural tube closure defect: MR imaging evaluation. Childs Nerv Syst 2001; 17:405.
232. Thorne A, Pierre-Kahn A, Sonigo P. Antenatal diagnosis of spinal lipomas. Childs Nerv Syst 2001; 17:697.
233. Park SH, Huh JS, Cho KH, et al. Teratoma in human tail lipoma. Pediatr Neurosurg 2005. 41:158.
234. Vajtai I, Varga Z, Hackel J. Neuromuscular choristoma. Orv Hetil 1999; 140:1743.
235. Alston SR, Fuller GN, Boyko OB, et al. Ectopic immature renal tissue in a lumbosacral lipoma: pathologic and radiologic findings. Pediatr Neurosci 1989; 15:100.
236. Kanev PM, Lemire RJ, Loeser JD, et al. Management and long-term follow-up review of children with lipomyelomeningocele, 1952–1987. J Neurosurg 1990; 73:48,
237. Koyanagi I, Iwasaki Y, Hida K, et al. Surgical treatment supposed natural history of the tethered cord with occult spinal dysraphism. Childs Nerv Syst 1997; 13:268.
238. Van Calenbergh F, Vanvolsem S, Verpoorten C, et al. Results after surgery for lumbosacral lipoma: the significance of early and late worsening. Childs Nerv Syst 1999; 15:439.
239. Cochrane DD, Finley C, Kestle J, et al. The patterns of late deterioration in patients with transitional lipomyelomeningocele. Eur J Pediatr Surg 2000; 10:13.

Neural fibrolipoma (lipofibromatous hamartoma of nerves)

240. Toms AP, Anastakis D, Bleakney RR, et al. Lipofibromatous hamartoma of the upper extremity: a review of the radiologic findings for 15 patients. AJR Am J Roentgenol 2006; 186:805.
240a. Bisceglia M, Vigilante E, Ben-Dor D. Neural lipofibromatous hamartoma. A report of two cases and review of the literature. Adv Anat Pathol 2007; 14:46.
241. Walbaum R, Van de Velde-Staquet MF, Bahon-Le Capon J, et al. Neurolipomatosis with encephalo-oculo-cutaneous dysplasia. Pediatrie (Bucur) 1979; 34:717.
242. Silverman TA, Enzinger FM. Fibrolipomatous hamartoma of nerve. A clinicopathologic analysis of 26 cases. Am J Surg Pathol 1985; 9:7.
243. Watt AJ, Chung KC. Macrodystrophia lipomatosa: a reconstructive approach to gigantism of the foot. J Foot Ankle Surg 2004; 43:51.
244. De Maeseneer M, Jaovisidha S, Lenchik L, et al. Fibrolipomatous hamartoma: MR imaging findings. Skeletal Radiol 1997; 26:155.
245. Marom EM, Helms CA. Fibrolipomatous hamartoma: pathognomonic on MR imaging. Skeletal Radiol 1999; 28:260.
246. Drut R. Ossifying fibrolipomatous hamartoma of the ulnar nerve. Pediatr Pathol 1988; 8:179.
247. Patel ME, Silver JW, Lipton DE, et al. Lipofibroma of the median nerve in the palm and digits of the hand. J Bone Joint Surg [Am] 1979; 61:393.
248. Sondergaard G, Mikkelsen S. Fibrolipomatous hamartoma of the median nerve. J Hand Surg [Br] 1987; 12:224.

Diffuse lipomatosis

249. Greiss ME, Williams DH. Macrodystrophia lipomatosis in the foot. A case report and review of the literature. Arch Orthop Trauma Surg 1991; 110:220.
250. Arslan A, Alic B, Uzunlar AK, et al. Diffuse lipomatosis of thyroid gland. Auris Nasus Larynx 1999; 26:213.
251. Coode PE, McGuinness FE, Rawas MM, et al. Diffuse lipomatosis involving the thoracic and abdominal wall: CT features. J Comput Assist Tomogr 1991; 15:341.
252. Punia RS, Nanda A, Bakshi A, et al. Recurrent diffuse lipomatosis of the neck – a case report. Indian J Pathol Microbiol 2004; 47:41.
253. Zargar AH, Laway BA, Masoodi SR, et al. Diffuse abdominal lipomatosis. J Assoc Physicians India 2003; 51:621.
254. Berdou R, Osterhage HR. Pelvic lipomatosis – what to do? Urologe A 2003; 42:1244.
255. Nixon HH, Scobie WG. Congenital lipomatosis: a report of four cases. J Pediatr Surg 1971; 6:742.
256. Kindblom LG, Moller-Nielsen J. Diffuse lipomatosis in the leg after poliomyelitis. Acta Pathol Microbiol Scand [A] 1975; 83:339.
257. Alcazar JD, Ramos R, Verdugo J. Dorsal transthoracic diffuse lipomatosis in a patient with familial tuberous sclerosis. Arch Bronconeumol 1998; 34:468.
258. Klein JA, Barr RJ. Diffuse lipomatosis and tuberous sclerosis. Arch Dermatol 1986; 122:1298.

Symmetric lipomatosis

259. Madelung OW. Die aetiologie und die operative behandlung der dupuytren'schen fingerverkrumung. Berl Klin Wochenschr 1875; 12:191.
260. Launois PE, Bensaude R. De l'adenolipomatose symmetrique. Soc Med Hosp Paris Bull Mem 1889; 15:298.
261. Brodie BC. Clinical lectures on surgery delivered at St. George's Hospital. Philadelphia: Lea & Blanchard; 1846:275.
262. Guilemany JM, Romero E, Blanch JL. An aesthetic deformity: Madelung's disease. Acta Otolaryngol (Stockh) 2005; 125:328.
263. Lee MS, Lee MH, Hur KB. Multiple symmetric lipomatosis. J Korean Med Sci 1988; 3:163.
264. Kise Y, Shimoji M, Toda T, et al. Benign symmetric lipomatosis in a 73-year-old man: a case report with a brief review of the literature. Rinsho Byori 2004; 52:824.
265. Gonzalez-Garcia R, Rodriguez-Campo FJ, Sastre-Perez J, et al. Benign symmetric lipomatosis (Madelung's disease): case reports and current management. Aesthetic Plast Surg 2004; 28:108.
266. Morelli F, De Benedetto A, Toto P, et al. Alcoholism as a trigger of multiple symmetric lipomatosis? J Eur Acad Dermatol Venereol 2003; 17:367.

267. Naumann M, Schalke B, Klopstock T, et al. Neurological multisystem manifestation in multiple symmetric lipomatosis: a clinical and electrophysiological study. Muscle Nerve 1995; 18:693.

268. Fernandez-Vozmediano J, Armario-Hita J. Benign symmetric lipomatosis (Launois-Bensaude syndrome). Int J Dermatol 2005; 44:236.

269. Preisz K, Karpati S, Horvath A. Launois-Bensaude syndrome and Bureau-Barriere syndrome in a psoriatic patient: successful treatment with carbamazepine. Eur J Dermatol 2002; 12:267.

270. Saiz Hervas E, Martin Llorens M, Lopez Alvarez J. Peripheral neuropathy as the first manifestation of Madelung's disease. Br J Dermatol 2000; 143:684.

271. Berkovic SF, Andermann F, Shoubridge EA, et al. Mitochondrial dysfunction in multiple symmetrical lipomatosis. Ann Neurol 1991; 29:566.

272. Chalk CH, Mills KR, Jacobs JM, et al. Familial multiple symmetric lipomatosis with peripheral neuropathy. Neurology 1990; 40:1246.

273. Ruzicka T, Vieluf D, Landthaler M, et al. Benign symmetric lipomatosis Launois-Bensaude. Report of ten cases and review of the literature. J Am Acad Dermatol 1987; 17:663.

274. Stopar T, Jankovic VN, Casati A. Four different airway-management strategies in patient with Launois-Bensaude syndrome or Madelung's disease undergoing surgical excision of neck lipomatosis with a complicated postoperative course. J Clin Anesth 2005; 17:300.

275. Borges A, Torrinha F, Lufkin RB, et al. Laryngeal involvement in multiple symmetric lipomatosis: the role of computed tomography in diagnosis. Am J Otolaryngol 1997; 18:127.

276. Enzi G. Multiple symmetric lipomatosis: an updated clinical report. Medicine (Baltimore) 1984; 63:56.

277. Ahuja AT, King AD, Chan ES. Ultrasound, CT and MRI in patients with multiple symmetric lipomatosis. Clin Radiol 2000; 55:79.

278. Busetto L, Strater D, Enzi G, et al. Differential clinical expression of multiple symmetric lipomatosis in men and women. Int J Obes Relat Metab Disord 2003; 27:1419.

279. Kratz C, Lenard HG, Ruzicka T, et al. Multiple symmetric lipomatosis: an unusual cause of childhood obesity and mental retardation. Eur J Paediatr Neurol 2000; 4:63.

280. Nisoli E, Regianini L, Briscini L, et al. Multiple symmetric lipomatosis may be the consequence of defective noradrenergic modulation of proliferation and differentiation of brown fat cells. J Pathol 2002; 198:378.

281. Nielsen S, Levine J, Clay R, et al. Adipose tissue metabolism in benign symmetric lipomatosis. J Clin Endocrinol Metab 2001; 86:2717.

282. Zancanaro C, Sbarbati A, Morroni M, et al. Multiple symmetric lipomatosis. Ultrastructural investigation of the tissue and preadipocytes in primary culture. Lab Invest 1990; 63:253.

283. Klopstock T, Naumann M, Schalke B, et al. Multiple symmetric lipomatosis: abnormalities in complex IV and multiple deletions in mitochondrial DNA. Neurology 1994; 44:862.

284. Naumann M, Kiefer R, Toyka KV, et al. Mitochondrial dysfunction with myoclonus epilepsy and ragged-red fibers point mutation in nerve, muscle, and adipose tissue of a patient with multiple symmetric lipomatosis. Muscle Nerve 1997; 20:833.

285. Verhelle NA, Nizet JL, Van den Hof B, et al. Liposuction in benign symmetric lipomatosis: sense or senseless? Aesthetic Plast Surg 2003; 27:319.

286. Adamo C, Vescio G, Battaglia M, et al. Madelung's disease: case report and discussion of treatment options. Ann Plast Surg 2001; 46:43.

287. Faga A, Valdatta LA, Thione A, et al. Ultrasound assisted liposuction for the palliative treatment of Madelung's disease: a case report. Aesthetic Plast Surg 2001; 25:181.

288. Lee HW, Kim TH, Cho JW, et al. Multiple symmetric lipomatosis: Korean experience. Dermatol Surg 2003; 29:235.

289. Enzi G, Busetto L, Ceschin E, et al. Multiple symmetric lipomatosis: clinical aspects and outcome in a long-term longitudinal study. Int J Obes Relat Metab Disord 2002; 26:253.

Pelvic lipomatosis

290. Engels EP. Sigmoid colon and urinary bladder in high fixation: Roentgen changes simulating pelvic tumor. Radiology 1959; 72:419.

291. Klein FA, Smith MJ, Kasenetz I. Pelvic lipomatosis: 35-year experience. J Urol 1988; 139:998.

292. Werboff LH, Korobkin M, Klein RS. Pelvic lipomatosis: diagnosis using computed tomography. J Urol 1979; 122:257.

293. Quirino L, Izzo A, Niglio E, et al. Pelvic lipomatosis complicating ovarian cyst removal: a case report. Eur J Gynaecol Oncol 2004; 25:517.

294. Honecke K, Butz M. Pelvic lipomatosis in a female: diagnosis and initial therapy. Urol Int 1991; 46:93.

295. Heyns CF. Pelvic lipomatosis: a review of its diagnosis and management. J Urol 1991; 146:267.

296. Yamaguchi T, Shimizu Y, Ono N, et al. A case of pelvic lipomatosis presenting with edema of the lower extremities. Jpn J Med 1991; 30:559.

297. Gajic O, Sprung J, Hall BA, et al. Fatal acute pulmonary embolism in a patient with pelvic lipomatosis after surgery performed after transatlantic airplane travel. Anesth Analg 2004; 99:1032.

298. Sharma S, Nabi G, Seth A, et al. Pelvic lipomatosis presenting as uraemic encephalopathy. Int J Clin Pract 2001; 55:149.

299. Tong RS, Larner T, Finlay M, et al. Pelvic lipomatosis associated with proliferative cystitis occurring in two brothers. Urology 2002; 59:602.

300. Masumori N, Tsukamoto T. Pelvic lipomatosis associated with proliferative cystitis: case report and review of the Japanese literature. Int J Urol 1999; 6:44.

301. Farina LA. Re: Pelvic lipomatosis associated with cystitis glandularis and adenocarcinoma of the bladder. J Urol 1992; 147:1380.

302. Bhatia RS, Chopda N, Devarbhavi H, et al. Pelvic lipomatosis. Indian J Pediatr 1995; 62:746.

303. Gordon NS, Sinclair RA, Snow RM. Pelvic lipomatosis with cystitis cystica, cystitis glandularis and adenocarcinoma of the bladder: first reported case. Aust NZ J Surg 1990; 60:229.

304. Sauty L, Ravery V, Toublanc M, et al. Florid glandular cystitis: study of 3 cases and review of the literature. Prog Urol 1998; 8:561.

305. Sozen S, Gurocak S, Uzum N, et al. The importance of re-evaluation in patients with cystitis glandularis associated with pelvic lipomatosis: a case report. Urol Oncol 2004; 22:428.

306. Torigian DA, Siegelman ES. CT findings of pelvic lipomatosis of nerve. AJR Am J Roentgenol 2005; 184:S94.

307. Beluffi G, DiGiulio G, Fiori P. Pelvic lipomatosis in the Proteus syndrome: a further diagnostic sign. Eur J Pediatr 1990; 149:866.

308. Costa T, Fitch N, Azouz EM. Proteus syndrome: report of two cases with pelvic lipomatosis. Pediatrics 1985; 76:984.

309. Andac N, Baltacioglu F, Cimsit NC, et al. Fat necrosis mimicking liposarcoma in a patient with pelvic lipomatosis. CT findings. Clin Imaging 2003; 27:109.

310. Halachmi S, Moskovitz B, Calderon N, et al. The use of an ultrasonic assisted lipectomy device for the treatment of obstructive pelvic lipomatosis. Urology 1996; 48:128.

Steroid lipomatosis

311. Shukla LW, Katz JA, Wagner ML. Mediastinal lipomatosis: a complication of high dose steroid therapy in children. Pediatr Radiol 1988; 19:57.

312. Mulrow CD, Corey GR. Pericardial pseudoeffusion due to steroid-induced lipomatosis. N C Med J 1985; 46:179.

313. Glickstein MF, Miller WT, Dalinka MK, et al. Paraspinal lipomatosis: a benign mass. Radiology 1987; 163:79.

314. Siskind BN, Weiner FR, Frank M, et al. Steroid-induced mesenteric lipomatosis. Comput Radiol 1984; 8:175.

315. Gilsanz V, Brill PW, Wolf BS. Increased retroperitoneal fat: a sign of corticosteroid therapy. Radiology 1977; 123:147.

316. Kotilainen E, Hohenthal U, Karhu J, et al. Spinal epidural lipomatosis caused by corticosteroid treatment in ulcerative colitis. Eur J Intern Med 2006; 17:138.

317. Salehian B, Bilas J, Bazargan M, et al. Prevalence and incidence of diabetes in HIV-infected minority patients on protease inhibitors. J Natl Med Assoc 2005; 97:1088.

318. Connolly N, Manders E, Riddler S. Suction-assisted lipectomy for lipodystrophy. AIDS Res Hum Retroviruses 2004; 20:813.

319. De Luca A, Murri R, Damiano F, et al. "Buffalo hump" in HIV-1 infection. Lancet 1998; 352:320.

Nevus lipomatosus cutaneous superficialis

320. Hoffman E, Zurhelle E. Ueber einen naevus lipomatosus cutaneous superficialis der linken glutaealgegend. Arch Dermatol 1921; 130:327.

321. Takashima H, Toyoda M, Ikeda Y, et al. Nevus lipomatosus cutaneous superficialis with perifollicular fibrosis. Eur J Dermatol 2003; 13:584.

322. Lane JE, Clark E, Marzec T. Nevus lipomatosus cutaneous superficialis. Pediatr Dermatol 2003; 20:313.

323. Knuttel R, Silver EA. A cerebriform mass on the right buttock. Dermatol Surg 2003; 29:780.

324. Dotz W, Prioleau PG. Nevus lipomatosus cutaneous superficialis. A light and electron microscopic study. Arch Dermatol 1984; 120:376.

325. Chanoki M, Sugamoto I, Suzuki S, et al. Nevus lipomatosus cutaneous superficialis of the scalp. Cutis 1989; 43:143.

326. Finley AG, Musso LA. Naevus lipomatosus cutaneous superficialis (Hoffman-Zurhelle). Br J Dermatol 1972; 87:557.

327. Wilson-Jones E, Marks R, Pongshirun D. Naevus superficialis lipomatosus. Br J Dermatol 1975; 93:121.

328. Eyre SP, Hebert AA, Rapini RP. Rubbery zosteriform nodules on the back. Nevus lipomatosus cutaneous superficialis

(Hoffmann-Zurhelle). Arch Dermatol 1992; 128:1395.

329. Weitzner S. Solitary nevus lipomatosus cutaneous superficialis of scalp. Arch Dermatol 1968; 97:540.

330. Sawada Y. Solitary nevus lipomatosus superficialis on the forehead. Ann Plast Surg 1986; 16:356.

331. Hann SK, Yang DS, Lee SH. Giant nevus lipomatosus superficialis associated with cavernous hemangioma. J Dermatol 1988; 15:543.

332. Park HJ, Park CJ, Yi JY, et al. Nevus lipomatosus superficialis on the face. Int J Dermatol 1997; 36:435.

333. Kaw P, Carlson A, Meyer DR. Nevus lipomatosus (pedunculated lipofibroma) of the eyelid. Ophthal Plast Reconstr Surg 2005; 21:74.

Hibernoma

334. Gery L. Discussions. Bull Mem Soc Anat (Paris) 1914; 89:111.

335. Furlong MA, Fanburg-Smith JC, Miettinen M. The morphologic spectrum of hibernoma: a clinicopathologic study of 170 cases. Am J Surg Pathol 2001; 25:809.

336. Cox RW. Hibernoma: the lipoma of immature adipose tissue. J Pathol Bacteriol 1954; 68:511.

337. Baskurt E, Padgett DM, Matsumoto JA. Multiple hibernomas in a 1-month-old female infant. AJNR Am J Neuroradiol 2004; 25:1443.

338. Baldi A, Santini M, Mellone P, et al. Mediastinal hibernoma: a case report. J Clin Pathol 2004; 57:993.

339. Ong SY, Maziak DE, Shamji FM, et al. Intrathoracic hibernoma. Can J Surg 2002; 45:145.

340. Gardner-Thorpe D, Hirschowitz L, Maddox PR. Mammary hibernoma. Eur J Surg Oncol 2000; 26:430.

341. Schwartz BF, Wasson L. Hibernoma arising from the adrenal gland. Urology 2003; 61:1035.

342. Kindblom LG, Save-Soderbergh J. The ultrastructure of liposarcoma. A study of 10 cases. Acta Pathol Microbiol Scand [A] 1979; 87A:109.

343. Wright C, Berry BH Jr, Patterson PJ, et al. Radiologic case study. Hibernoma. Orthopedics 2003; 26:1194.

344. Kallas KM, Vaughan L, Haghighi P, et al. Hibernoma of the left axilla; a case report and review of MR imaging. Skeletal Radiol 2003; 32:290.

345. Saqi A, Yu GH, Marshall MB. Fine-needle aspiration of hibernoma. Diagn Cytopathol 2003; 29:44.

346. Lemos MM, Kindblom LG, Meis-Kindblom JM, et al. Fine-needle aspiration characteristics of hibernoma. Cancer 2001; 93:206.

347. Zancanaro C, Pelosi G, Accordini C, et al. Immunohistochemical identification of the uncoupling protein in human hibernoma. Biol Cell 1994; 80:75.

348. Dal Cin P, Van Damme B, Hoogmartens M, et al. Chromosome changes in a case of hibernoma. Genes Chromosomes Cancer 1992; 5:178.

349. Meloni AM, Spanier SS, Bush CH, et al. Involvement of 10q22 and 11q13 in hibernoma. Cancer Genet Cytogenet 1994; 72:59.

350. Mertens F, Rydholm A, Brosjo O, et al. Hibernomas are characterized by rearrangements of chromosome bands 11q13-21. Int J Cancer 1994; 58: 503.

351. Mrozek K, Karakousis CP, Bloomfield CD. Band 11q13 is nonrandomly rearranged in hibernomas. Genes Chromosomes Cancer 1994; 9:145.

352. Gisselsson D, Hoglund M, Mertens F, et al. Hibernomas are characterized by homozygous deletions in the multiple endocrine neoplasia type I region. Metaphase fluorescence in situ hybridization reveals complex rearrangements not detected by conventional cytogenetics. Am J Pathol 1999; 155:61.

353. Maire G, Forus A, Foa C, et al. 11q13 alterations in two cases of hibernoma: large heterozygous deletions and rearrangement breakpoints near GARP in 11q13.5. Genes Chromosomes Cancer 2003; 37:389.

LIPOSARCOMA

Liposarcoma is one of the most common soft tissue sarcomas of adult life, with an annual incidence estimated to be 2.5 per million in a Swedish population[1] and the relative incidence among other sarcomas ranging from 9.8% to 16.0%.[2,3] Included in the general category of liposarcoma is a number of subtypes that are histologically, biologically, cytogenetically, and by molecular analyses[2,4–6] distinct from one another (Table 16–1). These subtypes range in behavior from nonmetastasizing neoplasms (e.g., atypical lipomatous neoplasm/well differentiated liposarcoma (ALN/WDL) to high-grade sarcomas with full metastatic potential (e.g., pleomorphic liposarcoma). So impressed were Enzinger and Winslow by the diversity of this group of lesions that they wrote in their seminal work on liposarcoma in 1962, "Among mesenchymal tumors, liposarcomas are probably unsurpassed by their wide range in structure and behavior. In fact the variations are striking that it seems more apt [sic] to regard them as groups of closely related tumors rather than as a well defined entity."[7] In no other group of sarcomas does the pathologist receive such a strong mandate to subclassify these lesions, as accurate subtyping translates into grade and biologic behavior.

Although the World Health Organization (WHO) divides liposarcomas into four subtypes (ALN/WDL, myxoid/round cell, dedifferentiated, pleomorphic),[4] it is useful to think of liposarcomas as three large groups from a conceptual point of view. ALN/WDL (WDL), also

termed atypical lipomatous neoplasm (ALN) when it occurs in superficial soft tissue or in the muscles of the extremity because of its low-grade behavior, and dedifferentiated liposarcoma comprise one subgroup. Widely disparate in terms of biologic behavior, they are closely related from a pathogenetic point of view, as a subset of ALN/WDL histologically progresses to dedifferentiated sarcomas. With dedifferentiation, the tumor acquires metastatic potential, a phenomenon accompanied by additional cytogenetic abnormalities. The second group is myxoid liposarcoma which ranges in appearance from pure myxoid tumors at one extreme to poorly differentiated round cell (poorly differentiated myxoid) tumors at the other. Pleomorphic liposarcomas are rare, poorly characterized tumors. Many, but not all, are virtually indistinguishable from malignant fibrous histiocytoma except for the presence of pleomorphic lipoblasts. Finally, a small number of liposarcomas exhibits unusual features or combines patterns not accounted for in the above classification (liposarcomas of mixed type). Such lesions are best individualized and diagnosed as liposarcomas of mixed or miscellaneous type until refinements in the current classification account for these nosologic oddities.

Certain generalizations should be kept in mind when considering the diagnosis of liposarcoma. First, most liposarcomas occur in deep soft tissue, in contrast to lipomas, which occur in superficial soft tissue. This implies that subcutaneous ALN/WDL are rare and that the diagnosis should be made only after the more common mimics (e.g., spindle cell lipoma, pleomorphic lipoma, chondroid lipoma, cellular forms of angiolipoma) are excluded from the differential diagnosis. Second, there is little, if any, evidence that lipomas undergo malignant transformation to liposarcomas, an axiom that derives strong support from the marked difference in location of lipomas and liposarcomas. Most likely, lesions suggesting malignant transformation of a lipoma are in reality liposarcomas in which inadequate sampling led to underdiagnosis of malignancy in the original material. Third, liposarcomas rarely occur in children. Liposarcoma-like lesions in this age group usually represent lipoblastomas, a fetal form of lipoma.

TABLE 16–1	COMPARISON OF LIPOSARCOMA SUBTYPES			
Liposarcoma	Age (years)	Location	Cytogenetic abnormality	Behavior
WDL	50–70	Extremity (75%); retroperitoneum	Giant marker + ring chromosome	Local recurrence high; no metastasis 5–15% dedifferentiate
DL	50–70	Retroperitoneum (75%)	Giant marker + ring + additional abnormalities t(12;16)	High local recurrence; metastasis
MRCL	25–45	Extremity (75%)	t(12;16)	Recurrence + metastasis (determined by round cell component)

WDL, well-differentiated liposarcoma; DL, dedifferentiated liposarcoma; MRCL, myxoid/round cell liposarcoma.

There have been great strides in our understanding of liposarcomas during the last several years largely as a result of cytogenetic studies. The reciprocal translocation between chromosomes 12 and 16, which characterizes most myxoid-round cell liposarcomas, results in expression of a number of fusion transcripts, which appear to play a direct role in oncogenesis. The large group of ALN/WDL, on the other hand, have an entirely different abnormality in the form of giant and ring chromosomes, derived at least in part from chromosome 12, resulting in amplification of a number of genes (e.g., *MDM2, CDK4*) which represent a recurring motif in a number of mesenchymal tumors. Liposarcoma cells have recently been shown to express the peroxisome proliferator-activated receptor gamma (PPAR gamma) which, when bound to its ligand pioglitazone, terminally differentiate.[8] Binding is associated with withdrawal from the cell cycle, induction of adipocyte specific genes, intracellular accumulation of lipid, and, in three patients treated with the ligand, tumor differentiation.[9] This suggests that pharmacologically induced differentiation may be a viable approach in the treatment of some sarcomas.

Interestingly, liposarcomas are seldom induced by radiation. Like other sarcomas, liposarcoma may also be associated with various signs and symptoms. Dedifferentiated liposarcomas have been associated with a leukemoid blood reaction,[10] and there has been one unillustrated report of an acquired Factor VII deficiency associated with a pleural liposarcoma that vanished and then reappeared with remission and relapse of the tumor, respectively.[11]

CRITERIA AND IMPORTANCE OF LIPOBLASTS

Traditionally, great emphasis has been placed on the identification of lipoblasts for diagnosing liposarcoma. Although it is certainly an appropriate task for pathologists to search for these cells in some situations, their importance in other situations has been overemphasized. For example, sclerosing ALN/WDL usually have few lipoblasts. In such cases the overall pattern and cellular components become more important determinants when making the diagnosis. On the other hand, imprecise criteria for the recognition of lipoblasts often lead to an erroneous diagnosis of liposarcoma.

Defined in the context of liposarcoma, the lipoblast is a neoplastic cell that to some extent recapitulates the differentiation cascade of normal fat. The earliest cells arise as pericapillary adventitial cells that closely resemble fibroblasts. These spindled cells, endowed with ample endoplasmic reticulum, slowly acquire fat droplets first at the poles of the cell and later throughout the cytoplasm. As fat accumulates in the cytoplasm, the cell loses its endoplasmic reticulum and assumes a round shape. Gradually, the nucleus becomes indented and pushed to one side of the cell. A similar range of changes can be identified in lipoblasts of some liposarcomas, notably the myxoid/round cell type (Fig. 16–1). In addition, pleomorphic cells with the features of lipoblasts can be identified in ALN/WDL and pleomorphic liposarcomas (Fig. 16–2), but these cells have no equivalent in the differentiation sequence of normal fat. The task for the pathologist is to decide at what point in the differentiation scheme the cell becomes sufficiently diagnostic to warrant the designation "lipoblast."

Criteria that have proved useful for identifying *diagnostic* lipoblasts include the following: (1) a hyperchromatic indented or sharply scalloped nucleus; (2) lipid-rich (neutral fat) droplets in the cytoplasm; and (3) an appropriate histologic background. The importance of the last criterion cannot be overemphasized, as lipoblast-like cells may be seen in a variety of conditions, and failure to take into consideration the overall appearance of a lesion can lead to an erroneous diagnosis of liposarcoma. For example, lipomas with fat necrosis (Fig. 16–3), fat with atrophic changes (Fig. 16–4), hibernomatous change in lipomas (Fig. 16–5), foreign body reaction to silicone (Fig. 16–6), non-specific accumulation of intracytoplasmic stromal mucin (Fig. 16–7), fixation artifact (Fig. 16–8), or signet ring melanoma, carcinoma and lymphoma (Fig. 16–9) all have cells that to some extent resemble lipoblasts. In each instance, other features indicate that the diagnosis of liposarcoma is not appropriate. Silicone reactions, for example, exhibit numerous multivacuolated histiocytes that fulfill some of the criteria of lipoblasts, yet the histologic background of foreign body giant cells and inflammation

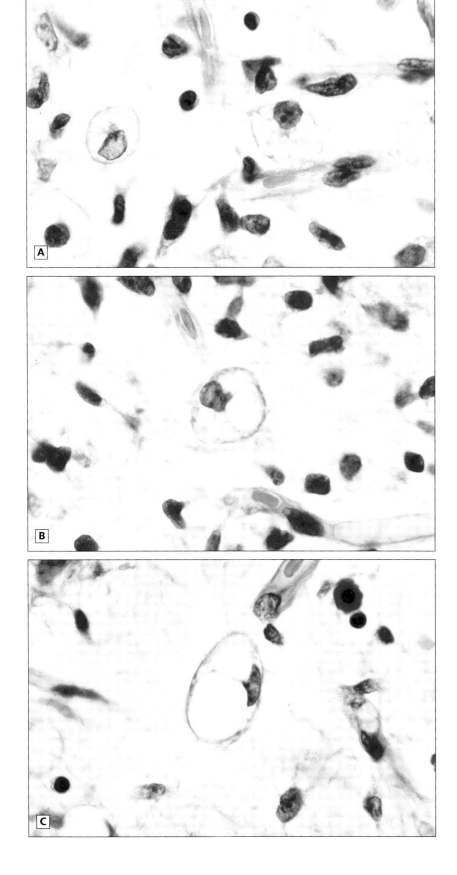

FIGURE 16–1 Developing lipoblasts from a myxoid liposarcoma, with an early stage **(A)** with fine vacuoles, an intermediate stage **(B, C)**, and a late stage **(D)** resembling mature white fat.

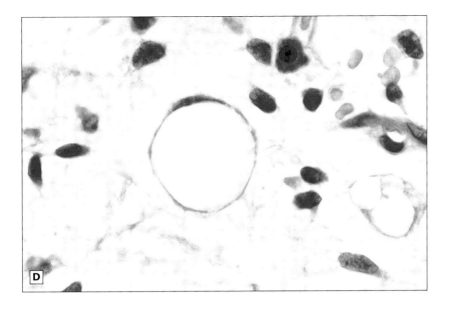

FIGURE 16–1 Continued.

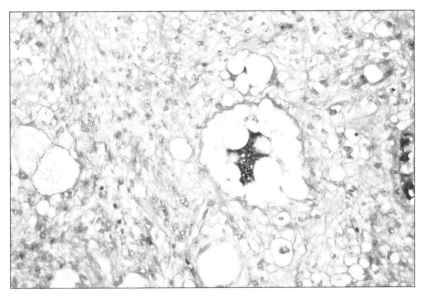

FIGURE 16–2 Pleomorphic lipoblast from a pleomorphic liposarcoma.

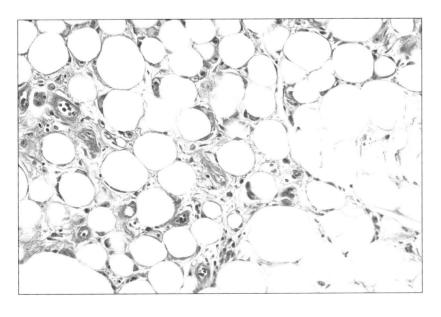

FIGURE 16–3 Fat necrosis in a lipoma. Scattered macrophages may be confused with atypical stromal cells of liposarcoma.

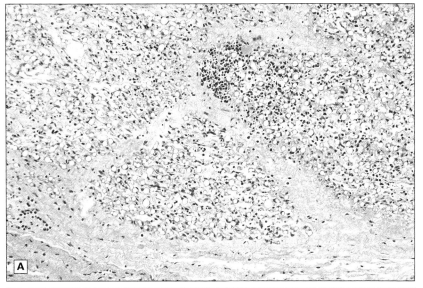

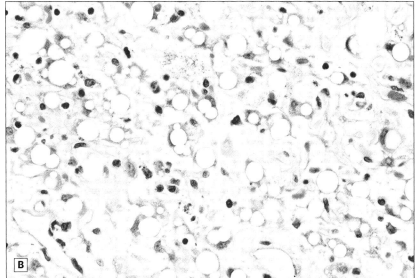

FIGURE 16–4 Atrophic fat occurring with malnutrition. Cells are arranged in lobules (A) and are uniformly small with lipofuscin pigment in the cytoplasm (B).

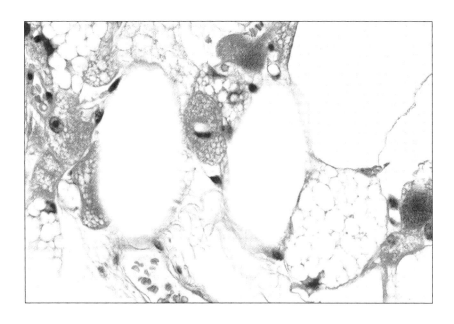

FIGURE 16–5 Finely vacuolated brown fat cells in a lipoma with hibernomatous changes mimicking lipoblasts.

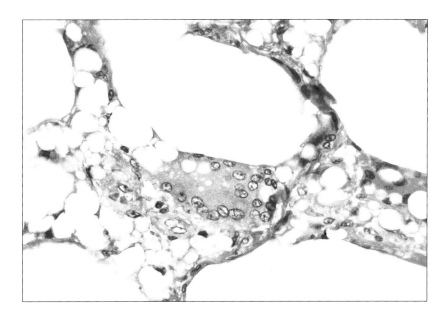

FIGURE 16–6 Silicone granuloma with multivacuolated histiocytes resembling lipoblasts.

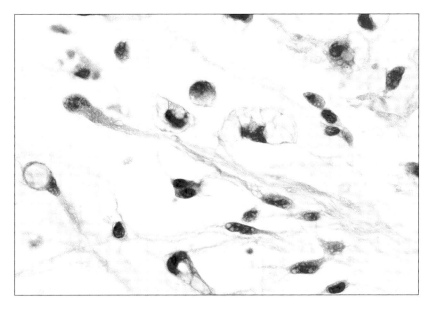

FIGURE 16–7 Cells of a myxoid malignant fibrous histiocytoma distended with hyaluronic acid. These cells are commonly misidentified as lipoblasts.

should alert the pathologist to the fact that the lesion is not a liposarcoma.

ATYPICAL LIPOMATOUS NEOPLASM/ALN/WDL

Clinical findings

ALN/WDL liposarcoma is the most common form of liposarcoma encountered in late adult life. It reaches a peak incidence during the sixth and seventh decades of life. Men and women are equally affected, although at certain sites (e.g., groin) there appears to be a predilection for men. In the collective experience of the Armed Forces Institute of Pathology (AFIP) and the Mayo Clinic, 75%

of cases developed in the deep muscles of the extremities and 20% in the retroperitoneum, with the remainder divided between the groin, spermatic cord, and miscellaneous sites.[12,13] Rarely do these tumors develop in the subcutis or in miscellaneous parenchymal sites.

Symptoms related to these tumors are dependent on the anatomic site. Those in the extremities develop as slowly growing masses that are present months or even several years before the patient seeks medical attention, whereas those in the retroperitoneum are associated with the usual symptoms of an intra-abdominal mass. Because ALN/WDL contain a significant component of mature fat, they present as fat density masses,[14-16] with mottled or streaky zones of higher density corresponding to the fibrous or sclerotic zones. They also tend to have less-well-defined borders than lipomas (Fig. 16–10).

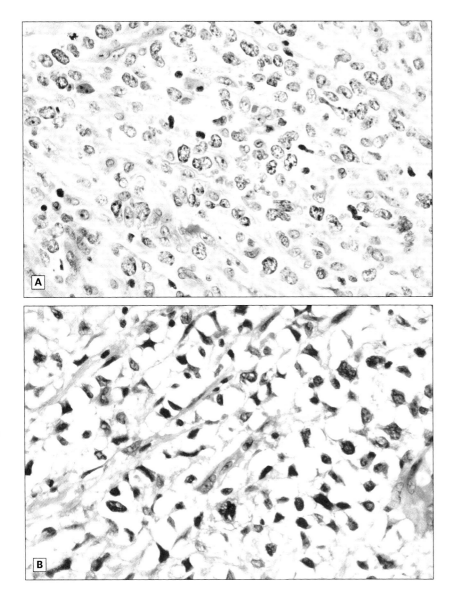

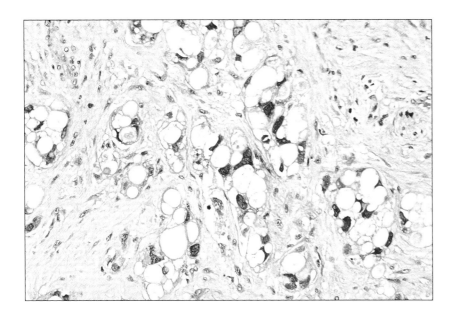

FIGURE 16–8 Large-cell lymphoma **(A)** with poorly fixed areas **(B)** in which the retraction artifact led to an erroneous diagnosis of liposarcoma.

FIGURE 16–9 Adenocarcinoma arising in Barrett's mucosa showing a treatment effect with pseudolipoblasts.

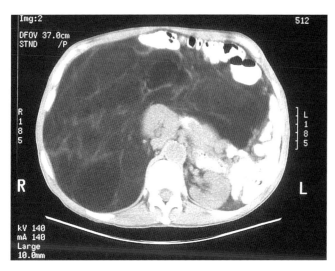

FIGURE 16–10 Computer tomography (CT) scan of ALN/WDL of the abdominal cavity and retroperitoneum. The mass, with a low attenuation value, replaces abdominal contents.

Gross and microscopic features

Grossly, ALN/WDL are large multilobular lesions that range in color from deep yellow to ivory (Figs 16–11, 16–12). Many could be mistaken for a lipoma except for their extremely large size and their tendency to have more fibrous bands, gelatinous zones, or punctate hemorrhage.

ALN/WDL have traditionally been divided into three subtypes: (1) lipoma-like; (2) sclerosing; and (3) inflammatory. Because many ALN/WDL combine features of both lipoma-like and sclerosing subtypes, the distinction between these two types is often arbitrary and of limited practical importance. We rarely subclassify these lesions in our daily practice, although these designations serve to draw attention to the range of appearances these tumors may assume. In the typical lipoma-like ALN/WDL, the tumor consists predominantly of mature fat with a variable number of spindled cells with hyperchromatic nuclei and multivacuolated lipoblasts (Figs 16–13 to 16–15). In some cases these atypical spindle cells are numerous, whereas in other cases the cells are so rare as to require extensive sampling of the tissue. Sclerosing forms of ALN/WDL, prevailing in the groin and retroperitoneum, have dense fibrotic zones alternating with mature adipocytes (Figs 16–16 to 16–19). In some cases the fibrotic zones consist of trabeculae intersecting fat, and in others the fibrous areas consist of broad sheets (Figs 16–17, 16–19). The fibrotic areas contain collagen fibrils of varying thickness in which are embedded scattered spindle and multipolar stromal cells with hyperchromatic nuclei. Similar cells may also be present between the mature adipocytes. Although lipoblasts may be present, they are usually rare. Thus, the diagnosis for this pattern of liposarcoma is more dependent on the identification of stromal cells with a requisite degree of atypia than on

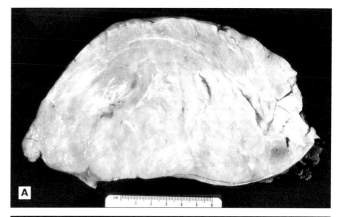

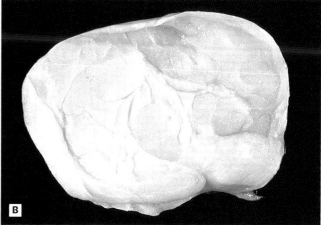

FIGURE 16–11 ALN/WDL closely resembling normal fat except for fibrous bands **(A)**. Others have a more gelatinous appearance **(B)**.

the identification of diagnostic lipoblasts. The inflammatory form of ALN/WDL occurs almost exclusively in the retroperitoneum and consists of a dense lymphocytic or plasmacytic infiltrate superimposed on a lipoma-like or sclerosing form of ALN/WDL (Fig. 16–20).[17] Because of the intense inflammatory infiltrate these tumors may be confused with lipogranulomatous inflammation.

An unusual feature that has received recent attention is the coexistence of smooth muscle tissue in ALN/WDL (Figs 16–21, 16–22).[18–23] These so-called *lipoleiomyosarcomas* are dual-lineage sarcomas in which both the lipomatous and smooth muscle components are low grade. Biologically, they have a behavior identical to ALN/WDL including the ability to dedifferentiate[22] and are recognized by areas of ALN/WDL blending with fascicles, nodules, or broad expanses of smooth muscle tissue having mild to moderate nuclear atypia and low levels of mitotic activity. In some cases, the smooth muscle appears to extend out from the walls of large vessels which similarly contain atypical smooth muscle cells (Fig. 16–22). The amount of smooth muscle varies considerably from case to case with some tumors showing only occasional foci and others broad expanses. It is important that this

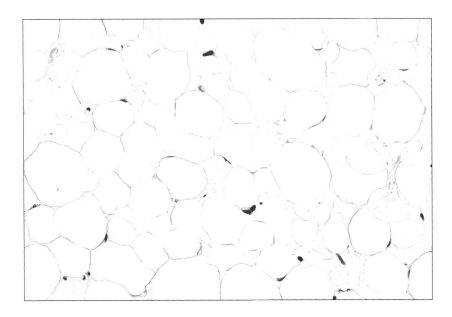

FIGURE 16–12 Well-differentiated (lipoma-like) liposarcoma showing only a rare atypical stromal cell amid a mature lipomatous backdrop.

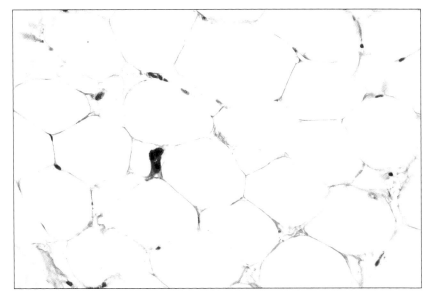

FIGURE 16–13 Atypical stromal cell in an ALN/WDL illustrating nuclear hyperchromatism.

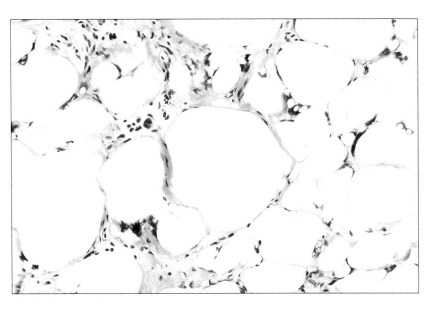

FIGURE 16–14 ALN/WDL with a larger number of atypical stromal cells and lipoblasts than in Figure 16–13.

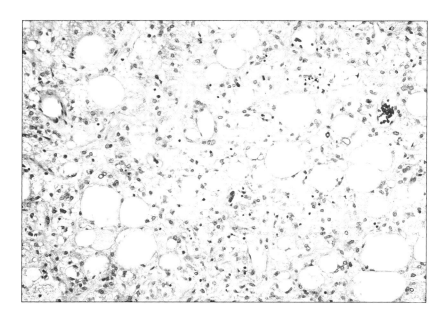

FIGURE 16–15 Well-differentiated (lipoma-like) liposarcoma with numerous lipoblasts.

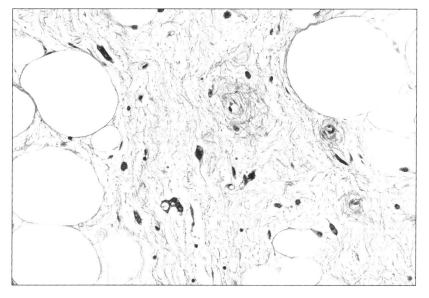

FIGURE 16–16 Sclerosing ALN/WDL.

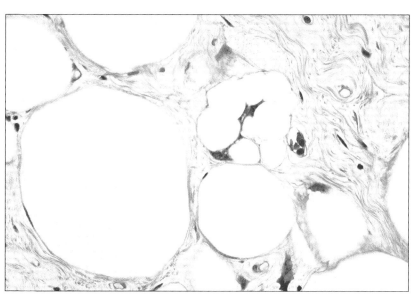

FIGURE 16–17 Well-differentiated (sclerosing) liposarcoma showing sheet-like areas of collagen and fat. Note the multivacuolated lipoblast in this lesion. Such cells are typically rare.

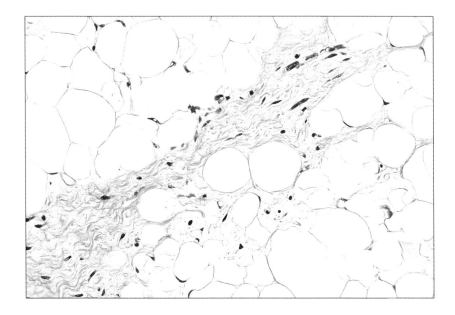

FIGURE 16–18 Well-differentiated (sclerosing) liposarcoma with fibrous bands containing atypical cells.

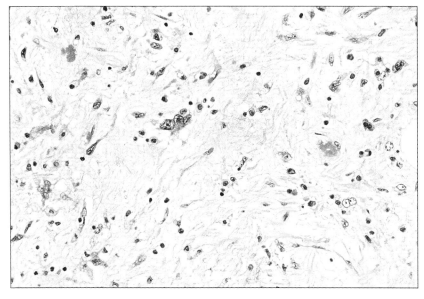

FIGURE 16–19 Nonlipogenic zone in a well-differentiated (sclerosing) liposarcoma. Note that the cellularity is far less than in nonlipogenic zones of dedifferentiated liposarcoma. Small-needle biopsies providing specimens from such areas can lead to the erroneous conclusion that the tumor is not a liposarcoma.

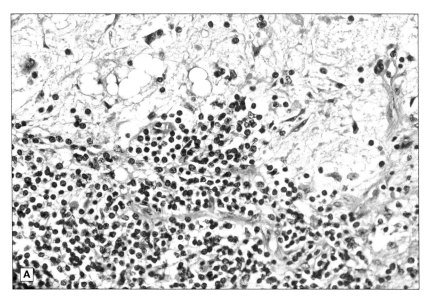

FIGURE 16–20 ALN/WDL of the inflammatory type with a dense lymphocytic infiltrate **(A)** and areas of lipoblastic differentiation **(B)**.

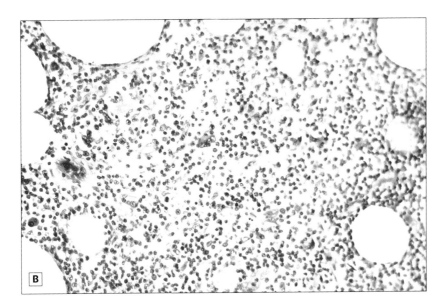

FIGURE 16–20 Continued.

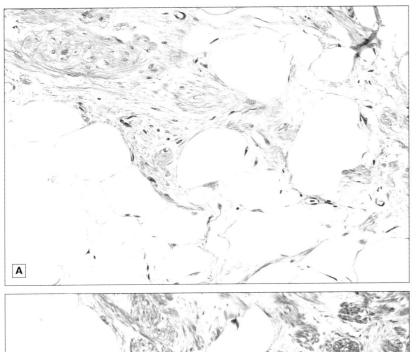

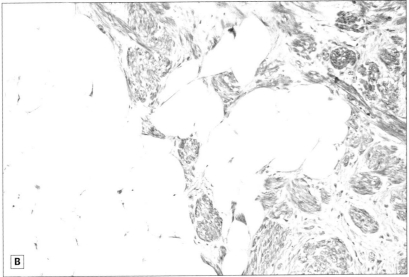

FIGURE 16–21 ALN/WDL with smooth muscle differentiation (lipoleiomyosarcoma) **(A)** and stained with Masson trichrome **(B)**.

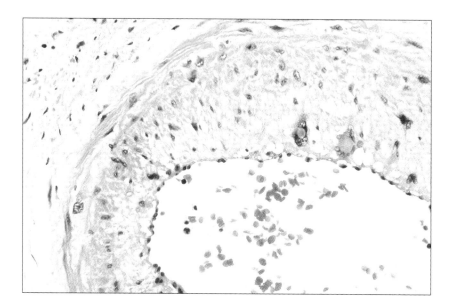

FIGURE 16–22 Lipoleiomyosarcoma showing atypia in vessel wall.

variant of ALN/WDL be clearly distinguished from ALN/WDL with low-grade dedifferentiation since the biologic behavior of the latter is more aggressive than that of lipoleiomyosarcoma.

Occasionally, ALN/WDL may have a predominantly myxoid appearance, a phenomenon which has led to the conjecture that such tumors represent either a variant of myxoid liposarcoma or a mixed type of liposarcoma. Several studies have shown that these tumors lack the TLS-CHOP fusion and therefore are unrelated to myxoid liposarcoma.[24-25]

Differential diagnosis

Various neoplastic and nonneoplastic lesions enter the differential diagnosis of ALN/WDL (Table 16-2). For most of these conditions, none of the available histochemical or immunohistochemical stains is useful. Rather, careful sampling of the material and thin, well-stained hematoxylin and eosin sections comprise the mainstay of accurate diagnosis. Lipid stains, although obviously positive in ALN/WDLs, also disclose lipid-positive deposits in the vast panorama of reactive lesions in fat and a variety of tumors.

Normal Fat with Lochkern. Normal white fat consists of spherical cells containing one large lipid vacuole that displaces the thin oval nucleus to one side. On routine sections the nucleus of most fat cells is barely perceptible. From time to time, a section grazes an adipocyte nucleus such that it is viewed en face, displaying its characteristic central vacuole, termed *lochkern* (German: hole in the nucleus) (Fig. 16-23). Nuclei *lochkern* are viewed more frequently in thick sections and, therefore, are sometimes misinterpreted as evidence of lipoblastic differentiation and hence a liposarcoma.

TABLE 16-2	LESIONS SIMULATING ALN/WDL
Lipoma with fat necrosis	
Lipoma with *lochkern*	
Fatty atrophy	
Silicone reaction	
Diffuse lipomatosis	
Spindle cell lipoma / pleomorphic lipoma	
Myolipoma	
Cellular angiolipoma	
Angiomyolipoma	
Lipomatous hemangiopericytoma	

Fat Necrosis. In areas of fat necrosis, finely granular or vacuolated macrophages are located in the vicinity of damaged fat characterized by diminished cell size, dropout of adipocytes, and chronic inflammation (Fig. 16-3). Unlike lipoblasts, these macrophages are of uniform size and have small, evenly dispersed vacuoles that do not indent the nucleus. The nucleus has a rounded shape with delicate staining. In thick sections, the nuclei of macrophages may overlap one another, giving the impression of hyperchromatism, which typifies the atypical stromal cells in ALN/WDL. It is important when making such distinctions to have suitably thin histologic sections.

Atrophy of Fat. Starvation, malnutrition, and local trauma result in atrophy of fat. Atrophy is accompanied by a loss of intracellular lipid such that the cell shrinks dramatically and assumes an epithelioid shape (Fig. 16-4). With loss of lipid, the nuclei become more prominent, and the cells superficially resemble lipoblasts. Important observations include the fact that such cells appear to be of uniform size and maintain their arrangement in lobules. With extreme atrophy the cells may contain lipofuscin.

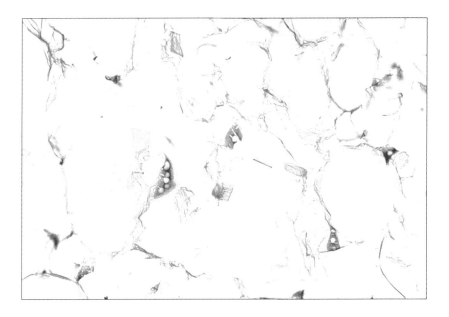

FIGURE 16–23 Nuclear vacuoles *(lochkern)* in normal fat.

Such changes are particularly noticeable in subcutaneous tissue and omentum.

Localized Massive Lymphedema. Massive forms of lymphedema restricted to a portion of the body may be confused clinically and histologically with ALN/WDL.[26] These lesions develop in morbidly obese individuals and appear to be the result of lymphedema secondary to chronic dependency of a fatty panniculus. Not surprisingly, these lesions develop in the proximal extremities and may be aggravated by underlying factors such as lymphadenectomy. Grossly and microscopically, the lesions exhibit the changes of lymphedema, including thickening of overlying skin, dermal fibrosis, ectasia and proliferation of lymphatics with focal cysts, and expansion of connective tissue septa (Fig. 16–24). A misdiagnosis of liposarcoma is attributable to the fact that the expanded connective tissue septa are believed to be part of a sclerosing liposarcoma. The septa contain mild to moderately atypical fibroblasts and delicate collagen fibrils separated by edema. In addition, there is often striking vascular proliferation at the interface between the expanded connective tissue septa and lobules of fat.

Silicone Reaction. Injection of silicone for various therapeutic and cosmetic purposes results in sheets of massively distended multivacuolated histiocytes that are disarming replicas of lipoblasts (Fig. 16–6). Lipoblasts of such quality and number are rarely encountered in true liposarcomas. Silicone reactions are also accompanied by a modest inflammatory and giant cell reaction and a large cyst with eosinophilic borders. Most silicone reactions in clinical practice are encountered around silicone breast implants but occasionally are seen on the face and in the abdomen. Free silicone can also migrate under gravitational effect and therefore is found at sites distant from the original introduction site.

Intramuscular Lipoma with Atrophic Muscle. Infrequently, atrophic skeletal muscle fibers are seen in intramuscular lipomas (Fig. 16–25). When these collections retain a clustered arrangement and have identifiable eosinophilic cytoplasm, this phenomenon is easily recognized. Isolated degenerating myofibers with barely perceptible cytoplasm understandably can be misidentified as atypical stromal cells of ALN/WDL. Positive identification can be accomplished with desmin immunostains.

Cytogenetic studies

ALN/WDL are characterized by giant marker and ring chromosomes,[27,28] sometimes as a sole finding or occasionally in association with other numerical or structural alterations.[4] The giant marker and ring chromosomes contain amplified sequences of 12q13-15, the site of several genes (e.g., MDM2, GLI, SAS, CDK4, and HMGIC). This structural abnormality results in the consistent amplification of MDM2 and the frequent amplification of the adjacent genes, SAS, CDK4, and HMG1C. Immunostaining for MDM2 and CDK4 has recently been shown to be a relatively sensitive and specific means of identifying and separating ALN/WDL from various benign lipomatous lesions.[29,30] Immunoreactivity can be detected within the nuclei of atypical spindled cells in nearly all ALN/WDL but not within deep lipomas. It should be noted, however, that a small percentage of spindle cell-pleomorphic lipomas express MDM2 and CDK4. Interestingly, nuclear MDM2 and CDK4 can also be detected by immunohistochemistry in a number of nonlipomatous sarcomas (e.g., malignant peripheral nerve sheath tumor).

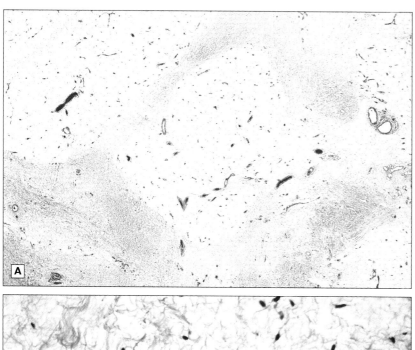

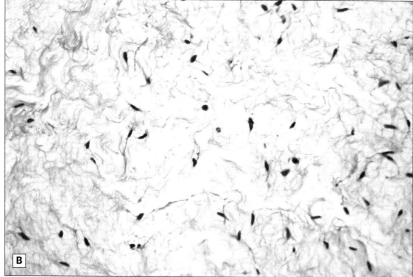

FIGURE 16–24 Changes of lymphedema that may mimic an ALN/WDL. Connective tissue septa are expanded **(A)**, with mildly atypical fibroblasts in the septa **(B)**.

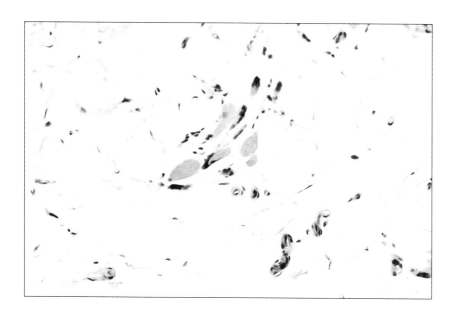

FIGURE 16–25 Atrophic muscle in an intramuscular lipoma. Degenerating myofibers are occasionally mistaken for atypical cells in liposarcomas.

Clinical behavior

ALN/WDL are nonmetastasizing lesions that are either ungraded or accorded a grade I in grading schemes. Their rate of local recurrence and disease-related mortality are strongly influenced by location,[12,13,31] however. As depicted in Table 16–3, tumors in the extremities have significantly lower rates of local recurrence than those in the retroperitoneum. Extremity lesions recur in nearly one-half of cases, whereas in the retroperitoneum recurrence rates approach 100%.[13] One could legitimately argue that ALN/WDL of the retroperitoneum is basically an incurable lesion. About one-third of patients die as a direct result of their disease, but this figure increases with longer follow-up periods owing to the indolent growth of these lesions. On the other hand, those rare ALN/WDL that occur in the subcutaneous tissues are generally cured by limited excisions. Although the data reported by Azumi et al.[32] and Evans et al.[31] indicate essentially no recurrences of ALN/WDL of the subcutis, it should be noted that some of the tumors included in this group were spindle cell and pleomorphic lipomas, which are known to have a benign course. Nonetheless, the thrust of their collective data appears accurate.

Lest well-differentiated ALN/WDL be dismissed as little more than benign but locally aggressive lesions, a small percentage of these tumors over time dedifferentiate or progress histologically to a higher grade lesion (dedifferentiated liposarcoma).[12,13,33] Although this phenomenon occurs most frequently with retroperitoneal liposarcomas, it also occurs with deep extremity lesions; it is rare in subcutaneous tumors. It, therefore, does not appear to be a site-specific phenomenon as was formerly believed but a time-dependent phenomenon encountered in those locations in which there is a high likelihood of clinical persistence of disease. With retroperitoneal tumors, for which complete excision is a veritable impossibility, there is a substantial risk of dedifferentiation (about 10–15%); it is somewhat lower for extremity lesions (5%). In ALN/WDL that have been followed longitudinally, dedifferentiation occurs after an average of 7–8 years but may be seen as long as 16–20 years after the original diagnosis. Once dedifferentiation occurs, the lesions can usually be considered fully malignant sarco-mas. An exception is the rare tumor in which dedifferentiation is restricted to an extremely small focus (see Minimal dedifferentiation, below).

Because of site-dependent differences in behavior of "well-differentiated liposarcoma," "atypical lipoma" was a term originally introduced in 1979 by Evans et al. and used by others[34] for WDL of the subcutis and deep muscles of the extremity.[31] At that time, these authors suggested retention of the term "ALN/WDL" for lesions in the retroperitoneum, but later recommended that this term be abandoned altogether in favor of the term "atypical lipomatous tumor." To avoid confusion, the WHO has endorsed the combined term ALN/WDL for all lesions previously diagnosed as atypical lipoma, atypical lipomatous neoplasm, or ALN/WDL. We believe there is merit in retaining the term WDL for retroperitoneal, mediastinal or body cavity lesions to emphasize the life-threatening nature of these tumors in these locations, to assure adequate therapy and follow-up care, and to acknowledge the risk of dedifferentiation over time. However, implied in the foregoing discussion is the understanding that *atypical lipomatous neoplasm and ALN/WDL are synonyms, and the choice of one over the other in the past has been based on the location of the lesion rather than a constellation of subtle histologic differences.*

Unfortunately, it has not been possible to predict in the individual case which ALN/WDL will dedifferentiate. Comparison of ALN/WDL with the ALN/WDL component of dedifferentiated liposarcomas discloses no significant differences in immunohistochemical expression patterns for P53, MDM2, p21WAF1, and MIB1,[35,36] although overexpression is more prevalent in the dedifferentiated components. Comparison of gene expression profile between pure ALN/WDL and ALN/WDL that have dedifferentiated disclose differences, but those differences have not been applied prospectively to identify lesions at greatest risk to dedifferentiate.[37] Analysis of P53 mutations by molecular methods disclosed abnormalities in this gene in fewer than 10% of cases, but there were *MDM2* gene abnormalities in well over half of the dedifferentiated liposarcomas in both the well differentiated and nonlipogenic areas, suggesting that P53 inactivation occurs via the *MDM2* pathway.[38] For the moment, all ALN/WDLs of deep soft tissues should be considered at

TABLE 16–3	BEHAVIOR OF 83 ALN/WDLs			
Site	Recurrence (%)	Died of disease (%)	Dedifferentiation (%)	Years of follow-up range and median
Extremity	43	0	6	2–25 (9)
Retroperitoneum	91	33	17	1–35 (10)
Groin	79	14	28	2–25 (8)
Total	63	11	13	

From Weiss SW, Rao VK. ALN/WDL (atypical lipoma) of deep soft tissue of the extremities, retroperitoneum and miscellaneous sites: a follow-up study of 92 cases with analysis of the incidence of "dedifferentiation." Am J Surg Pathol 1992; 16:1051.

risk to dedifferentiate, although that risk varies with the location and duration of disease.

DEDIFFERENTIATED LIPOSARCOMA

Dedifferentiation or histologic progression to a higher-grade, less well-differentiated neoplasm was first described by Dahlin as a late complication in the natural history of well-differentiated chondrosarcoma, but it is now known to occur in other low-grade mesenchymal tumors including parosteal osteosarcoma, chordoma, and ALN/WDL.[39-41] Traditionally, dedifferentiated liposarcomas were defined as ALN/WDL juxtaposed to areas of high-grade nonlipogenic sarcoma, usually resembling either a fibrosarcoma or malignant fibrous histiocytoma. Dedifferentiation was believed to occur after a latent period of several years. These views have now been modified. Whereas most dedifferentiated liposarcomas display high-grade dedifferentiation, a small number contain exclusively low-grade areas or a combination of low- and high-grade areas.[40,42,43] Second, in most dedifferentiated liposarcomas encountered in clinical practice, the dedifferentiated foci are seen at the original excision (primary dedifferentiation, dedifferentiation ab initio). Arguably, they could be examples of secondary dedifferentiation that were biopsied late in their course.

Clinical features

Dedifferentiated liposarcomas develop in approximately the same age group as ALN/WDL, reaching a peak during the early seventh decade.[40-42] The sexes are affected approximately equally. Unlike ALN/WDL, location in the retroperitoneum is favored over deep soft tissues of the extremities by a margin of nearly 3 : 1. Fewer than 20% of dedifferentiated liposarcomas occur collectively in the head, neck, trunk, and spermatic cord and less than 1% in subcutaneous sites.[44] Radiographically, they have areas characteristic of ALN/WDL but have, in addition, mass-like areas of nonfatty tissue. The latter have imaging characteristics similar to other sarcomas, with prolonged T1 and T2 relaxation by MRI and attenuation coefficients higher than that for normal fat on CT scans.[45]

Gross and microscopic features

The lesions present as large multinodular masses ranging in color from yellow to yellow-tan admixed with firm tan-gray areas that correspond to the dedifferentiated foci. Microscopically, the lesions consist of areas of ALN/WDL that display the range of changes described above and a nonlipogenic (dedifferentiated) component. The interface between the two zones is typically abrupt (Fig. 16–26), although in some cases there is a gradual transition between the two (Fig. 16–27). Rarely, the two patterns co-mingle, giving the impression of mosaicism (Fig. 16–28).

In about 90% of cases, the dedifferentiated zones have the appearance of a high-grade fibrosarcoma or malignant fibrous histiocytoma (pleomorphic undifferentiated sarcoma) (Figs 16–29, 16–30). Those areas resembling malignant fibrous histiocytoma may display the full range of subtypes, from the common storiform pleomorphic and myxoid types (high-grade myxofibrosarcoma) to the less common giant cell and inflammatory forms, including some with a dense lymphoid component.[46] Dedifferentiated areas resembling inflammatory malignant fibrous histiocytoma have been associated with leukemoid blood reactions.[10] In fact, based on a combi-

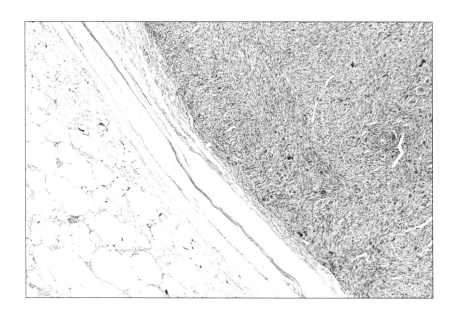

FIGURE 16–26 Dedifferentiated liposarcoma with sharp abutment of two zones.

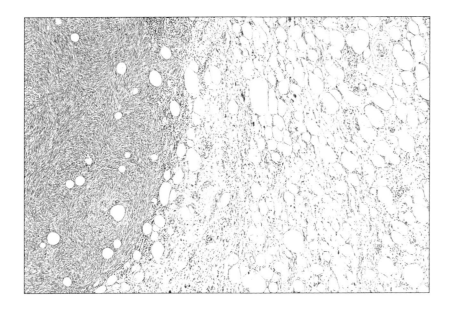

FIGURE 16–27 Dedifferentiated liposarcoma with an indistinct margin between well-differentiated and dedifferentiated zones.

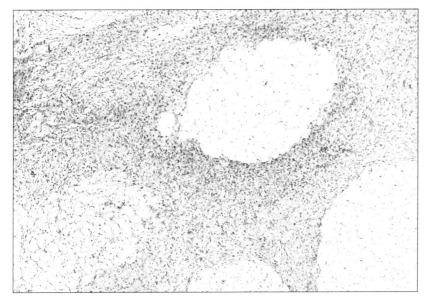

FIGURE 16–28 Mosaic pattern of a dedifferentiated liposarcoma.

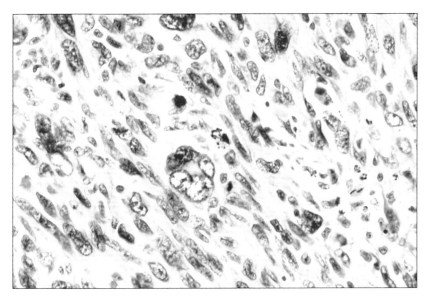

FIGURE 16–29 Dedifferentiated liposarcoma with areas resembling high-grade malignant fibrous histiocytoma.

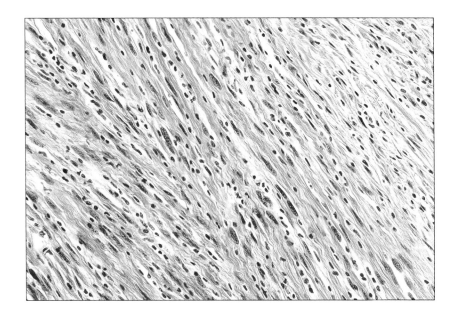

FIGURE 16–30 Dedifferentiated liposarcoma with areas having the appearance of a fibrosarcoma.

nation of genomic profiling and MDM2 and CDK4 status, it has recently been suggested that most so-called inflammatory malignant fibrous histiocytomas are, in fact, dedifferentiated liposarcomas.[47,48] Some dedifferentiated areas depart from the foregoing description and resemble a low-grade fibrosarcoma or fibromatosis. Usually, these areas coexist with areas of high-grade dedifferentiation, but in about 10% of cases only low-grade areas are present (Fig. 16–31). A number of unusual patterns are seen in dedifferentiated zones (Figs 16–32 to 16–34). They include undifferentiated large round cells in areas resembling a carcinoma or melanoma (Fig. 16–33), spindle cell areas containing whorled structures reminiscent of a meningioma or nerve sheath tumor (Fig. 16–32),[40,49,50] areas with a pericytic pattern, amianthoid fibers (Fig. 16–34), and divergent rhabdomyosarcomatous,[51] osteosarcomatous, or leiomyosarcomatous elements (Figs 16–35, 16–36).[40]

Ultrastructurally, the dedifferentiated zones display little lipogenic differentiation. The cells have well-developed rough endoplasmic reticulum, primitive cell junctions, and prominent lysosomes. Occasional cells have a small amount of cytoplasmic lipid.[52]

Differential diagnosis

Sarcoma Infiltrating Fat. The most common problem in the differential diagnosis is distinguishing between a pleomorphic sarcoma infiltrating fat and a dedifferentiated liposarcoma. We believe there should be clear-cut evidence of ALN/WDL some distance from the dedifferentiated areas for the diagnosis of dedifferentiated liposarcoma. Evaluating a high-grade sarcoma at its interface with normal fat results in an inappropriately low threshold for the diagnosis of dedifferentiated liposarcoma.

Minimal Dedifferentiation. A relatively rare problem with the diagnosis is finding a microscopic focus of dedifferentiation in an otherwise typical ALN/WDL. We have adopted the position that dedifferentiation ought to be macroscopically visible (>1.0 cm) before the label "dedifferentiated liposarcoma" is applied. Even so, it is likely that small foci of dedifferentiation (1–2 cm), which we have termed "minimal" or "early" dedifferentiation, are associated with a prolonged clinical course. For example, we have followed a patient with a 3 cm focus of dedifferentiation that evolved into a fully dedifferentiated tumor over a 25-year course. Nonetheless, the above case serves to illustrate the fact that even tumors with minimal dedifferentiation can progress to full-fledged dedifferentiated liposarcomas. We believe such cases should be individualized and signed out in a descriptive fashion, indicating the size of the dedifferentiated focus, until additional data are available.

Clinical behavior

The behavior of dedifferentiated liposarcomas appears to be similar to, but perhaps slightly better than, that of other pleomorphic high-grade sarcomas in adults.[40] Altogether, 41% of patients experience local recurrences and 17% metastasis, with 28% dying of their tumors. These figures reflect the accelerated tempo of the disease once dedifferentiation occurs. Whereas the metastatic rate might appear low compared to that of some high-grade sarcomas, two points should be emphasized. First, most patients die of the local effects of their tumor before distant metastasis becomes apparent; and second, it is difficult to determine accurately which criteria differentiate between local (contiguous) intra-abdominal spread and local metastasis. For these reasons the

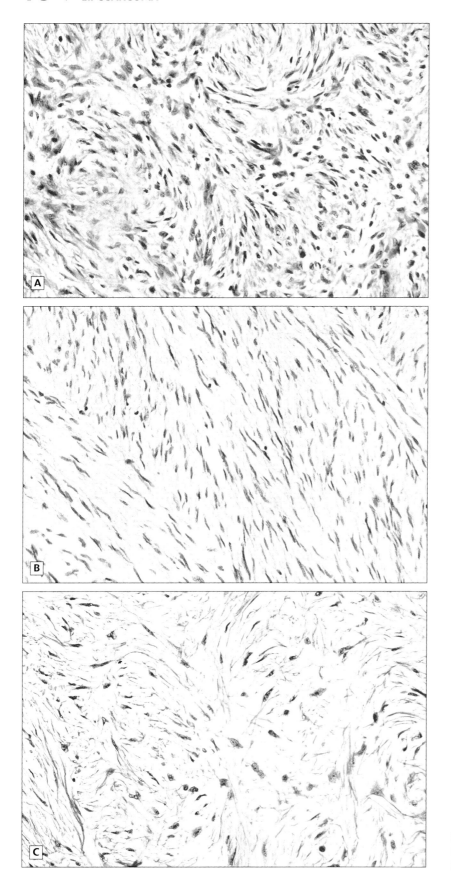

FIGURE 16–31 Dedifferentiated liposarcoma with low-grade dedifferentiation, ranging from grade II **(A)** to grade I **(B, C)**.

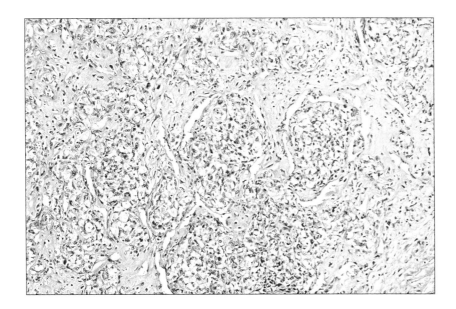

FIGURE 16–32 Dedifferentiated liposarcoma with areas of whorled structures.

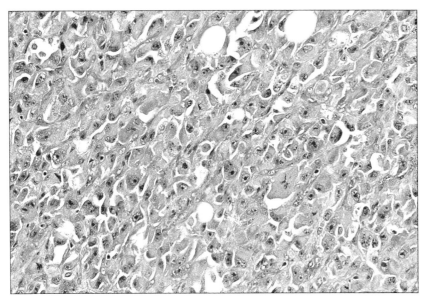

FIGURE 16–33 Dedifferentiated liposarcoma composed of undifferentiated large round cells.

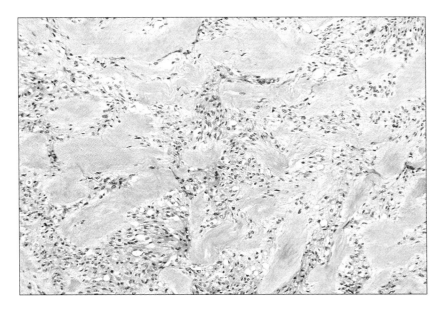

FIGURE 16–34 Dedifferentiated liposarcoma with amianthoid fibers.

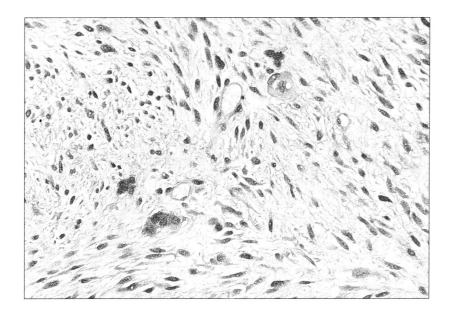

FIGURE 16–35 Dedifferentiated liposarcoma with rhabdomyosarcomatous differentiation in dedifferentiated areas.

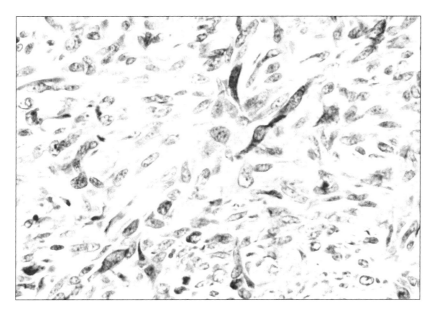

FIGURE 16–36 Dedifferentiated liposarcoma with rhabdomyosarcomatous differentiation in dedifferentiated areas. Desmin immunostain decorates rhabdomyoblasts.

metastatic rate, determined with an average follow-up of 3 years, represents a conservative estimate of metastatic potential.[40]

Among the various prognostic factors, site appears to be the most significant. As with ALN/WDL, the dedifferentiated liposarcomas located in the retroperitoneum have the worst prognosis. Although one might anticipate that the extent and grade of dedifferentiation would affect outcome, it does not appear to be true for the range of tumors commonly encountered in clinical practice.[40] What this seems to imply is that once these tumors are clinically apparent the amount of dedifferentiation is already so significant that quantitating and grading these zones does not provide any additional stratification that can identify good and poor prognosis subgroups. Furthermore, the fact that patients with low-grade dedifferentiation may suffer the same untoward consequences as those with high-grade dedifferentiation indicates that the traditional definition of dedifferentiation (high-grade nonlipogenic sarcoma) should be expanded to include low-grade nonlipogenic sarcomas as well.

MYXOID LIPOSARCOMA

Myxoid liposarcoma embraces a continuum of lesions which includes at one extreme highly differentiated myxoid tumors with ample lipoblastic differentiation to poorly differentiated round cell tumors in which lipoblastic differentiation is inconspicuous at best, the latter endpoint sometimes referred to as "round cell liposarcoma." Evidence supporting the idea that these two histologic extremes represent the same tumor category is derived from their similarity in terms of age, location, and cytogenetic abnormalities and by the identification of tumors with transitional or hybrid features.[53–55] Because of the range in observed behavior of this tumor, it is essential that some measure of biologic aggressiveness be given either in the form of a grade or an estimate of round cell areas (see below).

Clinical features

Myxoid liposarcomas account for about one-third to one-half of all liposarcomas. Unlike ALN/WDL and dedifferentiated liposarcomas, this form occurs in a younger age group, with a peak incidence during the fifth decade. It develops preferentially in the lower extremity (75%), particularly the medial thigh and popliteal area, and less frequently in the retroperitoneum (Fig. 16–37). Radiographically, these lesions are quite varied. Typically they appear as nonhomogeneous masses on CT scans. The attenuation values of highly myxoid lesions exceed those of normal fat but are less than that of the surrounding soft tissue. Less-differentiated round cell areas have attenuation values similar to those of other soft tissue sarcomas.[14]

Gross and microscopic features

Grossly, pure or predominantly myxoid liposarcomas are multinodular, gelatinous masses usually devoid of necrosis, although occasionally hemorrhage is encountered (Fig. 16–38). Those tumors with discrete areas of round cell liposarcoma have corresponding opaque white nodules situated in the myxoid mass, whereas those that are predominantly round cell have a white fleshy appearance similar to that of other high-grade sarcomas.

Histologically pure myxoid liposarcomas bear a marked similarity to developing fetal fat (Figs 16–39 to 16–44). At low power, the lesion is a multinodular mass of low cellularity with enhanced cellularity at the periphery (Fig. 16–40). Each nodule is composed of bland fusiform or round cells that lie suspended individually in a myxoid matrix composed of hyaluronic acid. Mitotic figures are typically rare or absent altogether. A delicate plexiform capillary vascular network is present throughout these tumors and provides an important clue for distinguishing them from myxomas. The proliferating neoplastic cells recapitulate, albeit imperfectly, the sequence of adipocyte differentiation. Immature spindled cells lacking obvious lipogenesis may be seen next to multivacuolar and univacuolar lipoblasts. Although lipoblasts are usually easy to identify in these liposarcomas, they may be especially prominent at the periphery of the tumor nodules (Fig. 16–41).

The hyaluronic acid-rich (Alcian blue-positive; hyaluronidase-sensitive)[56] stroma (Figs 16–45 to 16–47) is

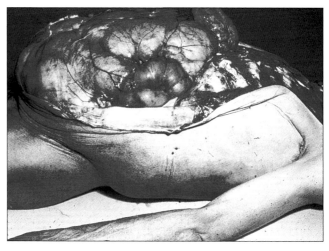

FIGURE 16–37 Myxoid liposarcoma massively replacing the abdominal contents.

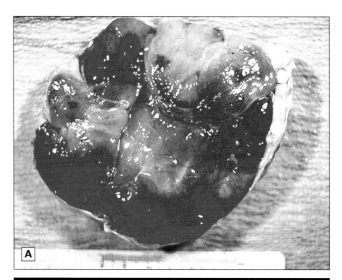

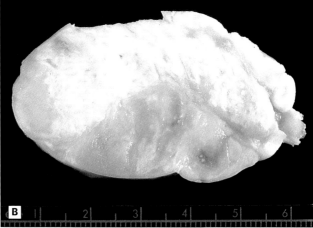

FIGURE 16–38 Gross specimen of a pure myxoid liposarcoma with a gelatinous cut surface **(A)** compared to a liposarcoma that contains myxoid (gelatinous) and round cell (opaque) areas **(B)**.

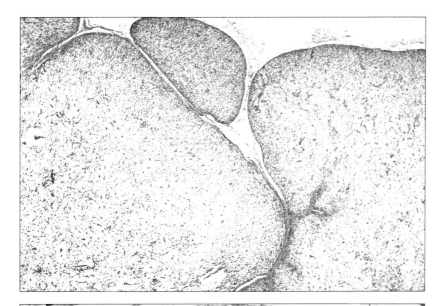

FIGURE 16–39 Multinodular appearance of a myxoid liposarcoma.

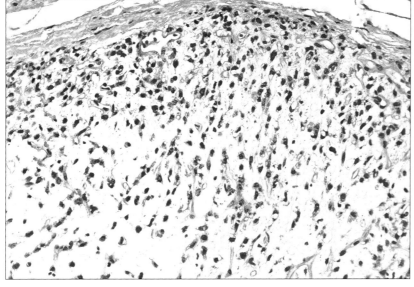

FIGURE 16–40 Enhanced cellularity at the periphery of nodules in a myxoid liposarcoma.

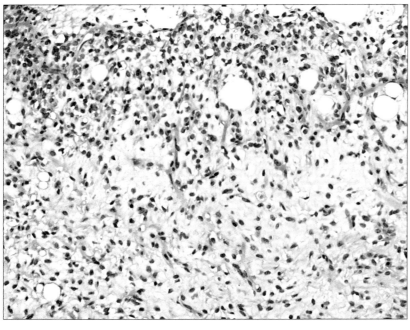

FIGURE 16–41 Myxoid liposarcoma with characteristic lipoblastic differentiation at the periphery.

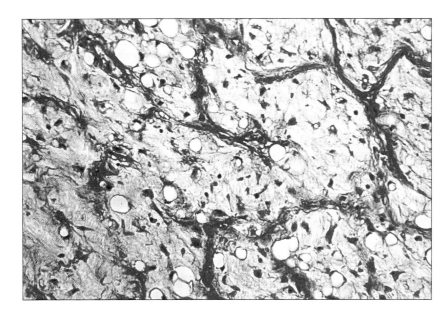

FIGURE 16–42 Typical appearance of a myxoid liposarcoma.

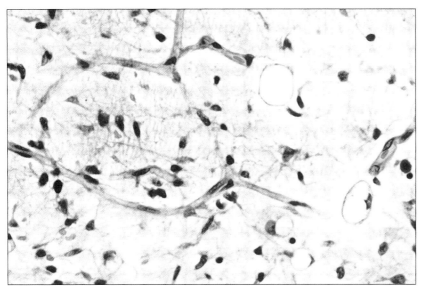

FIGURE 16–43 Myxoid liposarcoma with arborizing vasculature and lipoblasts at varying stages.

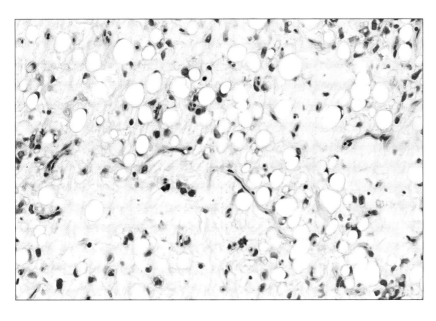

FIGURE 16–44 Myxoid liposarcoma with a larger number of mature lipoblasts than seen in Figure 16–43.

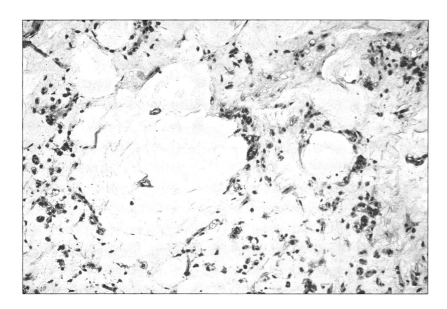

FIGURE 16–45 Small pools of stromal mucin in myxoid liposarcoma.

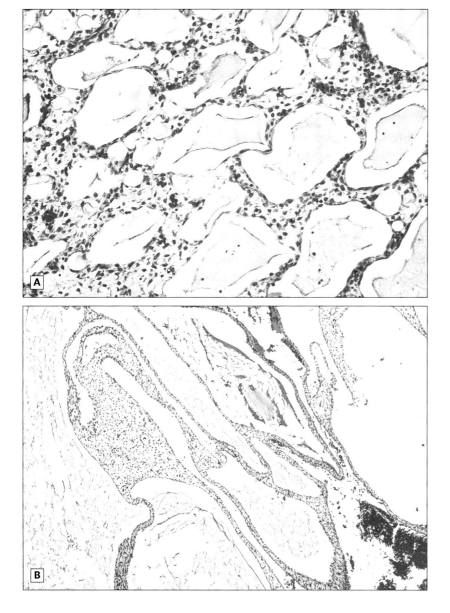

FIGURE 16–46 (A) Pools of stromal mucin in a myxoid liposarcoma forming a sieve pattern. **(B)** Pools of stromal mucin forming cysts.

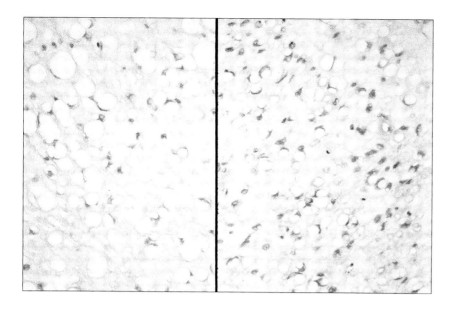

FIGURE 16–47 Alcian blue staining of myxoid liposarcoma before **(left)** and after **(right)** hyaluronidase digestion. Stromal mucin staining is abolished following enzyme treatment, indicating the presence of hyaluronic acid.

present primarily in the extracellular space but may also be found in individual tumor cells. Frequently, the extracellular mucin forms large pools, creating a cribriform or lace-like pattern in the tumor and infrequently gross cysts (Figs 16–45, 16–46). The cellular condensation at the rim of these pools produces a pseudoacinar pattern. In others, the weak staining of accumulated mucin and the flattened tumor cells mimic a lymphangioma. Interstitial hemorrhage is common and may be so prominent that the tumor is confused with a hemangioma. Focal cartilaginous,[57,58] leiomyomatous, or osseous differentiation occurs in myxoid liposarcomas. These elements do not appear to affect the prognosis. The significance of rhabdomyosarcomatous differentiation (Figs 16–48 to 16–50), which we have encountered once and which has been reported anecdotally in the literature, is uncertain.[59]

As myxoid liposarcomas lose their differentiation, they assume an increasingly round cell appearance, which is expressed in one of two ways. Amid a myxoid backdrop one may encounter a pure round cell nodule (Fig. 16–51) characterized by sheets of primitive round cells with a high nuclear/cytoplasmic ratio and a prominent nucleolus. In these areas, the cells are so numerous that essentially they lie back to back with no intervening myxoid stroma; and the capillary vascular pattern, though present, cannot be visualized easily. More commonly, however, the progression toward round cell areas is reflected in a more gradual fashion; and, instead, one encounters areas with transitional features (Fig. 16–52). In these areas the cellularity is clearly greater, and the cells are usually larger with a more rounded shape. At what point one applies the label "round cell" has been problematic. Smith et al. suggested that for a threshold definition for round cell differentiation there should be

areas in which the cells acquire a rounded shape and have overlapping nuclei such that one can easily identify clusters of cells sitting back to back.[60] On the other hand, they did not regard areas of enhanced cellularity with cells lying individually in a myxoid background as sufficient for a diagnosis of round cell differentiation, as these "transitional areas" did not correlate with an adverse outcome (Fig. 16–52A).

Occasionally, round cell areas are characterized by branching cords and rows of primitive small rounded cells (Figs 16–53, Fig 16–54) or large cells with an eosinophilic granular or multivacuolar cytoplasm resembling malignant brown fat cells. Solidly cellular round cell areas, out of context, can be difficult to recognize as a liposarcoma unless an occasional lipoblast is identified. In fact, in the absence of a lipoblast one might entertain a diagnosis of another round cell sarcoma or a lymphoma. Finally, there have been a few exceptional myxoid/round cell liposarcomas that have displayed dedifferentiated areas similar to those seen in ALN/WDLs.[61]

Ancillary studies

The diagnosis of myxoid/round cell liposarcoma continues to be based primarily on review of routine histologic sections, although ultrastructural studies effectively demonstrate lipogenic differentiation. The cells in myxoid liposarcoma display a range of differentiation from primitive mesenchymal cells with high nuclear/cytoplasmic ratios, few organelles, and discontinuous basal lamina to identifiable lipoblasts containing nonmembrane-bound lipid. In the less differentiated round cell areas the cells tend have more mitochondria, numerous polyribosomes, and fewer lipid vacuoles (Figs 16–55, 16–56).[62–66]

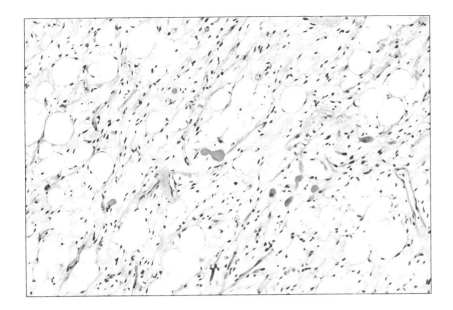

FIGURE 16–48 Unusual myxoid liposarcoma with rhabdomyoblastic differentiation.

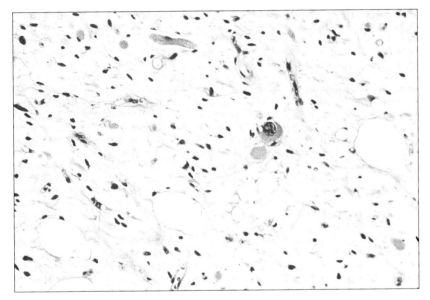

FIGURE 16–49 Rhabdomyoblasts in a myxoid liposarcoma.

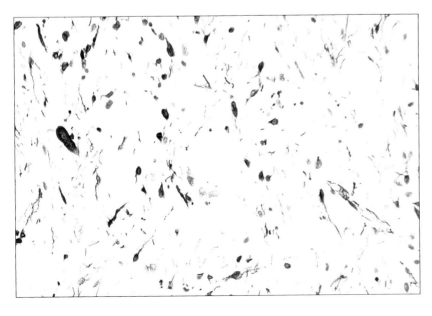

FIGURE 16–50 Desmin-positive rhabdomyoblasts in myxoid liposarcoma.

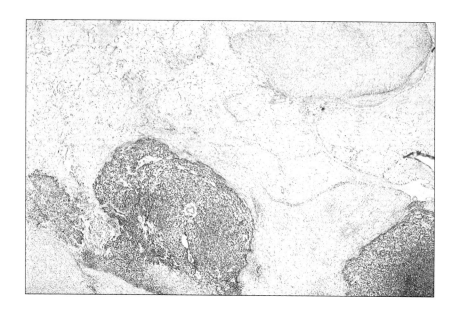

FIGURE 16–51 Myxoid liposarcoma with sharply demarcated nodules of round cell liposarcoma.

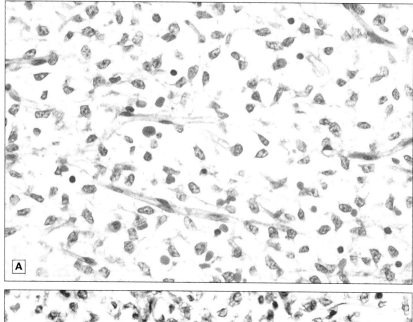

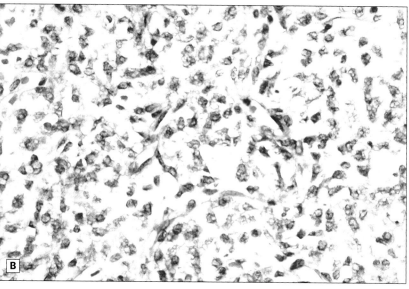

FIGURE 16–52 Myxoid/round cell liposarcoma with progressive transition, from somewhat cellular myxoid areas **(A)** to borderline areas **(B)** to round cell liposarcoma **(C, D)** where cells have overlapping nuclei and some residual myxoid stroma. Round cell areas without myxoid stroma **(E)** may be impossible to diagnose as liposarcoma.

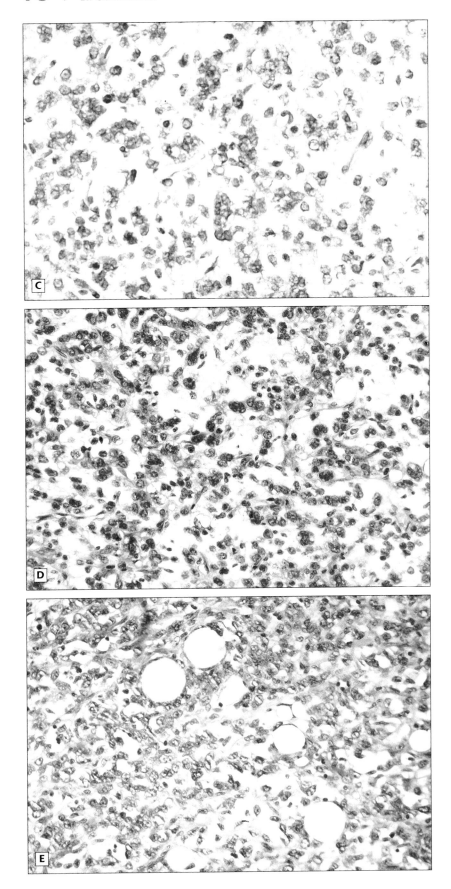

FIGURE 16–52 Continued.

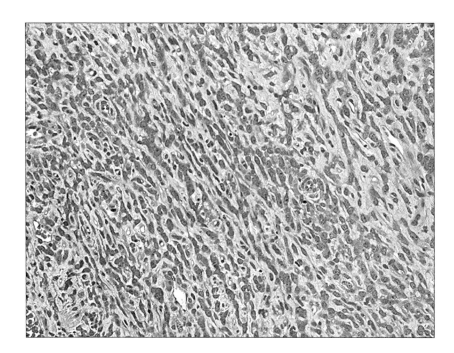

FIGURE 16–53 Cord-like pattern in a round cell liposarcoma.

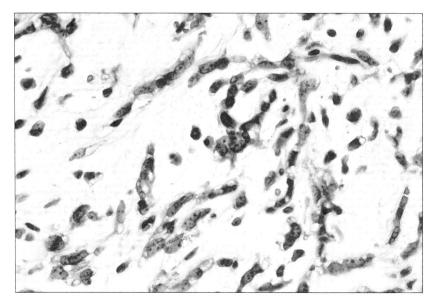

FIGURE 16–54 Cord-like pattern and stromal hyalinization in a round cell liposarcoma.

Differential diagnosis

The differential diagnosis of myxoid liposarcoma includes a wide range of lesions that appear myxoid (Table 16–4). The two most common myxoid sarcomas of adults that are confused with myxoid liposarcoma are myxoid malignant fibrous histiocytoma and myxoid chondrosarcoma. The former is characterized by a significant degree of nuclear atypia and a coarser vasculature than is encountered in myxoid liposarcomas. It is tempting to interpret the pleomorphic vacuolated cells encountered in these tumors as lipoblasts and to draw the erroneous conclusion that the tumor is a liposarcoma (Fig. 16–7). The vacuoles of these pseudolipoblasts are large, poorly defined, and filled with hyaluronic acid rather than lipid.

Myxoid chondrosarcomas are composed of small, distinctly eosinophilic cells typically arranged in small clusters, cords, or pseudoacini, unlike the single cell arrangement in pure myxoid liposarcomas. The myxoid background in well-stained hematoxylin and eosin sections usually has a pale blue appearance in contrast to the clear appearance of the stroma in myxoid liposarcomas. Extremely myxoid forms of dermatofibrosarcoma protuberans occasionally closely mimic myxoid liposarcoma, but the superficial location of such lesions and the lack of lipoblastic differentiation are important observations that alert one to the correct diagnosis.

The diagnosis of myxoid liposarcoma with predominantly round cell areas fundamentally rests on finding unequivocal areas of myxoid liposarcoma or lipoblasts in

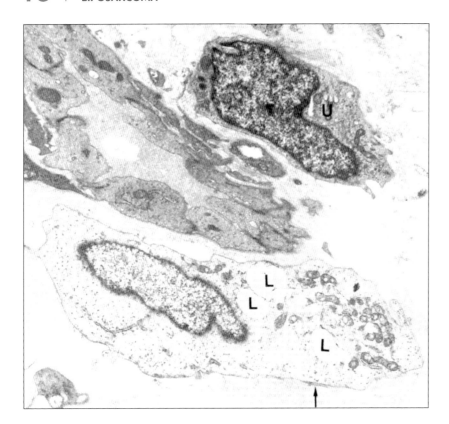

FIGURE 16–55 Electron micrograph of a myxoid liposarcoma showing an undifferentiated mesenchymal cell (U) and lipoblasts with multiple non-membrane-bound lipid inclusions (L). Note the basal lamina (arrow). (From Taxy JB, Battifora H. The electron microscope in the study and diagnosis of soft tissue tumors. In: Trump BF, Jones RT, eds. Diagnostic electron microscopy. New York: Wiley; 1980, with permission.)

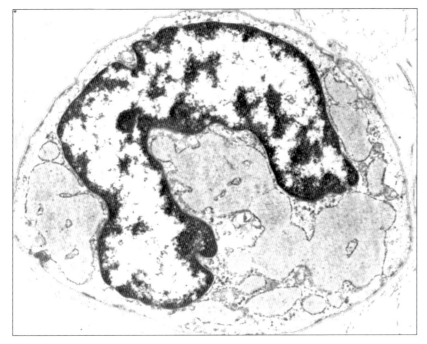

FIGURE 16–56 Electron micrograph of an undifferentiated mesenchymal cell from a myxoid liposarcoma. The cell has dilated endoplasmic reticulum filled with granular material suggestive of mucopolysaccharide and is surrounded by a basal lamina. (From Taxy JB, Battifora H. The electron microscope in the study and diagnosis of soft tissue tumors. In: Trump BF, Jones RT, eds. Diagnostic electron microscopy. New York: Wiley; 1980, with permission.)

TABLE 16–4	LESIONS SIMULATING MYXOID LIPOSARCOMA

Myxoma (intramuscular and cutaneous forms)
Angiomyxoma
Myxoid dermatofibrosarcoma protuberans
Myxoid chondrosarcoma
Myxoid malignant fibrous histiocytoma, low grade (myxofibrosarcoma)

the lesion. Fortunately, pure round cell liposarcomas are extraordinarily rare, and one can almost always find at least a few better differentiated diagnostic zones. Obviously, ancillary studies to exclude other round cell sarcomas such as rhabdomyosarcoma, poorly differentiated (round cell) synovial sarcoma, and Ewing's sarcoma/primitive neuroectodermal tumors are important in selected cases (see Chapter 31).

Cytogenetic and molecular studies

Nearly all myxoid/round cell liposarcomas are characterized by a reciprocal translocation between chromosomes 12 and 16: t(12;16)(q13; p11).[54,57,67–69] This molecular event results in fusion of the *CHOP* gene on chromosome 12 with the *FUS* gene on chromosome 16. Rarely, a translocation between chromosomes 12 and 22,[70,71] t(12;22)(q13; p11), or an insertion between chromosomes 12 and 16, (12;16)(q13; p11.2p13), occurs.[72] The normal *CHOP* gene encodes a DNA transcription factor, whereas the *FUS* gene encodes an RNA binding protein with an affinity for steroid, thyroid hormone, and retinoid receptors.[73] The chimeric *FUS-CHOP* gene gives rise to at least three fusion transcripts,[74–76] one of which (type II) has been identified in most myxoid/round cell liposarcomas. When introduced experimentally into preadipocyte cell lines, this transcript renders them unresponsive to adipogenic stimulation and adipocytic genes.[75] These cells also lose the property of contact inhibition and are capable of generating tumors in nude mice. Interestingly, it has also been possible to detect chimeric *FUS/CHOP* DNA in peripheral blood of patients with myxoid/round cell liposarcoma by means of the polymerase chain reaction. Detection of genomic DNA in peripheral blood has not been correlated with clinical outcome on the basis of the few cases studied, however.[71]

A number of studies has focused on the integrity of the P53 pathway in this group of neoplasms.[77,78] Unlike ALN/WDL, in which only a small percentage demonstrate aberrations in this pathway, about 30% of myxoid/round cell liposarcomas have mutations in this gene, indicating differences among subsets of liposarcoma in terms of molecular oncogenic events.

Clinical course

In the past it has been difficult to assess the behavior of myxoid liposarcomas because of the lack of common criteria for making the diagnosis, the failure to distinguish the pure myxoid forms of the tumor from those having a significant round cell component, and the inability to compare outcome based on common therapeutic strategies.[5] There seems to be general agreement now that the amount of round cell differentiation figures prominently into metastasis and survival, the question centering on the appropriate threshold levels one should use. Kilpatrick et al. have employed a three-tiered system (0–5%; 5–25%; >25% round cell component),[53] whereas Antonescu et al. proposed a two-tiered system (< or ≥5% round cell component).[79] Either way, tumors should be well sampled (utilizing one section per centimeter tumor diameter) and the proportion of round cell component qualitatively estimated. This approach deals only with the percentage of round cell component, not the absolute amount. Therefore, it does not allow for disparities that might occur between a small liposarcoma containing a large proportion of round cells and a large liposarcoma containing a low proportion of round cells.

Despite the shortcomings, both a two- and three-tiered system show excellent correlation with survival and metastasis (Table 16–5). In the Mayo Clinic experience, 35% of patients with myxoid liposarcoma developed metastasis, and 31% died of their tumors. Using a multivariate analysis, age (>45 years), the percentage of round cell differentiation (< or >25%) and the presence of spontaneous necrosis were significantly associated with a poor prognosis (Table 16–6).[53] In the study by Antonescu et al., high histologic grade defined as ≥5% round cell component, necrosis (≥5% of tumor mass) and overexpression of P53 immunostaining correlated significantly with reduced metastasis-free survival (Figs 16–57, 16–58). Interestingly, there was no correlation between *FUS-CHOP* fusion type and grade or disease-specific survival.[79]

Although myxoid/round cell liposarcoma metastasizes to usual sites, such as lung and bone, it displays a curious tendency, unlike all other liposarcomas, to metastasize to other soft tissue sites. Of the 16 metastatic myxoid liposarcomas reported by Evans, 12 metastasized to soft tissue sites, 7 to lung, and 8 to bone.[80]

TABLE 16–5	MYXOID/ROUND CELL LIPOSARCOMA: CORRELATION OF ROUND CELL DIFFERENTIATION WITH CLINICAL OUTCOME	
Round cell population (%)		**Metastasis**
0–5		11/48 (23%)
5–10		5/14 (35%)
>25%		14/24 (58%)

From Kilpatrick SE, Doyon J, Choong PF, et al. The clinicopathologic spectrum of myxoid and round cell liposarcoma: a study of 95 cases. Cancer 1996; 77:1450.

TABLE 16–6	MYXOID/ROUND CELL LIPOSARCOMA: CORRELATION OF CLINICAL AND HISTOLOGIC FEATURES WITH SURVIVAL	
Feature	**5-year survival (%)**	**10-year survival (%)**
Age (years)		
<45	88	80
>45	72	50
Necrosis		
Yes	25	0
No	90	70
Round cell (%)		
<25	89	66
>25	79	40

From Kilpatrick SE, Doyon J, Choong PF, et al. The clinicopathologic spectrum of myxoid and round cell liposarcoma: a study of 95 cases. Cancer 1996; 77:1450.

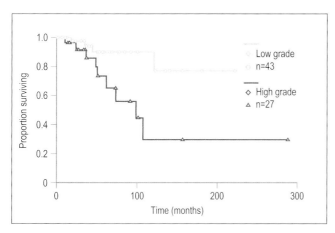

FIGURE 16–57 Disease-free survival in myxoid liposarcoma based on amount of round cell component. Low-grade lesion have <5% round cell component; whereas high-grade lesions have ≥5%. (From Antonescu et al. Clin Cancer Res 2001, with permission).

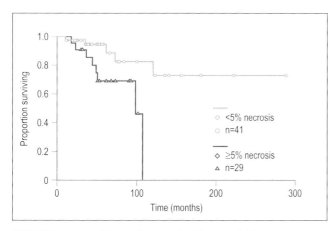

FIGURE 16–58 Disease-free survival in myxoid liposarcoma based on amount of necrosis. (From Antonescu et al. Clin Cancer Res 2001, with permission).

PLEOMORPHIC LIPOSARCOMA

Pleomorphic liposarcoma is the least common and consequently the least well understood of the various liposarcomas. It represents less than 15% of all liposarcomas,[1,2,7,81,82] develops during late adult life, and is equally distributed between the retroperitoneum and deep somatic soft tissues of the extremities. About one-quarter develop in skin or subcutis.[83]

Pleomorphic liposarcomas display two related but clearly distinguishable histologic patterns which may coexist within the same tumor. Both share a disorderly growth pattern and an extreme degree of cellular pleomorphism, including bizarre giant cells, but they differ in their content of intracellular lipid material. The more common pattern resembles a malignant fibrous histiocytoma but contains, in addition, giant lipoblasts with bizarre hyperchromatic, scalloped nuclei, many of which have a deeply acidophilic cytoplasm with eosinophilic hyaline droplets (Fig. 16–59). In the absence of these characteristic univacuolated or multivacuolated lipoblasts (which may require careful sampling to identify), these lesions are routinely diagnosed as malignant fibrous histiocytoma or rhabdomyosarcoma.

The second pattern in pleomorphic liposarcoma is less common. It consists mainly of sheets of large pleomorphic giant cells associated with smaller mononuclear forms (Figs 16–60 to Fig. 16–62). Both cell types are highly vacuolated and lipid rich, and lipoblasts are easy to identify (in contrast to those in the first type of pleomorphic liposarcoma). Depending on the relative proportions of the two cell populations, this form of liposarcoma can be a highly anaplastic tumor or a small round clear-cell tumor resembling a carcinoma or melanoma. Tumors with a plethora of small round clear cells have been termed "epithelioid" variant of pleomorphic liposarcoma and are important because of their close mimicry of adrenal cortical carcinoma. Although these tumors can focally express keratin, actin, desmin, and S-100 protein[83,84] they neither express inhibin nor manifest ultrastructural features of steroid-producing tumors (i.e., smooth endoplasmic reticulum).[85]

Based on several recent studies, pleomorphic liposarcomas are fully malignant high-grade sarcomas with local recurrence and metastatic rates of 30–40% and overall 5-year survival of 55–65%.[83,84] Superficial lesions have a far better prognosis. In multivariate analyses, age, size, and central location were predictive of adverse outcome in pleomorphic liposarcoma.

Given the rarity of these lesions, there are far fewer cytogenetic and molecular data pertaining to this form of liposarcoma. Although pleomorphic and dedifferentiated liposarcoma share overlapping histologic features, cytogenetic and expression profiling studies indicate that these two tumors are quite different,[86,87] and there is certainly no morphologic evidence of pleomorphic liposarcomas arising from a low-grade precursor lesion. A recent case study, however, identified a FUS-CHOP transcript within a pleomorphic liposarcoma, raising the question as to whether some may be variants of myxoid liposarcoma.[88]

SPINDLE CELL LIPOSARCOMA

A very rare and unusual form of liposarcoma consisting almost entirely of loosely arranged fibroblast-like spindle cells oriented along a single plane and surrounded by a delicate reticulin meshwork has been termed spindle cell liposarcoma.[89] At low power, the lesion bears a superficial similarity to spindle cell lipoma, although it is far more cellular (Figs 16–63 to 16–65). The cellularity of these lesions coupled with the uniformity of the spindle cells

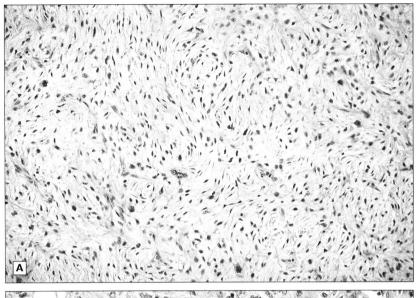

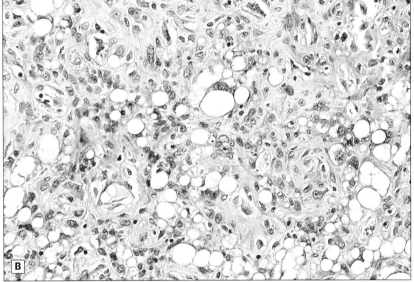

FIGURE 16–59 Pleomorphic liposarcoma with areas of undifferentiated pleomorphic sarcoma **(A)** and areas containing pleomorphic lipoblasts **(B)**.

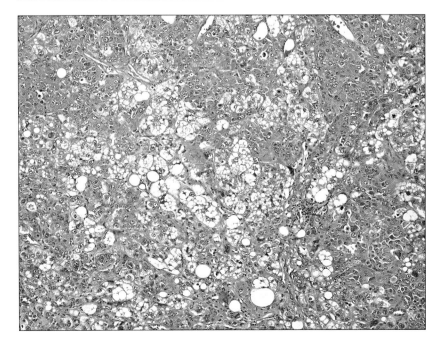

FIGURE 16–60 Pleomorphic liposarcoma showing sheets of epithelioid cells with scattered pleomorphic lipoblasts.

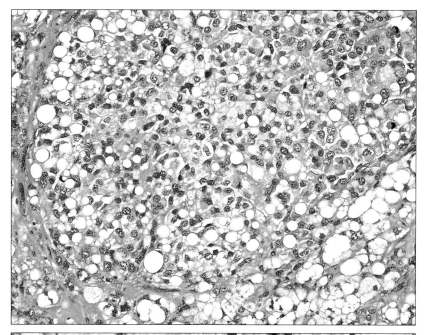

FIGURE 16–61 Pleomorphic liposarcoma showing sheets of vacuolated epithelioid lipoblasts.

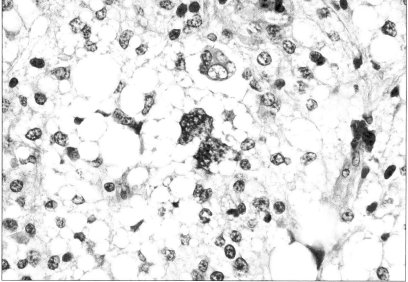

FIGURE 16–62 Pleomorphic liposarcoma showing pleomorphic lipoblasts.

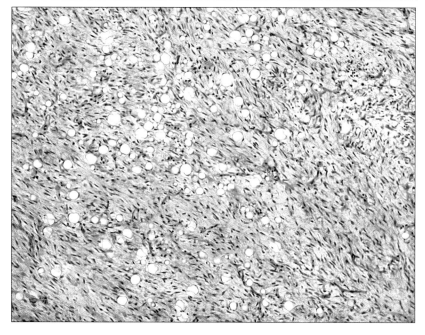

FIGURE 16–63 Spindle cell liposarcoma with prominent spindled tumor cells.

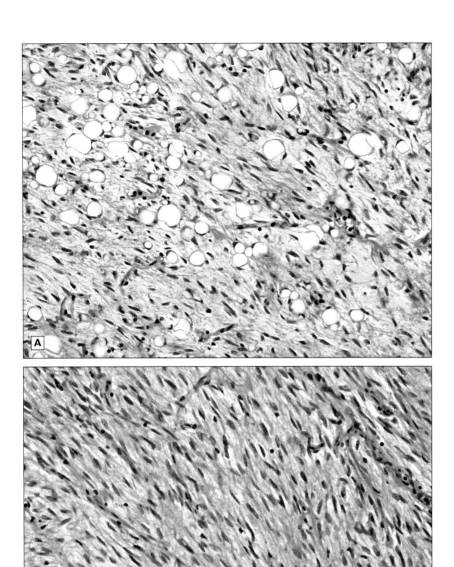

FIGURE 16–64 Spindle cell liposarcoma with scattered lipoblasts **(A)**. The presence of lipoblasts and the variably sized spindle cells with hyperchromatic nuclei help distinguish this tumor from spindle cell lipoma. Area of spindle cell liposarcoma devoid of lipoblasts **(B)**.

and their parallel orientation distinguish this tumor from the usual form of well-differentiated sclerosing liposarcoma. It is not yet clear whether these lesions are variants of ALN/WDL, a spindled version of myxoid liposarcoma, (low-grade) dedifferentiated liposarcoma, or a unique form of liposarcoma.

LIPOSARCOMA OF MIXED AND MISCELLANEOUS TYPE

Approximately 5% of liposarcomas do not fit easily into any of the foregoing categories,[90] or they exhibit an unusual combination of patterns. For example, myxoid liposarcomas occasionally display areas of ALN/WDL,

dedifferentiated liposarcoma, or rhabdomyosarcoma. Some liposarcomas, although appearing highly myxoid, display an inordinate degree of nuclear atypia such that they resemble a myxoid malignant fibrous histiocytoma. The WHO has recommended that these unusual cases be diagnosed as liposarcomas of mixed type. More importantly, the combination of patterns along with their relative proportions and grade should be noted so their biologic behavior can be assessed.

LIPOSARCOMA IN CHILDREN

Although most liposarcomas occur in patients older than 15 years, rare bone fide liposarcomas in patients 10–15

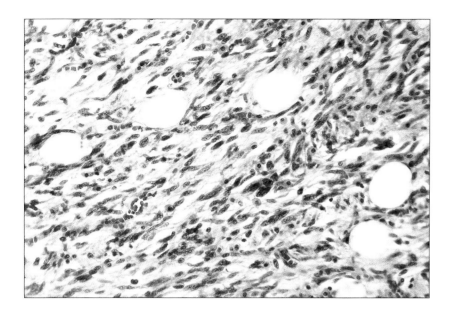

FIGURE 16–65 Spindle cell liposarcoma with more atypia of spindled cells than in Figure 16–64A.

years of age are on record.[91,92] Liposarcomas in infants and children are vanishingly uncommon, and nearly all such tumors are lipoblastomas or lipoblastomatosis.[93,94] We have encountered unequivocal examples in an 8-month-old boy with a massive tumor in the scapular region and a 3-year-old girl with a tumor of the knee. The former had a tumor of the round cell type and the latter one of the myxoid type. It is remarkable that both were well over 2 years of age at the initial diagnosis. In fact, the youngest patient in a series of 17 children with liposarcoma who died of the disease was an 11-year-old boy with a myxoid liposarcoma of the right axilla that was treated by local excision and postoperative radiotherapy.[92] Many of the reported cases are poorly illustrated and difficult to evaluate.[95,96] Castleberry et al. reviewed the reported cases of childhood liposarcoma in 1984.[97]

SO-CALLED MULTICENTRIC LIPOSARCOMA

The concept of multicentric liposarcoma was suggested in the early literature by the observation that the interval

between first and second liposarcomas in some patients was unusually long.[98,99] Whereas it is difficult to discount this idea completely, the majority of multifocal liposarcomas probably represents metastatic lesions, based on the histologic similarity of the tumors and development of metastases in conventional sites such as the lung. Recent molecular evidence in a case of "multifocal" myxoid liposarcoma indicated clonality of all lesions consistent with metastasis.[100]

LIPOSARCOMA ARISING IN A LIPOMA

The concept that lipomas can undergo malignant transformation to liposarcomas is no longer accepted. The striking demographic differences between lipomas and liposarcomas support the distinctness of the two lesions. Histologic variability of some ALN/WDL and/or poor sampling of the original tumor are the most common explanations for the apparent "transformation" of a lipoma to ALN/WDL.

REFERENCES

General

1. Kindblom LG, Angervall L, Svendsen P. Liposarcoma: a clinicopathologic, radiographic and prognostic study. Acta Pathol Microbiol Scand 1975; 253:1.
2. Hashimoto H, Enjoji M. Liposarcoma: a clinicopathologic subtyping of 52 cases. Acta Pathol Jpn 1982; 32:933.
3. Russell WO, Cohen J, Enzinger FM, et al. A clinical and pathological staging system for soft tissue sarcomas. Cancer 1977; 40: 1562.

4. Fletcher CDM, Unni KK, eds. Pathology and genetics: tumours of soft tissue and bone. World Health Organization Classification of Tumors. Lyon: IARC Press; 2002:35–46.
5. Weiss SW. Lipomatous tumors. In: Weiss SW, Brooks JJ, eds. Soft tissue tumors. Baltimore: Williams & Wilkins; 1996.
6. Dei Tos AP. Liposarcoma: new entities and evolving concepts. Ann Diag Pathol 2000; 4:252.
7. Enzinger FM, Winslow DJ. Liposarcoma: a study of 103 cases. Virchows Arch [Pathol Anat] 1962; 335:367.
8. Tontonoz P, Singer S, Forman BM, et al. Terminal differentiation of human liposarcoma

cells induced by ligands for peroxisome proliferator-activator receptor gamma and the retinoid X receptor. Proc Natl Acad Sci USA 1997; 94:237.
9. Demetri GD, Fletcher CD, Mueller E, et al. Induction of solid tumor differentiation by the peroxisome proliferator-activator receptor-gamma ligand troglitazone in patients with liposarcoma. Proc Natl Acad Sci USA 1999; 96:3951.
10. Hisaoka M, Tsuji S, Hashimoto H, et al. Dedifferentiated liposarcoma with an inflammatory malignant fibrous histiocytoma-like component presenting a leukemoid reaction. Pathol Int 1997; 47:642.

11. de Raucourtz E, Dumont MD, Tourani JM, et al. Acquired factor VII deficiency associated with pleural liposarcoma. Blood Coagul Fibrinolysis 1994; 5:833.

ALN/WDL

12. Lucas DR, Nascimento AG, Sanjay KSS, et al. Well-differentiated liposarcoma: the Mayo Clinic experience with 58 cases. Am J Clin Pathol 1994; 102:677.
13. Weiss SW, Rao VK. Well-differentiated liposarcoma (atypical lipoma) of deep soft tissue of the extremities, retroperitoneum and miscellaneous sites: a follow-up study of 92 cases with analysis of the incidence of "dedifferentiation." Am J Surg Pathol 1992; 16:1051.
14. Arkun R, Memis A, Akalin T, et al. Liposarcoma of soft tissue: MRI findings with pathologic correlation. Skeletal Radiol 1997; 26:167.
15. Ehara S, Rosenberg AE, Kattapuram SV. Atypical lipomas, liposarcomas, and other fat containing sarcomas: CT analysis of the fat element. Clin Imaging 1995; 19:50.
16. Jelinek JS, Kransdorf MJ, Schmookler BM, et al. Liposarcoma of the extremities: MR and CT findings in the histologic subtypes. Radiology 1993; 186:455.
17. Kraus MD, Guillou L, Fletcher CD. Well-differentiated inflammatory liposarcoma: an uncommon and easily overlooked variant of a common sarcoma. Am J Surg Pathol 1997; 21:518.
18. Evans HL. Smooth muscle in atypical lipomatous tumors: a report of three cases. Am J Surg Pathol 1990; 14:714.
19. Gomez-Roman JJ, Val-Bernal JF. Lipoleiomyosarcoma of the mediastinum. Pathology 1997; 29:428.
20. Suster S, Wong TY, Moran CA. Sarcomas with combined features of liposarcoma and leiomyosarcoma: study of two cases of an unusual soft-tissue tumor showing dual lineage differentiation. Am J Surg Pathol 1993; 17:905.
21. Tallini G, Erlandson RA, Brennan MF, et al. Divergent myosarcomatous differentiation in retroperitoneal liposarcoma. Am J Surg Pathol 1993; 17:546.
22. Folpe AL, Weiss SW. Lipoleiomyosarcoma (well-differentiated liposarcoma with leiomyosarcomatous differentiation): a clinicopathologic study of nine cases including one with dedifferentiation. Am J Surg Pathol 2002; 26:742.
23. Womack C, Turner AG, Fisher C. Paratesticular liposarcoma with smooth muscle differentiation mimicking angiomyolipoma. Histopathology 2000; 36:221.
24. Antonescu CR, Elahi A, Humphrey M, et al. Specificity of TLS-CHOP rearrangement for classic myxoid/round cell liposarcoma: absence in predominantly myxoid well-differentiated liposarcomas. J Mol Diagn 2000; 2:132.
25. Meis-Kindblom JM, Sjogren H, Kindblom LG, et al. Cytogenetics and molecular genetic analyses of liposarcoma and its soft tissue simulators: recognition of new variants and differential diagnosis. Virchows Archiv 2001; 439:41.
26. Farshid G, Weiss SW. Massive localized lymphedema in the morbidly obese simulating liposarcoma. Mod Pathol 1997; 10:9A.
27. Fletcher CDM, Akerman M, Dal Cin P, et al. Correlation between clinicopathological features and karyotype in lipomatous tumors: a report of 178 cases from the chromosomes and morphologic (CHAMP) collaborative study group. Am J Pathol 1996; 148:623.
28. Rosai J, Akerman M, Dal Cin P, et al. Combined morphologic and karyotypic study of 59 atypical lipomatous tumors: evaluation of their relationship and differential diagnosis with other adipose tissue tumors (a report of the CHAMP study group). Am J Surg Pathol 1996; 20:1182.
29. Binh MB, Sastre-garau X, Guillou L, et al. MDM2 and CDK4 immunostaining are useful adjuncts in diagnosing well differentiated and dedifferentiated liposarcoma subtypes: a comparative analysis of 559 soft tissue neoplasms with genetic data. Am J Surg Pathol 2005; 29:1340.
30. Hostein I, Pelmus M, Aurias A, et al. Evaluation of MDM2 and CDK4 amplification by real time PCR on paraffin wax-embedded material: a potential tool for the diagnosis of atypical lipomatous tumours/well-differentiated liposarcomas. J Pathol 2004; 202:95.
31. Evans HL, Soule EH, Winkelman RK. Atypical lipoma, atypical intramuscular lipoma, and well differentiated retroperitoneal liposarcoma. Cancer 1979; 43:574.
32. Azumi N, Curtis J, Kempson RL, et al. Atypical and malignant neoplasms showing lipomatous differentiation: a study of 111 cases. Am J Surg Pathol 1987; 11:161.
33. Brooks JJ, Connor AM. Atypical lipoma of the extremities and peripheral soft tissues with dedifferentiation: implications for management Surg Pathol 1990; 3:169.
34. Kindblom LG, Angervall L, Fassina AS. Atypical lipoma. Acta Pathol Microbiol Scand 1982; 90A:27.
35. Goldblum JR, Poy ES, Frank TS, et al. p53 mutations and histologic progression in well-differentiated liposarcoma and dermatofibrosarcoma protuberans. Int J Surg Pathol 1995; 3:35.
36. Adachi T, Oda Y, Sakamoto A, et al: Immunoreactivity of p53, mdm2, and p21WAF1 in dedifferentiated liposarcoma: special emphasis on the distinct immunophenotype of the well differentiated component. Int J Surg Pathol 2001; 9:99.
37. Shimoji T, Kanda H, Kitagawa T, et al. Clinico-molecular study of dedifferentiation in well-differentiated liposarcoma. Biochemical Biophys Res Comm 2004; 314:1133.
38. Dei Tos AP, Doglioni C, Piccinin S, et al. Molecular abnormalities of the p53 pathway in dedifferentiated liposarcoma. J Pathol 1997; 181:8.

Dedifferentiated liposarcoma

39. Coindre JM, de Loynes B, Bui NB, et al. Dedifferentiated liposarcoma: a clinicopathologic study of 6 cases. Ann Pathol 1992; 12:20.
40. Henricks WH, Chu Y-C, Goldblum JR, et al. Dedifferentiated liposarcoma: a clinicopathological analysis of 155 cases with a proposal for an expanded definition of dedifferentiation. Am J Surg Pathol 1997; 21:271.
41. McCormick D, Mentzel T, Beham A, et al. Dedifferentiated liposarcoma: clinicopathologic analysis of 32 cases suggesting a better prognostic group among pleomorphic sarcomas. Am J Surg Pathol 1994; 18:1213.
42. Elgar F, Goldblum JR. Well-differentiated liposarcoma of the retroperitoneum: a clinicopathologic analysis of 20 cases, with particular attention to the extent of low grade dedifferentiation. Mod Pathol 1997; 10:113.
43. Huang H-Y, Brennan MF, Singer S, et al. Distant metastasis in retroperitoneal dedifferentiated liposarcoma is rare and rapidly fatal: a clinicopathological study with emphasis on the low grade myxofibrosarcoma-like pattern as an early sign of dedifferentiation. Mod Pathol 2005; 18:976.
44. Yoshikawa H, Ueda T, Mori S, et al. Dedifferentiated liposarcoma of the subcutis. Am J Surg Pathol 1996; 20:1525.
45. Kransdorf MJ, Meis JM, Jelinek JS. Dedifferentiated liposarcoma of the extremities: imaging findings in four patients. AJR Am J Roentgenol 1993; 161:127.
46. Kuhnen C, Mentzel T, Sciot R, et al. Dedifferentiated liposarcoma with extensive lymphoid component. Pathol Res Prac 2005; 201:347.
47. Coindre JM, Odette M, Mairal F, et al. Most malignant fibrous histiocytomas developed in the retroperitoneum are dedifferentiated liposarcomas: a review of 25 cases initially diagnosed as malignant fibrous histiocytoma. Mod Pathol 2003; 16:256.
48. Coindre JM, Hostein I, Gaire G, et al. Inflammatory malignant fibrous histiocytomas and dedifferentiated liposarcomas: histological review, genomic profile and MDM2 and CDK4 status favor a single entity. J Pathol 2004; 203:822.
49. Fanburg-Smith JC, Miettinen M. Liposarcoma with meningothelial-like whorls: a study of 17 cases of a distinctive histological pattern associated with dedifferentiated liposarcoma. Histopathology 1998; 33:414.
50. Nascimento AG, Kurtin PJ, Guillou L, et al. Dedifferentiated liposarcoma: a report of nine cases with a peculiar neurallike whorling pattern associated with metaplastic bone formation. Am J Surg Pathol 1998; 22:945.
51. Salzano RP, Tomkiewicz Z, Africano WA. Dedifferentiated liposarcoma with features of rhabdomyosarcoma. Conn Med 1991; 55:200.
52. Chorneyko K. The ultrastructure of liposarcomas with attention to "dedifferentiation." Ultrastruct Pathol 1997; 21:545.

Myxoid/round cell liposarcoma

53. Kilpatrick SE, Doyon J, Choong PF, et al. The clinicopathologic spectrum of myxoid and round cell liposarcoma: a study of 95 cases. Cancer 1996; 77:1450.
54. Orndal C, Mandahl N, Rydholm A, et al. Chromosomal evolution and tumor progression in a myxoid liposarcoma. Acta Orthop Scand 1990; 61:99.
55. Tallini G, Akerman M, Dal Cin P, et al. Combined morphologic and karyotypic study of 28 myxoid liposarcomas: implications for a revised morphologic typing (a report from the CHAMP Group). Am J Surg Pathol 1996; 20:1047.
56. Winslow DJ, Enzinger FM. Hyaluronidase-sensitive acid mucopolysaccharides in liposarcomas. Am J Pathol 1960; 37:497.
57. Dijkhuizen T, Molenaar WM, Hoekstra HJ, et al. Cytogenetic analysis of a case of myxoid liposarcoma with cartilaginous differentiation. Cancer Genet Cytogenet 1996; 92:141.
58. Siebert JDS, Williams RP, Pulitzer DR. Myxoid liposarcoma with cartilaginous differentiation. Mod Pathol 1996; 9:249.
59. Shanks JH, Banerjee SS, Eyden BP. Focal rhabdomyosarcomatous differentiation in primary liposarcoma. J Clin Pathol 1996; 49:770.
60. Smith TA, Easley KA, Goldblum JR. Myxoid/round cell liposarcoma of the extremities: a clinicopathologic study of 29 cases with particular attention to the extent of round cell liposarcoma. Am J Surg Pathol 1996; 17:171.
61. Mentzel T, Fletcher CD. Dedifferentiated myxoid liposarcoma: a clinicopathological study suggesting a closer relationship between myxoid and well-differentiated liposarcoma. Histopathology 1997; 30:457.
62. Battifora H, Nunez-Alonso C. Myxoid liposarcoma: study of 10 cases. Ultrastruct Pathol 1980; 1:157.

63. Fu YS, Parker FG, Kaye GI, et al. Ultrastructure of benign and malignant adipose tissue tumors. Pathol Annu 1980; 15:67.

64. Gould VE, Wellington J, Gould NS. Electron microscopy of adipose tissue tumors: comparative features of hibernomas, myxoid and pleomorphic liposarcomas. Pathobiol Annu 1979; 9:339.

65. Kindblom LG, Save-Soderbergh J. The ultrastructure of liposarcoma: a study of 10 cases. Acta Pathol Microbiol Scand [A] 1979; 87:109.

66. Rossouw DJ, Cinti S, Dickersin GR. Liposarcoma: an ultrastructural study of 15 cases. Am J Clin Pathol 1985; 85:649.

67. Gibas Z, Miettinen M, Limon J, et al. Cytogenetic and immunohistochemical studies were performed in nine myxoid liposarcomas. Am J Clin Pathol 1995; 103:20.

68. Knight JC, Renwick PJ, Cin PD, et al. Translocation t(12;16)(q13; p11) in myxoid liposarcoma and round cell liposarcoma: molecular and cytogenetic analysis. Cancer Res 1995; 55:24.

69. Panagopoulos I, Hoglund M, Mertens F, et al. Fusion of the EWS and CHOP genes in myxoid liposarcoma. Oncogene 1996; 12:489.

70. Dal Cin P, Sciot R, Panagopoulos I, et al. Additional evidence of a variant translocation t(12;22) with EWS/CHOP fusion in myxoid liposarcoma: clinicopathologic features. J Pathol 1997; 182:437.

71. Panagopoulos I, Aman P, Mertens F, et al. Genomic PCR detects tumor cells in peripheral blood from patients with myxoid liposarcoma. Genes Chromosomes Cancer 1996; 17:102.

72. Mrozek K, Szumigala J, Brooks JS, et al. Round cell liposarcoma with the insertion (12;16)(q13; p11.2p13). Am J Clin Pathol 1997; 108:35.

73. Powers CS, Mathur M, Raaka BM, et al. TLS (translocated in-liposarcoma) is a high affinity interactor for steroid, thyroid hormone, and retinoid receptors. Mol Endocrinol 1998; 12:4.

74. Kuroda M, Ishida T, Horiuchi H, et al. Chimeric TLS/FUS-CHOP gene expression and the heterogeneity of its junction in human myxoid and round cell liposarcoma. Am J Pathol 1995; 147:1221.

75. Kuroda M, Ishida T, Takanashi M, et al. Oncogenic transformation and inhibition of adipocytic conversion of preadipocytes by TLS/FUS-CHOP type II chimeric protein. Am J Pathol 1997; 151:735.

76. Yang X, Nagasaki K, Egawa S, et al. FUS/TLS-CHOP chimeric transcripts in liposarcoma tissues. Jpn J Clin Oncol 1995; 25:234.

77. Dei Tos AP, Piccinin S, Doglioni C, et al. Molecular aberrations of the G_1-S checkpoint in myxoid and round cell liposarcoma. Am J Pathol 1997; 151:1531.

78. Smith TA, Goldblum JR. Immunohistochemical analysis of p53 protein in myxoid/round cell liposarcoma of the extremities. Appl Immunohistochem 1996; 4:228.

79. Antonescu CR, Tschernyavsky SJ, Decuseara R, et al. Prognostic impact of P53 status, TLS-CHOP fusion transcript structure and histological grade in myxoid liposarcoma; a molecular and clinicopathologic study of 82 cases. Clin Cancer Res 2001; 7:3977.

80. Evans HL. Liposarcomas and atypical lipomatous tumors: a study of 66 cases followed for a minimum of 10 years. Surg Pathol 1988; 1:41.

Pleomorphic liposarcoma

81. Enterline HT, Culberson JD, Rochlin DB, et al. Liposarcoma: a clinical and pathological study of 53 cases. Cancer 1960; 13:932.

82. Oliveira AM, Nascimento AG. Pleomorphic liposarcoma. Sem Diag Pathol 2001; 18:274.

83. Hornick JL, Bosenberg MW, Mentzel T, et al. Pleomorphic liposarcoma: clinicopathologic analysis of 57 cases. Am J Surg Pathol 2004; 28:1257.

84. Gebhard S, Coindre JM, Michels JJ, et al. Pleomorphic liposarcoma: clinicopathologic, immunohistochemical, and follow up analysis of 63 cases: a study from the French Federation of Cancer Centers Sarcoma Group. Am J Surg Pathol 2002; 26:601.

85. Huang H-Y, Antonescu CR. Epithelioid variant of pleomorphic liposarcoma: a comparative immunohistochemical and ultrastructural analysis of six cases with emphasis on overlapping features with epithelial malignancies. Ultrastruct Path 2002; 26:299.

86. Fritz B, Schubert F, Wrobel G, et al. Microarray based copy number and expression profiling in dedifferentiated and pleomorphic liposarcoma. Cancer Res 2002; 62:2993.

87. Rieker RJ, Joos S, Bartsch C, et al. Distinct chromosomal imbalances in pleomorphic and in high grade dedifferentiated liposarcomas. Int J Cancer 2002; 99:68.

88. DeCecco L, Gariboldi M, Reid JF, et al. Gene expression profile identifies a rare epithelioid variant case of pleomorphic liposarcoma

carrying FUS-CHOP transcript. Histopathology 2005; 46:334.

Spindle cell liposarcoma

89. Dei Tos AP, Mentzel T, Newman PL, et al. Spindle cell liposarcoma: a hitherto unrecognized variant of well-differentiated liposarcoma: an analysis of six cases. Am J Surg Pathol 1994; 18:913.

Liposarcoma of mixed and miscellaneous type

90. Menon M, Velthoven PM. Liposarcoma of the breast. Arch Pathol 1974; 98:370.

Liposarcoma in children

91. Ferrari A, Casanova M, Spreafico F, et al. Childhood liposarcoma: a single institutional twenty-year experience. Pediatr Hematol Oncol 1999; 16:415.

92. Shmookler BM, Enzinger FM. Liposarcoma occurring in children: an analysis of 17 cases and review of the literature. Cancer 1983; 52:567.

93. Hanada M, Tokuda R, Ohnishi Y, et al. Benign lipoblastoma and liposarcoma in children. Acta Pathol Jpn 1986; 36:605.

94. Kauffman SL, Stout AP. Lipoblastic tumors of children. Cancer 1959; 12:912.

95. Kretschmer HL. Retroperitoneal lipofibrosarcoma in a child. J Urol 1940; 43:61.

96. Peeples WJ, Hazra T. Retroperitoneal liposarcoma in a child. Urology 1976; 7:89.

97. Castleberry RP, Kelly DR, Wilson ER, et al. Childhood liposarcoma: report of a case and review of the literature. Cancer 1984; 54:579.

So-called multicentric liposarcoma

98. Ackerman LV. Multiple primary liposarcomas. Am J Pathol 1944; 20:789.

99. Barkhof F, Melkert P, Meyer S, et al. Derangement of adipose tissue: a case report of multicentric retroperitoneal liposarcoma, retroperitoneal lipomatosis, and multiple subcutaneous lipomas. Eur J Oncol 1991; 17:547.

100. Antonescu CR, Humphrey H, Elahi A, et al. Monoclonality of multifocal myxoid liposarcoma: molecular confirmation by analysis of TLS-CHOP or EWS-CHOP rearrangements. Clin Cancer Res 2000; 67:2788.

CHAPTER 17

BENIGN TUMORS OF SMOOTH MUSCLE

To a large extent the distribution of benign smooth muscle tumors parallels the distribution of smooth muscle tissue in the body. The tumors tend to be relatively common in the genitourinary and gastrointestinal tracts, less frequent in the skin, and rare in deep soft tissue. In the experience of Farman,[1] based on 7748 leiomyomas, approximately 95% occurred in the female genital tract, and the remainder were scattered over various sites, including the skin (230 cases), gastrointestinal tract (67 cases), and bladder (5 cases). This study, based on surgical material, probably underestimates the large number of asymptomatic gastrointestinal and genitourinary lesions documented only in autopsy material. In general, soft tissue leiomyomas cause little morbidity; hence, there are few studies in the literature concerning their presentation, diagnosis, and therapy. For purposes of classification these tumors can be divided into several groups.

Cutaneous leiomyomas (leiomyoma cutis) comprise the most common group and are of two types. Those arising from the pilar arrector muscles of the skin are often multiple and associated with significant pain. Those arising from the network of muscle fibers that lie in the deep dermis of the scrotum (dartoic muscles), labia majora, and nipple are almost always solitary and are collectively referred to as genital leiomyomas. The second group of benign smooth muscle tumors includes the angiomyomas (vascular leiomyomas), which are distinctive, painful, subcutaneous tumors composed of a con-

glomerate of thick-walled vessels associated with smooth muscle tissue. They differ from cutaneous leiomyomas in their anatomic distribution, predominantly subcutaneous location, and predilection for women. The third group constitutes leiomyomas of deep soft tissue, lesions whose very existence has been questioned (see below). Although recent studies provide reasonable evidence that soft tissue leiomyomas exist, they are, indeed, rare and should be diagnosed using only the most stringent criteria. Leiomyomatosis peritonealis disseminata and intravenous leiomyomatosis are also included, although they are not strictly soft tissue tumors. The first can be conceptualized as a diffuse metaplastic response of the peritoneal surfaces in which multiple smooth muscle nodules form. The second is a uterine tumor that extends into the uterine or pelvic veins. Both may be confused with metastatic leiomyosarcoma because of their unusual growth patterns. Lastly, a number of lesions are discussed in this chapter (palisaded myofibroblastoma, myofibroblastoma of the breast, angiomyofibroblastoma), which although linked in name to the myofibroblast, may, in fact, be more closely related to a type of smooth muscle cell.[2]

STRUCTURE AND FUNCTION OF SMOOTH MUSCLE CELLS

Smooth muscle cells are widely distributed throughout the body and contribute to the wall of the gastrointestinal, genitourinary, and respiratory tracts. They constitute the muscles of the skin, erectile muscles of the nipple and scrotum, and iris of the eye. Their characteristic arrangements in these organs determine the net effect of contraction. For instance, the circumferential arrangement in blood vessels results in narrowing of the lumen during contraction, whereas contraction of the longitudinal and circumferential muscle layers in the gastrointestinal tract causes the propulsive peristaltic wave.

Smooth muscle cells are fusiform in shape and have centrally located cylindrical nuclei with round ends that develop deep indentations during contraction. The length of the muscle cell varies depending on the organ, achieving its greatest length in the gravid uterus, where it may measure as much as 0.5 mm. The cells are usually arranged in fascicles in which the nuclei are staggered so the tapered end of one cell lies in close association with the thick nuclear region of an adjacent cell. Typically, there are no connective tissue cells between individual muscle fibers, although a delicate basal lamina and small connective tissue fibers, presumably synthesized by the muscle cells,[3] can be seen as a thin periodic acid-Schiff (PAS)-positive rim around individual cells in light microscopic preparations.

Ultrastructurally, the cells are characterized by clusters of mitochondria, rough endoplasmic reticulum, and free ribosomes, which occupy the zone immediately adjacent to the nucleus. The remainder of the cytoplasm (sarcoplasm) is filled with myofilaments oriented parallel to the long axis of the cell.[4-7] There are three types of filaments in the cell.[8-10] Thick myosin filaments (12 nm) are surrounded by seven to nine thin actin filaments (6-8 nm). Thick and thin filaments are aggregated into larger groups, or units, which correspond by light microscopy to linear myofibrils. In addition to the contractile proteins, intermediate filaments, measuring 10 nm and forming part of the cytoskeleton, are centered around the dense bodies or plaques, which are believed to be the smooth muscle analogue of the Z-band. The plasma membrane is dotted with tiny pinocytotic vesicles; and overlying the surface of the cell is a delicate basal lamina. Although the basal lamina separates individual cells, limited areas exist between cells in which the substance is lacking and in which the plasma membranes lie in close proximity, separated by a space of about 2 nm. This area, known as a gap junction or nexus, may allow spread of electrical impulses between adjacent cells.

Smooth muscle cells display diversity in their content of contractile and intermediate filament proteins, depending on their location and function. It is useful to be aware of some of the regional variations when evaluating neoplasms. For example, the gamma isoform of muscle actin is present along with desmin in most smooth muscle cells, whereas in vascular smooth muscle the alpha isoform of muscle actin and vimentin predominate.

CUTANEOUS LEIOMYOMA (LEIOMYOMA CUTIS)

Superficial, or cutaneous, leiomyomas are of two types. Those arising from the pilar arrector muscles of the skin may be solitary or multifocal and are often associated with considerable pain and tenderness.[11-22] The other form, the genital leiomyoma, arises from the diffuse network of muscle in the deep dermis of the genital zones (e.g., scrotum, nipple, areola, vulva).[23-26] In the scrotum they arise from the dartoic muscles (dartoic leiomyoma) and in the nipple from the muscularis mamillae and areolae. This form is nearly always solitary and rarely causes significant pain.

Leiomyoma of pilar arrector origin

Although formerly believed to be the more common form of cutaneous leiomyoma, leiomyomas of pilar arrector origin are probably far less common than previously thought and are probably outnumbered by those arising in genital sites. They may be solitary or multiple. Most develop during adolescence or early adult life, although occasional cases appear at birth or during early childhood. Some occur on a familial basis.[12,21] Recent evidence suggests that the majority of patients presenting with cutaneous leiomyomas have germline mutations of the fumarate hydratase gene, mapped to chromosome 1q43 and encoding an enzyme in the Krebs cycle.[27,28] This disease, known as cutaneous leiomyomatosis (MCL), also predisposes to early-onset uterine leiomyomas in women and to early-onset renal cell carcinoma of the collecting duct and papillary type in both men and women (hereditary leiomyomatosis and renal cell cancer; HLRCC).[28] Sporadic leiomyomas and leiomyosarcomas seemingly do not harbor somatic mutations of this gene very frequently, however.[29,30]

Typically, cutaneous leiomyomas develop as small brown-red to pearly discrete papules that in the incipient stage can be palpated more readily than they can be seen (Fig. 17-1). Eventually they form nodules that coalesce into a fine linear pattern following a dermatome distribution. The extensor surfaces of the extremities are most often affected. The lesions often produce significant pain that can be triggered by exposure to cold. In one unusual case reported by Fisher and Helwig,[13] the patient claimed that strong emotions evoked pain in the lesions. It is not clear whether the pain produced by these tumors is the result of contraction of the muscle tissue or compression of nearby nerves by the tumors. Usually, the tumors grow slowly over a period of years, with new lesions forming as older lesions stabilize. The slowly progressive nature of the disease probably accounts for the fact that patients often seek medical attention only after a number of years.

Most pilar leiomyomas are 1-2 cm in diameter. They lie in the dermal connective tissue and are separated from the overlying atrophic epidermis by a grenz zone. The lesions are less well defined than the angiomyoma and blend in an irregular fashion with the surrounding dermal collagen and adjacent pilar muscle (Fig. 17-2). The central portions of the lesions are usually devoid of connective tissue and consist exclusively of packets or bundles of smooth muscle fibers. They usually intersect in an orderly fashion and often create the impression of hyperplasia or overgrowth of the pilar arrector muscle. The cells resemble normal smooth muscle cells, and myofibrils can be easily demonstrated with special stains such as the Masson trichrome stain, in which they appear as red linear streaks traversing the cytoplasm in a longitudinal fashion. Muscle antigens are readily identified by immu-

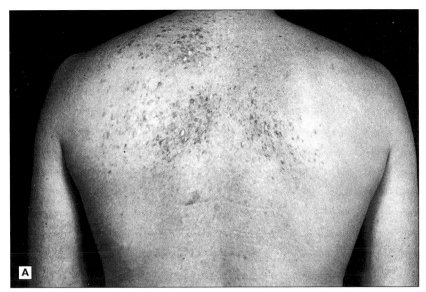

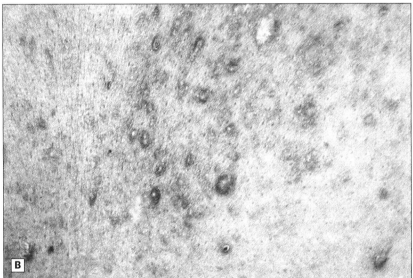

FIGURE 17–1 (A, B) Clinical appearance of multiple cutaneous leiomyomas.

nohistochemistry (Fig. 17–3). Ultrastructurally, the cells have myofilaments, surface pinocytotic vesicles, and investing basal laminae.[18]

Diagnosis is rarely difficult in the typical case, particularly one with a characteristic history. Occasionally, solitary forms of the disease are mistaken for other benign tumors such as the cutaneous fibrous histiocytoma (dermatofibroma). The cells in the fibrous histiocytoma are slender, less well ordered, and lack myofibrils. Secondary elements such as inflammatory cells, giant cells, and xanthoma cells, common to the cutaneous fibrous histiocytoma, are lacking in the cutaneous leiomyoma. Distinction of cutaneous leiomyomas from lesions reported as smooth muscle hamartomas of the skin is less clear-cut and may relate more to differences in clinical presentation than histologic features. Smooth muscle hamartomas are typically described as a single lesion measuring several centimeters in diameter and occurring in the lumbar region during childhood or early adult life.[20] Consisting of well-defined smooth muscle bundles in the dermis, these lesions are sometimes associated with hyperpigmentation and hypertrichosis (Becker's nevus).[20] Since leiomyosarcomas also occur in the skin, care should be taken to ensure that neither atypia nor mitotic activity is encountered in a presumptive cutaneous leiomyoma. In this regard, we do not subscribe to the view that atypia in dermal smooth muscle tumors is equivalent to atypia in uterine smooth muscle tumors and that such lesions can be comfortably labeled "symplastic leiomyomas." In our experience, cutaneous smooth muscle tumors with significant atypia (even in the absence of mitotic activity) recur and progress over time, indicating that they should be considered leiomyosarcomas.

Cutaneous leiomyomas do not undergo malignant transformation; nonetheless, they may be difficult to treat. The lesions are often so numerous that total surgical

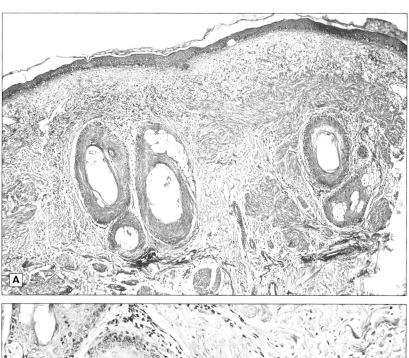

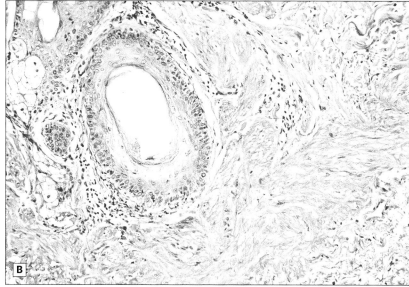

FIGURE 17–2 (A) Cutaneous leiomyoma of pilar arrector origin. **(B)** Smooth muscle bundles are closely associated with hair follicles and consist of well-differentiated, highly oriented cells.

excision is not possible. Laser therapy has been used with some success.

Genital leiomyomas

Early studies based on referred consultations suggested that genital leiomyomas were far less common than those of pilar arrecti origin.[13] Judging from more recent hospital-based series, genital leiomyomas may outnumber pilar ones by a margin of 2 : 1.[22] Affected sites include the areola of the nipple, scrotum, labium, penis, and vulva. The tumors are small, seldom exceeding 2 cm, and pain is not a prominent symptom. Histologically, genital leiomyomas, with the exception of the nipple lesions, differ from pilar leiomyomas in that they tend to be more circumscribed and more cellular, and they display a greater range of histologic appearances.[14] For example, Tavassoli

and Norris,[26] in a review of 32 vulvar leiomyomas, noted myxoid change and an epithelioid phenotype of the cells, features not encountered in pilar leiomyomas.

ANGIOMYOMA (VASCULAR LEIOMYOMA)

The angiomyoma, a solitary form of leiomyoma that usually occurs in the subcutis, is composed of numerous thick-walled vessels. In the early literature, little attempt was made to distinguish these lesions from cutaneous leiomyomas, and the two were collectively termed tuberculum dolorosum because of their pain-producing properties.[31–37] Stout[31] later designated them vascular leiomyomas to contrast them with the cutaneous leiomyoma that has inconspicuous thin-walled vessels. These

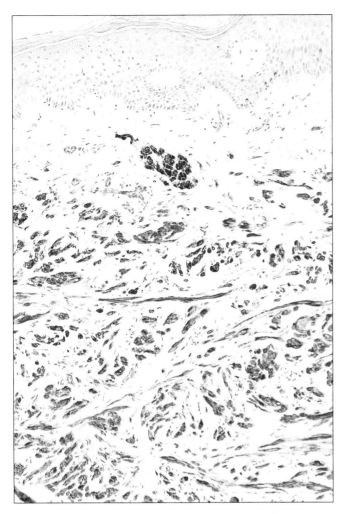

FIGURE 17–3 Actin immunostain of a cutaneous leiomyoma showing irregular packets and fascicles of spindle cells.

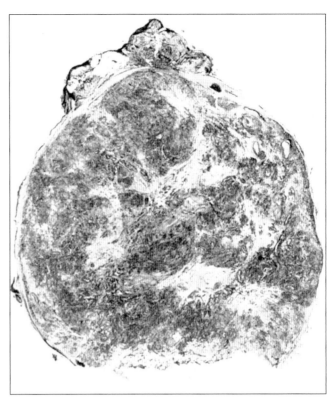

FIGURE 17–4 Angiomyoma of subcutaneous tissue. Congeries of thick-walled vessels constitute a major portion of the lesion and blend with surrounding smooth muscle tissue and focal myxoid stroma (Masson trichrome).

lesions account for about 5% of all benign soft tissue tumors[32] and one-fourth to one-half of all superficial leiomyomas. They occur more frequently in women,[33] except for those in the oral cavity where the reverse is true.[34] Unlike cutaneous leiomyomas, these tumors develop later in life, usually between the fourth and sixth decades, as solitary lesions.[32,33] They occur preferentially on the extremities, particularly the lower leg. In the series reported by Hachisuga et al., 375 of 562 occurred in the lower extremity, 125 on the upper extremity, 48 on the head, and 14 on the trunk.[32] Most were less than 2 cm in diameter.

Affected patients complain most often of a small, slowly enlarging mass usually of several years' duration. Pain is a prominent feature in about half of the patients,[35] and in some cases it is exacerbated by pressure, change in temperature, pregnancy,[33] or menses.[35] The prevalence of pain has led some to suggest that these tumors are probably derived from arteriovenous anastomoses, similar to the glomus tumor.[36] They differ in appearance from the glomus tumor and are almost never encountered in a subungual location, however. The tumors are usually located in the subcutis and less often in the deep dermis, where they produce overlying elevations of the skin but without surface changes of the epidermis. Grossly, the tumors are circumscribed, glistening, white-gray nodules. Occasional they are blue or red, and rarely calcium flecks are visible grossly. The leiomyomas that visibly contract or writhe when touched or surgically manipulated are probably of this type.

Microscopically, the tumors have a characteristic appearance that varies little from case to case. The usual appearance is of a well-demarcated nodule of smooth muscle tissue punctuated with thick-walled vessels with partially patent lumens (Figs 17–4, 17–5). Typically, the inner layers of smooth muscle of the vessel are arranged in an orderly circumferential fashion, and the outer layers spin or swirl away from the vessel, merging with the less well-ordered peripheral muscle fibers. Areas of myxoid change (Fig. 17–6), hyalinization, calcification, and fat are seen. The vessels in these tumors are difficult to classify because they are not altogether typical of veins or arteries. Their thick walls and small lumens are reminiscent of arteries, but they consistently lack internal and external elastic laminae. In the experience of Hachisuga et al., a small number of angiomyomas are composed of predominantly cavernous-type vessels.[32] Nerve fibers are

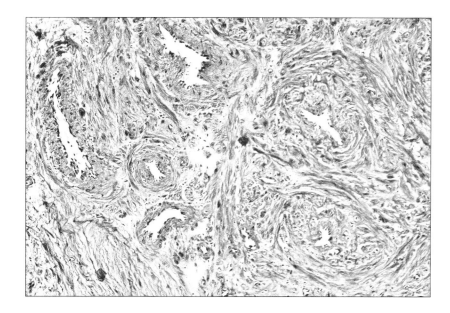

FIGURE 17–5 Thick-walled vessel of an angiomyoma. Inner layer of muscle is usually arranged circumferentially, and outer layer blends with less well-ordered smooth muscle tissue of tumors.

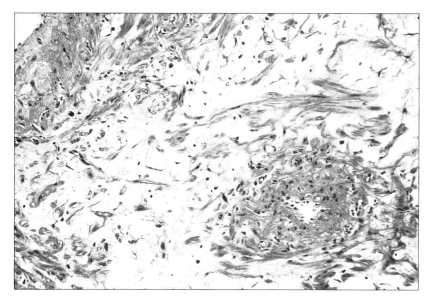

FIGURE 17–6 Focal myxoid change in an angiomyoma.

usually difficult to demonstrate but undoubtedly are present, accounting for the exquisite sensitivity of these lesions to manipulation. Rarely, angiomyomas display degenerative nuclear atypia similar to that seen in symplastic leiomyomas.[37] The angiomyoma is a benign tumor, causing few problems apart from pain. Simple excision is adequate. None of the patients reported by Duhig and Ayer[33] developed recurrence following excision. In the series of Hachisuga et al.,[32] only two patients had a recurrence, although their follow-up data were incomplete.

LEIOMYOMA OF DEEP SOFT TISSUE

Unequivocal leiomyomas of deep soft tissue are exceptionally rare compared to their malignant counterpart, and until recently there has been no consensus as to how

one separated soft tissue leiomyomas from leiomyosarcomas. In fact, the observation that some tumors that were initially labeled "leiomyoma" ultimately proved to be malignant enhanced the impression that it was nearly impossible to establish a minimum threshold for malignancy, leading inevitably to the conclusion that all smooth muscle tumors of deep soft tissue should be considered malignant.[38,39] Recent studies have presented convincing evidence that leiomyomas of deep soft tissue exist but are rare and should be diagnosed using strict criteria derived empirically from the evaluation of soft tissue smooth muscle tumors.[40–43] Soft tissue leiomyomas are of two distinct types (somatic and gynecologic) which differ in their clinical presentation and in the criteria of malignancy.

The less common *somatic leiomyoma* arises in the deep somatic soft tissue of the extremities and affects the sexes equally.[40] Measuring several centimeters at the time of presentation, about one-third also contain calcification (Fig. 17–7), probably a reflection of long duration and a feature that occasionally leads to a number of radiologic diagnoses including "calcifying schwannoma," "synovial sarcoma," or "myositis ossificans." Histologically, these lesions are composed of fascicles of well-differentiated smooth muscle cells with abundant eosinophilic cytoplasm similar to vascular smooth muscle (Figs 17–8 to 17–10). Rarely somatic leiomyomas may have a predominantly clear cell appearance or display psammoma bodies (Figs 17–11, 17–12).

By definition, somatic leiomyomas should harbor no necrosis, at most mild atypia, and virtually no mitotic activity (<1 mitoses/50 high-power fields [HPF]). The number of somatic leiomyomas with extended follow-up information is still quite small but in the largest series reported by Billings et al., all 11 patients were alive and well from 5 to 97 months (median 67 months) after diagnosis.[40]

The more common *leiomyoma of gynecologic (or uterine) type* occurs almost exclusively in women, usually in the perimenopausal period. They are situated predominantly in the pelvic retroperitoneum, although other peritoneal sites may be affected.[40,41] Although in the past, some of these lesions have undoubtedly been interpreted as autoamputated uterine leiomyomas, recent experience showing origin at sites clearly distinct from the uterus or in women without uterine fibroids suggests that they are more likely de novo soft tissue lesions.

Grossly and histologically, they bear an unmistakable similarity to uterine leiomyomas, thereby accounting for the term "leiomyoma of gynecologic type" (Figs 17–13 to 17–17). Grossly, they are well circumscribed, gray-

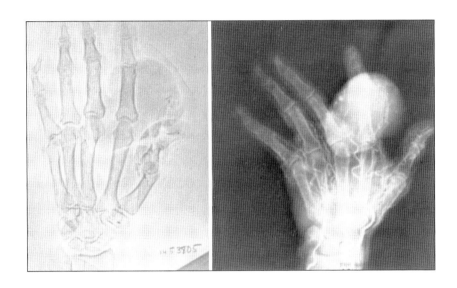

FIGURE 17–7 Radiograph showing calcification of a soft tissue leiomyoma.

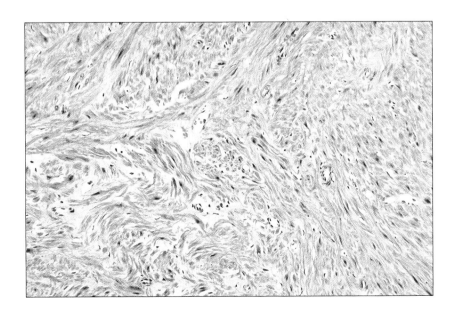

FIGURE 17–8 Somatic leiomyoma of deep soft tissue. Fascicles of smooth muscle tend to be less well oriented than in cutaneous leiomyomas.

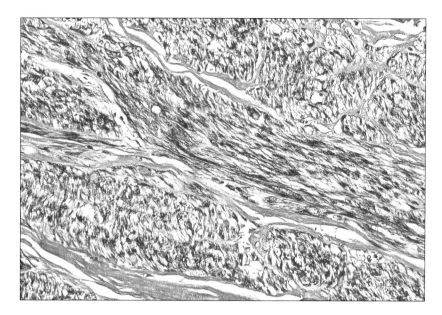

FIGURE 17–9 Masson trichrome stain of a deep leiomyoma. Cells are deeply fuchsinophilic with linear striations.

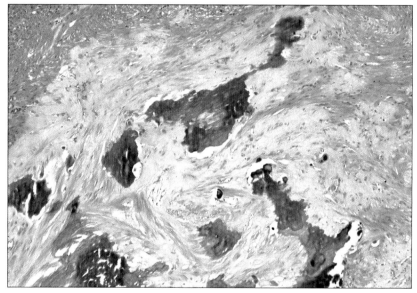

FIGURE 17–10 Somatic leiomyoma of soft tissue with calcification.

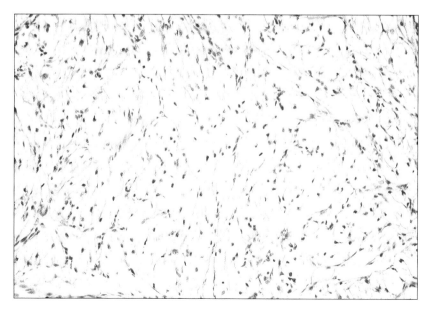

FIGURE 17–11 Clear-cell change of the cytoplasm in a somatic leiomyoma of soft tissue.

white lesions which range greatly in size from a few centimeters to more than 10 cm and consist of intersecting fascicles of slender tapered smooth muscle cells with less cytoplasm than their somatic counterparts. The stroma contains vessels often with striking mural hyalinization (Fig. 17–13). Other features of uterine leiomyomas are also encountered, such as hydropic (Fig. 17–14) and myxoid change, hyaline necrosis, and an epithelioid or cord-like arrangement of the cells (Fig. 17–16). Fatty change is quite common (Fig. 17–17) and has led to the use of alternative terms (e.g., lipoleiomyoma, myolipoma).[44,45]

Unlike somatic leiomyomas, gynecologic leiomyomas typically display both nuclear estrogen and progesterone receptor protein (Fig. 17–18) suggesting that they arise from hormonally sensitive smooth muscle of the retroperitoneum. Not surprisingly, the criteria of malignancy for evaluating this group of lesions seems to approximate those used for uterine lesions (see below). Although, by definition, neither necrosis nor more than mild atypia should be allowed in making this diagnosis, mitotic activity occurs frequently and does not seem to imply any adverse outcome. In two large studies, mitotic activity of 5/10 HPF was encountered in about one-quarter of cases

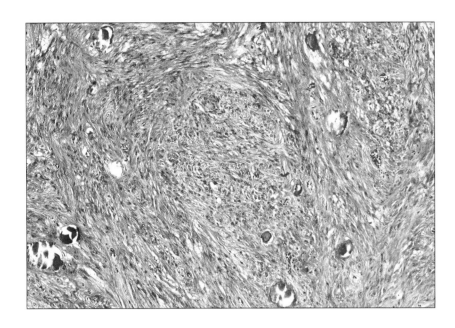

FIGURE 17–12 Somatic leiomyoma with psammomatous calcification.

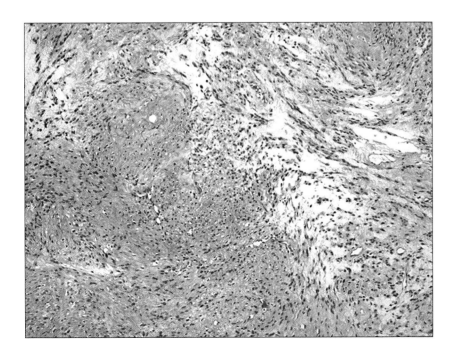

FIGURE 17–13 Gynecologic-type leiomyoma. Note prominent vessels and hyalinization.

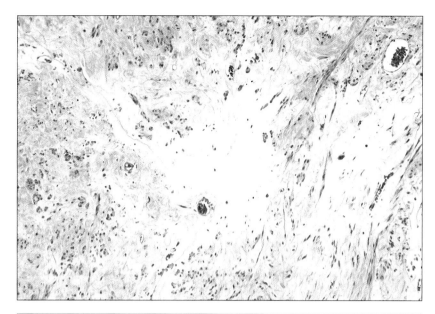

FIGURE 17–14 Gynecologic-type leiomyoma with hydropic change.

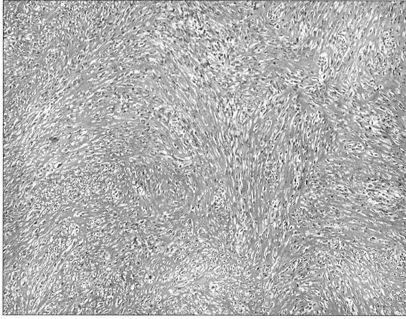

FIGURE 17–15 Prominent hyalinization within gynecologic-type leiomyoma.

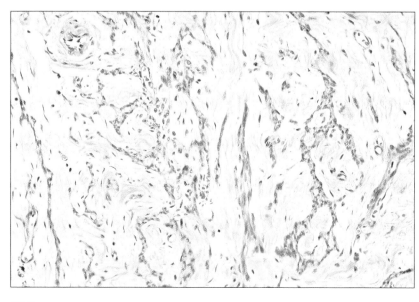

FIGURE 17–16 Gynecologic leiomyoma with cord-like arrangement of cells.

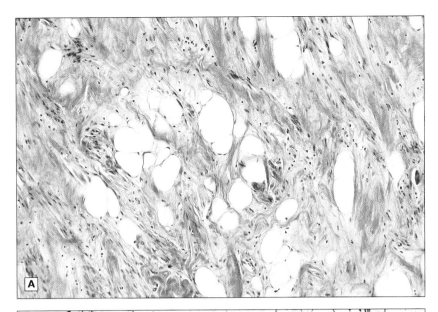

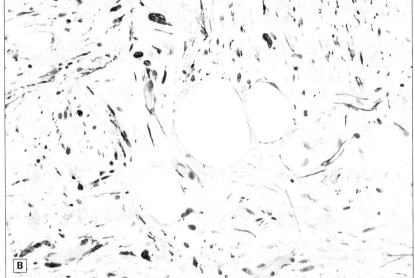

FIGURE 17–17 Leiomyoma with fat (myolipoma) **(A)**. Desmin immunostain illustrates muscle cells between adipocytes **(B)**.

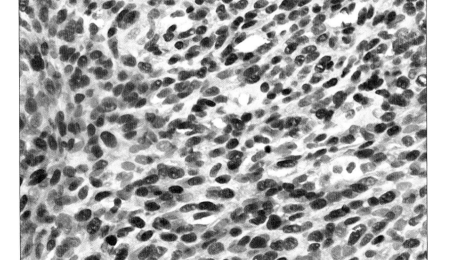

FIGURE 17–18 Estrogen receptor protein staining in gynecologic leiomyoma of retroperitoneum.

with no observed adverse event. Although higher levels of mitotic activity may still be compatible with a benign diagnosis, the experience with such lesions is limited and they are best labeled as "uncertain malignant potential" until further data are accrued (Fig. 17–19). Given the similarity to uterine lesions, the question might also be raised as to whether there is a soft tissue analogue to a symplastic leiomyoma of the uterus (Fig. 17–20). Regrettably, there is no published information on this point. Until such time as there is, we recommend that such lesions be considered of uncertain malignant potential. These criteria of benignancy have been validated in two recent large studies. Of the 54 patients reported collectively by Billings et al. and Paal and Miettinen,[40,41] 20% experienced local recurrence, but no metastasis within an average follow-up period of 42 months in the former

study and 142 months in the latter. Finally, even though hormone receptor proteins are characteristic of soft tissue leiomyomas of the gynecologic type, they may be expressed in leiomyosarcomas from women. Therefore, identification of positive receptor status in a deep smooth muscle tumor does not per se identify it as a leiomyoma but that feature should be assessed in the context of traditional histologic features.

INTRAVENOUS LEIOMYOMATOSIS

Intravenous leiomyomatosis is a rare condition in which gross nodules of benign smooth muscle tissue grow in the veins of the myometrium and occasionally extend for a variable distance into the uterine and hypogastric veins. In about 10% of patients, cardiac symptoms predominate owing to the presence of tumor in the vena cava and heart. This condition develops as a result of extensive vascular invasion by a leiomyoma.

The lesion develops primarily in premenopausal middle-aged women, and prior pregnancy is noted in about half of the patients. The common presenting symptoms are abnormal vaginal bleeding and pelvic pain. In more than half of the patients, the uterus is enlarged. Grossly, the lesion is distinctive, characterized by coiled masses in the myometrium and in some cases by serpiginous extensions of the process into the uterine veins of the broad ligament (Figs 17–21, 17–22). The masses have a rubbery texture and a pink to white-gray color similar to an ordinary uterine myoma. Histologically, the smooth muscle proliferations in leiomyomatosis may show the same spectrum of changes as those in ordinary leiomyo-

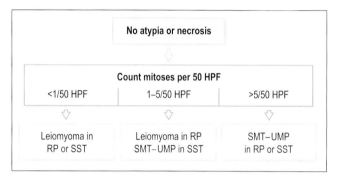

FIGURE 17–19 A schematic diagram showing the approach to evaluation of differentiated smooth muscle tumors of soft tissue. (HPF, high power field; RP, retroperitoneum; SST, somatic soft tissue; SMT, smooth muscle tumour; UMP, uncertain malignant potential.)

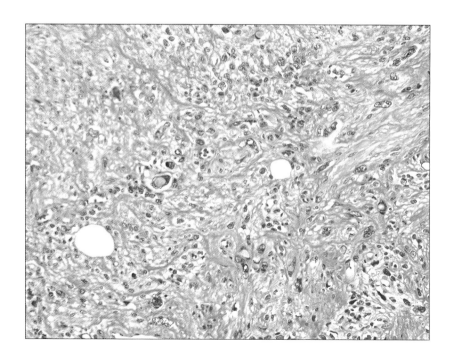

FIGURE 17–20 Localized area of atypia within an otherwise typical gynecologic-type leiomyoma. Whether these should be regarded as the equivalent to symplastic leiomyomas of uterus is uncertain.

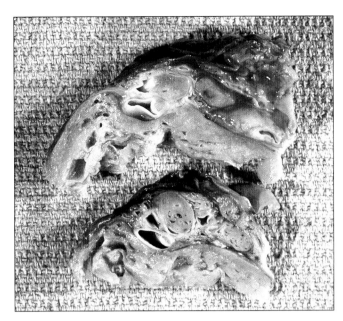

FIGURE 17–21 Gross specimen of intravenous leiomyomatosis showing intravascular growth of the neoplasm.

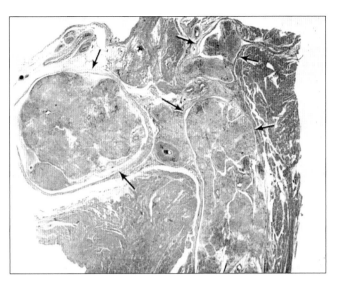

FIGURE 17–22 Intravenous leiomyomatosis with plugs of smooth muscle tissue in uterine veins (×60). (Courtesy of Dr. H.J. Norris.)

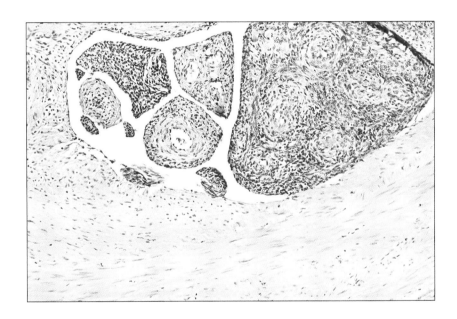

FIGURE 17–23 Intravenous leiomyomatosis with intraluminal protrusions or growths.

mas (Figs 17–23, 17–24). The lesions may vary from highly cellular smooth muscle proliferations to less cellular ones marked by fibrosis, hydropic change, and perivascular hyalinization. A characteristic feature is the presence of thick-walled vessels in the plugs of intravascular smooth muscle tissue, creating a "vessel within a vessel" appearance. Unusual features in this condition include epithelioid change of the cells, fat, or endometrial glands in association with smooth muscle cells[46] and bizarre nuclear changes similar to those of symplastic leiomyoma.[46] Despite the intravascular location, the smooth muscle cells are well differentiated, showing in nearly all cases no or only a modest degree of nuclear hyperchromatism. Mitotic figures are rare, with an incidence well below that associated with borderline (5–9 mitoses/10 HPF) or malignant (≥10 mitoses/10 HPF) smooth muscle tumors of the uterus (see Chapter 18). Thus, from a purely morphologic point of view, the tumor would be classified as "leiomyoma."

Two mechanisms have been proposed to explain the pathogenesis. In most cases there are associated uterine leiomyomas, supporting the notion that extensive angio-invasion by one or more myometrial tumors results in this condition. An alternative mechanism is that the

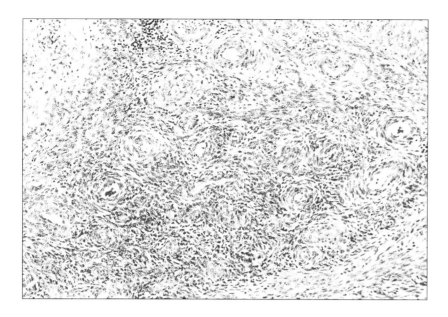

FIGURE 17–24 Intravenous leiomyomatosis.

lesions arise de novo from the vessel wall. This explanation has recently been questioned due to the fact there are discrepancies in immunostaining for hormone receptors in the intravascular growths compared to the native vessel wall.[47] Recent molecular studies provide evidence that intravenous leiomyomatosis may also be the source of retroperitoneal leiomyomas in some patients.[48]

Despite the intravascular location, the prognosis in most cases is good. About 70% of patients can be cured by hysterectomy; the remaining 30% have persistence or recurrence of the disease.[49] Unfortunately, recurrence rates have not correlated well with the presence of extra-uterine extension noted at the time of the original surgery. In a small percentage of patients, the disease may be fatal because of extension into the hepatic veins, the heart, and even the lungs.[49-51] Resection of these cardiac and caval extensions, if technically feasible, is compatible with prolonged survival.[46,49,52,53] Because some patients with intravenous leiomyomatosis have steroid receptors,[50,54] it has been suggested that oophorectomy or estrogen antagonists can play a therapeutic role in those in whom tumor excision has been incomplete. It is likely that some "benign metastasizing leiomyomas" of the lung evolve by way of "intravenous leiomyomatosis."[51] Others may evolve as a result of microscopic showers of tumor emboli occurring at the time of myomectomy; and still others may represent well-differentiated leiomyosarcomas in which the original tumor or the metastasis was misdiagnosed as a leiomyoma.[55]

The best name for this condition is debatable, as the ability of a tumor to invade the bloodstream and grow in foreign tissue satisfies a minimum definition of malignancy for some. On the other hand, the condition is compatible with long survival and differs histologically from most leiomyosarcomas of venous origin. The latter are usually high-grade tumors composed of smooth muscle cells with easily recognized mitotic figures. They arise preferentially in the vena cava, particularly the upper portion, and are usually associated with a poor prognosis because of their unresectability (see Chapter 18).

LEIOMYOMATOSIS PERITONEALIS DISSEMINATA

Leiomyomatosis peritonealis disseminata is a rare condition in which multiple smooth muscle or smooth muscle-like nodules develop in a subperitoneal location throughout the abdominal cavity. The lesion occurs exclusively in women, usually during the childbearing years. Most cases reported in the United States have been in African-American women. More than half have occurred in pregnant women. Others have occurred in women taking oral contraceptives, and one patient had a functioning ovarian tumor.[56] These observations and the fact that the lesion regresses following pregnancy[57] provide circumstantial evidence for the involvement of hormonal factors in its pathogenesis. The rarity of the condition suggests that other unknown factors must also be important. In most instances, leiomyomatosis is discovered incidentally at the time of surgery for other medical or obstetric conditions, although vague abdominal pain is often an accompanying symptom.

Grossly, the disease has an alarming appearance. The peritoneal surfaces, including the surfaces of the bowel, urinary bladder, and uterus, are studded with firm white-gray nodules of varying size (Fig. 17–25). The smallest nodules may be only a few millimeters in diameter whereas the largest are several centimeters. Although the diffuseness of the process initially suggests an intra-abdominal malignancy, the lesions lack hemorrhage and necrosis. Moreover, they do not violate the parenchyma of the affected organs, nor are they found in extra-abdominal sites such as the lung or in lymph nodes. Leiomyomas of the uterus have been identified in some but not all cases of leiomyomatosis, indicating that the lesions do not represent localized spread of an intra-uterine lesion.

Microscopic findings

Although the term leiomyomatosis indicates the similarity to normal smooth muscle and to benign leiomyomas, reports in the literature coupled with cases reviewed at the Armed Forces Institute of Pathology (AFIP)[58] suggest that there is a range of histologic changes perhaps not fully appreciated when the term was coined. In the classic case the earliest nodules develop as microscopic foci of proliferating smooth muscle immediately subjacent to the peritoneum (Figs 17–26 to 17–29). With progressive growth they may remain nodular or may, in addition, dissect through the underlying soft tissue in a more permeative fashion. The slender cells are arranged in close, compact fascicles oriented perpendicular to each other. The cells may show a minimal degree of nuclear pleomorphism that falls far short of being a leiomyosarcoma. Mitotic figures may be seen, but they are infrequent. Bundles of longitudinally oriented myofibrils can be identified in the cells by means of conventional special stains (Masson trichrome). In some cases, endometriosis has been present in the smooth muscle nodules.[59,60]

In a significant number of cases, the histologic appearance of these subperitoneal nodules is more fibroblastic or "myofibroblastic." Cases of this type have been described by Parmley et al.,[61] Winn et al.,[62] and Pieslor et al.[63] The proliferating cell is usually large, has plump eosinophilic cytoplasm, and is usually not arranged in well-defined fascicles. Round decidual cells with an eosinophilic or foamy cytoplasm are usually scattered amid the spindled cells; and at times it is impossible to delimit these cells clearly from spindle cells by light microscopy. In such cases the cells lack distinct longitudinal striations, as are seen in the foregoing type. Hyalinization of the nodules is seen in cases of regressing or regressed leiomyomatosis (Fig. 17–29). The one case in the literature allegedly representing lipomatous differentiation in the cells is dubious, judging from the photomicrographs.[64] Glandular inclusions or sex cord-like structures may be seen infrequently in these lesions.[65,66]

Ultrastructural findings

In view of the range of changes observed by light microscopy, it is not surprising that electron microscopy has produced conflicting reports regarding the histogenesis of

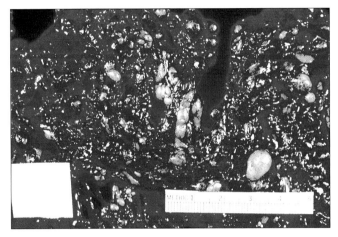

FIGURE 17–25 Gross appearance of leiomyomatosis peritonealis disseminata.

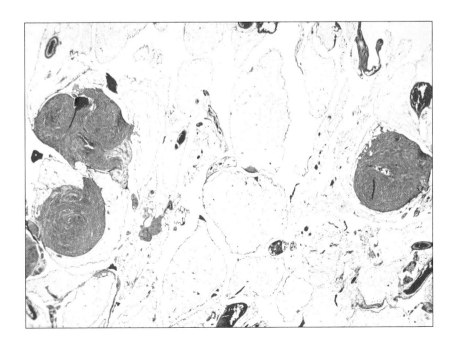

FIGURE 17–26 Leiomyomatosis peritonealis disseminata with numerous smooth muscle nodules of varying size arising underneath the peritoneal surface and involving underlying fat. Early nodules are present as microscopic foci.

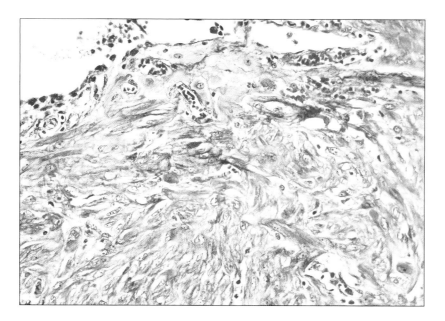

FIGURE 17–27 Subperitoneal nodule of leiomyomatosis peritonealis disseminata with decidualization.

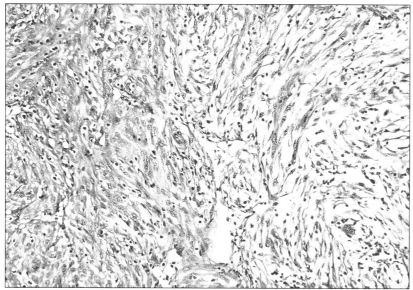

FIGURE 17–28 Leiomyomatosis peritonealis disseminata with a myofibroblastic appearance.

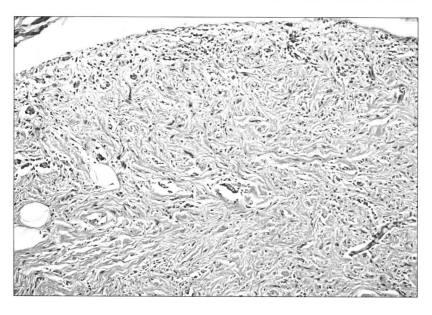

FIGURE 17–29 End-stage of leiomyomatosis peritonealis disseminata with extensive interstitial fibrosis.

this condition. In the studies of Nogales et al.,[67] Kuo et al.,[68] and Goldberg et al.,[69] most of the cells resembled mature smooth muscle cells and had an investiture of basal lamina, surface-oriented pinocytotic vesicles, and abundant longitudinally oriented myofilaments. In contrast, Parmley et al.[61] and Winn et al.[62] believed the predominant cells were fibroblastic and, based on the close relation with the decidual cells, suggested that leiomyomatosis is a reparative fibrosis occurring in a preexisting decidual reaction (fibrosing deciduosis). Others have documented a variety of cell types, including fibroblasts, myofibroblasts, and smooth muscle cells[63] and suggested a close interrelation of all three.[58] The theory that leiomyomatosis represents metaplasia or differentiation of pluripotential cells of the serosa or subserosal tissue along several closely related cell lines is supported by the experimental work of Fujii et al.[70] Estrogen administered to guinea pigs induces peritoneal nodules similar to those of leiomyomatosis peritonealis. These nodules are composed of fibroblasts and myofibroblasts in animals receiving estrogen only, whereas smooth muscle differentiation and decidualization occurs if estrogen plus progesterone are administered.

Behavior and treatment

In view of the benign nature of this condition, no particular therapy is warranted once the diagnosis has been firmly secured. In fact, there seems to be some evidence that the lesions regress following pregnancy or removal of the estrogenic source,[63] although with subsequent pregnancy progression or recrudescence occurs.[60] The case reported by Aterman et al.[71] documented partial regression of lesions 5 months after the initial surgery without any intervening therapy and regression of another lesion within 12 weeks.[72] Gonadotropin-releasing hormone antagonists (e.g., leuprolide acetate) and megestrol acetate[73] have been used with some success to treat this disease.[74] There have been a few cases purporting to show malignant degeneration of the condition. The cases reported by Akkersdijk et al.[75] and Abulafia et al.[76] are scantily illustrated, and autopsies were not performed in either case. The case reported by Rubin et al.[77] is better documented.

In the past leiomyomatosis peritonealis disseminata was regarded as a diffuse metaplastic process of the peritoneum. Quade et al., however, demonstrated clonality of multiple lesions in a given patient by assessing X-linked inactivation of the androgen receptor gene with the human androgen receptor assay (HUMARA).[72] Although the authors believe that this indicates metastasis from a unicentric disease, they are careful to point out that their data are also consistent with multicentric clones selected for an X-linked gene.

INTRANODAL PALISADED MYOFIBROBLASTOMA

Reported simultaneously by Weiss et al.[78] and Suster and Rosai,[79] the palisaded myofibroblastoma is a distinctive benign spindle cell tumor arising exclusively from the lymph nodes and bearing an unmistakable similarity to a schwannoma.[80,81] In fact, so striking is the resemblance that these lesions were originally regarded as schwannoma of the lymph node.[82,83] Based on immunohistochemistry, they have features of a modified smooth muscle cell or myofibroblast. The tumor may develop at any age but typically presents as a localized swelling in the region of the groin. A few cases have been reported in submandibular lymph nodes,[84,85] and we have also reviewed a consultation case in the mediastinal nodes.

On cut section, the tumors are gray-white, focally hemorrhagic masses that usually obscure the nodal landmarks (Fig. 17–30). It is usually possible to identify a rim of residual node at the periphery of the tumor (Fig. 17–31). The tumors are composed of differentiated spindle cells arranged in short intersecting or crisscrossed fascicles with foci vaguely palisaded nuclei (Figs 17–32, 17–33). In some areas, the cells form broad sheets with slit-like extracellular spaces containing erythrocytes similar to those of Kaposi's sarcoma (Fig. 17–34). The cells usually have little atypia and only a rare mitotic figure. They seem to represent an unusual myofibroblastic (or myoid) cell in that they strongly express actin and vimentin but not desmin. Linear striations, which are

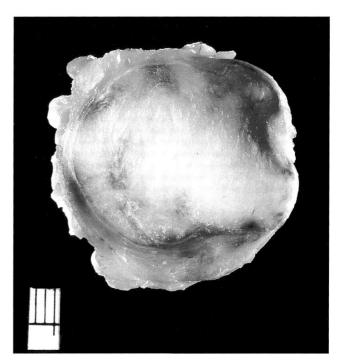

FIGURE 17–30 Gross specimen of a palisaded myofibroblastoma. Note the focal hemorrhages.

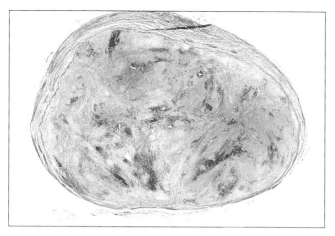

FIGURE 17–31 Palisaded myofibroblastoma with nearly complete effacement of a lymph node.

easily identified in conventional benign smooth muscle cells, cannot be demonstrated with Masson trichrome stain, although in many cases fuchsinophilic bodies, representing accumulations of actin, are prominent.

The most distinctive feature of the tumor is the "amianthoid" fibers or thick collagen mats that are nearly always present. These structures appear as broad eosinophilic bands, ellipses, or circular profiles, depending on the plane of the section. They contain a central collagen-rich zone surrounded by a paler collagen-poor zone containing actin and other materials extruded from nearby degenerating cells. Immunohistochemically, type I collagen can be identified throughout the amianthoid fibers, and type III collagen is localized peripherally.[86] Although the name "amianthoid" was used by Suster and Rosai for these distinctive bodies, it has recently been pointed out that these structures do not meet the strict definition of

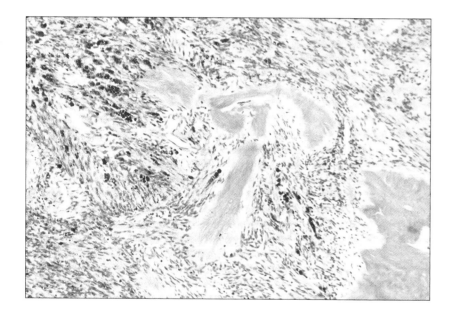

FIGURE 17–32 Palisaded myofibroblastoma with amianthoid fibers. It has a deeply eosinophilic core and lighter periphery.

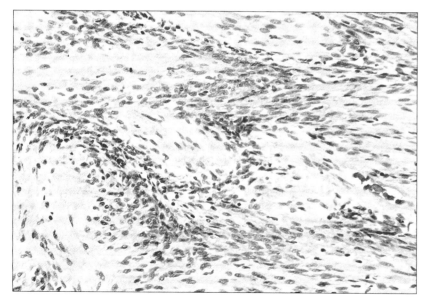

FIGURE 17–33 Palisaded myofibroblastoma with vague palisading of cells.

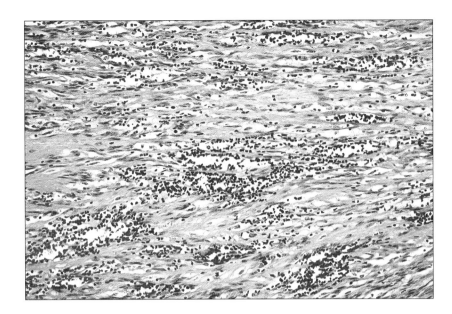

FIGURE 17–34 Kaposi-like areas in a palisaded myofibroblastoma.

amianthoid fibers.[87] The latter are thick collagen fibers measuring 280–1000 nm, whereas the fibers in these structures have the width of normal collagen fibers. The mechanism of formation of these unusual bodies is not clear. Some have suggested that they represent a degenerative change around vessels[84] to which the tumor cells and their contents become adherent.[78,87] These lesions appear to arise from modified smooth muscle cells that normally are found in the lymph node capsule and stroma. The predilection of this tumor to occur in the groin probably reflects the relative frequency with which smooth muscle cells are found in this location relative to other lymph node chains.[78]

All of the cases reported in the literature have behaved in a benign fashion, with no recurrence or metastasis.[78,79] It is important to recognize that this lesion represents a primary benign mesenchymal lesion and not a metastatic sarcoma. These tumors are quite well differentiated and have extremely low levels of mitotic activity, in contrast to most metastatic sarcomas. Moreover, sarcomas infrequently metastasize to lymph nodes, and when they do so it is usually an expression of disseminated disease and rarely an initial presentation.

MAMMARY-TYPE MYOFIBROBLASTOMA

Myofibroblastoma of the breast is an uncommon but highly characteristic mesenchymal tumor that occurs more frequently in men.[88–91] Since similar lesions have also been identified in soft tissue the term mammary-type myofibroblastoma[89] is used for both mammary and extramammary lesions. Of the 16 original mammary cases reported by Wargotz et al.,[88] 11 were in men, with an average age of 63 years. Rare cases have occurred bilaterally.[91] The tumor develops as a discrete, well-marginated mass that does not infiltrate the surrounding breast tissue (Fig. 17–35), although fat trapping may

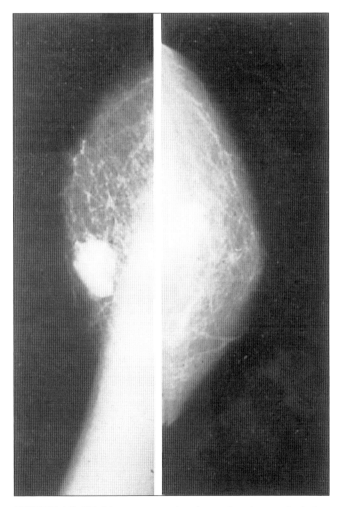

FIGURE 17–35 Mammogram showing a sharply marginated myofibroblastoma.

be seen in the middle of the tumor. The tumors contain slender fibroblast-like spindle cells arranged in sheets or short packets separated by thick collagen bundles. Mast cells may be scattered throughout the lesions (Figs 17–36, 17–37). Rarely, chondroid metaplasia is seen. On electron microscopy and immunohistochemistry the proliferating cells seem most closely related to myofibroblasts or modified smooth muscle cells. They express desmin[88,90] and actin and contain collections of actin filaments, dense bodies, basal lamina, and surface-oriented pinocytotic vesicles.[92] Interestingly, they also express CD34, an antigen expressed by spindle cell lipoma, a lesion which bears an unmistakable similarity to myofibroblastoma.

Once familiar with the pattern of this tumor, most pathologists have little difficulty identifying it. Those unfamiliar with the lesion have a tendency to regard it as a well-differentiated metaplastic carcinoma of the breast or a stromal sarcoma. Perhaps the most helpful feature seen at low power is the impressive circumscription of this lesion compared to malignant spindle cell lesions of the breast. It is also helpful to note that the lesion does not insinuate itself in the substance of the breast, as one would see with carcinomas or stromal sarcomas. The presence of short fascicles of plump cells interrupted by collagen bundles is also at variance with fibromatosis, which consists of long, sweeping fascicles of attenuated fibroblastic cells.

These tumors are entirely benign. None of the original patients described by Wargotz et al.[88] developed recurrence or metastasis. Thus, once the correct diagnosis is established, simple excision is adequate.

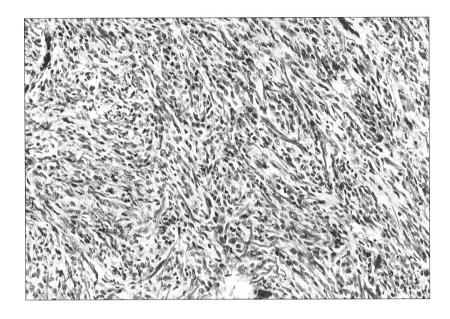

FIGURE 17–36 Mammary-type myofibroblastoma.

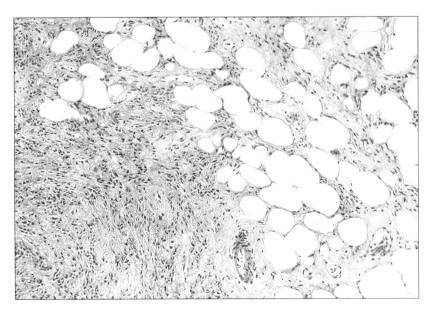

FIGURE 17–37 Fat trapping in a mammary-type myofibroblastoma.

BENIGN GENITAL STROMAL TUMORS

A number of benign mesenchymal tumors arising from or differentiating along the lines of specialized stroma of the female genital tract has been reported over the last two decades. This family of lesions includes angiomyofibroblastoma,[93] cellular angiofibroma,[94] angiomyofibroblastoma of male genital tract,[95] angiomyxoma, and superficial cervicovaginal myofibroblastoma.[96] We regard them as closely related lesions as evidenced by their overlapping histologic and immunophenotypic features. Even among experts, distinction of these lesions may not be clear cut. For example, the lesion reported by Laskin et al.[95] as "angiomyofibroblastoma-like tumor of male genital tract" and regarded as a hybrid between classic angiomyofibroblastoma and spindle cell lipoma was described by Fletcher et al.[93] as "cellular angiofibroma." Although we have endeavored to use the appropriate labels in typical cases, we have found the term "benign genital stromal tumor" very useful for hybrid or ambiguous cases, especially since these various distinctions have little clinical or biologic import.

Angiomyofibroblastoma

Angiomyofibroblastoma is a distinctive tumor that usually involves the vulva[93,94,97–100] but can involve the vagina and rarely the scrotum. These tumors develop as slowly growing, marginated masses in the subcutaneous tissues. Because of their preferential location on the vulva they may be confused with a Bartholin's cyst. The tumors contain prominent, sometimes ectatic vessels surrounded by clusters of eosinophilic epithelioid cells, some of which blend or fan out from the muscular walls of the vessels. The prominence of the eosinophilic cytoplasm has lead to the term "plasmacytoid" for these distinctive cells which lie in small chains, cords, or singly in a matrix that varies from myxoid to hyaline (Figs 17–38, 17–39).

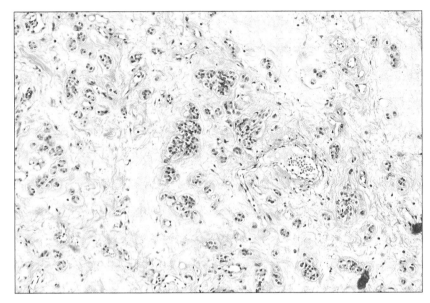

FIGURE 17–38 Angiomyofibroblastoma of the vulva.

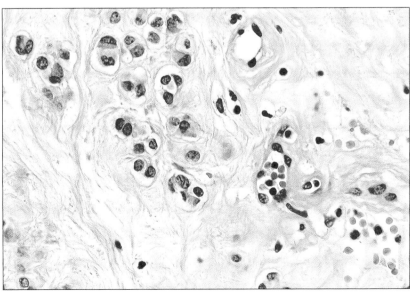

FIGURE 17–39 Epithelioid cells in an angiomyofibroblastoma.

In some cases the cells spindle, and in others they separate from the stroma, creating pseudovascular spaces (Figs 17–40, 17–41). Lesions having a spindled appearance closely resemble cellular angiofibroma. Mature fat is occasionally encountered within these lesions and when prominent has led to the proposed term "lipomatous variant of angiomyofibroblastoma."[101] Immunohistochemically, the cells of angiomyofibroblastoma express vimentin, desmin, and hormone receptor proteins but usually not actin or CD34. Recently, fibroblast growth factor, vascular endothelial growth factor and stem cell factor have been identified in neoplastic cells.

The overwhelming majority of angiomyofibroblastomas are benign with recurrences occurring in those which are less marginated and, therefore, difficult to excise. Histologically malignant forms of angiomyofibroblastoma have been reported.[102,103] These tumors may either resemble an angiomyofibroblastoma except that the cells possess marked atypia and mitotic activity or they may assume a totally different appearance with areas resembling a leiomyosarcoma or undifferentiated sarcoma similar in nature to dedifferentiation in other mesenchymal tumors. None of these rare malignant tumors has metastasized to date, possibly due to their superficiality and ease of resection.

Cellular angiofibroma (angiomyofibroblastoma-like tumor of male genital tract)

The cellular angiofibroma was initially described in 1997 and later in a more extended form by Iwasa and Fletcher[104] in a series of 51 cases. As intimated above, the lesion referred to as angiomyofibroblastoma of the male genital tract[104] is considered a similar, if not identical, tumor. Cel-

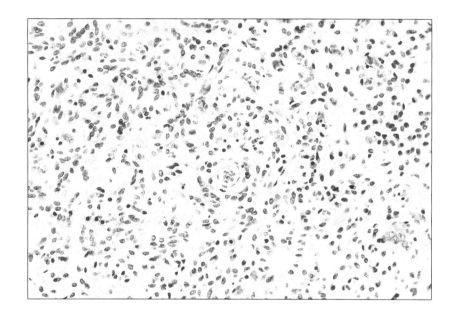

FIGURE 17–40 Angiomyofibroblastoma with more cellularity and spindling than is seen in Figure 17–38.

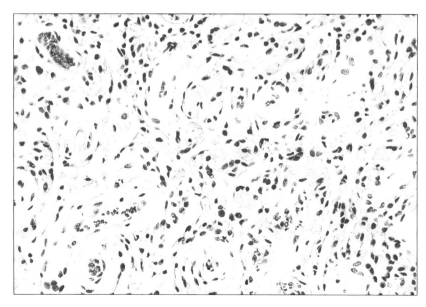

FIGURE 17–41 Pseudovascular spaces in an angiomyofibroblastoma.

lular angiofibroma occurs almost exclusively in the vulvo-vaginal region of women or in the inguinal–scrotal region of males. Unlike the angiomyofibroblastoma which is seen nearly exclusively in women, this lesion affects the sexes in roughly equal proportion and presents as a circumscribed dermal or subcutaneous tumor measuring a few centimeters in diameter. The lesions consist of two components, a cellular spindle cell component arranged randomly or in short fascicles, vague palisades, or swirls around a prominent vasculature (Figs 17–42, 17–43). The cells are either spindled or fusiform in shape with bland cytologic features and usually low mitotic activity

(<1/10 HPF). The stroma contains evenly dispersed small- to medium-sized vessels with mural hyalinization and delicate pale collagen interspersed with short, thicker ones. As in angiomyofibroblastoma, mature fat is seen in about one-quarter of cases. In one highly unusual case reported by Iwasa and Fletcher,[104] a focus of pleomorphic liposarcoma was noted in the center of an otherwise typical cellular angiofibroma. These tumors are notable for strong and diffuse expression for CD34 (60%) with relatively less expression of smooth muscle actin (21%) and desmin (8%). Both estrogen and progesterone receptor proteins can be seen in a subset of cases, but

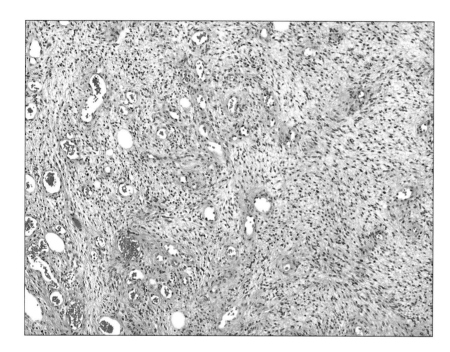

FIGURE 17–42 Cellular angiofibroma.

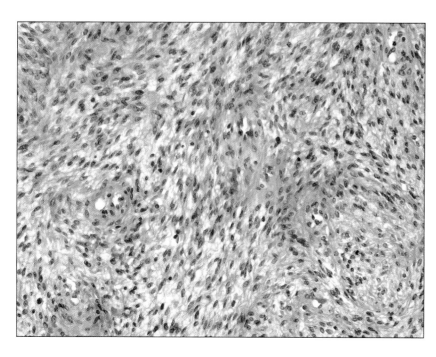

FIGURE 17–43 Cellular angiofibroma.

more often in tumors removed from women than men. Follow-up in 40 cases disclosed no recurrences or metastases within the mean follow-up period of 31 months.[104]

Differential diagnosis of benign genital stromal tumors

The differential diagnosis of benign genital stromal tumors has become a confusing topic largely because of the tendency to split these lesions into subcategories on the basis of subtle differences and the fact that there is considerable overlap in immunophenotype among them (Table 17–1). The challenge is to make an assessment of the predominant histologic features and use the immunohistochemistry in a confirmatory fashion, recognizing that ambiguous cases can be labeled simply as benign genital stromal tumor.

Both angiomyofibroblastoma and cellular angiofibroma present as circumscribed superficial nodules with the latter having the greater propensity to occur in males and in sites outside the gynecologic tract. The most distinctive feature of angiomyofibroblastoma is the characteristic nests or cords of distinctly epithelioid cells arranged around a vasculature of small vessels. In contrast to cellular angiofibroma, it is a uniformly cellular, epithelioid lesion that lacks the epithelioid arrangement of cells around vessels. Its strong expression of CD34 in a majority of cases contrasts with the only rare occurrence in angiomyofibroblastoma.

MISCELLANEOUS LESIONS CONFUSED WITH LEIOMYOMAS

Although the diagnosis of leiomyoma is seldom difficult, occasionally hamartomatous or choristomatous deposits of smooth muscle tissue suggest leiomyoma. Examples include accessory scrotal (Fig. 17–44) or areolar tissue.

TABLE 17–1 BENIGN GENITAL STROMAL TUMORS					
Tumor	Sex predilection	Desmin	Actin	CD 34	ER/PR
Angiomyofibroblastoma	Females	+	±	Rare	+
Angiomyofibroblastoma-like tumor of male genital tract	Males	+	++	+++	+
Cellular angiofibroma	Females = males	Rare	+	+++	+
Angiomyxoma	Females	+	+	+	++

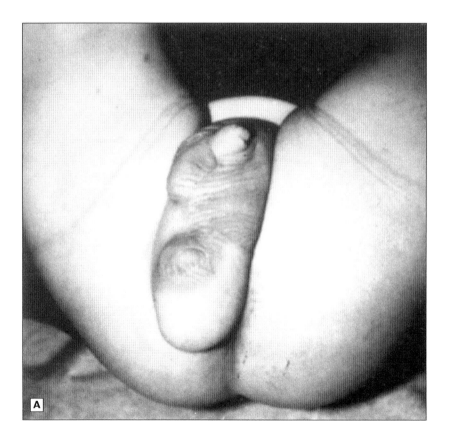

FIGURE 17–44 (A) Accessory scrotum in an infant.

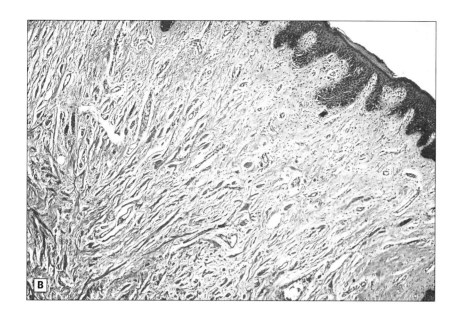

FIGURE 17–44 Continued. **(B)** Microscopic section shows well-differentiated smooth fibers oriented perpendicular to the skin surface.

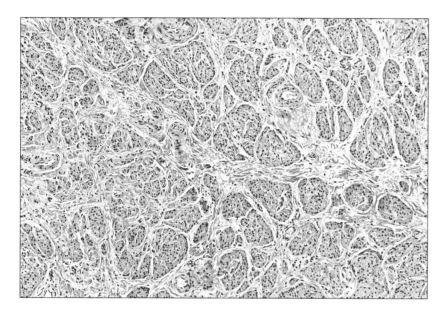

FIGURE 17–45 Round ligament removed at the time of inguinal herniorrhaphy. Cells are distinctly rounded with small centrally placed nuclei.

The clinical appearance and location of the lesions usually suggest the correct diagnosis. The round ligament, when removed incidentally during repair of an inguinal hernia, may also be misinterpreted as a leiomyoma. The round ligament is composed of distinctive, closely packed, polygonal muscle cells with small, dark, centrally placed nuclei (Fig. 17–45)

REFERENCES

General

1. Farman AG. Benign smooth muscle tumors. S Afr Med J 1974; 48:1214.
2. Eyden B. Electron microscopy in the study of myofibroblastic lesions. Sem in Diag Pathol 2003; 20:13.

Structure and function of smooth muscle cells

3. Ross R. The smooth muscle cell. II. Growth of smooth muscle in culture and formation of elastic fibers. J Cell Biol 1971; 50:172.

4. Harman JW, O'Hegarty MT, Byrnes CK. The ultrastructure of human smooth muscle. I. Studies of cell surface and connections in normal and achalasia esophageal smooth muscle. Exp Mol Pathol 1962; 1:204.
5. Hashimoto H, Komori A, Kosaka M, et al. Electron microscopic studies on smooth muscle of the human uterus. J Jpn Obstet Gynecol Soc 1960; 7:115.
6. Morales AR, Fine G, Pardo V, et al. The ultrastructure of smooth muscle tumors with a consideration of the possible relationship of glomangiomas, hemangiopericytomas, and cardiac myxomas. Pathol Annu 1975; 10:65.

7. Rosenbluth J. Smooth muscle: an ultrastructural basis for the dynamics of its contraction. Science 1965; 148:1337.
8. Schuerch LW, Skalli O, Seemeyer TA, et al. Intermediate filament proteins and actin isoforms as markers for soft tissue tumor differentiation and origin. 1. Smooth muscle tumors. Am J Pathol 1987; 128:91.
9. Skalli O, Ropraz P, Trzeciak A, et al. A monoclonal antibody against alpha smooth muscle actin: a new probe for smooth muscle differentiation. J Cell Biol 1986; 103:2787.
10. Uehara Y, Campbell GR, Burnstock G. Cytoplasmic filaments in developing and adult

vertebrate smooth muscle. J Cell Biol 1971; 50:484.

Cutaneous leiomyoma

11. Archer CB, Whittaker S, Greaves MW. Pharmacological modulation of cold-induced pain in cutaneous leiomyomata. Br J Dermatol 1988; 118:255.
12. Auckland G. Hereditary multiple leiomyoma of the skin. Br J Dermatol 1967; 79:63.
13. Fisher WC, Helwig EB. Leiomyomas of the skin. Arch Dermatol 1963; 88:510.
14. Fox SR. Leiomyomatosis cutis. N Engl J Med 1960; 263:1248.
15. Gagne EJ, Su WPD. Congenital smooth muscle hamartoma of the skin. Pediatr Dermatol 1993; 10:142.
16. Jansen LH, Driessen FML. Leiomyoma cutis. Br J Dermatol 1958; 70:446.
17. Kloepfer HW, Krafchuk J, Derbes V, et al. Hereditary multiple leiomyoma of the skin. Am J Hum Genet 1958; 10:48.
18. Mann PR. Leiomyoma cutis: an electron microscope study. Br J Dermatol 1970; 82: 463.
19. Montgomery H, Winkelmann RK. Smooth muscle tumors of the skin. Arch Dermatol 1959; 79:32.
20. Urbanek RW, Johnson WC. Smooth muscle hamartoma associated with Becker's nevus. Arch Dermatol 1978; 114:104.
21. Verma KC, Chawdhry SD, Rathi KS. Cutaneous leiomyomata in two brothers. Br J Dermatol 1973; 90:351.
22. Yokayama R, Hashimoto H, Daimaru Y, et al. Superficial leiomyomas: a clinicopathologic study of 34 cases. Acta Pathol Jpn 1987; 37:1415.
23. Nascimento AG, Karas M, Rosen PP, et al. Leiomyoma of the nipple. Am J Surg Pathol 1979; 3:151.
24. Newman PL, Fletcher CDM. Smooth muscle tumours of the external genitalia: clinicopathologic analysis of a series. Histopathology 1991; 8:523.
25. Siegel GP, Gaffey TA. Solitary leiomyomas arising from the tunica dartos scrotis. J Urol 1976; 116:69.
26. Tavassoli FA, Norris HJ. Smooth muscle tumors of the vulva. Obstet Gynaecol 1979; 53:213.
27. Alam NA, Olpin S, Leigh IM. Fumarate hydratase mutations and predisposition to cutaneous leiomyomas, uterine leiomyomas and renal cancer. Br J Dermatol 2005; 153:11.
28. Kiruru M, Launonen V. Hereditary leiomyomatosis and renal cell cancer (HLRCC). Curr Mol Med 2004; 4:869.
29. Barker KT, Bevan S, Wang R, et al. Low frequency of somatic mutations in FH/multiple cutaneous leiomyomatosis gene in sporadic leiomyosarcomas and uterine leiomyomas. Br J Cancer 2002; 87:446.
30. Lehtonen R, Kiuru M, Vanharanta S, et al. Biallelic inactivation of fumarate hydratase (FH) occurs in nonsyndromic uterine leiomyomas but is rare in other tumors. Am J Pathol 2004; 164:17.

Angiomyoma (vascular leiomyoma)

31. Stout AP. Solitary cutaneous and subcutaneous leiomyoma. Am J Cancer 1937; 24:435.
32. Hachisuga T, Hashimoto H, Enjoji M. Angioleiomyoma: a clinicopathologic reappraisal of 562 cases. Cancer 1984; 54:126.
33. Duhig JJ, Ayer JP. Vascular leiomyoma: a study of 61 cases. Arch Pathol 1959; 68:424.
34. Gutmann J, Cifuentes C, Balzarini MA, et al. Angiomyoma of the oral cavity. Oral Surg Oral Med Oral Pathol 1974; 38:269.
35. Bardach H, Ebner H. Das Angioleiomyom der Haut. Hautarzt 1975; 26:638.

36. Ekestrom S. Comparison between glomus tumour and angioleiomyoma. Acta Pathol Microbiol Scand 1950; 27:86.
37. Carla TG, Filotico R, Filotico M. Bizarre angiomyomas of superficial soft tissues. Pathologica 1991; 83:237.

Leiomyoma of deep soft tissue

38. Kilpatrick SE, Mentzel T, Fletcher CDM. Leiomyoma of deep soft tissue: clinicopathologic analysis of a series. Am J Surg Pathol 1994; 18:576.
39. Fletcher CDM, Kilpatrick SE, Mentzel T. The difficulty of predicting behavior of smooth muscle tumors in deep soft tissue. Am J Surg Pathol 1995; 19:116.
40. Billings SD, Folpe AL, Weiss SW. Do leiomyomas of deep soft tissue exist? An analysis of highly differentiated smooth muscle tumors of deep soft tissue supporting two distinct subtypes. Am J Surg Pathol 2001; 25:1134.
41. Paal E, Miettinen M. Retroperitoneal leiomyoma: a clinicopathologic study of 56 cases. Am J Surg Pathol 2001; 25:1355.
42. Miettinen M, Fetsch JF. Evaluation of the biologic potential of smooth muscle tumors. Histopathology 2006; 48:97.
43. Weiss SW. Smooth muscle tumors of soft tissue: an overview. Adv Anat Pathol 2002; 9:351.
44. Meis JM, Enzinger FM. Myolipoma of soft tissue. Am J Surg Pathol 1991; 15:121.
45. Scurry JP, Carey MP, Targett CS, et al. Soft tissue lipoleiomyoma. Pathology 1991; 23:360.

Intravenous leiomyomatosis

46. Clement PH, Young RH, Scully RE. Intravenous leiomyomatosis of the uterus: a clinicopathological analysis of 16 cases with unusual histologic features. Am J Surg Pathol 1988; 12:932.
47. Kir G, Kir M, Gurbuz A, et al. Estrogen and progesterone expression of vessel walls with intravascular leiomyomatosis, discussion of histogenesis. Eur J Gynecol Oncol 2004; 25:362.
48. Quade BJ, Dal Cin P, Neskey DM, et al. Intravenous leiomyomatosis: molecular and cytogenetic analysis of a case. Mod Pathol 2002; 15:351.
49. Clement PH. Intravenous leiomyomatosis of the uterus. Pathol Annu 1988; 23:153.
50. Heinonen PK, Taina E, Nerdrum T, et al. Intravenous leiomyomatosis. Ann Chir Gynaecol 1984; 73:100.
51. Norris HJ, Parmley TH. Mesenchymal tumors of the uterus. V. Intravenous leiomyomatosis: a clinical and pathologic study of 14 cases. Cancer 1975; 36:2164.
52. Shida T, Yoshimura M, Chihara H, et al. Intravenous leiomyomatosis of the pelvis and re-extension into the heart. Ann Thorac Surg 1986; 42:104.
53. Suginami H, Kaura R, Ochi H, et al. Intravenous leiomyomatosis with cardiac extension: successful surgical management and histopathologic study. Obstet Gynecol 1990; 76:527.
54. Tierney WM, Ehrlich CE, Bailey JC, et al. Intravenous leiomyomatosis of the uterus with extension into the heart. Am J Med 1980; 69:471.
55. Wolff M, Silva F, Kaye G. Pulmonary metastases (with admixed epithelial elements) from smooth muscle neoplasms: report of nine cases including three males. Am J Surg Pathol 1979; 3:325.

Leiomyomatosis peritonealis disseminata

56. Willson JR, Peale AR. Multiple peritoneal leiomyomas associated with a granulosa-cell

tumor of the ovary. Am J Obstet Gynecol 1952; 64:204.
57. Crosland DB. Leiomyomatosis peritonealis disseminata: a case report. Am J Obstet Gynecol 1973; 117:179.
58. Tavassoli FA, Norris HJ. Peritoneal leiomyomatosis (leiomyomatosis peritonealis disseminata). Int J Gynecol Pathol 1982; 1:59.
59. Kaplan C, Bernirschke K, Johnson KC. Leiomyomatosis peritonealis disseminata with endometrium. Obstet Gynecol 1980; 55:119.
60. Lim OW, Segal A, Ziel HK. Leiomyomatosis peritonealis disseminata associated with pregnancy. Obstet Gynecol 1980; 55:122.
61. Parmley TH, Woodruff JD, Winn K, et al. Histogenesis of leiomyomatosis peritonealis disseminata (disseminated fibrosing deciduosis). Obstet Gynecol 1975; 46:511.
62. Winn KJ, Woodruff JD, Parmley TH. Electron microscopic studies of leiomyomatosis peritonealis disseminata. Obstet Gynecol 1976; 48:225.
63. Pieslor PC, Orenstein JM, Hogan DL, et al. Ultrastructure of myofibroblasts and decidualized cells in leiomyomatosis peritonealis disseminata. Am J Clin Pathol 1979; 72:875.
64. Kitazawa S, Shiraishi N, Maeda S. Leiomyomatosis peritonealis disseminata with adipocytic differentiation. Acta Obstet Gynecol Scand 1992; 71:482.
65. Chen KT, Hendricks EJ, Freeburg B. Benign glandular inclusion of the peritoneum associated with leiomyomatosis peritonealis disseminata. Diagn Gynecol Obstet 1982; 4:41.
66. Ma KF, Chow LT. Sex cord-like pattern leiomyomatosis peritonealis disseminata: a hitherto undescribed feature. Histopathology 1992; 21:389.
67. Nogales FF, Matilla A, Carrascal E. Leiomyomatosis peritonealis disseminata: an ultrastructural study. Am J Clin Pathol 1978; 69:452.
68. Kuo T, London SN, Dinh TV. Endometriosis occurring in leiomyomatosis peritonealis disseminata: ultrastructural study and histogenetic consideration. Am J Surg Pathol 1980; 4:197.
69. Goldberg MF, Hurt WG, Frable WJ. Leiomyomatosis peritonealis disseminata: report of a case and review of the literature. Obstet Gynecol 1977; 49:46.
70. Fujii S, Nakashima N, Okamura H, et al. Progesterone-induced smooth muscle-like cells in subperitoneal nodules produced by estrogen: experimental approach to leiomyomatosis peritonealis disseminata. Am J Obstet Gynecol 1981; 139:164.
71. Aterman K, Fraser GM, Lea RH. Disseminated peritoneal leiomyomatosis. Virchows Arch [Pathol Anat] 1977; 374:13.
72. Quade BJ, McLachlin CM, Soto-Wright V, et al. Disseminated peritoneal leiomyomatosis: clonality analysis by X chromosome inactivation and cytogenetics of a clinically benign smooth muscle proliferation. Am J Pathol 1997; 150:2153.
73. Hovnck van Papendrecht HPCM, Gratam S. Leiomyomatosis peritonealis disseminata. Eur J Obstet Reprod Biol 1983; 14:251.
74. Parente JT, Levy J, Chinea E, et al. Adjuvant surgical and hormonal treatment of leiomyomatosis peritonealis disseminata: a case report. J Reprod Med 1995; 40:468.
75. Akkersdijk GJ, Flu PK, Giard RW, et al. Malignant leiomyomatosis peritonealis disseminata. Am J Obstet Gynecol 1990; 163:591.
76. Abulafia O, Angel C, Sherer DM, et al. Computed tomography of leiomyomatosis peritonealis disseminata with malignant transformation. Am J Obstet Gynecol 1993; 169:52.

77. Rubin SC, Wheeler JE, Mikuta JJ. Malignant leiomyomatosis peritonealis disseminata. Obstet Gynecol 1986; 68:126.

Intranodal palisaded myofibroblastoma

78. Weiss SW, Gnepp DR, Bratthauer GL. Palisaded myofibroblastoma: a benign mesenchymal tumor of lymph node. Am J Surg Pathol 1989; 13:341.
79. Suster S, Rosai J. Intranodal hemorrhagic spindle-cell tumor with "amianthoid" fibers: report of six cases of a distinctive mesenchymal neoplasm of the inguinal region that simulates Kaposi's sarcoma. Am J Surg Pathol 1989; 13:347.
80. Lee JY-Y, Abell E, Shevechek GJ. Solitary spindle cell tumor with myoid differentiation of lymph node. Arch Pathol Lab Med 1989; 113:547.
81. Michal M, Chlumska A, Povysilova V. Intranodal "amianthoid" myofibroblastoma: report of six cases with immunohistochemical and electron microscopical study. Pathol Res Pract 1992; 188:199.
82. Katz D. Neurilemmoma with calcerosiderotic nodules. Isr J Med Sci 1974; 10:1156.
83. Deligdish L, Loewenthal M, Friedlaender E. Malignant neurilemmoma (schwannoma) in the lymph nodes. Int Surg 1968; 49:226.
84. Alguacil-Garcia A. Intranodal myofibroblastoma in a submandibular lymph node: a case report. Am J Clin Pathol 1992; 97:69.
85. Fletcher CD, Stirling RW. Intranodal myofibroblastoma presenting in the submandibular region: evidence of a broader clinical and histological spectrum. Histopathology 1990; 16:287.
86. Skalova A, Michal M, Chlumska A, et al. Collagen composition and ultrastructure of the so-called amianthoid fibres in palisaded myofibroblastoma: ultrastructural and immunohistochemical study. J Pathol 1992; 167:335.
87. Bigotti G, Coli A, Mottolese M, et al. Selective location of palisaded myofibroblastoma with amianthoid fibres. J Clin Pathol 1991; 44:761.

Mammary-type myofibroblastoma

88. Wargotz ES, Weiss SW, Norris HJ. Myofibroblastoma of the breast: sixteen cases of a distinctive benign mesenchymal tumor. Am J Surg Pathol 1987; 11:493.
89. McMenamin ME, Fletcher CD. Mammary-type myofibroblastoma of soft tissue: a tumor closely related to spindle cell lipoma. Am J Surg Pathol 2001; 25:1022.
90. Lee AH, Sworn MJ, Theaker JM, et al. Myofibroblastoma of breast: immunohistochemical study. Histopathology 1993; 22:75.
91. Hamele-Bena D, Cranor ML, Sciotto C, et al. Uncommon presentation of mammary myofibroblastoma. Mod Pathol 1996; 9:786.
92. Amin MB, Gottlieb CA, Fitzmaurice M, et al. Fine-needle aspiration cytologic study of myofibroblastoma of the breast: immunohistochemical and ultrastructural findings. Am J Clin Pathol 1993; 99:593.

Benign genital stromal tumor

93. Fletcher CD, Tsang WY, Fisher C, et al. Angiomyofibroblastoma of the vulva: a benign neoplasm distinct from aggressive angiomyxoma. Am J Surg Pathol 1992; 16:373.
94. Granter SR, Nucci MR, Fletcher CDM. Aggressive angiomyxoma: reappraisal of its relationship with angiomyofibroblastoma in a series of 16 cases. Histopathology 1997; 30:3.
95. Laskin WB, Fetsch JF, Mostofi FK. Angiomyofibroblastoma-like tumor of the male genital tract: analysis of 11 cases with comparison to female angiomyofibroblastoma and spindle cell lipoma. Am J Surg Pathol 1998; 22:6.
96. McCluggage WG. A review and update of morphologically bland vulvovaginal mesenchymal lesions. Int J Gynec Path 2005; 24:26.
97. Horiguchi H, Matsui-Horiguchi M, Fujiwara M, et al. Angiomyofibroblastoma of the vulva: report of a case with immunohistochemical and molecular analysis. Int J Gynecol Pathol 2003; 22:277.
98. Hiruki T, Thomas MJ, Clement PB. Vulvar angiomyofibroblastoma. Am J Surg Pathol 1993; 17:423.
99. Hisaoka M, Kouho H, Aoki T, et al. Angiomyofibroblastoma of the vulva: a clinicopathologic study of seven cases. Pathol Int 1995; 45:487.
100. Nielsen GP, Rosenberg AE, Young RH, et al. Angiomyofibroblastoma of the vulva and vagina: a clinicopathologic study of 12 cases. Mod Pathol 1996; 9:284.
101. Cao D, Srodon M, Montgomery et al. Lipomatous variant of angiomyofibroblastoma: report of two cases and review of the literature. Int J Gynecol Pathol 2005; 24:196.
102. Nielsen GP, Young RH, Dickersin GR, et al. Angiomyofibroblastoma of the vulva with sarcomatous transformation ("angiomyofibrosarcoma"). Am J Surg Pathol 1997; 21:1104.
103. Folpe AL, Tworek JA, Weiss SW. Sarcomatous transformation in angiomyofibroblastomas: a clinicopathological and immunohistochemical study of eleven cases (abstract). Mod Pathol 2001; 14:12A.
104. Iwasa Y, Fletcher CD. Cellular angiofibroma: clinicopathologic and immunohistochemical analysis of 51 cases. Am J Surg Pathol 2004; 28:1426.

LEIOMYOSARCOMA

Leiomyosarcomas account for 5–10% of soft tissue sarcomas.[1,2] They are principally tumors of adult life but are far outnumbered by the more common adult sarcomas such as liposarcoma and pleomorphic undifferentiated sarcoma (malignant fibrous histiocytoma). Likewise, they are less common than leiomyosarcomas of uterine or gastrointestinal origin, and only some of the data gleaned from the collective experience with tumors in these two sites are directly applicable to the soft tissue counterpart. Few predisposing or etiologic factors are recognized for this disease. In general, these tumors are more common in women than men. About two-thirds of all retroperitoneal leiomyosarcomas[3,4] and more than three-quarters of all vena caval leiomyosarcomas occur in women.[5] The significance of this observation is not clear, although growth and proliferation of smooth muscle tissue in women have been noted to coincide with pregnancy and estrogenic stimulation (see Chapter 17). Children rarely develop these tumors,[6,7] and there is conflicting evidence as to whether leiomyosarcomas in children have a better prognosis.[6,8,9]

Leiomyosarcomas also rarely occur following radiation[10–12] but may develop as a second malignancy in the setting of bilateral (hereditary) retinoblastoma.[13] Because these tumors may occur at sites distant from their irradiated site, their pathogenesis is directly attributable to the *Rb1* mutation and not to irradiation. A study by Stratton et al. indicated that deletions or mutations of the *Rb1* locus can be identified in a small number of leiomyosarcomas that occur on a sporadic basis as well.[14] There is no evidence that leiomyomas undergo malignant transformation with any degree of regularity. Well-differentiated areas resembling leiomyoma are often found in a leiomyosarcoma, but this by no means proves that malignant transformation occurred. In fact, the predilection of leiomyosarcomas for deep soft tissue, in contrast to the superficial location of leiomyomas, provides some evidence to the contrary. Interestingly, there is growing evidence that as a group leiomyosarcomas may have a poorer prognosis than other sarcomas when matched for other variables,[15,16] an observation which may warrant type-specific modifications of current grading systems.

It is useful to divide leiomyosarcomas into several site-related subgroups because of significant clinical and biologic differences. In fact, site alone is one of the most important prognostic factors in assessing outcome in this disease. Leiomyosarcomas of retroperitoneum and abdominal cavity are the most common subgroup and are associated with an aggressive clinical course. Leiomyosarcomas of somatic soft tissue are a second but less common subgroup associated with a better prognosis. There is increasing evidence that many, if not most, arise from small vessels, a relationship which may be important for defining the behavior and risk of metastasis. Although technically such lesions could be referred to as "vascular leiomyosarcomas," this designation usually refers to a tumor arising from a major vessel such that clinical symptoms, radiographic findings, or both suggest the relationship preoperatively. Cutaneous leiomyosarcomas comprise a third subgroup which has a good prognosis because of its superficial location. They can be likened to atypical fibroxanthoma and superficial forms of malignant fibrous histiocytoma (see Chapter 14), which have a highly atypical appearance but a favorable clinical course because of their limited clinical stage. The last subgroup comprises leiomyosarcomas of vascular origin. As implied above, in this chapter we use this designation to refer to tumors arising from medium-size or large veins, in contrast to leiomyosarcomas in which the vascular origin is identified on the basis of microscopic examination. Defined in this fashion these tumors are rare. Leiomyosarcomas may occur in an unusual soft tissue site such as the head and neck and paratesticular region[17,18] but these are decidedly uncommon.

RETROPERITONEAL/ABDOMINAL LEIOMYOSARCOMAS

About one-half to three-quarters of all soft tissue leiomyosarcomas arise in the retroperitoneum and a smaller number in the abdominal cavity or mediastinum. Two-thirds of affected patient are women. The peak incidence occurs in the seventh decade. The presenting signs and symptoms are relatively non-specific and include an abdominal mass or swelling, pain, weight loss, nausea, or vomiting.

Gross and microscopic findings

Virtually all retroperitoneal tumors are more than 5 cm and most larger than 10 cm when first detected,[3,4,19] in striking contrast to the majority of somatic soft tissue leiomyosarcomas.[20] They commonly involve other structures, such as the kidney, pancreas, and vertebral column by direct extension. Grossly, some have a white-gray whorled appearance resembling a leiomyoma on cut section (Fig. 18–1) whereas others are fleshy white-gray masses with foci of hemorrhage and necrosis and are, therefore, indistinguishable from other sarcomas (Fig. 18–2).

Histologically, the typical cell of a leiomyosarcoma is elongated and has abundant cytoplasm that varies tinctorially from pink to deep red in sections stained with hematoxylin-eosin. The nucleus is usually centrally located and blunt-ended or "cigar-shaped" (Fig. 18–3).

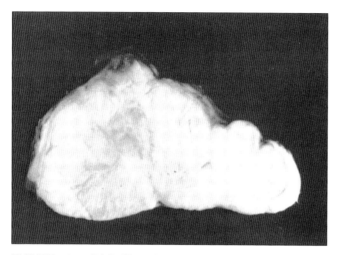

FIGURE 18–1 Well-differentiated leiomyosarcoma with a whorled appearance similar to that of a leiomyoma on cut section.

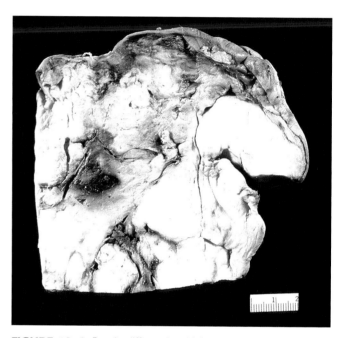

FIGURE 18–2 Poorly differentiated leiomyosarcoma characterized by fleshy white tissue with hemorrhage and necrosis.

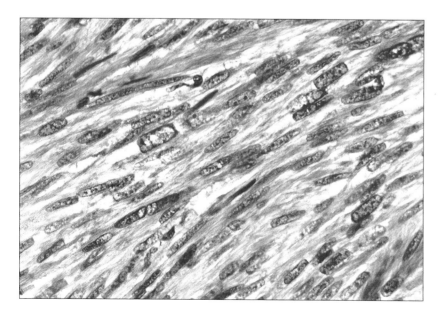

FIGURE 18–3 Cytologic features of leiomyosarcoma showing eosinophilic cytoplasm and blunt-ended nuclei. Occasional cells have perinuclear vacuoles.

In some smooth muscle cells a vacuole is seen at one end of the nucleus, causing a slight indentation, so the nucleus assumes a concave rather than a convex contour (Fig. 18–3). In less well-differentiated tumors the nucleus is larger and more hyperchromatic and often loses its central location. Multinucleated giant cells are common. Likewise, depending on the degree of differentiation, the appearance of the cytoplasm varies. Differentiated cells have numerous well-oriented myofibrils that are demonstrable as deep red, longitudinally placed parallel lines running the length of the cell as seen with a Masson trichrome stain (Fig. 18–4). In poorly differentiated cells the longitudinal striations are less numerous, poorly oriented, and therefore more difficult to identify. In some tumors the cytoplasm has a "clotted" appearance as a result of clumping of the myofilamentous material (Fig.

18–5). When this phenomenon occurs it may be difficult to identify linear striations. They are composed of slender or slightly plump cells arranged in fascicles of varying size (Figs 18–6 to 18–9). In well-differentiated areas the fascicles intersect at right angles so it is possible to see transverse and longitudinal sections side by side, similar to the pattern of a uterine myoma. In many areas the pattern is not that orderly, however, and it more closely resembles the intertwining fascicular growth of a fibrosarcoma (Fig. 18–10). In occasional leiomyosarcomas the nuclei align themselves to create palisades, similar to a schwannoma (Fig. 18–11). Hyalinization is a relatively common, but usually focal, feature of many leiomyosarcomas (Fig. 18–12).[21]

About 10% of retroperitoneal leiomyosarcomas are anaplastic tumors (Figs 18–13, 18–14), which in the

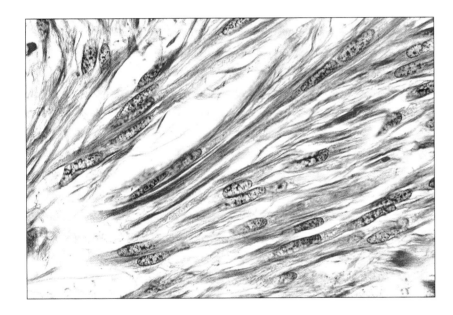

FIGURE 18–4 Masson trichrome stain illustrating longitudinal striations in a leiomyosarcoma. Striations appear as red, hair-like streaks in the cytoplasm.

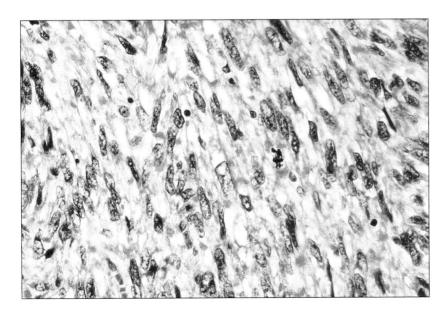

FIGURE 18–5 Leiomyosarcoma with "clotted" or clumped myofilamentous material in the cytoplasm.

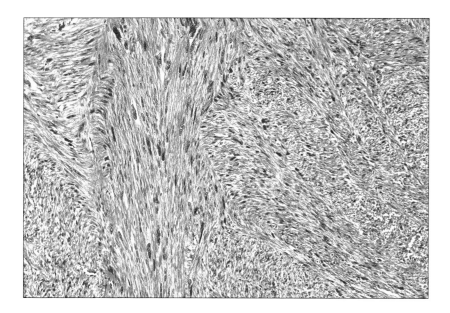

FIGURE 18–6 Moderately differentiated leiomyosarcoma composed of deeply eosinophilic fascicles intersecting at right angles.

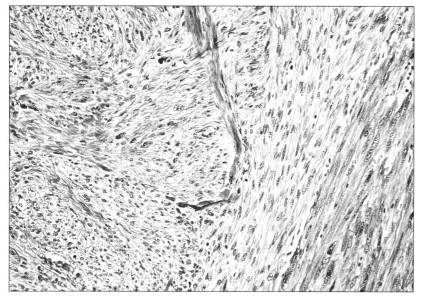

FIGURE 18–7 Moderately differentiated leiomyosarcoma composed of intersecting fascicles, some having a deeply eosinophilic hue and others a clear-cell appearance.

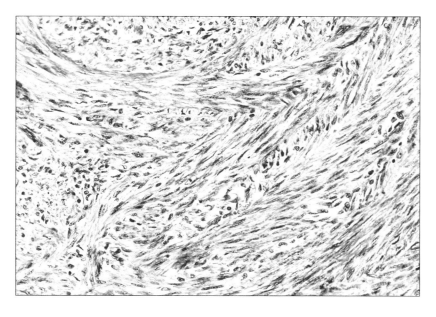

FIGURE 18–8 Well-differentiated leiomyosarcoma with a fascicular growth pattern.

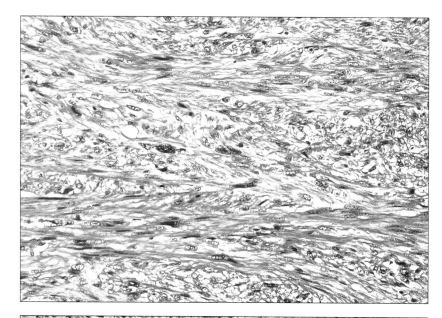

FIGURE 18–9 Moderately differentiated leiomyosarcoma with a fascicular growth pattern.

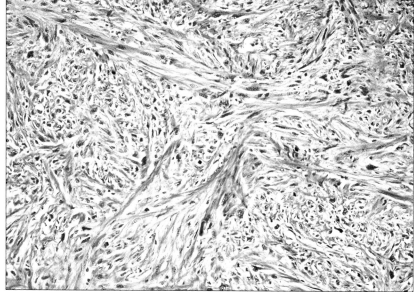

FIGURE 18–10 Leiomyosarcoma with a pattern of short intersecting fascicles.

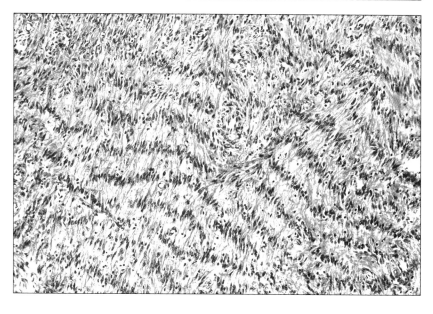

FIGURE 18–11 Leiomyosarcoma with nuclear palisading.

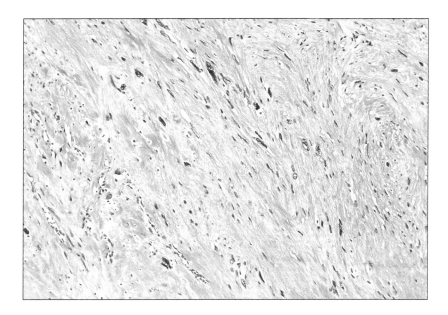

FIGURE 18–12 Hyalinization in a leiomyosarcoma.

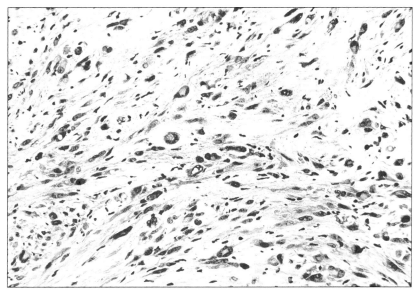

FIGURE 18–13 Pleomorphism in a leiomyosarcoma.

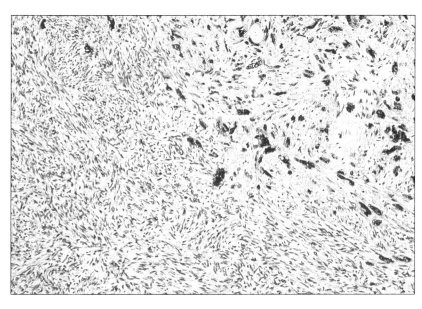

FIGURE 18–14 Leiomyosarcoma with pleomorphic areas that resemble malignant fibrous histiocytoma (top right).

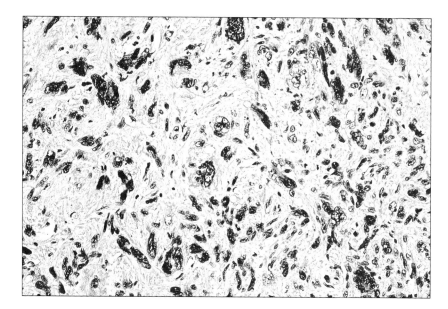

FIGURE 18-15 Pleomorphic area in leiomyosarcoma resembling malignant fibrous histiocytoma.

extreme case resemble a malignant fibrous histiocytoma.[22] They contain numerous pleomorphic giant cells with deeply eosinophilic cytoplasm intimately admixed with a complement of more uniform-appearing spindle and round cells (Figs 18–15 to 18–17). In contrast to malignant fibrous histiocytoma, these tumors have less interstitial collagen and few inflammatory cells. In addition, it is usually possible to document myogenic differentiation in the less pleomorphic areas. Necrosis, hemorrhage, and mitotic figures are frequent in these pleomorphic tumors. Osteoclastic giant cells, with histiocytic (CD68), but not myogenic markers,[23] are an uncommon feature of leiomyosarcomas.[23-26] Based on their distinct immunophenotypic profile, they may well represent an unusual host response to the tumor, rather than an intrinsic part of the lesion. Unusually, leiomyosarcomas with liposarcoma[27] or rhabdomyosarcomas have been reported.[28]

Histologic variants of leiomyosarcoma

Myxoid change may occur in leiomyosarcomas. When extensive, these tumors appear grossly gelatinous and are referred to as *myxoid leiomyosarcoma*. Although most common in the uterus,[29,30] they develop in conventional soft tissue locations as well.[31] The spindled muscle cells are separated by pools of hyaluronic acid, and in cross-section the fascicles may resemble the cords of tumor seen in a myxoid chondrosarcoma (Figs 18–18, 18–19). Because these tumors are quite hypocellular relative to conventional leiomyosarcomas, mitotic rates estimated by counting high-power fields are usually deceptively low, giving the false impression of a benign tumor. In general, myxoid leiomyosarcomas segregate toward the low-grade end of a grading spectrum. Of the 18 cases reported by Rubin and Fletcher[31], 9 were considered grade 1, 8 grade

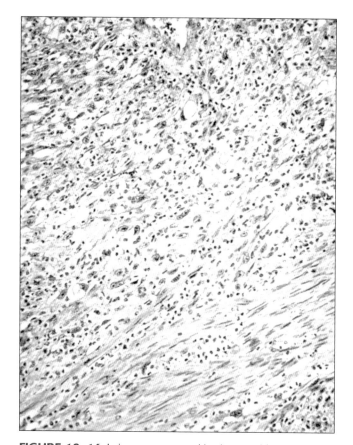

FIGURE 18-16 Leiomyosarcoma with pleomorphic areas resembling the inflammatory form of malignant fibrous histiocytoma. (×160)

2, and only 1 grade 3. In their series, 5 of 13 patients experienced recurrences, often repeated, and 2, metastases. It is quite possible that spillage of the gelatinous matrix at the time of surgery contributes to the common phenomenon of local recurrence.

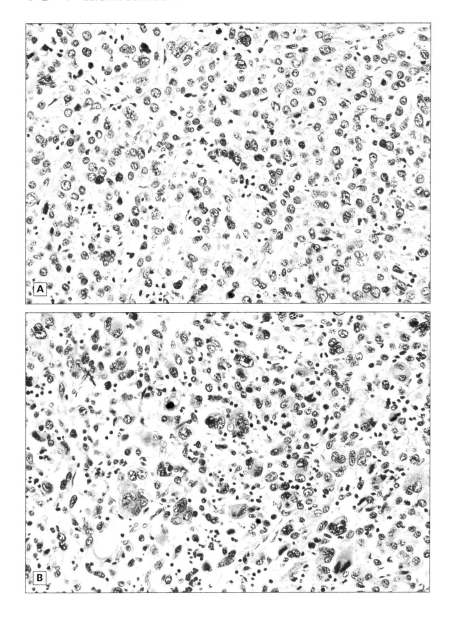

FIGURE 18–17 Leiomyosarcoma with round cell **(A)**, and pleomorphic **(B)** areas.

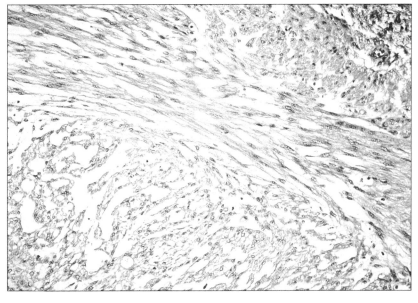

FIGURE 18–18 Myxoid leiomyosarcoma.

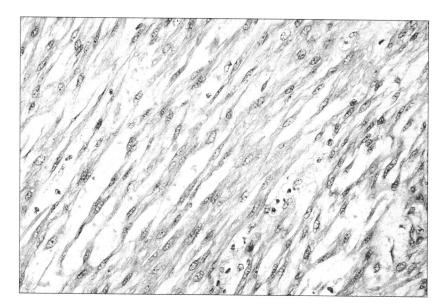

FIGURE 18–19 Myxoid leiomyosarcoma showing separation of spindle cells.

So-called *"inflammatory leiomyosarcoma"* is a rare entity defined as a leiomyosarcoma containing xanthoma cells and a prominent inflammatory infiltrate (usually lymphocytes but occasionally neutrophils).[32] They do not occur in any specific location and may be associated with constitutional or paraneoplastic symptoms such as anorexia, fever, night sweats, and diarrhea. Interestingly, whereas these tumors express desmin to a significant degree they lack or only focally express other muscle markers including muscle specific actin, alpha smooth muscle actin, and caldesmon leading to the recent suggestion that these lesions may not be true smooth muscle tumors.[33] Most cases that have been analyzed have displayed a near-haploid karyotype. Although originally associated with an excellent prognosis, recent cases have been reported with metastases.

Rarely, leiomyosarcomas contain cells with granular eosinophilic cytoplasm[34] (*granular cell leiomyosarcomas*). This change corresponds to the presence of numerous granules that stain positively with PAS and are resistant to diastase. Ultrastructurally, they are similar to the phagolysosomes seen in granular cell tumors.

Ultrastructural and immunohistochemical findings

Leiomyosarcomas are characterized by many of the same features as normal smooth muscle cells, but in general they are less developed. Differentiated leiomyosarcomas have deeply clefted nuclei and numerous well-oriented, thin (6–8 nm) myofilaments and dense bodies that occupy a large portion of the cell (Fig. 18–20). Pinocytotic vesicles and intercellular connections are conspicuous, and basal lamina invests the entire cell membrane. The presence of these features is diagnostic of smooth muscle differentiation even without the benefit of light

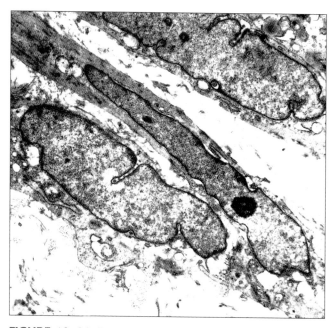

FIGURE 18–20 Electron micrograph of metastatic leiomyosarcoma. Cells are characterized by an elongated shape, deeply grooved nuclei, and numerous thin filaments with dense bodies.

microscopic findings. On the other hand, poorly differentiated tumors show a loss of myofilaments as rough endoplasmic reticulum, and free ribosomes assume greater prominence.[35] Pinocytotic vesicles and intercellular attachments are sparse, and basal lamina may be incomplete or lacking altogether. All of these features must be evaluated in toto in these tumors and interpreted in conjunction with the light microscopic findings for diagnostic purposes. It should be emphasized that the mere presence of thin myofilaments with dense bodies does not identify a smooth muscle cell. Thin myofilaments are a non-specific finding and can be seen in a variety of tumors where they typically occur underneath the cytoplasmic membrane.

Localization of muscle antigens by means of immuno-histochemistry has assumed more importance in diagnosis than electron microscopy over the past several years due in part to a larger number of high-performance antibodies. Although seldom required when the light microscopic features of smooth muscle differentiation are apparent, it is quite useful in the diagnosis of poorly differentiated leiomyosarcomas whose features approximate those of many malignant fibrous histiocytomas (pleomorphic undifferentiated sarcoma), recognizing that the distribution and intensity of muscle markers in highly pleomorphic areas of leiomyosarcoma are generally diminished compared to classic-appearing areas.[22]

Smooth muscle actin and muscle-specific actin (HHF35)[36] can be detected in most leiomyosarcomas.[7,22,37,38] Desmin, more variable, has been documented in one-half to nearly 100% of tumors,[22,38,39] depending on the series. Although there seems to be general agreement that the presence of desmin diffusely throughout a tumor is usually indicative of myoid differentiation, the presence of actin or desmin focally should not necessarily be equated with myoid lineage, as myofibroblasts in a variety of neoplastic and nonneoplastic conditions also display this phenotype. H-caldesmon, regarded as a muscle marker which can discriminate between smooth muscle cells and myofibroblasts, is present in about 40% of leiomyosarcomas and seems to vary not only with tumor site but degree of differentiation.[39] Thus, it is becoming increasingly common to employ a panel of several muscle markers to assess whether on balance a given tumor is displaying smooth muscle differentiation. Smooth muscle tumors comprise one of the mesenchymal lesions in which keratin immunoreactivity has been reported,[40–43] and, along with EMA, may be encountered in about 40% of cases.[44] The immunoreactivity is usually localized to a perinuclear zone and is due to the presence of keratins 8 and 18.[42] Other antigens sporadically identified in leiomyosarcomas are S-100 protein, and estrogen and progesterone receptor protein.[38,45]

Criteria of malignancy

Criteria of malignancy in smooth muscle tumors have been alluded to in Chapter 17. In general, the finding of significant nuclear atypia even of a focal nature is a cause for concern in soft tissue smooth muscle tumors and should lead to an evaluation of mitotic activity. By definition, leiomyosarcomas possess some degree of nuclear atypia but mitotic activity varies considerably. However, we accept even very low levels of mitotic activity (<1/10HPF) in the face of significant atypia as sufficient evidence of malignancy. In retroperitoneal lesions coagu-

lative necrosis is usually also present and can be quite impressive.

Differential diagnosis

The differential diagnosis of leiomyosarcomas traditionally includes other sarcomas composed of fascicles of moderately differentiated spindle cells, such as fibrosarcoma and malignant peripheral nerve sheath tumor. Although the low-power appearance of all three can be similar, there is a greater tendency to see a close juxtaposition of longitudinally and transversely cut fascicles in a leiomyosarcoma. The cytologic features play a more important role in the differential diagnosis. Compared with the cells of leiomyosarcoma, those of a fibrosarcoma tend to be tapered, and those of a malignant peripheral nerve sheath tumor are wavy, buckled, and distinctly asymmetric. Usually, neither malignant peripheral nerve sheath tumors nor fibrosarcomas contain glycogen; and although both occasionally display fuchsinophilia of the cytoplasm, neither has longitudinal striations. There are, in addition to the above lesions, reactive fibroblastic lesions in the submucosa of various parenchymal organs that are commonly confused with leiomyosarcomas or even rhabdomyosarcomas. Many of these lesions have been reported in the bladder, where some have been associated with prior instrumentation. We have also encountered them in the vagina, endometrium, larynx, and oral cavity. They have been termed postoperative spindle cell nodule,[46] inflammatory pseudotumor,[47] and pseudosarcomatous fibromyxoid tumor.[48] They are composed of bipolar or stellate fibroblasts with bizarre nuclei and a light basophilic cytoplasm set in a myxoid stroma containing inflammatory cells (see Chapter 9). Mitotic figures may be encountered, although atypical mitotic figures are not seen. The principal features we have found helpful for distinguishing these bizarre reactive lesions from leiomyosarcoma are the less-ordered arrangement of the cells with respect to one another, the basophilic hue of the cytoplasm, and the absence of distinct linear striations. In the limited number of cases we have studied, the cells have been strongly positive for vimentin but negative for desmin; interestingly, they may express cytokeratin and ALK-1 protein.

Clinical behavior

Retroperitoneal leiomyosarcomas are aggressive lesions which cause death not only by distant metastasis but also by local extension. The survival figures differ among series and are obviously influenced by the criteria of malignancy, proportion of high-grade versus low-grade tumors, and length of the follow-up. Early studies reflected mortality rates of 80–90% within a 2–5 year follow-up period.[4,19,20] However, a recent multi-institutional study published by the FNCLCC detailing experience with 165 retroperitoneal sarcomas of all types indicates that an improvement in complete resection rates in retroperitoneal sarcomas has reduced local recurrence to 50% and improved survival rates to 50%. Factors which influence outcome in (nonliposarcomatous) retroperitoneal sarcomas include size, grade, and whether extension to bone and nerve is present.[49]

The importance of genetic and molecular analysis in assessing prognosis is becoming apparent. As a group, leiomyosarcomas display complex karyotypic alterations,[50] but certain genomic imbalances suggest that both a loss of tumor suppressor genes and activation of oncogenes play a role in tumorigenesis of these lesions.[51] For example, large tumors and those with metastases commonly display 10q deletions and high-grade lesions 5p gains,[51] and Wang et al. identified loss of 13q14-q21 and gain of 5p14pter in the progression of leiomyosarcoma.[52] Inactivation of cancer-related genes (e.g., RASSF1A, p16INK4a) secondary to hypermethylation have also been associated with poor prognosis.[53,54] Analysis of cyclin-dependent kinase inhibitors by immunohistochemistry has been proposed as a useful prognostic tool.[55] Specific gene expression signature patterns may offer the ability to further predict outcome.[56,57]

LEIOMYOSARCOMAS OF SOMATIC SOFT TISSUE

Compared with retroperitoneal lesions, tumors arising from the soft tissues of the extremities and trunk are far less common and affect the sexes equally. Only 48 cases were identified by Gustafson et al.[1,58] in a 22-year review of a Swedish population in Lund, and we have studied 42 cases largely based on referred consultations. These tumors present as an enlarging mass, usually in the lower extremity. About half develop in the subcutis and the remainder in muscle. They have a circumscribed multinodular appearance and are significantly smaller (6 cm) than those in the retroperitoneum. When examined microscopically, at least one-third arise from a small vein causing expansion of the wall and protrusion into the lumen. Since many remain partially or completely confined by the adventitia they give the impression of being discrete, encapsulated lesions, a feature that often leads to an inadvertent enucleation by the surgeon. Despite their vascular origin, few are associated with symptoms of vascular compromise as occurs with leiomyosarcomas arising from major vessels. The histologic features and criteria of malignancy in this group of leiomyosarcomas are similar to those in the retroperitoneum with some minor exceptions. Although, by definition, all display some degree of atypia, the range of mitotic activity can be quite wide with levels as low as <1/10HPF. Necrosis is rarely encountered to the extent as that seen in retroperitoneal leiomyosarcomas.

The behavior of somatic soft tissue leiomyosarcomas has been poorly defined owing to the relatively small number of reported cases. Our experience,[58] combined with that of Gustafson et al.[1] for a total of 90 cases, indicates that these lesions are aggressive but do not have nearly the accelerated disease tempo as do retroperitoneal lesions. Local recurrence rates range from 10% to 25% and metastatic rates from 44% to 45%, with a 5-year survival of 64%. Most metastases develop in lung and rarely in lymph nodes.

A number of variables affects the prognosis in this subgroup of leiomyosarcomas, but their relative importance differs depending on the study. Gustafson et al. found that age over 60 years and vascular invasion were independent risk factors for death from the tumor,[1] whereas others have reported depth, tumor size and stage as independent factors.[59,60] In our experience, factors which were predictive of metastasis at 36 months in a multivariate analysis were grade (FNCLCC system) and whether the tumor had been violated surgically (i.e., disruption). However, disruption also correlated with size and depth and therefore could represent a surrogate marker for both.[58] On the other hand, this group of soft tissue sarcomas requires special scrutiny, as their frequent origin from vessels may grant them greater accessibility to the bloodstream and hematogenous dissemination. This phenomenon was underscored by Berlin et al., who reported metastasis from all six extremity leiomyosarcomas that originated from veins.[61] One patient with a small (3 cm) mass arising from the saphenous vein died 1 month after surgery with liver and lung metastases.

CUTANEOUS LEIOMYOSARCOMAS

Although in the past the term cutaneous leiomyosarcoma referred to tumors arising in the dermis or subcutis, we believe this designation should be restricted to lesions that arise from the dermis and only secondarily invade the subcutis. The reason for this change resides in the fact that leiomyosarcomas based exclusively in the subcutis, in many instances, arise from vessels and therefore have far more in common with soft tissue leiomyosarcomas with respect to their origin, access to the bloodstream, and ultimate prognosis. Unfortunately, this definition has not been routinely employed in the past, and so the distinction between these two potentially different diseases has been blurred.

Cutaneous leiomyosarcomas occur at almost any age but are most common between the fifth and seventh decades. Although Stout and Hill[62] originally commented on the predilection of the tumors for women, more recent reports indicate that the disease is far more common in men, by a ratio of 2:1 or 3:1.[12] Like their benign counterparts, they usually occur on the extremities and show a predilection for the hair-bearing extensor surfaces.[12]

Unlike subcutaneous leiomyomas, most are solitary lesions; and the presence of multiple superficial leiomyosarcomas always suggests the possibility of metastasis from another soft tissue site such as the retroperitoneum.[2] In a few cases the tumor has developed at a site of previous irradiation.[12,63]

Cutaneous tumors are usually small, averaging less than 2 cm when first detected.[64] They often produce surface changes in the overlying epidermis such as discoloration, umbilication, and ulceration. Because of their rarity these lesions are seldom correctly diagnosed preoperatively.

Gross and microscopic findings

Grossly, these leiomyosarcomas usually have a gray-white whorled appearance and a varying degree of circumscription. Those in the dermis appear ill defined by virtue of the intricate blending of tumor fascicles with the surrounding collagen and pilar arrector muscle. Those with extensions into the subcutis, in contrast, appear more circumscribed owing to the fact that they compress the surrounding tissue, creating a pseudocapsule. Most superficial leiomyosarcomas resemble retroperitoneal leiomyosarcomas in basic organization (Fig. 18–21).

Most are moderately well-differentiated tumors, differing principally by a lack of regressive or degenerative change. Hemorrhage, necrosis, hyalinization, and myxoid change are rarely encountered, which is probably a reflection of the smaller size of these lesions. Giant cells may be present, but, as in retroperitoneal tumors, it is uncommon to encounter a tumor that has a predominantly pleomorphic appearance. Mitotic figures, including atypical forms, are easily identified in these tumors. In the largest series, reported by Fields and Helwig,[12] 80% of these tumors had more than 2 mitoses/10 HPF. We have generally employed the same criteria of histologic malignancy for these tumors as was proposed earlier for retroperitoneal tumors, recognizing that the better course of these tumors is directly attributable to the superficial location and small size, rather than to intrinsic histologic differences. Muscle actin is present in virtually all tumors, although desmin is variably expressed and when present may be seen only focally.[64] A small number of cutaneous leiomyosarcomas contain cytokeratin.[64]

Clinical behavior

The behavior of cutaneous leiomyosarcomas is excellent and is analogous to that of other sarcomas restricted to the superficial soft tissue (see Chapter 14). Although recurrences develop in almost half of patients,[12] metastases are infrequent and seem to correlate well with the depth of the original tumor: tumors confined to the dermis do not metastasize,[12,64,65] whereas those involving the subcutis metastasize in approximately 30–40% of cases.[12,64,65] The high rate of metastasis (50%) noted in the early report of Stout and Hill[62] reflects the fact that most of their cases were subcutaneous lesions, and some even penetrated deep soft tissue, a phenomenon that substantially alters the outcome for the worse. As indicated above, tumors of this type are better classified as soft tissue leiomyosarcomas rather than cutaneous ones. Other factors that correlate with outcome include the size of the tumor and the histologic grade. Both of these parameters correlate with depth. For example, nearly all intradermal leiomyosarcomas are small (<2 cm) and are of low histologic grade (I–II), although even those

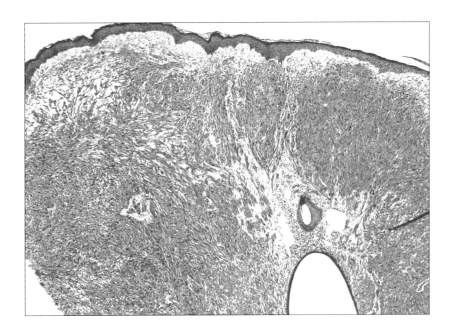

FIGURE 18–21 Superficial leiomyosarcoma arising from dermis.

unusual intradermal leiomyosarcomas that are high grade have behaved in a benign fashion.[64] Metastatic spread occurs hematogenously to the lung, although regional lymph nodes were involved in about 25% of Stout and Hill's cases[62] and have been noted in sporadic case reports.[62,66]

Because many of these lesions are potentially curable, every effort should be made to eradicate the tumor initially with wide excision. Lesions allowed to recur run an increased risk of eventual metastasis because there is a distinct tendency for recurrent lesions to be larger and to involve deeper structures.[12] Mohs' surgery has recently been used in the treatment of this disease[67,68] with a reported recurrence rate of 14%.[68]

LEIOMYOSARCOMAS OF VASCULAR ORIGIN

Leiomyosarcomas of vascular origin comprise a seemingly rare group of tumors illustrated by the fact that only a few hundred cases have been reported in the literature and only isolated instances are recorded in several large autopsy series. Hallock et al.[69] noted one case in 34 000 autopsies from the University of Minnesota; Abell[70] reported two in 14 000 autopsies at the University of Pennsylvania; and Dorfman and Fisher[71] found none in 30 000 autopsies at the Johns Hopkins Hospital. Yet it should be emphasized that several features of this disease probably significantly affect its detection, diagnosis, and incidence. Lesions arising from major vessels such as the vena cava are likely to produce symptoms leading to their detection. Conversely, tumors arising from small vessels, vessels subserved by ancillary tributaries, or vessels in deep locations probably go unrecognized in a significant percentage of cases. It is difficult, therefore, to be certain what percentage of leiomyosarcomas of the retroperitoneum or other deep soft tissue sites may actually be of vascular origin. Hashimoto et al.[2] recently documented that at least one-fourth of leiomyosarcomas of peripheral soft tissue in their experience arose from or involved a vessel; and we have observed this in at least one-third of cases.[58] Thus, the recorded experience with vascular leiomyosarcomas is a biased one, which probably underestimates the true incidence and possibly also conveys a false impression concerning clinical behavior.

Clinical findings

The distribution of vascular leiomyosarcomas parallels in a crudely inverse fashion the pressure in the vascular bed. Leiomyosarcomas are most common in large veins such as the vena cava, far less common in the pulmonary artery, and rare in systemic arteries. In an extensive review by Kevorkian and Cento[5] of cases reported up to the early 1970s, a total of 33 cases arose in the inferior vena cava,

and 35 collectively affected other medium-size or large veins; 10 occurred in the pulmonary artery alone, and 8 arose in systemic arteries. One report has indicated the unique occurrence of a leiomyosarcoma in a surgically created arteriovenous fistula.[72] The symptoms related to these tumors are diverse and are determined by the location of the tumor, rate of growth, and degree of collateral blood flow or drainage in an affected part.

Inferior vena cava leiomyosarcoma

Inferior vena cava leiomyosarcomas occur during middle or late adult life, at an average age of about 50 years; 80–90% of patients are women.[73–75] The location of the tumor in the vessel is significant because it determines the symptoms and surgical resectability. Based on material submitted to the International Registry of Inferior Vena Cava Leiomyosarcomas, most tumors arise in the lower (44.2%) or middle (50.8%) portion, with only a small number (4.2%) arising from the upper third or suprahepatic region.[76] Patients with upper segment tumors develop Budd-Chiari syndrome, with hepatomegaly, jaundice, and massive ascites. Nausea, vomiting, and lower extremity edema may also be present. These tumors are surgically unresectable. Tumors of the middle segment involve the region between the renal veins and hepatic veins; they produce symptoms of right upper quadrant pain and tenderness, frequently mimicking biliary tract disease. Extension into the hepatic veins may cause some of the symptoms of the Budd-Chiari syndrome, whereas extension into the renal veins results in varying degrees of renal dysfunction, from mild elevation of blood urea nitrogen to nephrotic syndrome. Some of these lesions are surgically resectable. Lesions arising below the renal veins cause lower leg edema; but unless they have spread extensively beyond the confines of the vessel, they are often amenable to surgical excision. In a few cases of vena cava leiomyosarcoma, abnormalities of red blood cell morphology and consumption coagulopathy have been observed.[77] Although previously an antemortem diagnosis of these lesions was difficult, selective arteriography and vena cavography can now be used to define the presence and extent of the mass.[78]

To date, the long-term outlook for this disease is poor. A large study comparing the effect of caval wall resection with more extended segmental resection of the vessel demonstrated no significant difference in either 5-year (55% versus 37%) or 10-year (42% versus 23%) survival. This seems to indicate that at the time of clinical detection the disease is relatively advanced and not curable by surgery. This conjecture is supported by the relatively large size of these tumors and the predominantly extraluminal growth in both groups. Metastatic disease is seen most commonly in lung, kidney, pleura, chest wall, liver, and bone.[79]

Leiomyosarcomas of other veins

Unlike vena cava lesions, those in other veins affect the sexes equally and most often arise in the veins of the lower extremity, including the saphenous, iliac, and femoral veins. They usually present as mass lesions of variable duration that occasionally produce lower leg edema. Pressure on nerves coursing close to the affected vessel may produce additional symptoms of numbness. Angiographically, the lesions are highly vascular and create compression of the accompanying artery. The compression appears to be the result of entrapment of the artery that resides in the same preformed fibrous sheath (conjunctiva vasorum) as the vein. Because incisional biopsy of intravascular sarcomas can give rise to considerable seeding of tumor by hemorrhage, it has been suggested that thorough radiographic evaluation be followed by needle biopsy in selected cases. The behavior of this group of leiomyosarcomas has been a controversial topic.[80] Although one series suggested that small intravascular leiomyosarcomas might have a relatively good prognosis,[80] all six patients reported by Berlin et al.[61] developed metastases, even those with relatively low mitotic rates. However, all but one of the tumors exceeded 4 cm in diameter.

Pulmonary artery leiomyosarcoma

Pulmonary artery leiomyosarcomas are the most common form of arterial leiomyosarcoma. They occur in adults and display no predilection for either sex. Their symptoms are referable to decreased pulmonary outflow and include chest pain, dyspnea, palpitations, dizziness, syncopal attacks, and eventual right heart failure. Until recently, the diagnosis was inevitably made at autopsy. Most of these tumors arise at the base of the heart and grow distally into the left and right main pulmonary arteries.

Gross and microscopic findings

In almost all reported cases, vascular leiomyosarcomas are described as polypoid or nodular masses that are firmly attached to the vessel at some point and have spread for a variable extent along its surface (Fig. 18–22). The rare cases describing extensive spread along the vena cava into the right heart, however, may represent intravenous leiomyomatosis that was originally misdiagnosed (see Chapter 16).[81] In the case of thin-walled veins, extension to the adventitial surfaces and adjacent structures is a relatively early event, whereas in arteries the integrity of the internal elastic lamina is often preserved so there is no spread outside the vessel. Histologically, the tumors are similar to those in the retroperitoneum, although they usually do not exhibit as prominent a degree of hemorrhage or necrosis (Fig. 18–23). Mitoses, in our

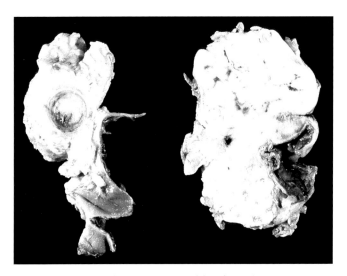

FIGURE 18–22 Leiomyosarcoma arising from the vena cava. Tumor occludes the lumen and extends into soft tissue **(left)**. Adjacent section of tumor shows a close relation to the duodenal wall **(right)**.

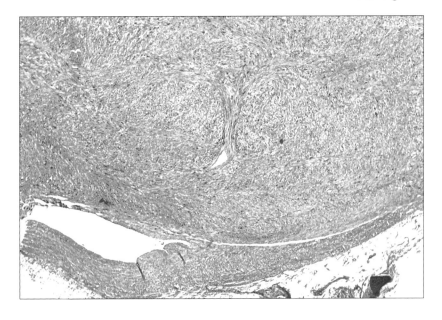

FIGURE 18–23 Leiomyosarcoma arising from a vein. Tumor protrudes into the vessel lumen.

experience, are rather easy to identify in these tumors; and the histologic criteria of malignancy previously discussed are equally applicable to these lesions. In fact, true leiomyomas arising from vessels are rare, and this diagnosis should be made with extreme caution and only after the lesion has been sampled extensively.

Behavior and treatment

The morbidity and mortality associated with these tumors are primarily a result of direct extension of the tumor along vessels, compromising the circulation. In only about half of the patients are metastases documented at the time of surgery or autopsy; they occur mainly in the liver or lung and less often in regional lymph nodes or intra-abdominal organs. Unfortunately, owing to the fact that only about half of the cases were diagnosed antemortem in the past, there is little information concerning the results of therapy. It may be anticipated that more sophisticated angiographic techniques leading to earlier diagnosis and therapy will improve survival rates, which thus far have been poor. In 1973 Stuart and Baker[82] analyzed 10 such tumors in the vena cava that were treated surgically; they noted that all five patients who were followed longer than 1 year died. In a more recent series by Burke and Virmani,[79] only 7 of 13 inferior vena cava sarcomas developed metastases.

One of the greatest problems when treating this disease is that the location itself may preclude surgical resection. This is true of suprahepatic lesions, where ligation of the cava and partial hepatectomy have never been accomplished. Middle caval lesions may be resected with difficulty but require removal of one kidney and pelvic transplantation of the other if irradiation is contemplated.

MISCELLANEOUS SARCOMAS OF VASCULAR ORIGIN

Nonmyogenic sarcomas arising from vessels are a veritable potpourri of lesions that are difficult to classify.[70,83–87] In contrast to the foregoing group, most of these peculiar hybrid lesions occur more often in the arterial system, particularly the pulmonary artery, where they tend to present during middle age with a constellation of symptoms associated with right ventricular outflow obstruction or pulmonary emboli.[79] Most of the tumors in this location probably arise from the base of the heart, although it is difficult to exclude an origin from the valve or even the heart itself. Aortic sarcomas tend to develop in older patients and involve the lower portion of the vessel. They are associated with myriad symptoms related to systemic embolization.[79] Arterial sarcomas grow in an intraluminal fashion similar to leiomyosarcomas, but there is a tendency for such lesions to creep along the

vessel wall, splitting apart the layers of intima and media in their paths. This form of spreading was termed intimal sarcomatosis by Hedinger.[88] Histologically, a variety of terms have been applied to these tumors, including pleomorphic sarcoma, intimal sarcoma, undifferentiated sarcoma,[89] fusocellular sarcoma, malignant mesenchymoma,[90] chondrosarcoma,[85] and osteosarcoma.[76,91,92] The terms serve to emphasize the fact that these tumors are, in general, highly pleomorphic tumors composed of haphazardly arranged giant cells and spindle cells.

The largest institutional review of arterial sarcomas was reported by the AFIP which analyzed 11 and 16 cases from the aorta and pulmonary artery, respectively.[79] Histologically, the sarcomas in both locations were for the most part pleomorphic, intima-based lesions. Of the 17 cases reported, 3 had the pattern of angiosarcoma and 3 osteosarcoma; the remainder were pleomorphic sarcomas that were difficult to classify. Other reports have documented the presence of cartilage or skeletal muscle differentiation in these tumors.[86,90]

The fact that these tumors occur in a different set of vessels, exhibit a strikingly different histologic appearance, and often remain confined to the superficial portions of the vessel suggests the possibility that they are intimal sarcomas, in contrast to the previous group, which are more properly considered sarcomas of medial or adventitial origin. Because of their location the diagnosis is rarely made antemortem, and death from local tumor extension, particularly to the lungs, is the rule.

EPSTEIN-BARR VIRUS-ASSOCIATED SMOOTH MUSCLE TUMORS

Smooth muscles tumors occur in immunocompromised patients with greater frequency than in the general population. Reported initially as a complication of renal transplantation and immunosuppression during the 1970s,[93,94] these smooth muscle tumors have been associated more recently with acquired immunodeficiency syndrome (AIDS)[95–102] and with cardiac and liver transplantation. However, it was not until 1995 that a causal link between these tumors and EBV infection was established.[99,100] These tumors may be associated with either of the two EBV strains.

Most EBV smooth muscle tumors (EBVSMT) occur in children and interestingly develop in organs not traditionally considered preferred sites for leiomyosarcomas (soft tissue, liver, lung, spleen, dura). About 50% of patients will have multiple lesions at the time of presentation and often small tumor seedlings can be seen adjacent to small vessels, suggesting vascular smooth muscle as a site of infection (Fig. 18–24).

Although most reported tumors are scantily illustrated and have been variously diagnosed as "leiomyoma," "leiomyosarcoma," and "smooth muscle tumor of uncer-

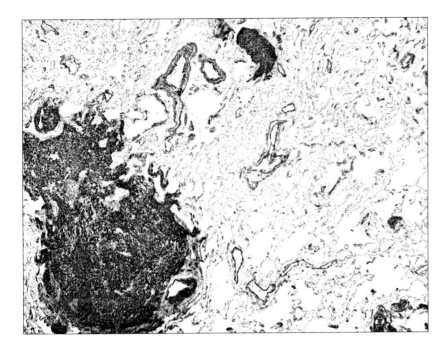

FIGURE 18–24 Actin immunostain of EBVSMT highlighting multifocal disease occurring within the lung.

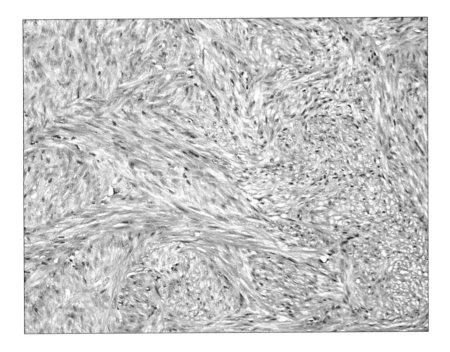

FIGURE 18–25 EBVSMT illustrating differentiated smooth muscle cells with some nuclear atypia.

tain malignant potential," all possess some level of mitotic activity. Histologically, these lesions differ somewhat from classic leiomyosarcomas in several respects. Consisting of intersecting fascicles of differentiated smooth muscle cells, they never achieve the level of atypia noted in classic leiomyosarcomas, yet all display some level of mitotic activity (Fig. 18–25). In about one-half of cases nodules of primitive rounded cells, representing an unusual altered smooth muscle cell, can be identified (Figs 18–26; 18–27). Intralesional T lymphocytes are also a common feature (Fig. 18–28). Usually, the clinical setting in association with the foregoing features suggests the diagnosis of an EBVSMT, but the diagnosis can be confirmed by in situ hybridization of Epstein-Barr virus early RNA (EBER) (Fig. 18–29) if PCR-based methods for viral identification are not available.

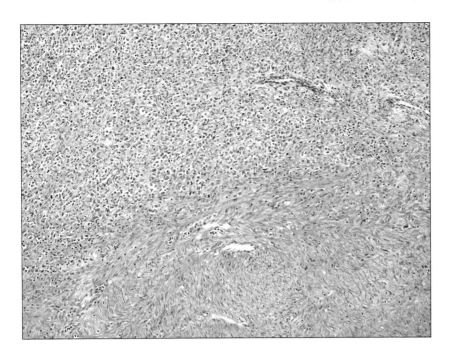

FIGURE 18–26 EBVSMT showing classic-appearing smooth muscle areas abutting round cell myoid areas (upper left).

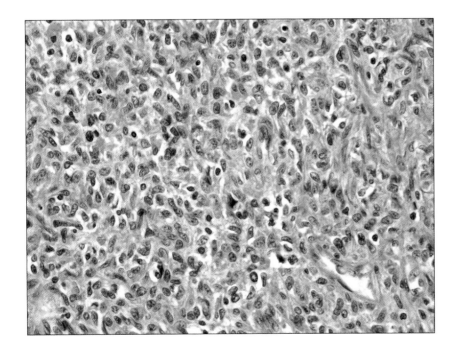

FIGURE 18–27 Round cell myoid areas within an EBVSMT.

In our experience with 18 patients, over three-quarters were alive at the end of the follow-up period (mean 25 months) with most having persistent disease. Only one patient succumbed directly to tumor. These data raise the question as to whether multiple lesions are the result of metastasis in the traditional sense (spread from a primary site) or multifocality due to multiple independent infection events. Based on viral episomal analysis of lesions, we and others have shown that multiple lesions are derived from separate viral clones and therefore likely to be multiple infection events.[103]

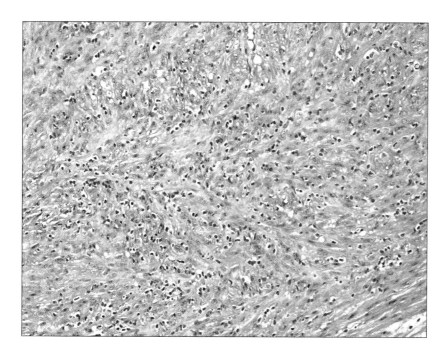

FIGURE 18–28 Intralesional lymphocytes in EBVSMT.

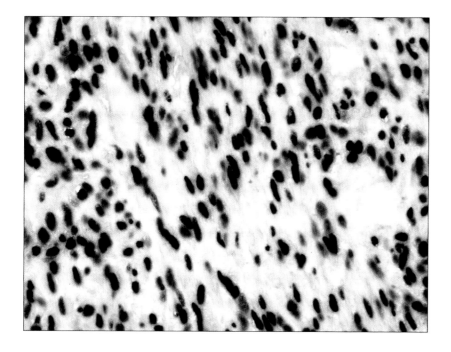

FIGURE 18–29 In situ hybridization for EBER (Epstein-Barr virus early RNA) in an EBVSMT.

REFERENCES

General

1. Gustafson P, Willen H, Baldetorp B, et al. Soft tissue leiomyosarcoma: a population-based epidemiologic and prognostic study of 48 patients, including cellular DNA content. Cancer 1992; 70:114.
2. Hashimoto H, Daimaru Y, Tsuneyoshi M, et al. Leiomyosarcoma of the external soft tissues. Cancer 1986; 57:2077.
3. Hashimoto H, Tsuneyoshi M, Enjoji M. Malignant smooth muscle tumors of the retroperitoneum and mesentery: a clinicopathologic analysis of 44 cases. J Surg Oncol 1985; 28:177.
4. Shmookler BM, Lauer DH. Retroperitoneal leiomyosarcoma: a clinicopathologic analysis of 36 cases. Am J Surg Pathol 1983; 7:269.
5. Kevorkian J, Cento JP. Leiomyosarcoma of large arteries and veins. Surgery 1973; 73:39.
6. Botting AJ, Soule EH, Brown AL. Smooth muscle tumors in children. Cancer 1965; 18:711.
7. Swanson PE, Wick MR, Dehner LP. Leiomyosarcoma of somatic soft tissues in childhood: an immunohistochemical analysis of six cases with ultrastructural correlation. Hum Pathol 1991; 22:569.
8. De Saint Aubain Somerhausen N, Fletcher CDM. Leiomyosarcoma of soft tissue in children: clinicopathologic analysis of 20 cases. Am J Surg Pathol 1999; 23:755.
9. Lack EE. Leiomyosarcomas in childhood: a clinical and pathologic study of 10 cases. Pediatr Pathol 1986; 6:181.
10. Laskin WB, Silverman TA, Enzinger FM. Postradiation soft tissue sarcomas: an analysis of 53 cases. Cancer 1988; 62:2330.
11. Robinson E, Neugut AI, Wylie P. Clinical aspects of postirradiation sarcomas. J Natl Cancer Inst 1988; 80:233.
12. Fields JP, Helwig EB. Leiomyosarcoma of the skin and subcutaneous tissue. Cancer 1981; 47:156.
13. Font RL, Jurco S, Brechner RJ. Postradiation leiomyosarcoma of the orbit complicating bilateral retinoblastoma. Arch Ophthalmol 1983; 101:1557.

14. Stratton MR, Williams S, Fisher C, et al. Structural alterations of the RB1 gene in human soft tissue tumours. Br J Cancer 1989; 60:202.
15. Koea JB, Leung D, Lewis JJ, et al. Histopathologic type: an independent prognostic factor in primary soft tissue sarcoma of the extremity? Ann Surg Oncol 2003; 10:432.
16. Deyrup AT, Haydon RC, Huo D, et al. Myoid differentiation and prognosis in adult pleomorphic sarcomas of the extremity. Cancer 2003; 98:805.
17. Fisher C, Goldblum JR, Epstein JI, et al. Leiomyosarcoma of the paratesticular region: a clinicopathologic study. Am J Surg Pathol 2001; 25:1143.
18. Montgomery E, Goldblum JR, Fisher C. Leiomyosarcoma of the head and neck: a clinicopathologic study. Histopathology 2002; 40:518.

Retroperitoneal/abdominal leiomyosarcomas

19. Ranchod M, Kempson RL. Smooth muscle tumors of the gastrointestinal tract and retroperitoneum. Cancer 1977; 39:255.
20. Wile AG, Evans HL, Romsdahl MM. Leiomyosarcoma of soft tissue: a clinicopathologic study. Cancer 1981; 48:1022.
21. Karroum JE, Zappi EG, Cockerell CJ. Sclerotic primary cutaneous leiomyosarcoma. Am J Dermatopathol 1995; 17:292.
22. Oda Y, Miyajima K, Kawaguchi K, et al. Pleomorphic leiomyosarcoma: clinicopathologic and immunohistochemical study with special emphasis on its distinction from ordinary leiomyosarcoma and malignant fibrous histiocytoma. Am J Surg Pathol 2001; 25:1030.
23. Mentzel T, Calonje E, Fletcher CD. Leiomyosarcoma with prominent osteoclast-like giant cells. Am J Surg Pathol 1995; 19:487.
24. Matthews TJ, Fisher C. Leiomyosarcoma of soft tissue and pulmonary metastasis, both with osteoclast-like giant cells. J Clin Pathol 1994; 47:370.
25. Mentzel T, Calonje E, Fletcher CD. Leiomyosarcoma with prominent osteoclast-like giant cells: analysis of eight cases closely mimicking the so-called giant cell variant of malignant fibrous histiocytoma. Am J Surg Pathol 1994; 18:258.
26. Wilkinson N, Fitzmaurice RJ, Turner PG, et al. Leiomyosarcoma with osteoclast-like giant cells. Histopathology 1992; 20:446.
27. Suster S, Wong TY, Moran CA. Sarcomas with combined features of liposarcoma and leiomyosarcoma: study of two cases of an unusual soft-tissue tumor showing dual lineage differentiation. Am J Surg Pathol 1993; 17:905.
28. Roncaroli F, Eusebi V. Rhabdomyoblastic differentiation in a leiomyosarcoma of the retroperitoneum. Hum Pathol 1996; 27:310.
29. King ME, Dickersin GR, Scully RE. Myxoid leiomyosarcoma of the uterus: a report of six cases. Am J Surg Pathol 1982; 6:589.
30. Salm R, Evans DJ. Myxoid leiomyosarcoma. Histopathology 1985; 9:159.
31. Rubin BP, Fletcher CD. Myxoid leiomyosarcoma of soft tissue: an underrecognized variant. Am J Surg Pathol 2000; 24:927.
32. Merchant W, Calonje E, Fletcher CD. Inflammatory leiomyosarcoma: a morphological subgroup within the heterogeneous family of so-called inflammatory malignant fibrous histiocytoma. Histopathology 1995; 27:525.
33. Chang A, Schuetze SM, Conradd EU, et al. So-called "inflammatory leiomyosarcoma": a series of 3 cases providing additional insights into a rare entity. Int J Surg Pathol 2005; 13:185.
34. Nistal M, Raniagua R, Picazo ML, et al. Granular changes in vascular leiomyosarcoma. Virchows Arch [Pathol Anat] 1980; 386:239.

35. Ferenczy A, Richart RM, Okagaki T. A comparative ultrastructural study of leiomyosarcoma, cellular leiomyoma, and leiomyoma of the uterus. Cancer 1971; 28:1004.
36. Tsukada T, Tippens D, Mar H, et al. HHF35, a muscle-actin-specific monoclonal antibody. I. Immunocytochemical and biochemical characterization. Am J Pathol 1987; 125:51.
37. Rangdaeng S, Truong LD. Comparative immunohistochemical staining for desmin and muscle-specific actin: a study of 576 cases. Am J Clin Pathol 1991; 96:32.
38. Swanson PE, Stanley MW, Scheithauer BW, et al. Primary cutaneous leiomyosarcoma: a histologic and immunohistochemical study of 9 cases with ultrastructural correlations. J Cutan Pathol 1988; 15:129.
39. Hisaoka M, Wei-Qui S, Jian W, et al. Specific but variable expression of h-caldesmon in leiomyosarcomas: an immunohistochemical reassessment of a novel myogenic marker. Appl Imm Mol Morph 2001; 9:302.
40. Brown DC, Theaker JM, Banks PM, et al. Cytokeratin expression in smooth muscle and smooth muscle tumours. Histopathology 1987; 11:477.
41. Meredith RF, Wagman LD, Piper JA, et al. Beta-chain human chorionic gonadotropin-producing leiomyosarcoma of the small intestine. Cancer 1986; 58:131.
42. Miettinen M. Immunoreactivity for cytokeratin and epithelial membrane antigen in leiomyosarcomas. Arch Pathol Lab Med 1988; 112:637.
43. Miettinen M. Keratin subsets in spindle cell sarcomas: keratins are widespread but synovial sarcoma contains a distinctive keratin polypeptide pattern and desmoplakins. Am J Pathol 1991; 138:505.
44. Iwata J, Fletcher C. Immunohistochemical detection of cytokeratin and epithelial membrane antigen in leiomyosarcoma: a systematic study of 100 cases. Pathol Internat 2000; 5:7.
45. Kelley TW, Borden EC, Goldblum JR. Estrogen and progesterone receptor expression in uterine and extrauterine leiomyosarcomas: an immunohistochemical study. Appl Immunohistochem Mol Morphol 2004; 12:338.
46. Proppe KH, Scully RE, Rosai J. Postoperative spindle cell nodules of genitourinary tract resembling sarcomas: a report of eight cases. Am J Surg Pathol 1984; 8:101.
47. Nochomovitz LE, Orenstein JM. Inflammatory pseudotumor of the urinary bladder: possible relationship to nodular fasciitis: two case reports, cytologic observations, and ultrastructural observations. Am J Surg Pathol 1985; 9:366.
48. Ro JY, Ayala AG, Ordonez NG, et al. Pseudosarcomatous fibromyxoid tumor of the urinary bladder. Am J Clin Pathol 1986; 86:583.
49. Stoeckle E, Coindre JM, Bonvalot S, et al. Prognostic factors in retroperitoneal sarcoma: a multivariate analysis of a series of 165 patients of the French Federation Sarcoma Group. Cancer 2001; 92:359.
50. Mandahl N, Fletcher CD, Dal Cin P, et al. Comparative cytogenetic study of spindle cell and pleomorphic leiomyosarcomas of soft tissues: a report from the CHAMP Study Group. Cancer Genet Cytogen 2000; 116:66.
51. Hu J, Rao UN, Jasani S, et al. Loss of DNA copy number of 10q is associated with aggressive behavior of leiomyosarcomas: a comparative genomic hybridization study. Cancer Genet Cytogen 2005; 161:20.
52. Wang R, Titley JC, Lu YJ, et al. Loss of 13q14-q21 and gain of 5p14-pter in the progression of leiomyosarcoma. Mod Pathol 2003; 16:778.

53. Kawaguchi K, Oda Y, Saito T, et al. Mechanisms of inactivation of the p16INK4a gene in leiomyosarcoma of soft tissue: decreased p16 expression correlates with promoter methylation and poor prognosis. J Pathol 2003; 201:487.
54. Seidel C, Bartel R, Rastetter M, et al. Alterations of cancer-related genes in soft tissue sarcomas: hypermethylation of RASSF1A is frequently detected in leiomyosarcoma and associated with poor prognosis in sarcoma. Int J Cancer 2005; 114:442.
55. Dobashi Y, Noguchi T, Nasuno S, et al. CDK-inhibitors-associated kinase activity: a possible determinant of malignant potential in smooth muscle tumors of the external soft tissue. Int J Cancer 2001; 94:353.
56. Lee YF, Falconer JM, Edwards S, et al. A gene expression signature associated with metastatic outcome in human leiomyosarcomas. Cancer Res 2004; 64:7201.
57. Ren B, Yu YP, Jing L, et al. Gene expression analysis of human soft tissue leiomyosarcoma. Hum Pathol 2003; 34:549.

Leiomyosarcomas of somatic soft tissue

58. Farshid G, Pradhan M, Goldblum J, et al. Leiomyosarcomas of somatic soft tissues: a tumor of vascular origin with multivariate analysis of outcome in 42 cases. Am J Surg Pathol 2002; 26:14.
59. Miyajima K, Oda Y, Oshiro Y, et al. Clinicopathologic prognostic factors in soft tissue leiomyosarcoma: a multivariate analysis. Histopathology 2002; 40:353.
60. Mankin HJ, Casas-Ganem J, Kim JI, et al. Leiomyosarcoma of somatic soft tissues: Clinical Orthopaed Rel Res 2004; 421:225.
61. Berlin O, Stener B, Kindblom L, et al. Leiomyosarcoma of venous origin in the extremities: a correlated clinical, roentgenologic, and morphologic study with diagnostic and surgical implications. Cancer 1984; 54:2147.

Cutaneous leiomyosarcomas

62. Stout AP, Hill WT. Leiomyosarcoma of the superficial soft tissue. Cancer 1964; 11:844.
63. Hietanen A, Sakai Y. Leiomyosarcoma in an old irradiated lupus lesion. Acta Dermatol Venereol 1960; 40:167.
64. Jensen ML, Myhre Jensen O, Michalski W, et al. Intradermal and subcutaneous leiomyosarcoma: a clinicopathological and immunohistochemical study of 451 cases. J Cutan Pathol 1996; 23:458.
65. Dahl I, Angervall L. Cutaneous and subcutaneous leiomyosarcoma: a clinicopathologic study of 47 patients. Pathol Eur 1974; 9:307.
66. Rising JA, Booth E. Primary leiomyosarcoma of the skin with lymphatic spread. Arch Pathol 1966; 81:94.
67. Humphreys TR, Finkelstein DH, Lee JB. Superficial leiomyosarcoma treated with Mohs' micrographic surgery. Dermatol Surg 2004; 30:108.
68. Huether MJ, Zitelli JA, Brodland DG. Mohs' micrographic surgery for the treatment of spindle cell tumors of the skin. J Am Acad Dermatol 2001; 44:656.

Leiomyosarcomas of vascular origin

69. Hallock P, Watson CJ, Berman L. Primary tumor of inferior vena cava with clinical features suggestive of Chari's disease. Arch Intern Med 1940; 66:50.
70. Abell MR. Leiomyosarcoma of inferior vena cava: review of literature and report of two cases. Am J Clin Pathol 1957; 28:272.

71. Dorfman HD, Fisher ER. Leiomyosarcoma of the greater saphenous vein. Am J Clin Pathol 1963; 39:73.

72. Weinreb W, Steinfeld A, Rodil J, et al. Leiomyosarcoma arising in an arteriovenous fistula. Cancer 1983; 52:390.

73. Demers ML, Curley SA, Romsdahl MM. Inferior vena cava leiomyosarcoma. J Surg Oncol 1992; 51:89.

74. Griffin AS, Sterchi JM. Primary leiomyosarcoma of the inferior vena cava: a case report and review of the literature. J Surg Oncol 1987; 34:53.

75. Jurayj MN, Midell AJ, Bederman S, et al. Primary leiomyosarcoma of the inferior vena cava: report of a case and review of the literature. Cancer 1970; 26:1349.

76. Mingoli A, Sapienza P, Cavallaro A, et al. The effect of extent of caval resection in the treatment of inferior vena cava leiomyosarcoma. Anticancer Res 1997; 17:3877.

77. Wackers FJT, Vander Schoot JB, Hampe JF. Sarcoma of the pulmonary trunk associated with hemorrhagic tendency: a case report and review of the literature. Cancer 1969; 23:339.

78. Brewster DC, Athanasoulin CA, Darling RC. Leiomyosarcoma of the inferior vena cava: diagnosis and surgical management. Arch Surg 1976; 111:1081.

79. Burke AP, Virmani R. Sarcomas of the great vessels: a clinicopathologic study. Cancer 1993; 71:1761.

80. Leu HJ, Makek M. Intramural venous leiomyosarcomas. Cancer 1986; 57:1395.

81. Jonasson D, Pritchard J, Long L. Intraluminal leiomyosarcoma of the inferior vena cava. Cancer 1966; 19:1311.

82. Stuart FP, Baker WH. Palliative surgery for leiomyosarcoma of the inferior vena cava. Ann Surg 1973; 177:237.

Miscellaneous sarcomas of vascular origin

83. Haber IM, Truong L. Immunohistochemical demonstration of the endothelial nature of aortic intimal sarcoma. Am J Surg Pathol 1988; 12:798.

84. Hayata T, Sato I. Primary leiomyosarcoma arising in the trunk of pulmonary artery: a case report and review of the literature. Acta Pathol Jpn 1977; 27:137.

85. Hohbach C, Mall W. Chondrosarcoma of the pulmonary artery. Beitr Pathol 1977; 160:298.

86. McGlennen RC, Manivel JC, Stanley SJ, et al. Pulmonary artery trunk sarcoma: a clinicopathological, ultrastructural, and immunohistochemical study of four cases. Mod Pathol 1989; 2:486.

87. Wright EP, Virmani R, Glick AD, et al. Aortic intimal sarcoma with embolic metastasis. Am J Surg Pathol 1985; 9:890.

88. Hedinger E. Ueber Intima Sarkomatose von Venen und Arterien in sarkomatoesen Strumen. Virchows Arch [Pathol Anat] 1901; 164:199.

89. Shmookler BM, Marsh HB, Roberts WC. Primary sarcoma of the pulmonary trunk and of left main pulmonary artery: a rare cause of obstruction to right ventricular outflow. Am J Med 1977; 63:263.

90. Hagstrom L. Malignant mesenchymoma in pulmonary artery and right ventricle. Acta Pathol Microbiol Scand 1961; 51:87.

91. McConnel TH. Bony and cartilaginous tumor of the heart and great vessels. Cancer 1970; 25:611.

92. Murphy MSN, Meckstroth GV, Merkel BH, et al. Primary intimal sarcoma of pulmonary valve and trunk with osteogenic sarcomatous elements. Arch Pathol Lab Med 1976; 100:649.

Epstein-Barr virus-associated smooth muscle tumors

93. Shen SC, Yunis EJ. Leiomyosarcoma developing in a child during remission of leukemia. J Pediatr 1976; 89:780.

94. Walker D, Gill TJ III, Corson JM. Leiomyosarcoma in a renal allograft recipient treated with immunosuppressive drugs. JAMA 1971; 215:2084.

95. Bluhm JM, Yi ES, Diaz G, et al. Multicentric endobronchial smooth muscle tumors associated with the Epstein-Barr virus in an adult patient with the acquired immunodeficiency syndrome. Cancer 1997; 80:1910.

96. Boman F, Gultekin H, Dickman PS. Latent Epstein-Barr virus infection demonstrated in low-grade leiomyosarcomas of adults with acquired immunodeficiency syndrome, but not in adjacent Kaposi's lesion or smooth muscle tumors in immunocompetent patients. Arch Pathol Lab Med 1997; 121:834.

97. Chadwick EG, Connor EJ, Guerra Hanson C, et al. Tumors of smooth-muscle origin in HIV infected children. JAMA 1990; 263:3182.

98. Kingma DW, Shad A, Tsokos M, et al. Epstein-Barr virus (EBV)-associated smooth muscle tumor arising in a post-transplant patient treated successfully for two PT-EBV associated large-cell lymphomas: case report. Am J Surg Pathol 1996; 20:1511.

99. Lee E, Locker J, Nalesnik M, et al. The association of Epstein-Barr virus with smooth muscle tumors occurring after organ transplantation. N Engl J Med 1995; 332:19.

100. McClain KL, Leach CT, Jenson HB, et al. Association of Epstein-Barr virus with leiomyosarcomas in young people with AIDS. N Engl J Med 1995; 332:12.

101. McLoughlin LC, Nord KS, Joshi VV, et al. Disseminated leiomyosarcoma in a child with acquired immune deficiency syndrome. Cancer 1991; 67:2618.

102. Ross JS, Del Rosario A, Bui HX, et al. Primary hepatic leiomyosarcoma in a child with the acquired immunodeficiency syndrome. Hum Pathol 1992; 23:69.

103. Deyrup AT, Lee VK, Hill CE, et al. Epstein Barr virus associated smooth muscle tumors are distinctive mesenchymal tumors reflecting multiple infection events: a clinicopathologic and molecular analysis of 29 tumors from 19 patients. Am J Surg Path 2006; 30:75.

EXTRAGASTROINTESTINAL STROMAL TUMORS

CHAPTER CONTENTS

Gastrointestinal stromal tumors (GIST) arise within the wall of the gut and recapitulate the phenotype of the interstitial cell of Cajal, the gastrointestinal pacemaker cell of the Auerbach plexus, which is responsible for generation of the slow peristaltic wave. Because of the important biologic and therapeutic implications for this group of lesions they should be clearly distinguished from intramural tumors showing true smooth muscle differentiation as well as the occasional tumor showing other forms of lineage-specific differentiation. A small number of GIST arise in soft tissues of the mesentery or retroperitoneum and are referred to as extragastrointestinal stromal tumor (EGIST). By definition, they display no connection, however tenuous, to the wall or serosal surface of the viscera. There is far less published information that specifically relates to EGIST, but it is generally presumed that most of the basic principles and features of GIST are applicable to EGIST.

GIST were first described by Martin[1] and Stout[2] who described several unusual tumors of the stomach characterized by rounded epithelioid cells. Stout coined the term "leiomyoblastoma" for these lesions in the belief they were primitive smooth muscle tumors. Unfortunately, the term leiomyoblastoma implied little about biologic behavior, and it was not until the classic paper by Appelman and Helwig[3] that a rigorous attempt was made to separate them into benign and malignant forms. These authors considered the lesions variants of smooth muscle tumors and employed the terms "epithelioid leiomyoma" and "epithelioid leiomyosarcoma." A significant nomenclatural change occurred in 1983 when Mazur and Clark[4] published a seminal paper which documented the

absence of muscle markers in most of these lesions and the unexpected finding of neural markers in some as detected by immunohistochemistry. They postulated that these lesions displayed different lines of differentiation, reflecting the various elements of the gut wall (e.g., muscle, autonomic nerve), and proposed the unifying term "stromal tumor," which has since been modified to "gastrointestinal stromal tumor" (GIST) to ensure distinction from stromal tumors of other sites (e.g., uterus, breast). During the ensuing decade, however, many pathologists, ignoring the original morphologic description of Stout, loosely and inappropriately applied the term GIST to any mesenchymal tumor of the gut, resulting in a confusing array of lesions reported under this rubric.

The 1998 paper by Hirota[5] et al., however, radically changed our thinking of GIST. Extrapolating from the observation that the proto-oncogene c-KIT, a type III tyrosine kinase receptor, was required for normal development of interstitial cells of Cajal and its loss resulted in their depletion, Hirota et al. questioned whether gain of function mutations might result in neoplasms with a phenotype similar to the interstitial cells of Cajal. They further theorized that GIST represented the product of this neoplastic event and in support of this idea documented gain of function mutations in several of these tumors. Nearly simultaneous publications by others confirmed this hypothesis and resulted in a strict definition for these tumors, requiring the presence of *KIT* mutations.

Despite the general agreement that standardized diagnosis of GIST requires immunohistochemistry and in some cases molecular confirmation, there continue to be lingering issues as to how one should approach the question of malignancy in this group of lesions. The prevailing view, namely that all GIST should be considered potentially malignant, is implied in the recent consensus statement which proposes the use of a risk stratification scheme applicable to GIST of all locations.[6] However, it is still not entirely clear to what extent site-specific factors should be incorporated into a risk assessment scheme and whether factors such as mutational status also should be included. Undoubtedly, the current scheme will undergo modifications but for the moment this scheme appears to be the most reasonable approach to providing some assessment of malignant potential.

CLINICAL FINDINGS

Although originally believed to be a very rare disease, there may be as many as 6000 new cases in the United States annually.[7,8] In large part this reflects the more accurate recognition and diagnosis of these tumors, a fact well illustrated by a recent Icelandic study that reported an increased incidence of GIST from 2.1 cases to 12.6 cases/million inhabitant in the 8 years since the advent of immunohistochemistry.[9] EGIST are uncommon compared to their gastrointestinal counterparts. In the early study of Pizzimbono et al., fewer than 5% of leiomyoblastomas arose in the soft tissues of the abdomen,[10] whereas in a recent study from the Armed Forces Institute of Pathology (AFIP) of 1004 cases, 7% of tumors arose in the soft tissues of the omentum, mesentery, and retroperitoneum.[11] The latter study, however, makes no clearcut distinction between tumors with true smooth muscle differentiation and those with features of a stromal tumor. Putative cases have also been reported outside the abdominal cavity, but, in our experience, such tumors are so rare that the diagnosis should be questioned or the possibility of a metastasis from an intra-abdominal primary tumor should be raised. Gastrointestinal stromal tumors have been associated with Carney's triad (multiple gastric stromal tumors, pulmonary chondroma, paraganglioma),[12,13] neurofibromatosis 1,[14–16] and in families with germline mutations of *KIT*.[17–19]

EGISTs usually present during adult life as enlarging masses of variable duration, although occasionally such tumors are discovered incidentally at the time of laparotomy. Approximately 80% are located in the omentum or mesentery, and the remainder develop in the retroperitoneum (Fig. 19–1). Unlike their gastrointestinal counterpart, these lesions tend to be large when first detected, with most measuring more than 10 cm.[20] Most are firm, fleshy gray-red masses lacking the whorled appearance that is often seen with conventional smooth muscle tumors (Fig. 19–2). A significant subset undergo cystic change as a result of extensive hemorrhage or necrosis.

MICROSCOPIC FINDINGS

The histologic appearance of EGISTs is variable, but in general there are two patterns: epithelioid and spindle cell. In a given tumor one pattern usually predominates, although in about 10% of cases the patterns coexist in roughly equal proportions. The epithelioid pattern corresponds to most of the older descriptions of leiomyoblastoma in which the tumor is composed of round cells

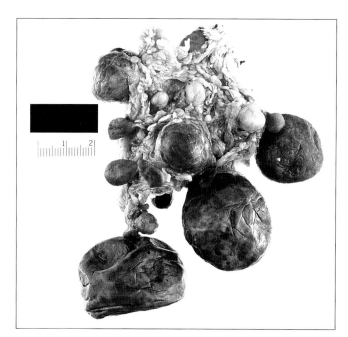

FIGURE 19–1 Stromal tumor of the omentum, presenting as multiple pedunculated masses.

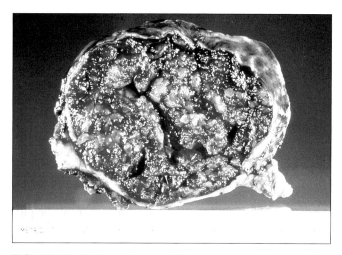

FIGURE 19–2 Stromal tumor of the omentum with a partially hemorrhagic red-gray appearance.

that vary from small uniform cells to large pleomorphic cells with eosinophilic cytoplasm (Figs 19–3 to 19–6). In some cases there is a striking population of epithelioid cells with multiple, peripherally oriented nuclei (Fig. 19–6). Although the hyperchromatism of the nuclei sometimes suggests malignancy, these multinucleated cells are more likely to be encountered in benign than malignant stromal tumors. Another characteristic feature of these tumors is the prominent cytoplasmic vacuole, which in extreme instances results in a signet ring cell appearance (Figs 19–4, 19–5). Tumors composed of a predominance of signet ring-like cells may be mistaken for liposarcoma or mucinous carcinoma by those

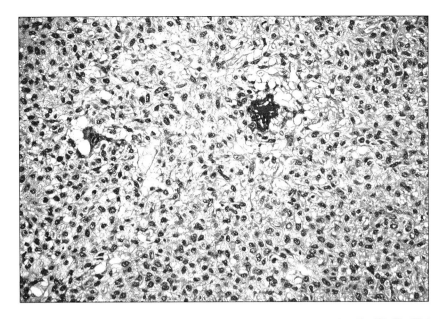

FIGURE 19–3 Stromal tumor composed of sheets of dispersed epithelioid cells.

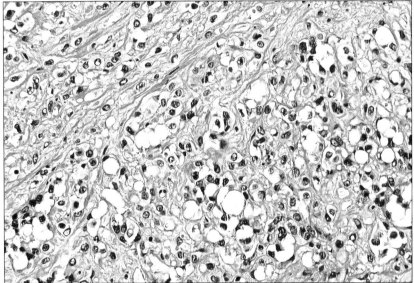

FIGURE 19–4 Stromal tumor composed of epithelioid cells with focal vacuolar (signet ring) change.

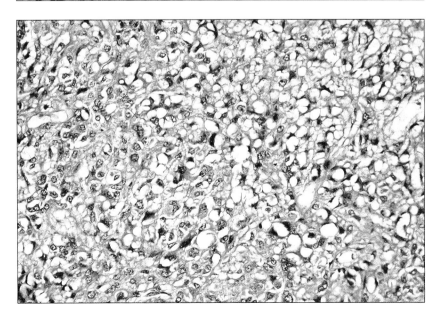

FIGURE 19–5 Stromal tumor with epithelioid cells with extensive signet ring change.

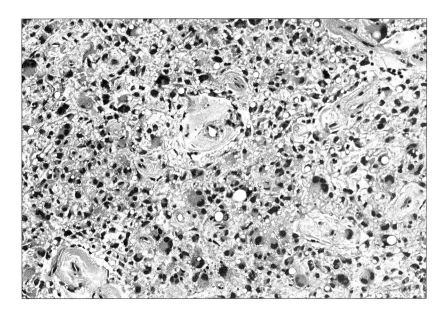

FIGURE 19–6 Stromal tumor with numerous hyperchromatic cells with multiple peripherally oriented nuclei. These cells are typically seen in benign stromal tumors.

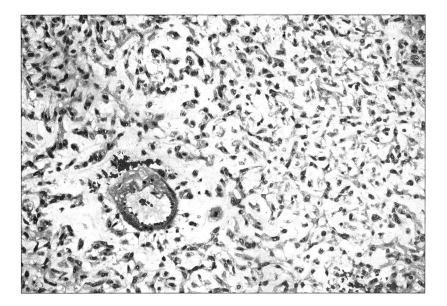

FIGURE 19–7 Stromal tumor with myxoid change.

unfamiliar with their appearance. As emphasized originally by Stout, the vacuoles of these signet ring-like cells do not stain for fat, mucosubstances, or glycogens and therefore can be readily distinguished from those of liposarcoma or carcinoma. In fact, these vacuoles seem to represent an artifact of formalin fixation because they are not present in frozen sections or in material fixed for electron microscopy. The cells in epithelioid stromal tumors are commonly arranged in small groups or nests separated by a matrix of dense or fibrillary collagen, pools of stromal mucin, or both (Figs 19–7 to 19–9). In some instances, mucin collections are striking enough to form microscopic cysts.

Tumors with a spindled pattern more closely resemble conventional smooth muscle tumors but nonetheless can be distinguished from them by the fact that the cells usually have a short fusiform shape in contrast to the elongated cells of leiomyomas and leiomyosarcomas (Figs 19–10 to 19–14). They have an oval, centrally placed nucleus and lightly staining cytoplasm in which it is usually not possible to identify distinct myofibrils with hematoyxlin-eosin or trichrome stain. At best, a few wisps of fuchsinophilic material may be seen. The neoplastic cells, furthermore, are not arranged in long well-oriented fascicles like a smooth muscle tumor but consist of short ill-defined fascicles, sometimes in a storiform pattern. Nuclear palisading is occasionally seen and in some cases is so striking as to suggest the diagnosis of a schwannoma (Figs 19–13, 19–14). The stroma is typically composed of mats of fine, hair-like collagen interrupted by a delicate vasculature. As in epithelioid stromal tumors, microcystic change is also observed.

A number of features may be encountered in these tumors independent of pattern. Extensive hyaline change

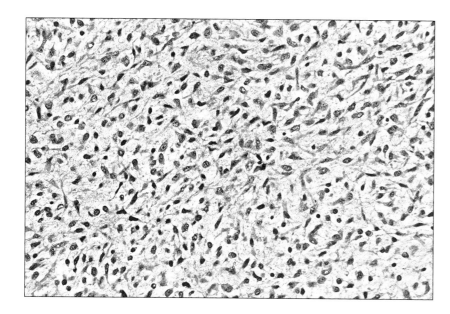

FIGURE 19–8 Stromal tumor with myxoid change.

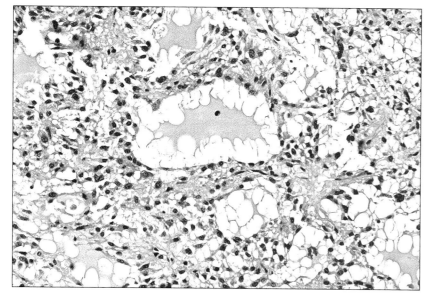

FIGURE 19–9 Stromal tumor with microcysts.

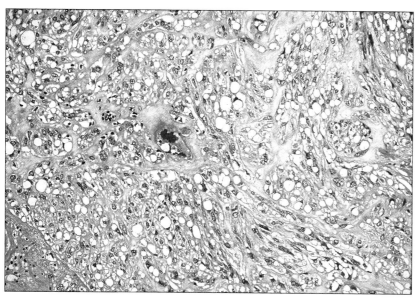

FIGURE 19–10 Stromal tumor with transition between epithelioid and spindled areas.

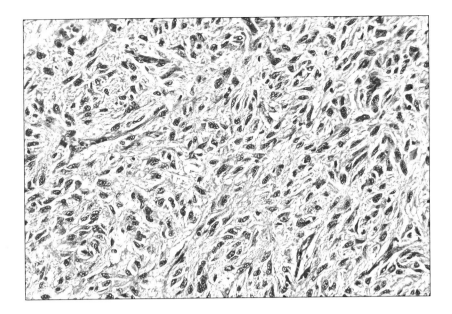

FIGURE 19–11 Stromal tumor with a spindled pattern composed of short fusiform cells in a fine fibrillary background.

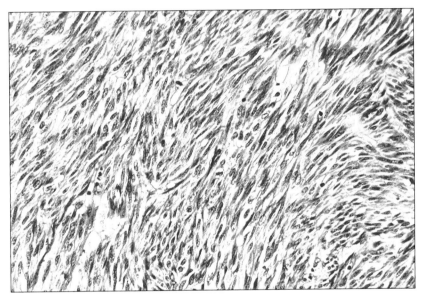

FIGURE 19–12 Stromal tumor with a spindled pattern composed of cells arranged in distinct fascicles.

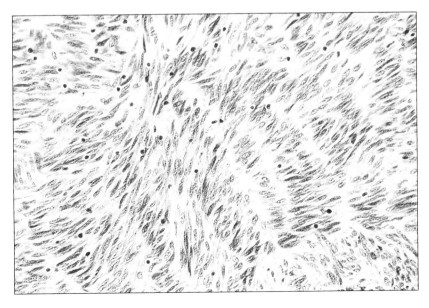

FIGURE 19–13 Stromal tumor with nuclear palisading.

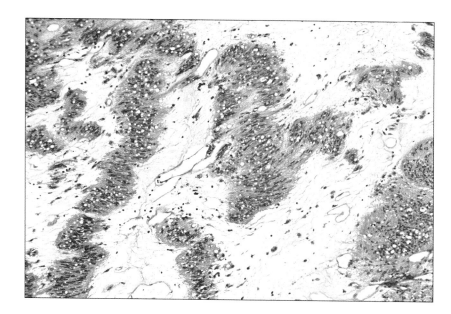

FIGURE 19–14 Stromal tumor with nuclear palisading.

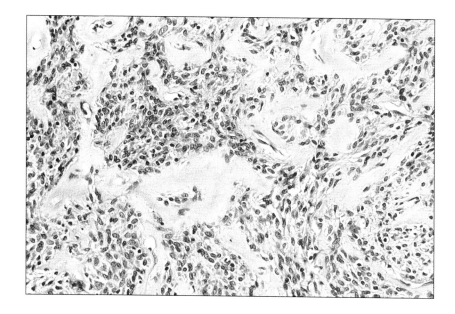

FIGURE 19–15 Stromal tumor with prominent hyalinization.

is seen in about 20% of cases and can result in striking perivascular hyalinization as in a hemangiopericytoma (Fig. 19–15), extensive intratumoral hyaline change as in uterine leiomyomas, or bands of hyaline material creating a secondary trabecular pattern (Fig. 19–16). Skeinoid fibers (extracellular collagen-containing eosinophilic globules),[21,22] reported occasionally in small intestinal stromal tumors and originally believed to reflect neural differentiation, are usually absent in EGISTs (Fig. 19–17).

Usually, metastases from extragastrointestinal stromal tumors resemble the parent growth, although mitotic rates sometimes differ. Occasionally, isolated metastases in the liver or lymph node are difficult to diagnose because of their similarity to metastatic carcinoma or metastatic neuroendocrine tumors. This situation most frequently arises in patients from whom tumors were resected previously and in whom metastatic disease supervenes years later.

Assessing the level of malignancy in EGIST presents problems similar to GIST. Although consensus guidelines have been recommended for GIST of all locations (see below), it is not clear to what extent these guidelines will be predictive of outcome for EGIST.[6] In our experience, the most important histologic criteria of malignancy for EGIST are cellularity, mitotic activity, and necrosis (Figs 19–18 to 19–21). Lesions at high risk to produce metastasis have high cellularity (as defined by areas with frequent overlapping nuclei), mitotic activity in excess of 2 mitoses/50 high-power fields (HPF), and any amount of coagulative necrosis. Such lesions can comfortably be labeled malignant. Lesions lacking these features have a

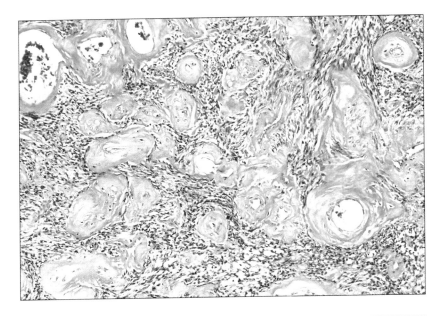

FIGURE 19-16 Stromal tumor with perivascular hyalinization.

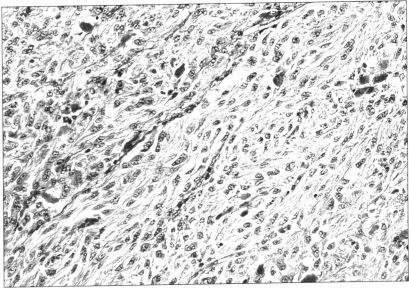

FIGURE 19-17 Skeinoid fibers in a stromal tumor appear as interstitial eosinophilic blobs.

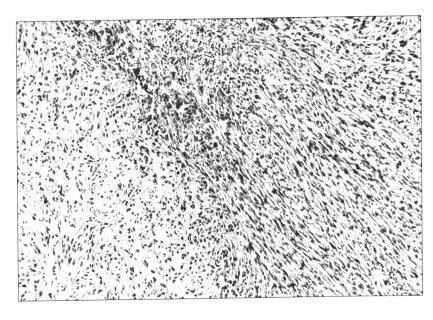

FIGURE 19-18 Stromal tumor with a transition between more differentiated **(left)** and more aggressive- **(right)** appearing areas.

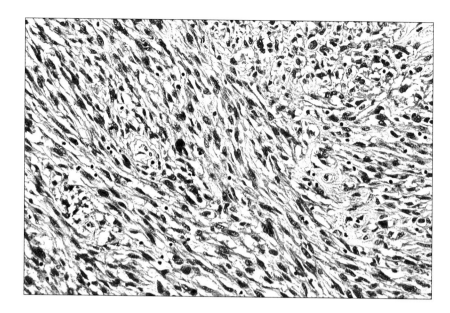

FIGURE 19–19 Stromal tumor with malignant features. Tumor is highly cellular with significant atypia.

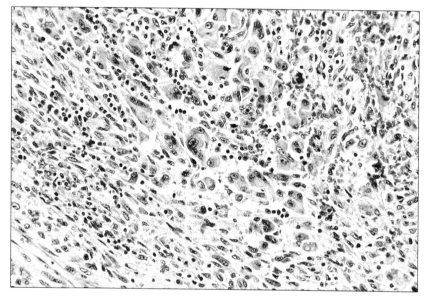

FIGURE 19–20 Stromal tumor with malignant features. Tumor is highly cellular with marked atypia.

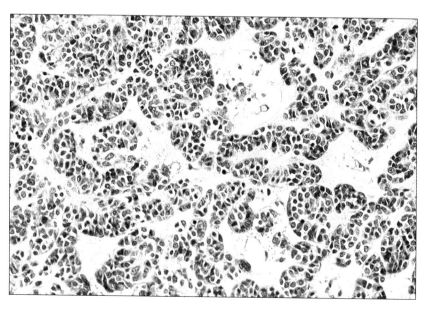

FIGURE 19–21 Stromal tumor with malignant features. Tumor is composed of nests of small, round, primitive-appearing cells.

lower risk of metastasis, although it is not possible to guarantee benignancy.

IMMUNOHISTOCHEMICAL FINDINGS

Immunohistochemical findings in extragastrointestinal lesions (Table 19–1) generally parallel those of GIST. Nearly all GIST are KIT-positive (CD117), making this antigen the most sensitive and specific means of confirming the diagnosis.[23,24] KIT immunoreactivity is usually strong and diffuse and is observed in a cytoplasmic, membranous, or dot-like paranuclear (golgi-like) pattern (Fig. 19–22). One-half to two-thirds of GIST are CD34 positive and one-quarter, SMA positive. Desmin and keratin are rarely present (<5%). There have been questionable reports of *KIT* positivity in abdominal fibromatosis, a lesion that enters the differential diagnosis of GIST. In our experience when technical conditions are carefully controlled, fibromatoses are *KIT*-negative. However, *KIT* staining may be seen in a number of tumors notably, melanoma, angiosarcoma, seminoma, and mast cell tumors and these should be kept in mind when evaluating tumors metastatic to the gut or retroperitoneum.

Approximately 5% of GIST are *KIT*-negative and tend to be located in the stomach and omentum/peritoneum and have an epithelioid appearance. Most harbor platelet-derived growth factor A (PDGFA) mutations while a minority (20%) harbor *KIT* mutations,[25,26] but not both. In the evaluation of a KIT-negative tumor presumed on histologic ground to be a GIST, CD34 becomes an important secondary immunostain, particularly if molecular analysis for KIT or PDGFRA mutations is not readily available.

TABLE 19–1 STROMAL TUMORS: IMMUNOHISTOCHEMICAL FINDINGS			
	Extragastrointestinal (%)	Gastrointestinal (%)	
Immunohistochemical profile	Reith et al.[20] (25 cases)	Kindblom et al.[23] (78 cases)	Erlandson et al.[29] (56 cases)
c-kit	100	100	ND
CD34	48	75	59
SMA	24	15	23
Desmin	4	0	16
S-100 protein	8	0	9
MSA	ND	0	50
NSE	31	0	59
NFP	ND	0	3
Chromogranin	0	0	3
Synaptophysin	ND	ND	ND
Keratin	0	ND	2

NSE, neuron-specific enolase; SMA, smooth muscle actin; MSA, muscle-specific actin; ND, not done.

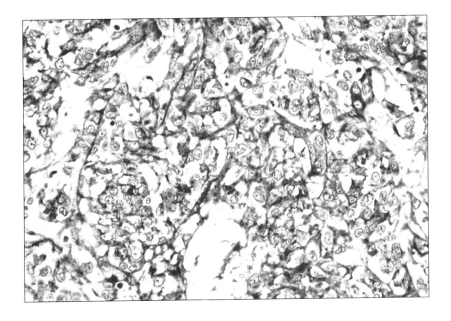

FIGURE 19–22 Immunostain for c-KIT receptor in a stromal tumor. The tumor displays strong linear surface and, to a lesser extent, cytoplasmic immunoreactivity.

Gene expression profiling studies have recently identified two proteins which are strongly expressed in GIST: protein kinase C theta, a signaling molecule important in T-cell activation,[27] and DOG1 (discovered on GIST-1), a protein of unknown function which is expressed in GIST, irrespective of mutational status.[28] Unfortunately, commercial antibodies are only available for protein kinase C theta.

ULTRASTRUCTURAL FINDINGS

These tumors may have features of smooth muscle cells (as evidenced by parallel arrays of intracytoplasmic thin [actin] filaments with or without dense bodies, micropinocytotic vesicles, and discontinuous basal lamina) or neural cells (with thin interdigitating cytoplasmic processes connected by primitive junctions and containing microtubules and dense-core granules).[29] In the past, stromal tumors with neural (synaptic) differentiation were classified as gastrointestinal autonomic nerve tumors (GANT),[30-39] although the rationale for this distinction has recently been questioned (see gastrointestinal autonomic tumor). Still other tumors display few if any features of specific differentiation, having cytoplasmic processes without any diagnostic structures.[29]

The range of features noted in these tumors has led some to suggest an ultrastructural classification system.[29] Others, noting the presence of *KIT* receptor and *KIT* mutations in all tumors regardless of ultrastructural features,[23,40] have suggested the ultrastructural differences are relatively unimportant and simply reflect the same range of differentiation as the interstitial cell of Cajal, which may display both neural and smooth muscle features.[23]

CYTOGENETIC AND MOLECULAR FINDINGS

KIT mutations occur in approximately 80–95% of GIST and lead to ligand-independent phosphorylation and constitutional activation of the KIT signaling pathway to the nucleus.[5,41-43] The fact that these mutations are observed even in small, incidental tumors[44] and in patients with germline KIT mutations who develop GISTs provides strong evidence that KIT mutation is an early, if not primary, tumorigenic event. Mutations cluster within four regions of the KIT gene.[43] Approximately 70% occur within exon 11 encoding the juxtramembrane portion of the protein, 10% in exon 9 encoding the extramembranous domain, and the remainder in exon 13 and 17 of the kinase domains (Fig. 19–23). Approximately 5% of GIST have mutations within PDGFRA, another receptor tyrosine kinase. These tumors do not possess KIT mutations, indicating that mutations in the two genes are

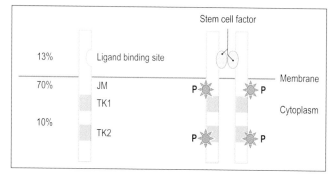

FIGURE 19–23 Schematic version of unbound kit receptor **(left)** showing incidence of kit mutations by location. Majority occur in the JM (juxtamembrane portion) with a minority in the extracellular or tyrosine kinase (TK1 and TK2) domains. Dimerization and phosphorylation (P) occur following binding of ligand, stem cell factor **(right)**.

mutually exclusive. In those GIST that lack both KIT and PDGFRA mutations, it is presumed that mutations in other tyrosine kinase receptors or downstream effectors are operational.[45] Although there are more limited data related to EGIST, it appears that they possess mutations essentially similar to GIST.[46]

Secondary cytogenetic changes occur in GIST and are likely responsible for tumor progression.[47-52] Loss of chromosome 14, 22q, 1p, 9p, and 11p and gains in chromosomes 5p, 20q, 8q, and 17q have been most frequently reported. The chromosomal losses presumably correspond to loss of tumor suppressor genes whereas gains correspond to amplification of oncogenes. Although the pattern of gains and losses varies from tumor to tumor, highly malignant GIST usually have three or more cytogenetic alternations.[8]

BEHAVIOR AND TREATMENT

An inordinate amount of study has focused on histologic criteria to separate benign from malignant GIST. Although this approach usually distinguishes lesions with high metastatic potential from those with low potential, it is at best imperfect. Lesions designated as benign histologically metastasized whereas not all of those labeled histologically malignant prove fatal. For this reason the trend has shifted to one of "risk assessment,"[20,53-56] a method that analyzes a number of features independently and correlates them with an adverse or nonadverse outcome. By combining features, high-risk versus low-risk groups can be identified. The features generally accorded prognostic significance in various studies are tumor size, nuclear grade, mitotic activity, cellularity, and necrosis, although the relative importance of these features varies from site to site and from study to study. The level of cellularity has been one of the most consistent prognostic

TABLE 19–2	ADVERSE PROGNOSTIC INDICATORS IN STROMAL TUMORS

	Indicator, by Tumor Site					
Parameter	Stomach[2,30]	Duodenum[19]	Jejunum/ileum[55]	Colon[56]	Rectum[57]	Soft tissues[43]
High cellularity	+	+	+	+		+
Mitoses	>10/50 HPF, 100% metastasis	>2/50 HPF	>5/50 HPF	High		>2/50 HPF
Size	>6 cm	>4.5 cm	>9 cm		>5 cm	
Necrosis						+
Mucosal invasion	+		+	+		
Growth pattern		Nonorganoid	Epithelioid (>50%)			
Infiltration of muscularis propria				+		

HPF, high-power field.

TABLE 19–3	EXTRAGASTROINTESTINAL STROMAL TUMOR: INCIDENCE OF ADVERSE OUTCOME BY NUMBER OF HISTOLOGIC RISK FACTORS

Risk factors (no.)	Patients with adverse outcome/ total in group (no.)	Incidence of adverse outcomes per person-year*
0–1	1/19 (5%)	0.02
2–3	11/12 (95%)	0.54

HPF, high power field.
*Risk factors are cellularity, necrosis, and mitotic activity (>2 mitoses/10 HPF).
Data from Reith J, Goldblum JR, Weiss SW. Extragastrointestinal (soft tissue) stromal tumors: an analysis of 48 cases with emphasis on histologic predictors of outcome. Mod Pathol 2000; 13:577.

indicators (Table 19–2). Tumors with high cellularity, as defined by frequent areas with overlapping nuclei, have been associated with a statistically higher risk of an adverse outcome in several studies of both gastrointestinal and extragastrointestinal lesions. Likewise, mitotic activity is usually an important prognostic indicator, although the threshold level reported from site to site differs with threshold levels as low as 2 mitoses/50 HPF in the duodenum.[57]

To date, only one study has dealt exclusively with EGISTs.[20] In other studies, extragastrointestinal lesions are either absent or comprise only a small proportion.[11] In view of the site-dependent criteria of malignancy, it may not be appropriate to apply data gleaned from the gastrointestinal experience to stromal tumors arising from the omentum, mesentery, and retroperitoneum. In our experience of 32 patients with follow-up information, 41% developed metastasis or died of tumor during a follow-up period of 24 months. Because the follow-up was relatively short, it is expected that this figure may increase significantly with time. In a univariate analysis, cellularity (high versus low), mitotic activity (<2 or >2 mitoses/50 HPF), and necrosis (present or absent) correlated with an adverse outcome as defined by metastasis or death due to the tumor. In a multivariate analysis, both mitotic activity and necrosis displayed a trend toward an independent predictive value. Despite this, stratification of patients with EGIST into those with one

or more adverse histologic factor versus those with two or three factors offers the advantage of grouping patients into two categories with markedly different risk of an adverse outcome in the short term (Table 19–3). No correlation was noted between tumor type (spindled versus epithelioid appearance) or immunophenotypic profile. Miettinen et al. suggested that omental lesions are associated with a better prognosis than mesenteric lesions, but the number of cases in each group was small.[58]

A recent consensus conference convened under the auspices of the National Institutes of Health was charged to develop guidelines for assessing malignancy in GIST. To simplify the situation, the consensus group proposed that GIST from all sites be stratified based on size and mitotic activity, the two most important variables in GIST.[6] Using threshold values of <5 and >5 cm and mitotic count of <5 and >5/50 HFP and combining the various subgroups, four risk groups were proposed (Table 19–4). This system has become increasingly popular because it is easy to use and reproducible. Its principal drawback is that it is not clear whether the cutoff points for each variable are equally applicable to GIST in all sites. In other words, does a 5 cm lesion with <5 mitoses/50 HPF in the small bowel have the same risk of metastasizing as a comparable lesion in the omentum?

Imatinib mesylate (Gleevec), originally developed to inhibit the Abl-kinase of chronic myelogenous leukemia, is an ATP analogue that binds to KIT and, by inhibiting its signaling, negates the effect of the activating KIT mutation. In clinical studies, over 50% of patients with GIST respond to oral administration of this drug,[59] with differential sensitivity noted depending on mutational status. Because resistance to this drug occurs through secondary mutations,[60-62] guidelines for the responsible use of the drug are still evolving. There is general agreement that it should be used in metastatic, unresectable disease. Following successful response to imatinib, GIST display loss of cellularity, hyalinization, and cyst formation (Fig. 19–24).[63]

GASTROINTESTINAL AUTONOMIC NERVE TUMOR

First described in 1984 by Herrera et al. as "plexosarcoma," the gastrointestinal autonomic nerve tumor is a GIST that exhibits neuronal differentiation at the ultrastructural level.[64] These tumors have demographic, histologic, immunohistochemical, molecular, and behavioral similarities to conventional GIST.[40] Like other gastrointestinal stromal tumors, they too have been associated with Carney's syndrome and neurofibromatosis 1.[39,65] When examined ultrastructurally, these tumors has elongated processes containing dense-core neurosecretory granules, microtubules, intermediate filaments, and a bulbous synapse-like structure (Figs 19–25, 19–26). Since the majority of GIST are not examined ultrastructurally, the diagnosis of GANT is seldom made in routine practice.

CHILDHOOD GIST AND GIST SYNDROMES

Familial GIST

Familial gastrointestinal stromal tumor is a rare autosomal dominant genetic disease. Patients with this condition manifest germline mutations in KIT and develop diffuse and nodular hyperplasia of the ICC (Fig. 19–27) leading to intestinal diverticulosis and perforation.[17,18,66] Some patients have also developed dysphagia, hyperpigmentation, and urticaria pigmentosa. The GIST are

TABLE 19–4	CONSENSUS GUIDELINES FOR RISK ASSESSMENT OF GIST	
	Size*	Mitotic count
Very low risk	<2 cm	<5/50 HPF
Low risk	2–5 cm	<5/50 HPF
Intermediate risk	<5 cm	6–10/50 HPF
Intermediate risk	5–10 cm	<5/50 HPF
High risk	>5 cm	>5/50 HPF
High risk	>10 cm	Any mitotic rate
High risk	Any size	>10 HPF

HPF, high power field.
*Single largest dimension. The threshold for aggressive behavior perhaps should be reduced by 1–2 cm in the small bowel.
From Fletcher et al. Diagnosis of gastrointestinal stromal tumors: a consensus approach. Hum Pathol 2002; 33:459.

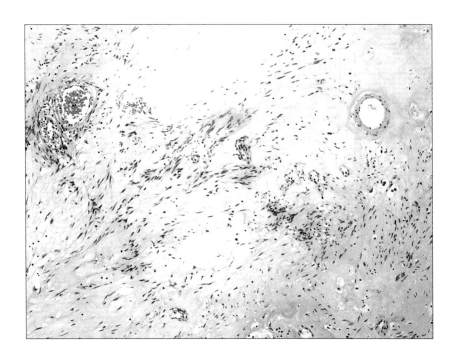

FIGURE 20–24 GIST following treatment with imatinib illustrating hyalinization and cyst formation.

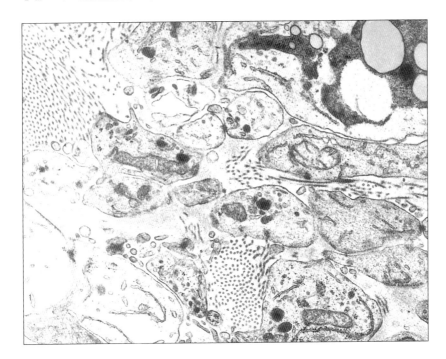

FIGURE 19–25 Electron micrograph of a gastrointestinal autonomic nerve tumor with neuronal and synapse-like structures containing dense-core neurosecretory granules and microtubules (×17 700). (Courtesy of Dr. Robert Erlandson.)

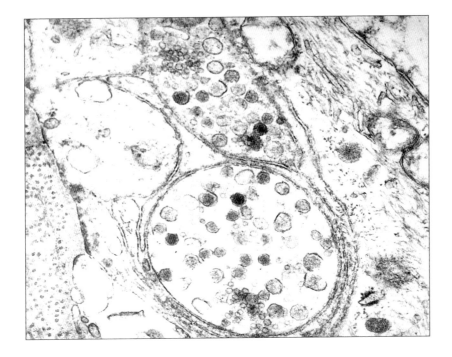

FIGURE 19–26 Electron micrograph of a gastrointestinal autonomic nerve tumor illustrating details of the synapse-like structures. Note the neurosecretory granules and vesicles. A portion of a neurite is also present (×35 700). (Courtesy of Dr. Robert Erlandson.)

typically multifocal and vary in size (Fig. 19–28). Heterozygosity for the KIT mutation can be documented in small tumors, whereas large tumors show loss of the remaining wild-type KIT allele, supporting its importance in tumor progression.[18]

NF1 and GIST

Approximately 7% of patients with NF1 develop GIST which are typically located in the jejunum or ileum in association with ICC hyperplasia.[16] Typically multiple, they are small, mitotically inactive, and express S-100 protein to a significant degree. In the largest series to date published from the AFIP, most patient were alive and well at the end of a long follow-up period.[16] The five patients (of 35) who died of metastatic disease had tumors greater than 5 cm or with mitotic activity >5/50 HPF or both. In contrast to sporadic GIST and familial GIST, less than 10% of NF1 patients with GIST display mutations in either KIT or PDGFRA.[14–16]

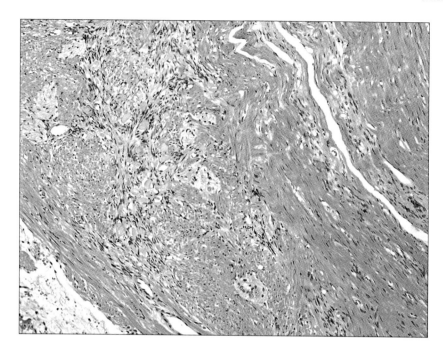

FIGURE 19–27 Familial GIST showing hyperplasia of interstitial cells of Cajal.

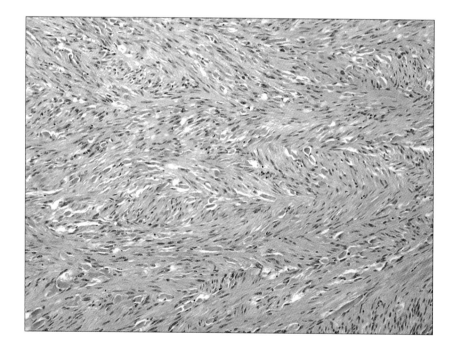

FIGURE 19–28 Jejunal GIST arising in a patient with germline mutation of KIT. Tumor possesses abundant skeinoid fibers.

Carney's syndrome

Although it has been recognized for some time that patients with Carney's syndrome develop multifocal GIST of the stomach in association with pulmonary chondroma and functioning paragangliomas, limited reports indicated that KIT mutations are not present.[8]

Childhood GIST

GIST occurring in children and young adults are rare. Experience from the Armed Forces Institute of pathology identified 44 patients under the age of 21 with this tumor.[67] All patients under the age of 16 years were female and only one patient had Carney's syndrome. The tumors were predominantly gastric and KIT-positive. Curiously, none harbored the common KIT or PDGFRA mutations noted in adults.

REFERENCES

1. Martin JF, Bazin P, Feroldi J, et al. Tumeurs myoides intra-murales de l'estomac: considerations microscopiques a propos de 6 cas. Ann Anat Pathol (Paris) 1960; 5:484.
2. Stout AP. Bizarre smooth muscle tumors of the stomach. Cancer 1962; 15:400.
3. Appelman HD, Helwig EB. Gastric epithelioid leiomyoma and leiomyosarcomas (leiomyoblastoma). Cancer 1976; 38:708.
4. Mazur MT, Clark HB. Gastric stromal tumors: reappraisal of histogenesis. Am J Surg Pathol 1983; 7:507.
5. Hirota S, Isozaki K, Moriyama Y, et al. Gain-of-function mutations of c-KIT in human gastrointestinal stromal tumors. Science 1998; 279:577.
6. Fletcher CD, Berman JJ, Corless C, et al. Diagnosis of gastrointestinal stromal tumors: a consensus approach. Hum Pathol 2002; 33:459.

Clinical findings

7. Kindblom LG, Meis-Kindblom JM, Bumming P, et al. Incidence, prevalence phenotype, and biologic spectrum of gastrointestinal stromal cell tumors (GIST) a population based study of 600 cases. Ann Oncol 2002; 13 suppl (5):157.
8. Rubin BP. Gastrointestinal stromal tumours: an update. Histopathology 2006; 49:1.
9. Tryggvason G, Gislason HG, Magnusson MK, et al. Gastrointestinal stromal tumors in Iceland, 1990–2003: the Icelandic GIST study, a population based incidence and pathologic risk stratification study. Int J Cancer 2005; 117:289.
10. Pizzimbono CA, Higa E, Wise L. Leiomyoblastoma of the lesser sac: case report and review of the literature. Am Surg 1973; 39:692.
11. Emory TS, Sobin LH, Lukes L, et al. Prognosis of gastrointestinal smooth-muscle (stromal) tumors. Am J Surg Pathol 1999; 23:82.
12. Carney JA. The triad of gastric epithelioid leiomyosarcomas, functioning extraadrenal paraganglioma, and pulmonary chondroma. Cancer 1979; 43:374.
13. Carney JA. The triad of gastric epithelioid leiomyosarcomas, pulmonary chondroma, and functioning extraadrenal paraganglioma: a five year review. Medicine 1983; 62:159.
14. Andersson J, Sihto H, Meis-Kindblom JM, et al. NF-1 associated gastrointestinal stromal tumors have unique clinical phenotypic and genotypic characteristics. Am J Surg Pathol 2005; 29:1170.
15. Takazawa Y, Sakurai S, Sakuma Y, et al. Gastrointestinal stromal tumors of neurofibromatosis type I (von Recklinghausen's disease). Am J Surg Pathol 2005; 29:755.
16. Miettinen M, Fetsch JF, Sobin LH, et al. Gastrointestinal stromal tumors in patients with neurofibromatosis 1: a clinicopathologic and molecular genetic study of 45 cases. Am J Surg Pathol 2006; 30:90.
17. Hirota S, Okazaki T, KITamura Y, et al. Cause of familial and multiple gastrointestinal autonomic nerve tumors with hyperplasia of interstitial cells of Cajal is germline mutation of the c-KIT gene. Am J Surg Pathol 2000; 24:326.
18. O'Riain C, Corless CL, Heinrich MC, et al. Gastrointestinal stromal tumours: insights from a new familial GIST kindred with unusual genetic and pathologic features. Am J Surg Pathol 2005; 29:1680.
19. Li FP, Fletcher JA, Heinrich MC, et al. Familial gastrointestinal stromal tumor syndrome: phenotypic and molecular features of a kindred. J Clin Oncol 2005; 23:2735.
20. Reith J, Goldblum JR, Weiss SW. Extragastrointestinal (soft tissue) stromal tumors: an analysis of 48 cases with emphasis on histologic predictors of outcome. Mod Pathol 2000; 13:577.

Microscopic findings

21. Matsukuma S, Doi M, Suzuki M, et al. Numerous eosinophilic globules (skeinoid fibers) in a duodenal stromal tumor: an exceptional case showing smooth muscle differentiation. Pathol Int 1997; 47:789.
22. Min K-W. Small intestinal stromal tumors with skeinoid fibers: clinicopathological, immunohistochemical, and ultrastructural investigations. Am J Surg Pathol 1992; 16:145.

Immunohistochemical findings

23. Kindblom LG, Remotti HE, Aldenborg F, et al. Gastrointestinal pacemaker cell tumor (GIPACT): gastrointestinal stromal tumors show phenotypic characteristics of the interstitial cells of Cajal. Am J Pathol 1998; 152:12459.
24. Sarlomo-Rikala M, Kovatich AJ, Barusevicius A, et al. CD117: a sensitive marker for gastrointestinal stromal tumors that is more specific than CD34. Mod Pathol 1998; 11:728.
25. Medeiros F, Corless CL, Duensing A, et al. KIT-negative gastrointestinal stromal tumors: proof of concept and therapeutic implications. Am J Surg Pathol 2004; 28:889.
26. Debiec-Rychter M, Wasag B, Stul M, et al. Gastrointestinal stromal tumors (GISTs) negative for KIT (CD117) immunoreactivity. J Pathol 2004; 202:430.
27. Blay P, Astudillo A, Buesa JM, et al. Protein kinase C theta is highly expressed in gastrointestinal stromal tumors but not in other mesenchymal neoplasias. Clin Cancer Res 2004; 10:4089.
28. West RB, Corless CL, Chen X, et al. The novel marker, DOG1 is expressed ubiquitously in gastrointestinal stromal tumors irrespective of KIT or PDGFRA mutation status. Am J Pathol 2004; 165:107.

Ultrastructural findings

29. Erlandson RA, Klimstra DS, Woodruff JM. Subclassification of gastrointestinal stromal tumors based on evaluation by electron microscopy and immunohistochemistry. Ultrastruct Pathol 1996; 20:373.
30. Kodet R, Snajdauf J, Smelhous V. Gastrointestinal autonomic nerve tumor: a case report with electron microscopic and immunohistochemical analysis and review of the literature. Pediatr Pathol 1994; 14:1005.
31. Lam KY, Law SY, Chu KM, et al. Gastrointestinal autonomic nerve tumor of the esophagus: a clinicopathologic immunohistochemical, ultrastructural, study of a case and review of the literature. Cancer 1996; 79:1651.
32. Lauwers GY, Erlandson RA, Casper ES, et al. Gastrointestinal autonomic nerve tumor: a clinicopathologic, immunohistochemical, and ultrastructural study of 12 cases. Am J Surg Pathol 1993; 17:887.
33. MacLeod CB, Tsokos M. Gastrointestinal autonomic nerve tumor. Ultrastruct Pathol 1991; 15:49.
34. Matsumoto K, Min W, Yamada N, et al. Gastrointestinal autonomic nerve tumors: immunohistochemical and ultrastructural studies in cases of gastrointestinal nerve tumors. Pathol Int 1997; 47:308.
35. Ojanguren I, Ariza A, Navas-Palacios JJ. Gastrointestinal autonomic nerve tumor: further observations regarding an ultrastructural and immunohistochemical analysis of six cases. Hum Pathol 1996; 27:1311.
36. Segal A, Carello S, Carterina P, et al. Gastrointestinal autonomic nerve tumors: a clinicopathological, immunohistochemical and ultrastructural study of 10 cases. Pathology 1994; 26:439.
37. Shanks JH, Harris M, Banerjee SS, et al. Gastrointestinal autonomic nerve tumours: a report of nine cases. Histopathology 1996; 29:111.
38. Shek TW, Luk IS, Loong F, et al. Inflammatory cell-rich gastrointestinal autonomic nerve tumor: an expansion of its histologic spectrum. Am J Surg Pathol 1996; 20:325.
39. Tortella BJ, Matthews JB, Antonioli DA, et al. Gastric autonomic nerve (GAN) tumor and extra-adrenal paraganglioma in Carney's triad: a common origin. Ann Surg 1987; 205:221.
40. Lee JR, Joshi V, Griffin JW, et al. Gastrointestinal autonomic nerve tumor: immunohistochemical and molecular identify with gastrointestinal stromal tumor. Am J Surg Pathol 2001; 25:979.

Cytogenetic and molecular findings

41. Rubin BP, Singer S, Tsao C, et al. KIT activation is a ubiquitous feature of gastrointestinal stromal tumors. Cancer Res 2001; 61:8118.
42. Nakahara M, Isozaki K, Hirota S, et al. A novel gain of function mutation of c-KIT gene in gastrointestinal stromal tumors. Gastroenterology 1998; 115:1090.
43. Lux M, Rubin BP, Biase TL. KIT extracellular and kinase domain mutations in gastrointestinal stromal tumors. Am J Pathol 2000; 156:791.
44. Corless CL, McGreevey L, Haley A, et al. KIT mutations are common in incidental gastrointestinal stromal tumors one centimeter or less in size. Am J Pathol 2002; 160:1567.
45. Rubin BP, Lux M, Singer S, et al. Correlation of c-KIT mutations status with c-KIT protein expression in gastrointestinal stromal tumors. Mod Pathol 1999; 12:83A.
46. Yamamoto H, Oda Y, Kawaguchi K, et al. C-KIT and PDGFRA mutations in extragastrointestinal stromal tumors. Am J Surg Pathol 2004; 28:479.
47. Bergmann F, Gunawan B, Hermanns B, et al. Cytogenetic and morphologic characteristics of gastrointestinal stromal tumors: recurrent rearrangements of chromosome 1 and losses of chromosomes 14 and 22 as common anomalies. Verh Dtsch Ges Pathol 1998; 82:275.
48. Debiec-Rychter M, Lasota J, Sarlomo-Rikala, et al. Chromosomal aberrations in malignant gastrointestinal stromal tumors: correlation with c-KIT gene mutation. Cancer Genet Cytogenet 2001; 128:24.
49. Fukasawa T, Chong, Sakurai S, et al. Allelic loss of 14q and 22q, NF2 mutations, and genetic instability occur independently of c-KIT mutation in gastrointestinal stromal tumor. Jpn J Cancer Res 2000; 91:1241.
50. Kim NG, Kim JJ, Ahn JY, et al. Putative chromosomal deletions on 9p,9q,22q occur preferentially in malignant gastrointestinal stromal tumors. Int J Cancer 2000; 85:633.
51. El-Rifai W, Sarlomo-Rikala M, Miettinen M, et al. DNA copy number losses in chromosome 14: an early change in gastrointestinal stromal tumors. Cancer Res 1996; 56:3230.
52. Marci V, Casorzo L, Sarotto I, et al. Gastrointestinal stromal tumor, uncommitted type, with monosomies 14 and 22 as the only chromosomal abnormalities. Cancer Genet Cytogenet 1998; 102:135.

Behavior and treatment

53. Franquemont DW. Differentiation and risk assessment of gastrointestinal stromal tumors. Am J Clin Pathol 1995; 103:41.
54. Tworek JA, Appelman HD, Singleton TP, et al. Stromal tumors of the jejunum and ileum. Mod Pathol 1997; 10:200.

55. Tworek JA, Goldblum JR, Weiss SW, et al. Stromal tumors of the abdominal colon: a clinicopathologic study of 20 cases. Am J Surg Pathol 1999; 23:937.

56. Tworek JA, Goldblum JA, Weiss SW, et al. Stromal tumors of the anorectum: a clinicopathologic study of 22 cases. Am J Surg Pathol 1999; 23:946.

57. Goldblum JR, Appelman HD. Stromal tumors of the duodenum: a histologic and immunohistochemical study of 20 cases. Am J Surg Pathol 1995; 19:71.

58. Miettinen M, Monihan JM, Sarlomo-Rikala M, et al. Gastrointestinal stromal tumors/ smooth muscle tumors (GISTs) primary in the omentum and mesentery: clinicopathologic and immunohistochemical study of 26 cases. Am J Surg Pathol 1999; 23:1109.

59. Heinrich MC, Corless CL, Demetri GD, et al. Kinase mutations and imatinib response in patients with metastatic gastrointestinal stromal tumor. J Clin Oncol 2002; 21:4342.

60. Antonescu CR, Besmer P, Guo T, et al. Acquired resistance to imatinib in gastrointestinal stromal tumor occurs through secondary gene mutation. Clin Cancer Res 2005; 11:4182.

61. Chen LL, Trent JC, Wu EF, et al. A missense mutation in KIT kinase domain 1 correlates with imatinib resistance in gastrointestinal stromal tumors. Cancer Res 2004; 63:5913.

62. Wardelmann E, Thomas N, Merkelbach-Bruse S, et al. Acquired resistance to imatinib in gastrointestinal stromal tumours caused by multiple KIT mutations. Lancet Oncol 2005; 6:249.

63. Pauwels P, Debiec Rychter M, Stul M, et al. Changing phenotype of gastrointestinal stromal tumours under imatinib mesylate treatment: a potential diagnostic pitfall. Histopathology 2005; 47:41.

Gastrointestinal autonomic nerve tumor

64. Herrera GA, Pinto de Moraes H, Grizzle WE, et al. Malignant small bowel neoplasm of enteric plexus derivation (plexosarcoma): light and electron microscopic study confirming the origin of the neoplasm. Dig Dis Sci 1984; 29:275.

65. Walsh NMG, Bodurtha A. Auerbach's myenteric plexus: a possible site of origin for gastrointestinal stromal tumors in von Recklinghausen's neurofibromatosis. Arch Pathol Lab Med 1990; 114:522.

Childhood GIST and GIST syndromes

66. Nishida T, Hirota S, Taniguchi M, et al. Familial gastrointestinal stromal tumours with germline mutation of the KIT gene. Nature Genet 1998; 19:323.

67. Miettinen M, Lasota J, Sobin LH. Gastrointestinal stromal tumors of the stomach in children and young adults: a clinicopathologic, immunohistochemical and molecular genetic study of 44 cases with long-term follow-up and review of the literature. Am J Surg Pathol 2005; 29:1373.

RHABDOMYOMA

CHAPTER CONTENTS

STRIATED MUSCLE TISSUE: DEVELOPMENT AND STRUCTURE

Skeletal muscle is formed primarily within myotomes, which are arranged in segmental pairs along the spine and make their first appearance in the cephalic region during the third week of intrauterine life. In the region of the anterior head and neck, skeletal muscle may also develop from mesenchyme derived from the neural crest (mesectoderm).

At the earliest stage of muscle development, primitive mesenchymal cells differentiate along two lines: (1) as fibroblasts, which are loosely arranged spindle-shaped cells with the capacity to form collagen; and (2) as myoblasts, which are round or oval cells with single, centrally positioned nuclei and granular eosinophilic cytoplasm. Over the next few weeks the individual myoblasts assume a more elongated bipolar shape with slender, symmetrically arranged processes and nonstriated longitudinal myofibrils that are laid down first in the peripheral portion of the cytoplasm; this phase is followed by successive alignment and fusion of the individual myoblasts into myotubes with multiple centrally placed nuclei (myotubular stage). During the seventh to tenth weeks of intrauterine development, as differentiation progresses, the myofibrils become thicker and more numerous by longitudinal division, and they develop increasingly distinct cross-striations. Finally, during the eleventh to fifteenth weeks the nucleus is moved from its initial central position toward the periphery of the muscle fiber. Muscles derived from the cervical and thoracic myotomes mature earlier than those arising more distally.

Ultrastructurally, the individual myofibrils are composed of two types of myofilaments: thin (actin) filaments measuring 50–70 nm in diameter and thick (myosin) filaments measuring 140–160 nm in diameter. The thin filaments are laid down first in a random fashion, but later they become rearranged and form parallel bundles together with thick filaments and polyribosomes. In cross-section the thin filaments are seen to surround the thick filaments in distinct, evenly spaced hexagonal patterns.

Mature striated muscle consists of parallel arrays of closely packed myofibrils embedded within sarcoplasm and enveloped by a thin sarcolemmal sheath. Each of the myofibrils shows distinct cross-banding, light and dark bands caused by the periodic arrangement and interdigitation of the thin and thick myofilaments. In this arrangement, isotropic (I) bands, anisotropic (A) bands, and H bands can be distinguished. The I band consists solely of thin (actin) filaments and is divided at its center by the Z line or disc, which is thought to serve as an attachment site for the sarcomeres, the repeating individual units of the muscle fiber. The adjacent A band is a zone of overlapping thin and thick (actin and myosin) filaments; it is separated by the H band, which consists only of thick myofilaments. The width of the individual bands and sarcomeres varies and depends on the state of muscle contraction (Fig. 20–1).

Closely associated with the parallel arrays of myofilaments and the surrounding sarcoplasm are mitochondria, a canalicular network of endoplasmic reticulum, a small Golgi complex, ribosomes, and glycogen and lipid granules. These organelles are confined by a sarcolemmal membrane that measures approximately 70 nm in thickness and is covered by a basal lamina. The sarcolemmal nuclei measure 6–12 mm in greatest diameter and contain one or two small nucleoli; they are located at the periphery of the myofibrils underneath the sarcolemmal membrane. Satellite cells – reserve cells and possible precursors of myoblasts that play a role in the regeneration of striated muscle tissue – are situated in the endomysium between the sarcolemmal membrane and basal lamina.

CLASSIFICATION OF RHABDOMYOMAS

Although as a general rule benign soft tissue neoplasms outnumber malignant neoplasms by a sizable margin, this does not hold true for the neoplasms of striated muscle tissue. Rhabdomyomas (benign tumors of striated muscle tissue) are considerably less common than rhabdomyosarcomas and account for no more than 2% of all striated muscle tumors.

There are two broad categories of rhabdomyomas – cardiac and extracardiac. Among the extracardiac rhabdomyomas, three clinically and morphologically different subtypes can be distinguished: (1) the *adult type*, a slowly growing lesion that is nearly always found in the head and neck area of elderly persons; (2) the *fetal type*, a rare tumor that also principally affects the head and neck region but occurs in both children and adults; and (3) the *genital type*, a polypoid mass found almost exclusively in the vagina and vulva of middle-aged women. A related lesion is the *rhabdomyomatous mesenchymal hamartoma*, a peculiar striated muscle proliferation that occurs chiefly in the periorbital and perioral region of infants and young children (Table 20–1).

CARDIAC RHABDOMYOMA

Cardiac rhabdomyoma occurs almost exclusively in the hearts of infants and young children, often as multiple intramural lesions in the right and left ventricles, although the interventricular septum and atria may be involved as well.[1,2] It often occurs in the setting of tuberous sclerosis and in association with other congenital abnormalities.[3,4] Bosi et al. studied 33 patients with cardiac rhabdomyoma, 30 (91%) of whom had tuberous sclerosis.[5] Similarly, Bader and colleagues found that 25 of 26 patients with a prenatal diagnosis of cardiac rhabdomyoma had evidence of this complex.[6] Patients with a cardiac rhabdomyoma and a family history of tuberous sclerosis and those with multifocal lesions are far more likely to have tuberous sclerosis.[7] In studies that have examined patients with tuberous sclerosis by repeated echocardiograms, 47%[8] to 67%[9] of patients harbor one or more cardiac rhabdomyomas.

Clinically, the lesion may be asymptomatic or may cause cardiac arrhythmia, tachycardia, ventricular outflow obstruction, Wolff-Parkinson-White syndrome, or even sudden death.[10–13] To our knowledge, the concurrence of cardiac and extracardiac rhabdomyomas in the same patient has not been observed, although rare examples of adult rhabdomyoma may occur in the heart.[14,15] These lesions tend to be more cellular, composed of smaller cells, and have fewer spider cells. Extracardiac rhabdomyoma has not been found in association with manifestations of the tuberous sclerosis complex.

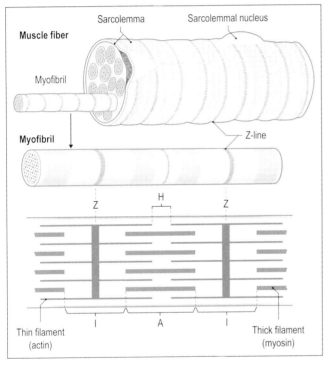

FIGURE 20–1 Muscle fiber, myofibril, and sliding actin and myosin filaments during the rest phase of muscle contraction.

TABLE 20–1	CLINICAL FEATURES OF VARIOUS RHABDOMYOMAS					
Parameter	Cardiac type	Adult type	Fetal myxoid type	Fetal intermediate type	Genital type	RMH
Peak age	Infants	>40 years	Infants	Children and adults	Young to middle-aged adults	Newborns
Gender (M/F)	1:1	3:1	3:1	3:1	Almost all female	Almost all male
Favored site(s)	Ventricles	Head and neck	Head and neck	Head and neck	Vagina, vulva	Chin
Associated conditions	Tuberous sclerosis	None	Nevoid BCC syndrome	Nevoid BCC syndrome	None	Congenital anomalies
Spontaneous regression	Yes	No	No	No	No	No

RMH, rhabdomyomatous mesenchymal hamartoma; BCC, basal cell carcinoma.

Histologically, the lesions are usually small and are composed predominantly of large polygonal "spider cells" with large cytoplasmic vacuoles secondary to loss of glycogen during processing (Figs 20–2, 20–3).[1] The cells stain for muscle markers, including muscle-specific actin and desmin. Some authors have also reported HMB-45 immunoreactivity, supporting a relation with angiomyolipoma and lymphangioleiomyomatosis as components of the tuberous sclerosis complex.[16] More recently, it has also been noted that the neoplastic cells lose expression of tuberin (protein coded for by the *TSC2* gene on chromosome 16) and hamartin (protein coded for by the *TSC1* gene on chromosome 9).[17]

Treatment of this lesion is reserved for those with life-threatening obstructive symptoms or arrhythmias refractory to medical therapy.[18] The lesions have a tendency to regress spontaneously over time.[19] Many of these lesions can be detected by prenatal ultrasound or magnetic resonance imaging (MRI).[20,21]

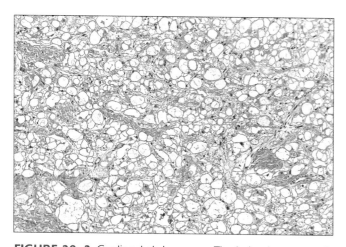

FIGURE 20–2 Cardiac rhabdomyoma. The lesion is composed predominantly of large polygonal "spider cells" with large cytoplasmic vacuoles.

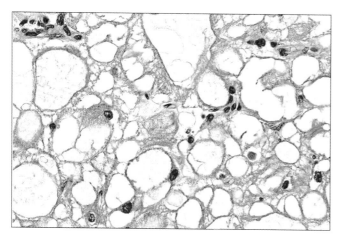

FIGURE 20–3 Cardiac rhabdomyoma with vacuolated spider cells. Cross-striations are rare but can be identified.

ADULT RHABDOMYOMA

The adult type of rhabdomyoma is the most common subtype of extracardiac rhabdomyoma, but it is still rare. There is no etiologic relation between adult rhabdomyoma and *granular cell tumor.*

Clinical findings

The lesion usually presents as a solitary round or polypoid mass in the head and neck region that causes neither tenderness nor pain; it may compress or displace the tongue or may protrude into and partially obstruct the pharynx or larynx. As a consequence, it may cause hoarseness or progressive difficulty with breathing or swallowing.[22,23] It has also been reported as an incidental finding at autopsy or during radical neck dissection for an unrelated cause. It is a slowly growing process, and several of the reported cases were present for many years. Most cases occur in adults older than 40 years (median age 60 years); few cases arise in children.[24] Men are affected three to four times more commonly than women, but apparently there is no predilection for any particular race.[23] The principal site of involvement is the neck, where the tumor arises from the branchial musculature of the third and fourth branchial arches. It is found most frequently in the region of the pharynx, oral cavity including the floor of the mouth or base of the tongue, and the larynx.[23] It may also involve the soft palate and the uvula, usually as an extension of a pharyngeal rhabdomyoma.[25] Rare tumors have been described outside the head and neck region, including the stomach,[26] esophagus,[27] mediastinum[28] and muscles of the extremity.[29] Yu et al. described a typical adult rhabdomyoma that arose in the right atrium of a 42-year-old woman.[15] Most adult rhabdomyomas are solitary, but about 20% are multifocal, mostly involving the general area of the neck.[30]

Pathologic findings

As a rule, the tumor is well defined, rounded, or coarsely lobulated and ranges from 0.5 to 10.0 cm in greatest diameter (median 3.0 cm). Some are multinodular, and others form sessile or pedunculated polypoid submucosal masses. On cut section it has a finely granular, gray-yellow to red-brown appearance.

Microscopically, it is composed of tightly packed, large, round or polygonal cells 15–150 μm in diameter and separated from one another by thin fibrous septa and narrow vascular channels. The cells have deeply acidophilic, finely granular cytoplasm, one or (rarely) two centrally or peripherally placed vesicular nuclei, and one or more prominent nucleoli (Figs 20–4, 20–5). Many of the cells are vacuolated because intracellular glycogen has been removed during processing;[31] some of the vacuolated cells, in fact, contain merely a small central acido-

FIGURE 20–4 Low-power view of adult rhabdomyoma composed of an admixture of deeply eosinophilic polygonal cells and cells with vacuolated cytoplasm.

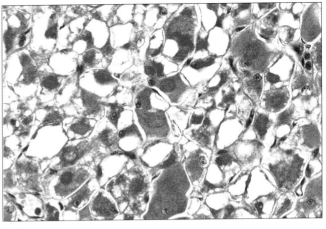

FIGURE 20–6 Adult rhabdomyoma with rare "jackstraw"-like crystalline structures within the cytoplasm of some of the eosinophilic polygonal cells.

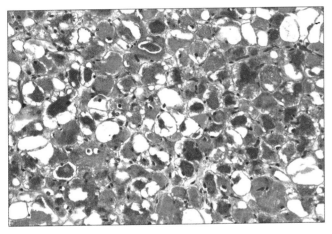

FIGURE 20–5 Adult rhabdomyoma composed of variously sized, deeply eosinophilic polygonal cells with small, peripherally placed nuclei and occasional intracellular vacuoles.

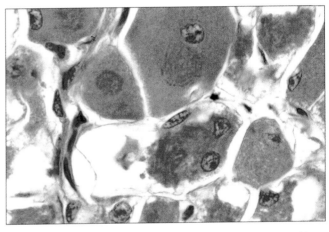

FIGURE 20–7 High-power view of adult rhabdomyoma with crystalline intracellular structures, probably representing Z-band material.

philic cytoplasmic mass connected by thin strands of cytoplasm to a condensed rim of cytoplasm at the periphery (spider cells), but these cells are much more conspicuous in cardiac than extracardiac rhabdomyomas. Mitotic figures are nearly always absent. Cross-striations can be discerned in most cases, but sometimes they are detected only after a prolonged search; additional features present in many cases are intracytoplasmic rod-like or "jackstraw"-like crystalline structures (Figs 20–6, 20–7).[32] Both cross-striations and crystalline structures are identified much more readily with the phosphotungstic acid-hematoxylin (PTAH) stain than with hematoxylin-eosin; moreover, many cells contain intracellular lipid demonstrable with oil red O.

Immunohistochemical, ultrastructural and cytogenetic findings

Immunohistochemically, the cells also stain positively for desmin (Fig. 20–8) and muscle-specific actin; they are

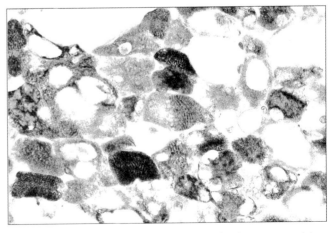

FIGURE 20–8 Adult rhabdomyoma showing immunoreactivity for desmin. Note accentuation of cross-striations.

positive less commonly for vimentin, S-100 protein, and Leu-7.[23,33] Some cases also show focal staining for smooth muscle actin.[23]

There is agreement among most observers as to the ultrastructure of adult rhabdomyoma.[34–36] The cytoplasm contains, in addition to a variable number of mitochondria with linear cristae and deposits of glycogen, thin and thick myofilaments showing a varying degree of differentiation and measuring 50–70 nm and 135–150 nm in diameter, respectively. Distinct Z lines are readily discernible within the I band, but sometimes A, H, M, and N bands are also apparent (Fig. 20–9). Crystalline intracytoplasmic inclusions may be seen and have been identified as hypertrophied Z bands.[37] There are also "triads," trigonal arrays of actin and myosin filaments that can be seen in cross-section,[38] and parallel rows of electron-dense particles within the mitochondria.[39,40]

Very few cytogenetic data are available pertaining to rhabdomyoma. Gibas and Miettinen, in a cytogenetic study of a recurrent peripharyngeal rhabdomyoma in a 64-year-old man, found a reciprocal translocation of chromosomes 15 and 17 and abnormalities in the long arm of chromosome 10.[41]

Differential diagnosis

Problems in diagnosis are unlikely for anyone familiar with the characteristic picture of the tumor (Table 20–2).

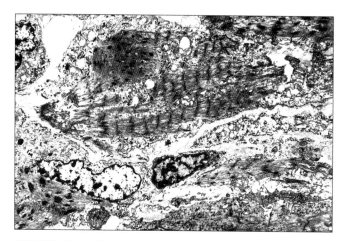

FIGURE 20–9 Electron micrograph of adult rhabdomyoma. Clearly discernible Z-lines are present, along with bundles of actin and myosin filaments.

Yet in the earlier literature, *granular cell tumor* and adult rhabdomyoma were often confused. Granular cell tumor most often involves the skin, tongue or larynx. The cells of a granular cell tumor tend to be less well defined and lack the characteristic vacuolation caused by intracellular glycogen; they are also devoid of cross-striations and usually are associated with more collagen. Moreover, the cells of granular cell tumors contain numerous periodic acid-Schiff (PAS)-positive, diastase-resistant granules that are related to the numerous intracytoplasmic phagolysosomes. Although S-100 protein is focally expressed in some cases of adult rhabdomyoma, its expression is more constant and diffuse in granular cell tumors, which are composed of Schwann cells.

Hibernoma also enters the differential diagnosis because of its frequent intracytoplasmic vacuoles and the presence of intracellular lipid. This tumor, however, is composed of small deeply eosinophilic granular cells that frequently contain distinct, variably sized lipid droplets in the cytoplasm. Clinically, hibernoma is most often found in the interscapular region of patients who are usually younger than 40 years of age. *Reticulohistiocytoma*, another lesion that must be included in the differential diagnosis, usually consists of an intimate mixture of deeply acidophilic histiocytes and fibroblasts intermingled with xanthoma cells, multinucleated giant cells, and chronic inflammatory elements. Typically, none of these cells contains glycogen, and the cells do not express myogenic antigens.

Crystal-storing histiocytosis associated with lymphoplasmacytic neoplasms may also simulate adult rhabdomyoma. In this lesion, however, the crystal-storing cells and histiocytes stain positively for CD68 but are negative for skeletal muscle markers and S-100 protein.[42] Moreover, the associated lymphoplasmacytic infiltrate demonstrates monoclonality with immunostains for kappa and lambda chains (see Chapter 12).

Cardiac rhabdomyoma bears a close resemblance to adult rhabdomyoma, but its cells show a greater number of vacuolated spider cells and a more prominent population of giant cells. Cardiac rhabdomyoma is frequently encountered in association with tuberous sclerosis of the brain, sebaceous adenomas, and various other hamartomatous lesions of the kidney and other organs. Unlike adult rhabdomyoma, it has a propensity for spontaneous regression.

TABLE 20–2	DIFFERENTIAL DIAGNOSIS OF ADULT-TYPE RHABDOMYOMA			
Parameter	**Adult rhabdomyoma**	**Granular cell tumor**	**Hibernoma**	**Paraganglioma**
Favored site	Head and neck	Skin, tongue	Interscapular	Extra-adrenal ganglia
Electron microscopy	Thin/thick filaments	Phagolysosomes	Mitochondria	Neurosecretory granules
S-100 protein	Rare, focal	Diffuse	Diffuse	Sustentacular cells
Muscle-specific actin	Diffuse	Negative	Negative	Negative
Chromogranin	Negative	Negative	Negative	Diffuse

Rhabdomyosarcoma is composed of poorly differentiated and pleomorphic round or spindle-shaped cells associated with varying numbers of rhabdomyoblasts. Mitotic figures are common in rhabdomyosarcomas but are absent or rare in adult rhabdomyomas. *Oncocytoma* is an epithelial neoplasm of salivary gland origin composed of mitochondria-rich polyhedral cells with finely granular, eosinophilic cytoplasm. The cells stain for epithelial markers but do not express actin or desmin. *Paraganglioma* is a neuroendocrine neoplasm composed of cells arranged in an organoid pattern (Zellballen). As seen by immunohistochemistry, the cells express neuroendocrine markers, including neuron-specific enolase, synaptophysin, and chromogranin. S-100 protein outlines the sustentacular cells, and the cells lack myogenic antigens. Neurosecretory granules can be demonstrated by electron microscopy.

Prognosis and therapy

The tumor is readily amenable to therapy but may recur locally if incompletely excised. In one series of 19 cases with follow-up information, the tumor recurred in 8 (42%) of the cases.[23] Examples of multiple and late recurrences have also been described.[23,43] Spontaneous regression, as is seen with some cardiac rhabdomyomas, has not been observed.[44]

FETAL RHABDOMYOMA

Fetal rhabdomyoma is even rarer in our experience than adult-type rhabdomyoma, and only a small number of cases have been recorded in the medical literature. Awareness of the existence of this tumor, however, is of considerable importance because of its resemblance to embryonal rhabdomyosarcoma. The lesion has a variable histological pattern, with a spectrum of skeletal muscle differentiation that ranges from immature, predominantly myxoid tumors to those showing a high degree of cellular differentiation and hardly any myxoid matrix. The former have been described as *myxoid*[43] or *classic*[45] *fetal rhabdomyomas*; the latter are variously described as *intermediate*,[45,46] *cellular*,[43] or *juvenile*[47] *fetal rhabdomyomas*. Intermediate forms between these two types are not uncommon. There is also a third, still ill-defined morphologic variant of this tumor that is marked by prominent neural involvement showing some similarities to neuromuscular hamartoma.[48–50]

Clinical features

The age incidence varies slightly according to the prevailing histologic type. Tumors of the predominantly *myxoid type* mainly affect boys during the first year of life and are rare in older patients. In the series of Kapadia et al.,[45] six of the eight patients were infants younger than 1 year of age. The favorite sites of the myxoid type are the subcutaneous tissue and the submucosa of the head and neck, especially the pre- and postauricular regions.[45,51] The *intermediate type* affects adults more often than children. It occurs almost exclusively in the region of the head and neck, including the orbit, tongue, nasopharynx, and soft palate.[52,53] Rare cases of fetal rhabdomyoma have been described outside the head and neck region, including the chest wall/axilla,[54] abdominal wall,[39] spermatic cord,[55] extremity,[56] retroperitoneum,[57] and perianal region.[58] For both types, males outnumber females by a ratio of approximately 3 : 1.

There are several reports in the literature of fetal rhabdomyoma associated with the nevoid basal cell carcinoma syndrome.[49,59–62] This syndrome is an autosomal dominant disorder characterized by multiple basal cell carcinomas that appear early during childhood, various skeletal abnormalities, and odontogenic keratocysts, among other findings. Mutations in the *PTCH* tumor suppressor gene have been implicated in the development of this syndrome.[63]

Pathologic findings

On gross examination the tumors are generally well circumscribed and average 2–6 cm in greatest diameter, although lesions as large as 12.5 cm have been reported.[45] Mucosal lesions tend to be smooth and polypoid or pedunculated. On sectioning they are gray-white to pink, often with a mucoid, glistening surface. Unlike rhabdomyosarcoma, fetal rhabdomyoma is primarily a superficial tumor and is found more often in the subcutis or submucosa than in muscle. Most are solitary, but multicentric fetal rhabdomyomas have been reported in association with the nevoid basal cell carcinoma syndrome.[59]

Two closely related types can be distinguished by microscopy. The *myxoid type* is chiefly composed of primitive oval or spindle-shaped cells with indistinct cytoplasm, interspersed immature skeletal muscle fibers reminiscent of fetal myotubes seen during the seventh to tenth weeks of intrauterine life, and a richly myxoid matrix (Figs 20–10, 20–11). The immature skeletal muscle cells have small uniform nuclei with delicate chromatin and inconspicuous nucleoli with bipolar or sometimes unipolar, finely tapered eosinophilic cytoplasmic processes. Cross-striations are rare and often difficult to discern; they are best seen with PTAH or Masson trichrome stains or with immunohistochemical stains for desmin or muscle-specific actin. The cells may be arranged in short bundles or isolated within the myxoid matrix. Sometimes, focal proliferation of abundant muscle fibers makes it difficult to draw a sharp line between tumor and normal muscle tissue. The primitive undifferentiated cells have oval nuclei with slight nuclear hyperchromasia and scanty, indistinct cytoplasm.

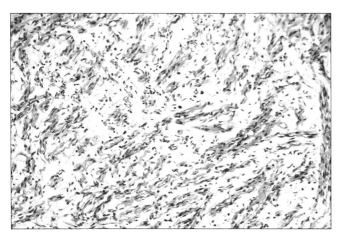

FIGURE 20–10 Fetal rhabdomyoma, myxoid type. The lesion is composed of an intimate mixture of primitive, round and spindle-shaped mesenchymal cells and differentiated myofibrils within a richly myxoid background.

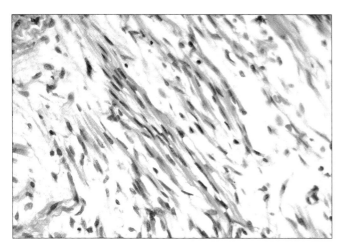

FIGURE 20–11 Fetal rhabdomyoma, myxoid type. Unlike embryonal rhabdomyosarcoma, the muscle cells vary little in size and shape, and there is no mitotic activity. The cells are deposited in an abundant myxoid matrix.

The *intermediate type* is characterized by the presence of numerous differentiated muscle fibers, less conspicuous or absent spindle-shaped mesenchymal cells, and little or no myxoid stroma (Fig. 20–12). In any given case, there may be a wide spectrum of skeletal muscle differentiation. The predominant cells are broad, strap-shaped muscle cells with abundant eosinophilic cytoplasm, centrally located vesicular nuclei, and frequent cross-striations reminiscent of the cells seen in adult rhabdomyomas; many of the cells contain glycogen and are often vacuolated. Others have prominent ganglion-like rhabdomyoblasts with large vesicular nuclei and prominent nucleoli. Mucosa-based lesions tend to have the widest spectrum of rhabdomyoblastic differentiation and the most mature-appearing cells.[45] In some cases there is mild cellular pleomorphism, but marked cellular atypia is not a feature of the disease, as it is with embryo-

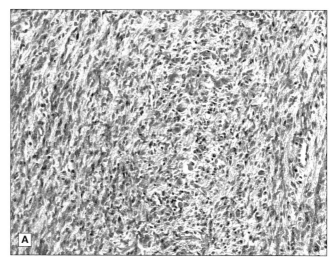

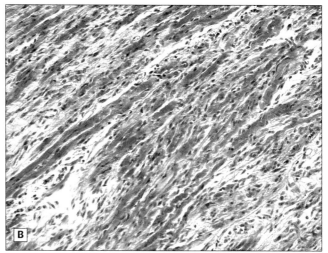

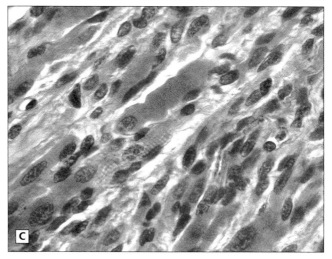

FIGURE 20–12 (A) Fetal rhabdomyoma, intermediate (cellular) type, consisting of intersecting bundles of differentiated eosinophilic myofibrils containing cross-striations. Myofibrils separated by small undifferentiated spindle cells. **(B)** Higher-magnification view of interspersed spindled cells with differentiated myofibrils. **(C)** High-magnification view of fetal rhabdomyoma, intermediate (cellular) type. (Case courtesy of Dr. Cyril Fisher, Royal Marsden Hospital, London, England.)

nal rhabdomyosarcoma. Transitional forms between the myxoid and intermediate types are not rare. In fact, age and duration may play a role in the maturation of some tumors, as suggested by the older mean age of patients with the intermediate (cellular) type and the reported long duration of some cases. In both types, mitotic figures are rare or absent.

In addition to the myxoid and intermediate types there are sporadic fetal rhabdomyoma-like tumors that are intimately associated with peripheral nerves reminiscent of neuromuscular choristoma (benign Triton tumor). We have seen two such cases in the head and neck region; others have reported similar lesions associated with the trigeminal nerve,[64] and facial nerve.[50] By immunohistochemistry, the muscle cells stain positively for desmin and muscle-specific actin, with only rare and focal staining for vimentin, S-100 protein, Leu-7, glial fibrillary acidic protein, and smooth muscle actin.[45]

Ultrastructurally, the differentiated muscle cells consist of organized bundles of thick (myosin) and thin (actin) myofilaments with the characteristic banding in some of the more differentiated muscle cells. Rod-like cytoplasmic inclusions or hypertrophied Z-band materials have been described but seem to be much less common than with adult rhabdomyoma.[47] The differentiated cells also contain considerable amounts of intracellular glycogen and a small number of mitochondria. The intervening small spindle cells are devoid of any specific cellular differentiation.

Differential diagnosis

Distinction from *embryonal* and *spindle cell rhabdomyosarcoma* is the principal issue (Table 20–3); unlike rhabdomyosarcoma, fetal rhabdomyoma tends to be fairly well circumscribed and is superficially located. Mitotic figures are rare, and the tumor lacks a significant degree of cellular pleomorphism and areas of necrosis; considerable cellularity, a mild degree of cellular pleomorphism, and occasional mitotic figures do not rule out this diagnosis.

Caution must also be exercised in the differential diagnosis because of the possible malignant transformation of fetal rhabdomyoma. We have encountered one case in which the initial lesion, biopsied at 3 weeks of age, seemed to be characteristic of fetal rhabdomyoma, whereas the recurrent tumor, excised at 23 months, showed a much greater degree of cellularity and mitotic activity and was indistinguishable from embryonal rhabdomyosarcoma. Another possible case of "cellular fetal rhabdomyoma with malignant transformation" was reported by Kodet et al. in the tongue of an 18-month-old infant.[65]

Infantile fibromatosis may bear a close resemblance to fetal rhabdomyoma, especially if the tumor diffusely infiltrates muscle tissue and contains numerous residual muscle fibers that have been entrapped by the proliferating fibroblasts. Fetal rhabdomyoma, however, is better circumscribed than fibromatoses, is situated in the subcutis rather than in muscle tissue, and lacks the fasciculated spindle cell pattern. In addition, interspersed fat cells, a frequent feature of diffuse infantile fibromatosis, are absent in fetal rhabdomyoma. The "neural variant of fetal rhabdomyoma" may be difficult to distinguish from a neuromuscular choristoma (benign Triton tumor). However, the latter tends to be more lobular and has a more distinct mature skeletal muscle and Schwann cell population, with clear macroscopic attachment to a nerve.

Prognosis and therapy

Fetal rhabdomyoma, a benign lesion, is readily curable by local excision, with only rare reports of local recurrence.[39,45] It is a slowly growing process, and there are reports of lesions having been present for years with little change in size or histologic picture except for interstitial fibrosis. Whether it is a neoplasm or a hamartoma is unclear; it has been known to be associated with the nevoid basal cell carcinoma syndrome. There is no valid support for the contention that fetal rhabdomyoma is an early stage in the development of adult rhabdomyoma.

GENITAL RHABDOMYOMA

Although genital rhabdomyoma bears some resemblance to both adult and fetal rhabdomyomas, it is sufficiently different in its clinical and microscopic manifestations to qualify as a separate entity. So far only a small number of cases have been described, including some that were reported as fetal rhabdomyoma.[43] Almost all arise as a slowly growing "polypoid" mass or "cyst" in the vagina or vulva of young or middle-aged women.[66–69] Rare cases have been described in the cervix[70] and male urogenital tract including the prostate,[71] testicular tunica vaginalis,[72] epididymis[73,74] and spermatic cord.[75] Most are asymptomatic and are found on routine physical examination; some cause dyspareunia or vaginal bleeding secondary to mucosal erosion.

TABLE 20–3	DISTINGUISHING FEATURES OF FETAL RHABDOMYOMA AND EMBRYONAL RHABDOMYOSARCOMA	
Parameter	**Fetal rhabdomyoma**	**Embryonal rhabdomyosarcoma**
Gross appearance	Well circumscribed	Infiltrative
Depth	Superficial	Deep
Mitotic figures	Absent or rare	Easily identified
Pleomorphism	Absent or slight	Moderate or marked
Necrosis	Absent	Often present

Microscopically, the excised tumor usually forms a polypoid or cauliflower-like mass covered by epithelium and rarely measures more than 3 cm in greatest diameter. It consists of scattered, more or less mature muscle fibers showing distinct cross-striations and a matrix containing varying amounts of collagen and mucoid material (Figs 20–13 to 20–15). As with other rhabdomyomas, the cells are immunoreactive for desmin and muscle-specific actin.[68] Electron microscopic examination of the lesion reveals a large nucleus with a prominent dense nucleolus and arrays of thick and thin myofilaments with Z lines and A and I bands, together with intracytoplasmic bodies and basal lamina. There are also attachment plaques or peripheral couplings.[76]

The differential diagnosis includes benign *vaginal polyps* and *botryoid embryonal rhabdomyosarcoma (sarcoma botryoides)*. Benign vaginal polyps are characterized by atypical single or multinucleated stromal cells, but they lack classic strap cells with cross-striations. Botryoid

embryonal rhabdomyosarcoma usually occurs in young children who present with a rapidly growing lesion that frequently ulcerates the overlying epithelium. In contrast, genital rhabdomyoma usually occurs in middle-aged women and is generally a slowly growing tumor associated with an intact overlying epithelium. The subepithelial "cambium layer" characteristic of botryoid embryonal rhabdomyosarcoma is not found in genital rhabdomyomas. In addition, nuclear pleomorphism and mitotic figures are more prominent in rhabdomyosarcomas than in rhabdomyomas (Table 20–4).

The lesion, which pursues a benign course, is adequately treated by local excision. As with other types of rhabdomyoma, it is still undecided whether the lesion is a hamartoma or a neoplasm.

RHABDOMYOMATOUS MESENCHYMAL HAMARTOMA OF SKIN

Originally described in 1986 by Hendrick et al. as *striated muscle hamartoma*,[77] rhabdomyomatous mesenchymal hamartoma of skin, which occurs principally in the

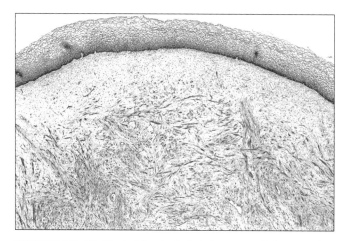

FIGURE 20–13 Genital (vaginal) rhabdomyoma. Submucosal proliferation of striated muscle cells separated by varying amounts of myxoid material and collagen.

TABLE 20–4	DISTINGUISHING FEATURES OF GENITAL RHABDOMYOMA AND BOTRYOID RHABDOMYOSARCOMA	
Parameter	**Genital rhabdomyoma**	**Botryoid rhabdomyosarcoma**
Peak age	Young to middle-aged adults	Birth to 15 years
Gender (M/F)	Almost all females	1 : 1
Growth	Slowly growing	Rapidly growing
Epithelial ulceration	Absent	Often present
Cambium layer	Absent	Present
Mitotic figures	Absent or rare	Easily identified
Pleomorphism	Absent or slight	Moderate or marked

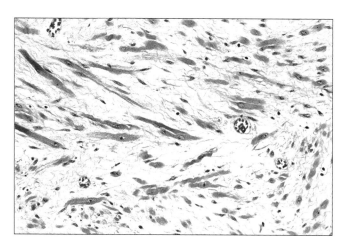

FIGURE 20–14 Genital rhabdomyoma composed of loosely arranged striated muscle cells and fibroblasts.

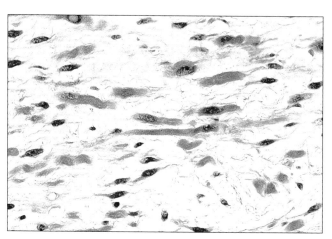

FIGURE 20–15 High-power view of genital rhabdomyoma showing rare striated muscle cells with cross-striations.

face and neck of newborns, is rare, with fewer than 30 cases reported in the literature. The lesion typically presents as a small dome-shaped papule or a polypoid pedunculated lesion in newborns. There are case reports of this lesion in adults, although it is not clear if these lesions were present since childhood.[78,79] The lesions range in size from a few millimeters to 1–2 cm. The most common location appears to be the chin, followed by the periorbital, periauricular, and anterior mid-neck region.[80] Other unusual locations where these lesions have been reported include the oral cavity[81] and nares.[82] Almost all lesions occur in males, with only rare cases having been described in females.[82,83] Virtually all are solitary; Sahn et al. described multiple pedunculated lesions arising in the periorbital and periauricular region in a newborn boy.[84] Some patients have associated congenital anomalies.[85] For example, Takeyama and colleagues described a case of rhabdomyomatous mesenchymal hamartoma associated with a nasofrontal meningocele and a dermoid cyst.[86] One of the patients in the original report by Hendrick et al. had a cleft lip and cleft gum as well as circumferential amniotic bands around the head and distal left leg.[77] Sahn et al. described one patient with bilateral diffuse sclerocorneas with probable retinal dysplasia.[84]

Grossly, most lesions are polypoid and attached to the skin by a long stalk, with circumferential constriction of the distal attachment site. Other lesions are more globular in shape, occasionally with central umbilication. Histologically, the lesions are covered by normal-appearing squamous epithelium. More centrally, single or small groups of mature-appearing skeletal muscle fibers are found within the subcutaneous tissue and dermis.[87–91] The fibers frequently are deposited in a collagenous stroma admixed with mature adipose tissue and adnexal structures, often aligned perpendicular to the surface epithelium. Blood vessels and nerves may also be found admixed among the mature skeletal muscle fibers. Rare cases show central calcification or ossification.

The differential diagnosis includes *nevus lipomatosis superficialis*, which shows mature adipose tissue within the dermis but lacks skeletal muscle elements. Similarly, *fibrous hamartoma of infancy* contains an admixture of mature adipose tissue, collagenous bundles, and more cellular areas deposited in a myxoid stroma but lacks the skeletal muscle fibers. *Neuromuscular choristoma (benign Triton tumor)*, a rare subcutaneous lesion found in association with peripheral nerves, is composed of mature skeletal muscle fibers and neural tissue. Finally, rhabdomyomatous mesenchymal hamartoma must be distinguished from the rare and much less differentiated *cutaneous embryonal rhabdomyosarcoma*.[92]

This congenital hamartomatous lesion is adequately treated by local excision, and recurrences have not been described. The identification of these lesions in female patients suggests that this entity is not an X-linked disorder, as previously suggested.[93]

MISCELLANEOUS LESIONS MIMICKING BENIGN STRIATED MUSCLE TUMORS

Various benign lesions of striated muscle may be confused with rhabdomyoma. Supernumerary muscles in the popliteal fossa and ankle region of young adults presenting as a tumor-like mass have been described.[94] Similar accessory muscles may occur in the hand, fingers, and other portions of the body; some are bilateral. Likewise, unilateral or bilateral hypertrophy of the masseter muscle may be mistaken for a muscle tumor.[95] This condition occurs chiefly in young adults and is often accompanied by bony overgrowth or a spur at the angle of the mandible.[96] Benign skeletal muscle differentiation has also been observed in the uterus and in a uterine leiomyoma.[97]

REFERENCES

Cardiac rhabdomyoma

1. Burke AP, Virmani R. Cardiac rhabdomyoma: A clinicopathologic study. Mod Pathol 1991; 4:70.
2. Isaacs H Jr. Fetal and neonatal cardiac tumors. Pediatr Cardiol 2004; 25:252.
3. Kelekci S, Yazicioglu HF, Yilmaz B, et al. Cardiac rhabdomyoma with tuberous sclerosis: a case report. J Reprod Med 2005; 50:550.
4. Habbu JH, Hayman R, Roberts LJ. Tuberous sclerosis in an antenatally diagnosed cardiac rhabdomyoma. J Obstet Gynaecol 2005; 25:193.
5. Bosi G, Lintermans JP, Pellegrino PA, et al. The natural history of cardiac rhabdomyoma with and without tuberous sclerosis. Acta Paediatr 1996; 85:928.
6. Bader RS, Chitayat D, Kelly E, et al. Fetal rhabdomyoma: Prenatal diagnosis, clinical outcome, and incidence of associated tuberous sclerosis complex. J Pediatr 2003; 143:620.
7. Gamzu R, Achiron R, Hegesh J, et al. Evaluating the risk of tuberous sclerosis in cases with prenatal diagnosis of cardiac rhabdomyoma. Prenat Diagn 2002; 22:1044.
8. Jozwiak S, Kawalec W, Dluzewska J, et al. Cardiac tumours in tuberous sclerosis: Their incidence and course. Eur J Pediatr 1994; 153:155.
9. DiMario FJ Jr, Diana D, Leopold H, et al. Evolution of cardiac rhabdomyoma in tuberous sclerosis complex. Clin Pediatr (Phila) 1996; 35:615.
10. Venugopalan P, Babu JS, Al-Bulushi A. Right atrial rhabdomyoma acting as the substrate for Wolff-Parkinson-White syndrome in a 3-month-old infant. Acta Cardiol 2005; 60:543.
11. Abdel-Rahman U, Ozaslan F, Esmaeili A, et al. A giant rhabdomyoma with left ventricular inflow occlusion and univentricular physiology. Thorac Cardiovasc Surg 2005; 53:259.
12. Friedberg M, Silverman NH. Right ventricular outflow tract obstruction in an infant. Heart 2005; 91:748.
13. Kagan KO, Schmidt M, Kuhn U, et al. Ventricular outflow obstruction, valve aplasia, bradyarrhythmia, pulmonary hypoplasia and non-immune fetal hydrops because of a large rhabdomyoma in a case of unknown tuberous sclerosis: A prenatal diagnosed cardiac rhabdomyoma with multiple symptoms. BJOG 2004; 111:1478.
14. Burke AP, Gatto-Weis C, Griego JE, et al. Adult cellular rhabdomyoma of the heart: a report of 3 cases. Hum Pathol 2002; 33:1092.
15. Yu GH, Kussmaul WG, DiSesa VJ, et al. Adult intracardiac rhabdomyoma resembling the extracardiac variant. Hum Pathol 1993; 24:448.
16. Weeks DA, Chase DR, Malott RL, et al. HMB-45 staining in angiomyolipoma, cardiac rhabdomyoma, other mesenchymal processes, and tuberous sclerosis-associated brain lesions. Int J Surg Pathol 1994; 1:191.
17. Vinaitheerthan M, Wei J, Mizuguchi M, et al. Tuberous sclerosis: immunohistochemistry expression of tuberin and hamartin in a 31-week gestational fetus. Fetal Pediatr Pathol 2004; 23:241.

18. Padalino MA, Basso C, Milanesi O, et al. Surgically treated primary cardiac tumors in early infancy and childhood. J Thorac Cardiovasc Surg 2005; 129:1358.

19. Fesslova V, Villa L, Rizzuti T, et al. Natural history and long-term outcome of cardiac rhabdomyomas detected prenatally. Prenat Diagn 2004; 24:241.

20. Zhou QC, Fan P, Peng QH, et al. Prenatal echocardiographic differential diagnosis of fetal cardiac tumors. Ultrasound Obstet Gynecol 2004; 23:165.

21. Chen X, Hoda SA, Edgar MA. Cardiac rhabdomyoma. Arch Pathol Lab Med 2002; 126:1559.

Adult rhabdomyoma

22. Johansen EC, Illum P. Rhabdomyoma of the larynx: A review of the literature with a summary of previously described cases of rhabdomyoma of the larynx and a report of a new case. J Laryngol Otol 1995; 109:147.

23. Kapadia SB, Meis JM, Frisman DM, et al. Adult rhabdomyoma of the head and neck: A clinicopathologic and immunophenotypic study. Hum Pathol 1993; 24:608.

24. Solomon MP, Tolete-Velcek F. Lingual rhabdomyoma (adult variant) in a child. J Pediatr Surg 1979; 14:91.

25. Bock D, Bock P. Rhabdomyoma of the soft palate. Fine structural details of a highly differentiated muscle tumor. Histol Histopathol 1987; 2:285.

26. Tuazon R. Rhabdomyoma of the stomach. Report of a case. Am J Clin Pathol 1969; 52:37.

27. Roberts F, Kirk AJ, More IA, et al. Oesophageal rhabdomyoma. J Clin Pathol 2000; 53:554.

28. Sidhu JS, Nicolas MM, Taylor W. Mediastinal rhabdomyoma: A case report and review of the literature. Int J Surg Pathol 2002; 10:313.

29. Cronin CT, Keel SB, Grabbe J, et al. Adult rhabdomyoma of the extremity: a case report and review of the literature. Hum Pathol 2000; 31:1074.

30. Liess BD, Zitsch RP 3rd, Lane R, et al. Multifocal adult rhabdomyoma: A case report and literature review. Am J Otolaryngol 2005; 26:214.

31. Favia G, Lo Muzio L, Serpico R, et al. Rhabdomyoma of the head and neck: clinicopathologic features of two cases. Head Neck 2003; 25:700.

32. Moran JJ, Enterline HT. Benign rhabdomyoma of the pharynx. A case report, review of the literature, and comparison with cardiac rhabdomyoma. Am J Clin Pathol 1964; 42:174.

33. Helliwell TR, Sissons MC, Stoney PJ, et al. Immunochemistry and electron microscopy of head and neck rhabdomyoma. J Clin Pathol 1988; 41:1058.

34. Fukuda Y, Okamura HO, Nemoto T, et al. Rhabdomyoma of the base of the tongue. J Laryngol Otol 2003; 117:503.

35. Silverman JF, Kay S, Chang CH. Ultrastructural comparison between skeletal muscle and cardiac rhabdomyomas. Cancer 1978; 42:189.

36. Cleveland DB, Chen SY, Allen CM, et al. Adult rhabdomyoma. A light microscopic, ultrastructural, virologic, and immunologic analysis. Oral Surg Oral Med Oral Pathol 1994; 77:147.

37. Cornog JL Jr, Gonatas NK. Ultrastructure of rhabdomyoma. J Ultrastruct Res 1967; 20:433.

38. Warner TF, Goell W, Sundharadas M, et al. Adult rhabdomyoma: ultrastructure and immunocytochemistry. Arch Pathol Lab Med 1981; 105:608.

39. Konrad EA, Meister P, Hubner G. Extracardiac rhabdomyoma: report of different types with light microscopic and ultrastructural studies. Cancer 1982; 49:898.

40. Blaauwgeers JL, Troost D, Dingemans KP, et al. Multifocal rhabdomyoma of the neck. Report of a case studied by fine-needle aspiration, light and electron microscopy, histochemistry, and immunohistochemistry. Am J Surg Pathol 1989; 13:791.

41. Gibas Z, Miettinen M. Recurrent parapharyngeal rhabdomyoma. Evidence of neoplastic nature of the tumor from cytogenetic study. Am J Surg Pathol 1992; 16:721.

42. Kapadia SB, Enzinger FM, Heffner DK, et al. Crystal-storing histiocytosis associated with lymphoplasmacytic neoplasms. Report of three cases mimicking adult rhabdomyoma. Am J Surg Pathol 1993; 17:461.

43. Di Sant'Agnese PA, Knowles DM 2nd. Extracardiac rhabdomyoma: a clinicopathologic study and review of the literature. Cancer 1980; 46:780.

44. Andersen CB, Elling F. Adult rhabdomyoma of the oropharynx recurring three times within thirty-five years. Acta Pathol Microbiol Immunol Scand [A] 1986; 94:281.

Fetal rhabdomyoma

45. Kapadia SB, Meis JM, Frisman DM, et al. Fetal rhabdomyoma of the head and neck: a clinicopathologic and immunophenotypic study of 24 cases. Hum Pathol 1993; 24:754.

46. Fernandez JM, Medlich MA, Lopez LH, et al. Fetal intermediate rhabdomyoma of the lip: case report. J Clin Pediatr Dent 2005; 29:179.

47. Crotty PL, Nakhleh RE, Dehner LP. Juvenile rhabdomyoma. An intermediate form of skeletal muscle tumor in children. Arch Pathol Lab Med 1993; 117:43.

48. Hardisson D, Nistal M. The origin of striated muscle cells in non-neoplastic lung tissue. Hum Pathol 2001; 32:763.

49. Watson J, Depasquale K, Ghaderi M, et al. Nevoid basal cell carcinoma syndrome and fetal rhabdomyoma: a case study. Ear Nose Throat J 2004; 83:716.

50. Vandewalle G, Brucher JM, Michotte A. Intracranial facial nerve rhabdomyoma. Case report. J Neurosurg 1995; 83:919.

51. Dehner LP, Enzinger FM, Font RL. Fetal rhabdomyoma. An analysis of nine cases. Cancer 1972; 30:160.

52. Myung J, Kim IO, Chun JE, et al. Rhabdomyoma of the orbit: a case report. Pediatr Radiol 2002; 32:589.

53. Bozic C. Fetal rhabdomyoma of the parotid gland in an infant: histological, immunohistochemical, and ultrastructural features. Pediatr Pathol 1986; 6:139.

54. Seidal T, Kindblom LG, Angervall L. Myoglobin, desmin and vimentin in ultrastructurally proven rhabdomyomas and rhabdomyosarcomas. An immunohistochemical study utilizing a series of monoclonal and polyclonal antibodies. Appl Pathol 1987; 5:201.

55. Kurzrock EA, Busby JE, Gandour-Edwards R. Paratesticular rhabdomyoma. J Pediatr Surg 2003; 38:1546.

56. Osgood PJ, Damron TA, Rooney MT, et al. Benign fetal rhabdomyoma of the upper extremity. A case report. Clin Orthop Rel Res 1998; 349:200.

57. Whitten RO, Benjamin DR. Rhabdomyoma of the retroperitoneum. A report of a tumor with both adult and fetal characteristics: a study by light and electron microscopy, histochemistry, and immunochemistry. Cancer 1987; 59:818.

58. Lapner PC, Chou S, Jimenez C. Perianal fetal rhabdomyoma: case report. Pediatr Surg Int 1997; 12:544.

59. Dahl I, Angervall L, Save-Soderbergh J. Foetal rhabdomyoma. Case report of a patient with two tumours. Acta Pathol Microbiol Scand [A] 1976; 84:107.

60. DiSanto S, Abt AB, Boal DK, et al. Fetal rhabdomyoma and nevoid basal cell carcinoma syndrome. Pediatr Pathol 1992; 12:441.

61. Gorlin RJ. Nevoid basal-cell carcinoma syndrome. Medicine (Baltimore) 1987; 66:98.

62. Schweisguth O, Gerard-Marchant R, Lemerle J. Basal cell nevus syndrome. Association with congenital rhabdomyosarcoma. Arch Fr Pediatr 1968; 25:1083.

63. Hahn H, Wicking C, Zaphiropoulous PG, et al. Mutations of the human homolog of drosophila patched in the nevoid basal cell carcinoma syndrome. Cell 1996; 85:841.

64. Zwick DL, Livingston K, Clapp L, et al. Intracranial trigeminal nerve rhabdomyoma/choristoma in a child: a case report and discussion of possible histogenesis. Hum Pathol 1989; 20:390.

65. Kodet R, Fajstavr J, Kabelka Z, et al. Is fetal cellular rhabdomyoma an entity or a differentiated rhabdomyosarcoma? A study of patients with rhabdomyoma of the tongue and sarcoma of the tongue enrolled in the Intergroup Rhabdomyosarcoma Studies I, II, and III. Cancer 1991; 67:2907.

Genital rhabdomyoma

66. Lin GY, Sun X, Badve S. Pathologic quiz case. Vaginal wall mass in a 47-year-old woman. Vaginal rhabdomyoma. Arch Pathol Lab Med 2002; 126:1241.

67. Iversen UM. Two cases of benign vaginal rhabdomyoma. Case reports. APMIS 1996; 104:575.

68. Lopez Varela C, Lopez de la Riva M, La Cruz Pelea C. Vaginal rhabdomyomas. Int J Gynaecol Obstet 1994; 47:169.

69. Willis J, Abdul-Karim FW, di Sant'Agnese PA. Extracardiac rhabdomyomas. Semin Diagn Pathol 1994; 11:15.

70. Urbanke A. True rhabdomyoma of the uterus. Zentralbl Allg Pathol 1962; 103:241.

71. Morra MN, Manson AL, Gavrell GJ, et al. Rhabdomyoma of prostate. Urology 1992; 39:271.

72. Tanda F, Rocca PC, Bosincu L, et al. Rhabdomyoma of the tunica vaginalis of the testis: a histologic, immunohistochemical, and ultrastructural study. Mod Pathol 1997; 10:608.

73. Wehner MS, Humphreys JL, Sharkey FE. Epididymal rhabdomyoma: report of a case, including histologic and immunohistochemical findings. Arch Pathol Lab Med 2000; 124:1518.

74. Matsunaga GS, Shepherd DL, Troyer DA, et al. Epididymal rhabdomyoma. J Urol 2000; 163:1876.

75. Maheshkumar P, Berney DM. Spermatic cord rhabdomyoma. Urology 2000; 56:331.

76. Chabrel CM, Beilby JO. Vaginal rhabdomyoma. Histopathology 1980; 4:645.

Rhabdomyomatous mesenchymal hamartoma of skin

77. Hendrick SJ, Sanchez RL, Blackwell SJ, et al. Striated muscle hamartoma: description of two cases. Pediatr Dermatol 1986; 3:153.

78. Chang CP, Chen GS. Rhabdomyomatous mesenchymal hamartoma: A plaque-type variant in an adult. Kaohsiung J Med Sci 2005; 21:185.

79. Rosenberg AS, Kirk J, Morgan MB. Rhabdomyomatous mesenchymal hamartoma: an unusual dermal entity with a report of two cases and a review of the literature. J Cutan Pathol 2002; 29:238.

80. Kim HS, Kim JY, Kim JW, et al. Rhabdomyomatous mesenchymal hamartoma. J Eur Acad Dermatol Venereol 2007; 21:564.

81. Magro G, Di Benedetto A, Sanges G, et al. Rhabdomyomatous mesenchymal hamartoma of oral cavity: an unusual location for such a rare lesion. Virchows Arch 2005; 446:346.

82. Farris PE, Manning S, Vuitch F. Rhabdomyomatous mesenchymal hamartoma. Am J Dermatopathol 1994; 16:73.

83. Hayes M, van der Westhuizen N. Congenital rhabdomyomatous mesenchymal hamartoma. Am J Dermatopathol 1992; 14:64.
84. Sahn EE, Garen PD, Pai GS, et al. Multiple rhabdomyomatous mesenchymal hamartomas of skin. Am J Dermatopathol 1990; 12:485.
85. Read RW, Burnstine M, Rowland JM, et al. Rhabdomyomatous mesenchymal hamartoma of the eyelid: report of a case and literature review. Ophthalmology 2001; 108:798.
86. Takeyama J, Hayashi T, Sanada T, et al. Rhabdomyomatous mesenchymal hamartoma associated with nasofrontal meningocele and dermoid cyst. J Cutan Pathol 2005; 32:310.
87. Ashfaq R, Timmons CF. Rhabdomyomatous mesenchymal hamartoma of skin. Pediatr Pathol 1992; 12:731.

88. Elgart GW, Patterson JW. Congenital midline hamartoma: Case report with histochemical and immunohistochemical findings. Pediatr Dermatol 1990; 7:199.
89. Katsumata M, Keong CH, Satoh T. Rhabdomyomatous mesenchymal hamartoma of skin. J Dermatol 1990; 17:384.
90. Mills AE. Rhabdomyomatous mesenchymal hamartoma of skin. Am J Dermatopathol 1989; 11:58.
91. White G. Congenital rhabdomyomatous mesenchymal hamartoma. Am J Dermatopathol 1990; 12:539.
92. Chang Y, Dehner LP, Egbert B. Primary cutaneous rhabdomyosarcoma. Am J Surg Pathol 1990; 12:731.
93. Mills E. Congenital rhabdomyomatous mesenchymal hamartoma. Am J Dermatopathol 1991; 13:429.

Miscellaneous lesions mimicking benign striated muscle tumors

94. Durm AW. Anomalous muscle simulating soft tissue tumors on the lower extremities. J Bone Joint Surg [Am] 1965; 47:1397.
95. Wade WM Jr, Roy EW. Idiopathic masseter muscle hypertrophy: report of case. J Oral Surg 1971; 29:196.
96. Waldhart E, Lynch JB. Benign hypertrophy of the masseter muscles and mandibular angles. Arch Surg 1971; 102:115.
97. Martin-Reay DG, Christ ML, LaPata RE. Uterine leiomyoma with skeletal muscle differentiation. Report of a case. Am J Clin Pathol 1991; 96:344.

RHABDOMYOSARCOMA

The concept of what constitutes rhabdomyosarcoma has been the subject of considerable change over the years. During the 1930s and 1940s, the diagnosis of adult or pleomorphic rhabdomyosarcoma gained in popularity, and most of the rhabdomyosarcomas reported during this period were of this type.[1,2] These tumors occurred mainly in the muscles of the lower extremity and affected patients 50–70 years of age. They displayed a striking degree of cellular pleomorphism, but cells with cross-striations were absent in most instances. It was soon realized that most of these tumors were in fact other types of pleomorphic sarcoma. With the redefinition and acceptance of "malignant fibrous histiocytoma," most lesions that had formerly been labeled "pleomorphic rhabdomyosarcoma" were placed in the category of "malignant fibrous histiocytoma," such that the very existence of pleomorphic rhabdomyosarcoma was questioned.

It also became gradually evident that many childhood sarcomas formerly diagnosed merely as round cell or spindle cell sarcomas were rhabdomyosarcomas of alveolar or embryonal type. Knowledge of these tumors was fostered by the introduction of newer, more effective modes of therapy. Before 1960, childhood rhabdomyosarcoma was known as an almost uniformly fatal neoplasm that recurred and metastasized in a high percentage of cases. During the last four decades, however, it has been shown that this tumor responds well to multimodality therapy – encompassing biopsy or conservative surgery, multiagent chemotherapy, and radiotherapy – and that many children treated by these modalities remain free of recurrent and metastatic disease. The numerous reports of the Intergroup Rhabdomyosarcoma Studies (IRS) have greatly contributed to our understanding of childhood rhabdomyosarcomas and especially the effect of the various treatment modalities on the survival of patients with this tumor.[3–9]

As with other sarcomas, there is little to suggest that rhabdomyosarcoma arises from skeletal muscle cells. These tumors often arise at sites in which striated muscle tissue is normally absent (e.g., common bile duct, urinary bladder) or in areas in which striated muscle is scant (e.g., nasal cavity, middle ear, vagina).

Little is known about the underlying cause of the rhabdomyoblastic proliferations and the stimulus that induces such growth. Genetic factors are implicated by the rare occurrence of the disease in siblings,[10] the occasional presence of the tumor at birth,[11] and the association of the disease with other neoplasms in the same patient. Rhabdomyosarcoma has been described in conjunction with congenital retinoblastoma,[12,13] familial polyposis,[14] multiple lentigines syndrome,[15] type 1 neurofibromatosis,[16] Costello syndrome,[17] Beckwith-Wiedemann syndrome,[18] and a variety of congenital anomalies.[19,20] There appears to be an increased risk of a familial cancer syndrome when embryonal rhabdomyosarcoma (or other soft tissue sarcoma) is diagnosed during the first 2 years of life, especially in a male child.[21,22] Savasan et al. reported two children with alveolar rhabdomyosarcoma with constitutional balanced translocations, with peripheral blood lymphocytes harboring the same cytogenetic abnormality as that of the tumor cells.[23]

INCIDENCE

Rhabdomyosarcoma is not only the most common soft tissue sarcoma in children under 15 years of age but also one of the most common soft tissue sarcomas of adolescents and young adults. It is estimated that rhabdomyosarcoma accounts for about 8% of cancer in children, with an annual incidence of 6.4 cases per million neonates and infants each year and 4.5 cases per million children and adolescents each year.[24] It is rare in persons older than 45 years; it has been estimated to account for between 2% and 5% of all adult sarcomas.[25]

HISTOLOGIC CLASSIFICATION

Arthur Purdy Stout was the first to delineate rhabdomyosarcoma as a distinct entity,[2] and Horn and Enterline devised the first classification scheme in 1958 based on the clinical and pathologic features of these tumors.[26] This scheme, also known as the "conventional scheme," recognized embryonal, botryoid, alveolar, and pleomorphic subtypes. Most patients in that series died of rhabdomyosarcoma, and the authors were unable to identify any prognostic differences among the four histologic subtypes. This scheme was adopted by the World Health Organization (WHO) Classification of Soft Tissue Tumors and served as the basis for the numerous IRS studies to follow, with minor modifications (Table 21–1).[27]

Subsequently, Palmer et al. devised a new classification scheme based on tumor cytology rather than tumor architecture.[28,29] This scheme, known as the cytohistologic scheme, identified two major unfavorable histologic subtypes: the monomorphous round cell type and the anaplastic type. This was the only classification that was not based on the Horn and Enterline scheme but, rather, was devised solely on nuclear morphology.

In 1989, the International Society for Pediatric Oncology (SIOP), including collaborators from 30 European countries, developed a classification scheme that emphasized the relation between clinical behavior and cellular differentiation in rhabdomyosarcoma subtypes with and without alveolar morphology (Table 21–2).[30] Based on a review of 513 rhabdomyosarcomas from the SIOP tumor registry, they found that an alveolar architecture was not independently prognostically significant. Loose botryoid and dense well-differentiated rhabdomyosarcomas had a better prognosis than loose nonbotryoid and dense poorly differentiated and alveolar rhabdomyosarcomas. This group also delineated "embryonal sarcoma" as a spindle cell tumor composed of peripheral mesenchymal cells with no evidence of myoblastic differentiation.

In 1992, collaborators at the Pediatric Branch of the National Cancer Institute (NCI) developed a modification of the conventional scheme based on their review of 159 rhabdomyosarcomas (Table 21–3).[31] This scheme recognized the favorable prognosis of conventional embryonal rhabdomyosarcoma and three subtypes (pleomorphic, leiomyomatous, and those with aggressive histologic features) and the unfavorable prognosis of alveolar

TABLE 21–1	MODIFIED CONVENTIONAL (HORN AND ENTERLINE) CLASSIFICATION USED BY INTERGROUP RHABDOMYOSARCOMA STUDIES I AND II

Embryonal
Botryoid
Alveolar
Pleomorphic
Sarcoma, not classified
Small round-cell sarcoma, type indeterminate
Extraosseous Ewing's sarcoma

TABLE 21–2	INTERNATIONAL SOCIETY FOR PEDIATRIC ONCOLOGY CLASSIFICATION FOR RHABDOMYOSARCOMA

Embryonal sarcoma
Embryonal rhabdomyosarcoma
  Loose
    Botryoid
    Nonbotryoid
  Dense
    Well-differentiated
    Poorly differentiated
Alveolar rhabdomyosarcoma
Adult (pleomorphic) rhabdomyosarcoma
Other specified soft tissue tumors
Sarcoma, not otherwise specified

TABLE 21–3	NATIONAL CANCER INSTITUTE CLASSIFICATION OF RHABDOMYOSARCOMA

Embryonal rhabdomyosarcoma (favorable)
  Conventional
  Pleomorphic
  Leiomyomatous
  Aggressive histologic features
Alveolar rhabdomyosarcoma (unfavorable)
  Conventional
  Solid alveolar
Pleomorphic rhabdomyosarcoma
Rhabdomyosarcoma, "other"

rhabdomyosarcoma. It also delineated the "solid alveolar rhabdomyosarcoma," composed of round tumor cells identical to those in conventional alveolar rhabdomyosarcoma but lacking the characteristic alveolar architecture. These authors found that tumors with any degree of alveolar architecture or cytology had an unfavorable prognosis, regardless of extent.

From 1987 to 1991, the IRS committee conducted a comparative study of the various rhabdomyosarcoma classification systems to determine the reproducibility and prognostic significance of each of these systems.[32] Eight hundred representative rhabdomyosarcomas were reviewed by 16 pathologists and classified using the conventional, SIOP, NCI, and cytohistologic classification systems; survival rates for all subtypes were compared.

The highest degree of interobserver and intraobserver reproducibility was achieved using a modification of the conventional system, with fair to good observer agreement (Table 21–4). In addition, the histologic subtypes of the modified conventional system demonstrated a highly significant relation to survival. Based on the reproducibility and prognostic significance of this system, this group proposed a classification scheme, known as the International Classification of Rhabdomyosarcoma (ICR), which essentially was a modification of the conventional scheme with elements of the SIOP and NCI systems (Table 21–5).[33] The botryoid and spindle cell variants of embryonal rhabdomyosarcoma were found to have a superior prognosis, conventional embryonal rhabdomyosarcoma an intermediate prognosis, and alveolar rhabdomyosarcoma and undifferentiated sarcoma a poor prognosis. In addition, this classification scheme included those rhabdomyosarcoma subtypes in which the prognosis was yet to be determined (rhabdomyosarcoma with rhabdoid features). Similar to the NCI scheme, the ICR classified a tumor as the alveolar subtype if there was any degree of alveolar architecture or cytology. Pleomorphic rhabdomyosarcoma was excluded from the ICR given its extreme rarity in children. The classification has been recently modified to include the anaplastic variant of rhabdomyosarcoma.[34,35] Anaplasia is a histologic feature that may be found in any histologic subtype of rhabdomyosarcoma but is most common in embryonal rhabdomyosarcoma.[35]

AGE AND GENDER INCIDENCE

Despite the striking diversity in location, clinical presentation, and histologic picture, rhabdomyosarcoma has a fairly uniform age incidence; it occurs predominantly in infants and children and somewhat less frequently in adolescents and young adults. In the series of Ragab et al.,[36] 5% of 1561 patients with rhabdomyosarcomas were younger than 1 year of age. About 2% of tumors are present at birth.[37] Each of the rhabdomyosarcoma subtypes occurs in a characteristic age group. For example, embryonal rhabdomyosarcomas and the botryoid and spindle cell subtypes affect mainly, but not exclusively, children between birth and 15 years of age. On the other hand, alveolar rhabdomyosarcoma tends to affect older patients, with a peak age of 10–25 years. The median age of 440 patients with embryonal rhabdomyosarcomas diagnosed at the AFIP during a 10-year period was 8 years; the median age of 118 patients with alveolar rhabdomyosarcomas seen during the same period was 16 years (Fig. 21–1).

Rhabdomyosarcomas are uncommon in patients older than 40 years.[25,38,39] Rhabdomyosarcomas in adults are often of the pleomorphic subtype, with a reported median age range of 50–56 years, although embryonal and alveolar subtypes may also arise in adult patients.[25,40] There is some correlation between tumor location and age; for example, rhabdomyosarcomas of the urinary

TABLE 21–4	INTEROBSERVER AND INTRAOBSERVER VARIATION IN THE DIAGNOSIS OF RHABDOMYOSARCOMA SUBTYPES	
System	Interobserver average Kappa (K)	Intraobserver average Kappa (K)
Modified conventional	0.451	0.605
SIOP	0.406	0.573
NCI	0.384	0.579
Cytohistologic	0.328	0.508
ICR	0.525	0.625

Modified from Asmar L, Gehan EM, Newton WA Jr, et al. Agreement among and within groups of pathologists in the classification of rhabdomyosarcoma and related childhood sarcomas: report of an international study of four pathology classifications. Cancer 1994; 74:2579.
SIOP, International Society for Pediatric Oncology; NCI, National Cancer Institute; ICR, International Classification of Rhabdomyosarcoma.

TABLE 21–5	INTERNATIONAL CLASSIFICATION OF RHABDOMYOSARCOMA

Superior prognosis
  Botryoid rhabdomyosarcoma
  Spindle cell rhabdomyosarcoma
Intermediate prognosis
  Embryonal rhabdomyosarcoma
Poor prognosis
  Alveolar rhabdomyosarcoma
  Undifferentiated sarcoma
Subtypes whose prognosis is not presently evaluable
  Rhabdomyosarcoma with rhabdoid features

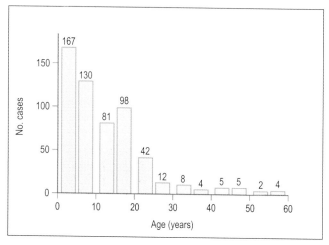

FIGURE 21–1 Age distribution of 558 rhabdomyosarcomas reviewed at the Armed Forces Institute of Pathology (AFIP) during a 10-year period. More than half of the cases occurred during the first 10 years of life, and most of these tumors were of the embryonal type. The second peak lies at 15–20 years of age, a result of the preponderance of alveolar rhabdomyosarcomas in this age group.

bladder, prostate, vagina, and middle ear tend to occur at a younger age (median: 4 years) than those in the paratesticular region (median: 14 years) or the extremities (median: 14 years). Each of the histologic subtypes of rhabdomyosarcoma occurs in a typical age group, and this will be further addressed later in this chapter.

Males are affected more commonly than females by a ratio of approximately 1.3:1.0, but the male predominance is less pronounced during adolescence and young adulthood and for rhabdomyosarcomas of the alveolar type. African-Americans seem to be less commonly affected than Caucasians.

CLINICAL FEATURES

Although rhabdomyosarcomas may arise anywhere in the body, they occur predominantly in three regions: the head and neck, genitourinary tract and retroperitoneum, and upper and lower extremities. Each rhabdomyosarcoma histologic subtype may occur in virtually any location, but each subtype has a site predilection, as will be discussed in the specific sections. Table 21–6 shows the anatomic distribution of rhabdomyosarcomas reviewed and diagnosed at the AFIP during a 10-year period. Table 21–7 shows the anatomic distribution of these tumors from the IRS-I, IRS-II, and IRS-III studies between 1972 and 1991.[4,7,8]

The head and neck is the principal location of rhabdomyosarcoma; 246 (44%) of 558 tumors diagnosed at the AFIP, and 970 (35%) of 2747 tumors from the IRS-I, IRS-II, and IRS-III studies occurred in this location. In the head and neck, parameningeal tumors are the most common, accounting for 16% of all tumors in the IRS

studies. Parameningeal rhabdomyosarcomas are distinguished from the other rhabdomyosarcomas arising in the head and neck because of their potential intracranial extension and seeding – hence their less favorable clinical course.[41,42]

The orbit is the second most common site of rhabdomyosarcoma in the head and neck, accounting for 9% of cases from the IRS series. Most rhabdomyosarcomas in this location are of the embryonal subtype.[43-45] For example, 221 (90%) of 245 orbital tumors from the IRS-I through IRS-IV studies were of the embryonal subtype, although rare botryoid-type embryonal rhabdomyosarcomas and alveolar rhabdomyosarcomas also arise in the orbit.[46]

Rhabdomyosarcoma may also involve a variety of other sites in the head and neck, including the nasal cavity and nasopharynx, followed in frequency by the ear and ear canal, paranasal sinuses, soft tissues of the face and neck, and the oral cavity including the tongue, lip, and palate.[47-49]

After the head and neck, the genitourinary tract is the second most common site for rhabdomyosarcoma.[50] In the IRS series, 650 (24%) of 2747 cases arose in this general region. Histologically, most tumors arising in this location are of the embryonal subtype. The tumors in this region most commonly arise in a paratesticular location and occur predominantly in adolescents. The spindle cell subtype of embryonal rhabdomyosarcoma has a propensity to arise in the paratesticular region.[51-53] They may also involve the spermatic cord and epididymis but usually are separate from the testis proper. There is a high incidence of retroperitoneal or para-aortic lymph node involvement.[54,55]

The retroperitoneum and pelvis are not uncommon sites of involvement. Approximately 45% of tumors in these sites are of the embryonal subtype, and up to 15% are alveolar rhabdomyosarcomas.[8,56,57] In general, effective therapy of rhabdomyosarcomas in the retroperitoneum and pelvic region is more difficult than that of paratesticular rhabdomyosarcomas.[58]

TABLE 21–6	ANATOMIC DISTRIBUTION OF RHABDOMYOSARCOMA (AFIP, 558 CASES)	
Anatomic location	**No.**	**%**
Head and neck	**246**	44.0
Orbit, eyelid, skull	109	19.5
Nasal cavity, nasopharynx, palate, mouth, pharynx	73	13.1
Sinuses, cheek, neck	47	8.4
Ear, mastoid	17	3.1
Trunk	**231**	41.4
Paratesticular region	114	20.4
Retroperitoneum, pelvis	46	8.2
Chest wall, back, flank, abdominal wall	41	7.3
Urinary bladder, prostate	25	4.5
Vagina, vulva	5	0.9
Extremities	**81**	14.6
Upper extremity	41	7.4
Lower extremity	40	7.2
Total	558	100.0

AFIP, Armed Forces Institute of Pathology.

TABLE 21–7	ANATOMIC DISTRIBUTION OF RHABDOMYOSARCOMA FROM INTERGROUP RHABDOMYOSARCOMA GROUP STUDIES (IRS-I, IRS-II, IRS-III), 1972–1991	
Anatomic location	**No.**	**%**
Head and neck	970	35
Parameningeal	437	16
Miscellaneous sites	276	10
Orbit	257	9
Genitourinary	650	24
Extremities	511	19
Other sites	616	22
Total	2747	100

Modified from Pappo AS, Shapiro DN, Crist WM, et al. Biology and therapy of pediatric rhabdomyosarcoma. J Clin Oncol 1995; 13:2123.

Approximately 5% of rhabdomyosarcomas arise in the urinary bladder or prostate. In fact, rhabdomyosarcoma is the most common bladder tumor in children under 10 years of age. Almost all tumors arising in this location are embryonal or botryoid rhabdomyosarcomas.[59-62] Those with a botryoid histology typically grow into the lumen of the urinary bladder as a grape-like, richly mucoid, multinodular or polypoid mass with a broad base that not infrequently causes obstruction of the internal urethral orifice and prostatic urethra. This in turn results in incontinence and difficulty with urination. Rarely, rhabdomyosarcomas arise in other genitourinary sites, including the fallopian tube,[63] uterus,[64] cervix,[10] vagina,[65] labium and vulva,[66] and the perineum and perianal region.[67] Tumors in these locations are often (but not always) of the botryoid subtype. Rhabdomyosarcomas which arise in gynecologic organs in adults are morphologically similar to those arising in pediatric patients, but they seem to behave more aggressively.[67a]

Unlike adult soft tissue sarcomas, rhabdomyosarcomas involve the extremities much less commonly. As shown in Table 21-6, only 14.6% of cases from the AFIP series occurred in this location, with a similar incidence in the upper and lower extremities; alveolar rhabdomyosarcomas outnumbered embryonal rhabdomyosarcomas by a ratio of 4:3, similar to that found in the IRS-I and IRS-II studies.[8] Although rare, most pleomorphic rhabdomyosarcomas arise in the deep soft tissues of the extremities of adults.

Unusual rhabdomyosarcomas arise outside the head and neck, the genitourinary tract and retroperitoneum, and extremities. Tumors originating in the hepatobiliary tract have been described and usually arise from the submucosa of the common bile duct.[68,69] Most are botryoid type with typical myxoid grape-like gross and microscopic appearances.

GROSS FINDINGS

Macroscopically, there is little that is characteristic of this tumor; as with other rapidly growing sarcomas, the gross appearance reflects the degree of cellularity, the relative amounts of collagenous or myxoid stroma, and the presence and extent of secondary changes such as hemorrhage, necrosis, and ulceration. In general, tumors growing into body cavities, such as those in the nasopharynx and urinary bladder, are fairly well circumscribed, multinodular, or distinctly polypoid with a glistening, gelatinous, gray-white surface that on cross-section often shows patchy areas of hemorrhage or cyst formation. Deep-seated tumors involving or arising in the musculature are usually less well defined and nearly always infiltrate the surrounding tissues. They are more firm and rubbery and have a mottled gray-white to pink-tan, smooth or finely granular, often bulging surface. They rarely become large, averaging 3–4 cm in greatest diameter. There are often areas of focal necrosis and cystic degeneration.

RHABDOMYOSARCOMA SUBTYPES

Embryonal rhabdomyosarcoma

Embryonal rhabdomyosarcoma (without other distinguishing features) accounts for approximately 49% of all rhabdomyosarcomas.[33] It mostly affects children younger than 10 years of age (mean age: near 7 years), but it also occurs in adolescents and young adults; it is uncommon in patients older than 40 years of age. The most common site of embryonal rhabdomyosarcoma is the head and neck, particularly the orbit and parameninges (Table 21-8). After the head and neck, this tumor is most commonly found in the genitourinary tract, followed by the deep soft tissues of the extremities and the pelvis and retroperitoneum.

Histologically, embryonal rhabdomyosarcoma bears a close resemblance to various stages in the embryogenesis of normal skeletal muscle, but its pattern is much more variable, ranging from poorly differentiated tumors that are difficult to diagnose without immunohistochemical or electron microscopic examination to well-differentiated neoplasms that resemble fetal muscle. Features common to most are: (1) varying degrees of

TABLE 21–8	**DISTRIBUTION OF ANATOMIC SITES OF RHABDOMYOSARCOMA SUBTYPES FOR 1626 IRS-I AND IRS-II PATIENTS**					
Site	Embryonal	Alveolar	Botryoid	Pleomorphic	Other	Total no.
Head and neck	411 (71%)	76 (13%)	13 (2%)		77 (13%)	577
Genitourinary	246 (71%)	8 (2%)	70 (20%)	1 (<1%)	23 (7%)	348
Extremities	76 (24%)	156 (50%)		5 (2%)	74 (24%)	311
Trunk	27 (19%)	43 (30%)		3 (2%)	71 (49%)	144
Pelvis	45 (48%)	19 (20%)			29 (31%)	93
Retroperitoneum	44 (59%)	14 (19%)		1 (1%)	16 (21%)	75
Perineum/anus	13 (33%)	19 (48%)	1 (2%)	1 (2%)	6 (15%)	40
Other sites	15 (39%)	9 (24%)	4 (11%)		10 (26%)	38

Modified from Newton WA Jr, Soule EH, Hamoudi AB, et al. Histopathology of childhood sarcomas, Intergroup Rhabdomyosarcoma Studies I and II: clinicopathologic correlation. J Clin Oncol 1988; 6:67.

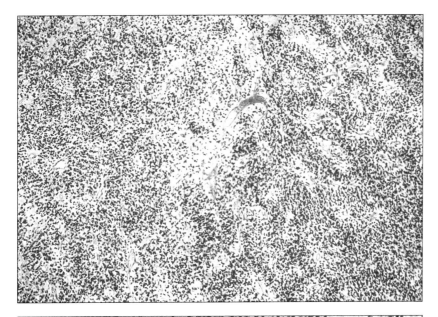

FIGURE 21–2 Low-power view of embryonal rhabdomyosarcoma with alternating cellular and myxoid areas, a characteristic feature of this tumor.

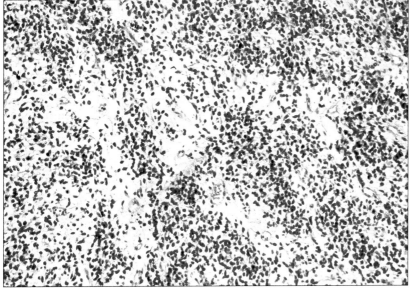

FIGURE 21–3 Alternating cellular and myxoid zones in an embryonal rhabdomyosarcoma.

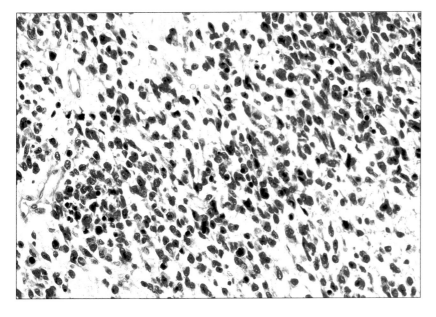

FIGURE 21–4 High-power view of an embryonal rhabdomyosarcoma composed predominantly of primitive ovoid cells.

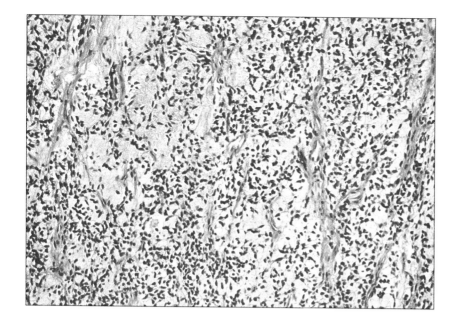

FIGURE 21–5 Primitive spindle-shaped cells deposited in an abundant myxoid stroma in an embryonal rhabdomyosarcoma.

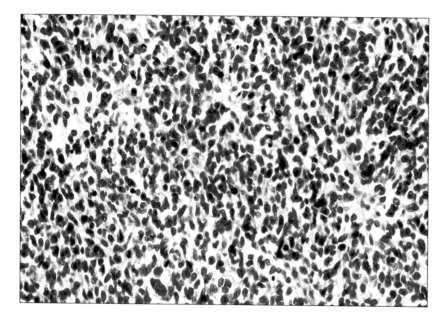

FIGURE 21–6 Embryonal rhabdomyosarcoma composed almost exclusively of primitive cells devoid of rhabdomyoblastic differentiation.

cellularity with alternating densely packed, hypercellular areas and loosely textured myxoid areas (Figs 21–2 to 21–5); (2) a mixture of poorly oriented, small, undifferentiated, hyperchromatic round or spindle-shaped cells (Fig. 21–6) and a varying number of differentiated cells with eosinophilic cytoplasm characteristic of rhabdomyoblasts; and (3) a matrix containing little collagen and varying amounts of myxoid material. Cross-striations are discernible in 50–60% of cases.

The least well-differentiated examples of this tumor correspond in appearance to developing muscle at 5–8 weeks' gestation. They consist for the most part of small, round or spindle-shaped cells with darkly staining hyperchromatic nuclei and indistinct cytoplasm. The nuclei vary slightly in size and shape (more so than those of alveolar rhabdomyosarcoma), have one or two small nucleoli, and usually exhibit a high rate of mitotic activity. Differentiated rhabdomyoblasts are either absent entirely or are confined to a few small areas, making it mandatory to examine multiple sections from different portions of the tumor; adjunctive diagnostic procedures are required to confirm the diagnosis in virtually all cases.

Better-differentiated examples have, in addition to the primitive or undifferentiated cellular areas, larger round or oval eosinophilic cells characteristic of rhabdomyoblasts (Figs 21–7 to 21–9); the cytoplasm of these cells contains granular material or deeply eosinophilic masses of stringy or fibrillary material concentrically arranged near or around the nucleus. Cross-striations are rare in the round cells, and if present they are usually confined to narrow bundles of concentrically arranged

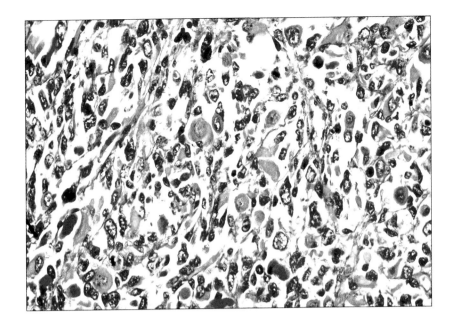

FIGURE 21-7 Embryonal rhabdomyosarcoma. Note the scattered cells with eosinophilic cytoplasm.

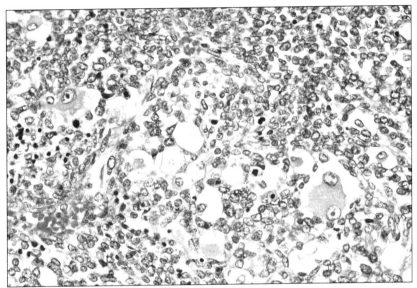

FIGURE 21-8 Embryonal rhabdomyosarcoma composed predominantly of primitive ovoid cells with scattered rhabdomyoblasts. The rhabdomyoblasts in this case have eccentric vesicular nuclei and abundant densely eosinophilic cytoplasm.

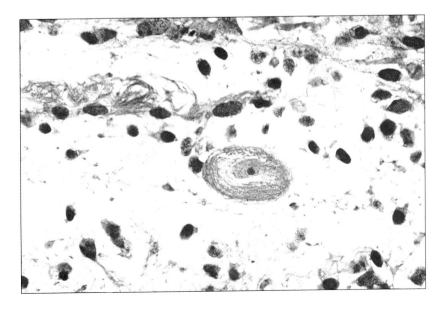

FIGURE 21-9 Characteristic rhabdomyoblast in an embryonal rhabdomyosarcoma. Deeply eosinophilic fibrillar material is concentrically arranged around the nucleus.

myofibrils at the circumference of the rhabdomyoblast. Degenerated rhabdomyoblasts with a glassy or hyalinized deeply eosinophilic cytoplasm and pyknotic nuclei but without cross-striations are a frequent feature of this tumor.

Cross-striations are more readily discernible in embryonal rhabdomyosarcomas with a more prominent spindle cell component (Figs 21–10, 21–11), tumors that might be regarded as the morphologic equivalent of normal muscle at 9–15 weeks of intrauterine development; these neoplasms are composed mainly of a mixture of undifferentiated cells and differentiated fusiform or elongated cells that are readily identifiable as rhabdomyoblasts by light microscopy. The rhabdomyoblasts range from slender spindle-shaped cells with a small number of peripherally placed myofibrils to large eosinophilic cells with a strap, ribbon, tadpole, or racquet shape and one or two centrally positioned nuclei and prominent nucle-

oli, with or without cross-striations. Cross-striations in neoplastic cells differ from those in residual or entrapped muscle cells by their more irregular distribution and the fact that they often traverse only part of the tumor cell. Intracellular granules may be confused with cross-striations, but their granular nature is readily apparent after careful examination of the cell under oil immersion. Sometimes, the strap-shaped cells are sharply angulated and form a diagnostically useful "zigzag," or "broken straw," pattern. Most of these tumors have only a moderate degree of cellular pleomorphism.

Embryonal rhabdomyosarcomas with a prominent degree of cellular pleomorphism ("anaplasia") are rare and, in some cases, are difficult to distinguish from adult pleomorphic rhabdomyosarcomas (Fig. 21–12), except for the more frequent occurrence of cross-striations in childhood tumors and the identification of areas of more typical embryonal rhabdomyosarcoma.

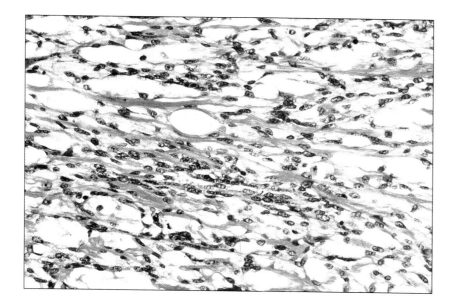

FIGURE 21–10 Embryonal rhabdomyosarcoma composed predominantly of atypical spindle-shaped cells with scattered elongated rhabdomyoblasts.

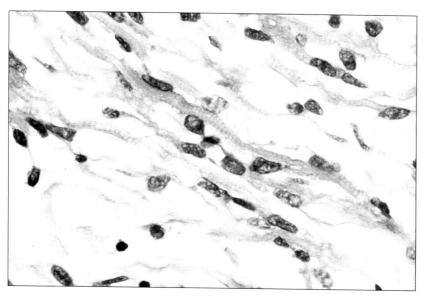

FIGURE 21–11 High-power view of elongated rhabdomyoblasts with distinct cross-striations in an embryonal rhabdomyosarcoma.

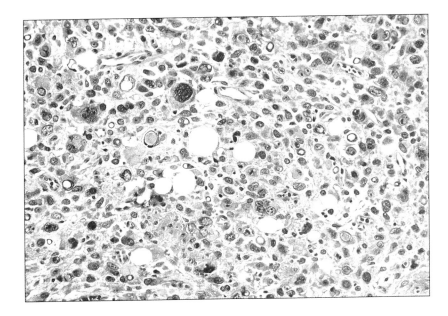

FIGURE 21-12 Embryonal rhabdomyosarcoma with anaplastic features arising in a 3-year-old child.

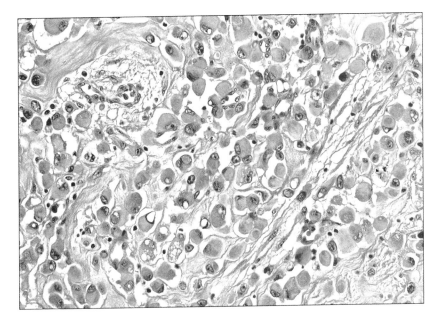

FIGURE 21-13 Embryonal rhabdomyosarcoma consisting almost entirely of differentiated rhabdomyoblasts, a feature occasionally encountered in recurrent tumors following therapy.

According to Kodet et al.,[70] survival in patients with diffuse anaplasia in embryonal rhabdomyosarcoma is similar to the unfavorable survival of patients with alveolar rhabdomyosarcoma.

There are also extremely well-differentiated embryonal rhabdomyosarcomas that consist almost entirely of well-differentiated rounded, spindle-shaped, or polygonal rhabdomyoblasts with abundant eosinophilic cytoplasm and frequent cross-striations. Some of these differentiated tumors are found in recurrent or metastatic neoplasms after prolonged therapy (Fig. 21–13), possibly due to the "selective destruction of undifferentiated tumor cells."[71,72]

Glycogen is demonstrable in most rhabdomyosarcomas regardless of type; when the glycogen is removed during fixation, multivacuolated cells or "spider cells"

result, which are large multivacuolated rhabdomyoblasts with narrow strands of cytoplasm connecting the center of the cell with its periphery. The centrally located nuclei and the irregular shape of the cytoplasmic vacuoles help distinguish these cells from the more rounded lipid-filled vacuoles of lipoblasts. In contrast to alveolar rhabdomyosarcoma, multinucleated giant cells are rare in embryonal rhabdomyosarcomas.

Occasionally, the embryonal rhabdomyosarcoma displays, in addition to its rhabdomyoblastic component, foci of immature cartilaginous (Fig. 21–14) or osseous tissue, or both. These tumors occur at any age and any location but seem to be more common in the genitourinary tract and the retroperitoneum. Daya and Scully[73] observed cartilaginous differentiation in 45% of rhabdomyosarcomas of the uterine cervix.

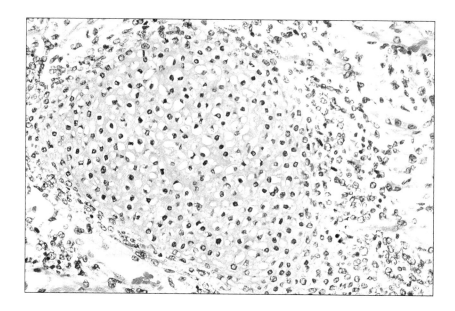

FIGURE 21-14 Embryonal rhabdomyosarcoma with foci of immature cartilage.

Cytogenetic findings

The cytogenetic abnormalities of embryonal and alveolar rhabdomyosarcomas are distinct. Embryonal rhabdomyosarcoma is characterized by a consistent loss of heterozygosity (LOH) for multiple closely linked loci at chromosome 11p15.5.[74] This loss of heterozygosity may result in activation of a tumor suppressor gene or genes, including the human tyrosine hydroxylase gene,[75] or GOK.[76] Others have reported trisomy 8 as a consistent finding in embryonal rhabdomyosarcomas.[77]

Embryonal rhabdomyosarcoma, spindle cell type

In 1992, Cavazzana et al. reported 21 embryonal rhabdomyosarcomas composed predominantly (>80%) of elongated spindle cells mimicking fetal myotubes at a late stage of cellular differentiation.[51] In this study, there was a striking predilection for this tumor to arise in males, particularly in a paratesticular location. By immunohistochemistry and electron microscopy, the cells showed a high degree of skeletal muscle differentiation. The authors coined the term *spindle cell rhabdomyosarcoma* to distinguish this entity from the usual embryonal rhabdomyosarcoma because of its more favorable clinical course. Subsequent studies have confirmed the distinctive clinical and pathologic features of this rhabdomyosarcoma subtype.[52,78,79]

Spindle cell rhabdomyosarcoma is a rare subtype of rhabdomyosarcoma, accounting for 21 (4.4%) of 471 rhabdomyosarcomas retrieved from the files of the German-Italian Cooperative Soft Tissue Sarcomas Study Group.[51] Of 800 randomly selected rhabdomyosarcomas from the IRS, this variant accounted for 3% of all rhabdomyosarcomas.[33] Like other forms of embryonal rhabdomyosarcoma, the spindle cell type tends to arise in young patients (mean age: approximately 7 years), but

TABLE 21-9	ANATOMIC DISTRIBUTION OF SPINDLE CELL RHABDOMYOSARCOMAS	
Anatomic location	**No.**	**%**
Paratesticular	30	38
Head and neck	21	27
Extremities	8	10
Genitourinary	8	10
Other	11	15
Total	78	100

Data are from references 51 and 52.

rare cases have been described in adults.[78,80,80a] There appears to be a striking male predilection with males being affected about six times more commonly than females. The most common site of involvement is the paratesticular soft tissue (38%), followed by the head and neck (27%) (Table 21-9), but rare examples have also been described in the urinary bladder, abdomen, retroperitoneum, and soft tissues of the extremities.

Histologically, the tumor is composed almost exclusively of elongated fusiform cells with cigar-shaped nuclei and prominent nucleoli (Figs 21-15 to 21-17). The tumor cells have eosinophilic fibrillar cytoplasm with distinct cellular borders, closely resembling late-stage fetal myoblasts. Cytoplasmic cross-striations may be observed. The collagen-rich form is characterized by spindle cells separated by abundant collagen fibers arranged in a storiform or whorled growth pattern. The collagen-poor form is a more cellular proliferation of cells arranged in bundles or fascicles, reminiscent of leiomyosarcoma.

Immunohistochemically, the tumor cells consistently express myogenic antigens, including muscle-specific actin and desmin. However, this rhabdomyosarcoma subtype more consistently expresses myogenic antigens

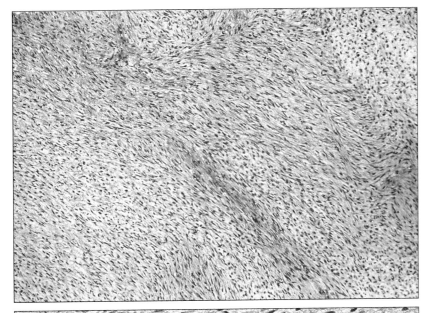

FIGURE 21–15 Low-power view of spindle cell type of embryonal rhabdomyosarcoma arising in the urinary bladder.

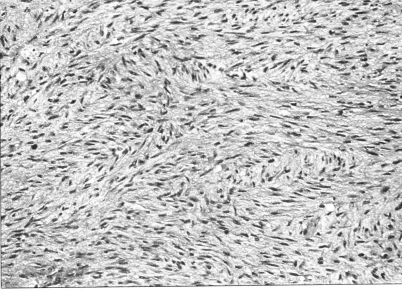

FIGURE 21–16 Spindle cell type of embryonal rhabdomyosarcoma composed of relatively uniform spindle-shaped cells deposited in a myxoid stroma. Cells are arranged in an irregular fascicular pattern reminiscent of leiomyosarcoma.

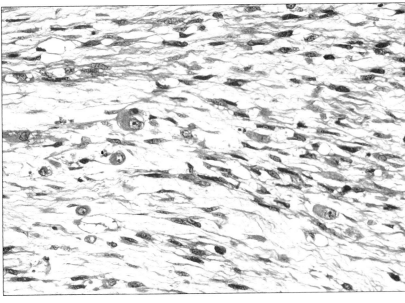

FIGURE 21–17 Scattered rhabdomyoblasts are apparent in this spindle cell type of embryonal rhabdomyosarcoma.

which are generally expressed at a late stage of myogenesis (titin and troponin D), supporting a greater degree of differentiation of these spindle-shaped cells.[51,81]

Few cases of spindle cell rhabdomyosarcoma have been evaluated by cytogenetics. Debiec-Rychter and colleagues described one case arising in the cheek of an 18-year-old girl with a der (2)t(2;7), with apparent involvement of 2q36–37.[82] Gil-Benso et al. reported a case with structural rearrangements of chromosomes 8, 12, 21, and 22.[83]

Embryonal rhabdomyosarcoma, botryoid type

Botryoid rhabdomyosarcoma accounts for approximately 6% of all rhabdomyosarcomas.[33] The word *botryoid* is derived from the Greek word for grapes; this variant is characterized grossly by its polypoid (grape-like) growth and microscopically by its relative sparsity of cells and abundance of mucoid stroma, often resulting in a myxoma-like picture. Most botryoid rhabdomyosarcomas are found in mucosa-lined hollow organs, such as the nasal cavity, nasopharynx, bile duct, urinary bladder, and vagina (Fig. 21–18; Table 21–8); tumors of this type may also be encountered in areas where the expanding neoplasm reaches the body surface, as in some rhabdomyosarcomas of the eyelid or the anal region. Obviously, its unrestricted growth in body cavities or on body surfaces accounts for its characteristic edematous and grape-like appearance.

Although a grape-like configuration has traditionally been a defining feature of the botryoid variant, the ICR scheme does not require this characteristic gross appearance.[33] According to the ICR criteria, a "cambium layer," characterized by a subepithelial condensation of tumor cells separated from an intact surface epithelium by a zone of loose stroma, must be present to recognize this

variant (Figs 21–19 to 21–21). The tumor cells should form a distinct zone that is several layers thick, although the thickness of this layer may vary in extent in different areas of the tumor. The cells range from primitive small cells to cells with clear-cut myoblastic differentiation (Fig. 21–22). Cells with stellate cytoplasmic processes are often prominent. The stroma is typically loosely cellular with a myxoid appearance, including a hypocellular zone that separates the surface epithelium from the underlying cambium layer. The surface epithelium may be hyperplastic or may undergo squamous changes, sometimes mimicking a carcinoma.

Immunohistochemically, there is usually strong staining for myogenic antigens, particularly in cells showing light microscopic evidence of myoblastic differentiation. By cytogenetics, Palazzo et al. reported deletion of the short arm of chromosome 1 and trisomies

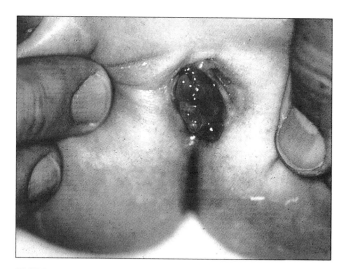

FIGURE 21–18 Botryoid-type embryonal rhabdomyosarcoma of the vagina.

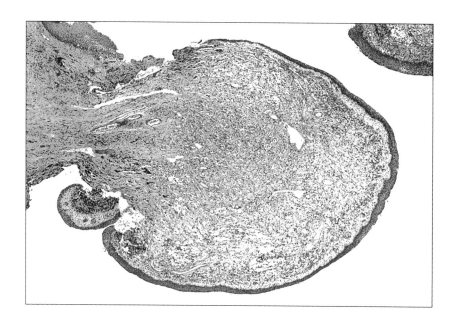

FIGURE 21–19 Polypoid fragment lined by squamous mucosa in a botryoid-type embryonal rhabdomyosarcoma of the vagina.

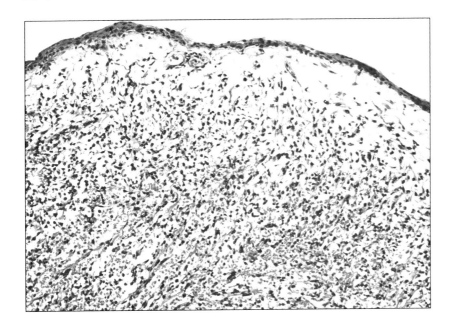

FIGURE 21–20 Botryoid-type embryonal rhabdomyosarcoma with the characteristic "cambium" layer, a submucosal zone of markedly increased cellularity.

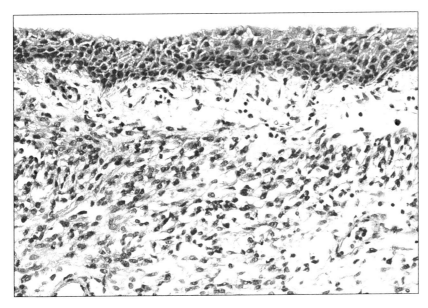

FIGURE 21–21 Primitive spindle-shaped and ovoid cells in the cambium layer of this botryoid-type embryonal rhabdomyosarcoma.

of chromosomes 13 and 18.[84] A second reported case showed a hyperdiploid clone with a complex karyotype, including numerous chromosomal gains.[85]

Alveolar rhabdomyosarcoma

Alveolar rhabdomyosarcoma is the second most common subtype, accounting for approximately 31% of all rhabdomyosarcomas.[33] This variant tends to arise at a slightly older age than embryonal, botryoid, and spindle cell rhabdomyosarcomas, with a peak incidence at 10–25 years of age. It has a predilection for the deep soft tissues of the extremities, although the tumor may arise in many other sites, including the head and neck, trunk, perineum, pelvis, and retroperitoneum (Table 21–8).

Histologically, alveolar rhabdomyosarcoma is composed largely of ill-defined aggregates of poorly differentiated round or oval tumor cells that frequently show central loss of cellular cohesion and formation of irregular "alveolar" spaces (Figs 21–23 to 21–25). The individual cellular aggregates are separated and surrounded by a framework of dense, frequently hyalinized fibrous septa that surround dilated vascular channels. Characteristically, the cells at the periphery of the alveolar spaces are well preserved and adhere in a single layer to the fibrous septa in a manner somewhat reminiscent of an adenocarcinoma or papillary carcinoma. The cells in the center of the alveolar spaces tend to be more loosely arranged, or "freely floating" (Figs 21–25, 21–26); they are often poorly preserved and show evidence of degeneration and

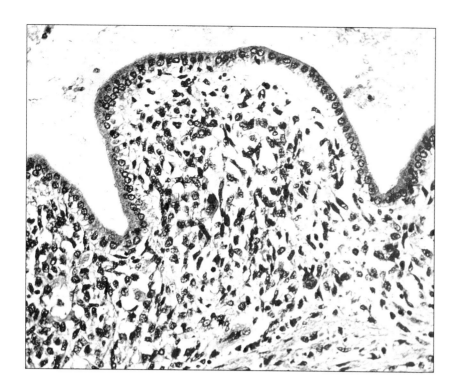

FIGURE 21–22 Embryonal rhabdomyosarcoma of the biliary tract with botryoid features. Scattered rhabdomyoblasts are apparent.

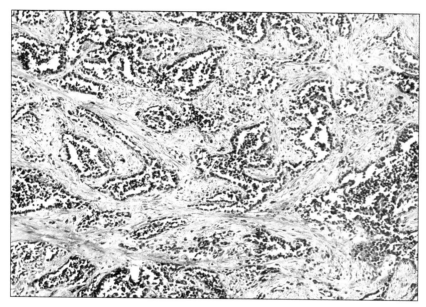

FIGURE 21–23 Alveolar rhabdomyosarcoma with the characteristic "alveolar" growth pattern.

necrosis. In rare instances viable cells are virtually absent, and the tumor consists merely of a coarse sieve-like or honeycomb-like meshwork of thick fibrous trabeculae surrounding small, loosely textured groups of severely degenerated cells with pyknotic nuclei and necrotic cellular debris.[27]

There are also "solid" forms of this tumor that lack an alveolar pattern entirely and are composed of densely packed groups or masses of tumor cells resembling the round cell areas of embryonal rhabdomyosarcoma but with a more uniform cellular picture with little or no fibrosis (Fig. 21–27).[31] These solidly cellular areas are more commonly encountered at the periphery of the tumor and probably represent the most active and most cellular stage of growth. It is important not to confuse the solid form of alveolar rhabdomyosarcoma with the undifferentiated form of embryonal rhabdomyosarcoma, as the former carries a less favorable prognosis. This distinction may be difficult; in most cases, examination of the solid tumor shows, in addition to the uniform cellular pattern, incipient alveolar features. Even in the solid areas there is a regular arrangement of fibrous septa that surround the primitive round cells. As discussed below, cytogenetic/molecular studies may aid in this distinction.

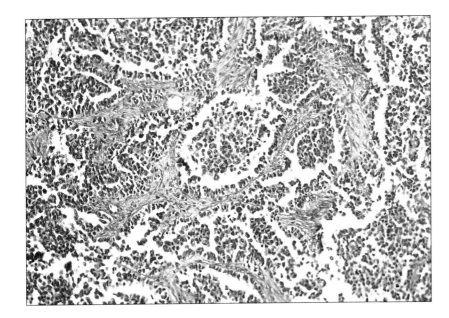

FIGURE 21–24 Alveolar rhabdomyosarcoma. A single layer of neoplastic cells adheres to dense fibrous septa with central loss of cellular cohesion.

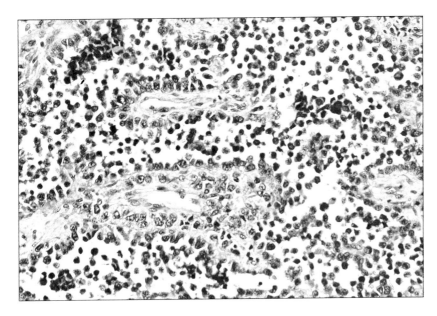

FIGURE 21–25 High-power view of alveolar rhabdomyosarcoma. Fibrovascular septa are lined by a single layer of round cells. There is loss of cellular cohesion and individual tumor cell necrosis between the fibrous septa.

There are also rare cases in which the cells have abundant pale-staining, glycogen-containing cytoplasm and vaguely resemble clear cell carcinoma or clear cell malignant melanoma (*clear cell rhabdomyosarcoma*).[86,87]

The individual cells in both alveolar and solid portions of the tumor have round or oval hyperchromatic nuclei with scant amounts of indistinct cytoplasm. Bulbous or club-shaped cells, sometimes with deeply eosinophilic cytoplasm, are often seen protruding from the fibrous walls into the lumen of the alveolar spaces. Mitotic figures are common. Neoplastic rhabdomyoblasts with pronounced stringy or granular eosinophilic cytoplasm are less common in alveolar than in embryonal rhabdomyosarcomas and are present in no more than about 30% of cases. Most of the rhabdomyoblasts in the alveolar spaces have a round or oval configuration (Fig. 21–28); those located in or attached to the fibrous septa tend to be strap-shaped or spindle-shaped. If cross-striations are present, they are almost exclusively found in the spindle-shaped cells.

Multinucleated giant cells are a prominent and diagnostically important feature (Figs 21–29, 21–30). Usually, the giant cells have multiple, peripherally placed nuclei and pale-staining or weakly eosinophilic cytoplasm, without cross-striations. Transitional forms between rhabdomyoblasts and giant cells suggest that the latter are formed by cellular fusion. Collagen formation is usually confined to the intervening septa, but occasionally large portions of the tumor are obliterated by extensive fibroplasia. As already mentioned, mixed types with embryonal and alveolar features should be classified as alveolar rhabdomyosarcomas.[33]

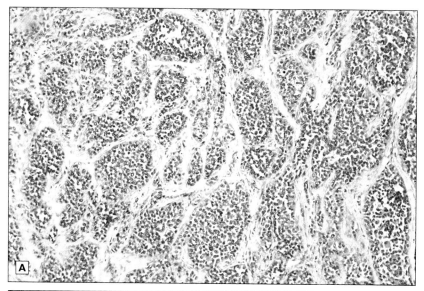

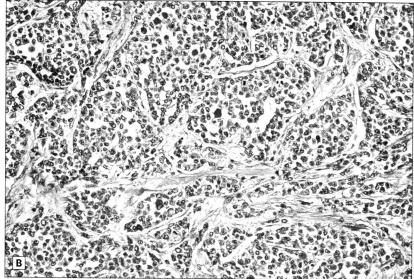

FIGURE 21–26 (A) Low-power view of alveolar rhabdomyosarcoma with incipient loss of cellular cohesion in cellular nests. **(B)** Masson trichrome-stained section of an alveolar rhabdomyosarcoma accentuating fibrous trabeculae between cellular nests.

Most alveolar rhabdomyosarcomas originate in muscle tissue, and entrapment of normal muscle fibers is common. These fibers are apt to be mistaken for neoplastic rhabdomyoblasts with cross-striations, a feature that sometimes results in the correct diagnosis for the wrong reason.

Metastatic alveolar rhabdomyosarcomas in lymph nodes, lung, and other viscera also display a distinct alveolar pattern (Fig. 21–31), making it unlikely that this pattern is merely the result of infiltrative growth along the fibrous framework of the involved musculature. Diffuse bone marrow metastases may be mistaken for leukemia.[88]

The immune profile of alveolar rhabdomyosarcoma is similar to that for other rhabdomyosarcomas. Because the differential diagnosis includes numerous other "small round cell tumors," a large battery of immunostains is often required to exclude other entities, as discussed below.

Alveolar rhabdomyosarcoma is characterized by distinctive cytogenetic abnormalities that allow its distinction from other rhabdomyosarcoma subtypes and other round cell neoplasms in the differential diagnosis. Most of these tumors have a t(2;13)(q35;q14) translocation,[89,90] which results in the generation of two derivative chromosomes: a shortened chromosome 13 and an elongated chromosome 2. The breakpoints occur within the *PAX3* gene on chromosome 2 and the *FKHR* gene (also known as *FOXO1a*) on chromosome 13,[91] resulting in a *PAX3-FKHR* fusion gene on chromosome 13 and a *FKHR-PAX3* fusion gene on chromosome 2. Both of these genes encode transcription factors that regulate the expression of specific target genes. The chimeric gene that results from this translocation encodes for a chimeric protein that acts as an aberrant transcription factor that excessively activates expression of genes with *PAX3* binding sites.[92,93] The *PAX3-FKHR* fusion appears to be more sensitive

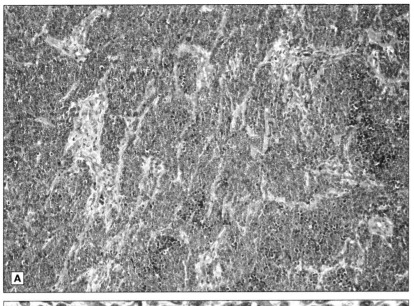

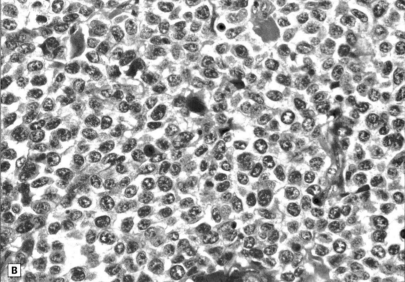

FIGURE 21–27 **(A)** Low-power view of a solid variant of alveolar rhabdomyosarcoma. Although the characteristic alveolar structures are not present, cellular nests are still separated by fibrovascular septa, characteristic of this tumor. **(B)** High-power view of a solid variant of alveolar rhabdomyosarcoma. The cytologic features are identical to those of the usual type of alveolar rhabdomyosarcoma. Cells are round with large nuclei and little cytoplasm.

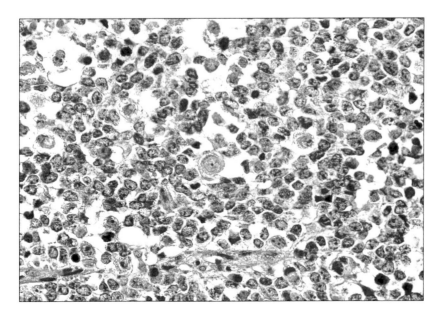

FIGURE 21–28 High-power view of an alveolar rhabdomyosarcoma with rare rhabdomyoblasts.

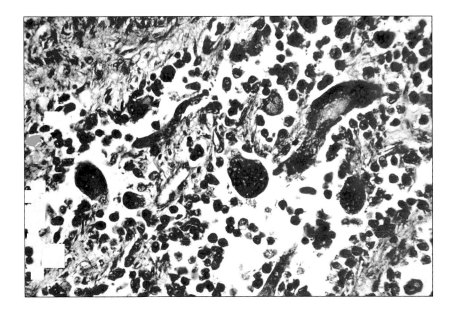

FIGURE 21–29 Multinucleated giant cells in an alveolar rhabdomyosarcoma.

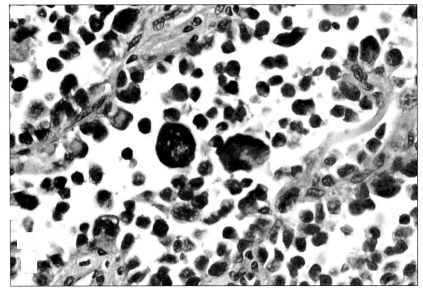

FIGURE 21–30 Alveolar rhabdomyosarcoma with multinucleated giant cells. These cells have peripherally placed "wreath-like" nuclei and are usually free-floating in alveolar structures.

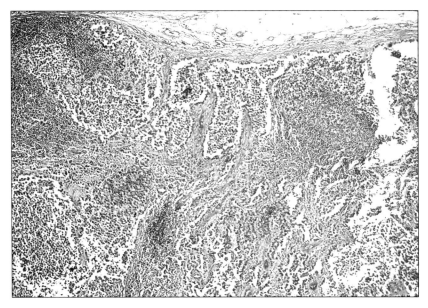

FIGURE 21–31 Metastatic alveolar rhabdomyosarcoma to a lymph node. The alveolar pattern is present in the metastasis as well.

and specific than the *FKHR-PAX3* fusion in detecting this tumor.[94]

A subset of alveolar rhabdomyosarcomas is associated with a variant translocation, t(1;13)(p36;q14), which juxtaposes the *PAX7* gene on 1p36 with the *FKHR* gene on 13q14.[95,96] There is a high degree of homology between *PAX3* and *PAX7*, and it is likely that the fusion proteins that result from the translocations involving these genes aberrantly regulate a common set of target genes involved in the pathogenesis of alveolar rhabdomyosarcoma.

In addition to cytogenetic examination, these molecular abnormalities can be detected by reverse transcriptase-polymerase chain reaction (RT-PCR) or fluorescence in situ hybridization (FISH) using either frozen or paraffin-embedded tissues. Recently, Barr and colleagues evaluated 78 formalin-fixed, paraffin-embedded alveolar rhabdomyosarcomas derived from the IRS-III clinical trial by RT-PCR.[97] Satisfactory results were obtained in 59 (76%) samples. Thirty-five cases (59%) had a *PAX3-FKHR* fusion, 11 (19%) had a *PAX7-FKHR* fusion, and 13 (22%) cases were fusion-negative. Nishio et al. analyzed 75 paraffin-embedded specimens by FISH and RT-PCR, including 40 alveolar rhabdomyosarcomas, 16 embryonal rhabdomyosarcomas, 8 mixed embryonal/alveolar tumors and 11 non-rhabdomyosarcomas.[98] *PAX-FKHR* classification results were concordant using these two techniques in 53 of 56 (94.6%) cases. The authors also utilized probes for *PAX3* and *PAX7* and demonstrated a high degree of sensitivity and specificity when comparing FISH results to RT-PCR and conventional karyotyping. Overall, about 80% of tumors diagnosed histologically as alveolar rhabdomyosarcoma are found to have the *PAX3-FKHR* or *PAX7-FKHR* fusions (Table 21–10). Solid variants of alveolar rhabdomyosarcoma seem to be more likely than non-solid types to be fusion negative.[98a] Kelly et al. found that tumors with the *PAX7-FKHR* fusion tend to arise in younger patients, more often arise in the extremities, are usually localized, and are associated with significantly longer event-free survival (discussed later in this chapter).[99] There appears to be a significant genetic heterogeneity among the fusion-negative alveolar rhabdomyosarcomas. Closer evaluation of such cases by Barr et al. revealed low expression of standard fusions or variant fusions in some cases, but over 50% of these were found to be truly fusion-negative.[100]

Pleomorphic rhabdomyosarcoma

Pleomorphic rhabdomyosarcoma is a rare variant of rhabdomyosarcoma that almost always arises in adults older than 45 years of age.[101-103] Given its extreme rarity in children,[104] this subtype was not included in the ICR. The concept of pleomorphic rhabdomyosarcoma has changed considerably since its inclusion in the Horn and Enterline classification scheme reported in 1958.[26] One-third of the 39 tumors in their study were designated pleomorphic rhabdomyosarcomas, most of which arose in the deep soft tissues of the extremities of adults. Studies published in the 1960s described the clinical and pathologic features of pleomorphic rhabdomyosarcoma,[105,106] and this tumor was reported to account for between 9% and 14% of all soft tissue sarcomas.[1] However, with the emergence of the concept of malignant fibrous histiocytoma (MFH), many pleomorphic rhabdomyosarcomas were subsequently reclassified as storiform-pleomorphic variants of MFH,[107] and as such, pleomorphic rhabdomyosarcoma became regarded as rare[108] or nonexistent.[109] Subsequently, with the advent of immunohistochemistry and refinement in recognizing tumors with skeletal muscle differentiation, studies confirmed the existence of pleomorphic rhabdomyosarcoma and delineated criteria by which this sarcoma could be distinguished from other pleomorphic sarcomas.[102,110,111]

Most of these tumors arise in adults with a peak incidence in the fifth decade of life. The youngest patient in the study by Gaffney et al. was 27 years of age;[102] Hollowood and Fletcher recorded encountering this tumor in a 13-year-old.[103] Most series have shown a predilection for this tumor to arise in males. In the study of 38 cases of pleomorphic rhabdomyosarcoma culled from the AFIP, 28 arose in males.[101] The tumor most commonly arises in the skeletal muscle of the extremities, particularly the thigh. Less commonly, these tumors arise in the abdomen/retroperitoneum, chest/abdominal wall, spermatic cord/testes, and upper extremities.[101] Most present with a rapidly growing, painless mass of several months' duration; some present with pulmonary metastases.[103]

TABLE 21–10	FREQUENCY OF *PAX3-FKHR* AND *PAX7-FKHR* FUSION TRANSCRIPTS IN ALVEOLAR AND EMBRYONAL RHABDOMYOSARCOMAS			
	Alveolar		**Embryonal**	
Study	**PAX3-FKHR**	**PAX7-FKHR**	**PAX3-FKHR**	**PAX7-FKHR**
Barr[196]	16/21 (76%)	2/21 (10%)	1/30 (3%)	1/30 (3%)
De Alava[197]	7/13 (54%)	2/13 (15%)	0/9 (0%)	0/9 (0%)
Downing[198]	20/23 (87%)		2/12 (17%)	
Arden[199]	8/13 (62%)	1/13 (8%)	0/11 (0%)	0/11 (0%)
Total	51/70 (73%)	5/47 (11%)	3/62 (5%)	1/50 (2%)

The tumor is usually large (>10 cm), and most are fleshy, well-circumscribed, intramuscular masses with focal hemorrhage and extensive necrosis. Histologically, pleomorphic rhabdomyosarcoma can be distinguished from embryonal and alveolar rhabdomyosarcoma by the association of loosely arranged, haphazardly oriented, large, round or pleomorphic cells with hyperchromatic nuclei and deeply eosinophilic cytoplasm (Figs 21–32, 21–33). As in embryonal rhabdomyosarcomas, there are racket-shaped and tadpole-shaped rhabdomyoblasts, but they are generally larger with more irregular outlines. Cells with cross-striations are commonly found in embryonal rhabdomyosarcomas with focal pleomorphic features[70] but are rare in adult pleomorphic rhabdomyosarcomas.[101,102] The tumor cells may be arranged in a haphazard pattern, but arrangement in a storiform pattern or a fascicular pattern reminiscent of leiomyosarcoma may be present (Fig. 21–34). The most helpful light microscopic feature suggesting this diagnosis is the presence of large bizarre tumor cells with deeply eosinophilic cytoplasm (Fig. 21–35). Rare lesions have cells with a rhabdoid morphology characterized by the presence of a peripherally located vesicular nucleus, with a prominent nucleolus and an intracytoplasmic eosinophilic hyaline inclusion.[102] Other features include phagocytosis by tumor cells, the presence of intracytoplasmic glycogen, and a moderately dense lymphohistiocytic infiltrate.

Ancillary techniques are required to confirm the diagnosis of pleomorphic rhabdomyosarcoma. Immunohistochemical detection of sarcomeric differentiation using antibodies to desmin (Fig. 21–36), muscle-specific actin, myoglobin, and sarcomeric α-actin, is extremely useful. Several studies have reported a high sensitivity and specificity for MyoD1 and/or myogenin in recognizing pleomorphic rhabdomyosarcoma and its distinction from other adult pleomorphic soft tissue sarcomas.[112-114] However, Furlong and colleagues reported sensitivities of MyoD1 and myogenin of only 53% and 56%, respectively, in cases of pleomorphic rhabdomyosarcoma.[101] This discrepancy may be related to differences in antibodies and antigen retrieval techniques.[115]

The ultrastructural features of pleomorphic rhabdomyosarcomas are similar to those of other rhabdomyosarcoma subtypes.[101] The tumor cells range from undifferentiated cells to those showing alternating thin and thick filaments with Z-band material to cells with well-defined sarcomeres.[116]

By cytogenetics, pleomorphic rhabdomyosarcoma does not have any characteristic aberration. Most have a highly complex karyotype. In a study of 46 pleomorphic sarcomas with Mertens and colleagues from the CHAMP Study Group,[117] karyotyping was not found to be useful in determining the line of differentiation in pleomorphic sarcomas.

The differential diagnosis includes a variety of other pleomorphic sarcomas and many other tumors that may simulate a pleomorphic sarcoma. First, pleomorphic rhabdomyosarcoma should be distinguished from the other rhabdomyosarcoma subtypes, all of which may have foci of pleomorphic cells. Adequate sampling of the latter usually reveals more typical areas of embryonal or alveolar rhabdomyosarcoma. Furthermore, pleomorphic rhabdomyosarcoma occurs in adults, whereas the other subtypes are seen mostly in children or adolescents. Pleomorphic rhabdomyosarcoma may be arranged in a fascicular growth pattern reminiscent of that seen in *pleomorphic leiomyosarcoma*. However, most cases of pleomorphic leiomyosarcoma have lower-grade areas that display a well-defined fascicular pattern composed of cells with typical smooth muscle features. Both tumors are immunoreactive for actin and desmin, but immunostains for

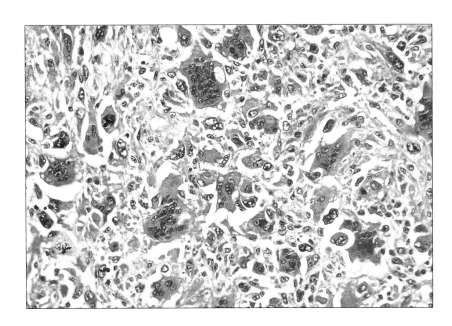

FIGURE 21–32 Pleomorphic rhabdomyosarcoma. This tumor was found in the deep soft tissues of the thigh in a 69-year-old man.

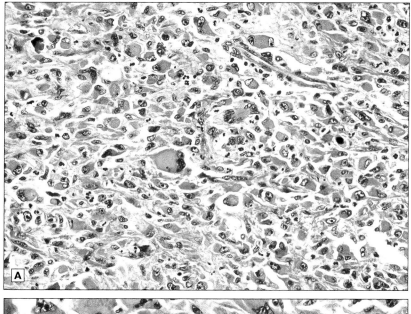

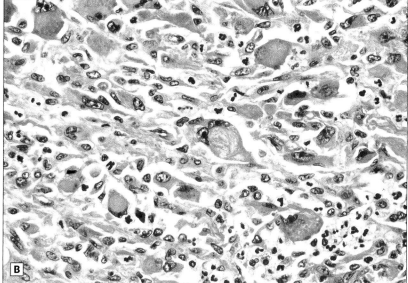

FIGURE 21–33 **(A)** Pleomorphic rhabdomyosarcoma composed predominantly of spindle-shaped cells with scattered large cells containing deeply eosinophilic cytoplasm. **(B)** Large cells with eosinophilic stringy cytoplasm in a pleomorphic rhabdomyosarcoma.

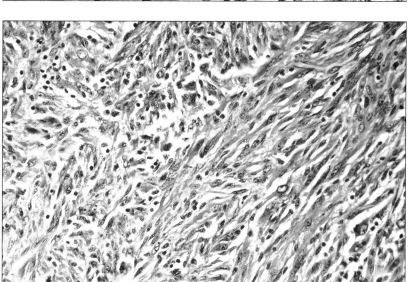

FIGURE 21–34 Pleomorphic rhabdomyosarcoma composed of spindle-shaped cells arranged in a fascicular pattern reminiscent of leiomyosarcoma.

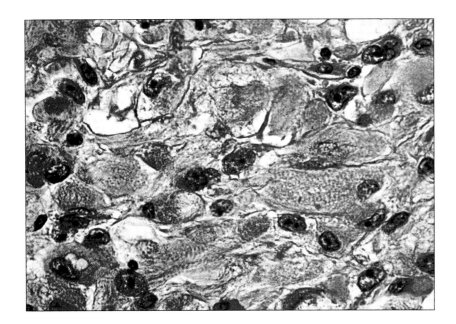

FIGURE 21–35 Unusual pleomorphic rhabdomyosarcoma. This focus was composed of numerous cells with eosinophilic fibrillar cytoplasm and cross-striations. Other portions of this tumor more closely resembled malignant fibrous histiocytoma.

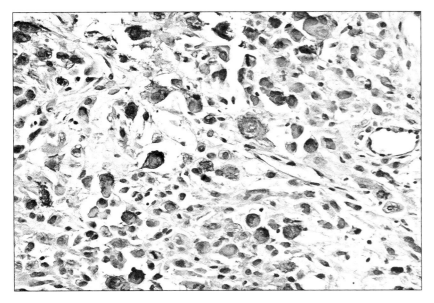

FIGURE 21–36 Desmin immunoreactivity in large eosinophilic cells in a pleomorphic rhabdomyosarcoma.

myoglobin, MyoD1, and myogenin are useful for recognizing pleomorphic rhabdomyosarcomas. These markers are also useful in distinguishing pleomorphic rhabdomyosarcoma from all other types of pleomorphic sarcoma, including pleomorphic undifferentiated sarcoma. Ultrastructurally, the identification of ribosome-myosin complexes and hexagonal arrays of thick and thin filaments help identify a tumor as a pleomorphic rhabdomyosarcoma.

Like other pleomorphic sarcomas, pleomorphic rhabdomyosarcoma is a clinically aggressive neoplasm that frequently metastasizes early in its course.[103] In the series by Gaffney et al.,[102] seven of eight patients for whom follow-up information was available died of disease, including five patients within 8 months of diagnosis. The AFIP study reported that 70% of patients died of disease, with a mean survival of only 20 months.[101]

Sclerosing rhabdomyosarcoma

In 2002, Folpe and colleagues described four cases of an unusual hyalinizing, matrix-rich variant of rhabdomyosarcoma which could be easily confused with an osteosarcoma, chondrosarcoma, or angiosarcoma.[118] All four of these tumors arose in adults whose ages ranged from 18 to 50 years, including three males and one female. These authors reported these lesions as sclerosing rhabdomyosarcomas, which they noted to be histologically similar, if not identical, to the two cases reported by Mentzel and Katenkamp as "sclerosing, pseudovascular rhabdomyosarcoma in adults."[119] Subsequently, there have been several additional reports of sclerosing rhabdomyosarcoma that have contributed to our understanding of the clinical, histologic, and molecular genetic spectrum of this tumor.[120–123]

Clinically, sclerosing rhabdomyosarcoma does not appear to have a unique presentation, as most patients present with a slowly enlarging mass. Although the four cases reported by Folpe et al. arose in adults,[118] subsequent reports have documented this tumor in children.[120,121] Chiles and colleagues from the Intergroup Rhabdomyosarcoma Study reported 13 cases of sclerosing rhabdomyosarcoma in children and adolescents; these cases were identified from 1207 pediatric rhabdomyosarcomas.[120] There are too few cases to determine if there is a gender predilection, but tumors have been reported in both males and females.

Grossly, sclerosing rhabdomyosarcoma ranges in size from 3 cm to up to 8 cm. On gross examination, the tumor is tan to yellow, rubbery in consistency, and typically infiltrates the surrounding soft tissues.

Histologically, sclerosing rhabdomyosarcoma has a characteristic constellation of features. The neoplastic cells are divided into lobules, small nests, microalveoli and even single-file arrays by an abundantly hyalinized, eosinophilic to basophilic matrix that closely resembles primitive osteoid or chondroid material (Figs 21–37, 21–38). Overall, the tumors are usually of moderate cellularity and are composed of primitive-appearing nuclei with a small amount of eosinophilic cytoplasm, irregular nuclear contours, coarse nuclear chromatin and small and occasionally multiple nucleoli. Wreath-like giant cells characteristic of alveolar rhabdomyosarcoma are not found. It is also unusual to identify rhabdomyoblasts, although strap cells may occasionally be seen. The mitotic rate is typically high. The hyalinized stroma is a dominant feature and often comprises up to 50% of the entire neoplasm.

The immunohistochemical features of this variant of rhabdomyosarcoma are somewhat unique. Folpe et al. described focal and dot-like desmin staining in their four cases,[118] a pattern of desmin staining that is quite different from that seen in other variants of rhabdomyosarcoma. Although MyoD1 staining tends to be strong and diffuse, myogenin staining is usually only focal and can be quite weak.

A small number of cases of sclerosing rhabdomyosarcoma have been studied at the molecular level. Folpe et al. only had adequate RNA for RT-PCR evaluation in one of their cases, and there was no evidence of a *PAX3/FKHR* or *PAX7/FKHR* fusion in this case.[118] In the study by Chiles and colleagues,[120] one case was found to harbor a *PAX3/FKHR* fusion, but five other cases were negative for *PAX3/FKHR* and *PAX7/FKHR* fusions.

The exact relationship between sclerosing rhabdomyosarcoma and embryonal or alveolar rhabdomyosarcoma is uncertain at this time, given the small number of cases reported. From a morphologic standpoint, sclerosing rhabdomyosarcoma does share overlapping features with alveolar rhabdomyosarcoma. However, sclerosing rhabdomyosarcoma lacks well-formed alveoli and lacks the wreath-like giant cells characteristic of alveolar rhabdomyosarcoma. An obvious difference is the more extensive hyalinized matrix characteristic of sclerosing rhabdomyosarcoma, as opposed to the fibrovascular septa found in alveolar rhabdomyosarcoma. Immunohistochemically, alveolar rhabdomyosarcoma virtually always shows strong nuclear staining for myogenin.[124,125] In contrast, sclerosing rhabdomyosarcoma tends to show much stronger immunoreactivity for MyoD1 and only focal nuclear staining for myogenin.[118]

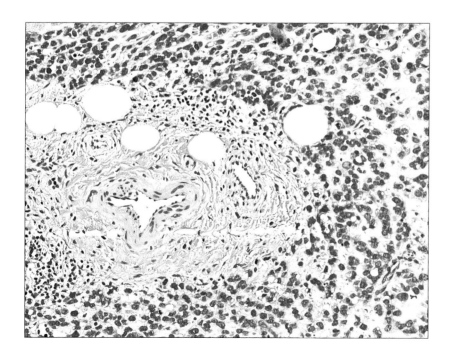

FIGURE 21–37 Sclerosing rhabdomyosarcoma composed of small nests and microalveoli of primitive round cells deposited in an abundantly hyalinized matrix. (Case courtesy of Dr. Andrew Folpe, Mayo Clinic, Rochester MN.)

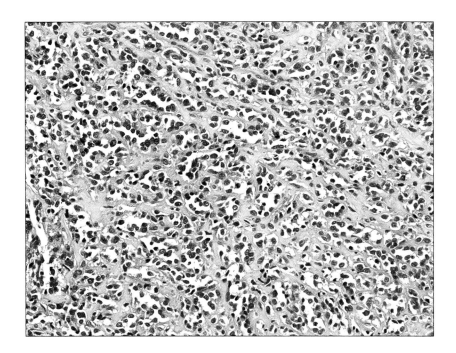

FIGURE 21–38 High-magnification view of sclerosing rhabdomyosarcoma composed of cords of primitive round cells arranged around a blood vessel and deposited in a densely hyalinized matrix. (Case courtesy of Dr. Andrew Folpe, Mayo Clinic, Rochester MN.)

Folpe and colleagues suggested the possibility that sclerosing rhabdomyosarcoma is an unusual variant of embryonal rhabdomyosarcoma or possibly even a new subtype of rhabdomyosarcoma.

The differential diagnosis includes *sclerosing osteosarcoma*, although the latter can be distinguished from sclerosing rhabdomyosarcoma by virtue of matrix calcification, the frequent presence of osteoclasts, the typical coexistence of other patterns of osteosarcoma, and the epithelioid morphology of the osteoblasts. *Extraskeletal myxoid chondrosarcoma* is composed of cords and chains of eosinophilic cells deposited in a myxoid matrix and lacks the densely hyalinized matrix of sclerosing rhabdomyosarcoma. *Mesenchymal chondrosarcoma* shows an admixture of primitive round cells and nodules of well-differentiated cartilage, often with a prominent hemangiopericytoma-like vascular pattern. Cases of sclerosing rhabdomyosarcoma showing cords of cells embedded in a hyalinized stroma may also simulate *sclerosing epithelioid fibrosarcoma*. However, the latter usually shows at least focal areas of typical fibrosarcoma or low-grade fibromyxoid sarcoma. Immunohistochemical analysis is extremely useful in distinguishing sclerosing rhabdomyosarcoma from *angiosarcoma*, since the latter typically shows strong membranous CD31 immunoreactivity and an absence of staining for MyoD1 and myogenin.

SPECIAL DIAGNOSTIC PROCEDURES

Special stains

Although many rhabdomyosarcomas can be diagnosed with routine sections, many poorly differentiated sarcomas masquerade as rhabdomyosarcomas (and visa versa),

and ancillary diagnostic procedures are often essential for a reliable diagnosis. During the past two decades, conventional special stains, such as the periodic acid-Schiff (PAS) preparation or the Masson trichrome stain, have become much less important for diagnosis and have been largely replaced by immunohistochemical procedures. Despite the greatly diminished role of conventional stains, Masson trichrome stain, phosphotungstic acid hematoxylin (PTAH), and iron-hematoxylin stain complement the morphologic findings and facilitate scanning multiple sections for the presence of differentiated cells (rhabdomyoblasts) among poorly differentiated cellular elements. These stains, however, lack specificity and stain both myofibrils and other cellular and extracellular structures. Most rhabdomyosarcomas contain considerable amounts of intracellular PAS-positive glycogen; in many tumors the glycogen is irregularly distributed and as a rule is much more conspicuous in well-differentiated than poorly differentiated tumor cells. Extracellular mucinous material stains positively with colloidal iron and Alcian blue and is removed by prior treatment with hyaluronidase.

Immunohistochemical procedures

Many immunohistochemical markers have been applied to the diagnosis of rhabdomyosarcoma, but their diagnostic value, sensitivity, and specificity vary substantially (Table 21–11);[125a] not all of the reported markers are even commercially available. Of the various markers, antibodies against desmin (for the muscle type of intermediate filaments), muscle-specific actin (HHF35), and myoglobin have been the most widely used for diagnostic purposes. These markers can be used with frozen and

TABLE 21–11	IMMUNOHISTOCHEMICAL EXPRESSION OF VARIOUS MYOGENIC MARKERS IN 95 RHABDOMYOSARCOMAS				
Rhabdomyosarcoma subtype	**Positive staining (%)**				
	Desmin	**Actin (HHF-35)**	**Sarcomeric actin**	**Troponin-T**	**Smooth muscle actin**
Embryonal (n = 61)	95	95	73	87	14
Alveolar (n = 19)	100	100	61	67	11
Botryoid (n = 9)	100	100	63	89	0
Spindle cell (n = 6)	100	100	83	83	0

Modified from Wijnaendts LCD, van der Linden JC, van Unnik AJM, et al. The expression pattern of contractile and intermediate filament proteins in developing skeletal muscle and rhabdomyosarcoma of childhood: diagnostic and prognostic utility. Am J Pathol 1994; 174:283.[125a]

alcohol-fixed material as well as with formalin-fixed tissue, even after years in paraffin.

Desmin is a reasonably sensitive marker of rhabdomyosarcoma (Fig. 21–39) although tumors composed predominantly of primitive cells may not stain for this antigen.[126] Furthermore, this marker is not useful for distinguishing rhabdomyosarcoma from leiomyosarcoma. Desmin is not entirely specific; it has been detected in a number of nonmyogenic tumors, including Ewing's sarcoma/primitive neuroectodermal tumor (ES/PNET), neuroblastoma, and malignant mesothelioma. Similarly, muscle-specific actin, although a sensitive marker of rhabdomyosarcoma, is not useful for distinguishing this tumor from leiomyosarcoma. This antigen is more resistant to formalin fixation than desmin but may also be negative in poorly differentiated rhabdomyosarcomas. Smooth muscle actin is an excellent marker of tumors with smooth muscle differentiation, but it may be found in up to 13% of rhabdomyosarcomas.[127]

Sarcomeric α-actin has also been reported to be a specific marker of rhabdomyosarcoma.[127] Monoclonal antibodies recognize both cardiac and skeletal α-actin; however, Schürch et al. found that all variants of rhabdomyosarcoma express cardiac α-actin transcripts but not skeletal α-actin mRNA by Northern blot hybridization.[127] Because cardiac α-actin is present in embryonic skeletal muscle,[128] these authors suggested that rhabdomyosarcomas follow normal skeletal myogenesis but do not complete the final step of skeletal α-actin mRNA expression.

Myoglobin, although a specific marker of skeletal muscle tumors, is not particularly sensitive.[126,129] For example, Parham et al. reported staining for myoglobin in only 17 (46%) of 37 formalin-fixed rhabdomyosarcomas.[126] Furthermore, staining tends to be restricted to the more differentiated cells, and this antigen may also be detected in nonmuscle cells as a result of diffusion.[130]

Other somewhat less sensitive markers that have been used in the diagnosis of rhabdomyosarcoma include antibodies for fast, slow, and fetal myosin, creatine kinase (isoenzymes MM and BB), β-enolase, Z-protein, titin, and vimentin. Vimentin, although entirely non-specific, is co-expressed in virtually all rhabdomyosarcomas but is more prominent in undifferentiated than well-differentiated tumors. Cytokeratin and S-100 protein have also been demonstrated in occasional undifferentiated tumor cells and rhabdomyoblasts, respectively.[131,132] Of course, many malignant peripheral nerve sheath tumors with rhabdomyoblastic differentiation (so-called malignant Triton tumor) contain, in addition to rhabdomyoblasts, nerve sheath elements that stain positively for S-100 protein. Neural cell adhesion molecules and isoforms of neurofilament protein have also been detected in some rhabdomyosarcomas.[133]

Immunohistochemical expression of myoregulatory proteins has been found to be an excellent marker of all rhabdomyosarcoma subtypes, showing both high sensitivity and specificity (Table 21–12). MyoD1, the best-studied member of a family of myogenic regulatory genes, which includes myf-5 and mrf-4-herculin/myf-6, acts as a nodal point for the initiation of skeletal muscle differentiation by binding to enhancer sequences of muscle-specific genes.[134,135] These genes are expressed at an early stage of skeletal muscle differentiation and are capable of converting multipotential murine fibroblasts into myoblasts.[136] Although originally detected only using frozen tissues,[113,137,138] antigen retrieval techniques have allowed detection of MyoD1 in formalin-fixed, paraffin-embedded tissues.[114] Detection of this nuclear antigen is useful in the differential diagnosis of pediatric small round cell tumors[114] and for distinguishing pleomorphic rhabdomyosarcoma from other pleomorphic sarcomas of adulthood.[112,113] Using formalin-fixed, paraffin-embedded tissues and antigen retrieval techniques, Wang et al. detected nuclear expression of MyoD1 in 30 (91%) of 33 rhabdomyosarcomas, with no significant differences in sensitivity among the various histologic subtypes.[114] Furthermore, none of the ES/PNETs or neuroblastomas demonstrated nuclear immunoreactivity for this antigen. These authors found a similar percentage of lesions to stain with antibodies to myogenin. The anti-myogenin antibody was found to have technical advantages over the anti-MyoD1 antibody in that there was an absence of non-specific cytoplasmic immunoreactivity, which was sometimes seen with

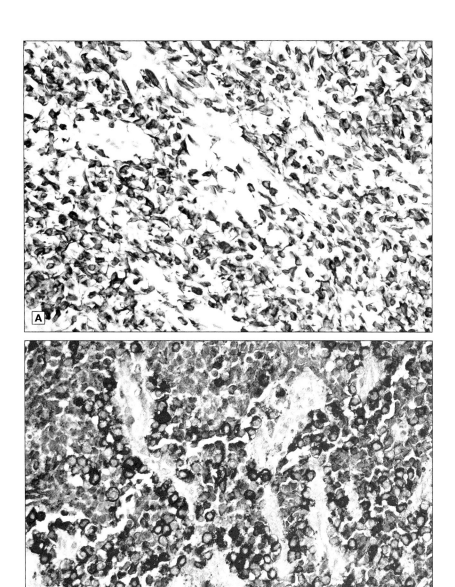

FIGURE 21–39 Diffuse, strong immunoreactivity for desmin in an embryonal rhabdomyosarcoma **(A)** and an alveolar rhabdomyosarcoma **(B)**.

TABLE 21–12	IMMUNOREACTIVITY FOR MYOGENIC MARKERS IN RHABDOMYOSARCOMA AND OTHER PEDIATRIC ROUND CELL TUMORS					
Tumor	**Myogenin**	**MyoD1**	**Actin (HHF-35)**	**Sarcomeric Actin**	**Desmin**	**Myoglobin**
Rhabdomyosarcomas	30/33	30/33	30/33	21/33	33/33	8/28
Embryonal	22/25	23/25	22/25	18/25	25/25	6/20
Spindle cell	1/1	1/1	1/1	1/1	1/1	0/1
Alveolar	4/4	3/4	4/4	3/4	4/4	1/4
Pleomorphic	3/3	3/3	3/3	2/3	3/3	1/3
EWS/PNET	0/26	0/26	0/26	0/6	3/26	0/6
Neuroblastomas	0/12	0/12	0/12	0/12	0/12	0/12

Modified from Wang NP, Marx J, McNutt MA, et al. Expression of myogenic regulatory proteins (myogenin and MyoD1) in small blue round cell tumors of childhood. Am J Pathol 1995; 147:1799. pPNET, peripheral primitive neuroectodermal tumors.

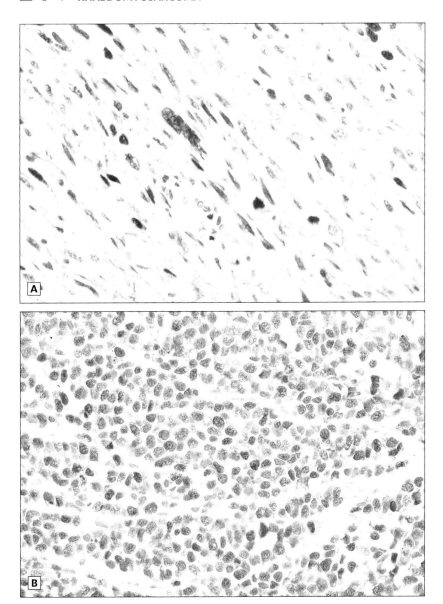

FIGURE 21–40 Nuclear staining for myogenin in an embryonal rhabdomyosarcoma **(A)** and an alveolar rhabdomyosarcoma **(B)**.

the anti-MyoD1 antibody (Fig. 21–40). In this study, expression of both MyoD1 and myogenin was reciprocally related to the degree of cellular differentiation, with more primitive-appearing cells staining and decreased or absent immunoreactivity in large differentiated rhabdomyoblasts. In general, both myogenin and MyoD1 are expressed to a greater degree in alveolar rhabdomyosarcoma than embryonal subtypes.[138a]

Ultrastructural findings

The ultrastructure of rhabdomyosarcoma bears a striking resemblance to that of embryonal muscle tissue in varying stages of development, but there is a much wider spectrum in the appearance of the tumor cells, which range from primitive undifferentiated cells with few organelles to highly differentiated cells with abundant but often incomplete sarcomeres. The least differentiated cells contain only scattered or parallel bundles of thin (actin) myofilaments measuring 6–8 nm in diameter; this is a non-specific finding that does not permit a reliable diagnosis of rhabdomyosarcoma; better-differentiated cells are characterized by distinct bundles of thick (myosin) filaments 12–15 nm in diameter, with attached ribosomes having an Indian-file arrangement (ribosome and myosin complex), a feature characteristic of rhabdomyoblastic differentiation. Further cellular maturation is marked by alternating thin (actin) and thick (myosin) filaments in a parallel arrangement, with a characteristic hexagonal pattern seen on cross-sections and rod-like structures or disks composed of Z-band material. In many tumors there are also well-differentiated rhabdomyoblasts with distinct sarcomeres, including the characteristic A and I banding and clearly discernible Z lines (Fig. 21–41).[116,139]

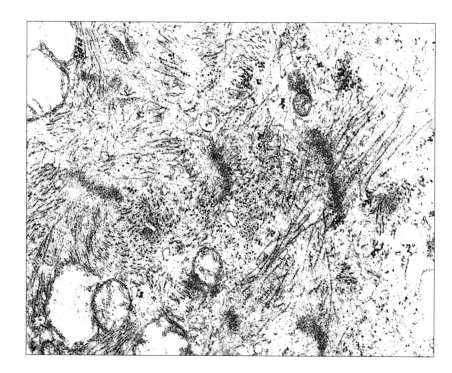

FIGURE 21–41 Ultrastructure of an embryonal rhabdomyosarcoma with a typical mixture of thick (myosin) and thin (actin) fibrils in longitudinal and cross-section with distinct Z banding in several places.

In addition to myofilaments, the cytoplasm of the rhabdomyoblasts contains a prominent Golgi apparatus and varying numbers of mitochondria and glycogen particles. There are also small lysosomes, droplets of lipid, occasional pinocytotic vesicles, and complete or incomplete basal lamina. The multinucleated giant cells, characteristic of the alveolar type, have neither myofilaments nor basal laminae.[140]

DIFFERENTIAL DIAGNOSIS

Poorly differentiated round and spindle cell sarcomas, especially in children or young adults, constitute the most common problem in differential diagnosis. Included in this group are neuroblastomas, ES/PNETs, poorly differentiated angiosarcomas, synovial sarcomas, malignant melanomas, melanotic neuroectodermal tumors of infancy, granulocytic sarcomas, and malignant lymphomas. Small cell carcinoma must also be considered when the tumor occurs in a patient older than 45 years. The differential diagnosis requires not only careful evaluation of clinical data, patient age, and tumor location, but also painstaking examination of multiple sections for specific features such as rhabdomyoblasts, rosettes, biphasic cellular or vascular differentiation, and intracellular pigment, as well as immunohistochemical assessment with multiple markers, and possibly cytogenetic/molecular testing.

Immunohistochemical analysis using a battery of stains is indispensable, including stains for muscle markers such as desmin, muscle-specific actin, and MyoD1 or myogenin. It must also be kept in mind that CD99, although a highly sensitive marker of ES/PNET, is sometimes detected in embryonal or alveolar rhabdomyosarcoma.[141,142]

Infantile rhabdomyofibrosarcoma, described by Lundgren et al. in 1993,[143] is a rare tumor that resembles infantile fibrosarcoma but has ultrastructural and immunohistochemical evidence of rhabdomyoblastic differentiation. The spindle-shaped cells in this tumor express vimentin, desmin, smooth muscle actin, and sarcomeric actin; electron microscopy reveals fibroblastic and myofibroblastic features. The tumor shows cytogenetic alterations (monosomy 19 and monosomy 22) distinct from those found in either infantile fibrosarcoma or embryonal or alveolar rhabdomyosarcoma.

Rhabdomyosarcoma with rhabdoid features is uncommon but well described.[144,145] These lesions have cells with cytoplasmic hyaline inclusions composed of intermediate filaments. A battery of immunostains, including stains for cytokeratins and myoregulatory proteins, is often necessary to distinguish this variant of rhabdomyosarcoma from other tumors with rhabdoid features including *malignant extrarenal rhabdoid tumor*.

Problems in diagnosis may also be caused by benign reactive and neoplastic lesions such as polypoid cystitis, polyps and pseudosarcomatous myofibroblastic proliferations of the genitourinary tract, infectious granuloma, proliferative myositis, skeletal muscle regeneration, granular cell tumor, and fetal rhabdomyoma. Conversely, we have also encountered sparsely cellular botryoid-type rhabdomyosarcomas that were initially misinterpreted as *myxomas*. In these cases, consideration of age and location usually allows for the correct diagnosis, as myxomas are virtually nonexistent in children and almost never occur in visceral organs.

Some tumors have *heterologous rhabdomyoblastic components*. Focal rhabdomyoblastic differentiation occurs in a variety of malignant neoplasms, including those with only sarcomatous differentiation, those with epithelial or germ cell elements, and tumors of neuroectodermal derivation (Table 21–13).[146] Identification of such elements may be obvious on light microscopic examination alone, but in some cases the use of immunohistochemical or electron microscopic techniques is required to support rhabdomyoblastic differentiation. In addition, sarcomas with a propensity for undergoing dedifferentiation, including chondrosarcomas and liposarcomas, may have areas of divergent rhabdomyoblastic differentiation.[147]

Epithelial tumors may also exhibit rhabdomyoblastic differentiation, including malignant mixed mesodermal tumors of the uterus, cervix, or ovary, carcinosarcomas of the breast and stomach, pulmonary blastomas, nephroblastomas, and mixed-type hepatoblastomas. The rhabdomyoblastic component may even dominate the microscopic picture. Rhabdomyoblastic differentiation is also encountered in malignant or immature teratomas, but rarely as a major element. In most of these tumors the rhabdomyoblastic component is accompanied by malignant epithelial and other mesenchymal elements such as cartilage and bone. Rare ovarian Sertoli-Leydig cell tumors contain heterologous rhabdomyoblastic foci.[148]

Lastly, rhabdomyoblastic elements may be found in various neuroectodermal neoplasms, notably the malignant peripheral nerve sheath tumor (malignant Triton tumor), ganglioneuroma (ectomesenchymoma), medulloepithelioma, and medulloblastoma. Malignant peripheral nerve sheath tumors with rhabdomyoblastic differentiation chiefly occur in patients older than 30 years who have manifestations of neurofibromatosis.[149-151] Malignant ectomesenchymoma is primarily a tumor of children and is not known to be associated with neurofibromatosis; it consists of a mixture of rhabdomyoblastic elements, mature ganglion cells, and neuroma-like structures.[152,153] We have observed one case in which the initial tumor had features of an embryonal rhabdomyosarcoma and the recurrent tumor was indistinguishable from a ganglioneuroma save for a few peripherally located groups of rhabdomyoblasts. We have also reviewed concurrent rhabdomyosarcoma of the retroperitoneum and pheochromocytoma in a 46-year-old woman.

DISCUSSION

During the past 40 years, the prognosis of rhabdomyosarcoma has improved dramatically. Prior to 1960 the prognosis was extremely poor, and there were few survivors even after radical, often destructive and disfiguring, surgical therapy. An AFIP study in 1963 based on 147 cases showed that 90% of patients died of disease within a period of 5 years.[154] In another AFIP study devoted exclusively to alveolar rhabdomyosarcomas,[27] the 5-year mortality rate was an astronomic 98%.

Since the early 1960s there has been marked improvement in the survival rates of patients with rhabdomyosarcoma because of a multidisciplinary therapeutic approach that consists of biopsy or surgical removal of the neoplasm and multiagent chemotherapy with or without radiotherapy.[4,9] As a rule, treatment is carried out after biopsy or resection and careful, comprehensive assessment of tumor stage or tumor group with radiography, computed tomographic (CT) scans, magnetic resonance imaging (MRI), bone scans and, if necessary, angiograms. Recommendations for therapy chiefly depend on the stage or clinical group of the disease and the site of the tumor following accurate microscopic diagnosis. Because rhabdomyosarcomas tend to metastasize to bone marrow, bilateral bone marrow aspiration/biopsy should be part of the staging process.

The IRS-II study, confined to patients younger than 21 years with a confirmed diagnosis of rhabdomyosarcoma, distinguished four clinical groups based on the amount of tumor remaining after initial surgery (Table 21–14). Because this approach is influenced by the variable practices of surgeons, the IRS Committee adopted a modification of the tumor-node-metastasis (TNM) system, which

---

TABLE 21–13	**TUMORS WITH HETEROLOGOUS RHABDOMYOBLASTIC COMPONENTS**

Tumors with epithelial components
  Carcinosarcoma (especially of breast, stomach, urinary bladder)
  Malignant mixed Müllerian tumor (uterus, cervix, ovary)
  Wilms' tumor
  Hepatoblastoma
  Pulmonary blastoma
  Thymoma
Tumors with germ cell or sex cord elements
  Germ cell tumors (seminoma, teratoma)
  Sertoli-Leydig cell tumor
Tumors with only sarcomatous elements
  Malignant mesenchymoma
  Dedifferentiated chondrosarcoma
  Dedifferentiated liposarcoma
Tumors of neuroectodermal derivation
  Malignant peripheral nerve sheath tumor (malignant Triton tumor)
  Ectomesenchymoma
  Medulloepithelioma
  Medulloblastoma
  Congenital pigmented nevus (giant nevus)

Modified from Woodruff JM, Perino G. Non-germ-cell or teratomatous malignant tumors showing additional rhabdomyoblastic differentiation, with emphasis on the malignant Triton tumor. Semin Diagn Pathol 1994; 11:69.

relies on pretreatment assessment of tumor extent.[155,156] This system includes evaluation of the site of the primary tumor, the maximum diameter of the tumor, determination of tumor invasion into adjacent structures, status of regional lymph nodes, and the presence or absence of distant metastases (Table 21–15). More recent studies of rhabdomyosarcoma rely on both the IRS clinical grouping system and the TNM stage to determine therapy. Both IRS clinical group and TNM stage have been found to have major prognostic significance (Table 21–16). Low-risk patients generally have localized embryonal histology tumors. Most of these patients have resected (group I or II) tumors, as well as group III tumors arising in favorable sites. Patients with embryonal tumors that are group III, stage 2 or 3, and all patients with nonmetastatic alveolar tumors are intermediate-risk. Patients with

metastatic tumors (regardless of subtype) are treated with high-risk protocols. Based on data from the IRS-IV study, overall survival rates were 95%, 75%, and 27% for low-risk, intermediate-risk, and high-risk patients, respectively.[9] Similar results were reported from the European Cooperative Group studies using a four-tier risk system.[157,158]

Additional factors that influence the clinical course of the disease and necessitate more intensive therapy include the anatomic site and histologic subtype of the tumor. Tumors of the orbit have the best prognosis (92% 5-year survival) followed by tumors of the head and neck and nonbladder/prostate genitourinary tumors (about 80% 5-year survival).[9,157,158] A less favorable prognosis is found in patients whose tumors are located in a parameningeal location, bladder and prostate, and the extremities, with approximately 70% 5-year survivals for each. The poorest prognosis occurs in patients with tumors at other sites, including the retroperitoneum, biliary tract, and peritoneum. Late detection and large tumor size, difficulties encountered during removal, extension into the meninges with or without spinal fluid spread, and an increased rate of lymph node metastasis are primarily responsible for the prognostic differences related to the anatomic sites.

Anatomic site is a major factor when determining the mode of therapy. For example, for rhabdomyosarcomas of the orbit, control is typically accomplished with biopsy, systemic chemotherapy, and irradiation alone.[43] Excellent results are achieved with rhabdomyosarcomas of the paratesticular region using radical orchiectomy with clear margins, radical retroperitoneal lymph node resection, and chemotherapy.[159] Tumors in parameningeal and paraspinal regions require extended irradiation and intrathecal chemotherapy to reduce local failure and spread of the disease. Preoperative radiotherapy or chemotherapy for rhabdomyosarcomas of the urinary bladder and prostate usually allow less-extensive surgical therapy and better functional preservation.[60,61] Total excision of the tumor is part of the recommended therapy for rhabdomyosarcomas in the trunk and extremities.[44]

TABLE 21–14	CLINICAL STAGING OF PATIENTS WITH RHABDOMYOSARCOMA (INTERGROUP RHABDOMYOSARCOMA STUDIES CLASSIFICATION)

Group I
  Localized disease, completely resected (regional nodes not involved)
  Confined to muscle or organ of origin
  Contiguous involvement with infiltration outside the muscle or organ of origin, as through fascial planes
Group II
  Grossly resected tumor with microscopic residual disease
  No evidence of gross residual tumor; no evidence of regional node involvement
  Regional disease, completely resected (regional nodes involved, extension of tumor into an adjacent organ, or both); all tumor completely resected with no microscopic residual tumor
  Regional disease with involved nodes, grossly resected, but with evidence of microscopic residual disease
Group III
  Incomplete resection or biopsy with gross residual disease
Group IV
  Distant metastatic disease present at onset (lung, liver, bones, bone marrow, brain, distant muscle and nodes)

From Maurer HM, Beltangady M, Gehan EA, et al. The Intergroup Rhabdomyosarcoma Study I: a final report. Cancer 1988; 61:209, with permission.

TABLE 21–15	TNM STAGING CLASSIFICATION FOR RHABDOMYOSARCOMA, AS MODIFIED BY THE IRS COMMITTEE					
Stage	Sites	T*	Size*	N†	M‡
1	Orbit, head and neck (excluding parameningeal sites); genitourinary (nonbladder/nonprostate)	T1 or T2	a or b	N0 or N1 or Nx	M0
2	Bladder/prostate; extremity; cranial parameningeal sites; other (e.g., trunk, retroperitoneum)	T1 or T2	a	N0 or Nx	M0
3	Bladder/prostate; extremity; cranial parameningeal sites; other (e.g., trunk, retroperitoneum)	T1 or T2	a	N1	M0
			b	N0 or N1 or Nx	M0
4	All	T1 or T2	a or b	N0 or N1	M1

Modified from Pappo AS, Shapiro DN, Crist WM, et al. Biology and therapy of pediatric rhabdomyosarcoma. J Clin Oncol 1995; 13:2123.
*Tumor: T (site) 1, confined to anatomic site of origin; (a) ≤5 cm, (b) >5 cm. T (site) 2, extension and/or fixation to surrounding tissue; (a) ≤5 cm, (b) >5 cm.
†Regional nodes: N0, regional nodes not clinically involved; N1, regional nodes clinically involved by neoplasm; Nx, status of regional nodes unknown.
‡Metastasis: M0, no distant metastasis; M1, distant metastasis.

TABLE 21-16	FAVORABLE AND UNFAVORABLE FACTORS FOR RHABDOMYOSARCOMAS

Prognostically favorable factors

Age: infants and children

Orbital or genitourinary (nonbladder/prostate) location

Small size (<5 cm)

Botryoid or spindle cell type

Localized noninvasive tumor without regional lymph node involvement or distant metastasis

Complete initial resection

Prognostically unfavorable factors

Age: adults

Location in head and neck (nonorbital), paraspinal region, abdomen, biliary tract, retroperitoneum, perineum, or extremities

Large size (>5 cm)

Alveolar (especially *PAX3/FKHR* fusion transcript-positive) or pleomorphic type

Diploid DNA content

Local tumor invasion, especially parameningeal or paraspinal region, sinuses, or skeleton

Local recurrence

Local recurrence during therapy

Regional lymph node involvement or distant metastasis

Incomplete initial excision or unresectability

Histologic subtype has been found to be an important independent prognostic variable.[33] Newton et al. found histologic subtype to be strongly predictive of survival by multivariate analysis, in addition to the known prognostic factors of primary site, clinical group, and tumor size.[33] The latter study established that the botryoid and spindle cell subtypes of embryonal rhabdomyosarcoma have a superior prognosis (95% and 88% 5-year survivals, respectively); classic embryonal rhabdomyosarcoma has an intermediate prognosis (66% 5-year survival); and the alveolar subtype has a poor prognosis, with a 54% 5-year survival.

The degree of cellular differentiation (i.e., tumor cells resembling skeletal muscle cells) has been found by some to be of major prognostic significance. Wijnaendts et al. found that a greater degree of cellular maturation was associated with prolonged survival, independent of histologic subtype.[160] In addition, it has been repeatedly documented that tumor cells may undergo therapy-induced cytodifferentiation.[71,161] Botryoid and embryonal rhabdomyosarcoma subtypes are more likely to exhibit therapy-induced cytodifferentiation than other rhabdomyosarcoma subtypes.[161]

Age at diagnosis is also an independent predictor of outcome in patients with rhabdomyosarcoma.[3,162] Age has its greatest prognostic effect on patients with invasive but nonmetastatic tumors.[162]

The mitotic rate is of little value for predicting therapeutic response and outcome of the disease.[163] The prognostic value of flow cytometric DNA analysis is not clear, since conflicting data have been published.[164,165] San

Miguel-Fraile and colleagues evaluated 45 cases of childhood rhabdomyosarcoma and found DNA ploidy to be an independent prognostic factor by multivariate analysis.[166] DNA hyperdiploid and triploid tumors had a favorable prognosis, whereas DNA diploid and polyploid tumors had a poor prognosis. However, Pohar-Marinsek et al. only found a correlation between DNA ploidy and histologic subtype, patient age, and gender.[167] A hyperdiploid DNA pattern was associated with an embryonal subtype, whereas alveolar tumors tended to be tetraploid. In their review of the literature of 12 studies evaluating the relationship between DNA ploidy and survival, six studies found a correlation, whereas six did not. They suggested that difference in therapy (chemotherapy versus no chemotherapy), differences in grouping DNA histograms and low number of patients studied likely account for the discrepancies reported in the literature. Similarly inconsistent results have been reported on the prognostic impact of proliferative activity, as measured by Ki-67 index.[168–171]

The possible prognostic impact of various molecular alterations has been an area of intensive research in recent years. Accumulated intranuclear p53 protein has been detected by immunohistochemical techniques in a proportion of rhabdomyosarcomas.[169] Although some of these tumors harbor *p53* gene mutations, it appears that *MDM2* gene overexpression with subsequent *MDM2*-*p53* complex formation constitutes an alternative mechanism of inactivation of wild-type *p53* in some rhabdomyosarcomas.[172–174] The prognostic significance of *p53* alterations is still unknown. The *MYCN* oncogene, formerly known as N-*myc*, is amplified in some rhabdomyosarcomas, including both embryonal and alveolar subtypes, but seems to be significantly more common in the latter.[175–177] However, there is no clear relationship between *MYCN* amplification and clinical outcome. P-glycoprotein, a product of the multiple drug resistance (*MDR*) gene, functions as a membrane transport system associated with chemotherapy resistance. P-glycoprotein immunoreactivity and/or the expression of *MDR* gene correlate with decreased survival of rhabdomyosarcoma patients in some studies[178,179] but not in others.[180] Klunder et al. found the expression of *MDR* gene, particularly lung resistance-related protein (LRP) to be related to therapy-induced maturation.[181] Finally, techniques such as RT-PCR and FISH to detect gene fusion subtype may emerge as important tools for determining prognosis in this group of patients. Several studies have found the *PAX7/FKHR* fusion transcript to be associated with a better prognosis than the *PAX3/FKHR* fusion in patients with alveolar rhabdomyosarcoma.[99,182] For example, Sorensen et al. evaluated 171 childhood rhabdomyosarcomas and found *PAX3/FKHR* and *PAX7/FKHR* fusions in 55% and 22% of alveolar rhabdomyosarcomas, respectively.[182] Twenty-three percent of patients with alveolar tumors were fusion negative. Although fusion status was not correlated with outcome in patients with locoregional disease, there was a striking difference in outcome in patients presenting with metastatic disease, with estimated 4-year overall survivals of 75% and 8% for *PAX7/FKHR* and *PAX3/FKHR* fusions, respectively.

Long-term complications resulting from therapy depend on the location of the primary tumor. On occasion, treatment causes cataracts, xerophthalmia and craniofacial deformities, enteritis, acute or chronic diarrhea, intestinal obstruction, cystitis, hematuria, neutropenia, and excessive weight loss, among others.[57,183,184] Radiation therapy may affect growth and induce secondary tumors, including osteosarcoma and leukemia.[185]

RECURRENCE

Inadequately treated tumors grow in an infiltrative, destructive manner and recur in a high percentage of cases. Recurrence may herald metastasis, but by no means do all recurrent tumors metastasize. Bone does not constitute an effective barrier to growth of the tumor, and bone invasion is a frequent finding, particularly with rhabdomyosarcomas in the head and neck region and in the hands and feet. In the head and neck, the tumors tend to erode and destroy the bony walls of the orbit and sinuses, the temporal or mastoid bone, and the base of the skull; they may prove fatal because of extensive meningeal spread (parameningeal rhabdomyosarcomas) and spinal cord "drop metastases."[42,186-188] Meningeal spread may also occur with rhabdomyosarcomas at other sites.

METASTASIS

Metastases develop during the course of the disease and are present at the time of diagnosis in about 20% of cases. Major metastatic sites include the lung, lymph nodes, and bone marrow followed by the heart, brain, meninges, pancreas, liver, and kidney. The lungs are involved in at least two-thirds of patients with metastasis.[189,190] The incidence of lymph node metastasis largely depends on the location of the tumor. It is higher with rhabdomyosarcomas of the prostate, paratesticular region, and extremities than with those of the orbit and head and neck.[191] In fact, exploration and biopsy of ipsilateral retroperitoneal lymph nodes is recommended when assessing paratesticular rhabdomyosarcomas.[192] It is also useful to keep in mind that alveolar rhabdomyosarcoma is one of the few soft tissue tumors in which lymph node metastasis may antedate discovery of the primary mass. There is a surprisingly high incidence of cardiac metastasis. Pratt and colleagues found 8 of 23 fatal cases to have metastases to the heart.[193] There are also reports of multiple skin metastases as the primary manifestation of the disease.[194,195]

Microscopically, the recurrent and metastatic lesions may be less well differentiated than the primary growth; but unlike most other types of sarcoma, some recurrent or metastatic lesions for unknown reasons show a higher degree of differentiation. We have observed several cases where a definitive diagnosis of rhabdomyosarcoma was possible only after rhabdomyoblasts with cross-striations were found in the pulmonary metastases. In addition, cytologic differentiation in rhabdomyosarcomas following polychemotherapy, probably due to "selective destruction of undifferentiated tumor cells,"[72] has been demonstrated.[71]

REFERENCES

1. Pack GT, Everhart WF. Rhabdomyosarcoma of skeletal muscle; report of 100 cases. Surgery 1952; 32:1023.
2. Stout AP. Rhabdomyosarcoma of the skeletal muscles. Ann Surg 1946; 123:447.
3. Crist WM, Garnsey L, Beltangady MS, et al. Prognosis in children with rhabdomyosarcoma: a report of the Intergroup Rhabdomyosarcoma Studies I and II. Intergroup Rhabdomyosarcoma Committee. J Clin Oncol 1990; 8:443.
4. Crist W, Gehan EA, Ragab AH, et al. The third Intergroup Rhabdomyosarcoma Study. J Clin Oncol 1995; 13:610.
5. Gaiger AM, Soule EH, Newton WA Jr. Pathology of rhabdomyosarcoma: experience of the Intergroup Rhabdomyosarcoma Study, 1972–78. Natl Cancer Inst Monogr 1981; 56:19.
6. Maurer HM, Beltangady M, Gehan EA, et al. The Intergroup Rhabdomyosarcoma Study-I. A final report. Cancer 1988; 61:209.
7. Maurer HM, Gehan EA, Beltangady M, et al. The Intergroup Rhabdomyosarcoma Study-II. Cancer 1993; 71:1904.
8. Newton WA Jr, Soule EH, Hamoudi AB, et al. Histopathology of childhood sarcomas. Intergroup Rhabdomyosarcoma Studies I and II: Clinicopathologic correlation. J Clin Oncol 1988; 6:67.
9. Crist WM, Anderson JR, Meza JL, et al. Intergroup Rhabdomyosarcoma Study-IV: results for patients with nonmetastatic disease. J Clin Oncol 2001; 19:3091.
10. Villella JA, Bogner PN, Jani-Sait SN, et al. Rhabdomyosarcoma of the cervix in sisters with review of the literature. Gynecol Oncol 2005; 99:742.
11. Corapcioglu F, Memet Ozek M, Sav A, et al. Congenital pineoblastoma and parameningeal rhabdomyosarcoma: concurrent two embryonal tumors in a young infant. Childs Nerv Syst 2006; 22:533.
12. Caglar K, Varan A, Akyuz C, et al. Second neoplasms in pediatric patients treated for cancer: a center's 30-year experience. J Pediatr Hematol Oncol 2006; 28:374.
13. Hwang JC, Ko JY, Hsiao CC, et al. Intraosseous embryonal rhabdomyosarcoma as a second neoplasm following retinoblastoma. Pathology 2005; 37:552.
14. Armstrong SJ, Duncan AW, Mott MG. Rhabdomyosarcoma associated with familial adenomatous polyposis. Pediatr Radiol 1991; 21:445.
15. Heney D, Lockwood L, Allibone EB, et al. Nasopharyngeal rhabdomyosarcoma and multiple lentigines syndrome: a case report. Med Pediatr Oncol 1992; 20:227.
16. Oguzkan S, Terzi YK, Guler E, et al. Two neurofibromatosis type 1 cases associated with rhabdomyosarcoma of bladder, one with a large deletion in the NF1 gene. Cancer Genet Cytogenet 2006; 164:159.
17. Estep AL, Tidyman WE, Teitell MA, et al. HRAS mutations in Costello syndrome: detection of constitutional activating mutations in codon 12 and 13 and loss of wild-type allele in malignancy. Am J Med Genet A 2006; 140:8.
18. Smith AC, Squire JA, Thorner P, et al. Association of alveolar rhabdomyosarcoma with the Beckwith-Wiedemann syndrome. Pediatr Dev Pathol 2001; 4:550.
19. Lollis SS, Hug EB, Gladstone DJ, et al. Acquired Chiari malformation type I following fractionated radiation therapy to the anterior skull base in a 20-month-old boy. Case report. J Neurosurg 2006; 104:133.
20. Doladzas T, Arvelakis A, Karavokyros IG, et al. Primary rhabdomyosarcoma of the lung

arising over cystic pulmonary adenomatoid malformation. Pediatr Hematol Oncol 2005; 22:525.

21. Avigad S, Peleg D, Barel D, et al. Prenatal diagnosis in Li-Fraumeni syndrome. J Pediatr Hematol Oncol 2004; 26:541.

22. Lampe AK, Seymour G, Thompson PW, et al. Familial neurofibromatosis microdeletion syndrome complicated by rhabdomyosarcoma. Arch Dis Child 2002; 87:444.

23. Savasan S, Lorenzana A, Williams JA, et al. Constitutional balanced translocations in alveolar rhabdomyosarcoma. Cancer Genet Cytogenet 1998; 105:50.

Incidence

24. Gurney JG, Ross JA, Wall DA, et al. Infant cancer in the U.S.: histology-specific incidence and trends, 1973 to 1992. J Pediatr Hematol Oncol 1997; 19:428.

25. Hawkins WG, Hoos A, Antonescu CR, et al. Clinicopathologic analysis of patients with adult rhabdomyosarcoma. Cancer 2001; 91:794.

Histologic classification

26. Horn RC, Enterline HT. Rhabdomyosarcoma: a clinicopathological study of 39 cases. Cancer 1958; 11:181.

27. Enzinger FM, Shiraki M. Alveolar rhabdomyosarcoma. An analysis of 110 cases. Cancer 1969; 24:18.

28. Palmer NF, Sachs N, Foulkes M. Histopathology and prognosis in rhabdomyosarcoma. Proc Int Soc Pediatr Oncol 1981; 1:113.

29. Palmer NF, Sachs N, Foulkes M. Histopathology and prognosis in rhabdomyosarcoma (IRS-1). Proc Am Clin Oncol 1982; 1:170.

30. Caillaud JM, Gerard-Marchant R, Marsden HB, et al. Histopathological classification of childhood rhabdomyosarcoma: a report from the International Society of Pediatric Oncology Pathology Panel. Med Pediatr Oncol 1989; 17:391.

31. Tsokos M, Webber BL, Parham DM, et al. Rhabdomyosarcoma. A new classification scheme related to prognosis. Arch Pathol Lab Med 1992; 116:847.

32. Asmar L, Gehan EA, Newton WA, et al. Agreement among and within groups of pathologists in the classification of rhabdomyosarcoma and related childhood sarcomas. Report of an international study of four pathology classifications. Cancer 1994; 74:2579.

33. Newton WA Jr, Gehan EA, Webber BL, et al. Classification of rhabdomyosarcomas and related sarcomas. Pathologic aspects and proposal for a new classification – an Intergroup Rhabdomyosarcoma Study. Cancer 1995; 76:1073.

34. Qualman SJ, Bowen J, Parham DM, et al. Protocol for the examination of specimens from patients (children and young adults) with rhabdomyosarcoma. Arch Pathol Lab Med 2003; 127:1290.

35. Qualman SJ, Coffin CM, Newton WA, et al. Intergroup Rhabdomyosarcoma Study: update for pathologists. Pediatr Dev Pathol 1998; 1:550.

Age and gender incidence

36. Ragab AH, Heyn R, Tefft M, et al. Infants younger than 1 year of age with rhabdomyosarcoma. Cancer 1986; 58:2606.

37. Lobe TE, Wiener ES, Hays DM, et al. Neonatal rhabdomyosarcoma: the IRS experience. J Pediatr Surg 1994; 29:1167.

38. Little DJ, Ballo MT, Zagars GK, et al. Adult rhabdomyosarcoma: outcome following multimodality treatment. Cancer 2002; 95:377.

39. Hulse N, Raja S, Kumar A, et al. Rhabdomyosarcoma of the extremities in adults. Acta Orthop Belg 2006; 72:199.

40. Esnaola NF, Rubin BP, Baldini EH, et al. Response to chemotherapy and predictors of survival in adult rhabdomyosarcoma. Ann Surg 2001; 234:215.

Clinical features

41. Michalski JM, Meza J, Breneman JC, et al. Influence of radiation therapy parameters on outcome in children treated with radiation therapy for localized parameningeal rhabdomyosarcoma in Intergroup Rhabdomyosarcoma Study group trials II through IV. Int J Radiat Oncol Biol Phys 2004; 59:1027.

42. Meazza C, Ferrari A, Casanova M, et al. Evolving treatment strategies for parameningeal rhabdomyosarcoma: the experience of the Istituto Nazionale Tumori of Milan. Head Neck 2005; 27:49.

43. Yock T, Schneider R, Friedmann A, et al. Proton radiotherapy for orbital rhabdomyosarcoma: clinical outcome and a dosimetric comparison with photons. Int J Radiat Oncol Biol Phys 2005; 63:1161.

44. Punyko JA, Mertens AC, Baker KS, et al. Long-term survival probabilities for childhood rhabdomyosarcoma. A population-based evaluation. Cancer 2005; 103:1475.

45. Buwalda J, Blank LE, Schouwenburg PF, et al. The AMORE protocol as salvage treatment for non-orbital head and neck rhabdomyosarcoma in children. Eur J Surg Oncol 2004; 30:884.

46. Kodet R, Newton WA Jr, Hamoudi AB, et al. Orbital rhabdomyosarcomas and related tumors in childhood: relationship of morphology to prognosis – an Intergroup Rhabdomyosarcoma Study. Med Pediatr Oncol 1997; Oncol 29:51.

47. Gillespie MB, Marshall DT, Day TA, et al. Pediatric rhabdomyosarcoma of the head and neck. Curr Treat Options Oncol 2006; 7:13.

48. Buwalda J, Freling NJ, Blank LE, et al. AMORE protocol in pediatric head and neck rhabdomyosarcoma: descriptive analysis of failure patterns. Head Neck 2005; 27:390.

49. Pappo AS, Meza JL, Donaldson SS, et al. Treatment of localized nonorbital, nonparameningeal head and neck rhabdomyosarcoma: lessons learned from Intergroup Rhabdomyosarcoma Studies III and IV. J Clin Oncol 2003; 21:638.

50. Kaefer M, Rink RC. Genitourinary rhabdomyosarcoma. Treatment options. Urol Clin North Am 2000; 27:471.

51. Cavazzana AO, Schmidt D, Ninfo V, et al. Spindle cell rhabdomyosarcoma. A prognostically favorable variant of rhabdomyosarcoma. Am J Surg Pathol 1992; 16:229.

52. Leuschner I. Spindle cell rhabdomyosarcoma: histologic variant of embryonal rhabdomyosarcoma with association to favorable prognosis. Curr Top Pathol 1995; 89:261.

53. Leuschner I, Newton WA Jr, Schmidt D, et al. Spindle cell variants of embryonal rhabdomyosarcoma in the paratesticular region. A report of the Intergroup Rhabdomyosarcoma Study. Am J Surg Pathol 1993; 17:221.

54. Stewart RJ, Martelli H, Oberlin O, et al. Treatment of children with nonmetastatic paratesticular rhabdomyosarcoma: results of the malignant mesenchymal tumors studies (MMT 84 and MMT 89) of the International

Society of Pediatric Oncology. J Clin Oncol 2003; 21:793.

55. Ferrari A, Bisogno G, Casanova M, et al. Is alveolar histotype a prognostic factor in paratesticular rhabdomyosarcoma? The experience of Italian and German Soft Tissue Sarcoma Cooperative Group. Pediatr Blood Cancer 2004; 42:134.

56. Cecchetto G, Bisogno G, Treuner J, et al. Role of surgery for nonmetastatic abdominal rhabdomyosarcomas: a report from the Italian and German Soft Tissue Cooperative Group's studies. Cancer 2003; 97:1974.

57. Spunt SL, Sweeney TA, Hudson MM, et al. Late effects of pelvic rhabdomyosarcoma and its treatment in female survivors. J Clin Oncol 2005; 23:7143.

58. Raney RB, Stoner JA, Walterhouse DO, et al. Results of treatment of fifty-six patients with localized retroperitoneal and pelvic rhabdomyosarcoma: a report from the Intergroup Rhabdomyosarcoma Study-IV, 1991–1997. Pediatr Blood Cancer 2004; 42:618.

59. Kumar N, Hegarty PK, Johal N, et al. Transpubic radical prostatectomy: a novel approach for rhabdomyosarcoma of the prostate in children. Pediatr Surg Int 2006; 22:453.

60. Soler R, Macedo A Jr, Bruschini H, et al. Does the less aggressive multimodal approach of treating bladder-prostate rhabdomyosarcoma preserve bladder function? J Urol 2005; 174:2343.

61. Nigro KG, MacLennan GT. Rhabdomyosarcoma of the bladder and prostate. J Urol 2005; 173:1365.

62. Ferrer FA. Re: Does bladder preservation (as a surgical principle) lead to retaining bladder function in bladder/prostate rhabdomyosarcoma? Results from Intergroup Rhabdomyosarcoma Study IV. J Urol 2004; 172:2084.

63. Buchwalter CL, Jenison EL, Fromm M, et al. Pure embryonal rhabdomyosarcoma of the fallopian tube. Gynecol Oncol 1997; 67:95.

64. Reynolds EA, Logani S, Moller K, et al. Embryonal rhabdomyosarcoma of the uterus in a postmenopausal woman. Case report and review of the literature. Gynecol Oncol 2006; 103(2):736.

65. Filipas D, Fisch M, Stein R, et al. Rhabdomyosarcoma of the bladder, prostate or vagina: the role of surgery. Br J Urol Int 2004; 93:125.

66. Martelli H, Oberlin O, Rey A, et al. Conservative treatment for girls with nonmetastatic rhabdomyosarcoma of the genital tract: a report from the Study Committee of the International Society of Pediatric Oncology. J Clin Oncol 1999; 17:2117.

67. Okamura K, Yamamoto H, Ishimaru Y, et al. Clinical characteristics and surgical treatment of perianal and perineal rhabdomyosarcoma: analysis of Japanese patients and comparison with IRSG reports. Pediatr Surg Int 2006; 22:129.

67a. Ferguson SE, Gerald W, Barakat RR, et al. Clinicopathologic features of rhabdomyosarcoma of gynecologic origin in adults. Am J Surg Pathol 2007; 31:382.

68. Roebuck DJ. Interventional radiology in children with hepatobiliary rhabdomyosarcoma. Med Pediatr Oncol 1998; 31:187.

69. Roebuck DJ, Yang WT, Lam WW, et al. Hepatobiliary rhabdomyosarcoma in children: diagnostic radiology. Pediatr Radiol 1998; 28:101.

Rhabdomyosarcoma subtypes

70. Kodet R, Newton WA Jr, Hamoudi AB, et al. Childhood rhabdomyosarcoma with

anaplastic (pleomorphic) features. A report of the Intergroup Rhabdomyosarcoma Study. Am J Surg Pathol 1993; 17:443.

71. Coffin CM, Lowichik A, Zhou H. Treatment effects in pediatric soft tissue and bone tumors: practical considerations for the pathologist. Am J Clin Pathol 2005; 123:75.

72. Molenaar WM, Oosterhuis JW, Kamps WA. Cytologic "differentiation" in childhood rhabdomyosarcomas following polychemotherapy. Hum Pathol 1984; 15:973.

73. Daya DA, Scully RE. Sarcoma botryoides of the uterine cervix in young women: a clinicopathological study of 13 cases. Gynecol Oncol 1988; 29:290.

74. Besnard-Guerin C, Newsham I, Winqvist R, et al. A common region of loss of heterozygosity in Wilms' tumor and embryonal rhabdomyosarcoma distal to the D11S988 locus on chromosome 11p15.5. Hum Genet 1996; 97:163.

75. Besnard-Guerin C, Cavenee WK, Newsham I. A new highly polymorphic DNA restriction site marker in the 5′ region of the human tyrosine hydroxylase gene (TH) detecting loss of heterozygosity in human embryonal rhabdomyosarcoma. Hum Genet 1994; 93:349.

76. Sabbioni S, Barbanti-Brodano G, Croce CM, et al. GOK: A gene at 11p15 involved in rhabdomyosarcoma and rhabdoid tumor development. Cancer Res 1997; 57:4493.

77. Afify A, Mark HF. Trisomy 8 in embryonal rhabdomyosarcoma detected by fluorescence in situ hybridization. Cancer Genet Cytogenet 1999; 108:127.

78. Edel G, Wuisman P, Erlemann R. Spindle cell (leiomyomatous) rhabdomyosarcoma, a rare variant of embryonal rhabdomyosarcoma. Pathol Res Pract 1993; 189:102.

79. Nascimento AF, Fletcher CD. Spindle cell rhabdomyosarcoma in adults. Am J Surg Pathol 2005; 29:1106.

80. Rubin BP, Hasserjian RP, Singer S, et al. Spindle cell rhabdomyosarcoma (so-called) in adults: report of two cases with emphasis on differential diagnosis. Am J Surg Pathol 1998; 22:459.

80a. Mentzal T, Kuhnen C. Spindle cell rhabdomyosarcoma in adults: clinicopathological and immunohistochemical analysis of seven new cases. Virchows Arch 2006; 449:554.

81. Leuschner I, Harms D, Mattke A, et al. Rhabdomyosarcoma of the urinary bladder and vagina: a clinicopathologic study with emphasis on recurrent disease: a report from the Kiel pediatric tumor registry and the German CWS study. Am J Surg Pathol 2001; 25:856.

82. Debiec-Rychter M, Hagemeijer A, Sciot R. Spindle-cell rhabdomyosarcoma with 2q36 approximately q37 involvement. Cancer Genet Cytogenet 2003; 140:62.

83. Gil-Benso R, Carda-Batalla C, Navarro-Fos S, et al. Cytogenetic study of a spindle-cell rhabdomyosarcoma of the parotid gland. Cancer Genet Cytogenet 1999; 109:150.

84. Palazzo JP, Gibas Z, Dunton CJ, et al. Cytogenetic study of botryoid rhabdomyosarcoma of the uterine cervix. Virchows Arch A Pathol Anat Histopathol 1993; 422:87.

85. Kadan-Lottick NS, Stork L, Ruyle SZ, et al. Cytogenetic abnormalities in a case of botryoid rhabdomyosarcoma. Med Pediatr Oncol 2000; 34:293.

86. Boman F, Champigneulle J, Schmitt C, et al. Clear cell rhabdomyosarcoma. Pediatr Pathol Lab Med 1996; 16:951.

87. Govender D, Chetty R. Clear cell (glycogen-rich) rhabdomyosarcoma presenting as cervical lymphadenopathy. ORL J Otorhinolaryngol Relat Spec 1999; 61:52.

88. Kahn DG. Rhabdomyosarcoma mimicking acute leukemia in an adult: report of a case with histologic, flow cytometric, cytogenetic, immunohistochemical, and ultrastructural studies. Arch Pathol Lab Med 1998; 122:375.

89. Douglass EC, Valentine M, Etcubanas E, et al. A specific chromosomal abnormality in rhabdomyosarcoma. Cytogenet Cell Genet 1987; 45:148.

90. Turc-Carel C, Lizard-Nacol S, Justrabo E, et al. Consistent chromosomal translocation in alveolar rhabdomyosarcoma. Cancer Genet Cytogenet 1986; 19:361.

91. Barr FG. Gene fusions involving PAX and FOX family members in alveolar rhabdomyo-sarcoma. Oncogene 2001; 20:5736.

92. Xia SJ, Barr FG. Analysis of the transforming and growth suppressive activities of the PAX3-FKHR oncoprotein. Oncogene 2004; 23:6864.

93. Tomescu O, Xia SJ, Strzelecki D, et al. Inducible short-term and stable long-term cell culture systems reveal that the PAX3-FKHR fusion oncoprotein regulates CXCR4, PAX3, and PAX7 expression. Lab Invest 2004; 84:1060.

94. Frascella E, Toffolatti L, Rosolen A. Normal and rearranged PAX3 expression in human rhabdomyosarcoma. Cancer Genet Cytogenet 1998; 102:104.

95. Davis RJ, D'Cruz CM, Lovell MA, et al. Fusion of PAX7 to FKHR by the variant t(1;13)(p36;q14) translocation in alveolar rhabdomyosarcoma. Cancer Res 1994; 54:2869.

96. Biegel JA, Meek RS, Parmiter AH, et al. Chromosomal translocation t(1;13)(p36;q14) in a case of rhabdomyosarcoma. Genes Chromosomes Cancer 1991; 3:483.

97. Barr FG, Smith LM, Lynch JC, et al. Examination of gene fusion status in archival samples of alveolar rhabdomyosarcoma entered on the Intergroup Rhabdomyosarcoma Study-III trial: a report from the Children's Oncology Group. J Mol Diagn 2006; 8:202.

98. Nishio J, Althof PA, Bailey JM, et al. Use of a novel FISH assay on paraffin-embedded tissues as an adjunct to diagnosis of alveolar rhabdomyosarcoma. Lab Invest 2006; 86:547.

98a. Parham DM, Qualman SJ, Teot L, et al. Correlation between histology and PAX/FKHR fusion status in alveolar rhabdomyosarcoma. A report from the Children's Oncology Group. Am J Surg Pathol 2007; 31:895.

99. Kelly KM, Womer RB, Sorensen PH, et al. Common and variant gene fusions predict distinct clinical phenotypes in rhabdomyosarcoma. J Clin Oncol 1997; 15:1831.

100. Barr FG, Qualman SJ, Macris MH, et al. Genetic heterogeneity in the alveolar rhabdomyosarcoma subset without typical gene fusions. Cancer Res 2002; 62:4704.

101. Furlong MA, Mentzel T, Fanburg-Smith JC. Pleomorphic rhabdomyosarcoma in adults: a clinicopathologic study of 38 cases with emphasis on morphologic variants and recent skeletal muscle-specific markers. Mod Pathol 2001; 14:595.

102. Gaffney EF, Dervan PA, Fletcher CD. Pleomorphic rhabdomyosarcoma in adulthood. Analysis of 11 cases with definition of diagnostic criteria. Am J Surg Pathol 1993; 17:601.

103. Hollowood K, Fletcher CD. Rhabdomyosarcoma in adults. Semin Diagn Pathol 1994; 11:47.

104. Furlong MA, Fanburg-Smith JC. Pleomorphic rhabdomyosarcoma in children: four cases in the pediatric age group. Ann Diagn Pathol 2001; 5:199.

105. Linscheid RL, Soule EH, Henderson ED. Pleomorphic rhabdomyosarcomata of the extremities and limb girdles: a clinicopathological study. J Bone Joint Surg [Am] 1965; 47:715.

106. Patton RB, Horn RC Jr. Rhabdomyosarcoma: clinical and pathological features and comparison with human fetal and embryonal skeletal muscle. Surgery 1962; 52:572.

107. Weiss SW, Enzinger FM. Malignant fibrous histiocytoma: an analysis of 200 cases. Cancer 1978; 41:2250.

108. Weiss SW. Malignant fibrous histiocytoma. A reaffirmation. Am J Surg Pathol 1982; 6:773.

109. Seidal T. Rhabdomyosarcoma. Histopathology 1990; 17:482.

110. Fletcher CD. Pleomorphic malignant fibrous histiocytoma: fact or fiction? A critical reappraisal based on 159 tumors diagnosed as pleomorphic sarcoma. Am J Surg Pathol 1992; 16:213.

111. Schürch W, Begin LR, Seemayer TA, et al. Pleomorphic soft tissue myogenic sarcomas of adulthood. A reappraisal in the mid-1990s. Am J Surg Pathol 1996; 20:131.

112. Wesche WA, Fletcher CD, Dias P, et al. Immunohistochemistry of MyoD1 in adult pleomorphic soft tissue sarcomas. Am J Surg Pathol 1995; 19:261.

113. Tallini G, Parham DM, Dias P, et al. Myogenic regulatory protein expression in adult soft tissue sarcomas. A sensitive and specific marker of skeletal muscle differentiation. Am J Pathol 1994; 144:693.

114. Wang NP, Marx J, McNutt MA, et al. Expression of myogenic regulatory proteins (myogenin and MyoD1) in small blue round cell tumors of childhood. Am J Pathol 1995; 147:1799.

115. Folpe AL. MyoD1 and myogenin expression in human neoplasia: a review and update. Adv Anat Pathol 2002; 9:198.

116. Erlandson RA. The ultrastructural distinction between rhabdomyosarcoma and other undifferentiated "sarcomas." Ultrastruct Pathol 1987; 11:83.

117. Mertens F, Fletcher CD, Dal Cin P, et al. Cytogenetic analysis of 46 pleomorphic soft tissue sarcomas and correlation with morphologic and clinical features: a report of the CHAMP study group. Chromosomes and Morphology. Genes Chromosomes Cancer 1998; 22:16.

118. Folpe AL, McKenney JK, Bridge JA, et al. Sclerosing rhabdomyosarcoma in adults: report of four cases of a hyalinizing, matrix-rich variant of rhabdomyosarcoma that may be confused with osteosarcoma, chondrosarcoma, or angiosarcoma. Am J Surg Pathol 2002; 26:1175.

119. Mentzel T, Katenkamp D. Sclerosing, pseudovascular rhabdomyosarcoma in adults. Clinicopathological and immunohistochemical analysis of three cases. Virchows Arch 2000; 436:305.

120. Chiles MC, Parham DM, Qualman SJ, et al. Sclerosing rhabdomyosarcomas in children and adolescents: a clinicopathologic review of 13 cases from the Intergroup Rhabdomyosarcoma Study Group and Children's Oncology Group. Pediatr Dev Pathol 2004; 7:583.

121. Vadgama B, Sebire NJ, Malone M, et al. Sclerosing rhabdomyosarcoma in childhood: case report and review of the literature. Pediatr Dev Pathol 2004; 7:391.

122. Croes R, Debiec-Rychter M, Cokelaere K, et al. Adult sclerosing rhabdomyosarcoma: cytogenetic link with embryonal rhabdomyosarcoma. Virchows Arch 2005; 446:64.

123. Knipe TA, Chandra RK, Bugg MF. Sclerosing rhabdomyosarcoma: a rare variant with predilection for the head and neck. Laryngoscope 2005; 115:48.

124. Kumar S, Perlman E, Harris CA, et al. Myogenin is a specific marker for

rhabdomyosarcoma: an immunohistochemical study in paraffin-embedded tissues. Mod Pathol 2000; 13:988.

125. Dias P, Chen B, Dilday B, et al. Strong immunostaining for myogenin in rhabdomyosarcoma is significantly associated with tumors of the alveolar subclass. Am J Pathol 2000; 156:399.

125a. Wijnaendts LCD, van der Linden JC, van Unnik AJM, et al. The expression pattern of contractile and intermediate filaments proteins in developing skeletal muscle and rhabdomyosarcoma of childhood: diagnostic and prognostic utility. Am J Surg Pathol 1994; 174:283.

Special diagnostic procedures

126. Parham DM, Webber B, Holt H, et al. Immunohistochemical study of childhood rhabdomyosarcomas and related neoplasms. Results of an Intergroup Rhabdomyosarcoma Study Project. Cancer 1991; 67:3072.

127. Schürch W, Bochaton-Piallat ML, Geinoz A, et al. All histological types of primary human rhabdomyosarcoma express alpha-cardiac and not alpha-skeletal actin messenger RNA. Am J Pathol 1994; 144:836.

128. Sassoon DA. Myogenic regulatory factors: dissecting their role and regulation during vertebrate embryogenesis. Dev Biol 1993; 156:11.

129. Tsokos M. The role of immunocytochemistry in the diagnosis of rhabdomyosarcoma. Arch Pathol Lab Med 1986; 110:776.

130. Eusebi V, Bondi A, Rosai J. Immunohistochemical localization of myoglobin in nonmuscular cells. Am J Surg Pathol 1984; 8:51.

131. Coindre JM, de Mascarel A, Trojani M, et al. Immunohistochemical study of rhabdomyosarcoma. Unexpected staining with S100 protein and cytokeratin. J Pathol 1988; 155:127.

132. Miettinen M, Rapola J. Immunohistochemical spectrum of rhabdomyosarcoma and rhabdomyosarcoma-like tumors. Expression of cytokeratin and the 68-kD neurofilament protein. Am J Surg Pathol 1989; 13:120.

133. Molenaar WM, Muntinghe FL. Expression of neural cell adhesion molecules and neurofilament protein isoforms in skeletal muscle tumors. Hum Pathol 1998; 29:1290.

134. Tapscott SJ, Davis RL, Thayer MJ, et al. MyoD1: a nuclear phosphoprotein requiring a myc homology region to convert fibroblasts to myoblasts. Science 1988; 242:405.

135. Davis RL, Cheng PF, Lassar AB, et al. The MyoD DNA binding domain contains a recognition code for muscle-specific gene activation. Cell 1990; 60:733.

136. Miller JB. Myogenic programs of mouse muscle cell lines: expression of myosin heavy chain isoforms, MyoD1, and myogenin. J Cell Biol 1990; 111:1149.

137. Dias P, Parham DM, Shapiro DN, et al. Monoclonal antibodies to the myogenic regulatory protein MyoD1: epitope mapping and diagnostic utility. Cancer Res 1992; 52:6431.

138. Dias P, Parham DM, Shapiro DN, et al. Myogenic regulatory protein (MyoD1) expression in childhood solid tumors: diagnostic utility in rhabdomyosarcoma. Am J Pathol 1990; 137:1283.

138a. Morotti RA, Nicol KK, Parham DM, et al. An immunohistochemical algorithm to facilitate diagnosis and subtyping of rhabdomyosarcoma: the Children's Oncology Group Experience. Am J Surg Pathol 2006; 30:962.

139. Franchi A, Massi D, Santucci M. The comparative role of immunohistochemistry and electron microscopy in the identification of myogenic differentiation in soft tissue pleomorphic sarcomas. Ultrastruct Pathol 2005; 29:295.

140. Churg A, Ringus J. Ultrastructural observations on the histogenesis of alveolar rhabdomyosarcoma. Cancer 1978; 41:1355.

Differential diagnosis

141. Scotlandi K, Serra M, Manara MC, et al. Immunostaining of the p30/32MIC2 antigen and molecular detection of EWS rearrangements for the diagnosis of Ewing's sarcoma and peripheral neuroectodermal tumor. Hum Pathol 1996; 27:408.

142. Hess E, Cohen C, DeRose PB. Nonspecificity of p30/32MIC2 immunolocalization with the 013 monoclonal antibody in the diagnosis of Ewing's sarcoma: application of an algorithmic immunohistochemical analysis. Appl Immunohistochem 1997; 5:94.

143. Lundgren L, Angervall L, Stenman G, et al. Infantile rhabdomyofibrosarcoma: a high-grade sarcoma distinguishable from infantile fibrosarcoma and rhabdomyosarcoma. Hum Pathol 1993; 24:785.

144. Suarez-Vilela D, Izquierdo-Garcia FM, Alonso-Orcajo N. Epithelioid and rhabdoid rhabdomyosarcoma in an adult patient: a diagnostic pitfall. Virchows Arch 2004; 445:323.

145. Kodet R, Newton WA Jr, Hamoudi AB, et al. Rhabdomyosarcomas with intermediate-filament inclusions and features of rhabdoid tumors. Light microscopic and immunohistochemical study. Am J Surg Pathol 1991; 15:257.

146. Woodruff JM, Perino G. Non-germ-cell or teratomatous malignant tumors showing additional rhabdomyoblastic differentiation, with emphasis on the malignant triton tumor. Semin Diagn Pathol 1994; 11:69.

147. Henricks WH, Chu YC, Goldblum JR, et al. Dedifferentiated liposarcoma: a clinicopathological analysis of 155 cases with a proposal for an expanded definition of dedifferentiation. Am J Surg Pathol 1997; 21:271.

148. Prat J, Young RH, Scully RE. Ovarian Sertoli-Leydig cell tumors with heterologous elements. II. Cartilage and skeletal muscle: a clinicopathologic analysis of twelve cases. Cancer 1982; 50:2465.

149. Ordonez NG, Tornos C. Malignant peripheral nerve sheath tumor of the pleura with epithelial and rhabdomyoblastic differentiation: report of a case clinically simulating mesothelioma. Am J Surg Pathol 1997; 21:1515.

150. Velagaleti GV, Miettinen M, Gatalica Z. Malignant peripheral nerve sheath tumor with rhabdomyoblastic differentiation (malignant Triton tumor) with balanced t(7;9)(q11.2;p24) and unbalanced translocation der(16)t(1;16)(q23;q13). Cancer Genet Cytogenet 2004; 149:23.

151. Huang L, Espinoza C, Welsh R. Malignant peripheral nerve sheath tumor with divergent differentiation. Arch Pathol Lab Med 2003; 127:e147.

152. Weiss E, Albrecht CF, Herms J, et al. Malignant ectomesenchymoma of the cerebrum. Case report and discussion of therapeutic options. Eur J Pediatr 2005; 164:345.

153. Oppenheimer O, Athanasian E, Meyers P, et al. Malignant ectomesenchymoma in the wrist of a child: case report and review of the literature. Int J Surg Pathol 2005; 13:113.

Discussion

154. Enzinger FM, Lattes R, Torloni H. Histological typing of soft tissue tumours. In: International histological classification of tumors, No. 3. Geneva: World Health Organization; 1969.

155. Pappo AS, Shapiro DN, Crist WM, et al. Biology and therapy of pediatric rhabdomyosarcoma. J Clin Oncol 1995; 13:2123.

156. Lawrence W Jr, Anderson JR, Gehan EA, et al. Pretreatment TNM staging of childhood rhabdomyosarcoma: a report of the Intergroup Rhabdomyosarcoma Study Group. Children's Cancer Study Group. Pediatric Oncology Group. Cancer 1997; 80:1165.

157. Stevens MC, Rey A, Bouvet N, et al. Treatment of nonmetastatic rhabdomyosarcoma in childhood and adolescence: Third study of the International Society of Paediatric Oncology – SIOP malignant mesenchymal tumor 89. J Clin Oncol 2005; 23:2618.

158. Carli M, Colombatti R, Oberlin O, et al. European Intergroup studies (MMT4-89 and MMT4-91) on childhood metastatic rhabdomyosarcoma: final results and analysis of prognostic factors. J Clin Oncol 2004; 22:4787.

159. Mondaini N, Palli D, Saieva C, et al. Clinical characteristics and overall survival in genitourinary sarcomas treated with curative intent: a multicenter study. Eur Urol 2005; 47:468.

160. Wijnaendts LC, van der Linden JC, Van Unnik AJ, et al. Histopathological features and grading in rhabdomyosarcomas of childhood. Histopathology 1994; 24:303.

161. Coffin CM, Rulon J, Smith L, et al. Pathologic features of rhabdomyosarcoma before and after treatment: a clinicopathologic and immunohistochemical analysis. Mod Pathol 1997; 10:1175.

162. La Quaglia MP, Heller G, Ghavimi F, et al. The effect of age at diagnosis on outcome in rhabdomyosarcoma. Cancer 1994; 73:109.

163. Hawkins HK, Camacho-Velasquez JV. Rhabdomyosarcoma in children. Correlation of form and prognosis in one institution's experience. Am J Surg Pathol 1987; 11:531.

164. Pappo AS, Crist WM, Kuttesch J, et al. Tumor-cell DNA content predicts outcome in children and adolescents with clinical group III embryonal rhabdomyosarcoma. The Intergroup Rhabdomyosarcoma Study Committee of the Children's Cancer Group and the Pediatric Oncology Group. J Clin Oncol 1993; 11:1901.

165. Kilpatrick SE, Teot LA, Geisinger KR, et al. Relationship of DNA ploidy to histology and prognosis in rhabdomyosarcoma. Comparison of flow cytometry and image analysis. Cancer 1994; 74:3227.

166. San Miguel-Fraile P, Carrillo-Gijon R, Rodriguez-Peralto JL, et al. Prognostic significance of DNA ploidy and proliferative index (MIB-1 index) in childhood rhabdomyosarcoma. Am J Clin Pathol 2004; 121:358.

167. Pohar-Marinsek Z, Bracko M, Lavrencak J, et al. DNA ploidy as a prognostic factor in rhabdomyosarcoma. Analysis of 35 cases with image cytometry. Anal Quant Cytol Histol 2003; 25:235.

168. San Miguel-Fraile P, Carrillo-Gijon R, Rodriguez-Peralto JL, et al. DNA content and proliferative activity in pediatric genitourinary rhabdomyosarcoma. Pediatr Pathol Mol Med 2003; 22:143.

169. Staibano S, Franco R, Tranfa F, et al. Orbital rhabdomyosarcoma: relationship between DNA ploidy, p53, bcl-2, MDR-1 and Ki67 (MIB1) expression and clinical behavior. Anticancer Res 2004; 24:249.

170. Noguchi S, Tamiya S, Nagoshi M, et al. The prognostic importance of nuclear morphometry and the MIB-1 index in rhabdomyosarcoma. Mod Pathol 1996; 9:253.

171. De Zen L, Sommaggio A, d'Amore ES, et al. Clinical relevance of DNA ploidy and proliferative activity in childhood rhabdomyosarcoma: a retrospective analysis of patients enrolled onto the Italian Cooperative Rhabdomyosarcoma Study RMS88. J Clin Oncol 1997; 15:1198.

172. Takahashi Y, Oda Y, Kawaguchi K, et al. Altered expression and molecular abnormalities of cell-cycle-regulatory proteins in rhabdomyosarcoma. Mod Pathol 2004; 17:660.

173. Leuschner I, Langhans I, Schmitz R, et al. p53 and mdm-2 expression in rhabdomyosarcoma of childhood and adolescence: clinicopathologic study by the Kiel pediatric tumor registry and the German Cooperative Soft Tissue Sarcoma Study. Pediatr Dev Pathol 2003; 6:128.

174. Xia SJ, Pressey JG, Barr FG. Molecular pathogenesis of rhabdomyosarcoma. Cancer Biol Ther 2002; 1:97.

175. Williamson D, Lu YJ, Gordon T, et al. Relationship between MYCN copy number and expression in rhabdomyosarcomas and correlation with adverse prognosis in the alveolar subtype. J Clin Oncol 2005; 23:880.

176. Toffolatti L, Frascella E, Ninfo V, et al. MYCN expression in human rhabdomyosarcoma cell lines and tumour samples. J Pathol 2002; 196:450.

177. Lu YJ, Williamson D, Clark J, et al. Comparative expressed sequence hybridization to chromosomes for tumor classification and identification of genomic regions of differential gene expression. Proc Natl Acad Sci USA 2001; 98:9197.

178. Gallego S, Llort A, Parareda A, et al. Expression of multidrug resistance-1 and multidrug resistance-associated protein genes in pediatric rhabdomyosarcoma. Oncol Rep 2004; 11:179.

179. Komdeur R, Klunder J, van der Graaf WT, et al. Multidrug resistance proteins in rhabdomyosarcomas: comparison between children and adults. Cancer 2003; 97:1999.

180. Kuttesch JF, Parham DM, Luo X, et al. P-glycoprotein expression at diagnosis may not be a primary mechanism of therapeutic failure

181. Klunder JW, Komdeur R, Van Der Graaf WT, et al. Expression of multidrug resistance-associated proteins in rhabdomyosarcomas before and after chemotherapy: the relationship between lung resistance-related protein (LRP) and differentiation. Hum Pathol 2003; 34:150.

182. Sorensen PH, Lynch JC, Qualman SJ, et al. PAX3-FKHR and PAX7-FKHR gene fusions are prognostic indicators in alveolar rhabdomyosarcoma: a report from the Children's Oncology Group. J Clin Oncol 2002; 20:2672.

183. Paulino AC. Late affects of radiotherapy for pediatric extremity sarcomas. Int J Radiat Oncol Biol Phys 2004; 60:265.

184. Raney B Jr, Heyn R, Hays DM, et al. Sequelae of treatment in 109 patients followed for 5 to 15 years after diagnosis of sarcoma of the bladder and prostate. A report from the Intergroup Rhabdomyosarcoma Study Committee. Cancer 1993; 71:2387.

185. Heyn R, Haeberlen V, Newton WA, et al. Second malignant neoplasms in children treated for rhabdomyosarcoma. Intergroup Rhabdomyosarcoma Study Committee. J Clin Oncol 1993; 11:262.

186. Raney RB. Spinal cord "drop metastases" from head and neck rhabdomyosarcoma: Proceedings of the Tumor Board of the Children's Hospital of Philadelphia. Med Pediatr Oncol 1978; 4:3.

187. Meazza C, Ferrari A, Casanova M, et al. Rhabdomyosarcoma of the head and neck region: experience at the pediatric unit of the Istituto Nazionale Tumori, Milan. J Otolaryngol 2006; 35:53.

188. Mazzoleni S, Bisogno G, Garaventa A, et al. Outcomes and prognostic factors after recurrence in children and adolescents with nonmetastatic rhabdomyosarcoma. Cancer 2005; 104:183.

189. Raney RB Jr, Tefft M, Maurer HM, et al. Disease patterns and survival rate in children with metastatic soft-tissue sarcoma. A report from the Intergroup Rhabdomyosarcoma Study (IRS)-I. Cancer 1988; 62:1257.

190. Williams BA, Williams KM, Doyle J, et al. Metastatic rhabdomyosarcoma: a retrospective review of patients treated at the hospital for sick children between 1989 and 1999. J Pediatr Hematol Oncol 2004; 26:243.

191. Wharam MD, Meza J, Anderson J, et al. Failure pattern and factors predictive of local failure in rhabdomyosarcoma: a report of group III patients on the third Intergroup Rhabdomyosarcoma Study. J Clin Oncol 2004; 22:1902.

192. Ferrari A, Bisogno G, Casanova M, et al. Paratesticular rhabdomyosarcoma: report from the Italian and German Cooperative Group. J Clin Oncol 2002; 20:449.

193. Pratt CB, Hustu HO, Kumar APM, et al. Treatment of childhood rhabdomyosarcoma at St. Jude Children's Research Hospital 1962–1978. Natl Cancer Inst Monogr 1981; 56:93.

194. Setterfield J, Sciot R, Debiec-Rychter M, et al. Primary cutaneous epidermotropic alveolar rhabdomyosarcoma with t(2;13) in an elderly woman: case report and review of the literature. Am J Surg Pathol 2002; 26:938.

195. Rodriguez-Galindo C, Hill DA, Onyekwere O, et al. Neonatal alveolar rhabdomyosarcoma with skin and brain metastases. Cancer 2001; 92:1613.

196. Barr FG, Chatten J, D'Cruz CM, et al. Molecular assays for chromosomas translocations in the diagnosis of pediatric soft tissue sarcomas. JAMA 1995; 273:553.

197. De Alava E, Ladanyi M, Rosai J, et al. Detection of chimeric transcripts in desmoplastic small round cell tumor and related developmental tumors by reverse transcriptase polymerase chain reaction: a specific diagnostic assay. Am J Pathol 1995; 147:1584.

198. Downing JR, Khandeker A, Shurtleff SA, et al. Multiplex RT-PCR assay for the differential diagnosis of alveolar rhabdomyosarcoma and Ewing's sarcoma. Am J Pathol 1995; 146:626.

199. Arden KC, Anderson MJ, Finckenstein FG, et al. Detection of the t(2;13) translocation in alveolar rhabdomyosarcoma using the reverse transcriptase-polymerase chain reaction. Genes Chromosomes Cancer 1996; 16:254.

BENIGN TUMORS AND TUMOR-LIKE LESIONS OF BLOOD VESSELS

CHAPTER CONTENTS

Hemangiomas are benign lesions that closely resemble normal vessels. So faithfully is this facsimile reproduced that it is difficult to distinguish clearly hamartomas, malformations, and tumors. These taxonomic distinctions are complicated by the fact that classifications of vascular lesions as proposed by clinicians, pathologists, and radiologists are based on different parameters.[1,2] For example, clinicians emphasize clinical presentation and growth characteristics and contend that lesions present at birth are malformations, whereas actively growing lesions presenting shortly after birth are neoplastic (e.g., juvenile hemangioma). Although scientific evidence supports the idea that congenital and noncongenital lesions may be fundamentally different, there are problematic aspects to this generalization.[2] For example, some congenital malformations may not become apparent until later in life (e.g., angiomatosis) depending on their location and rate of growth and those "hemangiomas" that regress with time may not be neoplasms at all. The pathologist, lacking detailed clinical and radiologic information, classifies vascular lesions by vessel type (e.g., capillary, venous) such that lesions with different clinical or radiologic features might well earn the same pathologic designation. Some vascular lesions have been linked recently to specific genetic defects,[3–7] suggesting that with time the classification of vascular lesions will embrace an even more sophisticated level of information (Table 22–1).

In this chapter we have utilized a classification based on pathologic features but indicate in specific situations the unique clinical and radiographic features that accompany the lesion. "Hemangioma" is used in the broadest sense as a benign, nonreactive process in which there is an increase in the number of normal or abnormal-appearing vessels, recognizing that many of these lesions represent tissue malformations rather than true tumors.

There are two principal forms of hemangioma: those localized to one area and those that involve large segments of the body, such as an entire extremity. The latter type, known as *angiomatosis*, deserves specific mention because of the inherent problems it poses in diagnosis and therapy. Localized hemangiomas, however, are far more common and account for most of the vascular tumors encountered in daily practice.

NORMAL STRUCTURE AND FUNCTION

Vascular development

Vasculogenesis refers to the *de novo* development of blood vessels from stem cells or primitive endothelial cells and contrasts with *angiogenesis*, a term that implies the formation of new microvessels from differentiated endothelium.[8] Vasculogenesis is largely restricted to early embryogenesis, whereas angiogenesis occurs during embryogenesis and in the postnatal state. Angiogenesis is also the mechanism whereby tumors derive their blood supply.

On a molecular level, embryonic vasculogenesis and angiogenesis are the result of a series of genetic events that depend on the orderly expression of at least two sets of tyrosine kinase receptors, one set largely influencing endothelial differentiation and proliferation and the other governing vascular wall formation and vascular bed morphogenesis.[9]

The embryonic vascular system develops during the third week of fetal life from mesodermal cells of the "blood islands." Initially located in the region of the yolk sac, these cells eventually populate the mesenchyme throughout the fetus. Early events in vasculogenesis are dependent on fibroblast growth factor (FGF) and vascular endothelial growth factors A and B (VEGF A and B). Under their influence, angioblasts differentiate from mesoderm of the blood islands, proliferate, migrate, and ultimately form primitive vascular tubes. The pattern of endothelial differentiation is further determined by VEGF C and its receptor (VEGFR3) which are expressed on

TABLE 22–1	HEREDITARY VASCULAR MALFORMATIONS				
Malformation		Locus	Locus name	Mutated gene	Type of mutation
Hereditary capillary malformation (CM)		5q13-15	CMC	?	
Cerebral cavernous (or capillary) malformation (CCM)		7q11-22	CCM1	KRIT1	Inactivating?
		7p13-35	CCM2	?	
		3q25.2-27	CCM3	?	
Hyperkeratotic cutaneous capillary venous malformation (HCCVM)		7q11-22	CCM1	KRIT1	Inactivating?
Arteriovenous malformation		5q13-15?	CMC1	?	
Hereditary hemorrhagic telangiectasia (HHT)		9q33-34	HHT1	ENG	Inactivating
		12q11-14	HHT2	ALK1	Inactivating
Venous malformation (VM)		9p21	VMCM1	TIE2 (TEK)	Activating
Glomuvenous malformation		1p21-22	VMGLOM	GLOMULIN	Inactivating?
Primary congenital lymphedema (Milroy's disease)		5q34-35	?	FLT4 (VEGFR3)	Inactivating?

Modified from Brouillard P, Vikkula M. Vascular malformations: localized defects in vascular morphogenesis. Clin Genet 2003; 63:340.

endothelial cells destined to become veins and lymphatics.[9] Mesenchymal cells, recruited to the surface of the newly formed vascular tubes, differentiate into pericytes and smooth muscle cells. This process is likely mediated by platelet-derived growth factor (PDGF) which is secreted from the basal surface of the immature endothelium and which finds ready targets on the surface of muscle cell progenitors. Abolishing either PDGF or its receptor at this stage results in pericyte-poor vessels that hemorrhage easily. Continued growth of endothelial cells and modeling of vascular walls is dependent on the expression of an additional set of receptor tyrosine kinases (Tie1 and Tie2) and angiopoietin 1 (Ang1) and angiopoietin 2 (Ang2), the ligands for Tie2. Although the function of Ang1 and Ang2 are contextual and vary from organ to organ, they can, under certain circumstances, function as antagonists. Ang1, produced by mural cells, stabilizes nascent vessels by making them leak resistant, whereas Ang2, in the absence of VEGF, destabilizes vessels and allows their regression. Recently it has been shown that mutations in either Ang1 or its receptor Tie2 result in defective vessels with vascular malformations characterized by poorly formed muscle walls and microaneurysms.

In contrast to formation of blood vessels in the embryo, new vessel formation in the postnatal state occurs largely as a result of microvessel formation from differentiated endothelial cells. Angiogenesis is governed by a complex interaction of proangiogenic and antiangiogenic factors[10,11] (Table 22–2) which are under tight control so that there is little, if any, increase in vessels in the normal state.[9] However, in response to stimuli such as tissue injury or hypoxia, this balance is perturbed and angiogenesis occurs. These substances therefore serve as "signals" that influence growth, migration, and the permeability of endothelial cells. During angiogenesis, endothelial cells acquire protease, which permits them to digest basal lamina and move in the direction of the signal. Foremost among the signaling substances are VEGF and FGF. Once separated from a parent vessel, endothelial cells acquire small vacuoles or primitive lumens, which fuse with

TABLE 22–2	PROANGIOGENIC AND ANTIANGIOGENIC MOLECULES

Proangiogenic molecules
Basic fibroblast growth factor (FGF)
Vascular endothelial growth factor (VEGF)
Prostaglandin E_2
Hepatocyte growth factor
Nitric oxide
Integrins
Interleukin-8
Platelet-derived growth factor

Antiangiogenic molecules
Angiostatin
Endostatin
Curcumin
Thalidomide
Nitric oxide inhibitors
Interferon-α
Glucocorticoids
Retinoids

Modified from Arbiser JL. Angiogenesis: relevance for pathogenesis and treatment of dermatologic disease. Adv Dermatol 1999; 15:31.

lumens of adjacent endothelium to form capillary channels. Although the mechanism by which these signals are processed by the endothelial cells is still the subject of intense inquiry, it appears that endothelial junctions (adherens junctions) play a pivotal role.[12] This specialized apparatus, consisting of a transmembrane protein VE (vascular endothelial) cadherin bound in its intracellular domain to catenin and in its extracellular domain to VE cadherins of adjacent cells, localizes or traps extracellular signaling molecules. The extracellular signals, in turn, alter the cadherin-catenin complex, thereby modifying the confluence and permeability of the endothelial cell. The cadherin-catenin complex is also involved in intracellular signaling from the cytoplasm to the nucleus such that gene expression is affected.

In addition to the above generalizations there is firm evidence that tissues play a critical role in determining both the diversity of endothelial cells and organ-specific variations of the capillary bed and that in reciprocal fashion endothelial cells may communicate by signaling pathways with tissues. Impressive differences have been documented between endothelium of small and large vessels, between endothelium of veins and arteries, and between endothelium of neoplastic and non-neoplastic vessels by both DNA microarray analysis and *in vivo* phage display. These findings have led to the concept that each type of endothelium bears a destination address or "zip code" and that elucidating these differences may lead to organ-specific therapeutic targeting.[13]

Normal structure

The vasculature is divided into arterial and venous components joined by a network of capillaries. The arteries represent a system of dichotomously branching conduits that regulate pressure and deliver blood to the capillary bed; the thin-walled veins return blood to the heart under lower pressures. The capillaries along with the terminal venules are the principal sites of gas exchange. Larger venules (postcapillary venules) are sensitive to vasoactive amines; hence they represent the most permeable portions of the vascular tree. The capillaries represent the smallest vessels, but it is often difficult to determine morphologically the exact point of transition between the smallest vein (or artery) and the capillary. Indeed, the current definition of *capillary* as a vessel, the diameter of which approximates that of the normal erythrocyte (8 nm), is based not only on morphologic but also physiologic observations.[14] The vessels are composed of a single flattened endothelial cell surrounded by basal lamina and occasional pericytes. The basal lamina is not appreciated by light microscopy but can be inferred by the periodic acid-Schiff (PAS)-positive staining material underneath the endothelium. Although this basic pattern pertains to all capillaries, electron microscopy has demonstrated various alterations from organ to organ. For instance, capillaries consisting of a continuous layer of endothelium and basal lamina are typical of capillaries in skeletal and smooth muscle. Fenestrated capillaries, with small pores closed by flaps or diaphragms, are found in endocrine organs, the renal glomerulus, and other sites where there is rapid exchange of solute material.

Veins parallel the arterial system but are more numerous and appear as partially collapsed structures in tissue sections as a result of their inelasticity. In large and medium-sized veins most of the wall is composed of adventitia made up of muscle fibers and elastic tissue arranged in a less orderly fashion than in the arteries. Small veins have no elastic tissue and only a small investiture of smooth muscle. The smallest veins are difficult to distinguish from small arteries, and the distinction at times is best made by the topographic relation to the capillary.

Ultrastructure of the vascular membrane

The endothelial cell has an elongated shape and measures 25–50 nm in length. It is covered on its luminal aspect by a fine coat of carbohydrate-rich material. Underneath the fine cell coat, the luminal surface is thrown into small folds or projections. Small micropinocytotic vesicles (60–70 nm) dot both the luminal and antiluminal surfaces of the cell and are believed important in the transport of fluid across the cell.[15] The cytoplasm usually contains a small amount of smooth and rough endoplasmic reticulum, free ribosomes, and mitochondria. A variety of filaments are present in the endothelium, including thin (actin), intermediate (vimentin), and thick (myosin) filaments. Rod-shaped bodies (Weibel-Palade bodies), a relatively specific feature of the endothelial cell, measure 0.1–0.3 nm in length and contain an internal structure of parallel tubules. They vary in number depending on the type of vessel; and on rare occasions they are also found in pericytes. Von Willebrand factor has been localized to these organelles by means of immunoelectron microscopy.[16] Intercellular attachments are typically prominent in the endothelial cell. Arterioles have elaborate attachments, whereas venules have less prominent ones, a feature that correlates with the observation that the venules represent preferred sites of permeability changes.

Vascular endothelium rests on a thin basal lamina (50 nm) of nonperiodic collagen, which is synthesized at least in part by the endothelial cells. In some areas in the vascular tree, the basal lamina may have a multilayered appearance. External to the endothelium but enveloped within the basal lamina are the pericytes. These mesenchymal cells have few distinguishing features apart from their branched processes, their close contacts with the endothelial cell, and their investiture by basal lamina. These cells are probably derived from fibroblasts of the surrounding connective tissue and in turn may differentiate into smooth muscle cells of the vessel wall.

Normal function

In additional to its traditional lining, or barrier, role the endothelium engages in a variety of other functions including vasoregulation, coagulation, and mediation of the immune response. The specific function and phenotype of a given endothelial cell are dependent on the tissue in question, the local microenvironment, and the activation by cytokines. Basic properties of endothelial metabolism include its ability to transport macromolecules through its system of pinocytotic vesicles, its receptor-mediated uptake of low-density lipoproteins, and its uptake of sugars and amino acids. Endothelium has both procoagulant and anticoagulant properties, but under normal conditions it represents a nonthrombogenic surface. It synthesizes von Willebrand factor,[16] factor V, and plasminogen activator, which promote coagulation, whereas thrombomodulin, a surface endothelial protein, indirectly causes proteolyisis of von Willebrand factor and factor V. When appropriately stimulated, endothelial cells produce prostacyclin, a potent inhibitor of platelet aggregation. By virtue of its interactions with various mediators, the endothelium, particularly that of the microcirculation, is an important regulator of vascular tone and permeability. It produces both vasodilators (e.g., nitric oxide) and vasoconstrictors (e.g., angiotensin-converting enzyme and endothelin). Finally, endothelium participates in the immune and inflammatory responses by facilitating cell adhesion and transmigration. The selectins and the immunoglobulin gene superfamily are the two most important groups of cellular adhesion molecules expressed by endothelium. Many are constitutively expressed by endothelium but can also be upregulated by inflammatory cytokines. For example, intercellular adhesion molecule-1 (ICAM-1) is normally expressed by endothelium but increases during the inflammatory response and is responsible for leukocyte adhesion and transendothelial migration.

HEMANGIOMAS

Hemangioma is one of the most common soft tissue tumors (7% of all benign tumors) and is the most common tumor during infancy and childhood.[17-22] Most hemangiomas are superficial lesions that have a predilection for the head and neck region, but they may also occur internally, notably in organs such as the liver (Table 22–3). The common capillary and cavernous hemangiomas of adults are more frequently encountered in women and may fluctuate in size with pregnancy and menarche; this suggests that the endothelial cells of these tumors

TABLE 22–3	DISTRIBUTION OF 570 HEMANGIOMAS
Location	No. of cases
Cutaneous or mucosal hemangiomas	370
Oral cavity	80
Face	75
Arm	60
Leg	50
Scalp	46
Vulva and scrotum	5
Other	54
Liver	109
Central nervous system	43
Heart	16
Bone	12
Gastrointestinal tract, kidney, mesentery	10
Muscle	10
Total	**570**

Data modified from Geshickter CF, Keasbey LE. Tumors of blood vessels. Am J Cancer 1935; 23:568.

may be responsive to circulating hormones. Although some vascular tumors regress altogether (e.g., juvenile hemangioma), most persist if untreated but have limited growth potential. Hemangiomas virtually never undergo malignant transformation; likewise, the concept of a benign metastasizing hemangioma is no longer accepted. Most prove to be angiosarcomas with well-differentiated areas.

Capillary (lobular) hemangioma

Capillary hemangiomas comprise the largest single group of hemangiomas. Architecturally, virtually all are composed of nodules of small capillary-sized vessels, each of which is subserved by a "feeder" vessel and for this reason they are often referred to as lobular hemangiomas. This lobular or grouped arrangement of vessels is a helpful feature for distinguishing benign and malignant vascular proliferations.[23] There are several variants of capillary hemangioma discussed below.

Capillary hemangiomas usually appear during the first few years of life (with the notable exception of the senile or cherry angioma) and are located in the skin or subcutaneous tissue. Rare cases are familial; linkage analysis has localized the mutation to chromosome 5[24] although the candidate gene has not been identified. However, sporadic hemangiomas also exhibit loss of heterozygosity in the region of 5q, which includes the FLT4 (VEGFR3)[25] gene. Typically elevated and red to purple in color, they are composed of a proliferation of capillary-sized vessels lined by flattened endothelium (Fig. 22–1).

Juvenile hemangioma

The juvenile hemangioma is a form of capillary hemangioma[24,26-37] which occurs during infancy at a rate of about 1 in every 200 live births.[38] About one-fifth of the cases are multiple. During the early stage it may resemble a common birthmark in that it is a flat, red lesion that intensifies in color when the infant strains or cries. With time it acquires an elevated, protruding appearance that distinguishes it from birthmarks and has earned it the fanciful designation of *strawberry nevus* (Fig. 22–2). Deeply situated lesions impart little color to the overlying skin and consequently may be misdiagnosed preoperatively. These tumors may be located on any body surface but are most common in the region of the head and neck, particularly the parotid, where they seemingly follow the distribution of cutaneous nerves and arteries.

The evolution of these lesions is characteristic. Although described as congenital they actually appear within a few weeks after birth[38] and rapidly enlarge over a period of several months, achieving the largest size in about 6–12 months; they regress over a period of a few years. Regression is usually accompanied by fading of the lesion from scarlet to dull red-gray and by concomitant

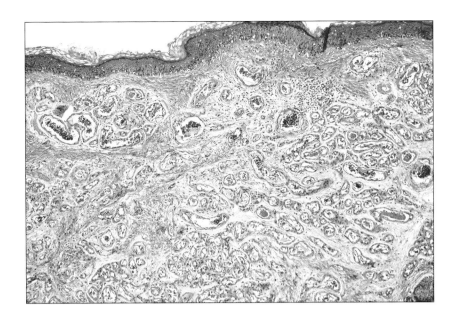

FIGURE 22–1 Adult form of capillary hemangioma consisting of small vessels lined by flattened mature endothelium.

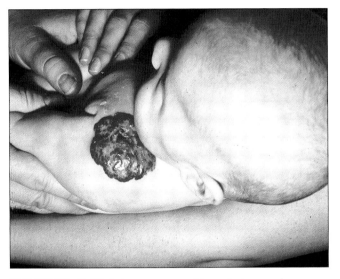

FIGURE 22–2 Clinical appearance of juvenile hemangioma.

wrinkling of the once-taut skin. It has been estimated that by age 7 years, 75–90% have involuted, leaving a small pigmented scar. In the lesions that have ulcerated, the cosmetic defect may be more significant. The clinical phases of juvenile hemangioma have distinctive physiologic differences elegantly detailed by Takahashi et al.[39] (see below).

The tumors are multinodular masses fed by a single normally occurring arteriole (Fig. 22–3).[38] Histologically, the tumor varies with its age. Early lesions are characterized by plump endothelial cells that line vascular spaces with small inconspicuous lumens (Figs 22–4 to 22–6). Mitotic figures may be present in moderate numbers. Mast cells and factor XIII-positive interstitial cells are a consistent feature of these tumors. The former may be

important in the production of angiogenic factors that regulate the growth of these tumors.[31] At this early stage of development the vascular nature of the tumor may not be readily apparent unless a reticulin preparation is done that demonstrates connective tissue fibers encircling myriad tiny vessels. As the lesions mature and blood flow through the lesion commences, the endothelium becomes flattened and resembles that seen in adult forms of capillary hemangioma (Fig. 22–5). Maturation usually begins at the periphery of the tumors but ultimately involves all zones. Regression of the juvenile hemangioma is accompanied by a progressive, diffuse interstitial fibrosis and is believed to be mediated by way of apoptosis. In unusual cases infarction of the tumor may occur, presumably as a result of thrombosis.

Electron microscopy and immunohistochemistry can be helpful for defining the vascular nature of these tumors.[34,35,40] Solid nests of endothelium are surrounded by basal lamina and are encircled by a cuff of pericytes (Fig. 22–6). More mature areas, of course, display canalization of the vessels. Weibel-Palade bodies may be present but tend to be scarce in less mature areas. A peculiar crystalline structure has been identified in the endothelium of these tumors.[41,42] Measuring about 0.5–2.0 mm, they have a substructure consisting of parallel lamellar bands with a periodicity of 18–30 nm. Their exact significance is unknown, although it is believed that they reflect the immaturity of the endothelium, as similar structures have been noted in human fetal endothelium.

The clinical phases of juvenile hemangiomas have been correlated with a distinctive immunophenotypic profile.[36,37,39,43–46] During the early proliferative phase (0–12 months) the tumors can be shown immunohistochemically to express proliferating cell nuclear antigen (PCNA), VEGF, and type IV collagenase, the former two

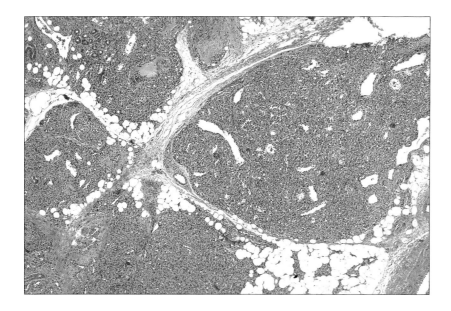

FIGURE 22-3 Low-power view of juvenile hemangioma illustrating lobular growth. Lobules contain central "feeding" vessels.

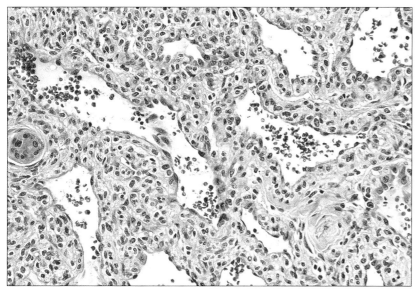

FIGURE 22-4 Juvenile form of capillary hemangioma showing combination of well-canalized and poorly-canalized vessels.

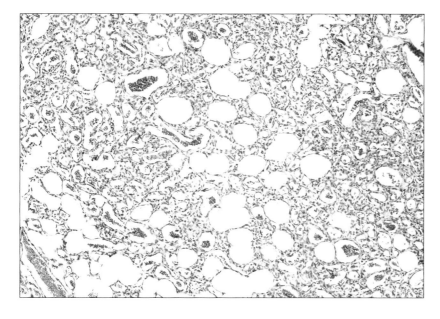

FIGURE 22-5 Juvenile hemangioma showing canalization of most vessels.

localized to both endothelium and pericytes and the last to endothelium. All of these substances are associated with proliferation and growth of vessels. The adjacent epidermis potentially contributes to the production of angiogenic factors.[43] During the involuting phase (1–5 years) these substances are dramatically reduced, whereas the tissue inhibitors of metalloproteinases (TIMP), anti-angiogenic factors, are markedly elevated. The traditional vascular markers CD31, von Willebrand factor (vWF), and smooth muscle actin (a pericyte marker) are present during the proliferative and involuting phases but are lost after the lesion is fully involuted. These findings contrast with congenital vascular lesions and malformations, which remain static throughout their natural history, and do not express PCNA, VEGF, and type IV collagenase. Juvenile hemangiomas also express GLUT1, a glucose transport receptor.[46] The expression of this receptor is independent of proliferative activity and is not found in other forms of hemangioma, although it is present rarely in angiosarcomas. This protein is also expressed by human placenta and has led to the novel hypothesis that the proliferative component of juvenile hemangiomas may be derived from embolized placental vascular cells.[46]

Treatment of these lesions must be individualized and depends on factors such as the location and rate of growth. When this tumor is in the rapid growth phase, there is often a tendency to be overzealous in therapy. It has been suggested that these lesions be approached with a policy of masterful neglect. Most can be followed clinically with little or no intervention. Large, life-threatening lesions impinging on critical structures (e.g., airway) are usually treated with systemic glucocorticoids until a clinical response is achieved. A second option is interferon-α (INFα) which retards endothelial proliferation. Both glucocorticoids[47] and INFα require long-term administra-

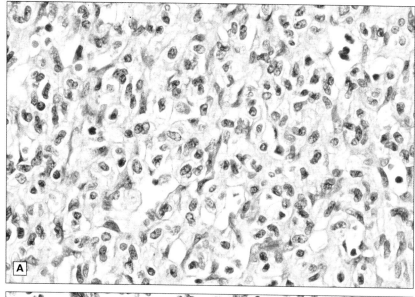

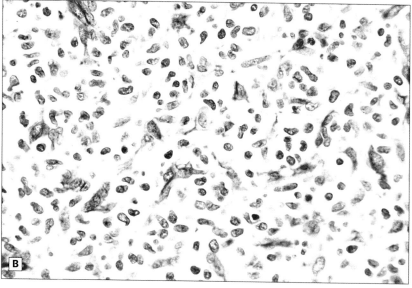

FIGURE 22–6 (A) High power view of cellular areas of juvenile hemangioma. **(B)** Immunostain for von Willebrand factor (vWF) illustrates a network of mature endothelial cells. Note the population of nonreactive cells representing a combination of immature endothelial cells and pericytes.

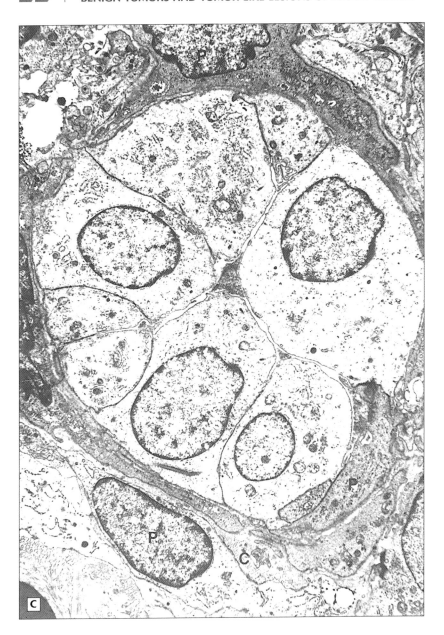

FIGURE 22-6 Continued. **(C)** Electron micrograph of juvenile hemangioma. Prominent endothelial cells eclipse the lumen. Vessels are surrounded by basal lamina, pericytes (P), and collagen (C). (From Taxy JB, Battifora H. In: Trump BF, Jones RT, eds. Diagnostic electron microscopy. New York: Wiley; 1980.)

tion with some attendant side effects. INFα, in particular, has been associated with spastic diplegia.[11]

North et al. recently demonstrated that juvenile hemangiomas have nonrandom X-inactivation patterns suggesting they are monoclonal proliferations. Two of the 15 cases studied also harbored somatic mutations of VEGFR2 (FLK1/KDR) or VEGFR3 (FLT4) which the authors suggest represent gain of function mutations that account for tumorigenesis.[46]

Pyogenic granuloma (granulation tissue-type hemangioma)

The pyogenic granuloma is a polypoid form of capillary hemangioma occurring on the skin and mucosal surfaces. Its pathogenesis is controversial, some considering them neoplasms and others a reactive hyperplasia. Their lobular architecture has been used to justify their inclusion with other capillary hemangiomas, but conversely their appearance following trauma, during pregnancy (see granuloma gravidarum), and during retinoid therapy[48] mounts a compelling counterargument.

The pyogenic granuloma bears a striking resemblance to granulation tissue, and, in fact, most early pathologists considered them infectious. Poncet and Dor, credited with the first description, believed these lesions were secondary to infection by *Botryomyces* organisms, whereas others implicated pyogenic bacteria, specifically staphylococci. Uncomplicated lesions, however, lack ulceration and inflammation and resemble other capillary (lobular) hemangiomas.

These tumors occur on either the skin or the mucosal surfaces, although the latter accounts for about 60% of all cases.[49] In the extensive review of 289 cases by Kerr,[49] the following were the most common sites, in descending order of frequency: gingiva (64 cases), finger (44 cases), lips (40 cases), face (28 cases), and tongue (20 cases). The genders are affected approximately equally, and the disease is evenly distributed over all decades. Approximately one-third develop following minor trauma. Multiple lesions may develop simultaneously, but this phenomenon almost always occurs in the cutaneous form rather than the mucosal form of the disease. There have been a few reports of disseminated (eruptive) forms of pyogenic granuloma,[50-52] with one following surgical removal of a solitary pyogenic granuloma. Disseminated pyogenic granulomas progress for a limited time and ultimately stabilize or regress. The mechanism for these initially alarming presentations is not clear, although some have suggested the release of angiogenic factors by the tumors. In the ordinary case, the tumors develop rapidly and achieve their maximal size of several milli-

meters to a few centimeters within a few weeks or months. The well-established lesion is a polypoid, friable, purple-red mass that bleeds easily and frequently ulcerates. Sessile forms of this tumor also occur, but they tend to be recurrent lesions.

The appearance of these lesions at low magnification immediately suggests the diagnosis. They are a distinctly exophytic growth connected to the skin by a stalk of varying diameter (Figs 22-7 to 22-11) and occasionally are surrounded by a heaped-up collar of normal tissue. The adjacent epithelium is hyperkeratotic or acanthotic, but the epithelium overlying the lesion itself is flattened, atrophic, or ulcerated. The basic lesion is a lobular (cellular) hemangioma[53] set in a fibromyxoid matrix. Each lobule of the hemangioma is made up of a larger vessel, often with a muscular wall and surrounded by congeries of small capillaries. Most lesions, however, are altered by secondary inflammatory changes; as a result, they have

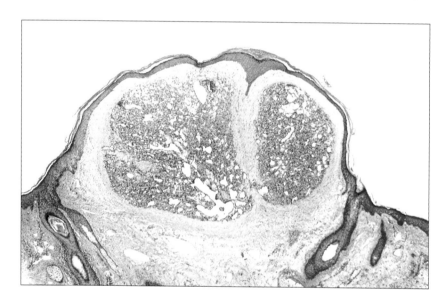

FIGURE 22-7 Granulation tissue-type hemangioma (pyogenic granuloma). Lesion is characterized by exophytic growth.

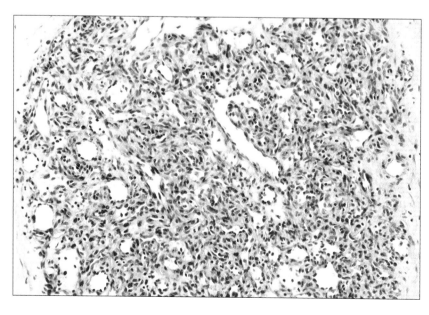

FIGURE 22-8 Lobular growth of vessels in a pyogenic granuloma.

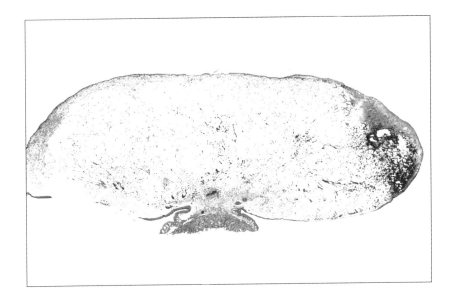

FIGURE 22–9 Pyogenic granuloma with ulceration of surface and marked stromal edema.

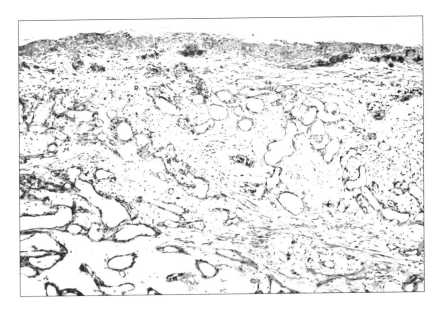

FIGURE 22–10 Stromal edema widely separating vessels of a pyogenic granuloma. (Same case as Fig. 22–41.)

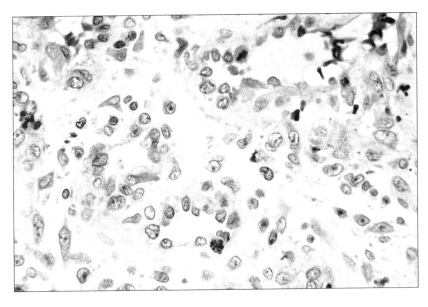

FIGURE 22–11 Mitotic activity in stromal and endothelial cells of a pyogenic granuloma.

been likened to granulation tissue. Both acute and chronic inflammatory cells are scattered throughout the lesion but, not unexpectedly, are most numerous at the surface. Secondary invading microorganisms are occasionally present in the superficial reaches of ulcerated lesions. Stromal edema may separate the capillary lumens and obscure the lobular arrangement of the tumor (Fig. 22–10). Mitotic activity may be brisk in the endothelium and stromal fibroblasts when secondary changes such as edema and inflammation are present. In lesions that involute, there is evidence to suggest they develop a progressive stromal and perivascular fibrosis. Rarely, the pyogenic granuloma has areas in which the endothelium has an epithelioid appearance.

The clinical appearance of these lesions is quite characteristic and can serve as a useful diagnostic adjunct to the pathologist in difficult situations where a distinction between lesions, must be made (e.g., between a well-differentiated angiosarcoma or an angiomatous form of Kaposi sarcoma). In these situations it is useful to recall that the pyogenic granuloma is a more or less circumscribed lesion, often with a lobular arrangement, in contrast to the rambling, poorly confined nature of malignant vascular neoplasms. In particular, the manner in which even well-differentiated angiosarcomas dissect through connective tissue and create irregular vascular spaces contrasts sharply with the pyogenic granuloma. Likewise, Kaposi sarcoma is not well circumscribed and contains, in addition, at least focal cellular zones of spindled cells, which form the classic slit-like vascular spaces. However, these diagnostic areas are often located in the central or deep areas of the tumor, whereas the well-differentiated angiomatous component is seen peripherally or superficially. Thus, in certain instances it is evident that a superficial biopsy of a vascular neoplasm may not be an adequate means to exclude malignancy.

Although the pyogenic granuloma is a benign lesion, 16% were noted to recur in one large series of tumors treated conservatively.[54] A significantly lower recurrence rate was noted in a series of 74 cases reported by Mills et al.[53] Recurrent disease may present as a solitary nodule or as multiple small satellite nodules around the site of the original lesion.[55-59] The phenomenon of *satellitosis* in this disease was analyzed by Warner and Wilson-Jones,[58] who found that most of these lesions occurred on the trunk, particularly the scapular area; and most had been incompletely excised initially. In contrast to the original tumors, the satellites are usually not pedunculated but, rather, are sessile and have an intact surface epithelium. In these respects they may grossly resemble ordinary hemangiomas. Although the rapid development of numerous satellite lesions often causes considerable alarm on the part of the clinician, these lesions usually respond to reexcision and in some instances have even regressed spontaneously. Therapy for these lesions

includes electrodesiccation, curettage, sclerotherapy, or laser therapy.[48]

Pregnancy-related pyogenic granuloma (granuloma gravidarum)

Granuloma gravidarum is a pyogenic granuloma that occurs on the gingival surface during pregnancy.[60] It is estimated that gingival changes occur in about 50% of pregnant women, but that only about 1% of this group develop localized tumors.[60] Typically, these lesions develop abruptly during the first trimester and arise from the interdental area of the gum. They are grossly and histologically indistinguishable from the ordinary form of pyogenic granuloma. They usually regress dramatically following parturition, although many persist as small mucosal nodules capable of renewed growth at the time of subsequent pregnancies. This unusual tumor has provided some of the most compelling evidence that the pyogenic granuloma lacks the degree of autonomous growth that characterizes most vascular tumors of adulthood. In fact, hormone sensitivity manifested by granuloma gravidarum has led many to conclude these are not neoplastic lesions.

Intravenous pyogenic granuloma

An intravenous counterpart of pyogenic granuloma was recognized by Cooper et al.[61] This tumor is most common on the neck and upper extremity. It presents as a red-brown intravascular polyp that can be easily mistaken for an organizing thrombus (Fig. 22–12). The tumor arises

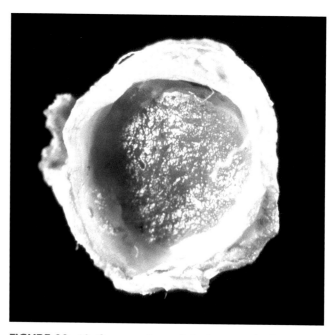

FIGURE 22–12 Gross specimen of the intravascular form of pyogenic granuloma.

from the vein wall and protrudes deeply into the lumen but remains anchored to the wall by means of a narrow stalk containing the "feeder" vessels. The tumor is covered by a lining of endothelium, and the stroma often contains smooth muscle fibers, presumably remnants of the vein wall. Histologically, they are identical to uncomplicated pyogenic granulomas in that these tumors display no inflammatory or ulcerative change (Fig. 22–13). Like other pyogenic granulomas they are benign and display no tendency to spread in the bloodstream.

Cherry angioma (senile angioma, Campbell de Morgan spots)

Cherry angioma is one of the most common acquired vascular lesions of adult life. Lesions present as ruby red papules with a pale halo which measure a few millimeters in diameter[62] and a predilection for the trunk and extremity. These lesions may increase in number over time, and some have been noted to occur in crops in nursing homes, in association with infections, and with exposure to various chemicals.[63–66] The lesions, located in the superficial corium, consist of dilated thin-walled capillaries, which create an elevation and mild atrophy of the overlying skin. Some lesions have a collarette similar to a pyogenic granuloma.

Epithelioid hemangioma (angiolymphoid hyperplasia with eosinophilia, histiocytoid hemangioma)

Epithelioid hemangioma is an unusual but distinctive vascular tumor that was first described by Wells and Whimster[67] as *angiolymphoid hyperplasia with eosinophilia* and subsequently by others as *inflammatory angiomatous nodule, atypical or pseudopyogenic granuloma,*[68,69] and *histiocytoid hemangioma.*[70,71] The lesions reported in the Japanese literature as *Kimura's disease*[39,72–80] represent a different entity, however.

Epithelioid hemangiomas typically occur during early to mid-adult life (age 20–40 years) and affect women more often than men. Most are situated superficially in the head and neck, particularly the region around the ear. As a result, they can be detected relatively early as small, dull red, pruritic plaques. Crusting, excoriation, bleeding, and coalescence of lesions are common secondary features. About half of the patients develop multiple lesions, generally in the same area. Affected patients appear relatively well, although occasionally significant regional lymph node enlargement and eosinophilia of the peripheral blood accompany the lesions. These signs have suggested the possibility of an infectious agent, but to date none has been identified.

These tumors are circumscribed lesions of the subcutis or dermis (Figs 22–14, 22–15), but occasionally they involve deep soft tissue, vessels, or parenchymal organs.[81] Intravascular forms of this tumor have been termed *intravenous atypical vascular proliferation.*[82] Like other capillary hemangiomas, epithelioid hemangiomas consist of lobules of small capillary-sized vessels centered around a larger parent vessel (Fig. 22–16). In most cases the capillary vessels are well-formed, multicellular channels with perceptible lumina. However, in epithelioid hemangiomas that are large and deep, the canalization of the vessels may be poor and give the impression that the lesion consists of solid sheets of epithelioid to slightly spindled cells (Figs 22–17, 22–18). Solid forms of epithelioid hemangioma are problematic for pathologists and occasionally are diagnosed as epithelioid sarcoma or epithelioid angiosarcoma (see below).

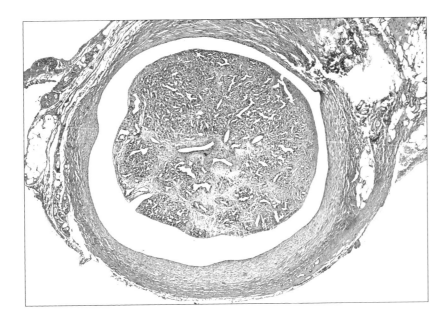

FIGURE 22–13 Intravascular pyogenic granuloma with preservation of the lobular arrangement of vessels.

The hallmark of these lesions are the epithelioid endothelial cells (Figs 22–19 to 22–22) that line a majority, but not necessarily all, of the vessels and protrude deeply into the lumen in a manner that has been likened to "tombstones." The epithelioid endothelial cells have rounded or lobated nuclei and abundant acidophilic cytoplasm containing occasional vacuoles that represent primitive vascular lumen formation. Although they have many of the ultrastructural features of endothelium, including micropinocytotic vesicles, antiluminal basal lamina, and Weibel-Palade bodies, they manifest certain modifications. Adjacent cells are often separated by rather large gaps and interdigitate only along their lateral basal

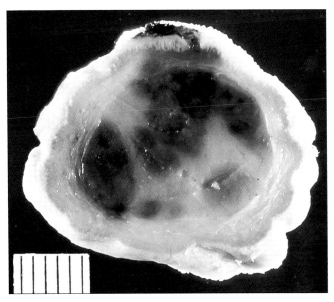

FIGURE 22–14 Gross appearance of a subcutaneous epithelioid hemangioma.

borders by means of tight junctions. Organelles are more abundant in these cells and include increased numbers of mitochondria, smooth and rough endoplasmic reticulum, free ribosomes, and thin cytofilaments.

Epithelioid hemangiomas are typically associated with a prominent inflammatory component. Eosinophils are particularly characteristic of these tumors, but lymphocytes, mast cells, and plasma cells are also present. Lymphoid aggregates replete with germinal centers are occasionally present but are believed by some to be a feature of longstanding lesions or a peculiar host response.

Although about one-third of these lesions recur, virtually none has produced metastasis. One case reported by Reed and Terazakis[83] evidently gave rise to microscopic metastases in a regional lymph node, but this appears to be a unique event.[83] Rare lesions have been noted to regress spontaneously, but usually surgical excision is required. About 80% of reported patients have responded at least partially to superficial radiotherapy,[73] but cryotherapy and injection of intralesional steroids have not met with success.[83]

Despite their benign nature, considerable controversy still exists as to the basic nature of these lesions; some authors consider them reactive and others neoplastic. In our experience based on 96 epithelioid hemangiomas, more than 60% were intimately associated with a large vessel that showed mural damage, rupture, or both.[84] These observations suggest that some soft tissue epithelioid hemangiomas are reactive lesions (Fig. 22–23). In this regard a rather impressive epithelioid hemangioma was reported to occur in a patient following a popliteal arteriovenous fistula.[85] Others have commented on the association with arteriovenous shunts, particularly in deeply situated forms of epithelioid hemangioma.

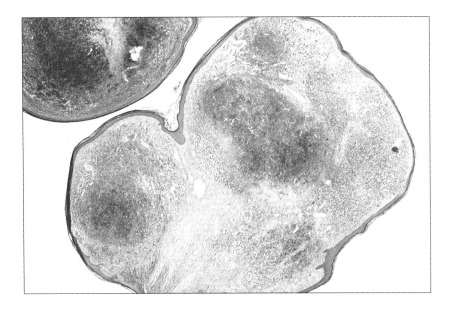

FIGURE 22–15 Low-power view of an epithelioid hemangioma with nodules of vessels surrounded by a prominent lymphoid cuff.

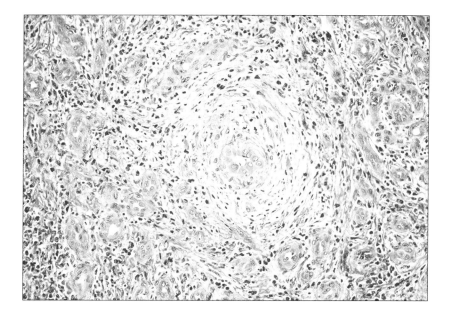

FIGURE 22–16 Epithelioid hemangioma with a central "parent" vessel surrounded by small vessels and dense inflammation.

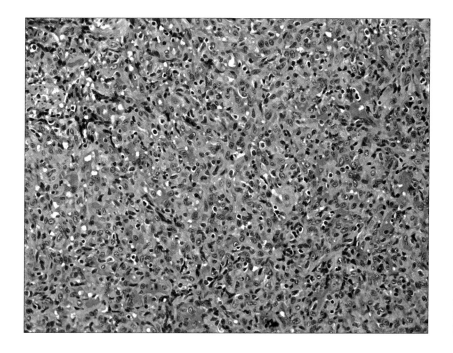

FIGURE 22–17 Solid form of epithelioid hemangioma in which luminal differentiation is subtle or inapparent.

Although sharing many common histologic features and a benign clinical course, the lesions may be pathogenetically heterogeneous.

Many have speculated on the nature and significance of the epithelioid endothelial cell. It probably represents an altered functional state of endothelium that may be encountered in benign and malignant vascular tumors as well as in reactive vascular lesions. Because of their lobated nuclei, decreased alkaline phosphatase, and the increased acid phosphatase compared with normal endothelium, these cells have also been termed *histiocytoid*.

Differential diagnosis

Epithelioid hemangioendothelioma and angiosarcoma. The differential diagnosis of epithelioid hemangioma includes the full spectrum of epithelioid vascular lesions, most often epithelioid hemangioendothelioma, and occasionally other epithelioid tumors. In contrast to epithelioid hemangiomas, epithelioid hemangioendotheliomas are angiocentric tumors having a distinctive myxohyaline or chondroid background. The cells are arranged in short cords or chains rather than multicellular vascular channels and rarely do they have a prominent inflammatory

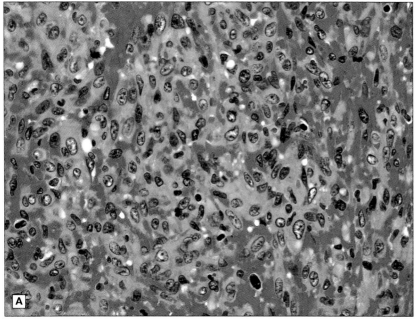

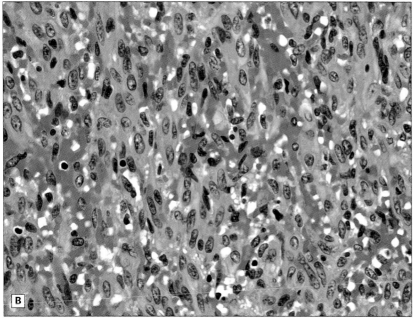

FIGURE 22–18 Solid form of epithelioid hemangioma showing epithelioid areas **(A)** and spindled areas **(B)**.

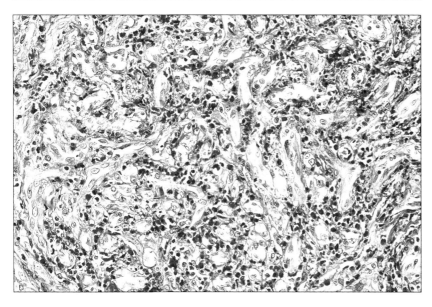

FIGURE 22–19 Epithelioid hemangioma. Vessels are lined by pale-staining cuboidal endothelial cells admixed with inflammatory elements, predominantly eosinophils.

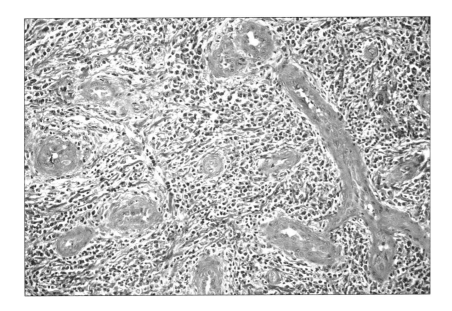

FIGURE 22–20 Epithelioid hemangioma in which some areas display more conventional-appearing endothelial cells interspersed with chronic inflammatory cells.

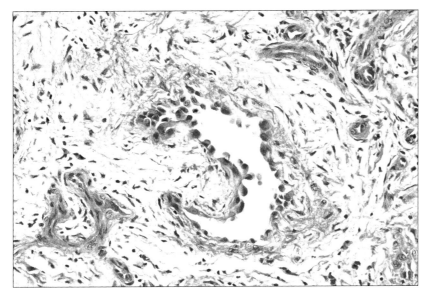

FIGURE 22–21 "Tombstone"-like appearance of cells in large vessels of epithelioid hemangioma.

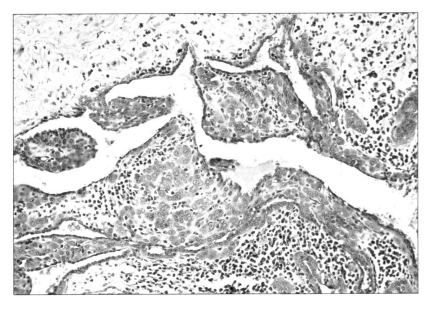

FIGURE 22–22 Epithelioid hemangioma involving the wall of a large vessel. This phenomenon should not be equated with malignancy.

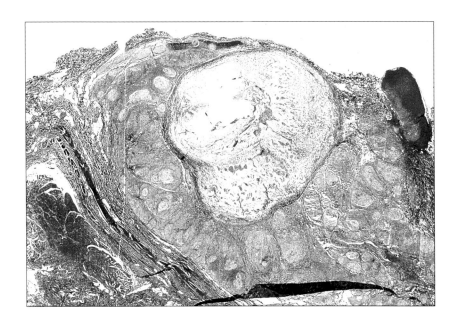

FIGURE 22–23 Changes of an epithelioid hemangioma arising from the walls of traumatized vessels. Note the prominent lymphocytic infiltrate around the lesions.

component. Those epithelioid hemangiomas that have solid or medullary zones may be mistaken for epithelioid angiosarcomas. The single most important observation in this regard is the nuclear grade of the cells. Epithelioid angiosarcomas are invariably high-grade lesions composed of large cells with prominent nuclei and nucleoli that sharply contrast with the nuclei of epithelioid hemangioma.

The recently described *epithelioid angiomatous nodule* may be a variant of epithelioid hemangioma having a predominantly solid growth pattern.[86] Like epithelioid hemangioma, they present as dermal nodules, occasionally display multicellular vascular channel formation and inflammation, and pursue a benign course.

The lesion first described by Kim in the Chinese literature and later by Kimura et al.[76] in the Japanese literature as *Kimura's disease* is a chronic inflammatory condition that appears to be endemic in the Asian population and occurs only infrequently in Westerners. Although formerly thought to be identical to epithelioid hemangioma (angiolymphoid hyperplasia), many data indicate that they are two entirely unrelated lesions bearing only a few superficial histologic similarities.[72,74,77,80] Kimura's disease is often confused with angiolymphoid hyperplasia (epithelioid hemangioma) largely because the term was inappropriately applied to classic examples of angiolymphoid hyperplasia. In fact, the two lesions are clinically and histologically quite different. Kimura's disease presents as lymphadenopathy with or without an associated soft tissue mass. Peripheral eosinophilia is nearly always present. Increased serum immunoglobulin E (IgE), proteinuria, and nephrotic syndrome may also occur as part of the disease.[79,87,88] Lesions are most frequent in the

subcutis of the head and neck area, although lesions have been noted in the groin, extremities, and chest wall. There is a striking male predilection in this disease. The lesions are characterized by dense lymphoid aggregates containing prominent germinal centers (Fig. 22–24). Within the germinal centers one occasionally identifies nuclear debris, polykaryocytes, and a delicate eosinophilic matrix. Immunohistochemical procedures reveal that IgE-bearing cells, corresponding to the distribution of dendritic reticulum cells, populate the germinal center. Thin-walled vessels, with the characteristics of postcapillary venules, reside adjacent to the germinal centers, occasionally dipping into the centers. Dense infiltrates of eosinophils adjacent to the lymphoid aggregates occasionally form "eosinophilic abscesses." During the late stages of the disease a dense hyaline fibrosis supervenes. The adherence of the mass to the surrounding structures often triggers alarm on the part of the surgeon regarding the possibility of malignancy. In affected lymph nodes, there is exuberant follicular hyperplasia with preservation of the architecture. The changes in the germinal center are as described above for soft tissue lesions.

The etiology of this condition is unknown, although the peripheral eosinophilia and elevated serum IgE suggest an immunologic reaction to an unknown stimulus. The lesions are benign, but recurrence may develop after surgical excision. There are no instances of malignancy supervening on these peculiar lymphoid proliferations.

Although Kimura's disease and angiolymphoid hyperplasia have in common a lymphoid infiltrate with eosinophils, there are rather striking differences. The vascular proliferation in Kimura's disease is relatively minor and

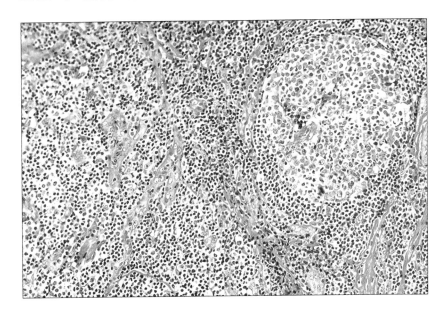

FIGURE 22–24 Kimura's disease. Lesion differs from epithelioid hemangioma in that the lymphoid component overshadows the minor vascular component.

is eclipsed by the inflammatory component. Moreover, the vessels in Kimura's disease are not lined by epithelioid endothelium but by more attenuated endothelial cells.

Cavernous hemangioma

Cavernous hemangiomas are less frequent than capillary hemangiomas but share common age and anatomic distributions. They are most common during childhood and are located in the upper portion of the body. As a result, some suggest they simply represent massively engorged capillary hemangiomas, a contention supported by the fact that some hemangiomas have a capillary component at the surface and a cavernous component in the deeper portion. They differ from capillary hemangiomas in several important respects. They are usually larger and less circumscribed, and they more frequently involve deep structures. They show essentially no tendency to regress and may even be locally destructive by virtue of the pressure they exert on neighboring structures. Consequently, most cavernous hemangiomas require surgery, in contrast to their capillary counterparts.

The color and surface appearance of these lesions relate to the location. Superficial lesions are blue, puffy masses with an irregular surface caused by dilatation of the vessels (Fig. 22–25). Deep lesions may impart little or no color to the overlying skin. Radiographically, the large deep lesions appear as localized or diffuse nonhomogeneous water density masses. Tortuous water density channels representing the afferent and efferent blood supplies are occasionally seen in adjacent fat. Calcification is common and may be of several types (Fig. 22–26). Amorphous or curvilinear calcification is non-specific, whereas phlebolith formation is not only more frequent but also a more specific finding. Both are the result of dystrophic calcification in organizing thrombi.[89] Cavern-

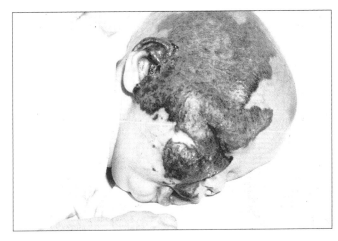

FIGURE 22–25 Cavernous hemangioma of the face.

ous hemangiomas are composed of large, dilated, blood-filled vessels lined by flattened endothelium (Fig. 22–27). The vessels may be arranged in a roughly lobular arrangement or in a diffuse haphazard pattern. The walls are occasionally thickened by an adventitial fibrosis, and inflammatory cells may be scattered throughout the stroma. Mature bone is occasionally present (Fig. 22–28). Some deep cavernous hemangiomas have overlapping features with venous hemangioma (malformation).

Sinusoidal hemangioma is a variant of cavernous hemangioma that differs from the latter in several respects.[89] It occurs as a solitary acquired lesion in adults, usually women, and is relatively well demarcated (Figs 22–29, 22–30). The thin-walled cavernous vessels ramify with one another to a much greater extent than in a conventional cavernous hemangioma. Papillary infoldings of the endothelium are usually identified; and in two cases reported by Calonje and Fletcher,[89] central infarction of the tumors occurred.

syndrome occurs with kaposiform hemangioendothelioma,[94] angiomatosis, and rarely angiosarcoma. Typically, the syndrome occurs during infancy, and the onset of purpura is heralded by rapid enlargement of the tumor. The patients develop numerous cutaneous petechiae and ecchymoses, not only in the skin but also in internal organs, due to intravascular coagulation and sequestration of platelets in the tumor. Patients with this syndrome usually require therapy because death from hemorrhage and infection approaches 30%, and spontaneous regression of these tumors cannot be anticipated. In most cases surgery is not possible because of the precarious hematologic status of the patient and the large size of the tumor. In the past, steroids, irradiation, or both were the mainstay of treatment. Several new strategies include the administration of recombinant interferon alpha-2a[10,11] and pentoxifylline.[91]

A distinctive form of cavernous hemangioma of the skin in association with similar gastrointestinal tract lesions was delineated by Bean in 1958 as *blue rubber bleb nevus syndrome.*[62] The term aptly describes the blue cutaneous lesions, which look and feel like rubber nipples. They compress easily with pressure, leaving a flaccid wrinkled appearance to the skin, and then regain their shape with cessation of pressure. Hyperhidrosis may occur over these lesions probably as a result of increased surface temperature. In addition, most patients have gastrointestinal hemangiomas, usually in the small intestine. These internal lesions commonly bleed, so chronic anemia complicates the course of the disease. Some cases are inherited in an autosomal dominant fashion, although most appear to be sporadic. Because of the diffuse nature of the disease, therapy is aimed at resecting only bleeding lesions from the intestine.

Maffucci syndrome (dyschondroplasia with vascular hamartomas) is a rare mesodermal dysplasia characterized by multiple hemangiomas and enchondromas (Fig. 22–31). The vascular tumors are usually noted at birth and are of the cavernous type,[62] although the question has been raised as to whether many of these cavernous hemangiomas are really spindle cell hemangiomas. Other vascular lesions including lymphangiomas and phlebectasias may also be present. The cartilaginous tumors typically develop after the vascular lesions and are the result of a defect in endochondral ossification, so there is a marked overgrowth in the cartilage plates. The bones are shortened and have numerous enchondromas and exostoses. Pathologic fractures are common; and in about 20% of the patients malignant tumors, usually chondrosarcomas (or rarely angiosarcomas), develop.

Cerebral cavernous malformations consisting of abnormal cavernous vessels without intervening brain parenchyma occur in about 0.5% of the general population. Affected patients present with seizures, hemorrhage and focal neurologic deficits. Cavernous malformations in other sites (e.g., retina) may also occur. Some cases are

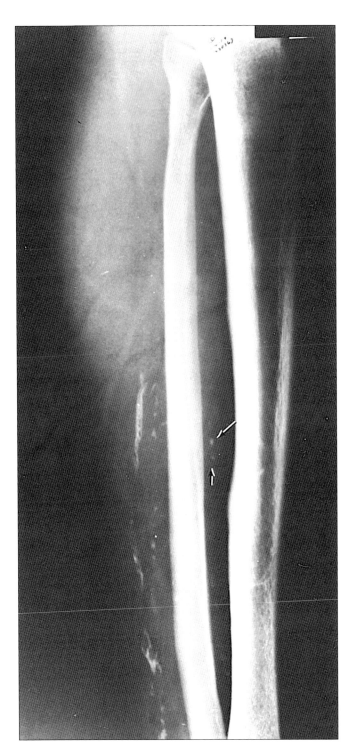

FIGURE 22–26 Radiograph of a hemangioma with both cavernous and venous features histologically. Note the long curvilinear calcifications in addition to phleboliths (arrows). The latter are highly characteristic of cavernous hemangiomas. (Courtesy of Dr. John Madewell.)

Several syndromes may be associated with cavernous hemangiomas. Thrombocytopenia purpura complicating giant hemangiomas is known as *Kasabach-Merritt syndrome.*[90–93] Most of these hemangiomas are large solitary cavernous lesions located on an extremity, although the

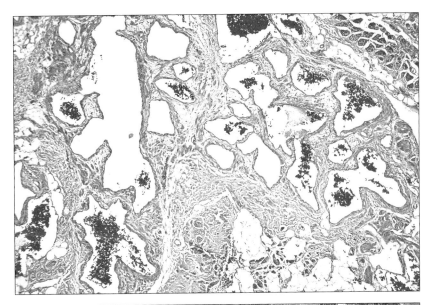

FIGURE 22–27 Cavernous hemangioma with large, thin-walled veins.

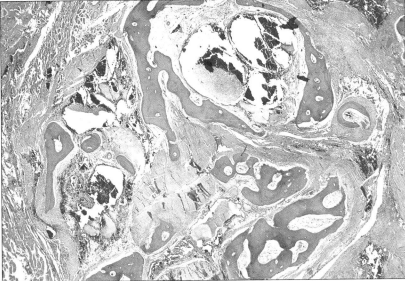

FIGURE 22–28 Cavernous hemangioma with bone.

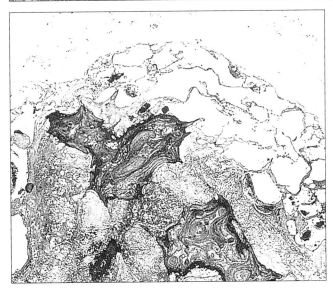

FIGURE 22–29 Sinusoidal hemangioma. (×25) (Case courtesy of Dr. C.D.M. Fletcher.)

sporadic, but others are inherited in an autosomal dominant pattern and have been localized to chromosomes 7q21.2 (CCM1), 7p15-p13 (CCM2), and 3q25.2-qq27(CCM3). In families with CCM1, mutations in the *KRIT1* gene (*KREV interaction trapped 1*), leading to premature truncation of KRIT1 protein, have been identified and suggest a loss of function mutation.[7]

MISCELLANEOUS HEMANGIOMAS

Verrucous hemangioma (hyperkeratotic vascular stain)

Verrucous hemangioma is a variant of capillary or cavernous hemangioma that undergoes reactive hyperkeratosis of the overlying skin and consequently may be confused with a wart or keratosis.[95-97] Some authors regard these as malformations (hyperkeratotic vascular stain).[48] Ver-

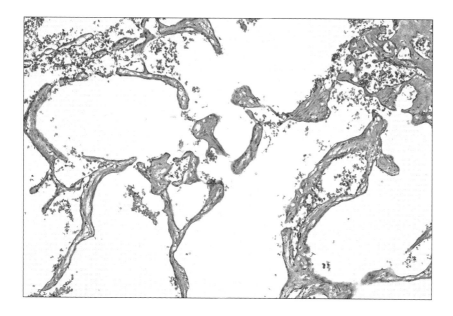

FIGURE 22–30 Sinusoidal hemangioma. (Case courtesy of Dr. C.D.M. Fletcher.)

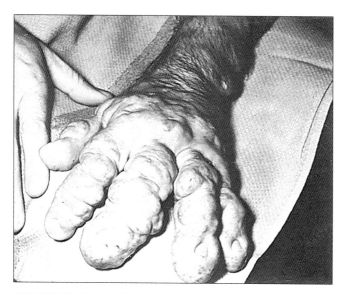

FIGURE 22–31 Multiple enchondromas in a patient with Maffucci syndrome. Patients also develop hemangiomas.

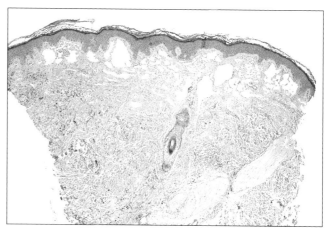

FIGURE 22–32 Hobnail hemangioma (targetoid hemosiderotic hemangioma).

rucous hemangiomas may occur as part of Cobb's syndrome (cutaneous vascular lesion and spinal cord vascular malformation within a segment or two of involved dermatome).[98]

The lesions begin during childhood as unilateral lesions in the dermis of the lower extremity. Grossly and histologically, they resemble conventional hemangiomas during their early stage of development. With time, the overlying epidermis displays hyperkeratosis, acanthosis, and papillomatosis, features that obscure the vascular nature of the lesions. The vessels, a mixture of dilated capillaries and veins, involve superficial and deep dermis and sometimes extend into the subcutis. Because of their deep extension, complete excisions can be difficult and recurrences and satellite lesions may develop. Angiokeratomas resemble these lesions clinically and histologically but are distinguished by a lack of a deep component.

Hobnail hemangioma (targetoid hemosiderotic hemangioma)

Hobnail hemangioma, described by Guillou et al.,[99] represents the benign counterpart of retiform hemangioendothelioma. It usually develops on the skin of the extremities in young adults as an angiomatous/pigmented or exophytic mass and has a distinctive biphasic appearance (Figs 22–32, 22–33). The superficial portion of the lesion consists of dilated vessels lined by hobnail endothelial cells (see Chapter 24) containing occasional intraluminal papillary tufts similar to the Dabska tumor. The deep portion consists of attenuated, slit-like capillaries that ramify in the dermis. Although the pattern is sugges-

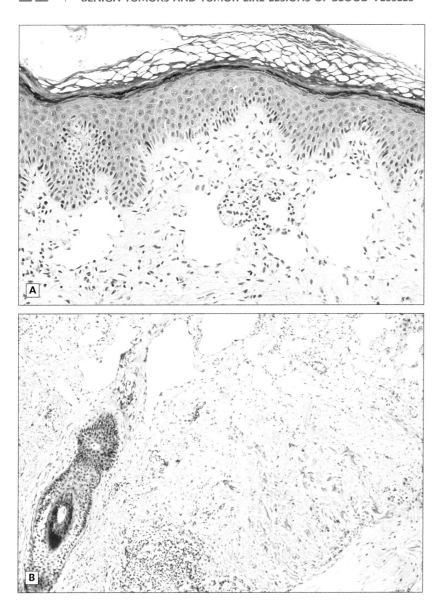

FIGURE 22–33 Hobnail hemangioma (targetoid hemosiderotic hemangioma) showing ectatic vessels at the surface **(A)** and in deeper regions illustrating the interface of ectatic vessels with attenuated slit-like vessels **(B)**.

tive of an angiosarcoma, the vessels have an innocuous appearance. Hemorrhage, hemosiderin deposits, lymphocytes, and dermal sclerosis can accompany the lesions. The endothelial cells in hobnail hemangiomas are CD31, VEGFR3[+], and D2–40[100] positive and CD34 negative[101] indicating a lymphatic phenotype similar to retiform hemangioendothelioma. The lesional vessels lack a pericytic cuff as would be expected for lymphatic vessels. Microshunts between small blood and lymphatic vessels have been imputed as the explanation for the frequent microaneurysms, hemorrhage, inflammatory changes and scarring that are so typical of these lesions.[101] The more than 50 cases that have been reported have had a benign clinical course.[99,100]

Hobnail hemangiomas correspond to some lesions originally termed targetoid hemosiderotic hemangioma by Santa Cruz and Aronberg.[102,103] However, targetoid hemosiderotic hemangioma is a clinical term referring to

the presence of an ecchymotic halo surrounding a violaceous papule, and it is unclear whether these clinically defined lesions have a common pathologic appearance. The term hobnail hemangioma has, therefore, proven to be more useful to pathologists.

Acquired tufted angioma (angioblastoma of Nakagawa)

Described by Wilson-Jones and Orkin[104] as "acquired tufted angioma" and by Japanese authors as "angioblastoma of Nakagawa,"[105] this vascular lesion shares some features of juvenile hemangiomas,[104,106,107] but is more likely identical to or a closely related variant of kaposiform hemangioendothelioma. Evidence supporting this includes the following. Most cases of acquired tufted hemangiomas reported in children are impossible to distinguish from kaposiform hemangioendothelioma based on published photomicrographs.[105,108–111] Both occur principally in children, are characterized by infiltrating nodules of tumor with focal glomeruloid structures, display a lymphatic component (see Chapter 23), and have a similar immunophenotype (Fig. 22–34). Several reports even comment on the fact that some lesions have features of both tumors or show transformation between the two.[108,109,112] Many patients with acquired tufted angioma also develop Kasabach-Merritt syndrome (KMS), but apparently less frequently than patients with kaposiform hemangioendothelioma. The relatively minor differences observed between the two lesions are best explained by the bias to label lesions occurring in an adult without manifestations of KMS as acquired tufted angioma and in children with KMS as kaposiform hemangioendothelioma. Although we have used the term kaposiform hemangioendothelioma for all lesions, there may be merit to retain the term acquired tufted hemangioma

for indolent cutaneous lesions in adults. Recently, a familial predisposition to acquired tufted hemangioma, suggesting a monogenic autosomal dominant pattern of inheritance linked to three possible candidate genes, *EDR*, *ENG* and *FLT4*,[113] has been reported. Similar observations have not yet been made in kaposiform hemangioendothelioma.

Spindle cell hemangioma

First described in 1986[114] as "spindle cell hemangioendothelioma," the spindle cell hemangioma is an acral vascular tumor characterized by cavernous blood vessels and spindled areas reminiscent of Kaposi sarcoma. Although originally believed to be a tumor with limited metastatic potential, it is regarded as a benign, but frequently multifocal, lesion. The tumor usually occurs in young adults and affects the subcutis of the distal extremities, particu-

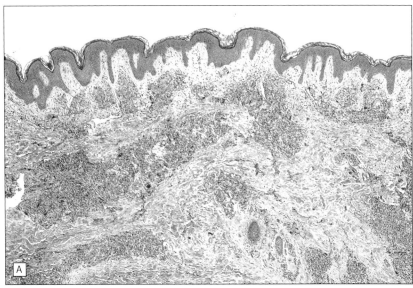

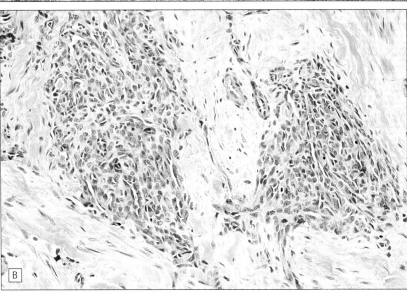

FIGURE 22–34 Acquired tufted hemangioma illustrating "cannonball" nests of tumor in the dermis **(A)**. High-power view depicts irregular groups of capillary-sized vessels **(B)**. (Case courtesy of Dr. Philip Allen.)

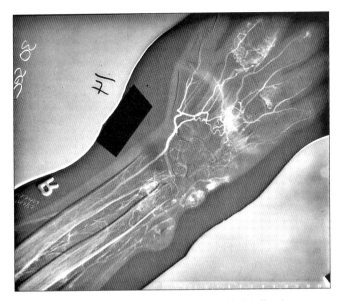

FIGURE 22–35 Radiograph of a patient with Maffucci syndrome and multiple spindle cell hemangiomas (some with phleboliths) on the lateral portion of the wrist and hand. Patient also has an enchondroma of the phalanx of the forefinger.

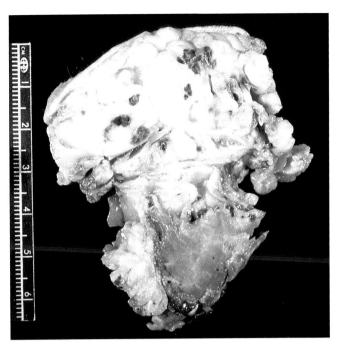

FIGURE 22–36 Gross specimen of a spindle cell hemangioma showing multiple lesions in the subcutis.

larly the hand. The lesions produce so few symptoms that patients may delay seeking medical attention for several years. The tumor is occasionally associated with Maffucci syndrome (Fig. 22–35);[116] and it appears that many of the lesions originally described as cavernous hemangiomas in Maffucci syndrome may well be spindle cell hemangiomas. In addition, spindle cell hemangiomas are also seen in Klippel-Trénaunay syndrome,[115] early-onset varicosities, congenital lymphedema, and rarely in association with epithelioid hemangioendothelioma. Most begin as a solitary nodule but have a remarkable tendency to give rise to multiple lesions in the same general area (Figs 22–36, 22–37). Approximately one-half of cases are intravascular; it appears that intravascular growth is the mechanism by which they give rise to multiple lesions in the same general area.

Histologically, the lesions are composed of thin-walled cavernous vessels lined by flattened endothelial cells and containing a mixture of erythrocytes and thrombi. Between the cavernous spaces are bland spindled areas reminiscent of Kaposi sarcoma (Figs 22–38 to 22–40). Unlike Kaposi sarcoma, however, they contain distinctive round or epithelioid cells containing vacuoles or intracytoplasmic lumens similar to those in an epithelioid hemangioendothelioma (Fig. 22–41). In the extreme case, these clusters of vacuolated cells in the spindled stroma can be mistaken for entrapped fat (Fig. 22–42). Von Willebrand factor can be identified in the endothelium lining of the cavernous spaces and in the epithelioid endothelium of the stroma. The spindled areas appear to be made up of collapsed vessels, pericytes, and fibroblastic cells, indicating that architecturally

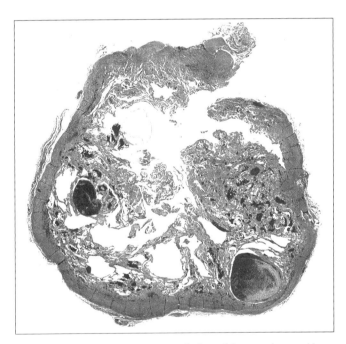

FIGURE 22–37 Subcutaneous spindle cell hemangioma with relative circumscription.

they are complex and have all the elements of the vessel wall.

About 60% of spindle cell hemangiomas recur,[116] although as stated above, the mechanism of recurrence appears to be growth in vessels to discontinuous regional sites in contrast to true local regrowth or local metastasis. There is no evidence that these lesions have the ability to

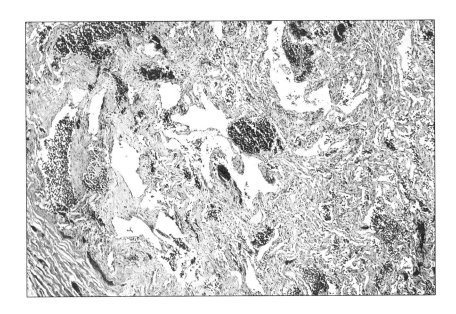

FIGURE 22–38 Spindle cell hemangioma with juxtaposition of the cellular and cavernous areas.

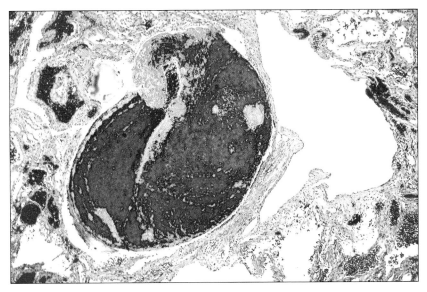

FIGURE 22–39 Spindle cell hemangioma with blood-filled cavernous spaces.

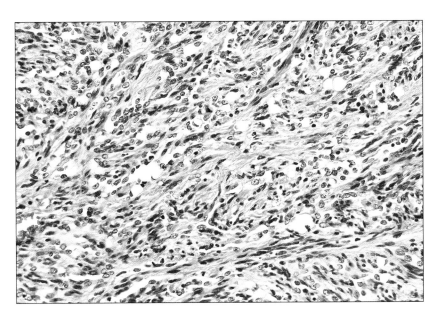

FIGURE 22–40 Spindle cell hemangioma with cellular (Kaposi-sarcoma-like) areas.

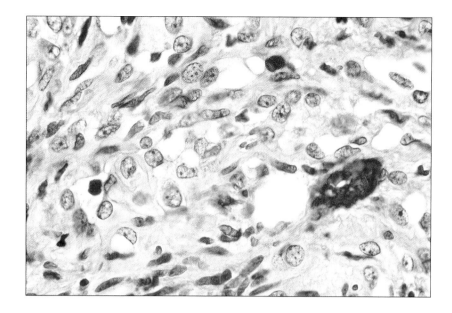

FIGURE 22–41 Spindle cell hemangioma with round "epithelioid" endothelial cells within cellular areas. Some show vacuolation.

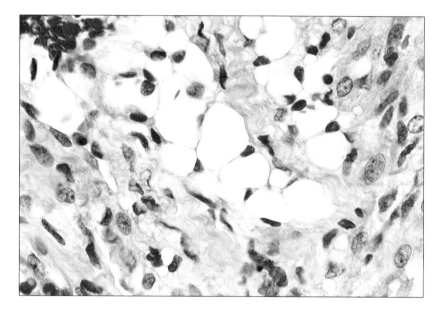

FIGURE 22–42 Spindle cell hemangioma with prominent vacuolation of endothelial cells. Such areas are frequently confused with fat.

metastasize either distantly or regionally, however. There has been considerable debate as to whether these lesions are reactive or neoplastic. The lesions arise in the vicinity of what are clearly abnormal vessels, supporting the idea that the spindle cell hemangioma is most likely a vascular malformation in which variation in blood flow gives rise to alternating areas of vascular expansion and collapse. The fact that the cellular zones appear to have all the elements of the vessel wall suggest that they are fundamentally similar to the cavernous areas but represent areas of vascular collapse.

Venous hemangioma (venous malformation)

Venous hemangiomas, collections of large, slow-flow venous vessels, are considered by most as malformations and have been linked in a few patients to mutations in the VMCM1 locus on chromosome 9 which results in ligand-independent autophosphorylation of the TIE-2 receptor with resultant downstream alterations.[117,118] Venous hemangiomas range from superficial varicosities to large, complex masses that infiltrate soft tissues. They are formed by congeries of venous vessels (Fig. 22–43) which are often not visualized on arteriography but require venography or direct injection to identify their presence and extent (Fig. 22–44).[88] Venous hemangiomas consist principally of large veins with irregularly attenuated or disorganized walls (Fig. 22–45). Due to slow flow, the vessels develop intraluminal thrombi, calcification, and phleboliths. Some contain areas of cavernous hemangioma, suggesting that cavernous and venous hemangiomas are related lesions. Some cases of diffuse

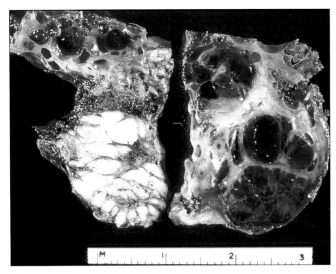

FIGURE 22–43 Gross specimen of a venous hemangioma.

hemangioma (angiomatosis) have the appearance of a venous hemangioma. Venous hemangiomas have also been reported in Turner syndrome. These rather distinctive forms of venous hemangioma may represent one of the various cardiovascular abnormalities associated with this genetic syndrome.

Arteriovenous hemangioma (arteriovenous malformation)

Arteriovenous hemangioma is a term used in the past to describe deeply situated vascular lesions composed of both veins and arteries, often associated with arteriovenous shunting documented radiologically or clinically (Fig. 22–46). Most lesions designated as arteriovenous hemangiomas by clinicians and radiologists have the features of intramuscular hemangioma or angiomatosis. For this reason the term "arteriovenous hemangioma" is seldom used as a pathologic diagnosis but does transmit useful clinical and physiologic information.

The majority of arteriovenous hemangiomas (malformations) occurs sporadically, although a few are familial. The CMC1 locus on 5q,[7] important in the pathogenesis of capillary hemangiomas (malformations), has been targeted as a possible locus in this condition as well. This suggests that similar mutations could have different phenotypic expressions depending of the vessels affected. Of importance is the fact that cutaneous manifestations of arteriovenous malformations can crudely simulate the appearance of Kaposi sarcoma (see Chapter 24). These changes have been referred to as *kaposiform angiodermatitis* or *pseudo-Kaposi sarcoma*[119-121] These changes consist of a proliferation of small capillary-sized vessels with thickened walls in association with fibroblasts and hemosiderin deposits (Fig. 22–47).

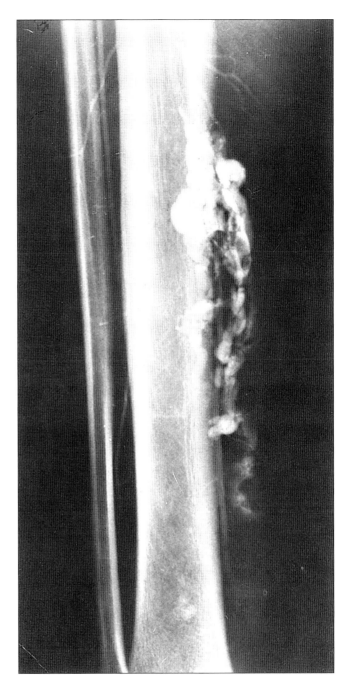

FIGURE 22–44 Hemangioma with venous and cavernous features (same case as in Fig. 22–8). Venous phase of the arteriogram portrays large saccular structures that correspond to tortuous thick-walled muscular veins. (Courtesy of Dr. John Madewell.)

DEEP HEMANGIOMAS OF MISCELLANEOUS SITES

Compared with cutaneous hemangiomas, those involving deep soft tissue structures are uncommon (Table 22–2), yet these tumors deserve special mention because it is their unorthodox locations and different clinical presentations that create concern on the part of clinician and pathologist as to the possibility of malignancy.

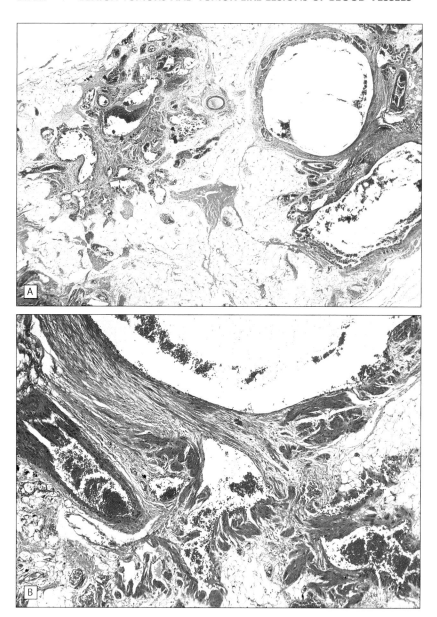

FIGURE 22–45 Large, thick-walled veins of a venous hemangioma.

Intramuscular hemangioma

The skeletal muscle hemangioma is probably the most common form of hemangioma of deep soft tissue, but it is nonetheless rare if one considers the spectrum of benign vascular neoplasms.[122–127] Watson and McCarthy[22] estimated that these lesions account for 0.8% of all benign vascular tumors, a figure that varies depending on the frequency with which incidental hemangiomas are excised at a given institution. Most intramuscular hemangiomas occur in young adults, with 80–90% manifesting before the age of 30 years.[122] The young age of affected patients and the long duration of symptoms in some cases raise the possibility that many of these lesions are congenital tumors that slowly give rise to symptoms during late childhood or early adult life. Unlike cutaneous hemangiomas, this form does not show a striking predilection for females and affects the genders in roughly equal numbers. Although any muscle can be affected, most intramuscular hemangiomas are located in the lower extremity, particularly the muscles of the thigh. There is some evidence that intramuscular hemangiomas of the capillary type have a greater predilection for the head and neck musculature and in this respect have a distribution similar to the juvenile form of capillary hemangiomas.

Clinically, these lesions are more likely to pose diagnostic problems than are superficial hemangiomas. They present as enlarging soft tissue masses with few signs or symptoms to reveal their vascular nature. In particular, there is rarely any overlying discoloration of the skin, visible pulsation, or audible bruit. Radiography and arteriography are far more helpful for suggesting the diagnosis. Plain films may reveal phleboliths in addition to a

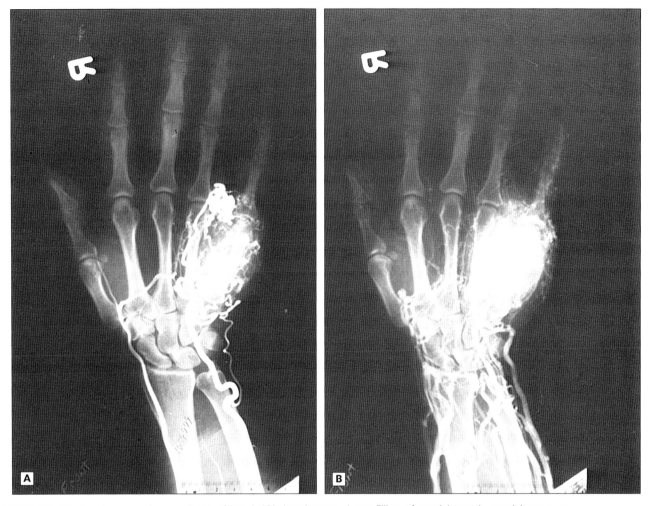

FIGURE 22–46 Arteriovenous hemangioma of hand. **(A)** Arteriogram shows filling of arterial vessels supplying tumor. **(B)** Opacification of tumor in the region of the fifth metacarpal and filling of draining veins while still in the arterial phase. (Courtesy of Dr. John Madewell.)

soft tissue mass, and arteriography may demonstrate a highly vascular lesion with early venous runoff. Moreover, the vessels are oriented parallel to one another in a "striated" pattern.[123] This pattern, created by the orderly entry and proliferation of vessels between fascicles of muscle, is considered a helpful feature in support of the benignancy of the lesion. Pain is a frequent but not invariable symptom and is said to be more common with tumors involving long, narrow muscles where stretching of the muscle and nerve fibers by the tumor is more intense. Occasionally, function is impaired or anatomic deformity occurs. Although a history of trauma is given in about one-fifth of cases, there is no evidence that the lesions are caused by trauma; it appears more likely that trauma merely aggravates the underlying tumor.

Intramuscular hemangiomas vary greatly in their gross and microscopic appearances, depending on whether they are of the capillary, cavernous, or mixed type. In many cases it is not possible to sharply classify these types because they are all part of the same histologic spectrum.

Intramuscular hemangiomas of the capillary type are most common and are also likely to be confused with a malignant tumor. Grossly, they do appear vascular because they vary from tan to yellow or red (Fig. 22–48). They are composed of a myriad of small capillary-sized vessels with plump nuclei that extend between individual muscle fibers (Figs 22–49 to 22–51). Well-developed lumen formation is apparent in most areas, although occasional tumors have a solidly cellular appearance similar to the early stage of the juvenile hemangioma. In occasional cases, mitotic activity, intraluminal papillary tufting, and a proliferation of capillary vessels in perineural sheaths are present. Although seemingly disturbing features, none of these features is indicative of malignancy.

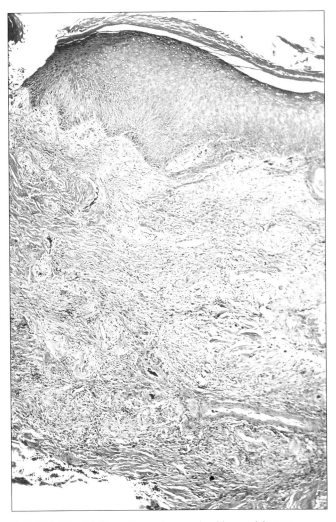

FIGURE 22–47 Kaposiform changes in skin overlying an arteriovenous fistula.

In contrast, the cavernous form of intramuscular hemangioma is easily recognized as a benign vascular tumor. Grossly, these lesions are blue-red masses composed of large vessels lined by bland, markedly attenuated endothelium, which seldom shows a significant degree of pleomorphism. The presence of adipose tissue in these tumors is common, and at times it may be so conspicuous as to suggest a diagnosis of lipoma. Tumors described in the early literature as *infiltrating angiolipomas of muscle* or *benign mesenchymoma* are examples of intramuscular hemangiomas with striking fatty overgrowth.

The most important consideration in the differential diagnosis of these lesions is the distinction from an angiosarcoma of skeletal muscle. Angiosarcomas of deep soft

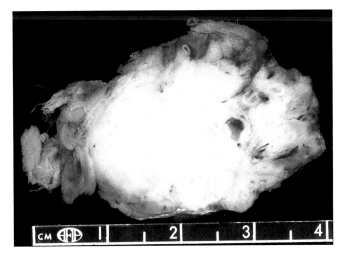

FIGURE 22–48 Gross appearance of an intramuscular hemangioma involving the medial thigh. Lesions often have a solid, nonhemorrhagic appearance.

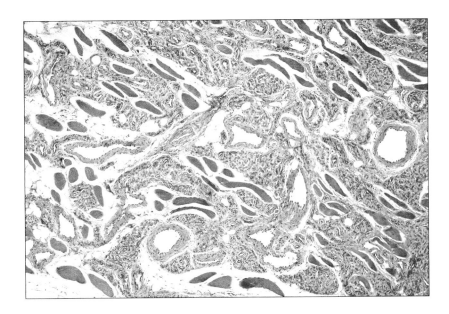

FIGURE 22–49 Intramuscular hemangioma with separation of muscle fibers by proliferating vessels. This pseudoinfiltrative pattern is often mistaken for evidence of malignancy.

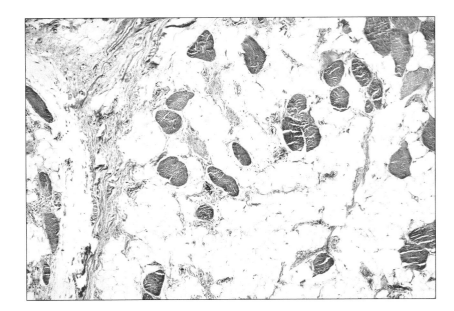

FIGURE 22–50 Intramuscular hemangioma with a significant admixture of fat. Such tumors have sometimes been classified as "angiolipomas" of muscle.

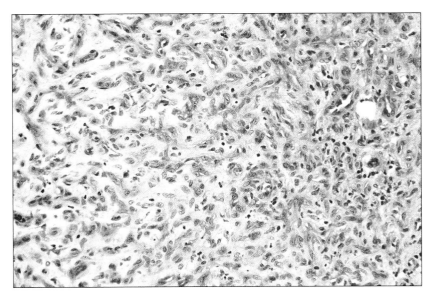

FIGURE 22–51 Small vessel (capillary) type of intramuscular hemangioma.

tissue, specifically skeletal muscle, are rare (see Chapter 24); thus a vascular tumor of skeletal muscle is statistically more likely to be benign than malignant. Moreover, intramuscular hemangiomas do not develop the freely anastomosing sinusoidal pattern encountered in most angiosarcomas, nor do they exhibit nuclear pleomorphism and hyperchromatism. As indicated earlier, some hemangiomas of skeletal muscle contain significant lipomatous components and therefore are occasionally confused with liposarcomas. Although well-differentiated liposarcomas contain an intricate vascular pattern, they rarely have the gaping vessels characteristic of hemangiomas, and they contain, in addition, hyperchromatic stromal cells. Finally, diffuse forms of hemangiomas (angiomatosis) involving skeletal muscle are histologically indistinguishable from intramuscular hemangiomas. The distinction of the two disorders is based on clinical parameters. In contrast to the intramuscular hem-

angioma, angiomatosis is usually a congenital or childhood lesion that involves an extensive body area, including muscle, skin, and bone. Intramuscular hemangiomas are best considered benign tumors with a small but definite risk of local recurrence attributable to the ease and adequacy of the initial excision. In our experience, 18% of patients develop local recurrences,[122] although other investigators have reported recurrences of more than 50%.[125] Metastases have not been recorded. Treatment is therefore best aimed at complete excision without resorting to radical surgery. Prior embolization of the tumor has been used as a means to facilitate surgical excision.[126]

Synovial hemangioma

Synovial hemangioma is a well-recognized but rare entity. Theoretically, it can arise from any synovium-lined surface and therefore may be found along the course of tendons or in a joint space.[128-135] In the former location these lesions present in the same fashion as tenosynovial giant cell tumor, that is, as painless soft tissue swellings. The origin from synovium in these cases is only assumed because they may also involve superficial structures, and confinement by synovium is often not apparent. Thus, the most characteristic form of synovial hemangioma is the intra-articular variety in which the tumor consists of a more or less discrete mass lined by a synovial membrane.[129,130,134] These tumors almost invariably involve the knee joint and classically present as recurrent episodes of pain, swelling, and joint effusion. The symptoms usually begin during childhood and persist several years before the time of diagnosis. In most instances a spongy compressible mass that decreases in size with elevation can be palpated over the joint. Plain films of the joint show non-specific changes, including capsular thickening and vague soft tissue density and rarely erosion of bone or invasion of adjacent muscle. Arteriography is more diagnostic in that the pooling of blood over the mass suggests a vascular tumor. The tumor grows either as a discrete pedunculated lesion or as a diffuse process.

Histologically, the tumors are cavernous hemangiomas in which the vessels are separated by an edematous, myxoid, or focally hyalinized matrix occasionally containing inflammatory cells and siderophages (Fig. 22–52). The synovium overlying the tumor is sometimes thrown into villous projections, and its cells contain moderate to marked amounts of hemosiderin pigment (Figs 22–52, 22–53). These synovial changes appear to be secondary phenomena but sometimes are so striking they raise the possibility of primary synovitis. Proper evaluation depends on the recognition that the underlying vessels are far too numerous and large for the area in question.

It has been suggested that these lesions are not neoplasms but represent a reaction to trauma, although such a history is given in only a small number of cases. On the other hand, the young age of most afflicted patients again raises the question as to whether these lesions represent congenital malformations or tumors, especially because occasional patients have been noted to have hemangiomas elsewhere.

Treatment of local or pedunculated tumors is relatively easy, consisting of simple extirpation. Diffuse lesions are more difficult to eradicate surgically.

Hemangioma of peripheral nerves

Hemangiomas arising within the confines of the epineurium are rare. Of the few cases described in the literature several are probably unacceptable because they appear to involve nerve secondarily. Of the acceptable cases[136-140] there appears to be no characteristic age or anatomic distribution, although most occur in patients under the age of 40 years. Pain is a common symptom and may be accompanied by numbness and muscle wasting in the affected region. In one case, symptoms of carpal tunnel syndrome were noted as a result of the location of the tumor in the median nerve. Involved nerves have included the trigeminal, ulnar, median, posterior tibial, and peroneal nerves. Histologically, most of the tumors have been cavernous hemangiomas with no histologic features suggesting malignancy.

Treatment of these benign tumors must be individualized. The benefits of total resection must be balanced against the morbidity of the procedure. Complete removal of an intraneural hemangioma has been accomplished by intrafascicular dissection using dissecting microscopy.[140] Such an approach offers complete removal with minimal morbidity.

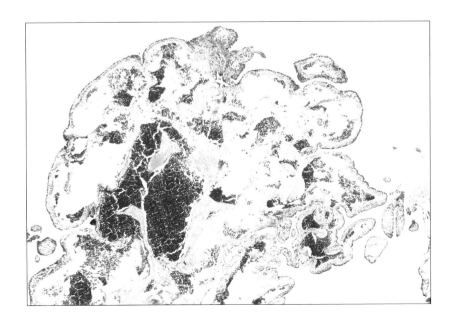

FIGURE 22–52 Synovial hemangioma depicting cavernous blood spaces located immediately subjacent to the synovial membrane.

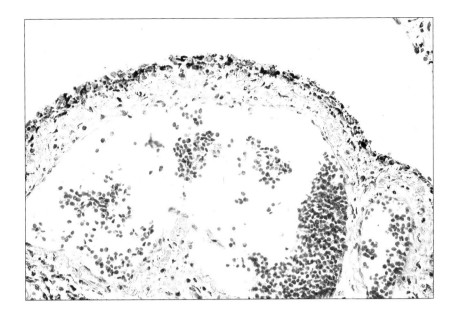

FIGURE 22–53 Synovial hemangioma. Pigmentation of synovial cells is a result of the presence of hemosiderin.

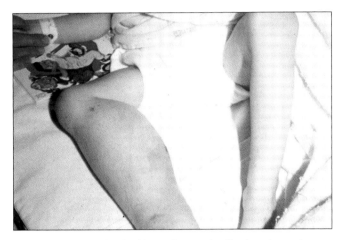

FIGURE 22–54 Child with angiomatosis affecting the entire lower leg.

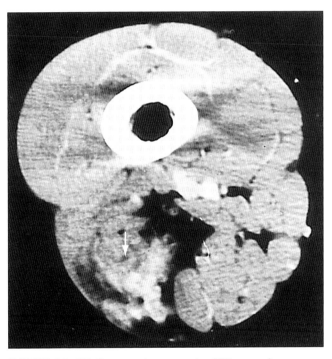

FIGURE 22–55 Computed tomography (CT) scan of angiomatosis illustrating diffuse nonhomogeneous regions in muscle. Serpiginous areas (arrow) represent tortuous vessels. (From Rao VK, Weiss SW. Angiomatosis of soft tissue: an analysis of the histologic features and clinical outcome in 51 cases. Am J Surg Pathol 1992; 16:764.)

ANGIOMATOSIS (DIFFUSE HEMANGIOMA)

Angiomatosis is a rare, benign but clinically extensive vascular lesion of soft tissue that almost invariably becomes symptomatic during childhood.[141–145] These lesions probably begin during early intrauterine life when the limb buds form, grow proportionately with the fetus, and consequently affect large areas of the trunk or extremity (Fig. 22–54). We propose a combined clinicopathologic definition for this condition requiring that such lesions be histologically benign and affect a large segment of the body in a contiguous fashion.[145] Involvement may be of two types: either extensive vertical involvement of multiple tissue planes (e.g., subcutis, muscle, and bone) or extensive involvement of tissue of the same type (e.g., multiple muscles). More than half of patients present within the first two decades of life, usually with symp-

toms of diffuse persistent swelling sometimes associated with pain and discoloration. Only rarely is hypertrophy, gigantism, or clinical evidence of arteriovenous shunting present. On computed tomography (CT) scans the lesions appear as ill-defined nonhomogeneous masses that may resemble sarcoma except for the presence of serpiginous dense areas that correspond to thick-walled, tortuous vessels (Fig. 22–55). Because of the presence of large amounts of fat, these tumors often appear as predominantly fatty tumors (Fig. 22–56).

Histologically, angiomatosis may assume one of two patterns. The first and more common pattern seen in most of the 50 cases we reviewed consisted of a mélange of large venous, cavernous, and capillary-sized vessels scattered haphazardly throughout soft tissue (Fig. 22–57). The venous vessels are remarkable for their irregular, thick walls that have occasional attenuations and herniations (Figs 22–58, 22–59). A rather characteristic feature of these veins is the presence of small vessels clustered just adjacent to or in the wall of a large vein (Fig. 22–58). The second pattern, which occurs in a small number of cases, is virtually identical to that of a capillary hemangioma, except that the nodules of tumor diffusely infiltrate the surrounding soft tissue. The prominent amount of fat present in these lesions has led previous authors to use the term *infiltrating angiolipoma*, suggesting that angiomatosis is probably best regarded as a more generalized mesenchymal proliferation. One unique case, which featured a diffuse proliferation of glomus cells in addition to the vessels, offers some support to the foregoing idea.[145]

In the study by Rao and Weiss,[145] nearly 90% of patients experienced recurrences, and 40% had more than one recurrence within a 5-year period. A somewhat lower recurrence rate was reported by Howat and Campbell.[144] This behavior contrasts with the recurrence rate of intramuscular hemangiomas, which is usually less than 50%. Although there has been speculation that recurrence rates may be higher in young children affected with this condition, it appears not to be true. There is no evidence that such lesions ever progress to frank malignancy, so the goal of therapy is to treat the lesions as conservatively as possible, balancing the need for complete surgical extirpation with the morbidity of the procedure.

Diagnosis of these unusual tumors may prove difficult. As indicated in the discussion of intramuscular hemangiomas, the distinction between angiomatosis and an intramuscular hemangioma is fundamentally based on clinical rather than pathologic criteria. However, we believe that the irregular venous channels with clustered small vessels in their walls are characteristic of angiomatosis and should certainly in small biopsy specimens prompt a dialogue with the clinician concerning the extent of the lesion.

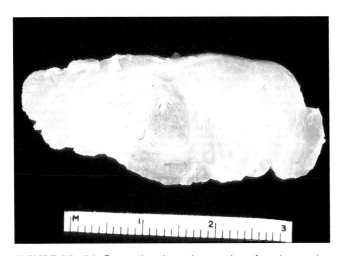

FIGURE 22–56 Cut section through a portion of angiomatosis. Pale appearance of muscle is typical and indicates replacement of fibers by vessels and fat.

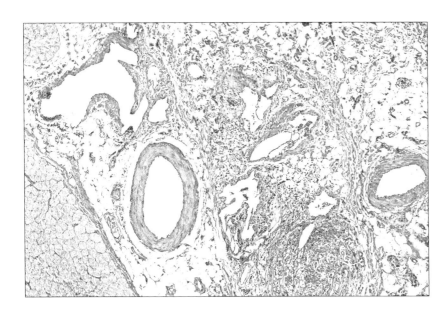

FIGURE 22–57 Angiomatosis with variously sized vessels involving muscle and fat.

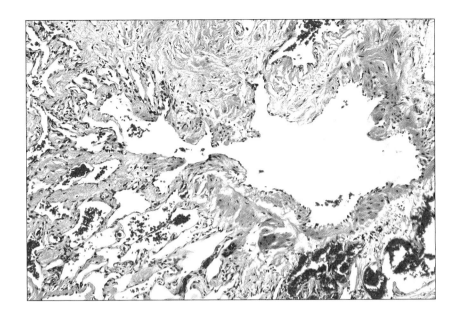

FIGURE 22–58 Angiomatosis with small vessels residing adjacent to and in the wall of a larger vessel.

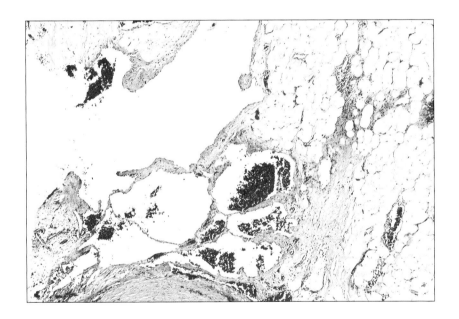

FIGURE 22–59 Venous vessel in angiomatosis illustrating irregular wall and herniations.

VASCULAR ECTASIAS

Vascular ectasias are collectively a common group of lesions characterized by localized dilatation of preformed vessels.[62,146–156] Although most are cutaneous and share certain common histologic features, the clinical presentation and etiology are different. In many instances, a precise diagnosis depends on complete knowledge of the clinical history and gross appearance of the lesion in question. Of the many types of vascular ectasias, only the more significant ones are mentioned. The reader is referred to an excellent review of the subject for detailed discussions of the less common forms.[62]

Nevus flammeus (nevus telangiectaticus)

The most common form of ectasia is the *nevus flammeus*, or ordinary birthmark. These lesions are most common on the mid-forehead, eyelids, and nape of the neck.[155,156] It has been estimated that about half of all infants have a *nevus flammeus* in the neck, which suggests an autosomal dominant mode of inheritance. Typically, the birthmark is a mottled macular lesion ranging in color from light pink to deep purple. Most are dull pink and are referred to as "salmon patches," or facetiously as "the affectionate peck of a stork." Most lesions eventually regress. Those on the forehead and eyelids are evanescent and disappear within the first year of life. Lesions on the nape of the neck fade more slowly, and their vestiges are documented in about 20% of the adult population.

The *port-wine stain* (*nevus vinosus*) is a specialized form of *nevus flammeus*. It differs from the latter in several respects; it grows proportionately with the child and demonstrates no tendency to fade. Although it begins as a smooth red to purple macular lesion on the face or extremity, it often acquires an elevated thickened surface that is more reminiscent of a true hemangioma. Dilatation of vessels in the mid and deep dermis is the principal alteration, and in the early lesion even this change may not be pronounced. Comparison of port-wine stains with normal skin has not indicated any differences in immunostaining for von Willebrand factor, basement membrane protein, fibronectin, or various monoclonal antibodies specific for endothelium (e.g., PAL-E, ICAM-1, ELAM-1).[152] There does, however, appear to be a decrease in the number of perivascular nerves, suggesting that lack of neural control of the vascular bed results in their progressive dilatation.[154] Treatment of port-wine stains by laser therapy has been used.[149]

Aside from the cosmetic problems it poses, the port-wine stain may indicate the presence of more extensive vascular malformation. Port-wine stains of the face that occur in the distribution of the trigeminal nerve may be associated with ipsilateral vascular malformations of the leptomeninges and occasionally of the retina (*Sturge-Weber syndrome, encephalotrigeminal angiomatosis*). Seizures, hemiplegia, and mental retardation, which characterize the full-blown syndrome, are the result of cerebral atrophy induced by the meningeal malformation. *Klippel-Trénaunay syndrome* includes a port-wine stain associated with varicosities and hypertrophy (gigantism) of an extremity.[157,158] In most instances of this rare condition the lower extremity is affected, and the extensive varicosities and edema appear to be the result of agenesis of the deep venous structures. In a small number of patients there may be, in addition, a congenital arteriovenous fistula. It has been suggested that this subgroup be separately designated as *Parkes-Weber syndrome* because the problems with management are different.[157,158] In Parkes-Weber syndrome the major therapeutic thrust must be directed toward reducing or eliminating the arteriovenous fistula to prevent supervening congestive heart failure.

A small number of port-wine stains are inherited as an autosomal dominant trait. Preliminary data suggest locus heterogeneity for these lesions with one locus, CMC1, identified on 5q13–22.[159,160]

Arterial spiders

Arterial spiders (*nevus araneus*) represent another common form of ectasia, but unlike the nevus flammeus they are rarely found at birth. Instead, they represent acquired lesions associated with altered physiologic states (e.g., pregnancy, liver disease, hyperthyroidism); the lesions often regress with restoration of the normal state.[62] Grossly, they are characterized by a small central arteriole or "punctum" from which tiny radial vessels emanate. With application of pressure over the punctum the entire lesion blanches. With release of pressure the lesion reddens in a centrifugal direction. The vascular spider consists of a thick-walled arteriole, which dilates, branches as it approaches the surface epithelium, and eventually anastomoses with small capillaries of the dermis.

Hereditary hemorrhagic telangiectasia (Osler-Weber-Rendu disease)

Hereditary hemorrhagic telangiectasia (HHT) is characterized by vascular anomalies consisting of dilated capillaries and veins of the skin and mucosal membranes.[153] It is inherited as an autosomal dominant disease. Linkage analysis has identified two loci, *HHT1* on 9q33–34 and *HHT2* on 12q11–14. Premature stop codons of the endoglin (*ENG*) and activin receptor-like kinase 1 (*ALK-1*) genes, important for the TGF-beta receptor complex in vascular endothelial cells, suggest loss of function mutations.[7]

The disease commences with the development of numerous small red papules on the skin and mucosa, particularly in the region of the face, lips, oral mucosa, and tongue. Similar lesions may be found in the gastrointestinal, genitourinary, and pulmonary systems. The lesions usually appear during childhood, increase with age, and in the elderly may have an appearance similar to that of the vascular spider. In contrast to the spider, the lesions are prone to bleeding, so the course of the disease is marked by repeated bouts of hemorrhage. Treatment must be supportive because treatment of ectasias by such modalities as electrocoagulation can result in the formation of satellite lesions.

REACTIVE VASCULAR PROLIFERATIONS

Papillary endothelial hyperplasia (vegetant intravascular hemangioendothelioma, intravascular angiomatosis)

Papillary endothelial hyperplasia is an exuberant, usually intravascular, endothelial proliferation that in many respects mimics an angiosarcoma.[161–168] It was first described by Masson, who designated it *vegetant intravascular hemangioendothelioma*.[167] He regarded it as a true neoplasm that displays degenerative changes including necrosis and thrombosis as it outgrows its blood supply, although now they are simply regarded as an exuberant form of organizing thrombus. Why only some thrombi display this form of organization is not clear.

Although this process may occur in virtually any vessel in the body, only those lesions that present as detectable masses are likely to come to the attention of the surgical pathologist. In our experience such lesions are most commonly located in veins on the head, neck, fingers, and trunk, where they appear as small, firm, superficial (deep dermis or subcutis) masses imparting a red to blue discoloration to the overlying skin (Fig. 22–60).[162] Usually, a history of trauma is not elicited. Both the appearance and symptoms are non-specific, so a biopsy is ultimately required to establish the identity of the lesion. In addition to its occurrence in a pure form in a dilated vessel, this lesion may be engrafted on

a preexisting vascular lesion such as a hemangioma, pyogenic granuloma, or vascular malformation. In these cases the symptoms, appearance, and ultimate prognosis are related to the underlying lesion. In fact, most deeply situated papillary endothelial hyperplasias occur in intramuscular hemangiomas.

In its pure form the lesion is a small (average 2 cm), purple-red, multicystic mass containing clotted blood and surrounded by a fibrous pseudocapsule containing residual smooth muscle or elastic tissue of the preexisting vessel wall (Fig. 22–61). In vessels of small caliber that are markedly dilated, little or no muscle is demonstrable in the pseudocapsule. Rarely, rupture of the vessel of origin permits spilling over of the process into surrounding soft tissue. In the early lesion, the ingrowth of endothelium along the contours of the thrombus partitions it into coarse papillae with fibrin cores (Fig. 22–62). In the well-established or typical lesion, myriad small delicate papillae project into the lumen and closely simulate the tufting growth of the hemangiosarcoma. These papillae are composed of a single layer of endothelium surrounding a collagenized core. The endothelial cells appear plump or swollen but lack significant pleomorphism and mitotic figures. During the late stage, clumping and fusing of the papillae give rise to an anastomosing network of vessels embedded in a loose mesh-like stroma of connective tissue (Fig. 22–62D).

Ultrastructurally, the cells lining the papillae appear to be differentiated endothelial cells with numerous micropinocytotic vesicles at the luminal aspect, tight junctions along the lateral boundaries, and occasional intracytoplasmic Weibel-Palade bodies. Basal lamina invests the antiluminal surface of the cell. In addition, pericytes and undifferentiated cells can be identified on the antiluminal aspects of the endothelial cells.[164] The participation of several cell types is similar to the situation encountered

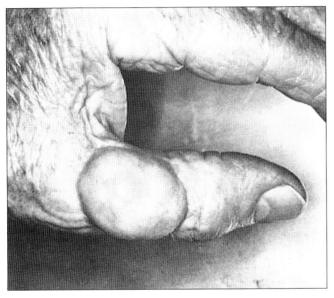

FIGURE 22–60 Papillary endothelial hyperplasia presenting as a localized nodule on the thumb.

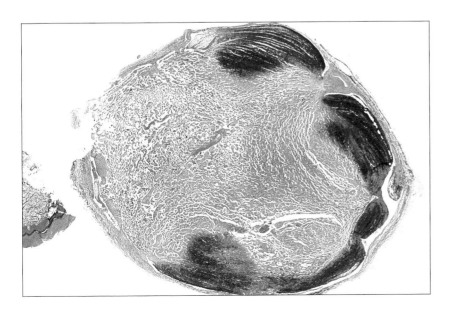

FIGURE 22–61 Organizing thrombus in a vessel showing early stages of papillary endothelial hyperplasia at the bottom of the picture.

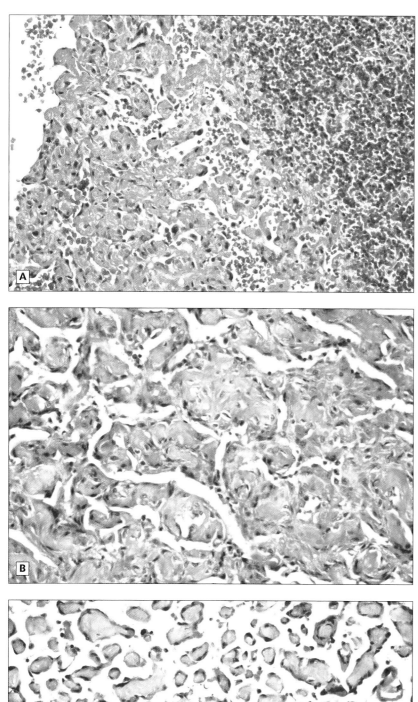

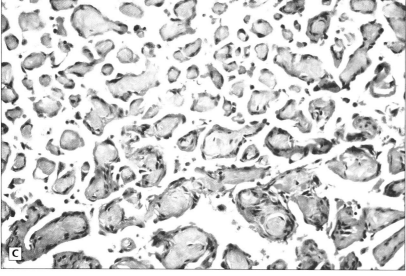

FIGURE 22–62 Stages of papillary endothelial hyperplasia. **(A)** Early stage is characterized by a thrombus with ingrowth of endothelial cells. Endothelium gradually subdivides the partially collagenized thrombus into coarse clumps **(B)** followed by papillae **(C)**.

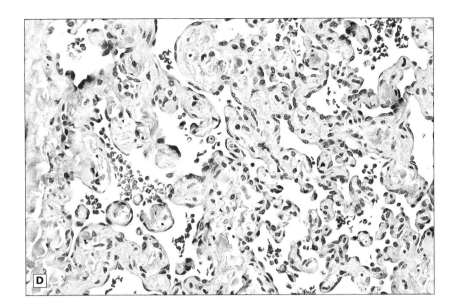

FIGURE 22–62 Continued. **(D)** At the end stage, papillae fuse to form a loosely anastomotic "secondary" vascular pattern.

in human granulation tissue and is further evidence of the reactive nature of this process.

The most significant aspect of this lesion is the regularity with which it is confused with an angiosarcoma. A helpful point in the differential diagnosis is its intravascular location, as angiosarcomas are almost never confined to a vascular lumen. As mentioned earlier, passive extension of this process into soft tissue may occur following vessel rupture. However, even in these cases the intravascular location of most of the lesion, coupled with the reactive changes in the vessel wall suggesting rupture, aid in the proper identification. On rare occasions papillary endothelial hyperplasia occurs extravascularly as a result of organization of a hematoma,[167] but this diagnosis should be made with caution. Apart from the usual intravascular location, papillary endothelial hyperplasia lacks the frank tissue necrosis, marked pleomorphism, and high mitotic rate that characterize many angiosarcomas.

The prognosis of this lesion is excellent. Essentially all cases are cured by simple excision. Those that do recur are usually those that are superimposed on vascular tumors. The therapy in these cases should be dictated by the nature of the underlying lesions.

Vascular transformation of lymph nodes (nodal angiomatosis)

First described as *vascular transformation of lymph nodes*[169] and later as *nodal angiomatosis*,[170] this reactive change of lymph node occurs secondary to lymphatic or venous obstruction, or both, and has been observed particularly in axillary lymph nodes removed at the time of radical mastectomy for breast carcinoma.[169–172] The change may also occur in lymph nodes removed for a variety of other diagnostic or therapeutic reasons. Typically, the change involves the subcapsular space and sinuses in either a segmental or diffuse fashion. In the most readily recognized case, the small, ectatic, capillary-sized vessels are well formed (Figs 22–63, 22–64). Chan et al.[171] emphasized a greater range of changes in this condition than was previously appreciated. In extreme examples of vascular transformation the vessels may be closely packed and slightly attenuated so the resemblance to Kaposi sarcoma is more than fleeting. Usually, however, there is maturation of the vessels toward the periphery of the lymph node such that ectatic capillaries are present immediately subjacent to the capsule. Extravasation of erythrocytes occurs; and in exceptional cases hyaline droplets, similar to those in Kaposi sarcoma, are identified.

There are a number of features that serve to distinguish this lesion from Kaposi sarcoma, including the overall preservation of lymph node architecture despite the expansion of the subcapsular and medullary sinuses, the peripheral maturation of the vessels, the lack of vessels arranged in distinct fascicles, and the presence of secondary sclerosis. However, the earliest stages of Kaposi sarcoma of lymph nodes, as seen in the patient with acquired immunodeficiency syndrome (AIDS), may prove exceptionally difficult and at some times impossible to distinguish from vascular transformation of the lymph node.

Glomeruloid hemangioma

Glomeruloid hemangioma is a descriptive term coined by Chan et al.[173] for the reactive vascular proliferations that occur in *POEMS syndrome* (Takatsuki syndrome and Crowe-Fukase syndrome).[173–176] This syndrome is characterized by *p*olyneuropathy (peripheral neuropathy, papilledema), *o*rganomegaly (hepatosplenomegaly,

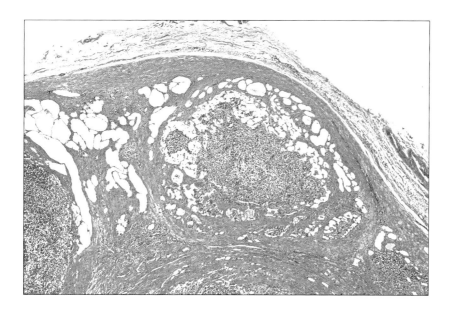

FIGURE 22–63 Vascular transformation in a lymph node (nodal angiomatosis). Vessels surround but preserve lymph follicles. Lymph node was removed as part of the regional lymph node dissection for carcinoma.

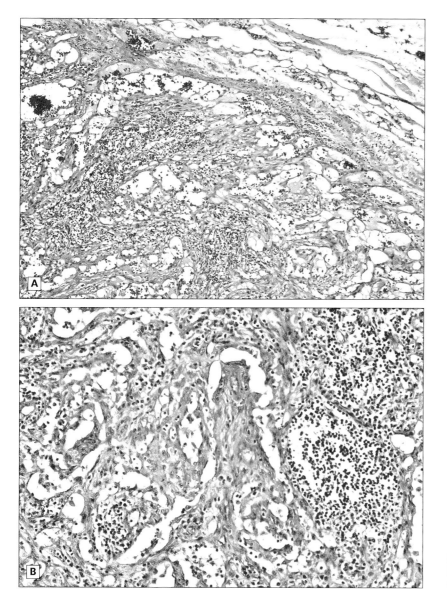

FIGURE 22–64 Vascular transformation of lymph node showing a subcapsular location (A) and prominent proliferation of vessels (B).

lymphadenopathy), *e*ndocrinopathy (amenorrhea, gynecomastia, impotence, adrenal insufficiency, hypothyroidism, glucose intolerance), *M*-protein (plasmacytosis, paraproteinemia, bone lesions), and *s*kin lesions (hyperpigmentation, hypertrichosis, angiomas); and, in some instances, it overlaps with multicentric Castleman's disease.[177]

The vascular lesions develop within the dermis underneath an intact, essentially normal epidermis. In the classic case, glomeruloid nests of capillaries lie in ectatic capillaries, creating a "vessel within a vessel" appearance (Figs 22–65, 22–66). The intravascular capillaries are lined by normal-appearing endothelium and are filled with erythrocytes. A distinctive feature of the intravascular proliferation is the large round cells filled with eosinophilic globules corresponding to polytypic immunoglobulin (Fig. 22–67). Chan et al.[173] suggested that these cells,

which reside principally outside the basal lamina, are closely related to endothelial cells rather than pericytes or smooth muscle cells. Their unusual appearance is probably induced by the presence of cytoplasmic immunoglobulin, which is derived from serum. In some cases of POEMS syndrome the vascular lesions are indistinguishable from an ordinary capillary hemangioma, and in other cases the lesions have features intermediate between a capillary hemangioma and the classic glomeruloid hemangioma, suggesting that they represent stages of the same process.

Bacillary (epithelioid) angiomatosis

Bacillary (epithelioid) angiomatosis is a pseudoneoplastic vascular proliferation, caused by *Bartonella* (formerly *Rochalimaea*), that occurs almost exclusively in immuno-

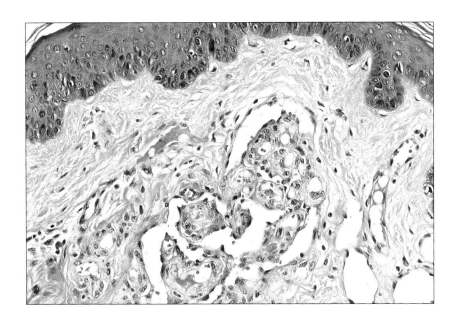

FIGURE 22–65 Glomeruloid hemangioma. (Case courtesy of Dr. C.D.M. Fletcher.)

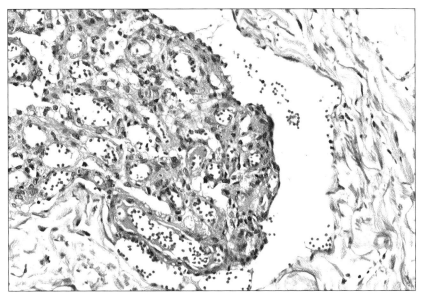

FIGURE 22–66 Glomeruloid hemangioma. (Case courtesy of Dr. C.D.M. Fletcher.)

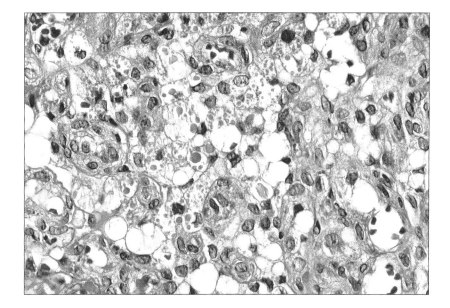

FIGURE 22–67 Hyaline droplets of immunoglobulin in a glomeruloid hemangioma. (Case courtesy of Dr. C.D.M. Fletcher.)

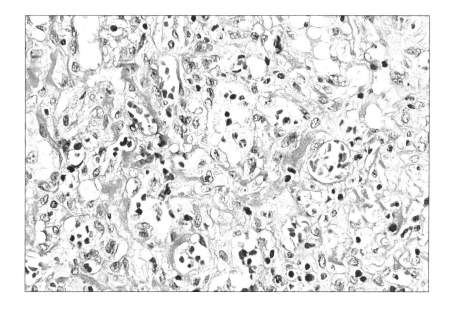

FIGURE 22–68 Bacillary angiomatosis showing endothelial cells with clear cytoplasm set in an inflammatory background.

compromised hosts.[178-186] *Bartonella* is a family of small Gram-negative bacilli that includes a number of species pathogenic for humans: *B. henselae, B. quinitana, B. bacilliformis*, and *B. elizabethae. Bartonella henselae* and *quintana* have been shown to be the causative agents for bacillary angiomatosis and bacillary peliosis, as well as for *Bartonella* bacterial endocarditis and classic cat-scratch disease.[185,186]

Most cases of bacillary angiomatosis occur in men in the setting of AIDS. Bacillary angiomatosis usually presents as multiple pink, elevated skin lesions that may resemble a pyogenic granuloma. Usually, their pink color distinguishes them from the dusky violaceous lesions of Kaposi sarcoma. In some cases, there are also liver, spleen, lymph node, bone, and soft tissue lesions.[178-181,184] In the classic case, bacillary angiomatosis consists of lobules of capillary-sized vessels lined by plump (epithelioid) endothelium with clear cytoplasm (Fig. 22–68). Mild atypia and occasional mitotic figures may be present in the endothelial cells. Although the strikingly clear cytoplasm of the endothelial cells bears some similarity to the endothelial changes in epithelioid hemangioma, there is a neutrophilic infiltrate in the interstitium along with collections of pink coagulum containing clusters of the organisms that are easily identified with the Warthin-Starry stain (Fig. 22–69). Unfortunately, some bacillary angiomatosis does not display the foregoing distinctive changes and may be virtually indistinguishable from granulation tissue.[186] Obviously, if the clinical setting suggests the diagnosis, one is obligated to rule out the diagnosis by means of special stains. On electron microscopy, the organisms appear as bacillary forms with a tri-

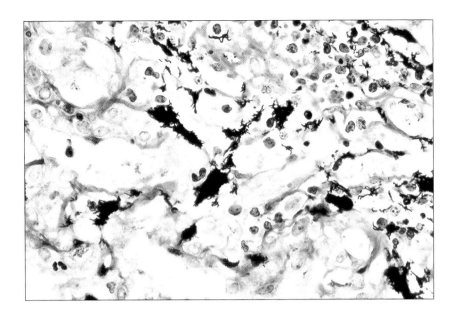

FIGURE 22–69 Warthin-Starry staining of bacillary angiomatosis showing numerous clumped rod-shaped organisms.

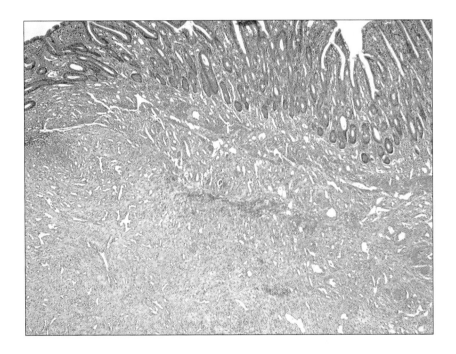

FIGURE 22–70 Florid vascular proliferation of the colon secondary to intussusception and colonic prolapse.

laminar cell wall. In the liver the organisms induce peliotic changes. Large numbers of organisms can be identified around the peliotic zones in the liver. Treatment of bacillary angiomatosis is effectively accomplished with erythromycin.

Florid vascular proliferation of the colon secondary to intussusception and prolapse

A florid vascular proliferation occurring in adult patients with intussusception and prolapse has recently been reported by Bavikatty et al.[187] The lesion, consisting of a lobular proliferation of small capillary-sized vessels, extends from the submucosa through the entire bowel wall and is associated with mucosal ischemia and ulceration (Figs 22–70, 22–71) Although the vascular proliferation dissects muscle fibers, the vessels are well formed and display minimal nuclear atypia. In two of the five cases reported, an underlying vascular malformation was identified. The excellent follow-up in the reported cases underscores the reactive nature of these proliferations.

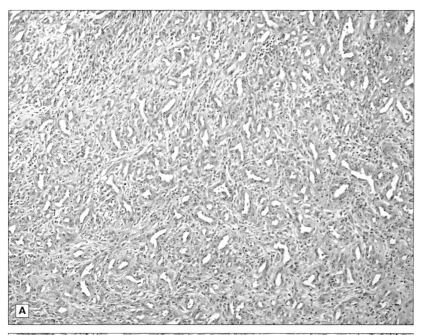

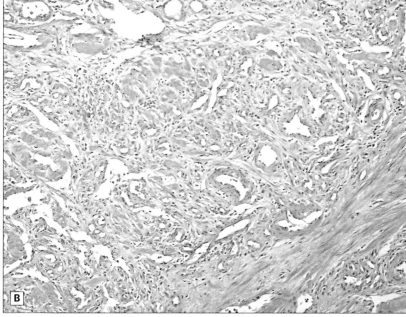

FIGURE 22–71 Florid vascular proliferation of the colon secondary to intussusception and colonic prolapse showing well-formed vessels **(A)** which involve muscularis propria **(B)**.

REFERENCES

General

1. Enjolras O. Vascular tumors and vascular malformations: are we at the dawn of a better knowledge. Pediatr Dermatol 1994; 16:238.
2. North PE, Mizeracki JR, Thomas R, et al. Intramuscular "hemangiomas" are vascular malformations immunodistinctive from juvenile hemangiomas [abstract 61]. Mod Pathol 2000; 13:14A.
3. Blei F, Walter J, Orlow SJ, et al. Familial segregation of hemangiomas and vascular malformations as an autosomal dominant trait. Arch Dermatol 1998; 134:718.
4. Laubauge P, Laberge S, Brunereau L, et al. Hereditary cerebral cavernous angiomas:

clinical and genetic features in 57 French families. Lancet 1998; 352:1892.
5. Nichols GE, Gaffey MJ, Mills SE, et al. Lobular capillary hemangioma: an immunohistochemical study including steroid hormone receptor status. Am J Clin Pathol 1992; 97:77.
6. Wawro NM, Fredrickson RW, Tennant RW. Hemangioma of the parotid gland in the newborn and in infancy. Cancer 1955; 8:595.
7. Brouillard P, Vikkula M. Vascular malformations: localized defects in vascular morphogenesis. Clin Genet 2003; 63:340.

Normal structure and function

8. Isner JM, Asahara T. Angiogenesis and vasculogenesis as therapeutic strategies for

postnatal neovascularization. J Clin Invest 1999; 103:1231.
9. Cines DB, Pollak ES, Buck CA, et al. Endothelial cells in physiology and in the pathophysiology of vascular disorders. Blood 1998; 91:3527.
10. Folkman J. Clinical application of research on angiogenesis. N Engl J Med 1995; 333:1757.
11. Arbiser JL. Angiogenesis: relevance for pathogenesis and treatment of dermatologic disease. Adv Dermatol 1999; 15:31.
12. Dejana E. Endothelial adherens junctions: implications in the control of vascular permeability and angiogenesis. J Clin Invest 1996; 98:1949.
13. Cleaver O, Melton DA. Endothelial signaling during development. Nature Med 2003; 9:661.

14. Messmer K, Hammersen F, eds. Structure and function of endothelial cells. Basel: Karger; 1983.

15. Thorgeirsson G, Robertson AL Jr. The vascular endothelium – pathobiologic significance. Am J Pathol 1978; 93:801.

16. Hoyer LW. The factor VIII complex: structure and function. Blood 1981; 58:1.

Hemangiomas

17. Coffin CM, Dehner LP. Vascular tumors in children and adolescents: a clinicopathologic study of 228 tumors in 222 patients. Pathol Annu 1993; 1:97.

18. Enjolras O, Mulliken JB. Vascular tumors and vascular malformations. Adv Dermatol 1998; 13:375.

19. Esterly NB. Cutaneous hemangiomas, vascular stains, and malformations, and associated syndromes. Curr Probl Dermatol 1995; 3:69.

20. Powell J. Update on hemangiomas and vascular malformations. Curr Opin Pediatr 1999; 11:457.

21. Requena L, Sangueza OP. Cutaneous vascular anomalies. Part I. Hamartomas, malformations, and dilatations of preexisting vessels. Am Acad Dermatol 1997; 37:523.

22. Watson WL, McCarthy WD. Blood and lymph vessel tumors. Surg Gynecol Obstet 1940; 71:569.

23. Weiss SW. Vascular tumors: a deductive approach to diagnosis. Surg Pathol 1989; 2:185.

24. Walter JW, Blei F, Anderson JL, et al. Genetic mapping of a novel familial form of infantile hemangioma. Am J Med Genet 1999; 82:77.

25. Berg JN, Walter JW, Thisanagayam U, et al. Evidence for the loss of heterozygosity of 5q in sporadic hemangiomas: are somatic mutations involved in hemangioma formation. J Clin Pathol 2001; 54:249.

26. Bowers RE, Graham EA, Tomlinson KM. Spontaneous cure of strawberry nevi. Arch Dermatol 1960; 82:667.

27. Campbell JS. Congenital capillary hemangiomas of the parotid gland: a lesion characteristic of infancy. N Engl J Med 1956; 254:56.

28. Goldman RL, Perzik SL. Infantile hemangioma of the parotid gland: a clinicopathological study of 15 cases. Arch Otolaryngol 1969; 90:605.

29. Gonzalez-Crussi F, Hull MT, Grosfeld JL, et al. Congenital hemangioendothelioma: immunologic and ultrastructural studies. Lab Invest 1978; 38:387A.

30. Gonzalez-Crussi F, Reyes-Mugica M. Cellular hemangiomas (hemangioendotheliomas) in infants: light microscopic, immunohistochemical, and ultrastructural observations. Am J Surg Pathol 1991; 15:769.

31. Jang YC, Arumugam S, Ferguson M, et al. Changes in matrix composition during the growth and regression of human hemangiomas. J Surg Res 1998; 80:9.

32. Lister WA. The natural history of strawberry nevi. Lancet 1938; 1:1429.

33. McFarland J. A congenital capillary angioma of the parotid gland: considerations of similar cases in the literature. Arch Pathol 1930; 9:820.

34. Pasyk KA, Grabb WC, Cherry GW. Cellular hemangioma: light and electron microscopic studies of two cases. Virchows Arch [Pathol Anat] 1982; 396:103.

35. Taxy JB, Gray SR. Cellular angiomas of infancy: an ultrastructural study of two cases. Cancer 1979; 43:2322.

36. Verkarre V, Patey-Mariaud de Serre N, Vazeux R, et al. ICAM-3 and E-selectin endothelial cell expression differentiate two phases of angiogenesis in infantile hemangiomas. J Cutan Pathol 1999; 26:17.

37. Yusunaga C, Sueshi K, Ohgami H, et al. Heterogeneous expression of endothelial cell markers in infantile hemangioendothelioma: immunohistochemical study of two solitary cases and one multiple one. Am J Clin Pathol 1989; 91:673.

38. Walsh TS, Tompkins VN. Some observations on the strawberry nevus of infancy. Cancer 1956; 9:869.

39. Takahashi K, Mulliken JB, Kozakewich HPW, et al. Cellular markers that distinguish the phases of hemangioma during infancy and childhood. J Clin Invest 1994; 93:2357.

40. Walter JW, North PE, Waner M, et al. Somatic mutation of vascular endothelial growth factor receptors in juvenile hemangioma. Genes Chromosomes Cancer 2002; 33:295.

41. Pasyk KA, Grabb WC, Cherry GW. Crystalloid inclusions in endothelial cells of cellular and capillary hemangiomas. Arch Dermatol 1983; 119:134.

42. Kumakiri M, Muramoto F, Tsukinaga T, et al. Crystalline lamellae in the endothelial cells of a type of hemangioma characterized by the proliferation of immature endothelial cells and pericytes. J Am Acad Dermatol 1983; 8:68.

43. Bielenberg DR, Bucana CD, Sanchez R, et al. Progressive growth of infantile cutaneous hemangioma is directly correlated with hyperplasia and angiogenesis of adjacent epidermis and inversely correlated with expression of endogenous angiogenesis inhibitor, IFN-beta. Int J Oncol 1999; 14:401.

44. Pasyk KA, Grabb WC, Cherry GW. Ultrastructure of mast cells in growing and involuting stages of hemangiomas. Hum Pathol 1983; 14:174.

45. Razon MJ, Kraling BM, Mulliken JB, et al. Increasing apoptosis coincides with onset of involution in infantile hemangioma. Microcirculation 1998; 5:189.

46. North PE, Waner M, Mizerack A, et al. A unique microvascular phenotype shared by juvenile hemangiomas and human placenta. Arch Dermatol 2001; 137:559.

47. Ezekowitz RA, Mulliken JB, Folkman J. Interferon alpha-2a therapy for life-threatening hemangiomas of infancy. N Engl J Med 1992; 326:1456.

48. Sangueza OP, Requena L. Pathology of vascular skin lesions: clincopathologic correlations. Totowa, NJ: Human Press; 2003:47.

49. Kerr DA. Granuloma pyogenicum. Oral Surg Oral Med Oral Pathol 1951; 4:158.

50. De Kaminsky AR, Otero AC, Kaminsky CA, et al. Multiple disseminated pyogenic granuloma. Br J Dermatol 1978; 98:461.

51. Juhlin L, Sven-Olaf H, Ponten J, et al. Disseminated granuloma pyogenicum. Acta Dermatotvener (Stockh) 1970; 50:134.

52. Wilson BB, Greer KE, Cooper PH. Eruptive disseminated lobular capillary hemangioma (pyogenic granuloma). J Am Acad Dermatol 1989; 21:391.

53. Mills SE, Cooper PH, Fechner RE. Lobular capillary hemangioma: the underlying lesion of pyogenic granuloma. Am J Surg Pathol 1980; 4:471.

54. Bhaskar SN, Jacoway JR. Pyogenic granuloma: clinical features, incidence, histology, and result of treatment: report of 242 cases. J Oral Surg 1966; 24:391.

55. Coskey RJ, Mehregan AH. Granuloma pyogenicum with multiple satellite recurrences. Arch Dermatol 1967; 96:71.

56. Grupper C, Pastel A. Pyogenic granuloma with multiple satellites. Bull Soc Fr Dermatol Syphilogr 1969; 76:496.

57. Nagashima N, Niizuma K. Multiple satellite granuloma telangiectaticum. Jpn J Dermatol 1972; 82:1.

58. Warner J, Wilson-Jones E. Pyogenic granuloma recurring with multiple satellites: a report of 11 cases. Br J Dermatol 1968; 80:218.

59. Zaynoun ST, Juljulian HH, Kurban AK. Pyogenic granuloma with multiple satellites. Arch Dermatol 1974; 9:689.

60. McDonald RH. Granuloma gravidarum. Am J Obstet Gynecol 1956; 72:1132.

61. Cooper PH, McAllister HA, Helwig EB. Intravenous pyogenic granuloma: a study of 18 cases. Am J Surg Pathol 1979; 3:221.

62. Bean WB. Vascular spiders and related lesions of the skin. Springfield, IL: Charles C Thomas; 1958.

63. Honish A, Grimsrud K, Miedzinski L, et al. Outbreak of Campbell de Morgan spots in a nursing home – Alberta. Can Dis Wkly Rep 1988; 14:211.

64. Raymond LW, Williford LS, Burke WA. Eruptive cherry angiomas and irritant symptoms after one acute exposure to the glycol ether solvent 2-butoxyethanol. J Occup Environ Med 1998; 40:1059.

65. Firooz A, Komeili A, Dowlati Y. Eruptive melanocytic nevi and cherry angiomas secondary to exposure to sulfur mustard gas. J Am Acad Dermatol 1999; 40:646.

66. Cohen AD, Cagnano E, Vardy DA. Cherry angiomas associated with exposure to bromides. Dermatology 2001; 202:52.

67. Wells GC, Whimster I. Subcutaneous angiolymphoid hyperplasia with eosinophilia. Br J Dermatol 1969; 81:1.

68. Eady RAJ, Cowen T, Wilson-Jones E. Pseudopyogenic granuloma: the histopathogenesis in the light of ultrastructural studies. Br J Dermatol 1976; 95(Suppl):14.

69. Eady RAJ, Wilson-Jones E. Pseudopyogenic granuloma: enzyme histochemical and ultrastructural study. Hum Pathol 1977; 8:653.

70. Rosai J, Gold J, Landy R. The histiocytoid hemangiomas: a unifying concept embracing several previously described entities of skin, soft tissue, large vessels, bone, and heart. Hum Pathol 1979; 10:707.

71. Waldo E, Sidhu GS, Stahl R, et al. Histiocytoid hemangioma with features of angiolymphoid hyperplasia and Kaposi's sarcoma: a study by light microscopy, electron microscopy, and immunologic techniques. Am J Dermatopathol 1983; 5:525.

72. Googe PB, Harris NL, Mihm MC. Kimura's disease and angiolymphoid hyperplasia with eosinophils: two distinct histopathological entities. J Cutan Pathol 1987; 14:263.

73. Kitabatake T, Kurokawa H, Kurokawa S, et al. Radiotherapy for eosinophilic granuloma of the soft tissue (Kimura's disease). Strahlentherapie 1972; 144:407.

74. Chan JKC, Hui PK, Ng CS, et al. Epithelioid hemangioma (angiolymphoid hyperplasia with eosinophilia) and Kimura's disease in Chinese. Histopathology 1989; 15:557.

75. Hui PK, Chan JKC, Ng CS, et al. Lymphadenopathy of Kimura's disease. Am J Surg Pathol 1989; 13:177.

76. Kimura T, Yoshimura S, Ishikawa E. Unusual granulation combined with hyperplastic change of lymphatic tissue. Trans Soc Pathol Jpn 1948; 37:179.

77. Kung ITM, Gibson JB, Bannatyne PM. Kimura's disease: a clinicopathological study of 21 cases and its distinction from angiolymphoid hyperplasia with eosinophilia. Pathology 1984; 16:39.

78. Kuo TT, Shih L-Y, Chan H-L. Kimura's disease: involvement of regional lymph nodes and distinction from angiolymphoid hyperplasia with eosinophilia. Am J Surg Pathol 1988; 12:843.

79. Quinibi WY, Al-Sibai MB, Akhtar M. Mesangioproliferative glomerulonephritis associated with Kimura's disease. Clin Nephrol 1988; 30:111.

80. Urabe A, Tsuneyoshi M, Enjoji M. Epithelioid hemangioma versus Kimura's disease: a

comparative clinicopathologic study. Am J Surg Pathol 1987; 11:758.

81. Fetsch JF, Sesterhenn IA, Miettinen et al. Epithelioid hemangioma of the penis: a clinicopathologic and immunohistochemical analysis of 19 cases, with special reference to exuberant examples often confused with epithelioid hemangioendothelioma and epithelioid angiosarcoma. Am J Surg Pathol 2004; 28:523.

82. Rosai J, Ackerman LR. Intravenous atypical vascular proliferation: a cutaneous lesion simulating a malignant blood vessel tumor. Arch Dermatol 1974; 109:714.

83. Reed RJ, Terazakis N. Subcutaneous angioblastic lymphoid hyperplasia with eosinophilia (Kimura's disease). Cancer 1972; 29:489.

84. Fetsch JF, Weiss SW. Observations concerning the pathogenesis of epithelioid hemangioma (angiolymphoid hyperplasia). Mod Pathol 1991; 4:449.

85. Moesner J, Pallesen R, Sorensen B. Angiolymphoid hyperplasia with eosinophilia (Kimura's disease): a case with dermal lesions in the knee and a popliteal arteriovenous fistula. Arch Dermatol 1981; 117:650.

86. Brenn T, Fletcher CDM. Cutaneous epithelioid angiomatous nodule: a distinct lesion in the morphologic spectrum of epithelioid vascular tumors. Am J Dermatopath 2004; 26:14.

87. Yamada A, Mitsuhashi K, Miyakawa Y, et al. Membranous glomerulonephritis associated with eosinophilic folliculitis of the skin (Kimura's disease): report of a case and review of the literature. Clin Nephrol 1982; 18:211.

88. Madewell JE, Sweet DE. Tumors and tumorlike lesions in or about joints. In: Resnick D, Niwayama G, eds. Diagnosis of bone and joint disorders, vol 3. Philadelphia: WB Saunders; 1981.

89. Calonje E, Fletcher CDM. Sinusoidal hemangioma: a distinctive benign vascular neoplasm within the group of cavernous hemangiomas. Am J Surg Pathol 1991; 15:1130.

90. Brizel HE, Raccuglia G. Giant hemangioma with thrombocytopenia: radioisotope demonstration of platelet sequestration. Blood 1965; 26:751.

91. De Prost Y, Teillac D, Bodemer C, et al. Successful treatment of Kasabach-Merritt syndrome with pentoxifylline. J Am Acad Dermatol 1991; 25:854.

92. Inceman S, Tangu Y. Chronic defibrination syndrome due to a giant hemangioma associated with microangiopathic hemolytic anemia. Am J Med 1969; 46:997.

93. Kasabach HH, Merritt KK. Capillary hemangioma with extensive purpura: report of a case. Am J Dis Child 1961; 59:1063.

94. Sarkar M, Mulliken JB, Koazakewich HP, et al. Thrombocytopenic coagulopathy (Kasabach-Merritt phenomenon) is associated with kaposiform hemangioendothelioma and not with common infantile hemangioma. Plast Reconstruct Surg 1997; 100:1377.

Miscellaneous hemangiomas

95. Imperial R, Helwig EB. Verrucous hemangioma: a clinicopathologic study of 21 cases. Arch Dermatol 1967; 96:247.

96. Chan JKC, Tsang WYW, Calonje E, et al. Verrucous hemangioma: a distinctive but neglected variant of cutaneous hemangioma. Int J Surg Pathol 1995; 2:171.

97. Calduch L, Ortega C, Navarro V, et al. Verrucous hemangioma: report of two cases and review of the literature. Pediatro Dermatol 2000; 17:213.

98. Clinton TS, Cooke LM, Graham BS. Cobb syndrome associated with a verrucous (angiokeratoma-like) vascular malformation. Cutis 2003; 71:283.

99. Guillou L, Calonje E, Speight P, et al. Hobnail hemangioma: a pseudomalignant vascular lesions with a reappraisal of targetoid hemosiderotic hemangioma. Am J Surg Pathol 1999; 23:97.

100. Mentzel TP, Partanen TA, Kutzner H. Hobnail hemangioma ("targetoid hemosiderotic hemangioma"): clinicopathologic and immunohistochemical analysis of 62 cases. J Cutan Pathol 1999; 26:279.

101. Franke FE, Steger K, Marks A, et al. Hobnail hemangioma (targetoid hemosiderotic hemangiomas) are true lymphangiomas. J Cutan Pathol 2004; 31:362.

102. Santa Cruz DJ, Aronberg J. Targetoid hemosiderotic hemangioma. J Am Acad Dermatol 1988; 19:550.

103. Vion B, Frenk E. Targetoid hemosiderotic hemangioma. Dermatology 1992; 184:300.

104. Wilson-Jones E, Orkin M. Tufted angioma (angioblastoma): a benign progressive angioma, not to be confused with Kaposi's sarcoma or low-grade angiosarcoma. J Am Acad Dermatol 1989; 20:214.

105. Okada E, Tamura A, Ishikawa O, et al. Tufted angioma (angioblastoma): case report and review of 41 cases in the Japanese literature. Clin Exp Dermatol 2000; 25:627.

106. Kumakiri M, Muramoto LE, Tsukinga I, et al. Crystalline lamellae in the endothelial cells of a type of hemangioma characterized by the proliferation of immature endothelial cells and pericytes-angioblastoma (Nakagawa). J Am Acad Dermatol 1983; 8:68.

107. Padilla RS, Orkin M, Rosai J. Acquired tufted angioma (progressive capillary hemangioma): a distinctive clinicopathologic entity related to lobular capillary hemangioma. Am J Dermatopathol 1987; 9:292.

108. Brasanac D, Janic D, Boricic I, et al. Retroperitoneal kaposiform hemangioendothelioma with tufted angioma-like features in an infant with Kasabach-Merritt syndrome. Pathol Int 2003; 53:627.

109. Chu CY, Cheng HC, Hsien-Ching. Transformation between kaposiform hemangioendothelioma and tufted angioma. Dermatology 2003; 206:334.

110. Herron MD, Coffin CM, Vanderhooft SL. Tufted angioma: variability of the clinical morphology. Pediatr Dermatol 2002; 19:394.

111. Browning J, Frieden I, Baselga E, et al. Congenital self-regressing tufted angioma. Arch Dermatol 2006; 142:749.

112. Haisley-Royster C, Enjoiras O, Frieden IJ, et al. Kasabach-Merritt phenomenon: a retrospective study of treatment with vincristine. J Pediat Hemat Oncol 2002; 24:459.

113. Tille JC, Morris MA, Brundler MA, et al. Familial predisposition to tufted angioma: identification of blood and lymphatic vascular components. Clin Genet 2003; 63:393.

114. Weiss SW, Enzinger FM. Spindle cell hemangioendothelioma: a low grade angiosarcoma resembling a cavernous hemangioma and Kaposi's sarcoma. Am J Surg Pathol 1986; 10:521.

115. Perkins P, Weiss SW. Spindle cell hemangioendothelioma: an analysis of 78 cases with reassessment of its pathogenesis and biologic behavior. Am J Surg Pathol 1996; 20:1196.

116. Fletcher CDM, Beham A, Schmid C. Spindle cell hemangioendothelioma: a clinicopathological and immunohistochemical study indicative of a non-neoplastic lesion. Histopathology 1991; 18:291.

117. Gallione CJ, Pasyk KA, Boon LM, et al. A gene for familial venous malformations maps to chromosome 9p in a second large kindred. J Med Genet 1995; 32:197.

118. Vikkula M, Boon LM, Carraway KL, et al. Vascular dysmorphogenesis caused by an activating mutation in the receptor tyrosine kinase TIE2. Cell 1996; 87:1181.

119. Bluefarb SM, Adams LA. Arteriovenous malformation with angiodermatitis: stasis dermatitis simulating Kaposi's sarcoma. Arch Dermatol 1967; 96:176.

120. Earhart RN, Aeling JA, Nuss DD, et al. Pseudo-Kaposi's sarcoma: a patient with arteriovenous malformation and skin lesions simulating Kaposi's sarcoma. Arch Dermatol 1974; 110:907.

121. Strutton G, Weedon D. Acro-angiodermatitis: a simulant of Kaposi's sarcoma. Am J Dermatopathol 1987; 9:85.

122. Allen PW, Enzinger FM. Hemangiomas of skeletal muscle: an analysis of 89 cases. Cancer 1972; 29:8.

123. Angervall L, Nielsen JM, Stener B, et al. Concomitant arteriovenous vascular malformation in skeletal muscle. Cancer 1979; 44:232.

124. Angervall L, Nilsson L, Stener B, et al. Angiographic, microangiographic, and histologic study of vascular malformation in striated muscle. Acta Radiol 1968; 7:65.

125. Beham A, Fletcher CDM. Intramuscular angioma: a clinicopathologic analysis of 74 cases. Histopathology 1991; 18:53.

126. Cohen AJ, Youkey JR, Clagett GP. Intramuscular hemangioma. JAMA 1983; 249:2680.

127. Godanich IF, Capanacci M. Vascular hamartomata and infantile angioectatic osteohyperplasia of the extremities. J Bone Joint Surg [Am] 1962; 44:815.

128. Bate TH. Hemangioma of the tendon sheath. J Bone Joint Surg [Am] 1954; 36:104.

129. Bennett GE, Cobey MC. Hemangioma of joints: report of five cases. Arch Surg 1939; 38:487.

130. Burman MS, Milgram JE. Hemangioma of tendon and tendon sheath. Surg Gynecol Obstet 1930; 50:397.

131. Cobey MC. Hemangioma of joints. Arch Surg 1943; 46:465.

132. Harkins HN. Hemangioma of a tendon sheath: report of a case with a study of 24 cases from the literature. Arch Surg 1937; 34:12.

133. Lichtenstein L. Tumors of synovial joints, bursae, and tendon sheath. Cancer 1955; 8:816.

134. Osgood RB. Tuberculosis of the knee joint: angioma of the knee joint. Surg Clin North Am 1921; 1:665.

135. Webster GV, Geschickter DF. Benign capillary hemangioma of digital flexor tendon sheath: case report. Ann Surg 1945; 122:444.

136. Kojima T, Ide Y, Marumo E, et al. Hemangioma of median nerve causing carpal tunnel syndrome. Hand 1976; 8:62.

137. Losli EJ. Intrinsic hemangiomas of the peripheral nerves. Arch Pathol 1952; 53:226.

138. Sato S. Uber das cavernose Angiom des peripherischen Nerven system. Arch Klin Chir 1913; 100:553.

139. Sommer R. Uber cavernose Angiome am peripheren Nervensystem. Dtsch Z Chir 1922; 173:65.

140. Wood MB. Intraneural hemangioma: report of a case. Plast Reconstr Surg 1980; 65:74.

Angiomatosis (diffuse hemangioma)

141. Devaney K, Vinh TN, Sweet DE. Skeletal-extraskeletal angiomatosis: a clinicopathological study of fourteen patients and nosological considerations. J Bone Joint Surg [Am] 1994; 76:878.

142. Doederlein H. An unusually extensive hemangioma of diaphragm and of internal thoracic and abdominal wall as a cause of death in newborn. Zentralbl Allg Pathol 1938; 71:193.

143. Holden KR, Alexander E. Diffuse neonatal hemangiomatosis. Pediatrics 1970; 46:411.

144. Howat AJ, Campbell PE. Angiomatosis: a vascular malformation of infancy and childhood. Pathology 1987; 19:377.
145. Rao VK, Weiss SW. Angiomatosis of soft tissue: an analysis of the histologic features and clinical outcome in 51 cases. Am J Surg Pathol 1992; 16:764.

Vascular ectasias

146. Alderson MR. Spider naevi: their incidence in healthy school children. Arch Dis Child 1963; 38:286.
147. Barsky SH, Rosen S, Geer DE, et al. The nature and evolution of port wine stains: a computer-assisted study. J Invest Dermatol 1980; 74:154.
148. Buecker JW, Ratz JL, Richfield DF. Histology of port-wine stain treated with carbon dioxide laser. J Am Acad Dermatol 1984; 10:14.
149. Finley JL, Arndt KA, Noe J, et al. Argon laser port-wine stain interaction. Arch Dermatol 1984; 120:613.
150. Finley JL, Clark RAF, Colvin RB, et al. Immunofluorescent staining with antibodies to factor VIII, fibronectin, and collagenous basement membrane protein in normal skin and port-wine stains. Arch Dermatol 1982; 118:971.
151. Finley JL, Noe JM, Arndt KA, et al. Port wine stains: morphologic variations and developmental lesions. Arch Dermatol 1984; 120:1453.
152. Neumann R, Leonhartsberger H, Knobler R, et al. Immunohistochemistry of port wine stains and normal skin with endothelium-specific antibodies PAL-E, anti-ICAM, anti-ELAM, and anti-factor VIIIrAG. Arch Dermatol 1994; 130:879.
153. Osler W. On a family form of recurring epistaxis associated with multiple telangiectases of the skin and mucous membranes. Bull Johns Hopkins Hosp 1901; 12:333.
154. Smoller B, Rosen S. Port-wine stains: a disease of altered neural modulation of blood vessels. Arch Dermatol 1986; 122:177.
155. Tan KL. Nevus flammeus of the nape, glabella, and eyelids. Clin Pediatr 1972; 11:112.
156. Wenzl JE, Burgert EO. The spider nevus in infancy and childhood. Pediatrics 1964; 33:227.
157. Letts RM. Orthopedic treatment of hemangiomatous hypertrophy of the lower extremity. J Bone Joint Surg [Am] 1977; 59:777.
158. Lindenauer SM. The Klippel-Trénaunay syndrome: varicosity, hypertrophy, and hemangioma with arteriovenous fistula. Ann Surg 1965; 162:303.

Reactive vascular proliferations

159. Eerola I, Boon LM, Watanabe S, et al. Locus for susceptibility for familial capillary malformation ("port wine stain") maps to 5q. Eur J Hum Genet 2002; 10:375.
160. Breugem CC, Alders M, Salieb-Beugelaar GB, et al. A locus for hereditary capillary malformations mapped on chromosomes 5q. Hum Genet 2002; 110:343.
161. Barr RJ, Graham JH, Sherwin LA. Intravascular papillary endothelial hyperplasia: a benign lesion mimicking angiosarcoma. Arch Dermatol 1978; 114:723.
162. Clearkin KP, Enzinger FM. Intravascular papillary endothelial hyperplasia. Arch Pathol Lab Med 1976; 100:441.
163. Hashimoto H, Daimaru Y, Enjoji M. Intravascular papillary endothelial hyperplasia: a clinicopathologic study of 91 cases. Am J Dermatopathol 1983; 5:539.
164. Kreutner A Jr, Smith RM, Trefny FA. Intravascular papillary endothelial hyperplasia: light and electron microscopic observations of a case. Cancer 1978; 42:2305.
165. Kuo T, Sayers P, Rosai J. Masson's "vegetant intravascular hemangioendothelioma": a lesion often mistaken for angiosarcoma. Cancer 1976; 38:1227.
166. Masson P. Hemangioendotheliome vegetant intravasculaire. Bull Soc Anat (Paris) 1923; 93:517.
167. Pins MR, Rosenthal DI, Springfield DS, et al. Florid extravascular papillary endothelial hyperplasia (Masson's pseudoangiosarcoma) presenting as a soft tissue sarcoma. Arch Pathol Lab Med 1993; 117:259.
168. Salyer WR, Salyer DC. Intravascular angiomatosis: development and distinction from angiosarcoma. Cancer 1975; 36:995.
169. Haferkamp O, Rosenau W, Lennert K. Vascular transformation of lymph node sinuses due to venous obstruction. Arch Pathol 1971; 92:81.
170. Fayemi AO, Toker C. Nodal angiomatosis. Arch Pathol 1975; 99:170.
171. Chan JKC, Warnke RA, Dorfman R. Vascular transformation of sinuses in lymph nodes: a study of its morphological spectrum and distinction from Kaposi's sarcoma. Am J Surg Pathol 1991; 15:732.
172. Ostrowski ML, Siddiqui T, Barnes RE, et al. Vascular transformation of lymph node sinuses: a process displaying a spectrum of histologic features. Arch Pathol Lab Med 1990; 114:656.
173. Chan JKC, Fletcher CDM, Hicklin GA, et al. Glomeruloid haemangioma: a distinctive cutaneous lesion of multicentric Castleman's disease associated with POEMS syndrome. Am J Surg Pathol 1990; 14:1036.

174. Ishikawa AO, Nihei Y, Ishikawa H. The skin changes of POEMS syndrome. Br J Dermatol 1987; 117:523.
175. Kanitakis J, Roger H, Soubrier M, et al. Cutaneous angiomas in POEMS syndrome: an ultrastructural and immunohistochemical study. Arch Dermatol 1988; 124:695.
176. Zak FG, Solomon A, Fellner MJ. Viscerocutaneous angiomatosis with dysproteinemia phagocytosis: its relationship to Kaposi's sarcoma and lymphoproliferative disorders. J Pathol 1966; 92:594.
177. Yang SG, Cho KH, Bang YJ, et al. A case of glomeruloid hemangioma associated with multicentric Castleman's disease. Am J Dermatol 1998; 20:266.
178. Baron AL, Steinbach LS, LeBoit PE, et al. Osteolytic lesions and bacillary angiomatosis in HIV infection: radiologic differentiation from AIDS-related Kaposi's sarcoma. Radiology 1990; 177:77.
179. Chan JKC, Lewin KJ, Lombard CM, et al. Histopathology of bacillary angiomatosis of lymph node. Am J Surg Pathol 1991; 15:430.
180. Cockerell CJ, Bergstresser PR, Myrie-Williams C, et al. Bacillary epithelioid angiomatosis occurring in an immunocompetent individual. Arch Dermatol 1990; 126:787.
181. LeBoit PE, Berger TG, Egbert BM, et al. Bacillary angiomatosis: the histopathology and differential diagnosis of a pseudoneoplastic infection in patients with human immunodeficiency virus disease. Am J Surg Pathol 1989; 13:909.
182. Reed JA, Brigati DJ, Flynn SD, et al. Immunocytochemical identification of Rochalimaea henselae in bacillary (epithelioid) angiomatosis, parenchymal bacillary peliosis, and persistent fever with bacteremia. Am J Surg Pathol 1992; 16:650.
183. Relman DA, Loutit JS, Schmidt TM, et al. The agent of bacillary angiomatosis: an approach to the identification of uncultured pathogens. N Engl J Med 1990; 323:1573.
184. Schnella RA, Greco MA. Bacillary angiomatosis presenting as a soft-tissue tumor without skin involvement. Hum Pathol 1990; 21:567.
185. Spach DH, Koehler JE. Bartonella-associated infections. Infect Dis Clin North Am 1998; 12:137.
186. Wong R, Tappero J, Cockerell CJ. Bacillary angiomatosis and other Bartonella species infections. Semin Cutan Med Surg 1997; 16:186.
187. Bavikatty NR, Goldblum FR, Abdul-Karim FW, et al. Florid vascular proliferation of the colon related to intussusception and mucosal prolapse: potential diagnostic confusion with angiosarcoma. Mod Pathol 2001; 14:1114.

HEMANGIOENDOTHELIOMA: VASCULAR TUMORS OF INTERMEDIATE MALIGNANCY

CHAPTER CONTENTS

The term *hemangioendothelioma* has become a useful designation for vascular tumors that have a biologic behavior intermediate between a hemangioma and a conventional angiosarcoma. Tumors included in this group have the ability to recur locally and have some ability to metastasize, but at a far reduced level compared to angiosarcoma. The risk of metastasis varies from tumor to tumor within this group. For example, the epithelioid hemangioendothelioma, the most aggressive member of this family, produces distant metastasis and death in a small but definite number of cases, whereas the retiform and Dabska-type hemangioendotheliomas, two closely related tumors, are rarely associated with regional lymph node metastasis.

EPITHELIOID HEMANGIOENDOTHELIOMA

The epithelioid hemangioendothelioma, an angiocentric vascular tumor, can occur at almost any age but rarely occurs during childhood;[1,2] it affects the sexes about equally. To date no predisposing factors have been identified. The tumor develops as a solitary, slightly painful mass in either superficial or deep soft tissue, although in rare instances it occurs multifocally in a localized region of the body (Fig. 23–1). At least half of cases are closely associated with or arise from a vessel, usually a vein (Fig. 23–2). In some cases, occlusion of the vessel accounts for more profound symptoms, such as edema or thrombophlebitis. Those tumors that arise from vessels usually have a variegated, white-red color and superficially resemble organizing thrombi, except that they are firmly attached to the surrounding soft tissue. Those that do not arise from vessels are white-gray and offer little hint of

their vascular nature on gross inspection. Calcification is occasionally seen in large deeply situated tumors (Fig. 23–1).

Microscopic features

Lesions that arise from vessels have a characteristic appearance when seen at low power. They expand the vessel, usually preserving its architecture as they extend centrifugally from the lumen to the soft tissue (Figs 23–3, 23–4). The lumen is filled with a combination of tumor, necrotic debris, and dense collagen. Unlike the epithelioid hemangioma (see Chapter 22), in which vascular differentiation proceeds through the formation of multicellular, canalized vascular channels, vascular differentiation in these tumors is more primitive and is expressed primarily at the cellular level. The tumors are composed of short strands or solid nests of rounded to slightly spindled endothelial cells (Figs 23–5 to 23–9). Rarely are large, distinct vascular channels seen, except in the more peripheral portions of the tumor (Fig. 23–7). Instead, the tumor cells form small intracellular lumens, which are seen as clear spaces, or "vacuoles," that distort or "blister" the cell (Figs 23–8, 23–9). Frequently confused with the mucin vacuoles of adenocarcinoma, these miniature lumens occasionally contain erythrocytes. The stroma varies from highly myxoid to hyaline. The myxoid areas are light blue on hematoxylin-eosin staining, and conventional histochemical treatment with aldehyde fuchsin pH 1.0 may reveal sulfated acid mucopolysaccharides. This staining pattern should not be equated with cartilaginous differentiation; it simply reflects the tendency of some vascular tumors to produce sulfated acid mucins similar to the ground substance of vessel walls. Although occasional tumors do contain eosinophils and lymphocytes, rarely is this feature as pronounced as it is in the epithelioid hemangioma.

In most cases the tumors appear quite bland, and there is virtually no mitotic activity. In about one-fourth of cases the tumors contain areas with significant atypia, mitotic activity (more than 1 mitosis per 10 high-power fields [HPF]), focal spindling of the cells, or necrosis (Figs 23–10 to 23–12). Such features can be correlated with a

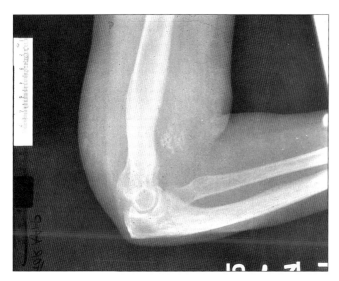

FIGURE 23-1 Plain film of arm showing an epithelioid hemangioendothelioma of the distal arm that has created erosion of bone. The mass is also partially calcified.

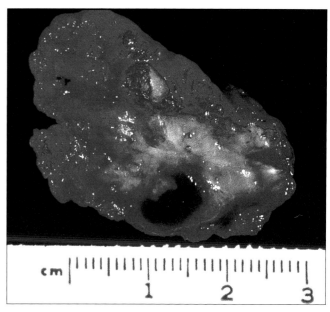

FIGURE 23-2 Gross specimen of epithelioid hemangioendothelioma. The tumor resembles an organizing thrombus in a small vein.

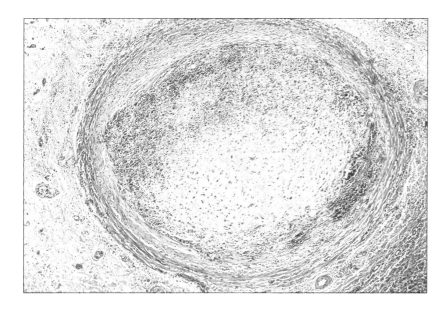

FIGURE 23-3 Epithelioid hemangioendothelioma.

more aggressive course, as discussed below. When metastases occur in this disease, they usually develop from tumors with these atypical features. Not unexpectedly, metastases also contain these features. In rare instances both primary and metastatic lesions appear bland cytologically.

Differential diagnosis

The differential diagnosis of this tumor includes metastatic carcinoma (or melanoma) and various sarcomas, which can assume an epithelioid appearance. In general, *carcinomas* and *melanomas* metastatic to soft tissue display far more nuclear atypia and mitotic activity than the epithelioid hemangioendothelioma and are rarely angiocentric. *Epithelioid angiosarcomas* are composed of solid sheets of highly atypical, mitotically active, epithelioid endothelial cells. Necrosis is common, and vascular differentiation is expressed primarily by the formation of irregular sinusoidal vascular channels. Occasional tumors have an architectural pattern (i.e., cords of epithelioid cells in a myxohyaline background) of an epithelioid hemangioendothelioma in some areas but solid sheets of epithelioid angiosarcoma in others. In our opinion these lesions should be regarded as conventional angiosarcomas, reserving the term epithelioid hemangioendothelioma

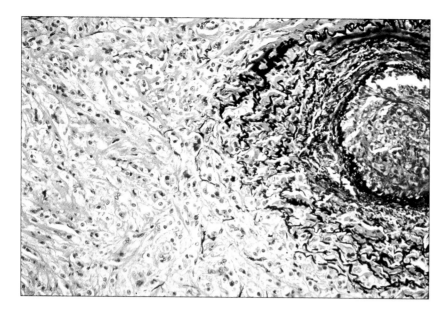

FIGURE 23-4 Epithelioid hemangioendothelioma arising in a small artery and extending centrifugally into soft tissue.

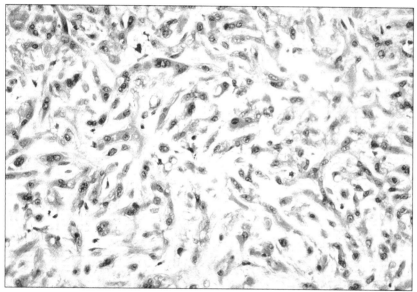

FIGURE 23-5 Epithelioid hemangioendothelioma composed of cords and chains of epithelioid endothelial cells in a myxoid background.

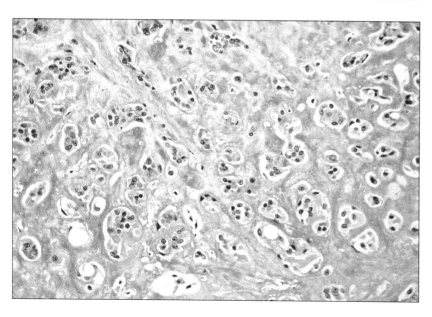

FIGURE 23-6 Epithelioid hemangio-endothelioma with nests of cells in a hyalinized background.

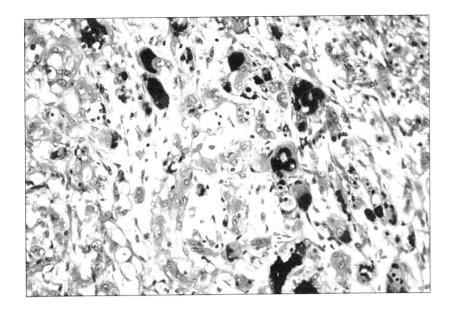

FIGURE 23–7 Peripheral areas of epithelioid hemangioendothelioma showing well-formed capillary-sized vessels.

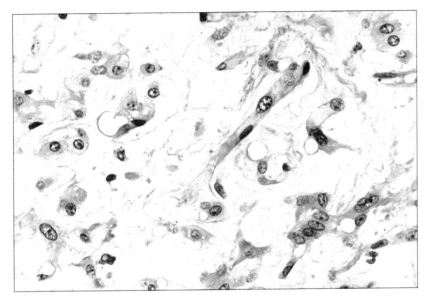

FIGURE 23–8 Cells of epithelioid hemangioendothelioma with characteristic intracytoplasmic vacuoles that "blister" the cell.

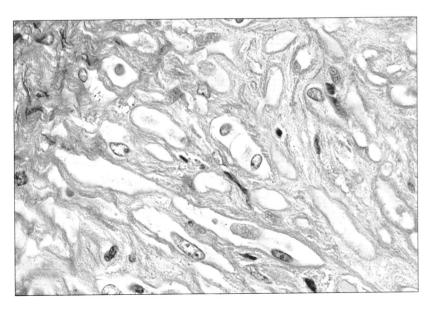

FIGURE 23–9 Epithelioid hemangioendothelioma with cytoplasmic vacuoles that "blister" the cell.

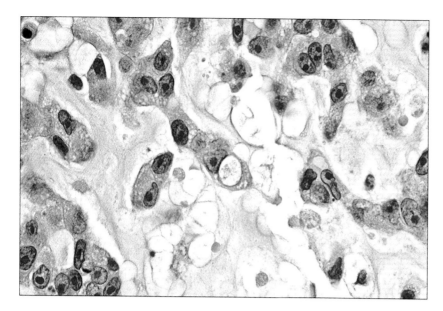

FIGURE 23–10 Malignant epithelioid hemangioendothelioma showing cells with marked atypia.

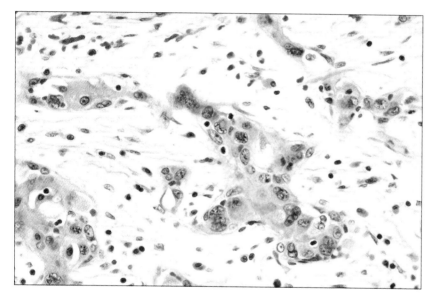

FIGURE 23–11 Malignant epithelioid hemangioendothelioma with cohesive nests of markedly atypical cells.

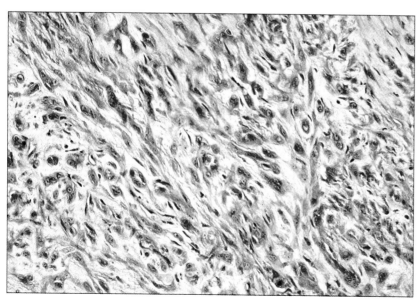

FIGURE 23–12 Marked spindling of cells in a malignant epithelioid hemangioendothelioma.

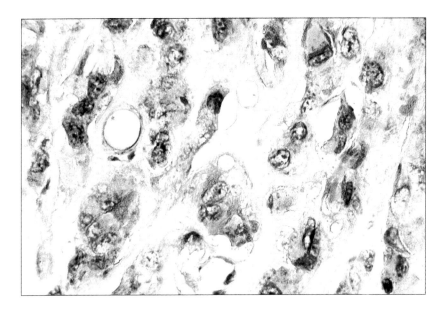

FIGURE 23-13 Positive von Willebrand factor (vWf: factor VIII-associated protein) immunostaining in an epithelioid hemangioendothelioma.

for tumors that display the typical architectural pattern throughout.

Epithelioid sarcoma is perhaps the closest mimic of this tumor. Composed of nodules of rounded eosinophilic cells that surround cores of necrotic debris and collagen, epithelioid sarcoma develops primarily as a distal extremity lesion in young individuals. The polygonal cells usually blend and merge with the collagen in a close interplay between cell and stroma. In ambiguous cases, immunohistochemistry and electron microscopy may provide the most reliable clues for differentiation. With appropriate "cocktails" of monoclonal antibodies directed against a broad spectrum of cytokeratins, immunostaining is positive in virtually all carcinomas and epithelioid sarcomas. About one-fourth of epithelioid hemangioendotheliomas express cytokeratin,[3] but usually the staining is less intense and focal compared to epithelioid sarcoma. With optimal material, von Willebrand factor can be demonstrated in the cytoplasm of most epithelioid hemangioendotheliomas (Fig. 23-13). Accentuation of the staining is often noted around the cytoplasmic mini-lumens. The cells of epithelioid hemangioendothelioma express CD31 and CD34 (Fig. 23-7). By electron microscopy, the cells have the characteristics of endothelium, including well-developed basal lamina, pinocytotic vesicles, and occasional Weibel-Palade bodies (Figs 23-14, 23-15).[1,4] They differ from normal endothelium principally by the superabundance of intermediate filaments that crowd the cytoplasm.

Behavior and treatment

Although this tumor is capable of producing regional and distant metastasis, it does so far less frequently than conventional angiosarcoma. In our experience with 46 patients followed up for an average of 48 months, 6

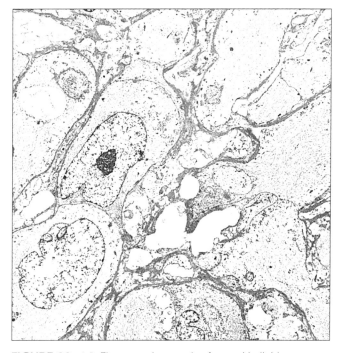

FIGURE 23-14 Electron micrograph of an epithelioid hemangioendothelioma showing complete investiture of cells with basal lamina, numerous intermediate filaments, and surface-oriented pinocytotic vesicles (×2200).

(13%) developed a local recurrence, and 14 (31%) developed metastasis in regional lymph nodes, lung, liver, and bone (Table 23-1).[2] Fewer than half of the patients who developed metastases died of their disease, however. This is explained by the fact that half of all metastases are in regional lymph nodes, and excision of these structures may result in cure or at least long-term disease-free survival. Mentzel et al. have reported similar findings.[5]

Because the metastatic rate of epithelioid hemangio-endotheliomas is higher than that for other "hemangioendotheliomas," the World Health Organization has recently grouped epithelioid hemangioendothelioma as a variant of angiosarcomas.[6] Since the majority of epithelioid hemangioendotheliomas have innocuous histologic features and have a good clinical course, we continue to regard them as tumors of intermediate malignancy. It must be emphasized, however, that for this designation to be meaningful the diagnosis should be restricted to lesions that demonstrate features of epithelioid hemangioendothelioma throughout and which lack atypical features such as marked cellular atypia, mitotic activity (>1 mitosis per 10 HPF), necrosis, extensive spindling, or solid areas of overt angiosarcoma. Compared to lesions lacking these features, atypical epithelioid hemangioendotheliomas have a more aggressive course with a higher rate of metastasis and shorter interval between diagnosis and metastasis. Mentzel et al. have shown in a univariate analysis that similar features correlate with poor outcome.[5] For these reasons we have adopted the approach of identifying lesions with the above features as "atypical" or "malignant" epithelioid hemangioendotheliomas.

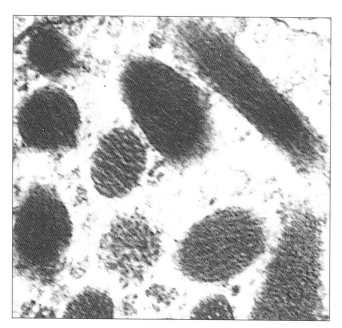

FIGURE 23–15 Weibel-Palade body in an epithelioid hemangioendothelioma. In longitudinal section the body has linear substructure; in cross-section a dot matrix pattern is seen (×75 200).

A small percentage of benign-appearing epithelioid hemangioendotheliomas metastasize and cause the death of the patient. In our experience this occurs in 10–15% of cases and seems to occur when the lesion acquires more atypical features over time. Because of the low-grade nature of these tumors, complete and, ideally, wide local excision without adjuvant radiotherapy or chemotherapy is the treatment of choice. Histologically malignant forms are treated similarly to other sarcomas with at least radical local excision. Because the regional lymph nodes represent a common metastatic site, these structures should be evaluated as part of the treatment of this disease.

An identical t(1;3)(p36.3;q25), and apparently specific, translocation has been identified in two epithelioid hemangioendotheliomas.[7] The genes participating in this translocation have not yet been identified.

Epithelioid hemangioendotheliomas in other sites

Epithelioid hemangioendotheliomas occur in sites other than soft tissue.[8-17] In epithelial organs there is an even greater tendency for these tumors to be confused with carcinomas (Table 23–2). For example, in the lung they were initially believed to be an unusual form of intravascular bronchioloalveolar carcinoma[8,9] (Fig. 23–16) and in the liver a sclerosing form of cholangiocarcinoma. Their vascular nature has been confirmed in numerous reports. Identical tumors have also been reported in bone.[13] They occur infrequently in the skin,[16,18] lymph nodes, brain and meninges[15] (Fig. 23–17), and peritoneum. Although the basic features of the tumor are similar in the various organs, the clinical presentation and disease-related signs and symptoms differ. In the liver and lung the tumor occurs primarily in women and has a striking tendency to present in a multifocal fashion because of extensive growth along small vessels. The death rates from the disease in the lung and liver vary from 40% to 65%,[2,19] respectively, compared with a 13% death rate in soft tissues (Table 23–1).[2] In a study by Marino et al.,[14] the projected 5-year survival rate of patients undergoing orthotopic liver transplantation was 76%, a figure that compares favorably with that for patients undergoing the procedure for nonmalignant disease.

	Soft tissue		Bone	Liver
Behavior	**Weiss et al.[2] (46 cases)**	**Mentzel et al.[5] (24 cases)**	**Kleer et al.[13] (26 cases)**	**Makhlouf et al.[19] (60 cases)**
Local recurrence	6 (13%)	3 (12%)		
Metastasis	14 (31%)	5 (21%)	8 (31%)	37 (61%)
Mortality	6 (13%)	4 (18%)	8 (31%)	26 (43%)

TABLE 23–1 **BEHAVIOR OF EPITHELIOID HEMANGIOENDOTHELIOMAS BY SITE**

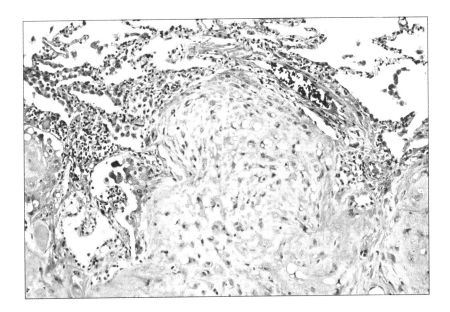

FIGURE 23–16 Epithelioid hemangioendothelioma of the lung (intravascular bronchioloalveolar tumor).

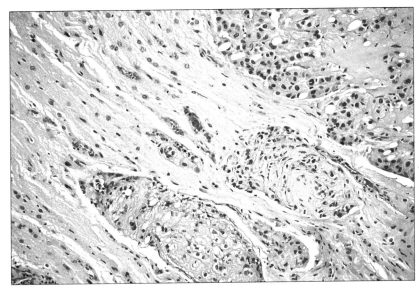

FIGURE 23–17 Epithelioid hemangioendothelioma of the meninges with brain involvement.

TABLE 23–2	COMPARISON OF EPITHELIOID HEMANGIOENDOTHELIOMAS IN VARIOUS ORGANS			
Organ	**Age**	**Gender**	**Multifocal**	**Angiocentricity**
Soft tissue	2nd to 9th decades	M = F	Rarely	One-half
Bone	2nd to 8th decades	M = F	>50%	
Lung	Median 40 years	F > M	Common	Intravascular spread common
Liver	Median 46 years	F > M	Common	Intravascular spread common

M, males; F, females.

KAPOSIFORM HEMANGIOENDOTHELIOMA

The kaposiform hemangioendothelioma is a rare tumor that occurs nearly exclusively during the childhood and teenage years; one-half occurring during the first year of life alone.[20,21] It has features common to both capillary hemangioma and Kaposi sarcoma and for that reasons many terms were used in the past for these tumors including "kaposi-like infantile hemangioendothelioma" and "hemangioma with Kaposi sarcoma-like features." Although many were probably mistaken in the past for juvenile hemangiomas, there are compelling reasons for distinguishing between the two. The lesions occur in either superficial or deep soft tissue, although those in the latter sites, particularly the retroperitoneum, are associated with consumption coagulopathy and thrombocytopenia (Kasabach-Merritt phenomenon). Interestingly, it now appears that most cases of Kasabach-Merritt phenomenon (KMP) occur with kaposiform hemangioendotheliomas and not with hemangiomas of the usual type as was previously assumed.[22,23] A subset of cases are associated with lymphangiomatosis,[21] and one unique case supervened on congenital lymphedema.[24]

On the skin they present as an ill-defined violaceous plaque (Fig. 23–18). In deep soft tissue the tumor infiltrates as multiple coarse nodules which often evoke a striking desmoplasia. Alternating between areas resembling a capillary hemangioma and Kaposi sarcoma (Figs 23–19 to 23–24), the nodules are punctuated by glomeruloid structures, a signature feature of the lesion.

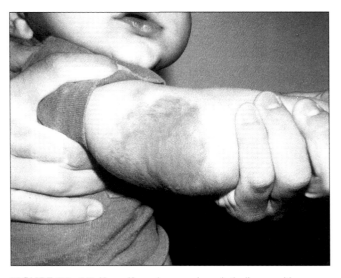

FIGURE 23–18 Kaposiform hemangioendothelioma with a violaceous plaque-like appearance on the arm of a child.

Consisting of small CD31-positive vessels surrounded by actin-positive pericytes, the glomeruloid structures seem to be specialized zones of platelet and red cell destruction as evidenced by the presence of red blood cell fragments, hyaline droplets, finely granular hemosiderin and CD61-positive fibrin microthrombi. When carefully studied, most kaposiform hemangioendotheliomas have an impressive lymphatic component consisting of thin-walled vessels surrounding the vascular tumor nodules or in the extreme case by a discrete lymphangioma (Fig. 23–25).

Immunohistochemically, these tumors have a profile suggesting participation of both blood vascular and lymphatic components. Most cells within the tumors express the vascular markers CD31, CD34, and FLI1 protein whereas the peripheral lymphatic component noted above express lymphatic markers (e.g., D2-40)[25,26] (Fig. 23–26). GLUT1, a member of a family of facilitative glucose transporter proteins which is strongly expressed in juvenile hemangiomas, is absent in kaposiform hemangioendothelioma and provides yet another contrasting point between these two tumors.

In contrast to juvenile hemangiomas, these lesions show no tendency to regress and the eventual outcome is strongly influenced by site, clinical extent, and the development of consumption coagulopathy. A majority of patients can be cured following surgical excision of the tumor. Medical intervention is required when surgery is not possible or when KMP is present. Treatment of KMP has proven to be the most challenging issue in the disease and may require a multimodality approach using steroids, cytotoxic agents, and interferon.[27,28] Unfortunately, there is evidence that kaposiform hemangioendothelioma may be less responsive to interferon than the common juvenile hemangioma. Death occurs in about 10% of patients either from the local effects of disease or

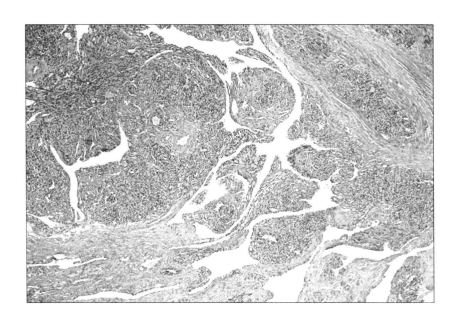

FIGURE 23–19 Kaposiform hemangioendothelioma with irregular nodules of tumor coursing through soft tissue.

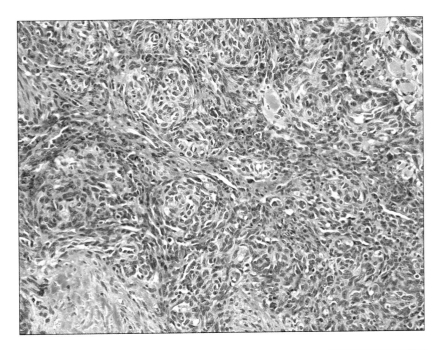

FIGURE 23–20 Kaposiform hemangioendothelioma with spindled zones merging with glomeruloid nests of rounded or epithelioid endothelial cells.

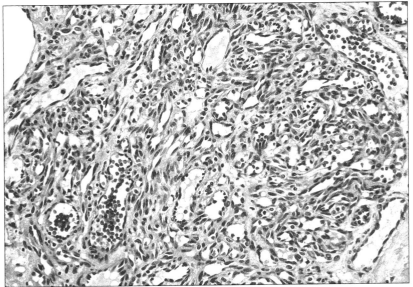

FIGURE 23–21 Capillary hemangioma-like areas in a kaposiform hemangioendothelioma.

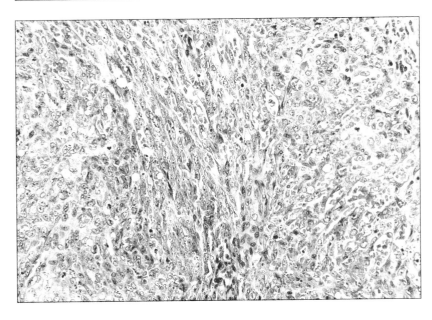

FIGURE 23–22 Kaposi-sarcoma-like areas in a kaposiform hemangioendothelioma.

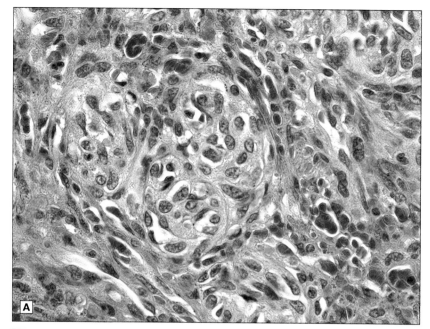

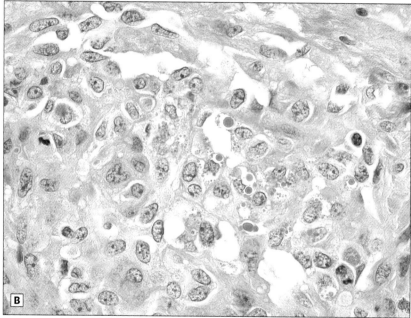

FIGURE 23–23 High-power view of glomeruloid-like areas in a kaposiform hemangioendothelioma **(A)** illustrating hyaline globules and hemosiderin **(B)**.

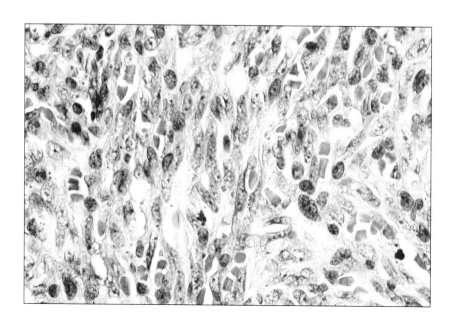

FIGURE 23–24 High-power view of Kaposi-sarcoma-like areas in a kaposiform hemangioendothelioma.

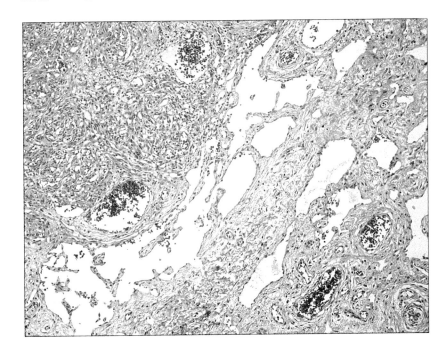

FIGURE 23–25 Kaposiform hemangioendothelioma associated with lymphangiomatosis.

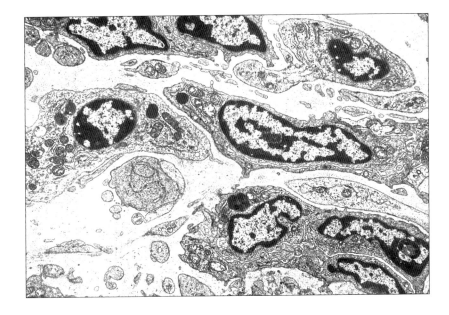

FIGURE 23–26 Electron micrograph of a kaposiform hemangioendothelioma illustrating primitive endothelial cells.

from complications of KMP. Regional lymph node metastases are rare (Fig. 23–27) and, to date, no distant metastases have been reported. However, given the fact that fewer than 100 cases have been reported, it is not inconceivable that the potential for distant metastasis exists but at a very low and as yet undetectable rate.

It is still not clear why this tumor, above all others, should be so closely associated with KMP. It does not appear to be strictly related to size since far larger vascular tumors, and even metastatic angiosarcomas are rarely associated with KMP. More likely it is related to unique attributes of vascular architecture and/or endothelium.

As implied, the two most important differential considerations in this disease are capillary (cellular) heman-

gioma of infancy and Kaposi sarcoma. Capillary hemangiomas are composed of distinct nodules of small capillary-sized vessels. Although canalization can be imperfect during the early phase of growth, capillary hemangiomas do not display spindling of the cells, nor do they contain the signature glomeruloid structures of kaposiform hemangioendothelioma. Kaposi sarcoma is an exceptionally rare tumor during childhood with the exception of lymphadenopathic forms described in Africa. It is characterized by uniform spindling of the cells and often a striking inflammatory infiltrate peripherally. Although portions of kaposiform hemangioendothelioma may be indistinguishable from Kaposi sarcoma, the former shows much greater variation from area to

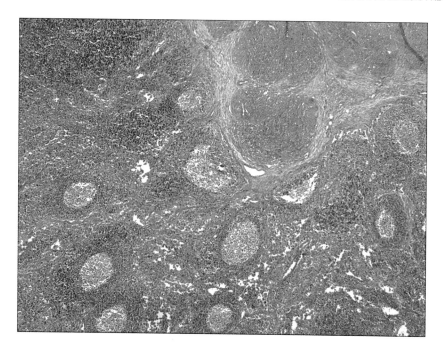

FIGURE 23-27 Kaposiform hemangioendothelioma metastatic to lymph node.

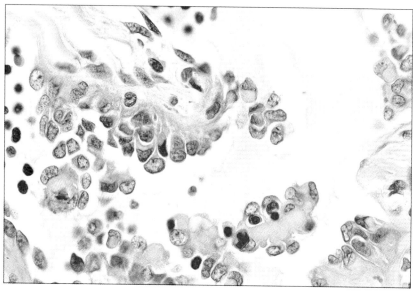

FIGURE 23-28 Hobnail, or "matchstick," endothelium, which characterizes the retiform and Dabska forms of hemangioendothelioma.

area. Human papillomavirus 8 (HHV8) has not been associated with kaposiform hemangioendothelioma and thus staining for this antigen can distinguish between the tumors fairly readily. Acquired tufted hemangioma, a skin lesion reported initially in adults, bears an unmistakable histologic and immunophenotypic similarity to kaposiform hemangioendothelioma and is, in our opinion, a closely related, if not identical, tumor (see Chapter 22).

HOBNAIL (DABSKA-RETIFORM) HEMANGIOENDOTHELIOMA

Hobnail hemangioendothelioma is a term we employ for two closely related tumors, the retiform hemangioendo-thelioma and Dabska-type hemangioendothelioma, both of which are characterized by a hobnail or cuboidal endothelial cell (Fig. 23-28). This cell is characterized by a high nuclear/cytoplasmic ratio and an apically placed, occasionally grooved nucleus that produces a surface bulge, accounting for the term "hobnail" or "matchstick." Hobnail endothelial cells vary in size and shape, from small lymphocytoid cells to larger cuboidal cells and in the extreme case tall columnar cells which appear to be of lymphatic lineage.[25,29] The two tumors have similar biologic behavior but display minor clinical and pathologic differences (Table 23-3). For purposes of clarity, the classic features of each are presented, but one must recognize that tumors with overlapping features occur and patients falling outside the normal age range for each tumor may be encountered.

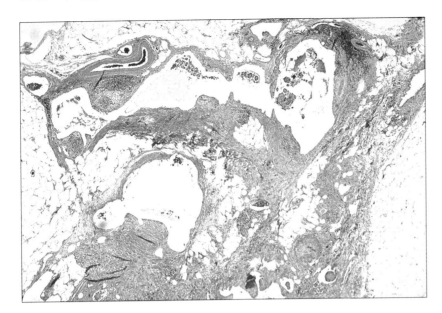

FIGURE 23–29 Dabska-type hobnail hemangioendothelioma with a lymphangiomatous background with intraluminal papillary growth.

TABLE 23–3	COMPARISON OF DABSKA AND RETIFORM HEMANGIOENDOTHELIOMAS	
Parameter	**Dabska**	**Retiform**
Age	Children (25% adult)	Adults (15% child)
Location	Distal extremities (50%)	Distal extremities (50%)
Local recurrence	≈40%	≈60%
Lymph node metastasis	<10%	<10%
Distant metastasis	One case	None
Associations	Vascular/lymphatic malformation of tumor	Lymphedema, radiation

Dabska-type hemangioendotheliomas were first described in 1969 in a small series of six patients.[30,31] All occurred in the skin or subcutis of infants and young children and were characterized by a distinctive small cuboidal or hobnail endothelial cell lining vascular spaces and forming intravascular glomeruloid papillations. Termed "endovascular papillary angioendothelioma," these rare tumors have never lent themselves to extensive studies. It has even been intimated that these lesions might not represent a distinct entity. More recently, another low-grade angiosarcoma, also characterized by hobnail endothelial cells but occurring in adults and forming long retiform vessels largely without intravascular papillations, has been described as "retiform hemangioendothelioma."[32]

Clinical features

Hobnail hemangioendotheliomas may be seen in a broad age range, although lesions with classic features of the Dabska tumor typically occur in children, whereas retiform ones more commonly occur in adults (mean, fourth decade) (Table 23–3). Both, however, develop as ill-defined or plaque-like lesions of the skin and subcutaneous tissue sometimes associated with overlying violaceous discoloration. About one-half of cases occur in the distal portion of the extremity, but other sites may be affected. Rare cases of the Dabska type have been recorded in the spleen and in deep locations.[33,34]

Microscopic features

The Dabska-type hemangioendothelioma is characterized by well-formed vessels lined by cuboidal endothelium and featuring intraluminal growth of papillary endothelial structures (Figs 23–29 to 23–33; Table 23–4). The vessels are often flanked by dense hyaline zones containing lymphocytes (Figs 23–30, 23–33). The papillations are lined by a hobnail endothelial cell with central hyaline cores (Fig. 23–31) composed of accumulated basement membrane material presumably synthesized by the tumor cells.[35] These structures have been compared to renal glomeruli. Intracytoplasmic vacuolation of the endothelium may be observed, a phenomenon seen in epithelioid vascular tumors. In some cases there is a close intermingling of endothelial cells with the intravascular

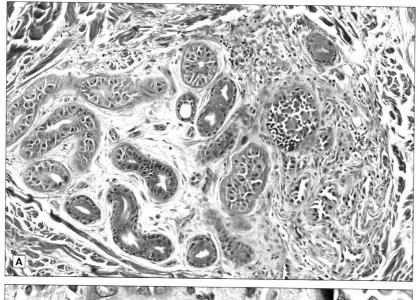

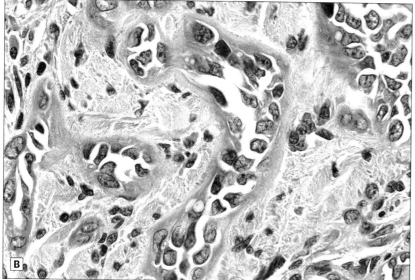

FIGURE 23–30 Dabska-type hemangioendothelioma with vessels lined by cuboidal-columnar endothelium **(A)** and surrounded by hyaline material **(B)**.

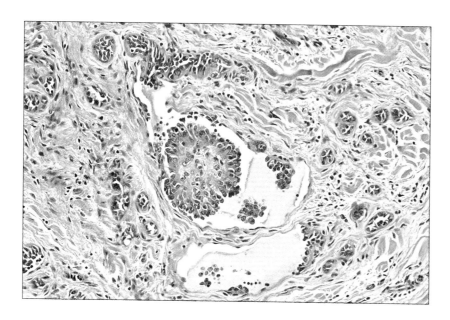

FIGURE 23–31 Intravascular papillations in a Dabska-type hemangioendothelioma.

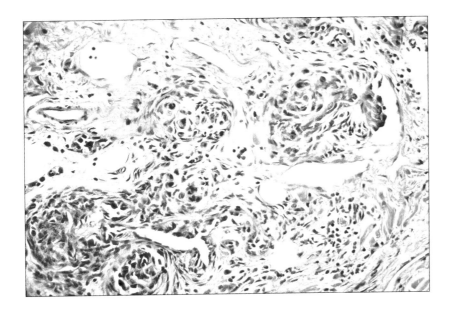

FIGURE 23–32 Solid areas of intravascular growth in a Dabska-type hemangioendothelioma.

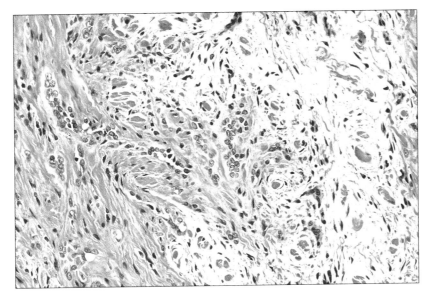

FIGURE 23–33 Dense hyaline sclerosis around vessels in a Dabska tumor.

lymphocytes, an observation that has led some to suggest that the tumor cells express some of the properties of the "high" endothelial cell of the postcapillary venule.[36] Although the intravascular papillations are admittedly the most spectacular part of the tumor, there is usually an underlying lesion, which may range from a lymphangioma to a more complex tumor with areas of hemangioma and lymphangioma (Fig. 23–29). Two cases in the literature have documented Dabska tumors arising in preexisting benign vascular tumors/malformations.[33,37]

The typical retiform hemangioendothelioma, on the other hand, consists of numerous elongated vessels, resembling the shape of the rete testis, that replace the dermis and extend into the subcutis (Table 23–4). These vessels are lined by a single layer of hobnail endothelial cells (Figs 23–34, 23–35). In the vicinity of the epidermal junction, the vessels may become ectatic such that the retiform pattern is lost. The vessels, often surrounded by

TABLE 23–4	**HISTOLOGIC COMPARISON OF DABSKA AND RETIFORM HEMANGIOENDOTHELIOMAS**	
Feature	**Dabska**	**Retiform**
Hobnail endothelium	+++	+++
Lymphocytes	+++	+++
Perivascular hyalinization	+++	+++
Intravascular papillary tufts	+++	+
Retiform vessels	–	+++
Lymphangioma areas	++	–

hyaline sclerosis and lymphocytes, intercommunicate with one another; but dissection of the collagen planes by small groups of endothelial cells, as is seen in a conventional angiosarcoma, does not occur. Intraluminal papillary tufts of endothelial cells similar to the Dabska-type hemangioendothelioma can be identified, but are usually infrequent (Fig. 23–36).

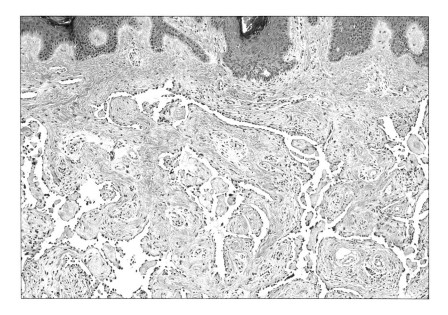

FIGURE 23–34 Retiform hemangio-endothelioma involving the dermis.

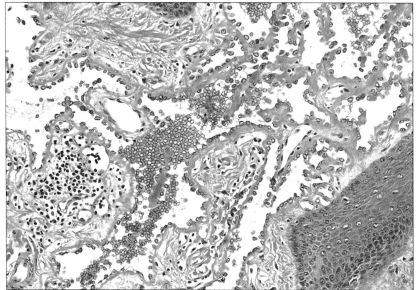

FIGURE 23–35 Retiform hemangio-endothelioma with elongated vessels lined by cuboidal endothelium.

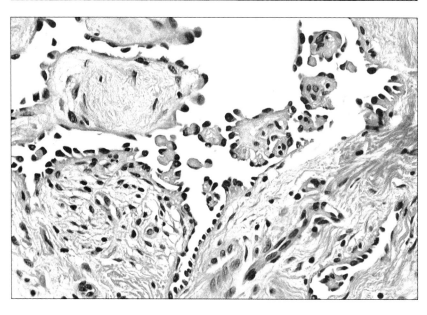

FIGURE 23–36 Retiform hemangio-endothelioma with small intravascular papillations similar to a Dabska tumor.

Although the foregoing descriptions seemingly depict two different lesions, one occasionally encounters hybrid tumors that defy precise classification. Such tumors may be made up of vessels lined by hobnail endothelium but not arranged in a retiform pattern and with only rare intraluminal papillations and no underlying vascular malformation. Such tumors underscore the need to create a designation that embraces all of the lesions under discussion.

Immunohistochemical findings

The immunohistochemistry of the Dabska and retiform lesions is remarkably similar. The neoplastic endothelial cells usually express von Willebrand factor, CD31, and CD34, although staining of the first two is usually significantly less intense than that of the last. In addition, these lesions strongly express lymphatic markers (Fig. 23–37).[25,29] For this reason Fanburg-Smith et al. suggested that the Dabska-type hemangioendothelioma be termed "papillary intralymphatic angioendothelioma" (PILA).[29] The lymphocytic infiltrate usually shows a mixture of B (CD20+) and T (CD3+) cells, although the intraluminal ones are predominantly T cells.[32]

Discussion

Hobnail hemangioendotheliomas, regardless of whether they are of the Dabska or retiform type, appear to be low-grade lesions with a capacity to extend to regional lymph nodes. Of the six patients reported by Dabska, two developed regional lymph node metastasis, and one eventually died of metastasis (as cited by Argani and Athanasian[33]). In the experience of Calonje et al. nearly 60% of patients developed local recurrence and one of 14 patients developed a lymph node metastasis.[32] In our experience with 10 cases including both Dabska and retiform types, four developed local recurrences and one patient, with a tumor of an exclusively retiform pattern, developed a regional lymph node metastasis. In the series of Dabska-type hemangioendotheliomas reported by Fanburg-Smith et al., none of eight patients developed recurrence or metastasis during a median follow-up of 9 years.[29]

It should be emphasized that these data are based on tumors that fulfill a strict definition. Specifically, hobnail hemangioendotheliomas are composed of (hobnail) endothelium of low nuclear grade with an overall architectural pattern as described above. Intravascular tufts of atypical endothelium occur in angiosarcomas, but such lesions do not qualify as Dabska-type hemangioendotheliomas. There are also rare angiosarcomas characterized by high-grade hobnail cells growing in solid sheets or as permeative vessels. These, too, should be designated angiosarcomas, rather than hobnail hemangioendotheliomas.

EPITHELIOID SARCOMA-LIKE HEMANGIOENDOTHELIOMA

The epithelioid sarcoma-like hemangioendothelioma is a rare vascular tumor which develops in either the superficial or deep soft tissues of the extremities and is characterized by nodules of deeply eosinophilic, cytokeratin-positive cells reminiscent of an epithelioid sarcoma (Figs 23–38 to 23–41). Measuring up to a few centimeters in diameter these tumors consist of nodules of glassy, eosinophilic epithelioid cells which show frequent transitions to spindled and multipolar cells with little cellular cohesion. The atypia within the lesions

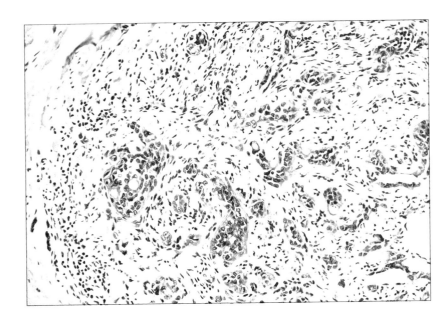

FIGURE 23–37 VEGFR-3 immunostaining in a Dabska tumor suggesting lymphatic differentiation.

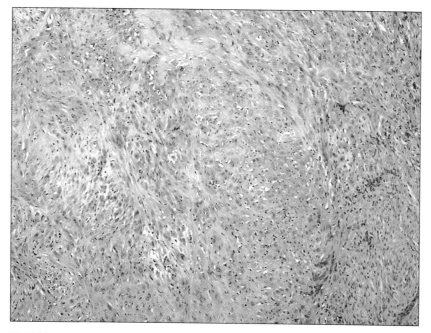

FIGURE 23–38 Low-power view of epithelioid sarcoma-like hemangioendothelioma.

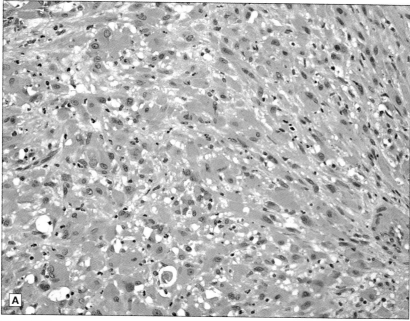

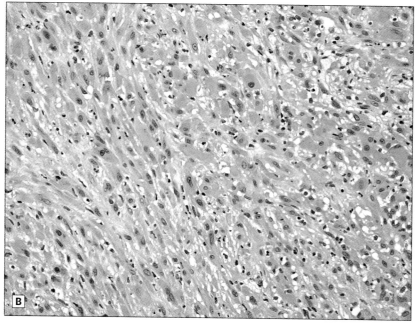

FIGURE 23–39 Epithelioid endothelial cells within an epithelioid sarcoma-like hemangioendothelioma **(A)**. Transition between epithelioid and spindled endothelial cells within an epithelioid sarcoma-like hemangioendothelioma **(B)**.

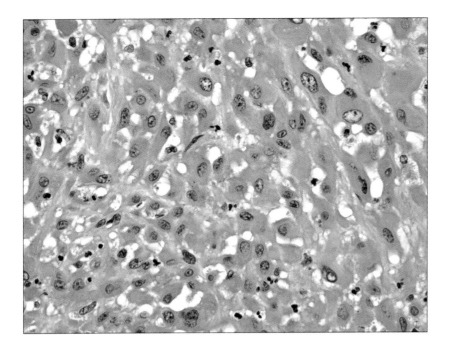

FIGURE 23–40 High-power view of epithelioid endothelial cells within an epithelioid sarcoma-like hemangioendothelioma.

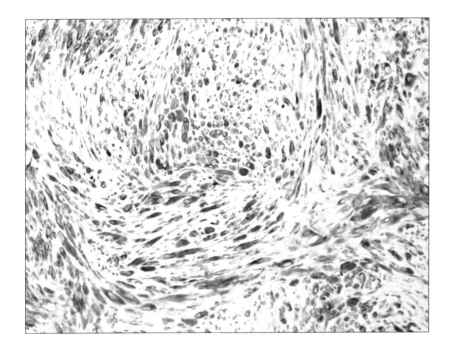

FIGURE 23–41 Diffuse keratin immunoreactivity within epithelioid sarcoma-like hemangioendothelioma.

varies from mild to moderate but mitotic activity is usually low (<5/50 HPF). The diagnosis of a vascular tumor is seldom suspected because these lesions do not recreate multicellular vascular channels or manifest the cytoplasmic vacuolization so typical of epithelioid vascular tumors in general (see epithelioid hemangioendothelioma). However, all strongly express CD31 and the fli1 protein, but CD34 has not been identified thus far in these tumors. Thus, their immunophenotypic profile sets them apart from both epithelioid hemangioendothelioma and epithelioid sarcoma. However, the classic

features of an epithelioid hemangioendothelioma such as angiocentricity, cord-like pattern, and myxochondroid background are lacking in this tumor (Table 23–5).[38]

The data related to this tumor are limited, but they are presumed to fit best within the category of hemangioendothelioma. Based on the original seven cases, two patients presented with regional soft tissue metastasis; two additional patients developed recurrences and one regional soft tissue metastasis within the follow-up period of 39 months (3–72 months).

TABLE 23-5 COMPARISON OF EPITHELIOID SARCOMA-LIKE HEMANGIOENDOTHELIOMA AND ITS MIMICKS

	EHE	ES-like HE	ES
Cord-like growth pattern	+++	–	–
Coarse nodules often with central necrosis	+ (in malignant forms)	–	+++
Intracytoplasmic vacuoles	Common	Rare	Rare
Myxochondroid background	+++	–	–
Origin from vessel	More than 50%	No	No
Keratin	+/++	+++	+++
CD31	+++	+++	–
CD34	+++	None so far	60%

EHE, epithelioid hemangioendothelioma; ES-like HE, epithelioid sarcoma-like hemangioendothelioma; ES, epithelioid sarcoma.

POLYMORPHOUS HEMANGIOENDOTHELIOMA

Although previously considered an intermediate vascular tumor of lymph nodes,[39] the WHO has recently deleted polymorphous hemangioendothelioma from its classification of soft tissue tumors based on the rarity of the lesion, the lack of precise criteria for diagnosis, and observed metastases in some cases.[6]

REFERENCES

Epithelioid hemangioendothelioma

1. Weiss SW, Enzinger FM. Epithelioid hemangioendothelioma: a vascular tumor often mistaken for a carcinoma. Cancer 1982; 50:970.
2. Weiss SW, Ishak KG, Dail DH, et al. Epithelioid hemangioendothelioma and related lesions. Semin Diagn Pathol 1986; 3:259.
3. Gray MH, Rosenberg AE, Dickersin GR, et al. Cytokeratin expression in epithelioid vascular neoplasms. Hum Pathol 1990; 21:212.
4. Vasquez M, Ordonez NG, English GW, et al. Epithelioid hemangioendothelioma of soft tissue: report of a case with ultrastructural observations. Ultrastruct Pathol 1998; 22:73.
5. Mentzel T, Beham A, Calonje E, et al. Epithelioid hemangioendothelioma of skin and soft tissues: clinicopathologic and immunohistochemical study of 30 cases. Am J Surg Pathol 1997; 21:363.
6. Fletcher CDM, Unni KK, Mertens F. Pathology and genetics tumours of soft tissue and bone. World Health Organization Classification of Tumours. Other intermediate vascular neoplasm. 2002:173.
7. Mendlick MR, Nelson M, Pickering D, et al. Translocation t(1;3)(p36.3q25) is a nonrandom aberration in epithelioid hemangioendothelioma. Am J Surg Pathol 2001; 25:684.
8. Bhagavan BS, Dorfman HD, Murthy MSN, et al. Intravascular bronchioloalveolar tumor (IVBAT): a low-grade sclerosing epithelioid angiosarcoma of lung. Am J Surg Pathol 1982; 6:41.
9. Dail DH, Liebow AA, Gmelich JT, et al. Intravascular, bronchiolar, and alveolar tumor of the lung (IVBAT): an analysis of twenty cases of a peculiar sclerosing endothelial tumor. Cancer 1983; 51:451.
10. Dean PJ, Haggitt RC, O'Hara CJ. Malignant epithelioid hemangioendothelioma of the liver in young women: relationship to oral contraceptive use. Am J Surg Pathol 1985; 9:695.
11. Ishak KG, Sesterhenn IA, Goodman ZD, et al. Epithelioid hemangioendothelioma of the liver: a clinicopathologic and follow-up study of 32 cases. Hum Pathol 1984; 15:839.
12. Kelleher MB, Iwatsuki S, Sheahan DG. Epithelioid hemangioendothelioma of the liver: clinicopathological correlation of 10 cases treated with orthotropic liver transplantation. Am J Surg Pathol 1989; 13:999.
13. Kleer CG, Unni KK, McLeod RA. Epithelioid hemangioendothelioma of bone. Am J Surg Pathol 1996; 20:1301.
14. Marino I, Todo S, Tzakis AG, et al. Treatment of hepatic epithelioid hemangioendothelioma with liver transplantation. Cancer 1988; 62:2079.
15. Nora FE, Scheithauer BW. Primary epithelioid hemangioendothelioma of the brain. Am J Surg Pathol 1996; 20:707.
16. Quante M, Patel NK, Hill S, et al. Epithelioid hemangioendothelioma presenting in the skin: a clinicopathologic study of eight cases. Am J Dermatopathol 1998; 20:541.
17. Tsuneyoshi M, Dorfman HD, Bauer TW. Epithelioid hemangioendothelioma of bone: a clinicopathologic, ultrastructural, and immunohistochemical study. Am J Surg Pathol 1986; 10:754.
18. Kato N, Tamura A, Okushiba M. Multiple cutaneous epithelioid hemangioendothelioma: a case with spindle cells. J Dermatol 1998; 25:453.
19. Makhlouf HR, Ishak KG, Goodman ZD. Epithelioid hemangioendothelioma of the liver: a clinicopathologic study of 137 cases. Cancer 1999; 85:562.

Kaposiform hemangioendothelioma

20. Zukerberg LR, Nickoloff BJ, Weiss SW. Kaposiform hemangioendothelioma of infancy and childhood: an aggressive neoplasm associated with Kasabach-Merritt syndrome and lymphangiomatosis. Am J Surg Pathol 1993; 17:321.
21. Lyons LL, North PE, Mac-Moune Lai F, et al. Kaposiform hemangioendothelioma: a study of 33 cases emphasizing its pathologic, immunophenotypic, and biologic uniqueness from juvenile hemangiomas. Am J Surg Pathol 2004; 28:559.
22. Enjolras O, Wassef M, Mazoyer E, et al. Infants with Kasabach-Merritt syndrome do not have "true" hemangiomas. J Pediatr 1997; 130:631.
23. Sarkar M, Mulliken JB, Kozakewich HP, et al. Thrombocytopenic coagulopathy (Kasabach-Merritt phenomenon) is associated with kaposiform hemangioendothelioma and not with common infantile hemangioma. Plast Reconstruct Surg 1997; 100:1377.
24. Mendez R, Capdevila A, Tellado MG. Kaposiform hemangioendothelioma associated with Milroy's disease (primary hereditary lymphedema). J Pediatr Surg 2003; 38:E9.
25. Folpe AL, Veikkola T, Valtola R, et al. Vascular endothelial growth factor receptor-3 (VEGFR-3): a marker of vascular tumors with presumed lymphatic differentiation, including Kaposi's sarcoma, kaposiform and Dabska-type hemangioendotheliomas, and a subset of angiosarcomas. Mod Pathol 2000; 13:180.
26. Debelenko LV, Perez-Atade AR, Mulliken JB, et al. D2-40 immunohistochemical analysis of pediatric vascular tumors reveals positivity in kaposiform hemangioendothelioma. Mod Pathol 2005; 18:1454.
27. Deb G, Jenker A, DeSio L, et al. Spindle cell (kaposiform) hemangioendothelioma with Kasabach-Merritt syndrome in an infant: successful treatment with alpha-2A interferon. Med Pediatr Oncol 1997; 28:358.
28. Haisley-Royster C, Enjoiras O, Frieden IJ. Kasabach-Merritt phenomenon: a retrospective study of treatment with vincristine. J Pediatr Hemato Oncol 2002; 24:459.

Hobnail (Dabska-retiform) hemangioendothelioma

29. Fanburg-Smith JC, Michal M, Partanen TA, et al. Papillary intralymphatic angioendothelioma (PILA): a report of twelve cases of a distinctive vascular tumor with phenotypic feature of lymphatic vessels. Am J Surg Pathol 1999; 23:1004.
30. Dabska M. Malignant endovascular papillary angioendothelioma of the skin in childhood. Cancer 1969; 24:503.
31. Schartz RA, Dabski C, Dabska M. The Dabska tumor: a thirty year retrospect. Dermatology 2001; 201:1.
32. Calonje E, Fletcher CDM, Wilson-Jones E, et al. Retiform hemangioendothelioma: a distinctive form of low-grade angiosarcoma delineated in a series of 15 cases. Am J Surg Pathol 1994; 18:115.
33. Argani P, Athanasian E. Malignant endovascular papillary angioendothelioma (Dabska tumor) arising within a deep intramuscular hemangioma. Arch Pathol Lab Med 1997; 121:992.

34. Katz JA, Mahoney DH, Shukla LW, et al. Endovascular papillary angioendothelioma in the spleen. Pediatr Pathol 1988; 8:185.

35. Patterson K, Chandra RS. Malignant endovascular papillary angioendothelioma: a cutaneous borderline tumor. Arch Pathol Lab Med 1985; 109:671.

36. Manivel JC, Wick MR, Swanson PE, et al. Endovascular papillary angioendothelioma of childhood: a vascular lesion possibly characterized by "high" endothelial cell differentiation. Hum Pathol 1986; 17:1240.

37. Quecedo E, Martinez-Escribano JA, Febrer I, et al. Dabska tumor developing within a preexisting vascular malformation. Am J Dermatopathol 1996; 18:303.

Epithelioid sarcoma-like hemangioendothelioma

38. Billings SD, Folpe AL, Weiss SW. Epithelioid sarcoma-like hemangioendothelioma. Am J Surg Pathol 2003; 27:4857.

Polymorphous hemangioendothelioma

39. Nascimento AG, Keeney GL, Sciot R, et al. Polymorphous hemangioendothelioma: a report of two cases, one affecting extranodal soft tissues, and review of the literature. Am J Surg Pathol 1997; 21:1083.

MALIGNANT VASCULAR TUMORS

ANGIOSARCOMA

Angiosarcomas are malignant tumors that recapitulate many of the functional and morphologic features of normal endothelium. They may vary from highly differentiated tumors that resemble hemangiomas to those in which anaplasia makes them difficult to distinguish from carcinomas or melanomas. Consequently, the literature is replete with terms such as hemangioendothelioma, lymphangioendothelioma, hemangioblastoma, lymphangiosarcoma, and hemangiosarcoma, attesting to the wide morphologic spectrum. Since it is usually impossible to determine which tumors display lymphatic versus vascular differentiation, all are referred to as angiosarcoma, even those that arise in the setting of lymphedema. The ability to define specific differences between lymphatic and vascular endothelium by molecular and immunophenotypic methods may in time result in refinements in the classification of angiosarcomas, and, in fact, already there is evidence that some angiosarcomas have a mixed phenotype.[1] In contrast to the term "angiosarcoma," the term "hemangioendothelioma" is used exclusively for vascular tumors of borderline malignancy (see Chapter 23), thereby implying that the risk of metastatic disease is significantly lower than for angiosarcoma.

Incidence

Angiosarcomas are collectively one of the rarest forms of soft tissue neoplasm. They account for a vanishingly small proportion of all vascular tumors, and they comprise less than 1% of all sarcomas. Although they may occur at any location in the body, they rarely arise from major vessels and have a decided predilection for skin and superficial soft tissue, a phenomenon which contrasts sharply with the deep location of most soft tissue sarcomas. These tumors infrequently occur during childhood, but when they do they seem to occur in an epidemiologic pattern different from that of adults. For example, there is a greater tendency for them to develop in internal organs or with various disease states (e.g., Klippel-Trénaunay syndrome).[2] Analysis of 366 angiosarcomas reviewed at the Armed Forces Institute of Pathology (AFIP) during a 10-year period (Table 24–1) showed that one-third (121 cases) occurred in the skin, about one-fourth (89 cases) in soft tissue, and the remainder at other sites (e.g., breast, liver, bone, spleen).

The presentation and behavior of these tumors differ depending on location. Hence, angiosarcomas are more properly considered as several closely related tumors rather than as a single entity and can be divided into several clinical groups: cutaneous angiosarcoma of the usual type unassociated with lymphedema; cutaneous angiosarcoma associated with lymphedema (so-called lymphangiosarcoma); angiosarcoma of the breast; radiation-induced angiosarcoma; and angiosarcoma of deep soft tissue. There are also rare angiosarcomas that develop adjacent to foreign material, in the vicinity of arteriovenous fistulas in renal transplant patients, in other tumors, or in association with rare genetic syndromes. Although eclipsed in number by the other forms of angiosarcoma, these unusual associations suggest more than a fortuitous occurrence (see below).

Etiologic factors and pathogenesis

Chronic lymphedema is the most widely recognized predisposing factor for angiosarcomas of skin and soft tissue, yet in the AFIP experience only about 10% of tumors have been associated with this condition (Table 24–1). Typically, lymphedema-associated angiosarcomas occur in women who have undergone radical mastectomy for breast carcinoma and have suffered chronic severe lymphedema for years. Chronic lymphedema occurring on a congenital, idiopathic, traumatic, or infectious basis also predisposes to angiosarcoma.

Several theories have been advanced to explain the association of lymphedema and angiosarcoma. Some have suggested that the growth and proliferation of obstructed lymphatics eventually fail to respond to normal control mechanisms. Others have subscribed to the idea that carcinogens in lymphatic fluid induce the neoplastic change or that the lymphedematous extremity

TABLE 24-1	ANATOMIC DISTRIBUTION OF ANGIOSARCOMAS: 1966–1976 (366 CASES)	
Location	No. of cases	%
Skin	121	33
without lymphedema	101	
with lymphedema	20	
Soft tissue	89	24
Breast	30	8
Liver	31	8
Bone	20	6
Spleen	16	4
Heart and great vessels	10	3
Orbit	10	3
Pharynx/oral cavity	13	4
Other	26	7
Total	366	100

Data are from the Armed Forces Institute of Pathology (AFIP).

represents an "immunologically privileged site"[3] that is unable to perform immunologic surveillance of normally occurring mutant cell populations.

In the past it has been difficult to evaluate the role of radiation in the pathogenesis of angiosarcoma, as many patients who had undergone irradiation also had chronic lymphedema. There is now little doubt that there are bona fide postirradiation angiosarcomas.[4] To be considered radiation-induced, these tumors must be biopsy-proven angiosarcomas arising in the radiation field after an interval of several years, and they must not be associated with chronic lymphedema. More than half of the cases qualifying as postirradiation angiosarcomas have occurred following radiotherapy for another malignant tumor such as carcinoma of the cervix, ovary, endometrium, or breast and Hodgkin's disease after an interval of more than 10 years. Briefer intervals are noted in patients developing angiosarcomas following lumpectomy and radiation for breast carcinoma and longer intervals in patients receiving low-dose radiation for various benign conditions.

A number of angiosarcomas have developed at the site of defunctionalized arteriovenous fistulas[5–7] in renal transplant patients. All of these patients were immunosuppressed, and it seems likely that the altered immune status plays a major role in tumorigenesis. However, it does not explain why these tumors, all angiosarcomas, occur in the immediate vicinity of the fistulas. Angiosarcomas also have been reported adjacent to foreign material introduced into the body iatrogenically or accidentally. In an extensive review of the literature by Jennings et al.,[8] nine angiosarcomas associated with foreign material were identified. Common to all was a long latent period between the time of introduction of the foreign material and the development of the tumor. Although one case occurred within 3 years, the remainder appeared more than a decade later. A variety of solid materials were implicated, including shrapnel, steel, plastic and synthetic (usually Dacron) vascular graft material, surgical sponges, and bone wax.[2,8] The authors suggest that an exuberant host response in the form of a fibrous tissue capsule around the foreign material may represent an important intermediate step in the development of the sarcoma. An angiosarcoma occurring in a long-standing gouty tophus suggests that urate deposits may function as the equivalent of foreign material.[9]

Angiosarcomas supervening on other tumors such as port-wine stains, hemangiomas, lymphangiomas,[2,10] benign and malignant nerve sheath tumors,[11–15] malignant germ cell tumors,[16] and leiomyomas[17] have been well documented but are extraordinarily rare. In addition, angiosarcomas may develop in association with other diseases such as neurofibromatosis,[2] Maffucci syndrome associated with spindle cell hemangioma,[2] bilateral retinoblastoma (Rb1 deletion),[18] Klippel-Trénaunay syndrome,[2] xeroderma pigmentosum,[19] and Aicardi syndrome.[20] The latter is an X-linked disorder associated with multiple congenital abnormalities including agenesis of the corpus callosum.

Unfortunately, there is little information concerning the possible role of environmental carcinogens in the pathogenesis of soft tissue angiosarcomas. That such factors exist is suggested by the relatively strong evidence linking various substances to the induction of hepatic angiosarcomas (Kupffer cell sarcomas). About one-fourth of hepatic angiosarcomas[21] occur in patients who have received thorium dioxide (Thorotrast) for cerebral angiography, in vineyard workers exposed to AsO_3-containing insecticides, or in industrial workers exposed to vinyl chloride during the production of synthetic rubber.[21,22] A few cases have been recorded in patients receiving long-term androgenic anabolic steroids and one in a patient taking estrogen. Mutations of the K-*ras-2* gene have been detected in both sporadic and Thorotrast-induced hepatic angiosarcomas.[23]

Vascular endothelial growth factor (VEGF), an angiogenic cytokine, has become a recent focus in the study of tumor angiogenesis. This 45 000 dalton glycoprotein, normally produced by macrophages and stromal cells, stimulates growth and enhances permeability of endothelial cells. VEGF may also be produced by various tumors including some angiosarcomas, which express both VEGF and its receptors.[24,25] This observation implies that growth of angiosarcomas can occur by both autocrine and paracrine loops.

Cutaneous angiosarcoma not associated with lymphedema

Cutaneous angiosarcoma without lymphedema is the most common angiosarcoma. It primarily affects elderly persons (Tables 24–2, 24–3) and more often males than females. They are typically located on the head and neck, particularly the area of the scalp (Table 24–4) and upper forehead. Whether sun exposure is important in the pathogenesis of cutaneous angiosarcoma is uncertain. Clinically, the appearance of these lesions is variable. Most begin as ill-defined bruise-like areas with an indurated border, and, for this reason, they are apt to be considered benign. In a small number of cases a diagnosis of facial edema is entertained. Large, advanced lesions are elevated, nodular, and occasionally ulcerated (Fig. 24–1). It is difficult to determine the extent of these lesions clinically. This fact, coupled with multifocality in about half of the cases, seriously complicates therapy and probably results in suboptimal initial therapy in a large number of cases. Preoperative mapping of angiosarcoma using grid-pattern biopsies or Mohs' surgery has resulted in better delineation of tumor extent and treatment planning.[26]

Grossly, the tumors consist of ill-defined hemorrhagic areas (Fig. 24–2) that may flatten or ulcerate the overlying skin. Rarely, the epidermis displays verrucous hyperplasia. On cut section, the tumors have a microcystic or sponge-like quality due to the presence of blood-filled spaces. The tumors extensively involve the dermis and extend well beyond their apparent gross confines. In poorly differentiated, rapidly growing tumors, deep structures such as the subcutis and fascia may also be invaded. The periphery of the tumors contains a fringe of dilated lymphatic vessels surrounded by chronic inflammatory cells and usually small capillaries in which piling up and tufting of the endothelium suggests incipient malignant change.

Many cutaneous angiosarcomas are well to moderately differentiated lesions that form distinct vascular channels, albeit of irregular size and shape (Figs 24–3 to 24–8). Such tumors at first may suggest poorly confined hemangiomas because of the numerous channels and the flattened, innocuous appearance of the cells. Yet in contrast to true hemangiomas, the vascular channels seem to create their own tissue planes, dissecting through the dermal collagen (Fig. 24–6) and fascia or splitting apart groups of subcutaneous fat cells. Moreover, there is a tendency for the channels to communicate with each other, forming an anastomosing network of sinusoids (Figs 24–4, 24–5). Although the cells resemble normal endothelium to some extent, they usually have larger, more chromatic nuclei and often pile up along the lumens, creating the papillations so typical of angiosarcomas (but which may also be seen in reactive vascular proliferations such as papillary endothelial hyperplasia).

TABLE 24–2	**AGE DISTRIBUTION OF CUTANEOUS ANGIOSARCOMAS WITHOUT LYMPHEDEMA: 1966–1976 (101 CASES)**	
Age (years)	**No. of cases**	**%**
0–11	11	11
11–20	9	9
21–30	6	6
31–40	5	5
41–50	18	18
51–60	10	10
61–70	17	17
>70	22	22
Unspecified	3	2
Total	101	100

Data are from the AFIP.

TABLE 24–3	**GENDER DISTRIBUTION OF CUTANEOUS ANGIOSARCOMAS WITHOUT LYMPHEDEMA: 1966–1976 (101 CASES)**	
Gender	**No. of cases**	**%**
Male	62	62
Female	31	31
Unknown	8	7
Total	101	100

Data are from the AFIP.

TABLE 24–4	**ANATOMIC DISTRIBUTION OF CUTANEOUS ANGIOSARCOMAS WITHOUT LYMPHEDEMA: 1966–1976 (101 CASES)**	
Location	**No. of cases**	**%**
Head and neck	52	52
Leg	13	13
Trunk	13	13
Arm	8	8
Generalized	2	1
Not specified	13	13
Total	101	100

Data are from the AFIP.

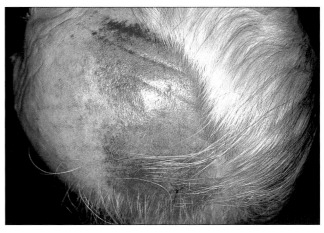

FIGURE 24–1 Angiosarcoma of the scalp in an elderly man. (Case courtesy of Dr. Vernon Sondak.)

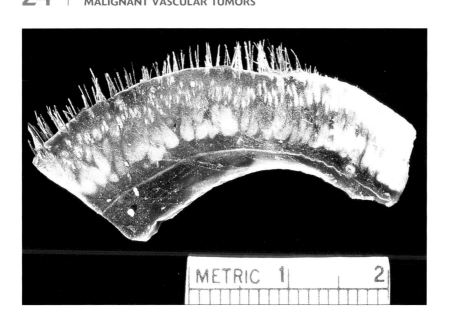

FIGURE 24–2 Angiosarcoma of the scalp. Hemorrhagic appearance frequently suggests a diagnosis of dissecting hemorrhage or hematoma.

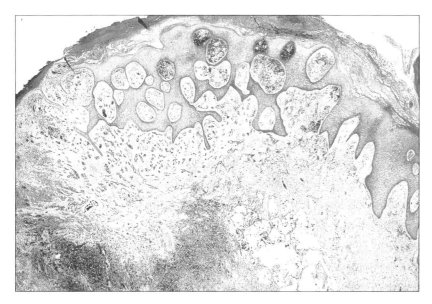

FIGURE 24–3 Cutaneous angiosarcoma composed of irregular vascular channels infiltrating the dermis. Some areas resemble a pyogenic granuloma.

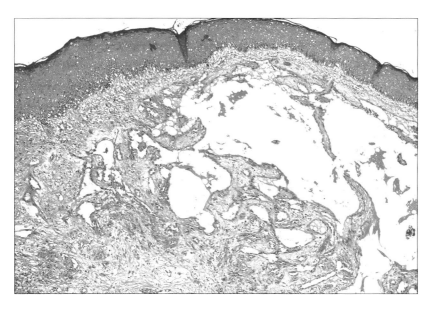

FIGURE 24–4 Cutaneous angiosarcoma with an irregular or sinusoidal pattern of vessels.

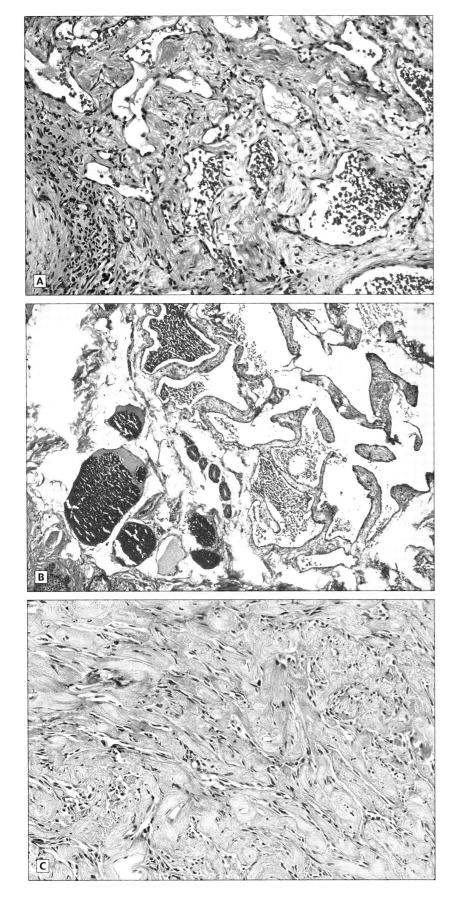

FIGURE 24–5 Varying patterns in cutaneous angiosarcomas. **(A)** Irregular ectatic vessels dissecting the dermis. **(B)** Large cavernous vascular spaces resembling a cavernous hemangioma. **(C)** Slit-like vessels dissecting collagen.

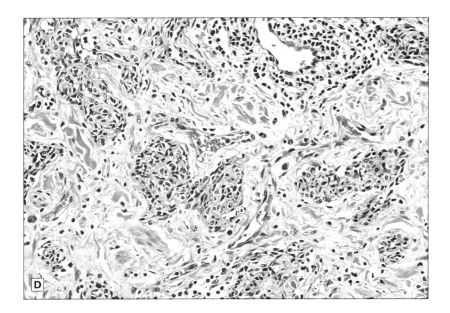

FIGURE 24–5 Continued. **(D)** Small clusters of slit-like vessels surrounded by chronic inflammatory cells.

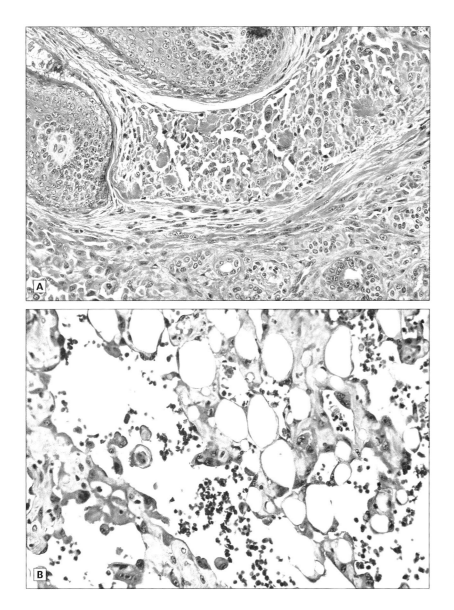

FIGURE 24–6 Infiltrative growth of an angiosarcoma around a hair shaft **(A)**, within fat **(B)** and between collagen bundles **(C)**.

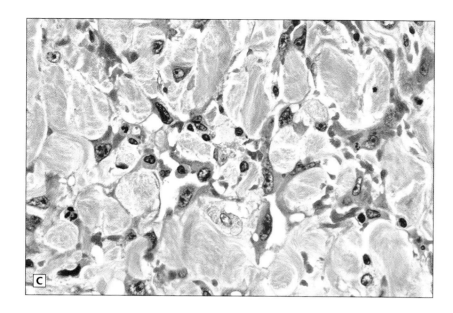

FIGURE 24–6 Continued.

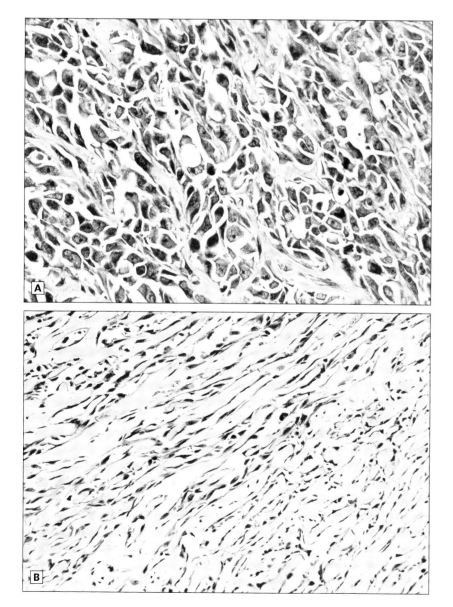

FIGURE 24–7 Variety of patterns in a high-grade angiosarcoma, including a solid or medullary focus **(A)** and marked spindling of the cells **(B, C)**.

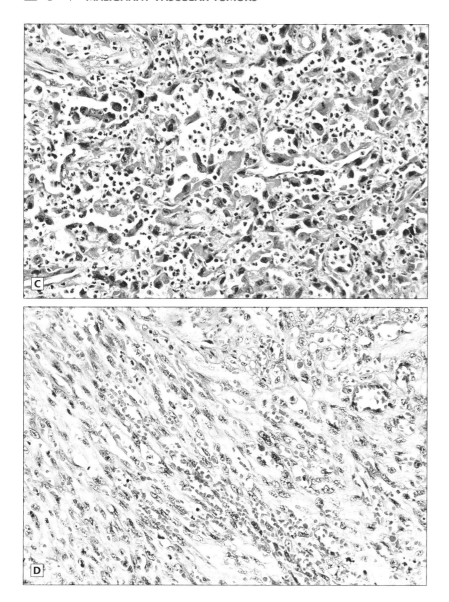

FIGURE 24-7 Continued. **(D)** Highly pleomorphic tumor with rudimentary lumen formation.

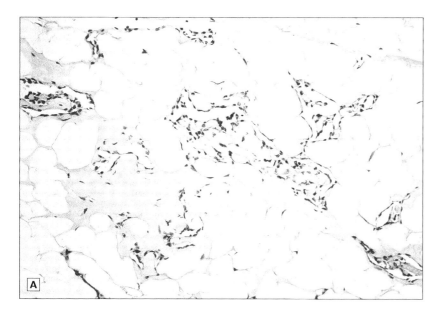

FIGURE 24-8 Low-grade angiosarcoma with bland vessels dissecting fat **(A)**, some with small intravascular papillations **(B)**.

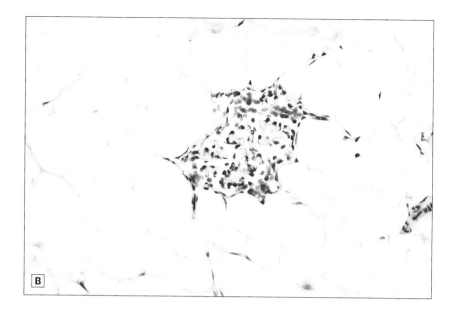

FIGURE 24–8 Continued.

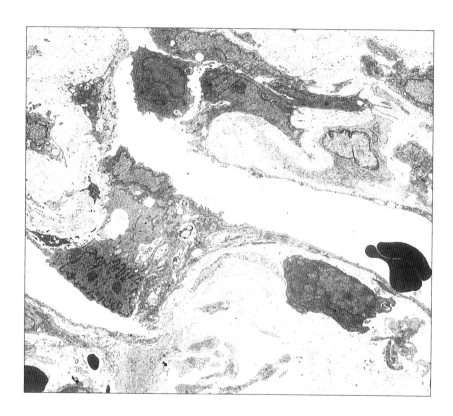

FIGURE 24–9 Electron micrograph of an angiosarcoma. An irregularly shaped blood vessel is lined by neoplastic endothelial cells with segments of basal lamina. Several perithelial cells and their processes are present outside the vessel wall. (Courtesy of Dr. Jerome B. Taxy.)

A small number of cutaneous angiosarcomas are relatively high-grade tumors that are difficult to distinguish from carcinomas or high-grade fibrosarcomas (Fig. 24–7). These tumors may have occasional well-differentiated areas, as described earlier, that facilitate diagnosis. Others are composed exclusively of poorly differentiated areas. The cells in the poorly differentiated tumors may be pleomorphic and usually display prominent mitotic activity. A small number of angiosarcomas have a low-grade appearance consisting of innocuous vessels infiltrating soft tissue and containing intraluminal papillations (Fig.

24–8). The diagnosis in these cases is based more on the pattern of growth than on the degree of cytologic atypia and mitotic activity.

Ultrastructural findings

The best-differentiated areas of these tumors have many of the features of normal endothelium, including a partial investiture of basal lamina along the antiluminal borders (Fig. 24–9), tight junctions between cells, pinocytotic vesicles, and occasional cytofilaments.[27,28] Weibel-Palade bodies, tubular structures found in normal endothelium, are present in a disappointingly small number of angiosarcomas[2,29,30] and, when present, are few in number. Poorly differentiated tumors, however, lack many and sometimes all of the foregoing features. However, in an ultrastructural study of 47 angiosarcomas, Mackay et al.[29] pointed out that poorly differentiated areas still display topographic features that suggest vascular differentiation, including a close relation between tumor cells and erythrocytes such that the latter lie between or sometimes within the cytoplasm of the former. Ramifying clefts between the cells suggest primitive or abortive vascular (luminal) differentiation. The authors did not note any ultrastructural differences between angiosarcomas arising in lymphedema and those that did not.

Immunohistochemical findings

Immunohistochemical confirmation of the diagnosis of angiosarcoma, even those that are poorly differentiated, can usually be accomplished using a panel of vascular markers. In recent years a number of new antibodies directed against various structural and protein products of endothelium has gradually replaced von Willebrand factor in diagnostic importance (see Chapter 7). Antibodies directed against CD34 and CD31 identify nearly all angiosarcomas, including poorly differentiated ones, although there are a few caveats to be noted. Although CD34 is expressed by many angiosarcomas and Kaposi sarcoma, it is also seen in some soft tissue tumors (e.g., epithelioid sarcoma) that may enter into the differential diagnosis of angiosarcoma. CD31 (platelet-endothelial cell adhesion molecule), on the other hand, seems to be the more sensitive and more specific antigen for endothelial differentiation (Fig. 24–10). In the context of soft tissue neoplasia, virtually all benign and malignant vascular tumors express this membrane protein, whereas more than 100 soft tissue tumors of nonvascular lineage do not.[31,32] The most prudent approach to the diagnosis of angiosarcomas, therefore, is to use immunohistochemical studies to rule out other diagnoses that may legitimately enter the differential diagnosis in a given case coupled with a panel of vascular markers (e.g., CD31, CD34) that, if positive, support the diagnosis of angiosarcoma.

Antibodies to thrombomodulin, an antagonist of factor VIII-AG, decorate most angiosarcomas but also react with various carcinomas, mesotheliomas, and trophoblastic tumors.[32–34] Although seldom required for diagnostic purposes, immunostains for laminin outline vascular channels by highlighting the basal lamina investing groups of neoplastic cells, and actin decorates pericytes occasionally present around neoplastic endothelium.[2] Additional newer markers for vascular and lymphatic endothelial tumors are discussed in Chapter 7.

Cytogenetic findings

Only a few angiosarcomas have been studied cytogenetically.[35–37] The chromosome number ranges from hypodiploid to hypertriploid. The most common abnormalities are gains in chromosomes 5, 8, and 20 and losses of chromosomes 4, 7, and 22 and the Y chromosome.

Behavior and treatment

The prognosis of cutaneous angiosarcomas is poor,[30,38,39] partly because of the delay in seeking medical advice by patients, who are often elderly, and the tendency to underestimate and undertreat the tumors initially. The overall survival varies from 10% to 34%[30,38,40] with most patients dying within 2–3 years of metastases to lung, liver, and lymph node.[30]

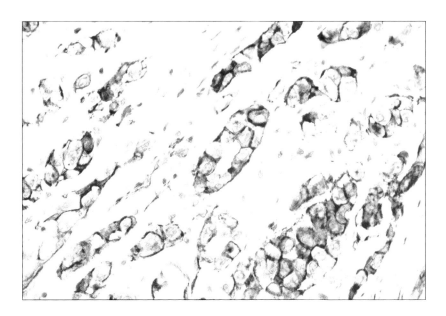

FIGURE 24–10 Immunostain for CD31 shows intense staining of most angiosarcoma cells.

Prognosis can be related to a number of clinical parameters. Size is the parameter most consistently linked to outcome. Tumors measuring <5 cm in diameter (T1) have a significantly better prognosis than those that are larger (T2).[30,38–41] Mark et al.[38] reported a 5-year survival of 32% for lesions <5 cm compared to 13% for those >5 cm, and Pawlik et al.[39] noted a mortality of less than 10% in patients with lesions less than 5 cm, and 75% in those greater than 5 cm. Predicting outcome is more accurate when based on pathologic, as opposed to clinical, size as the latter commonly underestimates the extent of the lesion. Unfortunately, only a minority of patients with cutaneous angiosarcomas present with T1 lesions, however.

A number of other features have been linked to outcome and these include depth of tumor, margin status, local recurrence, and metastasis. Negative margin status is highly correlated with improved survival, but it should be noted that it is not only difficult to achieve negative margins in angiosarcoma, but it is also difficult to accurately assess these margins at the time of frozen section. At one institution as many as two-thirds of margins interpreted as negative at the time of frozen section were judged to be positive on permanent section.[39] For this reason, definitive reconstruction surgery should be postponed until the results of permanent sections are available.

Treatment of angiosarcomas consists of surgery, when technically feasible, and in the majority of cases subsequent radiotherapy,[38,39] since the latter substantially prolongs survival.[39] The role of adjuvant chemotherapy is less well defined, although some dramatic results with paclitaxol have been reported.[42]

Angiosarcoma associated with lymphedema

In 1949 Stewart and Treves[43] reported six patients who developed vascular sarcomas following radical mastectomy and axillary lymph node dissection for breast carcinoma. Although some of the patients had also undergone radiotherapy, the common denominator in each of the cases appeared to be the presence of chronic lymphedema, which usually supervened shortly after mastectomy. Since this original description, many cases of vascular sarcomas complicating chronic lymphedema have been recorded. Not unexpectedly, most have occurred in women following mastectomy, although tumors have been documented on the abdominal wall following lymph node dissection for carcinoma of the penis and the arm or leg affected by congenital, idiopathic, or traumatic lymphedema. Other reports have noted the association of angiosarcoma with filarial lymphedema.[3,44–51] The pathogenesis of these unusual tumors is far from understood. It has been suggested that chronic lymphatic obstruction results in an abortive attempt at collateralization that eventually goes awry.

Other explanations obviously must be considered, and localized defects in cellular immunity may play a role.[3] Moreover, it is possible that radiotherapy plays a secondary role in some cases by enhancing or aggravating the lymphedema.

Clinical findings

About 90% of all angiosarcomas associated with chronic lymphedema occur after mastectomy for breast carcinoma,[52] although the frequency of this complication has been estimated by Shirger[49] as only 0.45% of all women who survive 5 years after mastectomy. These patients are typically women in their seventh decade who have developed a significant degree of lymphedema, usually within a year of mastectomy. The tumors develop within 10 years of the original surgery, although the interval may be as short as 4 years or as long as 27 years. In rare instances the tumor has been reported in postmastectomy patients who have experienced little or no lymphedema. Whether some patients truly have no lymphedema must be questioned because minor degrees of lymphedema in obese patients could go undetected clinically.

When these tumors occur in congenital or idiopathic lymphedema, the affected patients are usually younger, the lymphedema is of longer duration, and any extremity may be affected. Most patients are in their fourth or fifth decade and have experienced lymphedema for 19–20 years. There has been one case of congenital lymphedema and angiosarcoma associated with Maffucci syndrome.

Regardless of the clinical setting, the onset of cancer is heralded by the development of one or more polymorphic lesions superimposed on the brawny nonpitting edema of the affected extremity. Deeply situated lesions in the subcutis may impart only a mottled purple-red hue to the overlying skin, whereas superficial lesions can be palpated as distinct nodules that coalesce to form large polypoid growths (Fig. 24–11). Ulceration, accompanied by a serosanguinous discharge, characterizes late lesions. Repeated healing and breakdown give rise to lesions of various stages which spread distally to the hands and feet or proximally to the chest wall or trunk in advanced cases.

Microscopic findings

Despite the fact that the term *lymphangiosarcoma* is commonly used, these lesions appear essentially identical to those of the head and neck described in the preceding sections. The hallmark of the lesion is the presence of small capillary-sized vessels composed of obviously malignant cells that infiltrate soft tissue and skin. The lumens may be empty, filled with clear fluid, or engorged with erythrocytes, a finding that has made it difficult to classify these tumors as to blood vessel or lymphatic origin and has led to the suggestion that two lines of differentiation may be present. Lymphocytes are occasionally found around the neoplastic vessels, but because this feature is also seen in other angiosarcomas it does not provide sufficient evidence of lymphatic differentiation.

Perhaps the only feature that sets this tumor apart from the conventional angiosarcomas discussed in this chapter and provides some support for lymphatic differentiation is its association with areas of so-called lymphangiomatosis.[52] These changes appear to represent premalignant changes of small vessels, presumably lymphatics. The vessels become dilated and appear to form a diffuse ramifying network throughout the soft tissue (Fig. 24–12). They are lined by plump endothelial cells with hyperchromatic nuclei. These areas may merge imperceptibly with areas of frank angiosarcoma or may exist alone in patients who have not yet developed discrete clinical lesions.

Therapy for this premalignant lesion is problematic. Such patients probably are at risk of developing angiosarcoma and deserve scrupulous follow-up care. It seems best to recommend therapy only for patients who have developed distinct clinical lesions.

Electron microscopic findings

One of the most significant contributions of electron microscopy to the understanding of this disease has been to eradicate any lingering doubt concerning the possibility that these tumors represent carcinomas, specifically late recurrence of the original breast carcinoma.[45,50] Ultrastructurally, the best-differentiated areas of this tumor have features of capillary endothelial cells, including numerous pinocytotic vesicles, lateral desmosome-like attachments, and occasionally paranuclear filaments.[45] The cells are, furthermore, surrounded by basal lamina outside of which pericytes may be identified. Weibel-Palade bodies have also been identified.[45] There appear to be no differences ultrastructurally between the tumors that arise in lymphedema and those that do not,[29] although in one case reported by Kindblom et al.[45] the authors believed that some areas showed lymphatic as well as vascular differentiation. Although electron microscopy can document subtle degrees of endothelial differentiation not appreciated by light microscopy, poorly differentiated tumors understandably contain few ultrastructural features that would permit their recognition. In these areas, the cells resemble primitive mesenchymal cells containing abundant rough endoplasmic reticulum, glycogen, few intercellular attachments, and no luminal differentiation.[50]

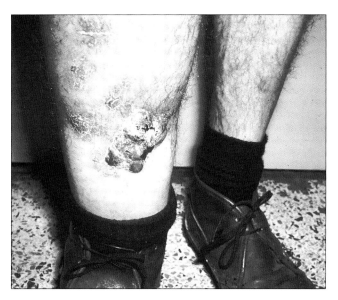

FIGURE 24–11 Angiosarcoma in a lymphedematous extremity.

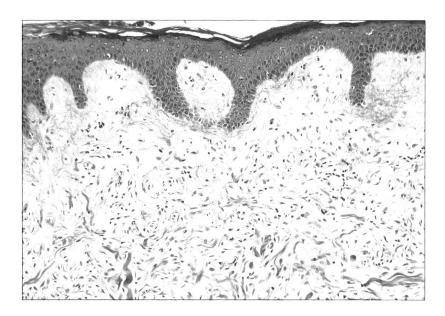

FIGURE 24–12 Diffuse proliferation of dermal lymphatic vessels (lymphangiomatosis) containing atypical endothelium. Lesion occurred in a patient a few years after mastectomy for breast carcinoma. Minimal lymphedema was present. Such changes have been considered "premalignant" and may herald the onset of frank angiosarcoma (lymphangiosarcoma) (×160).

Behavior and treatment

It is difficult to interpret survival data reliably because of the paucity of cases and the fact that early cases were treated suboptimally by modern standards. Woodward et al.[52] attempted a retrospective analysis of these tumors based on their experience at the Mayo Clinic and that reported in the literature. The mean (actuarial) survival time of patients with (lymph)angiosarcoma following mastectomy was 19 months, compared with 34 months for those developing the tumor outside this setting. The median survival time of patients with angiosarcoma and lymphedema in the experience of the Memorial Sloan-Kettering Cancer Center is 31 months.[53] Only six of the 40 patients survived 5 years or longer. The salient point in both studies is that long-term survivors have usually been treated by initial radical ablative surgery, either limb disarticulation or hindquarter or forequarter amputation. Patients treated by less radical surgery or by irradiation run an unacceptably high risk of local recurrence. It is probable that "local recurrence" of this disease is an expression of extensive multifocal disease, a phenomenon that underscores the need to excise the lesions radically. Metastases to the lung, pleura, and chest wall are common and account for essentially all of the disease-related deaths.

Angiosarcoma of the breast

Angiosarcoma of breast parenchyma is a rare tumor which is clinically different from cutaneous angiosarcomas of the breast following breast conserving surgery and radiation. It accounts for approximately 1 in 1700–2000 primary malignant tumors of the breast. Despite its aggressive course, it may have a deceptively bland appearance, a phenomenon that has led to underdiagnosis in almost half of the reported cases. Unlike other angiosarcomas, this type occurs exclusively in women, usually during the third or fourth decade. Only occasional cases have been reported during the postmenopausal period. Several cases have been reported in pregnant women.[54]

These lesions usually develop as rapidly growing masses that cause diffuse enlargement of the breast associated with blue-red discoloration of the skin (Fig. 24–13). Patients often have concurrent metastatic disease at the time of presentation.[55] Despite the appreciable size at the time of biopsy, the classic signs of ordinary mammary carcinoma, such as skin retraction, nipple discharge, and axillary node enlargement, are absent. The tumors are invariably located deep in the substance of the breast. They usually spread to involve the skin but seldom extend into the pectoral fascia. The tumors are ill-defined, hemorrhagic, spongy masses surrounded by a rim of vascular engorgement. The rim corresponds to a zone of well-differentiated but nonetheless neoplastic capillary-sized vessels that can be compared with areas of a hemangioma

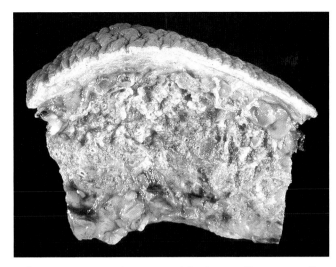

FIGURE 24–13 Angiosarcoma of the breast with a sponge-like quality.

except that their growth is more permeative. The main tumor mass shows the same changes that characterize other angiosarcomas. Likewise, metastasis may resemble the parent lesion or may show less differentiation.

Differential diagnosis

The differential diagnosis of this lesion lies principally in distinguishing it from *benign hemangioma* or *angiolipoma*, two *nonpalpable* breast lesions which are increasingly detected and biopsied as a result of more sophisticated imaging techniques. Angiosarcomas of the breast are ill-defined lesions that almost always contain cellular areas with atypia, mitotic activity, and necrosis. It is the presence of these features that ultimately distinguishes these tumors from hemangiomas. However, because some areas of an angiosarcoma can be well differentiated, it is advisable to totally embed small histologically benign or borderline lesions. Large lesions presenting the same diagnostic problem should be generously sampled. True hemangiomas or angiolipomas of the breast are usually sharply demarcated from normal breast tissue. The vessels of a hemangioma are regular in shape, whereas those of angiolipoma have typical microthrombi.

Behavior and treatment

Angiosarcomas of the breast are highly aggressive. In the past, 90% of patients died of the disease within 2 years of diagnosis. Metastasis occurred relatively rapidly after diagnosis and most frequently involved the lungs, skin, and bone. In some instances massive bleeding from metastatic lesions appears to be the immediate cause of death. A more recent study from a large cancer center indicates an overall 3-year survival of approximately 50%.[55] Some studies suggest that grading of these lesions adds prognostic value to the diagnosis. In one study more three-quarters of patients with grade I lesions were alive compared with fewer than one-fifth with grade III lesions.[56] A similar trend was noted for 15 patients with breast angiosarcoma entered into the Connecticut Tumor Registry.[57] The best chance of survival is among patients who present shortly after the onset of symptoms with relatively small lesions and who undergo prompt mastectomy. Less radical procedures almost always lead to local recurrence. Axillary lymph node dissection is not essential for management of this disease because metastasis to these structures, even in the face of large primary lesions, is rare.

Angiosarcoma of soft tissue

Angiosarcomas arising from and essentially restricted to deep soft tissue are uncommon. The estimate that one-fourth of angiosarcomas are of this type (Table 24–1) likely overestimates their frequency, as many are probably cutaneous angiosarcomas with deep extension. Even allowing for the difficulty of ascertaining acceptable cases, it appears that these tumors do not display the relatively homogeneous clinical characteristics of other angiosarcomas. Rather, these tumors occur at any age and are evenly distributed throughout all decades (Tables 24–5, 24–6). About one-third develop in association with other conditions such as inherited diseases (neurofibromatosis, Klippel-Trénaunay syndrome, Maffucci syndrome), synthetic vascular grafts, and other neoplasms. Like the more common soft tissue sarcomas, this form of angiosarcoma has a propensity to occur on the extremities or in the abdominal cavity (Table 24–7), where it presents as a large, markedly hemorrhagic mass (Fig. 24–14). It is not unusual for these tumors to be confused with a chronic hematoma, even after biopsy of the tumor, if the biopsy

TABLE 24–6	GENDER DISTRIBUTION OF ANGIOSARCOMAS OF SOFT TISSUE: 1966–1976 (89 CASES)	
Gender	**No. of cases**	**%**
Male	58	66
Female	28	32
Unknown	3	2
Total	89	100

Data are from the AFIP.

TABLE 24–5	AGE DISTRIBUTION OF ANGIOSARCOMAS OF SOFT TISSUE: 1966–1976 (89 CASES)	
Age (Years)	**No. of cases**	**%**
0–10	12	12
11–20	14	16
21–30	16	18
31–40	12	13
41–50	8	10
51–60	11	12
>60	16	19
Total	89	100

Data are from the AFIP.

TABLE 24–7	ANATOMIC DISTRIBUTION OF ANGIOSARCOMAS OF SOFT TISSUE: 1966–1976 (89 CASES)	
Location	**No. of cases**	**%**
Leg	34	38
Arm	17	19
Trunk	22	25
Head and neck	13	15
Unknown	3	3
Total	89	100

Data are from the AFIP.

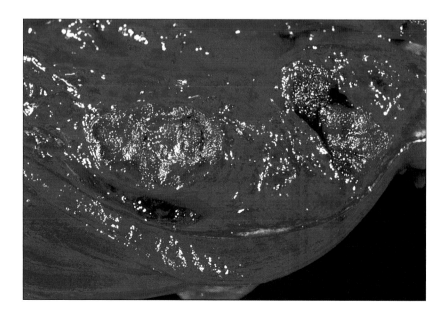

FIGURE 24–14 Angiosarcoma in deep soft tissue with prominent hemorrhage.

material is limited or nonrepresentative. In the very young, the large size of this tumor may result in hematologic abnormalities, such as thrombocytopenia, high-output cardiac failure from arteriovenous shunting, or even death due to massive exsanguination. Unlike angiosarcomas of the skin, deep angiosarcomas more commonly have an epithelioid appearance consisting of nests and clusters of round cells of high nuclear grade (Figs 24–15, 24–16).[2,10,58] These so-called epithelioid angiosarcomas consist of sheets of highly atypical round cells with prominent nuclei, some of which contain intracytoplasmic lumens. In addition to von Willebrand factor, about one-third of cases also express cytokeratin,[2,10] a finding that may make distinction from a carcinoma problematic. The presence of CD31 therefore becomes an essential adjunctive stain.

Based on the largest series thus far, soft tissue angiosarcomas are aggressive neoplasms.[2] Altogether, 53% of patients were dead of the disease within 1 year; another 31% had no evidence of disease at 46 months. Overall, 20% of patients experienced local recurrences and 49% distant metastasis, most often to the lung followed by lymph node, bone, and soft tissue. The features statistically associated with poor outcome included older age, retroperitoneal location, large size, and high Ki67 values (>10%). In a smaller series of epithelioid angiosarcomas four of six patients died of the disease.[10]

Radiation-induced angiosarcoma

Although not a common postirradiation sarcoma, angiosarcomas have been documented following therapeutic irradiation for tumors of diverse types. In previous decades postirradiation angiosarcomas commonly presented as intra-abdominal or abdominal wall masses following irradiation for carcinoma of the cervix, ovary, or uterus,

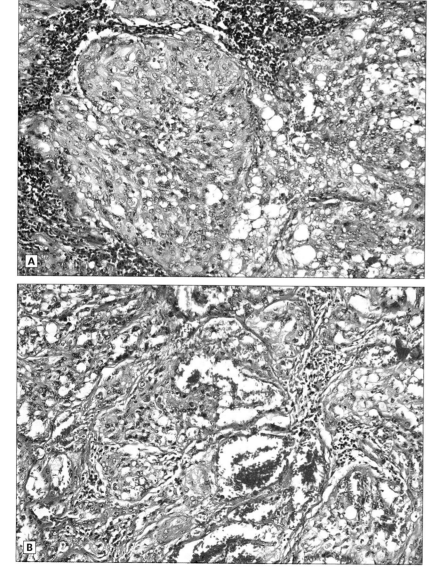

FIGURE 24–15 Angiosarcoma of deep soft tissue with a solid medullary pattern **(A)** with focal luminal differentiation **(B)**.

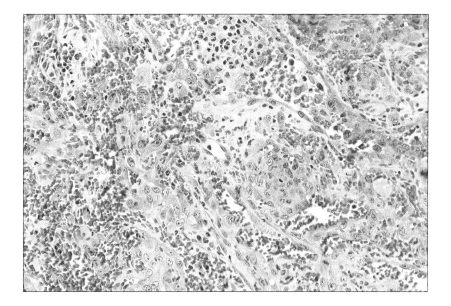

FIGURE 24–16 Epithelioid angiosarcoma of deep soft tissue.

with a small number of cases occurring after irradiation for various other malignant or benign conditions.[59-61] During the last several years, however, the clinical profile seems to be changing. More than 100 angiosarcomas involving the skin overlying the breast have been reported in women who have had breast-sparing surgery and whole breast irradiation for mammary carcinoma often coupled with axillary lymph node dissection.[62-73] The incidence of this complication has been estimated at 0.05–0.14% of all patients.[66,74]

Most develop within 5 years following high doses of radiation (median 50 Gy), but a significant subset occur with a latency as short as 3 years.[75] The onset of these lesions is heralded by ecchymoses or thickening of the skin with one or more elevated lesions (Fig. 24–17) that develop in the background of little or no lymphedema but with changes of radiation damage in the epidermis (Fig. 24–18). Typically multifocal, they vary greatly in size (0.4–20 cm) but on an average are significantly larger than the atypical vascular lesion described below. Histologically, they involve dermis and rarely extend into the underlying breast parenchyma. Their features are similar to other cutaneous angiosarcomas. Approximately 50% of patients experience recurrences and 40% metastases which occur most commonly in the lung, contralateral breast, and bone. To date, histologic features have not been especially helpful in predicting outcome. Although there have a few reports suggesting that tumors with "low-grade" features have a good prognosis, there have been too few cases of this type for statistical analysis.[75]

This form of postirradiation angiosarcoma differs from others by the relatively short interval between radiation and the development of tumor. The reason for this shorter latency is not well understood, but the large volume of skin encompassed in the radiation field has been suggested as one explanation.[75]

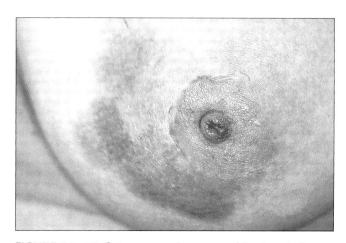

FIGURE 24–17 Cutaneous angiosarcoma of the breast after breast-conserving surgery and irradiation for carcinoma.

Atypical vascular lesion

Atypical vascular lesion is a term that refers to a continuum of cutaneous lesions which may develop following radiation and which have some, but not all, the features of angiosarcoma.[76-79] The term was first used by Fineberg and Rosen[64] to refer to small, sharply circumscribed intradermal vascular lesions which resembled a lymphangiectasia or lymphangioma and pursued a benign course. It is now evident that the spectrum of changes that occur in this clinical setting is more diverse than originally appreciated and that some lesions, while not diagnostic of angiosarcoma, are nonetheless quite worrisome and therefore deserving of careful scrutiny.

Clinically, atypical vascular lesions are small pink-brown cutaneous papules (<1 cm) which are frequently multifocal and usually develop within 3 years of radiation. In the most banal cases, they consist of a sharply circumscribed lesion in the superficial dermis containing dilated vessels lined by relatively bland endothelium which is typically one layer thick and of low nuclear grade (Fig. 24–19). More atypical lesions display less circumscription and a more complex architectural pattern of anastomosing vessels involving the dermis but rarely extending into the subcutis (Figs 24–20, 24–21). Such lesions are somewhat reminiscent of progressive lymphangiomas. Features that should not be encountered in atypical vascular lesions and which should raise concern about angiosarcoma include significant cytologic atypia,

prominent nucleoli, sheet-like growth of cells, and blood lakes (Table 24–8).[77]

Most atypical vascular lesions are benign. However, the extended outlook, particularly for the more atypical cases, is uncertain. That these lesions in some instances may represent a precursor to angiosarcoma is suggested by common occurrence of these changes adjacent to angiosarcoma and by their rare progression to angiosarcoma.[78] Consequently, these lesions should be completely excised with clear margins and new lesions immediately re-biopsied.

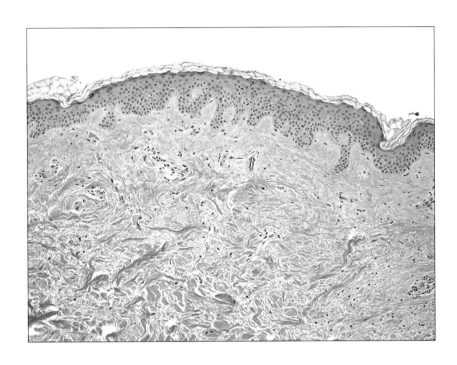

FIGURE 24–18 Radiation changes in the epidermis in a patient who had angiosarcoma following lumpectomy and radiation. Note homogenized, eosinophilic appearance of superficial dermis.

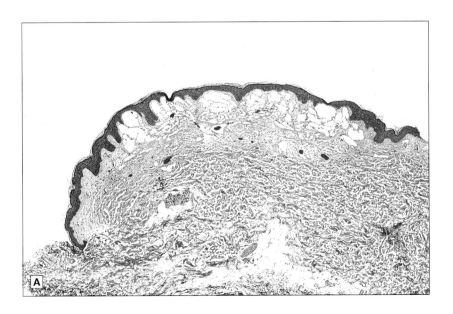

FIGURE 24–19 Atypical vascular lesion of the breast after breast-conserving surgery and irradiation for carcinoma. This lesion is a circumscribed dermal nodule **(A)** with minimal endothelial atypia but some anastomotic growth **(B)**. Lesions of this type thus far have proved to be benign.

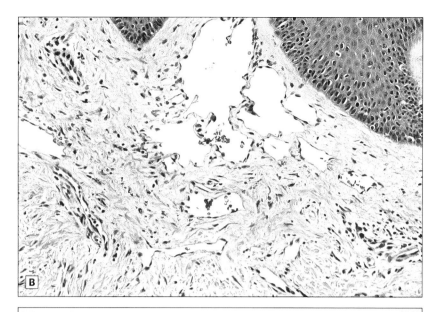

FIGURE 24–19 Continued.

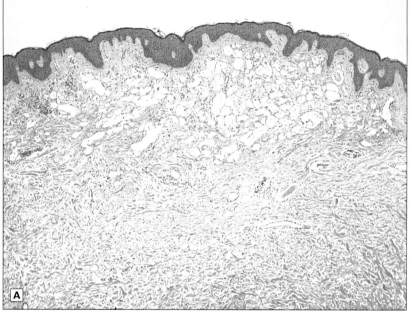

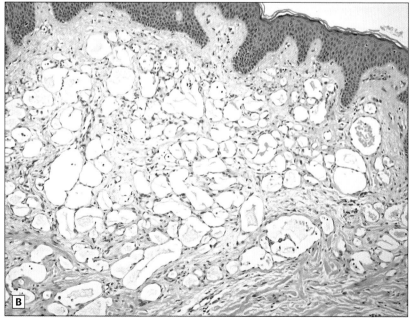

FIGURE 24–20 Atypical vascular lesion of the breast showing more irregular vascular proliferation in the dermis **(A)** consisting of anastomosing vessels **(B)**.

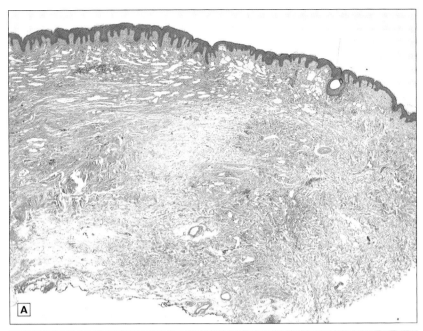

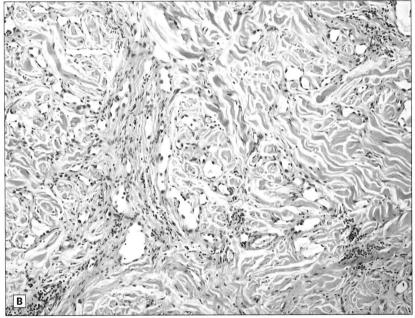

FIGURE 24–21 Atypical vascular lesion of breast with involvement of deep dermis **(A)** and more permeative growth of vessels **(B)**.

KAPOSI SARCOMA

In 1872 Kaposi[80] described five cases of an unusual tumor that principally affected the skin of the lower extremities of elderly men in a multifocal, often symmetrical fashion. Termed "idiopathic multiple pigmented sarcoma of the skin," by Kaposi, this form of the disease later became known as "sporadic" or "classic" Kaposi sarcoma. Other forms were subsequently recognized and included an "endemic" form prevalent in sub-Saharan Africa, a rapidly progressive or "epidemic" form associated with AIDS, and an "iatrogenic" form following organ transplanta-tion. Despite these apparent differences, epidemiologic data strongly pointed to an infectious etiology for all. Cytomegaloinclusion virus was originally considered the probable agent until a seminal study by Chang et al. identified DNA fragments within Kaposi sarcoma tissue that shared a sequence identity to Epstein-Barr virus (EBV) and herpesvirus saimurai (HVS).[81] The agent, sub-sequently classified as a gamma 2 herpesvirus, is known as Kaposi sarcoma-associated herpesvirus (KSHV) or human herpesvirus 8 (HHV8). This virus is also respon-sible for primary effusion lymphoma and multifocal Castleman disease.

TABLE 24–8	COMPARISON OF ATYPICAL VASCULAR LESION AND POSTIRRADIATION ANGIOSARCOMA	
	Atypical vascular lesion	Angiosarcoma
Size	Usually <1 cm	Typically >1 cm Average about 4.0 cm
Multifocality	Common	Common
Circumscription	++	–
Subcutaneous extension	Rare	Common
Anastomotic vessels	++	+++
Cytologic atypia and prominent nucleoli	–	+++
Multilayered endothelium	–	+++
Blood lakes	–	++

Modified from Reference 78.

HHV8 is now considered the causative agent for all forms of Kaposi sarcoma based on a number of key observations:[82,83] (1) the incidence of Kaposi sarcoma mirrors the prevalence of HHV8 in all populations studied; (2) HHV8 seroconversion is a predictor of Kaposi sarcoma and occurs before clinically evident lesions in all forms of the disease; (3) HHV8 can be identified in Kaposi sarcoma cells and is capable of transforming endothelial cells;[84–86] and (4) the genome of HHV8 contains homologues of cellular genes (e.g., v-*cyclin*) which can stimulate cell growth and angiogenesis. HHV8 infection, alone, is not considered sufficient, however. The marked variation in the incidence of Kaposi sarcoma in the various risk groups implies the importance of other cofactors in tumorigenesis. For example, Kaposi sarcoma is quite common in male homosexuals with AIDS, but is less common in organ transplant recipients, observations that support the potentiating effects of HIV-1 (see below).

Transmission of HHV8 through sexual and close, non-sexual contact is implied by a variety of epidemiologic observations, although the precise details of transmission are not well understood. Once introduced, the virus appears capable of infecting a number of cell types including B lymphocytes and endothelium where it establishes a latent infection. Reactivation of latent virus, believed to be pivotal in the development of Kaposi sarcoma, results in the expression of a number of viral genes which dysregulate the immune response and signaling pathways. These genes, which bear homology to cellular genes of humans, include cyclins, inhibitors of apoptosis, and cytokines and receptors. Tumor growth is further enhanced by HIV co-infection. HIV-1 induces various inflammatory cytokines and growth factors (e.g., fibroblast growth factor) that enhance tumor growth, and the HIV-1 Tat protein, secreted extracellularly, stimulates Kaposi sarcoma cells to produce metalloproteinase that promotes tumor invasion and angiogenesis. Finally, Kaposi sarcoma cells themselves produce a number of cytokines (e.g., VEGF) which through their own receptors autoregulate growth.[87]

Clinical findings

Classic Kaposi sarcoma

The chronic or classic form occurs primarily in men (90%) during late adult life (peak incidence sixth and seventh decades). The disease is prevalent in certain parts of the world including Poland, Russia, Italy, and the central equatorial region of Africa. In the latter region it accounts for up to 9% of all reported cancers.[88] It is rare in the United States and accounts for only 0.02% of all cancers. This form is statistically and significantly associated with a second malignant tumor or altered immune state.[89]

The disease commences with the development of multiple cutaneous lesions, usually on the distal portion of the lower extremity. Less commonly, the lesions occur on the upper extremity and rarely in a visceral organ in the absence of cutaneous manifestations. The initial lesion is a blue-red nodule often accompanied by edema of the extremity. The latter sign has been interpreted by some as indicating deep soft tissue or lymphatic involvement by the tumor. The lesions slowly increase in size and number, spreading proximally and coalescing into plaques or polypoid growths that may resemble pyogenic granuloma. Occasional lesions even ulcerate. In some patients the early lesions regress while others evolve so that many stages of the disease are present at the same time. The course of the disease is characteristically indolent and prolonged.

Endemic (African) Kaposi sarcoma

Prior to the development of the AIDS pandemic, African Kaposi sarcoma was a disease primarily encountered in young males and very young children who presented with bulky lymph node disease. Its prevalence, furthermore, coincided with that of podoconiosis, a form of lymphedema associated with barefoot exposure to soil containing silica, a substance thought to result in localized immune suppression.[82] With the advent of AIDS, it has become increasingly difficult to delineate a pure (non-AIDS) endemic form of Kaposi sarcoma. Kaposi sarcoma in this region is more frequent in women and children than anywhere else in the world and occurs in several forms, one of which resembles classic Kaposi sarcoma and the others of which resembles the progressive Kaposi sarcoma of AIDS. One of the latter forms, in particular, occurs in very young children (<3 years), who present with localized or generalized lymphadenopathy and occasionally ocular and salivary gland disease. Skin lesions are usually minimal. The fulminant course of the disease is attributed to a tendency for internal involvement.

Iatrogenic (transplantation-associated) Kaposi sarcoma

The development of Kaposi sarcoma in transplant patients is well established, although the incidence varies depending on the patient population, suggesting again the importance of co-factors. It occurs almost exclusively in renal transplant recipients and not recipients of solid organ or bone marrow transplants. Renal transplant recipients who are seropositive for HHV8 prior to the transplant or who receive cyclophosphamide as part of their immunosuppressive regime are also more likely to develop Kaposi sarcoma than others. The disease develops several months to a few years after the transplant (average 16 months), and the extent of the disease can be correlated directly with the loss of cellular immunity.

The clinical course of this form of Kaposi sarcoma depends on the stage of the disease and the ability to manipulate the immunosuppressive dosage successfully. Patients with disease restricted to the skin who could tolerate a 50% reduction in the immunosuppression dosage had a 100% response rate. Patients who develop organ or internal involvement succumb to their disease.[90]

AIDS-related Kaposi sarcoma

Caused by HIV-1, AIDS produces profound immunodeficiency and susceptibility to opportunistic infections and various tumors. AIDS originated in Africa, where its epidemic proportions have been attributed to heterosexual transmission and to transmission via contaminated medical equipment (e.g., syringes). In the United States most cases occur in the male homosexual population, although other risk groups, including intravenous drug users and hemophiliacs receiving factor VIII-enriched blood fractions, are also well recognized. During the zenith of the AIDS epidemic, approximately 30% of patients with AIDS developed Kaposi sarcoma but this incidence has been markedly reduced with the advent of highly active antiretroviral therapy (HAART). Kaposi sarcoma, however, does not affect the known risk groups equally. At one time as many as 40% of homosexual patients with AIDS developed Kaposi sarcoma compared with less than 5% in the other recognized risk groups. It has only rarely occurred in transfusion recipients. The typical presentation is a young adult male who presents with multiple small, flat, pink patches (Fig. 24–22) which later acquire the classic blue-violet papular appearance (Fig. 24–23). They occur in almost any location but have

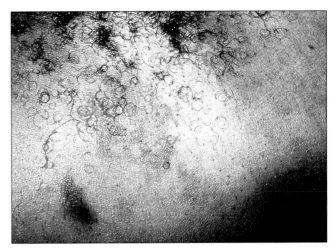

FIGURE 24–22 Early patch stage of Kaposi sarcoma as seen in a patient with acquired immunodeficiency syndrome (AIDS). Lesion is flat and mottled. (Courtesy of Dr. Abe Macher.)

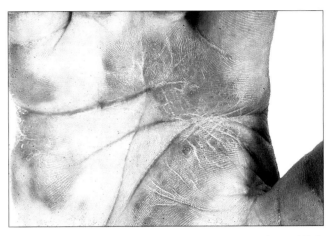

FIGURE 24–23 Advanced stage of Kaposi sarcoma in an AIDS patient with a combination of patch, plaque, and nodular lesions. (Courtesy of Dr. Abe Macher.)

a predilection for lines of cleavage, mucosal surfaces and internal organs.

Microscopic findings

There appears to be no fundamental difference in the appearance of Kaposi sarcoma among the various clinical groups. In our experience, the early lesions of Kaposi sarcoma are seen most commonly now in the AIDS patient, and the subtlety of changes in many cases presents an ongoing challenge to the surgical pathologist.

The earliest (*patch*) stage of Kaposi sarcoma is a flat lesion characterized by a proliferation of miniature vessels surrounding larger ectatic vessels. A slightly more advanced patch lesion displays, in addition, a loosely ramifying network of jagged vessels in the upper dermis (Figs 24–24, 24–25). In some respects this stage resem-

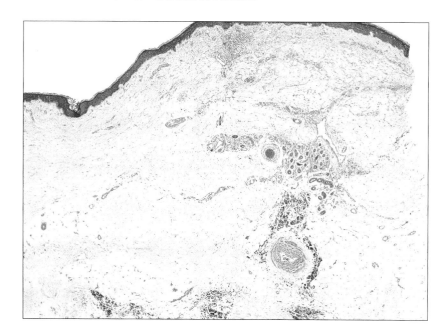

FIGURE 24–24 Early lesion of Kaposi sarcoma in an AIDS patient. Lesions are flat or slightly elevated.

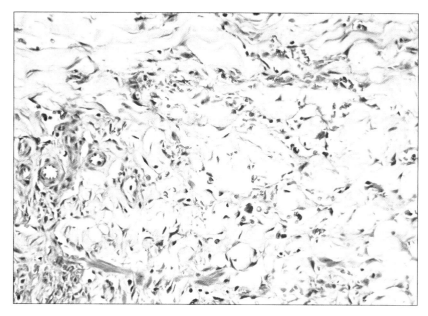

FIGURE 24–25 Early lesion of Kaposi sarcoma illustrating irregular proliferation of miniature vessels in the dermis somewhat reminiscent of the pattern of an angiosarcoma.

bles a well-differentiated angiosarcoma, except that the cells are so bland they closely resemble normal capillary or lymphatic endothelium. There is also a sparse infiltrate of lymphocytes and plasma cells surrounding the patch lesion. The histologic changes seen in patch lesions have also been noted in clinically normal areas of skin in patients who have Kaposi sarcoma elsewhere. This observation underscores the diffuseness of the disease process.

The more advanced (*plaque*) stage of the disease produces slight elevation of the skin; it is at this point that the vascular proliferation usually involves most of the dermis and may extend to the subcutis. A discernible but relatively bland spindle cell component, initially cen-

tered around the proliferating vascular channels, appears at this stage. In time, the spindle cell foci coalesce and produce the classic nodular lesions of Kaposi sarcoma. Diagnosis of the well-established case is seldom difficult. Graceful arcs of spindle cells intersect one another in the manner of a well-differentiated fibrosarcoma (Figs 24–26 to 24–30); but unlike fibrosarcoma, slit-like spaces containing erythrocytes separate the spindle cells and vascular channels (Fig. 24–27). In cross-section, these arcs of spindle cells are equally diagnostic by virtue of the sieve-like or honeycomb pattern they create. Inflammatory cells (lymphocytes and plasma cells), hemosiderin deposits, and dilated vessels are commonly seen at the periphery of nodular lesions (Fig. 24–26). A characteristic, but

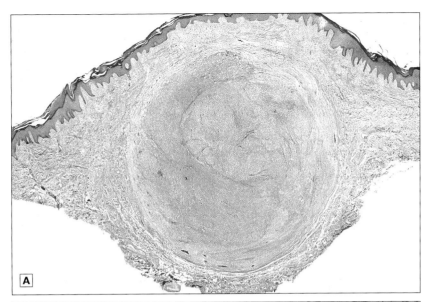

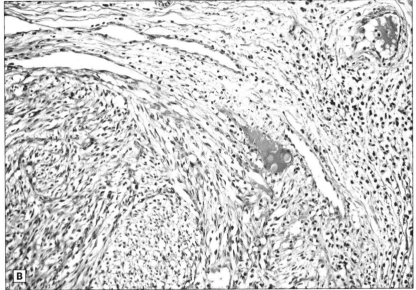

FIGURE 24–26 (A) Well established lesion of Kaposi sarcoma. **(B)** Tumor nodule is circumscribed by lymphocytes and ectatic or crescentic vessels.

not specific feature of the well-established lesion is the presence of the hyaline globule. These periodic acid-Schiff (PAS)-positive, diastase-resistant spherules may be located both intracellularly and extracellularly (Fig. 24–30).[91] Some of the hyaline globules are effete erythrocytes, an idea that derives support from the finding of erythrocytes in phagolysosomes by ultrastructural analysis and by certain common histochemical features (positive for toluidine blue and endogenous peroxidase).[92]

Although the typical lesions of Kaposi sarcoma are devoid of pleomorphism and a significant number of mitotic figures, histologically aggressive forms of Kaposi sarcoma can be seen. They may result from progressive histologic dedifferentiation in otherwise typical cases. This phenomenon was observed in 5 of 14 autopsy cases reviewed by Cox and Helwig.[93] In our experience, poorly differentiated tumors may also arise ab initio and seem to be more common in cases of Kaposi sarcoma originating in Africa. In these tumors the cells not only appear more pleomorphic but there may be a brisk level of mitotic activity. Kaposi sarcoma, particularly in the setting of AIDS, may show transitional areas that appear more akin to angiosarcoma. These areas may contain large ectatic vascular spaces similar to a hemangioma or lymphangioma and, in addition, have papillary tufts lined by atypical endothelial cells (Fig. 24–29). The former feature was addressed in the literature, and such tumors were termed "lymphangioma-like Kaposi sarcoma."[94,95]

Just as the early changes of Kaposi sarcoma in the skin present a diagnostic challenge, so do early changes of this tumor in other organs (Fig. 24–31). A particularly common problem is the evaluation of lymph nodes in the AIDS patient. The earliest changes in lymph nodes may be represented by a mild angiectasia and proliferation of

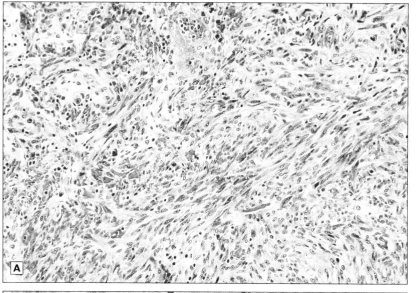

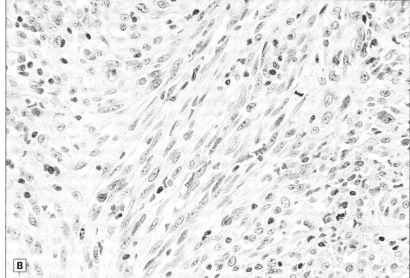

FIGURE 24–27 (A) Kaposi sarcoma illustrating monomorphic spindle cells arranged in ill-defined fascicles. **(B)** Cells are separated by slit-like vessels containing erythrocytes.

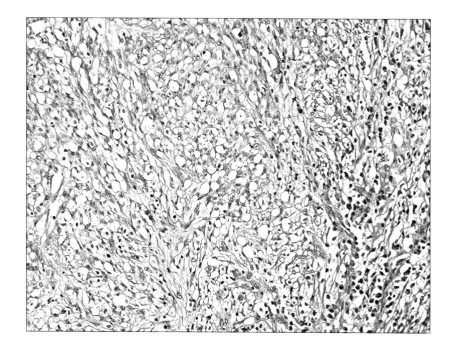

FIGURE 24–28 Transverse section through a fascicle of Kaposi sarcoma illustrating the sieve-like pattern.

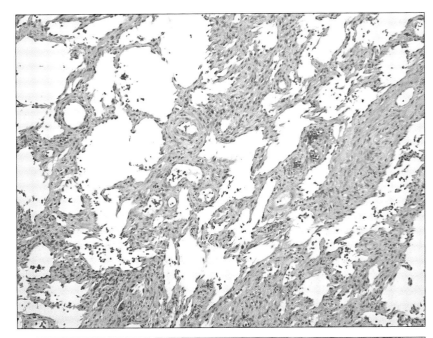

FIGURE 24–29 Kaposi sarcoma with lymphangioma-like areas.

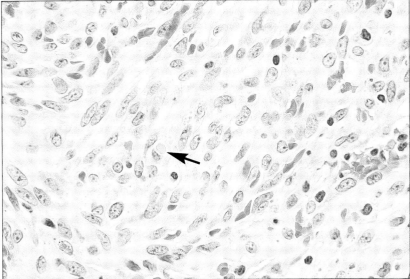

FIGURE 24–30 High-power view of Kaposi sarcoma with hyaline globules (H&E).

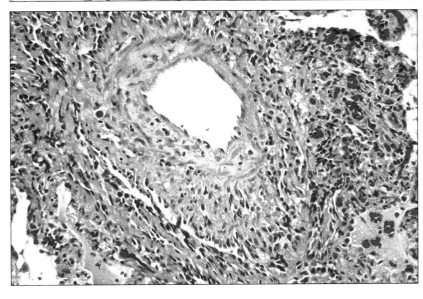

FIGURE 24–31 Kaposi sarcoma involving lung. Note permeation of the septa and perivascular connective tissue.

vessels in the subcapsular sinus. The interfollicular sinuses are gradually involved and expanded. The earliest stages may closely resemble the reactive lymph node condition known variously as nodal angiomatosis and vascular transformation of the subcapsular sinus, which occurs as a result of lymph node obstruction. Others have noted the similarity of these lymph nodes to Castleman disease, when the proliferating vessels are centered around the follicles. Accurate diagnosis of these histologically ambiguous lymph nodes should include complete sectioning of the block. This tactic often reveals more solidly cellular spindled foci, which confirm the diagnosis. Well-advanced cases of Kaposi sarcoma involving lymph nodes do not present a problem of the same magnitude, as they exhibit partial or complete lymph node effacement by a monotonous spindle cell proliferation. Because patients with AIDS are prone to develop mycobacterial pseudotumors of the lymph node, special stains may be needed to distinguish these changes from Kaposi sarcoma of the node (see Chapter 13).

Immunohistochemical findings

Identification of HHV8 as the causative agent of Kaposi sarcoma has made possible the targeting of viral antigens as markers for the diagnosis of Kaposi sarcoma. Latency-associated nuclear antigen (LANA-1), encoded by the open reading frame 73 of HHV8, is responsible for anchoring viral DNA to host heterochromatin and is constitutively expressed in infected tissues. Commercially available antibodies to this protein have high sensitivity and specificity for identifying Kaposi sarcoma. Over 90% of Kaposi sarcoma of all types display strong nuclear immunoreactivity for this protein in both the endothelium and spindled component (Fig. 24–32B)[96-99] whereas other vascular tumors, even those from HIV-infected patients, are negative for this antigen. Although usually not needed to diagnose classic examples of Kaposi sarcoma, LANA-1 antibodies have proved to be useful for diagnosing the early or subtle lesions of Kaposi sarcoma or for discriminating spindled cell angiosarcomas from Kaposi sarcoma.

CD31, a pan-endothelial marker, is expressed by both the spindled and endothelial component of Kaposi lesions (Fig. 24–32A). In addition, VEGFR-3, podoplanin, and D2-40, generally considered markers of lymphatic endothelium, are strongly expressed by these tumors[100-103] and collectively provide support for the idea that Kaposi sarcoma is a tumor of lymphatic lineage.

Ultrastructural observations

Electron microscopy has traditionally supported the idea of endothelial differentiation in these tumors. In the early lesions, slender endothelial cells with oval nuclei and small nucleoli line slit-like lumens (Fig. 24–33). Few intercellular junctions are noted, and focally gaps may be present between the cells. Fragmented basal lamina encircles the abluminal surface of the cells, and few if any pericytes are observed.[104] The latter observations seem to be more compatible with lymphatic than vascular differentiation. Advanced lesions not unexpectedly contain cells that have been variously described as "perithelial" or "fibroblastic," although immunohistochemical observations indicate that they are actually modified endothelial cells. Ultrastructurally, the spindled "perithelial" cells

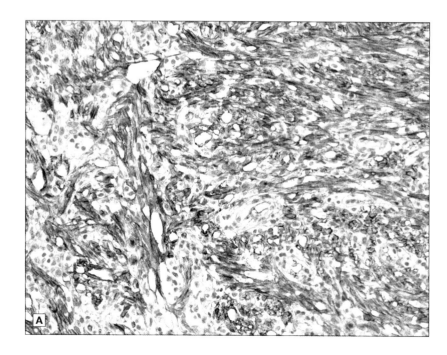

FIGURE 24–32 CD 31 immunostaining of Kaposi sarcoma illustrating immunoreactivity of majority of spindled cells **(A)**. Immunostaining for LANA1 of HHV8 decorates most nuclei within lesional cells of Kaposi sarcoma **(B)**.

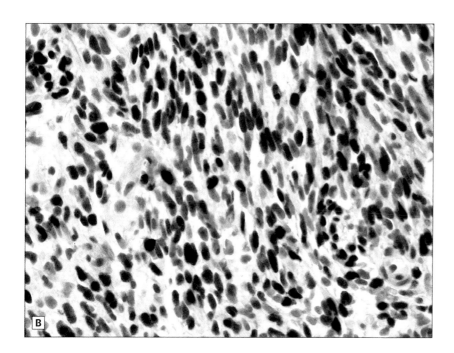

FIGURE 24–32 Continued.

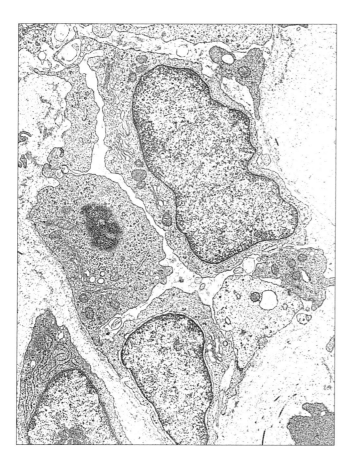

FIGURE 24–33 Electron micrograph of Kaposi sarcoma. Cells exhibit endothelial characteristics and are surrounded by fragmented basal lamina. Pericytes are absent or greatly reduced (×9000). (From McNutt NS, Fletcher V, Conant MA. Early lesions of Kaposi sarcoma in homosexual men: an ultrastructural comparison with other vascular proliferations in the skin. Am J Pathol 1983; 111:62. With permission.)

have lysosomes and ferritin and appear to be actively phagocytic.

Differential diagnosis

As indicated, recognition of the early changes of Kaposi sarcoma, especially in the AIDS patient, remains one of the most difficult diagnostic problems. The irregular infiltrative pattern of the endothelial cells in early lesions is more helpful for the diagnosis than the degree of cytologic atypia, although the changes may be virtually indistinguishable from those in a well-differentiated angiosarcoma. An accurate clinical history becomes of paramount importance for establishing the diagnosis. The well-advanced case may be confused with a fibrosarcoma. Features that distinguish a highly cellular form of Kaposi sarcoma from a fibrosarcoma include the presence of ectatic vessels and inflammatory cells at the periphery of the lesions, the more curvilinear fascicles, and the presence of hyaline globules.

Arteriovenous malformations occasionally give rise to cutaneous lesions that clinically duplicate the picture of Kaposi sarcoma. Such lesions have been termed "pseudo-Kaposi sarcoma."[105] Histologically, these lesions consist of a proliferation of small capillary-sized vessels occasionally surrounded by extravasated erythrocytes and hemosiderin. Frank spindling and formation of slit-like lumens are not seen. Arteriographic studies documenting the presence of an underlying arteriovenous malformation and the clinical findings of a bruit in the area of the lesions provide additional contrasting points.

The spindle cell hemangioendothelioma (see Chapter 23) is frequently confused with Kaposi sarcoma. The

TABLE 24–9   REVISED AIDS CLINICAL TRIALS GROUP STAGING CLASSIFICATION FOR KAPOSI SARCOMA*

	Good risk (0; all of the following)	Poor risk (1; any of the following)
Tumor (T)	Confined to skin and/or lymph nodes	Tumor associated edema or ulceration; extensive oral KS; gastrointestinal KS; KS in other non-nodal visceral locations
Immune system (I; Not included if HIV sensitive to HAART)*	CD4 cells >150 μL	CD4 cells <150 μL.
Systemic illness (S)	No history of opportunistic infection or thrush; no "B" symptoms (unexplained fever, night sweats, >10% involuntary weight loss, or diarrhea) persistent more than 2 weeks; performance status >70 (Karnofsky)	History of opportunistic infections and/or thrush; "B" symptoms present; performance status <70; other HIV-related illness (e.g., lymphoma)

KS, Kaposi sarcoma; HAART, highly active antiretroviral therapy.
*CD4 cutoff of 200 μL previously proposed has been revised to 150 μL.
From References 106, 107.

presence of cavernous vessels and epithelioid endothelial cells (which are not seen in Kaposi sarcoma) are the most reliable features for distinguishing the two tumors.

Behavior and treatment

The behavior of Kaposi sarcoma is dependent on a number of interrelated factors, such as the form of the disease, clinical stage, immunocompetence of the host, and presence or absence of opportunistic infections.

In the classic or chronic form of the disease, which occurs in more immunocompetent individuals who present with limited cutaneous disease, the disease-related mortality rate is 10–20%. Even in patients in this group who die of their disease the duration of the disease is 8–10 years, although an additional 25% of patients die of a second malignancy. Local therapy, consisting of cryotherapy, intralesional injections and radiation therapy is usually sufficient for limited mucocutaneous disease. Surgery is used principally to provide diagnostic biopsy material prior to therapy.

Kaposi sarcoma arising in patients with AIDS has a far more aggressive course, however. In the past the mortality in this population was as high as 90% particularly if opportunistic infections supervened. The advent of highly active antiretroviral therapy (HAART) has decreased the mortality to less than 50%. HAART appears to act both by reducing the risk of developing Kaposi sarcoma and by a direct effect on tumors.[106,107] It is now recommended that patients with AIDS-associated Kaposi sarcoma receive HAART and that those with advanced symptomatic disease receive chemotherapy as well. To evaluate the efficacy of various drug combinations accurately, the AIDS Clinical Trials Group Oncology Committee has devised specific definitions of "clinical response" along with a staging system unique for AIDS-related Kaposi sarcoma.[107] This staging system replaces traditional ones and encompasses a number of parameters including extent of tumor (T), status of the immune system (I) and severity of the illness (S) (Table 24–9). Good risk is designated with subscript 0 following the criteria and poor risk with 1. In the pre-HAART era, poor risk in any category denoted poor risk overall. With the advent of HAART, CD4 level does not seem to provide additional prognostic information. Thus, two risk groups are currently recognized: good (T0S0, T1S0, T0S1) and poor (T1S1).

REFERENCES

Angiosarcoma

1. Breiteneder-Geleff S, Soleiman A, Kowalski H. Angiosarcomas express mixed endothelial phenotypes of blood and lymphatic capillaries: podoplanin as a specific marker for lymphatic endothelium. Am J Pathol 1999; 154:385.
2. Meis-Kindblom JM, Kindblom LG. Angiosarcoma of soft tissue: a study of 80 cases. Am J Surg Pathol 1998; 22:683.
3. Schreiber H, Barry FM, Russell WC, et al. Stewart-Treves syndrome: a lethal complication of postmastectomy lymphedema and regional immune deficiency. Arch Surg 1979; 114:82.
4. Cafiero F, Gipponi M, Peressini A, et al. Radiation-associated angiosarcoma: diagnostic and therapeutic implications: two cases reports and review of the literature. Cancer 1996; 77:2496.

5. Bessis D, Sotto A, Roubert P, et al. Endothelin-secreting angiosarcoma occurring at the site of an arteriovenous fistula for haemodialysis in a renal transplant recipient. Br J Dermatol 1998; 138:361.
6. Byers RJ, McMahon RFT, Freemont AJ, et al. Epithelioid angiosarcoma arising in an arteriovenous fistula. Histopathology 1992; 21:87.
7. Wehrli BM, Janzen DL, Shokeir O, et al. Epithelioid angiosarcoma arising in a surgically constructed arteriovenous fistula: a rare complication of chronic immunosuppression in the setting of renal transplantation. Am J Surg Pathol 1998; 22:1154.
8. Jennings TA, Peterson L, Axiotis CA, et al. Angiosarcoma associated with foreign body material: a report of three cases. Cancer 1988; 62:2436.
9. Folpe AL, Johnston CA, Weiss SW. Cutaneous angiosarcoma arising in a gouty tophus: report

of a unique case and a review of foreign material-associated angiosarcoma. Am J Dermatopathol 2000; 22:418.
10. Fletcher CDM, Beham A, Bekir S, et al. Epithelioid angiosarcoma of deep soft tissue: a distinctive tumor readily mistaken for an epithelial neoplasm. Am J Surg Pathol 1991; 15:915.
11. Brown RW, Tornos C, Evans HL. Angiosarcoma arising from malignant schwannoma in a patient with neurofibromatosis. Cancer 1992; 70:1141.
12. Chaudhuri B, Ronan SG, Manaligod JR. Angiosarcoma arising in a plexiform neurofibroma. Cancer 1980; 46:605.
13. Meis JM, Kindblom L-G, Enzinger FM. Angiosarcoma arising in von Recklinghausen's disease (NF1): report of five additional cases. Mod Pathol 1994; 7:8A.
14. Morphopoulos GD, Banerjee SS, Ali HH, et al. Malignant peripheral nerve sheath tumour with

vascular differentiation: a report of four cases. Histopathology 1996; 28:401.

15. Trassard M, LeDoussal V, Bui BN, et al. Angiosarcoma arising in a solitary schwannoma (neurilemoma) of the sciatic nerve. Am J Surg Pathol 1996; 20:1412.

16. Ulbright TM, Clark SA, Einhorn LH. Angiosarcoma associated with germ cell tumors. Hum Pathol 1985; 16:268.

17. Tallini G, Price FV, Carcangiu ML. Epithelioid angiosarcoma arising in uterine leiomyomas. Am J Clin Pathol 1993; 100:514.

18. Dunkel IJ, Gerald WL, Rosenfield NS, et al. Outcome of patients with history of bilateral retinoblastoma treated for a second malignancy: the Memorial Sloan Kettering experience. Med Pediatr Oncol 1998; 30:59.

19. Leake J, Sheehan MP, Rampling D, et al. Angiosarcoma complicating xeroderma pigmentosum. Histopathology 1992; 21:179.

20. Tso CY, Sommer A, Hamoudi AB. Aicardi syndrome, metastatic angiosarcoma of the leg, and scalp lipoma. Am J Med Genet 1993; 45:594.

21. Popper H, Thomas LB, Telles NC, et al. Development of hepatic angiosarcoma in man induced by vinyl chloride, Thorotrast, and arsenic. Am J Pathol 1978; 92:349.

22. Makk L, Delorme F, Creech J, et al. Clinical and morphologic features of hepatic angiosarcoma in vinyl chloride workers. Cancer 1976; 37:149.

23. Przygodski RM, Finkelstein SD, Keohayong P, et al. Sporadic and Thorotrast-induced angiosarcoma of the liver manifest frequent and multiple point mutations in K-ras-2. Lab Invest 1997; 76:153.

24. Brown LF, Tognazzi K, Dvorak HF, et al. Strong expression of kinase insert domain-containing receptor, a vascular permeability factor/vascular endothelial growth factor receptor in AIDS-associated Kaposi sarcoma and cutaneous angiosarcoma. Am J Pathol 1996; 148:1065.

25. Hashimoto M, Ohsawa A, Onhnishi A, et al. Expression of vascular endothelial growth factor and its receptor mRNA in angiosarcoma. Lab Invest 1995; 73:859.

26. Bullen R, Larson PO, Landeck AE, et al. Angiosarcoma of the head and neck managed by a combination of multiple biopsies to determine tumor margin and radiation therapy: report of three cases and review of the literature. Dermatol Surg 1998; 24:1105.

27. Waldo ED, Vuletin JC, Kaye GI. The ultrastructure of vascular tumors: additional observations and a review of the literature. Pathol Ann 1977; 12:278.

28. Rosai J, Sumner HW, Kostianovsky M, et al. Angiosarcoma of the skin: a clinicopathologic and fine structural study. Hum Pathol 1976; 7:83.

29. Mackay B, Ordoñez NG, Huang W-L. Ultrastructural and immunocytochemical observations on angiosarcomas. Ultrastruct Pathol 1989; 13:97.

30. Holden CA, Spittle MF, Jones EW. Angiosarcoma of the face and scalp: prognosis and treatment. Cancer 1987; 59:1046.

31. DeYoung BR, Wick MR, Fitzgibbon JF, et al. CD31: an immunospecific marker for endothelial differentiation in human neoplasms. Appl Immunohistochem 1993; 1:97.

32. Orchard GE, Zelger B, Jones EW, et al. An immunocytochemical assessment of 19 cases of cutaneous angiosarcoma. Histopathology 1996; 28:235.

33. Appleton MA, Attonoos RL, Jasnai B. Thrombomodulin as a marker of vascular and lymphatic tumors. Histopathology 1996; 29:153.

34. Yonezawa S, Maruyama I, Sakae K, et al. Thrombomodulin as a marker for vascular tumors: comparative study with factor VIII and Ulex europaeus I lectin. Am J Clin Pathol 1987; 88:405.

35. Mandahl N, Jin Y, Heim S, et al. Trisomy 5 and loss of the Y chromosome as the sole cytogenetic anomalies in a cavernous hemangioma/angiosarcoma. Genes Chromosomes Cancer 1990; 1:315.

36. Molina A, Bangs CD, Donlon T. Angiosarcoma of the scalp with a complex hypotetraploid karyotype. Cancer Genet Cytogenet 1989; 41:268.

37. Schuborg C, Mertens F, Rydholm A, et al. Cytogenetic analysis of four angiosarcomas from deep and superficial soft tissue. Cancer Genet Cytogenet 1998; 100:52.

38. Mark RJ, Poen JC, Tran LM, et al. Angiosarcoma: a report of 67 patients and a review of the literature. Cancer 1996; 77:2400.

39. Pawlik TM, Paulino AF, McGinn CJ, et al. Cutaneous angiosarcoma of the scalp: a multidisciplinary approach. Cancer 2003; 98:1716.

40. Morgan MB, Swann M, Somach S, et al. Cutaneous angiosarcoma: a case series with prognostic correlation. J Am Acad Dermatol 2004; 50:867.

41. Maddox JC, Evans HL. Angiosarcoma of skin and soft tissue: a study of 44 cases. Cancer 1981; 48:1907.

42. Fata F, O'Reilly E, Ilson D, et al. Paclitaxel in the treatment of patients with angiosarcoma of the scalp or face. Cancer 1999; 86:2034.

43. Stewart FW, Treves N. Lymphangiosarcoma in postmastectomy lymphedema. Cancer 1949; 1:64.

44. Devi L, Bahuleyan CK. Lymphangiosarcoma of the lower extremity associated with chronic lymphedema of filarial origin. Int J Cancer 1977; 14:176.

45. Kindblom L-G, Stenman G, Angervall L. Morphological and cytogenetic studies of angiosarcoma in Stewart-Treves syndrome. Virchows Arch [Pathol Anat Histopathol] 1991; 419:439.

46. Mackenzie DH. Lymphangiosarcoma arising in chronic congenital and idiopathic lymphoedema. J Clin Pathol 1971; 24:524.

47. Merrick T, Erlandson RA, Hajdu SI. Lymphangiosarcoma of a congenitally lymphedematous extremity. Arch Pathol 1971; 91:365.

48. Muller R, Hajdu SI, Brennan MF. Lymphangiosarcoma associated with chronic filarial lymphedema. Cancer 1987; 59:174.

49. Shirger A. Postoperative lymphedema: etiologic and diagnostic factors. Med Clin North Am 1962; 46:1045.

50. Silverberg SG, Kay S, Koss LG. Postmastectomy lymphangiosarcoma: ultrastructural observations. Cancer 1971; 27:100.

51. Sordillo EM, Sordillo PP, Hajdu SI, et al. Lymphangiosarcoma after filarial infection. J Dermatol Surg Oncol 1981; 7:235.

52. Woodward AH, Ivins JC, Soule EH. Lymphangiosarcoma arising in chronic lymphedematous extremities. Cancer 1972; 30:562.

53. Sordillo PP, Chapman R, Hajdu SI, et al. Lymphangiosarcoma. Cancer 1981; 48:1674.

54. Steingaszner LC, Enzinger FM, Taylor HB. Hemangiosarcoma of the breast. Cancer 1965; 18:352.

55. Vorburger SA, Xing Yan, Hunt KK, et al. Angiosarcoma of the breast. Cancer 2005; 104:2682.

56. Donnell RM, Rosen PP, Lieberman PH, et al. Angiosarcoma and other vascular tumors of the breast: pathologic analysis as a guide to prognosis. Am J Surg Pathol 1981; 5:629.

57. Merino MJ, Carter D, Berman M. Angiosarcoma of breast. Am J Surg Pathol 1983; 7:53.

58. Maiorana A, Fante R, Fano RA, et al. Epithelioid angiosarcoma of the buttock: case report with immunohistochemical study on the expression of keratin polypeptides. Surg Pathol 1991; 4:325.

59. Girard C, Johnson WC, Graham JH. Cutaneous angiosarcoma. Cancer 1970; 26:868.

60. Hodgkinson DJ, Soule EH, Woods JE. Cutaneous angiosarcoma of the head and neck. Cancer 1979; 44:1106.

61. Wovlov RB, Sato N, Azumi N, et al. Intraabdominal "angiosarcomatosis": report of two cases after pelvic irradiation. Cancer 1991; 67:2275.

62. Cancellieri A, Eusebi V, Mambellin V, et al. Well-differentiated angiosarcoma of the skin following radiotherapy. Pathol Res Pract 1991; 187:301.

63. Edeiken S, Russo DP, Knecht J, et al. Angiosarcoma after tylectomy and radiation therapy for carcinoma of the breast. Cancer 1992; 70:644.

64. Fineberg S, Rosen PP. Cutaneous angiosarcoma and atypical vascular lesions of the skin and breast after radiation therapy for breast carcinoma. Am J Clin Pathol 1994; 102:757.

65. Givens SS, Ellerbroek NA, Butler JJ, et al. Angiosarcoma arising in an irradiated breast: a case report and review of the literature. Cancer 1989; 64:2214.

66. Marchal C, Weber B, de Lafontan B. Nine breast angiosarcomas after conservative treatment for breast carcinoma: a survey from French comprehensive cancer centers. Int J Radiat Oncol Biol Phys 1999; 44:113.

67. Moskaluk CA, Merino MJ, Danforth DN, et al. Low-grade angiosarcoma of the skin of the breast: a complication of lumpectomy and radiation therapy for breast carcinoma. Hum Pathol 1992; 23:710.

68. Otis CN, Peschel R, McKhann C, et al. The rapid onset of cutaneous angiosarcoma after radiotherapy for breast cancer. Cancer 1986; 57:2130.

69. Parham DM, Fisher C. Angiosarcomas of the breast developing post radiotherapy. Histopathology 1997; 31:189.

70. Rubin E, Maddox WA, Mazur MT. Cutaneous angiosarcoma of the breast 7 years after lumpectomy and radiation therapy. Radiology 1990; 174:258.

71. Sessions SC, Smenk RD. Cutaneous angiosarcoma of the breast after segmental mastectomy and radiation therapy. Arch Surg 1992; 127:1362.

72. Shaikh NA, Beaconsfield T, Walker M, et al. Postirradiation angiosarcoma of the breast: a case report. Eur J Surg Oncol 1988; 14:449.

73. Stokkel MPM, Peterse HL. Angiosarcoma of the breast after lumpectomy and radiation therapy for adenocarcinoma. Cancer 1992; 69:1965.

74. Fodor J, Orosz Z, Szabo E, et al. Angiosarcoma after conservation treatment for breast carcinoma: our experience and a review of the literature. J Am Acad Dermatol 2006; 54:499.

75. Billings SD, McKenney JK, Folpe AL, et al. Cutaneous angiosarcoma following breast-conserving surgery and radiation: an analysis of 27 cases. Am J Surg Pathol 2004; 28:781.

76. Requena L, Kutzner H, Mentzel T, et al. Benign vascular proliferations in irradiated skin. Am J Surg Pathol 2002; 26:328.

77. Brenn T, Fletcher CDM. Postradiation vascular proliferations: an increasing problem. Histopathology 2006; 48:106.

78. Brenn T, Fletcher CD. Radiation-associated cutaneous atypical vascular lesions and angiosarcoma: clinicopathologic analysis of 42 cases. Am J Surg Pathol 2005; 29:983.

79. Sener SF, Milos S, Feldman JL, et al. The spectrum of vascular lesions in the mammary skin including angiosarcoma after breast conservation treatment for breast cancer. J Am Coll Surg 2001; 193:22.

Kaposi sarcoma

80. Kaposi M. Idiopathisches multiples Pigmentsarkom der Haut. Arch Dermatol Syph 1872; 4:265.

81. Chang Y, Cesarman E, Pessin MS, et al. Identification of herpesvirus-like DNA sequences in AIDS-associated Kaposi sarcoma. Science 1994; 266:1865.

82. Dourmishev L, Dourmishev AL, Paleri D, et al. Molecular genetics of Kaposi sacoma-associated herpesvirus (human herpesvirus 8) epidemiology and pathogenesis. Microbiol Mol Biol Rev 2003; 67:175.

83. Pantanwitz L, Dezube BJ. Advances in the pathobiology and treatment of Kaposi sarcoma. Curr Opin Oncol 2004; 16:443.

84. Dictor M, Rambech E, Way D, et al. Human herpesvirus 8 (Kaposi sarcoma-associated herpesvirus) DNA in Kaposi sarcoma lesions, AIDS Kaposi sarcoma cell lines, endothelial Kaposi sarcoma simulators, and the skin of immunosuppressed patients. Am J Pathol 1996; 148:2009.

85. Li JJ, Huang YQ, Cockrell CJ, Friedman-Kien AE. Localization of human herpes-like virus type 8 in vascular endothelial cells and perivascular spindle-shaped cells of Kaposi sarcoma lesions by in situ hybridization. Am J Pathol 1996; 148:1741.

86. Flore O, Rafii S, Ely S, et al. Transformation of primary human endothelial cells by Kaposi sarcoma-associated herpes virus. Nature 1998; 394:588.

87. Masood R, Cai J, Zheng T, et al. Vascular endothelial growth factor/vascular permeability factor is an autocrine growth factor for AIDS-Kaposi sarcoma. Proc Natl Acad Sci USA 1997; 94:979.

88. Bluefarb SM. Kaposi sarcoma. Springfield, IL: Charles C Thomas; 1966.

89. Safai B, Mike V, Giraldo G, et al. Association of Kaposi sarcoma with second primary malignancies: possible etiopathogenic implications. Cancer 1980; 45:1472.

90. Qunibi WY, Barri Y, Alfurayh O, et al. Kaposi sarcoma in renal transplant recipients: a report of 26 cases from a single institution. Transplant Proc 1993; 25:1402.

91. Fukunaga M, Silverberg S. Hyaline globules in Kaposi sarcoma: a light microscopic and immunohistochemical study. Mod Pathol 1991; 4:187.

92. Kao GF, Johnson FB, Sulica VI. The nature of the hyaline (eosinophilic) globules and vascular slits of Kaposi sarcoma. Am J Dermatopathol 1990; 12:256.

93. Cox FH, Helwig EB. Kaposi sarcoma. Cancer 1959; 12:289.

94. Cossu S, Satta R, Cottoni F, et al. Lymphangioma-like variant of Kaposi sarcoma: clinicopathologic study of seven cases with review of the literature. Am J Dermatopathol 1997; 19:16.

95. Gange RW, Wilson-Jones E. Lymphangioma-like Kaposi sarcoma: a report of 3 cases. Br J Dermatol 1979; 100:327.

96. Cheuk WW, Wong KO, Wong SC, et al. Immunostaining for human herpesvirus 8 latent nuclear antigen-1 helps distinguish Kaposi sarcoma from its mimickers. Am J Clin Pathol 2004; 121:335.

97. Hammock L, Reisenauer A, Wang W, et al. Latency associated nuclear antigen expression and human herpesvirus 8 polymerase chain reaction in the evaluation of Kaposi sarcoma and other vascular tumors in HIV positive patients. Mod Pathol 2005; 18:463.

98. Patel RM, Goldblum JR, His ED. Immunohistochemical detection of human herpesvirus-8 latent nuclear antigen-1 is useful in the diagnosis of Kaposi sarcoma. Mod Pathol 2004; 17:456.

99. Schwartz EJ, Dorfman RF, Kohler S. Human herpesvirus 8 latent nuclear antigen 1 in endemic Kaposi sarcoma: an immunohistochemical study of 16 cases. Am J Surg Pathol 2003; 27:1546.

100. Kahn HJ, Bailey D, Marks A. Monoclonal antibody D2-40, a new marker of lymphatic endothelium, reacts with Kaposi sarcoma and a subset of angiosarcomas. Mod Pathol 2002; 15:434.

101. Folpe AL, Veikkola T, Valtola R, et al. Vascular endothelial growth factor receptor-3 (VEGFR-3): a marker of vascular tumors with presumed lymphatic differentiation, including Kaposi sarcoma, kaposiform and Dabska-type hemangioendotheliomas, and a subset of angiosarcomas. Mod Pathol 2000; 13:180.

102. Weninger W, Partanen TA, Breiteneder-Geleff S, et al. Expression of vascular endothelial growth factor receptor-3 and podoplanin suggests a lymphatic endothelial cell origin of Kaposi sarcoma tumor cells. Lab Invest 1999; 79:243.

103. Fukunaga M. Expression of D2-40 in lymphatic endothelium of normal tissues and in vascular tumors. Histopathology 2005; 46:396.

104. McNutt NS, Fletcher V, Conant MA. Early lesions of Kaposi sarcoma in homosexual men: an ultrastructural comparison with other vascular proliferations in the skin. Am J Pathol 1983; 111:62.

105. Marshall ME, Hatfield ST, Hatfield DR. Arteriovenous malformation simulating Kaposi sarcoma (pseudo Kaposi sarcoma). Arch Dermatol 1985; 121:99.

106. Nasti G, Talamini R, Antinori A, et al. AIDS-related Kaposi sarcoma: evaluation of potential new prognostic factors and assessment of the AIDS Clinical Trial Group staging system in the HAART era – the Italian Cooperative Group on AIDS and Tumors and the Italian Cohort of Patients naïve from antiretrovirals. J Clin Oncol 2003; 21:2876.

107. Krown SE, Testa MA, Huang J. AIDS-related Kaposi sarcoma: prospective validation of the AIDS Clinical Trials Group staging classification. AIDS Clinical Trials Group Oncology Committee. J Clin Oncol 1997; 15:3085.

TUMORS OF LYMPH VESSELS

The lymphatics are an extensive unidirectional system of blunt-ending vessels which regulate normal tissue pressure by retrieving excess fluid from the interstitium, transporting it to regional lymph nodes, and returning it to the venous system by way of the thoracic duct. The system also absorbs protein and lipid from the small intestine and liver and serves as a conduit for immune cells between the skin and lymph nodes. These small vessels are nearly ubiquitous but are conspicuously absent in the brain, anterior chamber of the eye, and portions of organs served by an "open," or sinusoidal, blood system such as bone marrow and red pulp of spleen. The smallest lymphatic vessels approximate the size of the blood capillary and are made up of fragile endothelial channels situated in a background of reticulum fibers and ground substance. Larger collecting channels contain, in addition, valves, muscle fibers, and elastic tissue, although the latter two are never developed to the extent observed in veins.

Based on the classic injection studies of Sabin on graded pig embryos, the lymphatic system makes its appearance during the sixth week of human embryonic development as an outgrowth from the venous system, although in some species de novo differentiation of lymph vessels from mesenchyme seems to occur. On a molecular level, lymphangiogenesis is heralded by the polarized expression of the homeobox transcription factor Prox 1 in a subpopulation of endothelial cells located within the cardinal vein.[1,2] This event is accompanied by budding of the endothelium from primitive veins and by the induction of lymphatic specific genes, LYVE1 and VEGFR3. Expression of PROX1 appears to be a "master" event in lymphangiogenesis, for in its absence there is agenesis of the entire lymphatic system. VEGFR3, in turn, is largely responsible for the migration and for-

mation of primary lymphatic sacs which through budding growth give rise to the lymphatic vasculature. Once lymphatic sacs are formed, the lymphatic and blood vasculature develop independently and only remain connected at certain specific points to allow return of the lymph fluid. The molecular events underlying late lymphangiogenesis are less well understood. One gene, FOXC2, which is mutated in inherited lymphedema, appears highly associated with the morphogenesis of lymphatic valves, and deficiencies in angiopoietin 2 are associated with defects in both patterning and function of the lymphatic system.

At the level of light microscopy the small lymphatics closely resemble capillaries and sometimes are only tentatively identified by the nature of their contents. Fine structural analysis, however, has documented rather significant differences. Although the basic conformation of the endothelial cell of the lymphatic system is similar to that of the blood capillary, it is invested by neither a basement membrane nor pericytes, with the exception of large collecting lymphatic channels. The former finding is also borne out by immunohistochemical analysis. Whereas antibodies to type IV collagen and laminin demonstrate a linear pattern of immunoreactivity around vascular capillary endothelium, this pattern is lacking around lymphatic capillary endothelium.[3] Thus, lymphatic endothelium is in direct contact with the interstitial space. This topographic relation is believed important for the expeditious recovery of fluid because a basement membrane serves as a partial diffusion barrier. In addition, there are thin "anchoring filaments" that terminate directly on the abluminal surface of the cell membrane and probably serve to maintain patency of the lymphatics during periods of increased interstitial pressure. The intercellular contacts between lymphatic endothelia are variable. Although tight junctions (zonula adherens), macula adherens, and desmosomes are present, there are many areas of simple overlapping of cells with no junctions.[4,5] This arrangement creates a "swinging door" effect so fluid can passively enter the lymphatic space during periods of increased interstitial pressure. Pinocytotic vesicles, thin cytofilaments, modest numbers of mitochondria, and endoplasmic reticulum, similar to those in capillaries, are also present in lymphatic cells.

Further differences between vascular and lymphatic capillary endothelium can be demonstrated by means of immunohistochemistry using antibodies targeted against lineage-specific substances, basal lamina, and pericytes. Lymphatic endothelium typically expresses PROX1, LYVE1, VEGFR3, but usually lack CD34 and do not possess an investiture of actin-positive pericytes. In contrast the reverse phenotype is observed in blood vascular endothelium.[3,6,7]

LYMPHANGIOMAS

As with hemangiomas, it is often difficult to state whether lymphangiomas are true neoplasms, hamartomas, or lymphangiectasias. In actuality, this distinction is of little practical value because they are all benign lesions, and therapy is largely dictated by their location and clinical extent. Most regard lymphangiomas as malformations that arise from sequestrations of lymphatic tissue that fail to communicate normally with the lymphatic system (Fig. 25–1). These remnants may have some capacity to proliferate, but more importantly they accumulate vast amounts of fluid, which accounts for their cystic appearance. The fact that most lymphangiomas manifest clinically during childhood and develop in areas where the primitive lymph sacs occur (e.g., neck, axilla) provides presumptive evidence for this hypothesis. Some early workers such as Goetsch considered these lesions to be true neoplasms capable of locally aggressive behavior, whereas others have suggested that they arise when inflammation causes fibrosis and obstruction of lymphatic channels. Although it is probable that some lymphangiomas are acquired lesions arising on an obstructive basis following surgery, irradiation, or infection,[8,9] most seem to represent developmental lesions that appear relatively early in life.

Histologic classification of lymphangiomas into capillary, cavernous or cystic subtypes based on the size of the vessels is not longer used. Instead, the all-inclusive term "lymphangioma" is preferred since this distinction is of little practical importance. In fact, many lymphangiomas have both cystic and cavernous components, a fact which raises the possibility that the cystic lymphangioma is merely a long-standing cavernous lymphangioma in which the cavernous spaces have been converted to cystic spaces. Bill and Sumner[10] suggested that histologic differences are attributable to differences in anatomic location. Cystic lymphangiomas arise in areas such as the neck and axilla, where loose connective tissue allows expansion of the endothelium-lined channels; cavernous lymphangiomas develop in the mouth, lips, cheek, tongue, or other areas where dense connective tissue and muscle prevent expansion. Cystic and cavernous lymphangiomas are not sufficiently distinct to be treated separately and differences between the two are mentioned only as necessary.

Clinical findings

Compared with hemangiomas, lymphangiomas are relatively rare. Anderson,[11] reviewing 768 benign tumors at Babies Hospital in New York over a 15-year period, identified only 48 lymphangiomas; and Bill and Sumner[10] estimated that they accounted for five of 3000 admissions at Children's Orthopedic Hospital. Kindblom and Angervall[12] reported 100 lymphangiomas over a 5-year period at the Sahlgren Hospital. The gender incidence is roughly equal,[10,12] although a slight male predominance is often recorded. It is estimated that 50–65% of these tumors are present at birth, and as many as 90% manifest by the end of the second year of life.[10,13–16] In some series nearly one-third were documented during adult life.[12] Those that present during adult life are the superficial cutaneous lymphangiomas (lymphangioma circumscriptum),[8,9,17] some of which are acquired lymphangiectasias which follow radiation[18,19] and intra-abdominal lymphangiomas that present after long symptom-free intervals. Lymphangiomas affect almost any part of the body served by the lymphatic system but show a predilection for the head, neck, and axilla (Figs 25–2, 25–3), sites that account for one-half to three-fourths of all lymphangiomas (Table 25–1). They also occur sporadically in various parenchymal organs including lung, gastrointestinal tract, spleen, liver, and bone. In the last three locations they occasionally signify the presence of diffuse or multifocal disease (see Lymphangiomatosis, below). Lymphangiomas also occur in association with hemangiomas in Maffucci syndrome.

The most common presentation of lymphangioma is that of a soft fluctuant mass that enlarges, remains static,

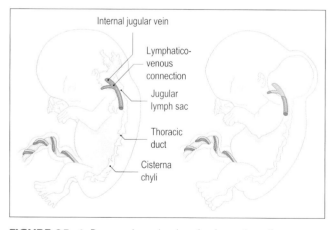

FIGURE 25–1 Proposed mechanism for formation of a lymphangioma. Lymphatic system in a normal fetus **(left)** with a patent connection between the jugular lymph sac and the internal jugular vein and a cystic hygroma from a failed lymphaticovenous connection **(right)**. (Modified from Chervenak FA, Issacson G, Blakemore KJ. Fetal cystic hygroma: cause and natural history. N Engl J Med 1983; 309:822.)

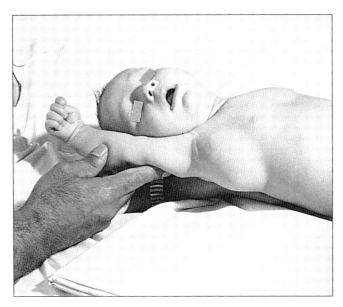

FIGURE 25–2 Lymphangioma (cystic hygroma) of the axilla.

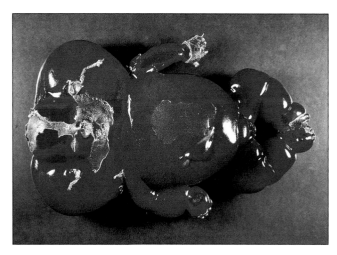

FIGURE 25–4 Abortus with Turner syndrome (XX/XO). A large cystic hygroma had been detected in utero by ultrasonography.

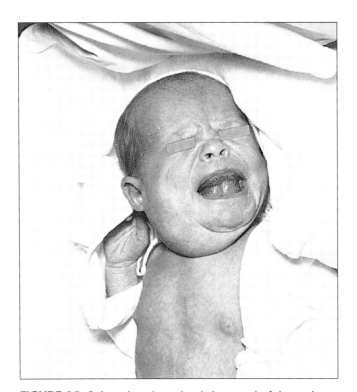

FIGURE 25–3 Lymphangioma (cystic hygroma) of the neck.

TABLE 25–1	ANATOMIC LOCATION OF LYMPHANGIOMAS (61 PATIENTS)
Anatomic location	**No.**
Head	35
Tongue	8
Cheek	7
Floor of the mouth	7
Parotid	5
Other	8
Neck	25
Trunk and extremities	43
Axilla	15
Pectoral	10
Arm	6
Scapula	5
Other	7
Internal	6
Mediastinum	5
Abdomen	1

Modified from Bill AH, Sumner DS. A unified concept of lymphangioma and cystic hygroma. Surg Gynecol Obstet 1965; 120:79.
There are more than 61 tumors owing to the fact that large tumors were tabulated under several locations.

or waxes and wanes during the period of clinical observation. In a few cases rapid enlargement can be related to an upper respiratory tract infection, which apparently causes obstruction in the lymphatics draining the lesion.

Lymphangioma (cystic hygroma) may also be detected in utero by ultrasonography. Such cases merit special comment, as they have been shown to be associated with hydrops fetalis and Turner syndrome, and they are asso-ciated with a high death rate (Figs 25–4, 25–5).[20,21] Chervenak et al.[21] reported on 15 intrauterine cystic hygromas and found that 11 were associated with the cytogenetic abnormalities of Turner syndrome (45,X/O or 46,XO/46,XX). Of the 15 fetuses, 13 had severe hydrops, and none of the 15 ultimately survived. Thus, it seems that defects in the lymphatic and vascular systems comprise part of Turner syndrome. The authors suggested that severe aberrations of the lymphatic system in this condition are incompatible with life; milder forms are compatible with survival but give rise to webbing of the neck and edema of the hands and feet, which characterize the Turner syndrome infantile phenotype (Fig. 25–6).

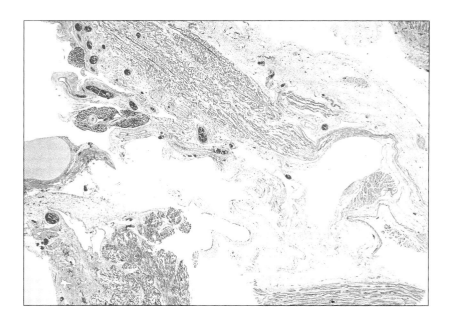

FIGURE 25–5 Section of a cystic hygroma from a fetus with Turner syndrome.

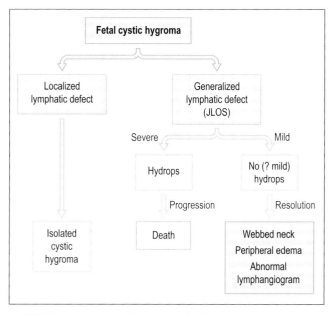

FIGURE 25–6 Natural history of a fetal nuchal cystic hygroma. Generalized lymphatic defect results from the jugular lymphatic obstruction sequence (JLOS). Depending on the severity of the obstruction, varying degrees of hydrops are noted. (Modified from Chervenak FA, Issacson G, Blakemore KJ. Fetal cystic hygroma: cause and natural history. N Engl J Med 1983; 309:822.)

Other syndromes may also be associated with fetal cystic hygroma, including Noonan syndrome, familial pterygium colli, fetal alcohol syndrome, and several chromosomal aneuploidies.[22] Because aneuploidic conditions may recur during subsequent pregnancies, cytogenetic analysis of fetuses born with cystic hygroma is indicated.

Lymphangiomas of the head and neck

Lymphangiomas are most common in the neck, where they typically lie in the supraclavicular fossa of the posterior cervical triangle or extend toward the crest of the shoulder. Less frequently, they are located in the anterior cervical triangle just below the angle of the jaw. Tumors in this location are the ones most apt to present with significant airway or feeding problems.[23] About 10% of lymphangiomas of the neck extend into the mediastinum, illustrating the need for preoperative chest radiographs prior to planning a surgical approach. Grossly, these tumors are unicystic or multicystic masses that involve the superficial soft tissue and tend to bulge outward rather than extend inward (Fig. 25–3). Consequently, they usually do not compromise vital structures such as the trachea and esophagus unless they are large. In contrast to lymphangiomas of the neck, those involving the soft tissues of the lips, cheek, tongue, and mouth are usually of the cavernous type, frequently involve deep soft tissue structures, and cause functional impairment depending on their size.

Intra-abdominal lymphangiomas

Intra-abdominal tumors are rare (Fig. 25–7), as evidenced by the fact that Galifer et al.[24] tabulated only 139 cases from the English literature. Although 60% are present in patients under the age of 5 years, a significant percentage does not manifest until adult life.[15] The most common location is the mesentery, followed by the omentum, mesocolon, and retroperitoneum (Table 25–2). In addition to a palpable mass, patients with tumors in the first three locations often develop symptoms of an acute condition in the abdomen caused by the common complica-

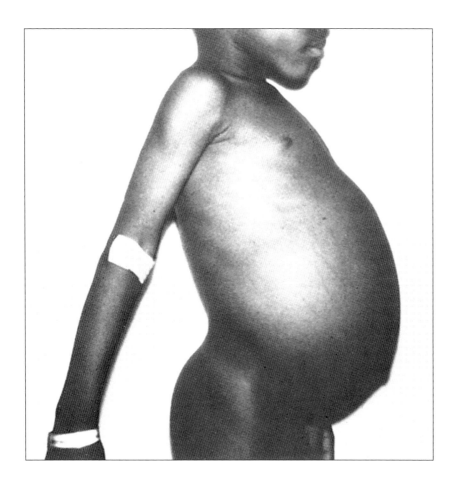

FIGURE 25–7 Large intra-abdominal lymphangioma.

TABLE 25–2	LOCATION OF 139 INTRA-ABDOMINAL LYMPHANGIOMAS	
Anatomic location	**No. of cases**	**%**
Mesentery	96	69
Jejunum	25	
Ileum	44	
Root of mesentery	5	
Not specified	22	
Omentum	21	15
Mesocolon	15	11
Retroperitoneum	7	5
Total	139	100

Modified from Galifer RB, Pous JG, Juskiewenski S, et al. Intra-abdominal cystic lymphangiomas in childhood. Prog Pediatr Surg 1978; 11:173.

tions of intestinal obstruction, volvulus, and infarction. In fact, a provisional diagnosis of acute appendicitis is frequently entertained because of the common occurrence of right lower quadrant pain. In contrast, retroperitoneal tumors produce few acute symptoms but ultimately are diagnosed by virtue of a large palpable mass causing displacement of one or more organs. Most arise in the lumbar area and cause displacement of the kidney, usually without urinary tract obstruction. Those arising in the superior portion of the retroperitoneum shift the pancreas and duodenum anteriorly.

In the past an abdominal lymphangioma was seldom diagnosed preoperatively. The diagnosis can usually be suspected with a combination of radiologic studies.[25] Ultrasonography is useful for localizing and determining the cystic nature of the tumors. As seen by arteriography, the lesions are poorly vascularized; and in a few reported cases connections between lower extremity lymphatics and the tumors can be demonstrated with lymphography. On CT scans the tumors appear as multiple, homogeneous, nonenhancing areas with variable attenuation values, depending on whether the fluid is chylous or serous.

Cutaneous lymphangiomas

Cutaneous lymphangiomas can be divided into superficial and deep forms. The latter form is histologically and clinically identical to the usual cavernous lymphangioma and does not require additional elaboration (Fig. 25–8). The superficial intradermal form, sometimes referred to as *lymphangioma circumscriptum*,[9] has rather characteristic features. These lesions develop as multiple small vesicles or wart-like nodules that cover localized areas of skin (Fig. 25–9), although in some cases large areas of the body are affected. Histologically, dilated irregular lymphatic channels fill the papillary dermis and protrude

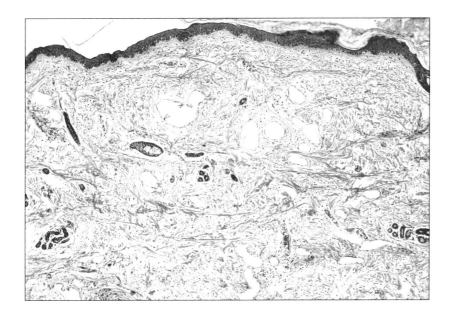

FIGURE 25–8 Cutaneous lymphangioma of the deep type. Dilated lymphatic channels extend over large areas of skin and involve superficial and deep dermis.

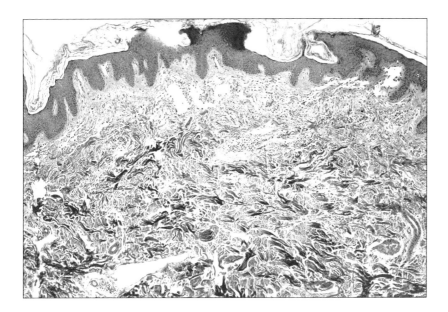

FIGURE 25–9 Cutaneous lymphangioma of superficial type (lymphangioma circumscriptum). Lymphatic vessels are localized and restricted to superficial dermis.

into the epidermis, giving the impression of being "intraepidermal." The overlying epidermis is acanthotic and thrown into papillae. Generally, the lesions are asymptomatic unless they become irritated. They may arise de novo or be secondary to surgery or irradiation. In the latter setting some prefer to classify the lesions as "lymphangiectasis,"[8,18,19] although they are clinically and histologically indistinguishable from the de novo lesions.

Another form of cutaneous lymphangioma deserves special mention because of its mimicry of well-differentiated angiosarcoma. The *acquired progressive lymphangioma (lymphangioendothelioma)* is a slowly growing cutaneous lymphangioma that occurs spontaneously in children and usually following surgery, irradiation, or minor forms of injury[26–30] in adults (Figs 25–10 to 25–12). Because of their association with irradiation some have also employed the term "benign lymphangiomatous papules following radiotherapy."[26] Some of the lesions referred to as "atypical vascular lesion" following radiation are examples of this. Clinically, the lesion appears as one or more erythematous, white-tan or translucent vesicles. Those seen following irradiation occur after an interval of several months to years in the irradiated area. One of the most important clues to the diagnosis is the ectatic lymph vessels in the subpapillary region of the upper dermis that create the papular or vesicular appearance. The vessels ramify in the dermis and occasionally extend into the subcutis. The vessels, filled with clear fluid, are lined by attenuated endothelial cells that do not exhibit atypia, mitotic activity, or solid areas of growth. Lymphoid aggregates accompany the lymphatic channels.

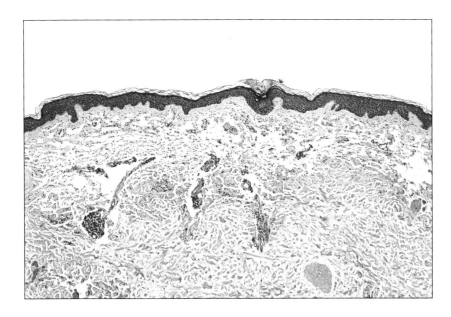

FIGURE 25–10 Acquired progressive lymphangioma with superficial proliferation of lymphatic vessels.

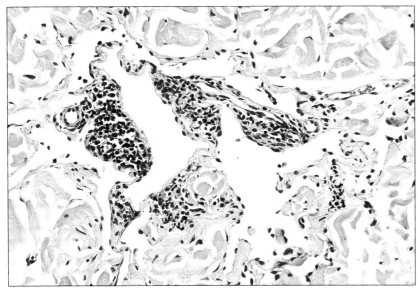

FIGURE 25–11 Acquired progressive lymphangioma with dissection of dermis by well-differentiated lymphatic vessels.

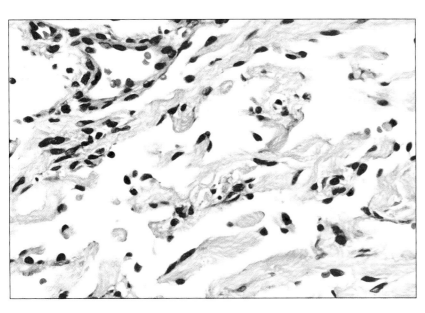

FIGURE 25–12 Acquired progressive lymphangioma with a single layer of endothelial cells without atypia.

Follow-up of a limited number of cases has indicated a benign clinical course with no evidence of metastasis. In particular, three of the five patients reported following irradiation by Diaz-Cascajo et al. had follow-up of more than 3 years and were alive and well with neither recurrence nor metastasis.[26] In the series by Guillou and Fletcher, one of nine patients developed a recurrence.[27] Nonetheless, we believe the diagnosis of acquired progressive lymphangioma should be employed cautiously when dealing with postirradiation lesions in adults, as this situation is well recognized as a precursor to the development of angiosarcoma. In this setting it has been our approach to sample such lesions well, correlate the pathologic findings closely with the clinical features, and recommend close follow-up care.

Gross and microscopic findings

Lymphangiomas vary from well-circumscribed lesions made up of one or more large interconnecting cysts to ill-defined, sponge-like compressible lesions (Figs 25–13 to 25–19) composed of microscopic cysts. The former were traditionally termed as *cystic lymphangiomas (cystic hygroma)* and the latter as *cavernous lymphangiomas*. Tumors often combine features of the two, and their differences are offset by their overall similarities. Regardless of the size of the lymphatic spaces, both lesions are lined by attenuated endothelium resembling that in normal lymphatics. Small lymphatic spaces have only an inconspicuous adventitial coat surrounding them, whereas large lymphatic spaces have, in addition, fascicles of poorly developed smooth muscle. The lymphatic spaces classically are filled with proteinaceous fluid containing lymphocytes, although occasionally erythrocytes are present as well. The stroma is composed of a delicate meshwork of collagen punctuated by small lymphoid aggregates (Fig. 24–16). With repeated bouts of infection, the stroma of a lymphangioma becomes inflamed, edematous (Fig. 25–19), and ultimately fibrotic.

In most cases there is little difficulty establishing the correct diagnosis. However, lymphangiomas with secondary hemorrhage are sometimes confused with cavernous hemangiomas. Histologic features that favor the diagnosis of lymphangioma over hemangioma include the presence of lymphoid aggregates in the stroma and more irregular lumens with widely spaced nuclei. Immunohistochemistry for lymphatic lineage markers

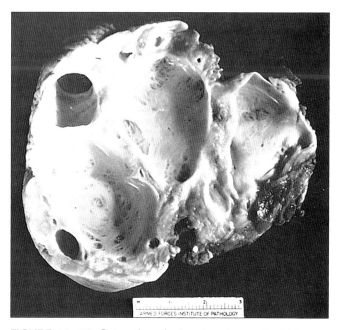

FIGURE 25–13 Cut section of a lymphangioma with thick-walled cysts of various sizes.

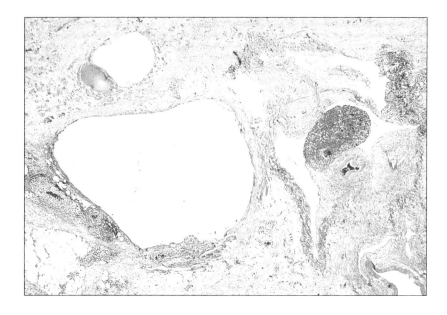

FIGURE 25–14 Low-power view of lymphangioma.

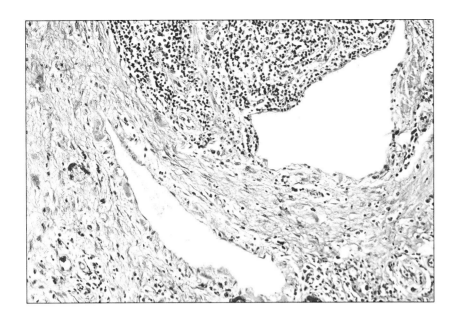

FIGURE 25–15 High-power view of lymphangioma.

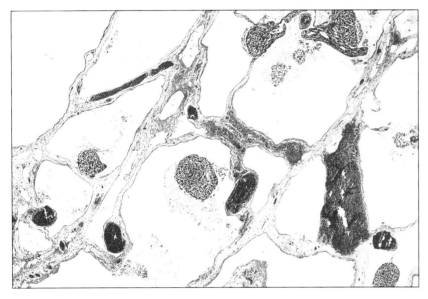

FIGURE 25–16 Lymphangioma containing dense lymphoid aggregates.

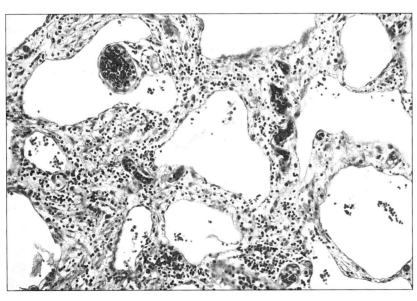

FIGURE 25–17 Lymphangioma with engorged vascular spaces.

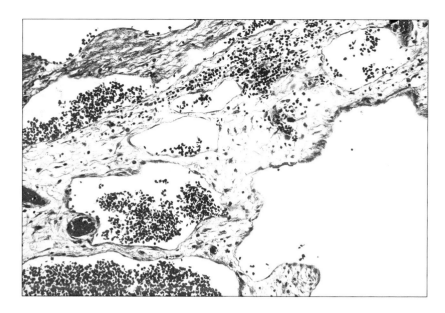

FIGURE 25–18 Lymphangioma with stromal hemorrhage.

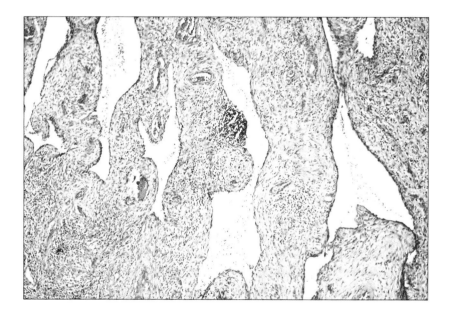

FIGURE 25–19 Inflamed intra-abdominal lymphangioma.

(e.g., VEGFR3, D2-40) can also assist in this distinction.[6,31]

It is more important to distinguish an intra-abdominal lymphangioma from a cystic form of mesothelioma or microcystic adenoma of the pancreas. The cystic mesothelioma presents as a multicystic mass that affects a large area of peritoneum and requires repeated surgery for control (see Chapter 29). The clinical extent of the lesion is at variance with the lymphangioma, which usually involves a localized area of peritoneum. Cystic mesotheliomas are composed of gland-like spaces that show greater variation in size than the vascular spaces of the lymphangioma. Moreover, there is a transition from normal or reactive mesothelium to the glandular spaces of the mesothelioma. Out of context, however, the cells may look surprisingly similar. The cells of mesotheliomas have numerous microvilli, whereas those of lymphangiomas are smoothly contoured and resemble normal lymphatic endothelia. In ambiguous situations immunohistochemical procedures are easy, reliable means to make this distinction, as the cells of multicystic mesothelioma, like other mesothelial tumors but unlike lymphatic tumors, express cytokeratin and epithelial membrane antigen. Microcystic adenomas of the pancreas are composed of cystic spaces lined by cuboidal or low columnar, keratin-positive epithelium. The glandular spaces are more regular in shape than in lymphangioma and rest on a stroma containing a rich network of small blood capillaries, a feature usually not encountered in lymphangiomas.

Behavior and treatment

Although the lymphangioma is a benign lesion, it may cause significant morbidity because of its large size, critical location, or proclivity to become secondarily infected. Only rare cases are known to have regressed spontaneously, and eventually virtually all lesions require some form of therapy. In the past, surgery has been the mainstay of treatment. The best results were achieved in cystic lymphangiomas that were well circumscribed and amenable to complete excision. Higher recurrence rates accompanied surgery performed for cavernous hemangiomas which were infiltrative of surrounding structures. Postsurgical nerve palsies appeared in one-third of the patients.[23] A staged surgical excision was often required to eradicate these tumors. More recently, treatment with the sclerosing agent OK-432 has been successfully used in some lymphangiomas.[32–34] Approximately one-third of all lymphangiomas respond to this therapy. Factors which predict good response include head and neck location, size less than 5 cm, and macrocystic architecture.[34,35]

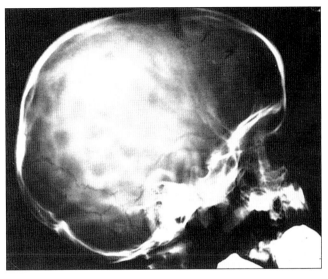

FIGURE 25–20 Male child with lymphangiomatosis affecting multiple bones and soft tissue sites. Multiple osteolytic lesions are present in the skull.

LYMPHANGIOMATOSIS

Lymphangioma affecting soft tissue or parenchymal organs in a diffuse or multifocal fashion is termed *lymphangiomatosis*. This rare disease can be conceptualized as the lymphatic counterpart of angiomatosis (see Chapter 22). It should be emphasized, however, that it is not always possible to distinguish angiomatosis from lymphangiomatosis clearly because overlap occurs between the two. By convention, the term lymphangiomatosis is reserved for lesions with predominantly, if not exclusively, lymphatic differentiation.

Like angiomatosis, this disease occurs principally in children and rarely manifests after age 20. Diagnosis of this condition at birth is uncommon because it seems that a latent period is required for these lesions to achieve sufficient size to become symptomatic. There is no gender predilection. The presenting symptoms are varied and depend on the site and extent of involvement. More than three-fourths of patients have multiple bone lesions. These well-delimited osteolytic lesions with a variable degree of sclerosis (Figs 25–20 to 25–22) are usually asymptomatic, are often discovered incidentally, and are frequently diagnosed as fibrous dysplasia or bone changes associated with hyperparathyroidism. Acute symptoms more often relate to the presence of lymphangiomas in soft tissue, mediastinum, liver, spleen, or lung. The prognosis is determined by the extent of the disease.[36] Patients with liver, spleen, lung, and thoracic duct involvement usually have a poor prognosis,[36] as the lesions tend to be diffuse and are not amenable to surgical excision. On the other hand, patients with soft tissue involvement with or without skeletal involvement enjoy an excellent progno-

sis[37] because in most cases the bone lesions eventually stabilize and the soft tissue lesions respond to limited surgical resection. In contrast, patients with lesions in the vertebrae may develop cord compression and ultimately die of their disease.

Lymphangiomatosis affecting principally soft tissue and bone presents with fluctuant brawny swelling of an extremity that corresponds on the lymphangiogram to numerous interconnecting lymphatic channels (Fig. 25–23). The skin is thickened, and the soft tissue has a brown sponge-like quality due to the extensive replacement by proliferating lymphatic channels (Fig. 25–24). The proliferating vessels are lined by a single layer of flattened endothelium that ramifies in the soft tissue in a pattern analogous to a well-differentiated angiosarcoma. Stromal hemosiderin deposits in the absence of active hemorrhage can be seen. Atypical features such as endothelial tufting, atypia, and mitotic activity of the lymphatic endothelium are not present. In these respects lymphangiomatosis is similar histologically to the deep portions of acquired progressive lymphangioma. The diagnosis of lymphangiomatosis may be difficult to establish when only bone biopsy is undertaken. To the unsuspecting pathologist the bland dilated lymph channels devoid of cells may appear so innocuous as to be overlooked altogether, and more emphasis may be placed on the surrounding bone resorption and atrophy. One or more vascular markers can be detected in the lymphatic endothelium, although CD31 seems to be the most sensitive.

The differential diagnosis of lymphangiomatosis includes angiomatosis, acquired progressive lymphangioma, and, most importantly, angiosarcoma. Although the infiltrative appearance at low power usually

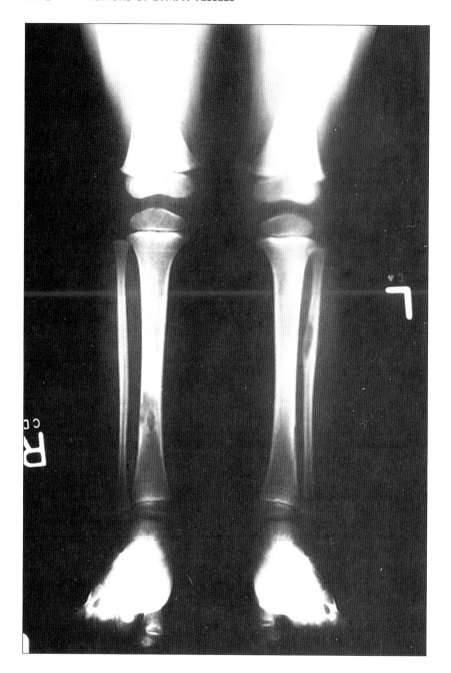

FIGURE 25–21 Lymphangiomatosis (same case as in Figure 25–18) with multiple, bilateral osteolytic lesions in long bones.

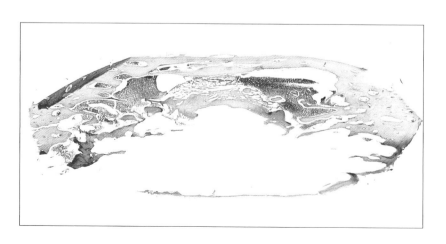

FIGURE 25–22 Section of lymphangioma removed from the rib of a patient with lymphangiomatosis. Note the delicate lining of lymphatic cells around the defect (same case as in Figure 25–20).

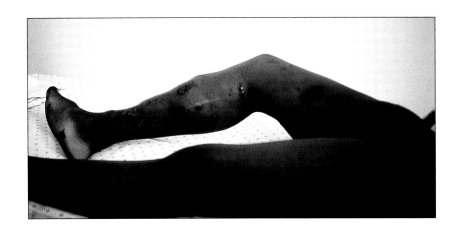

FIGURE 25–23 Lymphangiomatosis affecting one lower extremity.

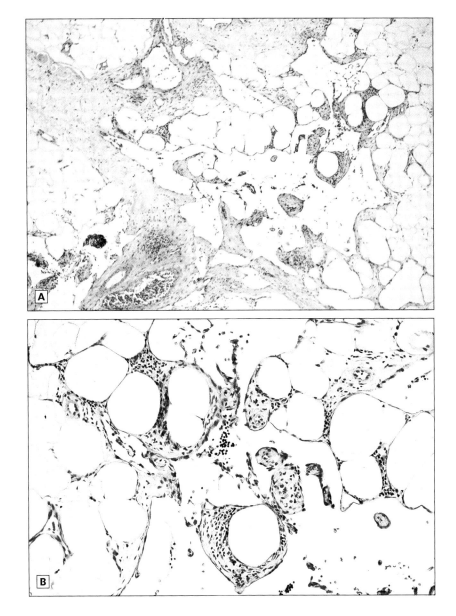

FIGURE 25–24 Persistently recurring lymphangiomatosis of the leg. Lymphatic channels diffusely involve soft tissue **(A)** and are composed of cells with little atypia **(B)**.

immediately suggests angiosarcoma, one is always struck by the apparent discordance between the infiltrative pattern, which suggests an aggressive process, and the relatively innocuous appearance of the lymphatic endothelium. Features such as endothelial redundancy and nuclear atypia, which are the hallmark of virtually all angiosarcomas, are absent in lymphangiomatosis and provide an important clue to the correct diagnosis. Angiomatosis is typically composed of vessels of varying size and mural complexity (see Chapter 22). Although some have a prominent capillary vascular component, the capillary vessels do not dissect and ramify throughout the soft tissue to the extent seen in lymphangiomatosis. The distinction between acquired progressive lymphangioma and lymphangiomatosis is more problematic. In our experience, portions of acquired progressive lymphangioma are virtually indistinguishable from lymphangiomatosis. Therefore, one could conceptualize the acquired progressive lymphangioma in some cases as a limited or superficial form of lymphangiomatosis. The distinction between the two is therefore best made based on presentation and clinical extent, a situation analogous to the distinction between hemangioma and angiomatosis.

LOCALIZED MASSIVE LYMPHEDEMA

Localized areas of massive lymphedema develop in morbidly obese individuals and frequently simulate a well-differentiated liposarcoma.[38] The pathogenetic mechanism of this pseudoneoplastic condition appears to be localized lymphatic obstruction due to the weight of large dependent folds of fat. In some cases the condition is probably exacerbated by previous surgery that has interrupted lymphatics and contributes to obstruction.

Patients with this condition usually weigh in excess of 300 pounds and develop lesions preferentially in the medial portion of the extremities. Clinically, the lesions are pendulous masses with a thickened hyperkeratotic or peau d'orange-like appearance of skin (Fig. 25–25). Radiologically, the mass corresponds to expanded subcutaneous tissue with soft tissue "streaking" but without a discrete mass lesion. On cut section one is impressed by the amount of fibrous tissue traversing the fat and by the presence of cysts of various sizes that "weep" serous fluid (Fig. 25–26).

Histologically, the changes are those of chronic lymphedema. The overlying skin is thickened and occasionally hyperkeratotic (Fig. 25–27), whereas the underlying dermis is hyalinized and contains numerous small lymphatic channels surrounded by clusters of lymphocytes (Fig. 25–28). In the subcutis, the interlobular septa are markedly expanded by edema fluid and mildly atypical fibroblasts such that the lobules of fat appear minimized (Figs 25–29, 25–30). At the interface of the septa and the residual fat one occasionally finds a fringe of reactive capillary-sized vessels.

Although these lesions represent a reactive condition involving the lymphatic system, they are commonly confused with liposarcoma (see Chapter 16) because the expanded interlobular septa are misinterpreted as the fibrous bands of a sclerosing well-differentiated liposarcoma. The salient observations when making this distinction are the overall preservation of the architecture of normal subcutaneous fat and the lack of significant atypia in the fibrous bands separating the fat. Because the underlying cause of the condition is morbid obesity, persistence or even recurrence of these lesions is to be expected following surgery. None has behaved in an aggressive manner.

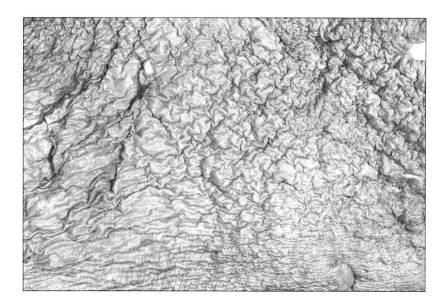

FIGURE 25–25 Localized massive lymphedema showing thickened pebble-like skin.

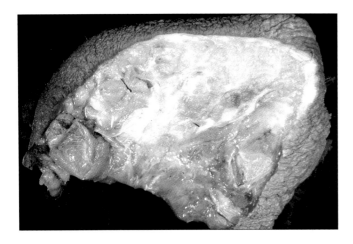

FIGURE 25–26 Localized massive lymphedema with multiple cysts of the subcutis and exaggerated fibrous trabeculae.

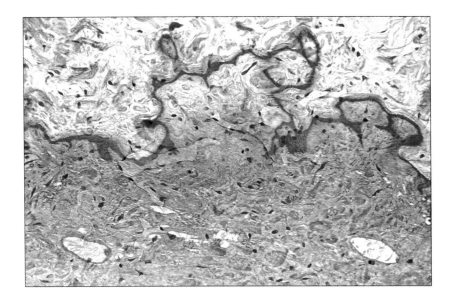

FIGURE 25–27 Thickened hyperkeratotic skin in localized massive lymphedema.

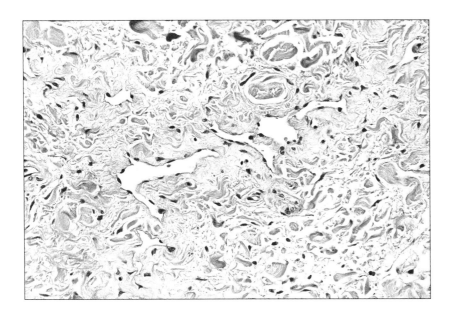

FIGURE 25–28 Irregular lymphatic channels in sclerotic dermis in localized massive lymphedema.

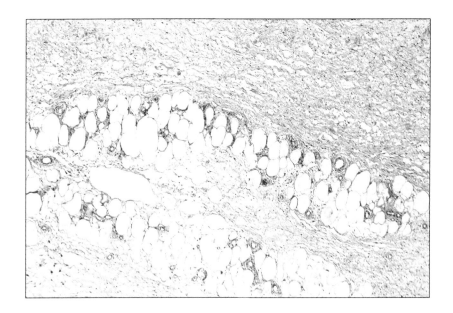

FIGURE 25–29 Widened fibrous trabeculae in the subcutis in massive localized lymphedema. Note fringe of capillaries of interface of fat and fibrous trabeculae.

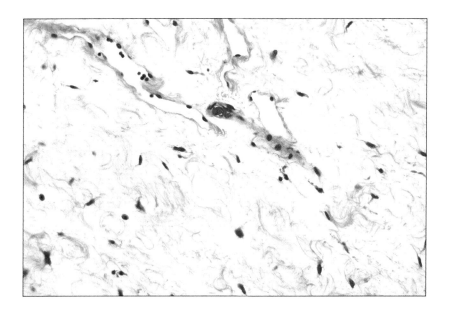

FIGURE 25–30 Mildly atypical fibroblasts in fibrous trabeculae within massive localized lymphedema.

LYMPHANGIOSARCOMA

Traditionally, lymphangiosarcoma is defined as a vascular sarcoma arising in the setting of chronic lymphedema. Most occur in patients with postsurgical lymphedema, particularly as a result of radical mastectomy for breast carcinoma (Stewart-Treves syndrome), but they may develop in chronic lymphedema from almost any cause. Although the clinical setting suggests that these tumors arise from proliferating lymphatic endothelium, it is difficult to distinguish them histologically from other forms of angiosarcoma and they are discussed in Chapter 24.

LYMPHANGIOMYOMA AND LYMPHANGIOMYOMATOSIS

Lymphangiomyoma and its diffuse form, lymphangiomyomatosis, are perilymphatic proliferations of the perivascular epithelioid cell (PEC), a distinctive cell co-expressing muscle and melanocytic markers. These two lesions are considered with other members of the PEComa family in Chapter 36.

REFERENCES

1. Tammela T, Petrova TV, Alitalo K. Molecular lymphangiogenesis: new players. Trends Cell Biol 2005; 15:434.
2. Hong Y-K, Detmar M. Prox1, master regulator of the lymphatic vascular phenotype. Cell Tissue Res 2003; 314:85.
3. Barsky SH, Baker A, Siegel OP. Use of anti-basement membrane antibodies to distinguish blood vessel capillaries from lymphatic capillaries. Am J Surg Pathol 1983; 7:667.
4. Fraley EE, Weiss L. An electron microscopic study of lymphatic vessels in the penile skin of the rat. Am J Anat 1961; 109:85.
5. Leak LV, Burke JF. Fine structure of the lymphatic capillary and the adjoining connective tissue area. Am J Anat 1966; 118:785.
6. Fugunaga M. Expression of D2-40 in lymphatic endothelium of normal tissues and in vascular tumors. Histopathology 2005; 46:396.
7. Folpe AL, Veikkola T, Valtola R, et al. Vascular endothelial growth factor receptor-3 (VEGFR-3): a marker of vascular tumors with presumed lymphatic differentiation, including Kaposi's sarcoma, kaposiform and Dabska-type hemangioendotheliomas, and a subset of angiosarcomas. Mod Pathol 2000; 13:180.

Lymphangiomas

8. Fisher I, Orkin M. Acquired lymphangioma (lymphangiectasis). Arch Dermatol 1970; 101:230.
9. Peachy RO, Limm CC, Whimster IW. Lymphangioma of skin: a review of 65 cases. Br J Dermatol 1970; 83:519.
10. Bill AH, Sumner DS. A unified concept of lymphangioma and cystic hygroma. Surg Gynecol Obstet 1965; 120:79.
11. Anderson DH. Tumors of infancy and childhood. Cancer 1951; 4:890.
12. Kindblom L-G, Angervall L. Tumors of lymph vessels. Contemp Issues Surg Pathol 1991; 18:163.
13. Alqahtani A, Nguyen LT, Flageole H, et al. 25 years' experience with lymphangiomas in children. J Pediatr Surg 1999; 34:1164.

14. Castanon M, Margarit J, Carrasco R, et al. Long term follow up of nineteen cystic lymphangiomas treated with fibrin sealant. J Pediatr Surg 1999; 34:1276.
15. Chung JH, Suh YL, Park IA, et al. A pathologic study of abdominal lymphangiomas. J Korean Med Sci 1999; 14:257.
16. Fonkalsrud EW. Congenital malformations of the lymphatic system. Semin Pediatr Surg 1994; 3:62.
17. Whimster IW. The pathology of lymphangioma circumscriptum. Br J Dermatol 1974; 10:35.
18. Prioleau PG, Santa Cruz DJ. Lymphangioma circumscripta following radical mastectomy and radiation therapy. Cancer 1978; 42:1989.
19. Wagamon K, Ranchoff RE, Rosenberg AS, et al. Benign lymphangiomatous papules of the skin. J Am Acad Dermatol 2005; 52:912.
20. Byrne J, Blanc WA, Warburton D, et al. The significance of cystic hygroma in fetuses. Hum Pathol 1984; 15:61.
21. Chervenak FA, Isaacson G, Blakemore KJ. Fetal cystic hygroma: cause and natural history. N Engl J Med 1983; 309:822.
22. Fryns JP, Kleczkowska K, Vandenberghe F, et al. Cystic hygroma and hydrops fetalis in dup(11p) syndrome. Am J Med Genet 1985; 22:287.
23. Emery PJ, Bailey CM, Evans JNG. Cystic hygroma of the head and neck: a review of 37 cases. J Laryngol Otol 1984; 98:613.
24. Galifer RB, Pous JG, Juskiewenski S, et al. Intraabdominal cystic lymphangiomas in childhood. Prog Pediatr Surg 1978; 11:173.
25. Koshy A, Tandon RK, Kapur BML, et al. Retroperitoneal lymphangioma. Am J Gastroenterol 1978; 69:485.
26. Diaz-Cascajo C, Borghi S, Weyers W, et al. Benign lymphangiomatous papules of the skin following radiotherapy: a report of five new cases and review of the literature. Histopathology 1999; 35:319.
27. Guillou L, Fletcher CD. Benign lymphangioendothelioma (acquired progressive lymphangioma): a lesion not to be confused with well-differentiated angiosarcoma and patch stage Kaposi's sarcoma: clinicopathologic analysis of a series. Am J Surg Pathol 2000; 24:1047.

28. Kato H, Kadoya A. Acquired progressive lymphangioma occurring following femoral arteriography. Clin Exp Dermatol 1996; 21:159.
29. Meunier L, Barneon G, Meynadier J. Acquired progressive lymphangioma. Br J Dermatol 1994; 131:706.
30. Wilson-Jones E, Winkelmann RK, Zachary CB, et al. Benign lymphangioendothelioma. J Am Acad Dermatol 1990; 23:229.
31. Galambos C, Nodit L. Identification of lymphatic endothelium in pediatric vascular tumors and malformations. Ped Dev Pathol 2005; 8:181.
32. Wheeler JS, Morreau P, Mahadevan M, et al. OK-432 and lymphatic malformations in children: the Starship Children's Hospital experience. A NZ J Surg 2004; 74:855.
33. Sichel JY, Udassin R, Gozal D, et al. OK-432 therapy for cervical lymphangioma. Laryngoscope 2004; 114:1805.
34. Banieghbal B, Davies MRQ. Guidelines for the successful treatment of lymphangioma with OK-432. European J Ped Surg 2003; 13:103.
35. Hall N, Ade-Ajayi N, Brewis C, et al. Is intralesional injection of OK-432 effective in the treatment of lymphangioma in children? Surgery 2003; 133:238.

Lymphangiomatosis

36. Ramani P, Shah A. Lymphangiomatosis: histologic and immunohistochemical analysis of four cases. Am J Surg Pathol 1993; 17:329.
37. Gomez CS, Calonje E, Ferrar DW, et al. Lymphangiomatosis of the limbs: clinicopathologic analysis of a series with a good prognosis. Am J Surg Pathol 1995; 19:125.

Localized massive lymphedema

38. Farshid G, Weiss SW. Massive localized lymphedema in the morbidly obese: a histologically distinct reactive lesion simulating liposarcoma. Am J Surg Pathol 1998; 22:1277.

PERIVASCULAR TUMORS

Perivascular tumors recapitulate the appearance of the modified myoid cells that support or invest blood vessels (i.e., glomus cell and pericyte). Sometimes referred to as perivascular myoid tumors, they include the glomus tumor and its variants, myopericytoma, and the hemangiopericytoma-like tumor of the nasal passages. The so-called hemangiopericytoma, while a distinctive lesion histologically, does not display true pericytic differentiation but shares many histologic, immunophenotypic and cytogenetic features with the solitary fibrous tumor. Since there is a consensus that hemangiopericytoma and solitary fibrous tumor are part of the same spectrum of lesions that are of uncertain lineage, they are covered in Chapter 36.

CLASSIC (SPORADIC) GLOMUS TUMOR

The glomus tumor is a distinctive neoplasm that resembles the normal glomus body. It was originally considered a form of angiosarcoma until Masson[1] published his classic paper on the subject in 1924. His work was based on observations of three patients who had experienced strikingly similar symptoms. Each suffered paroxysms of lancinating pain in the upper extremity that abated abruptly after removal of the tumor. Masson compared the tumors to the normal glomus body and suggested that the lesion represented hyperplasia or overgrowth of this structure.

The normal glomus body is a specialized form of arteriovenous anastomosis which regulates heat. It is located in the stratum reticularis of the dermis and is most fre-

quently encountered in the subungual region, the lateral areas of the digits, and the palm.[2] Glomus bodies are also identified in the precoccygeal soft tissue as one or more grouped structures (glomus coccygeum) varying in diameter from <1 to 4 mm. According to Popoff,[2] the structure does not develop until several months after birth and gradually undergoes atrophy during late adult life. Although it may be damaged in certain disease states, there is evidence that it may regenerate, probably as a result of differentiation of perivascular cells. The glomus body is made up of an afferent arteriole derived from the small arterioles supplying the dermis and branching into two or four preglomic arterioles (Figs 26–1 to 26–3). These arterioles are endowed with the usual complement of muscle cells and an internal elastic lamina, but they blend gradually into a thick-walled segment with an irregular lumen known as the Sucquet-Hoyer canal. This region is the arteriovenous anastomosis proper. It is lined by plump cuboidal endothelial cells, which in turn are surrounded by longitudinal and circular muscle fibers but no elastic tissue. Scattered throughout the muscle fibers are the rounded, epithelioid "glomus" cells. These canals drain into a series of thin-walled collecting veins. The entire glomic complex is encompassed by lamellated collagenous tissue containing small nerves and vessels.

Clinical findings

Glomus tumors are uncommon, with an estimated incidence of 1.6% among the 500 consecutive soft tissue tumors reported from the Mayo Clinic.[3] The tumor is about equally common in both genders, although there is a striking female predominance (3:1) among patients with subungual lesions.[3] Multiple subungual glomus tumors have been reported in neurofibromatosis 1.[4,5] Most glomus tumors are diagnosed during adult life (20–40 years of age), although often symptoms have been present for several years before the diagnosis. The lesions develop as small blue-red nodules that are usually located in the deep dermis or subcutis of the upper or lower extremity. The single most common site is the subungual region of the finger, but other common sites include the palm, wrist, forearm, and foot (Table 26–1). Glomus tumors probably also occur in the subcutaneous tissue

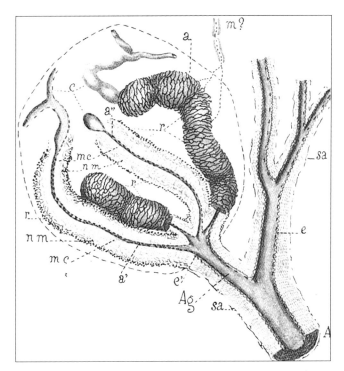

FIGURE 26–1 Normal glomus body according to Masson.[1] Afferent arteriole (Ag) gives rise to four preglomic arterioles, which blend with an irregular, thick-walled segment known as the Sucquet-Hoyer canal containing the arteriovenous anastomosis. It terminates in the collecting veins (c). (From Masson P. Le glomus neuromyoarterial des regions tactiles et ses tumeurs. Lyon Chir 1924; 21:257.)

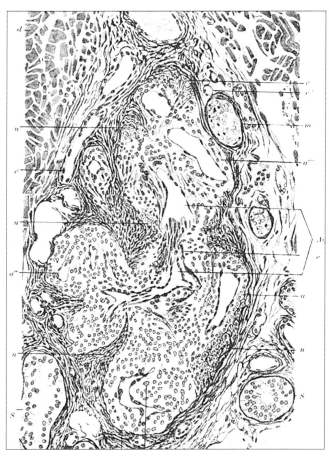

FIGURE 26–2 Histologic cross section through a glomus body according to Masson.[1] Glomic arterioles of Sucquet-Hoyer canal (a, a," a′ ,") contain glomus cells in their walls. Collecting veins are located at the periphery (c). Small nerves and collagen fibers encircle the glomus body. (From Masson P. Le glomus neuromyoarterial des regions tactiles et ses tumeurs. Lyon Chir 1924; 21:257.)

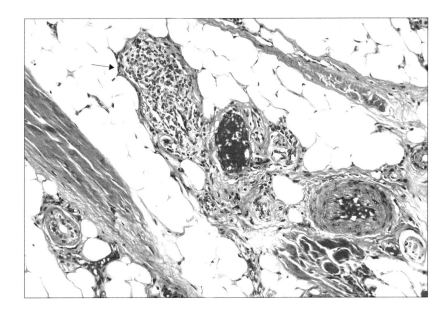

FIGURE 26–3 Normal glomus body from the foot. Arrow indicates the Sucquet-Hoyer canal with glomus cells.

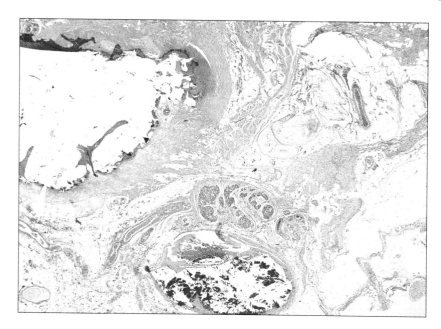

FIGURE 26-4 Glomus coccygeum located at the ventral tip of the coccyx.

TABLE 26-1	**ANATOMIC DISTRIBUTION OF GLOMUS TUMORS ACCORDING TO HISTOLOGIC SUBTYPE: AFIP, 506 CASES**					
	Glomus tumor		**Glomangioma**		**Glomangiomyoma**	
Anatomic location	**No. cases**	**%**	**No. cases**	**%**	**No. cases**	**%**
Upper extremities	176	34	45	9	16	3
Finger	81		9		3	
Lower extremities	98	19	29	6	14	3
Head and neck	29	6	6	1	5	1
Trunk	24	5	8	2	0	0
Other	45	9	4	1	7	1
Total	372	73	92	19	42	8

AFIP, Armed Forces Institute of Pathology.

near the tip of the spine, where they presumably arise from the glomus coccygeum (Fig. 26-4). However, many "incidental" glomus tumors arising in the region of the coccyx may well represent the normal glomus coccygeum[6,7] as this structure can reach several millimeters in diameter in the absence of clinical symptoms suggesting a neoplasm.[8] These tumors also develop in sites where the normal glomus body may be sparse or even absent. Unusual locations have included the bone, stomach, colon, and trachea, vagina, cervix, and mesentery.

Classic glomus tumors are typically solitary. The symptoms produced by glomus tumors are characteristic and often well out of proportion to the size of the neoplasm. Paroxysms of pain radiating away from the lesion are the most common complaint. These episodes can be elicited by changes in temperature, particularly exposure to cold, and tactile stimulation of even minor degree. In some patients the pain is accompanied by additional signs of hypesthesia, muscle atrophy, or osteoporosis of the affected part. In unusual instances disturbances of autonomic function (e.g., Horner syndrome) have been reported.[1] Although the mechanism of pain production has not been fully elucidated, identification of nerve fibers containing immunoreactive substance P (a pain-associated vasoactive peptide) in glomus tumors suggests pain mediation through release of this substance.[9]

Gross findings

Grossly, the lesions are small blue-red nodules (usually <1 cm) which are immediately apparent on clinical examination. Subungual lesions may be more difficult to detect, and care should be taken to look for ridging of the nail or discoloration of the nail bed. Radiographs are helpful when they demonstrate a small scalloped osteolytic defect with a sclerotic border in the terminal phalanx, as this finding is highly characteristic of a glomus tumor and epidermal inclusion cyst (Fig. 26-5). The more recent

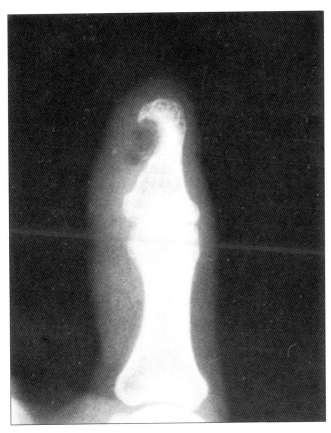

FIGURE 26–5 Postoperative radiograph showing a defect in the distal phalanx created by a subungual glomus tumor.

use of high-resolution magnetic resonance imaging (MRI) offers the promise of detecting extremely small soft tissue-based lesions.[10]

Classic glomus tumors are most common in the upper extremity and have a marked predilection for the finger, particularly the subungual region. The common form of *glomus tumor* accounts for about three-fourths of all cases in our material (Table 26–1). It is a well-circumscribed lesion consisting of tight convolutes of capillary-sized vessels surrounded by collars of glomus cells set in a hyalinized or myxoid stroma (Fig. 26–6). Rarely, it appears as a poorly circumscribed, diffuse lesion. Depending on the size of the nests of glomus cells, the tumor may have a vascular appearance reminiscent of a hemangiopericytoma or paraganglioma or a cellular appearance suggestive of an epithelial tumor (Fig. 26–7).[11] The glomus cell is distinctive, and its appearance is one of the most reliable means of distinguishing this tumor from others with similar growth patterns. The cell has a rounded, regular shape with a sharply punched-out rounded nucleus set off from the amphophilic or eosinophilic cytoplasm (Fig. 26–8). The outlines of the cells are not fully appreciated on routine hematoxylin-eosin-stained sections but can be accentuated with a periodic acid-Schiff (PAS) or toluidine blue stain on 1 μm sections. In these preparations a "chicken-wire" network of matrix material is present between the cells.

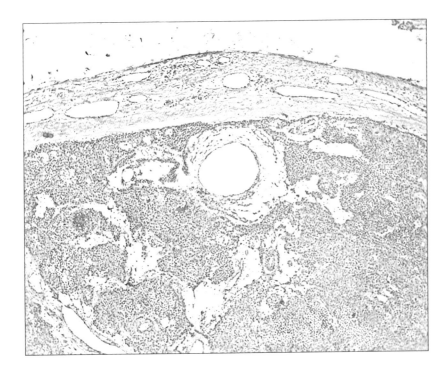

FIGURE 26–6 Common form of glomus tumor with a dense fibrous pseudocapsule surrounding solid sheets of cells (×15).

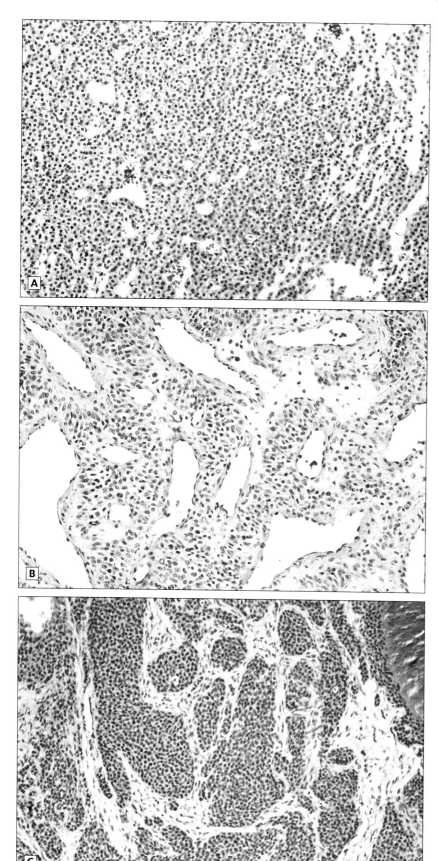

FIGURE 26–7 Variable patterns in glomus tumors. Most tumors are composed of solid sheets of cells interrupted by vessels of varying size **(A, B)**. Some areas have an organoid or epithelioid pattern of growth **(C)**.

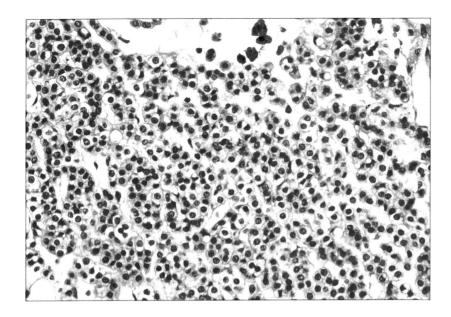

FIGURE 26–8 Glomus tumor with round cells exhibiting punched-out nuclei, pale cytoplasm, and a lacework of basement membrane material around the cells.

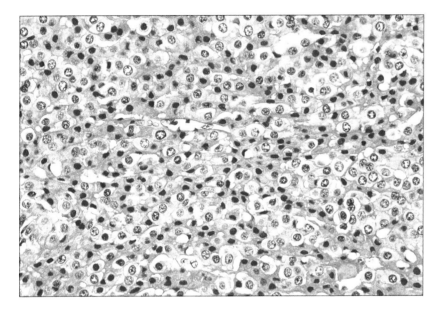

FIGURE 26–9 Oncocytic change in a glomus tumor.

Only rarely do glomus cells deviate from the foregoing description, but, when they do, alterations in either the nucleus or the cytoplasm may be seen. Large hyperchromatic nuclei, probably representing a degenerative change, may replace the typical round, regular nuclei. If this change is present as an isolated finding in an otherwise typical glomus tumor, it should not be equated with malignancy. Such tumors are referred to as "symplastic glomus tumors" (see below). A less common phenomenon is the acquisition of abundant granular, eosinophilic cytoplasm such that portions of the tumor appear "oncocytic" (Fig. 26–9).[12,13] Intravascular growth and signet-ring changes in the cells have been noted in a multifocal gastric glomus tumor.[14]

Although the cells are regarded as variants of smooth muscle cells, the cytoplasm is usually devoid of glycogen, and there is only minimal fuchsinophilia observed on staining with the Masson trichrome stain, two features that contrast with the staining reactions of conventional smooth muscle cells. Peripherally, the tumors have an ill-defined rim of collagen containing small nerves and vessels. This rim seldom serves as a complete or totally confining capsule, as isolated nests of glomus cells can be identified outside its boundaries and occasionally in the walls of small vessels surrounding the main tumor mass (Fig. 26–10). Vascular invasion is rarely seen in benign glomus tumors and does not appear to be predictive in and of itself of malignancy.

Because glomus tumors are quite distinctive by virtue of their characteristic cells, location, and symptoms, errors in diagnosis are infrequent. Nonetheless, it has been our experience that highly cellular glomus tumors are occasionally mistaken for adnexal tumors or less frequently intradermal nevi. In the former instance, it is

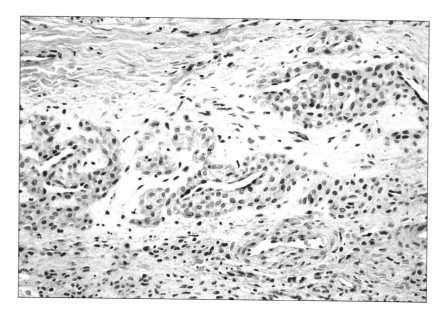

FIGURE 26–10 Proliferation of glomus cells in vessels at the periphery of a glomus tumor. This feature may be helpful for distinguishing solid glomus tumors from adnexal tumors.

important to note the intimate relation of glomus cells around small vessels at the periphery of the tumor (Fig. 26–10) and the total lack of ductular differentiation or epithelial mucin production. Immunohistochemistry can reliably discriminate glomus tumors from solid forms of hidradenoma (the adnexal tumor most closely resembling a glomus tumor).[15] Virtually all hidradenomas contain immunoreactive keratin, whereas glomus tumors do not. In addition, hidradenomas frequently also express carcinoembryonic and epithelial membrane antigens, which are not encountered in glomus tumors. Likewise, S-100 protein is a reliable marker for distinguishing nevi from glomus tumors.[16] Although electron microscopy can serve as a diagnostic adjunct, it is seldom needed, given the reliability of immunohistochemistry in most cases.

Ultrastructural and immunohistochemical findings

The glomus cell is rounded or polygonal in shape and measures 8–12 μm with a rounded nucleus with occasional clefts and prominent nucleoli (Fig. 26–11). The cells are closely spaced and often interdigitate with each other along their short, knobby processes. Their surfaces are invested by a thick, often continuous, basal lamina. The cytoplasm contains modest numbers of mitochondria and endoplasmic reticulum but is most notable for the bundles of thin (8 nm) actin-like filaments that fill the cytoplasm. The bundles are well oriented, have typical dense bodies, and occasionally terminate in dense attachment plaques on the cytoplasmic membrane.[17] In the glomus tumors with oncocytic features, not surprisingly the cytoplasm is filled with numerous mitochondria, making it more difficult to identify microfilaments.[13] Originally, glomus cells were thought to be pericytes on

the basis of certain morphologic similarities noted in tissue culture. However, as a result of determining the foregoing ultrastructural features, the glomus tumor is generally considered more closely related to the smooth muscle cell. Certainly, the quantity of myofilaments present in these cells exceeds that normally encountered in the pericyte, and the cell processes are less well developed than those of the latter cell. Vimentin and muscle actin isoforms can be identified in nearly all glomus tumors (Fig. 26–12A).[2,18–22] Desmin is highly variable, however.[21,22] In concert with the ultrastructural features of the neoplasm, laminin and type IV collagen, two constituents of basal lamina, outline the cells or small groups of cells (Fig. 26–12B).[14] Nerve growth factor receptor and myelin-associated glycoprotein can be identified in some glomus tumors, although the meaning of this finding is not clear.[21]

Behavior and treatment

Most glomus tumors are benign and can be treated adequately by simple excision. Only 10% recur following conservative excision.[23] Infrequent local recurrences probably represent persistence of tumor following inadequate excision or infrequently a benign glomus tumor growing in a diffuse or infiltrative fashion[24,25] (see below).

GLOMUVENOUS MALFORMATION (GLOMANGIOMA, FAMILIAL GLOMANGIOMA)

Glomuvenous malformations, formerly called glomangioma and considered variants of classic glomus tumor, comprise only about one-fifth of glomus lesions.[26] Recent genetic studies have demonstrated that they arise

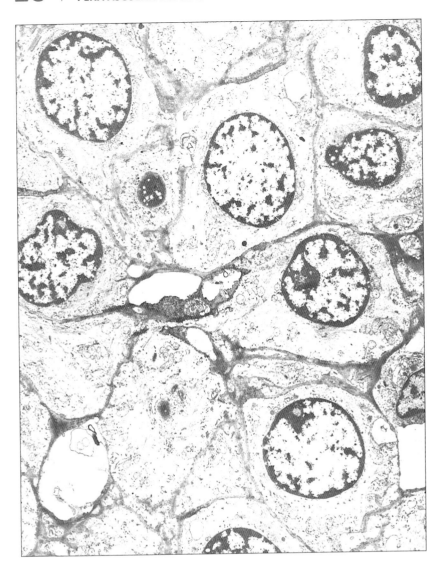

FIGURE 26–11 Electron micrograph of a glomus tumor. Cells are invested by dense basal lamina, have pinocytic vesicles along their surfaces, and contain cytoplasmic myofilaments with dense bodies (Magnification reduced from ×5000). (Courtesy of the Department of Pathology, Veterans Administration Hospital, Hines, IL.)

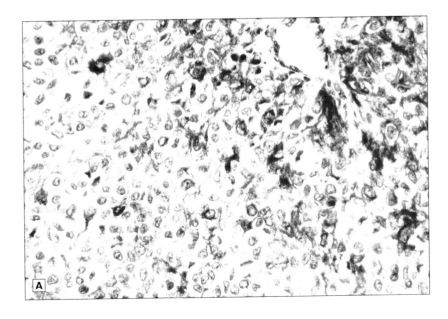

FIGURE 26–12 (A) Immunostains for actin reveal strong cytoplasmic positivity in glomus cells.

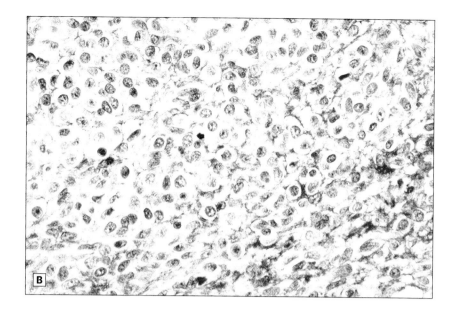

FIGURE 26–12 Continued.
(B) Immunostains for type IV collagen in a glomus tumor show intricate chicken-wire pattern between cells.

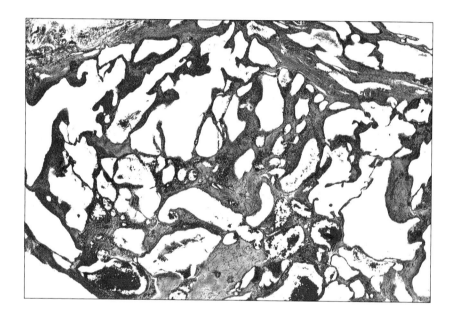

FIGURE 26–13 Partially collapsed glomangioma with dilated cavernous blood spaces.

secondary to truncating mutations of the glomulin gene located at 1p21-22 and are likely malformations.[27] Although glomulin is a normal component of vascular smooth muscle during embryogenesis, it is not yet understood how its functional absence relates to the development of these malformations. Based on analysis of several families with paradominantly inherited lesions, four principal germline mutations have been identified. Random post-zygotic mutations may explain both the variation in the number and distribution of lesions in familial cases and the occurrence of nonfamilial cases.

Unlike classic glomus tumor, glomuvenous malformations occur more often during childhood, are rarely subungual, and are less likely to be painful or symptomatic. Most predominate on the hand and forearm. Histologically, they are usually poorly circumscribed, occasionally

plaque-like lesions that resemble cavernous hemangiomas,[28] in contrast to the classic glomus tumor, which is usually better circumscribed and more cellular. Grossly and microscopically, they resemble cavernous hemangiomas (Figs 26–13 to 26–15). They are composed of gaping veins with small clusters of glomus cells in their walls. Secondary thrombosis and phlebolith formation may occur in these lesions just as they would in an ordinary hemangioma.

GLOMANGIOMYOMA

Glomangiomyoma are glomus lesions that display focal or partial smooth muscle differentiation. In actuality, most probably represent variations in either a classic

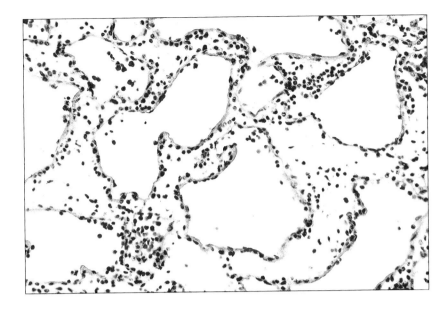

FIGURE 26–14 Glomangioma with cuffs of cells around dilated vessels.

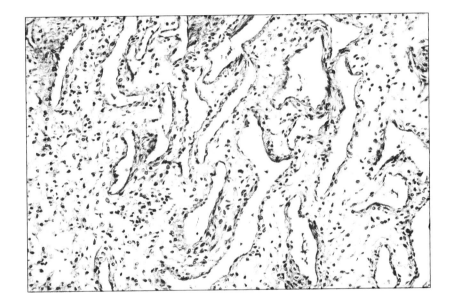

FIGURE 26–15 Glomangioma with marked hyalinization.

glomus tumor or glomuvenous malformation. Those glomangiomyomas with the architectural pattern of classic glomus tumor show transitions between glomus cells and cells with partial smooth muscle features as evidenced by their fusiform shape and cytoplasmic eosinophilia. Usually, these transitional areas comprise only a small portion of the lesions. In glomangiomyomas with the architectural features of a glomuvenous malformation, the glomus cells intermingle with the mature smooth muscle of the large vessels. Many cases reported in the pediatric literature as glomangiomyoma are examples of this form, and, hence, glomuvenous malformations (Figs 26–16, 26–17).[29,30] The term *glomangiopericytoma* has been used recently for glomus tumors with prominent thin and thick-walled vessels and slight spindling of the glomus cells (Fig. 26–18).

GLOMANGIOMATOSIS (DIFFUSE GLOMUS TUMOR)

Glomus tumors can present as diffusely infiltrating lesions similar to some vascular tumors and malformations. We refer to them as "glomangiomatosis" and conceptualize them as the glomoid counterpart of angiomatosis. Glomangiomatosis is rare, accounting for only 5% of glomus tumors with unusual or atypical features and a vanishingly smaller percentage of all glomus tumors. This form of glomus tumor may be more prevalent among patients who present during childhood.[31] Others have been reported in the literature.[25,32–34] Typically, such lesions are extensive, deep, and often pain-producing. Like angiomatosis, they consist of well-formed vessels of varying size that grow in a diffuse or infiltrative

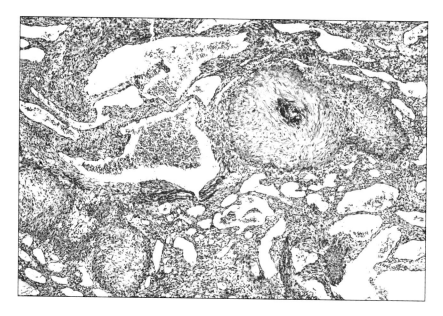

FIGURE 26–16 Glomangiomyoma. Note the blending of muscle in the vessels with tumor (Masson trichrome stain).

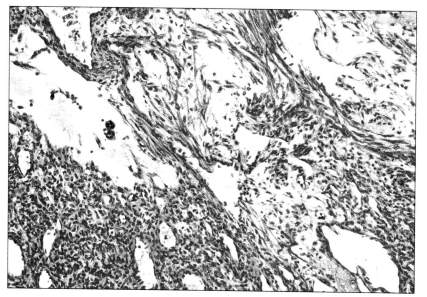

FIGURE 26–17 Glomangiomyoma. Glomus cells undergo transition to smooth muscle cells (Masson trichrome stain).

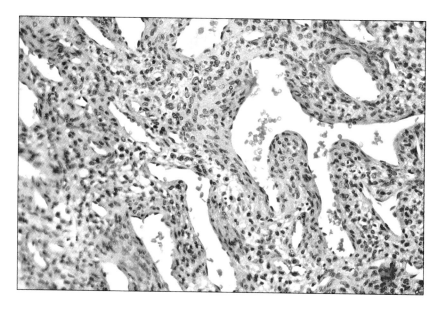

FIGURE 26–18 Glomus tumor that recurred with predominantly pericytic features: a so-called glomangiopericytoma.

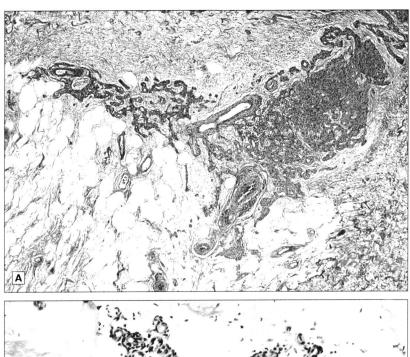

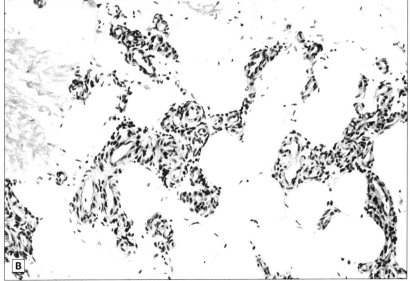

FIGURE 26–19 Diffuse glomus tumor (glomangiomatosis) with infiltrative growth of vessels **(A)**, which are encircled by glomus cells **(B)**.

fashion (Fig. 26–19). Mature fat sometimes accompanies the vessels. Clusters of glomus cells invest the vessels, particularly small vessels. There is no evidence that these lesions are malignant or undergo malignant transformation, but like angiomatosis they may be difficult to eradicate. In fact, we have seen one remarkable case in which microscopic residua of glomangiomatosis were associated with persistence of pain and required wide excision to alleviate symptoms. In general, the extent of excision is gauged by the symptomatic and cosmetic needs of the patient.

ATYPICAL AND MALIGNANT GLOMUS TUMORS

Over the years, the malignancy of glomus tumors has been more of a concept than a reality. Although several histologically malignant glomus tumors have been reported, biologic confirmation of malignancy in these cases was lacking,[24,35-41] probably because many were superficial and therefore cured by therapy. A second compounding factor was the fact that the rare malignant glomus tumors that produced metastases lacked a benign glomus component, and so the accuracy of the diagnosis was questioned. The tumor reported by Lumley and Stansfeld which produced metastases is an example of this phenomenon.[32] Two other reports, one by Brathwaite and Poppiti[42] and a second by Watanabe et al.,[43] detailed two patients with malignant glomus tumors clearly arising in the setting of a benign glomus tumor. The first case, a mitotically active glomus tumor of the nose in a patient with multiple glomus tumors, produced disseminated disease documented at autopsy. The second case was a glomangiomyoma, which produced pulmonary metastases in 2 years.

Based on our experience we believe that a malignant glomus tumor can be diagnosed in the absence of a benign glomus component provided ancillary immuno-histochemical data are available. In fact, only about one-half of malignant glomus tumors in our experience have a discernible benign component. The scheme in Table 26–2 is the one we propose for classifying glomus tumors with unusual features such as nuclear atypia and mitotic activity.

Malignant glomus tumor

Malignant glomus tumors are defined as those that are (1) large (>2 cm) and deeply located; (2) have marked

TABLE 26–2	**CLASSIFICATION OF GLOMUS TUMORS WITH ATYPICAL FEATURES**

Malignant glomus tumor
  Marked atypia + mitotic activity (>5/50 HPF) *or*
  Atypical mitotic figures *or*
  Large size (>2 cm) + deep location

Glomus tumor of uncertain malignant potential
  Superficial location + high mitotic activity (>5/50 HPF) or
  Large size only or
  Deep location only

Symplastic Glomus Tumor
  Lacks criteria for malignant glomus tumor and
  Marked nuclear atypia only

Glomangiomatosis
  Lacks criteria for malignant glomus tumor or glomus tumor of
    uncertain malignant potential and
  Diffuse growth resembling angiomatosis with prominent glomus
    component

From Folpe AL, Fanburg-Smith JC, Miettinen M, et al. Atypical and malignant glomus tumors: analysis of 53 cases with a proposal for the reclassification of glomus tumors. Am J Surg Pathol 2001; 25:1.

nuclear atypia and elevated mitotic rates (>5 mitoses/50 high-power fields [HPF]); or (3) display atypical mitotic figures.[44] A compressed rim of benign glomus tumor surrounding the malignant areas is seen in about one-half of cases (Fig. 26–20). The malignant areas can assume one of two patterns (Figs 26–21, 26–22). In the first, the tumor retains its architectural similarity to a benign glomus tumor and consists of sheets of round cells with a high nuclear/cytoplasmic ratio, high nuclear grade, and typical or atypical mitotic figures. At first glance these lesions resemble a round cell sarcoma such as Ewing sarcoma (Fig. 26–22). In the second pattern, the malignant areas differ cytoarchitecturally from a glomus tumor and are composed of spindle or fusiform cells arranged in short fascicles reminiscent of a fibrosarcoma or leiomyosarcoma (Fig. 26–21). In the absence of a benign glomus component, the diagnosis of malignant glomus tumor nearly always presupposes the use of immunohistochemistry. Identification of cytoplasmic actin and the lattice-work of type IV collagen at least focally is highly suggestive of the diagnosis. Of the 21 glomus tumors meeting the criteria of malignancy detailed above, 38% developed metastases, providing support for the validity of the criteria.[44]

Glomus tumor of uncertain malignant potential

Some glomus tumors fail to meet the minimum criteria of malignancy but display features that are clearly beyond the realm of an ordinary glomus tumor. We designate such lesions "glomus tumor of uncertain malignant potential." Most lesions falling into this category are superficial tumors with high mitotic activity and no significant nuclear atypia, or they are large or deep (Table 26–2). To date, the follow-up of glomus tumors of uncertain malignant potential has been uniformly good, but

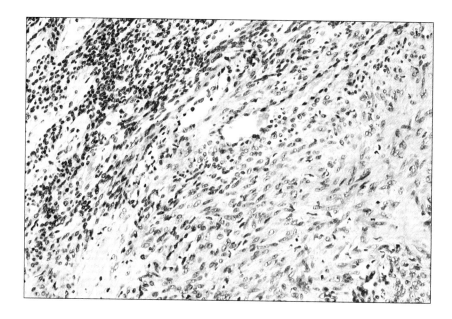

FIGURE 26–20 Malignant glomus tumor. There is a compressed rim of benign glomus tumor (upper left) next to a histologically malignant glomus tumor with a spindled pattern.

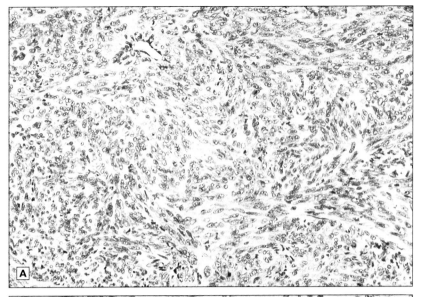

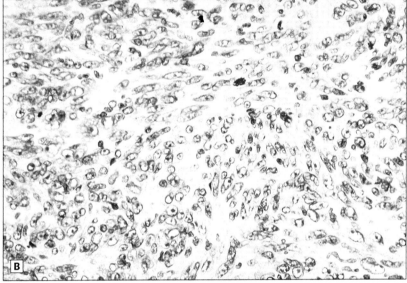

FIGURE 26–21 Malignant glomus tumor with a predominantly spindled pattern **(A)**. Cells have myoid features with marked atypia and mitotic activity **(B)**. Same case as in Figure 27–20.

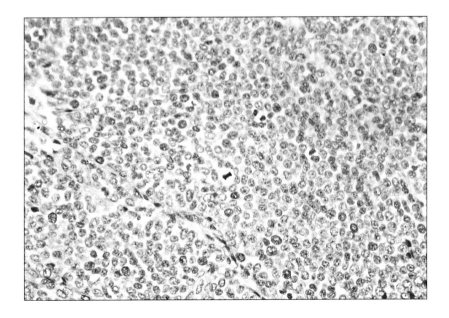

FIGURE 26–22 Malignant glomus tumor with the features of a predominantly round cell sarcoma. Such tumors may be confused with Ewing sarcoma or lymphoma.

the number of cases is small and the follow-up relatively short. We believe that affixing the label "uncertain malignant potential" guarantees adequate follow-up for this problematic group of lesions.

Symplastic glomus tumor

Glomus tumors that have marked nuclear atypia as their sole unusual feature can be labeled "symplastic glomus tumors" (Fig. 26–23). The marked nuclear atypia that characterizes tumors in this group appears to be a degenerative phenomenon that can be likened to symplastic change in uterine leiomyomas. To date, symplastic glomus tumors have a benign course, similar to ordinary glomus tumors.

MYOPERICYTOMA

Myopericytoma is a benign perivascular myoid tumor which has some overlapping features with glomus tumor and myofibroma.[45–47] It develops as a solitary, painless, slowly growing mass in the subcutaneous tissues of the lower extremity. Usually well marginated and measuring only a few centimeters in diameter, it is composed of oval to short fusiform cells which demonstrate a striking multilayered concentric growth around the vessels which may appear small and rounded or elongated and ectatic (Fig. 26–24). Architecturally, the close and intricate arrangement of myoid cells to vessels in this tumor brings to mind the arrangement of the angiomyoma except that the cells of the myopericytoma

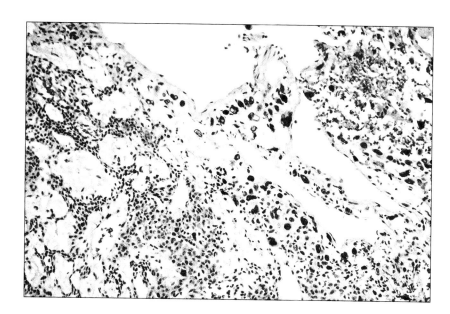

FIGURE 26–23 Glomus tumor with degenerative atypia ("symplastic glomus tumor").

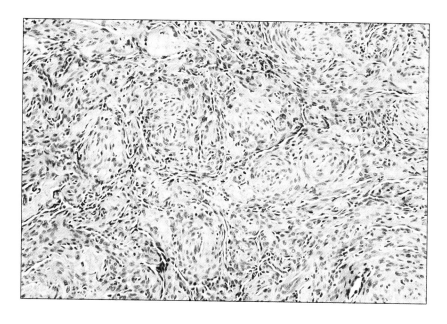

FIGURE 26–24 Myopericytoma. Muscle from the walls of small-caliber vessels spin off into the stroma of the lesion, giving it an appearance intermediate between a hemangiopericytoma and an angiomyoma.

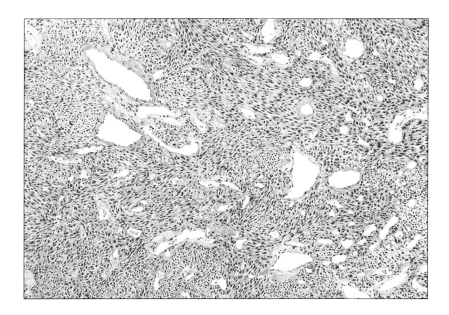

FIGURE 26–25 Hemangiopericytoma-like tumor of the nasal passage. The rounded to spindled myoid cells are arranged around an intricate vasculature.

do not display a mature muscle phenotype. A small subset of myopericytomas may reside intravascularly. By immunohistochemistry, the cells of myopericytomas have a distinct myoid phenotype and express smooth muscle actin, h-caldesmon, and, less frequently, desmin and CD34.

Myopericytomas are almost always benign. Most do not recur following excision; those that do are likely poorly marginated. Rare examples of malignant myopericytoma have been reported[46,47] and are recognized by deeply infiltrative growth, marked atypia, and increased proliferative activity.

HEMANGIOPERICYTOMA-LIKE TUMOR OF NASAL PASSAGES

First described by Compagno and Hyams in 1976, the hemangiopericytoma-like tumor of the nasal passages (HTNP) is a distinctive tumor characterized by spindled myoid cells which are arranged around a prominent vasculature (Fig. 26–25). Both features have led to the suggestion that this lesion has little in common with the classic hemangiopericytoma of soft tissue but is more closely related to other perivascular myoid lesions, specifically the glomus tumor.[48–51]

The HTNP appears unique to the nasal cavity and passages and seems to have no counterpart in soft tissue proper. Patients typically present with nasal obstruction or epistaxis. The majority are polypoid lesions which involve the nasal cavity or paranasal sinuses and grow as diffuse submucosal masses encircling minor salivary glands. Spindled to oval cells are arranged in short fascicular, storiform, whorled, or mixed patterns. The thin-walled vessels are occasionally staghorn shaped and hyalinized. Atypia is generally absent and mitotic activity low (1/10 HPF). Mast cells and eosinophils are noted in most cases.

The cells within HTNP have a distinctly myoid phenotype despite the fact they do not resemble mature smooth muscle cells. The vast majority express SMA and MSA, but not desmin. Only a minority of cases express CD34, the classic marker of the hemangiopericytoma/solitary fibrous tumor family of lesions. Most behaved in a benign manner.[49] In the largest experience reported to date, the 5- and 10-year disease-free survival was 74.2% and 64.4%, respectively. Patients at greatest risk to die of their disease are those with a long history of symptoms or those whose tumors display marked atypia or bone invasion.

REFERENCES

Classic (sporadic) glomus tumor

1. Masson P. Le glomus neuromyoarteriel des regions tactiles et ses tumeurs. Lyon Chir 1924; 21:257.
2. Popoff NW. The digital vascular system with reference to the state of the glomus in inflammation, arteriosclerotic gangrene, thromboangiitis obliterans, and supernumerary digits in man. Arch Pathol 1934; 18:295.
3. Shugart RR, Soule EH, Johnson EW. Glomus tumor. Surg Gynecol Obstet 1963; 117:334.

4. Okada O, Demitsu T, Manabe M, et al. A case of multiple subungual glomus tumors associated with neurofibromatosis type 1. J Dermatol 1999; 26:535.
5. Sawada S, Honda M, Kamide R, et al. Three cases of subungual glomus tumors with von Recklinghausen's neurofibromatosis. J Am Acad Dermatol 1995; 32:277.
6. Albrecht S, Zbieranowski I. Incidental glomus coccygeum: when a normal structure looks like a tumor. Am J Surg Pathol 1990; 14:922.
7. Duncan L, Halverson J, DeSchryver-Kecskemeti K. Glomus tumor of the coccyx: a curable cause

of coccygodynia. Arch Pathol Lab Med 1991; 115:78.
8. Gatalica Z, Wang L, Lucio ET, et al. Glomus coccygeum in surgical pathology specimens: small troublemaker. Arch Pathol Lab Med 1999; 123:905.
9. Kishimoto S, Nagatani H, Miyashita A, et al. Immunohistochemical demonstration of substance P-containing nerve fibres in glomus tumours. Br J Dermatol 1985; 113:213.
10. Idy-Peretti I, Cermakova E, Dion E, et al. Subungual glomus tumor: diagnosis based on high-resolution MR images. Am J Roentgenol 1992; 159:1351.

11. Pulitzer DR, Martin PC, Reed RJ. Epithelioid glomus tumor. Hum Pathol 1995; 26:1022.
12. Shin DLH, Park SS, Lee JH, et al. Oncocytic glomus tumor of the trachea. Chest 1990; 98:102l.
13. Slater DN, Cotton DWK, Azzopardi JG. Oncocytic glomus tumour: a new variant. Histopathology 1987; 11:523.
14. Haque S, Modlin IM, West AB. Multiple glomus tumors of the stomach with intravascular spread. Am J Surg Pathol 1992; 16:291.
15. Haupt HM, Stern JB, Berlin SJ. Immunohistochemistry in the differential diagnosis of nodular hidradenoma and glomus tumor. Am J Dermatopathol 1992; 14:310.
16. Kaye VM, Dehner LP. Cutaneous glomus tumor: a comparative immunohistochemical study with pseudoangiomatous intradermal melanocytic nevi. Am J Dermatopathol 1991; 13:2.
17. Venkatachalam MA, Greally JG. Fine structure of glomus tumor: similarity of glomus cells to smooth muscle. Cancer 1969; 23:1176.
18. Brooks JJ, Miettinen M, Virtanen I. Desmin immunoreactivity in glomus tumors. Am J Clin Pathol 1987; 87:292.
19. Dervan PA, Tobbia IN, Casey M, et al. Glomus tumours: an immunohistochemical profile of 11 cases. Histopathology 1989; 14:483.
20. Nuovo MA, Grimes MM, Knowles DM. Glomus tumors: clinicopathologic and immunohistochemical analysis of forty cases. Surg Pathol 1990; 3:31.
21. Porter PG, Bigler SA, McNutt M, et al. The immunophenotype of hemangiopericytoma and glomus tumors with special reference to muscle protein expression: an immunohistochemical study and review of the literature. Mod Pathol 1991; 4:46.
22. Schürch W, Skalli O, Lagace R, et al. Intermediate filament proteins and actin isoforms as markers for soft tissue tumor differentiation and origin. III. Hemangiopericytomas and glomus tumors. Am J Pathol 1990; 136:771.
23. Tsuneyoshi M, Enjoji M. Glomus tumor: a clinicopathologic and electron microscopic study. Cancer 1982; 50:1601.
24. Gould EW, Manivel JC, Albores-Saavedra J, et al. Locally infiltrative glomus tumors and glomangiosarcomas: a clinical, ultrastructural, and immunohistochemical study. Cancer 1990; 65:310.
25. Rao VK, Weiss SW. Angiomatosis of soft tissue: an analysis of the histologic features and clinical outcome in 51 cases. Am J Surg Pathol 1992; 16:764.

Glomuvenous malformation

26. Boon L, Mulliken JB, Enjoiras O, et al. Glomuvenous malformation (glomangioma) and venous malformation: distinct clinicopathologic and genetic entities. Arch Dermatol 2004; 1540:971.
27. Broullilard P, Boon LM, Mulliken JB, et al. Mutations in a novel factor, glomulin, are responsible for glomuvenous malformations ("glomangiomas"). Am J Hum Genet 2002; 70:866.
28. Eyster WH, Montgomery H. Multiple glomic tumors. Arch Dermatol Syph 1950; 62:893.

Glomangiomyoma

29. Yang JS, Ko JW, Suh KS, et al. Congenital multiple plaque-like glomangiomyoma. Am J Dermatopathol 1999; 21:454.
30. Calduch L, Monteagudo C, Martinez-Ruiz E, et al. Familial generalized multiple glomangiomyoma: report of a new family, with immunohistochemical and ultrastructural studies and review of the literature. Ped Dermatol 2002; 19:402.

Glomangiomatosis

31. Stout AP. Tumors of the neuromyoarterial glomus. Am J Cancer 1935; 24:255.
32. Lumley JSP, Stansfeld AG. Infiltrating glomus tumor of lower limb. Br Med J 1972; 1:484.
33. Negri G, Schulte M, Mohr W. Glomus tumor with diffuse infiltration of the quadriceps muscle: a case report. Hum Pathol 1997; 28:750.
34. Skelton HG, Smith KJ. Infiltrative glomus tumor arising from a benign glomus tumor: a distinctive immunohistochemical pattern in the infiltrative component. Am J Dermatopathol 1999; 21:562.

Atypical and malignant glomus tumors

35. Aiba M, Hirayama A, Kuramochi S. Glomangiosarcoma in a glomus tumor: an immunohistochemical and ultrastructural study. Cancer 1988; 61:1467.
36. Hegyi L, Cormack GC, Grant JW. Histochemical investigation into the molecular mechanisms of malignant transformation in a benign glomus tumour. J Clin Pathol 1998; 51:872.
37. Hirose T, Hasegawa T, Seki K, et al. Atypical glomus tumor in the mediastinum: a case report with immunohistochemical and ultrastructural studies. Ultrastruct Pathol 1996; 20:451.
38. Hiruta N, Kameda N, Tokudome T, et al. Malignant glomus tumor: a case report and review of the literature. Am J Surg Pathol 1997; 21:1096.
39. Lopez-Rios F, Rodriguez-Peralto JL, Castano E, et al. Glomangiosarcoma of the lower limb: a case report with a literature review. J Cutan Pathol 1997; 24:571.

40. Noer H, Krogdahl A. Glomangiosarcoma of the lower extremity. Histopathology 1991; 18:365.
41. Wetherington RW, Lyle WG, Sangueza OP. Malignant glomus tumor of the thumb: a case report. J Hand Surg [Am] 1997; 22:1098.
42. Brathwaite CD, Poppiti RJ. Malignant glomus tumor: a case report of widespread metastases in a patient with multiple glomus body hamartomas. Am J Surg Pathol 1996; 20:233.
43. Watanabe K, Sugino T, Saita A, et al. Glomangiosarcoma of the hip: report of a highly aggressive tumour with widespread distant metastases. Br J Dermatol 1998; 139:1097.
44. Folpe AL, Fanburg-Smith JC, Miettinen M, et al. Atypical and malignant glomus tumors: analysis of 53 cases with a proposal for the reclassification of glomus tumors. Am J Surg Pathol 2001; 25:1.

Myopericytoma

45. Grantner SR, Badizadegan K, Fletcher CDM. Myofibromatosis in adults, glomangiopericytoma, and myopericytoma: a spectrum of tumors showing perivascular myoid differentiation. Am J Surg Pathol 1998; 22:513.
46. McMenamin ME, Fletcher CDM. Malignant myopericytoma: expanding the spectrum of tumours with myopericytic differentiation. Histopathology 2002; 41:450.
47. Mentzel T, Dei Tos A, Sapi Z, et al. Myopericytoma of skin and soft tissues: clinicopathologic and immunohistochemical study of 54 cases. Am J Surg Pathol 2006; 30:104.

Hemangiopericytoma-like tumor of nasal passages

48. Fletcher CDM. Hemangiopericytoma-a dying breed? Reappraisal of an entity and its variant: a hypothesis. Curr Diagn Pathol 1994; 1:19.
49. Thompson LDR, Miettinen M, Wenig BM. Sinonasal-type hemangiopericytoma: a clinicopathologic and immunophenotypic analysis of 104 cases showing perivascular myoid differentiation. Am J Surg Pathol 2003; 27:737.
50. Tse LLY, Chang JKC. Sinonasal hemangiopericytoma-like tumour: a sinonasal glomus tumour or a haemangiopericytoma. Histopathology 2002; 40:510.
51. Kuo F-Y, Lin H-C, Eng H-L, et al. Sinonasal hemangiopericytoma-like tumor with true pericytic myoid differentiation: a clinicopathologic and immunohistochemical study of five cases. Head Neck 2005; 27:124.

BENIGN TUMORS AND TUMOR-LIKE LESIONS OF SYNOVIAL TISSUE

CHAPTER CONTENTS

The synovial membrane forms the lining of joints, tendons, and bursae. In addition, its cells synthesize hyaluronate, a major component of synovial fluid, and facilitate the exchange of substances between blood and synovial fluid. The synovial membrane varies considerably in appearance, depending on local mechanical factors and the nature of the underlying tissue. For instance, the synovial surface of joints subjected to high pressure is flat and acellular, whereas joints under less stress have a redundant surface lined by cells that resemble cuboidal or columnar epithelium.[1,2] Unlike epithelial lining cells, the synovial cells do not rest on a basal lamina but blend with the underlying stromal elements, occasionally forming only an incomplete layer at the surface.[3] Thus, joint fluid and blood vessels come in close contact with each other, a relationship that probably enhances solute exchange between the two compartments.

Electron microscopically, the synovial membrane is composed of two cell types.[4,5] Type A cells are found beneath the surface. Type A cells and are characterized by filopodia that extend upward and form a ramifying network of overlapping processes devoid of junctional attachments. In addition, they have a prominent Golgi apparatus, numerous vacuoles containing granular material, mitochondria, and pinocytotic vesicles. Under appropriate conditions these cells engage in phagocytosis. The surface synoviocytes are termed Type B cells. These cells have ovoid nuclei and long cytoplasmic processes that circumferentially surround the nucleus. The cytoplasmic processes contain ribosomes, a well-developed Golgi complex, flattened endoplasmic reticulum and subplasmalemmal pinocytotic vesicles. Although seemingly different, these cells probably represent functional modulations of the same cell because transitional forms are often seen.[1,4,5] Both cells are embedded in a collagen-rich extracellular matrix with pools of amorphous ground substance. Immunohistochemically, both synoviocyte types stain for vimentin and CD68. They are not labeled by antibodies to actins, desmin, CD34, CD45, S-100 protein or cytokeratins.

A number of benign tumors and tumor-like lesions arise from the synovium, such as chondroma of the tendon sheath, fibroma of the tendon sheath, synovial chondromatosis, and synovial hemangioma; yet only the giant cell tumor is considered prototypical. This tumor is the most common benign tumor of the tendon sheath and synovium and is the only one that generally recapitulates the appearance of the normal synovial cell.

During the twentieth century, concepts concerning the pathogenesis of these lesions underwent constant revision. The earliest descriptions of the giant cell tumor of the tendon sheath indicate that it was considered a sarcoma until the classic description by Heurteux,[6] who suggested it was benign and proposed the term *myeloma of the tendon sheath*. Subsequent authors have emphasized the presence of foam cells and have consequently grouped these tumors with true xanthomas occurring in the setting of hyperlipidemia. Giant cell tumors, however, almost always arise in normolipemic persons and bear only a superficial similarity to tendinous xanthomas.

The most significant contribution to the understanding of giant cell tumor of tendon sheath was made by Jaffe et al.,[7] who regarded the synovium of the tendon sheath, bursa, and joint as an anatomic unit that could give rise to a common family of lesions, including the giant cell tumor of tendon sheath (nodular tenosynovitis), localized and diffuse forms of pigmented villonodular synovitis, and rare cases of extra-articular pigmented villonodular synovitis arising from bursae (diffuse type giant cell tumor of tendon sheath). The differences in clinical extent and growth, these authors maintained, were influenced by the anatomic location. Lesions of the joints tended to expand inward and grow along the joint surface as the path of least resistance. Tumors of the tendon sheath, of necessity, grew outward, molded and confined by the shearing forces of the tendon. At present there has been no improvement of the elegant unifying concept of Jaffe et al. On the other hand, their hypothesis that these lesions are reactive in nature is probably incorrect, as the preponderance of evidence indicates that they are neoplastic.

Although a number of terms have been applied in the literature, including fibrous xanthoma of the synovium,[8] benign synovioma,[9] and nodular tenosynovitis,[10] we prefer the term *tenosynovial giant cell tumor* and divide the tumors into localized and diffuse forms, depending on their growth characteristics.[10a] The localized type primarily affects the digits and arises from the synovium of tendon sheaths or interphalangeal joints. The diffuse form occurs in areas adjacent to large weight-bearing joints such as the knee and ankle and in many instances represents an extra-articular extension of pigmented villonodular synovitis. A small number of diffuse giant cell tumors have no intra-articular component and probably take origin from bursae associated with large joints. Pigmented villonodular synovitis restricted to the joint proper is not specifically discussed in this chapter.

GIANT CELL TUMOR OF TENDON SHEATH, LOCALIZED TYPE (TENOSYNOVIAL GIANT CELL TUMOR, LOCALIZED TYPE)

The localized form of giant cell tumor of tendon sheath is characterized by a discrete proliferation of rounded synovial-like cells accompanied by a variable number of multinucleated giant cells, inflammatory cells, siderophages, and xanthoma cells. This tumor was first described by Chassaignac,[11] who referred to it as a "cancer of tendon sheath." It subsequently has been designated by other names, all of which underscore the lack of agreement concerning its basic nature and line of differentiation.

Clinical findings

Giant cell tumor of tendon sheath may occur at any age, but is most common in patients 30 to 50 years of age. Women area affected about twice as often as men.[12,13] The tumors occur predominantly on the hand, where they represent the most common neoplasm of that region (Figs 27–1, 27–2). Less common sites include the feet, ankles, and knees. In the study by Ushijima and colleagues (Table 27–1), 183 of 208 tumors occurred in the digits, most commonly one of the fingers (158 cases);[13] only 25 tumors were found in the larger joints, including the ankle/foot (10 cases), knee (8 cases), wrist (6 cases), and elbow (1 case). Finger lesions are typically located adjacent to the interphalangeal joint, although other sites may also be affected. Jaffe et al.[7] originally commented on the preference of these tumors to locate on the flexor surface, but subsequent workers have shown that the lesions are more evenly distributed between flexor and extensor tendons.[12,13] They may even be found in a lateral or circumferential location.

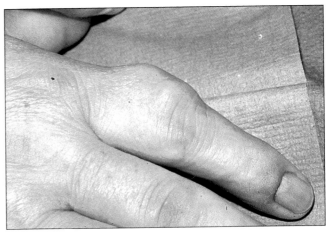

FIGURE 27–1 Localized giant cell tumor involving the proximal portion of the finger.

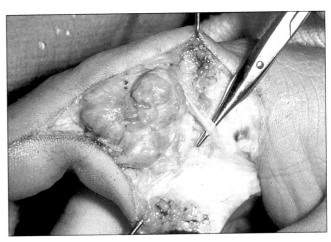

FIGURE 27–2 Localized giant cell tumor. Lobulated mass is present adjacent to the tendon (same case as in Figure 27–1).

TABLE 27–1	ANATOMIC DISTRIBUTION OF GIANT CELL TUMOR OF THE TENDON SHEATH	
Location		**No. of cases**
Digits		183
Fingers		158
Toes		25
Large joints		25
Ankle/foot		10
Knee		8
Wrist		6
Elbow		1

Modified from Ushijima M, Hashimoto H, Tsuneyoshi M, et al. Giant cell tumor of the tendon sheath (nodular tenosynovitis): a study of 207 cases to compare the large joint group with the common digit group. Cancer 1986; 57:875.

The tumors develop gradually over a long period of time and often remain the same size for several years. On physical examination they are fixed to deep structures but are usually not attached to skin unless the lesion occurs in the distal portion of the fingers where skin is closely related to tendon. Serum cholesterol levels are invariably normal. Antecedent trauma occurs in a variable number of patients, but its association with the lesions is likely fortuitous. Radiographic studies usually demonstrate a circumscribed soft tissue mass and occasionally degenerative changes of the adjacent joint.[14] In only a small portion of patients (perhaps 10%), however, is there cortical erosion of bone.[15,16] It has been suggested that giant cell tumors of the feet more frequently produce bone changes because the dense ligaments of that region are more likely to prevent outward growth of the tumor.[15] Invasion of adjacent bone is rare.[17]

Gross findings

Giant cell tumor of tendon sheath is a circumscribed lobulated mass that occasionally has shallow grooves along its deep surfaces created by the underlying tendons (Figs 27–3, 27–4).[1] They are usually relatively small, ranging from 0.5 to 3.0–4.0 cm in diameter. Those on the feet are often larger and more irregular in shape than those on the hands. On cut section the tumors have a mottled appearance: a pink-gray background flecked with yellow or brown, depending on the amount of lipid and hemosiderin. Tumors arising in the large joints are usually of greater size and more irregular in shape than tumors in the digits.

Microscopic findings

The earliest lesion is a villous structure that projects into the synovial space of the tendon sheath. Limited space prevents continued growth into the cavity so ultimately the tumor grows outward in a cauliflower fashion and compresses synovium-lined clefts into its substance. At the stage at which most lesions are surgically excised, they are exophytic masses attached to the tendon sheath and

have smooth but lobulated contours. They are partially invested by a dense collagenous capsule that penetrates the tumor, dividing it into vague nodules. The capsule is not totally confining, as isolated nests of tumor can be identified outside its bounds, especially at the deep margin where the tumor blends with the synovial membrane.

The histologic appearance of this tumor varies depending on the proportion of mononuclear cells, giant cells, xanthoma cells, hemosiderin and the degree of collagenization (Figs 27–5 to 27–7). Most tumors are moderately cellular and are composed of sheets of round or polygonal cells that blend with hypocellular collagenized zones in which the cells appear slightly spindled.

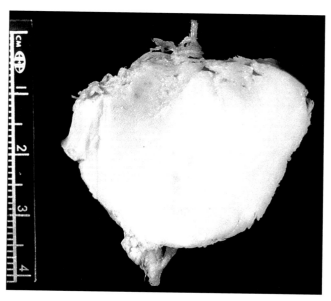

FIGURE 27–3 Gross appearance of giant cell tumor of the tendon sheath, localized type.

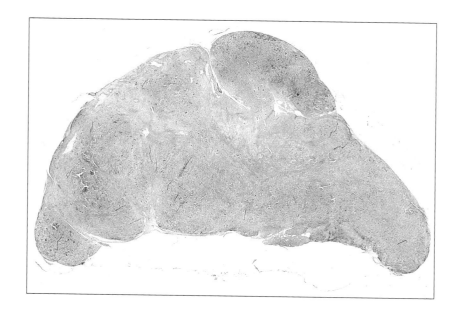

FIGURE 27–4 Localized giant cell tumor illustrating a late-stage lesion. Deep synovial clefts are obliterated and replaced by fibrous bands that impart a vague lobular pattern to the tumor. Concave surface at the bottom is created by underlying tendon.

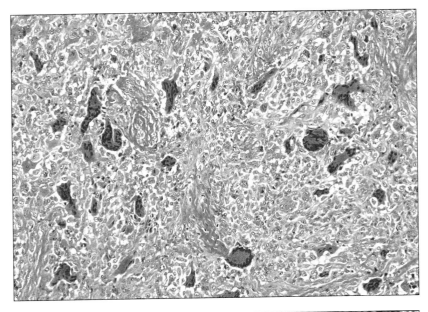

FIGURE 27–5 Localized form of giant cell tumor with a regular distribution of multinucleated giant cells admixed with round cells and collagen.

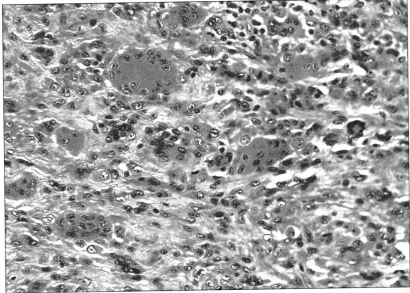

FIGURE 27–6 Giant cell-rich area of a localized form of giant cell tumor.

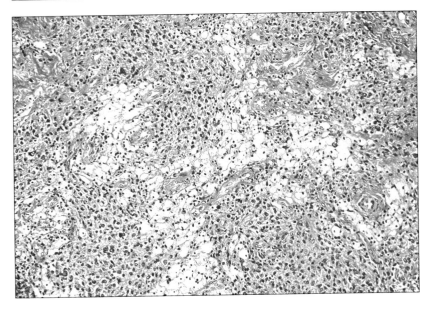

FIGURE 27–7 Localized form of giant cell tumor showing focal collections of xanthoma cells intermixed with round cells.

Cleft-like spaces are occasionally present, particularly in lesions arising near large joints. Some probably represent synovium-lined spaces, whereas others are artifactual spaces caused by shrinkage and loss of cellular cohesion. Multinucleated giant cells are scattered throughout the lesions. In the typical case they are relatively numerous but become sparse in highly cellular lesions, particularly recurrent ones (Fig. 27–8). These cells, which form by fusion of the more prevalent mononuclear cells, have a variable number of nuclei, ranging from as few as 3–4 to as many as 50–60.[18] Xanthoma cells are also frequent, tend to be located geographically in these tumors, and often contain fine hemosiderin granules and/or cholesterol clefts (Fig. 27–9). Cartilaginous and osseous metaplasia is a rare focal finding.

The diagnosis of giant cell tumor of tendon sheath is rarely difficult, but the evaluation of certain atypical features can be problematic. For instance, the presence of mitotic figures occasionally leads to a mistaken diagnosis of a malignant neoplasm. Rao and Vigorita documented three or more mitotic figures per 10 high-power fields (HPF) in more than 10% of their cases.[19] Although it may indicate an actively growing lesion that is likely to recur, we have no evidence to suggest such lesions are at increased risk to metastasize (Figs 27–10, 27–11). In about 1–5% of cases, tumor thrombi are observed in small veins draining these lesions (Fig. 27–12). Likewise, this feature does not correlate with the ability to produce metastasis based on follow-up information in our own cases. In fact, because of the extreme rarity of

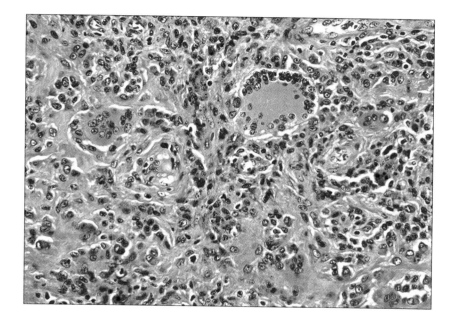

FIGURE 27–8 Rare giant cells admixed with round cells and areas of hemosiderin deposition in a giant cell-poor localized form of giant cell tumor.

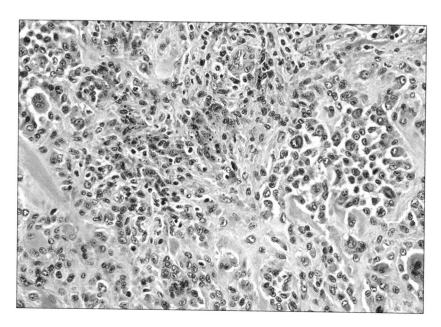

FIGURE 27–9 Abundant hemosiderin deposition in a localized giant cell tumor.

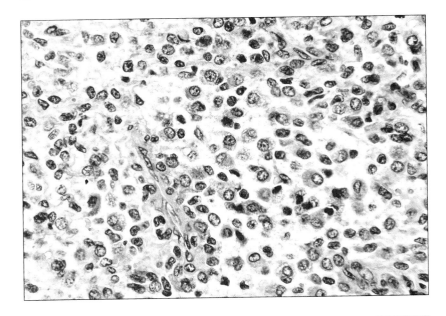

FIGURE 27–10 High-power view of round cells in a giant cell tumor with a paucity of giant cells. Some of the cells contain intracytoplasmic hemosiderin.

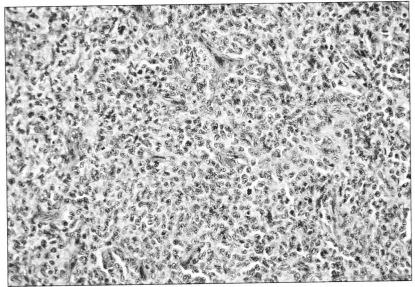

FIGURE 27–11 Cellular example of a localized form of giant cell tumor with a paucity of giant cells. Rare mitotic figures can be seen.

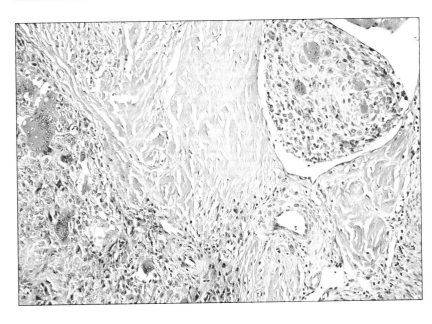

FIGURE 27–12 Focus of tumor in a vein in a localized giant cell tumor. This feature does not necessarily indicate malignancy.

metastasizing forms of giant cell tumor of tendon sheath, it is justifiable to adopt a conservative approach when interpreting these atypical features.

Differential diagnosis

Occasionally, benign lesions located in the vicinity of the tendon sheath are confused with giant cell tumors, including foreign body granulomas, necrobiotic granulomas, tendinous xanthomas, and fibromas of the tendon sheath. *Granulomatous lesions*, however, are less localized and have a greater complement of inflammatory cells. *Necrobiotic granulomas* are characterized by cores of degenerating collagen rimmed by histiocytes and a prominent zone of proliferating capillaries. Giant cells are usually scarce or nonexistent. The distinction of giant cell tumor of tendon sheath with a prominent xanthomatous compo-

nent (Fig. 27–13) and *tendinous xanthoma* formerly represented a problem in differential diagnosis. As a result of the recognition and early treatment of hyperlipidemia, it is seldom a practical problem for the surgical pathologist today. In contrast to giant cell tumors, tendinous xanthomas that arise in the setting of hyperlipidemia are often multiple and occur in the tendon proper. Histologically, they consist almost exclusively of xanthoma cells, with only a few multinucleated giant cells and chronic inflammatory cells. *Fibromas of the tendon sheath* bear some similarity to hyalinized forms of giant cell tumor (Fig. 27–14), and some believe that the former represents an end-stage of the latter.[20,21] In general, the cells of fibroma of the tendon sheath appear fibroblastic and are deposited in a more uniformly hyalinized stroma, although some lesions have areas reminiscent of giant cell tumors. Occasionally *epithelioid sarcomas* with numer-

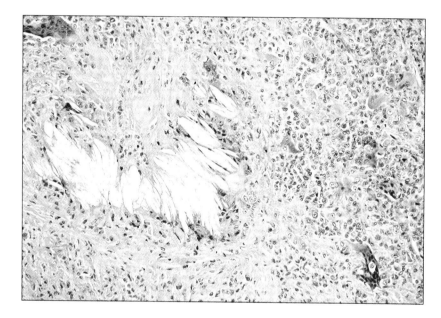

FIGURE 27–13 Cholesterol clefts in a localized giant cell tumor.

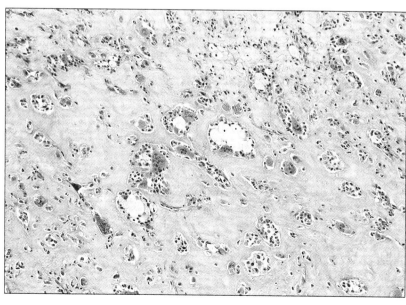

FIGURE 27–14 Localized giant cell tumor with extensive hyalinization bearing some resemblance to a fibroma of the tendon sheath.

ous giant cells mimic a giant cell tumor. The relatively monomorphic population of cells with dense cytoplasmic eosinophilia and strong and diffuse expression of keratin distinguish it from giant cell tumor. Clefted areas of a giant cell tumor may also suggest the glandular component of a *biphasic synovial sarcoma*, but the cells lining the spaces are identical to those found in the solid portion of the tumor and lack epithelial features, as determined by immunohistochemistry.

Immunohistochemical and ultrastructural findings

Immunohistochemically, the mononuclear cells in giant cell tumor of tendon sheath express "histiocytic" markers including CD68, HAM56, MAC387, and PG-M1 (Table 27–2).[1,22-24] Some authors have taken this as evidence of monocyte/macrophage differentiation, whereas others have suggested a synovial origin, given the overlapping immunophenotypic features with non-neoplastic synovium. A proportion of the mononuclear cells stain for factor XIIIa,[25] and rare cells also express actins.[24] About 50% of cases contain occasional desmin-positive dendritic cells, which may cause confusion with alveolar rhabdomyosarcoma.[26] Like their mononuclear counterparts, the multinucleated giant cells express CD68 and CD45. Several authors have suggested that these giant cells have features of osteoclasts, based on the immunohistochemical expression of tartrate-resistant acid phosphatase, vitronectin receptor, calcitonin receptor, and parathyroid hormone-related peptide and receptor.[27-30] Only the mononuclear cells express Ki67 and proliferating cell nuclear antigen (PCNA), suggesting that they are the actively proliferating cells.[31]

Ultrastructurally, the cells of these lesions have been compared with normal synovium, and the existence of both types of synovial cell has been used by some as support for a reactive process.[32] The predominant cell type has histiocyte-like features, with abundant electron-dense cytoplasm containing numerous ribosomes, a moderate number of mitochondria, and varying numbers of lysosomes.[33] These cells have a ruffled cell membrane, with pseudopodia and filopodia, and some show phagocytosis of erythrocytes or deposits of hemosiderin. A smaller proportion of cells are spindle-shaped fibroblast-like cells with well-developed endoplasmic reticulum; rare cells have intracytoplasmic filaments with focal dense bodies, suggesting focal myofibroblastic differentiation.

Cytogenetic findings and DNA ploidy

Several studies have reported clonal cytogenetic abnormalities in giant cell tumors of the tendon sheath. Dal Cin and co-workers found clonal abnormalities in five of six lesions, including three with t(1;2) (p11;q35-36), one with t(1;5)(p11;q22), and one with t(2;16)(q33;q24).[34] Others have also found that rearrangements of 1p11-13 are frequent in both localized and diffuse forms of giant cell tumor of tendon sheath.[35-38] Although the most common translocation partner is 2q35-37, others include 5q22-31, 11q11-12, and 8q21-22. Recently, *CSF-1* has been identified as the gene at the 1p13 breakpoint.[38a] In approximately 60–70% of cases of both giant cell tumor of tendon sheath and pigmented villonodular synovitis, there is evidence of a *CSF-1* fusion with COL6a3 on 2q35.[38b] High levels of *CSF-1* RNA expression by in situ hybridization and CSF-1 protein expression are present, even in cases with no evidence of a *CSF-1*.

Interestingly, Mertens et al. found cytogenetic aberrations in non-neoplastic synovial lesions, including hemorrhagic synovitis and rheumatoid synovitis.[39] These cytogenetic data must be reconciled with molecular diagnostic studies indicating that these lesions are polyclonal, as suggested by X chromosome inactivation analysis.[40,41] Cupp and colleagues found no evidence of a *CSF-1* translocation in non-neoplastic synovial conditions, but did find upregulation of CSF-1 RNA and protein expression in these conditions.[38b]

DNA ploidy analysis of a small group of tenosynovial giant cell tumors indicates that diploid patterns are invari-

TABLE 27–2	IMMUNOHISTOCHEMICAL FEATURES OF GIANT CELL TUMOR OF THE TENDON SHEATH AND REACTIVE SYNOVITIS			
	GCTTS		Reactive synovitis	
Factor	Mononuclear cells	Giant cells	Mononuclear cells	Giant cells
CD68	+	+	+	+
MAC387	+	−	+	−
HAM56	+	−	+	−
LCA	±	+	−	+
S-100 protein	±	−	+	−
Keratins	−	−	−	−
Actins	+	−	−	−
Desmin	±	±	−	−

Data are from Maluf et al.[24] and O'Connell et al.[23]
GCTTS, giant cell tumor of the tendon sheath.

ably present in the localized forms and in pigmented villonodular synovitis, whereas nearly half of diffuse tenosynovial giant cell tumors are aneuploid.[42] The latter group displays a higher proliferation index than the former two groups, a finding that may reflect rapid, uncontrolled growth.

Discussion

Giant cell tumor of tendon sheath is a benign lesion that nonetheless has a capacity for local recurrence in about 10–20% of cases.[12,13,19,43] However, recurrences are non-destructive and are easily controlled by re-excision. Recurrences seem to develop more often in highly cellular lesions with increased mitoses and in patients who undergo simple enucleation, as microscopic residua are invariably left behind at the deep margin. Local excision with a small cuff of normal tissue is usually considered adequate therapy, even for lesions with increased cellularity and mitotic activity. Most are cured by this approach, and more extended surgery can always be planned at a later time for persistently recurring lesions.

Since the detailed description by Jaffe et al.[7] there has been much controversy as to whether giant cell tumors of the tendon sheath are a reactive or neoplastic process. Observation that trauma precedes about one-half of the cases, that some cases are multifocal, and that similar lesions have been induced following intra-articular injections of blood in experimental animals[44] seem offset by cytogenetic studies indicating a clonal abnormality in these lesions, a finding that speaks strongly to a neoplastic process.[45] A neoplastic origin is also supported by the fact that this lesion is capable of a certain degree of autonomous growth, including local recurrence following surgical excision. Finally, as discussed later in the chapter, rare giant cell tumors have given rise to metastatic disease.

GIANT CELL TUMOR OF TENDON SHEATH, DIFFUSE TYPE (TENOSYNOVIAL GIANT CELL TUMOR, DIFFUSE TYPE; EXTRA-ARTICULAR PIGMENTED VILLONODULAR SYNOVITIS)

The diffuse tenosynovial giant cell tumor can be regarded as the soft tissue counterpart of pigmented villonodular synovitis of the joint space. In most instances the lesion represents extra-articular extension of a primary intra-articular process, a contention supported by the similarity in age, location, clinical presentation, and symptoms of the two processes. In rare instances this disease resides completely outside a joint, in which case its origin must be ascribed to the synovium of the bursa or tendon sheath.[42,46–48] In their original description of villonodular synovitis, Jaffe and colleagues described four extra-articular cases including two arising from the popliteal

bursa, one from the bursa anserina, and one from the ankle bursa.[7] Only one of 34 cases of pigmented villonodular synovitis reported by Atmore et al. was located extra-articularly,[49] and several of the cases reported by Arthaud would probably also qualify as diffuse forms of giant cell tumor.[50] In many instances it is difficult to define the origin of the tumor. Therefore, we have employed the term *tenosynovial giant cell tumor of the diffuse type* when there is a poorly confined soft tissue mass with or without involvement of the adjacent joint.

Compared with the localized giant cell tumor, this form is uncommon and exhibits certain clinical differences. There is a tendency for these lesions to occur in young persons. In the largest study to date of 50 cases, Somerhausen and Fletcher reported an age range of 4 to 76 years, with a median age of 41 years.[46] Females are affected slightly more often than males. Typically, symptoms are of relatively long duration, often several years, and include pain and tenderness in the affected extremity. The additional presence of joint effusion, hemarthrosis, limitation of joint motion, and locking signify articular involvement. Its anatomic distribution parallels that of pigmented villonodular synovitis and includes the knee followed by the ankle and foot (Table 27–3). Uncommon locations are the finger, elbow, toe, and temporomandibular and sacroiliac areas. Radiographically, a soft tissue mass is usually evident and may be accompanied by osteoporosis, widening of the joint space, and cortical erosion of the adjacent bone (Fig. 27–15).

At surgery the lesions are large, firm or sponge-like, multinodular masses. Color varies from white to yellow or brown, although usually staining with hemosiderin is less evident than in their articular counterparts, and they usually do not have grossly discernible villous patterns (Figs 27–16, 27–17).

In contrast to localized giant cell tumors, this form is not surrounded by a mature collagenous capsule but instead grows in expansive sheets (Figs 27–18, 27–19) interrupted by cleft-like or pseudoglandular spaces (Fig. 27–20). Many of the spaces represent residual synovial membrane, whereas others are probably artifactual. The

TABLE 27–3	ANATOMIC DISTRIBUTION OF DIFFUSE GIANT CELL TUMOR OF THE TENDON SHEATH (40 PATIENTS)	
Location		**No. of cases**
Knee		15
Ankle and foot		12
Wrist		5
Finger		3
Elbow		2
Hip and sacroiliac region		2
Toe		1
Total		40

Data are from the Armed Forces Institute of Pathology (AFIP).

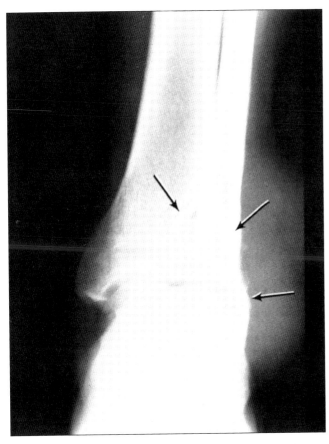

FIGURE 27–15 Radiograph of a diffuse form of giant cell tumor. Large soft tissue mass is present in the ankle region and has caused secondary destruction of the distal tibia and fibula (arrows). Minimal changes in the joint space suggest that the tumor arose in an extra-articular location.

predominant cell is round or polygonal (Fig. 27–21). Its cytoplasm may be clear or deeply brown when ladened with hemosiderin. Gradual transition between these cells, spindle cells, and xanthoma cells is common; and in some tumors the diagnosis of xanthoma is suggested.

Multinucleated giant cells and chronic inflammatory cells are intermingled so the net effect is that of a highly polymorphic population of cells. In general, giant cells are less numerous than in localized tumors. In cellular areas the collagenous stroma is delicate and inconspicuous, whereas in hypocellular areas the stroma may be quite hyalinized.

These lesions usually present greater diagnostic problems than their localized counterparts. The pronounced cellularity, coupled with the clinical findings of an extensive, destructive mass is likely to lead to a diagnosis of malignancy. Particular problems arise in the early lesions, which are characterized by a monomorphic population of round cells with a high nuclear to cytoplasmic ratio and a brisk mitotic rate (Figs 27–22, 27–23). Focal necrosis may be present if torsion of a pedunculated tumor nodule has occurred. In such cases, attention should be paid to the synovium-based location and to the apparent maturation of these tumor nodules at their periphery. In the peripheral zones the cells acquire a more prominent, slightly xanthomatous-appearing cytoplasm. Additional sections occasionally disclose focal giant cells, and iron staining may identify modest amounts of hemosiderin not discernible in routine sections. In more advanced lesions consisting of the classic polymorphic cellular population, other problems in differential diagnosis occur. For example, the pseudoglandular spaces are often misinterpreted as glandular spaces of a synovial sarcoma or the alveolar spaces of a rhabdomyosarcoma. The giant cell tumor shows great variation in type and arrangement of cells. Its geographic pattern of xanthomatous regions alternating with cellular hyalinized regions contrasts with the more uniform spindled appearance of most synovial sarcomas and the primitive round cells of alveolar rhabdomyosarcomas. Diffuse giant cell tumors with prominent xanthomatous components must also be distinguished from inflammatory or xanthomatous forms of malignant

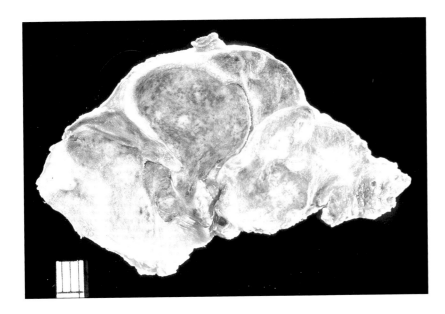

FIGURE 27–16 Diffuse form of giant cell tumor. The lesion has a multinodular appearance with variegated color. Shaggy villous projections, typical of pigmented villonodular synovitis, are not seen.

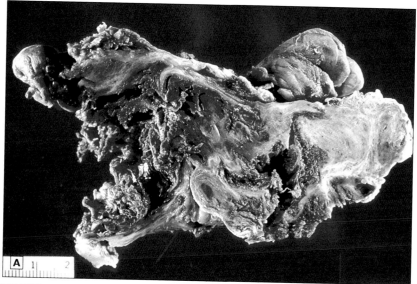

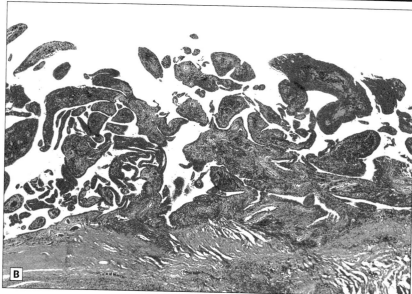

FIGURE 27–17 Intra-articular form of diffuse giant cell tumor (pigmented villonodular synovitis). Note the shaggy villous appearance in the gross **(A)** and microscopic **(B)** specimens.

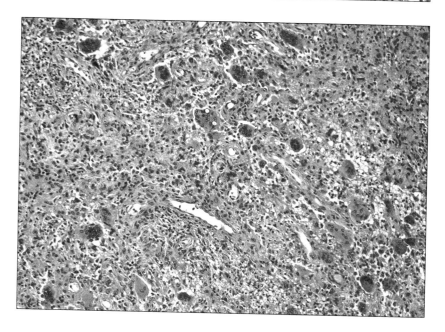

FIGURE 27–18 Diffuse form of giant cell tumor characterized by sheets of rounded synovial-like cells admixed with multinucleated giant cells and xanthoma cells with hemosiderin.

abstract form, Fanburg-Smith and Miettinen reported 27 histologically malignant giant cell tumors of the tendon sheath, six of which were clinically malignant.[63] The clinically malignant cases were characterized histologically by a diffuse infiltrative growth pattern, scant giant cells, nucleomegaly and macronucleoli, tumor cell dyscohesion, necrosis, and mitotic counts of more than 10 MF/10 HPF. Wide excision or amputation of true malignant forms of tenosynovial giant cell tumor/pigmented villonodular synovitis is indicated.

MISCELLANEOUS CONDITIONS RESEMBLING DIFFUSE GIANT CELL TUMOR

Occasionally, reactive synovial lesions mimic the appearance of a diffuse giant cell tumor, particularly lesions of the intra-articular type (pigmented villonodular synovi-

TABLE 27–4	CLINICAL FEATURES OF MALIGNANT GIANT CELL TUMOR OF THE TENDON SHEATH/ PIGMENTED VILLONODULAR SYNOVITIS AND PIGMENTED VILLONODULAR SYNOVITIS	
Parameter	**PVNS**	**MPVNS**
Age	50% < 40 years	12–79 years (peak: 6th decade)
Gender	Females > males	Females > males
Local recurrence (%)	25–50	60–70
Metastasis (%)		60–70
Died of tumor	None	40–50

PVNS, pigmented villonodular synovitis; MPVNS, malignant pigmented villonodular synovitis. Modified from Bertoni F, Unni KK, Beabout JW, et al. Malignant giant cell tumor of the tendon sheaths and joints (malignant pigmented villonodular synovitis). Am J Surg Pathol 1997; 21:153.

tis). Perhaps the most common condition that produces this picture is intra-articular hemorrhage (hemosiderotic synovitis). Long known to be associated with synovitis in hemophiliacs, intra-articular hemorrhage can give rise to hyperplastic changes of the synovium consisting of villous change and large deposits of hemosiderin.[1,64] However, only in the early stages of chronic hemarthrosis are the lesions reminiscent of pigmented villonodular synovitis. During the late stage the synovium is flattened and the subjacent tissue markedly fibrotic. A second condition that can histologically resemble pigmented villonodular synovitis is the synovitis associated with failed orthopedic prosthetic devices.[65] Collectively termed "detritic synovitis," these lesions are characterized by villous hyperplasia of the synovium (Fig. 27–26A). The subsynovial space is infiltrated with histiocytes, multinucleated giant cells, and a variable number of chronic inflammatory cells. The prosthetic material can be detected under polarized light as weakly birefringent intracellular or extracellular spicules (Fig. 27–26B). Usually, it can also be stained with oil red O, but it requires a long incubation period (up to 48 hours). In addition, histiocytic reactions in the lymph nodes draining the regions of prosthetic devices can occur.[66] Finally, we reviewed synovial tissue from a patient with α-mannosidase deficiency who developed bilateral destructive synovitis of the ankle region.[67] The hyperplastic villous-appearing synovium was infiltrated with clear-appearing histiocytes containing PAS-positive, diastase-resistant material representing partially degraded oligosaccharides in lysosomes (Figs 27–27 to 27–30). Although definitive diagnosis requires an adequate clinical history with confirmatory biochemical data, the presence of a systemic disease was suspected because of the bilaterally symmetric distribution of the lesions, a distribution seldom encountered in pigmented villonodular synovitis.

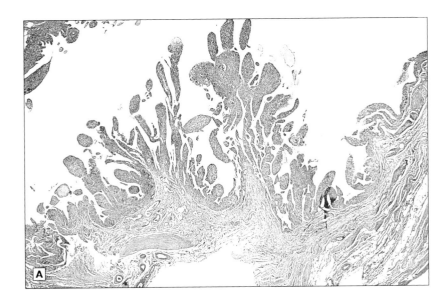

FIGURE 27–26 (A) Detritic synovitis showing villous configuration of the synovium.

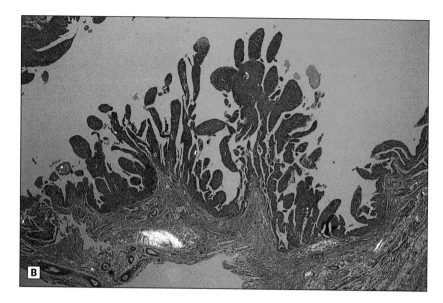

FIGURE 27–26 Continued. **(B)** Graft material is visible as birefringent particles in this partially polarized view.

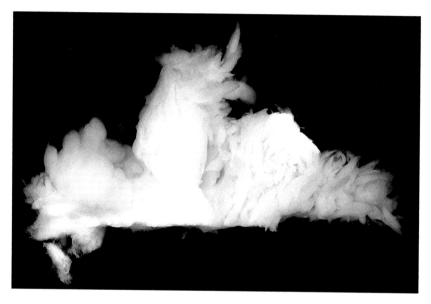

FIGURE 27–27 Gross appearance of synovium in a patient with α-mannosidase deficiency. Note that the synovium has delicate villous fronds.

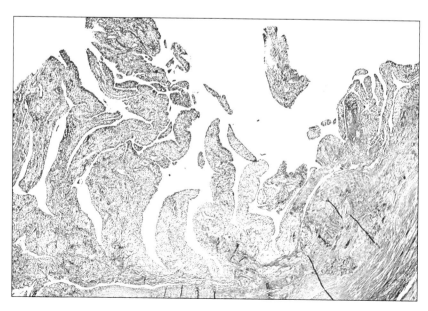

FIGURE 27–28 Synovitis due to α-mannosidase deficiency. At low power the lesion superficially resembles pigmented villonodular synovitis.

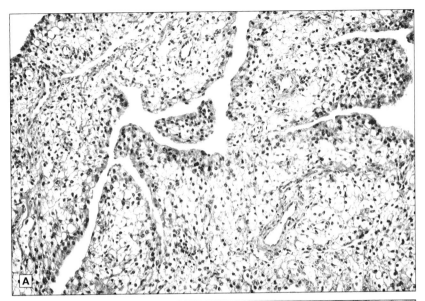

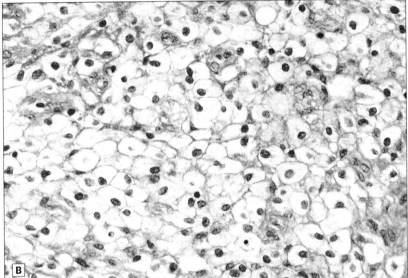

FIGURE 27–29 (A) Synovitis due to α-mannosidase deficiency composed of synovial-lined papillary projections with centrally located vacuolated cells. **(B)** At high power the infiltrate consists of clear-appearing histiocytes containing PAS-positive, diastase-resistant bodies representing partially degraded oligosaccharides. (From Weiss SW, Kelly WD. Bilateral destructive synovitis associated with alpha-mannosidase deficiency. Am J Surg Pathol 1983; 7:487.)

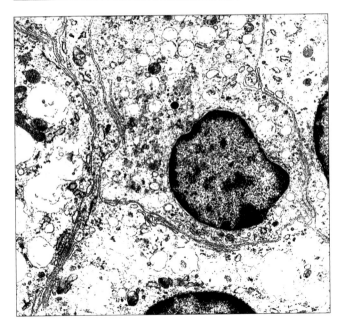

FIGURE 27–30 Electron micrograph of histiocytes from the synovium of a patient with α-mannosidase deficiency. Oligosaccharide is represented by granuloamorphous material in lysosomes. (From Weiss SW, Kelly WD. Bilateral destructive synovitis associated with alpha-mannosidase deficiency. Am J Surg Pathol 1983; 7:487.)

REFERENCES

1. O'Connell JX. Pathology of the synovium. Am J Clin Pathol 2000; 114:773.
2. Lever JD, Ford EH. Histological, histochemical and electron microscopic observations on synovial membrane. Anat Rec 1958; 132:525.
3. Cohen MJ, Kaplan L. Histology and ultrastructure of the human flexor tendon sheath. J Hand Surg 1987; 12:25.
4. Schmidt D, Mackay B. Ultrastructure of human tendon sheath and synovium: Implications for tumor histogenesis. Ultrastruct Pathol 1982; 3:269.
5. Steinberg PJ, Hodde KC. The morphology of synovial lining of various structures in several species as observed with scanning electron microscopy. Scanning Microsc 1990; 4:987.
6. Heurteux MA. Myelome des gaines tendineuses. Arch Gen Med 1891; 167:40.
7. Jaffe HL, Lichtenstein L, Sutro CJ. Pigmented villonodular synovitis, bursitis, and tenosynovitis: a discussion of the synovial and bursal equivalents of the tenosynovial lesions commonly denoted as xanthoma, xanthogranuloma, giant cell tumor, or myeloma of the tendon sheath, with some consideration of the tendon sheath lesion itself. Arch Pathol 1941; 31:731.
8. Jones FE, Soule EH, Coventry MB. Fibrous xanthoma of synovium (giant-cell tumor of tendon sheath, pigmented nodular synovitis). A study of one hundred and eighteen cases. J Bone Joint Surg 1969; 51:76.
9. Wright CJ. Benign giant-cell synovioma; an investigation of 85 cases. Br J Surg 1951; 38:257.
10. Baes H, Tanghe W. Nodular tenosynovitis. Benign giant cell synovioma. Dermatologica 1974; 149:149.
10a. Rubin BP. Tenosynovial giant cell tumor and pigmented villonodular synovitis: a proposal for unification of these clinically distinct but histologically and genetically identical lesions. Skeletal Radiol 2007; 36:267.

Giant cell tumor of tendon sheath, localized type

11. Chassaignac DME. Cancer de la gaine des tendons. Gaz Hosp Civ Milit 1852; 47:185.
12. Monaghan H, Salter DM, Al-Nafussi A. Giant cell tumour of tendon sheath (localised nodular tenosynovitis): clinicopathological features of 71 cases. J Clin Pathol 2001; 54:404.
13. Ushijima M, Hashimoto H, Tsuneyoshi M, et al. Giant cell tumor of the tendon sheath (nodular tenosynovitis). A study of 207 cases to compare the large joint group with the common digit group. Cancer 1986; 57:875.
14. Kitagawa Y, Ito H, Amano Y, et al. MR imaging for preoperative diagnosis and assessment of local tumor extent on localized giant cell tumor of tendon sheath. Skeletal Radiol 2003; 32:633.
15. Karasick D, Karasick S. Giant cell tumor of tendon sheath: spectrum of radiologic findings. Skeletal Radiol 1992; 21:219.
16. Moore JR, Weiland AJ, Curtis RM. Localized nodular tenosynovitis: Experience with 115 cases. J Hand Surg 1984; 9:412.
17. Uriburu IJ, Levy VD. Intraosseous growth of giant cell tumors of the tendon sheath (localized nodular tenosynovitis) of the digits: Report of 15 cases. J Hand Surg 1998; 23:732.
18. Hosaka M, Hatori M, Smith R, et al. Giant cell formation through fusion of cells derived from a human giant cell tumor of tendon sheath. J Orthop Sci 2004; 9:581.
19. Rao AS, Vigorita VJ. Pigmented villonodular synovitis (giant-cell tumor of the tendon sheath and synovial membrane). A review of eighty-one cases. J Bone Joint Surg 1984; 66:76.
20. Lukaszewski B. Clinical and pathomorphological aspects of nodular tenosynovitis of the hand. Chir Narzadow Ruchu Ortop Pol 1979; 44:583.
21. Satti MB. Tendon sheath tumours: a pathological study of the relationship between giant cell tumour and fibroma of tendon sheath. Histopathology 1992; 20:213.
22. Cavaliere A, Sidoni A, Bucciarelli E. Giant cell tumor of tendon sheath: immunohistochemical study of 20 cases. Tumori 1997; 83:841.
23. O'Connell JX, Fanburg JC, Rosenberg AE. Giant cell tumor of tendon sheath and pigmented villonodular synovitis: immunophenotype suggests a synovial cell origin. Hum Pathol 1995; 26:771.
24. Maluf HM, DeYoung BR, Swanson PE, et al. Fibroma and giant cell tumor of tendon sheath: A comparative histological and immunohistological study. Mod Pathol 1995; 8:155.
25. Silverman JS, Knapik M. Letter to the editor. Fibroma and giant cell tumor of tendon sheath: a comparative histological and immunohistological study. Mod Pathol 1996; 9:82.
26. Folpe AL, Weiss SW, Fletcher CD, et al. Tenosynovial giant cell tumors: evidence for a desmin-positive dendritic cell subpopulation. Mod Pathol 1998; 11:939.
27. Wood GS, Beckstead JH, Medeiros LJ, et al. The cells of giant cell tumor of tendon sheath resemble osteoclasts. Am J Surg Pathol 1988; 12:444.
28. Neale SD, Kristelly R, Gundle R, et al. Giant cells in pigmented villonodular synovitis express an osteoclast phenotype. J Clin Pathol 1997; 50:605.
29. Rickert RR, Shapiro MJ. Pigmented villonodular synovitis of the temporomandibular joint. Otolaryngol Head Neck Surg 1982; 90:668.
30. Darling JM, Goldring SR, Harada Y, et al. Multinucleated cells in pigmented villonodular synovitis and giant cell tumor of tendon sheath express features of osteoclasts. Am J Pathol 1997; 150:1383.
31. Seki K, Hirose T, Hasegawa T, et al. Giant cell tumor of tendon sheath. An immunohistochemical observation on the characteristics and the capacity of proliferation of tumor cells. Zentralbl Pathol. 1993; 139: 287
32. Alguacil-Garcia A, Unni KK, Goellner JR. Giant cell tumor of tendon sheath and pigmented villonodular synovitis: an ultrastructural study. Am J Clin Pathol 1978; 69:6.
33. Galliani I, Cassiani G, Valmori A, et al. Giant cell tumor of tendon sheath: A light and electron microscopic study. J Submicrosc Cytol Pathol 2000; 32:69.
34. Dal Cin P, Sciot R, Samson I, et al. Cytogenetic characterization of tenosynovial giant cell tumors (nodular tenosynovitis). Cancer Res 1994; 54:3986.
35. Sciot R, Rosai J, Dal Cin P, et al. Analysis of 35 cases of localized and diffuse tenosynovial giant cell tumor: a report from the chromosomes and morphology (CHAMP) study group. Mod Pathol 1999; 12:576.
36. Occhipinti E, Heinrich SD, Craver R. Giant cell tumor of tendon sheath arising in the toe. Fetal Pediat Pathol 2004; 23:171.
37. Nilsson M, Hoglund M, Panagopoulos I, et al. Molecular cytogenetic mapping of recurrent chromosomal breakpoints in tenosynovial giant cell tumors. Virchows Arch 2002; 441:475.
38. Brandal P, Bjerkehagen B, Heim S. Molecular cytogenetic characterization of tenosynovial giant cell tumors. Neoplasia 2004; 6:578.
38a. West RB, Rubin BP, Miller MA, et al. A landscape effect in tenosynovial giant cell tumor from activation of *CSF-1* expression by a translocation in a minority of tumor cells. PNAS 2006; 103:690.
38b. Cupp JS, Miller MA, Montgomery KD, et al. Translocation and expression of CSF-1 in pigmented villonodular synovitis, tenosynovial giant cell tumor, rheumatoid arthritis and other reactive synovitides. Am J Surg Pathol 2007; 31:970.
39. Mertens F, Orndal C, Mandahl N, et al. Chromosome aberrations in tenosynovial giant cell tumors and nontumorous synovial tissue. Genes Chromosomes Cancer 1993; 6:212.
40. Vogrincic GS, O'Connell JX, Gilks CB. Giant cell tumor of tendon sheath is a polyclonal cellular proliferation. Hum Pathol 1997; 28:815.
41. Sakkers RJ, de Jong D, van der Heul RO. X-chromosome inactivation in patients who have pigmented villonodular synovitis. J Bone Joint Surg 1991; 73:1532.
42. Abdul-Karim FW, el-Naggar AK, Joyce MJ, et al. Diffuse and localized tenosynovial giant cell tumor and pigmented villonodular synovitis: a clinicopathologic and flow cytometric DNA analysis. Hum Pathol 1992; 23:729.
43. Reilly KE, Stern PJ, Dale JA. Recurrent giant cell tumors of the tendon sheath. J Hand Surg 1999; 24:1298.
44. Hoaglund FT. Experimental hemarthrosis. The response of canine knees to injections of autologous blood. J Bone Joint Surg 1967; 49:285.
45. El-Nagger AK, Abdul-Karim FW. Tenosynovial giant cell tumors and other lesions traditionally considered to be reactive: further evidence for neoplastic etiology. Adv Anat Pathol 1995; 2:329.

Giant cell tumor of tendon sheath, diffuse type

46. Somerhausen NS, Fletcher CD. Diffuse-type giant cell tumor: clinicopathologic and immunohistochemical analysis of 50 cases with extra-articular disease. Am J Surg Pathol 2000; 24:479.
47. Horvath RR, Bostanche J, Altman MI. Diffuse type tenosynovial giant cell tumor of the ankle. J Am Podiatr Med Assoc 1993; 83:231.
48. Rowlands CG, Roland B, Hwang WS, et al. Diffuse-variant tenosynovial giant cell tumor: a rare and aggressive lesion. Hum Pathol 1994; 25:423.
49. Atmore WG, Dahlin DC, Ghormley RK. Pigmented villonodular synovitis; a clinical and pathologic study. Minn Med 1956; 39: 196.
50. Arthaud JB. Pigmented nodular synovitis: report of 11 lesions in non-articular locations. Am J Clin Pathol 1972; 58:511.
51. Gonzalez-Campora R, Salas Herrero E, Otal-Salaverri C, et al. Diffuse tenosynovial giant cell tumor of soft tissues. Report of a case with cytologic and cytogenetic findings. Acta Cytol 1995; 39:770.
52. Dahlen A, Broberg K, Domanski HA, et al. Analysis of the distribution and frequency of trisomy 7 in vivo in synovia from patients with osteoarthritis and pigmented villonodular synovitis. Cancer Genet Cytogenet 2001; 131:19.
53. Ofluoglu O. Pigmented villonodular synovitis. Orthop Clin North Am 2006; 37:23.
54. Bisbinas I, De Silva U, Grimer RJ. Pigmented villonodular synovitis of the foot and ankle: a 12-year experience from a tertiary orthopedic oncology unit. J Foot Ankle Surg 2004; 43:407.
55. Chin KR, Brick GW. Extra-articular pigmented villonodular synovitis: A cause for failed knee arthroscopy. Clin Orthop 2002; 404:330.

Malignant giant cell tumor of the tendon sheath/
pigmented villonodular synovitis

56. Myers BW, Masi AT. Pigmented villonodular
    synovitis and tenosynovitis: a clinical
    epidemiologic study of 166 cases and
    literature review. Medicine (Baltimore) 1980;
    59:223.
57. Castens HP, Howell RS. Malignant giant cell
    tumor of tendon sheath. Virchows Arch A
    [Pathol Anat Histol] 1979; 382:237.
58. Layfield LJ, Meloni-Ehrig A, Liu K, et al.
    Malignant giant cell tumor of synovium
    (malignant pigmented villonodular synovitis).
    Arch Pathol Lab Med 2000; 124:1636.
59. Kalil RK, Unni KK. Malignancy in pigmented
    villonodular synovitis. Skeletal Radiol 1998;
    27:392.

60. Ushijima M, Hashimoto H, Tsuneyoshi M,
    et al. Malignant giant cell tumor of tendon
    sheath. Report of a case. Acta Pathol Jpn 1985;
    35:699.
61. Bertoni F, Unni KK, Beabout JW, et al.
    Malignant giant cell tumor of the tendon
    sheaths and joints (malignant pigmented
    villonodular synovitis). Am J Surg Pathol 1997;
    21:153.
62. Nielsen AL, Kiaer T. Malignant giant cell tumor
    of synovium and locally destructive pigmented
    villonodular synovitis: ultrastructural and
    immunohistochemical study and review of the
    literature. Hum Pathol 1989; 20:765.
63. Fanburg-Smith JC, Miettinen M. Malignant
    giant cell tumors of tendon sheath: histologic
    classification with clinical correlation. Clin Exp
    Pathol 1998; 46:16A.

Miscellaneous conditions resembling diffuse giant
cell tumor

64. Nelson IW, Sivamurugan S, Latham PD, et al.
    Total hip arthroplasty for hemophilic
    arthropathy. Clin Orthop Rel Res 1992; 276:
    210.
65. Perlman MD, Schor AD, Gold ML. Implant
    failure with particulate silicone synovitis
    (detritic synovitis). J Foot Surg 1990; 29:584.
66. Zaloudek C, Treseler PA, Powell CB.
    Postarthroplasty histiocytic lymphadenopathy
    in gynecologic oncology patients. A benign
    reactive process that clinically may be mistaken
    for cancer. Cancer 1996; 78:834.
67. Weiss SW, Kelly WD. Bilateral destructive
    synovitis associated with alpha-mannosidase
    deficiency. Am J Surg Pathol 1983; 7:487.

Mesothelioma is by no means a new disease and has been recognized as a distinct clinicopathologic entity since the second half of the nineteenth century.[1] Adami is usually credited with coining the term *mesothelioma* in 1908,[2] but it was Klemperer and Rabin who first fully defined the epithelial and fibrous types of mesothelioma.[3] However, since Wagner and colleagues demonstrated a high incidence of mesotheliomas among asbestos workers in the Cape Province of South Africa in 1960, mounting attention has been paid to this tumor.[4]

The increasing reports over the past 20 years are not only a reflection of widespread interest in the etiology of the disease and evolution of diagnostic criteria, but also interest in the increased incidence over the past decades.[5] This steady increase in the number of newly observed cases parallels the steep rise in the output and use of asbestos fibers in industrial countries during the first half of the twentieth century. Because there is a 20- to 40-year time lag between exposure to asbestos and development of the disease, this trend is likely to persist for several more years; the recent worldwide reduction in the industrial and commercial use of asbestos fibers is bound to decrease the incidence of malignant mesothelioma, probably during the early twenty-first century.[5]

Mesothelioma arises from the mesothelial cells of serosal surfaces and is about five times more common in the pleural cavity than in the peritoneal cavity. Not infrequently it involves both pleura and peritoneum as the result of direct extension through the diaphragm. It also occurs as a primary tumor in the pericardium and tunica vaginalis testis, but the incidence at those two sites accounts for less than 5% of all cases.

The prognosis differs slightly according to type. It is grave with the diffuse epithelial and biphasic types and even less favorable with the fibrous (sarcomatoid) type;

nearly all patients with these tumors die of complications caused by the primary neoplasm within 6–18 months after diagnosis. Metastases do occur but usually at a late stage of the disease. There is still no effective mode of therapy, but multiagent chemotherapy and radiation therapy, in addition to surgery, seem to alleviate symptoms and prolong survival.

HISTOLOGIC CLASSIFICATION

There are three forms of malignant mesothelioma: (1) epithelial; (2) fibrous (sarcomatoid); and (3) biphasic or mixed, with both epithelial and spindled features in close association. These three forms present almost exclusively as diffuse lesions, and so these terms are essentially synonymous with "diffuse mesothelioma," although there are infrequent but well-documented tumors that develop as localized lesions.[6] Such lesions could represent an early form of what may develop into a diffuse disease. Epithelial and biphasic diffuse mesotheliomas display a wide range of growth patterns and cellular compositions, and vary from well-differentiated tubulopapillary lesions to poorly differentiated ones consisting merely of solid nests and sheets of tumor cells that may be uniform in appearance or may have considerable cellular pleomorphism. Recognition of the fibrous or sarcomatoid type frequently poses considerable diagnostic problems, requiring immunohistochemical analysis.

There is only limited information as to the incidence and distribution of the various types. Among *diffuse mesotheliomas*, the epithelial type is by far the most common. For example, in the study by Leigh et al. of 746 diffuse peritoneal mesotheliomas,[7] 44% were of the epithelial type, 22% were biphasic or mixed type, and 9% were of the fibrous (sarcomatoid) type; in 25% there was no agreement among the reviewers as to the histologic type. Of 819 tumors reported by Hillerdal,[8] 50%, 34%, and 16% were of the epithelial, mixed, and fibrous types, respectively.

Less aggressive forms of mesothelial tumors exist and include (1) the rare *well-differentiated papillary mesothelioma*; (2) *multicystic peritoneal mesothelioma*; and (3) *adenomatoid tumor*. Commensurate with their excellent

TABLE 28–1	CLASSIFICATION OF MESOTHELIAL TUMORS		
Tumor	Localized	Diffuse	Clinical behavior
Adenomatoid tumor	Virtually always		Benign
Well-differentiated papillary mesothelioma	Usually	Rarely	Benign/intermediate
Multicystic peritoneal mesothelioma	Usually	Sometimes	Intermediate
Malignant mesothelioma	Rare	Virtually always	Malignant

prognosis, the above lesions present with limited or localized disease and rarely are responsible for tumor-related death (Table 28–1).

DIFFUSE MALIGNANT MESOTHELIOMA

Clinical findings

Diffuse malignant mesothelioma is an uncommon tumor and is estimated to have an incidence of about 3000 cases per year (about 11 per million Americans per year).[9–11] The tumor is mainly found in adults 45–75 years of age, regardless of whether it originates in the pleural, pericardial, or peritoneal cavity or the scrotum. Data as to the gender incidence vary considerably, but in most reviews, especially those with a large number of industrial workers, men outnumber women by a considerable margin.[10,12,13] This is particularly true for pleural tumors, as women account for less than 20% of mesotheliomas in this location. Mesotheliomas arising in children are uncommon.

The clinical symptoms differ substantially and depend on the primary location of the neoplasm. *Diffuse pleural mesothelioma*, which accounts for about 85% of all mesotheliomas, usually manifests with chest pain, shortness of breath, and significant weight loss over a short period; it may also cause chronic cough, fever, and radiating pain in the shoulder or arm. Physical examination usually reveals decreased chest excursion, diminished or absent breath sounds, and in virtually all patients evidence of serous or hemorrhagic pleural effusion that accumulates rapidly and requires frequent aspiration. Pulmonary osteoarthropathy with arthritic pain and clubbing of the fingers or toes is encountered in 5–10% of cases. Laboratory studies are not helpful in the diagnosis; some patients develop leukocytosis and anemia, or there may be a thrombocytosis with thromboembolic episodes and pulmonary embolism.[14]

Patients with *diffuse peritoneal mesothelioma* usually give a history of nagging or burning abdominal or epigastric pain that is often more severe after meals. The pain is frequently accompanied by constipation, anorexia, nausea, or vomiting. Palpation of the abdomen discloses marked distension, increased density, and at times an ill-defined mass.[15–19] Ascites is often demonstrable; it may be massive and frequently persists despite repeated paracenteses. Regional lymph nodes may be palpable and on biopsy contain metastatic deposits. Pericardial mesotheliomas are associated with pericardial effusion, arrhythmia, or cardiac failure;[20] mesotheliomas of the tunica vaginalis are usually marked by a hydrocele or a scrotal mass.[21–23]

Radiographic findings and staging

Radiographic films, computed tomography (CT), and magnetic resonance imaging (MRI) examinations in patients with *diffuse pleural mesothelioma* show a rather distinct picture, but it rarely permits an unequivocal diagnosis (Fig. 28–1).[24] The outstanding features are marked effusion, sometimes with compression of the adjacent lung and atelectasis, diffuse or irregular nodular thickening of the pleura or interlobular fissure, and not infrequently an intrathoracic mass. Less commonly, widening or displacement of the mediastinum and a nodular infiltrate of the pulmonary parenchyma and pneumothorax secondary to invasion of the underlying visceral pleura and lung are present. Pulmonary fibrosis, however, is usually less severe than with asbestosis or carcinoma.

Radiographic films, CT and MRI scans of *diffuse peritoneal mesothelioma* reveal thickening of the visceral and parietal peritoneum and omentum or multiple small nodules, often in association with ascites, signs of gastrointestinal tract dysfunction, and intestinal obstruction.[25,26]

Refinements have been made in non-invasive staging techniques in recent years. CT and MRI improve detection of disease that may not be apparent by traditional techniques.[24,26,27] MRI appears to be superior to CT for accurate staging and is valuable for selection of patients for surgery.[28] Positron-emission tomography (PET) scanning, particularly when combined with CT, is superior to both CT or MRI alone for detecting occult extrathoracic disease and mediastinal lymph node involvement.[29,30] The group from MD Anderson Cancer Center recommend all patients undergo extended surgical staging since this technique identifies a subset of unresectable lesions that are not identified by imaging techniques.[31]

Pleural and ascitic fluid

Pleural or ascitic fluid is viscous (owing to the high content of hyaluronic acid), amber-colored, or frankly

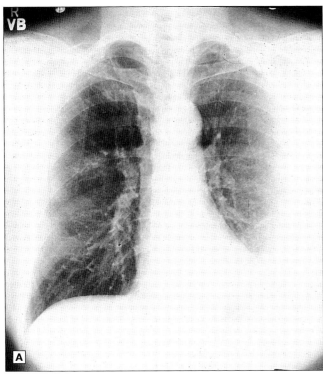

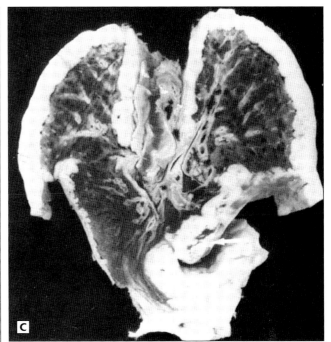

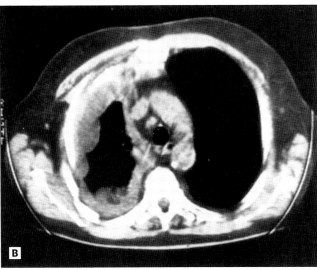

FIGURE 28–1 (A) Chest radiograph from a patient with diffuse pleural mesothelioma. There is evidence of a pleural effusion on the left side with obliteration of the left costophrenic angle. **(B)** Computed tomography (CT) scan of a diffuse pleural mesothelioma showing complete encasement of the right lung by tumor tissue. **(C)** Diffuse mesothelioma encasing and compressing both lungs of a 63-year-old man.

hemorrhagic with demonstrable malignant cells in slightly more than half of the cases.[32] Markedly elevated levels of hyaluronic acid have been observed in a high percentage of cases, but they are also seen, although much less frequently, with carcinomas and sarcomas.

Needle biopsy

Needle biopsy guided by ultrasonography or CT scan is diagnostic in a minority of cases, and thoracotomy and open biopsy may be necessary to establish the diagnosis.

However, this technique can be quite reliable for the diagnosis of local recurrence and distant metastases.

Mesothelioma and asbestos exposure

Although the association between pulmonary asbestosis and carcinoma was established during the early 1930s, the causal relation between asbestos exposure and mesothelioma was not recognized until 1960, when Wagner et al. gave a detailed account of 47 diffuse mesotheliomas observed within a 5-year period in the asbestos regions of South Africa.[4] Several years later, Selikoff and colleagues reported on "asbestos exposure and neoplasia" in insulation workers of the New York area.[33] Since publication of these reports, numerous studies carried out in England, Scotland, South Africa, Canada, the United States, and other parts of the world have confirmed these observations and have demonstrated an increased incidence of mesothelioma not only among asbestos miners but also among industrial workers with a prolonged history of asbestos exposure.

In their classic study of 17 800 asbestos insulation workers, Selikoff et al. found that among 2271 consecutive deaths, there were 175 mesotheliomas plus a large number of pulmonary carcinomas and carcinomas at other sites.[33] In fact, cancer was responsible for 44% of all deaths, in contrast to the expected rate of 19%. Of the 175 mesotheliomas, 63 (36%) involved the pleura and 112 (64%) the peritoneum; most became apparent 25–40 years after the worker had started employment and been exposed to asbestos. This time lag between exposure and emergence of symptoms serves to explain not only the rarity of mesothelioma in young persons but also the surge in its incidence following a period in which the output and use of asbestos had risen markedly, especially in highly industrialized countries.

Exposure to asbestos is an occupational hazard not only in the mining and milling industries but also in the process of manufacturing, repairing, and installing (and removing) asbestos products such as thermal and electrical insulations, floor and ceiling tiles, automobile brake and clutch linings, cement tiles and pipes, and numerous other applications. Domestic exposure appears to be less significant but has been observed in one or more relatives of asbestos workers and in persons and even animals living in the vicinity of asbestos mines and industries.

Multiple factors are important when determining the asbestos-related mesothelioma risk.[34] Asbestos fibers can be divided into two families: serpentine and amphibole (Table 28–2). Chrysotile is the main member of the serpentine family, whereas the amphibole family is composed of several members, including crocidolite, amosite, anthophyllite, tremolite, and actinolite. Several studies have showed a marked difference in the ability of these asbestos fiber types to induce mesothelioma. The highest

risk is with exposure to crocidolite, followed by amosite and tremolite. Chrysotile, the white asbestos found chiefly in Canada and Russia, accounts for more than 95% of the asbestos used commercially but rarely causes mesothelioma.[35] Exposure to more than one type of fiber is common, however, and it has been suggested that the tumorigenicity of chrysotile is due to contamination with noncommercial amphiboles such as actinolite, tremolite, and anthophyllite.[36] Hodgson and Darnton estimated the exposure-specific risk of mesotheliomas from the three principal commercial asbestos types to be in a ratio of 1 : 100 : 500 for chrysotile, amosite and crocidolite, respectively.[37]

There are other properties of the type of asbestos fiber that determine mesothelioma risk. For example, the length and diameter of the fiber appear to be inversely related to mesothelioma risk, as fibers longer than 8 μm and thinner than 0.25 μm are much more likely to be associated with mesothelioma.[38] After inhalation, these fibrils are capable of passing into the pleural cavity. They may also be able to penetrate the bowel wall and migrate to the peritoneum, as suggested by animal experiments.[39,40] The curlier fibrils of chrysotile are less penetrating and are more readily removed by macrophages and lymphatics.[41] Finally, the greater biopersistence and ability to generate active oxygen radicals of crocidolite compared to other asbestos fiber types probably contribute to its greater tumorigenicity.[42]

Duration and intensity of exposure are also major factors when determining mesothelioma risk. Asbestos-related mesotheliomas characteristically have long latency periods. Lanphear and Buncher found that 99% of patients with mesothelioma had a latent period of more than 15 years (median 32 years).[43] Furthermore, there appears to be a direct relation between the intensity of exposure and cancer risk.

Most of the asbestos fibers in the body are too small to be visualized by light microscopy, but they are readily recognized in the lung as "asbestos bodies," asbestos fibers coated with acid mucopolysaccharides and hemosiderin granules. These segmented, "nail-headed," golden-brown structures are difficult to distinguish from the ferruginous structures formed about a nonasbestos core, such as iron, talc, mica, carbon, and rutile. Assisting in the distinction of these fibers are the thin, transparent, usually straight central core of asbestos (Fig. 28–2), the refractile yellow core of talc and mica, and the black core of iron and rutile. Examination by electron and scanning microscopy reveals that most ferruginous bodies have asbestos cores.

More efficient ways of demonstrating and counting ferruginous bodies are examination of a lung juice smear and digestion of wet lung tissue with sodium hypochlorite and membrane filtration.[41] Using the latter method, Smith and Naylor found ferruginous bodies in 100% of consecutive autopsies, regardless of the cause of death.[44]

TABLE 28–2 CLASSIFICATION OF ASBESTOS FIBERS

Serpentines
    Chrysotile (white asbestos)
Amphiboles
    Crocidolite (blue asbestos)
    Amosite
    Anthophyllite
    Tremolite
    Actinolite

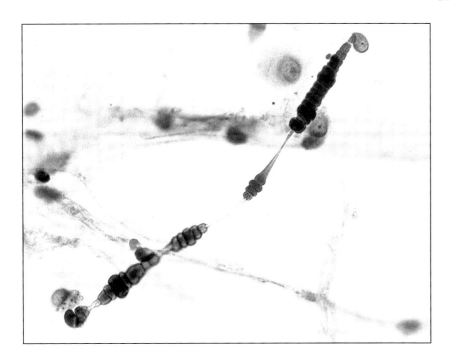

FIGURE 28–2 Ferruginous body with a thin, transparent, straight central core, consistent with an asbestos body.

Likewise, Churg et al. found asbestos bodies in nearly all of the cases examined, but they noted a considerable increase in concentration in workers in certain asbestos-related occupations and in patients with mesothelioma.[45] Counts of asbestos fibers by electron microscopy are even more reliable than those with tissue digestion.[46]

Although measures have been taken in recent years to reduce asbestos exposure of industrial workers and the general population, it is likely – considering the long latent period of the disease – that the high incidence of mesothelioma will continue over the coming years, at least in some parts of the world. It has been estimated that the incidence of mesothelioma will likely peak in Great Britain between 2011 and 2015, followed by a rapid decline. In contrast, data suggest the peak incidence in the United States may have already passed in the mid-1990s.[10] At particular risk are those who have been exposed to asbestos for several years, either as workers in the asbestos industry or by living in an asbestos-contaminated urban or industrial atmosphere. Also at risk are workers engaged in the demolition of buildings or refitting of ships containing asbestos packing around boilers and furnaces. Smoking does not seem to enhance the risk of developing the disease.

Although most mesotheliomas are related to asbestos exposure, other causes have also been proposed. Non-asbestos fibers, such as erionite, a naturally occurring mineral fiber found in central Turkey where it is used in the construction of houses, has been reported to be associated with a high prevalence of mesothelioma.[47,48] Pleural and peritoneal mesotheliomas have been associated with radiation exposure[49] and administration of thorium dioxide contrast (Thorotrast).[50] Pleural and peritoneal mesotheliomas have been associated with chronic empyema and peritonitis, respectively.[51,52]

Mesothelioma and SV40

Simian virus-40 (SV40), a DNA papovavirus, has been linked with mesothelioma, as several studies have found SV40 sequences in both animal and human mesotheliomas.[53-55] SV40 was found to be a contaminant of polio and adenovirus vaccines in the 1950s and 1960s. SV40 infection is highest among immunocompromised patients, can occur in adults and children, and is thought to be transmitted via maternal–fetal and oral–fecal routes.[56] The SV40 large tumor antigen (Tag) stimulates host cell proliferation, and its protein appears to bind and inactivate several important tumor suppressor genes including p53 and the retinoblastoma gene. SV40 Tag is found in a significant percentage of mesotheliomas. For example, in the study by Carbone and colleagues,[57] this antigen was detected in 29 of 48 human mesotheliomas (using the polymerase chain reaction), whereas Strickler et al. were unable to document these sequences in 50 mesotheliomas.[58] Similarly, Dhaene and colleagues were unable to detect nuclear expression of this viral oncoprotein in a large series of mesotheliomas.[59] SV40 may have its effect, at least in part, by methylating and inactivating regulatory pathway genes including *DcR1*, *cyclin D2* and *HIC1*, among others.[56,60,61] There have been several reports of mesothelioma arising in family members, although the relative roles of genetic and environmental influences are unclear.[62]

Gross findings

Initially, the disease is characterized by numerous small nodules or plaques covering visceral and parietal serosal surfaces. At a later stage the individual nodules fuse and form a diffuse, sheet-like thickening that frequently encases and compresses the lungs or intestines and sometimes the liver and spleen (Fig. 28–1). In the thoracic cavity the growth tends to be fairly uniform but often is more pronounced in the serosal coverings of the lower lobe and diaphragm; in the peritoneum, involvement is usually more variable, and the diffuse or multinodular growth is often associated with large localized masses or a conglomerate of tumor nodules of variable size. Massive involvement of the omentum is a common occurrence that clinically may simulate the presence of a solitary localized neoplasm. The final stages of the disease are marked by massive encasement of the viscera with matting of the affected structures, commonly causing complete obliteration of the pleural or peritoneal cavity and severe, often fatal, functional disturbances. In many cases the tumor tissue invades the adjacent lung or viscera, but in general invasion is more superficial than deep and is confined to the immediate subserosal tissues. Not infrequently the tumor extends through the chest or abdominal wall along a needle biopsy tract or a scar from a previous excision, a complication that must be given consideration when planning thoracoscopy, peritoneoscopy, or needle biopsy or when aspirating fluid for cytologic examination or to relieve symptoms. The excised tissue varies greatly in appearance and may be firm and rubbery or soft and gelatinous; on section it is generally gray-white and glistening, frequently with foci of hemorrhage or necrosis.

Microscopic findings

Although there is often a striking variation in different areas of the same neoplasm, most diffuse mesotheliomas are of the *epithelial type* and can be identified by their characteristic tubulopapillary pattern present at least focally. This pattern consists of papillary structures, branching tubules, and gland-like acinar and cystic spaces lined by rather uniform cuboidal or flattened epithelial-like cells with vesicular nuclei, one or two nucleoli, and abundant eosinophilic cytoplasm with distinct cytoplasmic borders (Figs 28–3, 28–4). Mitotic figures are absent or rare in well-differentiated neoplasms, but they may be numerous in poorly differentiated ones. The surrounding matrix varies from myxoid to densely fibrous with or without hyalinization. Some examples show a pronounced myxoid stroma and can be easily confused with other types of myxoid neoplasms.[63]

In addition to the typical tubulopapillary and tubuloglandular patterns, some tumors are composed of small uniform cells arranged in a delicate lace-like pattern, and others contain sheets of vacuolated cells vaguely reminiscent of liposarcoma (Fig. 28–5).[64,65] Others are marked by cleft-like structures or large, irregular, cystic spaces lined by a single layer of flattened epithelioid cells. In some of these cases fusion or rupture of the cystic spaces leads to the formation of large mucin-filled pools; in others the cystic structures are filled or replaced by multiple papillary projections with fibrous cores that bear a close resemblance to papillary carcinoma (Fig. 28–6).

There are also less-well-differentiated epithelial mesotheliomas in which the tubulopapillary pattern is largely inconspicuous or absent, and the tumor consists merely of small round or polygonal cells disposed in a linear or cord-like pattern or in clusters and solid nests and sheets (Figs 28–7, 28–8). These tumors may resemble poorly differentiated carcinoma and therefore require ancillary immunohistochemical or electron microscopic studies (or both) for accurate diagnosis (discussed below). Associated with these changes is often a striking loss of cellular cohesion, with rounded or polygonal cells freely floating in the mucinous pools or dispersed in a loosely textured, myxoid stroma. This loss of cellular cohesion constitutes a frequent and useful feature in the differential diagnosis of mesothelioma. Calcospherites or psammoma bodies occur in approximately 5% of mesotheliomas, notably in those of the tubulopapillary type. Several unusual variants of epithelial mesothelioma have been described, including sporadic tumors that consist of nests of small hyperchromatic cells (*small cell mesothelioma*),[66] pleomorphic variants, and those composed of cells with abundant glassy eosinophilic cytoplasm resembling a decidual reaction (*deciduoid mesothelioma*) (Fig. 28–9). Although the latter variant was initially believed to have a predilection for arising in the peritoneum of young adult females without a history of asbestos exposure,[67,68] subsequent reports have documented this tumor in the pleura of adults, some of whom had significant asbestos exposure.[69–72]

The second type, the *fibrous* or *sarcomatoid type* of diffuse mesothelioma, may be difficult to diagnose and is apt to be confused with fibrosarcoma, malignant hemangiopericytoma, malignant solitary fibrous tumor or some other type of high-grade sarcoma (Fig. 28–10). As a rule, however, there are well-oriented, spindle-shaped, fibroblast-like cells with nuclear hyperchromatism, pleomorphism, and occasional giant cells associated with areas of dense fibrosis, hyalinization, and necrosis. The presence of some of these fibrosing areas may cause confusion with a reactive fibrosing process (fibrous pleurisy); but as discussed below, the cellular atypia, increased mitotic activity, bland necrosis, and infiltrative growth are essential clues to the diagnosis.[73] There also may be a focal whorled, storiform, hemangiopericytoma-like or fibrosarcoma-like pattern. The term *desmoplastic diffuse mesothelioma* has been applied to richly collagenous

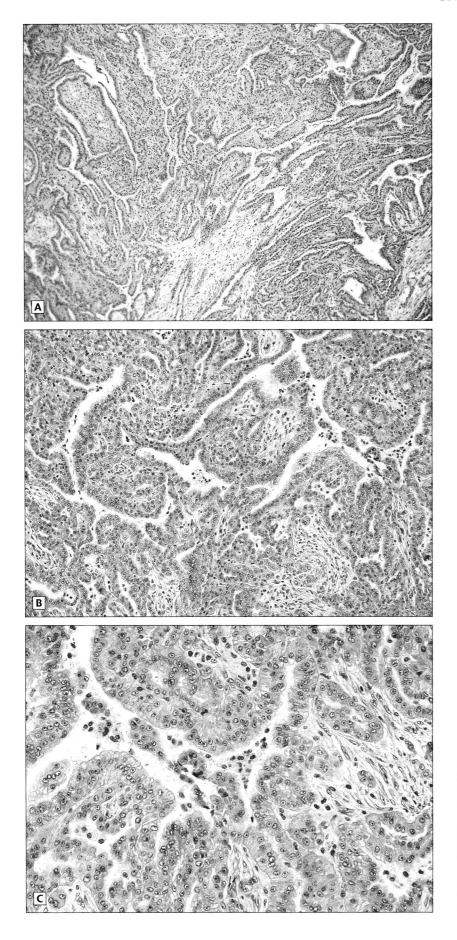

FIGURE 28–3 (A) Low-power view of a diffuse epithelial mesothelioma with a prominent tubulopapillary pattern. **(B)** Prominent tubulopapillary pattern composed of epithelioid cells with abundant eosinophilic cytoplasm in a diffuse epithelial mesothelioma. **(C)** Characteristic cytologic features of mesothelial cells in a diffuse epithelial mesothelioma with a prominent tubulopapillary pattern. The cells have vesicular nuclei with prominent nucleoli and abundant eosinophilic cytoplasm.

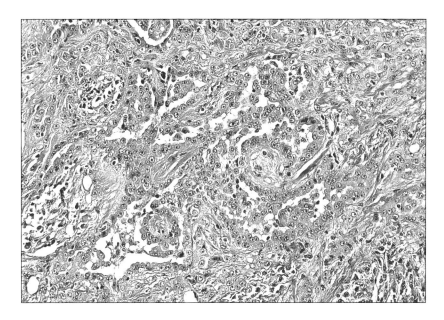

FIGURE 28–4 Papillary structures with fibrous cores are surrounded by malignant mesothelial cells.

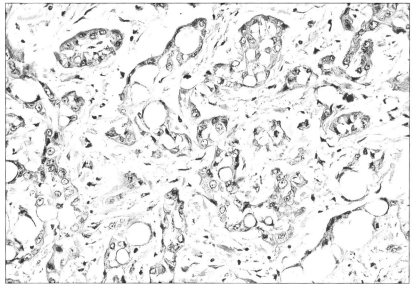

FIGURE 28–5 Diffuse epithelial mesothelioma with vacuolated malignant cells arranged in a lace-like growth pattern reminiscent of that seen in adenomatoid tumors.

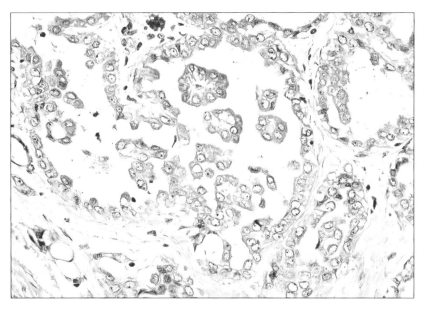

FIGURE 28–6 Multiple papillary projections with fibrous cores in a diffuse epithelial mesothelioma. These areas bear a close resemblance to papillary adenocarcinoma.

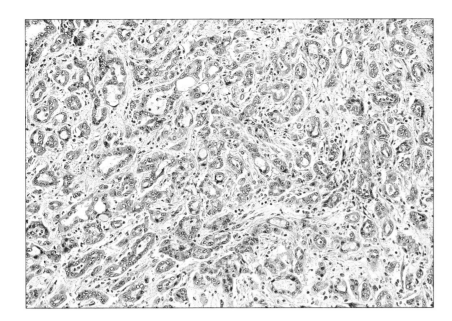

FIGURE 28–7 Diffuse epithelial mesothelioma composed predominantly of small tubules and cords.

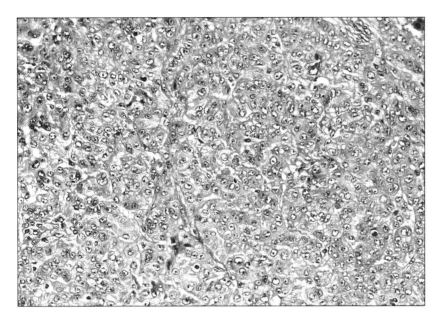

FIGURE 28–8 Solid sheet-like arrangement of malignant mesothelial cells with vesicular nuclei and macronucleoli.

tumors of this type (Fig. 28–11). Despite the extensive desmoplasia in these cases, the clinical course is that of a highly malignant neoplasm.[73–76] Osseous or cartilaginous metaplasia in some cases raises the question of chondrosarcoma or osteosarcoma.[77,78] Rare tumors are composed of histiocytoid cells admixed with a dense polymorphous infiltrate composed of lymphocytes, plasma cells, eosinophils, and xanthoma cells (*lymphohistiocytoid mesothelioma*).[79,80] Foci of epithelial differentiation are rare in the sarcomatoid type of diffuse mesothelioma and may be found only after careful scrutiny of multiple sections. In the absence of such areas, the diagnosis rests mainly on the presence of the diffuse and pleomorphic spindle cell pattern and the characteristic immunohistochemical and ultrastructural findings (discussed below).

The third type, the *mixed* or *biphasic type* of diffuse mesothelioma, consists of a mixture of epithelial and sarcomatous components that usually blend with one another such that transitional areas may be seen (Figs 28–12, 28–13). Rarely in our experience do the two components abut one another in an abrupt fashion, as one sees in synovial sarcoma or carcinosarcomas of various organs. As in the diffuse fibrous type, osseous and cartilaginous differentiation occasionally occurs. Several investigators have noted a prevalence of the mixed type among patients with an occupational history of asbestos exposure.[81] Although there is some debate about the incidence of localized forms of epithelial and biphasic mesothelioma, there appears to be good documentation in a few cases.[6,82] Many alleged cases represent diffuse lesions that are inadequately staged, and others probably

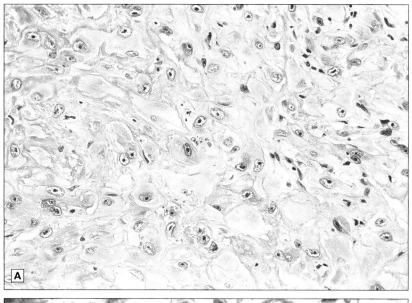

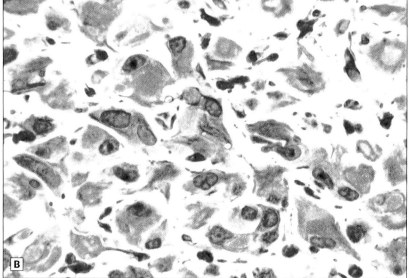

FIGURE 28-9 **(A)** Peritoneal deciduoid mesothelioma composed of cells with abundant glassy eosinophilic cytoplasm resembling a decidual reaction. **(B)** Diffuse cytokeratin immunoreactivity in a peritoneal deciduoid mesothelioma.

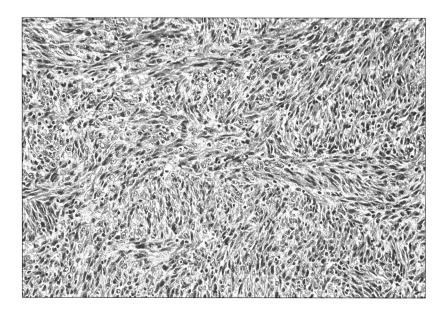

FIGURE 28-10 Fibrous (sarcomatoid) type of diffuse mesothelioma composed of spindle-shaped cells arranged in short fascicles.

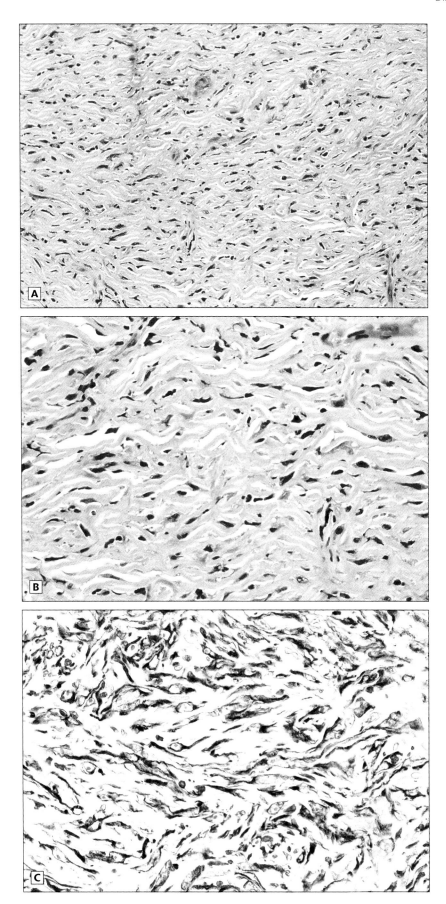

FIGURE 28–11 Low-power **(A)** and high-power **(B)** views of a desmoplastic diffuse mesothelioma. Such cases may be difficult to distinguish from pleural plaques. **(C)** Diffuse and strong immunoreactivity for low-molecular-weight cytokeratin (CAM5.2) in a desmoplastic diffuse mesothelioma.

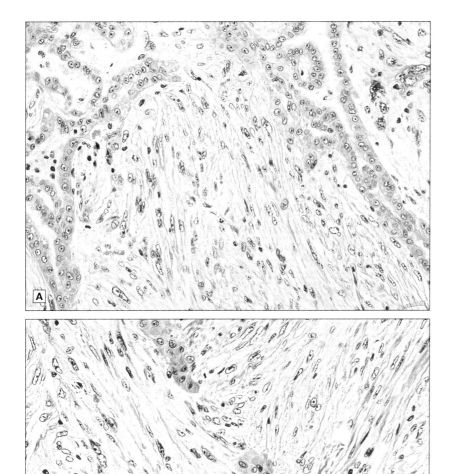

FIGURE 28–12 **(A)** Biphasic pleural mesothelioma. **(B)** High-power view of a biphasic pleural mesothelioma showing a gradual transition between epithelial and spindle-shaped cells.

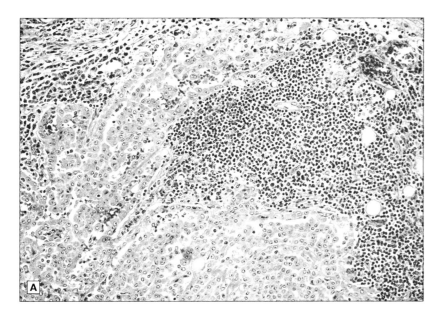

FIGURE 28–13 Unusual case of a biphasic pleural mesothelioma composed of roughly equal amounts of epithelial mesothelioma **(A)** and a high-grade malignant fibrous histiocytoma-like tumor.

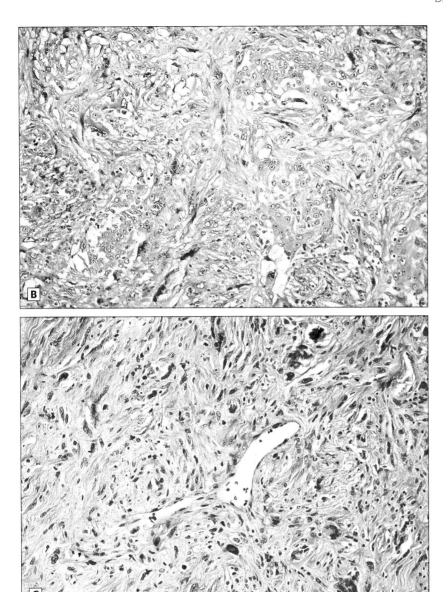

FIGURE 28–13 Continued. **(B)** Transitional area between epithelial mesothelioma and malignant fibrous histiocytoma-like area. **(C)** High-power view of a malignant fibrous histiocytoma-like area in this unusual pleural mesothelioma.

represent malignant forms of solitary fibrous tumor or biphasic tumors of other types (e.g., synovial sarcoma).

Staining characteristics

Special stains are helpful in the diagnosis of mesothelioma and particularly for differentiating this tumor from adenocarcinoma (Table 28–3). As in normal mesothelium, the occasional mucin droplets present in the tumor cells stain positively with Alcian blue and colloidal iron stains and lose their staining characteristics or stain less intensely after treating the sections with hyaluronidase. However, unlike adenocarcinoma – and many synovial sarcomas – the mucin droplets do not stain with periodic

TABLE 28–3	**DIFFERENTIAL DIAGNOSIS OF MESOTHELIOMA AND ADENOCARCINOMA BASED ON INTRACELLULAR MUCIN***	
Stain	**Malignant epithelial mesothelioma**	**Adenocarcinoma**
PAS[†]	–	+
PAS-diastase	–	+
Alcian blue	+	+
Alcian blue-hyaluronidase	±	+

*Including mucin in acinar spaces.
[†]Intracellular PAS-positive glycogen granules are present in many epithelial and biphasic mesotheliomas.

acid-Schiff (PAS) after diastase digestion. Glycogen granules positive for PAS and sensitive to diastase digestion are present in the cytoplasm of many tumor cells, however.[83,84] Many of the intracellular droplets also stain for mucicarmine. Unfortunately, mucin droplets that stain positively for Alcian blue (and negatively for PAS) are rare or entirely absent in at least half of the cases, especially in tumors that are less well differentiated.[85] The stromal mucin outside the tumor cells stains with Alcian blue (pH 2.5) and is removed by hyaluronidase, a finding that mesothelioma shares with other sarcomas. However, acid mucin can be lost during processing in aqueous fixatives, and rare adenocarcinomas have Alcian blue-positive stromal mucins.[86]

Immunohistochemical findings

Because of the lack of sensitivity and specificity of histochemical stains, immunostaining is indispensable for the diagnosis of mesothelioma. A completely specific marker for mesothelioma has not been found, and so a panel of antibodies is always used to allow discrimination of mesothelioma from other neoplasms, particularly adenocarcinoma (Table 28–4). There have been innumerable reviews on this subject, with each study proposing a different panel of antibodies.[87–95] Until the mid-1990s, most of these antibody panels were composed of antibodies that frequently reacted with adenocarcinomas but only rarely with mesotheliomas, including CEA, CD15 (Leu-M1), B72.3, Ber-Ep4, Bg8, E-cadherin and MOC-31. However, since then, a number of antibodies that commonly react with mesotheliomas but not with adenocarcinomas have become available, including calretinin, WT-1, podoplanin, D2-40, mesothelin, cytokeratin 5/6, thrombomodulin, OC-125 and HBME-1.[96–99] As noted by Ordonez,[88] there is general agreement that these immunohistochemical panels should be composed of both negative and positive mesothelioma markers, but there is

certainly no agreement on the optimal panel of markers. The antibody panel chosen depends upon the differential diagnosis (e.g., pleural epithelioid mesothelioma versus lung adenocarcinoma, peritoneal epithelioid mesothelioma versus ovarian or peritoneal serous carcinoma and sarcomatoid mesothelioma versus other spindle cell neoplasms). This discussion will focus on the most useful antibodies in these diagnostic settings, as opposed to serving as a comprehensive review of all of the positive and negative antibodies that have been evaluated. Further details regarding the immunohistochemical evaluation of mesothelioma are discussed in Chapter 7.

Pleural epithelioid mesothelioma versus lung adenocarcinoma

In the not-too-distant past, the distinction between pleural epithelioid mesothelioma and lung adenocarcinoma was based on the absence of expression of a number of proteins in mesothelioma. However, given the commercial availability of a number of "anti-mesothelioma" markers, it is clear that a panel of antibodies using both positive and negative markers is ideal. Recently, Ordonez performed a comparative study of 60 well-characterized pleural epithelioid mesotheliomas and 50 lung adenocarcinomas using 19 markers in an attempt to determine the optimal panel.[88] Table 28–5 summarizes the results of this study, which indicated that the best combination of markers to make this distinction included calretinin (Fig. 28–14) and cytokeratin 5/6 (or WT-1) for positive markers and CEA and MOC-31 (or B72.3, Ber-Ep4 or Bg8) for negative markers. Similarly, using logic regression statistical analysis, Yaziji and colleagues identified a three antibody panel including calretinin, Bg8 and MOC-31 to be optimal, providing over 96% sensitivity and specificity for distinguishing between these neoplasms.[100]

TABLE 28–4	DIFFERENTIAL DIAGNOSIS OF MESOTHELIOMA AND ADENOCARCINOMA BASED ON IMMUNOHISTOCHEMISTRY	
Marker/antibody	**Malignant mesothelioma**	**Adenocarcinoma**
Vimentin	+	Up to 50% +
Cytokeratin	+	+
Epithelial membrane antigen	+ (membranous)	+ (cytoplasmic)
Carcinoembryonic antigen	–	+
Leu-M1	–	+
Ber-EP4	Up to 25% +	+
B72.3	–	+
MOC-31	–	+
Calretinin	+	–
Cytokeratin 5/6	+	–

TABLE 28–5	SUMMARY OF IMMUNOHISTOCHEMICAL MARKERS IN EPITHELIOID MESOTHELIOMAS AND PULMONARY ADENOCARCINOMAS	
Antigen	**Epithelioid mesothelioma (%)**	**Pulmonary adenocarcinoma (%)**
Vimentin	60	20
Ber-Ep4	11	94
Leu-M1 (CD15)	5	85
B72.3	8	82
CEA	5	82
E-cadherin	52	96
MOC-31	20	98
CD44	72	54
Thrombomodulin	51	22
WT1	78	10
CK5/6	90	6
Calretinin	86	10

Modified from: Hammar SP. Ultrastruct Pathol 2006; 30:3, with data derived from Ordonez NG. Am J Surg Pathol 2003; 27:1031.

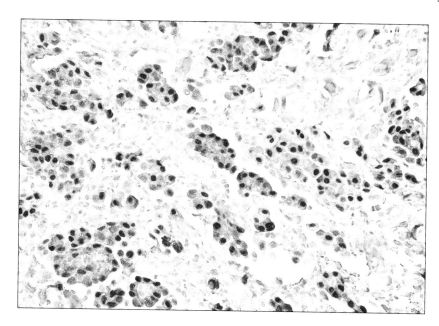

FIGURE 28–14 Diffuse immunoreactivity for calretinin in a diffuse epithelial mesothelioma of the pleura.

Peritoneal epithelioid mesothelioma versus ovarian or peritoneal serous carcinoma

The distinction between peritoneal epithelioid mesothelioma and either ovarian or primary peritoneal serous carcinoma can be extremely difficult due to overlapping morphologic features. Similar to the discussion above, panels of antibodies can be useful in assisting the pathologist in making this important distinction, especially if one utilizes both positive and negative markers. It must be kept in mind that markers that are useful in distinguishing pleural epithelioid mesothelioma from lung adenocarcinoma may be of limited utility in the setting of a peritoneal neoplasm. Ovarian and peritoneal serous carcinomas show a different immunoprofile than lung adenocarcinoma, and as such, it is only useful to compare the immunoprofile of peritoneal neoplasms to one another. In general, the "anti-mesothelioma" markers useful in recognizing pleural epithelioid mesotheliomas are also frequently expressed in peritoneal epithelioid mesotheliomas. These markers include calretinin,[101–103] thrombomodulin,[101,104] cytokeratin 5/6,[101,105] WT-1,[106] and D2-40.[107] However, because WT-1 is known to be frequently expressed in serous carcinomas, this marker has no value in this differential diagnosis.[108–110] Markers that are frequently expressed in serous carcinomas include estrogen and progesterone receptors,[111–113] MOC-31,[101,114] Ber-Ep4,[104,111] B72.3,[111,114] CD15 (Leu-M1),[104,111] Bg8,[111,115] CA19-9,[111,114] placental alkaline phosphatase (PLAP),[114] and CEA.[114] In his review of the literature, Ordonez found that a combination of MOC-31 (or Ber-Ep4), estrogen receptor and calretinin allowed for a clear distinction between these two peritoneal neoplasms in the vast majority of cases.[101]

Sarcomatoid (fibrous) mesothelioma versus other malignant spindle cell neoplasms

The diagnosis of sarcomatoid (fibrous) mesothelioma can be extremely challenging, especially since many of the "anti-mesothelioma" markers that stain epithelioid mesotheliomas are only focally positive or completely negative in sarcomatoid variants.[116,117] For example, in the study by Attanoos and colleagues, calretinin, thrombomodulin and cytokeratin 5/6 were expressed in only 39%, 29% and 29% of sarcomatoid mesotheliomas, respectively.[117] However, none of these markers was expressed in any of the spindled carcinomas. Broad-spectrum cytokeratins are expressed in most but not all sarcomatoid mesotheliomas. We have found antibodies to low-molecular-weight cytokeratins (CAM 5.2) to be more sensitive in recognizing sarcomatoid mesotheliomas, but of course these markers lack specificity, since most sarcomatoid carcinomas also express cytokeratins. The expression of cytokeratins may be useful in helping to distinguish sarcomatoid mesothelioma from other spindle cell sarcomas (for example, malignant solitary fibrous tumor).

Ultrastructural findings

Although mesotheliomas share some ultrastructural similarities with adenocarcinoma, they can be distinguished by the presence of abundant, long, slender, sometimes tortuous microvilli with a bush-like or shaggy appearance (Fig. 28–15).[118,119] The microvilli are found on the free surfaces of the tumor cells and in intracellular and intercellular lumens. The microvilli of adenocarcinoma are also located on the surface and inside cells but are

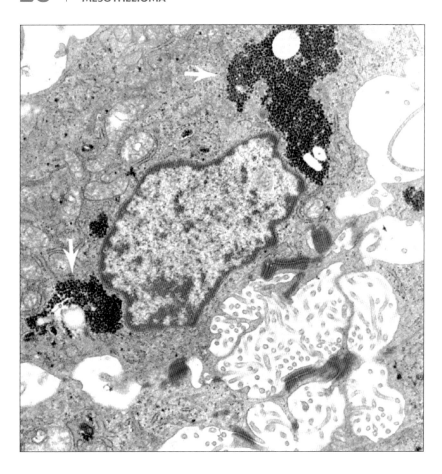

FIGURE 28–15 Electron microscopic view of a diffuse peritoneal mesothelioma in a 66-year-old woman. Note the intracellular and intercellular lumens with multiple slender microvilli and intracellular deposits of glycogen (arrows). (Courtesy Dr. Frederic I. Volini, West Suburban Hospital, Oak Park, IL.)

TABLE 28-6	DIFFERENTIAL DIAGNOSIS OF MESOTHELIOMA AND ADENOCARCINOMA BASED ON ULTRASTRUCTURAL FINDINGS	
Feature	**Malignant mesothelioma**	**Adenocarcinoma**
Microvilli	Numerous, long, slender, "bushy"	Fewer, short, blunt, "club-like"
Desmosomes	++	+ to ++
Intermediate filaments	+ to ++	0 to +
Basement membrane	++	++
Glycogen	++	0 to +

generally much shorter, less numerous, and have a more club-like appearance (Table 28–6).[120] The characteristic appearance of numerous, long, slender, microvilli is lost in poorly differentiated neoplasms.[119,121] The cells of a mesothelioma are further marked by large nuclei with prominent nucleoli, a moderate number of mitochondria enveloped by rough endoplasmic reticulum, and frequently glycogen granules and bundles of intermediate filaments. There are smooth-surfaced intracellular vacuoles, but the Golgi apparatus and the associated smooth endoplasmic reticulum are rather inconspicuous. Basal laminae are present but are often interrupted or incomplete. There are also junctional structures or desmosomes between adjoining cells and intermediate filaments or tonofilaments often limited to the apical portion of the cell or arranged circumferentially around the nucleus. There are no ultrastructural differences between pleural and peritoneal mesotheliomas.

Examination of the biphasic or mixed type of mesothelioma discloses a similar picture, but there are, in addition, fibroblast or myofibroblast-like cells with elongated nuclei and abundant rough endoplasmic reticulum and myofilaments with dense body formations and whorled aggregates of perinuclear intermediate filaments.[119] Forms transitional between the epithelial and spindle cells are not uncommon and can be recognized by the presence of intercellular microcavities with microvilli.[119] The latter feature has also been encountered in diffuse fibrous (sarcomatoid) mesotheliomas.

The extracellular spaces contain collagen fibers and colloidal iron-positive material, especially in close contact with the microvilli. None of the ultrastructural studies revealed asbestos fibers in the tumor cells, even in cases in which they were readily demonstrable in the surrounding pulmonary parenchyma.

Cytogenetic findings

Most mesotheliomas harbor multiple cytogenetic abnormalities. Karyotyping of a number of mesotheliomas has not revealed any specific diagnostic anomalies. Monosomy of chromosomes 4 and 22 and polysomy for chromosomes 5, 7, and 20 and loss at 1p21-22, 3p21, 6q15-21, 9p21-22, and 22q12 are the most common aberrations detected.[122–124] Studies utilizing FISH and comparative genomic hybridization (CGH) have also found losses at these loci to be among the most common in mesotheliomas.[125–127] A number of putative tumor suppressor genes have been implicated as being central to the pathogenesis of mesothelioma including *CDKN2A* (also known as *p16*, mapped to 9p),[128,129] *NF2* (mapped to 22q12),[130,131] *p53*,[132] *WT1*[133] MDM2[134] and *RB1*.[135]

Differential diagnosis

The differential diagnosis of diffuse mesothelioma depends on whether one is dealing with an epithelial, fibrous, or biphasic type. The differential diagnostic considerations for each of the types of diffuse mesothelioma are discussed below.

Epithelial mesothelioma

It is not always possible to distinguish well-differentiated epithelial mesothelial neoplasms from *reactive mesothelial proliferations* on the basis of a small biopsy specimen. In general, reactive or inflammatory mesothelial proliferations are limited to the serosal surfaces, where they may form small papillary structures, usually with gradual transitions between normal and hyperplastic mesothelium. These proliferations may arise in a variety of sites and settings. Rosai and Dehner described proliferations of mesothelial-like cells in hernial sacs.[136] They occurred in the inguinal region of children and followed hernial incarceration or some other mechanical injury. The lesions were marked by nodular proliferations of round or polygonal mesothelial cells associated with fibrin, hemosiderin, inflammatory cells, and a variable fibrovascular proliferation (Fig. 28–16). Similarly, nodular mesothelial proliferations of the pericardium can be seen and

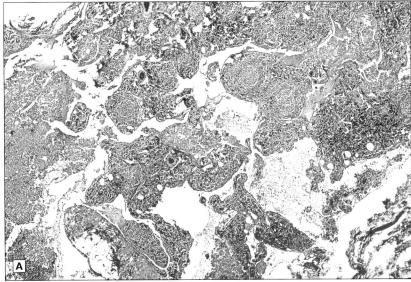

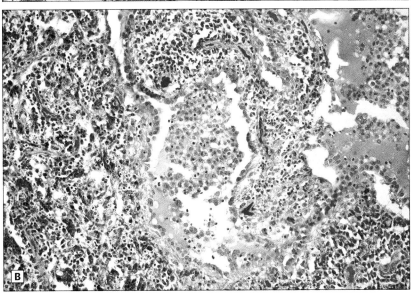

FIGURE 28–16 (A) Low-power view of reactive mesothelial hyperplasia in a hernial sac. **(B)** Reactive mesothelial proliferation admixed with chronic inflammatory cells and hemosiderin-laden macrophages.

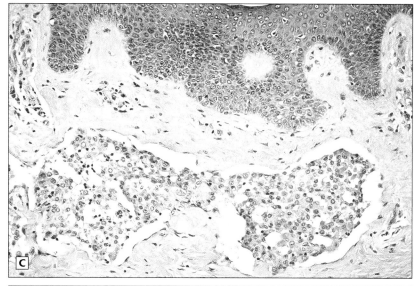

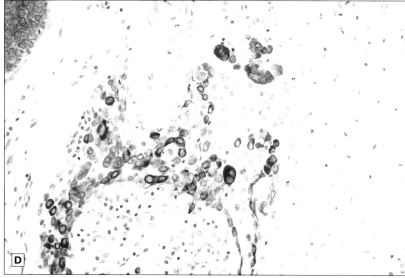

FIGURE 28–16 Continued. **(C)** Benign-appearing mesothelial cells within dermal lymphatics in the same case as that depicted in **A** and **B**. This lesion is easily mistaken for metastatic carcinoma. **(D)** Strong cytokeratin immunoreactivity in mesothelial cells in dermal lymphatic channels. The surrounding endothelial cells do not stain for this marker.

occasionally can lend consideration for a malignant mesothelioma.[137] These proliferations are composed of a mixed population of reactive mesothelial cells (cytokeratin-positive) and histiocytes (CD68-positive), with the relative proportion of each depending on the clinical setting.[138]

Several features are useful for distinguishing mesothelioma from reactive mesothelial hyperplasia (Table 28–7). Invasion into the underlying tissues is a useful indicator of mesothelioma but requires distinction from benign mesothelium, which may become entrapped in inflamed submesothelial connective tissue.[45,139,140] Entrapped benign mesothelial cells rarely extend deeper than the immediate subserosal fibrous layer, in contrast to mesothelioma, which shows more extensive and deeper invasion into the pleura (including subpleural adipose tissue), underlying chest wall, or lung, often accompanied by a desmoplastic stromal reaction. In

TABLE 28–7	FEATURES USEFUL IN THE SEPARATION OF REACTIVE MESOTHELIAL PROLIFERATIONS FROM MALIGNANT MESOTHELIOMA	
Feature	Reactive	Mesothelioma
Invasion	No stromal invasion (may have superficial entrapment)	Stromal invasion
Cellularity	May be densely cellular in pleural space but not in stroma	Dense cellularity in stroma
Zonation	Present, with progressive fibrosis toward chest wall	No zonation
Cytologic atypia	Minimal, confined to area of organization	Often present
Necrosis	Rare	May be present, usually a sign of malignancy

Modified from: Churg A, Colby TV, Cagle P, et al. Am J Surg Pathol 2000; 24:1183.

addition, malignant mesothelial cells show more nuclear atypia and more prominent nucleoli than is seen in reactive mesothelial cells. The presence of necrotic mesothelial cells also favors a diagnosis of mesothelioma. An excellent review of histologic features useful in separating benign and malignant mesothelial proliferations has been provided by the US-Canadian Mesothelioma Reference Panel.[45]

Immunohistochemical studies have found some differences between reactive mesothelial proliferations and mesothelioma, but the extent of overlap in the expression of these markers makes it difficult to endorse these stains for making this important distinction in the individual case. Most epithelial mesotheliomas exhibit extensive, strong linear membrane staining using antibodies to epithelial membrane antigen, in contrast to the weak or undetectable staining seen in reactive mesothelial hyperplasia.[141] However, a negative reaction does not exclude mesothelioma. Several studies have found a significant difference in frequency of p53 immunoreactivity in reactive and malignant mesothelial proliferations.[142,143] For example, Cagle et al.[142] found 19 of 40 mesotheliomas to be p53-positive, whereas all 13 areas of reactive mesothelial hyperplasia or organizing pleuritis were negative. Because only about 50% of mesotheliomas stain for p53 protein, a negative stain would be relatively meaningless in the individual case. Some have also found a higher percentage of proliferating cells detected by antibodies to proliferating cell nuclear antigen (PCNA) in mesotheliomas than in non-neoplastic mesothelium,[144] but again there is considerable overlap between reactive and malignant mesothelial proliferations.

Occasionally, collections of benign mesothelial cells are found in lymph nodes, mimicking metastatic mesothelioma. Although originally described in mediastinal lymph nodes,[145,146] benign mesothelial proliferations have also been described in abdominal lymph nodes found incidentally during staging procedures in patients with ovarian neoplasms.[147] In such cases there is also hyperplasia of peritoneal mesothelial cells, a common finding in patients with ovarian tumors. Collections of hyperplastic mesothelial cells have been reported in cervical and mediastinal lymph nodes in patients with pleural or pericardial effusions, presumably due to embolization via lymphatic channels.[148–151] Although metastatic mesothelioma in lymph nodes can occur in a sinusoidal distribution, features that suggest metastatic mesothelioma (rather than benign mesothelial proliferation) in lymph nodes include the identification of more than mild nuclear pleomorphism, tubulopapillary and alveolar patterns, and sclerosis.

Distinction of diffuse mesothelioma from *adenocarcinoma* and other primary or metastatic epithelial neoplasms is the most difficult diagnostic problem. Adenocarcinomas, particularly peripheral pulmonary adenocarcinomas, can show extensive pleural involvement and may be composed of large cells bearing a close resemblance to mesothelioma. These tumors, however, arise invariably in the pulmonary parenchyma, a feature that may be evident on CT scans. Moreover, in contradistinction to mesothelioma, the intracellular mucin produced by many of these tumors stains well with PAS; in most instances the cells stain positively with CEA, Ber-Ep4, Leu-M1, MOC-31 or B72.3. This also applies to metastases of occult carcinomas of the breast, ovary, and other visceral organs, which are usually multiple and involve both lungs. A detailed clinical history may prove helpful in some of these cases. In the peritoneal cavity, distinguishing epithelial peritoneal mesothelioma from *peritoneal* or *ovarian serous carcinomas* may also be difficult (Fig. 28–17). Again, a battery of immunostains including B72.3, Ber-Ep4, Leu-M1, calretinin, thrombomodulin,

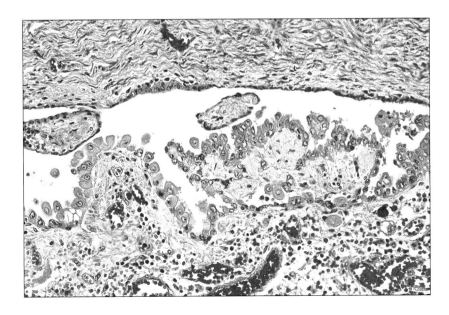

FIGURE 28–17 Diffuse epithelial mesothelioma attached to the surface of the ovary. Such tumors may be confused with ovarian or peritoneal serous adenocarcinoma.

and cytokeratin 5/6 is useful for this distinction, as previously discussed.

Fibrous (sarcomatoid) mesothelioma

The differential diagnosis of fibrous mesothelioma depends on the cellularity of the lesion. Hypocellular regions of desmoplastic mesothelioma may be difficult to distinguish from reactive *fibrosis* or *pleural plaques*, particularly in small biopsy specimens. Invasion of the subserosal connective tissues, chest wall, or lung parenchyma by neoplastic spindle cells is a highly sensitive, specific feature of desmoplastic malignant mesothelioma. In subtle cases, invasion of the underlying tissues may be highlighted by immunohistochemical stains for low-molecular-weight cytokeratins.[73] Because reactive submesothelial fibroblasts are frequently cytokeratin-positive, identification of staining in spindle cells in a thickened pleural lesion is of no diagnostic value. Bland necrosis characterized by necrotic foci accompanied by few if any inflammatory cells is a specific feature of desmoplastic malignant mesothelioma, but it lacks sensitivity, as this feature is found in the minority of cases.[73] The presence of frankly sarcomatoid areas, characterized by spindle cells with marked hyperchromasia and nuclear pleomorphism, may also be useful for this distinction. Features useful for recognizing fibrous pleurisy include cellular zonation, with the more cellular areas oriented toward the luminal side of the pleura, and a proliferation of capillaries oriented perpendicular to the pleural surface (Table 28–8). Certainly, radiographic studies may be extremely useful in this distinction.

More cellular examples of fibrous mesothelioma must be distinguished from benign and malignant variants of *solitary fibrous tumor*. Solitary fibrous tumor typically presents as a pedunculated, well-circumscribed mass composed of alternating hyper- and hypocellular zones with cytologically bland, patternless spindle cells deposited in a fibrous matrix. Immunohistochemically, the cells of solitary fibrous tumor uniformly express CD34 and rarely stain for cytokeratins. Malignant variants have a variable histologic appearance and may resemble a fibrosarcoma or a high-grade pleomorphic sarcoma. Immunostaining for CD34 is less consistent in these lesions, but stains for cytokeratins are typically negative. One must also consider the possibility of a sarcoma that has metastasized to the pleura; the clinical history and radiographic data are most useful in this regard.

Biphasic mesothelioma

The differential diagnosis for biphasic mesothelioma is limited, given the biphasic nature of this tumor. There is some resemblance to *biphasic synovial sarcoma*, but mesotheliomas are characterized by a mixture of epithelial and sarcomatous components that usually blend with one another such that transitional areas may be seen. Furthermore, it differs from most biphasic synovial sarcomas by the absence of intracellular PAS-positive mucin. In questionable cases, molecular genetic evaluation can be performed to detect the presence or absence of t(X;18), characteristic of synovial sarcoma.

Prognosis and therapy

The outlook is grave, and most patients with diffuse mesothelioma die of the disease within 1–2 years of diagnosis. The median survival in the Surveillance, Epidemiology and End Results (SEER) database is only 7 months, and this has not improved over the past two decades.[11] Survival rates vary slightly according to tumor type, as most studies have found slightly longer survival for patients with diffuse epithelial mesothelioma compared to those with biphasic or sarcomatoid tumors.[152,153] Survival periods are equally short or even shorter for those with diffuse fibrous (sarcomatoid) mesothelioma with extensive desmoplasia, with an even higher frequency of metastasis than found in non-desmoplastic tumors.[74] As the disease progresses, symptoms become increasingly severe, and many patients die of respiratory failure or intestinal obstruction. Additional complications are caused by extension of the tumor into neighboring tissues (e.g., lung, chest wall, diaphragm, intestinal wall, retroperitoneum) and by recurrence, sometimes along the needle tract of a previous aspiration or needle biopsy or the scar of a previous excision. Metastases do occur but at a relatively late stage of the disease. The most common sites of metastasis include the regional lymph nodes, especially those in the mediastinum, abdomen, and supraclavicular region, and the liver, lungs, adrenal glands, and bone marrow. Sometimes lymph node metastases are the first manifestation of the disease. Parameters aside from sarcomatoid histology which have been reported to be adverse prognostic indicators include male gender,[153] advanced age,[152,154] poor performance status,[153] high white blood cell count,[153,154] advanced stage,[154,155]

TABLE 28–8	FEATURES USEFUL IN THE SEPARATION OF FIBROUS PLEURISY FROM DESMOPLASTIC MESOTHELIOMA	
Feature	Fibrous pleurisy	Desmoplastic mesothelioma
Cellularity	Highest cellularity immediately beneath effusion	Paucicellular
Zonation	Present, with increased fibrosis away from effusion	Lacks zonation
Vascularity	Capillaries perpendicular to pleural surface	Capillaries not conspicuous
Invasion	No stromal invasion	Stromal invasion

Modified from: Churg A, Colby TV, Cagle P, et al. Am J Surg Pathol 2000; 24:1183.

TABLE 28–9	**REPORTED UNFAVORABLE PROGNOSTIC FACTORS FOR MALIGNANT PLEURAL MESOTHELIOMA**

Sarcomatoid type
High preoperative tumor volume
Poor performance status
Advanced age
Advanced stage
Male gender
High white blood cell count
Aneuploidy

TABLE 28–10	**BRIGHAM STAGING SYSTEM FOR MALIGNANT PLEURAL MESOTHELIOMA**

Stage	Definition
I	Confined to within capsule of parietal pleura: ipsilateral pleura, lung, pericardium, diaphragm, or chest wall disease limited to previous biopsy sites
II	Same as stage I plus positive intrathoracic lymph nodes
III	Local extension of disease into the chest wall or mediastinum, heart, or throughout the diaphragm or peritoneum; with or without extrathoracic or contralateral lymph node involvement
IV	Distant metastases

Modified from Sugarbaker DJ, Strauss GM, Lynch TJ, et al. Node status has prognostic significance in the multimodality therapy of diffuse, malignant mesothelioma. J Clin Oncol 1993; 11:1172.

pleural location,[152,154] and high preoperative tumor volume[156] (Tables 28–9, 28–10).

As is evident from the survival rates, treatment is rarely effective, although remissions have been achieved. Single-modality therapy has not influenced survival, although palliation may be provided by surgery, chemotherapy, or radiation therapy alone. Multimodality treatment with cytoreductive surgery (pleurectomy/decortication or extrapleural pneumonectomy) followed by chemotherapy and radiotherapy appears to prolong survival.[157–159] Several studies have also found that extrapleural pneumonectomy in combination with chemotherapy and postoperative radiation therapy in carefully selected patients results in a median survival of 24 months, and up to 20% show no evidence of disease at 5 years.[160,161] Furthermore, due to improvements in surgical techniques and postoperative management, surgical morbidity and mortality have decreased substantially over the past decade. For those patients who are not candidates for surgical resection, thorascopic talc poudrage has been found to be a safe primary palliative therapy with low morbidity.[162]

Although numerous chemotherapeutic agents have been evaluated in this setting, the combination of the anti-folate pemetrexed and cisplatin seems to be particularly active, and recent studies suggest an impact on survival.[163] Other regimens including the thymidelate synthase inhibitor raltitrexed have been similarly promising.[164,165] It is not clear whether these agents are best given in an adjuvant or neoadjuvant setting. The role of these chemotherapeutic agents in peritoneal mesothelioma is equally promising.[166]

The tendency for mesotheliomas to remain localized until late in their course and the relatively poor survival with conventional therapy has led to the unique opportunity to develop novel therapies that might affect survival. Mesothelioma cells secrete a variety of soluble factors, including transforming growth factor-β (TGFβ) and interleukin-6 (IL-6), which inhibit host immunity.[167–169] Attempts to inhibit secretion of these soluble factors, thereby allowing the host immune system to eradicate the tumor, have been attempted in vitro and in vivo, in some cases as part of multimodality therapy.[170] Mesotheliomas also overexpress the receptor tyrosine kinase *c-met* and EGFR, suggesting that specific small molecule inhibitors might have some role in the future treatment of this lethal disease.[171,172] Other potential targets include platelet-derived growth factors A and B (PDGF), vascular endothelial growth factor (VEGF) and mesothelin, a cell surface glycoprotein that is overexpressed in most epithelial mesotheliomas.[173,174] Recently, several serum tumor markers have been characterized which may have a role in monitoring response to treatment.[175,176] In a study from Australia of 44 patients with mesothelioma, 37 (84%) had elevated serum mesothelin-related protein levels compared with only 3 (2%) of 160 patients with other cancers or pleuropulmonary inflammatory disorders and 0 of 28 controls.[177] Even more potentially exciting, Pass and colleagues found serum osteopontin levels to separate patients with asbestos exposure with pleural mesothelioma from those with asbestos exposure without mesothelioma.[178]

WELL-DIFFERENTIATED PAPILLARY MESOTHELIOMA

The well-differentiated papillary mesothelioma, a rare mesothelial tumor, is sometimes referred to as *benign mesothelioma*, but given that some examples of this tumor pursue an aggressive clinical course, the more descriptive term *well-differentiated papillary mesothelioma* is preferred. The lesions are solitary or multifocal and are primarily located in the peritoneum of women in the third and fourth decades of life, with a predilection for the omentum, mesentery, and pelvis.[179,180] They may also arise from the tunica vaginalis,[181–184] pleura[185] and pericardium.[186] Many are incidental findings at autopsy or surgical exploration done for unrelated reasons.[187–189]

Histologically, the lesion is characterized by a proliferation of uniform, cuboidal cells with centrally placed nuclei and inconspicuous nucleoli that line well-formed papillary structures (Figs 28–18, 28–19). In some cases,

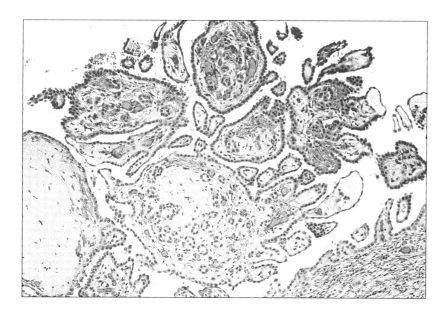

FIGURE 28–18 Low-power view of a well-differentiated papillary mesothelioma of the peritoneum. Papillary structures are lined by a single layer of cuboidal cells. Similar-appearing cells line tubules in the papillary cores.

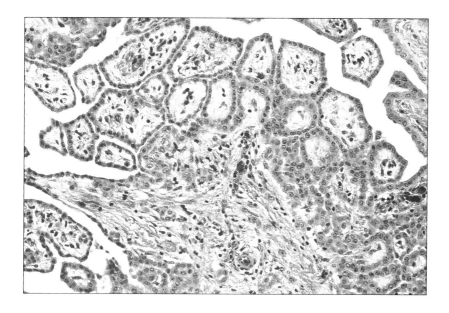

FIGURE 28–19 Cytologically bland mesothelial cells line papillary structures in a well-differentiated papillary mesothelioma of the peritoneum.

the neoplastic cells form solid nests, tubules, or cords in the connective tissue stroma. Rarely, the features of papillary mesothelioma are associated with those of an adenomatoid tumor.[190] Multinucleated stromal giant cells with nucleoli arranged in a floret-like fashion may be present.[191] Mitotic figures are absent or rare. Some cases show prominent myxoid change.[192] The immunohistochemical and electron microscopic features of the lining cells are typical of well-differentiated mesothelial cells.[193,194]

In our experience, localized, solitary tumors that have uniformly histologically benign features behave in a predictably benign fashion. Solitary tumors with slightly atypical cytologic features probably can also be expected to behave in a benign fashion if they are completely excised and are localized to one anatomic site.[191] Tumors that are widespread are much more likely to pursue a

progressive clinical course and cannot be reliably regarded as benign neoplasms.[195] Although there are reports of patients with widespread papillary mesotheliomas with histologically benign features that have behaved in a clinically benign fashion,[179] long-term follow-up is generally lacking in these cases. Some of these lesions recur, often after many years, or progress to malignant mesothelioma with occasional distant metastases. In the study of nine cases of well-differentiated papillary mesothelioma with complete follow-up by Butnor and colleagues, six had clinically indolent tumors, but one patient died 3 years after diagnosis with radiographic evidence of disease progression.[180] Areas resembling well-differentiated papillary mesothelioma may be seen in diffuse malignant mesothelioma, albeit as a focal finding, suggesting the possibility of tumor progression.

The presence of ascites and clinical symptoms other than those attributable to torsion of a pedunculated tumor should raise the possibility of a malignancy.

Unlike diffuse malignant mesothelioma, there is no clear link between asbestos exposure and the development of well-differentiated papillary mesothelioma. Of the 14 patients studied by Butnor et al, six (42%) had a history of asbestos exposure, including three patients with pleural plaques.[180]

Treatment depends upon the distribution of the lesions. Some patients can be adequately treated by laparoscopic resection, particularly those with small solitary lesions.[196] Patients with diffuse disease or those with atypical histologic features should be considered candidates for adjuvant chemotherapy.[197] Given the potentially aggressive clinical course, it is reasonable to consider this tumor to be of low malignant potential, as opposed to completely benign.

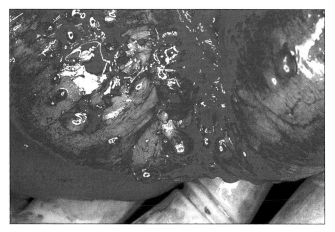

FIGURE 28–20 Multicystic mesothelioma diffusely involving the serosal surface of the intestine.

MULTICYSTIC PERITONEAL MESOTHELIOMA

"Multicystic peritoneal mesothelioma" has been used to describe an unusual mesothelial lesion that deserves separate consideration because of its characteristic histologic picture and its benign behavior. In the past this lesion was often confused with cystic lymphangioma, mesenteric lymphatic cyst in basal cell nevus syndrome (despite its different clinical course), diffuse mesothelioma or even a disseminated form of mucin-producing adenocarcinoma. First described by Plaut in 1928 as "loose cysts of the pelvis,"[198] this lesion has been referred to by a variety of names, including peritoneal inclusion cyst,[199] peritoneal cystosis,[200] benign cystic mesothelioma,[201] and multicystic mesothelial proliferation,[202,203] reflecting the controversial pathogenesis of this lesion.

Multicystic peritoneal mesothelioma occurs chiefly in adults, with a predilection for young and middle-aged women. It is usually noted because it produces vague lower abdominal pain or symptoms suggesting partial intestinal obstruction, such as distension, nausea, or vomiting. Rare patients present with an acute abdomen or ascites.[204,205] The symptoms of the disease are relatively non-specific, and a correct preoperative diagnosis is rarely rendered.

Exploratory laparotomy reveals a characteristic picture: numerous thin-walled transparent cysts are unevenly distributed in the serosal and subserosal tissues of the parietal and visceral peritoneum of the abdomen and pelvis, often forming multicystic masses (Fig. 28–20). The lesions have a propensity to arise on the surface of the uterus, cul-de-sac, bladder, or rectum. Rarely, these lesions can occur on the surface of the omentum,[206] pericardium,[207] appendix[208] or liver.[209] The cysts measure a few millimeters in diameter to several centimeters and contain clear

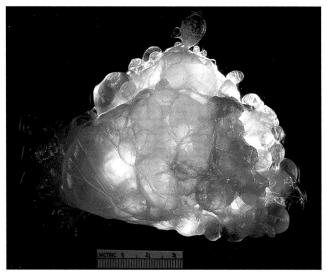

FIGURE 28–21 Multicystic peritoneal mesothelioma consisting of multiple transparent, fluid-filled cysts.

or blood-tinged fluid (Fig. 28–21). Occasionally, there are also multiple filamentous and string-like adhesions between the peritoneum, intestines, and viscera.[204]

Microscopic examination discloses one or more variously sized, round or irregularly shaped cystic spaces lined by a single layer of flattened or cuboidal mesothelial cells, sometimes displaying a brush border (Figs 28–22, 28–23). Less commonly, the cells are plump and protrude into the lumen in a hobnail or even papillary pattern. Focal squamous metaplasia is seen occasionally. The cystic spaces are separated by loose, edematous tissue often containing chronic inflammatory cells, fibrin deposits, and sometimes entrapped mesothelial cells resembling infiltrating carcinoma (so-called mural nodules) (Fig. 28–24). Transition between multicystic mesothelioma and adenomatoid tumor has been observed on several occasions (Fig. 28–25).[210,211] Unusual features

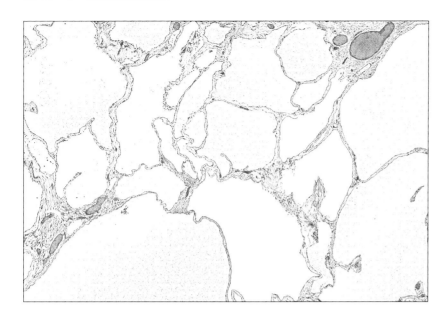

FIGURE 28–22 Multicystic mesothelioma composed of numerous mesothelial-lined cysts embedded in a delicate fibrovascular stroma.

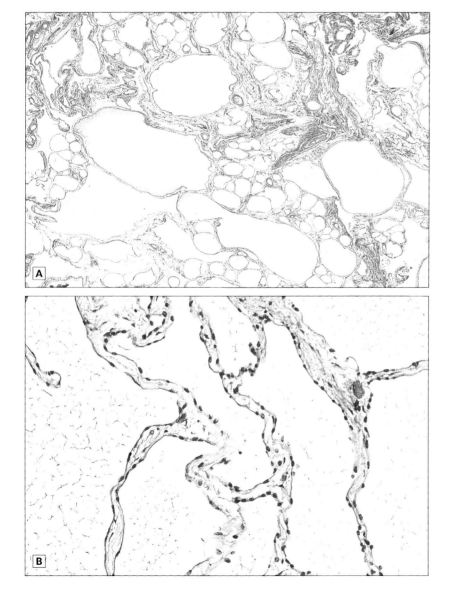

FIGURE 28–23 (A) Low-power view of a multicystic peritoneal mesothelioma mimicking a cystic lymphangioma. **(B)** Cysts are lined by cytologically bland flattened and cuboidal mesothelial cells.

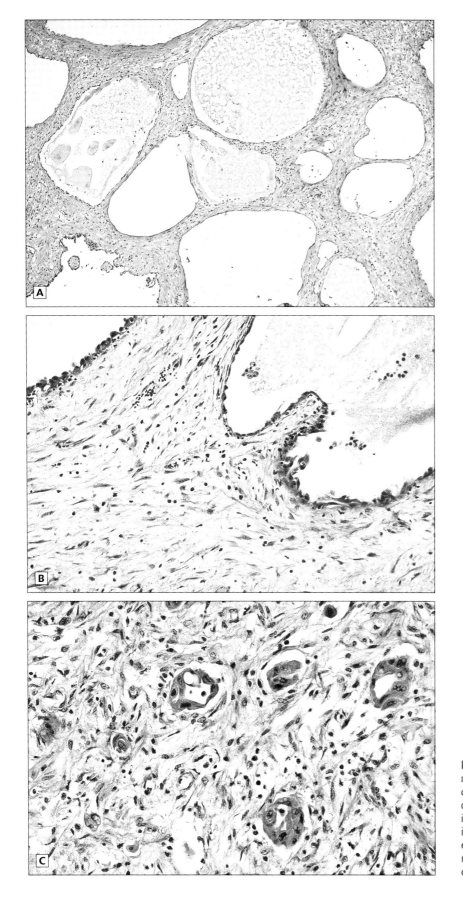

FIGURE 28–24 (A) Multicystic mesothelioma with secondary inflammatory changes. Rare cysts contain detached clumps of mesothelial cells. **(B)** Mesothelial spaces lie in an edematous, spindled stroma containing inflammatory cells. **(C)** Mesothelial cells entrapped in the wall of a multicystic mesothelioma closely mimicking infiltrating carcinoma.

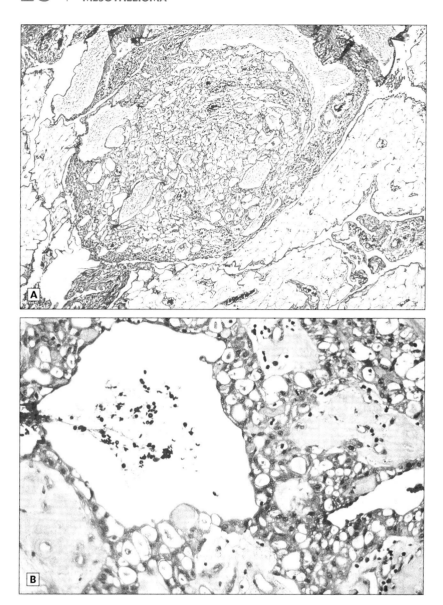

FIGURE 28–25 Low-power **(A)** and high-power **(B)** views of a multicystic mesothelioma with foci resembling adenomatoid tumor.

include the presence of extracellular or intracellular hyaline globules[212] and calcifications.[213] The secreted material in the spaces stains positively with Alcian blue and colloidal iron but negatively with PAS. Similarly staining material is found as a thin coating on the luminal surface of the tumor cells (Fig. 28–26) and rarely as small intracellular droplets.

Like other forms of mesothelioma the lining cells are immunoreactive for cytokeratins, epithelial membrane antigen, and a number of other markers which are typically expressed in mesothelial cells (cytokeratin 5/6, calretinin, thrombomodulin, among others).[202,214] The expression of these markers helps to exclude cystic lymphangioma as a diagnostic consideration. Moreover, cystic lymphangioma occurs chiefly in male children and adolescents and microscopically is characterized by stromal aggregates of lymphocytes and an endothelial lining

occasionally positive for factor VIII-related antigen and negative for cytokeratins. A layer of smooth muscle tissue may surround the vascular structures. Other conditions that must be considered in the differential diagnosis are reactive mesothelial proliferations, well-differentiated papillary mesothelioma, ovarian and extraovarian papillary serous carcinomas, endometriosis, and microcystic adenoma of the pancreas (Fig. 28–27).

Electron microscopic studies reveal the ultrastructural characteristics of mesothelial cells,[215] especially slender microvilli on the luminal surfaces of the lining cells, well-developed basal laminae, and tight desmosomal junctions (Fig. 28–28). There are also numerous intracytoplasmic filaments, ovoid mitochondria, and prominent rough endoplasmic reticulum (Fig. 28–29).

The clinical course is largely that of a benign lesion (Table 28–11). Among 25 patients with follow-up

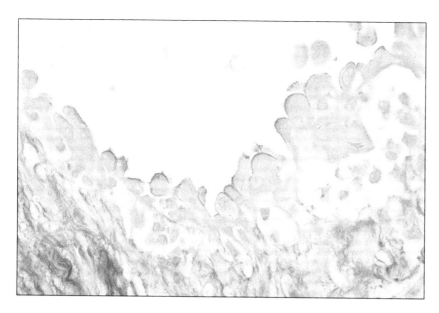

FIGURE 28–26 Colloidal iron stain showing a thin coating on the luminal surface of tumor cells in a multicystic mesothelioma.

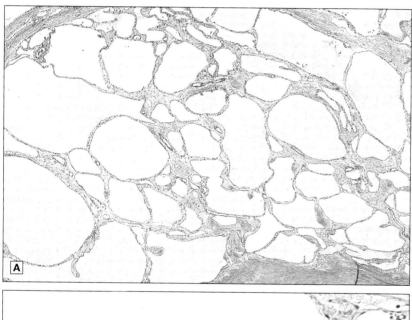

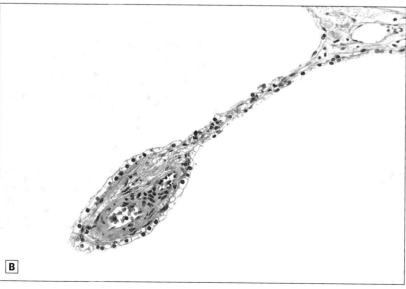

FIGURE 28–27 (A) Low-power view of a microcystic adenoma of the pancreas closely resembling multicystic mesothelioma. **(B)** Microcystic adenoma of the pancreas composed of cysts lined by cuboidal cells with vacuolated cytoplasm.

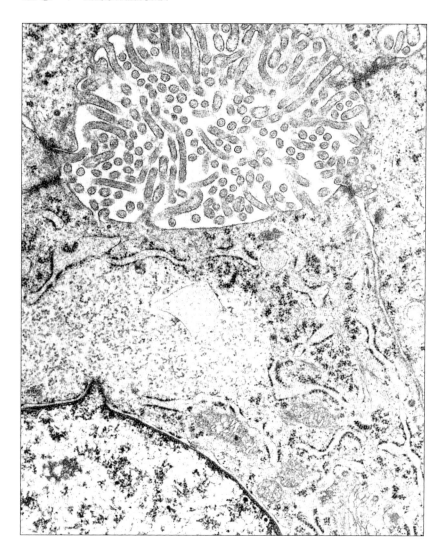

FIGURE 28–28 Electron microscopic view of a multicystic peritoneal mesothelioma showing intercellular space with numerous slender microvilli and deposits of intracellular glycogen. (From Mennemeyer R, Smith M. Multicystic, peritoneal mesothelioma: a report with electron microscopy of a case mimicking intra-abdominal cystic hygroma (lymphangioma). Cancer 1979; 44:692.)

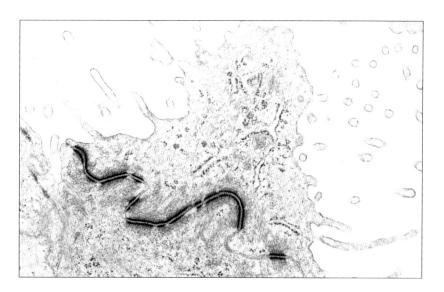

FIGURE 28–29 Electron microscopic view of a multicystic peritoneal mesothelioma with slender microvilli, prominent tight desmosomal junctions, and converging microfilaments. (From Mennemeyer R, Smith M. Multicystic, peritoneal mesothelioma: a report with electron microscopy of a case mimicking intra-abdominal cystic hygroma (lymphangioma). Cancer 1979; 44:692.)

TABLE 28–11	RELATION BETWEEN EXTENT OF MULTICYSTIC MESOTHELIOMA AT DIAGNOSIS AND CLINICAL OUTCOME				
Extent of disease	No. of patients	Alive	Died of disease	Died of other causes	No follow-up
Solitary	6	3	1*	0	2
Localized	15	7	0	8	0
Diffuse	16	11	1†	2	2
Total	37	21	2	10	4

*Combined cystic/epithelial mesothelioma.
†Patient refused therapy.
From Weiss SW, Tavassoli FA. Multicystic mesothelioma: an analysis of pathologic findings and biologic behavior in 37 cases. Am J Surg Pathol 1988; 12:737.

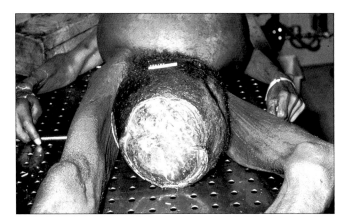

FIGURE 28–30 Multicystic peritoneal mesothelioma in a 47-year-old man. The patient refused therapy and died 12 years after initial detection of the tumor.

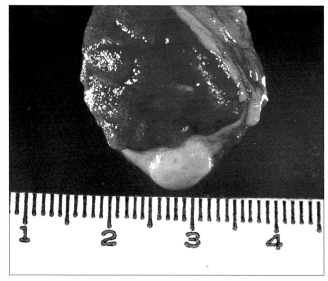

FIGURE 28–31 Adenomatoid tumor of the epididymis.

information reported by Weiss and Tavassoli,[204] 21 were alive, 2 died of other causes, and 2 died of the disease. The two patients who died were an infant who had a mixture of cystic and diffuse epithelial mesothelioma and a 47-year-old man who refused therapy and died 12 years after detection of the abdominal mass (Fig. 28–30).

The appropriate therapy seems to be total surgical excision for localized lesions and subtotal resection or debulking procedures for more extensive lesions.[204] Sometimes, the large number of lesions and their small size preclude complete resection, with further spread and recurrence years after the initial excision.[216] Rare cases have also been treated with laser therapy, sclerotherapy and transvaginal catheter drainage.[217,218]

The pathogenesis of this unusual lesion is not clear. The multiplicity of lesions, their spread and recurrence, and the transitions which may be seen with adenomatoid tumor and rarely diffuse malignant mesothelioma support the contention that this is a neoplasm, even though 30–50% of patients have a history of abdominal surgery, pelvic inflammatory disease, or endometriosis.[219,220] The fact that this tumor is rare in the pleura[203] and is only occasionally associated with occupational asbestos exposure suggests significant pathogenetic differences from the conventional form of diffuse malignant mesotheli-oma. Finally, it is possible that there is a genetic component, as this tumor has been described in siblings.[221]

ADENOMATOID TUMOR

Adenomatoid tumor is a clinically benign mesothelial neoplasm usually confined to the genital tract. In men it most commonly is found in the epididymis (Fig. 28–31) but may also be observed in the spermatic cord, testicular tunic, prostate, ejaculatory duct, and the parenchyma of the testis.[222–224] In women the lesion is most commonly seen in the uterus (Fig. 28–32) and fallopian tubes, but it may occur in the ovary.[225–227] This lesion can rarely arise in extragenital sites, including the small bowel mesentery,[228] heart,[229,230] pleura,[231,232] pancreas,[233] mediastinum,[234] lymph node,[235] and especially the adrenal gland.[236–238] Its mesothelial origin, first suggested by Masson et al. in 1942,[239] is now firmly established, but the earlier noncommittal term *adenomatoid tumor*, coined by Golden and Ash[240] in 1945, is still widely employed to distinguish this tumor from the rare papillary mesothelioma.

Clinical findings

The tumor presents as a small indurated mass or swelling that is painless and nontender. It is usually an incidental finding at routine examination, surgery for some other cause (hysterectomy), or autopsy. It rarely occurs before the age of 20 years and is chiefly encountered in patients 30–60 years of age. The tumor is usually solitary, but multiple nodular lesions have been observed. A small number of these lesions in the scrotum are associated with hydroceles.

Pathologic findings

Gross examination reveals a firm, well-circumscribed mass generally less than 2 cm in greatest dimension, which reveals a smooth, glistening, yellow-gray cut surface. On microscopic examination the tumor is seen to have a variable structural pattern ranging from irregularly arranged, dilated tubular channels and gland-like spaces lined by flattened or cuboidal cells to solid nests and strands of plump cells with abundant eosinophilic cytoplasm (Figs 28–33, 28–34). As in other mesothelial tumors, desquamated cells are often present in the dilated spaces. The fibrous stroma may be sparse or abundant and may contain aggregates of lymphocytes. The smooth muscle component, which is present and even conspicuous in some cases, is likely residual. Some cases show prominent cystic change and may even show features that overlap with those of multicystic mesothelioma.[234,241,242] Rarely, these tumors can show evidence of infarctive necrosis, which can obscure the characteristic features and even suggest malignancy.[243]

Ultrastructurally, the cells show characteristic features of mesothelial cells, including long, bushy microvilli on the luminal surfaces and intercellular spaces, irregular cytoplasmic protrusions, and desmosomes, often associated with tonofibrils.[244,245] Like mesothelial cells at other sites, the cells stain positively for cytokeratins, calretinin, thrombomodulin, D2-40, WT-1, HMBE-1, OC-125 and cytokeratin 5/6, among others (Fig. 28–35).[226,238,246–248] Otis reported Ber-Ep4 in 9 of 11 adenomatoid tumors and cautioned that staining with this antibody does not exclude an adenomatoid tumor.[249]

The tumor is benign, and local resection is adequate therapy. There are no reports of malignant transformation. As mentioned earlier in this chapter, some diffuse malignant mesotheliomas have a prominent adenomatoid growth pattern, but the cytologic features of the cells in such cases are overtly malignant.

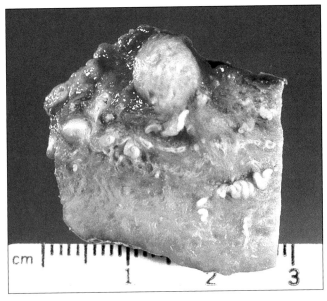

FIGURE 28–32 Adenomatoid tumor in the myometrium of a 44-year-old woman.

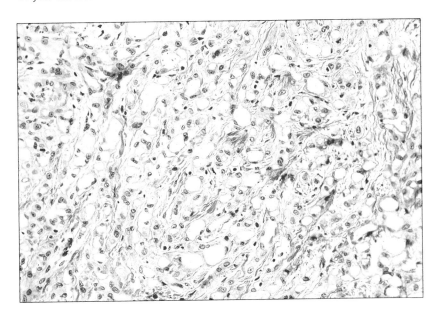

FIGURE 28–33 Benign mesothelioma of the genital tract (adenomatoid tumor) with a characteristic tubular pattern.

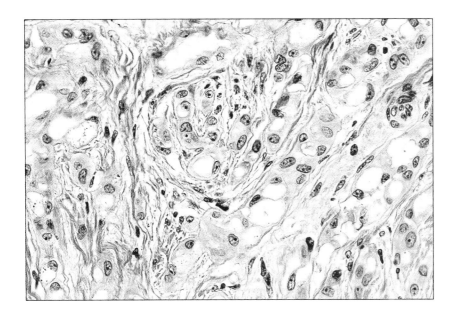

FIGURE 28–34 High-power view showing bland cytologic features of the mesothelial cells in an adenomatoid tumor.

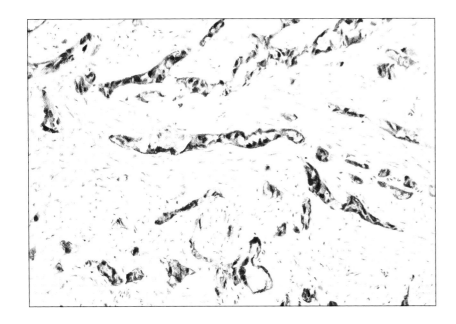

FIGURE 28–35 Diffuse calretinin immunoreactivity in an adenomatoid tumor of the fallopian tube.

REFERENCES

1. Geschickter CF. Mesothelial tumors. Am J Cancer 1936; 26:378.
2. Adami JG. Principles of pathology. Philadelphia: Lea & Febiger; 1908.
3. Klemperer P, Rabin CB. Primary neoplasms of the pleura: A report of five cases. Arch Pathol 1931; 11:385.
4. Wagner JC, Sleegs CA, Marchand P. Diffuse pleural mesothelioma and asbestos exposure in the North Western Cape Province. Br J Ind Med 1960; 17:260.
5. Burdorf A, Jarvholm B, Englund A. Explaining differences in incidence rates of pleural mesothelioma between Sweden and the Netherlands. Int J Cancer 2005; 113:298.

Histologic classification

6. Crotty TB, Myers JL, Katzenstein AL, et al. Localized malignant mesothelioma. A clinicopathologic and flow cytometric study. Am J Surg Pathol 1994; 18:357.
7. Leigh J, Rogers AJ, Ferguson DA, et al. Lung asbestos fiber content and mesothelioma cell type, site, and survival. Cancer 1991; 68:135.
8. Hillerdal G. Malignant mesothelioma 1982: Review of 4710 published cases. Br J Dis Chest 1983; 77:321.

Diffuse malignant mesothelioma

9. Price B, Ware A. Mesothelioma trends in the United States: an update based on surveillance, epidemiology, and end results program data for 1973 through 2003. Am J Epidemiol 2004; 159:107.
10. Edwards BK, Brown ML, Wingo PA, et al. Annual report to the nation on the status of cancer, 1975–2002, featuring population-based trends in cancer treatment. J Natl Cancer Inst 2005; 97:1407.
11. Antman K, Hassan R, Eisner M, et al. Update on malignant mesothelioma. Oncology (Williston Park) 2005; 19:1301.
12. Adams VI, Unni KK, Muhm JR, et al. Diffuse malignant mesothelioma of pleura. Diagnosis and survival in 92 cases. Cancer 1986; 58:1540.
13. Antman KH. Natural history and epidemiology of malignant mesothelioma. Chest 1993; 103:373S.
14. Sterman DH, Albelda SM. Advances in the diagnosis, evaluation, and management of malignant pleural mesothelioma. Respirology 2005; 10:266.
15. Baker PM, Clement PB, Young RH. Malignant peritoneal mesothelioma in women: a study of 75 cases with emphasis on their morphologic spectrum and differential diagnosis. Am J Clin Pathol 2005; 123:724.
16. Kerrigan SA, Turnnir RT, Clement PB, et al. Diffuse malignant epithelial mesotheliomas of the peritoneum in women: a clinicopathologic study of 25 patients. Cancer 2002; 94:378.

17. Kannerstein M, Churg J. Peritoneal mesothelioma. Hum Pathol 1977; 8:83.

18. Clement PB, Young RH, Scully RE. Malignant mesotheliomas presenting as ovarian masses. A report of nine cases, including two primary ovarian mesotheliomas. Am J Surg Pathol 1996; 20:1067.

19. Averbach AM, Sugarbaker PH. Peritoneal mesothelioma: treatment approach based on natural history. Cancer Treat Res 1996; 81:193.

20. Maruyama R, Sakai M, Nakamura T, et al. Triplet chemotherapy for malignant pericardial mesothelioma: a case report. Jpn J Clin Oncol 2006; 36:245.

21. Winstanley AM, Landon G, Berney D, et al. The immunohistochemical profile of malignant mesotheliomas of the tunica vaginalis: a study of 20 cases. Am J Surg Pathol 2006; 30:1.

22. Hassan R, Alexander R. Nonpleural mesotheliomas: mesothelioma of the peritoneum, tunica vaginalis, and pericardium. Hematol Oncol Clin North Am 2005; 19:1067.

23. Spiess PE, Tuziak T, Kassouf W, et al. Malignant mesothelioma of the tunica vaginalis. Urology 2005; 66:397.

24. Entwisle J. The use of magnetic resonance imaging in malignant mesothelioma. Lung Cancer 2004; 45(Suppl 1):S69.

25. Loggie BW. Malignant peritoneal mesothelioma. Curr Treat Options Oncol 2001; 2:395.

26. Puvaneswary M, Chen S, Proietto T. Peritoneal mesothelioma: CT and MRI findings. Australas Radiol 2002; 46:91.

27. Benamore RE, O'Doherty MJ, Entwisle JJ. Use of imaging in the management of malignant pleural mesothelioma. Clin Radiol 2005; 60:1237.

28. Stewart D, Waller D, Edwards J, et al. Is there a role for pre-operative contrast-enhanced magnetic resonance imaging for radical surgery in malignant pleural mesothelioma? Eur J Cardiothorac Surg 2003; 24:1019.

29. Ambrosini V, Rubello D, Nanni C, et al. Additional value of hybrid PET/CT fusion imaging vs. conventional CT scan alone in the staging and management of patients with malignant pleural mesothelioma. Nucl Med Rev Cent East Eur 2005; 8:111.

30. Flores RM. The role of PET in the surgical management of malignant pleural mesothelioma. Lung Cancer 2005; 49:S27.

31. Rice DC, Erasmus JJ, Stevens CW, et al. Extended surgical staging for potentially resectable malignant pleural mesothelioma. Ann Thorac Surg 2005; 80:1988.

32. Castro CY, Chhieng DC. Cytology and surgical pathology of pleural cavities. Adv Exp Med Biol 2005; 563:55.

33. Selikoff IJ, Churg J, Hammond EC. Asbestos exposure and neoplasia. JAMA 1964; 188:22.

34. Baas P, van 't Hullenaar N, Wagenaar J, et al. Occupational asbestos exposure: how to deal with suspected mesothelioma cases – the Dutch approach. Ann Oncol 2006; 17:848.

35. Price B, Ware A. Mesothelioma: risk apportionment among asbestos exposure sources. Risk Anal 2005; 25:937.

36. Carbone M, Rdzanek MA. Pathogenesis of malignant mesothelioma. Clin Lung Cancer 52004; (Suppl 2):S46.

37. Hodgson JT, Darnton A. The quantitative risks of mesothelioma and lung cancer in relation to asbestos exposure. Ann Occup Hyg 2000; 44:565.

38. Suzuki Y, Yuen SR, Ashley R. Short, thin asbestos fibers contribute to the development of human malignant mesothelioma: pathological evidence. Int J Hyg Environ Health 2005; 208:201.

39. Gibbs AR, Griffiths DM, Pooley FD, et al. Comparison of fibre types and size distributions in lung tissues of paraoccupational and occupational cases of malignant mesothelioma. Br J Ind Med 1990; 47:621.

40. Pooley FD, Ranson DL. Comparison of the results of asbestos fibre dust counts in lung tissue obtained by analytical electron microscopy and light microscopy. J Clin Pathol 1986; 39:313.

41. Dodson RF, Graef R, Shepherd S, et al. Asbestos burden in cases of mesothelioma from individuals from various regions of the United States. Ultrastruct Pathol 2005; 29:415.

42. Shukla A, Gulumian M, Hei TK, et al. Multiple roles of oxidants in the pathogenesis of asbestos-induced diseases. Free Radic Biol Med 2003; 34:1117.

43. Lanphear BP, Buncher CR. Latent period for malignant mesothelioma of occupational origin. J Occup Med 1992; 34:718.

44. Smith MJ, Naylor B. A method for extracting ferruginous bodies from sputum and pulmonary tissue. Am J Clin Pathol 1972; 58:250.

45. Churg A, Colby TV, Cagle P, et al. The separation of benign and malignant mesothelial proliferations. Am J Surg Pathol 2000; 24:1183.

46. Friedrichs KH, Brockmann M, Fischer M, et al. Electron microscopy analysis of mineral fibers in human lung tissue. Am J Ind Med 1992; 22:49.

47. Baris YI, Grandjean P. Prospective study of mesothelioma mortality in Turkish villages with exposure to fibrous zeolite. J Natl Cancer Inst 2006; 98:414.

48. Kokturk N, Firat P, Akay H, et al. Prognostic significance of bax and fas ligand in erionite and asbestos induced Turkish malignant pleural mesothelioma. Lung Cancer 2005; 50:189.

49. Jaurand MC, Fleury-Feith J. Pathogenesis of malignant pleural mesothelioma. Respirology 2005; 10:2.

50. van Kaick G, Dalheimer A, Hornik S, et al. The German thorotrast study: recent results and assessment of risks. Radiat Res 1999; 152:S64.

51. Minami M, Kawauchi N, Yoshikawa K, et al. Malignancy associated with chronic empyema: radiologic assessment. Radiology 1991; 178:417.

52. Gentiloni N, Febbraro S, Barone C, et al. Peritoneal mesothelioma in recurrent familial peritonitis. J Clin Gastroenterol 1997; 24:276.

53. Carbone M, Pass HI. Re: Debate on the link between SV40 and human cancer continues. J Natl Cancer Inst 2002; 94:229.

54. Carbone M, Kratzke RA, Testa JR. The pathogenesis of mesothelioma. Semin Oncol 2002; 29:2.

55. Carbone M, Rizzo P, Pass H. Simian virus 40: the link with human malignant mesothelioma is well established. Anticancer Res 2000; 20:875.

56. Hicks J. Mesothelioma, mesothelial proliferations, and their mimics: a multimodal approach. Ultrastruct Pathol 2006; 30:1.

57. Carbone M, Pass HI, Rizzo P, et al. Simian virus 40-like DNA sequences in human pleural mesothelioma. Oncogene 1994; 9:1781.

58. Strickler HD, Goedert JJ, Fleming M, et al. Simian virus 40 and pleural mesothelioma in humans. Cancer Epidemiol Biomarkers Prev 1996; 5:473.

59. Dhaene K, Verhulst A, Van Marck E. SV40 large T-antigen and human pleural mesothelioma. Screening by polymerase chain reaction and tyramine-amplified immunohistochemistry. Virchows Arch 1999; 435:1.

60. Suzuki M, Toyooka S, Shivapurkar N, et al. Aberrant methylation profile of human malignant mesotheliomas and its relationship to SV40 infection. Oncogene 2005; 24:1302.

61. Baldi A, Groeger AM, Esposito V, et al. Expression of p21 in SV40 large T antigen positive human pleural mesothelioma: relationship with survival. Thorax 2002; 57:353.

62. Bianchi C, Brollo A, Ramani L, et al. Familial mesothelioma of the pleura – a report of 40 cases. Ind Health 2004; 42:235.

63. Shia J, Qin J, Erlandson RA, et al. Malignant mesothelioma with a pronounced myxoid stroma: a clinical and pathological evaluation of 19 cases. Virchows Arch 2005; 447:828.

64. Chang HT, Yantiss RK, Nielsen GP, et al. Lipid-rich diffuse malignant mesothelioma: a case report. Hum Pathol 2000; 31:876.

65. Miyamoto Y, Nakano S, Shimazaki Y, et al. Pericardial mesothelioma presenting as left atrial thrombus in a patient with mitral stenosis. Cardiovasc Surg 1996; 4:51.

66. Mayall FG, Gibbs AR. The histology and immunohistochemistry of small cell mesothelioma. Histopathology 1992; 20:47.

67. Nascimento AG, Keeney GL, Fletcher CD. Deciduoid peritoneal mesothelioma. An unusual phenotype affecting young females. Am J Surg Pathol 1994; 18:439.

68. Orosz Z, Nagy P, Szentirmay Z, et al. Epithelial mesothelioma with deciduoid features. Virchows Arch 1999; 434:263.

69. Shia J, Erlandson RA, Klimstra DS. Deciduoid mesothelioma: A report of 5 cases and literature review. Ultrastruct Pathol 2002; 26:355.

70. Mourra N, de Chaisemartin C, Goubin-Versini I, et al. Malignant deciduoid mesothelioma: a diagnostic challenge. Arch Pathol Lab Med 2005; 129:403.

71. Ordonez NG. Epithelial mesothelioma with deciduoid features: report of four cases. Am J Surg Pathol 2000; 24:816.

72. Shanks JH, Harris M, Banerjee SS, et al. Mesotheliomas with deciduoid morphology: a morphologic spectrum and a variant not confined to young females. Am J Surg Pathol 2000; 24:285.

73. Mangano WE, Cagle PT, Churg A, et al. The diagnosis of desmoplastic malignant mesothelioma and its distinction from fibrous pleurisy: a histologic and immunohistochemical analysis of 31 cases including p53 immunostaining. Am J Clin Pathol 1998; 110:191.

74. Cantin R, Al-Jabi M, McCaughey WT. Desmoplastic diffuse mesothelioma. Am J Surg Pathol 61982; :215.

75. Crotty TB, Colby TV, Gay PC, et al. Desmoplastic malignant mesothelioma masquerading as sclerosing mediastinitis: a diagnostic dilemma. Hum Pathol 1992; 23:79.

76. Wilson GE, Hasleton PS, Chatterjee AK. Desmoplastic malignant mesothelioma: a review of 17 cases. J Clin Pathol 1992; 45:295.

77. Salgado RA, Corthouts R, Parizel PM, et al. Malignant pleural mesothelioma with heterologous osteoblastic elements: computed tomography, magnetic resonance, and positron emission tomography imaging characteristics of a rare tumor. J Comput Assist Tomogr 2005; 29:653.

78. Yousem SA, Hochholzer L. Malignant mesotheliomas with osseous and cartilaginous differentiation. Arch Pathol Lab Med 1987; 111:62.

79. Henderson DW, Attwood HD, Constance TJ, et al. Lymphohistiocytoid mesothelioma: a rare lymphomatoid variant of predominantly sarcomatoid mesothelioma. Ultrastruct Pathol 1988; 12:367.

80. Khalidi HS, Medeiros LJ, Battifora H. Lymphohistiocytoid mesothelioma. An often misdiagnosed variant of sarcomatoid malignant mesothelioma. Am J Clin Pathol 2000; 113:649.

81. McDonald JC, Armstrong B, Case B, et al. Mesothelioma and asbestos fiber type. Evidence

from lung tissue analyses. Cancer 1989; 63:1544.

82. Allen TC, Cagle PT, Churg AM, et al. Localized malignant mesothelioma. Am J Surg Pathol 2005; 29:866.

83. Silcocks PB, Herbert A, Wright DH. Evaluation of PAS-diastase and carcinoembryonic antigen staining in the differential diagnosis of malignant mesothelioma and papillary serous carcinoma of the ovary. J Pathol 1986; 149:133.

84. Bollinger DJ, Wick MR, Dehner LP, et al. Peritoneal malignant mesothelioma versus serous papillary adenocarcinoma. A histochemical and immunohistochemical comparison. Am J Surg Pathol 1989; 13:659.

85. Roggli VL, Kolbeck J, Sanfilippo F. Pathology of human mesothelioma: etiology and diagnostic considerations. Pathol Annu 1987; 22:91.

86. Leong AS, Stevens MW, Mukherjee TM. Malignant mesothelioma: cytologic diagnosis with histologic, immunohistochemical, and ultrastructural correlation. Semin Diagn Pathol 1992; 9:141.

87. King JE, Thatcher N, Pickering CA, et al. Sensitivity and specificity of immunohistochemical markers used in the diagnosis of epithelioid mesothelioma: A detailed systematic analysis using published data. Histopathology 2006; 48:223.

88. Ordonez NG. The immunohistochemical diagnosis of mesothelioma: a comparative study of epithelioid mesothelioma and lung adenocarcinoma. Am J Surg Pathol 2003; 27:1031.

89. Brockstedt U, Gulyas M, Dobra K, et al. An optimized battery of eight antibodies that can distinguish most cases of epithelial mesothelioma from adenocarcinoma. Am J Clin Pathol 2000; 114:203.

90. Comin CE, Novelli L, Boddi V, et al. Calretinin, thrombomodulin, CEA, and CD15: a useful combination of immunohistochemical markers for differentiating pleural epithelial mesothelioma from peripheral pulmonary adenocarcinoma. Hum Pathol 2001; 32:529.

91. Oates J, Edwards C. HBME-1, MOC-31, WT1 and calretinin: an assessment of recently described markers for mesothelioma and adenocarcinoma. Histopathology 2000; 36:341.

92. Carella R, Deleonardi G, D'Errico A, et al. Immunohistochemical panels for differentiating epithelial malignant mesothelioma from lung adenocarcinoma: a study with logistic regression analysis. Am J Surg Pathol 2001; 25:43.

93. Gonzalez-Lois C, Ballestin C, Sotelo MT, et al. Combined use of novel epithelial (MOC-31) and mesothelial (HBME-1) immunohistochemical markers for optimal first line diagnostic distinction between mesothelioma and metastatic carcinoma in pleura. Histopathology 2001; 38:528.

94. Roberts F, Harper CM, Downie I, et al. Immunohistochemical analysis still has a limited role in the diagnosis of malignant mesothelioma. A study of thirteen antibodies. Am J Clin Pathol 2001; 116:253.

95. Abutaily AS, Addis BJ, Roche WR. Immunohistochemistry in the distinction between malignant mesothelioma and pulmonary adenocarcinoma: A critical evaluation of new antibodies. J Clin Pathol 2002; 55:662.

96. Ordonez NG. Immunohistochemical diagnosis of epithelioid mesothelioma: an update. Arch Pathol Lab Med 2005; 129:1407.

97. Ordonez NG. D2-40 and podoplanin are highly specific and sensitive immunohistochemical markers of epithelioid malignant mesothelioma. Hum Pathol 2005; 36:372.

98. Ordonez NG. Application of mesothelin immunostaining in tumor diagnosis. Am J Surg Pathol 2003; 27:1418.

99. Ordonez NG. Immunohistochemical diagnosis of epithelioid mesotheliomas: a critical review of old markers, new markers. Hum Pathol 2002; 33:953.

100. Yaziji H, Battifora H, Barry TS, et al. Evaluation of 12 antibodies for distinguishing epithelioid mesothelioma from adenocarcinoma: identification of a three-antibody immunohistochemical panel with maximal sensitivity and specificity. Mod Pathol 2006; 19:514.

101. Ordonez NG. Value of immunohistochemistry in distinguishing peritoneal mesothelioma from serous carcinoma of the ovary and peritoneum: a review and update. Adv Anat Pathol 2006; 13:16.

102. Ordonez NG. The diagnostic utility of immunohistochemistry and electron microscopy in distinguishing between peritoneal mesotheliomas and serous carcinomas: A comparative study. Mod Pathol 2006; 19:34.

103. Doglioni C, Tos AP, Laurino L, et al. Calretinin: a novel immunocytochemical marker for mesothelioma. Am J Surg Pathol 1996; 20:1037.

104. Attanoos RL, Webb R, Dojcinov SD, et al. Value of mesothelial and epithelial antibodies in distinguishing diffuse peritoneal mesothelioma in females from serous papillary carcinoma of the ovary and peritoneum. Histopathology 2002; 40:237.

105. Reis-Filho JS, Simpson PT, Martins A, et al. Distribution of p63, cytokeratins 5/6 and cytokeratin 14 in 51 normal and 400 neoplastic human tissue samples using TARP-4 multi-tumor tissue microarray. Virchows Arch 2003; 443:122.

106. Trupiano JK, Geisinger KR, Willingham MC, et al. Diffuse malignant mesothelioma of the peritoneum and pleura: analysis of markers. Mod Pathol 2004; 17:476.

107. Chu AY, Litzky LA, Pasha TL, et al. Utility of D2-40, a novel mesothelial marker, in the diagnosis of malignant mesothelioma. Mod Pathol 2005; 18:105.

108. Al-Hussaini M, Stockman A, Foster H, et al. WT-1 assists in distinguishing ovarian from uterine serous carcinoma and in distinguishing between serous and endometrioid ovarian carcinoma. Histopathology 2004; 44:109.

109. Goldstein NS, Uzieblo A. WT1 immunoreactivity in uterine papillary serous carcinomas is different from ovarian serous carcinomas. Am J Clin Pathol 2002; 117:541.

110. Hashi A, Yuminamochi T, Murata S, et al. Wilms tumor gene immunoreactivity in primary serous carcinomas of the fallopian tube, ovary, endometrium, and peritoneum. Int J Gynecol Pathol 2003; 22:374.

111. Ordonez NG. Value of estrogen and progesterone receptor immunostaining in distinguishing between peritoneal mesotheliomas and serous carcinomas. Hum Pathol 2005; 36:1163.

112. Lindgren PR, Cajander S, Backstrom T, et al. Estrogen and progesterone receptors in ovarian epithelial tumors. Mol Cell Endocrinol 2004; 221:97.

113. Barnetson RJ, Burnett RA, Downie I, et al. Immunohistochemical analysis of peritoneal mesothelioma and primary and secondary serous carcinoma of the peritoneum: antibodies to estrogen and progesterone receptors are useful. Am J Clin Pathol 2006; 125:67.

114. Ordonez NG. Role of immunohistochemistry in distinguishing epithelial peritoneal mesotheliomas from peritoneal and ovarian serous carcinomas. Am J Surg Pathol 1998; 22:1203.

115. Riera JR, Astengo-Osuna C, Longmate JA, et al. The immunohistochemical diagnostic panel for epithelial mesothelioma: a reevaluation after heat-induced epitope retrieval. Am J Surg Pathol 1997; 21:1409.

116. King JE, Hasleton PS. Immunohistochemistry and the diagnosis of malignant mesothelioma. Histopathology 2001; 38:471.

117. Attanoos RL, Dojcinov SD, Webb R, et al. Anti-mesothelial markers in sarcomatoid mesothelioma and other spindle cell neoplasms. Histopathology 2000; 37:224.

118. Oury TD, Hammar SP, Roggli VL. Ultrastructural features of diffuse malignant mesotheliomas. Hum Pathol 1998; 29:1382.

119. Hammar SP. Macroscopic, histologic, histochemical, immunohistochemical, and ultrastructural features of mesothelioma. Ultrastruct Pathol 2006; 30:3.

120. Warhol MJ, Corson JM. An ultrastructural comparison of mesotheliomas with adenocarcinomas of the lung and breast. Hum Pathol 1985; 16:50.

121. Dardick I, Jabi M, McCaughey WT, et al. Diffuse epithelial mesothelioma: a review of the ultrastructural spectrum. Ultrastruct Pathol 1987; 11:503.

122. Sandberg AA, Bridge JA. Updates on the cytogenetics and molecular genetics of bone and soft tissue tumors. Mesothelioma. Cancer Genet Cytogenet 2001; 127:93.

123. Lee WC, Testa JR. Somatic genetic alterations in human malignant mesothelioma (review). Int J Oncol 1999; 14:181.

124. Ribotta M, Roseo F, Salvio M, et al. Recurrent chromosome 6 abnormalities in malignant mesothelioma. Monaldi Arch Chest Dis 1998; 53:228.

125. Balsara BR, Bell DW, Sonoda G, et al. Comparative genomic hybridization and loss of heterozygosity analyses identify a common region of deletion at 15q11.1-15 in human malignant mesothelioma. Cancer Res 1999; 59:450.

126. Scattone A, Pennella A, Gentile M, et al. Comparative genomic hybridization (CGH) in malignant deciduoid mesothelioma. J Clin Pathol 2006; 59:764.

127. Simon F, Johnen G, Krismann M, et al. Chromosomal alterations in early stages of malignant mesotheliomas. Virchows Arch 2005; 447:762.

128. Xiao GH, Beeser A, Chernoff J, et al. p21-activated kinase links Rac/Cdc42 signaling to merlin. J Biol Chem 2002; 277:883.

129. Lopez-Rios F, Chuai S, Flores R, et al. Global gene expression profiling of pleural mesotheliomas: overexpression of aurora kinases and P16/CDKN2A deletion as prognostic factors and critical evaluation of microarray-based prognostic prediction. Cancer Res 2006; 66:2970.

130. Xiao GH, Gallagher R, Shetler J, et al. The NF2 tumor suppressor gene product, merlin, inhibits cell proliferation and cell cycle progression by repressing cyclin D1 expression. Mol Cell Biol 2005; 25:2384.

131. Baser ME, De Rienzo A, Altomare D, et al. Neurofibromatosis 2 and malignant mesothelioma. Neurology 2002; 59:290.

132. Burmeister B, Schwerdtle T, Poser I, et al. Effects of asbestos on initiation of DNA damage, induction of DNA-strand breaks, P53-expression and apoptosis in primary, SV40-transformed and malignant human mesothelial cells. Mutat Res 2004; 558:81.

133. Scharnhorst V, van der Eb AJ, Jochemsen AG. WT1 proteins: functions in growth and differentiation. Gene 2001; 273:141.

134. Ungar S, Van de Meeren A, Tammilehto L, et al. High levels of MDM2 are not correlated with the presence of wild-type p53 in human

malignant mesothelioma cell lines. Br J Cancer 1996; 74:1534.

135. Papp T, Schipper H, Pemsel H, et al. Mutational analysis of N-ras, p53, p16INK4a, p14ARF and CDK4 genes in primary human malignant mesotheliomas. Int J Oncol 2001; 18:425.

136. Rosai J, Dehner LP. Nodular mesothelial hyperplasia in hernia sacs: a benign reactive condition simulating a neoplastic process. Cancer 1975; 35:165.

137. Luthringer DJ, Virmani R, Weiss SW, et al. A distinctive cardiovascular lesion resembling histiocytoid (epithelioid) hemangioma. Evidence suggesting mesothelial participation. Am J Surg Pathol 1990; 14:993.

138. Ordonez NG, Ro JY, Ayala AG. Lesions described as nodular mesothelial hyperplasia are primarily composed of histiocytes. Am J Surg Pathol 1998; 22:285.

139. Cagle PT, Churg A. Differential diagnosis of benign and malignant mesothelial proliferations on pleural biopsies. Arch Pathol Lab Med 2005; 129:1421.

140. Henderson DW, Shilkin KB, Whitaker D. Reactive mesothelial hyperplasia vs mesothelioma, including mesothelioma in situ: a brief review. Am J Clin Pathol 1998; 110:397.

141. Cury PM, Butcher DN, Corrin B, et al. The use of histological and immunohistochemical markers to distinguish pleural malignant mesothelioma and in situ mesothelioma from reactive mesothelial hyperplasia and reactive pleural fibrosis. J Pathol 1999; 189:251.

142. Cagle PT, Brown RW, Lebovitz RM. p53 immunostaining in the differentiation of reactive processes from malignancy in pleural biopsy specimens. Hum Pathol 1994; 25:443.

143. Mullick SS, Green LK, Ramzy I, et al. p53 gene product in pleural effusions. Practical use in distinguishing benign from malignant cells. Acta Cytol 1996; 40:855.

144. Ramael M, Jacobs W, Weyler J, et al. Proliferation in malignant mesothelioma as determined by mitosis counts and immunoreactivity for proliferating cell nuclear antigen (PCNA). J Pathol 1994; 172:247.

145. Brooks JS, LiVolsi VA, Pietra GG. Mesothelial cell inclusions in mediastinal lymph nodes mimicking metastatic carcinoma. Am J Clin Pathol 1990; 93:741.

146. Rutty GN, Lauder I. Mesothelial cell inclusions within mediastinal lymph nodes. Histopathology 1994; 25:483.

147. Clement PB, Young RH, Oliva E, et al. Hyperplastic mesothelial cells within abdominal lymph nodes: mimic of metastatic ovarian carcinoma and serous borderline tumor – a report of two cases associated with ovarian neoplasms. Mod Pathol 1996; 9:879.

148. Suarez-Vilela D, Izquierdo-Garcia FM. Hyperplastic mesothelial cells in mediastinal lymph node sinuses. Arch Pathol Lab Med 2000; 124:1749.

149. Suarez Vilela D, Izquierdo Garcia FM. Embolization of mesothelial cells in lymphatics: the route to mesothelial inclusions in lymph nodes? Histopathology 1998; 33:570.

150. Parkash V, Vidwans M, Carter D. Benign mesothelial cells in mediastinal lymph nodes. Am J Surg Pathol 1999; 23:1264.

151. Argani P, Rosai J. Hyperplastic mesothelial cells in lymph nodes: report of six cases of a benign process that can stimulate metastatic involvement by mesothelioma or carcinoma. Hum Pathol 1998; 29:339.

152. Herndon JE, Green MR, Chahinian AP, et al. Factors predictive of survival among 337 patients with mesothelioma treated between 1984 and 1994 by the cancer and leukemia group B. Chest 1998; 113:723.

153. Curran D, Sahmoud T, Therasse P, et al. Prognostic factors in patients with pleural mesothelioma: the European Organization for Research and Treatment of Cancer experience. J Clin Oncol 1998; 16:145.

154. Antman K, Shemin R, Ryan L, et al. Malignant mesothelioma: prognostic variables in a registry of 180 patients, the Dana-Farber Cancer Institute and Brigham and Women's Hospital experience over two decades, 1965–1985. J Clin Oncol 1988; 6:147.

155. Sugarbaker DJ, Flores RM, Jaklitsch MT, et al. Resection margins, extrapleural nodal status, and cell type determine postoperative long-term survival in trimodality therapy of malignant pleural mesothelioma: results in 183 patients. J Thorac Cardiovasc Surg 1999; 117:54.

156. Pass HI, Temeck BK, Kranda K, et al. Preoperative tumor volume is associated with outcome in malignant pleural mesothelioma. J Thorac Cardiovasc Surg 1998; 115:310.

157. Sugarbaker PH, Yan TD, Stuart OA, et al. Comprehensive management of diffuse malignant peritoneal mesothelioma. Eur J Surg Oncol 2006; 32:686.

158. Bueno R. Multimodality treatments in the management of malignant pleural mesothelioma: an update [review] [36 refs]. Hematol Oncol Clin North Am 2005; 19:1089.

159. Flores RM. Induction chemotherapy, extrapleural pneumonectomy, and radiotherapy in the treatment of malignant pleural mesothelioma: the Memorial Sloan-Kettering experience. Lung Cancer 2005; 49:S71.

160. Weder W, Kestenholz P, Taverna C, et al. Neoadjuvant chemotherapy followed by extrapleural pneumonectomy in malignant pleural mesothelioma. J Clin Oncol 2004; 22:3451.

161. Sugarbaker DJ, Jaklitsch MT, Bueno R, et al. Prevention, early detection, and management of complications after 328 consecutive extrapleural pneumonectomies. J Thorac Cardiovasc Surg 2004; 128:138.

162. Aelony Y, Yao JF. Prolonged survival after talc poudrage for malignant pleural mesothelioma: case series. Respirology 2005; 10:649.

163. Vogelzang NJ, Rusthoven JJ, Symanowski J, et al. Phase III study of pemetrexed in combination with cisplatin versus cisplatin alone in patients with malignant pleural mesothelioma. J Clin Oncol 2003; 21:2636.

164. Bottomley A. Gaafa R. Manegold C. et al. EORTC Lung-Cancer Group. National Cancer Institute, Canada. Short-term treatment-related symptoms and quality of life: results from an international randomized phase III study of cisplatin with or without raltitrexed in patients with malignant pleural mesothelioma: an EORTC Lung-Cancer Group and National Cancer Institute, Canada, Intergroup study. J Clin Oncol 2006; 24:1435.

165. Porta C. Adding raltitrexed to cisplatin improves overall survival in people with malignant pleural mesothelioma. Cancer Treat Rev 2006; 32:229.

166. Janne PA, Wozniak AJ, Belani CP, et al. Open-label study of pemetrexed alone or in combination with cisplatin for the treatment of patients with peritoneal mesothelioma: outcomes of an expanded access program. Clin Lung Cancer 2005; 7:40.

167. Bielefeldt-Ohmann H, Jarnicki AG, Fitzpatrick DR. Molecular pathobiology and immunology of malignant mesothelioma. J Pathol 1996; 178:369.

168. Fitzpatrick DR, Peroni DJ, Bielefeldt-Ohmann H. The role of growth factors and cytokines in the tumorigenesis and immunobiology of malignant mesothelioma. Am J Respir Cell Mol Biol 1995; 12:455.

169. Fitzpatrick DR, Manning LS, Musk AW, et al. Potential for cytokine therapy of malignant mesothelioma. Cancer Treat Rev 1995; 21:273.

170. Pass HI, Temeck BK, Kranda K, et al. Phase III randomized trial of surgery with or without intraoperative photodynamic therapy and postoperative immunochemotherapy for malignant pleural mesothelioma. Ann Surg Oncol 1997; 4:628.

171. Mukohara T, Civiello G, Davis IJ, et al. Inhibition of the met receptor in mesothelioma. Clin Cancer Res 2005; 11:8122.

172. Jagadeeswaran R, Ma PC, Seiwert TY, et al. Functional analysis of c-Met/hepatocyte growth factor pathway in malignant pleural mesothelioma. Cancer Res 2006; 66:352.

173. Nowak AK, Lake RA, Kindler HL, et al. New approaches for mesothelioma: biologics, vaccines, gene therapy, and other novel agents. Semin Oncol 2002; 29:82.

174. Hassan R, Bera T, Pastan I. Mesothelin: a new target for immunotherapy. Clin Cancer Res 2004; 10:3937.

175. Hassan R, Remaley AT, Sampson ML, et al. Detection and quantitation of serum mesothelin, a tumor marker for patients with mesothelioma and ovarian cancer. Clin Cancer Res 2006; 12:447.

176. Robinson BW, Creaney J, Lake R, et al. Soluble mesothelin-related protein – a blood test for mesothelioma. Lung Cancer 2005; 49(Suppl 1):S109.

177. Robinson BW, Creaney J, Lake R, et al. Mesothelin-family proteins and diagnosis of mesothelioma. Lancet 2003; 362:1612.

178. Pass HI, Lott D, Lonardo F, et al. Asbestos exposure, pleural mesothelioma, and serum osteopontin levels. N Engl J Med 2005; 353:1564.

Well-differentiated papillary mesothelioma

179. Daya D, McCaughey WT. Well-differentiated papillary mesothelioma of the peritoneum. A clinicopathologic study of 22 cases. Cancer 1990; 65:292.

180. Butnor KJ, Sporn TA, Hammar SP, et al. Well-differentiated papillary mesothelioma. Am J Surg Pathol 2001; 25:1304.

181. Chetty R. Well differentiated (benign) papillary mesothelioma of the tunica vaginalis. J Clin Pathol 1992; 45:1029.

182. Cabay RJ, Siddiqui NH, Alam S. Paratesticular papillary mesothelioma: a case with borderline features. Arch Pathol Lab Med 2006; 130:90.

183. Perez-Ordonez B, Srigley JR. Mesothelial lesions of the paratesticular region. Semin Diagn Pathol 2000; 17:294.

184. Xiao SY, Rizzo P, Carbone M. Benign papillary mesothelioma of the tunica vaginalis testis. Arch Pathol Lab Med 2000; 124:143.

185. Galateau-Salle F, Vignaud JM, Burke L, et al. Well-differentiated papillary mesothelioma of the pleura: a series of 24 cases. Am J Surg Pathol 2004; 28:534.

186. Sane AC, Roggli VL. Curative resection of a well-differentiated papillary mesothelioma of the pericardium. Arch Pathol Lab Med 1995; 119:266.

187. Hoekstra AV, Riben MW, Frumovitz M, et al. Well-differentiated papillary mesothelioma of the peritoneum: a pathological analysis and review of the literature. Gynecol Oncol 2005; 98:161.

188. Erkanli S, Kilicdag EB, Bolat F, et al. Well-differentiated papillary mesothelioma complicating endometrial carcinoma: a case report. Eur J Gynaecol Oncol 2004; 25:394.

189. Mangal R, Taskin O, Franklin R. An incidental diagnosis of well-differentiated papillary mesothelioma in a woman operated on for recurrent endometriosis. Fertil Steril 1995; 63:196.

190. Hanrahan JB. A combined papillary mesothelioma and adenomatoid tumor of the omentum; report of a case. Cancer 1963; 16:1497.

191. Goldblum J, Hart WR. Localized and diffuse mesotheliomas of the genital tract and

peritoneum in women. A clinicopathologic study of nineteen true mesothelial neoplasms, other than adenomatoid tumors, multicystic mesotheliomas, and localized fibrous tumors. Am J Surg Pathol 1995; 19:1124.

192. Diaz LK, Okonkwo A, Solans EP, et al. Extensive myxoid change in well-differentiated papillary mesothelioma of the pelvic peritoneum. Ann Diagn Pathol 2002; 6:164.

193. Gong Y, Ren R, Ordonez NG, et al. Fine needle aspiration cytology of well-differentiated papillary mesothelioma: A case report. Acta Cytol 2005; 49:537.

194. Hoekman K, Tognon G, Risse EK, et al. Well-differentiated papillary mesothelioma of the peritoneum: a separate entity. Eur J Cancer 1996; 32A:255.

195. Hejmadi R, Ganesan R, Kamal NG. Malignant transformation of a well-differentiated peritoneal papillary mesothelioma. Acta Cytol 2003; 47:517.

196. Porpora MG, Brancato V, D'Elia C, et al. Laparoscopic diagnosis and treatment of a well-differentiated papillary mesothelioma of the peritoneum. J Am Assoc Gynecol Laparosc 2002; 9:384.

197. Shukunami K, Hirabuki S, Kaneshima M, et al. Well-differentiated papillary mesothelioma involving the peritoneal and pleural cavities: successful treatment by local and systemic administration of carboplatin. Tumori 2000; 86:419.

Multicystic peritoneal mesothelioma

198. Plaut A. Multiple peritoneal cysts and their histogenesis. Arch Pathol 1928; 5:754.

199. Kagalwala DZ, Shankar S, Zota V, et al. Preoperative computed tomography-guided hookwire needle localization of a peritoneal multilocular inclusion cyst. J Comput Assist Tomogr 2005; 29:602.

200. Jacobson ES. Benign papillary peritoneal cystosis simulating serous cystadenocarcinoma of the ovary. Am J Obstet Gynecol 1974; 118:575.

201. Soreide JA, Soreide K, Korner H, et al. Benign peritoneal cystic mesothelioma. World J Surg 2006; 30:560.

202. De Rosa G, Donofrio V, Boscaino A, et al. Multicystic mesothelial proliferation: immunohistochemical, ultrastructural and DNA analysis of five cases. Virchows Arch A [Pathol Anat Histopathol] 1992; 421:379.

203. Ball NJ, Urbanski SJ, Green FH, et al. Pleural multicystic mesothelial proliferation. The so-called multicystic mesothelioma. Am J Surg Pathol 1990; 14:375.

204. Weiss SW, Tavassoli FA. Multicystic mesothelioma. An analysis of pathologic findings and biologic behavior in 37 cases. Am J Surg Pathol 1988; 12:737.

205. Moreira VF, Defarges V, Gonzalez Palacios F, et al. Benign peritoneal multicystic mesothelioma as a cause of ascites. Rev Clin Esp 1997; 197:384.

206. Horn LC, Schutz A, Heinemann K, et al. Multicystic peritoneal mesothelioma of the omentum. Eur J Obstet Gynecol Reprod Biol 2004; 116:246.

207. Drut R, Quijano G. Multilocular mesothelial inclusion cysts (so-called benign multicystic mesothelioma) of pericardium. Histopathology 1999; 34:472.

208. Bansal A, Zakhour HD. Benign mesothelioma of the appendix: an incidental finding in a case of sigmoid diverticular disease. J Clin Pathol 2006; 59:108.

209. Di Blasi A, Boscaino A, De Dominicis G, et al. Multicystic mesothelioma of the liver with secondary involvement of peritoneum and inguinal region. Int J Surg Pathol 2004; 12:87.

210. Chan JK, Fong MH. Composite multicystic mesothelioma and adenomatoid tumour of the uterus: different morphological manifestations of the same process? Histopathology 1996; 29:375.

211. Zamecnik M, Gomolcak P. Composite multicystic mesothelioma and adenomatoid tumor of the ovary: additional observation suggesting common histogenesis of both lesions. Cesk Patol 2000; 36:160.

212. Lamovec J, Sinkovec J. Multilocular peritoneal inclusion cyst (multicystic mesothelioma) with hyaline globules. Histopathology 1996; 28:466.

213. Hasan AK, Sinclair DJ. Case report: calcification in benign cystic peritoneal mesothelioma. Clin Radiol 1993; 48:66.

214. Datta RV, Paty PB. Cystic mesothelioma of the peritoneum. Eur J Surg Oncol 1997; 23:461.

215. Scucchi L, Mingazzini P, Di Stefano D, et al. Two cases of "multicystic peritoneal mesothelioma": description and critical review of the literature. Anticancer Res 1994; 14:715.

216. Bruni R, Nigita G, Pagani V, et al. Benign cystic mesothelioma with multiple recurrences: a clinical case. Chir Ital 2003; 55:757.

217. Rosen DM, Sutton CJ. Use of the potassium titanyl phosphate (KTP) laser in the treatment of benign multicystic peritoneal mesothelioma. Br J Obstet Gynaecol 1999; 106:505.

218. van der Klooster JM, Lambers MD, van Bommel EF, et al. Successful catheter drainage of recurrent benign multicystic mesothelioma of the peritoneum. Neth J Med 1997; 50:246.

219. McFadden DE, Clement PB. Peritoneal inclusion cysts with mural mesothelial proliferation. A clinicopathological analysis of six cases. Am J Surg Pathol 1986; 10:844.

220. Huter O, Brezinka C, Solder E, et al. Recurrent multicystic peritoneal mesothelioma in endometriosis of the pelvis. Geb Fran 1991; 51:856.

221. Tangjitgamol S, Erlichman J, Northrup H, et al. Benign multicystic peritoneal mesothelioma: case reports in the family with diverticulosis and literature review. Int J Gynecol Cancer 2005; 15:1101.

Adenomatoid tumor

222. Amin MB. Selected other problematic testicular and paratesticular lesions: Rete testis neoplasms and pseudotumors, mesothelial lesions and secondary tumors. Mod Pathol 2005; 18:S131.

223. Barry P, Chan KG, Hsu J, et al. Adenomatoid tumor of the tunica albuginea. Int J Urol 2005; 12:516.

224. Evans K. Rapidly growing adenomatoid tumor extending into testicular parenchyma mimics testicular carcinoma. Urology 2004; 64:589.

225. Ghossain MA, Chucrallah A, Kanso H, et al. Multilocular adenomatoid tumor of the ovary: ultrasonographic findings. J Clin Ultrasound 2005; 33:233.

226. Nogales FF, Isaac MA, Hardisson D, et al. Adenomatoid tumors of the uterus: an analysis of 60 cases. Int J Gynecol Pathol 2002; 21:34.

227. Sieunarine K, Cowie AS, Bartlett JD, et al. A novel approach in the management of a recurrent adenomatoid tumor of the uterus utilizing a Strassman technique. Int J Gynecol Cancer 2005; 15:671.

228. Craig JR, Hart WR. Extragenital adenomatoid tumor: evidence for the mesothelial theory of origin. Cancer 1979; 43:1678.

229. Groisman GM, Kerner H. Multicystic mesothelioma with endometriosis. Acta Obstet Gynecol Scand 1992; 71:642.

230. Natarajan S, Luthringer DJ, Fishbein MC. Adenomatoid tumor of the heart: report of a case. Am J Surg Pathol 1997; 21:1378.

231. Kaplan MA, Tazelaar HD, Hayashi T, et al. Adenomatoid tumors of the pleura. Am J Surg Pathol 1996; 20:1219.

232. Handra-Luca A, Couvelard A, Abd Alsamad I, et al. Adenomatoid tumor of the pleura. Case report. Ann Pathol 2000; 20:369.

233. Overstreet K, Wixom C, Shabaik A, et al. Adenomatoid tumor of the pancreas: a case report with comparison of histology and aspiration cytology. Mod Pathol 2003; 16:613.

234. Plaza JA, Dominguez F, Suster S. Cystic adenomatoid tumor of the mediastinum. Am J Surg Pathol 2004; 28:132.

235. Isotalo PA, Nascimento AG, Trastek VF, et al. Extragenital adenomatoid tumor of a mediastinal lymph node. Mayo Clin Proc 2003; 78:350.

236. Isotalo PA, Keeney GL, Sebo TJ, et al. Adenomatoid tumor of the adrenal gland: a clinicopathologic study of five cases and review of the literature. Am J Surg Pathol 2003; 27:969.

237. Fan SQ, Jiang Y, Li D, et al. Adenomatoid tumour of the left adrenal gland with concurrent left nephrolithiasis and left kidney cyst. Pathology 2005; 37:398.

238. Hamamatsu A, Arai T, Iwamoto M, et al. Adenomatoid tumor of the adrenal gland: case report with immunohistochemical study. Pathol Int 2005; 55:665.

239. Masson P, Riopelle JL, Simard LC. Le mesotheliome benin de la sphere genitale. Rev Can Biol 1942; 1:720.

240. Golden A, Ash JE. Adenomatous tumors of the genital tract. Am J Pathol 1945; 21:63.

241. Kim JY, Jung KJ, Sung NK, et al. Cystic adenomatoid tumor of the uterus. AJR Am J Roentgenol 2002; 179:1068.

242. Zamecnik M, Gomolcak P. Composite multicystic mesothelioma and adenomatoid tumor of the ovary: additional observation suggesting common histogenesis of both lesions. Cesk Patol 2000. 36:160.

243. Skinnider BF, Young RH. Infarcted adenomatoid tumor: a report of five cases of a facet of a benign neoplasm that may cause diagnostic difficulty. Am J Surg Pathol 2004; 28:77.

244. Hes O, Perez-Montiel DM, Alvarado Cabrero I, et al. Thread-like bridging strands: a morphologic feature present in all adenomatoid tumors. Ann Diagn Pathol 2003; 7:273.

245. Garg K, Lee P, Ro JY, et al. Adenomatoid tumor of the adrenal gland: a clinicopathologic study of 3 cases. Ann Diagn Pathol 2005; 9:11.

246. Schwartz EJ, Longacre TA. Adenomatoid tumors of the female and male genital tracts express WT1. Int J Gynecol Pathol 2004; 23:123.

247. Isotalo PA, Yazdi HM, Perkins DG, et al. Immunohistochemical evidence for mesothelial origin of paratesticular adenomatoid tumour. Histopathology 2000; 37:476.

248. Delahunt B, Eble JN, King D, et al. Immunohistochemical evidence for mesothelial origin of paratesticular adenomatoid tumour. Histopathology 2000; 36:109.

249. Otis CN. Uterine adenomatoid tumors: immunohistochemical characteristics with emphasis on ber-EP4 immunoreactivity and distinction from adenocarcinoma. Int J Gynecol Pathol 1996; 15:146.

CHAPTER
29

BENIGN TUMORS OF PERIPHERAL NERVES

Benign tumors of peripheral nerves are relatively common lesions that differ from most soft tissue tumors in several important respects. Most soft tissue tumors arise from mesodermally derived tissue and display a range of features consonant with that lineage. Nerve sheath tumors arise from tissues considered to be of neuroectodermal or neural crest origin and display a range of features that mirror the various elements of the nerve (e.g., Schwann cell, perineurial cell) and, in rare instances, even appear epithelioid (e.g., epithelioid schwannoma). Whereas most soft tissue tumors only seem to be encapsulated by virtue of the compression of surrounding tissues against their advancing border, benign nerve sheath tumors arising in a nerve are completely surrounded by epi- or perineurium

and, therefore, have a true capsule, a feature that facilitates their enucleation. Finally, benign nerve sheath tumors represent the most important group of benign soft tissue lesions in which malignant transformation is an acknowledged phenomenon. Malignant peripheral nerve sheath tumors develop in preexisting neurofibromas in a subset of patients with neurofibromatosis 1, thereby providing an excellent model in which to study the molecular pathway of malignant transformation.

This chapter discusses the two principal benign nerve sheath tumors – schwannoma (formerly neurilemoma) and neurofibroma, their variations, and associated syndromes. The schwannoma recapitulates in a more or less consistent fashion the appearance of the differentiated Schwann cell, whereas the neurofibroma displays a spectrum of cell types ranging from the Schwann cell to the fibroblast. Although the early literature often blurred or minimized the differences between schwannomas and neurofibromas, they are distinctive lesions that can be reproducibly distinguished from one another in most instances by their pattern of growth, cellular composition, associated syndromes, and cytogenetic alterations (Table 29–1). The perineurioma is a more recently recognized tumor that mirrors the normal perineurial cell, a barrier cell of the nerve sheath recognized by certain characteristic ultrastructural and immunophenotypic features. Several pseudotumorous lesions of nerve (e.g., traumatic neuroma, Morton's neuroma, nerve sheath ganglion) and two rare tumors, extracranial meningioma and pigmented neuroectodermal tumor of infancy, are also discussed in this chapter. The last two tumors are difficult to classify and are included because of their usually benign behavior and presumed neural crest lineage.

EMBRYOGENESIS AND NORMAL ANATOMY

The peripheral nervous system can be defined as nervous tissue outside the brain and spinal cord. It is an extensive system which includes somatic and autonomic nerves, end-organ receptors, and supporting structures. It develops when axons lying close to one another grow out from

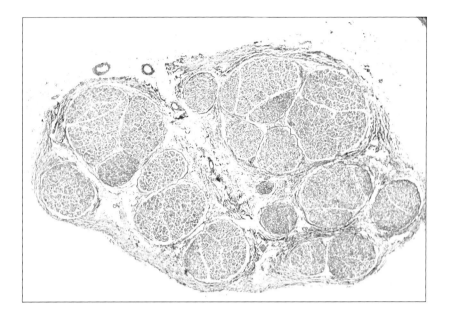

FIGURE 29–1 Normal sciatic nerve in cross-section. The entire nerve is surrounded by epineurium, and smaller nerve fascicles are encompassed by perineurium.

TABLE 29–1	COMPARISON OF SCHWANNOMA AND NEUROFIBROMA	
Parameter	**Schwannoma**	**Neurofibroma**
Age	20–50 years	20–40 years; younger in NF1
Common locations	Head-neck; flexor portion of extremities; less often retroperitoneum and mediastinum	Cutaneous nerves; deep locations in NF1
Encapsulation	Usually	Usually not
Growth patterns	Encapsulated tumor with Antoni A and B areas; plexiform type uncommon	Localized, diffuse and plexiform patterns
Associated syndromes	Most lesions sporadic; but some NF2, rarely NF1	Most lesions sporadic; some NF1
S-100 protein immunostaining	Strong and uniform	Variable staining of cells
Malignant transformation	Exceptionally rare	Rare in sporadic cases but occurs in 2–3% of NF1 patients

the neural tube and are gradually invested with Schwann cells. Schwann cells arise from the neural crest, a group of cells that arise from and lie lateral to the neural tube and underneath the ectoderm of the developing embryo. The major peripheral nerve trunks form by fusion and division of segmental spinal nerves and, therefore, often contain mixtures of sensory, motor, and autonomic elements. Precise identification of these elements is not always possible solely on morphologic grounds. As the peripheral nerves form, the Schwann cells migrate peripherally from the spinal ganglia, orient themselves parallel to the axons, and encase them with their cytoplasm. In myelinated fibers only one axon segment is encased by one Schwann cell, and synthesis and spiraling of the schwannian plasma membrane around the axon create the myelin sheath. However, discontinuities of the myelin sheath exist at those points where adjacent Schwann cells meet but where there is no lamination of the plasma membrane (nodes of Ranvier). In nonmyelinated nerves several axon segments are ensheathed by a common Schwann cell, but they are not enclosed beyond the initial stage of enfolding and therefore are invested with only a single or at most a few layers of schwannian plasma membrane. In humans the process of myelination commences during the eighteenth week of intrauterine life, is usually advanced by birth, and continues for several years postnatally.[1]

In the fully developed nerve a layer of connective tissue or epineurium surrounds the entire nerve trunk (Fig. 29–1). This structure varies in size depending of the location of the nerve, and it is composed of a mixture of collagen and elastic fibers along with mast cells. Several nerve fascicles lie within the confines of the epineurium, and each in turn is surrounded by a well-defined sheath known as the perineurium. These small nerve fascicles anticipate the subsequent division of the nerve into smaller branches, and for this reason the terms *epineurium* and *perineurium* can be used interchangeably when referring to small nerves. The smallest connective tissue unit of the nerve is the endoneurium, an intricate network of collagen, blood vessels, and fibroblasts encircling individual nerve fibers.

Considerable emphasis has been placed on the nature of the perineurium.[2] The outer portion of the perineurium consists of layers of connective tissue, and the inner portion is represented by a multilayered, concentrically arranged sheath of flattened cells. These cells, which are best defined by electron microscopy and immunohistochemistry, have been termed *perineurial fibroblasts, perineurial epithelium*, or simply *perineurial cells*. They are continuous with the pia-arachnoid of the central nervous system and appear to be important in maintaining a diffusion barrier for the peripheral nerve. It is not clear whether these cells are derived from Schwann cells, fibroblasts, or arachnoidal cells.[3,4] In contrast to Schwann cells, perineurial cells typically do not express S-100 protein but do express epithelial membrane antigen and claudin-1, a tight junction-associated protein, an immunophenotypic profile identical to pia-arachnoid cells. Ultrastructurally, they form close junctions with each other and have basal lamina along the endoneurial and perineurial aspects of the cell, features not encountered in the ordinary fibroblast and Schwann cell. The cytoplasm is rather poor in organelles except for the prominent, well-aligned pinocytotic vesicles along their surface and occasional myofilaments. Peculiar acellular, collagen-rich, whorled structures known as *Renaut's bodies* are occasionally found directly underneath the perineurium. Their significance is unknown, but their frequency near joints suggests a cushioning function.

Despite the undoubted importance of the investing connective tissue, the critical supporting element is the Schwann cell. It provides mechanical protection for the axon, produces and maintains the myelin sheath, and serves as a tube to guide regenerating nerve fibers. By light microscopy it is difficult to distinguish this cell from a fibroblast because their nuclei are similar. However, by electron microscopy a Schwann cell is easily identified by its intimate relation to its axons and by a continuous basal lamina that coats the surface of the cell facing the endoneurium. Current evidence suggests that the Schwann cell synthesizes this basal lamina and is capable of synthesizing collagen precursors.[5] Except for occasional 10 nm fibrils, microtubules, and mitochondria, other cytoplasmic organelles are not especially prominent except during periods of increased metabolism (e.g., myelin synthesis).[6] Pi granules, flattened lamellations of osmiophilic material, are occasionally present in a perinuclear location, but their significance is unknown. In routine preparations it is difficult to distinguish the axon from the myelin sheath. This distinction, however, is easily accomplished with special stains. Silver stains selectively stain the axon (Fig. 29–2), whereas stains such as Luxol fast blue stain myelin. The variation in diameter of axon and myelin sheath can be appreciated with these stains. In general, moderate or heavily myelinated fibers correspond to sensory and motor fibers with fast conduction speeds, whereas lightly myelinated or unmyelinated fibers correspond to autonomic fibers with slower conduction speeds.[6] Ultrastructurally, the cytoplasm of the axon is characterized by numerous cytoplasmic filaments, slender mitochondria, and a longitudinally oriented endoplasmic reticulum. Nissl substance, a feature of the nerve cell body, is not present in the axoplasm. In addition, small vesicles are observed occasionally; they may represent packets of neurotransmitter substance en route to the nerve terminal.

TRAUMATIC (AMPUTATION) NEUROMA

Traumatic neuroma is an exuberant but non-neoplastic proliferation of a nerve occurring in response to injury or surgery.[7–10] Under ideal circumstances the ends of a severed nerve re-establish continuity by an orderly growth of axons from proximal to distal stump through tubes of proliferating Schwann cells. However, if close apposition of the ends of nerve is not maintained or if there is no

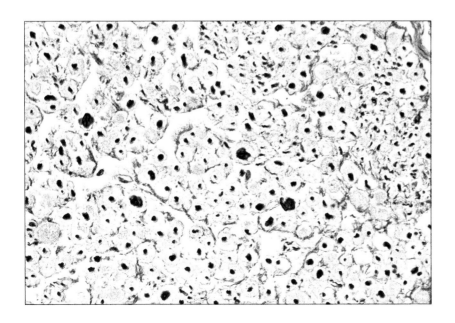

FIGURE 29–2 Normal peripheral nerve cut in cross-section and stained with Bodian (silver) stain. Individual axons stain positively; surrounding myelin sheath does not stain. The thickness of axons and the myelin sheath varies and determines the conduction speed.

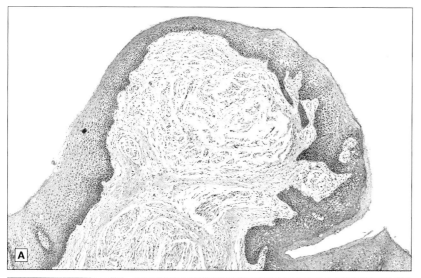

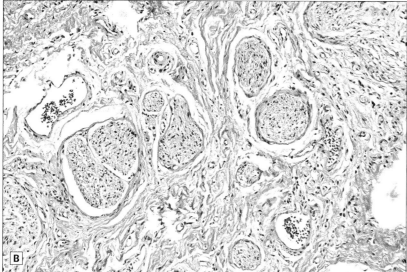

FIGURE 29–6 Mucosal neuroma from a patient with multiple endocrine neoplasia type IIb **(A)**. Irregular, convoluted nerves with prominent perineurium and focal myxoid change lie in submucosal tissue **(B)**.

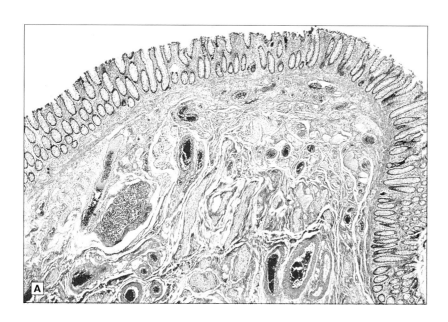

FIGURE 29–7 Ganglioneuromatosis of the gastrointestinal tract in a patient with MEN-IIb **(A)**.

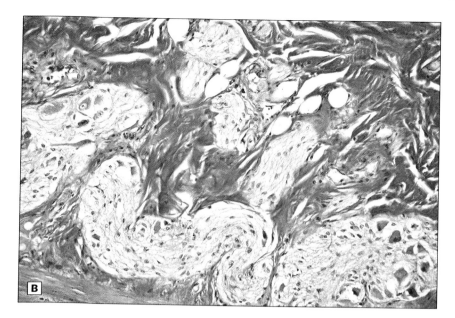

FIGURE 29–7 Continued. Autonomic nerves in the muscle wall are increased in size and number **(B)**.

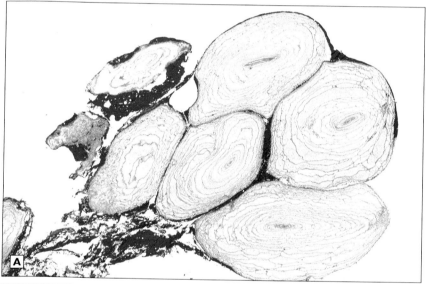

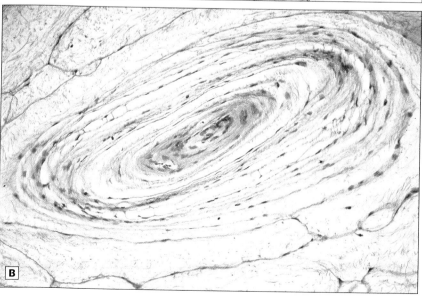

FIGURE 29–8 Pacinian neuroma **(A)**. High-power view **(B)**.

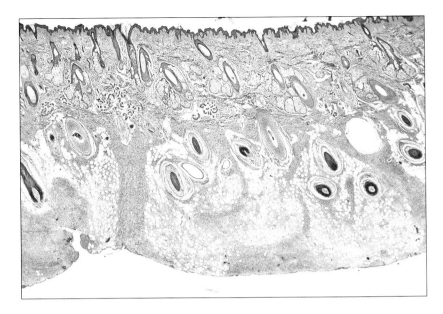

FIGURE 29–34 Diffuse neurofibroma with extensive permeation of subcutaneous tissue similar to a dermatofibrosarcoma protuberans.

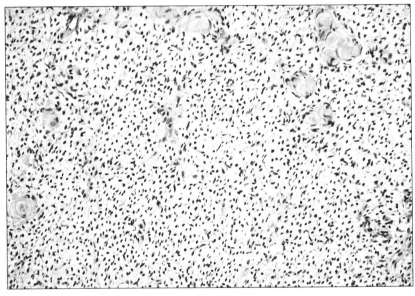

FIGURE 29–35 Diffuse neurofibroma showing the fine fibrillary collagenous background punctuated with Wagner-Meissner bodies.

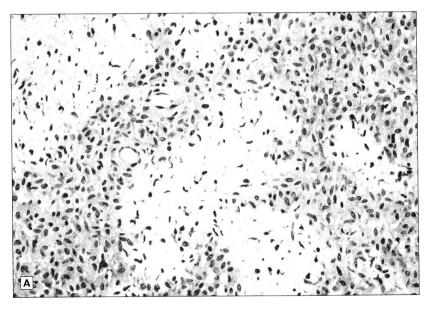

FIGURE 29–36 Diffuse neurofibroma with characteristic short fusiform or rounded Schwann cells. Shown at medium **(A)** and high power **(B)**.

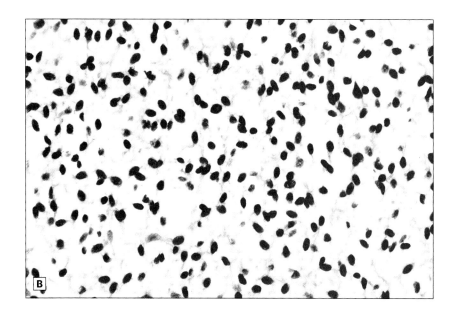

FIGURE 29–36 Continued.

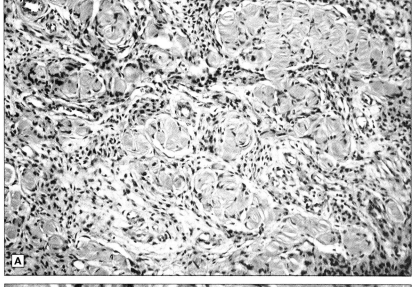

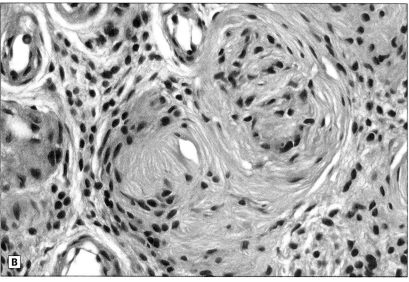

FIGURE 29–37 Wagner-Meissner bodies in a diffuse neurofibroma at medium **(A)** and high **(B)** power.

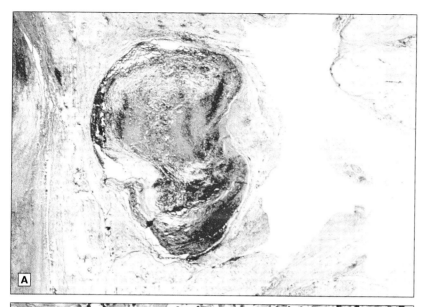

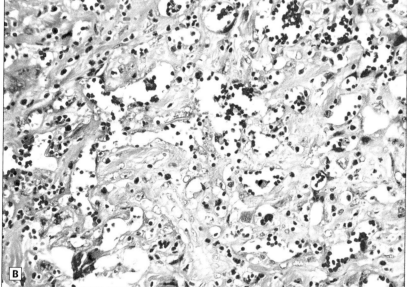

FIGURE 29–42 (A) Plexiform neurofibroma with an area of angiosarcoma (hemorrhagic zone). The tumor was an epithelioid angiosarcoma. **(B)** This pattern of malignant transformation is rare and is discussed in Chapter 31.

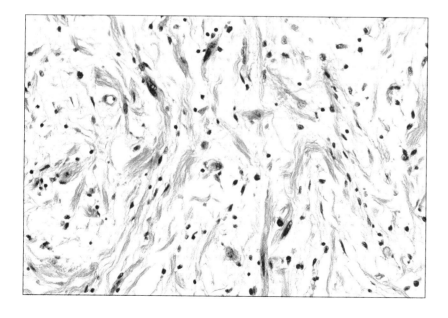

FIGURE 29–43 Neurofibroma with nuclear atypia of occasional cells without increased cellularity or mitotic activity.

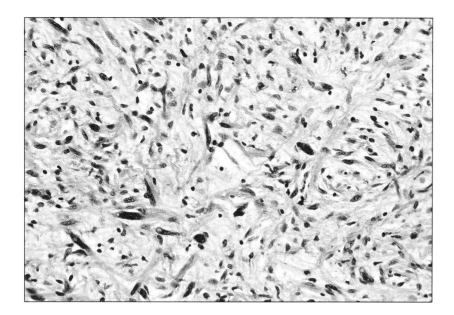

FIGURE 29–44 Neurofibroma with moderate cellularity and nuclear atypia. We use the designation neurofibroma with atypical features for changes of this type. This change was adjacent to areas of frank sarcoma.

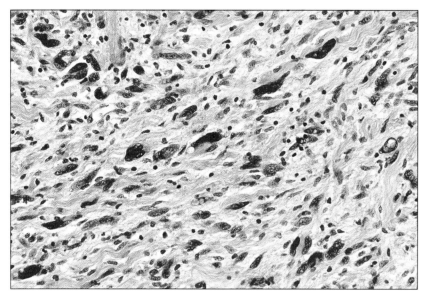

FIGURE 29–45 Low-grade malignant peripheral nerve sheath tumor arising in a neurofibroma. This "neurofibromatous" lesion is characterized by marked cellularity such that cells are nearly back-to-back. The nuclear atypia is marked and generalized.

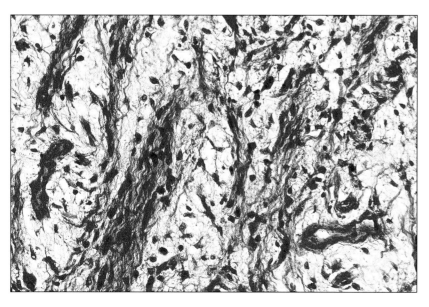

FIGURE 29–46 Low-grade malignant peripheral nerve sheath tumor arising in a neurofibroma. There is generalized marked atypia and increased cellularity such that the cells appear arranged in small fascicles. Low levels of mitotic activity were identified in the lesion.

TABLE 29–3	NEUROFIBROMAS WITH ATYPICAL AND MALIGNANT FEATURES			
Features			**Diagnostic terms**	
Nuclear atypia*	**Cellularity**	**Mitoses**	**Scheithauer et al.[66]**	**Weiss and Goldblum**
Usually focal; occasionally diffuse	–	–	Atypical neurofibroma	Neurofibroma
Absent	+	Absent	Cellular neurofibroma	Neurofibroma
Absent	+	+	Cellular neurofibroma	Neurofibroma with atypical features
Diffuse	+	–	Low-grade MPNST	Low-grade MPNST if cellularity is extreme with back-to-back cells or fascicles; otherwise neurofibroma with atypical features
Diffuse	+	+	Low-grade MPNST	Low-grade MPNST

MPNST, malignant peripheral nerve sheath tumor.
*Nuclear atypia is nuclear enlargement and hyperchromatism. Scheithauer et al. used nuclear enlargement of at least three times the normal Schwann cell for a diagnosis of malignancy.

following paragraphs represent our general approach to this problem, and Table 29–3 details the criteria and terms we and others employ.[66] In the final analysis, although labels are convenient, borderline neurofibromatous lesions require careful sampling, dialogue with the clinician, and potentially complete removal depending on the clinical setting.

Neurofibroma is used for conventional neurofibromas and those with nuclear atypia only (Fig. 29–43). The latter, as an isolated focal or diffuse change, is common in neurofibromas and does not correlate with malignancy. Although some use the term "atypical neurofibroma" for such lesions, we prefer not to use a term that could be misconstrued as reflecting concern about malignancy.

Neurofibroma with atypical features is the term used for neurofibromas that have any combination of atypical features that fall short of the minimum criteria for a diagnosis of low-grade MPNST (Fig. 29–44). This category excludes lesions characterized by nuclear atypia only.

Low-grade MPNST arising in neurofibroma is diagnosed when there is generalized nuclear atypia, increased cellularity, and usually low levels of mitotic activity (Figs 29–45, 29–46). Nuclear atypia consists of nuclear enlargement and hyperchromatism. Some suggest that nuclear enlargement should be at least three times the size of a normal Schwann cell nucleus.[66] If mitotic activity is not present, we diagnosis a low-grade MPNST if the cellularity (consisting of nearly back-to-back cells forming sheets or fascicles) and atypia are marked.

Discussion

Unlike solitary neurofibromas, those encountered in neurofibromatosis cause significant morbidity. The large number of lesions usually makes surgical therapy impossible. Therefore, surgery has traditionally been reserved for lesions that are large, painful, or located in strategic areas where continued expansion would compromise organ function. Even after attempted complete excision of these lesions, clinical recurrences occasionally develop, a phenomenon related to the ill-defined nature of the tumors. Targeted therapies, therefore, may prove to be extremely important. Treatment of plexiform neurofibromas with cis-retinoic acid, a maturational agent, and interferon-alpha, an antiangiogenic factor, have shown growth stabilization in a majority of patients.[67] Some patients have also responded to thalidomide, known to have antiangiogenic properties.[68]

A problem of greater importance is that of malignant transformation. The exact incidence is difficult to determine and has been estimated at 2–29% of patients with the disease,[50,58,69] but seems dependent on the severity of the disease among the population studied. A large follow-up study of a nationwide cohort of 212 Danish patients with neurofibromatosis found 9 sarcomas and 16 gliomas but noted the tumors occurred in the proband group (84 patients), who, by definition, required hospitalization and were probably more severely affected by the disorder.[70] The authors suggest that the natural history of neurofibromatosis may be more accurately reflected by the largest group of patients, relatives of the probands (128 patients) who did not require hospitalization and whose prognosis may have been better than previously thought. Both groups, however, had decreased survival rate after 40 years when compared with the general population. A more recent study by Evans et al.[71] documented a 8–13% lifetime risk for MPNST and de Raedt et al.[72] identified an association between large genomic deletions and malignancy in NF1 patients. The latter suggests that certain mutations may be more closely linked to the risk for malignant transformation.[73] In general, patients with NF1 and MPNST have had the disease for many years and present with rapid enlargement or pain in a preexisting neurofibroma.[74] Both symptoms, especially the former, should always lead to biopsy. Unfortunately, the prognosis for patients developing an MPNST in this setting is poor (see Chapter 31).

With the identification of the NF1 gene in 1990 it has become possible to examine the molecular events underlying tumorigenesis in this disease. Since conventional mice knockout models in which $Nf1$ is completely inactivated ($Nf1^{-/-}$) prove lethal in utero, conditional mice knockout models in which Schwann cell-specific $Nf1$ is inactivated have been employed.[55,75] In this system Zhu et al.[76] have shown that Schwann cell-specific knockout mice ($Nf1^{-/-}$) develop Schwann cell hyperplasias but rarely neurofibromas, whereas Schwann cell-specific knockout mice having one mutant and one wild type allele ($Nf1^{+/-}$) readily develop plexiform schwannomas containing $Nf1^{+/-}$ mast cells. These observations have led to the hypothesis that neurofibromin-deficient Schwann cells ($nf1^{-/-}$) require other haplo-insufficient ($nf1^{+/-}$) (e.g., mast cells, fibroblasts) cells in the microenvironment for tumorigenesis.[76,77] Progression of neurofibromas to malignant peripheral nerve sheath tumors requires additional mutational events involving mitogenic and cell cycle regulatory pathways. Mutations in $p53$, INK4 ($p16^{INK4a}$ and $p14^{ARF}$ genes),[78–81] $p27^{kip1}$ [79] and amplification of EGFR have been reported in malignant peripheral nerve sheath tumors and suggest a synergistic effect with NF.

SCHWANNOMA (NEURILEMOMA)

Schwannoma is an encapsulated nerve sheath tumor consisting of two components: a highly ordered cellular component (Antoni A area) and a loose myxoid component (Antoni B area). The presence of encapsulation and the two types of Antoni areas plus uniformly intense immunostaining for S-100 protein distinguish schwannoma from neurofibroma.

Clinical findings

Schwannomas occur at all ages but are most common in persons between the ages of 20 and 50 years.[45] They affect the genders in roughly equal numbers. The tumors have a predilection for the head, neck, and flexor surfaces of the upper and lower extremities.[82] Consequently, the spinal roots and the cervical, sympathetic, vagus, peroneal, and ulnar nerves are most commonly affected. Deeply situated tumors predominate in the posterior mediastinum and the retroperitoneum. Schwannomas are usually solitary sporadic lesions. In a population-based study of schwannomas, about 90% were sporadic, 3% occurred in patients with NF2, 2% in those with schwannomatosis, and 5% in association with multiple meningiomas in patients with or without NF2.[83] Rarely, schwannomas occur as part of NF1. Most schwannomas, whether sporadic or inherited, display inactivation mutations of the NF2 gene (see below).

Schwannoma is a slowly growing tumor that is usually present several years before diagnosis. When it involves small nerves, it is freely movable except for a single point of attachment. In large nerves, the tumor is movable except along the long axis of the nerve where the attachment restricts mobility.

Pain and neurologic symptoms are uncommon unless the tumor becomes large. In some instances the patient is vaguely aware that the tumor waxes and wanes in size,[82] a phenomenon that might be related to fluctuations in the amount of cystic change in the lesion. Of particular significance is the posterior mediastinal schwannoma, which often originates from or extends into the vertebral canal. Such lesions, termed dumbbell tumors, pose difficult management problems because patients may develop profound neurologic difficulties.

Gross findings

Because these tumors arise in nerve sheaths, they are surrounded by a true capsule consisting of the epineurium. Depending on the size of the involved nerve, the appearance of the tumor varies. Tumors of small nerves may resemble neurofibromas by virtue of their fusiform shape, and they often eclipse or obliterate the nerve of origin. In large nerves the tumors present as eccentric masses over which the nerve fibers are splayed.

On cut section these tumors have a pink, white, or yellow appearance and usually measure less than 5 cm (Figs 29–47, 29–48). Tumors in the retroperitoneum and mediastinum are considerably larger. As a result, these tumors are more likely to manifest secondary degenerative changes such as cystification and calcification (see discussion of the ancient schwannoma, below).

Microscopic findings

Most schwannomas are uninodular masses surrounded by a fibrous capsule consisting of epineurium and residual nerve fibers (Fig. 29–49). Neurites are generally not demonstrable in the substance of the tumor. In rare cases the schwannoma arises intradermally or, as mentioned above, manifests as a plexiform or multinodular growth similar to a plexiform neurofibroma.

The hallmark of a schwannoma is the pattern of alternating Antoni A and B areas (Figs 29–50 to 29–60). The relative amounts of these two components vary, and they may blend imperceptibly or change abruptly. Antoni A areas are composed of compact spindle cells that usually have twisted nuclei, indistinct cytoplasmic borders, and, occasionally, clear intranuclear vacuoles. They are arranged

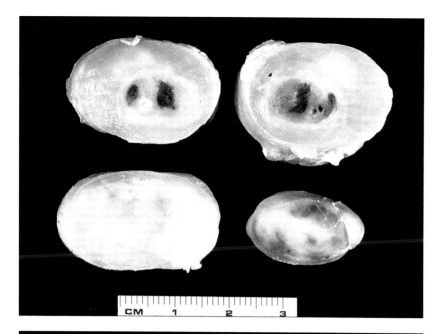

FIGURE 29–47 Multiple transverse sections through a schwannoma. Tumors are well circumscribed and commonly display foci of hemorrhage and cyst formation.

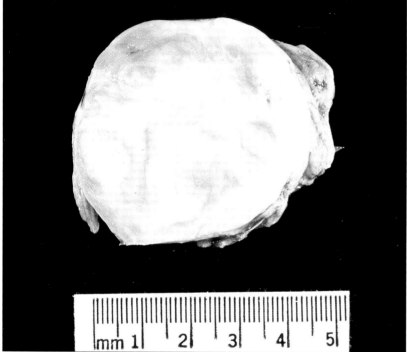

FIGURE 29–48 Mottled yellow-white appearance of a presacral schwannoma.

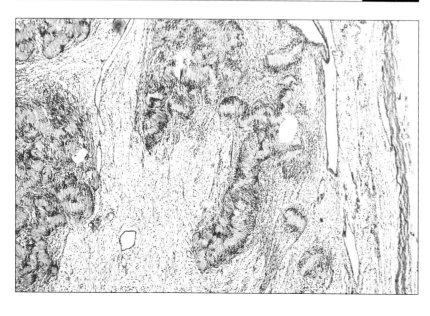

FIGURE 29–49 Schwannoma with a discrete, confining capsule.

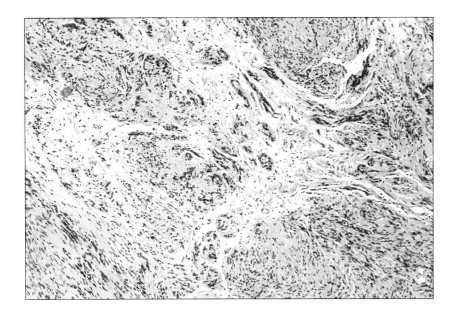

FIGURE 29–50 Schwannoma with alternating Antoni A and B areas.

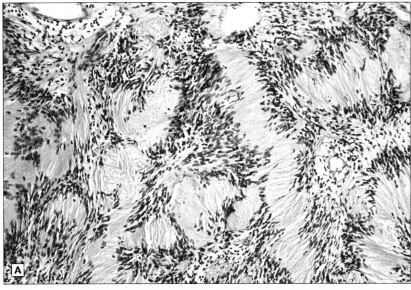

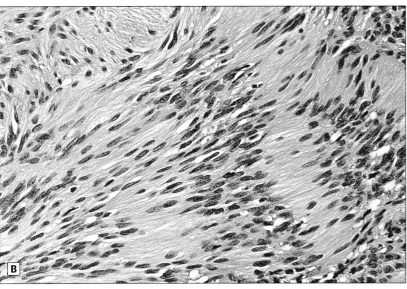

FIGURE 29–51 (A) Antoni A areas illustrating nuclear palisading with Verocay bodies. **(B)** High-power view shows nuclear palisading.

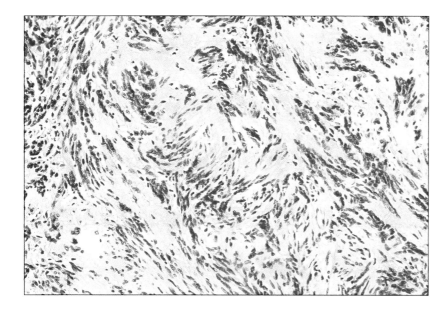

FIGURE 29–52 Antoni A areas with short fascicles and focal nuclear palisading.

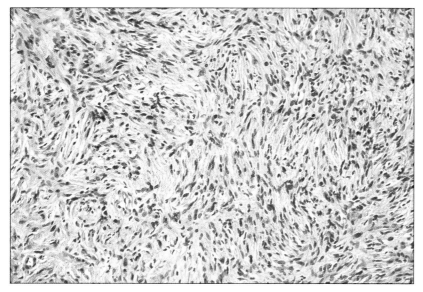

FIGURE 29–53 Antoni A areas with ill-defined fascicles without nuclear palisading.

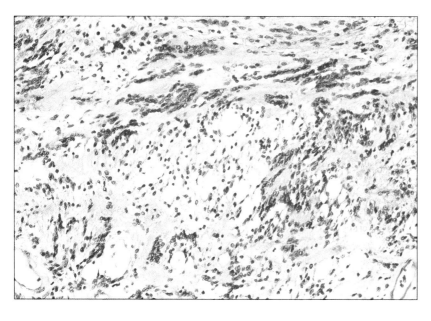

FIGURE 29–54 Transition between Antoni A areas and loosely textured Antoni B areas (center).

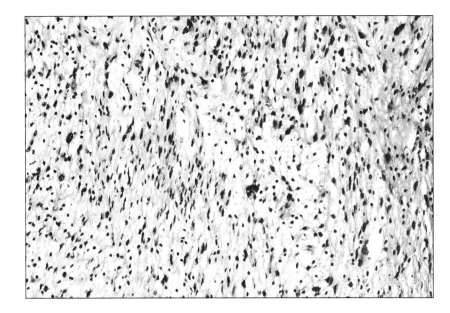

FIGURE 29–55 Antoni B areas in a schwannoma.

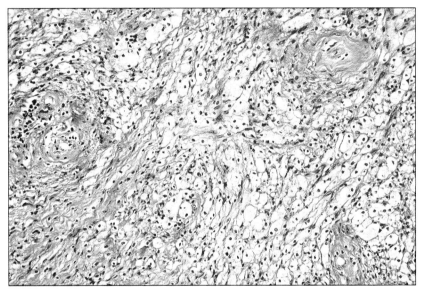

FIGURE 29–56 Antoni B areas with xanthomatous change.

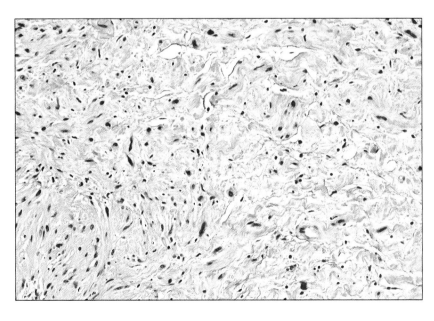

FIGURE 29–57 Antoni B areas with hyalinization.

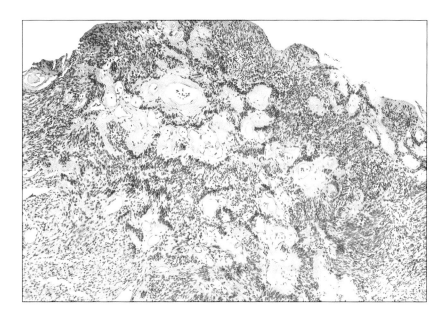

FIGURE 29–58 Ectatic irregularly shaped vessels with surrounding hyalinization are a common feature of schwannomas.

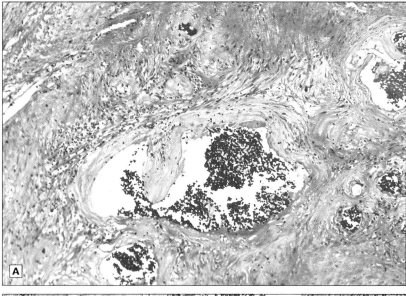

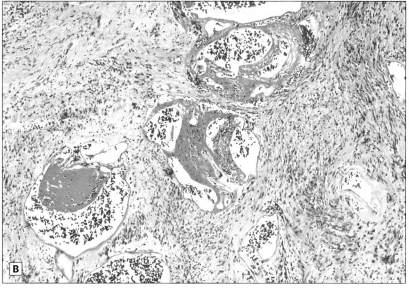

FIGURE 29–59 Hyalinized **(A)** and partially thrombosed **(B)** vessels in a schwannoma.

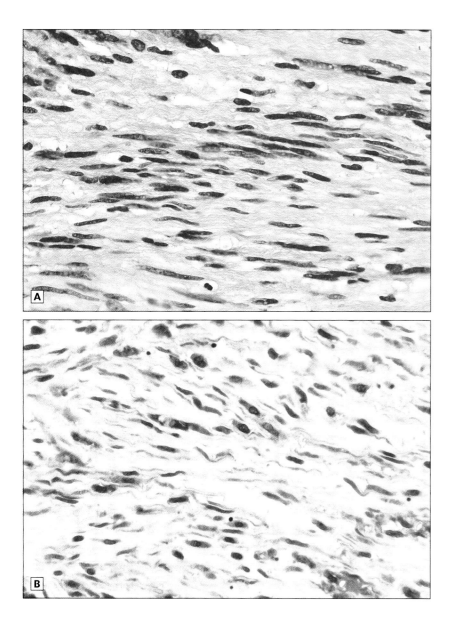

FIGURE 29–60 Differentiated Schwann cells **(A)** expressing S-100 protein **(B)** in a schwannoma.

in short bundles or interlacing fascicles (Figs 29–51 to 29–53). In highly differentiated Antoni A areas, there may be nuclear palisading, whorling of the cells (similar to meningioma), and Verocay bodies, formed by two compact rows of well-aligned nuclei separated by fibrillary cell processes (Fig. 29–51). Mitotic figures are occasionally present but can usually be dismissed if the lesion otherwise has all the hallmarks of schwannoma. S-100 protein, an acidic protein common to supporting cells of the central and peripheral nervous system, can be demonstrated in schwannomas, particularly in the Antoni A areas.

Antoni B areas are far less orderly and less cellular. The spindle or oval cells are arranged haphazardly in the loosely textured matrix, which is punctuated by microcystic change, inflammatory cells, and delicate collagen fibers (Figs 29–54 to 29–57). The large, irregularly spaced vessels, which are characteristic of schwannomas, become most conspicuous in the hypocellular Antoni B areas (Figs 29–58, 29–59). Their gaping, tortuous lumens are often filled with thrombus material in various stages of organization, and their walls are thickened by dense fibrosis. Glands and benign epithelial structures may occur in schwannoma (Fig. 29–61).[84,85] Judging from the number and type of glands, this seems to represent true epithelial differentiation in the tumor rather than entrapment or induced proliferation of normal structures. On occasion, schwannomas develop cystic spaces lined by Schwann cells that assume a round or epithelioid appearance. This change may be confused with true epithelial differentiation (Fig. 29–62). Such tumors have been referred to as pseudoglandular schwannomas.[86] Rarely, schwannomas contain a significant population of small lymphocyte-like Schwann cells arranged around collagen nodules forming giant rosettes (Figs 29–63, 29–64) or around vessels forming perivascular rosettes.[87]

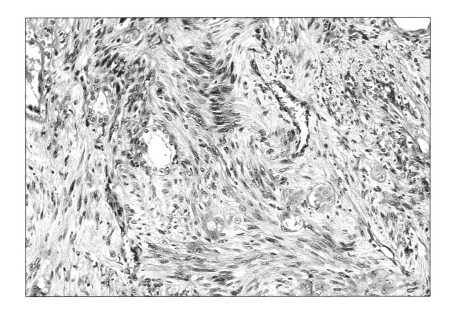

FIGURE 29–61 Schwannoma with benign glands and squamous islands.

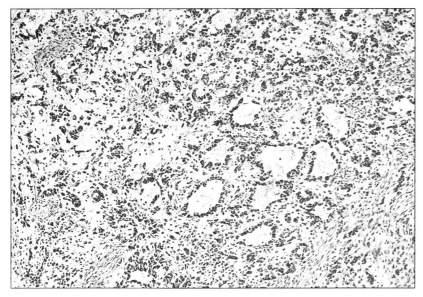

FIGURE 29–62 Schwannoma with cystic spaces resembling glands or dilated lymphatics (a so-called pseudoglandular schwannoma).

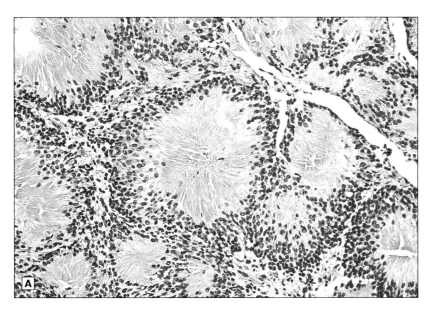

FIGURE 29–63 Neuroblastoma-like schwannoma composed of rounded Schwann cells forming rosettes **(A)**.

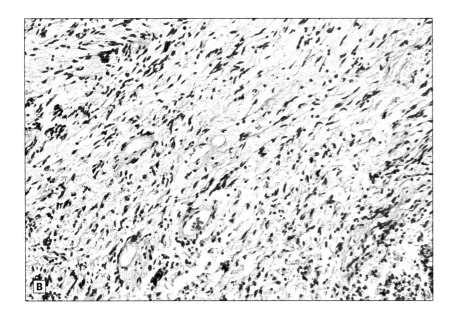

FIGURE 29–63 Continued. Other areas had a more conventional appearance **(B)**.

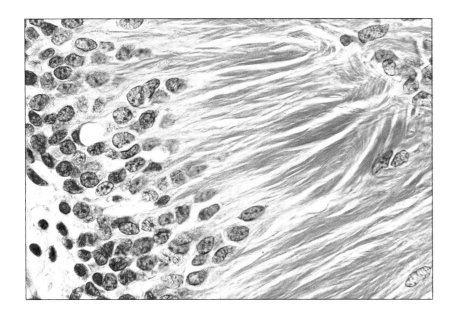

FIGURE 29–64 Giant rosette in a schwannoma formed by the radial arrangement of Schwann cells around a collagen core (Masson trichrome stain).

Ultrastructural and immunohistochemical findings

Electron microscopy has provided some of the best evidence in support of the separate natures of schwannomas and neurofibromas. In contrast to the neurofibroma, which contains a mixture of cell types, the schwannoma consists almost exclusively of Schwann cells.[62] These cells have attenuated cell processes that emanate from the cell body and lie in undulating layers adjacent to the cell body.[62,77–90] Basal lamina consisting of electron-dense material (measuring approximately 50 nm) coats the surface of the Schwann cell and lies in redundant stacks between the cells along with typical and long-spacing collagen (Fig. 29–65). The cytoplasm of the Schwann cell contains a flattened, occasionally invaginated nucleus,

microfibrils, occasional lysosomes, and scattered mitochondria. In Antoni B areas the Schwann cells have increased numbers of lysosomes and myelin figures with only a fragmented basal lamina, suggesting that these are degenerated Antoni A areas.

In concert with ultrastructural observations, most cells in schwannomas have the antigenic phenotype of Schwann cells. S-100 protein is strongly expressed by most cells in a schwannoma, in contrast to the cells of neurofibroma, which variably express the antigen. Leu-7 and occasionally glial fibrillary acidic protein are present in these tumors. Although the expression of S-100 protein is usually diminished in the Antoni B areas, immunostaining for this protein is so consistent and of such intensity that it serves as an important diagnostic tool. In our experience it is most valuable for diagnosing a severely

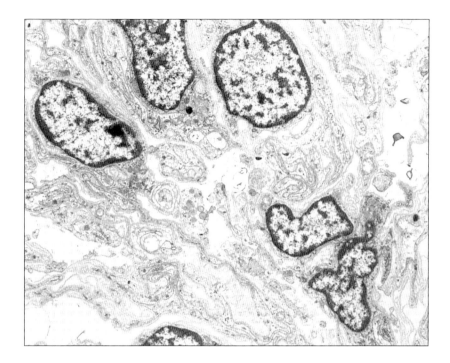

FIGURE 29–65 Electron micrograph of a schwannoma. Cells give off long cytoplasmic processes, which lie in layers adjacent to the cell body and are invested by well-formed continuous basal lamina. (From Taxy JB, Battifora H. In: Trump B, Jones RT, eds. Diagnostic electron microscopy. New York: Wiley; 1980.)

degenerated schwannoma in which the amount of myxoid change or fibrosis obscures the neoplastic nature of the lesion altogether. It usually also distinguishes deeply situated schwannomas from well-differentiated leiomyosarcomas. This important differential point is especially difficult in biopsy material from large intra-abdominal or retroperitoneal masses. The difficulty can be further compounded by the fact that schwannomas and leiomyosarcomas can display equivalent degrees of nuclear palisading. Whereas S-100 protein immunostaining is nearly always observed in schwannomas, it is seldom observed in leiomyosarcomas, in our experience.

Discussion

Schwannomas behave in a benign fashion. In Stout's series of 50 cases,[82] none recurred after simple or even incomplete excision. Malignant change is rare[91-93] and from a practical point of view can be discounted. Among the well over 1000 schwannomas we have seen, there has been only one instance of true malignant transformation. In that case, the original tumor had the features of a classic schwannoma, whereas the recurrent tumor, 8 years later, had areas of malignancy. The patient later succumbed to metastatic disease. Woodruff et al. presented nine acceptable cases,[94] including two of their own, in a comprehensive review of the literature. Others have subsequently been reported.[95] As a group, these tumors occur in adults without NF1 but with a longstanding mass. Unlike neurofibromas, in which supervening malignancy resembles a spindle cell sarcoma, malignancy in schwannomas often has an epithelioid appearance. Areas

of a conventional schwannoma are identified alongside confluent expanses of large, round, atypical eosinophilic cells (Fig. 29–66C,D).[96] McMenamin and Fletcher have noted microscopic collections of these epithelioid cells in schwannomas and suggested that they represent an early stage of malignant transformation (Fig. 29–66A,B).[95]

Schwannoma with degenerative change (ancient schwannoma)

Ancient schwannomas are those displaying marked nuclear atypia of a degenerative type.[97,98] They are usually large tumors of long duration, and a significant number are located in deep structures such as the retroperitoneum.[98] Degenerative changes include cyst formation, calcification, hemorrhage, and hyalinization (Figs 29–67 to 29–72). The tumor itself is usually infiltrated by large numbers of siderophages and histiocytes. One of the most treacherous aspects of this tumor is the degree of nuclear atypia encountered. The Schwann cell nuclei are large, hyperchromatic, and often multilobed but lack mitotic figures (Figs 29–68, 29–71). These tumors behave as ordinary schwannomas; therefore, the nuclear atypia can be regarded as a degenerative change.

Cellular schwannoma

Cellular schwannoma is a well-recognized variant of schwannoma[99-103] that, because of its cellularity, mitotic activity, and occasional presence of bone destruction, is diagnosed as malignant in more than one-fourth of cases.[104] Lesions reported as "plexiform MPNSTs of infancy

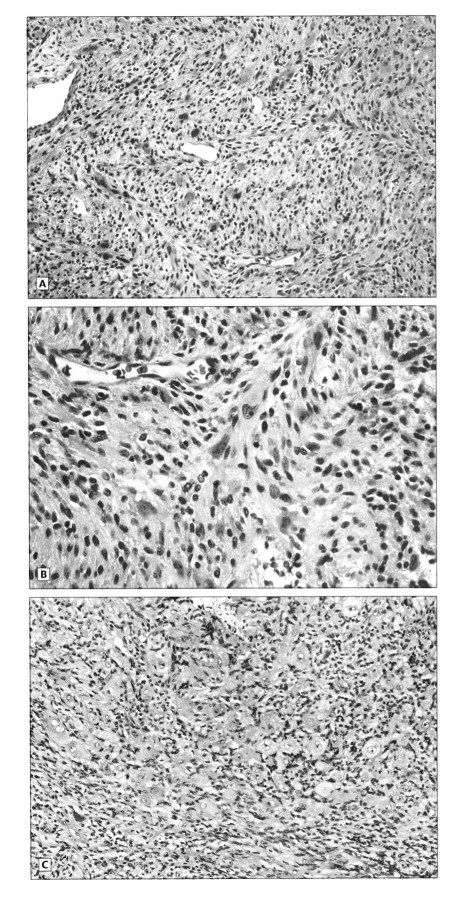

FIGURE 29–66 Schwannoma with scattered atypical **(A, B)** cells and frank malignant change **(C, D)**. Scattered atypical cells within otherwise benign schwannoma **(A, B)** have been described as the "precursor" lesion to frank malignancy which is diagnosed by confluent areas of obviously malignant cells **(C, D)**.

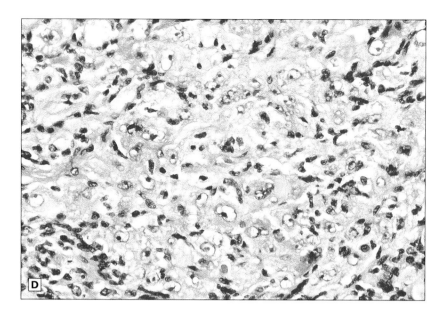

FIGURE 29–66 Continued.

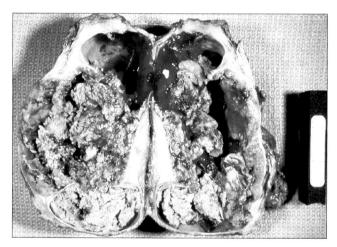

FIGURE 29–67 Gross specimen of a schwannoma of the retroperitoneum with extensive degenerative changes (ancient schwannoma). Tumors are characterized by areas of old and new hemorrhage, cyst formation, and calcification.

and childhood"[105] and congenital neural hamartoma (fascicular schwannoma)[106] are cellular schwannomas.[107] Defined as a schwannoma composed predominantly or exclusively of Antoni A areas that lack Verocay bodies, cellular schwannoma occurs in a similar age group as classic schwannoma but tends to develop more often in deep structures such as the posterior mediastinum and retroperitoneum. Only about one-fourth develop in the deep soft tissues of the extremities. It may present as a palpable asymptomatic mass noted radiographically or as a mass producing neurologic symptoms. Like classic schwannomas, the lesions appear circumscribed, if not encapsulated, and occasionally are multinodular or plexiform. Usually homogeneously tan in color, they commonly have hemorrhage but seldom display cystic degeneration (Fig. 29–73).[66] Underneath their capsule they may contain lymphoid aggregates. Antoni A areas dominate the histologic picture but small amounts of Antoni B may be present, usually not exceeding 10% of the lesion.[66] In addition to short, intersecting fascicles and whorls of Schwann cells, the Antoni A areas may display long, sweeping fascicles of Schwann cells sometimes arranged in a herringbone fashion (Figs 29–74, 29–75). The presence of this pattern often suggests the diagnosis of fibrosarcoma or leiomyosarcoma to those unfamiliar with cellular schwannomas. Mitotic activity may be observed but usually is low (<4 mitoses per 10 high-power fields [HPF]).[102] Focal areas of necrosis are seen in up to 10% of cases. The cells fringing the necrotic zones, however, are differentiated Schwann cells and lack the hyperchromatism and anaplasia so typical of those surrounding areas of zonal necrosis in MPNSTs. Like classic schwannomas, the cellular schwannoma displays diffuse, strong immunoreactivity for S-100 protein. Most cellular schwannomas are diploid with a low S-phase fraction (6–7%).[99]

Important factors that suggest a benign diagnosis include cellularity that is disproportionately high compared with the levels of mitotic activity and atypia, sharp circumscription if not encapsulation, perivascular hyalinization, occasionally focal Antoni B areas, and invariably strong, diffuse immunoreactivity for S-100 protein. Staining for S-100 protein is an invaluable adjunct for this diagnosis, particularly if one is dealing with material obtained by small-needle biopsies of large retroperitoneal or mediastinal masses. In fact, we rarely diagnose malignancy based on needle biopsies of differentiated spindle cell tumors if staining for S-100 protein is strongly positive because of the possibility of a cellular schwannoma.

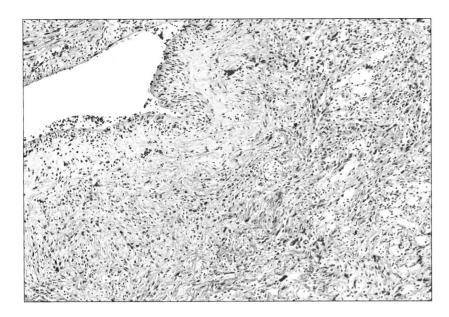

FIGURE 29–68 Ancient schwannoma with cyst formation and interstitial hyalinization.

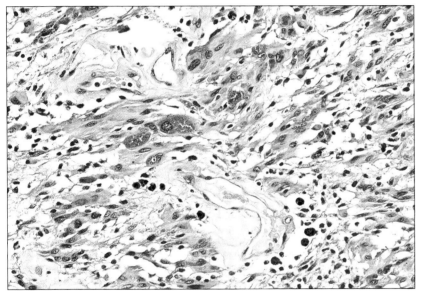

FIGURE 29–69 Ancient schwannoma with degenerative atypia and perivascular hyalinization. Note the lipofuscin-like pigment in the Schwann cells.

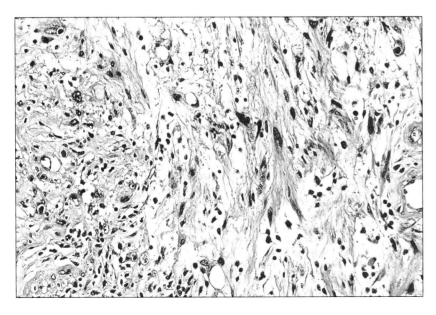

FIGURE 29–70 Ancient schwannoma.

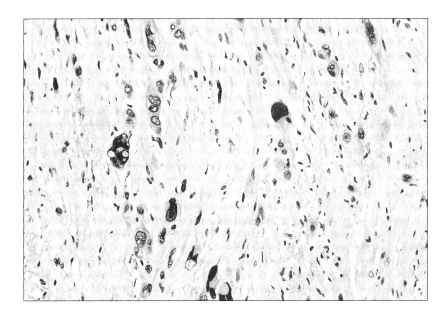

FIGURE 29–71 Ancient schwannoma with extensive hyalinization.

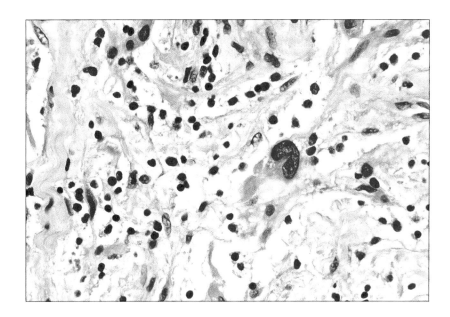

FIGURE 29–72 Degenerative atypia in an ancient schwannoma.

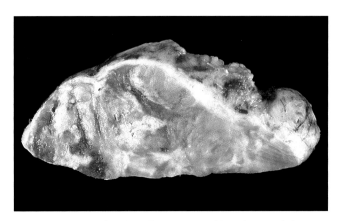

FIGURE 29–73 Cellular schwannoma with a characteristic tawny yellow color.

Although initial skepticism was expressed about the biologic behavior of cellular schwannomas, with some suggesting that they were in fact a low-grade MPNST, several large studies with extended follow-up information[99,101,102,108] have reaffirmed the initial findings of Woodruff et al. More than 100 cases have been reported, with nearly one-third having follow-up periods of more than 5 years. Fewer than 5% of patients have developed recurrences, and none has developed metastatic disease. In most of the cases reported by White et al.,[102] treatment was conservative and consisted of surgical excision only. That these truly represent variants of schwannoma is indicated not only by histologic but also by ultrastructural and cytogenetic similarities.[109]

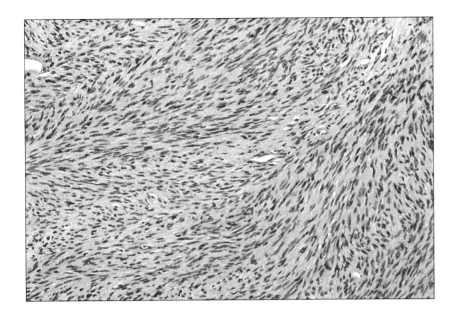

FIGURE 29–74 Cellular schwannoma with long fascicles of Schwann cells without Antoni B areas or Verocay bodies.

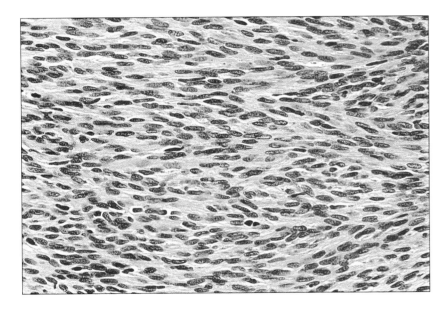

FIGURE 29–75 Cellular schwannoma consisting of differentiated Schwann cells without mitotic activity.

Plexiform schwannoma

About 5% of schwannomas grow in a plexiform or multinodular pattern,[110] which may or may not be apparent macroscopically (Figs 29–76 to 29–78). Unlike plexiform neurofibromas, which are considered nearly pathognomonic of NF1, the association of plexiform schwannomas with NF1 or NF2 is considerably weaker.[110] Of the approximately 50 cases reported in the literature, there have been only a few cases associated with NF1[108,111,112] or NF2.[113–115] Plexiform schwannomas usually occur in the skin and infrequently in deep sites. Like classic schwannoma, they are encapsulated but as a group are more cellular and therefore qualify also as cellular schwannomas. It is important to be aware of this fact, as there is a risk of misinterpreting a lesion as a sarcoma arising in a plexiform neurofibroma. Attention to the fact

that the lesion does not have a level of atypia commensurate with the mitotic activity, lacks geographic necrosis, and displays strong S-100 protein staining provides good support for benignancy in such cases.

Epithelioid schwannoma

Schwannomas consisting predominantly or exclusively of epithelioid Schwann cells have been described by Kindblom et al.[116] Like conventional schwannoma they develop as a circumscribed or encapsulated mass in the superficial soft tissues.[116,117] The tumor is composed of small rounded Schwann cells arranged singly, in small aggregates, or in cords within a collagenous or partially myxoid stroma (Fig. 29–79). Areas of conventional schwannoma may be seen in some tumors. The epithelioid Schwann cells are small and rounded with sharp

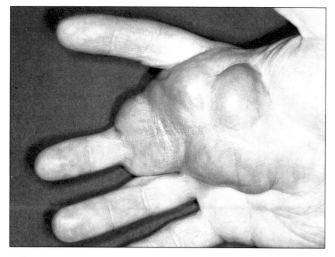

FIGURE 29–76 Plexiform schwannoma.

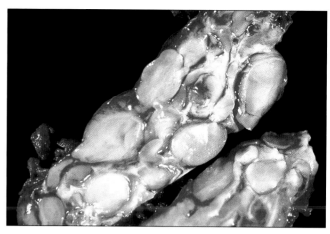

FIGURE 29–77 Gross specimen of a plexiform schwannoma illustrating a multinodular pattern of growth.

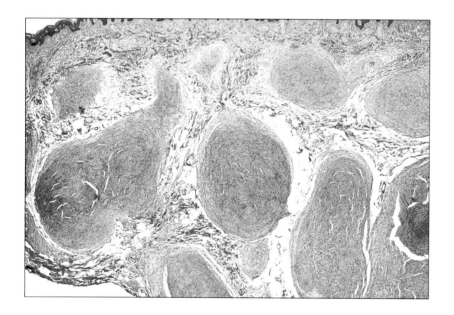

FIGURE 29–78 Plexiform schwannoma involving the dermis.

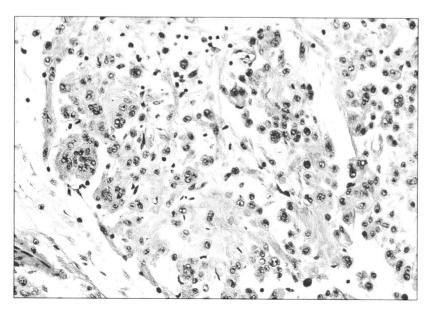

FIGURE 29–79 Epithelioid schwannoma. Note the cohesive nests of bland epithelioid cells.

cytoplasmic borders and occasionally intranuclear cytoplasmic (pseudo) inclusions. Although occasional atypical cells are seen, they seem to represent a degenerative change, as these tumors virtually always lack mitotic figures and have low proliferative activity as measured by Ki67 immunostaining.[116] The cells may be associated with dense collagen cores forming irregular collagen rosettes similar to those seen in the neuroblastoma-like schwannoma. Immunohistochemistry, electron microscopy, or both are helpful, if not essential, for establishing the diagnosis. Virtually all cells strongly express S-100 protein (Fig. 29–80A); immunostains for type IV collagen outlines a latticework of basement membrane material around individual cells and groups of cells (Fig. 29–80B). The combination of these two stains is highly suggestive of the diagnosis as few tumors co-express these two antigens to this degree. Electron microscopy shows that the cells resemble differentiated Schwann cells. Of the few cases reported, the behavior has been uniformly benign.

The differential diagnosis of these lesions includes notably epithelioid forms of MPNST. Although the two bear some similarity, epithelioid forms of MPNST should be diagnosed only when the constituent cells are cytologically malignant. Most have large nuclei with prominent macronuclei reminiscent of malignant melanoma.

NEUROFIBROMATOSIS 2 (BILATERAL VESTIBULAR SCHWANNOMAS)

Neurofibromatosis 2 is an autosomal dominant disease with an incidence of 1/30 000–40 000 live births which has as its hallmark bilateral vestibular schwannomas. It is the result of inactivating germline mutations of the tumor suppressor gene *NF2* located on chromosome 22

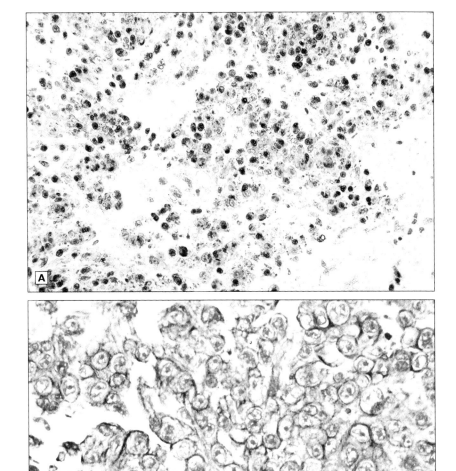

FIGURE 29–80 Epithelioid schwannoma with S-100 protein **(A)** and intricate pattern of type IV collagen immunoreactivity **(B)**. The latter is reflective of basal lamina material surrounding the cells.

which encodes the protein merlin or schwannomin, a 595 amino acid member of the moesin-ezrine-radixin cytoskeleton-associated proteins.[118] This protein is expressed in Schwann cells, meningeal cells, and the lens of the eye where it localizes to regions of the cell membrane engaged in cell contact and mobility. The mechanisms by which the loss of this protein results in tumorigenesis are not well understood. However, merlin appears to have several binding partners including cell surface, cytoskeletal, and ion transport proteins. The binding of one partner, CD44, a surface protein, appears to be important for cell growth arrest and reduced cell motility.[119]

The onset of NF2 is usually during adolescence or early adult life, with the development of tinnitus or hearing loss due to the presence of bilateral vestibular schwannomas which usually affect the vestibular portion of the VIII nerve. Café au lait spots and neurofibromas are rare or absent in this form of neurofibromatosis. In addition to vestibular schwannomas, other central nervous system tumors occur commonly, including schwannomas of other cranial nerves, meningioma, ependymoma, and glioma. Approximately one-half to two-thirds of patients with NF2 also develop cutaneous schwannomas, but schwannomas in the absence of bilateral vestibular schwannomas (schwannomatosis) is a different disease (see schwannomatosis). Since half of NF2 patients do not have a family history of NF2 and many present with meningiomas, spinal cord tumors, or peripheral schwannomas before the development of vestibular schwannomas, the NIH diagnostic criteria proposed in 1997 have recently been expanded under the less stringent Manchester system (Table 29–4).[118,120]

NF2-associated schwannomas are histologically similar to sporadic ones and do not undergo malignant transformation. Patients, nonetheless, experience significant morbidity and mortality. There appears to be some correlation between disease severity and mutational status. Patients with nonsense or frameshift mutations have severe disease whereas those with missense mutations, inframe deletions, and large deletions have a mild form.[121] However, by far the strongest predictor of mortality is age at diagnosis. In addition, patients referred to specialty centers have a significantly lower mortality.

SCHWANNOMATOSIS

Formerly considered by some an attenuated from of NF2, multiple schwannomas, or "schwannomatosis,"[122] is currently considered a completely different disease[123–125] not associated with germline mutations in either *NF1* or *NF2*. The majority of cases of schwannomatosis are sporadic, but there are well-documented familial cases that follow an autosomal dominant pattern of inheritance with reduced penetrance.[126] Men and women are equally affected. Patients present with multiple, often painful schwannomas involving skin or soft tissue. In some patients the schwannomas have a striking segmental distribution affecting the length of a nerve. Although some patients develop cranial or spinal nerve schwannomas, they do not develop the variety of central nervous system tumors seen in NF2, such as astrocytoma, ependymoma, and meningioma. Based on a large international clinical database, a revised set of criteria for schwannomatosis has been proposed (Table 29–5).[126]

By molecular and linkage analysis of familial cases, the schwannomatosis locus has been identified on chromosome 22 proximal to *NF2*. Interestingly, analysis of schwannomas in this disease has disclosed numerous truncating mutations of *NF2* even within different tumors from the same patient leading to the postulate that mutations in the schwannomatosis gene render *NF2* more susceptible to diverse somatic mutations.

Except for the multiplicity or segmental nature of the tumors, schwannomas in this disease resemble sporadic schwannomas histologically. Similarly, there are no instances of malignant transformation.

MELANOTIC SCHWANNOMA

A rare form of pigmented neural tumor commonly arising from the sympathetic nervous system was described in 1932 by Millar[127] as *malignant melanotic tumor of ganglion cells*, discussed under the term *melanocytic schwannoma* by Fu et al.,[128] and recently redesignated *psammomatous melanotic schwannoma* by Carney,[129] who noted its association with Carney syndrome. Based on our experience and that in the literature, the lesion is a distinctive neoplasm of adult life that differs significantly from classic schwannoma despite the similarity in names.[127–137] The tumor arises commonly from the spinal or autonomic nerves near the midline. However, a number of cases have been reported in the stomach and in bone and soft tissues. Unusual sites

TABLE 29–4	MANCHESTER CRITERIA FOR DIAGNOSIS OF NEUROFIBROMATOSIS 2

A. Bilateral vestibular schwannoma.
B. First-degree family relative with NF2 and unilateral vestibular schwannoma or any two* of the following: meningioma, schwannoma, glioma, neurofibroma, posterior subcapsular lenticular opacity.
C. Unilateral vestibular schwannoma and any two* of the following: meningioma, schwannoma, glioma, neurofibroma, posterior subcapsular lenticular opacity.
D. Multiple meningiomas (two or more) and unilateral vestibular schwannoma or any two* of the following: schwannoma, glioma, neurofibroma, cataract.

*Note any two means two individual tumors or cataracts.
From: Evans DGR et al. A clinical study of type 2 neurofibromatosis. Q J Med 1992; 84:603.

TABLE 29–5	REVISED CLINICAL CRITERIA FOR DIAGNOSIS OF SCHWANNOMATOSIS
Definite	**Possible**
Age >30 years AND	Age <30 years AND
two or more nonintradermal schwannomas, at least 1 with histologic confirmation AND	two or more nonintradermal schwannomas, at least 1 with histologic confirmation AND
no evidence of vestibular tumor on high quality MRI scan and no known constitutional *NF2* mutation	no evidence of vestibular tumor on high quality MRI scan AND no known constitutional *NF2* mutation
OR	OR
One pathologically confirmed nonvestibular schwannoma plus a first degree relative who meets above criteria	Age <45 years AND
	two or more nonintradermal schwannomas, at least 1 with histologic confirmation AND no symptoms of 8th nerve dysfunction AND no known constitutional *NF2* mutation
Segmental schwannomatosis	
Meets criteria for either definite or possible schwannomatosis but limited to one limb or five or fewer contiguous segments of the spine	

From MacCollin M et al. Diagnostic criteria for schwannomatosis. Neurology 2005; 64:1838.

include the heart, bronchus, liver, and skin.[129] More than half of patients with the tumor have evidence of *Carney syndrome*, which includes *myxomas* of the heart, skin, and breast, *spotty pigmentation* due to lentigenes, blue nevus, and the distinctive epithelioid blue nevus,[130] *endocrine overactivity* manifested by Cushing's disease (pigmented nodular adrenal disease), acromegaly (pituitary adenoma), or sexual precocity (Sertoli cell tumor). The tumor typically develops at an earlier age (average 22.5 years) in patients with Carney syndrome than in those without the syndrome (average 33.2 years).[129] About 20% of patients with melanotic schwannomas have multiple tumors, and in such patients there is an even higher probability that other manifestations of Carney's complex will be present.[129] The symptoms related specifically to the tumor depend on its location and rate of growth, but most commonly they are pain and neurologic symptoms in the affected part. Most striking is a case reported by Fu et al.,[128] in which the patient lost sympathetic nerve function in the ipsilateral lower extremity. In one of our cases, a well-encapsulated lesion of the mediastinum, the patient was symptom free, and the lesion was detected on a routine chest radiograph.

The tumors are usually circumscribed or encapsulated and vary from black-brown to gray-blue. It is often difficult to make out cellular detail in these tumors because of the heavy pigment deposits. Usually, there are at least focal areas with little or no pigment, so the character of the cells can be evaluated. The cells vary in shape from polygonal to spindled and blend gradually from one to another (Figs 29–81, 29–82). This feature, coupled with the ill-defined borders of the cytoplasm, often imparts a syncytial quality to the tumors that is somewhat reminiscent of a schwannoma. Likewise, the nuclei may display clear intranuclear cytoplasmic (pseudo) inclusions characteristic of Schwann cells. Nuclear chromatism may be marked, and the nucleoli are often prominent. Occasion-

ally, there is vague palisading or formation of whorled structures such that the tumor resembles a schwannoma or neurofibroma. Ganglion cell differentiation has not been observed in our material, although in the original reported case attenuated cytoplasmic processes led Millar[127] to conclude that the tumor cells were ganglionic. Psammoma bodies are present in most cases in our experience. Carney reported them in all of his cases but noted that extensive sampling was necessary to document them in some.[129]

The melanin pigment may be coarsely clumped or finely granular and varies from area to area. Tinctorially, it is similar to dermal melanin and stains positively with the Fontana stain and negatively for iron and periodic acid-Schiff (PAS). In this respect it differs from the faint and focal pigment seen in conventional schwannomas, which is neural melanin. On immunohistochemical studies, these tumors strongly express S-100 protein and a melanoma-associated antigen (HMB-45). Ultrastructurally there is a spectrum of maturation, including premelanosomes and melanosomes, which leads one to conclude that the pigment is synthesized by the tumor cell. Except for the presence of melanosomes, the cells resemble Schwann cells with elaborate cytoplasmic processes that interdigitate or spiral in the manner of mesaxons.

The biologic behavior of these tumors is difficult to predict, and metastases can occur in the absence of overt malignant features. Neither tumor size nor ploidy predicts malignant behavior. In the past it was thought that most of these lesions had a benign, indolent course. Metastases, for example, were reported in only 13% of patients with melanotic schwannomas and Carney syndrome.[129] A review of approximately 60 cases in the literature has disclosed metastasis in 26%.[137] Furthermore, only 53% of patients followed for more than 5 years were disease free, suggesting that long-term follow-up is required to fully judge metastatic risk. Although all may

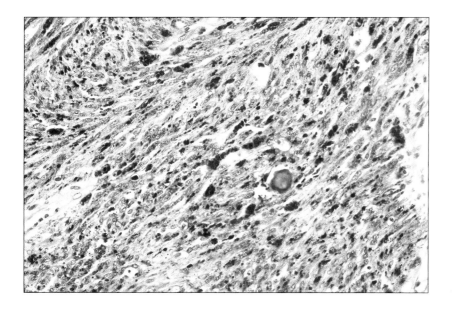

FIGURE 29–81 Melanotic schwannoma with heavy melanin deposits and a psammoma body.

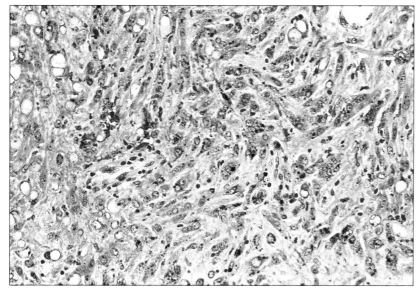

FIGURE 29–82 Melanotic schwannoma with a less pigmented area.

be potentially malignant, we have designated those with significant mitotic activity as malignant melanotic schwannomas. When metastases develop they too abound with melanin pigment.

The usual problem in differential diagnosis is distinguishing this tumor from a metastatic malignant melanoma. Primary melanotic schwannomas usually do not have the degree of nuclear atypia or mitotic activity expected in a metastatic melanoma. The peculiar syncytial quality of the cells and particularly the psammomatous calcification are important features of melanotic schwannoma that metastatic melanomas lack.

PERINEURIOMA

Perineurioma is a soft tissue tumor composed of cells resembling normal perineurium.[138-143] Since neurofibro-

mas contain a subpopulation of perineurial cells and rare nerve sheath tumors have hybrid features between neurofibroma and perineurioma,[144,145] the term perineurioma is used, strictly speaking, for tumors in which the vast majority of cells show perineurial differentiation. It was first described in 1978 by Lazarus and Trombetta[146] on the basis of ultrastructural findings. Although several cases were published after that early description,[138,147-149] the tumor was slow to gain wide recognition because of the inability to diagnose the lesion by light microscopy alone. Greater familiarity with its features coupled with additional immunohistochemical markers to document perineurial differentiation has resulted in more frequent and consistent diagnosis of this entity. Still, it appears that this lesion is far less common than neurofibromas and schwannomas. There are several forms of perineurioma: intraneural, extraneural (soft tissue), sclerosing, and reticular.

Intraneural perineurioma

Intraneural perineurioma is a rare condition that has recently been shown to be an intraneural clonal proliferation of perineurial cells. Many lesions formerly diagnosed as "localized hypertrophic neuropathy" are examples of intraneural perineurioma. The lesions usually develop in a nerve in the upper extremity of a young individual. Characteristic signs and symptoms include muscle weakness, denervation changes seen by electromyography, and, in extreme cases, muscle atrophy. The affected nerve displays a fusiform expansion extending several centimeters in length (Fig. 29–83). On cross-section the entire nerve is expanded by the formation of tiny "onion bulbs" consisting of concentric layers of perineurial cells ensheathing a central axon and Schwann cell (Fig. 29–84). The perineurial cells occasionally spin off the sheath and communicate with adjacent ones. Because of the highly organized nature of these lesions, the usual impression is that of a reactive or reparative process. However, with immunostains for epithelial membrane antigen (EMA) and S-100 protein, the striking preponderance of perineurial cells becomes readily apparent. Immunostains for EMA highlight the ensheathing perineurial cells, leaving the central portion of the "onion bulb" devoid of staining. With S-100 protein or neurofilament protein immunostains, highlighting Schwann cells and axons respectively, a reverse staining pattern is noted (Fig. 29–85).

The question of whether the intraneural perineurioma is a true neoplasm or an unusual reactive process has been debated and is reflected in the variety of terms employed for this lesion. The best evidence to date suggests that they are indeed neoplastic. These lesions are

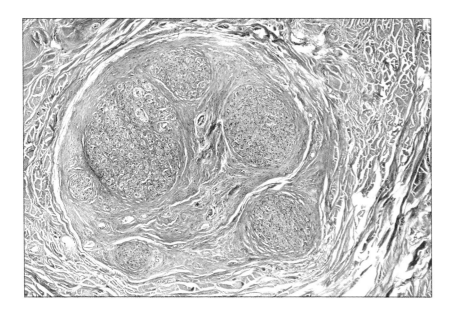

FIGURE 29–83 Intraneural perineurioma.

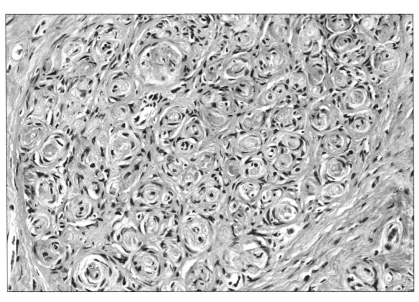

FIGURE 29–84 Intraneural perineurioma with "onion bulb" expansion of the nerve sheath.

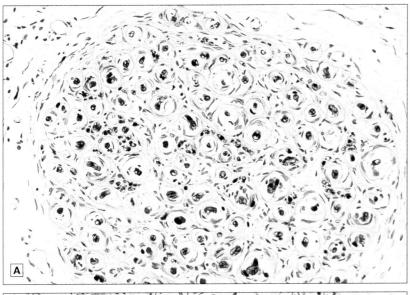

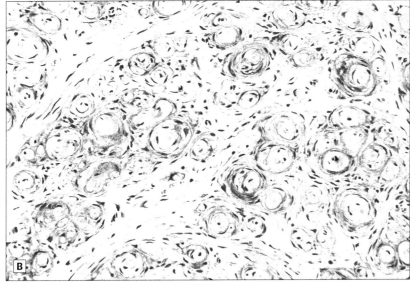

FIGURE 29–85 Intraneural perineurioma. S-100 protein immunostain decorates Schwann cells but not perineurial cells **(A)**. Epithelial membrane antigen (EMA) immunostain shows reverse pattern with positively staining perineurial component and no staining of Schwann cells **(B)**.

associated with significant proliferative activity (as reflected by MIB-1 and proliferating cell nuclear antigen [PCNA] immunoreactivity) and clonal alterations of chromosome 22.[150]

The behavior of intraneural perineurioma has been uniformly benign, with neither recurrences nor metastases reported. Nonetheless, there are no standard guidelines for the treatment of this condition. MRI has been successful in determining the extent of nerve involvement,[151] but because complete resection with nerve grafting does not completely restore function[152] this option should be carefully weighed against the degree of nerve compromise.

Soft tissue (extraneural) perineurioma

Soft tissue perineurioma, although more common than its intraneural counterpart, is still relatively uncom-

mon.[140,143,153–155] It occurs equally in the sexes and affects adults primarily. Most involve the superficial soft tissues of the extremities and trunk, but approximately 30% develop in deep soft tissue and rarely visceral locations.[143] They are not associated with NF1 or NF2. Although alterations of chromosome 22 have been reported, they have not been identified in NF2 locus per se.[140,156]

The lesions are circumscribed white masses ranging in size from 1 cm to nearly 20 cm with an average of about 4 cm.[143] The most common appearance of a soft tissue perineurioma is a spindle cell lesion composed of slender fibroblast-like cells with long streamer-like cell processes arranged in a storiform, whorled, pacinian, or short fascicular pattern (Figs 29–86 to 29–89). The lesions vary in their cellularity although most are hypocellular. Those with little stroma and a storiform pattern resemble dermatofibrosarcoma protuberans or benign fibrous histiocytoma whereas those with prominent myxoid stroma are

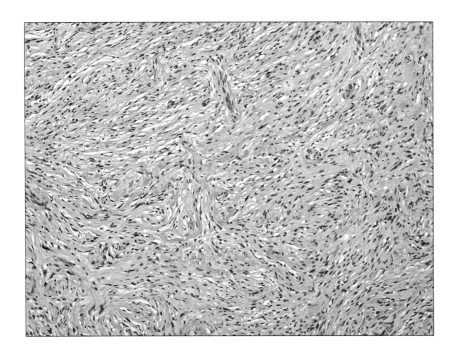

FIGURE 29–86 Extraneural (soft tissue) perineurioma with slender perineurial cells arranged in short fascicles.

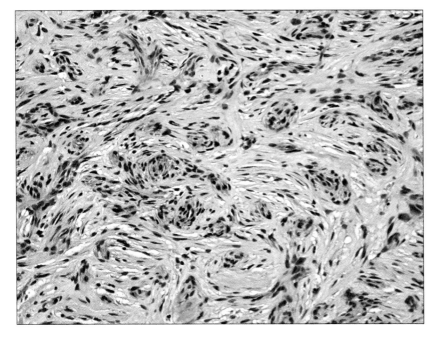

FIGURE 29–87 Whorled structures in a perineurioma.

often compared to myxoid neurofibromas. In highly collagenized perineuriomas, the slender processes may appear to ramify within or dissect through the matrix. Ossification occurs rarely.[142] Approximately 20% of perineuriomas have atypical features which include scattered atypical cells, low levels of mitotic activity (<13/30 HPF), increased cellularity, and infiltration of muscle. So far, these lesions have not pursued a significantly different course from typical cases.[143]

Definitionally, all benign perineuriomas are EMA-positive and usually S-100 protein-negative (Fig. 29–89), an immunophenotype that mirrors the normal perineurial cell.[138,157,158] In addition, the majority of perineurio-

mas also express claudin-1,[159] a tight junction-associated protein and GLUT1, human erythrocyte glucose transporter,[160] barrier function proteins present in normal perineurial cells.[149,161] Because EMA staining in perineuriomas is membranous, it may be difficult to appreciate if the cell processes are widely separated. Consequently, high-power examination of the tumor may be necessary. Claudin-1, on the other hand, stains perineuriomas more diffusely and robustly and, therefore, is easier to interpret. Type IV collagen and laminin, two components of the basement membrane, also decorate the abundant basal lamina elaborated by the perineurial cell. This finding, however, is not specific for perineurial tumors

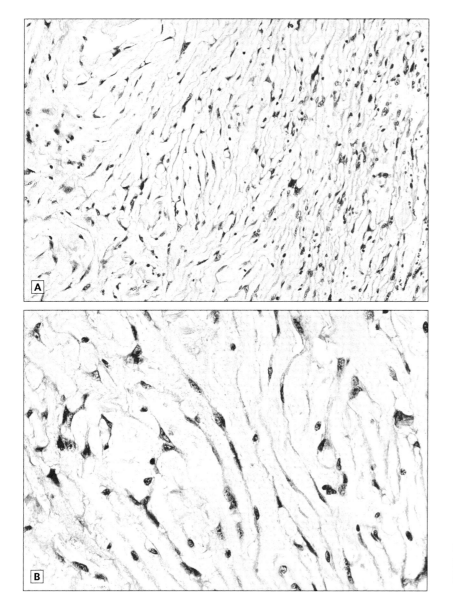

FIGURE 29–88 **(A)** Extraneural (soft tissue) perineurioma with cytologic atypia. **(B)** High-power view illustrating slender cell processes. The tumor behaved in an aggressive fashion.

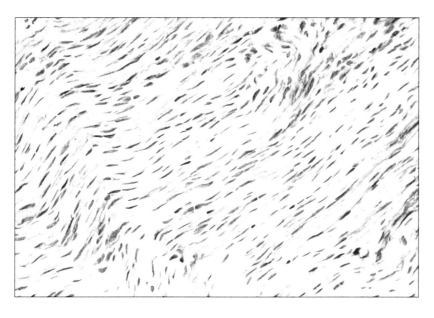

FIGURE 29–89 EMA immunostaining of a perineurioma.

and is seen in a variety of other soft tissue lesions, particularly conventional schwannomas. Electron microscopic identification may be used in lieu of immunohistochemistry, although the relative ease and low cost of immunohistochemistry has decreased its popularity. The attributes of perineurial cells include slender, nontapered processes containing large numbers of pinocytotic vesicles and partial investment with basal lamina (Figs 29–90, 29–91). Ribosome lamellar complexes were described in one perineurioma by Dhimes et al.[162]

Most perineuriomas possess little or no atypia and no mitotic activity; however, in the experience of Hornick and Fletcher,[143] 14 of 81 cases of perineuriomas had one or more atypical features, including mitotic activity (as high as 13/30 HPF), occasional pleomorphic cells, hypercellular foci, or infiltration of skeletal muscle (one case). Only two of 81 cases recurred and none metastasized within a mean follow-up period of 41 months, suggesting that none of these features per se predict malignancy.

Sclerosing perineurioma

An unusual variant of soft tissue perineurioma has been described by Fetsch and Miettinen as *sclerosing perineurioma*.[160,163,164] These lesions occur primarily in young men and affect the hand exclusively. Unlike the foregoing forms of perineurioma, the cells vary from spindled to distinctly rounded and are arranged in cords, trabeculae, and chains within a densely sclerotic stroma (Fig. 29–92). In addition to EMA and GLUT1[160] positivity, nearly half of the lesions also express smooth muscle or muscle-specific actin. The differential diagnosis includes a variety of epithelioid lesions (e.g., epithelioid hemangioendothelioma, adnexal tumors) and fibrosing lesions (fibroma

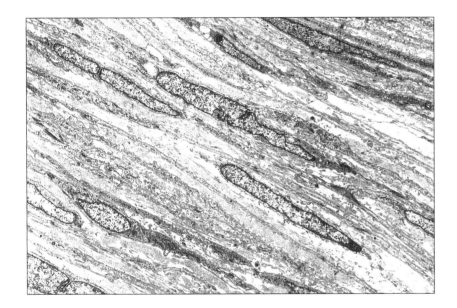

FIGURE 29–90 Electron micrograph of a perineurioma showing slender elongated cells invested with basal lamina.

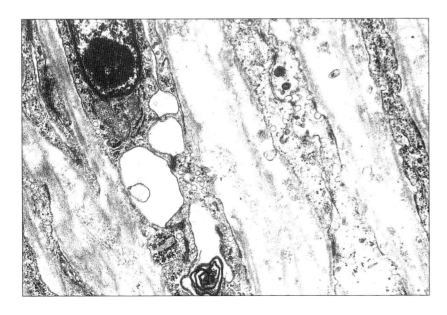

FIGURE 29–91 Electron micrograph of a perineurioma. A process of the perineurial cell is invested in basal lamina and has surface-oriented pinocytotic vesicles.

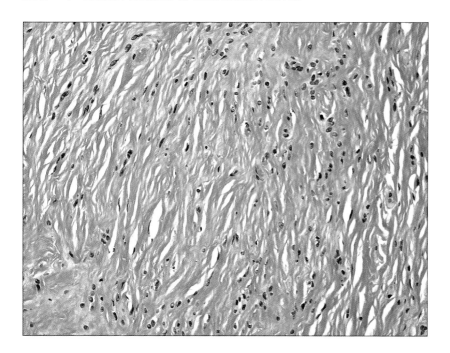

FIGURE 29–92 Sclerosing perineurioma.

of the tendon sheath, calcifying fibrous pseudotumor, fibrosing tenosynovial giant cell tumor). Because it is a recently recognized tumor, it is likely that many perineuriomas were previously diagnosed as fibrous histiocytoma, dermatofibrosarcoma protuberans, neurofibroma, or meningioma. Although it is occasionally possible to suspect the diagnosis of a perineurioma when distinct whorls are present in a tumor or when a presumed "neurofibroma" fails to stain for S-100 protein, the diagnosis must be confirmed with immunohistochemistry. Rearrangements/deletions of 10q[165] and deletions of *NF2* have been documented in this form of perineurioma.[165]

Reticular perineurioma

Reticular perineurioma is a variant of perineurioma characterized by a lace-like arrangement of cells that results in the formation of microscopic cysts (Fig. 29–93).[166–169] Aside from the unusual histologic appearance they appear to be similar to classic perineurioma.

Perineurial malignant peripheral nerve sheath tumor (malignant perineurioma)

By convention, the term perineurioma is used to refer to lesions with histologically benign or, at most, minimally atypical features as described above. However, tumors possessing the cytoarchitectural features of benign perineurioma, including cellular whorls and cells with thread-like cytoplasmic processes, but also significant atypia and mitotic activity that would qualify as overt malignancy have been recognized and designated perineurial malignant peripheral nerve sheath tumor (Figs 29–94,

29–95).[170] Seven such cases were recognized among 121 malignant peripheral nerve sheath tumors from the Mayo Clinic. Clinically, these tumors had a similar presentation similar to other malignant peripheral nerve sheath tumors, although none was associated with a neurofibroma or occurred in a patient with NF1. Four of the tumors were high grade and three low grade. Four of the seven cases recurred and two metastasized.

GRANULAR CELL TUMOR

The granular cell tumor is a benign neural tumor characterized by large granular-appearing eosinophilic cells. Although originally considered a muscle tumor by Abrikossoff[171] in 1926, its close association with nerve and immunohistochemical characteristics firmly identifies it as a neural lesion, but it is sufficiently distinctive to be separated from neurofibroma and schwannoma. Older terms for this tumor are *granular cell myoblastoma, granular cell neuroma, granular cell neurofibroma,* and *granular cell schwannoma.* Reactive granular lesions consisting of collections of granular-appearing histiocytes at sites of trauma comprise a separate, unrelated entity (see Chapter 12).[172]

Granular cell tumors are fairly common; for example, Vance and Hudson[173] found one case among 346 surgical specimens. The granular cell tumor generally occurs as a small, poorly circumscribed nodule that may be solitary or multiple and always pursues a benign clinical course. Malignant granular cell tumor is a well established but rare entity, with fewer than 100 reported cases. It is discussed separately below.

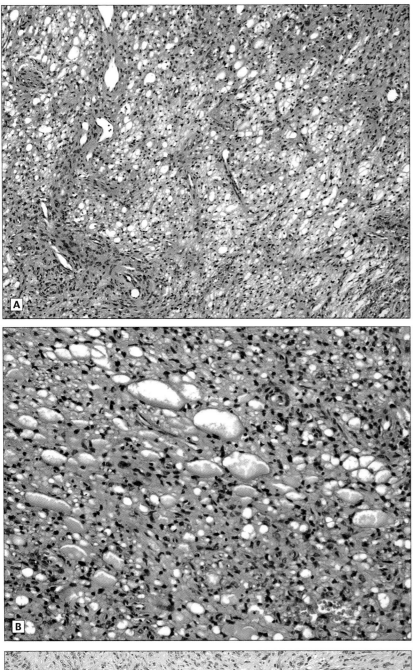

FIGURE 29–93 Reticular perineurioma **(A)** illustrating microscopic cysts **(B)**.

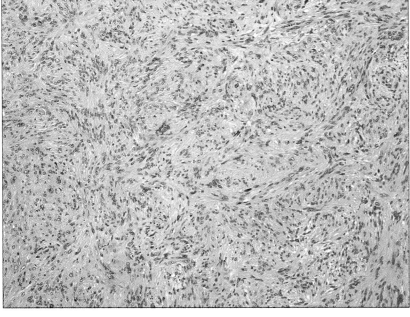

FIGURE 29–94 Perineurial malignant peripheral nerve sheath tumor illustrating generalized nuclear atypia.

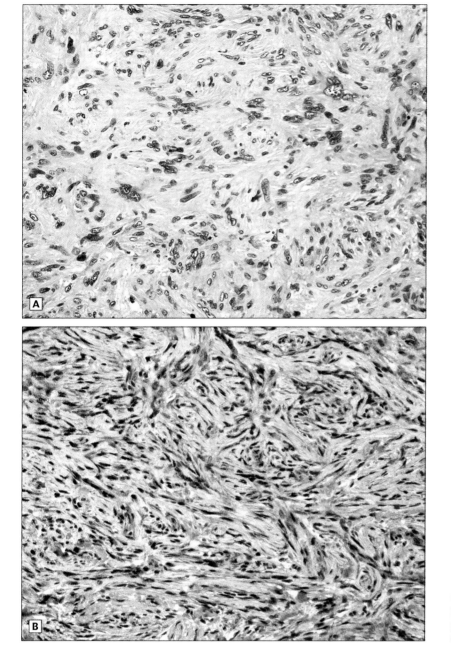

FIGURE 29–95 Perineurial malignant peripheral nerve sheath tumor (malignant perineurioma) **(A)**. Tumor was strongly and diffusely claudin-1-positive **(B)**.

Granular cell tumors occur in patients of any age but are most common in those in the fourth, fifth, and sixth decades of life; they are rare in children. It is about twice as common in women as in men. The lesion manifests as a solitary painless nodule located in the dermis or subcutis and less frequently in the submucosa, smooth muscle, or striated muscle (Fig. 29–96). It is also found in the internal organs, particularly the larynx, bronchus, stomach, and bile duct. Usually, the nodule is smaller than 3 cm and has been noted for less than 6 months.

Approximately 10–15% of patients with a granular cell tumor have lesions at multiple sites, frequently involving the subcutis, submucosa, and one or more visceral structures. The number of lesions varies greatly from patient to patient, but as many as 50 nodules have been counted in some cases. Multiple lesions may appear synchronously or over a period of many years. Increased familial incidence is extremely uncommon, but has been reported.

Pathologic findings

Granular cell tumors tend to be poorly circumscribed nodules measuring less than 3 cm in diameter, and on cut section are characteristically pale yellow-tan or yellow-gray. About two-thirds of the nodules are located in the dermal, subcutaneous, or submucosal tissues. Some are associated with marked acanthosis or pseudoepithelio-

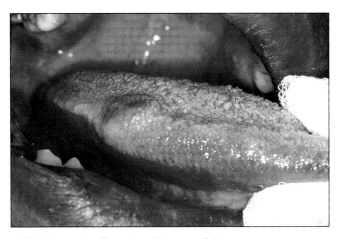

FIGURE 29–96 Granular cell tumor of the tongue.

matous hyperplasia of the overlying squamous epithelium, a striking feature that has repeatedly caused this process to be mistaken for squamous cell carcinoma (Fig. 29–97). Another important, histogenetically significant feature is the close association between granular cells and peripheral nerves. Frequently, the granular cells encompass small nerves or replace them almost entirely and are recognizable only by the residual neurites that can be demonstrated with the Bodian method or similar silver preparations (Fig. 29–98). At times, clusters of granular cells are also surrounded by circumferentially arranged spindle cells in the manner of perineurium.

The cells of granular cell tumor are rounded, polygonal, or slightly spindled in character, with nuclei ranging from small and dark to large with vesicular chromatin

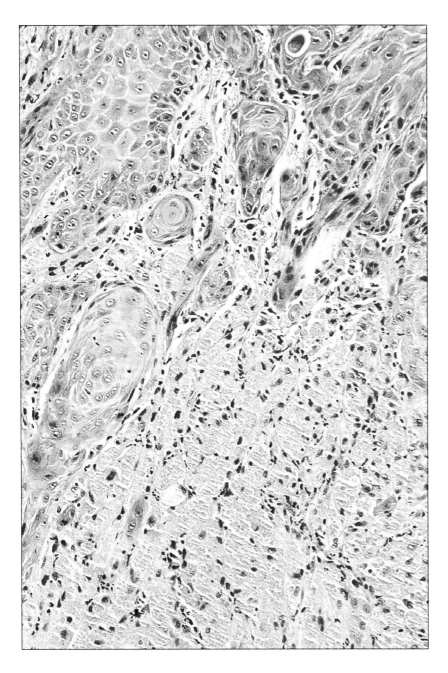

FIGURE 29–97 Granular cell tumor with pseudoepitheliomatous hyperplasia of the overlying skin.

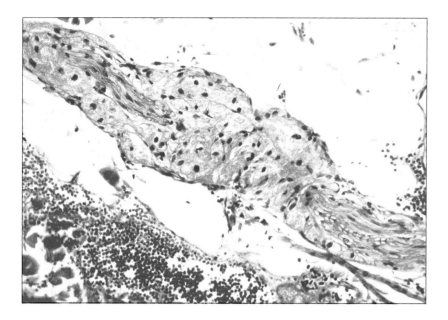

FIGURE 29–98 Granular cell tumor involving a small nerve.

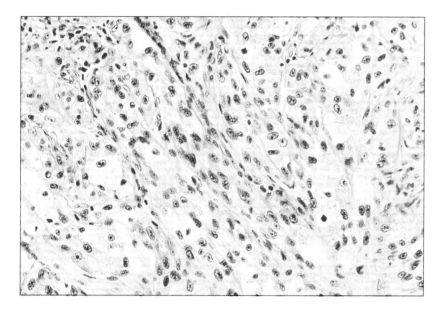

FIGURE 29–99 Granular cell tumor with spindled and rounded tumor cells.

(Figs 29–99, 29–100). Mild to moderate amounts of nuclear atypia may be seen but in and of itself is not indicative of malignancy (Fig. 29–101). The eosinophilic cytoplasm is fine to coarsely granular. The granules, representing phagolysosomes, are strongly PAS-positive, diastase-resistant (Fig. 29–102). Smaller cells containing coarse particles that are strongly PAS-positive are interspersed between the granular cells (interstitial cells, angulate body cells).

The growth pattern varies; the cells tend to be disposed in ribbons or nests divided by slender fibrous connective tissue septa or in large sheets with no particular cellular arrangement. Older lesions frequently exhibit marked desmoplasia, and some of these can be identified only by the presence of a few scattered nests of granular cells in a dense mass of collagen.

Less frequently, the granular cells involve or replace the musculature; they grow along the muscle fibers or even seem to extend within the sarcolemmal sheath. They may also be found in smooth muscle tissue, in fibrous tissue such as tendons, fascia, or ligaments, and rarely in small lymphoid aggregates or even lymph nodes, a feature that should not be confused with lymph node metastasis (Fig. 29–103).

The tumors are immunoreactive for S-100 protein (Fig. 29–104), neuron-specific enolase, laminin, and various myelin proteins. Because the characteristic granules are lysosomal in nature, it is not surprising that granular cell tumors are also strongly positive for the panmacrophage antigen CD68 (Kp1).[174,175] The cells do not react with antibodies for neurofilament proteins or glial fibrillary acidic protein (GFAP).[172,176,177]

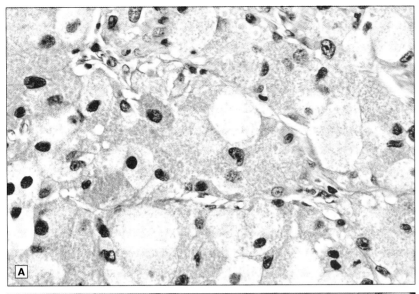

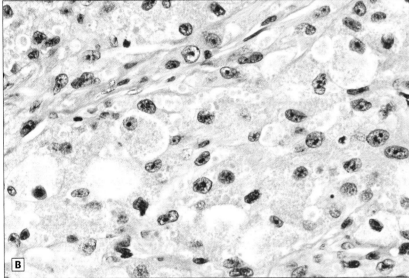

FIGURE 29–100 Granular cell tumor with a range of nuclear appearances. Some nuclei are small and dark **(A)**, and others are larger with a vesicular nuclear chromatin pattern **(B)**.

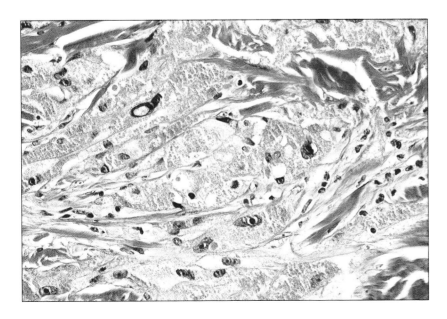

FIGURE 29–101 Benign granular cell tumor with atypical cells. This change does not per se indicate malignancy.

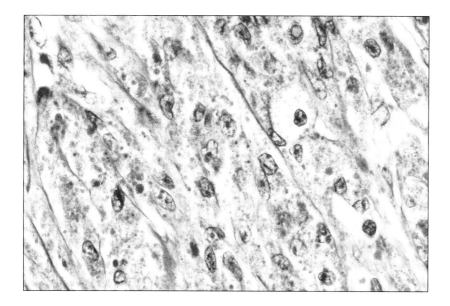

FIGURE 29–102 Periodic acid-Schiff (PAS)-positive diastase-resistant bodies in a granular cell tumor.

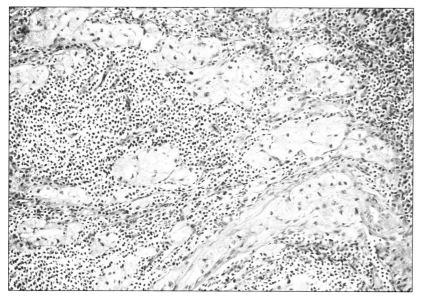

FIGURE 29–103 Granular cell tumor involving a lymph node.

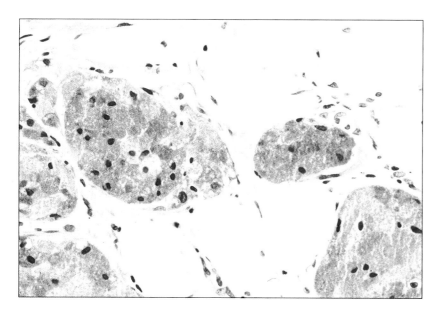

FIGURE 29–104 S-100 protein immunoreactivity in a granular cell tumor.

Ultrastructurally, the granular cell tumor contains intracellular granules consisting of membrane-bound, presumably autophagic, vacuoles containing myelin figures and fragmented rough endoplasmic reticulum and mitochondria. According to some authors, myelinated and nonmyelinated axon-like structures are also present (Figs 29–105, 29–106). There are also small interstitial cells with angulated bodies containing packets of parallel microtubules (Fig. 29–107), microfilaments, and lipid material as well as cells with multiple cytoplasmic processes, partly surrounded by incomplete basal laminae.

Differential diagnosis

A number of benign mesenchymal tumors have a granular appearance. The coarsely granular cytoplasm and the absence of cross-striations and glycogen distinguish the benign granular cell tumor from rhabdomyoma; the absence of lipid droplets distinguishes it from hibernoma and fibroxanthoma. Awareness of the frequent association of dermal granular cell tumor and marked acanthosis of the overlying squamous epithelium prevents a mistaken diagnosis of squamous cell carcinoma.

Finally, reactive changes that occur in association with surgical trauma or other types of injury may simulate a benign granular cell tumor. The granular cells in these lesions tend to be associated with inflammatory elements and areas of necrosis, and they stain more intensely with the Alcian blue stain and PAS preparation (see Chapter 12). This lesion also lacks the ribbon-like or nest-like cellular orientation of granular cell tumors. Sobel and Churg,[172,178] who gave a detailed account of this lesion, found several such examples in scars from cesarean sections. A massive granular reaction to epoxy polymer may also occur near prosthetic joint replacements (see Chapter 12).

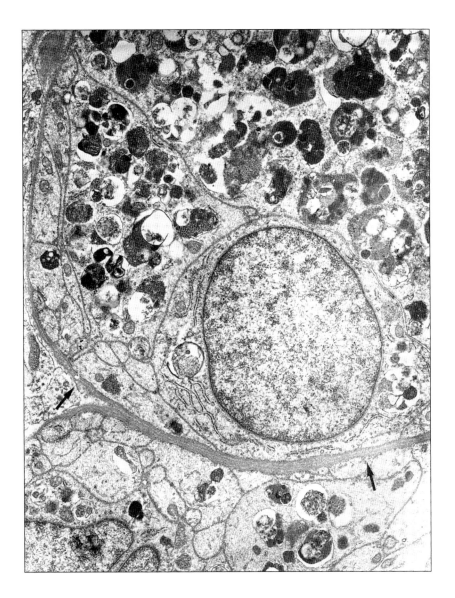

FIGURE 29–105 Ultrastructure of granular cell tumor. Large autophagic granules in the cytoplasm of the tumor cell are surrounded by a distinct basal lamina (arrows). (Courtesy of Dr. Zelma Molnar, Veterans Administration Hospital, Hines, IL.)

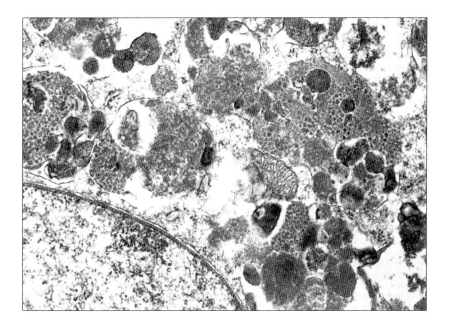

FIGURE 29–106 Large vacuoles containing finely granular structures and small masses of electron-dense material.

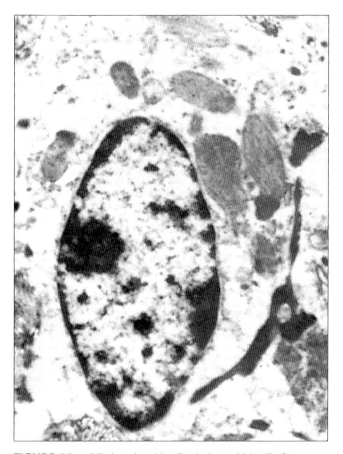

FIGURE 29–107 Angulated bodies in interstitial cell of a granular cell tumor (×7800).

Discussion

Early accounts uniformly regarded the granular cell tumor as one with muscle differentiation. This view gradually changed with the observation that nerves and neuromas occasionally display granular changes. In addition, electron microscopy and immunohistochemistry showed that the granular cell tumor had schwannian features. The tumors stain positively for S-100 protein, myelin proteins (PO and P2), and myelin-associated glycoproteins, suggesting that the granules are myelin or myelin breakdown products[176,179] The angular bodies in the interstitial cells are not marked by antibodies to S-100 protein, but they are positive on staining with antibodies to myelin protein.[176] Excluding the malignant tumors, recurrence is rare. Of 92 cases reported by Strong et al.,[180] six recurred, one of them after 10 years. Hence local surgical excision is curative in nearly all cases.

Malignant granular cell tumor

Malignant granular tumors constitute fewer than 2% of all granular cell tumors. Ravich et al.[181] are usually credited with the first account of this entity. It occurred in the wall of the urinary bladder of a 31-year-old woman who died of metastatic disease 17 months after the tumor was removed surgically and diagnosed as a malignant granular cell tumor. Since their report, about 80 additional cases have been described including the largest series of 46 cases reported by Fanburg-Smith et al.[182]

In most respects, malignant tumors are similar to benign ones except they are rarely encountered during childhood and tend to be, on average, larger than their benign counterparts. A history of long clinical duration and recent rapid growth has been observed in some cases, suggesting the possibility of malignant transformation from a preexisting benign granular cell tumor, analogous to the malignant transformation of neurofibromas.

Although in the earlier literature a variety of malignant soft tissue tumors were labeled malignant granular cell tumors (e.g., granular cell leiomyosarcoma), this diagnosis should be restricted to neoplasms that are histologically similar to benign granular cell tumors but that have a constellation of histologic features that portend an increased risk for metastasis.[182] Such features include necrosis, spindling, vesicular nuclei with prominent nucleoli, increased mitotic activity (>2 mitoses/10 HPF), high nucleocytoplasmic ratio, and pleomorphism. Tumors with three or more of these features are considered malignant and have an approximately 40% risk of causing death (Figs 29–108, 29–109). Tumors with fewer than three features (termed "atypical granular cell tumor") have an excellent outcome with no metastases. This system provides a systematic approach to identifying lesions with a significant risk of metastasis. When employing this system we usually require that features such as spindling and atypia be prominent in the tumor and not simply a focal change.

Frankly malignant granular cell tumors should be distinguished from other malignant tumors that display granular cytoplasm from time to time, such as leiomyosarcoma, malignant fibrous histiocytoma, and angiosarcoma. It is useful to keep in mind that granular cell tumors, even malignant ones, usually originate in superficial soft tissues, and their granularity tends to be a diffuse, uniform change as contrasted with the focal granularity in other malignant lesions.

Typically, the malignant form of granular cell tumor recurs before it metastasizes, usually within less than 1 year. Metastasis occurs through the lymphatics and bloodstream; and lymph node metastases and metastases to the lung, liver, and bone are common. The interval between excising the primary tumor and the appearance of metastasis is variable, but in most cases it takes several years before the metastatic lesions become apparent.

CONGENITAL (GINGIVAL) GRANULAR CELL TUMOR

The term *congenital (gingival) granular cell tumor* and its synonyms, *congenital epulis, congenital granular cell myoblastoma,* and *granular cell fibroblastoma,* have been applied to a variant of the granular cell tumor that is indistinguishable in its structure and staining characteristics from this tumor but differs by its exclusive occurrence in infants at or immediately after birth and by its characteristic location in the labial aspect of the dental ridge, with a predilection for the upper jaw.[183–193] It also differs from adult granular cell tumors by its prominent vascularity, the presence of scattered remnants of odontogenic epithelium, and the strong phosphatase activity of the tumor cells (Fig. 29–110). Moreover, it lacks interstitial cells with angulate bodies and does not show immunostaining for laminin or S-100 protein.[189] About 10% of these lesions are multiple, and approximately 90% afflict girls.[183,188] Characteristically, the condition manifests as a protruding, round or ovoid nodule covered by a smooth mucosal surface and firmly attached to the gum by a broad base or infrequently by a pedicle. Ulceration of the mucosa is uncommon, and microscopically there is no evidence of pseudoepitheliomatous hyperplasia of the overlying squamous epithelium.[188] Like other forms of granular cell tumor, the nodules are small, averaging 1–2 cm in greatest diameter.

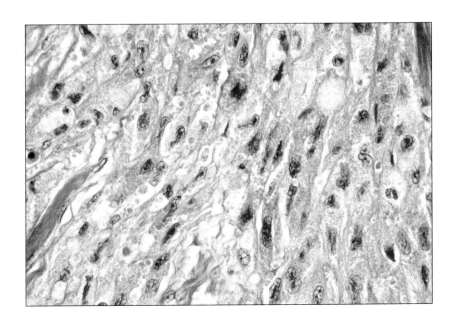

FIGURE 29–108 Malignant granular cell tumor with nuclear atypia, spindling, and prominent nucleoli.

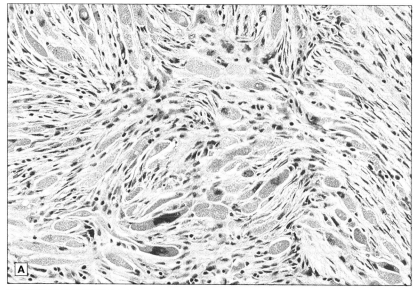

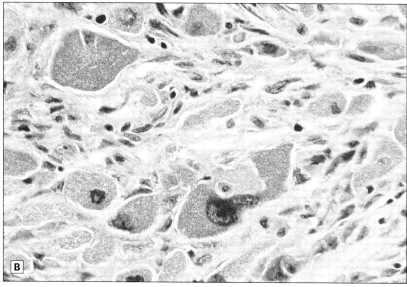

FIGURE 29–109 (A, B) Malignant granular cell minor illustrating profound nuclear atypia, prominent nucleoli, and spindling. Mitotic figures were also identified.

There is usually no further growth after birth and no tendency toward local recurrence. In fact, even without therapy, most congenital granular cell tumors cease to grow or regress spontaneously. Lack et al.[189] reported that lesions treated later in the neonatal period were smaller and exhibited some evidence of involution. There is no record of a malignant counterpart of this tumor. The exact nature of this condition is still not clear, and there is little support for an origin from odontogenic epithelial cells.

CLASSIC NEUROTHEKEOMA (NERVE SHEATH MYXOMA)

Neurothekeoma was first well described by Gallagher and Helwig[194] in a series of 53 cases although identical cases had been reported as *nerve sheath myxoma, dermal nerve sheath myxoma*,[195,196] and *bizarre cutaneous neurofibroma*.[197]

Some tumors, referred to as *pacinian neurofibromas*, are probably also neurothekeomas.

They usually arise during childhood and early adult life and have a predilection for the upper portion of the body, such as the head, neck, and shoulder. Mucous membranes are rarely involved. They are situated in the dermis and subcutis and in an exceptional instance occur in deep soft tissue.

At low power the lesion has a distinctive compartmentalized appearance due to the fibrous bands that subdivide the lesion into irregular lobules (Figs 29–111, 29–112). Each lobule consists of a variable mixture of cells and myxoid stroma (hyaluronic acid or sulfated acid mucin) (Figs 29–113, 29–114)[194] so that the overall tumor can appear myxoid or solid. The cells vary from round to spindled and typically have little atypia or mitotic activity. Giant cells are occasionally present in the lobules, and rarely neurites are identified among the

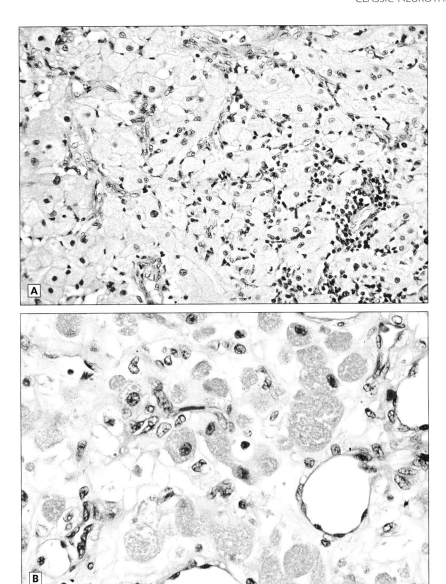

FIGURE 29–110 (A, B) Congenital granular cell tumor.

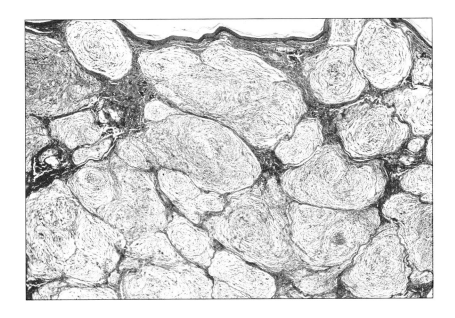

FIGURE 29–111 Neurothekeoma involving the dermis. Not the prominent septa.

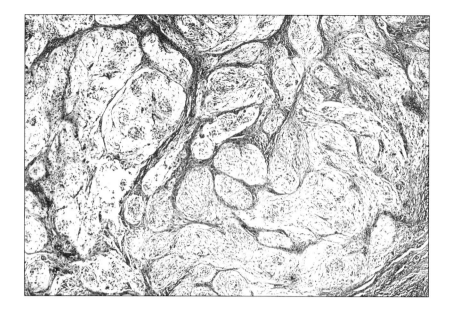

FIGURE 29–112 Neurothekeoma.

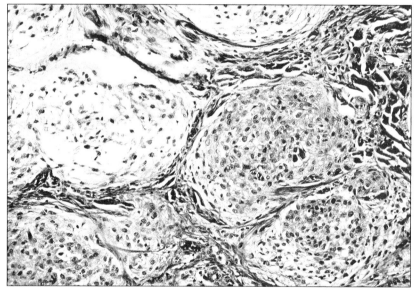

FIGURE 29–113 Myxoid and cellular nodules in a neurothekeoma.

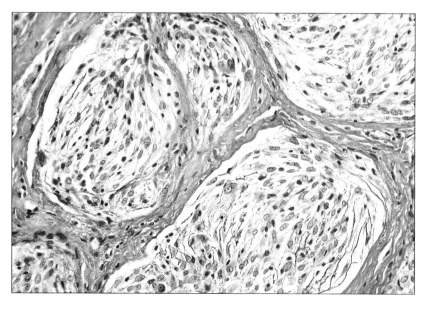

FIGURE 29–114 Cellular nodules in a neurothekeoma.

tumor cells. Although most tumors are quite myxoid, some are more cellular, with marked nuclear atypia, rare mitoses, extension into fat or skeletal muscle, or vascular invasion (Fig. 29–115). Known as *cellular neurotheke-oma*[198,199] or *cellular neurothekeoma with atypical features*,[200] they may be mistaken for sarcoma to those unfamiliar with the basic architectural pattern of the tumor (see below). The most helpful clues to the recognition of neurothekeomas with atypical features are the superficial dermal location and the distinctive septate architecture. Neurothekeoma is regarded as a benign neural tumor. Tumors typically express S-100 protein (Fig. 29–116)[201] and PGP9.5,[202] a broad neural marker. There is, however, controversy as to whether "cellular neurothekeoma" is a variant of classic neurothekeoma or not, due to differences in immunohistochemistry (Fig. 29–117).

The differential diagnosis of this unusual tumor includes notably focal mucinosis, myxoid malignant fibrous histiocytoma, and myxoid neurofibroma. Focal mucinosis does not display the degree of circumscription, lobulation, or cellularity seen in neurothekeoma. Myxoid malignant fibrous histiocytomas are poorly circumscribed, more pleomorphic lesions with a more elaborate and organized vasculature and no septations. Moreover, most develop as large, deeply situated tumors in adults in contrast to neurothekeoma, which occurs principally in the superficial soft tissues of young individuals. Distinction of this tumor from neurofibroma is more of an academic point, as they may well be related. In general, the multinodularity and the whorled arrangement of the cells of neurothekeoma contrast with most neurofibromas.

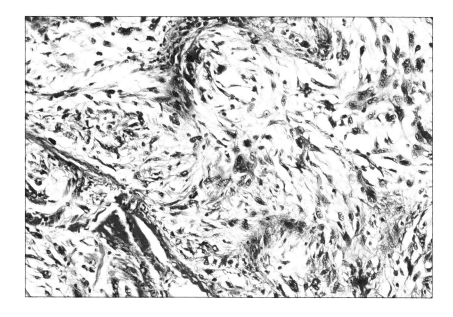

FIGURE 29–115 Nuclear atypia in a neurothekeoma, a feature not associated with aggressive behavior.

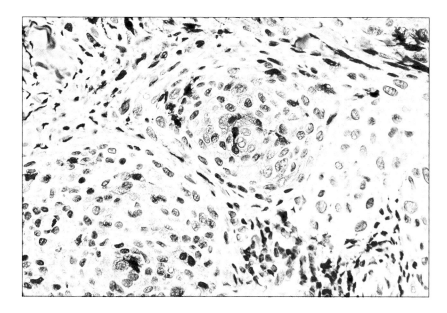

FIGURE 29–116 S-100 protein immunoreactivity in a neurothekeoma.

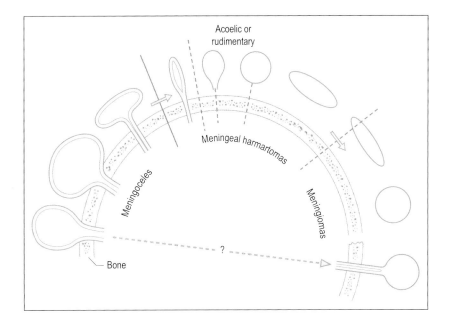

FIGURE 29–117 Histogenesis of cutaneous meningiomas. Note the possible relations between meningoceles, meningeal hamartomas, and type I extracranial meningiomas. The first retain their connections with the central nervous system and are predominantly cystic, whereas the last two lose the connections and are solid. (From Lopez DA, Silvers DN, Helwig EB. Cutaneous meningiomas: a clinicopathologic study. Cancer 1974; 34:728.)

Cellular neurothekeoma

In 1990 Barnhill and Mihm described the entity of "cellular neurothekeoma" and noted that, unlike classic neurothekeoma, it consistently lacked S-100 protein,[198] although this point has recently been contested.[201] Since that time, its similarity to classic neurothekeoma has been debated and some have considered it an epithelioid form of pilar leiomyoma.[199] In our opinion, the lesions that have been described as cellular neurothekeoma may well represent more than a single entity. Some probably represent classic neurothekeomas which lack a myxoid background and therefore appear cellular, whereas others may represent other tumor(s) altogether. The recent report that MiTF and NK1/3 (melanocytic markers) are strongly expressed in cellular neurothekeomas in the absence of S-100 protein and with the occasional presence of actin has led to the interesting proposal that the lesion might represent a member of the PEComa family (see chapter 36).[203]

EXTRACRANIAL MENINGIOMA

Extracranial meningiomas are rare tumors that occur in the skin or soft tissue of the scalp or along the vertebral axis.[204,205] By definition they are not associated with an underlying meningioma of the neuraxis, and extracranial extension of an intracranial tumor should always be considered before accepting a meningioma in soft tissue or skin as a primary tumor. Although true extracranial meningiomas probably arise from ectopic arachnoid lining cells, their precise presentation and localization suggest at least two pathogenetic mechanisms.[204]

One form of extracranial meningioma, termed type I by Lopez et al.,[204] arises in the skin of the scalp, forehead, and paravertebral areas and as a result may be mistaken clinically for cutaneous lesions, including epidermal inclusion cyst, skin tag, and nevus. The pathogenesis is probably similar to that of meningocele and is believed to be the result of abnormalities of neural tube closure with relocation of meningeal tissue in the surrounding skin and subcutis (Fig. 29–117). This proposal explains the congenital nature of the type I tumor and its distribution, which coincides with that of meningocele. The similarity of this tumor to meningocele is heightened by its histologic appearance. Although some consist of solid, isolated nests of meningothelial cells in the skin, others may contain a rudimentary stalk or cystic cavity (Fig. 29–118). Such lesions occupy an intermediate position in the spectrum between meningocele and extracranial meningioma and have been named *meningeal hamartomas*. The type I meningioma is benign, although persistence of a connection with the central nervous system can lead to postoperative meningitis or neurologic deficits.

The second form of extracranial meningioma (type II) (Fig. 29–119) may occur at any age, but adults are usually affected. These tumors are situated in the vicinity of the sensory organs (eye, ear, nose) or along the paths of the cranial and spinal nerves. Symptoms associated with the tumor are related to its size, location, and growth rate. Histologically, these lesions are indistinguishable from the ordinary intracranial meningioma. The solid nests of meningothelial cells are arranged in sheets or whorls and occasionally are punctuated by psammoma bodies (Fig. 29–120). In addition to surgical removal, appropriate studies to exclude an intracranial component are recommended for these more deeply situated tumors.

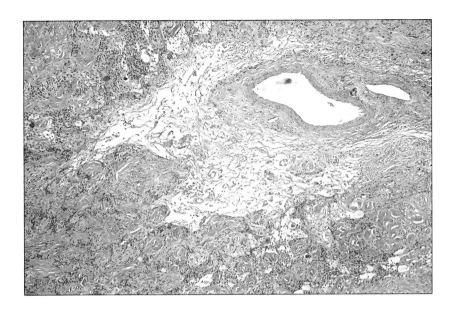

FIGURE 29–118 Type I ectopic meningioma from a child. Note the partially cystic central area.

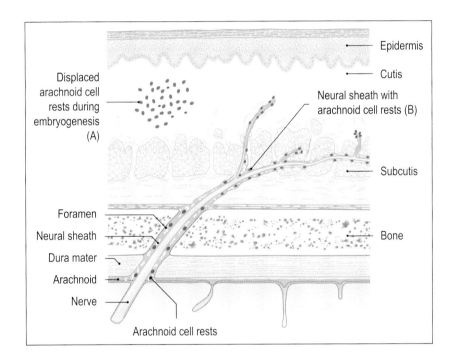

FIGURE 29–119 Primary cutaneous meningiomas. There are two possible origins of primary cutaneous meningiomas. **(A)** Type I may result from abnormalities of neural tube closure with resultant ectopic arachnoid cell rests. **(B)** Type II, which occurs in adults and follows the distribution of the sensory organs and nerves, probably is derived from arachnoid rests in nerve sheaths. (From Lopez DA, Silvers DN, Helwig EB. Cutaneous meningiomas: a clinicopathologic study. Cancer 1974; 34:728.)

GLIAL HETEROTOPIAS

Like ectopic meningeal rests, ectopic deposits of glial tissue occur occasionally on the scalp and rarely in other soft tissue sites.[206–208] Over the years they have been called a variety of names, including nasal glioma, glial hamartoma, and heterotopic glial tissue.[209] The common presentation of a glial heterotopia is that of a polypoid mass at the root of the nose or to one side of the bridge of the nose in an infant, which grows commensurately with the infant. In most cases the lesions lack a communication with the brain; in the few that do communicate with the brain, the connection occurs through the cribriform plate such that rhinorrhea may be an accompanying symptom. Histologically, the lesions consist of mats of mature glial tissue which, in addition to astrocytes, may also contain neurons (Fig. 29–121). Although most glial heterotopias may be viewed as variants of encephalocele, in which the communication with the brain is lost, we have encountered two glial heterotopias on the chest wall of adults, suggesting that other pathogenetic mechanisms allow the development of these unusual lesions.

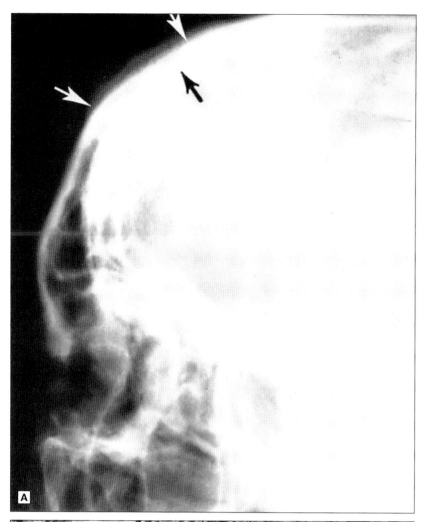

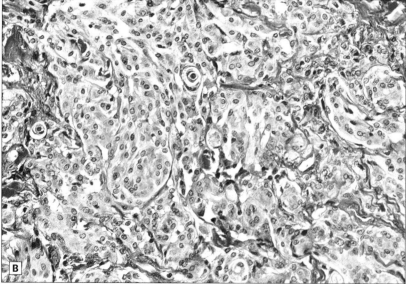

FIGURE 29–120 Primary cutaneous meningioma of the frontal area of the scalp. **(A)** Radiograph demonstrates extracranial location of frontal mass. The outer table of the skull is partly eroded (between the white arrows) whereas the inner table is intact (black arrow). **(B)** Tumor consists of whorls of plump epithelioid cells indistinguishable from cells of the intracranial form of meningioma.

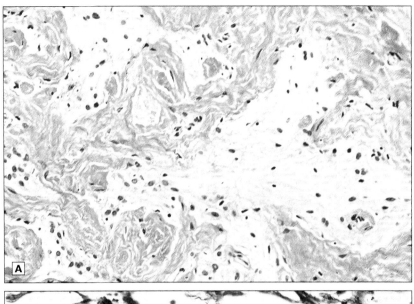

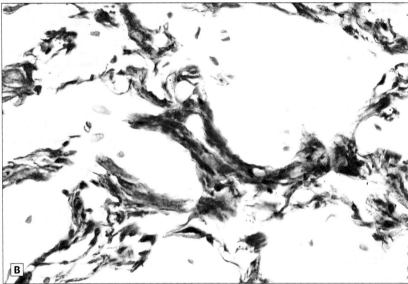

FIGURE 29–121 (A) Glial heterotopia with lightly staining glial tissue interspersed between collagen (dark areas). **(B)** Immunostaining for glial fibrillary acidic protein highlights glial tissue against the negatively staining backdrop of collagen.

MELANOTIC NEUROECTODERMAL TUMOR OF INFANCY (RETINAL ANLAGE TUMOR, MELANOTIC PROGONOMA)

First described in 1918 by Krompecher, the melanotic neuroectodermal tumor of infancy, a rare tumor of disputed histogenesis, has been referred to as *congenital melanocarcinoma, melanotic adamantinoma, retinal anlage tumor, melanotic progonoma,* and *pigmented epulis of infancy.*[210-233] Although most current studies support a neural crest origin of this tumor, there is little evidence that the tumor specifically represents retinal anlage. Therefore, we prefer the less fanciful term *melanotic neuroectodermal tumor of infancy.*

Clinical findings

The tumor usually develops during the first year of life and presents as a protruding mass in the upper or lower jaw. The skin or mucosa is tightly stretched over the lesion, but it is rarely if ever ulcerated. Radiographically, the tumor is a cystic radiolucent lesion with a capacity for local destruction and displacement of the developing teeth (Fig. 29–122). Patients with this tumor in unusual sites such as the anterior fontanelle, epididymis,[215,216,233] mediastinum,[226] and brain,[231] develop symptoms referable to those sites. The few cases reported in the uterus[226] and shoulder[225] and those in adults[224] should be disregarded because they represent different lesions altogether.

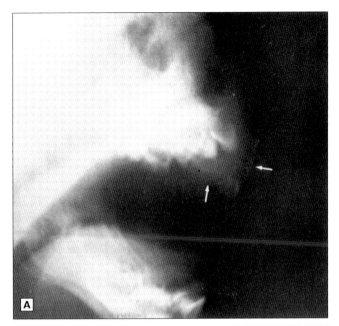

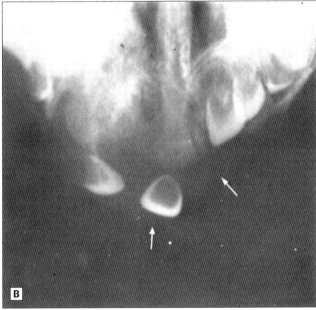

FIGURE 29–122 Radiograph of pigmented neuroectodermal tumor of infancy (retinal anlage tumor) in the maxilla. Tumor is a vaguely outlined soft tissue mass (arrows) with destruction of the maxilla **(A)** and displacement of teeth **(B)**.

We have encountered one of these tumors in the soft tissues of the extremity, and it has also been reported in long bone.

Gross and microscopic findings

Grossly, the tumor ranges in color from slate gray to blue-black, depending on the amount of melanin pigment. It is composed of irregular alveolar spaces lined by cuboidal cells containing varying amounts of melanin pigment

(Fig. 29–123). In addition, small, round, less well-differentiated cells resembling those of neuroblastoma lie in the alveolar space or as isolated nests in a fibrous stroma. Neurofibrillary material, resembling glial tissue, may be seen in association with these cells in the alveolar spaces. In two exceptional cases, glial tissue was found outside the epithelial islands. One case was a tumor arising in the brain in which the entire stroma was glial,[231] and the second was a tumor arising in a glial heterotopia of the oropharynx.[222]

The cuboidal cells have the electron microscopic features of epithelial and melanocytic cells.[213] They are bounded by basal laminae and elaborately interdigitate laterally with neighboring cells, forming desmosomes. Both mature and immature melanosomes similar to those of melanocytes and melanoma cells are present in the cytoplasm. Functionally, they share certain properties of the melanocyte in that melanization of these cells may be increased by agents that induce similar changes in melanocytes of animals.[213] Immunohistochemically, the cuboidal cells express cytokeratin and a melanoma-associated antigen (HMB-45). Neuron-specific enolase, Leu-7, and synaptophysin are variably present in the epithelial cells and the small neuroblastic element.

The round, less well-differentiated cells contain few organelles but are believed to be neuroblastic by virtue of their elongated cell processes, dense-core vesicles,[213] and intracytoplasmic neurofilamentous material.[213,217] Their association with glial-like areas and, in one case, with ganglioneuromatous areas[213] provides further support for this contention.

Discussion

Traditionally, this tumor was considered benign, but in a large series from the AFIP nearly half of those with follow-up information recurred, and 5–10% of cases reported in the literature have produced metastasis.[213,219,223] One case, a stillborn, was noted to have multiple metastases at delivery.[223] A second case, a tumor of the epididymis, produced micrometastases in regional lymph nodes;[219] and two others metastasized as primitive neuroblastic tumors devoid of melanin.[213,219] Although metastasis is a relatively uncommon event, attempts to eradicate the tumor at the time of initial surgery are endorsed. Unfortunately, it has not been possible to predict recurrence or metastasis in this disease by conventional parameters or by utilization of more sophisticated techniques such as flow cytometry.

The histogenesis of this tumor has been controversial. The concepts of a congenital melanoma and an odontogenic tumor are now obsolete for various reasons. The former does not account for the primitive neuroblastic component, and the latter does not take into consideration tumors at sites where there are no odontogenic rests. To date the most appealing theory is

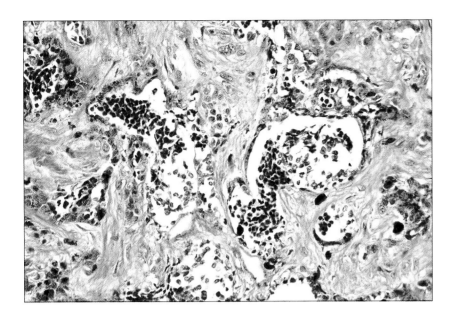

FIGURE 29–123 Pigmented neuroectodermal tumor of infancy with flattened pigmented epithelial cells lining alveolar spaces. Immature, nonpigmented rounded cells lie clumped in the spaces (×160).

that the tumor is derived from neural crest.[211,213] This concept allows latitude in the distribution of the lesions, accounts for the presence of pigmented and neuroblastic elements, and explains the rare tumor associated with increased levels of vanillylmandelic acid.[211,213] It does not seem necessary to compare this tumor specifically with the developing retina; in fact, the embryologic evidence against this possibility has been extensively summarized.[211] It seems more probable that this tumor merely reflects a primitive stage or degree of differentiation common to many types of pigmented neuroepithelium.

REFERENCES

Embryogenesis and normal anatomy

1. Asbury AK, Johnson PC. Pathology of peripheral nerve. In: Major problems in pathology, vol 9. Philadelphia: WB Saunders; 1978.
2. Burkel WE. The histological fine structure of perineurium Anat Rec 1967; 158:177.
3. Erlandson RA. The enigmatic perineural cell and its participation in tumors and in tumor-like entities. Ultrastruct Pathol 1991; 15:335.
4. Bunge MB, Wood PM, Tynan LB, et al. Perineurium originates from fibroblasts: demonstration in vitro with a retroviral marker. Science 1989; 243:229.
5. Church RL, Tanzer M, Pfeiffer SE. Collagen and procollagen production by a clonal line of Schwann cells. Proc Natl Acad Sci USA 1973; 70:1943.
6. Elvin LG. The structure and composition of motor, sensory, and autonomic nerves and nerve fibers. In: Bourne GH, ed. The structure and function of nervous tissue. Structure I, vol 1. San Diego: Academic Press; 1968:325.

Traumatic (amputation) neuroma

7. Cieslak AK, Stout AP. Traumatic and amputation neuromas. Arch Surg 1946; 53:646.
8. Das Gupta TW, Brasfield RD. Amputation neuromas in cancer patients. NY J Med 1969; 69:2129.
9. Huber CC, Lewis LD. Amputation neuroma: their development and prevention. Arch Surg 1920; 1:85.
10. Snyder CC, Knowles RP. Traumatic neuromas. J Bone Joint Surg [Am] 1965; 47:641.

11. Hume RH, Buxton RW. Post cholecystectomy amputation neuroma. Am Surg 1954; 20:698.
12. Shapiro L, Juhlin E, Brownstein MH. Rudimentary polydactyly: an amputation neuroma. Arch Dermatol 1973; 108:223.
13. Boldrey F. Amputation neuroma in nerves implanted in bone. Ann Surg 1943; 118:1052.

Mucosal neuroma

14. Williams ED, Pollack DJ. Multiple mucosal neuromata with endocrine tumors: a syndrome allied to von Recklinghausen's disease. J Pathol 1966; 91:71.
15. Carney JA, Hayles AB. Alimentary tract manifestations of multiple endocrine neoplasia, type 2b. Mayo Clin Proc 1977; 52:543.

Pacinian neuroma

16. Dembinski AS, Jones JW. Intra-abdominal pacinian neuroma: a rare lesion in an unusual location. Histopathology 1991; 19:89.
17. Fletcher CDM, Theaker JM. Digital pacinian neuroma: a distinctive hyperplastic lesion. Histopathology 1989; 15:249.
18. Fraitag S, Sherardi R, Wechsler J. Hyperplastic pacinian corpuscles: an uncommonly encountered lesion of the hand. J Cutan Pathol 1994; 21:457.
19. Hart WR, Thompson NW, Hildreth DH, et al. Hyperplastic pacinian corpuscles: a cause of digital pain. Surgery 1971; 70:730.
20. Rhode CM, Jennings WD Jr. Pacinian corpuscle neuroma of digital nerves. South Med J 1975; 68:86.

Palisaded encapsulated neuroma

21. Reed RJ, Fine RM, Meltzer HD. Palisaded encapsulated neuromas of the skin. Arch Dermatol 1972; 106:865.

22. Albrecht S, Kahn HJK, From L. Palisaded encapsulated neuroma: an immunohistochemical study. Mod Pathol 1989; 2:403.
23. Argenyi ZB, Cooper PH, Santa Cruz D. Plexiform and other unusual variants of palisaded encapsulated neuroma. J Cutan Pathol 1993; 20:34.
24. Dakin MC, Leppard B, Theaker JM. The palisaded encapsulated neuroma (solitary circumscribed neuroma). Histopathology 1992; 20:405.
25. Fletcher CDM. Solitary circumscribed neuroma of the skin (so-called palisaded, encapsulated neuroma): a clinicopathologic and immunohistochemical study. Am J Surg Pathol 1989; 13:574.
26. Argenyi ZB, Santa Cruz D, Bromley C. Comparative light-microscopic and immunohistochemical study of traumatic and palisaded encapsulated neuromas of the skin. Am J Dermatopathol 1992; 14:505.

Morton's interdigital neuroma

27. Bennett GL, Graham CE, Mauldin DM. Morton's interdigital neuroma: a comprehensive treatment protocol. J Foot Ankle Surg 1995; 16:760.
28. Lassmann G, Lassmann H, Stockinger L. Morton's metatarsalgia: light and electron microscopic observations and their relations to entrapment neuropathies. Virchows Arch [Pathol Anat] 1976; 370:307.
29. Reed RJ, Bliss BO. Morton's neuroma: regressive and productive intermetatarsal elastofibrositis. Arch Pathol 1973; 95:123.
30. Scotti TM. The lesion of Morton's metatarsalgia (Morton's toe). Arch Pathol 1957; 63:91.
31. Wu KK. Morton's interdigital neuroma: a clinical review of its etiology, treatment and results. J Foot Ankle Surg 1996; 35:112.

32. Young G, Lindsey J. Etiology of symptomatic recurrent interdigital neuromas. J Am Podiatr Med Assoc 1993; 83:255.

Nerve sheath ganglion

33. Barrett R, Cramer F. Tumors of the peripheral nerves and so-called ganglia of the peroneal nerve. Clin Orthop 1963; 27:135.
34. Cobb CA III, Moiel RN. Ganglion of the peroneal nerve: report of two cases. J Neurosurg 1974; 41:255.
35. Guardjian ES, Larsen RD, Lindner DW. Intraneural cyst of the peroneal and ulnar nerves: report of two cases. J Neurosurg 1965; 23:76.

Neuromuscular hamartoma

36. Van Dorpe JV, Sciot R, De Vos R, et al. Neuromuscular choristoma (hamartoma) with smooth and striated muscle component: case report with immunohistochemical and ultrastructural analysis. Am J Surg Pathol 1997; 21:1090.
37. Awasthi D, Kline DG, Beckman EN. Neuromuscular hamartoma (benign Triton tumor) of the brachial plexus. J Neurosurg 1991; 75:795.
38. Bonneau R, Brochu P. Neuromuscular choristoma: a clinicopathologic study of two cases. Am J Surg Pathol 1983; 7:521.
39. Louhimo I, Rapola J. Intraneural muscular hamartoma: report of two cases in small children. J Pediatr Surg 1972; 7:696.
40. Markel SF, Enzinger FM. Neuromuscular hamartoma: a benign "Triton tumor" composed of mature neural and striated muscle elements. Cancer 1982; 49:140.
41. Mitchell A, Scheithauer BW, Ostertag H, et al. Neuromuscular hamartoma. Am J Clin Pathol 1995; 103:460.
42. O'Connell JX, Rosenberg AE. Multiple cutaneous neuromuscular choristomas: report of a case and a review of the literature. Am J Surg Pathol 1990; 14:93.
43. Orlandi E. Sopra un caso di rhabdomioma del nervo ischiatico. Arch Sci Med (Torino) 1895; 19:113.
44. Zwick DL, Livingston K, Clapp L. Intracranial nerve rhabdomyoma/choristoma in a child: a case report and discussion of possible histogenesis. Hum Pathol 1989; 20:390.

Neurofibroma and NF1

45. Geschickter CF. Tumors of the peripheral nerves. Am J Cancer 1935; 25:377.
46. Friedman JM. Epidemiology of neurofibromatosis type 1. Am J Med Genet 1999; 89:1.
47. Mulvihill JJ, Parry DM, Sherman JL, et al. Neurofibromatosis 1 (Recklinghausen disease) and neurofibromatosis 2 (bilateral acoustic neurofibromatosis). Ann Intern Med 1990; 113:39.
48. Rasmussen SA, Friedman JM. NF1 gene and neurofibromatosis 1. Am J Epidemiol 2000; 151:33.
49. Gutmann DH, Aylsworth A, Carey JC, et al. The diagnostic evaluation and multidisciplinary management of neurofibromatosis 1 and neurofibromatosis 2. JAMA 1997; 278:71.
50. Brasfield RD, Das Gupta TK. Von Recklinghausen's disease: a clinicopathological study. Ann Surg 1972; 175:86.
51. Canale DJ, Bebin J. Von Recklinghausen disease of the nervous system. In: Vinken PJ, Bruyn GW, ed. Handbook of clinical neurology, vol 14. New York: Elsevier; 1972:132.
52. Barker D, Wright E, Nguyen L, et al. Gene for von Recklinghausen neurofibromatosis is in the pericentromeric region of chromosome 17. Science 1987; 236:1100.

53. Theos A, Korf BR. Pathophysiology of neurofibromatosis Type 1. Ann Intern Med 2006; 144:842.
54. Weiss B, Bollag G, Shannon K. Hyperactive Ras as a therapeutic target in neurofibromatosis type 1. Am J Med Genet 1999; 89:14.
55. Arun D, Gutmann DH. Recent advances in neurofibromatosis type 1. Curr Opin Neurol 2004; 17:101.
56. Jimbow K, Szabo G, Fitzpatrick TB. Ultrastructure of giant pigmented granules (macromelanosomes) in the cutaneous pigmented macules of neurofibromatosis. J Invest Dermatol 1973; 61:300.
57. Silvers DN, Greenwood RS, Helwig EG. Café-au-lait spots without giant pigment granules: occurrence in suspected neurofibromatosis. Arch Dermatol 1974; 110:87.
58. Crowe FW, Schull WJ, Neel JV. A clinical, pathological, and genetic study of multiple neurofibromatosis. Springfield, IL: Charles C Thomas; 1956.
59. Miller RM, Sparkes RS. Segmental neurofibromatosis. Arch Dermatol 1977; 113:837.
60. Riccardi VM. Von Recklinghausen neurofibromatosis. N Engl J Med 1981; 305:1617.
61. Chino F, Tsuruhara T. Electron microscopic study of von Recklinghausen's disease. Jpn J Med Sci 1968; 21:249.
62. Lassmann H, Jurecka W, Lassmann W, et al. Different types of benign nerve sheath tumors: light microscopy, electron microscopy, and autoradiography. Virchows Arch [Pathol Anat] 1977; 375:197.
63. Bird CC, Willis RA. The histogenesis of pigmented neurofibromas. J Pathol 1969; 97:631.
64. Fetsch JF, Michal M, Miettinen M. Pigmented (melanotic) neurofibroma: a clinicopathologic and immunohistochemical analysis of 19 lesions from 17 patients. Am J Surg Pathol 2000; 24:331.
65. Lin BT, Weiss LM, Medeiros LJ. Neurofibroma and cellular neurofibroma with atypia: a report of 14 tumors. Am J Surg Pathol 1997; 21:1443.
66. Scheithauer BW, Woodruff JM, Erlandson RA. Tumors of the peripheral nervous system. In: Atlas of tumor pathology. Washington, DC: American Registry of Pathology; 1999.
67. Packer RJ, Gutmann DH, Rubenstein A, et al. Plexiform neurofibromas in NF1: toward biologic-based therapy. Neurology 2002; 58:1461.
68. Gupta A, Cohen BH, Ruggieri P, et al. Phase I study of thalidomide for the treatment of plexiform neurofibroma in neurofibromatosis 1. Neurology 2003; 60:130.
69. Hosoi K. Multiple neurofibromatosis (von Recklinghausen's disease) with special reference to malignant transformation. Arch Surg 1931; 22:258.
70. Sorensen SA, Mulvihill JJ, Nielsen A. Long-term follow-up of von Recklinghausen neurofibromatosis: survival and malignant neoplasms. N Engl J Med 1986; 314:1010.
71. Evans DG, Baser ME, McGaughran J, et al. Malignant peripheral nerve sheath tumours in neurofibromatosis 1. J Med Genet 2002; 39:311.
72. de Raedt T, Brems H, Wolkenstein P, et al. Elevated risk for MPNST in NF1 microdeletion patients. Am J Hum Genet 2003; 72:1288.
73. Kluwe L, Friedrich RE, Peiper M, et al. Constitutional NF1 mutations in neurofibromatosis 1 patients with malignant peripheral nerve sheath tumors. Hum Mutat 2003; 22:420.
74. Guccion JG, Enzinger FM. Malignant schwannoma associated with von Recklinghausen's neurofibromatosis. Virchows Arch [Pathol Anat] 1979; 383:43.

75. Dasgupta B, Gutmann DH. Neurofibromatosis 1: closing the GAP between mice and men. Current Opin Genet Devel 2003; 13:20.
76. Zhu Y, Ghosh P, Charnay P, et al. Neurofibromas in NF1: Schwann cell origin and role of tumor environment. Science 2002; 296:920.
77. Yang FC, et al. Neurofibromin-deficient Schwann cells secrete a potent migratory stimulus for Nf1+/– mast cells. J Clin Invest 2003; 112:1851.
78. Perry A, Kunz S, Fuller CE, et al. Differential NF1, p16, and EGFR patterns by interphase cytogenetics (FISH) in malignant peripheral nerve sheath tumor (MPNST) and morphologically similar spindle cell neoplasms. J Neuropathol Exp Neurol 2002; 61:702.
79. Kourea HP, Cordon-Cardo C, Dudas M, et al. Expression of p27kip and other cell cycle regulators in malignant peripheral nerve sheath tumors and neurofibromas. Am J Pathol 1999; 155:1885.
80. Kourea HP, Orlow I, Scheithauer BW, et al. Deletions of the INK4A gene occur in malignant peripheral nerve sheath tumors but not in neurofibromas. Am J Pathol 1999; 155:1855.
81. Nielsen GP, Stemmer-Rachamimov AO, Ino Y, et al. Malignant transformation of neurofibromas in neurofibromatosis 1 is associated with CDKN2A/p16 inactivation. Am J Pathol 1999; 155:1879.

Schwannoma (neurilemoma)

82. Stout AP. The peripheral manifestations of specific nerve sheath tumor (neurilemoma). Am J Cancer 1935; 24:751.
83. Antiheimo J, Sankila R, Carpen O, et al. Population based analysis of sporadic and type 2 neurofibromatosis-associated meningiomas and schwannomas. Neurology 2000; 54:71.
84. Brooks JJ, Draffen RM. Benign glandular schwannoma. Arch Pathol Lab Med 1992; 116:192.
85. Fletcher CDM, Madziwa D, Heyderman E, et al. Benign dermal schwannoma with glandular elements – true heterology or a local "organizer" effect? Clin Exp Dermatol 1986; 11:475.
86. Chan JK, Fok KO. Pseudoglandular schwannoma. Histopathology 1996; 29:481.
87. Goldblum JR, Beals TF, Weiss SW. Neuroblastoma-like neurilemoma. Am J Surg Pathol 1994; 18:266.
88. Fisher ER, Vuzevski VD. Cytogenesis of schwannoma (neurilemoma), neurofibroma, dermatofibroma, and dermatofibrosarcoma as revealed by electron microscopy. Am J Clin Pathol 1968; 49:141.
89. Razzuk MA, Urschel HC, Martin JA, et al. Electron microscopical observations on mediastinal neurilemoma, neurofibroma, and ganglioneuroma. Ann Thorac Surg 1973; 15:73.
90. Waggener JD. Ultrastructure of benign peripheral nerve sheath tumors. Cancer 1966; 19:699.
91. Hanada M, Tanaka T, Kanayama S, et al. Malignant transformation of intrathoracic ancient neurilemoma in a patient without Von Recklinghausen's disease. Acta Pathol Jpn 1982; 32:527.
92. Nayler SJ, Leiman G, Omar T, et al. Malignant transformation in a schwannoma. Histopathology 1996; 29:189.
93. Rasbridge SA, Browse NL, Tighe JR, et al. Malignant nerve sheath tumor arising in a benign ancient schwannoma. Histopathology 1989; 14:525.
94. Woodruff JM, Selig AM, Crowley K, et al. Schwannoma with malignant transformation: a rare distinctive peripheral nerve tumor. Am J Surg Pathol 1994; 18:882.

95. McMenamin ME, Fletcher CDM. Epithelioid malignant change in benign schwannomas [abstract 54]. Mod Pathol 2000; 13:13A.
96. Carstens H, Schrodt G. Malignant transformation of a benign encapsulated neurilemoma. Am J Clin Pathol 1969; 51:144.
97. Ackerman LV, Taylor FH. Neurogenous tumors within the thorax. Cancer 1951; 4:669.
98. Dahl I. Ancient neurilemoma (schwannoma). Acta Pathol Microbiol Scand 1977; 85A:812.
99. Casadei GP, Scheithauer BW, Hirose T, et al. Cellular schwannoma: a clinicopathologic DNA flow cytometric and proliferation marker study of 71 cases. Cancer 1995; 75:1109.
100. Fletcher CDM, Davies SE, McKee PH. Cellular schwannoma: a distinct pseudosarcomatous entity. Histopathology 1987; 11:21.
101. Lodding L, Kindblom L-G, Angervall L, et al. Cellular schwannoma: a clinicopathologic study of 29 cases. Virchows Arch [Pathol Anat] 1990; 416:237.
102. White W, Shiu MH, Rosenblum MK, et al. Cellular schwannoma: a clinicopathologic study of 57 patients and 58 tumors. Cancer 1990; 66:1266.
103. Woodruff JM, Godwin TA, Erlandson RA, et al. Cellular schwannoma: a variety of schwannoma sometimes mistaken for a malignant tumor. Am J Surg Pathol 1981; 5:733.
104. Trassard M, LeDoussal V, Bui BN, et al. Angiosarcoma arising in a solitary schwannoma (neurilemoma) of the sciatic nerve. Am J Surg Pathol 1996; 20:1412.
105. Meis-Kindblom JM, Enzinger FM. Plexiform malignant peripheral nerve sheath tumor of infancy and childhood. Am J Surg Pathol 1994; 18:479.
106. Argeny Z, Goodenberger ME, Strauss JS. Congenital neural hamartoma ("fascicular schwannoma"): a light microscopic, immunohistochemical and ultrastructural study. Am J Dermatopathol 1990; 12:283.
107. Amr SS, LaQuaglia MP, Antonescu CR. Congenital and childhood plexiform (multinodular) cellular schwannoma: troublesome mimic of malignant peripheral nerve sheath tumor. Am J Surg Pathol 2003; 27:1321.
108. Fletcher CDM, Davies SE. Benign plexiform (multinodular) schwannoma: a rare tumor unassociated with neurofibromatosis. Histopathology 1986; 19:971.
109. Stenman G, Kindblom LG, Johansson M, et al. Clonal chromosome abnormalities and in vitro growth characteristics of classical and cellular schwannomas. Cancer Genet Cytogenet 1991; 57:121.
110. Woodruff JM, Marshall ML, Godwin TA, et al. Plexiform (multinodular) schwannoma: a tumor simulating the plexiform neurofibroma. Am J Surg Pathol 1983; 7:691.
111. Iwashita T, Enjoji M. Plexiform neurilemoma: a clinicopathologic and immunohistochemical analysis of 23 tumors from 20 patients. Virchows Arch [Pathol Anat] 1986; 422:305.
112. Kao GF, Laskin WB, Olsen TG. Solitary cutaneous plexiform neurilemoma (schwannoma): a clinicopathologic, immunohistochemical, and ultrastructural study of 11 cases. Mod Pathol 1989; 2:20.
113. Ishida T, Kuroda M, Motoi T, et al. Phenotypic diversity of neurofibromatosis 2: association with plexiform schwannoma. Histopathology 1998; 32:264.
114. Reith JD, Goldblum JR. Multiple cutaneous plexiform schwannomas: report of a case and review of the literature with particular reference to the association with types 1 and 2 neurofibromatosis and schwannomatosis. Arch Pathol Lab Med 1996; 120:399.
115. Val-Bernal JF, Figols J, Vazquez-Barquero A. Cutaneous plexiform schwannoma associated with neurofibromatosis type 2. Cancer 1995; 76:1181.

116. Kindblom LG, Meis-Kindblom JM, Havel G, et al. Benign epithelioid schwannoma. Am J Surg Pathol 1998; 22:762.
117. Smith K, Mezebish D, Williams JP, et al. Cutaneous epithelioid schwannomas: a rare variant of benign peripheral nerve sheath tumor. J Cutan Pathol 1998; 25:50.

Neurofibromatosis

118. Baser ME, Evans DGR, Gutmann DH. Neurofibromatosis 2. Curr Opin Neurol 2003; 16:27.
119. Morrison H, Sherman LS, Legg J, et al. The NF2 tumor suppressor gene product, merlin, mediates contact inhibition of growth through interactions with CD44. Gene Dev 2001; 15:968.
120. Evans DGR, Huson SM, Donnal D, et al. A clinical study of type 1 neurofibromatosis. Q J Med 1992; 84:603.
121. Evans DGR, Baser ME, O'Reilly BO, et al. Management of the patient and family with neurofibromatosis 2: a consensus conference statement. Br J Neurosurg 2005; 19:5.

Schwannomatosis

122. MacCollin M, Woodfin W, Kronn D, et al. Schwannomatosis: a clinical and pathologic study. Neurology 1996; 46:1072.
123. Buenger KM, Porter NC, Dozier SE, et al. Localized multiple neurilemomas of the lower extremity. Cutis 1993; 51:36.
124. Seppala MT, Sainio MA, Haltia MJ, et al. Multiple schwannomas: schwannomatosis or neurofibromatosis 2. J Neurosurg 1998; 89:36.
125. Shishiba T, Niimura M, Ohtsuka F, et al. Multiple cutaneous neurilemomas as a skin manifestation of neurilemomatosis. J Am Acad Dermatol 1984; 10:744.
126. MacCollin M, Chiocca EA, Evans DG, et al. Diagnostic criteria for schwannomatosis. Neurology 2005; 64:1838.

Melanotic schwannoma

127. Millar WG. A malignant melanotic tumor of ganglion cells arising from thoracic sympathetic ganglion. J Pathol Bacteriol 1932; 35:351.
128. Fu YS, Kaye GI, Lattes R. Primary malignant melanocytic tumors of the sympathetic ganglia with an ultrastructural study of one. Cancer 1975; 36:2029.
129. Carney JA. Psammomatous melanotic schwannoma: a distinctive heritable tumor with special associations including cardiac myxoma and the Cushing syndrome. Am J Surg Pathol 1990; 14:206.
130. Carney JA, Ferreiro JA. The epithelioid blue nevus: a multicentric familial tumor with important associations, including cardiac myxoma and psammomatous melanotic schwannoma. Am J Surg Pathol 1996; 20:259.
131. Font RL, Truong LD. Melanotic schwannoma of soft tissues: electron microscopic observations and review of the literature. Am J Surg Pathol 1984; 8:129.
132. Killeen RM, Davy CL, Bauserman SC. Melanocytic schwannoma. Cancer 1988; 62:174.
133. Krausz T, Azzopardi JG, Pearse E. Malignant melanoma of the sympathetic chain: with consideration of pigmented nerve sheath tumors. Histopathology 1984; 8:881.
134. Leger F, Vital C, Rivel J, et al. Psammomatous melanotic schwannoma of a spinal nerve root: relationship to the Carney complex. Pathol Res Pract 1996; 192:1142.
135. Lowman RM, LiVolsi VA. Pigmented (melanotic) schwannomas of the spinal canal. Cancer 1980; 46:391.
136. Mennenmeyer RP, Hammar SP, Tytus JS, et al. Melanotic schwannomas: clinical and ultrastructural studies of three cases with

evidence of intracellular melanin synthesis. Am J Surg Pathol 1979; 3:3.
137. Vallat-Decouvelacre AV, Wassef M, Lot G, et al. Spinal melanotic schwannoma: a tumour with poor prognosis. Histopathology 1999; 35:558.

Perineurioma

138. Ariza A, Bilbao JM, Rosai J. Immunohistochemical detection of epithelial membrane antigen in normal perineurial cells and perineurioma. Am J Surg Pathol 1988; 12:678.
139. Erlandson RA. The enigmatic perineurial cell and its participation in tumors and in tumorlike entities. Ultrastruct Pathol 1991; 15:335.
140. Giannini C, Scheithauer BW, Jenkins RB, et al. Soft tissue perineurioma: evidence for an abnormality of chromosome 22, criteria for diagnosis, and review of the literature. Am J Surg Pathol 1997; 21:164.
141. Mentzel T, Dei Tos AP, Fletcher CDM. Perineurioma (storiform perineural fibroma): clinicopathologic analysis of four cases. Histopathology 1994; 25:261.
142. Rank JP, Rostad SW. Perineurioma with ossification: a case report with immunohistochemical and ultrastructural studies. Arch Pathol Lab Med 1998; 122:366.
143. Hornick JL, Fletcher CDM. Soft tissue perineurioma: clinicopathologic analysis of 81 cases including those with atypical histologic features. Am J Surg Pathol 2005; 29:845.
144. Michal M, Kazakov DV, Belousova I, et al. A benign neoplasm with histopathologic feature of both schwannoma and retiform perineurioma (benign schwannoma-perineurioma): a report of six cases of a distinctive soft tissue tumor with a predilection for the fingers. Virchows Archiv 2004; 445:347.
145. Zamecnik M, Michal M. Perineurial cell differentiation in neurofibromas. Report of eight cases including a case with composite perineurioma-neurofibroma features. Pathol Res Pract 2001; 197:537.
146. Lazarus SS, Trombetta LD. Ultrastructural identification of a benign perineurial cell tumor. Cancer 1978; 41:1823.
147. Carneiro F, Brandao O, Correia AC, et al. Spindle cell tumor of the breast. Ultrastruct Pathol 1991; 15:335.
148. Ohno T, Park P, Akai M, et al. Ultrastructural study of a perineurioma. Ultrastruct Pathol 1988; 5:495.
149. Weidenheim KM, Campbell WG. Perineurial cell tumor: immunohistochemical and ultrastructural characterization: relationship to other peripheral nerve tumors with a review of the literature. Virchows Arch [Pathol Anat] 1986; 408:375.
150. Emory TS, Scheithauer BW, Horose T, et al. Intraneural perineurioma: a clonal neoplasm associated with abnormalities of chromosome 22. Am J Clin Pathol 1995; 103:696.
151. Simmons Z, Mahadeen ZI, Kothari MJ, et al. Localized hypertrophic neuropathy: magnetic resonance imaging findings and long term follow up. Muscle Nerve 1999; 22:28.
152. Jazayeri MA, Robinson JH, Legolvan DP. Intraneural perineurioma involving the median nerve. Plast Reconstr Surg 2000; 105:2089.
153. Sciot R, Cin PD, Hagemeijer A, et al. Cutaneous sclerosing perineurioma with cryptic NF2 gene deletion. Am J Surg Pathol 1999; 23:849.
154. Smith K, Skelton H. Cutaneous fibrous perineurioma. J Cutan Pathol 1998; 25:333.
155. Tsang WYW, Chan JKC, Chow LTC, et al. Perineurioma: an uncommon soft tissue neoplasm distinct from localized hypertrophic neuropathy and neurofibroma. Am J Surg Pathol 1992; 16:756.
156. Lasota J, Wozniak A, Debiec-Rychter M. Loss of chromosome 22q and lack of NF2 mutations in

perineuriomas [abstract 46]. Mod Pathol 2000; 13:11A.

157. Theaker JM, Fletcher CDM. Epithelial membrane antigen expression by the perineurial cell: further studies of peripheral nerve lesions. Histopathology 1989; 14:581.

158. Theaker JM, Gatter KC, Puddle J. Epithelial membrane antigen expression by the perineurium of peripheral nerve and in peripheral nerve tumors. Histopathology 1987; 13:171.

159. Folpe AF, Billings SD, McKenney JK, et al. Expression of claudin-1, a recently described tight junction-associated protein, distinguishes soft tissue perineurioma from potential mimics. Am J Surg Pathol 2002; 26:1620.

160. Yamaguchi U, Hasegawa T, Hirose T, et al. Sclerosing perineurioma: a clinicopathologic study of five cases and diagnostic utility of immunohistochemical staining for GLUT1. Virchows Arch 2003; 443:159.

161. Hirose T, Tani T, Shimada T, et al. Immunohistochemical demonstration of EMA/Glut1-positive perineurial cells and CD34-positive fibroblastic cells in peripheral nerve sheath tumors. Mod Pathol 2003; 16:293.

162. Dhimes P, Martizez-Gonzalez MA, Carabias E, et al. Ultrastructural study of a perineurioma with ribosome-lamella complexes. Ultrastruct Pathol 1996; 20:167.

163. Fetsch JF, Miettinen M. Sclerosing perineurioma: a clinicopathologic study of 19 cases of a distinctive soft tissue lesion with a predilection for the fingers and palms of young adults. Am J Surg Pathol 1997; 21:1433.

164. Burgues O, Monteagudo C, Noguera R, et al. Cutaneous sclerosing pacinian-like perineurioma. Histopathology 2001; 39:498.

165. Brock JE, Perez-Atayde AR, Kozakewich HP, et al. Cytogenetic aberrations in perineurioma: variation with subtype. Am J Surg Pathol 2005; 29:1164.

166. Graadt van Roggen JF, McMenamin ME, Belchis DA, et al. Reticular perineurioma: a distinctive variant of soft tissue perineurioma. Am J Surg Pathol 2001; 25:485.

167. Ushigome S, Takakuwa T, Hysuga M, et al. Perineurial cell tumor and the significance of the perineurial cells in neurofibroma. Acta Pathol Jpn 1986; 36:973.

168. Michal M. Extraneural retiform perineurioma: a report of 4 cases. Pathol Res Pract 1999; 195:759.

169. Mentzel T, Kutzner H. Reticular and plexiform perineurioma: clinicopathologic and immunohistochemical analysis of two cases and review of perineural neoplasms of skin and soft tissues. Virchows Arch 2005; 447:677.

170. Rosenberg AS, Langee CL, Sevens GL, et al. Malignant peripheral nerve sheath tumor with perineurial differentiation: "malignant perineurioma." J Cutan Pathol 2002; 29:362.

Granular cell tumor

171. Abrikossoff A. Ueber Myome ausgehened von der quergestreiften willkuerlichen Muskulatur. Virchows Arch [Pathol Anat] 1926; 260:215.

172. Sobel HJ, Arvin E, Marquet E, et al. Reactive granular cell in sites of trauma. Am J Clin Pathol 1974; 61:223.

173. Vance S, Hudson R. Granular cell myoblastoma. Am J Clin Pathol 1969; 52:208.

174. Filie AC, Lage JM, Azumi N. Immunoreactivity of S-100 protein, alpha-1 antitrypsin, and CD68 in adult and congenital granular cell tumors. Mod Pathol 1996; 9:888.

175. Kurtin PJ, Bonin DM. Immunohistochemical demonstration of the lysosome-associated glycoprotein CD68 (KP1) in granular cell tumors and schwannomas. Hum Pathol 1994; 25:1172.

176. Mukai M. Immunohistochemical localization of S-100 protein and peripheral nerve myelin proteins (P2 protein and PO protein) in granular cell tumors. Am J Pathol 1983; 112:139.

177. Nakazato Y, Ishizeki J, Takahashi K, et al. Immunohistochemical localization of S-100 protein in granular cell myoblastoma. Cancer 1982; 49:1624.

178. Sobel HJ, Churg J. Granular cells and granular cell lesions. Arch Pathol 1974; 77:132.

179. Smolle J, Konrad K, Kerl H. Granular cell minors contain myelin-associated glycoprotein: an immunohistochemical study using Leu-7 monoclonal antibody. Virchows Arch [A Pathol Anat Histopathol] 1985; 406:1.

180. Strong EW, McDivitt RW, Brasfield RD. Granular cell myoblastoma. Cancer 1970; 25:415.

181. Ravich A, Stout AP, Ravich RA. Malignant granular cell myoblastoma involving the urinary bladder. Ann Surg 1945; 121:361.

182. Fanburg-Smith JC, Meis-Kindblom JM, Fante R, et al. Malignant granular cell tumor of soft tissue: diagnostic criteria and clinicopathologic correlation. Am J Surg Pathol 1998; 22:779.

Congenital (gingival) granular cell tumor

183. Bhaskar SN, Akamine R. Congenital epulis (congenital granular cell fibroblastoma). J Oral Surg 1955; 8:517.

184. Cussen LJ, MacMahon RA. Congenital granular cell myoblastoma. J Pediatr Surg 1975; 10:249.

185. Fuhr AH, Krogh PHJ. Congenital epulis of the newborn: centennial review of the literature and a report of a case. J Oral Surg 1972; 30:30.

186. Henefer EP, Abaza NA, Anderson SP. Congenital granular cell epulis: report of a case. Oral Surg Oral Med Oral Pathol 1979; 47:515.

187. Koppang HS. Congenital gingival granular-cell myoblastoma. Oral Surg Oral Med Oral Pathol 1972; 34:98.

188. Lack E, Crawford BE, Worsham GF, et al. Gingival granular cell tumors of the newborn (congenital "epulis"): a clinical and pathologic study of 21 patients. Am J Surg Pathol 1981; 5:37.

189. Lack EE, Perez-Atayde AR, McGill TJ, et al. Gingival granular cell tumor of the newborn (congenital "epulis"): ultrastructural observations relating to histogenesis. Hum Pathol 1982; 13:686.

190. Lifshitz MS, Flotte TJ, Greco MA. Congenital granular cell epulis: immunohistochemical and ultrastructural observations. Cancer 1984; 53:1845.

191. Matthews JB, Mason GI. Oral granular cell myoblastoma: an immunohistochemical study. J Oral Pathol 1982; 11:343.

192. Slootweg P, de Wilde P, Vooijs P, et al. Oral granular cell lesions: an immunohistochemical study with emphasis on intermediate-sized filament proteins. Virchows Arch [Pathol Anat] 1983; 402:35.

193. Tucker JC, Rusnock EJ, Azumi N. Gingival granular cell tumors of the newborn: an ultrastructural and immunohistochemical study. Arch Pathol Lab Med 1990; 114:895.

Classic neurothekeoma

194. Gallagher RL, Helwig EB. Neurothekeoma: a benign cutaneous tumor of nerve sheath origin. Am J Clin Pathol 1980; 74:759.

195. Angervall L, Kindblom L, Haglid K. Dermal nerve sheath myxoma. Cancer 1984; 53:1752.

196. Aronson PJ, Fretzin DE, Potter BS. Neurothekeoma of Gallagher and Helwig (dermal nerve sheath myxoma variant): report of a case with electron microscopic and immunohistochemical studies. J Cutan Pathol 1985; 12:506.

197. King D, Barr R. Bizarre cutaneous neurofibromas. J Cutan Pathol 1980; 7:21.

198. Barnhill RL, Mihm MC Jr. Cellular neurothekeoma: a distinctive variant of neurothekeoma mimicking nevomelanocytic tumors. Am J Surg Pathol 1990; 14:113.

199. Calonje E, Wilson-Jones E, Smith NP, et al. Cellular "neurothekeoma": an epithelioid variant of pilar leiomyoma? Morphological and immunohistochemical analysis of a series. Histopathology 1992; 20:397.

200. Busam KJ, Mentzel T, Colpaert C, et al. Atypical or worrisome features in cellular neurothekeoma: a study of 10 cases. Am J Surg Pathol 1998; 22:1067.

201. Fullen DR, Lowe L, Su LD. Antibody to S100a6 protein is a sensitive immunohistochemical marker for neurothekeoma. J Cutan Pathol 2003; 30:118.

202. Wang AR, May D, Bourne P, et al. PGP: a marker for cellular neurothekeoma. Am J Surg Pathol 1999; 23:1401.

203. Page RN, King R, Mihm MC, et al. Microphthalmia transcription factor and NK1/C3 expression in cellular neurothekeoma. Mod Pathol 2003; 17:230.

Extracranial meningioma

204. Lopez DA, Silvers DN, Helwig EB. Cutaneous meningiomas: a clinicopathologic study. Cancer 1974; 34:728.

205. Theaker JM, Fleming KA. Meningioma of the scalp: a case report with immunohistochemical features. J Cutan Pathol 1987; 14:49.

Glial heterotopias

206. Rios JJ, Diaz-Cano SL, Rivera-Hueto F, et al. Cutaneous ganglion cell choristoma. J Cutan Pathol 1991; 18:469.

207. Shepherd NA, Coates PJ, Brown AA. Soft tissue gliomatosis-heterotopic glial tissue in the subcutis: a case report. Histopathology 1987; 11:655.

208. Skelton HG, Smith KJ. Glial heterotopia in the subcutaneous tissue overlying T-12. J Cutan Pathol 1999; 26:523.

209. Orkin M, Fisher I. Heterotopic brain tissue (heterotopic neural rest). Arch Dermatol 1966; 94:699.

Melanotic neuroectodermal tumor of infancy

210. Allen M, Harrison W, Jahrsdoerfer R. Retinal anlage tumors. Am J Clin Pathol 1969; 51:309.

211. Borello ED, Gorlin RJ. Melanotic neuroectodermal tumor of infancy: a neoplasm of neural crest origin. Cancer 1966; 19:196.

212. Cutler LS, Chaudhry AP, Topazian R. Melanotic neuroectodermal tumor of infancy: an ultrastructural, literature review, and reevaluation. Cancer 1981; 48:257.

213. Dehner LP, Sibley RK, Sauk JJ, et al. Malignant melanotic neuroectodermal tumor of infancy: a clinical, pathologic, ultrastructural, and tissue culture study. Cancer 1979; 43:1389.

214. Dooling EC, Chi JEG, Gilles FH. Melanotic neuroectodermal tumor of infancy: its histological similarities to fetal pineal gland. Cancer 1977; 39:1535.

215. Duckworth R, Seward GR. Amelanotic ameloblastic odontoma. Oral Surg Oral Med Oral Pathol 1965; 19:73.

216. Eaton WL, Ferguson JP. A retinoblastic teratoma of the epididymis. Cancer 1956; 9:718.

217. Frank GL, Koten HE. Melanotic hamartoma ("retinal anlage tumor") of the epididymis. J Pathol Bacteriol 1967; 93:549.

218. Hayward AF, Fickling BW, Lucas RB. An electron microscope study of a pigmented tumor of the jaw of infants. Br J Cancer 1969; 23:702.

219. Johnson RE, Scheithauer BW, Dahlin DC. Melanotic neuroectodermal tumor of infancy. Cancer 1983; 52:661.

220. Kapadia SH, Frisman DM, Hitchcock CL, et al. Melanotic neuroectodermal tumor of infancy. Am J Surg Pathol 1993; 17:566.

221. Koudstall J, Oldhoff J, Panders AK, et al. Melanotic neuroectodermal tumor of infancy. Cancer 1968; 22:151.

222. Lee SC, Henry MM, Gonzalez-Crussi F. Simultaneous occurrence of melanotic neuroectodermal tumor and brain heterotopia in the oropharynx. Cancer 1976; 38:249.

223. Lindahl F. Malignant melanotic progonoma: one case. Acta Pathol Microbiol Scand 1970; 78A:532.

224. Lurie HI. Congenital melanocarcinoma, melanocytic adamantinoma, retinal anlage tumor, progonoma, and pigmented epulis of infancy: summary and review of the literature and report of the first case in an adult. Cancer 1961; 14:1090.

225. Lurie HI, Isaacson C. A melanotic progonoma in the scapula. Cancer 1961; 14:1088.

226. Misugi K, Okajima H, Newton WA, et al. Mediastinal origin of a melanotic progonoma or retinal anlage tumor: ultrastructural evidence for neural crest origin. Cancer 1965; 18:477.

227. Navas Palacios JJ. Malignant melanotic neuroectodermal tumor: light and electron microscopic study. Cancer 1980; 46:529.

228. Pettinato G, Manivel C, d'Amore ESG, et al. Melanotic neuroectodermal tumor of infancy: an immunohistochemical study. Histopathology 1988; 12:425.

229. Schulz DM. A malignant melanotic neoplasm of the uterus resembling the retinal anlage tumor. Am J Clin Pathol 1957; 28:524.

230. Stirling RW, Powell G, Fletcher CDM. Pigmented neuroectodermal tumor of infancy: an immunohistochemical study. Histopathology 1988; 12:425.

231. Stowens D, Lin TH. Melanotic progonoma of the brain. Hum Pathol 1974; 5:105.

232. William AO. Melanotic ameloblastoma ("progonoma") of infancy showing osteogenesis. J Pathol Bacteriol 1967; 93:545.

233. Zone RM. Retinal anlage tumor of the epididymis: a case report. J Urol 1970; 103:106.

234. National Institutes of Health. Neurofibromatosis: National Institutes of Health Consensus Development Conference Statement, vol. 6(12). Bethesda, MD: US Department of Health and Human Services; July 13–15, 1987:1–9.

MALIGNANT TUMORS OF
THE PERIPHERAL NERVES

Malignant tumors arising from peripheral nerves or displaying differentiation along the lines of the various elements of the nerve sheath (e.g., Schwann cell, perineural cell, fibroblast) are collectively referred to as malignant peripheral nerve sheath tumors (MPNSTs). This term replaces the earlier terms *malignant schwannoma, neurofibrosarcoma,* and *neurogenic sarcoma.* Because MPNSTs recapitulate the appearance of various cells of the nerve sheath, they range in appearance from tumors that resemble a neurofibroma to those resembling a fibrosarcoma. Rarely, tumors arising from nerves or neurofibromas display aberrant lines of differentiation. For example, angiosarcomas may arise in nerves or in preexisting neurofibromas. By convention these tumors are not

considered MPNSTs but are classified according to their aberrant line of differentiation. Although primitive neuro-ectodermal tumors also arise from peripheral nerves, they are considered along with neuroblastic tumors and Ewing's sarcoma in Chapter 31.

The diagnosis of MPNSTs has traditionally been one of the most difficult and elusive among soft tissue diseases because of the lack of standardized diagnostic criteria. Although there is general agreement that if a sarcoma arises from a peripheral nerve or a neurofibroma it can usually be considered an MPNST, there has been less agreement about the diagnostic criteria for tumors occurring outside these settings. As a result, the incidence of this sarcoma has varied in the literature. In 1931 Stewart and Copeland,[1] reporting their experience from Memorial Hospital in New York, maintained that "neurogenic sarcomas" comprise most of the fibrosarcomas of soft tissue and that most occurred in patients without neurofibromatosis. Likewise, Geschickter,[2] in a review of cases from the Johns Hopkins Hospital, concluded that the tumor was among the most common of all soft tissue sarcomas. Both studies reflect a liberal diagnostic approach and willingness to accept many spindled collagen-producing sarcomas as neural, especially if they occur in certain locations or produce characteristic symptoms. On the other hand, Stout[3] proposed a stricter definition of the tumor. In his opinion, these tumors could not be distinguished from fibrosarcomas on histologic grounds, and their diagnosis rested on the documented origin from nerve or neurofibroma or association with von Recklinghausen's disease. The rarity of the tumor in Stout's experience and its high association with neurofibromatosis reflect in large part his stringent criteria.

A sarcoma is assumed to be an MPNST if one of three criteria can be met: (1) the tumor arises from a peripheral nerve; (2) it arises from a preexisting benign nerve sheath tumor, usually a neurofibroma; or (3) the tumor displays a constellation of histologic features that are seen in tumors arising in the foregoing situations and are generally accepted as reflecting Schwann cell differentiation by light microscopy. These features include the (1) dense and hypodense fascicles alternating in a "marble-like" pattern consisting of (2) asymmetrically tapered spindled cells with irregular buckled nuclei or (3) immunohisto-chemical or electron microscopic evidence of Schwann cell differentiation in the context of a fibrosarcomatous-appearing tumor. In addition, there are features that are less specific but frequently occur in Schwann cell tumors, including nuclear palisading, whorled structures that vaguely suggest large tactoid structures, peculiar "hyper-plastic" perivascular change, and occasionally heterolo-gous elements (e.g., cartilage, bone, skeletal muscle). Obviously, these criteria allow inclusion of only MPNST that are reasonably well differentiated or have not yet obscured their site of origin. Nonetheless, this approach offers an acceptable degree of diagnostic reproducibility and eliminates the potpourri of spindle cell tumors that have been diagnosed as MPNSTs in the past.

CLINICAL FINDINGS

The MPNST account for approximately 5–10% of all soft tissue sarcomas; about one-fourth to one-half occur in the setting of neurofibromatosis 1 (NF1).[4-6] The diagnos-tic criteria and type of pathologic material affect these figures, as illustrated by the fact that the association with NF1 varies from about one-fourth[2] to more than two-thirds in the literature. In large series in which there has been consistency in histologic diagnoses, the percentage of patients with MPNST having and not having NF1 is roughly equal.[5] Although the incidence of MPNST in NF1 has been estimated to be 3–5%,[4] the cumulative life-time risk is now considered to be 10%[7] and may be as high as 30% in those with symptomatic plexiform neurofibro-mas. There is some preliminary evidence that certain con-stitutional NF1 mutations are associated with an increased risk for MPNST, but that has not been confirmed by others.[8]

Patients with NF1 develop sarcomas usually after a relatively long latency (10–20 years[9]), and in some cases the MPNST are multiple. MPNSTs in childhood is recog-nized, but infrequent.[10-12]

The exact mechanism of malignant transformation or tumor progression in NF1 is not fully understood, but it seems to involve a multistep process in which genes other than the NF1 gene also participate (see below). Aside from the foregoing genetic predilection to develop MPNST, little is known about the pathogenesis of these tumors in humans. About 10–20% of cases occur as a result of therapeutic or occupational irradiation after a latent period of more than 15 years.[4,6,13-15] These tumors do not differ significantly from other MPNST.

Experimentally, these tumors can be induced in labo-ratory animals by transplacental injection of ethylnitro-sourea[16] or administration of methylcholanthrene.[17] As a result of these studies, it has been suggested that a search for chemical carcinogens in the environment might prove fruitful.

The MPNST is typically a disease of adult life, as most tumors occur in patients 20–50 years of age.[4,9,18-22] Patients with NF1 develop these tumors at an earlier age, how-ever. The average age at the time of diagnosis for patients with NF1 was 29 and 36 years in the Mayo Clinic[4] and Memorial Sloan-Kettering[5] studies, respectively, com-pared with 40 and 44 years, respectively, for patients without the disease. Our experience indicates an average age of 32 years for both groups but a wider age range among patients without NF1.[9] The gender ratio of patients with MPNST varies, depending on patient selection. Men predominate in studies that report a high percentage of patients with NF1 as a result of the bias toward men in this disease.[4,6,9,20] In studies of sporadic cases of MPNST, the gender ratio is roughly equal to or slightly biased toward women.[20,23] These observations parallel our expe-rience. Eighty percent of patients with NF1 and MPNST are men,[9] whereas only 56% of patients with sporadic MPNST are men.[9]

Like other sarcomas, these lesions present as enlarging masses that are usually noted several months before diag-nosis. Pain is variable but seems to be more prevalent in those with NF1. In fact, pain or sudden enlargement of a preexisting mass in this setting should lead to immedi-ate biopsy to exclude the possibility of malignant trans-formation of a neurofibroma. Fluorodeoxyglucose positron emission tomography (FDG PET), which allows visualization of glucose metabolism by cells, has been reasonably successful in identifying malignant change in plexiform neurofibromas,[24] and may give some indica-tion of the grade of the lesion.[25] MPNST that arise from major nerves typically give rise to a striking constellation of sensory and motor symptoms, including projected pain, paresthesias, and weakness. The symptoms rarely antedate the detection of a mass.

Most MPNST arise in association with major nerve trunks, including the sciatic nerve, brachial plexus, and sacral plexus. Consequently, the most common anatomic sites include the proximal portions of the upper and lower extremities and the trunk. Comparatively few arise in the head and neck, a feature that contrasts with the distribution of the schwannoma.

GROSS FINDINGS

In its classic form, an MPNST arises as a large fusiform or eccentric mass in a major nerve (Fig. 30–1). Thickening of the nerve proximally and distally to the main mass usually indicates spread of the neoplasm along the epi-neurium and perineurium. In NF1 patients MPNST may develop in a preexisting neurofibroma (Fig. 30–2). Most of these lesions are deeply situated; only rare ones arise from superficial neurofibromas. Regardless of the clinical setting, the gross appearance of the MPNST is essentially similar to that of other soft tissue sarcomas. It is usually large, averaging more than 5 cm in diameter, and has a fleshy, opaque, white-tan surface marked by areas of secondary hemorrhage and necrosis. This appearance contrasts with the white mucoid appearance of the typical neurofibroma.

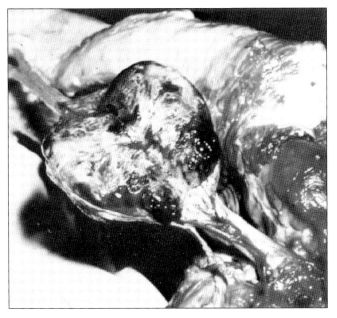

FIGURE 30–1 Malignant peripheral nerve sheath tumor (MPNST) arising as a large fusiform mass from the sciatic nerve. Cut section of tumor shows prominent hemorrhage and necrosis.

MICROSCOPIC FINDINGS

Most MPNST resemble fibrosarcomas in their overall organization (Figs 30–3 to 30–6) with certain modifications. Classically, the cells recapitulate the features of the normal Schwann cell. Unlike the symmetrically spindled cells of fibrosarcoma, they have markedly irregular contours. In profile, the nuclei are wavy, buckled, or comma-shaped, whereas when viewed en face they are asymmetrically oval (Fig. 30–7). The cytoplasm is lightly stained and usually indistinct. The cells can range from spindled in shape to fusiform or even rounded such that the lesion can mimic a fibrosarcoma or even a round cell sarcoma (Fig. 30–8).

The cells are arranged in sweeping fascicles, but there is greater variation in organization than in the fibrosarcoma. Densely cellular fascicles alternate with hypocellular, myxoid zones (Fig. 30–6), which swirl and interdigitate with one another, creating a marble-like effect (Fig. 30–3). Others display a peculiar nodular, curlicue, or whorled arrangement of spindled cells (Figs 30–9, 30–10) crudely suggesting tactoid differentiation. Nuclear palisading may be present, but in our cases it occurs in fewer than 10% of all MPNST and, when present, is usually of a focal nature (Fig. 30–11).

There are several other subtle features that are quite characteristic of MPNST. Because they are not completely specific, they must be evaluated in the context of the foregoing discussion before a given tumor is labeled MPNST. These features include hyaline bands (Fig.

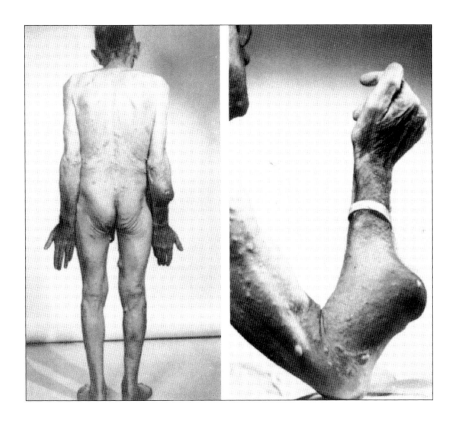

FIGURE 30–2 MPNST of the arm in a patient with long-standing neurofibromatosis.

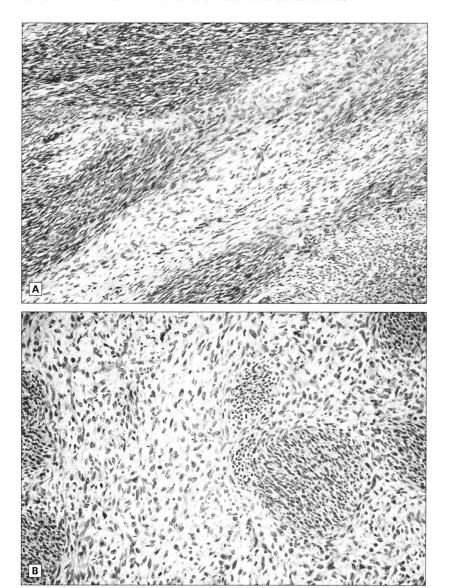

FIGURE 30–3 (A, B) Typical appearance of an MPNST with densely cellular areas alternating with less cellular ones, creating a marbleized appearance.

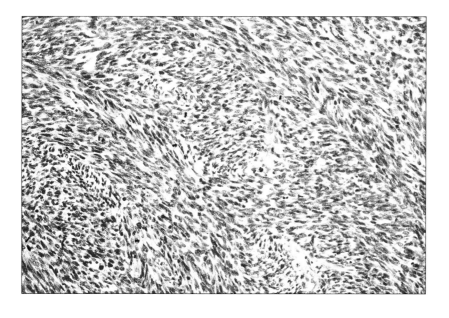

FIGURE 30–4 MPNST consisting exclusively of dense fascicles of spindled cells, similar to a fibrosarcoma.

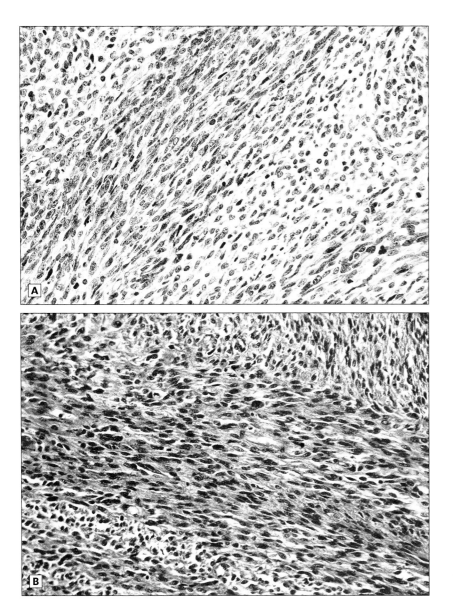

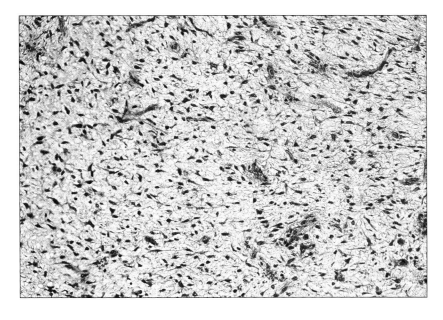

FIGURE 30–5 (A, B) Cellular fascicles of an MPNST.

FIGURE 30–6 Myxoid area in an MPNST showing randomly arranged Schwann cells.

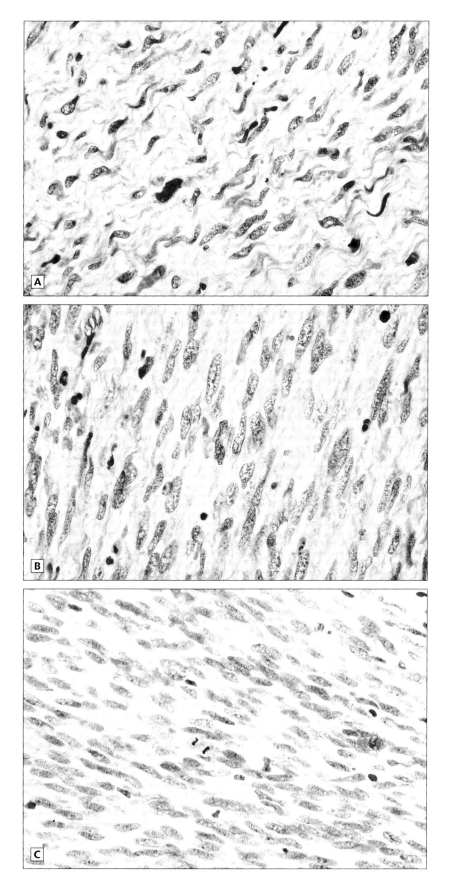

FIGURE 30–7 Cells in an MPNST with well-differentiated areas **(A)** in which cells have an irregular, buckled shape characteristic of Schwann cells to less differentiated areas **(B)**. **(C)** S-100 protein immunostain shows focal weak staining of cells in an MPNST.

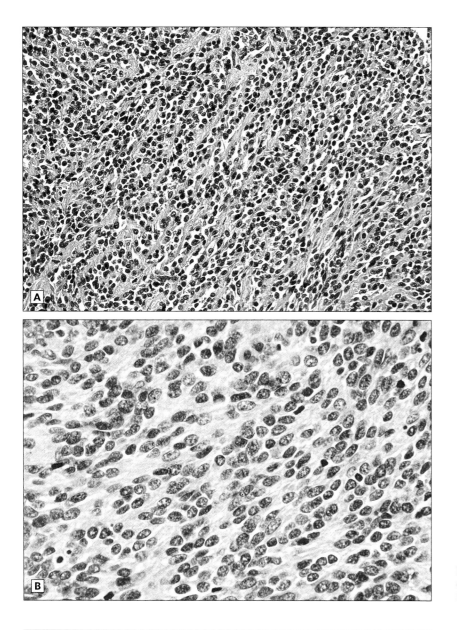

FIGURE 30–8 MPNST with areas composed of rounded **(A)** or short fusiform **(B)** cells. In (B), vague palisading of nuclei can be seen.

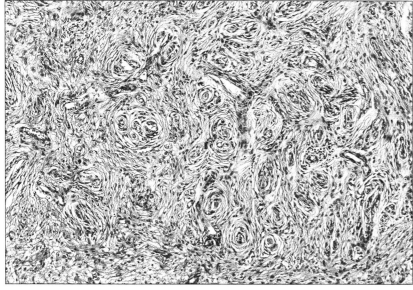

FIGURE 30–9 Low-grade MPNST with a curlicue arrangement of cells.

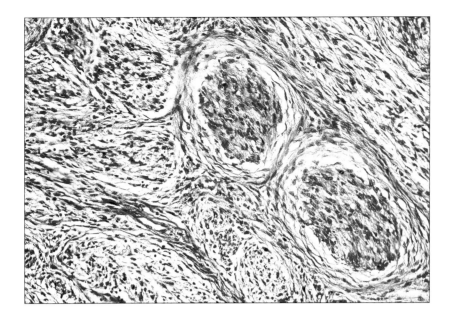

FIGURE 30–10 Whorled structures in an MPNST.

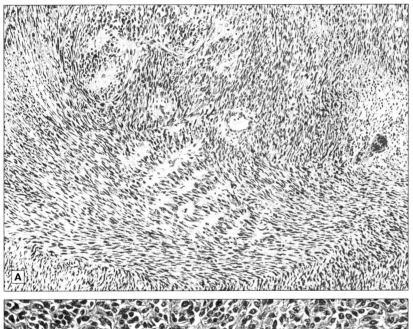

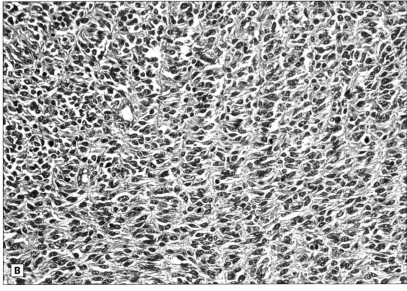

FIGURE 30–11 (A, B) Nuclear palisading is an uncommon feature in an MPNST. It may also be seen in schwannomas and some leiomyosarcomas.

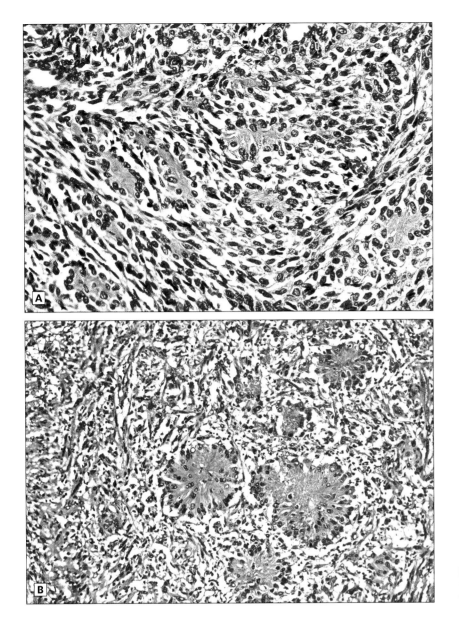

FIGURE 30–12 Hyalinized cords **(A)** and nodules **(B)** are uncommon but distinctive features of MPNSTs.

30–12) and nodules, which in cross-section can be likened to giant rosettes (Fig. 30–12B), extensive perineural and intraneural spread of tumor (Fig. 30–13), and a peculiar proliferation of tumor in the subendothelial zones of vessels so the neoplastic cells appear to herniate into the lumen (Fig. 30–14). Small vessels may also proliferate in the walls of or around large vessels (Fig. 30–14B). Likewise, heterologous elements, present in about 10–15% of MPNST, seem to be more common in MPNST than in other sarcomas.[12,26] Their presence may initially suggest the diagnosis in a tumor that otherwise resembles fibrosarcoma. Mature islands of cartilage and bone are the most common elements (Fig. 30–15), whereas skeletal muscle and mucin-secreting glands are rare. In addition, we have seen one MPNST with squamous differentiation.

Although most MPNST conform to this description, a small percentage appears quite different. Some of these tumors closely resemble neurofibromas except they manifest a greater degree of cellularity, pleomorphism, and mitotic activity. These MPNST are typically found in the setting of von Recklinghausen's disease and have sometimes been termed *malignant neurofibromas*. If the lesion fulfills the criteria of malignancy as detailed in Chapter 29, we refer to it as a *low-grade malignant peripheral nerve sheath tumor arising in a neurofibroma*. At the opposite end of the spectrum are anaplastic MPNST, which may be difficult to distinguish from other pleomorphic sarcomas (Fig. 30–16). They contain sheets of plump, spindled, and giant cells intermixed with areas of hemorrhage and necrosis. These pleomorphic tumors have been documented more often in the setting of von Recklinghausen's

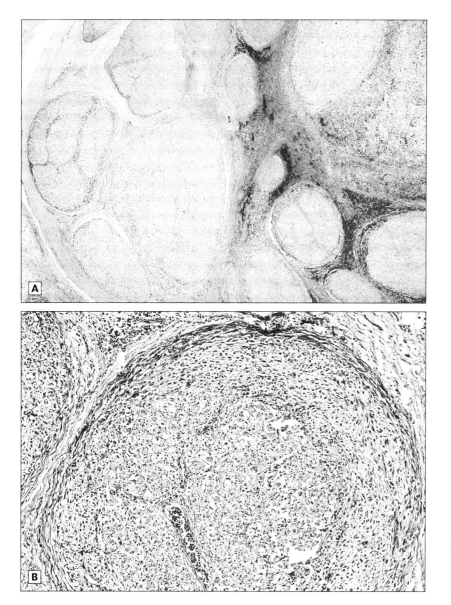

FIGURE 30–13 **(A)** Replacement of a peripheral nerve by an MPNST. **(B)** High-power view showing insinuation of a tumor between the nerve fascicles.

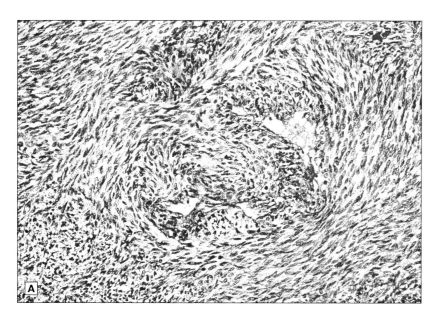

FIGURE 30–14 Peculiar changes around small vessels in MPNST. In **A** the tumor appears to herniate into lumens of vessels, whereas in **B** there is a small proliferation of small vessels in the walls of large vessels in MPNST.

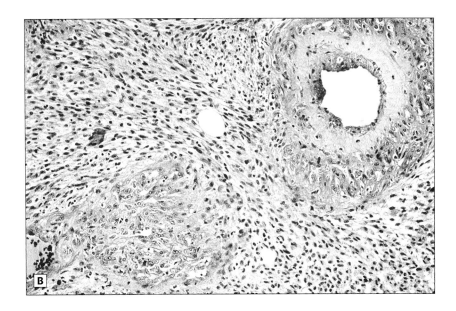

FIGURE 30–14 Continued.

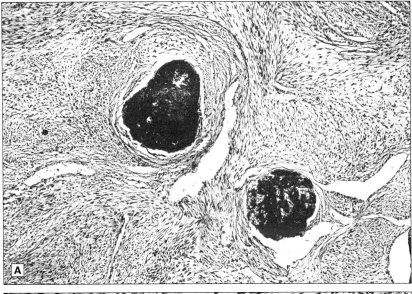

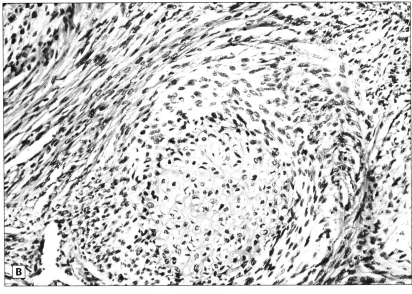

FIGURE 30–15 Heterologous elements in a malignant peripheral nerve sheath tumor are most often bone **(A)** and cartilage **(B)**.

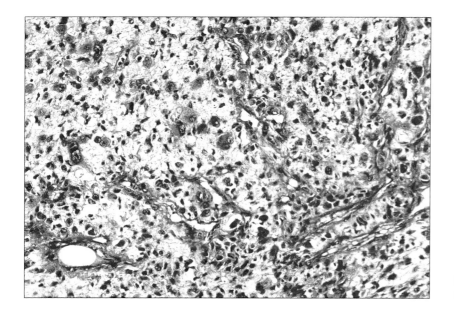

FIGURE 30–16 Pleomorphic areas in an MPNST.

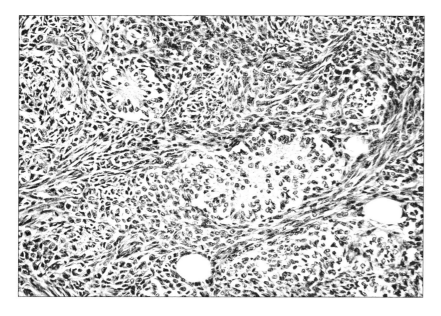

FIGURE 30–17 Primitive neuroectodermal differentiation in the form of a rosette in an MPNST.

disease. To some extent this may indicate the general reluctance to diagnose an anaplastic MPNST outside the setting of NF1. Diagnosis of these tumors depends on identifying areas of typical MPNST. Infrequently, MPNST contain areas of primitive neuroepithelial differentiation consisting of cords or nests of small round cells[27] and in extraordinary cases even rosettes (Fig. 30–17). Primitive neuroepithelial differentiation appears to be a more common feature of MPNST in children.[28]

IMMUNOHISTOCHEMICAL FINDINGS

A number of antigens are useful for identifying nerve sheath differentiation, including S-100 protein, Leu-7, PGP9.5, and myelin basic protein. Other antigens have also been studied in these tumors.[29,30] S-100 protein, the most widely used antigen for neural differentiation, can be identified in 50–90% of MPNSTs, although typically the staining is focal and limited to a small number of cells (Fig. 30–7C).[31–34] Because it is rare to encounter an MPNST with strong, diffuse immunoreactivity for S-100 protein, such a staining pattern always suggests reconsideration of various benign diagnoses, notably cellular schwannoma. Leu-7 and myelin basic protein are found in about 50% and 40% of MPNSTs, respectively.[34] Since none of these markers is specific for nerve sheath differentiation, use of panels is recommended, particularly if one wishes to distinguish MPNST from synovial sarcoma, the tumor with which it shares the most histologic overlap. Olsen et al. recently concluded using cluster analysis data from tissue microarrays that the combination of S-100 protein and nestin has a high predictive value for the diagnosis of MPSNT[35] and distinguishes it from synovial sarcoma which is EMA/CK7 positive. Smith et al.,[36] likewise, concluded that a combination of CK7/19, positive in synovial sarcoma, accurately distinguishes it from MPNST. HMGA proteins also appear to be differentially expressed in MPNST and synovial sarcomas. Significant immunoreactivity for HMGA2 is present in MPNST but not in synovial sarcoma.[37] CD34 is expressed in some MPNST and has been interpreted as focal perineurial differentiation. p53 immunoreactivity is also detected in more than half of MPNST, in contrast to its usual absence from neurofibromas.[38-40]

ELECTRON MICROSCOPIC FINDINGS

MPNSTs are characterized by many of the same features as benign nerve sheath tumors. Most significantly, the spindled or polygonal cells give off nontapered branching cytoplasmic processes that extend for appreciable distances from the cell body and contain microtubules and neurofilaments (Fig. 30–18). The processes usually lie close to one another and form junctional complexes.[41] In well-differentiated MPNST, the cells and processes are coated with basal lamina,[41-45] and occasional wisps of cytoplasm curl around themselves in the manner of mesaxon formation.[41] In less well-differentiated MPNST, the cell processes are broader,[44] and the basal laminae are poorly developed or incomplete.[41,44] The matrix contains collagen in various forms (e.g., typical, long spacing, and broad amianthoid fibers)[46] and wisps and scrolls of

basal lamina. One unique MPNST contained annulate lamellae.[47] Cells having both the ultrastructural and immunohistochemical features of perineurial cells are also identified within MPNST.[48-51] Malignant tumors showing pure perineurial differentiation are discussed in Chapter 29.

DIFFERENTIAL DIAGNOSIS

Most MPNST are easily diagnosed as malignant tumors, and the major challenge resides in distinguishing them from other sarcomas such as fibrosarcoma, monophasic synovial sarcoma, and leiomyosarcoma. As implied previously, fibrosarcoma and synovial sarcoma have a more uniform fascicular pattern, contain symmetric fusiform cells resembling fibroblasts, and obviously lack features of neural differentiation. Monophasic synovial sarcoma often contains densely hyalinized or calcified areas (or both) in combination with areas suggesting rudimentary epithelial differentiation in the form of clusters of round cells with clear cytoplasm. Immunostaining can be invaluable in the differential diagnosis (see above).

Leiomyosarcoma can usually be distinguished from MPNST without undue difficulty. Its cells have deeply eosinophilic cytoplasm, centrally placed blunt-ended nuclei, and juxtanuclear vacuoles. In a Masson trichrome stain its cytoplasm is fuchsinophilic with longitudinal striations. The cytoplasm of MPNST is usually less fuchsinophilic without longitudinal striations. An important diagnostic problem is the distinction of neurofibromas with one or more unusual features from an MPNST. This

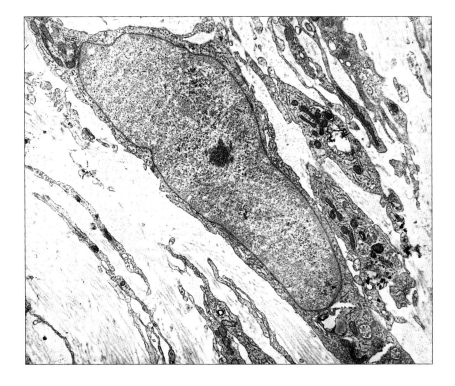

FIGURE 30–18 Electron micrograph of an MPNST illustrating an asymmetrically tapered cell with cell processes of adjacent cells lying parallel to it.

occurs typically with "borderline" neurofibromatous lesions of von Recklinghausen's disease. A diagnosis of malignancy depends on the findings of enhanced cellularity, diffuse atypia, and usually at least a low level of mitotic activity. This problem is discussed in greater detail in Chapter 29. In rare instances, one encounters a typical neurofibroma in which small foci may appear malignant by virtue of the foregoing criteria. We have interpreted such lesions as *neurofibroma with focal malignant change* and recommend conservative excision if the focus constitutes a small portion of the entire neurofibroma and the focus appears totally removed by the excision. Preliminary follow-up in these cases supports this conservative approach to management.

The criterion of mitotic activity paradoxically does not apply to schwannoma. Schwannoma displaying mitotic activity pursues a benign course, and rarely has this tumor been known to undergo malignant degeneration. Thus, when material from a small biopsy specimen is evaluated, it is hazardous to attempt to distinguish a cellular schwannoma from an MPNST solely on the basis of mitotic activity. In this situation, a larger sample of the mass is necessary to determine if the tumor in question has an Antoni A and B pattern, perivascular hyalinization, encapsulation, or other typical features of a schwannoma.

MOLECULAR AND CYTOGENETIC FINDINGS

The development of MPNST from neurofibroma appears to be a multistep process in which a number of genes participate, leading to gain in function of some and a loss of function of others. Patients with NF1 have germline inactivation of NF1. Evidence, furthermore, supports the view that both alleles are inactivated in neurofibromas[52] and MPNST,[53] and that Schwann cells derived from NF1-deleted (neurofibromin-deficient) animals acquire increased proliferative capacity and angioinvasive properties (see Chapter 29).[54,55] The progression of a neurofibroma to an MPNST is associated with a number of additional chromosomal alterations.[56–59] The most common alterations are genomic gains involving 17q, 7p, 5p, 8q, and 12q. Less common alterations are genomic losses of 9p, 13q, and 1p. 9p includes notably the *CDKN2* gene, a cyclin-dependent kinase inhibitor that is inactivated in more than 50% of MPNSTs but not in neurofibromas.[60,61] This gene produces two protein products, p16 and p19. The former negatively regulates cell cycling through the *Rb* pathway, whereas the latter negatively regulates cycling through the p53 pathway. Studies of sporadic and NF1-associated MPNST have demonstrated consistent absence of p16[62,63] in the face of normal expression of other cell cycle component proteins by Western blot analysis,[62] leading the authors to conclude that p16 inactivation is sufficient for abnormal stimulation of the cell cycle without involvement of other components.[62] However, others using immunohistochemical methods report diminished or absent expression of both p17 and p27,[64] but point out these alterations were not reliable in separating neurofibromas from low-grade peripheral nerve sheath tumors. That *p53* is ultimately affected in MPNST is suggested by positive immunostaining for p53 in a large number of MPNSTs, particularly high-grade ones, but not in neurofibromas.[38–40,64] Protein expression of the checkpoint with forkhead-associated domain and ring finger (CHFR), another mitotic checkpoint gene, is also reduced in MPNST and has been correlated with high mitotic activity.[65]

CLINICAL BEHAVIOR

Most MPNSTs are high-grade sarcomas, with a high likelihood of producing local recurrence and distant metastasis. Although the prognosis reported in the early literature for this disease was often dismal, the survival reported from large cancer referral centers in which patients have undergone sophisticated radiologic imaging and extensive surgery often coupled with adjuvant radiation or chemotherapy has improved. Based on three large studies from the Mayo Clinic and Memorial Sloan-Kettering Cancer Hospital,[5,6,15] the local recurrence rate varies from 40% to 65% and the metastatic rate from 40% to 68% (Table 30–1). The 5-year survival based on a study of 134 patients with tumors from all sites was 52%,[6] although lower survival rates (15%) are recorded when the lesions occur at sites for which it is difficult to achieve good margins (e.g., retroperitoneum, thoracic cavity).[5,15] There

TABLE 30–1	CLINICAL BEHAVIOR OF MALIGNANT PERIPHERAL NERVE SHEATH TUMORS BY SITE			
Location	No. of cases	Recurrence (%)	Metastasis (%)	5-year survival (%)
All sites	134	43	40	52
Lower extremity/buttock	43	40	63	39
Paraspinal	25	65	68	16
From references 5, 6, 15.				

appears to be a number of prognostic variables in this disease, including the size of the lesion, location, stage, grade, status of surgical margins, necrosis, and use of adjuvant radiation (Table 30–2). In a multivariate analysis, the status of surgical margins and a history of irradiation emerge as independent prognostic variables. Thus, patients who have positive surgical margins or who have radiation-induced sarcomas have a worse prognosis than the group as a whole.

In the past, a large body of literature indicated that tumors associated with NF1 have a particularly poor prognosis compared with those occurring on a sporadic basis. This was not surprising, because of the tendency of tumors in NF1 to be large, central, and deep. More recent large studies have not confirmed this finding, however.[5,66] In a large series from Memorial Hospital in which the authors compared tumors of roughly comparable size and location (buttock and leg) in patients with and without NF1, there was no significant difference in behavior. Approximately 40% of patients in both groups developed local recurrence, and it could be correlated with the type of surgery and the presence of positive margins.[5,66] Sixty-five percent of patients in both groups developed distant metastasis with a comparable interval between surgery and metastasis (14–18 months).[5] The overall 5-year survival rate in the experience of Wanebo et al. was 43.7%, with factors such as the age of the patient, size and location of tumor, and margins most influential for outcome.[66] Likewise, the most recent study by Wong et al. based on Mayo Clinic experience could not confirm that NF1 by itself was an independent variable for prognosis.[6]

The most common metastatic site for MPNST is the lung, followed by bone and pleura. Fewer than 10% of patients with metastasis developed regional node deposits, indicating that routine lymph node dissections do not play an important role in the treatment of this disease. This also emphasizes the fact that metastatic spindle cell lesions with Schwann cell-like features are apt to be metastatic desmoplastic or neurotropic melanomas or some other spindle cell tumor mimicking MPNST. However, in our experience, lymph node metastasis may be seen in the presence of widely metastatic disease. One should also be aware of the propensity of this tumor to spread for considerable distances along the nerve sheath, and there are reports of tumors entering the subarachnoid space of the spinal cord via this route. Therefore, it is wise to obtain a frozen section of the nerve margins to assess the adequacy of the excision.

Although MPNST does not occur often in the pediatric age group, it appears to have a course roughly comparable to adults. Meis et al., in a retrospective review based on consultation material, noted metastasis in 50% of patients at 2 years.[28] A report from two large centers, however, reported a 5-year survival of 51%[67] and 10-year survival of 41%.[67] Multivariate analysis identified absence of NF1, IRS groups I or II, and location on an extremity as independent favorable prognostic factors.[68] Others have related the prognosis closely to whether the patient underwent radical surgery. Survival at 10 years was 80% for patients who had undergone radical surgery compared to only 14% for those who did not.[67]

TABLE 30–2	**CORRELATION BETWEEN PROGNOSTIC VARIABLES AND SURVIVAL IN MALIGNANT PERIPHERAL NERVE SHEATH TUMORS**		
Prognostic factor	**5-year survival (%)**	**Univariate analysis (*p*)**	**Multivariate analysis (*p*)**
Size (cm)			
<5	70	<0.0001	0.24
5.1–10.0	57		
10.1–15	43		
>15			
Location			
Nonextremity	43	0.0064	0.20
Extremity	70		
History of NF1			
Yes	36	0.0074	0.075
No	57		
History of XRT			
Yes	58	0.0004	**0.023**
No			
Stage			
1	65	0.0340	
2	60		
3	46		
Grade			
1	65	0.0074	0.39
2	61		
3	35		
4	55		
Surgical margin			
Positive	22	0.0030	**0.0044**
Negative	67		
Close	43		
Unknown	37		
Use of IORT/BT			
Yes	72	0.039	0.32
No	50		
Necrosis			
Yes	37	37	
No	62	0.0099	

NF1, neurofibromatosis 1; XRT, x-irradiation; IORT/BT, intraoperative radiotherapy/brachytherapy.
The *p* values in boldface represent statistically significant parameters.
From Wong WW, Hirose T, Scheithauer BW, et al. Malignant peripheral nerve sheath tumor: analysis of treatment outcome. Int J Radiol Oncol Biol Phys 1998; 42:351.

MALIGNANT PERIPHERAL NERVE SHEATH TUMOR WITH RHABDOMYOBLASTIC DIFFERENTIATION (MALIGNANT TRITON TUMOR)

In the broadest sense, a Triton tumor is any neoplasm with both neural and skeletal muscle differentiation; included are the neuromuscular hamartoma (benign Triton tumor),[69–71] medulloblastoma with rhabdomyosarcoma,[72] rhabdomyosarcoma with ganglion cells (ectomesenchymoma), and MPNST with rhabdomyosarcoma.[26,73–75] The term *malignant Triton tumor* is usually applied only to the MPNST with rhabdomyosarcoma because it is the most widely recognized of the foregoing entities.[74,76–78] This composite neoplasm was first described in 1938 by Masson and Martin,[79] who suggested that the neural elements in the tumor induced differentiation of skeletal muscle in much the same fashion as normal nerve was believed to induce the regeneration of skeletal muscle in the Triton salamander. As a result, these tumors were eventually accorded the name of the amphibian.

A review of all reported cases of Triton tumors in the literature attests to their relative rarity and their tendency to occur in NF1.[80] Slightly more than half of the reported cases in the literature have occurred in conjunction with NF1.[73,81] However, our experience suggests the tumor may occur outside the setting of NF1 more often than is generally appreciated. Low estimates of sporadic cases seem to result from errors in diagnosis, as evidenced by the fact that most cases are referred to us with a diagnosis of fibrosarcoma or rhabdomyosarcoma, depending on the prominence of the muscle component. Because most reported cases occur in patients with von Recklinghausen's disease, affected individuals are usually young (average age 35 years). The tumors are widely distributed, but most occur on the head, neck, and trunk. Like other MPNST, symptoms are related to a progressively enlarging mass that may give rise to neurologic symptoms. The 5-year survival based on a literature review by Brooks et al. was 12%.[73]

The hallmark of this tumor is the presence of rhabdomyoblasts scattered throughout a stroma indistinguishable from an ordinary MPNST (Figs 30–19, 30–20). The number of rhabdomyoblasts varies greatly from tumor to

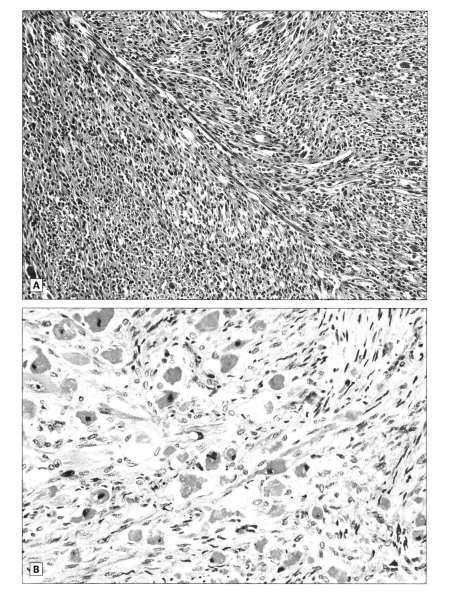

FIGURE 30–19 (A) Malignant peripheral nerve sheath tumor with rhabdomyoblastic differentiation (malignant Triton tumor). **(B)** Rounded or elongated large rhabdomyoblasts are scattered throughout the tumor.

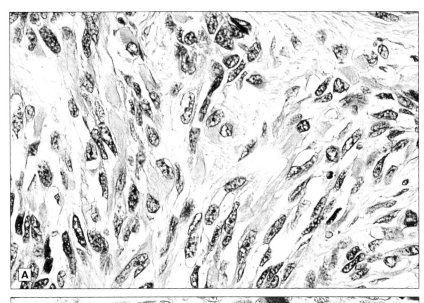

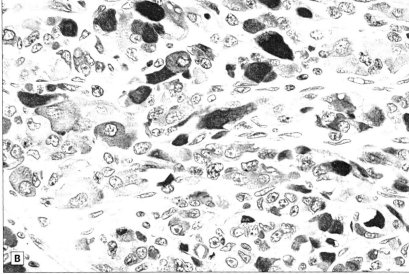

FIGURE 30–20 Rhabdomyoblasts in an MPNST **(A)** showing desmin immunoreactivity **(B)**.

tumor and even from area to area in the same tumor. They are usually relatively mature, and their abundant eosinophilic cytoplasm contrasts sharply with the pale-staining cytoplasm of the Schwann cells. Cross-striations can be identified but, as in rhabdomyosarcomas, are more readily identified in cells with elongated tapered cytoplasm. Both desmin and nuclear regulatory proteins (MyoD1 and myogenin) can be demonstrated in the rhabdomyoblasts (Fig. 30–20B).

The histogenesis of these unusual tumors has occasioned much discussion. Although Masson believed that one cell line induced the other, it seems more likely that both cell lines originate from less well-differentiated neural crest cells. Normally, the neural crest contributes to the formation of mesenchyme in certain vertebrates and ultimately forms portions of branchial cartilage, connective tissue, and muscle in the facial region.[82] Thus, these tumors recapitulate both the schwannian and the mesenchymal potentiality of the neural crest.

MALIGNANT PERIPHERAL NERVE SHEATH TUMOR WITH GLANDS (GLANDULAR MALIGNANT SCHWANNOMA)

In 1892, Garre[83] reported a patient with von Recklinghausen's disease and an MPNST of the sciatic nerve. Scattered throughout the schwannian background of the tumor were numerous well-differentiated glands. Since that time, very few additional tumors have been reported, probably making it among the rarest of MPNST with divergent differentiation.[36,84–88] Almost all of these tumors have occurred in patients with NF1, a fact that surely accounts for the young median age (about 30 years)[78] of affected patients. The tumors usually arise from major nerves, including the sciatic, median, brachial plexus, and spinal nerves.

Characteristically, they have a spindle-cell background indistinguishable from ordinary MPNST and may contain

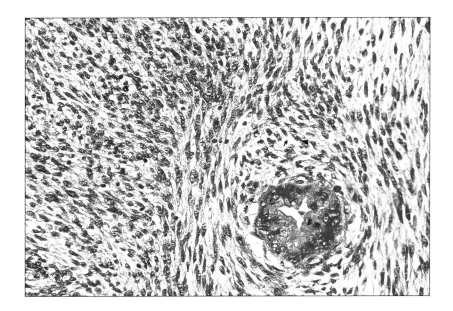

FIGURE 30–21 MPNST with glandular differentiation. Glands in this case appeared malignant.

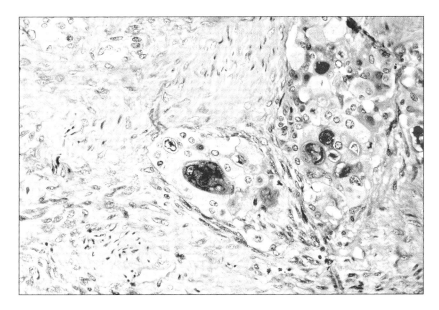

FIGURE 30–22 Glands in an MPNST containing carminophilic mucin.

other heterologous elements such as muscle, cartilage, and bone. The glands are usually few in number and are made up of well-differentiated, nonciliated cuboidal or columnar cells with clear cytoplasm and occasional goblet cells (Figs 30–21 to 30–23). Intracellular and extracellular mucin, which are histochemically identical to conventional epithelial mucins, can be demonstrated in the glands (Fig. 30–22). We have even encountered one that contained squamous islands in addition to glands (Fig. 30–23). By electron microscopy, the glands have features of intestinal epithelium with numerous well-oriented microvilli with core rootlets.[89] Some of the cells in the glands are argyrophilic and contain dense-core granules;[10] others have documented ependymal differentiation.[86] Somatostatin immunoreactivity was noted in the glands of one glandular schwannoma.[90] Rarely, the glands appear histologically malignant.

It may be difficult to distinguish these tumors from biphasic synovial sarcomas because the glandular elements may be virtually identical. It is principally the spindled element that distinguishes them, although obviously the presence of goblet cells or neuroendocrine differentiation favors the diagnosis of a glandular MPNST. In synovial sarcomas, the spindled element resembles a conventional fibrosarcoma and may be secondarily hyalinized or calcified. Subtle degrees of epithelial differentiation may also be evident in the spindled stroma of the synovial sarcoma. This feature is not present in glandular MPNST because the epithelial elements invariably arise rather abruptly from the stroma. The immunologic phenotypes of synovial sarcoma and glandular MPNST differ. The former often contains keratin-positive cells in the spindled zones (and occasionally S-100 protein-positive ones), whereas the latter displays only focal S-100 protein

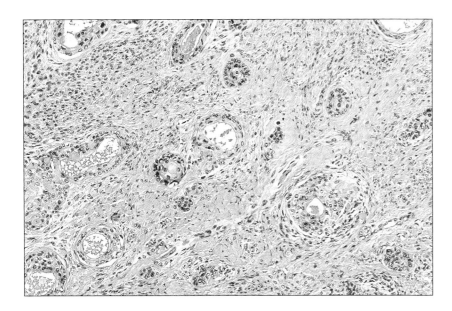

FIGURE 30–23 MPNST with glands and squamous islands.

positivity. The addition of other neural antigens such as nerve growth factor receptor (NGFR) and PGP9.5 may improve the sensitivity and specificity of the diagnosis.[91]

Although the glandular elements set this tumor apart as a peculiar histologic variant, they serve essentially no role in grading the tumor or predicting its biologic behavior. Tumors with a highly malignant schwannian component may be expected to do poorly regardless of the degree of differentiation of the glands. Most tumors reported in the literature seem to fall into this category. On the other hand, tumors with a low-grade schwannian element may do extremely well, as illustrated by the fact that the two patients with tumors of this type reported by Woodruff and Christensen[92] are alive and well. It should be noted in passing, however, that certain rare (benign) schwannomas with glandular elements should be clearly distinguished from glandular MPNST. Usually, they are superficial lesions with glands that resemble adnexal structures, leading some to question whether they are entrapped elements.

MALIGNANT PERIPHERAL NERVE SHEATH TUMOR WITH ANGIOSARCOMA

Slightly more than 20 angiosarcomas arising in nerve sheath tumors have been reported, making these tumors largely curiosities.[93–98] Most have developed in patients with NF1 and not surprisingly, therefore, were associated with either plexiform neurofibroma, MPNST, or both. Anecdotal reports attest to the fact that angiosarcoma may also occur in benign schwannomas,[96] normal nerves,[97] and sporadic MPNST.[98] Because of the strong association with NF1, these tumors usually occur in young individuals. They are indistinguishable from

MPNST and have conventional-appearing angiosarcomas that may be microscopic or macroscopic in size. The prognosis is poor, and most of the patients have succumbed to the disease.

EPITHELIOID MALIGNANT PERIPHERAL NERVE SHEATH TUMOR (EPITHELIOID MALIGNANT SCHWANNOMA)

Epithelioid MPNST is an unusual form of MPNST that closely resembles carcinoma or melanoma by virtue of the fact that the tumor is composed predominantly or exclusively of Schwann cells with a polygonal epithelioid appearance.[99–104] Although we estimated that 5% or fewer MPNST belong to this group, this estimate may be far too generous. In fact, for many years the exact nature of this unusual group of tumors was questioned, as indicated by Stewart and Copeland:[1] "We have observed tumors of deeper nerve trunks which looked like certain nonpigmented melanomas yet did not run the clinical course of melanoma. Are those melanomas or neurosarcomas?"

There is convincing evidence that these tumors represent nerve sheath tumors rather than melanomas or metastatic carcinomas. First, the tumors follow a distribution similar to that of the ordinary MPNST, with most occurring in patients 20–50 years of age. In our experience with 26 cases, the median age was 36 years; men were affected slightly more often than women. Most of the tumors reported in the literature originated in major nerves, including the sciatic, tibial, peroneal, facial, antebrachial cutaneous, and digital nerves. In our experience, 8 of 10 deeply situated epithelioid MPNST originated from a major nerve, including the sciatic nerve (three cases) and the brachial plexus, femoral, radial, and median nerves

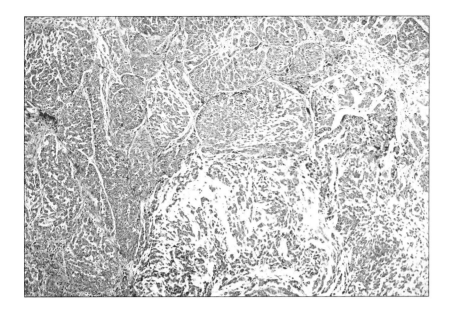

FIGURE 30–24 Epithelioid malignant peripheral nerve sheath tumor showing vague nodular growth. The tumor varies from slightly myxoid to cellular.

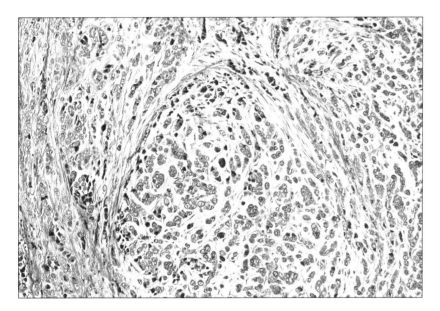

FIGURE 30–25 Epithelioid MPNST with cords of epithelioid cells.

(one case each). It is the cases in which origin from a nerve or neurofibroma cannot be documented that pose the most challenging and sometimes unresolvable problems in diagnosis. Although this form of MPNST may occur in NF1, it seems to occur less frequently than in ordinary MPNST. Lodding et al.[102] encountered one case in their series of 16, whereas none of our 26 patients had the disease.[101]

Histologically, the tumor is variable. In our cases, the most characteristic appearance is that of short cords of large epithelioid cells arranged in a vague nodular pattern (Figs 30–24 to 30–27). The cells in these tumors usually have large, round nuclei with prominent melanoma-like nucleoli (Fig. 30–26). The tumors may appear densely cellular or myxoid (Fig. 30–26B), depending on the accumulation of acid mucin between the cords, and there is often subtle blending of the epithelioid areas with spin-

dled areas resembling the conventional MPNST (Fig. 30–28). However, it is our belief that the term *epithelioid MPNST* should be reserved for tumors in which the predominant pattern is epithelioid. Although the combination of all of these features is usually sufficient to make the correct diagnosis, many tumors lack this distinctive appearance. In fact, most tumors reported in the literature have resembled melanomas or carcinomas and have consisted simply of small nests of epithelioid cells admixed with a spindled component.

There are a number of rather unusual forms of epithelioid MPNST that deserve comment. Some contain a predominance of clear cells, and others are made up of rhabdoid cells with a prominent glassy eosinophilic perinuclear zone corresponding ultrastructurally to the presence of whorls of intermediate filaments (Fig. 30–27). Still other tumors consist of sheets of rounded

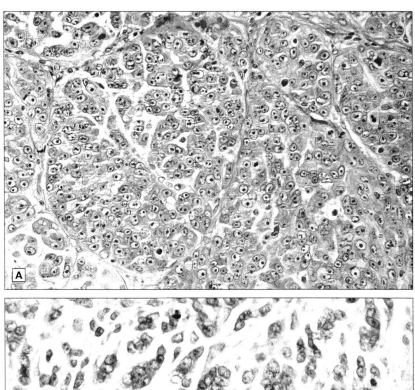

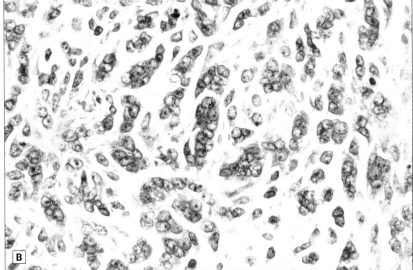

FIGURE 30–26 Epithelioid malignant peripheral nerve sheath tumor showing the polygonal shape of cells and prominent nucleoli **(A)**. In some areas, groups of cells are separated by myxoid stroma **(B)**.

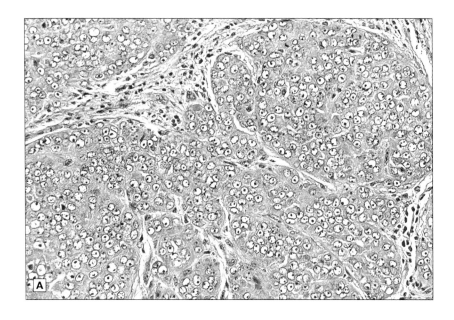

FIGURE 30–27 (A) Epithelioid malignant peripheral nerve sheath tumor with rhabdoid cells.

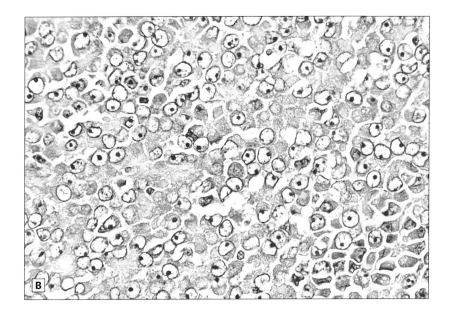

FIGURE 30–27 Continued. **(B)** High-power view of rhabdoid cells shows a glassy perinuclear zone.

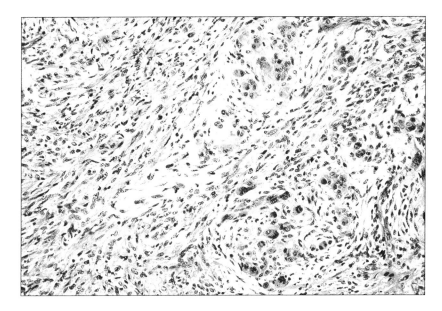

FIGURE 30–28 MPNST with focal epithelioid differentiation.

pleomorphic cells suggestive of a pleomorphic carcinoma (Fig. 30–29).

Consequently, the diagnosis has largely depended on an established origin from a nerve. In the absence of this feature, the diagnosis is sometimes suspected by a delicate "mesenchymal" pattern of collagenization and a transition to spindled "schwannian" areas (Fig. 30–28). Unlike many melanomas, neither melanin pigment nor glycogen can be demonstrated in the cytoplasm of these tumors. In one unique case we reviewed, the diagnosis of "malignant epithelioid schwannoma" was established by virtue of the presence of true rosettes in a tumor that otherwise resembled melanoma (Fig. 30–17). It should be emphasized that a clear-cut distinction from melanoma or carcinoma is not always possible on routine sections, a dilemma compounded by the fact that occa-

sionally metastatic spindled melanomas are virtually indistinguishable from MPNST.

In our experience, about 80% of these tumors are strongly and diffusely positive for S-100 protein, a pattern of immunoreactivity that contrasts with conventional MPNST (Fig. 30–30).[101] They do not express melanoma-associated antigen, and only rarely is keratin present. Therefore, the presence of either keratin or melanin-related antigens in a malignant epithelioid tumor argues against the diagnosis of epithelioid MPNST. Type IV collagen can be identified readily between individual cells and groups of cells with immunohistochemical procedures; regrettably, the pattern of basal lamina deposition does not help distinguish this tumor from melanoma, which also shares considerable overlap.[101]

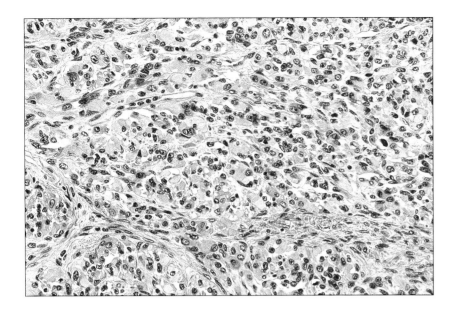

FIGURE 30–29 Epithelioid MPNST composed of pleomorphic epithelioid cells.

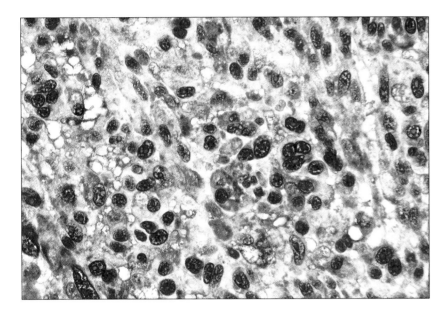

FIGURE 30–30 S-100 protein immunostaining in an epithelioid MPNST.

The ultrastructural features of epithelioid MPNST vary as a function of differentiation. Whereas it is possible to identify interlocking cell processes invested with basal lamina and displaying cell junctions, these features are not invariably present.

Despite the limited number of reported cases, there is no doubt that they are fully malignant tumors and should be treated accordingly. At least half of the patients reported in the literature developed distant metastases, usually in the lung. In our experience with 10 patients with tumors in deep soft tissue, three developed metastatic disease.[101] Because of the melanoma-like appearance of these tumors, the question has been raised as to whether they commonly spread to regional lymph nodes. Lodding et al. noted lymph node metastasis in three of their 14 cases,[102] but we had no instances of lymph node metas-

tasis in 16 cases.[101] Until additional cases adequately address the question, it seems prudent at least to evaluate these tumors clinically before deciding on definitive therapy.

SUPERFICIAL EPITHELIOID MALIGNANT PERIPHERAL NERVE SHEATH TUMOR

Epithelioid MPNST occurring in the superficial soft tissues are quite rare and many cases so reported are probably examples of epithelioid schwannoma (see Chapter 29). Only those epithelioid nerve sheath tumors with clear-cut malignant features should be considered in this category.

CLEAR CELL SARCOMA OF TENDON AND APONEUROSIS

Described by Enzinger in 1965,[105] the clear cell sarcoma is a rare melanin-producing soft tissue sarcoma. Although it is, unfortunately, also referred to as "malignant melanoma of soft parts," it is clinically, genetically, and biologically distinct from cutaneous melanoma despite certain histologic similarities. In contrast to cutaneous melanoma, clear cell sarcomas invariably arise in the deep soft tissue of the distal extremities, and 70% possess a consistent balanced translocation t(12;22)(q13;q12)[106-112] that is not found in melanoma and is believed to be an early, if not primary, event in tumorigenesis. This translocation fuses *EWS* on chromosome 22 with *ATF1*,[113] a member of the CREB transcription factor family on chromosome 12. This results in four fusion transcripts that are differentially expressed amongst tumors.[114] The fusion protein mimics the action of melanocyte stimulating hormone (MSH) by binding to and constitutively activating the promoter for MiTF, the melanocyte master transcription factor.[115] Recent evidence suggests that MiTF is a critical oncogenic target since it not only mediates melanin production in these tumors but also EWS-ATF1-induced tumor growth.[115,116]

Clinical findings

Clear cell sarcoma mainly affects young adults between the ages of 20 and 40 years with a median age of about 30 years. Approximately 40% of cases occur on the foot and ankle (Fig. 30–31) with another 30% on the knee, thigh, and hand.[117-120] The head and neck region and the trunk are distinctly unusual sites (Table 30–3). Clear cell sarcomas present as a slowly enlarging, occasionally painful mass, which is usually present about 2 years at the time of diagnosis, although a significant percentage have been present for 5 years or longer. They arise in deep soft tissue and unless the lesion is extremely large or distal, the overlying skin and dermis is usually not involved.

Pathologic findings

Macroscopically, the tumor consists of a lobulated or multinodular gray-white mass firmly attached to tendons or aponeuroses (Figs 30–32, 30–33) which averages between 2 and 6 cm. The cut surface may be marred by focal hemorrhage, necrosis, or cystic change. In a small proportion of cases the melanin may be prominent enough to be visualized as foci of dark brown or black discoloration (Fig. 30–33).

Histologically, tumors consist of compact nests or fascicles of predominantly fusiform or spindled cells with a clear cytoplasm bordered and defined by a delicate framework of fibrocollagenous tissue contiguous with adjacent

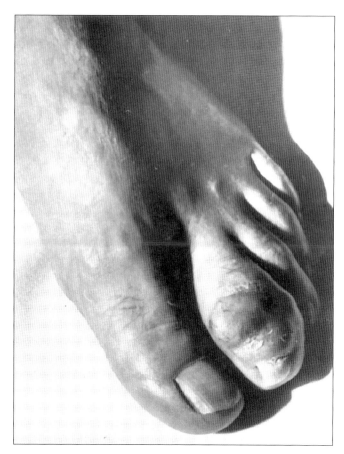

FIGURE 30–31 Clear cell sarcoma of the second toe.

TABLE 30–3	ANATOMIC DISTRIBUTION OF 141 CLEAR CELL SARCOMAS	
Location	**No. of patients**	**(%)**
Head and neck	1	0.8
Trunk	3	2.1
Upper extremity	31	22.0
Lower extremity (foot 28; knee 21; heel 15; ankle 11)	106	75.1
Total	141	100.00

Data are from Montgomery et al.[118]

tendons or aponeuroses (Figs 30–34 to 30–41). The cells have highly distinctive features consisting of nuclei with a vesicular nuclear chromatin pattern and prominent basophilic nucleoli reminiscent of malignant melanoma. The cytoplasm varies from clear to weakly eosinophilic (Fig. 30–42A) and contains large amounts of intracellular glycogen. Clear cells and eosinophilic cells coexist in different portions of the same neoplasm with focal transitions between the two (Fig. 30–40). A highly characteristic feature is the multinucleated tumor giant cells with 10–15 peripherally placed nuclei (Fig. 30–38). In general, clear cell sarcomas are neither pleomorphic nor mitotically highly active, although this

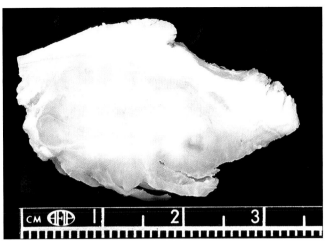

FIGURE 30–32 Clear cell sarcoma diffusely infiltrating a tendon (top) and skeletal muscle (bottom).

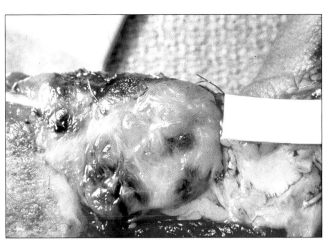

FIGURE 30–33 Clear cell sarcoma showing pigmented areas.

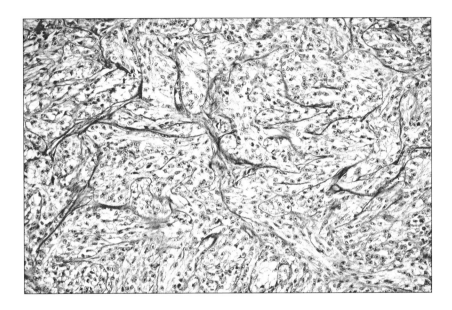

FIGURE 30–34 Clear cell sarcoma. Fibrous tissue septa divide the tumor into well-defined nests and groups of pale-staining tumor cells.

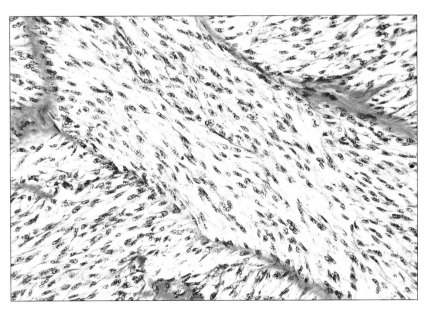

FIGURE 30–35 Clear cell sarcoma showing arrangement of the pale-staining tumor cells in short fascicles separated by dense fibrous septa.

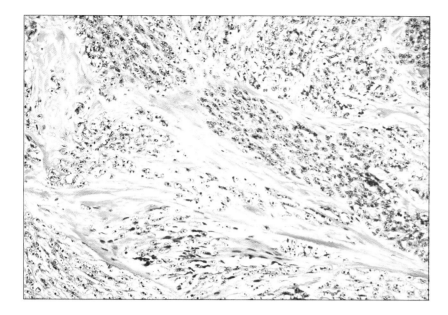

FIGURE 30–36 Clear cell sarcoma subdivided by dense fibrous bands.

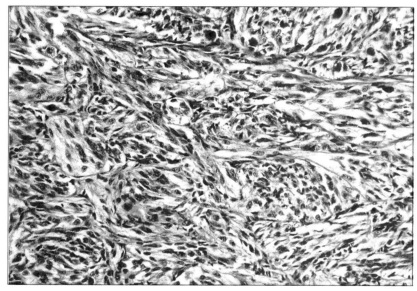

FIGURE 30–37 Clear cell sarcoma with cytoplasmic melanin pigment.

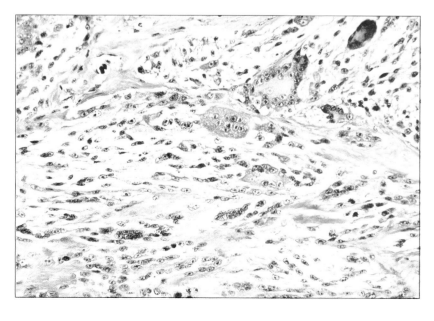

FIGURE 30–38 Clear cell sarcoma with scattered multinucleated giant cells. The giant cells have a wreath of peripherally placed nuclei of uniform size and shape.

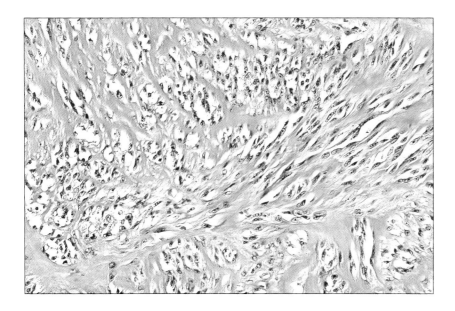

FIGURE 30–39 Clear cell sarcoma with areas of dense hyalinization.

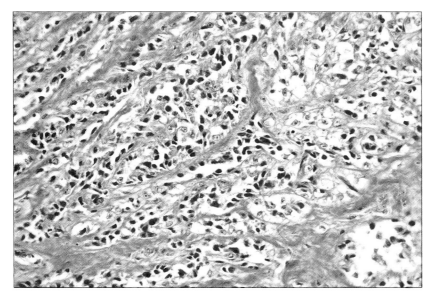

FIGURE 30–40 Clear cell sarcoma with degeneration. Cells can acquire a "small cell" appearance that is misleading.

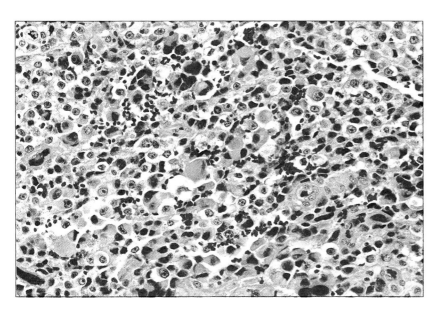

FIGURE 30–41 Metastatic clear cell sarcoma with marked pleomorphism and essentially no spindling. Metastatic deposits of this type resemble carcinoma or melanoma.

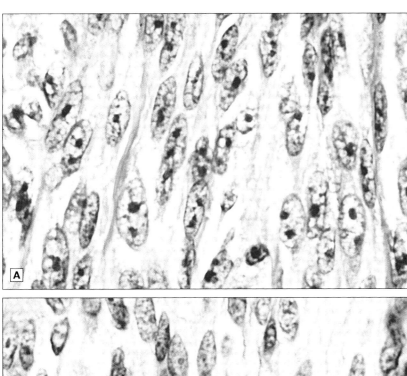

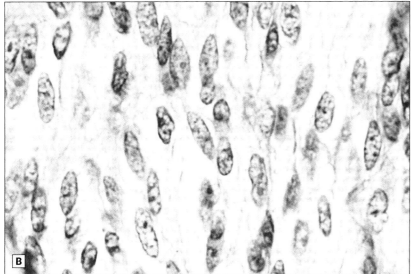

FIGURE 30–42 Comparison of cytologic features of clear cell sarcoma and a cellular blue nevus at the same magnification. **(A)** Clear cell sarcoma has prominent vesicular nuclei with a large single nucleolus. **(B)** Cellular blue nevus cells are smaller with a less vesicular nuclear chromatin pattern and small, pinpoint nucleoli.

observation does not necessarily apply to recurrent or metastatic lesions.

Melanin is present in over 50% of clear cell sarcomas but is usually not abundant enough to be seen on hematoxylin-eosin stain. It can be detected with appropriate histochemical (Fontana or Warthin-Starry) or immunohistochemical stains (Fig. 30–43). Virtually all clear cell sarcomas diffusely express S-100 protein (Fig. 30–44), and most also express antigens associated with melanin synthesis (HMB-45, Melan-A, Mel-CAM, MiTF).[121-123] Neuron-specific enolase, Leu-7, and LN3 have also been noted in these lesions.

Ultrastructurally, the tumor consists of oval or fusiform cells with rounded nuclei, evenly dispersed chromatin at the nuclear membrane, and a large, centrally placed, single nucleolus. The cytoplasm contains multiple, rounded and swollen mitochondria, membrane-bound vesicles, and ribosomes and polyribosomes in varying numbers. There are also aggregates of rough endoplasmic reticulum, scanty amounts of glycogen, and occasional lipid droplets. Mononuclear and multinuclear cells display similar ultrastructural characteristics. Melanosomes in varying stages of development are present in most cases.[120,124] Some show dense pigmentation, and others exhibit the typical lamellar, striated, or "barrelstave" internal structure of premelanosomes (Fig. 30–45). Basal laminae surround groups of closely apposed neoplastic cells. Collagen fibers are abundant in the extracellular spaces. Benson et al.[125] also described occasional cells with stubby or finger-like dendritic processes, a few of which contained longitudinally aligned filaments.

Differential diagnosis

Since cytologic features are of paramount importance in the diagnosis of clear cell sarcoma, care must be exercised to evaluate only optimally preserved areas. Poorly preserved or degenerated clear cell sarcomas having shriveled cells that cling to the fibrous bands are easily misconstrued as a round cell sarcoma, particularly alveolar rhabdomyosarcoma. In well-preserved material, however, the differential diagnosis typically includes, on the one hand, sarcomas with a predominant fascicular growth pattern such as fibrosarcoma, synovial sarcoma, and malignant peripheral nerve sheath tumor and, on the other hand, melanin-producing tumors such as cellular blue nevus and nodular malignant melanoma. The distinctive cytologic features of clear cell sarcoma including prominent melanoma-like nucleoli, clear cytoplasm, and immunophenotypic profile set this lesion apart from the spindle cell sarcomas noted above.

The distinction of clear cell sarcoma from other melanin-producing lesions can be more problematic and may require correlation of the histologic, clinical, and molecular data. In general, clear cell sarcomas originate in deep structures, rarely involve the dermis, and have a predominantly and relatively uniform spindle-cell appearance that contrasts with the epithelioid appearance of nodular melanomas. However, in ambiguous situations, molecular genetic analysis is highly recommended since the t(12;22) that characterizes clear cell sarcoma has not been identified in malignant melanoma. Cellular blue nevus can occur in a similar age and location and have certain common histologic features including spindled cells and giant cells with clear cytoplasm. Cellular blue nevi typically are dermal-based lesions with a peripheral zone that resembles a neurofibroma by virtue of the interdigitation of slender pigmented dendritic cells with surrounding collagen. The cells lack atypia and have small, pinpoint nucleoli (Fig. 30–42). Recurrent cellular blue nevi, however, can acquire more atypical cytologic features such that a distinction from clear cell sarcoma is not always possible. In these situations review of the original material and/or molecular genetic analysis is essential. The recently described paraganglioma-like dermal melanocytic tumor (PDMT), while having cells with a clear to eosinophilic cytoplasm, comprises zellballen-like nests of cells of distinctly low nuclear grade (Fig. 30–46A,B). These lesions, based in

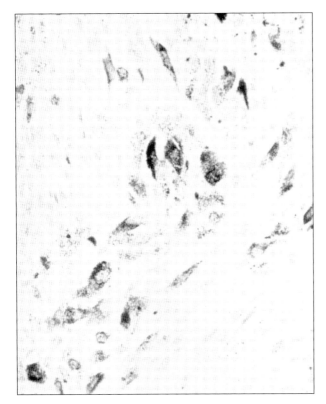

FIGURE 30–43 Clear cell sarcoma. Fontana's stain reveals melanin pigment in some of the tumor cells. (Fontana stain; ×400)

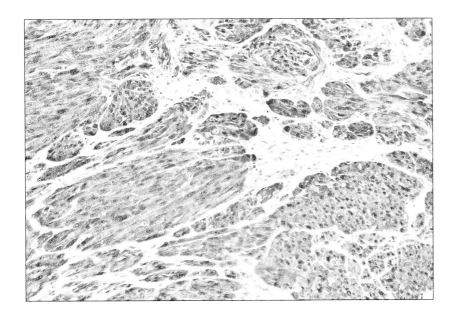

FIGURE 30–44 Strong S-100 protein immunostaining in a clear cell sarcoma.

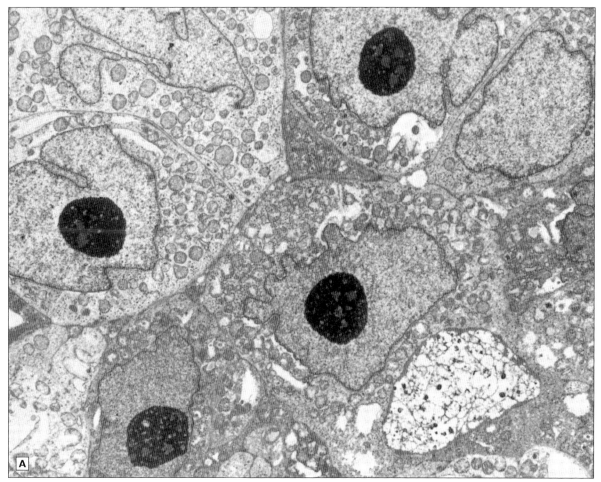

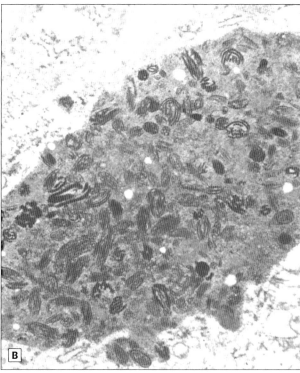

FIGURE 30–45 **(A)** Clear cell sarcoma (malignant melanoma of soft parts) showing tumor cells with irregular nuclear profiles, strikingly prominent nucleoli, and numerous mitochondria (×4600) (From Benson JD, Kraemer BB, Mackay B. Malignant melanoma of soft parts: an ultrastructural study of four cases. Ultrastruct Pathol 1985; 8:57.) **(B)** Melanosomes with typical lamellar or "barrel-stave" internal structure in a clear cell sarcoma. (×40 500)

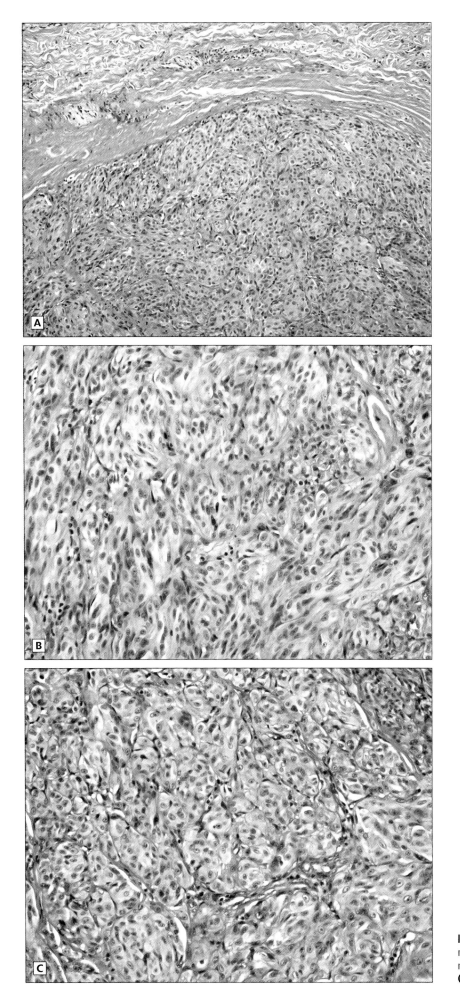

FIGURE 30–46 Paraganglioma-like dermal melanocytic tumor **(A)** showing zellballen-like nests of slightly spindled **(B)** to rounded cells **(C)**.

the dermis, rarely extend to deep structures. All thus far have behaved in a benign fashion.[126]

Discussion

Clear cell sarcoma is an extremely rare tumor for which it has been difficult to amass outcome and therapeutic data in a large patient population. For example, only 28 pediatric patients were referred to the Italian and German Soft Tissue Sarcoma Cooperative Group over a 20-year period from 1980 to 2000.[119] Nevertheless, there is agreement based on the largest studies that this is a high-grade sarcoma.[105,117–120,127] Recurrences, which reflect the adequacy of initial surgery, range from 14% to 39%, whereas metastases to lung or lymph node develop in approximately one-half of patients within an interval of 2–8 years. Late metastases after 10–20 years have been reported in patients with repeated local recurrences. Since patients who develop local recurrences or regional lymph node metastases eventually develop distant metastases, there is a clear need for controlling local disease and for long-term surveillance. Given the risk for regional lymph node metastases in this disease, there has been recent interest in performing sentinel lymph node biopsy. A recent report describes the feasibility of identifying and excising sentinel nodes,[128] but there is insufficient data on which to base a therapeutic recommendation.

Clear cell sarcoma has traditionally been considered an "ungradable" sarcoma and for that reason several studies have attempted to identify other prognostic factors. Size,[117,118,120] followed by necrosis,[117,118] have proved to be the most robust prognostic factors[117,118,120] with tumors >5 cm having a significantly worse outcome than those that are smaller. Other factors such as age, location, depth, or proliferation index have been found to be independent prognostic factors. Radical surgery is the mainstay of therapy, and chemotherapy has proven to have little efficacy.[119]

CLEAR CELL SARCOMA-LIKE TUMOR OF GASTROINTESTINAL TRACT

Tumors with many of the features of clear cell sarcoma and possessing the characteristic translocation have been reported as primary tumors of the gastrointestinal tract in recent years.[129–135] These tumors have arisen principally in the small bowel followed by stomach and colon. Most patients have been children or young adults. Histologically, these tumors are composed of nests and fascicles of clear cells that resemble classic clear cell sarcoma, but differ from the latter in often having a component of osteoclastic giant cells. All have expressed S-100 protein, but most have little or no evidence of melanin production. It has been suggested that this

variant of clear cell sarcoma possesses unique differences that account for its predilection for the gastrointestinal tract and lack of melanin production. Follow-up of a limited number of cases indicates the propensity for aggressive behavior with regional lymph node and liver metastases.

DESMOPLASTIC MELANOMA

Desmoplastic melanoma was a term coined by Conley et al.[136] for a distinctive fibrosing melanoma lacking pigmentation and having a predilection for the head and neck. Over the ensuing years the principal findings of the original study have been confirmed by many authors.[137–142] In 1979, the term "neurotropic" melanoma was introduced by Reed and Leonard[143] for a subset of desmoplastic melanomas that manifested a remarkable tendency to grow into and along nerves, a phenomenon that, they felt, accounted for the high rate of local recurrence. Because far more desmoplastic melanomas exhibit neurotropism than conventional melanoma,[144] the terms desmoplastic and neurotropic were often used together. However, desmoplastic melanoma is currently the most widely used term irrespective of the presence or absence of neurotropism. Although not, strictly speaking, a soft tissue lesion, the desmoplastic melanoma is discussed in this chapter because it is one of the most common non-mesenchymal lesions misdiagnosed as a nerve sheath tumor.[145]

Although early reports suggested an aggressive course similar to or worse than conventional melanoma, recent studies suggest the opposite. The reasons for these differences are accounted for by the heterogeneity of lesions reported under the rubric of desmoplastic melanoma and the failure to compare lesions of equivalent thickness and depth. For these reasons, Busam et al. have advocated a more standardized approach to the diagnosis of desmoplastic melanoma, and suggested they be divided into pure and mixed type.[146,147] "Pure desmoplastic melanomas" are those in which 80–90% of the invasive component is desmoplastic, whereas "mixed desmoplastic melanomas" have only partial desmoplasia.[146,148,149]

Clinical features

Desmoplastic melanomas are uncommon and account for less than 5% of all melanomas.[147,150] They present as firm plaques or nodules usually in the head and neck area (40–75%) (Figs 30–47, 30–48) of patients who are on average 10 years older than those with conventional malignant melanoma. The majority of desmoplastic melanomas are thick and deeply invasive at the time of clinical presentation (Fig. 30–49). Based on several large series, the average thickness of a desmoplastic melanoma ranges 2.5–6.5 mm,[146,151–153] and most involve Clark level IV or V.

Gross and microscopic features

The majority of desmoplastic melanomas are associated with an overlying in situ melanoma usually having the appearance of "lentigo maligna" and less often superficial spreading melanoma or acral lentiginous melanoma (Fig. 30–50). A small percentage (15–20%) lack an epidermal component and have been referred to as de novo desmoplastic malignant melanoma. Whether these tumors truly

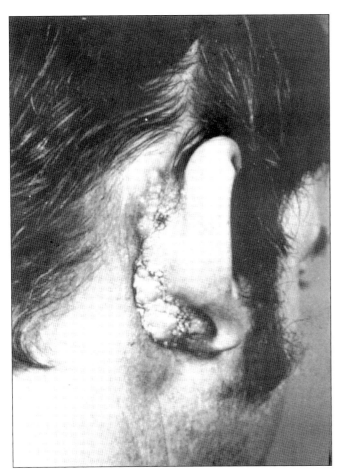

FIGURE 30–47 Neurotropic melanoma. Tumor arose in the posterior auricular region and produced a wart-like nonpigmented mass. Lesion recurred several times in the same region before metastasizing to the paraspinal area.

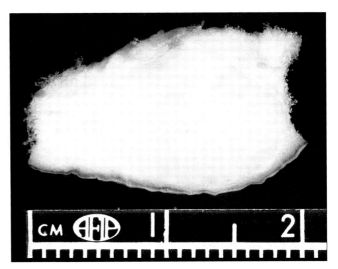

FIGURE 30–48 Neurotropic melanoma. Note the ill-defined, scar-like quality of this dermal tumor.

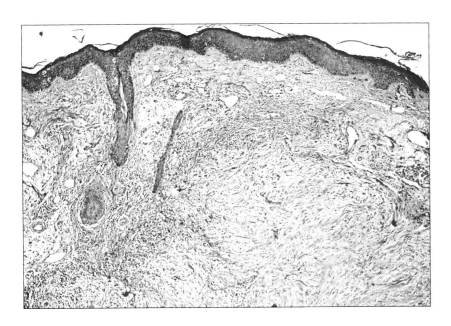

FIGURE 30–49 Neurotropic melanoma. This highly desmoplastic tumor was present in the mid and deep dermis. No epidermal lesion was present in the sections studied.

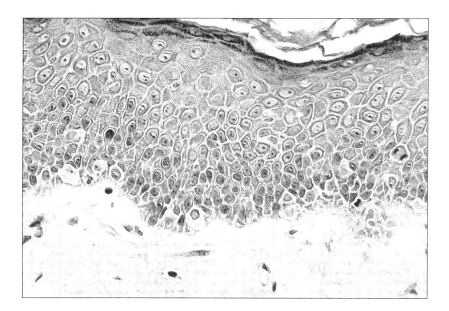

FIGURE 30–50 Neurotropic melanoma showing minimal melanocytic dysplasia at the surface of the lesion.

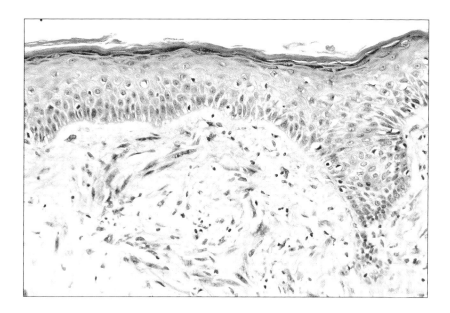

FIGURE 30–51 Neurotropic melanoma with subtle spindle-cell proliferation in the superficial dermis.

arise de novo or whether the precursor lesion has regressed or not been sampled is not clear.

On cut section the tumor has a firm, gray-white, scar-like appearance (Figs 30–48, 30–49) and is made up of spindled or fusiform cells that infiltrate the dermis as short packet-like fascicles or as individual tumor cells surrounded by fine and dense collagen deposits (Figs 30–51, 30–52). The cells range in appearance from those resembling fibroblasts to others resembling Schwann cells. Likewise, there is also a wide range of atypia within these lesions such that some can appear deceptively bland, like a scar, while recurrent or metastatic lesions may be highly pleomorphic. Neurotropism can be quite striking in some tumors and is manifested by encircle-ment or invasion of endoneurium or perineurium by neoplastic cells (Fig. 30–53), a feature believed to be one of the reasons for the high rate of local recurrence of this

lesion following conservative excision. Most tumors are associated with a lymphocytic reaction, a feature that can aid in separating these tumors from a benign or malignant nerve sheath tumor. Although the overlying precursor lesions display pigment, the invasive component of these lesions is almost always amelanotic.

Ultrastructural and immunohistochemical findings

Ultrastructurally, the cells in a neurotropic melanoma do not contain melanosomes or premelanosomes but express Schwann cell features to a variable degree.[142,154] Most des-moplastic melanomas exhibit positive immunostaining for S-100 protein and in these preparations the long, attenuated shape of these schwannian cells is easily appreciated (Fig. 30–54). Immunostains for gp100

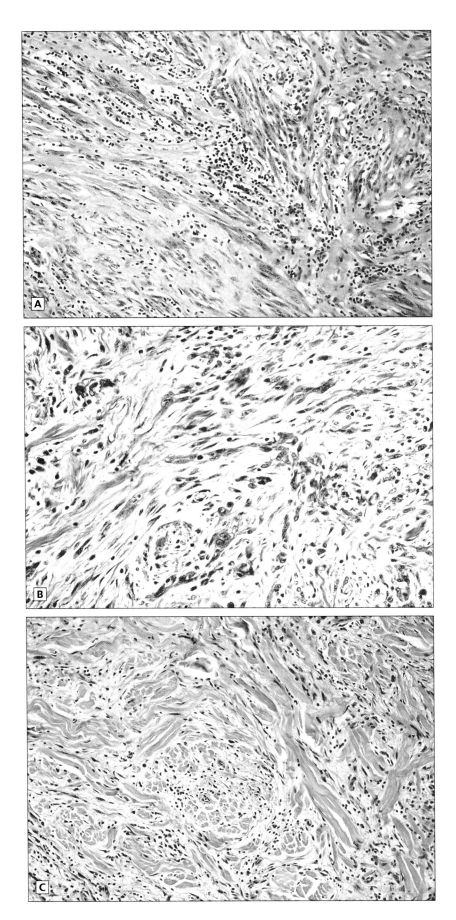

FIGURE 30–52 Various patterns in a neurotropic melanoma. Obvious areas of malignancy **(A)** have atypical cells arranged in short packets or fascicles. In other areas the spindled cells are arranged in slender packets or cords **(B)**. Desmoplasia can be marked with thick bands of collagen **(C)**.

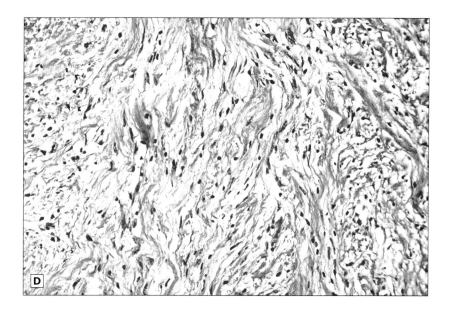

FIGURE 30–52 Continued. Areas with delicate collagen and widely separated neoplastic cells resemble neurofibroma **(D)**.

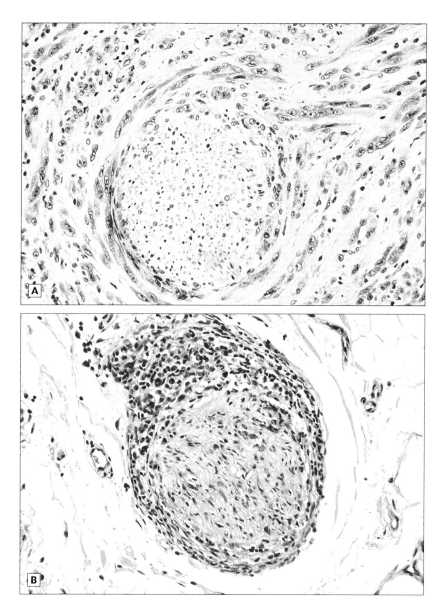

FIGURE 30–53 Neurotropic melanoma showing targeting of tumor cells around a nerve (neurotropism) **(A)**. Occasionally perineural deposits are associated with lymphocytic response, a subtle clue that the lesion may be a melanoma rather than a malignant Schwann cell tumor **(B)**.

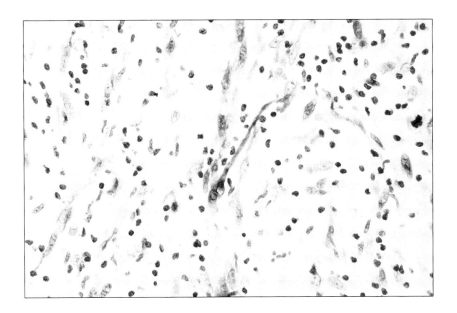

FIGURE 30–54 Immunostaining of neurotropic melanoma for S-100 protein, illustrating elongated schwannian cells.

(HMB-45) are almost always negative. MiTF, a nuclear regulatory protein found in melanin-producing cells, can be identified in about 40% of desmoplastic melanomas.[155] However, it is not restricted to tumors of melanocytic lineage and has been described occasionally in dermatofibroma, schwannoma, and leiomyosarcoma, emphasizing the need for caution in the interpretation of this stain.[156] Although the presence of S-100 protein immunostaining remains reliable for distinguishing desmoplastic melanoma from various reactive fibroblastic proliferations, S-100 protein-positive cells may be encountered in scars.[157,158] Therefore, it is important that an independent assessment of positive-staining cells be made prior to a diagnosis of desmoplastic melanoma. Features that favor a desmoplastic melanoma over a scar include an overlying precursor lesion, the presence of neurotropism in the lesion, and a prominent nodular lymphocytic infiltrate.

Clusterin, a protein implicated in metalloproteinase inhibition, has recently been identified in desmoplastic melanomas as a result of gene expression profiling studies. Using immunohistochemistry, this protein is expressed in desmoplastic melanomas and is absent or weakly expressed in conventional ones.[147] A significant percentage of desmoplastic melanomas express neurotrophin receptor, which mediates migration of Schwann cells along embryonic nerve. The strong correlation between expression of this protein and the desmoplastic phenotype is believed to explain the neurotropic properties of this tumor.[159]

Discussion

Mounting evidence supports the view that desmoplastic melanomas have a better outcome than conventional melanoma.[148,153] These differences are most significant when comparing "pure" desmoplastic melanomas to mixed-type or conventional melanomas and when comparing large, deep desmoplastic melanomas to similarly matched conventional melanomas. However, these differences become obscured when definitional criteria for desmoplastic melanoma become less stringent,[144,148] and likely explain the differences in outcome reported by various studies. Using criteria proposed by Busam et al.,[146,147] Hawkins et al.[148] reported a significantly lower 5-year melanoma-specific mortality for pure desmoplastic melanoma (11%) than mixed types (31%). The rates of local recurrence, however, are significantly higher for desmoplastic melanoma than conventional forms[148] and vary from 5% to 40%[144,149,150,160] depending on the patient population and adequacy of initial excision. Regional lymph node involvement varies from 0% to 15%,[135,148,151,161] and is extremely low in pure desmoplastic melanomas where it ranges 0–2.2%.[146,162] The low incidence of involvement in pure desmoplastic melanoma provides a strong argument against sentinel lymph node biopsies.[146] Distant metastases are noted primarily in the lung followed by liver, gastrointestinal tract, or bone where they can resemble an epithelial or Schwann cell tumor.

EXTRASPINAL (SOFT TISSUE) EPENDYMOMA

Soft tissue ependymomas are rare tumors that occur in subcutaneous locations dorsal to the sacrum and coccyx or in deep soft tissue anterior to the sacrum and posterior to the rectum.[163–174] Many that occur in the latter location represent ependymomas of the cauda equina that have extended through the sacral foramina to present as presacral masses.[174] Those situated dorsally to the sacrum represent the more significant group in terms of soft

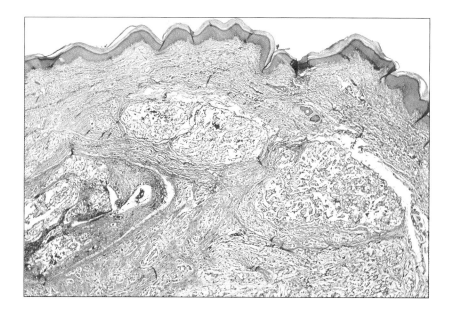

FIGURE 30–55 Extraspinal ependymoma presenting in a dorsococcygeal location.

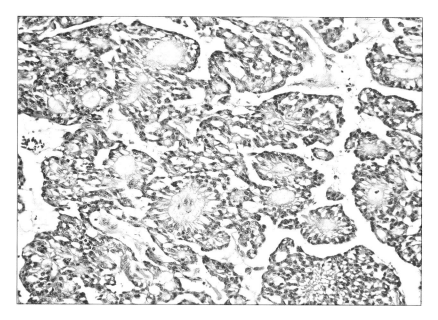

FIGURE 30–56 Extraspinal ependymoma. Tumor resembles a myxopapillary ependymoma of the cauda equina and contains perivascular pseudorosettes and papillary structures.

tissue tumors; consequently, this discussion is restricted to this group. Pathogenetically, the dorsal coccygeal ependymoma may arise from normal remnants of the neural tube (coccygeal medullary vestige) or from abnormal remnants resulting from embryologic malformations. The latter contention is supported by the fact that a significant proportion of patients with this tumor[164] have developmental abnormalities such as spina bifida.

Characteristically, these tumors present as long-standing masses that are often diagnosed preoperatively as pilonidal cysts, teratomas, or sweat gland tumors. Although a few have proved to be extensive at the time of initial surgery,[164] most are encapsulated and easily separated from the fascia overlying the sacrum and coccyx. Grossly, they are myxoid multilobulated masses with focal areas of hemorrhage and necrosis (Fig. 30–55).

Most resemble the ependymomas arising from the cauda equina and are of the "myxopapillary type." Cuboidal or columnar cells are arranged on fibrovascular stalks in a papillary configuration (Fig. 30–56). Secondary perivascular degenerative changes result in the peculiar myxoid and hyalinized appearance that characterizes the myxopapillary ependymoma. In cases where the degeneration is not marked, the tumor may resemble the more cellular papillary ependymoma of the brain. The cells are usually well differentiated with apically polarized nuclei. Occasionally, blepharoplasts are demonstrated by means of special stains (phosphotungstic acid-hematoxylin stain). Carminophilic intracytoplasmic mucin is not present in these cells despite its presence in the closely related "choroid plexus papilloma."[174] Ultrastructurally, these cells have many of the features of normal ependymal

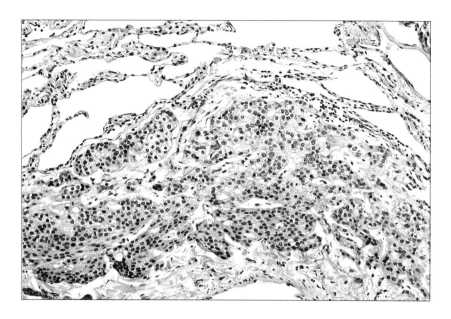

FIGURE 30–57 Extraspinal ependymoma metastatic to lung. Nests of tumor may mimic the pattern of carcinoma or carcinoid tumor.

cells. They contain microvilli and lateral desmosomes at their apical surfaces, whereas elaborate interdigitations of the plasma membrane and underlying basement membrane material characterize the basal surfaces. Parallel arrays of fine filaments and occasional microtubules are found in the cytoplasm.

Although ependymomas are, in general, low-grade neoplasms and usually pose only problems in control of local disease, dorsal coccygeal ependymomas have a greater propensity to metastasize than their intraspinal counterparts. This has been ascribed to their easier accessibility to lymphatic channels and to the longer survival time associated with these tumors. Thus, of 11 primary dorsal coccygeal ependymomas, three metastasized either to regional (inguinal) nodes or the lung. Metastasis to the lung may be mistaken for a carcinoid tumor (Fig. 30–57). Distant metastasis is a late event, usually occurring 10 years or more after diagnosis of the primary tumor. Adequate treatment of these tumors consists of wide local excision with irradiation for residual or inoperable disease. The protracted course of this disease underscores the need for extended follow-up care and even resection of isolated metastases if and when they appear.

REFERENCES

1. Stewart TW, Copeland MM. Neurogenic sarcoma. Am J Cancer 1931; 15:1235.
2. Geschickter CF. Tumors of the peripheral nerves. Am J Cancer 1935; 25:377.
3. Stout AP. The malignant tumors of the peripheral nerves. Am J Cancer 1935; 25:1.

Clinical findings

4. Ducatman BS, Scheithauer BW, Piepgras DG. Malignant peripheral nerve sheath tumors: a clinicopathologic study of 120 cases. Cancer 1986; 57:2006.
5. Hruban RH, Shiu MH, Senie RT, et al. Malignant peripheral nerve sheath tumors of the buttock and lower extremity. Cancer 1990; 66:1253.
6. Wong WW, Hirose T, Scheithauer BW, et al. Malignant peripheral nerve sheath tumor: analysis of treatment outcome. Int J Radiat Oncol Biol Phys 1998; 42:351.
7. Ferner RE, O'Doherty MJ. Neurofibroma and schwannoma. Curr Opin Neurol 2002; 15:679.
8. Upadhyaya M, Spurlock G, Majounie E, et al. The heterogeneous nature of germline mutations in NF1 patients with malignant peripheral nerve sheath tumours (MPNST). Hum Mutation 2006; 27:716.
9. Guccion JG, Enzinger FM. Malignant schwannoma associated with von Recklinghausen's neurofibromatosis. Virchows Arch [Pathol Anat] 1979; 383:43.
10. Carli M, Morgan M, Bisogno G, et al. Malignant peripheral nerve sheath tumors in childhood (MPNST): a combined experience of the Italian and German co-operative studies: SIOP XXVII meeting. Med Pediatr Oncol 1995; 25:243.
11. Coffin CM, Dehner LP. Peripheral neurogenic tumors of the soft tissues of children and adolescents: a clinicopathologic study of 139 cases. Pediatr Pathol 1989; 9:387.
12. De Cou JM, Rao BN, Parham DM, et al. Malignant peripheral nerve sheath tumors: the St. Jude Children's Research Hospital experience. Ann Surg Oncol 1995; 2:524.
13. Ducatman BS, Scheithauer BW. Port-irradiation neurofibrosarcoma. Cancer 1983; 51:1028.
14. Foley KM, Woodruff JM, Ellis F, et al. Radiation-induced malignant and atypical MPNST. Ann Neurol 1980; 7:311.
15. Kourea HP, Bilsky MH, Leung DH, et al. Subdiaphragmatic and intrathoracic paraspinal malignant peripheral nerve sheath tumors: a clinicopathologic study of 25 patients and 26 tumors. Am J Cancer 1998; 82:2191.
16. Koestner A, Swenberg JA, Wechslar W. Transplacental production of ethylnitrosourea of neoplasms of the nervous system in Sprague-Dawley rats. Am J Pathol 1971; 63:37.
17. Rigdon RH. Neurogenic tumors produced by methylcholanthrene in the white Pekin duck. Cancer 1955; 8:906.
18. Bojsen-Moller M, Myrhe-Jensen O. A consecutive series of 30 malignant schwannomas: survival in relation to clinicopathological parameters and treatment. Acta Pathol Microbiol Scand 1984; 92A:147.
19. D'Agostino AN, Soule EH, Miller RH. Primary malignant neoplasm of nerves (malignant neurilemomas) in patients without manifestations of multiple neurofibromatosis (von Recklinghausen's disease). Cancer 1963; 16:1003.
20. D'Agostino AN, Soule EH, Miller RH. Sarcomas of the peripheral nerves and somatic soft tissues associated with multiple neurofibromatosis (von Recklinghausen's disease). Cancer 1963; 16:1015.
21. Daimaru Y, Hashimoto H, Enjoji M. Malignant peripheral nerve-sheath tumors (malignant schwannomas): an immunohistochemical study of 29 cases. Am J Surg Pathol 1985; 9:434.
22. Sorensen SA, Mulvihill JJ, Nielsen A. Long-term follow-up of von Recklinghausen neurofibromatosis. N Engl J Med 1981; 305:1617.
23. Ghosh BC, Ghosh L, Huvos AG, et al. Malignant schwannoma: a clinicopathologic study. Cancer 1973; 31:184.
24. Ferner RE, Lucas JD, O'Doherty MJ, et al. Evaluation of fluorodeoxyglucose postiron emission tomography (FDG PET) in the detection of malignant peripheral nerve sheath

tumours arising from within plexiform neurofibromas in neurofibromatosis 1. J Neurol Neurosurg Psychiatry 2000; 68:353.

25. Brenner W, Friedrich RE, Karim G, et al. Prognostic relevance of FDGPET in patients with neurofibromatosis type-1 and malignant peripheral nerve sheath tumours. Eur J Nuc Med Mol Imaging 2006; 33:428.

Microscopic findings

26. Daimaru Y, Hashimoto H, Enjoji M. Malignant "Triton" tumors: a clinicopathologic and immunohistochemical study of nine cases. Hum Pathol 1984; 15:768.
27. Abe S, Imamura T, Partk P, et al. Small round-cell type of malignant peripheral nerve sheath tumor. Mod Pathol 1998; 11:747.
28. Meis JM, Enzinger FM, Martz KL, et al. Malignant peripheral nerve sheath tumors (malignant schwannoma) in children. Am J Surg Pathol 1992; 16:694.

Immunohistochemical findings

29. Gray MH, Rosenberg AE, Dickersin GR, et al. Glial fibrillary acidic protein and keratin expression by benign and malignant nerve sheath tumors. Hum Pathol 1989; 20:1089.
30. Johnson K, Glick AD, Davis BW. Immunohistochemical evaluation of Leu-7, myelin basic protein, S-100 protein, glial fibrillary acidic protein, and LN3 immunoreactivity in nerve sheath tumors and sarcomas. Arch Pathol Lab Med 1988; 112:155.
31. Matsunou H, Shimoda T, Kakimoto S, et al. Histopathologic and immunohistochemical study of malignant tumors of peripheral nerve sheath (malignant schwannoma). Cancer 1985; 56:2269.
32. Nakajima T, Watanaba S, Soto Y, et al. An immunoperoxidase study of S-100 protein distribution in normal and neoplastic tissues. Am J Surg Pathol 1982; 6:715.
33. Weiss SW, Langloss JM, Enzinger FM. The role of S-100 protein in the diagnosis of soft tissue tumors with particular reference to benign and malignant Schwann cell tumors. Lab Invest 1983; 49:299.
34. Wick MR, Swanson PE, Scheithauer BW, et al. Malignant peripheral nerve sheath tumor: an immunohistochemical study of 62 cases. Am J Clin Pathol 1987; 87:425.
35. Olsen SH, Thomas DG, Lucas DR. Cluster analysis of immunohistochemical profiles in synovial sarcoma, malignant peripheral nerve sheath tumor and Ewing sarcoma. Mod Pathol 2006; 19:659.
36. Smith TA, Machen SK, Fisher C, et al. Usefulness of cytokeratin subsets for distinguishing monophasic synovial sarcoma from malignant peripheral nerve sheath tumor. Am J Clin Pathol 1999; 112:641.
37. Hui P, Li N, Johnson C, et al. HMGA proteins in malignant peripheral nerve sheath tumor and synovial sarcoma: preferential expression of HMGA2 in malignant peripheral nerve sheath tumor. Mod Pathol 2005; 18:1519.
38. Halling KC, Scheithauer BW, Halling AC, et al. p53 expression in neurofibroma and malignant peripheral nerve sheath tumor: an immunohistochemical study of sporadic and NF-1 associated tumors. Am J Clin Pathol 1996; 106:282.
39. Kindblom LG, Ahlden M, Meis-Kindblom JM, et al. Immunohistochemical and molecular analysis of p53, MDM2, proliferating cell nuclear antigen and Ki67 in benign and malignant peripheral nerve sheath tumors. Virchows Arch 1995; 427:19.
40. McCarron KF, Goldblum JR. Plexiform neurofibroma with and without associated malignant peripheral nerve sheath tumor: a clinicopathologic and immunohistochemical analysis of 54 cases. Mod Pathol 1998; 11:612.

Electron microscopic findings

41. McKay B, Osborne BM. The contribution of electron microscopy to the diagnosis of tumors. Pathol Annu 1978; 8:359.
42. Chitale AR, Dickerson GR. Electron microscopy in the diagnosis of malignant schwannomas: a report of six cases. Cancer 1983; 51:1448.
43. Chiu HF, Troster M. Ultrastructure of malignant schwannomas. Lab Invest 1979; 40A:246.
44. Erlandson RA, Woodruff JM. Peripheral nerve sheath tumors: an electron microscopic study of 43 cases. Cancer 1982; 49:273.
45. Herrera GA, deMoraes HP. Neurogenic sarcomas in patients with neurofibromatosis (von Recklinghausen's disease): light, electron microscopy and immunohistochemistry study. Virchows Arch [Pathol Anat] 1984; 403:361.
46. Orenstein JM. Amianthoid fibers in synovial sarcoma and a malignant schwannoma. Ultrastruct Pathol 1983; 4:163.
47. Goodlad JR, Fletcher CDM. Malignant peripheral nerve sheath tumour with annulate lamellae mimicking pleomorphic malignant fibrous histiocytoma. J Pathol 1991; 164:23
48. Hirose T, Maeda T, Furuya K. Malignant peripheral nerve sheath tumor of the pancreas with perineural cell differentiation. Ultrastruct Pathol 1998; 22:227.
49. Hirose T, Scheithauer BW, Sano T. Perineural malignant peripheral nerve sheath tumor (MPNST): a clinicopathologic, immunohistochemical, and ultrastructural study of seven cases. Am J Surg Pathol 1998; 22:1368.
50. Maeda T, Furuya K, Kiyasu Y, et al. Malignant peripheral nerve sheath tumor of the pancreas with perineurial cell differentiation. Ultrastruct Pathol 1998; 22:227.
51. Takeuchi A, Ushigome S. Diverse differentiation in malignant peripheral nerve sheath tumours associated with neurofibromatosis-1: an immunohistochemical and ultrastructural study. Histopathology 2001; 39:298.

Molecular and cytogenetic findings

52. Sawada S, Florell S, Purandare SM, et al. Identification of NF1 mutations in both alleles of a dermal neurofibroma. Nat Genet 1996; 14:110.
53. Menon AG, Anderson KM, Riccardi VM, et al. Chromosome 17p deletions and p53 gene mutations associated with the formation of malignant neurofibrosarcomas in von Recklinghausen's neurofibromatosis. Proc Natl Acad Sci USA 1990; 87:5435.
54. Kim HA, Ling B, Ratner N. NF1 deficient mouse Schwann cells are angiogenic and invasive and can be induced to hyperproliferate reversion of some phenotypes by an inhibitor of farnesyl protein transferase. Mol Cell Biol 1997; 17:862.
55. Kim HA, Rosenbaum T, Marchionni MA, et al. Schwann cells from neurofibromin-deficient mice exhibit activation of p21-ras, inhibition of cell proliferation, and morphological changes. Oncogene 1995; 11:325.
56. Berner J-M, Sorlie T, Mertens F, et al. Chromosome band 9p21 is frequently altered in malignant peripheral nerve sheath tumors: studies of CDKN2A and other genes in the pRB pathway. Genes Chromosomes Cancer 1999; 26:151.
57. Mechtersheimer G, Otano-Joos M, Ohl S, et al. Analysis of chromosomal imbalances in sporadic and NF-1 associated peripheral nerve sheath tumors by comparative genomic hybridization. Genes Chromosomes Cancer 1999; 25:362.

58. Mertens F, Rydholm A, Bauer HF, et al. Cytogenetic findings in malignant peripheral nerve sheath tumors. Int J Cancer 1995; 61:793.
59. Schmidt H, Wuerl P, Taubert H, et al. Genomic imbalances of 7p and 17q in malignant peripheral nerve sheath tumors are clinically relevant. Genes Chromosomes Cancer 1999; 25:205.
60. Kourea HP, Cordon-Cardo C, Dudas M, et al. Expression of p27^{kip} and other cell cycle regulators in malignant peripheral nerve sheath tumors and neurofibromas. Am J Pathol 1999; 155:1885.
61. Kourea HP, Orlow I, Scheithauer BW, et al. Deletions of the INK4A gene occur in malignant peripheral nerve sheath tumors but not in neurofibromas. Am J Pathol 1999; 155:1855.
62. Agnesen TDH, Florenes VA, Molenaar WM, et al. Expression patterns of cell cycle components in sporadic and neurofibromatosis type 1-related malignant peripheral nerve sheath tumors. J Neuropathol Exp Neurol 2005; 64:74.
63. Sabah M, Cummins R, Leader M, et al. Loss of p16(INK4a) expression is associated with allelic imbalance/loss of heterozygosity of chromosome 9p21 in microdissected malignant peripheral nerve sheath tumors. Appl Imm Mol Morphology 2006; 14:97.
64. Zhou H, Coffin CM, Perkins S, et al. Malignant peripheral nerve sheath tumor: a comparison of grade immunophenotype and cell cycle/growth activation marker expression in sporadic and neurofibromatosis related lesions. Am J Surg Pathol 2003; 27:1337.
65. Kobayashi C, Oda Y, Takahira T, et al. Aberrant expression of CHFR in malignant peripheral nerve sheath tumors. Mod Pathol 2006; 19:524.

Clinical behavior

66. Wanebo JE, Malik JM, Vandenberg SR, et al. Malignant peripheral nerve sheath tumors: a clinicopathologic study of 28 cases. Cancer 1993; 71:1247.
67. Casanova M, Ferrari A, Spreafico F, et al. Malignant peripheral nerve sheath tumors in children: a single-institution twenty-year experience. J Pediatr Hematol Oncol 1999; 21:509.
68. Carli M, Ferrari A, Mattke A, et al. Pediatric malignant peripheral nerve sheath tumor: the Italian and German Soft Tissue Sarcoma Cooperative Group. J Clin Oncol 2005; 23:8422.

Malignant peripheral nerve sheath tumor with rhabdomyoblastic differentiation

69. Gratia. Une curieuse anomalie anatomique constituee par la presence de tissu musculaire strie dans la substance du nerf pneumogastrique. Ann Med Vet 1884; 33:649.
70. Orlandi E. Rhabdomyoma del nervo ischiatico. Arch Sci Med (Torino) 1895; 19:113.
71. Raney B, Schnaufer L, Ziegler M. Treatment of children with neurogenic sarcoma: experience at the Children's Hospital of Philadelphia 1958–1984. Cancer 1987; 59:1.
72. Zimmerman LE, Font RL, Andersen SR. Rhabdomyosarcomatous differentiation in malignant intraocular medulloepitheliomas. Cancer 1972; 30:817.
73. Brooks JS, Freeman M, Enterline HT. Malignant "Triton" tumors: natural history and immunohistochemistry of nine new cases with literature review. Cancer 1985; 55:2543.
74. Ordóñez NG, Tornos C. Malignant peripheral nerve sheath tumor of the pleura with epithelial and rhabdomyoblastic differentiation: report of a case clinically simulating

mesothelioma. Am J Surg Pathol 1997; 21:1515.

75. Woodruff JM, Chernik NL, Smith MC, et al. Peripheral nerve tumors with rhabdomyosarcomatous differentiation (malignant "Triton" tumors). Cancer 1973; 32:426.

76. Heffner DK, Gnepp DR. Sinonasal fibrosarcomas, malignant schwannomas, and "Triton" tumors: a clinicopathologic study of 67 cases. Cancer 1992; 70:1089.

77. Travis JA, Sandberg AA, Neff JR, et al. Cytogenetic findings in malignant Triton tumor. Genes Chromosomes Cancer 1994; 9:1.

78. Wong SY, Teh M, Tan YO, et al. Malignant glandular Triton tumor. Cancer 1991; 67:1076.

79. Masson P, Martin JF. Rhabdomyomes des nerfs. Bull Assoc Fr Etud Cancer 1938; 27:751.

80. Woodruff JM, Perino G. Non-germ cell or teratomatous malignant tumors showing rhabdomyoblastic differentiation with emphasis on the malignant Triton tumor. Semin Diagn Surg Pathol 1994; 11:69.

81. Ducatman BS, Scheithauer BW. Malignant peripheral nerve sheath tumor with divergent differentiation. Cancer 1984; 54:1049.

82. Weston JA. The migration and differentiation of neural crest cells. Adv Morphogen 1970; 8:41.

Malignant peripheral nerve sheath tumor with glands

83. Garre C. Uber sekundare Maligne Neurome. Beitr Z Chir Z 1892; 9:465.

84. Christensen WN, Strong EW, Bains MS, et al. Neuroendocrine differentiation in the glandular peripheral nerve sheath tumor: pathologic distinction form the biphasic synovial sarcoma with glands. Am J Surg Pathol 1988; 12:417.

85. Cross PA, Clarke NW. Malignant nerve sheath tumor with epithelial elements. Histopathology 1988; 12:547.

86. DeSchryver K, Santa Cruz DJ. So-called glandular schwannoma: ependymal differentiation in a case. Ultrastruct Pathol 1984; 6:167.

87. Foraker AG. Glandlike elements in a peripheral neurosarcoma. Cancer 1948; 1:286.

88. Michel SL. Epithelial elements in a malignant neurogenic tumor of the tibial nerve. Am J Surg 1967; 113:404.

89. Uri AK, Witzleben CL, Raney RB. Electron microscopy of glandular schwannoma. Cancer 1984; 53:493.

90. Warner TFCS, Louie R, Hafez GR, et al. Malignant nerve sheath tumor containing endocrine cells. Am J Surg Pathol 1983; 7:583.

91. Woodruff JM. Peripheral nerve tumors showing glandular differentiation (glandular schwannoma). Cancer 1976; 37:2399.

92. Woodruff JM, Christensen WN. Glandular peripheral nerve sheath tumors. Cancer 1993; 72:3618.

Malignant peripheral nerve sheath tumor with angiosarcoma

93. Bricklin AS, Rushton HW. Angiosarcoma of venous origin arising in radial nerve. Cancer 1977; 39:1556.

94. Brown RW, Tornos C, Evans HI. Angiosarcoma arising from malignant schwannoma in a patient with neurofibromatosis. Cancer 1992; 70:1141.

95. Chaudhuri B, Ronan SG, Manaligod JR. Angiosarcoma arising in a plexiform neurofibroma: a case report. Cancer 1980; 46:605.

96. Meis JM, Kindblom LG, Enzinger FM. Angiosarcoma arising in peripheral nerve sheath tumors: report of 5 additional cases. Lab Invest 1994; 70:80A.

97. Mentzel T, Katenkamp D. Intraneural angiosarcoma and angiosarcoma arising in benign and malignant peripheral nerve sheath tumours: clinicopathological and immunohistochemical analysis of four cases. Histopathology 1999; 35:114.

98. Morphopoulos GD, Banerjee SS, Ali HH, et al. Malignant peripheral nerve sheath tumor with vascular differentiation: a report of four cases. Histopathology 1996; 28:401.

Epithelioid malignant peripheral nerve sheath tumor

99. Alvira MM, Mandybur TI, Menefee MG. Light microscopic and ultrastructural observations of a metastasizing malignant epithelioid schwannoma. Cancer 1976; 38:1977.

100. Cohn I. Epithelial neoplasms of peripheral and cranial nerves: report of three cases: review of the literature. Arch Surg 1928; 17:117.

101. Laskin WB, Weiss SW, Bratthauer GL. Epithelioid variant of malignant peripheral nerve sheath tumor (malignant epithelioid schwannoma). Am J Surg Pathol 1991; 15:1136.

102. Lodding P, Kindblom LG, Angervall L. Epithelioid malignant schwannoma: a study of 14 cases. Virchows Arch [Pathol Anat] 1986; 409:433.

103. McCormick LJ, Hazard JB, Dickson JA. Malignant epithelioid neurilemoma (schwannoma). Cancer 1954; 7:725.

104. Taxy JB, Battifora HB. Epithelioid schwannoma: diagnosis by electron microscopy. Ultrastruct Pathol 1981; 2:19.

Clear cell sarcoma of tendon and aponeurosis

105. Enzinger FM. Clear cell sarcoma of tendons and aponeuroses: an analysis of 21 cases. Cancer 1965; 18:1163.

106. Bridge JA, Borek DA, Neff JR, et al. Choromosomal abnormalities in clear cell sarcoma: implication for histogenesis. Am J Clin Pathol 1990; 93:26.

107. Bridge JA, Sreekantaiah C, Neff JR, et al. Cytogenetic findings in clear cell sarcoma of tendons and aponeuroses: malignant melanoma of soft parts. Cancer Genet Cytogenet 1991; 52:101.

108. Reeves BR, Fletcher CD, Gusterson BA. Translocation t(12; 22)(q12; q13) is a nonrandom rearrangement in clear cell sarcoma. Cancer Genet Cytogenet 1992; 64:101.

109. Rodriquez E, Sreekantaiah C, Reuter VE, et al. t(12; 22)(q13; q13) and trisomy 8 are nonrandom aberrations in clear cell sarcoma. Cancer Genet Cytogenet 1992; 64:107.

110. Stenman G, Kindblom LG, Angervall L. Reciprocal translocation t(12; 22)(q13; q13) in clear cell sarcoma of tendons and aponeuroses. Genes Chromosomes Cancer 1992; 4:122.

111. Mrozek K, Karakousis CP, Perez-Mesa C, et al. Translocation t(12; 22)(q13; q12.2–12.3) in a clear cell sarcoma of tendons and aponeuroses. Genes Chromosomes Cancer 1993; 6:249.

112. Travis JA, Bridge JA. Significance of both numerical and structural chromosomal abnormalities in clear cell sarcoma. Cancer Genet Cytogenet 1992; 64:104.

113. Zucman J, Delattre O, Desmaze C, et al. EWS and ATF-gene fusion induced by t(12; 22) translocation in malignant melanoma of soft parts. Nat Genet 1993; 4:341.

114. Panagopoulos I, Mertens F, Isaksson M, et al. Absence of mutations of the BRAF gene in malignant melanoma of soft parts (clear cell sarcoma of tendons and aponeuroses). Cancer Genet Cytogenet 2005; 156:74.

115. Davis IJ, Kim JJ, Ozsolak F, et al. Oncogenic MITF dysregulation in clear cell sarcoma: defining the MiT family of human cancers. Cancer Cell 2006; 9:473.

116. Jishage M, Fujino T, Takashi Y, et al. Identification of target genes for EWS/ATF-1 chimeric transcription factor. Oncogene 2003; 22:41.

117. Lucas DR, Nascimento AG, Sim FH. Clear cell sarcoma of soft tissues: Mayo Clinic experience with 35 cases. Am J Surg Pathol 1992; 16:1197.

118. Montgomery EA, Meis JM, Ramos AG, et al. Clear cell sarcoma of tendons and aponeurosis: a clinicopathologic study of 58 cases with analysis of prognostic factors. Int J Surg Pathol 1993; 1:59.

119. Ferrari A, Casanova M, Bisogno G, et al. Clear cell sarcoma of tendons and aponeuroses in pediatric patients: a report from the Italian and German Soft Tissue Sarcoma Cooperative Group. Cancer 2002; 15:3269.

120. Sara AS, Evans HL, Benjamin RS. Malignant melanoma of soft parts (clear cell sarcoma): a study of 17 cases with emphasis on prognostic factors. Cancer 1990; 15:367.

121. Kindblom LG, Lodding P, Angervall L. Clear cell sarcoma of tendons and aponeuroses: an immunohistochemical and electron microscopic analysis indicating neural crest origin. Virchows Arch [Pathol Anat] 1983; 401:109.

122. Mechtersheimer G, Tilgen W, Klar E, et al. Clear cell sarcoma of tendons and aponeuroses: case presentation with special reference to immunohistochemical findings. Hum Pathol 1989; 20:914.

123. Swanson PE, Wick MR. Clear cell sarcoma: an immunohistochemical analysis of six cases and comparison with other epithelioid neoplasms of soft tissue. Arch Pathol Lab Med 1989; 113:55.

124. Kubo T. Clear cell sarcoma of patellar tendon studied by electron microscopy. Cancer 1969; 24:948.

125. Benson JD, Kraemer BB, Mackay B. Malignant melanoma of soft parts: an ultrastructural study of four cases. Ultrastruct Pathol 1985; 8:57.

126. Deyrup AT, Althof P, Zhou M, et al. Paraganglioma-like dermal melanocytic tumor: a unique entity distinct from cellular blue nevus, clear cell sarcoma, and cutaneous melanoma. Am J Surg Pathol 2004; 28:1579.

127. Chung EB, Enzinger FM. Malignant melanoma of soft parts: a reassessment of clear cell sarcoma. Am J Surg Pathol 1983; 7:405.

128. Picciotto F, Zaccagna A, Derosa G, et al. Clear cell sarcoma (malignant melanoma of soft parts) and sentinel lymph node biopsy. Eur J Dermatol 2005; 15:46.

Clear cell sarcoma-like tumor of gastrointestinal tract

129. Taminelli L, Zaman K, Gengler C, et al. Primary clear cell sarcoma of the ileum: an uncommon and misleading site. Virchows Arch 2005; 44:772.

130. Friedrichs N, Testi MA, Moiraghi L, et al. Clear cell sarcoma-like tumor with osteoclast-like giant cells in the small bowel: further evidence for a new tumor entity. Int J Surg Pathol 2005; 13:313.

131. Covinsky M, Gong S, Rajaram V, et al. EWS-ATF1 fusion transcripts in gastrointestinal tumors previously diagnosed as malignant melanoma. Hum Pathol 2005; 36:74.

132. Zambrano E, Reyes-Mugica M, Franchi A, et al. An osteoclast-rich tumor of the gastrointestinal tract with features resembling clear cell sarcoma of soft parts: reports of 6 cases of a GIST simulator. Int J Surg Pathol 2003; 11:75.

133. Ekfors TA, Kujari H, Isomaki M. Clear cell sarcoma of tendons and aponeurosis (malignant melanoma of soft parts) in the

duodenum: the first visceral cases. Histopathology 1993; 22:255.

134. Donner LE, Trompler RA, Dobin S. Clear cell sarcoma of the ileum: the crucial role of cytogenetics for the diagnosis. Am J Surg Pathol 1998; 22:121.

135. Pauwels P, Debiec-Richter M, Sciot R, et al. Clear cell sarcoma of the stomach. Histopathology 2002; 41:526.

Desmoplastic melanoma

136. Conley J, Lattes R, Orr W. Desmoplastic malignant melanoma: a rare variant of spindle cell melanoma. Cancer 1971; 28:914.

137. Bruijm JA, Mihm MC, Barnhill RL. Desmoplastic melanoma. Histopathology 1992; 20:197.

138. Egbert B, Kempson R, Sagebiel R. Desmoplastic malignant melanoma: a clinicopathologic study of 25 cases. Cancer 1988; 62:2033.

139. Jain S, Allen PW. Desmoplastic malignant melanoma and its variants. Am J Surg Pathol 1989; 13:358.

140. Longacre TA, Egbert BM, Rouse RV. Desmoplastic and spindle cell malignant melanoma: an immunohistochemical study. Am J Surg Pathol 1996; 20:1489.

141. Reiman HM, Goellner JR, Woods JE, et al. Desmoplastic melanoma of the head and neck. Cancer 1987; 60:2269.

142. Valensi Q. Desmoplastic malignant melanoma: a light and electron microscopic study of two cases. Cancer 1979; 43:1148.

143. Reed PJ, Leonard DD. Neurotropic melanoma: a variant of desmoplastic melanoma. Am J Surg Pathol 1979; 3:301.

144. Livestro DP, Muzikansky A, Kaine EM, et al. Biology of desmoplastic melanomas: a case-control comparison with other melanomas. J Clin Oncol 2005; 23:6739.

145. Arbiser ZK, Folpe AL, Weiss SW. Consultative expert second opinions in soft tissue pathology. Am J Clin Pathol 2001; 116:473.

146. Busam KJ, Mujumdar U, Hummer AG, et al. Cutaneous desmoplastic melanoma: reappraisal of morphologic heterogeneity and prognostic factors. Am J Surg Pathol 2004; 28:1518.

147. Busam KJ, Zhao H, Coit DG, et al. Distinction of desmoplastic melanoma from non-desmoplastic melanoma by gene expression profiling. J Invest Dermatol 2005; 124:412.

148. Hawkins WG, Busam KJ, Ben-Porat L, et al. Desmoplastic melanoma: a pathologically and clinically distinct form of cutaneous melanoma. Ann Surg Oncol 2005; 12:207.

149. Busam KJ. Cutaneous desmoplastic melanoma. Adv Anat Pathol 2005; 12:92.

150. Quinn MJ, Crotty KA, Thompson JF, et al. Desmoplastic and desmoplastic neurotropic melanoma: experience with 280 patients. Cancer 1998; 83:1128.

151. Su LD, Fullen DR, Lowe L, et al. Desmoplastic neurotropic melanoma: analysis of 33 patients with lymphatic mapping and sentinel lymph node biopsy. Cancer 2004; 100:598.

152. Dickersin GR, Sober AJ, Barnhill RL. Desmoplastic neurotropic melanoma: a clinicopathologic analysis of 28 cases. Cancer 1995; 75:2242.

153. Jaroszewski DE, Pockaj BA, DiCaudo DJ, et al. The clinical behavior of desmoplastic melanoma. Am J Surg 2001; 182:590.

154. DiMaio SM, Mackay B, Smith JL, et al. Neurosarcomatous transformation in malignant melanoma: an ultrastructural study. Cancer 1982; 50:2345.

155. Koch MB, Arbiser AK, Weiss SW, et al. Melanoma cell adhesion molecule (Mel-CAM) and microphthalmia transcription factor (MiTF) expression distinguish desmoplastic/sarcomatoid melanoma (DM) from morphological mimics [abstract 357]. Mod Pathol 2000; 13:63.

156. Grantner SR, Weilbaecher KN, Quigley C, et al. Microphthalmia transcription factor: not a sensitive or specific marker for the diagnosis of desmoplastic melanoma and spindle cell (non-desmoplastic) melanoma. Am J Dermatopathol 2001; 23:185.

157. Robson A, Allen P, Hollowood K. S100 protein expression in cutaneous scars: a potential diagnostic pitfall in the diagnosis of desmoplastic melanoma. Histopathology 2001; 38:135.

158. Kaneishi NK, Cockerell CJ. Histologic differentiation of desmoplastic melanoma from cicatrices. Am J Dermatopathol 1998; 20:128.

159. Iwamoto S, Odland PB, Piepkorn M, et al. Evidence that the p75 neurotrophin receptor mediates perineural spread of desmoplastic melanoma. J Am Acad Dermatol 1996; 35:725.

160. Posther KE, Selim MA, Mosca PJ, et al. Histopathologic characteristics, recurrence patterns, and survival of 129 patients with desmoplastic melanoma. Ann Surg Oncol 2006; 13:728.

161. Gyorki DE, Busam K, Panageas K, et al. Sentinel lymph node biopsy for patients with cutaneous desmoplastic melanoma. Ann Surg Oncol 2003; 10:403.

162. Pawlik TM, Ross MI, Prieto VG, et al. Assessment of the role of sentinel lymph node biopsy for primary cutaneous desmoplastic melanoma. Cancer 2006; 106:900.

Extraspinal (soft tissue) ependymoma

163. Adson AW, Moersch FP, Kernohan JW. Neurogenic tumors arising from the sacrum. Arch Neurol Psychiatry 1939; 41:535.

164. Anderson MS. Myxopapillary ependymomas presenting in the soft tissues over the sacrococcygeal region. Cancer 1966; 19:585.

165. Brindley GV. Sacral and presacral tumors. Ann Surg 1945; 121:721.

166. Heath MH. Presacral ependymoma: case report and review of the literature. Am J Clin Pathol 1963; 39:161.

167. Hendren TH, Hardin CA. Extradural metastatic ependymoma. Surgery 1963; 54:880.

168. Jackman RJ, Clark PL, Smith ND. Retrorectal tumors. JAMA 1951; 145:956.

169. Kernohan JW, Fletcher-Kernohan HA. Ependymomas: a study of 109 cases. Assoc Res Nerv Dis 1937; 16:182.

170. Lovelady SB, Dockerty MB. Extragenital pelvic tumors in women. Am J Obstet Gynecol 1949; 58:215.

171. Mallory FB. Three gliomata of ependymal origin: two in the fourth ventricle, one subcutaneous over the coccyx. J Med Res 1902; 8:1.

172. Ross ST. Sacral and presacral tumors. Am J Surg 1948; 76:687.

173. Vagaiwala MR, Robinson JS, Galicich JH, et al. Metastasizing extradural ependymoma of the sacrococcygeal area: case report and review of the literature. Cancer 1979; 44:326.

174. Wolff M, Santiago H, Duby MM. Delayed distant metastasis from a subcutaneous sacrococcygeal ependymoma: case report with tissue culture, ultrastructural observations, and review of the literature. Cancer 1972; 30:1046.

EWING'S SARCOMA/PNET TUMOR FAMILY AND RELATED LESIONS

CHAPTER CONTENTS

Neuroblastoma and the related tumors ganglioneuroblastoma and ganglioneuroma are derived from primordial neural crest cells that migrate from the mantle layer of the developing spinal cord and populate the primordia of the sympathetic ganglia and adrenal medulla. Cytogenetic and molecular genetic data have contributed to our understanding of this group of tumors and have been incorporated along with multiple other parameters into management decisions and prognostication for these patients. Although there are histologic similarities, extraskeletal Ewing's sarcoma and peripheral neuroepithelioma (also known as primitive neuroectodermal tumor) are clearly distinct from neuroblastoma. A number of lines of evidence suggest that extraskeletal Ewing's sarcoma and peripheral neuroepithelioma are closely related tumors, the former representing a less differentiated form of the latter. For the purposes of this chapter, these tumors are referred to as the Ewing's sarcoma/primitive neuroectodermal tumor (ES/PNET) family of tumors.

NEUROBLASTOMA AND GANGLIONEUROBLASTOMA

Neuroblastoma, ganglioneuroblastoma, and ganglioneuroma can be conceptualized as three maturational manifestations of a common neoplasm. Neuroblastoma, the least differentiated, resembles the fetal adrenal medulla and is composed of primitive neuroblasts. Ganglioneuroblastoma has primitive neuroblasts along with maturing ganglion cells; the number and arrangement of the cells vary so the tumor assumes a wide range of appearances and is associated with a wide range of biologic behavior. Ganglioneuroma, a fully differentiated tumor,

is characterized by a mixture of mature Schwann cells and ganglion cells. Neuroblastoma and ganglioneuroblastoma are discussed together because both are considered malignant. In contrast, pure ganglioneuromas, benign tumors requiring only conservative therapy, are considered separately.

Etiologic and genetic factors

Most neuroblastomas occur on a sporadic basis, but in a small number of patients there appears to be a genetic predisposition that follows an autosomal dominant pattern of inheritance.[1] There is one fascinating case of congenital neuroblastoma arising in monozygotic twins, but the authors raised the possibility of twin-to-twin metastasis rather than genetic predisposition.[2] There are rare reports of patients with neuroblastoma with a constitutional deletion or rearrangement of the distal short arm of chromosome 1 as the sole abnormality, suggesting the presence of a tumor-suppressor gene at this locus.[3,4] The tumor tends to be less common in African-Americans than whites; and in certain parts of the world, notably the Burkitt's lymphoma belt in Africa, it is practically nonexistent.[5] In situ neuroblastomas, small microscopic foci of neuroblastoma confined to the adrenal gland and discovered incidentally at autopsy, are rather common (1 in 200 infants dying of other causes), in dramatic contrast with the low incidence of clinical neuroblastoma.[6]

A number of cytogenetic abnormalities have been identified in neuroblastomas, although the exact manner in which they are etiologically linked to the tumor is not fully understood.[3] These will be discussed in great detail later in this chapter.

Clinical findings

Neuroblastoma is the third most common malignant tumor and the most common extracranial solid tumor in children; it occurs at a rate of about 1 per 10 000 live births.[7] At most large children's centers, neuroblastoma accounts for 10–12% of all malignant tumors, preceded in frequency by leukemias and brain tumors.[8] It develops at a relatively younger patient age than rhabdomyosarcoma and ES/PNET. About one-fourth of neuroblastomas are congenital, some of which are detected prenatally owing to the widespread use of ultrasonography.[9] In general, the tumors diagnosed prenatally are found in the adrenal gland, are often cystic, are of a favorable clinical stage, have favorable biologic features (lack of *MYCN* amplification), and have an excellent prognosis.[10] Half are diagnosed by the age of 2 years and 90% by the age of 5 years; only sporadic cases are seen during adolescence or adult life.[11–13] The peak age at the time of presentation is about 18 months, and there is a slight male predilection. The distribution of neuroblastomas and ganglioneuroblastomas generally follows the distribution of the sympathetic ganglia; hence they are found in a paramidline position at any point between the base of the skull and the pelvis, in addition to the adrenal medulla and organ of Zuckerkandl. Some cases possibly also arise from the dorsal root ganglia. This location would explain those dumbbell-shaped neuroblastomas in which significant enlargement of the intervertebral foramen occurs.[14] In the experience reported by DeLorimier et al.[15] based on the California Tumor Registry, 134 of 212 tumors occurred in the retroperitoneum, 33 in the mediastinum, 5 in the cervical region, and 6 in the sacral region. About half of all retroperitoneal tumors arise in the adrenal gland, although the difficulty determining the origin of large tumors must be acknowledged.

The constellation of symptoms varies depending on the age of the patient, location of the mass, and presence or absence of associated clinical syndromes. Usually, patients with neuroblastomas appear wasted and chronically ill and manifest a variety of non-specific signs and symptoms such as fever, weight loss, and gastrointestinal tract disturbances including watery diarrhea and anemia.[16] In half of the patients, a nodular fixed mass extending across the midline can be palpated on physical examination. So protean are the manifestations that half of neuroblastomas are misdiagnosed initially, and a significant number of patients are diagnosed as having rheumatic fever because of the frequent occurrence of fever and joint pain.[17] About one-third of neonates with neuroblastoma present with blue-red cutaneous metastases, which have been likened to blueberries (blueberry muffin baby).[18,19] Although hypertension is neither as common nor as severe as with pheochromocytomas, up to one-fifth of the patients have this symptom, which remits with tumor removal.[20] An uncommon presentation of neuroblastoma, usually associated with a good prognosis, is the "myoclonus-opsoclonus" syndrome. Characterized by rapid, alternating eye movements and myoclonic movements of the extremities, this symptom complex disappears following tumor eradication, suggesting that it is due to a circulating antitumor factor that cross-reacts with cerebellar cells.[21,22] Cases of neuroblastoma have been associated with myasthenia gravis,[23] Cushing syndrome,[24] von Recklinghausen's disease,[25] fetal hydantoin syndrome,[26] Hirschsprung's disease,[27] pediatric renal cell carcinoma associated with a translocation between Xp11.2 and *TFE3*,[28] and neurodevelopmental anomalies including focal cortical dysplasia.[29]

Radiographic findings

Retroperitoneal neuroblastomas cause anterior, lateral, and downward displacement of the kidney, usually without hydronephrosis or calyceal distortion. Calcification, a characteristic finding, occurs in about half of the tumors[30,31] and consists of finely stippled densities in the central portion of the tumor, although peripheral linear densities may also be seen. Metastatic lesions commonly occur in bone and result in osteolytic lesions that display a peculiar predilection for the skull, femur, and humerus; occasionally, they are bilaterally symmetric in their distribution. Radiolabeled metaiodobenzylguanidine (MIBG) is incorporated into catecholamine-secreting cells and has been used to detect bone and soft tissue involvement by neuroblastoma.[32]

According to the International Neuroblastoma Staging System (INSS),[33] extensive radiographic evaluation is required to define the extent of disease and identify metastatic foci. Computed tomography (CT), magnetic resonance imaging (MRI), and MIBG scans are used to evaluate the primary tumor, whereas bone radiography and scintigraphy, abdominal CT scans or MRI, chest radiography (with or without chest CT scans or MRI), in addition to bilateral posterior iliac crest bone marrow aspirates and biopsies, are required to determine the presence or absence of metastatic disease.

Laboratory findings

About 80–90% of patients with neuroblastoma have elevated levels of catecholamines (norepinephrine, epinephrine) and their metabolites (vanillylmandelic acid [VMA], homovanillic acid [HVA], and 3-methoxy-4-hydroxyphenylglycol [MHPG]) in their urine (Fig. 31–1).[17,34] This may reflect increased production or diminished storage of these substances by the tumor. Measurement of these substances has proved useful for the diagnosis and for monitoring the course of the disease during therapy. Persistent elevation following surgery suggests significant residual disease, and the metabolite levels are sometimes elevated before a recurrence is clinically evident. The VMA/HVA ratio may be of prognostic significance, as ratios of 1.5 or more are associated with an improved prognosis.[35,36] Neuropeptide Y, a biologically active polypeptide that co-localizes with catecholamines, is found in high levels in the serum of patients with neuroblastomas compared with the levels in those with ganglioneuroblastoma or ganglioneuroma. It is released during surgical manipulation of tumors, decreases following tumor removal, and reappears with recrudescence

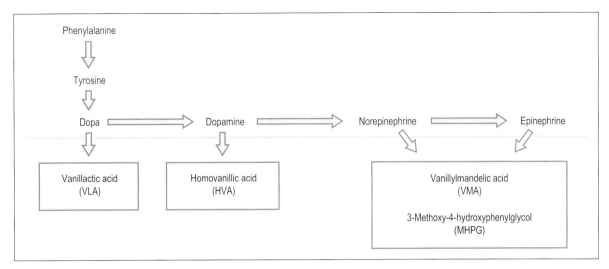

FIGURE 31–1 Metabolic pathway showing enzymatic conversion of phenylalanine to epinephrine. Catabolites below the dotted line are those that may be present in the urine of patients with neuroblastoma.

of disease, suggesting that it too may prove useful for monitoring the disease.[37]

Ferritin can be detected in the serum of patients with active disease and is also used as a prognostic indicator. This iron-binding protein, presumably synthesized by the tumor, is capable of coating the surface of T lymphocytes and is responsible for E rosette inhibition, a phenomenon observed in patients with advanced neuroblastoma. The presence of elevated serum neuron-specific enolase and lactate dehydrogenase has also been correlated with survival rates of patients with neuroblastoma.[38]

Gross findings

Neuroblastomas are lobulated masses averaging 6–8 cm in diameter; they are intimately related to the adrenal gland or sympathetic chain. At surgery, they often have delicate membranous capsules that are easily ruptured to yield the soft, fleshy, gray, partially hemorrhagic tumor. Tumors composed of large expanses of differentiated ganglioneuroma associated with neuroblastomatous foci (nodular ganglioneuroblastoma) have gray hemorrhagic nodules set in a firm white-gray tumor mass (Fig. 31–2).

Microscopic findings

The nomenclature of neuroblastomas has undergone significant revision. Old classification schemes utilizing terms such as "ganglioneuroblastoma" without further modification ignore the vast range of histology and behavior that can be encountered with tumors that have both neuroblastic and ganglionic elements. As described later in this chapter, the International Neuroblastoma Pathology Classification (INPC) has similarities to the systems proposed by Shimada et al.[39] and Joshi et al.[40–42]

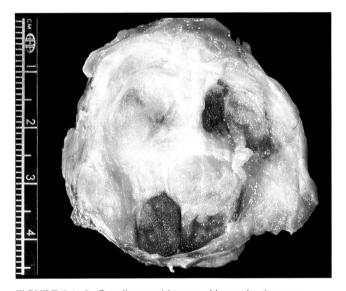

FIGURE 31–2 Ganglioneuroblastoma. Hemorrhagic areas corresponded to neuroblastoma, whereas the remainder of the tumor was ganglioneuroma.

and is an age-linked classification dependent on the degree of neuroblastic differentiation, cellular turnover index, and the presence or absence of schwannian stromal development.[43,44] Equivalent terms in old classification systems are indicated in Table 31–1 and depicted in Figure 31–3.

Neuroblastoma

The term "neuroblastoma" refers to a tumor that is composed chiefly of neuroblasts, which may display a variable degree of ganglionic differentiation (see below). These tumors are further subdivided into undifferentiated, poorly differentiated, and differentiating forms,

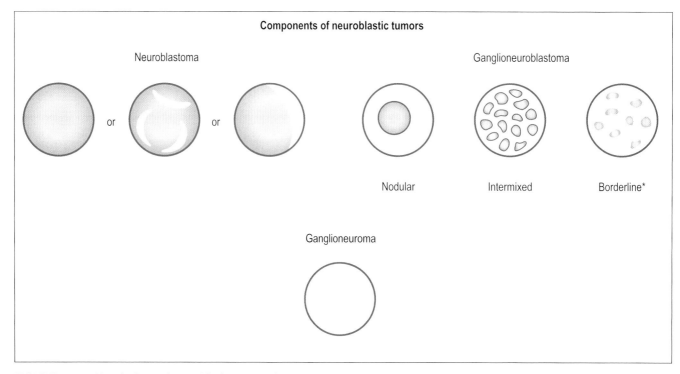

FIGURE 31–3 Terminology of neuroblastic tumors. Shaded areas represent the neuroblastomatous component. * Equivalent to maturing ganglioneuroma in INPC system. Unshaded areas are the ganglioneuromatous component. (Modified from Joshi VV, Cantor AB, Altshuler G, et al. Age-linked prognostic categorization based on a new histologic grading systems of neuroblastomas: a clinicopathologic study of 211 cases from the Pediatric Oncology Group. Cancer 1992; 69:2199.)

TABLE 31–1   NOMENCLATURE OF NEUROBLASTOMA

INPC system	Shimada system	Joshi system	Conventional system
Neuroblastoma (Schwannian stroma-poor)		Neuroblastoma	
Undifferentiated type	Stroma-poor, undifferentiated histology	Undifferentiated type	Neuroblastoma
Poorly differentiated type	Stroma-poor, undifferentiated histology	Poorly differentiated type	Neuroblastoma
Differentiating type	Stoma-poor, differentiated histology	Differentiating type	Ganglioneuroblastoma
Ganglioneuroblastoma, nodular (Composite Schwannian stroma/rich stroma-dominant and stroma-poor)	Stroma-rich, nodular type	Ganglioneuroblastoma Nodular type	Composite ganglioneuroblastoma
Ganglioneuroblastoma, intermixed (Schwannian stroma-rich)	Stroma-rich, intermixed type	Intermixed type	—
Ganglioneuroma (Schwannian stroma-dominant)			
Maturing	Stroma-rich, well-differentiated	Borderline type	Ganglioneuroblastoma
Mature	Ganglioneuroma	Ganglioneuroma	Ganglioneuroma

INPC, International Neuroblastoma Pathology Committee.

depending on the percentage of cells showing ganglionic differentiation. Undifferentiated forms display no ganglionic differentiation, whereas the other two forms display less than or more than 5% differentiating cells, respectively. Unlike ganglioneuroblastomas, schwannian stromal development comprises less than 50% of the neoplasm.

The most primitive neuroblastomas resemble the anlage of the developing sympathetic nervous system and adrenal medulla. They are composed of sheets of small round cells that are divided into small lobules by delicate fibrovascular stroma (Figs 31–4, 31–5). The cells, which are almost devoid of cytoplasm, have round to polygonal deeply staining nuclei similar to those of lymphocytes (Fig. 31–6). Out of context, poorly differentiated neuroblastoma may be mistaken for a number of round cell sarcomas (e.g., ES/PNET, lymphoma, or nucleated erythrocytes of erythroblastosis fetalis) (Fig. 31–7), especially if cellular preservation is poor and the cells are artifactually crushed. Some cases of poorly differentiated neuroblastoma (less than 8%) are composed of larger cells with sharply outlined nuclear membranes and one to four

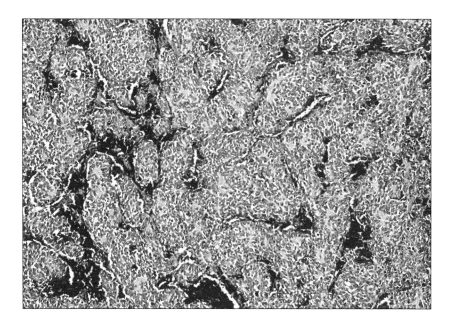

FIGURE 31–4 Poorly differentiated neuroblastoma with hemorrhagic fibrovascular septa that divide the tumor into small lobules.

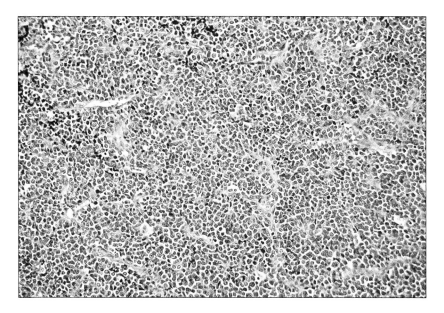

FIGURE 31–5 Poorly differentiated neuroblastoma composed of monotonous sheets of cells with little cytoplasm divided by fibrovascular septa.

prominent nucleoli (so-called large cell neuroblastoma).[45,46] These tumors virtually always reveal *MYCN* amplification.[45] Diagnosis of poorly differentiated neuroblastoma is sometimes suggested by the presence of calcification or morula-like clusters of cells that represent the earliest form of rosette formation or by ancillary immunohistochemical or ultrastructural studies documenting neuroblastic features (discussed below). With progressive differentiation, the neuroblasts acquire attenuated cytoplasmic processes (neurites) (Fig. 31–8), which are polarized toward a central point to form a rosette with a solid central core (Homer Wright rosette) (Fig. 31–9). In addition, the stroma contains mats of neuropil, which are tangled networks of cell processes. In the most differentiated neuroblastomas, some of the cells show partial or even complete ganglionic differentiation (Fig. 31–10).

Ganglionic differentiation is heralded by enlargement of the cells with acquisition of a discernible rim of eosinophilic cytoplasm. Binucleation occurs, and the nuclear chromatin pattern is distinctly vesicular.

Ganglioneuroblastoma

Ganglioneuroblastomas are tumors in which a portion of the lesion has the appearance of a neuroblastoma as described above and contains, in addition, a partial ganglioneuromatous stroma (see Ganglioneuroma, below). The exact amount and arrangement of this stroma further determines the subclassification of the ganglioneuroblastoma. Nodular ganglioneuroblastomas contain gross nodules of neuroblastoma abutting large expanses of ganglioneuroma (Figs 31–11, 31–12). This form of

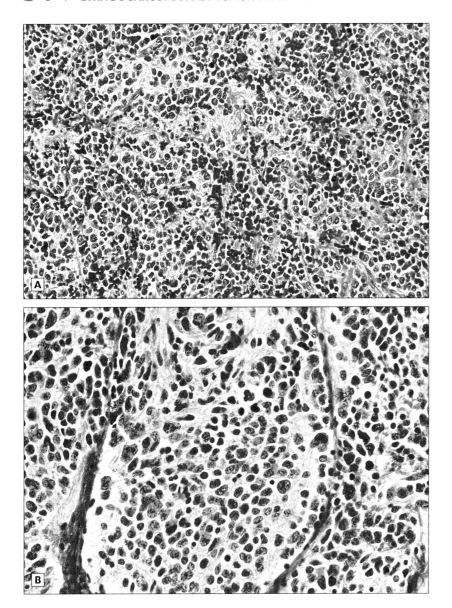

FIGURE 31–6 Low-power **(A)** and high-power **(B)** views of a poorly differentiated neuroblastoma composed of a sheet-like proliferation of monotonous small round cells with little cytoplasm.

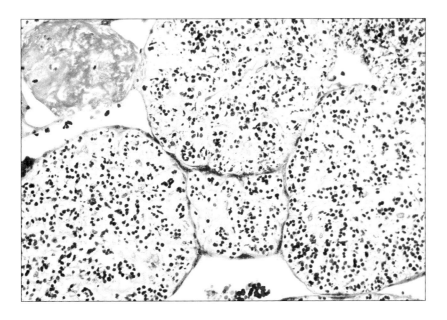

FIGURE 31–7 Congenital neuroblastoma involving the placenta. Tumor cells resemble nucleated erythrocytes and may be misinterpreted as evidence of erythroblastosis fetalis.

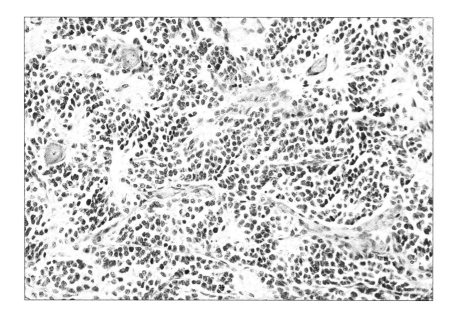

FIGURE 31–8 Poorly differentiated neuroblastoma. In this area of the tumor the neuroblasts have attenuated cytoplasmic processes that are polarized toward a central point to form Homer Wright rosettes.

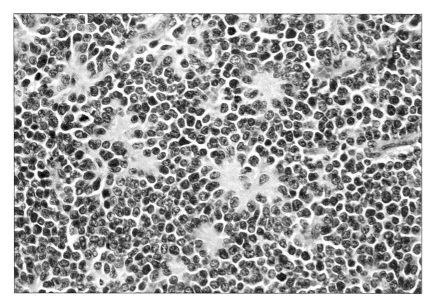

FIGURE 31–9 Homer Wright rosettes in a poorly differentiated neuroblastoma.

ganglioneuroblastoma was previously referred to as "ganglioneuroblastoma with focal complete differentiation" by Beckwith and Martin[47] and as "composite neuroblastoma" by Stout.[48] According to the International Neuroblastoma Pathology Classification (INPC), all nodular ganglioneuroblastomas have unfavorable histology. However, several studies have noted that a subtype of these tumors is associated with a more favorable prognosis.[49,50] The second, or intermixed, form of ganglioneuroblastoma consists of microscopic nests of neuroblastoma situated in a ganglioneuromatous stroma (Fig. 31–13). The nests of neuroblasts appear discrete but unencapsulated. According to the INPC, the subtype described as "stroma-rich, well-differentiated" ganglioneuroblastoma in the original Shimada classification and the "borderline-type" ganglioneuroblastoma in the Joshi system is now referred to as "ganglioneuroma, maturing subtype" (Figs 31–14 to 31–16).

Immunohistochemical findings

A number of neuroectodermal antigens can be identified in neuroblastomas, although generally the extent and intensity are related to the level of cellular differentiation.[51] Neuron-specific enolase (NSE) is probably the most sensitive but also the least specific marker for neuroblastomas. It can be identified at least focally in even poorly differentiated tumors and is identified with increasing intensity in differentiating tumors, ganglioneuroblastomas, and ganglioneuromas. Because it is present in many other small round cell tumors such as ES/PNET and rhabdomyosarcoma, it cannot be used alone to

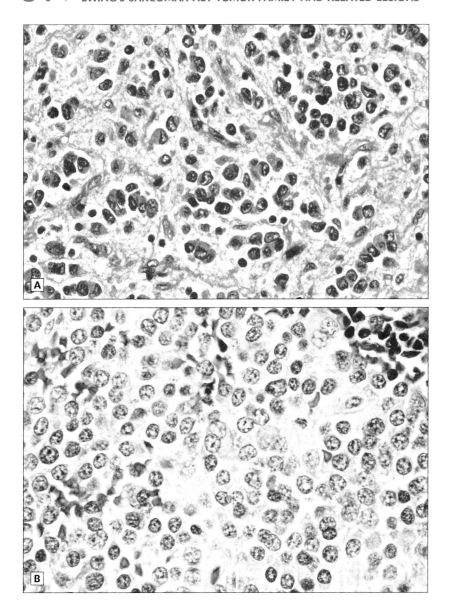

FIGURE 31–10 (A) Neuroblastoma composed predominantly of small round cells with little cytoplasm. Rare cells have a discernible rim of eosinophilic cytoplasm suggesting incipient ganglionic differentiation. **(B)** Neuroblastoma with focal ganglionic differentiation. A binucleated cell is apparent in the center of this photomicrograph.

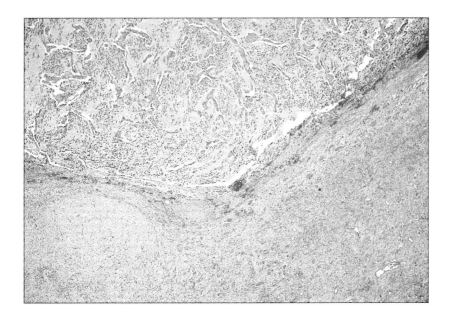

FIGURE 31–11 Low-power view of nodular ganglioneuroblastoma. Areas with neuroblastic differentiation are sharply circumscribed and separated from ganglioneuromatous zones.

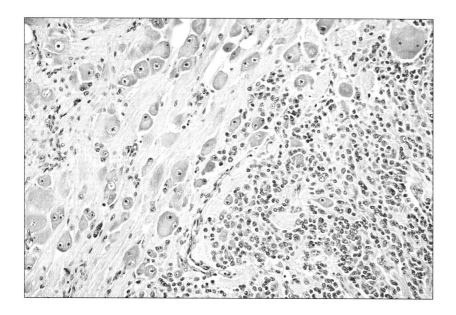

FIGURE 31–12 Nodular ganglioneuro-blastoma. Areas of ganglioneuroma abruptly give way to areas of neuroblastoma.

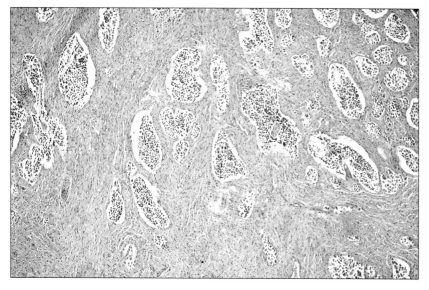

FIGURE 31–13 Ganglioneuroblastoma with patchy nodules of immature neuroblasts set in a mature ganglioneuromatous stroma.

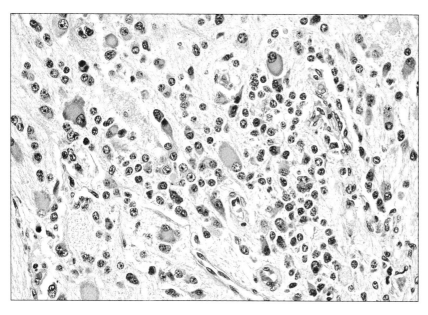

FIGURE 31–14 Ganglioneuroblastoma composed of an intimate admixture of neuroblasts and ganglion cells deposited in a fibrillary stroma.

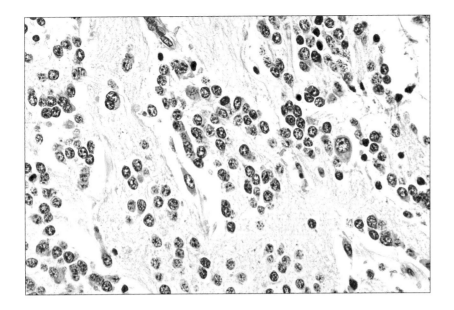

FIGURE 31–15 Ganglioneuroblastoma. This area is composed predominantly of neuroblasts in a fibrillary stroma. Rare binucleated forms and cells with obvious ganglionic differentiation are present.

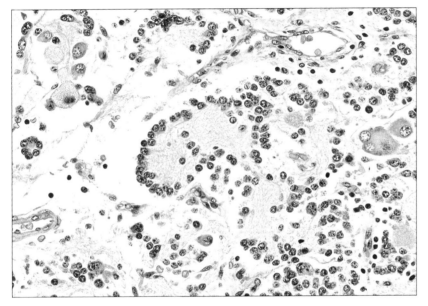

FIGURE 31–16 Homer Wright rosettes in a ganglioneuroblastoma.

distinguish among these tumors. Neurofilament protein (NFP), the intermediate filament characteristic of neuronal cells, can be identified in many neuroblastomas, although the immunoreactivity appears to depend greatly on the degree of differentiation and method of fixation.[52] S-100 protein is strongly expressed in the ganglioneuromatous portions of these tumors. Shimada et al. found that some neuroblastomas express S-100 protein in elongated spindle-shaped cells in the supportive stroma surrounding nests of tumor cells.[53] These cells likely represent precursor cells capable of producing a differentiated neuromatous stroma, as suggested by laser capture microdissection studies showing identical DNA content in the schwannian stromal cells and neuroblasts.[54] Several studies have found a favorable prognostic influence of S-100 protein staining in these tumors.[53,55] Other markers that have proved useful for diagnosing neuroblastoma

include protein gene product 9.5 (PGP9.5), chromogranin, CD56, vasoactive intestinal peptide (VIP), and synaptophysin.[56,57] All are best demonstrated in the more differentiated tumors. Glial fibrillary acidic protein (GFAP) and myelin basic protein are usually not identified in neuroblastomas unless they contain more-differentiated foci.[58] Although immunoreactivity for enzymes of catecholamine synthesis (tyrosine hydroxylase, dopamine decarboxylase) can be detected in neuroblastomas, the staining is usually weak.

A monoclonal antibody (NB-84) raised to neuroblastoma cells that recognizes a 57-kDa unknown antigen has been reported to be a sensitive marker of neuroblastomas.[59-61] Although this antibody is highly sensitive for recognizing neuroblastic tumors, it lacks complete specificity, as up to 20% of ES/PNETs are marked by this antibody.[62]

Ultrastructural findings

Ultrastructurally, neuroblastomas exhibit a wide range of cytologic differentiation.[63] The least differentiated cells may be difficult to distinguish from primitive cells in other types of tumors because they have a scant rim of cytoplasm, few organelles other than free ribosomes, and small numbers of heterogeneous granules measuring about 50 nm. More-differentiated cells can be clearly recognized as neural by virtue of attenuated cytoplasmic processes containing fine neurofilaments (8–12 nm) and microtubules (24–26 nm). Dense-core neurosecretory granules, presumably representing the site of conversion of dopamine to norepinephrine, vary in numbers. Although they typically occur in small clusters in the elongated cell processes, they may also be found in the cell body. The granules, measuring approximately 100 nm in diameter, contain central dense cores surrounded by clear halos and delicate outer membranes. Occasionally, clear vesicles are also noted. The significance of the latter structures is not certain, although they may contain acetylcholine or may be sites of exhausted catecholamine stores. Ganglionic differentiation in these tumors is accompanied by an increase in the cytoplasm, with concomitant increases in mitochondria, ribosomes, polysomes, and perinuclear Golgi apparatus. Small dense-core granules are found randomly throughout the cytoplasm (Fig. 31–17). In addition, large heterogeneous granules containing myelin figures are present in significant numbers and are believed to represent sites for storage of degraded catecholamines. Ganglioneuromatous areas contain, in addition to mature ganglion cells, a proliferation of Schwann cells characterized by long, tapered cytoplasmic processes invested with basal lamina.

Differential diagnosis

The young age of the patient, the location along the sympathetic chain, and elevated urinary catecholamines establish the diagnosis of neuroblastoma in most cases. Evaluation of needle biopsy specimens of poorly differentiated nonfunctioning tumors, however, may present diagnostic problems. The usual problem is the distinction of neuroblastoma from rhabdomyosarcoma or ES/PNET, but immunohistochemical, electron microscopic, and molecular diagnostic studies have greatly improved the accuracy of the diagnosis.

The clinical presentations of neuroblastoma and alveolar rhabdomyosarcoma may be similar. Both occur in young persons, often in intra-abdominal locations. Alveolar rhabdomyosarcomas usually show more variability in the size and shape of cells and nuclei. The cytoplasm is usually more abundant, more sharply outlined, and endowed with an eosinophilic hue. Careful search for differentiated areas often (but not always) reveals evidence of rhabdomyoblastic differentiation. Most rhabdomyosarcomas have moderate amounts of cytoplasmic glycogen, in contrast to neuroblastoma. The immunohistochemical detection of myogenic antigens, including actin, desmin, MyoD1, and myogenin, is extremely useful for confirming the diagnosis, as is evidence of a t(1;13) or t(2;13) characteristic of alveolar rhabdomyosarcoma.

Although patients with ES/PNET usually are older than those with neuroblastoma, we have found that the two tumors can be difficult to distinguish by light microscopy alone, particularly when cellular preservation is not optimal. In well-preserved specimens, ES/PNET has more regular nuclei, a more finely stippled chromatin pattern, and cytoplasm filled with glycogen. Usually, the cells are

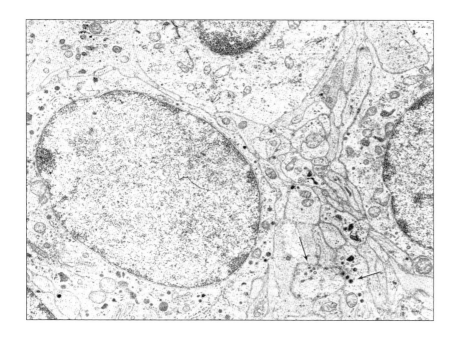

FIGURE 31–17 Electron micrograph of a neuroblastoma. Cells have numerous intertwining processes containing dense-core granules (arrows). Occasional dense-core granules are also present in the cell body. (Courtesy Dr. Tim Triche, National Cancer Institute, Bethesda, MD.)

arranged in sheets and lobules. However, the similarity between ES/PNET with Homer Wright rosettes and neuroblastoma may be striking. Neuroblastomas usually have a more fibrillary background, often have foci of calcification, and show evidence of ganglionic differentiation in many cases. Although CD99 can be detected immunohistochemically in almost all cases of ES/PNET, it is virtually never expressed in neuroblastomas. Detection of an *EWS* aberration is also extremely helpful in confirming a diagnosis of ES/PNET.

Behavior and treatment

Despite recent therapeutic advances, the survival rates of patients with neuroblastoma have remained relatively unchanged over the past two decades, a finding that contrasts with the prognosis of other childhood sarcomas. Survival rates depend on a number of partially interrelated factors (Tables 31–2, 31–3), including age at diagnosis, clinical stage (INSS stage), histopathologic features (International Neuroblastoma Pathology Classification),[43,44] presence of *MYCN* amplification, DNA ploidy, and possibly 1p deletions and other cytogenetic abnormalities, degree of trkA expression, and certain laboratory findings (e.g., serum ferritin, neuron-specific enolase, lactate dehydrogenase). Using these parameters, patients can be placed into low-, intermediate and high-risk groups and treated accordingly.

Age at diagnosis

Age at diagnosis is among the most important prognostic parameters. Most studies have evaluated the effect of age based upon whether the patient is less than or greater than 1 year of age at diagnosis.[64] However, more recent studies have found age to be a continuous variable. For example, Schmidt and colleagues studied patients with stage IV disease and nonamplification of *MYCN* and found that patients 12–18 months of age had longer event-free survival than those 18–24 months of age.[65] London et al. found better statistical separation of prognosis using an age cutoff of 460 days, as opposed to the usual 365 days.[66]

Clinical stage

The staging system used for neuroblastoma has evolved over the past 30 years. The system proposed by Evans et al.[67] in 1971 was adopted by the Children's Cancer Group. The surgicopathologic staging system proposed by Hayes et al.[68] and modified by the Pediatric Oncology Group[69] gained popularity during the 1980s. In 1993, the International Neuroblastoma Staging System (INSS) was established with elements borrowed from the staging systems of both Evans et al. and the Pediatric Oncology Group[33] (Table 31–4). Patients with stage I or II disease

TABLE 31–2	TWO-YEAR SURVIVAL RATES FOR NEUROBLASTOMA BY PROGNOSTIC FACTOR	
Factor	**No. of patients**	**Survival (%)**
Overall	124	60
Age		
<2 years	73	77
2+ years	51	38
Neuron-specific enolase		
Normal (1–100 ng/ml)	60	76
Abnormal (>100 ng/ml)	23	17
Ferritin		
Normal (0–150 ng/ml)	64	83
Abnormal (>150 ng/ml)	39	19
E rosette inhibition		
Normal (0–15%)	56	60
Abnormal (>15%)	27	54
VMA/HVA ratio		
High (>1)	28	84
Low (<1)	22	44
Stage		
I	15	100
II	27	82
III	18	42
IV	51	30
IV-S	13	100
Pathology (Shimada system)		
Favorable type	52	94
Unfavorable type	36	39

From Evans AE, Angio GJ, Propert K, et al. Prognostic factors in neuroblastoma. Cancer 1987; 59:1853.
VMA/HVA, vanillylmandelic acid/homovanillic acid.

TABLE 31–3	FAVORABLE PROGNOSTIC FACTORS FOR NEUROBLASTOMA

Young age (<1 year)
Favorable histologic type
Low stage (1, 2, 4S)
No *MYCN* amplification
Hyperdiploid or near-triploid DNA content
No allelic loss of 1p
High expression of TrKA
Normal serum ferritin, neuron-specific enolase, and lactate dehydrogenase
High urinary VMA/HVA ratio

have a significantly longer survival than do patients with stage III or IV disease. The location of the tumor, although important, is closely related to the stage of the disease. For instance, cervical, thoracic, and pelvic tumors have better prognoses than retroperitoneal and adrenal tumors but usually are detected at an earlier clinical stage.

A notable exception to the trend of decreasing survival rate with increasing clinical disease is a special group of stage IV lesions designated IVS. These tumors otherwise would be stage I or II, but there is also remote disease confined to the liver, skin, or bone marrow, without radiographic evidence of bone metastases. Despite tumor dissemination, these patients have a paradoxically favor-

TABLE 31–4	INTERNATIONAL NEUROBLASTOMA STAGING SYSTEM
Stage	**Definition**
1	Localized tumor confined to the area of origin; complete gross resection, with or without microscopic residual disease; representative ipsilateral lymph nodes negative for tumor
2A	Localized tumor with incomplete gross excision; representative ipsilateral nonadherent lymph nodes negative for tumor
2B	Localized tumor with or without complete gross excision, with ipsilateral nonadherent lymph nodes positive for tumor
	Enlarged contralateral lymph nodes negative for tumor
3	Unresectable unilateral tumor infiltrating across the midline, with or without regional lymph node involvement; or localized unilateral tumor with contralateral regional lymph node involvement; or midline tumor with bilateral extension by infiltration or by lymph node involvement
4	Any primary tumor with dissemination to distant lymph nodes, bone, bone marrow, liver, skin, and/or other organs except as defined for stage 4S
4S	Localized primary tumor (as defined for stage 1, 2A, or 2B), with dissemination limited to skin, liver, and/or bone marrow

Modified from Brodeur GM, Pritchard J, Berthold F, et al. Revisions in the international criteria for neuroblastoma diagnosis, staging and response to treatment. J Clin Oncol 1993; 11:1466.

TABLE 31–5	HISTOLOGIC TYPE OF NEUROBLASTOMA AND ITS EFFECT ON 2-YEAR SURVIVAL RATES	
Stromal character		**Survival (%)**
Stroma-rich		
Favorable histology		
Well-differentiated type		100
Intermixed type		92
Unfavorable histology		
Nodular type		18
Stroma-poor		
Favorable histology		84
Age <18 months; MKI <200/5000		
Age 18–60 months; MKI <100/5000 and differentiating		4.5
Unfavorable histology		
Age <18 months; MKI >200/5000		
Age 18–60 months; MKI >100/5000 or undifferentiated		
Age >5 years		

Modified from Shimada H, Chatten J, Newton WA Jr, et al. Histopathologic prognostic factors in neuroblastic tumors: definition of subtypes of ganglioneuroblastoma and an age-linked classification of neuroblastoma. J Natl Cancer Inst 1984; 73:405.
MKI, mitotic-karyorrhectic index.

able prognosis and a high rate of spontaneous tumor regression.[67,70,71] Van Noesel et al. reported on 119 patients with stage IVS neuroblastoma and found that 33 (28%) died, usually as a complication of hepatomegaly with renal failure, respiratory failure, or both.[72] All but one of the patients who died was diagnosed during the first 4 weeks of life. In addition, progression to stage IV disease and death were strongly related to *MYCN* amplification. Hachitanda and Hata found that most patients with stage IVS disease were less than 1 year of age, had favorable histology, and had an excellent outcome, although there was a subgroup with a poor prognosis who had unfavorable histopathologic and biologic features.[73] Thus, a thorough histologic evaluation and *MYCN* amplification are necessary to predict the outcome for this subgroup of patients.[74]

The reason for the excellent prognosis in patients with stage IVS disease is not completely understood.[75] Some authors have conceptualized stage IVS as multiple primary tumors rather than metastases;[76] others have hypothesized that stage IVS is a premalignant condition in which the final mutagenic event has not yet occurred.[77] In this respect, stage IVS could be considered comparable to in situ adrenal neuroblastoma, which regresses in most instances. Pritchard and Hickman suggested that a developmental time switch for apoptosis is the most likely mechanism for spontaneous regression of neuroblastoma.[78] Massive apoptosis of tumor cells, possibly mediated by caspase 3 activation,[79] may be important in tumor

regression, whereas inhibition of apoptosis by the Bcl-2 oncoprotein might be associated with tumor progression and resistance to therapy.[80]

Histopathology

In the past it has been difficult to correlate the degree of cellular differentiation with clinical outcome because, as indicated previously, terms such as "ganglioneuroblastoma" encompassed a broad range of tumors. In 1984, Shimada and associates proposed a new histologic system (Shimada classification) that replaced earlier systems for purposes of predicting the clinical course (Table 31–5).[39] This system divides neuroblastomas into those that have a differentiated stroma (stroma-rich) and those that do not (stroma-poor). The latter group, composed of pure neuroblastomas and some ganglioneuroblastomas, is further subdivided by the age of the patient, the degree of cellular maturation, and nuclear pathologic characteristics (mitosis-karyorrhexis index or MKI) into favorable and unfavorable subtypes.

The Shimada system identifies two groups of patients (unfavorable stroma-poor, nodular stroma-rich) with a notably poor prognosis.[81] This is a more complex system than earlier ones and introduces an entirely new nomenclature, with which pathologists are less familiar. The Joshi system[40–42] blends the basic observations of the Shimada system with more traditional terms.

In 1999, the International Neuroblastoma Pathology Classification (INPC) was established and represents a slight modification[82] of the original Shimada classification.[43,44] The major modifications include: (1) individual categories have corresponding grades of schwannian stromal development in parentheses (e.g., neuroblastoma [schwannian stroma-poor]); (2) there are three subtypes of neuroblastoma (undifferentiated, poorly differentiated, differentiating); and (3) there are two subtypes of ganglioneuroma (maturing and mature), as the *ganglioneuroblastoma, well-differentiated subtype* in the original Shimada classification renamed *ganglioneuroma, maturing subtype*. In the first large study evaluating the prognostic impact of the INPC, Shimada et al. confirmed the major differences in prognosis between favorable and unfavorable histology subgroups.[82]

MYCN amplification

Numerous studies have attested to the importance of *MYCN* amplification to the prognosis of neuroblastoma.[83,84] Approximately 20–25% of patients with neuroblastoma have *MYCN* amplification. (Table 31–6).[85] This gene may be amplified from 10 to more than 500-fold, but most are amplified in the 50–100-fold range. DNA sequence analyses have not revealed *MYCN* gene mutations, but amplification results in increased expression of the wild-type protein. There is an increased frequency of *MYCN* amplification with advanced stage of disease; there are relatively few reports of patients with low-stage disease and *MYCN* amplification.[86] In the study by Goto and colleagues from the Children's Cancer Group,[87] favorable INPC histology without and with *MYCN* amplification, and unfavorable INPC histology without and with *MYCN* amplification showed event-free survival rates of 92%, 37%, 41%, and 15%, respectively.

DNA ploidy

The presence or absence of *MYCN* amplification is closely linked to other biologic variables. Tumor cell ploidy seems to provide data complementary to *MYCN* amplification. Near-diploid or tetraploid levels of DNA are associated with advanced-stage disease, *MYCN* amplification, poor response to therapy, and a less favorable outcome. In contrast, hyperdiploidy is associated with lower-stage disease, better response to therapy, and a good prognosis.[88–90]

TABLE 31–6	CORRELATION AMONG N-*myc* AMPLIFICATION, STAGE, AND SURVIVAL	
Stage at diagnosis	MYCN amplification (%)	3-year survival (%)
1, 2	<5	90
4S	5–10	80
3, 4	30–35	30
Total	25–30	50

Modified from Brodeur GM, Maris JM, Yamashiro BJ, et al. Biology and genetics of human neuroblastomas. J Pediatr Hematol Oncol 1997; 19:93.

Cytogenetic aberrations

Loss of heterozygosity (LOH) of 1p (1p36) and 11q (11q23) is a relatively frequent event in neuroblastomas. Several studies have found an association between LOH at 1p36 and 11q23 and features of high-risk neuroblastoma.[91,92] 1p36 LOH has been found to be associated with *MYCN* amplification; Attiyeh and colleagues recently found LOH of 1p36 and unbalanced 11q LOH to be independently associated with a worse outcome.[93] Gain of 17q has also been found to be a prognostic variable that has been linked to 1p deletion, *MYCN* amplification, advanced tumor stage, and older patient age.[94–96]

TrkA

TrkA, also known as high-affinity nerve growth factor receptor, has been the subject of numerous studies since it is highly expressed in clinically favorable tumors.[97–99] Nakagawara and colleagues found a strong correlation between trkA expression and low tumor stage, younger patient age, nonamplification of *MYCN*, and a favorable prognosis.[99] In a recent study by Shimada et al.,[100] increased trkA expression was associated with favorable histology and nonamplification of *MYCN*. However, trkA expression did not add significant information above that which was provided by the combination of clinical stage, histopathology, and *MYCN* status.

Based on *MYCN* amplification, DNA ploidy, allelic loss of 1p, and trkA expression, three genetically distinct groups of neuroblastoma emerge (Table 31–7).[101] Hyperdiploid or near-triploid tumors virtually never show *MYCN* amplification, rarely show allelic loss of 1p, and have high trkA expression. These patients are usually younger than 1 year of age, generally have low-stage disease, and have an excellent prognosis. Most infants whose neuroblastomas are detected by screening studies fall into this category.[10,102] A second group of tumors have near-diploid or near-tetraploid DNA content, lack *MYCN* amplification, show allelic loss of 1p in 25–50% of cases, and usually have low trkA expression. These patients are more likely to be older than 1 year of age, have advanced stage disease, and have an intermediate prognosis. Patients with near-diploid or near-tetraploid tumors with *MYCN* amplification virtually always have allelic loss of 1p and low or absent trkA expression. These patients are almost always older than 1 year of age, have advanced-stage disease, and have a poor response to treatment with a rapidly progressive course.[3]

A number of other genes have also been implicated as having a prognostic impact in neuroblastoma, including other tumor-suppressor genes (e.g., *DCC*),[103] genes related to the multidrug resistance phenotype (*MDR1, MRP*),[104,105] genes related to invasion and metastasis (including *CD44*[106] and membrane-type matrix metalloproteinases[107]), genes related to apoptosis (e.g., caspase 8),[79,108]

TABLE 31–7	CLINICAL AND GENETIC TYPES OF NEUROBLASTOMA		
Feature	Type 1	Type 2	Type 3
DNA ploidy	Hyperdiploid or near-triploid	Near-diploid or near-tetraploid	Near-diploid or near-tetraploid
MYCN	Normal	Normal	Amplified
1p Allelic loss	<5%	25–50%	80–90%
TRK-A expression	High	Low	Low or absent
Age	<1 year	>1 year	>1 year
Stage	1, 2, or 4S	3 or 4	3 or 4
3-year survival	95%	25–50%	<5%

Modified from Brodeur GM, Maris JM, Yamashiro BJ, et al. Biology and genetics of human neuroblastomas. J Pediatr Hematol Oncol 1997; 19:93.

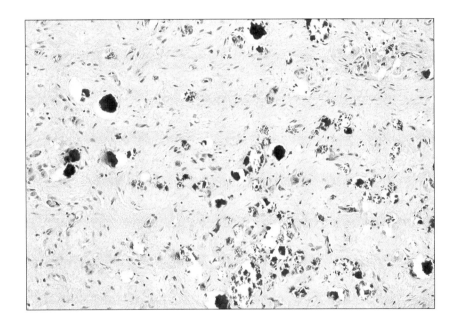

FIGURE 31–18 Zone of maturation in a neuroblastoma following therapy. There is extensive calcification of the neuromatous stroma, which is devoid of primitive neuroblasts.

and telomerase activity.[109,110] Elevated serum ferritin, neuron-specific enolase, lactate dehydrogenase, and the urinary VMA/HVA ratio also correlate with survival rates but not with the same level of statistical significance as the preceding factors.[36]

At the time of diagnosis, about two-thirds of patients harbor metastatic disease, a finding that emphasizes the need for thorough clinical evaluation before instituting therapy. Metastatic disease is most common in bone, lymph nodes, liver, and skin. Although the presence of metastasis does not necessarily portend death from disease, bone metastasis accompanied by overt radiologic changes is a notable exception, since this pattern of metastasis almost always signifies a fatal outcome.

A small number of tumors (1–2%) undergo spontaneous regression or maturation (Fig. 31–18), most often in children under 1 year of age.[111,112] It is generally believed that most clinical cures of neuroblastoma, particularly in patients with stage IVS disease, represent tumor regression rather than maturation.[113] Histologically, hypocellular zones with amorphic or plump degenerating cells

may be seen in tumors undergoing regression, as these changes have been described in resected tumors from untreated patients who were identified by a mass screening program.[114]

Management of patients with neuroblastoma is determined by the risk for recurrent disease based on age, INSS stage, and selected biologic features (mentioned above), resulting in low-, intermediate-, and high-risk groups.[17,34] Low-risk patients are generally managed by surgery or observation alone, and have up to 95% overall survival. The treatment of patients with stage IVS disease should be individualized. Because of the risk of respiratory failure secondary to hepatomegaly in patients with stage IVS disease who are less than 4 weeks of age, chemotherapy or irradiation prior to surgery has been recommended.[115] For patients with stage IVS disease who are more than 4 weeks of age, biologic markers can place the patients in low- and high-risk groups. Low-risk IVS patients can be treated with surgery alone, whereas adjuvant therapy has been recommended for patients with IVS disease who have unfavorable biologic markers.[72]

Intermediate-risk patients are generally treated with surgery and adjuvant chemotherapy of moderate intensity.[116] Patients with high-risk disease are generally treated with neoadjuvant regimens of dose-intensive induction chemotherapy with alkylating agents and platinum, delayed tumor resection, radiation therapy at the primary site, and myeloablative consolidation chemotherapy followed by autologous stem cell recovery.[117] These patients have less than 40% overall survival.[118,119]

Ganglioneuroma

Ganglioneuromas are fully differentiated tumors that contain no immature elements. They are rare compared with other benign neural tumors, such as schwannoma and neurofibroma, but they outnumber neuroblastomas along the sympathetic axis by about 3 to 1. In our experience, ganglioneuromas differ significantly in terms of age distribution and location compared with neuroblastomas. Most ganglioneuromas are diagnosed in patients older than 10 years and are most often located in the posterior mediastinum, followed by the retroperitoneum (Table 31–8). Only a minor proportion occur in the adrenal proper.[120] In the study by Geoerger and colleagues of 49 patients with this tumor,[121] the median age at diagnosis was 79 months (compared to 16 months for patients with neuroblastoma). Males and females were equally affected. Forty-one and a half percent of tumors arose in the thoracic cavity, followed by 37.5% in the abdomen outside of the adrenal gland; 21% arose within the adrenal parenchyma. The difference in distribution of neuroblastomas and ganglioneuromas support the idea that most ganglioneuromas develop de novo rather than by way of maturation in a preexisting neuroblastoma.

Ganglioneuromas may also be found at other sites, including the skin,[122] retro- or parapharynx,[123] the paratesticular region,[124] and gastrointestinal tract.[125] In the gastrointestinal tract, polypoid ganglioneuromas have been reported in association with several inherited diseases including Cowden syndrome,[126] tuberous sclerosis,[127] and juvenile polyposis.[128,129] Ganglioneuromatous polyposis has been described in patients with type 1 neurofibromatosis[130] and multiple endocrine neoplasia type IIb (MEN-IIb).[131]

Clinically, ganglioneuromas present as large masses in the retroperitoneum or mediastinum; they are usually present for a longer period of time than neuroblastomas prior to clinical detection. Most patients have normal levels of urinary catecholamine metabolites, although there is an increased incidence of elevated values in patients with extremely large tumors.[132] In the study by Geoerger et al., elevated serum and/or urine catecholamine levels were detected in 39% of patients.[121] However, extreme elevations should prompt careful evaluation for occult neuroblastomatous foci. On radiographic examination, about one-third of cases have intralesional calcification. CT, MRI, and positron emission tomography (PET) scans are useful in preoperative diagnosis, but lack specificity.[133-135] Clinically, patients may present with sweating, hypertension, virilization, and diarrhea.[136] Diarrheal symptoms in patients with these tumors may be related to the presence of vasoactive intestinal peptide, which can be localized to the cytoplasm of the ganglion cells by means of immunoperoxidase techniques.[137]

Grossly, the ganglioneuroma is a well-circumscribed tumor with a fibrous capsule. On cut section it is gray to yellow and sometimes displays a trabecular or whorled pattern similar to that of leiomyoma. Histologically, it has a uniform appearance throughout. The background consists of bundles of longitudinal and transversely oriented Schwann cells that crisscross each other in an irregular fashion (Figs 31–19, 31–20). Rarely, fat is present in the stroma.[138] Scattered throughout the schwannian backdrop are relatively mature ganglion cells (Figs 31–21 to 31–24). Although they may occur in an isolated fashion, usually they are found in small clusters or nests. In general, they are not fully mature and lack satellite cells and Nissl bodies. Typically, their voluminous cytoplasm is bright pink and contains one to three nuclei, which may exhibit a mild to moderate degree of atypia. Pigment is sometimes present in the ganglion cells and is believed to represent catecholamine products that undergo autooxidation to a melanin-like substance (neuromelanin).[139] Although the pigment has tinctorial properties of dermal melanin (Fontana-positive), ultrastructurally it does not have the regular subunit structure but consists instead of large lysosomal structures with myelin figures.[139] There are a number of reports in the literature of composite tumors composed of ganglioneuroma and paraganglioma/pheochromocytoma,[140,141] some of which have

TABLE 31–8	AGE AND ANATOMIC DISTRIBUTIONS OF GANGLIONEUROMA: 1970–1980 (88 CASES)	
Parameter		**No. of cases**
Age (years)		
0–4		5
5–9		9
10–19		23
20–29		22
30–39		12
40–49		4
50–59		6
60–69		4
>69		3
Location		
Mediastinal		34
Retroperitoneal		27
Adrenal		19
Pelvic		5
Cervical		2
Parapharyngeal		1

Data are from the Armed Forces Institute of Pathology (AFIP).

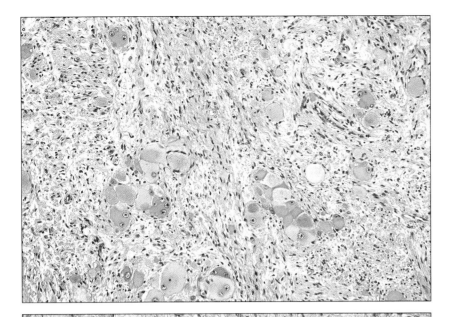

FIGURE 31–19 Ganglioneuroma composed of clusters of ganglion cells deposited in a neuromatous stroma.

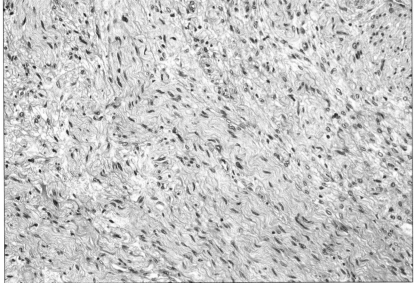

FIGURE 31–20 Neuromatous stroma devoid of ganglion cells in a ganglioneuroma.

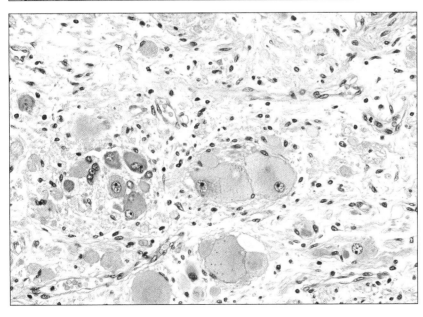

FIGURE 31–21 Ganglioneuroma with clusters of variably sized ganglion cells.

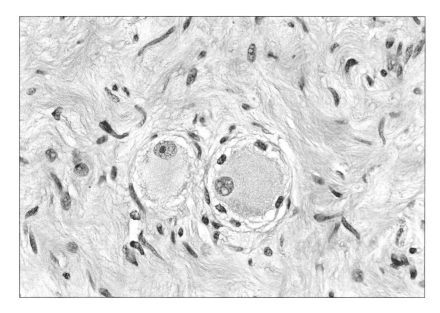

FIGURE 31–22 Mature ganglion cells with satellite cells in a ganglioneuroma.

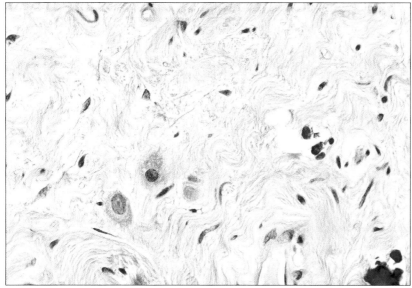

FIGURE 31–23 Ganglion cells from a ganglioneuroma having less Nissl substance and fewer satellite cells than their normal counterparts. Focal calcification is seen.

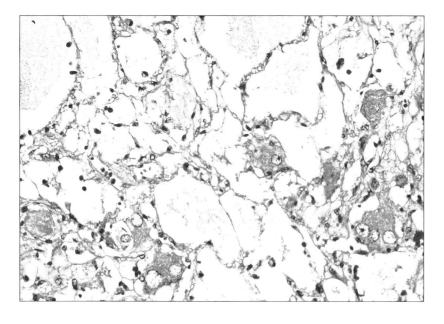

FIGURE 31–24 Cystic change in a ganglioneuroma obscuring the basic architecture of this lesion. Obvious ganglion cells can still be identified.

arisen in patients with type 1 neurofibromatosis[142] or MEN-II.[143]

Biologically, ganglioneuromas are benign tumors. However, it should be pointed out that rarely an apparent "metastatic" focus of ganglioneuroma is encountered in a lymph node adjacent to the main tumor mass or at a more distant site (Fig. 31–25).[121] It is assumed that these lesions represent neuroblastomas in which the metastasis and the primary tumor matured. Rare ganglioneuromas undergo malignant transformation,[144,145] including de novo ganglioneuromas as well as those derived from maturation in a neuroblastoma. Most commonly, the malignant component resembles a malignant peripheral nerve sheath tumor (Fig. 31–26).

GANGLION CELL CHORISTOMA

Collections of mature ganglion cells in the skin as an isolated, incidental finding have been termed "ganglion cell choristomas."[146–150] Rios et al. reported such a tumor in a 14-year-old child consisting of a poorly circumscribed collection of mature ganglion cells in the dermis.[146] The tumor was not associated with elevated levels of urinary VMA secretion, nor was the patient known to have a neuroblastoma. Lee et al. described a slightly different dermal lesion containing a superficial ganglionic component associated with a deep dermal neuromatous component.[149]

EXTRASKELETAL EWING'S SARCOMA/ PRIMITIVE NEUROECTODERMAL TUMOR FAMILY

There has been a remarkable evolution in the concepts regarding the histogenesis and relation of skeletal and extraskeletal Ewing's sarcoma and peripheral neuroepithelioma (also sometimes referred to as primitive neuroectodermal tumor). In 1918, Arthur Purdy Stout reported the case of a 42-year-old man with an ulnar nerve tumor composed of undifferentiated round cells that formed rosettes.[151] Three years later, James Ewing reported a round cell neoplasm in the radius of a 14-year-old girl, calling it a "diffuse endothelioma of bone" and proposed an endothelial derivation.[152] Over the next decades, there was much debate regarding the histogenesis of this neoplasm. Some authors challenged its very existence as a distinct entity,[153] whereas others believed the tumor was derived from Oberling's bone marrow reticular cell.[154] It was not until 1975 that Angervall and Enzinger described the first Ewing's sarcomas (ES) arising in soft tissue (extraskeletal ES).[155] Subsequent reports confirmed the clinical and pathologic features of extraskeletal ES.

At about the same time, Seemayer and colleagues described peripheral neuroectodermal tumors (PNET) arising in the soft tissues that were unrelated to structures of the peripheral or sympathetic nervous system;[156] subsequently Jaffe et al. reported identical tumors in bone.[157] In 1979, Askin and co-workers described the "malignant small cell tumor of the thoracopulmonary region" (Askin tumor) as having histologic features similar to those of PNET but with a unique clinicopathologic profile.[158] With the advent of immunohistochemical, cytogenetic, and molecular genetic techniques, it is almost universally regarded that these tumors represent ends of a morphologic spectrum known as the ES/PNET family of tumor.[159,160]

Identification of a common cytogenetic abnormality, t(11;22)(q24;q12), in Ewing's sarcoma[161] and PNET[162] clearly supports the contention that these neoplasms are histogenetically related. Since these early reports, numerous additional studies have found this translocation or variants involving 22q12, the site of the Ewing's sarcoma

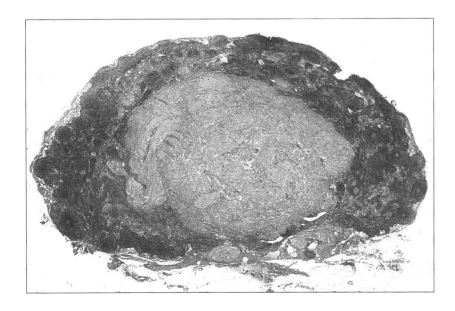

FIGURE 31–25 Apparent metastatic focus of a ganglioneuroma in a lymph node probably representing maturation of a neuroblastoma.

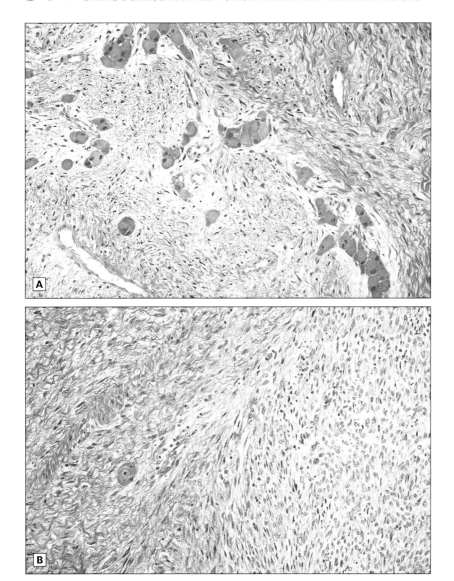

FIGURE 31–26 Rare example of malignant transformation of a ganglioneuroma to a malignant peripheral nerve sheath tumor. **(A)** Ganglioneuromatous portion of the tumor. **(B)** Interface between a ganglioneuroma and a malignant peripheral nerve sheath tumor.

(*EWS*) gene, in almost all ES/PNET.[163] It is clear that there is a spectrum of clinical and pathologic features in this group of tumors. The discussion below elaborates on this spectrum for tumors arising in extraskeletal locations.

Clinical features

Most patients with ES/PNET are adolescents or young adults, the majority of whom are less than 30 years of age.[164] In those studies which attempt to distinguish ES from PNET, there tends to be a broader age range in PNET, with a significant number of patients over the age of 40 years, although the mean ages are similar.[165–169] There is a slight male predilection, and the disease is very uncommon in non-Caucasians.[170] There is no evidence of familial predisposition or an association with environmental factors. Although some patients treated for ES/PNET develop secondary neoplasms (such as radiation-induced osteosarcoma or therapy-related acute myeloid leukemia),[171] ES/PNET rarely occurs as a second neoplasm after therapy for another tumor.[172]

ES/PNET may arise virtually anywhere but is most common in the deep soft tissues of the extremities. In our experience, the most common anatomic sites are the upper thigh and buttock followed by the upper arm and shoulder. Tumors that are intimately attached to a major nerve may give rise to signs and symptoms related to diminished neurologic function. Less commonly, the tumor arises in the paravertebral soft tissues or chest wall generally in close association with the vertebrae or the ribs (Fig. 31–27). Well-characterized examples of ES/PNET, often with molecular confirmation, have been reported in virtually every anatomic site (Table 31–9).

In general, the tumor presents as a rapidly growing, deeply located mass measuring 5–10 cm in greatest diameter. Superficially located cases do occur but are

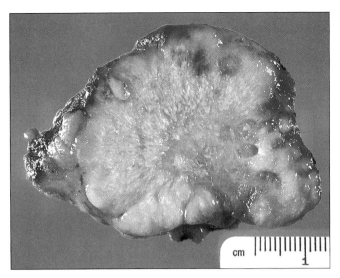

FIGURE 31–27 Gross photograph of a primitive neuroectodermal tumor from the chest wall of a 10-year-old boy. Foci of necrosis are apparent.

TABLE 31–9	UNUSUAL ANATOMIC SITES OF INVOLVEMENT OF ES/PNET	
Site	**Author (reference)**	**Year**
Pancreaticobiliary		
Pancreas	Movahedi-Lankarani[260]	2002
Biliary tract	O'Sullivan[261]	2001
Genitourinary		
Kidney	Jiminez[262]	2002
Bladder	Banerjee[263]	1997
Uterus	Karseladze[264]	2001
Ovary	Kim[265]	2004
Gastrointestinal		
Esophagus	Maesawa[266]	2002
Small bowel	Horie[267]	2000
Central nervous system		
Dura	Dedeurwaerdere[268]	2002
Cerebellopontine angle	Simmons[269]	2001
Cauda equina	Isotalo[270]	2000
Miscellaneous sites		
Adrenal gland	Kato[271]	2001
Lung	O'Sullivan[261]	2001
Heart	Charney[272]	1996
Parotid gland	Deb[273]	1998

uncommon.[173] The tumor is painful in about one-third of cases. If peripheral nerves or the spinal cord are involved, there may be progressive sensory or motor disturbances. As with other round cell sarcomas, the preoperative duration of symptoms is usually less than 1 year. Unlike neuroblastoma, catecholamine levels are within normal limits. CT, MRI, and PET scans are a routine part of the evaluation to determine anatomic relationships, presence of distant disease, and to evaluate the extent of therapeutic response to adjuvant therapy.[174,175]

Pathologic findings

The gross appearance of the tumor varies. In general, it is multilobulated, soft, and friable; it rarely exceeds 10 cm in greatest diameter. The cut surface has a gray-yellow or gray-tan appearance, often with large areas of necrosis, cyst formation, or hemorrhage. Despite the extensive necrosis, calcification is rare.

There is a spectrum of histologic change in this family of tumors, but criteria distinguishing Ewing's sarcoma, so-called atypical Ewing's sarcoma (large cell variant), and PNET are varied, as discussed below (Table 31–10). Because these lesions comprise a spectrum of histogenetically related tumors, the precise criteria for designating a tumor as an extraskeletal ES, atypical ES, or PNET are less critical. The morphologic spectrum of this family of tumors continues to expand to include "adamantinoma-like" cases,[176,177] cytokeratin-positive tumors,[177–179] and rare desmin-positive cases.[180] The morphologic and immunophenotypic diversity was the focus of a recent study of 66 genetically confirmed ES/PNET cases by Folpe and colleagues.[177] As discussed below, cases with classic morphologic features can be accurately diagnosed using light microscopy with ancillary immunohistochemistry. However, given the wide morphologic spectrum, genetic confirmation is essential for the diagnosis of unusual morphologic variants of ES/PNET.

The histologic features of typical ES include a solidly packed, lobular pattern of strikingly uniform round cells (Figs 31–28, 31–29). The individual cells have a round or ovoid nucleus measuring about 10–15 μm in diameter, with a distinct nuclear membrane, fine powdery

TABLE 31–10	SPECTRUM OF LIGHT MICROSCOPIC FEATURES ACROSS THE ES/PNET FAMILY OF TUMORS		
Feature	**Classic Ewing's sarcoma**	**Atypical Ewing's sarcoma**	**PNET**
Cell shape	Uniform, round	Irregular	Irregular
Chromatin	Fine	Coarse	Coarse
Nucleoli	Pinpoint	More prominent	Prominent
Glycogen	Abundant	Moderate	Scant
Rosettes	Absent	Absent	Present

Modified from Navarro S, Cavazanna AO, Llombart-Bosch A, et al. Comparison of Ewing's sarcoma of bone and peripheral neuroepithelioma: an immunocytochemical and ultrastructural analysis of two primitive neuroectodermal neoplasms. Arch Pathol Lab Med 1994; 118:608.

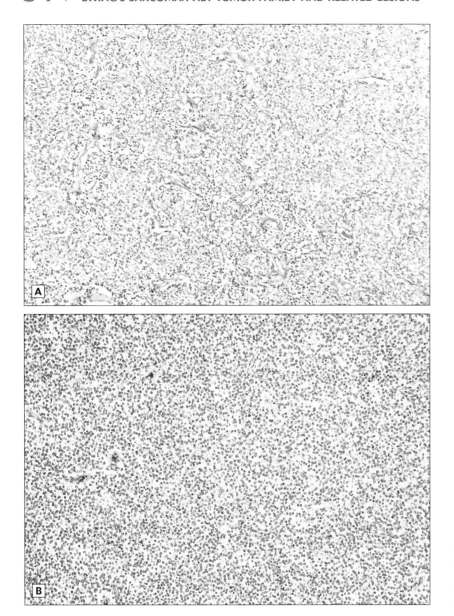

FIGURE 31–28 (A) Low-power view of extraskeletal Ewing's sarcoma characterized by a lobular round cell pattern of striking uniformity. **(B)** Typical low-power view of the monotonous appearance of this tumor.

chromatin, and one or two inapparent or small nucleoli. There are no multinucleated giant cells. The cytoplasm is ill-defined, scanty, and pale staining; and, in many cases, it is irregularly vacuolated as a result of intracellular deposits of glycogen (Figs 31–30, 31–31). Intracellular glycogen is present in most cases, but the amount varies from tumor to tumor and sometimes in different portions of the same neoplasm. In addition, glycogen droplets may compress and indent the nucleus (Fig. 31–32). The number of mitotic figures varies, and in many cases the paucity of mitotic figures contrasts with the immature appearance of the neoplastic cells.

Although the tumor is richly vascular, the thin-walled vessels are compressed and obscured by the closely packed tumor cells; the rich vascularity is often discernible only in areas of degeneration and necrosis (Fig. 31–33). In fact, the association of distinct vascular structures with degenerated or necrotic "ghost" cells is a common, striking feature ("filigree" pattern) (Fig. 31–34).[181] Aside from the prominent vascularity, there is occasionally a pseudo-vascular or pseudoalveolar pattern caused by small fluid-filled pools or blood lakes amid the solidly arranged tumor cells (Fig. 31–35), a feature occasionally misinterpreted as angiosarcoma or alveolar rhabdomyosarcoma by those unfamiliar with this secondary change. In the study by Folpe et al., 74% of cases had features of typical ES.[177]

In some cases, the cells show moderate nuclear enlargement, irregular nuclear contours, and frequent prominent nucleoli, corresponding to "atypical" or "large cell" ES (Fig. 31–36).[177,182–184]

ES/PNET with a prominent spindle-cell pattern can also be seen, albeit rarely. In such cases an elaborate hemangiopericytoma-like vascular pattern may be seen,

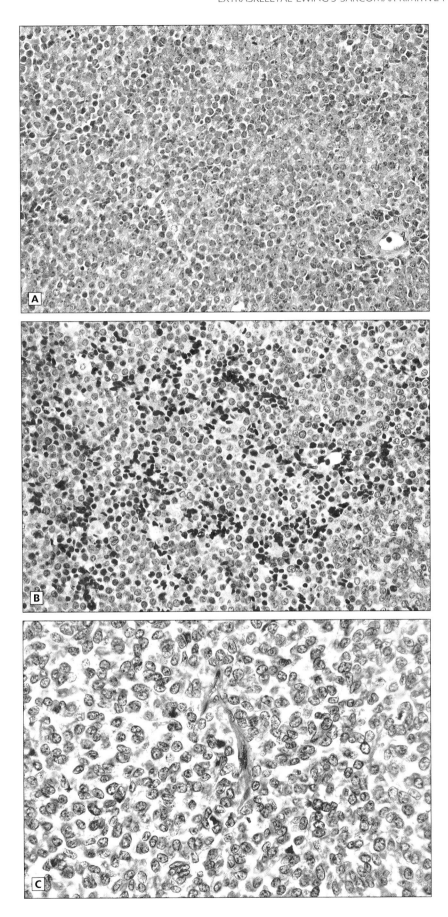

FIGURE 31–29 (A) Extraskeletal Ewing's sarcoma composed of a monotonous proliferation of round cells. Homer Wright rosettes are not seen. **(B)** Admixture of small round cells with crushed darker-staining cells. **(C)** High power view of round cell proliferation in an extraskeletal Ewing's sarcoma.

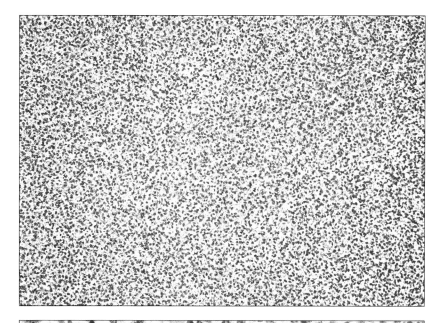

FIGURE 31–30 Low-power view of extraskeletal Ewing's sarcoma composed of cells with abundant cleared-out cytoplasm secondary to glycogen deposition.

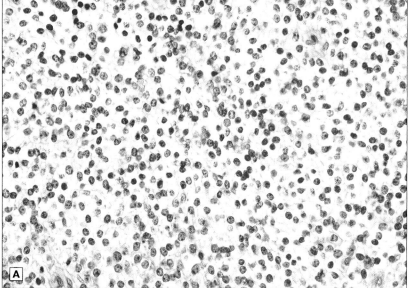

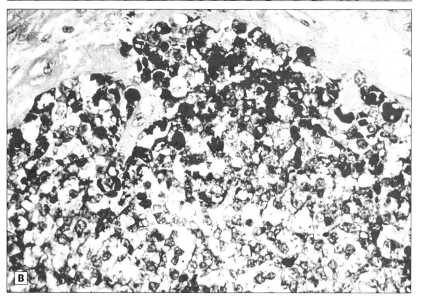

FIGURE 31–31 (A) Cells with abundant cleared-out cytoplasm and clearly defined cell borders in extraskeletal Ewing's sarcoma. (B) Extraskeletal Ewing's sarcoma. PAS preparation reveals intracellular glycogen, especially in the peripheral portion of the tumor.

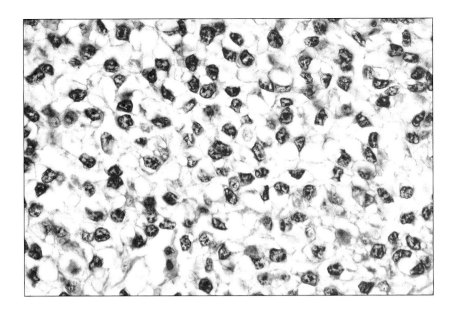

FIGURE 31–32 Extraskeletal Ewing's sarcoma. Cytoplasmic vacuoles secondary to the deposition of intracellular glycogen often indent the nuclei.

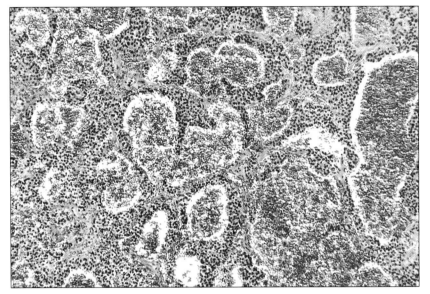

FIGURE 31–33 Hemorrhagic zone in extraskeletal Ewing's sarcoma resembling a vascular neoplasm.

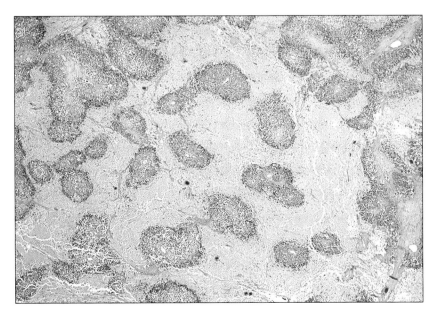

FIGURE 31–34 Extensive zones of necrosis in extraskeletal Ewing's sarcoma. There is maintenance of the tumor cells around blood vessels.

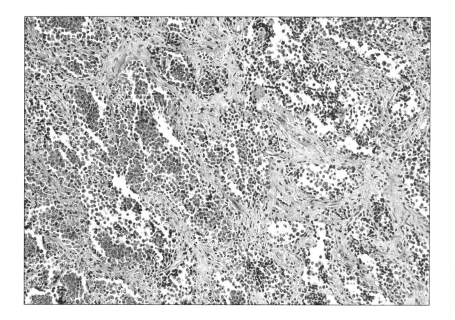

FIGURE 31–35 Pseudoalveolar pattern in an extraskeletal Ewing's sarcoma superficially resembling an alveolar rhabdomyosarcoma.

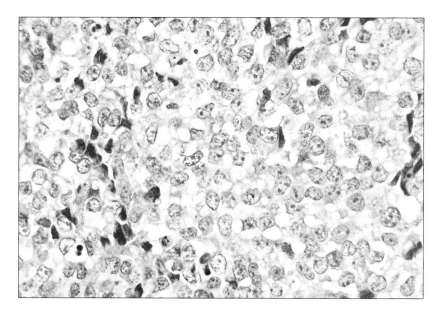

FIGURE 31–36 High-power view of large cells in an extraskeletal Ewing's sarcoma. The cells have vesicular chromatin and prominent nucleoli. Such tumors have been described as atypical or large-cell variants of Ewing's sarcoma.

thereby closely simulating a poorly differentiated synovial sarcoma.[177] Rarely, the stroma can be extensively hyalinized and densely eosinophilic, reminiscent of sclerosing epithelioid fibrosarcoma or sclerosing rhabdomyosarcoma.[177] Typical areas of ES/PNET are usually present and assist in their accurate classification.

One of the most difficult and least well-characterized variants of ES/PNET is the so-called "adamantinoma-like" variant, which accounted for 5% of the cases reported by Folpe and colleagues.[177] These tumors show a distinctly nested, epithelioid growth pattern with striking stromal desmoplasia (Fig. 31–37). The nests of tumor cells may display prominent peripheral nuclear palisading and contain large polygonal cells with irregularly contoured, hyperchromatic nuclei, prominent nucleoli, and moderate amounts of cytoplasm.[176,177,185] Rarely, squa-

mous pearls may be seen.[185] As discussed below, the immunophenotype of this variant is quite unusual, as they typically show strong, uniform expression of pancytokeratins and focal staining for high-molecular-weight cytokeratins.[177]

The typical PNET, comprising about 15% of cases, is composed of sheets or lobules of small round cells containing darkly staining, round or oval nuclei (Fig. 31–38). The cytoplasm is indistinct except in areas where the cells are more mature and the elongated hair-like cytoplasmic extensions coalesce to form rosettes (Figs 31–39, 31–40). Most of the rosettes are similar to those seen in neuroblastomas and contain a central solid core of neurofibrillary material (Homer Wright rosette). Rarely, the rosettes resemble those of retinoblastoma and contain a central lumen or vesicle (Flexner-Wintersteiner rosette). Some

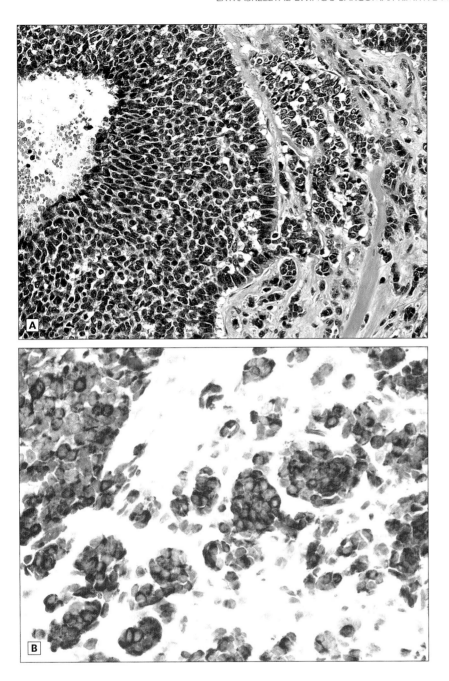

FIGURE 31–37 (A) Unusual case of an adamantinoma-like ES/PNET. **(B)** Strong cytokeratin immunoreactivity in an adamantinoma-like ES/PNET.

tumors are composed of cords or trabeculae of small round cells. These areas bear a resemblance to a carcinoid tumor or a small cell undifferentiated carcinoma, although histogenetically they are properly compared with primitive neuroepithelium. Rarely, ES/PNET may show evidence of cartilaginous or osseous differentiation.[186]

Ultrastructural features

Similar to the spectrum of histologic findings, there is also an ultrastructural spectrum of neural differentiation in the ES/PNET family (Table 31–11). Extraskeletal ES has primitive undifferentiated cells with uniform round

or ovoid nuclei, a smooth nuclear envelope, and finely granular chromatin with one or two small nucleoli (Fig. 31–41).[187,188] Characteristically, the cytoplasm contains few organelles, including a small number of mitochondria, a poorly developed Golgi complex, and abundant glycogen, sometimes containing small lipid droplets. There are also free ribosomes, inconspicuous rough endoplasmic reticulum, occasional membrane-bound dense bodies (presumably lysosomes), and bundles of intermediate filaments. The cells are closely apposed and are joined by infrequent, rudimentary cell junctions. Bundles of myofilaments, Weibel-Palade bodies, and distinct basal laminae are absent.

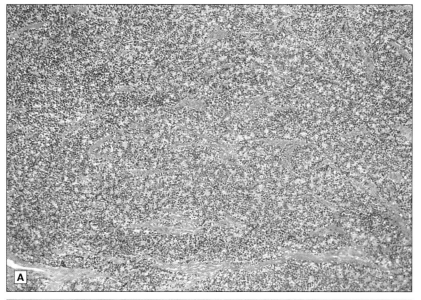

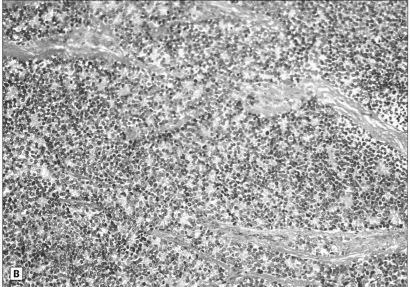

FIGURE 31-38 (A, B) Primitive neuroectodermal tumor (peripheral neuroepithelioma) with distinctive lobular architecture and numerous Homer Wright rosettes apparent at low magnification.

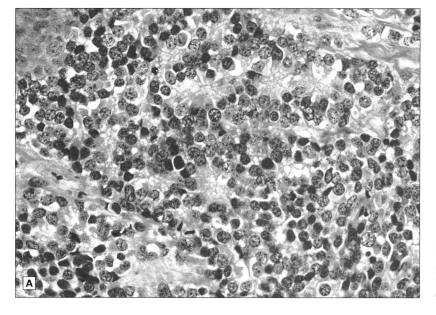

FIGURE 31-39 (A, B) Primitive neuroectodermal tumor (peripheral neuroepithelioma). Large cells with vesicular nuclei and prominent nucleoli surround a central fibrillary core (Homer Wright rosettes).

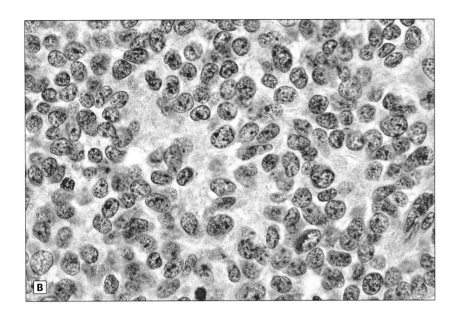

FIGURE 31–39 Continued.

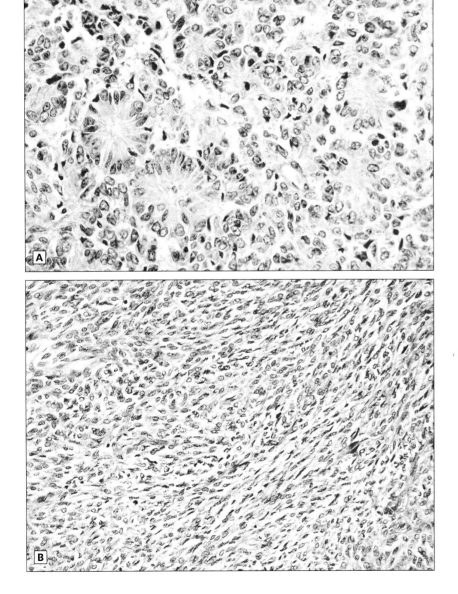

FIGURE 31–40 Primitive neuroectodermal tumor (peripheral neuroepithelioma) with round cell areas containing rosettes **(A)** and spindled areas **(B)** coexisting in the same tumor.

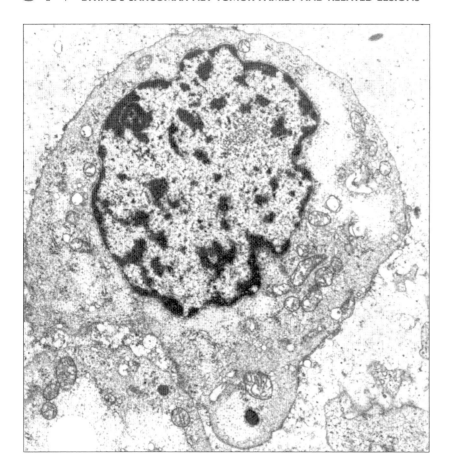

FIGURE 31–41 Electron microscopic view of a tumor in the extraskeletal Ewing's sarcoma/ primitive neuroectodermal tumor family. This cell has a prominent nucleus with marginated chromatin, few organelles, and abundant glycogen.

TABLE 31–11	SPECTRUM OF ULTRASTRUCTURAL FEATURES ACROSS THE ES/PNET FAMILY OF TUMORS		
Feature	**Classic Ewing's sarcoma**	**Atypical Ewing's sarcoma**	**PNET**
Organelles	Scarce	Moderate	Abundant
Dense-core granules	Absent	Rare	Abundant
Neurotubules	Absent	Rare	Abundant
Neuritic processes	Absent	Rare	Abundant

Modified from Navarro S, Cavazanna AO, Llombart-Bosch A, et al. Comparison of Ewing's sarcoma of bone and peripheral neuroepithelioma: an immunocytochemical and ultrastructural analysis of two primitive neuroectodermal neoplasms. Arch Pathol Lab Med 1994; 118:608.

On the other end of the spectrum, PNET is characterized by the presence of elongated cell processes that interdigitate with each other and contain small dense-core granules (neurosecretory granules) that measure 50–100 nm and occasionally contain microtubules.[187,189] The processes are most highly developed in the center of the rosette and in the neurofibrillary areas, where they form a tangled mass. They are also noted in areas that display little neurofibrillary differentiation by light microscopy.

Immunohistochemical findings

For many years, a diagnosis of ES/PNET was essentially an immunohistochemical diagnosis of exclusion. However, beginning in the early 1990s, numerous studies have confirmed the utility of the product of the *MIC2* gene (HBA71 antigen, glycoprotein p30/32, or CD99) in recognizing this group of tumors, confirming the high sensitivity of this marker for the ES/PNET family (Fig. 31–42).[177,190,191] The *MIC2* gene is a pseudoautosomal gene located on the short arms of the sex chromosomes; its product is a membranous glycoprotein (CD99) that can be detected immunohistochemically using a variety of antibodies, including 12E7 and O13. Although initially believed to be highly specific for the ES/PNET family, it is apparent that virtually all other round cell tumors in the differential diagnosis, on occasion, show membranous immunoreactivity for CD99 (Table 31–12), including lymphomas, particularly T-lymphoblastic lymphoma[192,193] and precursor B-lymphoblastic lymphoma,[194]

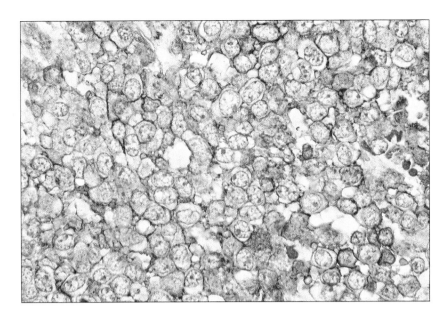

FIGURE 31–42 Strong membranous CD99 immunoreactivity in an extraskeletal Ewing's sarcoma/primitive neuroectodermal tumor.

TABLE 31–12	FREQUENCY OF CD99 IMMUNOREACTIVITY IN ES/PNET FAMILY AND OTHER SMALL ROUND CELL TUMORS	
Diagnosis		**Positive (%)**
ES/PNET		95
T-lymphoblastic lymphoma		92
Poorly differentiated synovial sarcoma		50
Small cell osteosarcoma		23
Rhabdomyosarcoma		21
Desmoplastic small round cell tumor		16
Small cell carcinoma		9
Merkel cell carcinoma		9
Neuroblastoma		0

Merkel cell carcinoma,[195] small cell carcinoma,[196] rhabdomyosarcoma,[197] small cell osteosarcoma,[198] desmoplastic small round cell tumor,[199] and mesenchymal chondrosarcoma.[200] Notably, childhood neuroblastomas have not been reported to stain for this antigen. Thus, although immunostains for CD99 are highly sensitive for recognizing the ES/PNET family of tumors, this marker should always be used as part of a panel of immunostains given the lack of complete specificity. Given the rarity of CD99 negativity in ES/PNET, suspected cases should be confirmed by molecular techniques prior to rendering a definitive diagnosis.

Many ES/PNET also stain for neural markers, including neuron-specific enolase, Leu-7, S-100 protein, synaptophysin, and PGP9.5.[57] Although PNET tend to express one or more of these neural markers with greater frequency than typical ES, there is significant overlap. It must be kept in mind that in many of the reported studies the immunohistochemical expression of neural markers is used as one of the criteria to differentiate cases of typical ES from PNET, leading to the above circular conclusion. Shanfeld et al. found that the degree of immunohistochemical expression of neural markers in tumors that lack light microscopic evidence of neural differentiation was not predictive of clinical behavior.[201] In addition, the extent of immunoexpression of these neural antigens has not been found to be related to the specific *EWS* gene fusion type.[202]

The recognition that ES/PNET may express epithelial markers has become increasingly acknowledged and is a recognized diagnostic pitfall. Folpe et al. found close to 25% of typical ES to be positive with the broad spectrum AE1/AE3 antibody, but these tumors did not express high-molecular-weight cytokeratins.[177] These findings are similar to those of Gu et al.[178] and Collini et al.,[179] who found cytokeratin staining in 20% (either AE1/AE3 or CAM5.2) and 32% (antibody not stated) of cases, respectively. This cytokeratin immunoreactivity is usually focal and often dot-like, but it may be strong and diffuse on occasion. The "adamantinoma-like" cells typically strongly express AE1/AE3, and may even stain with antibodies to high-molecular-weight cytokeratins,[177] probably reflecting the complex epithelial differentiation in this variant.

The expression of desmin is quite rare, being found in only one of 56 cases (2%) in the study by Folpe and colleagues.[177] Parham et al. also reported two cases of desmin positivity in ES/PNET, but these cases were not genetically confirmed.[180] Neither MyoD1 nor myogenin are expressed in ES/PNET, thereby reducing any potential confusion with rhabdomyosarcoma.

As described in detail below, *FLI1*, a member of the ETS family of DNA-binding transcription factors, is involved in the t(11;22) translocation frequently observed in ES/PNET. Polyclonal antibodies to the *FLI1* protein have been developed, and FLI1 nuclear positivity has been reported in 71% to 84% of ES/PNET cases.[203,204] Rossi et al., using a monoclonal antibody, found all 15 cases of ES/PNET stained for this antigen.[205] Folpe et al. found FLI1 positivity in 94% of ES/PNET with known *EWS-FLI1* fusions, as well as one case with an *EWS-ERG* fusion.[177] In the latter case, it was suggested that the polyclonal FLI1 antisera cross-reacted with a similar epitope found in the ERG protein since ERG and FLI1 show considerable homology.[206] Despite the sensitivity of this marker, FLI1 is also frequently positive in lymphoblastic and other non-Hodgkin lymphomas, and rare examples of melanoma, Merkel cell carcinoma, and neuroblastoma.[203-205]

Given the recent therapeutic success of imatinib mesylate (Gleevec) in the treatment of gastrointestinal stromal tumors, there has been some interest in evaluating the expression of CD117 in other tumors, including ES/PNET. Both CD117 and its ligand, stem cell factor, have been noted to be expressed in ES/PNET cell lines.[207,208] However, the frequency of CD117 in ES/PNET reported in the literature varies considerably, ranging from 20% to 71%.[209-211] Folpe et al. found CD117 staining in 24% of genetically confirmed ES/PNET.[212] There are few cases that have been evaluated for mutations in the *KIT* gene in ES/PNET; thus, the clinical and potentially therapeutic significance of CD117 staining in ES/PNET is not currently known.

Cytogenetic and molecular genetic findings

The defining feature of the ES/PNET family is the presence of nonrandom translocations leading to the fusion of the *EWS* gene on 22q12 with one of several members of the ETS family of transcription factors (Fig. 31–43).[206,212-215] The most frequent of these translocations is t(11;22)(q24;q12), detected in approximately 90% of cases,[216] resulting in fusion of the 3′ end of the *FLI* gene on 11q24 with the 5′ end of the *EWS* gene on 22q12.

The fusion gene encodes an oncoprotein (EWS-FLI fusion protein) domain of *FLI1* generating aberrantly active transcription factors capable of DNA binding and malignant transformation.[206] The second most common translocation is t(21;22)(q22;q12), leading to the fusion of *EWS* to *ERG* at 21q22.[217] Less common alterations (fewer than 5% of cases) result in the fusion of *EWS* to *ETV1* at 7p22,[218] *ETV4* (also known as *E1AF*) at 17q12,[219] *FEV* at 2q33,[220] and *ZSG*, resulting in an inv(22).[221] The translocation breakpoints are restricted to introns 7–10 of the *EWS* gene and introns 3–9 of the *ETS*-related genes.[222,223] Fusion of *EWS* exon 7 to *FLI1* exon 6 (type 1 fusion) and *EWS* exon 7 to *FLI1* exon 5 (type 2) account for about 85% of *EWS-FLI1* fusions.[223] The ability to detect these fusions by molecular genetic techniques (fluorescence in situ hybridization [FISH] and reverse transcriptase-polymerase chain reaction [RT-PCR]) using fixed, paraffin-embedded tissues has greatly facilitated the diagnosis of these tumors.[224,225] For example, in the recent study by Bridge et al.,[224] FISH (using fixed, paraffin-embedded tissue) showed a sensitivity and specificity of 91% and 100%, respectively. RT-PCR using fixed tissues showed sensitivity and specificity of only 59% and 85%, respectively. However, RT-PCR can provide additional information regarding fusion type, which may provide important prognostic information, as discussed below. Both techniques are complementary to one another.

Secondary cytogenetic abnormalities that occur in this group of tumors have been described, including trisomy 8,[226,227] trisomy 12,[228] and an unbalanced t(1;16) leading to gain of 1q and loss of 16q.[229] These cytogenetic abnormalities lack sufficient sensitivity and specificity for diagnostic purposes, but some have suggested a prognostic role.[230,231]

Differential diagnosis

Although a histogenetic relation between ES and PNET has been clearly established, the issue as to whether there is any clinical significance in differentiating between

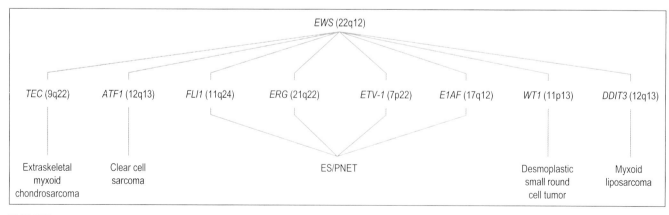

FIGURE 31–43 Critical role of the *EWS* gene (22q12) in the molecular genesis of sarcomas.

these lesions has been contentious. Part of the difficulty lies in the variability of criteria for classifying lesions as either ES or PNET. Whereas some studies require histologic evidence of rosette formation for a diagnosis of PNET, others require immunohistochemical evidence of neural differentiation, with or without rosettes. For example, in the study by Schmidt et al.,[169] a tumor was designated a PNET if it had Homer Wright rosettes on light microscopy or co-expressed two or more neural markers by immunohistochemistry. Using such criteria, the authors found that patients with PNET had a more aggressive clinical course than those with extraskeletal ES. Using identical criteria, however, others were unable to distinguish significant clinical differences between these tumors.[232,233] In the past, we diagnosed PNET if the tumor showed well-defined rosettes of the Homer Wright or Flexner-Wintersteiner type, if there were two or more positive neural markers, or if there was ultrastructural evidence of neural differentiation. Such arbitrary designations seem to be obsolete since recent studies, including those in which patients were uniformly treated, have failed to reveal significant clinical differences between these entities. Currently, we prefer to classify these tumors as members of the ES/PNET family, followed by a comment as to the presence or absence of light microscopic, immunohistochemical (Table 31–13), or ultrastructural features supporting neural differentiation.

Neuroblastoma enters the differential diagnosis because of the young age of some patients, the frequent paravertebral location of the tumor, and the presence of Homer Wright rosettes in some of the tumors. The average age of patients with ES/PNET is older than that of patients with neuroblastoma by a significant margin. Furthermore, patients with neuroblastoma often have elevated urinary catecholamine metabolite levels, a feature not found in patients with ES/PNET. The presence of mats of neuropil and ganglionic differentiation are usually features of primary or metastatic neuroblastoma. Intracellular glycogen is rare in neuroblastomas and may be discernible only by electron microscopy. Also, in contrast to neuroblastomas, the necrotic areas in ES/PNET rarely undergo calcification. Expression of CD99, as previously mentioned, all but excludes neuroblastoma as a diagnostic consideration. Although the monoclonal antibody NB-84 is a highly sensitive marker of neuroblastoma, it is found in up to 20% of ES/PNET. Finally, neuroblastoma is characterized by a consistent cytogenetic abnormality (deletion of the short arm of chromosome 1) and lacks the t(11;22) found in the ES/PNET family of tumors (Table 31–14).

Alveolar rhabdomyosarcoma may display similar densely packed cellular areas, especially at its periphery, but in general its nuclei contain more chromatin and tend to be more irregular in outline. When multiple sections are examined, the solid round cell areas are nearly always associated with areas showing loss of cellular cohesion and a distinct alveolar pattern, multinucleated giant cells with marginally placed nuclei, and, in about 20–30% of cases, eosinophilic cells characteristic of rhabdomyoblasts with or without cross-striations. Furthermore,

TABLE 31–13	IMMUNOHISTOCHEMICAL ANALYSIS OF ROUND CELL TUMORS							
Tumor	CD99	NB-84	NSE	S-100	Desmin	Myogenin/MyoD1	CK	LCA
ES/PNET	●	■	■	■			■	
Rhabdomyosarcoma	■	■	■	■	●	●	■	
Neuroblastoma		●	●	■				
Desmoplastic small round cell tumor	■	■	●	■	●		●	
Mesenchymal chondrosarcoma	●		●	■			■	
Lymphoblastic lymphoma	●							●

CK, cytokeratin; LCA, leukocyte common antigen; ● usually positive; ■ rarely positive.

TABLE 31–14	CYTOGENETIC FINDINGS IN ROUND CELL TUMORS	
Tumor	Cytogenetics	Genes
ES/PNET	t(11;22)(q24;q12)	*FLI1/EWS*
	t(21;22)(q22; q12)	*ERG/EWS*
	t(7;22)(p22;q12)	*ETV1/EWS*
	t(17;22)(q12;q12)	*E1AF/EWS*
	t(2;22)(q33;q12)	*FEV/EWS*
Alveolar rhabdomyosarcoma	t(2;13)(q35;q14)	*PAX3/FKHR*
	t(1;13)(p36;q14)	*PAX7/FKHR*
Neuroblastoma	1p⁻	
Desmoplastic small round cell tumor	t(11;22)(p13;q12)	*WT1/EWS*
Round cell liposarcoma	t(12;16)(q13;p11)	*DDIT3/FUS*
	t(12;22)(q13;q12)	*DDIT3/EWS*
Poorly differentiated synovial sarcoma	t(X;18)(p11;q11)	*SSX1 or SSX2/SYT*

most rhabdomyosarcomas show positive immunostaining for myogenic markers, including myogenin and MyoD1. It must also be kept in mind that some rhabdomyosarcomas exhibit membranous staining for CD99. Detection of t(2;13)(q35;q14) characteristic of alveolar rhabdomyosarcoma by cytogenetic or molecular genetic techniques is useful for distinguishing alveolar rhabdomyosarcoma from ES/PNET.

Malignant (non-Hodgkin) lymphoma is often suspected because of the undifferentiated appearance of the tumor cells. This diagnosis can be ruled out in most cases if attention is paid to the lobular arrangement and monotonous uniformity of the nuclei in ES/PNET and the presence of stainable intracellular glycogen. The presence or absence of lymph node involvement may be significant, as lymph node metastasis of ES/PNET is rare. Furthermore, malignant lymphomas almost always express leukocyte common antigen. Because CD99 is found in most T-cell lymphoblastic lymphomas and some lymphoblastic lymphomas do not express leukocyte common antigen, we routinely include a panel of antibodies that include T- and B-cell markers (e.g., CD20, CD79a, and TdT) to avoid an erroneous diagnosis.

Metastatic pulmonary small cell carcinoma and *cutaneous neuroendocrine carcinoma (Merkel cell carcinoma)* must be considered in the differential diagnosis, particularly when the tumor occurs in patients older than 45 years and is located superficially. In general, metastatic pulmonary small cell carcinoma can be ruled out if a thorough clinical history and radiographic studies fail to reveal pulmonary involvement. The cells of Merkel cell carcinoma have large, closely packed nuclei and little cytoplasm, and they are frequently arranged in a trabecular pattern. This tumor is chiefly located in the dermis or subcutis, and two-thirds occur in patients over 60 years of age. Although cutaneous ES/PNETs exist, they generally occur in much younger patients, with a peak incidence during the second decade of life. Immunohistochemically, virtually all Merkel cell carcinomas have a characteristic globular or punctate pattern of staining with CAM5.2. Furthermore, almost all of these tumors stain for cytokeratin 20, a marker generally absent in metastatic small cell carcinomas and ES/PNETs. Finally, most pulmonary small cell carcinomas and Merkel cell carcinomas are negative for CD99.

Mesenchymal chondrosarcoma is a rare neoplasm that typically occurs in young adults, with an extraosseous location in approximately 20% of cases. Histologically, the neoplasm is characterized by a biphasic appearance of small nests or nodules of well-differentiated cartilage intimately admixed with undifferentiated round cells, often arranged around a hemangiopericytoma-like vascular pattern. Although the biphasic appearance is characteristic, it may not be seen on a small biopsy specimen, making distinction from ES/PNET difficult. Immunohistochemically, mesenchymal chondrosarcoma

usually expresses neural markers such as neuron-specific enolase and S-100 protein. The diffuse membranous expression of CD99[200] and identification of the t(11;22) translocation in rare examples[234] raise the possibility that mesenchymal chondrosarcoma is part of the ES/PNET family of tumors.

Small cell osteosarcoma typically occurs in young patients and is composed of cells similar to those seen in ES/PNET. The diagnosis can be made only if osteoid is identified, but osteoid may be only focally present in the tumor and is often not identified in small biopsy specimens. Most tumors express neural markers, including neuron-specific enolase and Leu-7, and some express cytokeratins, actins, and rarely CD99. One small cell osteosarcoma with a t(11;22) translocation has been reported.[235]

Poorly differentiated synovial sarcoma is composed of small round cells often arranged around a hemangiopericytoma-like vasculature. However, unless one sees other areas of biphasic or monophasic synovial sarcoma, this lesion may be difficult to distinguish from malignant hemangiopericytoma or ES/PNET. Because only approximately 50% of poorly differentiated synovial sarcomas express cytokeratins and many show membranous CD99 immunoreactivity, the immunohistochemical distinction of poorly differentiated synovial sarcoma from ES/PNET is difficult in some cases. We have found cytokeratin subsets useful in this regard, as 60–70% of poorly differentiated synovial sarcomas stain for cytokeratins 7 and 19, whereas ES/PNET rarely if ever express these antigens.[236] Finally, detection of t(X;18) by conventional cytogenetics or the resultant *SSX1/SYT* or *SSX2/SYT* fusion by molecular techniques may serve as a diagnostic aid in these cases as well.

The *desmoplastic small round cell tumor* typically presents in young adults, usually men, as a large intra-abdominal mass with multiple peritoneal implants. Rare examples of this tumor have also been described in the pleura, central nervous system, and peripheral soft tissues. Histologically, it is composed of sharply outlined islands of tumor cells separated by a desmoplastic stroma containing myofibroblasts and prominent vascularity. The tumor nests often show peripheral palisading and central necrosis. The individual tumor cells are relatively uniform, small, and round to oval with hyperchromatic nuclei, inconspicuous nucleoli, and scanty cytoplasm. Immunohistochemically, these lesions have a polyphenotypic profile, with co-expression of cytokeratin, vimentin, desmin, and neuron-specific enolase. The pattern of desmin immunoreactivity is unique, with a characteristic perinuclear dot-like pattern of staining. The majority of cases also show nuclear WT1 protein expression. Up to 20% of these tumors can show membranous CD99 immunoreactivity. This tumor also has a unique cytogenetic abnormality: t(11;22)(p13;q22). The breakpoint on chromosome 22 is the same as that seen in the ES/PNET family of tumors, but the locus on chromosome 11 involves the Wilms' tumor gene (*WT1*), and thus detection of an *EWS/WT1* fusion by RT-PCR or FISH is quite helpful. In the case of FISH, using dual-color, breakapart probes for *EWS*, one must correlate the FISH results with the clinical, morphologic, and immunohistochemical features, since *EWS* aberrations are not specific for desmoplastic small round cell tumors.

Clinical behavior and therapy

Until the introduction of modern therapy, the outlook for patients with an ES/PNET was bleak, and only a small percentage of patients with this tumor survived. For instance, in the series of extraskeletal ES reported by Angervall and Enzinger in 1975,[155] 22 of the 35 patients with follow-up information died of metastatic disease, most commonly to the lung and skeleton. Similarly, many of the larger studies of PNET suggested that these tumors are highly aggressive neoplasms that rapidly give rise to metastatic disease and death. Jurgens et al. cited a survival rate of approximately 50% at 3 years,[237] whereas Kushner et al. found that only 25% of patients with tumors larger than 5 cm were alive at 24 months.[167] Although several older studies suggested that patients with PNET had a worse prognosis than those with extraskeletal ES,[166,168,169] others have not found this to be the case.[232,233,238] The data on this subject are difficult to interpret given the differences in diagnostic criteria for classifying tumors as extraskeletal ES or PNET.

Parham et al. studied 63 ES/PNET from patients who were treated uniformly to determine the prognostic significance of neuroectodermal differentiation.[232] Tumors were classified as PNET if they showed rosettes or immunohistochemical expression of at least two neural markers (or both). Using another classification scheme, tumors were classified as PNET if they showed rosettes or immunohistochemical expression of at least four neural markers (or both). Finally, using a third classification scheme, tumors that showed ultrastructural evidence of neural differentiation were classified as PNET. Using any of the above classification schemes, the authors were unable to show any significant difference in clinical outcome for patients with or without neuroectodermal differentiation.

The prognosis for patients with ES/PNET has steadily improved. About 75% of patients present with localized disease, and the combination of surgery and/or radiotherapy and systemic chemotherapy results in a cure rate near 75% in this group.[239–241] Preoperative chemotherapy using vincristine, doxorubicin, and cyclophosphamide alternating with ifosfamide and etoposide has allowed more conservative surgical procedures with better postsurgical function.[241,242] Krasin et al. reported 90% survival at 10 years for patients with localized disease treated with surgery and multiagent chemotherapy.[243] However,

patients with metastatic disease at presentation have a long-term cure rate of less than 30%, even with high-dose chemotherapy followed by stem cell reinfusion.[244-247] With increased understanding of the molecular pathways, opportunities for targeted therapy have emerged. Potential targets can be broadly classified into those related to the *EWS-ETS* gene fusion (e.g., STAT3,[248] laminin β3[249]), receptor tyrosine kinases and associated signaling pathways (e.g., IGFR,[250] PDGF[251]), the p53 and retinoblastoma pathways,[252] angiogenesis,[253] and apoptosis.[245] Minimal residual disease can be detected in peripheral blood or bone marrow by RT-PCR, and detection of fusion transcript-positive cells in the blood seems to predict disease progression.[254,255]

Key prognostic factors that adversely influence the outcome of the disease are the presence of metastatic disease at the time of initial diagnosis, large tumor size, extensive necrosis (filigree pattern), central axis tumors, and poor response to initial chemotherapy.[256,257] More recently, several studies have found that the type of *EWS/FLI1* fusion may be prognostically relevant, as patients with type 1 fusions appear to have longer disease-free survival than those with other fusion types. De Alava et al. found that patients with type 1 fusions have tumors with lower proliferative rates and generally respond better to chemotherapy.[258] However, Ginsberg et al.[259] found no significant clinical differences between those with *EWS/FLI1* or *EWS/ERG* fusions.

OLFACTORY NEUROBLASTOMA (ESTHESIONEUROBLASTOMA)

Described in 1924 by Berger and Luc,[274] olfactory neuroblastoma (also known as esthesioneuroblastoma) is a specialized form of malignant neuroectodermal tumor arising in the superior turbinate, cribriform plate, and upper one-third of the nasal cavity, including the superior nasal concha, the upper part of the nasal septum, the roof of the nose, and the cribriform plate of the ethmoid sinus.[275-277] Its origin has been debated and has been variously attributed to the neuroectodermal cells of the olfactory placode, sympathetic fibers (ganglionic loci of the nervus terminalis) in the anterior portion of the nasal cavity, the sphenopalatine ganglion, and the organ of Jacobson. Its location high in the nasal vault, however, and the fact that the tumor cells have ultrastructural features of olfactory nerve cells favor origin from the olfactory placode.[278,279]

Clinical features

Olfactory neuroblastoma accounts for less than 5% of all malignancies of the sinonasal tract. The majority of patients with this tumor are adults, although there seem to be two peaks. Most patients are in the fifth and sixth decades of life,[280] but there is a smaller peak in the second decade of life.[281,282] Men and women are equally affected. For localized lesions, the most common presentation is unilateral nasal obstruction and epistaxis, followed less frequently by lacrimation, rhinorrhea, and anosmia. Extensive lesions involving the sinuses are accompanied by frontal headache and diplopia. There are several reports of patients presenting with the syndrome of inappropriate antidiuretic hormone secretion.[283,284] Radiographically, spotty calcification may be detected in the tumor, although the specific bone changes depend on the extent of the tumor. MRI and CT are useful for delineating the anatomic extent of the tumor and determining resectability.[277,285]

Pathologic findings

Grossly, the lesions are fleshy, gray polypoid masses that may have areas of hemorrhage and necrosis. The cut surface has a gray-tan to pink-red hypervascular appearance. Histologically, there is a spectrum of morphologic alterations, with some tumors closely resembling childhood neuroblastoma and others resembling paragangliomas.[276] Low-grade tumors are composed of small round cells with hyperchromatic nuclei and scanty cytoplasm. True rosettes with a central lumen (Flexner-Wintersteiner or olfactory rosettes) and pseudorosettes containing a core of neurofibrillary material (Homer Wright rosettes) can be found. Such tumors span a spectrum from those with few mitotic figures, minimal nuclear pleomorphism, prominent fibrillary matrix, and an absence of necrosis to those with high-grade features including numerous mitotic figures, marked nuclear pleomorphism, minimal or absent fibrillary matrix, and extensive areas of necrosis.[276] Other tumors are composed of nodules of medium-sized polygonal cells with uniform ovoid

nuclei, inconspicuous nucleoli, and relatively abundant, slightly eosinophilic, granular cytoplasm, reminiscent of the cells seen in paragangliomas (Figs 31–44, 31–45). According to Hirose et al., most olfactory neuroblastomas have characteristics of both classic neuroblastoma and paraganglioma.[279] A prominent glomeruloid capillary network is often seen in the stroma.[286] Focal ganglionic differentiation is occasionally present.[287] Tumors are graded (grades I to IV) on the degree of cellular differentiation, presence of neural stroma, mitotic figures, and extent of necrosis (Table 31–15). As discussed below, tumor grading impacts prognosis.

Immunohistochemical and ultrastructural findings

Immunohistochemically, virtually all tumors express one or more markers of neuronal or neuroendocrine differentiation, including synaptophysin, neuron-specific enolase, neurofilament protein, CD56, and chromogranin.[276] Synaptophysin and chromogranin tend to be expressed more frequently by tumors with paraganglioma-like features (Fig. 31–46), whereas neurofilament protein is more commonly expressed by tumors that closely resemble neuroblastoma. A fine network of cells that are positive for S-100 protein and vimentin surround the cells in a diagnostically distinctive fashion, bringing to mind the S-100 protein-positive sustentacular network in paragangliomas.[288] Tumors with Flexner-Wintersteiner rosettes typically stain for cytokeratin and epithelial membrane antigen, but even tumors without such epithelial structures can exhibit focal cytokeratin immunoreactivity.[276,278] This is in contrast to the diffuse cytokeratin staining typical of neuroendocrine carcinomas. Unlike the ES/PNET family of tumors, olfactory neuroblastoma does not express CD99.[289]

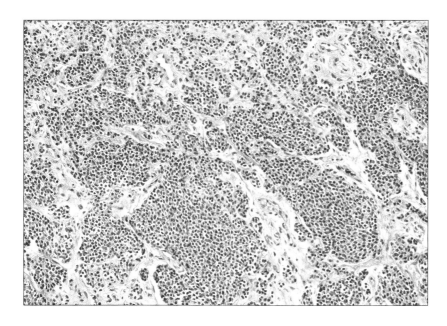

FIGURE 31–44 Low-power view of an olfactory neuroblastoma composed of nests of uniform ovoid cells in a fibrovascular stroma.

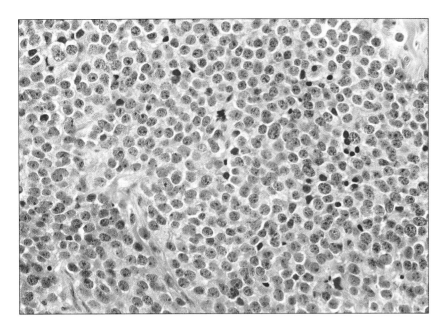

FIGURE 31–45 Olfactory neuroblastoma composed of uniform ovoid cells with powdery chromatin, small nucleoli, and eosinophilic granular cytoplasm.

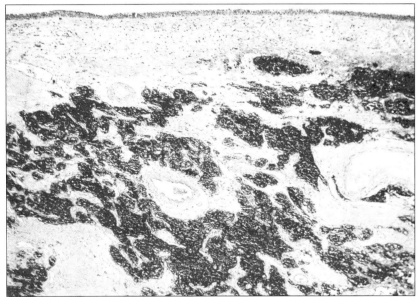

FIGURE 31–46 Diffuse synaptophysin immunoreactivity in an olfactory neuroblastoma.

TABLE 31–15	HYAMS'S GRADING SYSTEM FOR OLFACTORY NEUROBLASTOMA			
Feature	**Grade 1**	**Grade 2**	**Grade 3**	**Grade 4**
Architecture	Lobular	Lobular	Lobular	Lobular
Mitotic activity	Absent	Present	Prominent	Marked
Nuclear atypia	Absent	Moderate	Prominent	Marked
Rosettes	Homer Wright	Homer Wright	Flexner-Wintersteiner	Flexner-Wintersteiner
Matrix	Prominent	Present	Minimal	Absent
Necrosis	Absent	Absent	±	Common

Ultrastructurally, the cells have features of primitive neuroblasts, including dense-core (neurosecretory) granules and cell processes containing microtubules.[290] There are often numerous pleomorphic mitochondria and extensive paranuclear Golgi complexes. Sustentacular-like cells, with long, slender processes that encompass individual or groups of tumor cells, may be seen.[291]

Cytogenetic findings

Relatively few olfactory neuroblastomas have been evaluated cytogenetically; several have shown complex cytogenetic aberrations,[292,293] including deletions at 3p.[294] The t(11;22)(q24;q12) characteristic of the ES/PNET family of tumors has been reported in some tumors diagnosed as olfactory neuroblastoma,[295] but subsequent studies have been unable to detect the *EWS/FLI1* fusion transcript in primary olfactory neuroblastomas using either FISH or RT-PCR.[289,296]

Discussion

The initial management of an olfactory neuroblastoma usually involves multimodality therapy. This strategy has allowed improved survival, although late recurrences and metastases are still common. In more recent series, 5-year survival rates have ranged from 69% to 89%.[282,297-299] Treatment and survival are strongly dependent on tumor stage. The most widely used staging system was proposed by Kadish et al.[300] Stage A patients, with tumors limited to the nasal cavity, have a crude 5-year survival rate between 75% and 90%.[299] Stage B patients, with tumors involving the nasal cavity and one or more paranasal sinuses, have a survival rate between 68% and 71%. Stage C patients, with disease extending beyond the nasal cavity and sinuses, have a survival rate between 41% and 47%. Because of the frequency of endocranial invasion, a combined otolaryngologic and neurosurgical approach with bicoronal incision and frontal lobe exposure is often required.[297] However, several recent studies have shown excellent success with endoscopic-assisted cranionasal resection.[301-303] Several studies have validated the added survival advantage of radiation therapy, chemotherapy, or both.[304]

The differential diagnosis includes other sinonasal tumors composed of small round cells such as squamous cell carcinoma, sinonasal undifferentiated carcinoma, malignant melanoma, extranodal NK/T-cell lymphoma, rhabdomyosarcoma, and ES/PNET. Clinical features including age and anatomic site of origin of the tumor can be helpful. Histologic features such as cytologic atypia, necrosis, type of stroma, rosettes/pseudorosettes, and immunophenotype can usually resolve these issues. However, the diagnosis can be difficult in small biopsy specimens. For example, in a study from M.D. Anderson Cancer Center, only 2 of 12 cases referred for treatment for presumed olfactory neuroblastoma were ultimately felt to have a correct diagnosis.[305]

REFERENCES

Neuroblastoma and ganglioneuroblastoma

1. Kushner BH, Gilbert F, Helson L. Familial neuroblastoma. Case reports, literature review, and etiologic considerations. Cancer 1986; 57:1887.
2. Adaletli I, Kurugoglu S, Aki H, et al. Simultaneous presentation of congenital neuroblastoma in monozygotic twins: a case of possible twin-to-twin metastasis. AJR Am J Roentgenol 2006; 186:1172.
3. Brodeur GM, Maris JM, Yamashiro DJ, et al. Biology and genetics of human neuroblastomas. J Pediatr Hematol Oncol 1997; 19:93.
4. Biegel JA, White PS, Marshall HN, et al. Constitutional 1p36 deletion in a child with neuroblastoma. Am J Hum Genet 1993; 52:176.
5. Lopez-Ibor B, Schwartz AD. Neuroblastoma. Pediatr Clin North Am 1985; 32:755.
6. Shimada H. In situ neuroblastoma: an important concept related to the natural history of neural crest tumors. Pediatr Dev Pathol 2005; 8:305.
7. Gurney JG, Davis S, Severson RK, et al. Trends in cancer incidence among children in the U.S. Cancer 1996; 78:532.
8. Kim S, Chung DH. Pediatric solid malignancies: neuroblastoma and Wilms' tumor. Surg Clin North Am 2006; 86:469.
9. Jennings RW, LaQuaglia MP, Leong K, et al. Fetal neuroblastoma: prenatal diagnosis and natural history. J Pediatr Surg 1993; 28:1168.
10. Barrette S, Bernstein ML, Leclerc JM, et al. Treatment complications in children diagnosed with neuroblastoma during a screening program. J Clin Oncol 2006; 24:1542.
11. Esiashvili N, Goodman M, Ward K, et al. Neuroblastoma in adults: incidence and survival analysis based on SEER data. Pediatr Blood Cancer 2006; Epub ahead of print.

12. Conte M, Parodi S, De Bernardi B, et al. Neuroblastoma in adolescents: the Italian experience. Cancer 2006; 106: 1409.
13. Hasegawa T, Hirose T, Ayala AG, et al. Adult neuroblastoma of the retroperitoneum and abdomen: clinicopathologic distinction from primitive neuroectodermal tumor. Am J Surg Pathol 2001; 25:918.
14. Takeda S, Miyoshi S, Minami M, et al. Intrathoracic neurogenic tumors – 50 years' experience in a Japanese institution. Eur J Cardiothorac Surg 2004; 26:807.
15. DeLorimier AA, Bragg KU, Linden G. Neuroblastoma in childhood. Am J Dis Child 1969; 118:441.
16. Posner JB. Paraneoplastic syndromes in neuroblastoma. J Pediatr Hematol Oncol 2004; 26:553.
17. Castleberry RP. Neuroblastoma. Eur J Cancer 1997; 33:1430.
18. Evans AE, Chatten J, D'Angio GJ, et al. A review of 17 IV-S neuroblastoma patients at the Children's Hospital of Philadelphia. Cancer 1980; 45:833.
19. Holland KE, Galbraith SS, Drolet BA. Neonatal violaceous skin lesions: expanding the differential of the "blueberry muffin baby." Adv Dermatol 2005; 21:153.
20. Ehsani MA, Abouzari M, Rashidi A, et al. Unique role of enalapril in the treatment of severe hypertension in a child with an unusual form of neuroblastoma. J Pediatr Hematol Oncol 2005; 27:569.
21. Bell J, Moran C, Blatt J. Response to rituximab in a child with neuroblastoma and opsoclonus-myoclonus. Pediatr Blood Cancer 2006; Epub ahead of print.
22. Korfei M, Fuhlhuber V, Schmidt-Woll T, et al. Functional characterisation of autoantibodies from patients with pediatric opsoclonus-myoclonus-syndrome. J Neuroimmunol 2005; 170:150.
23. Muller KM, Nykyri E, Andersson LC. Effect of thymectomy and immunosuppressive therapy on anti-neuroblastoma antibody levels in

patients with myasthenia gravis. Acta Neurol Scand 1991; 83:336.
24. Espinasse-Holder M, Defachelles AS, Weill J, et al. Paraneoplastic Cushing syndrome due to adrenal neuroblastoma. Med Pediatr Oncol 2000; 34:231.
25. Origone P, Defferrari R, Mazzocco K, et al. Homozygous inactivation of NF1 gene in a patient with familial NF1 and disseminated neuroblastoma. Am J Med Genet A 2003; 118:309.
26. al-Shammri S, Guberman A, Hsu E. Neuroblastoma and fetal exposure to phenytoin in a child without dysmorphic features. Can J Neurol Sci 1992; 19:243.
27. Maris JM, Chatten J, Meadows AT, et al. Familial neuroblastoma: a three-generation pedigree and a further association with Zhirschsprung disease. Med Pediatr Oncol 1997; 28:1.
28. Altinok G, Kattar MM, Mohamed A, et al. Pediatric renal carcinoma associated with Xp11.2 translocations/TFE3 gene fusions and clinicopathologic associations. Pediatr Dev Pathol 2005; 8:168.
29. Blatt J, Hamilton RL. Neurodevelopmental anomalies in children with neuroblastoma. Cancer 1998; 82:1603.
30. Davidoff AM, Corey BL, Hoffer FA, et al. Radiographic assessment of resectability of locoregional disease in children with high-risk neuroblastoma during neoadjuvant chemotherapy. Pediatr Blood Cancer 2005; 44:158.
31. Henry MC, Tashjian DB, Breuer CK. Neuroblastoma update. Curr Opin Oncol 2005; 17:19.
32. Kushner BH, Cheung NK. Exploiting the MIBG-avidity of neuroblastoma for staging and treatment. Pediatr Blood Cancer 2006; Epub ahead of print.
33. Brodeur GM, Pritchard J, Berthold F, et al. Revisions of the international criteria for neuroblastoma diagnosis, staging, and response to treatment. J Clin Oncol 1993; 11:1466.

34. Castleberry RP, Pritchard J, Ambros P, et al. The international neuroblastoma risk groups (INRG): a preliminary report. Eur J Cancer 1997; 33:2113.

35. Strenger V, Kerbl R, Dornbusch HJ, et al. Diagnostic and prognostic impact of urinary catecholamines in neuroblastoma patients. Pediatr Blood Cancer 2006; Epub ahead of print.

36. Evans AE, D'Angio GJ, Propert K, et al. Prognostic factor in neuroblastoma. Cancer 1987; 59:1853.

37. Kitlinska J, Abe K, Kuo L, et al. Differential effects of neuropeptide Y on the growth and vascularization of neural crest-derived tumors. Cancer Res 2005; 65:1719.

38. Riley RD, Heney D, Jones DR, et al. A systematic review of molecular and biological tumor markers in neuroblastoma. Clin Cancer Res 2004; 10:4.

39. Shimada H, Chatten J, Newton WA Jr, et al. Histopathologic prognostic factors in neuroblastic tumors: definition of subtypes of ganglioneuroblastoma and an age-linked classification of neuroblastomas. J Natl Cancer Inst 1984; 73:405.

40. Joshi VV, Silverman JF, Altshuler G, et al. Systematization of primary histopathologic and fine-needle aspiration cytologic features and description of unusual histopathologic features of neuroblastic tumors: a report from the Pediatric Oncology Group. Hum Pathol 1993; 24:493.

41. Joshi VV, Cantor AB, Altshuler G, et al. Age-linked prognostic categorization based on a new histologic grading system of neuroblastomas. A clinicopathologic study of 211 cases from the Pediatric Oncology Group. Cancer 1992; 69:2197.

42. Joshi VV, Cantor AB, Altshuler G, et al. Recommendations for modification of terminology of neuroblastic tumors and prognostic significance of Shimada classification. A clinicopathologic study of 213 cases from the Pediatric Oncology Group. Cancer 1992; 69:2183.

43. Shimada H, Ambros IM, Dehner LP, et al. The international neuroblastoma pathology classification (the Shimada system). Cancer 1999; 86:364.

44. Shimada H, Ambros IM, Dehner LP, et al. Terminology and morphologic criteria of neuroblastic tumors: recommendations by the International Neuroblastoma Pathology Committee. Cancer 1999; 86:349.

45. Tornoczky T, Kalman E, Kajtar PG, et al. Large cell neuroblastoma: a distinct phenotype of neuroblastoma with aggressive clinical behavior. Cancer 2004; 100:390.

46. Kobayashi C, Monforte-Munoz HL, Gerbing RB, et al. Enlarged and prominent nucleoli may be indicative of MYCN amplification: a study of neuroblastoma (schwannian stroma-poor), undifferentiated/poorly differentiated subtype with high mitosis-karyorrhexis index. Cancer 2005; 103:174.

47. Beckwith JB, Martin RF. Observations on the histopathology of neuroblastoma. J Pediatr Surg 1968; 3:106.

48. Stout AP. Ganglioneuroma of the sympathetic nervous system. Surg Gynecol Obstet 1947; 84:101.

49. Peuchmaur M, d'Amore ES, Joshi VV, et al. Revision of the International Neuroblastoma Pathology Classification: confirmation of favorable and unfavorable prognostic subsets in ganglioneuroblastoma, nodular. Cancer 2003; 98:2274.

50. Umehara S, Nakagawa A, Matthay KK, et al. Histopathology defines prognostic subsets of ganglioneuroblastoma, nodular. Cancer 2000; 89:1150.

51. Wirnsberger GH, Becker H, Ziervogel K, et al. Diagnostic immunohistochemistry of neuroblastic tumors. Am J Surg Pathol 1992; 16:49.

52. Mukai M, Torikata C, Iri H, et al. Expression of neurofilament triplet proteins in human neural tumors. An immunohistochemical study of paraganglioma, ganglioneuroma, ganglioneuroblastoma, and neuroblastoma. Am J Pathol 1986; 122:28.

53. Shimada H, Aoyama C, Chiba T, et al. Prognostic subgroups for undifferentiated neuroblastoma: immunohistochemical study with anti-S-100 protein antibody. Hum Pathol 1985; 16:471.

54. Mora J, Cheung NK, Juan G, et al. Neuroblastic and schwannian stromal cells of neuroblastoma are derived from a tumoral progenitor cell. Cancer Res 2001; 61:6892.

55. Ambros IM, Zellner A, Roald B, et al. Role of ploidy, chromosome 1p, and Schwann cells in the maturation of neuroblastoma. N Engl J Med 1996; 334:1505.

56. Hachitanda Y, Tsuneyoshi M, Enjoji M. Expression of pan-neuroendocrine proteins in 53 neuroblastic tumors. An immunohistochemical study with neuron-specific enolase, chromogranin, and synaptophysin. Arch Pathol Lab Med 1989; 113:381.

57. Carter RL, al-Sams SZ, Corbett RP, et al. A comparative study of immunohistochemical staining for neuron-specific enolase, protein gene product 9.5 and S-100 protein in neuroblastoma, Ewing's sarcoma and other round cell tumours in children. Histopathology 1990; 16:461.

58. Molenaar WM, Baker DL, Pleasure D, et al. The neuroendocrine and neural profiles of neuroblastomas, ganglioneuroblastomas, and ganglioneuromas. Am J Pathol 1990; 136:375.

59. Miettinen M, Chatten J, Paetau A, et al. Monoclonal antibody NB84 in the differential diagnosis of neuroblastoma and other small round cell tumors. Am J Surg Pathol 1998; 22:327.

60. Thomas JO, Nijjar J, Turley H, et al. NB84: a new monoclonal antibody for the recognition of neuroblastoma in routinely processed material. J Pathol 1991; 163:69.

61. Sebire NJ, Gibson S, Rampling D, et al. Immunohistochemical findings in embryonal small round cell tumors with molecular diagnostic confirmation. Appl Immunohistochem Mol Morphol 2005; 13:1.

62. Folpe AL, Patterson K, Gown AM. Antineuroblastoma antibody NB-84 also identifies a significant subset of other small blue round cell tumors. Appl Immunohistochem 1997; 5:239.

63. Hachitanda Y, Tsuneyoshi M, Enjoji M. An ultrastructural and immunohistochemical evaluation of cytodifferentiation in neuroblastic tumors. Mod Pathol 1989; 2:13.

64. Evans AE, D'Angio GJ, Sather HN, et al. A comparison of four staging systems for localized and regional neuroblastoma: a report from the Children's Cancer Study Group. J Clin Oncol 1990; 8:678.

65. Schmidt ML, Lal A, Seeger RC, et al. Favorable prognosis for patients 12 to 18 months of age with stage 4 nonamplified MYCN neuroblastoma: a Children's Cancer Group study. J Clin Oncol 2005; 23:6474.

66. London WB, Boni L, Simon T, et al. The role of age in neuroblastoma risk stratification: the German, Italian, and Children's Oncology Group perspectives. Cancer Lett. 2005; 228:257.

67. Evans AE, D'Angio GJ, Randolph J. A proposed staging for children with neuroblastoma. Children's Cancer Study Group A. Cancer 1971; 27:374.

68. Hayes FA, Green A, Hustu HO, et al. Surgicopathologic staging of neuroblastoma: prognostic significance of regional lymph node metastases. J Pediatr 1983; 102:59.

69. Nitschke R, Smith EI, Altshuler G, et al. Postoperative treatment of nonmetastatic visible residual neuroblastoma: a Pediatric Oncology Group study. J Clin Oncol 1991; 9:1181.

70. Hufnagel M, Claviez A, Czech N, et al. Neuroblastoma stage 4S with 123I-MIBG-positive bone marrow involvement. Pediatr Blood Cancer 2006; 46:264.

71. Vandesompele J, Baudis M, De Preter K, et al. Unequivocal delineation of clinicogenetic subgroups and development of a new model for improved outcome prediction in neuroblastoma. J Clin Oncol 2005; 23:2280.

72. van Noesel MM, Hahlen K, Hakvoort-Cammel FG, et al. Neuroblastoma 4S: a heterogeneous disease with variable risk factors and treatment strategies. Cancer 1997; 80:834.

73. Hachitanda Y, Hata J. Stage IVS neuroblastoma: a clinical, histological, and biological analysis of 45 cases. Hum Pathol 1996; 27:1135.

74. Katzenstein HM, Bowman LC, Brodeur GM, et al. Prognostic significance of age, MYCN oncogene amplification, tumor cell ploidy, and histology in 110 infants with stage D(S) neuroblastoma: the Pediatric Oncology Group experience – a Pediatric Oncology Group study. J Clin Oncol 1998; 16:2007.

75. Matthay KK. Stage 4S neuroblastoma: what makes it special? J Clin Oncol 1998; 16:2003.

76. D'Angio GJ, Evans AE, Koop CE. Special pattern of widespread neuroblastoma with a favourable prognosis. Lancet 1971; 1:1046.

77. Knudson AG Jr, Meadows AT. Sounding board. Regression of neuroblastoma IV-S: a genetic hypothesis. N Engl J Med 1980; 302:1254.

78. Pritchard J, Hickman JA. Why does stage 4s neuroblastoma regress spontaneously? Lancet 1994; 344:869.

79. Koizumi H, Hamano S, Doi M, et al. Increased occurrence of caspase-dependent apoptosis in unfavorable neuroblastomas. Am J Surg Pathol 2006; 30:249.

80. Goldsmith KC, Hogarty MD. Targeting programmed cell death pathways with experimental therapeutics: opportunities in high-risk neuroblastoma. Cancer Lett 2005; 228:133.

81. Chatten J, Shimada H, Sather HN, et al. Prognostic value of histopathology in advanced neuroblastoma: a report from the Children's Cancer Study Group. Hum Pathol 1988; 19:1187.

82. Shimada H, Umehara S, Monobe Y, et al. International neuroblastoma pathology classification for prognostic evaluation of patients with peripheral neuroblastic tumors: a report from the Children's Cancer Group. Cancer 2001; 92:2451.

83. Brodeur GM, Seeger RC, Schwab M, et al. Amplification of N-myc in untreated human neuroblastomas correlates with advanced disease stage. Science 1984; 224:1121.

84. Seeger RC, Brodeur GM, Sather H, et al. Association of multiple copies of the N-myc oncogene with rapid progression of neuroblastomas. N Engl J Med 1985; 313:1111.

85. Schwab M, Westermann F, Hero B, et al. Neuroblastoma: biology and molecular and chromosomal pathology. Lancet Oncol 2003; 4:472.

86. Kushner BH, Cheung NK, LaQuaglia MP, et al. International neuroblastoma staging system stage 1 neuroblastoma: a prospective study and literature review. J Clin Oncol 1996; 14:2174.

87. Goto S, Umehara S, Gerbing RB, et al. Histopathology (International Neuroblastoma Pathology Classification) and MYCN status in patients with peripheral neuroblastic tumors:

a report from the Children's Cancer Group. Cancer 2001; 92:2699.

88. Bagatell R, Rumcheva P, London WB, et al. Outcomes of children with intermediate-risk neuroblastoma after treatment stratified by MYCN status and tumor cell ploidy. J Clin Oncol 2005; 23:8819.

89. Spitz R, Betts DR, Simon T, et al. Favorable outcome of triploid neuroblastomas: a contribution to the special oncogenesis of neuroblastoma. Cancer Genet Cytogenet 2006; 167:51.

90. Look AT, Hayes FA, Nitschke R, et al. Cellular DNA content as a predictor of response to chemotherapy in infants with unresectable neuroblastoma. N Engl J Med 1984; 311:231.

91. Maris JM, Guo C, Blake D, et al. Comprehensive analysis of chromosome 1p deletions in neuroblastoma. Med Pediatr Oncol 2001; 36:32.

92. White PS, Thompson PM, Gotoh T, et al. Definition and characterization of a region of 1p36.3 consistently deleted in neuroblastoma. Oncogene 2005; 24:2684.

93. Attiyeh EF, London WB, Mosse YP, et al. Chromosome 1p and 11q deletions and outcome in neuroblastoma. N Engl J Med 2005; 353:2243.

94. Bown N, Lastowska M, Cotterill S, et al. 17q gain in neuroblastoma predicts adverse clinical outcome. U.K. Cancer Cytogenetics Group and the U.K. Children's Cancer Study Group. Med Pediatr Oncol 2001; 36:14.

95. Lastowska M, Cotterill S, Bown N, et al. Breakpoint position on 17q identifies the most aggressive neuroblastoma tumors. Genes Chromosomes Cancer 2002; 34:428.

96. O'Neill S, Ekstrom L, Lastowska M, et al. MYCN amplification and 17q in neuroblastoma: evidence for structural association. Genes Chromosomes Cancer 2001; 30:87.

97. Brodeur GM. TRK-A expression in neuroblastomas: a new prognostic marker with biological and clinical significance. J Natl Cancer Inst 1993; 85:344.

98. Brodeur GM, Nakagawara A, Yamashiro DJ, et al. Expression of TrkA, TrkB and TrkC in human neuroblastomas. J Neurooncol 1997; 31:49.

99. Nakagawara A, Arima-Nakagawara M, Scavarda NJ, et al. Association between high levels of expression of the TRK gene and favorable outcome in human neuroblastoma. N Engl J Med 1993; 328:847.

100. Shimada H, Nakagawa A, Peters J, et al. TrkA expression in peripheral neuroblastic tumors: prognostic significance and biological relevance. Cancer 2004; 101:1873.

101. Brodeur GM, Nakagawara A. Molecular basis of clinical heterogeneity in neuroblastoma. Am J Pediatr Hematol Oncol 1992; 14:111.

102. Granata C, Fagnani AM, Gambini C, et al. Features and outcome of neuroblastoma detected before birth. J Pediatr Surg 2000; 35:88.

103. Desai A, Kisaalita WS, Keith C, et al. Human neuroblastoma (SH-SY5Y) cell culture and differentiation in 3-D collagen hydrogels for cell-based biosensing. Biosens Bioelectron 2006; 21:1483.

104. Flahaut M, Muhlethaler-Mottet A, Martinet D, et al. Molecular cytogenetic characterization of doxorubicin-resistant neuroblastoma cell lines: evidence that acquired multidrug resistance results from a unique large amplification of the 7q21 region. Genes Chromosomes Cancer 2006; 45:495.

105. Haber M, Smith J, Bordow SB, et al. Association of high-level MRP1 expression with poor clinical outcome in a large prospective study of primary neuroblastoma. J Clin Oncol 2006; 24:1546.

106. Combaret V, Gross N, Lasset C, et al. Clinical relevance of TRKA expression on neuroblastoma: comparison with N-MYC amplification and CD44 expression. Br J Cancer 1997; 75:1151.

107. Ebinger M, Senf L, Wachowski O, et al. Promoter methylation pattern of caspase-8, P16INK4A, MGMT, TIMP-3, and E-cadherin in medulloblastoma. Pathol Oncol Res 2004; 10:17.

108. Stupack DG, Teitz T, Potter MD, et al. Potentiation of neuroblastoma metastasis by loss of caspase-8. Nature 2006; 439:95.

109. Binz N, Shalaby T, Rivera P, et al. Telomerase inhibition, telomere shortening, cell growth suppression and induction of apoptosis by telomestatin in childhood neuroblastoma cells. Eur J Cancer 2005; 41:2873.

110. Isobe K, Yashiro T, Omura S, et al. Expression of the human telomerase reverse transcriptase in pheochromocytoma and neuroblastoma tissues. Endocr J 2004; 51:47.

111. Maris JM. The biologic basis for neuroblastoma heterogeneity and risk stratification. Curr Opin Pediatr 2005; 17:7.

112. Nuchtern JG. Perinatal neuroblastoma. Semin Pediatr Surg 2006; 15:10.

113. Nagasawa M, Kawamoto H, Tsuji Y, et al. Transient increase of serum granulysin in a stage IVs neuroblastoma patient during spontaneous regression: case report. Int J Hematol 2005; 82:456.

114. Ijiri R, Tanaka Y, Kato K, et al. Clinicopathologic study of mass-screened neuroblastoma with special emphasis on untreated observed cases: a possible histologic clue to tumor regression. Am J Surg Pathol 2000; 24:807.

115. Nickerson HJ, Matthay KK, Seeger RC, et al. Favorable biology and outcome of stage IV-S neuroblastoma with supportive care or minimal therapy: a Children's Cancer Group study. J Clin Oncol 2000; 18:477.

116. Matthay KK, Perez C, Seeger RC, et al. Successful treatment of stage III neuroblastoma based on prospective biologic staging: a Children's Cancer Group study. J Clin Oncol 1998; 16:1256.

117. Matthay KK, Villablanca JG, Seeger RC, et al. Treatment of high-risk neuroblastoma with intensive chemotherapy, radiotherapy, autologous bone marrow transplantation, and 13-cis-retinoic acid. Children's Cancer Group. N Engl J Med 1999; 341:1165.

118. Berthold F, Boos J, Burdach S, et al. Myeloablative megatherapy with autologous stem-cell rescue versus oral maintenance chemotherapy as consolidation treatment in patients with high-risk neuroblastoma: A randomised controlled trial. Lancet Oncol 2005; 6:649.

119. Pritchard J, Cotterill SJ, Germond SM, et al. High dose melphalan in the treatment of advanced neuroblastoma: results of a randomised trial (ENSG-1) by the European Neuroblastoma Study Group. Pediatr Blood Cancer 2005; 44:348.

120. Zografos GN, Markou A, Ageli C, et al. Laparoscopic surgery for adrenal tumors. A retrospective analysis. Hormones (Athens, Greece) 2006; 5:52.

121. Geoerger B, Hero B, Harms D, et al. Metabolic activity and clinical features of primary ganglioneuromas. Cancer 2001; 91:1905.

122. Wallace CA, Hallman JR, Sangueza OP. Primary cutaneous ganglioneuroma: a report of two cases and literature review. Am J Dermatopathol 2003; 25:239.

123. Starek I, Mihal V, Novak Z, et al. Pediatric tumors of the parapharyngeal space. Three case reports and a literature review. Int J Pediatr Otorhinolaryngol 2004; 68:601.

124. Pardalidis NP, Grigoriadis K, Papatsoris AG, et al. Primary paratesticular adult ganglioneuroma. Urology 2004; 63:584.

125. Al-Daraji WI, Abdellaoui A, Salman WD. Solitary polypoidal rectal ganglioneuroma: a rare presentation of a rare tumor. J Gastroenterol Hepatol 2005; 20:961.

126. Robinson S, Cohen AR. Cowden disease and Lhermitte-Duclos disease: an update. Case report and review of the literature. Neurosurg Focus 2006; 20:E6.

127. Devroede G, Lemieux B, Masse S, et al. Colonic hamartomas in tuberous sclerosis. Gastroenterology 1988; 94:182.

128. Kanter AS, Hyman NH, Li SC. Ganglioneuromatous polyposis: a premalignant condition. Report of a case and review of the literature. Dis Colon Rectum 2001; 44:591.

129. Mendelsohn G, Diamond MP. Familial ganglioneuromatous polyposis of the large bowel. Report of a family with associated juvenile polyposis. Am J Surg Pathol 1984; 8:515.

130. Shekitka KM, Sobin LH. Ganglioneuromas of the gastrointestinal tract. Relation to von Recklinghausen disease and other multiple tumor syndromes. Am J Surg Pathol 1994; 18:250.

131. Haggitt RC, Reid BJ. Hereditary gastrointestinal polyposis syndromes. Am J Surg Pathol 1986; 10:871.

132. Cronin EM, Coffey JC, Herlihy D, et al. Massive retroperitoneal ganglioneuroma presenting with small bowel obstruction 18 years following initial diagnosis. Ir J Med Sci 2005; 174:63.

133. Yamaguchi K, Hara I, Takeda M, et al. Two cases of ganglioneuroma. Urology 2006; 67:622.e1.

134. Tanaka O, Kiryu T, Hirose Y, et al. Neurogenic tumors of the mediastinum and chest wall: MR imaging appearance. J Thorac Imaging 2005; 20:316.

135. Ilias I, Shulkin B, Pacak K. New functional imaging modalities for chromaffin tumors, neuroblastomas and ganglioneuromas. Trends Endocrinol Metab 2005; 16:66.

136. Koch CA, Brouwers FM, Rosenblatt K, et al. Adrenal ganglioneuroma in a patient presenting with severe hypertension and diarrhea. Endocr Relat Cancer 2003; 10:99.

137. Reindl T, Degenhardt P, Luck W, et al. The VIP-secreting tumor as a differential diagnosis of protracted diarrhea in pediatrics. Klin Padiatr 2004; 216:264.

138. Duffy S, Jhaveri M, Scudierre J, et al. MR imaging of a posterior mediastinal ganglioneuroma: fat as a useful diagnostic sign. AJNR Am J Neuroradiol 2005; 26:2658.

139. Dundr P, Dudorkinova D, Povysil C, et al. Pigmented composite paraganglioma-ganglioneuroma of the urinary bladder. Pathol Res Pract 2003; 199:765.

140. Usuda H, Emura I. Composite paraganglioma-ganglioneuroma of the urinary bladder. Pathol Int 2005; 55:596.

141. de Montpreville VT, Mussot S, Gharbi N, et al. Paraganglioma with ganglioneuromatous component located in the posterior mediastinum. Ann Diagn Pathol 2005; 9:110.

142. Kimura N, Watanabe T, Fukase M, et al. Neurofibromin and NF1 gene analysis in composite pheochromocytoma and tumors associated with von Recklinghausen's disease. Mod Pathol 2002; 15:183.

143. Matias-Guiu X, Garrastazu MT. Composite phaeochromocytoma-ganglioneuroblastoma in a patient with multiple endocrine neoplasia type IIA. Histopathology 1998; 32:281.

144. Drago G, Pasquier B, Pasquier D, et al. Malignant peripheral nerve sheath tumor arising in a "de novo" ganglioneuroma: a case report and review of the literature. Med Pediatr Oncol 1997; 28:216.

145. de Chadarevian JP, MaePascasio J, Halligan GE, et al. Malignant peripheral nerve sheath tumor arising from an adrenal ganglioneuroma in a 6-year-old boy. Pediatr Dev Pathol 2004; 7:277.

Ganglion cell choristoma

146. Rios JJ, Diaz-Cano SJ, Rivera-Hueto F, et al. Cutaneous ganglion cell choristoma. Report of a case. J Cutan Pathol 1991; 18:469.
147. Argenyi ZB. Cutaneous neural heterotopias and related tumors relevant for the dermatopathologist. Semin Diagn Pathol 1996; 13:60.
148. Lena G, Dufour T, Gambarelli D, et al. Choristoma of the intracranial maxillary nerve in a child. Case report. J Neurosurg 1994; 81:788.
149. Lee JY, Martinez AJ, Abell E. Ganglioneuromatous tumor of the skin: a combined heterotopia of ganglion cells and hamartomatous neuroma: report of a case. J Cutan Pathol 1988; 15:58.
150. Radice F, Gianotti R. Cutaneous ganglion cell tumor of the skin. Case report and review of the literature. Am J Dermatopathol 1993; 15:488.

Extraskeletal Ewing's sarcoma/primitive neuroectodermal tumor family

151. Stout AP. Tumor of the ulnar nerve. Proc NY Pathol Soc 1918; 18:2.
152. Ewing J. Diffuse endothelioma of bone. Proc NY Pathol Soc 1921; 21:17.
153. Willis RA. Metastatic neuroblastoma in bone presenting the Ewing's syndrome, with a discussion of "Ewing's sarcoma." Am J Pathol 1940; 16:317.
154. Stout AP. A discussion of the pathology and histogenesis of Ewing's tumor of bone marrow. Am J Roentgenol 1943; 50:334.
155. Angervall L, Enzinger FM. Extraskeletal neoplasm resembling Ewing's sarcoma. Cancer 1975; 36:240.
156. Seemayer TA, Thelmo WL, Bolande RP, et al. Peripheral neuroectodermal tumors. Perspect Pediatr Pathol 1975; 2:151.
157. Jaffe R, Santamaria M, Yunis EJ, et al. The neuroectodermal tumor of bone. Am J Surg Pathol 1984; 8:885.
158. Askin FB, Rosai J, Sibley RK, et al. Malignant small cell tumor of the thoracopulmonary region in childhood: a distinctive clinicopathologic entity of uncertain histogenesis. Cancer 1979; 43:2438.
159. Dehner LP. Primitive neuroectodermal tumor and Ewing's sarcoma. Am J Surg Pathol 1993; 17:1.
160. Dehner LP. The evolution of the diagnosis and understanding of primitive and embryonic neoplasms in children: living through an epoch. Mod Pathol 1998; 11:669.
161. Aurias A, Rimbaut C, Buffe D, et al. Translocation involving chromosome 22 in Ewing's sarcoma. A cytogenetic study of four fresh tumors. Cancer Genet Cytogenet 1984; 12:21.
162. Whang-Peng J, Triche TJ, Knutsen T, et al. Chromosome translocation in peripheral neuroepithelioma. N Engl J Med 1984; 311:584.
163. de Alava E, Pardo J. Ewing tumor: tumor biology and clinical applications. Int J Surg Pathol 2001; 9:7.
164. Khoury JD. Ewing sarcoma family of tumors. Adv Anat Pathol 2005; 12:212.
165. Cavazzana AO, Ninfo V, Roberts J, et al. Peripheral neuroepithelioma: a light microscopic, immunocytochemical, and ultrastructural study. Mod Pathol 1992; 5:71.

166. Hartman KR, Triche TJ, Kinsella TJ, et al. Prognostic value of histopathology in Ewing's sarcoma. Long-term follow-up of distal extremity primary tumors. Cancer 1991; 67:163.
167. Kushner BH, Hajdu SI, Gulati SC, et al. Extracranial primitive neuroectodermal tumors. The Memorial Sloan-Kettering Cancer Center experience. Cancer 1991; 67:1825.
168. Marina NM, Etcubanas E, Parham DM, et al. Peripheral primitive neuroectodermal tumor (peripheral neuroepithelioma) in children. A review of the St. Jude experience and controversies in diagnosis and management. Cancer 1989; 64:1952.
169. Schmidt D, Herrmann C, Jurgens H, et al. Malignant peripheral neuroectodermal tumor and its necessary distinction from Ewing's sarcoma. A report from the Kiel Pediatric Tumor Registry. Cancer 1991; 68:2251.
170. Herzog CE. Overview of sarcomas in the adolescent and young adult population. J Pediatr Hematol Oncol 2005; 27:215.
171. Paulussen M, Ahrens S, Lehnert M, et al. Second malignancies after Ewing tumor treatment in 690 patients from a cooperative German/Austrian/Dutch study. Ann Oncol 2001; 12:1619.
172. Spunt SL, Rodriguez-Galindo C, Fuller CE, et al. Ewing sarcoma-family tumors that arise after treatment of primary childhood cancer. Cancer 2006; 107(1):201.
173. Hasegawa SL, Davison JM, Rutten A, et al. Primary cutaneous Ewing's sarcoma: immunophenotypic and molecular cytogenetic evaluation of five cases. Am J Surg Pathol 1998; 22:310.
174. Gyorke T, Zajic T, Lange A, et al. Impact of FDG PET for staging of Ewing sarcomas and primitive neuroectodermal tumours. Nucl Med Commun 2006; 27:17.
175. Hawkins DS, Schuetze SM, Butrynski JE, et al. [18F]fluorodeoxyglucose positron emission tomography predicts outcome for Ewing sarcoma family of tumors. J Clin Oncol 2005; 23:8828.
176. Bridge JA, Fidler ME, Neff JR, et al. Adamantinoma-like Ewing's sarcoma: genomic confirmation, phenotypic drift. Am J Surg Pathol 1999; 23:159.
177. Folpe AL, Goldblum JR, Rubin BP, et al. Morphologic and immunophenotypic diversity in Ewing family tumors: a study of 66 genetically confirmed cases. Am J Surg Pathol 2005; 29:1025.
178. Gu M, Antonescu CR, Guiter G, et al. Cytokeratin immunoreactivity in Ewing's sarcoma: prevalence in 50 cases confirmed by molecular diagnostic studies. Am J Surg Pathol 2000; 24:410.
179. Collini P, Sampietro G, Bertulli R, et al. Cytokeratin immunoreactivity in 41 cases of ES/PNET confirmed by molecular diagnostic studies. Am J Surg Pathol 2001; 25:273.
180. Parham DM, Dias P, Kelly DR, et al. Desmin positivity in primitive neuroectodermal tumors of childhood. Am J Surg Pathol 1992; 16:483.
181. Kissane JM, Askin FB, Foulkes M, et al. Ewing's sarcoma of bone: clinicopathologic aspects of 303 cases from the Intergroup Ewing's Sarcoma Study. Hum Pathol 1983; 14:773.
182. Navarro S, Noguera R, Pellin A, et al. Atypical pleomorphic extraosseous Ewing tumor/peripheral primitive neuroectodermal tumor with unusual phenotypic/genotypic profile. Diagn Mol Pathol 2002; 11:9.
183. Nascimento AG, Unii KK, Pritchard DJ, et al. A clinicopathological study of 20 cases of large-cell (atypical) Ewing's sarcoma of bone. Am J Surg Pathol 1980; 4:29.
184. Llombart-Bosch A, Pellin A, Carda C, et al. Soft tissue Ewing sarcoma–peripheral primitive

neuroectodermal tumor with atypical clear cell pattern shows a new type of EWS-FEV fusion transcript. Diagn Mol Pathol 2000; 9:137.
185. Fukunaga M, Ushigome S. Periosteal Ewing-like adamantinoma. Virchows Arch 1998; 433:385.
186. Oda Y, Kinoshita Y, Tamiya S, et al. Extraskeletal primitive neuroectodermal tumour with massive osteo-cartilaginous metaplasia. Histopathology 2000; 36:188.
187. Suh CH, Ordonez NG, Hicks J, et al. Ultrastructure of the Ewing's sarcoma family of tumors. Ultrastruct Pathol 2002; 26:67.
188. Navarro S, Cavazzana AO, Llombart-Bosch A, et al. Comparison of Ewing's sarcoma of bone and peripheral neuroepithelioma. An immunocytochemical and ultrastructural analysis of two primitive neuroectodermal neoplasms. Arch Pathol Lab Med 1994; 118:608.
189. Franchi A, Pasquinelli G, Cenacchi G, et al. Immunohistochemical and ultrastructural investigation of neural differentiation in Ewing sarcoma/PNET of bone and soft tissues. Ultrastruct Pathol 2001; 25:219.
190. Ambros IM, Ambros PF, Strehl S, et al. MIC2 is a specific marker for Ewing's sarcoma and peripheral primitive neuroectodermal tumors. Evidence for a common histogenesis of Ewing's sarcoma and peripheral primitive neuroectodermal tumors from MIC2 expression and specific chromosome aberration. Cancer 1991; 67:1886.
191. Stevenson AJ, Chatten J, Bertoni Jea. CD99 (p30/32^{MIC2}) neuroectoermal/Ewing's sarcoma antigen as an immunohistochemical marker: Review of more than 600 tumors and the literature experience. Appl Immunohistochem 1994; 2:231.
192. Ozdemirli M, Fanburg-Smith JC, Hartmann DP, et al. Differentiating lymphoblastic lymphoma and Ewing's sarcoma: lymphocyte markers and gene rearrangement. Mod Pathol 2001; 14:1175.
193. Lucas DR, Bentley G, Dan ME, et al. Ewing sarcoma vs lymphoblastic lymphoma. A comparative immunohistochemical study. Am J Clin Pathol 2001; 115:11.
194. Ozdemirli M, Fanburg-Smith JC, Hartmann DP, et al. Precursor B-lymphoblastic lymphoma presenting as a solitary bone tumor and mimicking Ewing's sarcoma: a report of four cases and review of the literature. Am J Surg Pathol 1998; 22:795.
195. Perlman EJ, Lumadue JA, Hawkins AL, et al. Primary cutaneous neuroendocrine tumors. Diagnostic use of cytogenetic and MIC2 analysis. Cancer Genet Cytogenet 1995; 82:30.
196. Lumadue JA, Askin FB, Perlman EJ. MIC2 analysis of small cell carcinoma. Am J Clin Pathol 1994; 102:692.
197. Hess E, Cohen C, DeRose PBea. Nonspecificity of p30/32^{MIC2} immunolocalization with the O13 monoclonal antibody in the diagnosis of Ewing's sarcoma: application of an algorithmic immunohistochemical analysis. Appl Immunohistochem 1997; 5:94.
198. Devaney K, Abbondanzo SL, Shekitka KM, et al. MIC2 detection in tumors of bone and adjacent soft tissues. Clin Orthop Relat Res 1995; 310:176.
199. Gerald WL, Ladanyi M, de Alava E, et al. Clinical, pathologic, and molecular spectrum of tumors associated with t(11;22)(p13;q12): desmoplastic small round-cell tumor and its variants. J Clin Oncol 1998; 16:3028.
200. Granter SR, Renshaw AA, Fletcher CD, et al. CD99 reactivity in mesenchymal chondrosarcoma. Hum Pathol 1996; 27:1273.
201. Shanfeld RL, Edelman J, Willis JE, et al. Immunohistochemical analysis of neural markers in peripheral primitive

neuroectodermal tumors (pPNET) without light microscopic evidence of neural differentiation. Appl Immunohistochem 1997; 5:78.

202. Amann G, Zoubek A, Salzer-Kuntschik M, et al. Relation of neurological marker expression and EWS gene fusion types in MIC2/CD99-positive tumors of the Ewing family. Hum Pathol 1999; 30:1058.

203. Folpe AL, Hill CE, Parham DM, et al. Immunohistochemical detection of FLI-1 protein expression: a study of 132 round cell tumors with emphasis on CD99-positive mimics of Ewing's sarcoma/primitive neuroectodermal tumor. Am J Surg Pathol 2000; 24:1657.

204. Llombart-Bosch A, Navarro S. Immunohistochemical detection of EWS and FLI-1 proteins in Ewing sarcoma and primitive neuroectodermal tumors: comparative analysis with CD99 (MIC-2) expression. Appl Immunohistochem Mol Morphol 2001; 9:255.

205. Rossi S, Orvieto E, Furlanetto A, et al. Utility of the immunohistochemical detection of FLI-1 expression in round cell and vascular neoplasm using a monoclonal antibody. Mod Pathol 2004; 17:547.

206. Janknecht R. EWS-ETS oncoproteins: the linchpins of Ewing tumors. Gene 2005; 363:1.

207. Ricotti E, Fagioli F, Garelli E, et al. c-kit is expressed in soft tissue sarcoma of neuroectodermic origin and its ligand prevents apoptosis of neoplastic cells. Blood 1998; 91:2397.

208. Landuzzi L, De Giovanni C, Nicoletti G, et al. The metastatic ability of Ewing's sarcoma cells is modulated by stem cell factor and by its receptor c-kit. Am J Pathol 2000; 157:2123.

209. Gonzalez I, Andreu EJ, Panizo A, et al. Imatinib inhibits proliferation of Ewing tumor cells mediated by the stem cell factor/KIT receptor pathway, and sensitizes cells to vincristine and doxorubicin-induced apoptosis. Clin Cancer Res 2004; 10:751.

210. Hornick JL, Fletcher CD. Immunohistochemical staining for KIT (CD117) in soft tissue sarcomas is very limited in distribution. Am J Clin Pathol 2002; 117:188.

211. Scotlandi K, Manara MC, Strammiello R, et al. C-kit receptor expression in Ewing's sarcoma: lack of prognostic value but therapeutic targeting opportunities in appropriate conditions. J Clin Oncol 2003; 21:1952.

212. Folpe AL, Goldblum JR, Rubin BP, et al. Morphologic and immunophenotypic diversity in Ewing family tumors: a study of 66 genetically confirmed cases. Am J Surg Pathol 2005; 29:1025.

213. Ladanyi M. EWS-FLI1 and Ewing's sarcoma: recent molecular data and new insights. Cancer Biol Ther 2002; 1:330.

214. Arvand A, Denny CT. Biology of EWS/ETS fusions in Ewing's family tumors. Oncogene 2001; 20:5747.

215. Delattre O, Zucman J, Melot T, et al. The Ewing family of tumors – a subgroup of small-round-cell tumors defined by specific chimeric transcripts. N Engl J Med 1994; 331:294.

216. Delattre O, Zucman J, Plougastel B, et al. Gene fusion with an ETS DNA-binding domain caused by chromosome translocation in human tumours. Nature 1992; 359:162.

217. Im YH, Kim HT, Lee C, et al. EWS-FLI1, EWS-ERG, and EWS-ETV1 oncoproteins of Ewing tumor family all suppress transcription of transforming growth factor beta type II receptor gene. Cancer Res 2000; 60:1536.

218. Jeon IS, Davis JN, Braun BS, et al. A variant Ewing's sarcoma translocation (7;22) fuses the EWS gene to the ETS gene ETV1. Oncogene 1995; 10:1229.

219. Kaneko Y, Kobayashi H, Handa M, et al. EWS-ERG fusion transcript produced by

chromosomal insertion in a Ewing sarcoma. Genes Chromosomes Cancer 1997; 18:228.

220. Peter M, Mugneret F, Aurias A, et al. An EWS/ERG fusion with a truncated N-terminal domain of EWS in a Ewing's tumor. Int J Cancer 1996; 67:339.

221. Mastrangelo T, Modena P, Tornielli S, et al. A novel zinc finger gene is fused to EWS in small round cell tumor. Oncogene 2000; 19:3799.

222. de Alava E, Kawai A, Healey JH, et al. EWS-FLI1 fusion transcript structure is an independent determinant of prognosis in Ewing's sarcoma. J Clin Oncol 1998; 16:1248.

223. Zoubek A, Pfleiderer C, Salzer-Kuntschik M, et al. Variability of EWS chimaeric transcripts in Ewing tumours: a comparison of clinical and molecular data. Br J Cancer 1994; 70:908.

224. Bridge RS, Rajaram V, Dehner LP, et al. Molecular diagnosis of Ewing sarcoma/primitive neuroectodermal tumor in routinely processed tissue: a comparison of two FISH strategies and RT-PCR in malignant round cell tumors. Mod Pathol 2006; 19:1.

225. Qian X, Jin L, Shearer BM, et al. Molecular diagnosis of Ewing's sarcoma/primitive neuroectodermal tumor in formalin-fixed paraffin-embedded tissues by RT-PCR and fluorescence in situ hybridization. Diagn Mol Pathol 2005; 14:23.

226. Brisset S, Schleiermacher G, Peter M, et al. CGH analysis of secondary genetic changes in Ewing tumors: correlation with metastatic disease in a series of 43 cases. Cancer Genet Cytogenet 2001; 130:57.

227. Sandberg AA, Bridge JA. Updates on cytogenetics and molecular genetics of bone and soft tissue tumors: Ewing sarcoma and peripheral primitive neuroectodermal tumors. Cancer Genet Cytogenet 2000; 123:1.

228. Maurici D, Perez-Atayde A, Grier HE, et al. Frequency and implications of chromosome 8 and 12 gains in Ewing sarcoma. Cancer Genet Cytogenet 1998; 100:106.

229. Stark B, Mor C, Jeison M, et al. Additional chromosome 1q aberrations and der(16)t(1;16), correlation to the phenotypic expression and clinical behavior of the Ewing family of tumors. J Neurooncol 1997; 31:3.

230. Ozaki T, Paulussen M, Poremba C, et al. Genetic imbalances revealed by comparative genomic hybridization in Ewing tumors. Genes Chromosomes Cancer 2001; 32:164.

231. Hattinger CM, Rumpler S, Strehl S, et al. Prognostic impact of deletions at 1p36 and numerical aberrations in Ewing tumors. Genes Chromosomes Cancer 1999; 24:243.

232. Parham DM, Hijazi Y, Steinberg SM, et al. Neuroectodermal differentiation in Ewing's sarcoma family of tumors does not predict tumor behavior. Hum Pathol 1999; 30:911.

233. Siebenrock KA, Nascimento AG, Rock MG. Comparison of soft tissue Ewing's sarcoma and peripheral neuroectodermal tumor. Clin Orthop Relat Res 1996; 329:288.

234. Sainati L, Scapinello A, Montaldi A, et al. A mesenchymal chondrosarcoma of a child with the reciprocal translocation (11;22)(q24;q12). Cancer Genet Cytogenet 1993; 71:144.

235. Noguera R, Navarro S, Triche TJ. Translocation (11;22) in small cell osteosarcoma. Cancer Genet Cytogenet 1990; 45:121.

236. Machen SK, Fisher C, Gautam RS, et al. Utility of cytokeratin subsets for distinguishing poorly differentiated synovial sarcoma from peripheral primitive neuroectodermal tumour. Histopathology 1998; 33:501.

237. Jurgens H, Bier V, Harms D, et al. Malignant peripheral neuroectodermal tumors. A retrospective analysis of 42 patients. Cancer 1988; 61:349.

238. Terrier P, Henry-Amar M, Triche TJ, et al. Is neuro-ectodermal differentiation of Ewing's

sarcoma of bone associated with an unfavourable prognosis? Eur J Cancer 1995; 31A:307.

239. Grier HE, Krailo MD, Tarbell NJ, et al. Addition of ifosfamide and etoposide to standard chemotherapy for Ewing's sarcoma and primitive neuroectodermal tumor of bone. N Engl J Med 2003; 348:694.

240. Rodriguez-Galindo C. Pharmacological management of Ewing sarcoma family of tumours. Expert Opin Pharmacother 2004; 5:1257.

241. Rodriguez-Galindo C, Spunt SL, Pappo AS. Treatment of Ewing sarcoma family of tumors: current status and outlook for the future. Med Pediatr Oncol 2003; 40:276.

242. Gururangan S, Marina NM, Luo X, et al. Treatment of children with peripheral primitive neuroectodermal tumor or extraosseous Ewing's tumor with Ewing's-directed therapy. J Pediatr Hematol Oncol 1998; 20:55.

243. Krasin MJ, Davidoff AM, Rodriguez-Galindo C, et al. Definitive surgery and multiagent systemic therapy for patients with localized Ewing sarcoma family of tumors: local outcome and prognostic factors. Cancer 2005; 104:367.

244. Meyers PA, Krailo MD, Ladanyi M, et al. High-dose melphalan, etoposide, total-body irradiation, and autologous stem-cell reconstitution as consolidation therapy for high-risk Ewing's sarcoma does not improve prognosis. J Clin Oncol 2001; 19:2812.

245. Kontny U. Regulation of apoptosis and proliferation in Ewing's sarcoma – opportunities for targeted therapy [review] [114 refs]. Hematol Oncol 2006; 24:14.

246. McAllister NR, Lessnick SL. The potential for molecular therapeutic targets in Ewing's sarcoma. Curr Treat Options Oncol 2005; 6:461.

247. Drabko K, Zawitkowska-Klaczynska J, Wojcik B, et al. Megachemotherapy followed by autologous stem cell transplantation in children with Ewing's sarcoma. Pediatr Transplant 2005; 9:618.

248. Lai R, Navid F, Rodriguez-Galindo C, et al. STAT3 is activated in a subset of the Ewing sarcoma family of tumours. J Pathol 2006; 208:624.

249. Irifune H, Nishimori H, Watanabe G, et al. Aberrant laminin beta3 isoforms downstream of EWS-ETS fusion genes in Ewing family tumors. Cancer Biol Ther 2005; 4:449.

250. Prieur A, Tirode F, Cohen P, et al. EWS/FLI-1 silencing and gene profiling of Ewing cells reveal downstream oncogenic pathways and a crucial role for repression of insulin-like growth factor binding protein 3. Mol Cell Biol 2004; 24:7275.

251. Zwerner JP, May WA. Dominant negative PDGF-C inhibits growth of Ewing family tumor cell lines. Oncogene 2002; 21:3847.

252. Huang HY, Illei PB, Zhao Z, et al. Ewing sarcomas with p53 mutation or p16/p14ARF homozygous deletion: a highly lethal subset associated with poor chemoresponse. J Clin Oncol 2005; 23:548.

253. Fuchs B, Inwards CY, Janknecht R. Vascular endothelial growth factor expression is up-regulated by EWS-ETS oncoproteins and Sp1 and may represent an independent predictor of survival in Ewing's sarcoma. Clin Cancer Res 2004; 10:1344.

254. Lin PP, Brody RI, Hamelin AC, et al. Differential transactivation by alternative EWS-FLI fusion proteins correlates with clinical heterogeneity in Ewing's sarcoma. Cancer Res 1999; 59:1428.

255. Fidelia-Lambert MN, Zhuang Z, Tsokos M. Sensitive detection of rare Ewing's sarcoma cells in peripheral blood by reverse transcriptase polymerase chain reaction. Hum Pathol 1999; 30:78.

256. Baldini EH, Demetri GD, Fletcher CD, et al. Adults with Ewing's sarcoma/primitive neuroectodermal tumor: adverse effect of older age and primary extraosseous disease on outcome. Ann Surg 1999; 230:79.

257. Cangir A, Vietti TJ, Gehan EA, et al. Ewing's sarcoma metastatic at diagnosis. Results and comparisons of two Intergroup Ewing's sarcoma studies. Cancer 1990; 66:887.

258. de Alava E, Antonescu CR, Panizo A, et al. Prognostic impact of P53 status in Ewing sarcoma. Cancer 2000; 89:783.

259. Ginsberg JP, de Alava E, Ladanyi M, et al. EWS-FLI1 and EWS-ERG fusion genes are associated with similar clinical phenotypes of Ewing's sarcoma. J Clin Oncol 1999; 17:1809.

260. Movahedi-Lankarani S, Hruban RH, Westra WH, et al. Primitive neuroectodermal tumors of the pancreas: a report of seven cases of a rare neoplasm. Am J Surg Pathol 2002; 26:1040.

261. O'Sullivan MJ, Perlman EJ, Furman J, et al. Visceral primitive peripheral neuroectodermal tumors: a clinicopathologic and molecular study. Hum Pathol 2001; 32:1109.

262. Jimenez RE, Folpe AL, Lapham RL, et al. Primary Ewing's sarcoma/primitive neuroectodermal tumor of the kidney: a clinicopathologic and immunohistochemical analysis of 11 cases. Am J Surg Pathol 2002; 26:320.

263. Banerjee SS, Eyden BP, McVey RJ, et al. Primary peripheral primitive neuroectodermal tumour of urinary bladder. Histopathology 1997; 30:486.

264. Karseladze AI, Filipova NA, Navarro S, et al. Primitive neuroectodermal tumor of the uterus. A case report. J Reprod Med 2001; 46:845.

265. Kim KJ, Jang BW, Lee SK, et al. A case of peripheral primitive neuroectodermal tumor of the ovary. Int J Gynecol Cancer 2004; 14:370.

266. Maesawa C, Iijima S, Sato N, et al. Esophageal extraskeletal Ewing's sarcoma. Hum Pathol 2002; 33:130.

267. Horie Y, Kato M. Peripheral primitive neuroectodermal tumor of the small bowel mesentery: a case showing perforation at onset. Pathol Int 2000; 50:398.

268. Dedeurwaerdere F, Giannini C, Sciot R, et al. Primary peripheral PNET/Ewing's sarcoma of the dura: a clinicopathologic entity distinct from central PNET. Mod Pathol 2002; 15:673.

269. Simmons MA, Luff DA, Banerjee SS, et al. Peripheral primitive neuroectodermal tumour (pPNET) of the cerebellopontine angle presenting in adult life. J Laryngol Otol 2001; 115:848.

270. Isotalo PA, Agbi C, Davidson B, et al. Primary primitive neuroectodermal tumor of the cauda equina. Hum Pathol 2000; 31:999.

271. Kato K, Kato Y, Ijiri R, et al. Ewing's sarcoma family of tumor arising in the adrenal gland – possible diagnostic pitfall in pediatric pathology: histologic, immunohistochemical, ultrastructural, and molecular study. Hum Pathol 2001; 32:1012.

272. Charney DA, Charney JM, Ghali VS, et al. Primitive neuroectodermal tumor of the myocardium: a case report, review of the literature, immunohistochemical, and ultrastructural study. Hum Pathol 1996; 27:1365.

273. Deb RA, Desai SB, Amonkar PP, et al. Primary primitive neuroectodermal tumour of the parotid gland. Histopathology 1998; 33:375.

Olfactory neuroblastoma (esthesioneuroblastoma)

274. Berger L, Luc R. L'esthesioneuroepithelioma olfactif. Bull Assoc Fr Etude Cancer 1924; 13:410.

275. Mills SE, Frierson HF Jr. Olfactory neuroblastoma. A clinicopathologic study of 21 cases. Am J Surg Pathol 1985; 9:317.

276. Mills SE. Neuroectodermal neoplasms of the head and neck with emphasis on neuroendocrine carcinomas. Mod Pathol 2002; 15:264.

277. Bradley PJ, Jones NS, Robertson I. Diagnosis and management of esthesioneuroblastoma. Curr Opin Otolaryngol Head Neck Surg 2003; 11:112.

278. Banerjee AK, Sharma BS, Vashista RK, et al. Intracranial olfactory neuroblastoma: evidence for olfactory epithelial origin. J Clin Pathol 1992; 45:299.

279. Hirose T, Scheithauer BW, Lopes MB, et al. Olfactory neuroblastoma. An immunohistochemical, ultrastructural, and flow cytometric study. Cancer 1995; 76:4.

280. Broich G, Pagliari A, Ottaviani F. Esthesioneuroblastoma: a general review of the cases published since the discovery of the tumour in 1924. Anticancer Res 1997; 17:2683.

281. Mishima Y, Nagasaki E, Terui Y, et al. Combination chemotherapy (cyclophosphamide, doxorubicin, and vincristine with continuous-infusion cisplatin and etoposide) and radiotherapy with stem cell support can be beneficial for adolescents and adults with esthesioneuroblastoma. Cancer 2004; 101:1437.

282. Kumar M, Fallon RJ, Hill JS, et al. Esthesioneuroblastoma in children. J Pediatr Hematol Oncol 2002; 24:482.

283. Freeman SR, Mitra S, Malik TH, et al. Expression of somatostatin receptors in arginine vasopressin hormone-secreting olfactory neuroblastoma – report of two cases. Rhinology 2005; 43:61.

284. Ferlito A, Rinaldo A, Rhys-Evans PH. Contemporary clinical commentary: esthesioneuroblastoma: an update on management of the neck. Laryngoscope 2003; 113:1935.

285. Das S, Kirsch CF. Imaging of lumps and bumps in the nose: a review of sinonasal tumours. Cancer Imaging 2005; 5:167.

286. Gaudin PB, Rosai J. Florid vascular proliferation associated with neural and neuroendocrine neoplasms. A diagnostic clue and potential pitfall. Am J Surg Pathol 1995; 19:642.

287. Miura K, Mineta H, Yokota N, et al. Olfactory neuroblastoma with epithelial and endocrine differentiation transformed into ganglioneuroma after chemoradiotherapy. Pathol Int 2001; 51:942.

288. Devaney K, Wenig BM, Abbondanzo SL. Olfactory neuroblastoma and other round cell lesions of the sinonasal region. Mod Pathol 1996; 9:658.

289. Argani P, Perez-Ordonez B, Xiao H, et al. Olfactory neuroblastoma is not related to the Ewing family of tumors: absence of EWS/FLI1 gene fusion and MIC2 expression. Am J Surg Pathol 1998; 22:391.

290. Min KW. Usefulness of electron microscopy in the diagnosis of "small" round cell tumors of the sinonasal region. Ultrastruct Pathol 1995; 19:347.

291. Vartanian RK. Olfactory neuroblastoma: an immunohistochemical, ultrastructural, and flow cytometric study. Cancer 1996; 77:1957.

292. Szymas J, Wolf G, Kowalczyk D, et al. Olfactory neuroblastoma: detection of genomic imbalances by comparative genomic hybridization. Acta Neurochir (Wien) 1997; 139:839.

293. Jin Y, Mertens F, Arheden K, et al. Karyotypic features of malignant tumors of the nasal cavity and paranasal sinuses. Int J Cancer 1995; 60:637.

294. Bockmuhl U, You X, Pacyna-Gengelbach M, et al. CGH pattern of esthesioneuroblastoma and their metastases. Brain Pathol 2004; 14:158.

295. Cavazzana AO, Navarro S, Noguera R, et al. Olfactory neuroblastoma is not a neuroblastoma but is related to primitive neuroectodermal tumor (PNET). Prog Clin Biol Res 1988; 271:463.

296. Mezzelani A, Tornielli S, Minoletti F, et al. Esthesioneuroblastoma is not a member of the primitive peripheral neuroectodermal tumour-Ewing's group. Br J Cancer 1999; 81:586.

297. Lund VJ, Howard D, Wei W, et al. Olfactory neuroblastoma: past, present, and future? Laryngoscope 2003; 113:502.

298. Constantinidis J, Steinhart H, Koch M, et al. Olfactory neuroblastoma: the University of Erlangen-Nuremberg experience 1975–2000. Otolaryngol Head Neck Surg 2004; 130:567.

299. Diaz EM Jr, Johnigan RH 3rd, Pero C, et al. Olfactory neuroblastoma: the 22-year experience at one comprehensive cancer center. Head Neck 2005; 27:138.

300. Kadish S, Goodman M, Wang CC. Olfactory neuroblastoma. A clinical analysis of 17 cases. Cancer 1976; 37:1571.

301. Yuen AP, Fan YW, Fung CF, et al. Endoscopic-assisted cranionasal resection of olfactory neuroblastoma. Head Neck 2005; 27:488.

302. Unger F, Haselsberger K, Walch C, et al. Combined endoscopic surgery and radiosurgery as treatment modality for olfactory neuroblastoma (esthesioneuroblastoma). Acta Neurochir (Wien) 2005; 147:595.

303. Casiano RR, Numa WA, Falquez AM. Endoscopic resection of esthesioneuroblastoma. Am J Rhinol 2001; 15:271.

304. Kim DW, Jo YH, Kim JH, et al. Neoadjuvant etoposide, ifosfamide, and cisplatin for the treatment of olfactory neuroblastoma. Cancer 2004; 101:2257.

305. Cohen ZR, Marmor E, Fuller GN, et al. Misdiagnosis of olfactory neuroblastoma. Neurosurg Focus 2002; 12:e3.

PARAGANGLIOMA

The paraganglia are widely dispersed collections of specialized neural crest cells that arise in association with the segmental or collateral autonomic ganglia throughout the body. This system includes the adrenal medulla, chemoreceptors (i.e., carotid and aortic bodies), vagal body, and small groups of cells associated with the thoracic, intra-abdominal, and retroperitoneal ganglia. Although the paraganglia are closely related structures, the present trend is to regard them as a large group of embryologically similar structures that manifest certain anatomic differences and functional specializations. For example, the adrenal medulla is a neuroendocrine organ that secretes large amounts of epinephrine and norepinephrine; its cells are chromaffin-positive, and tumors arising from this organ are often functionally active. On the other hand, the carotid and aortic bodies are chemoreceptors specialized to detect changes in the blood pH and oxygen tension. Although catecholamine storage can be documented in their chief cells by sensitive fluorometric techniques, their cells are usually chromaffin-negative, and tumors arising from these structures are usually nonfunctional.

According to Glenner and Grimley,[1] the extra-adrenal paraganglion system can be divided into several anatomic groups (Figs 32–1, 32–2). The *branchiomeric paraganglia* arise in association with arterial vessels and cranial nerves of the head and neck region, including the jugulotympanic, intercarotid (carotid body), subclavian, laryngeal, coronary, aorticopulmonary, and orbital paraganglia. Their cells are generally chromaffin-negative and are arranged in small cohesive nests (zellballen). Carotid body tumors epitomize the neoplasms arising from branchiomeric paraganglia.

The *intravagal paraganglia* are located in the perineurium of the vagus nerve, usually at the level of the jugular or nodose ganglion. The tumors arising from these structures are histologically and cytochemically indistinguishable from those arising in the branchiomeric paraganglia. In fact, those arising from the jugular ganglion and invading the temporal bone may be difficult to distinguish from glomus jugulare tumors.

Aorticosympathetic paraganglia arise in association with the sympathetic nervous system, particularly at the bifurcation of the aorta (Figs 32–2, 32–3, 32–4). They may also be found along the courses of the iliac and femoral vessels and in the thorax. Tumors arising from these structures vary in chromaffinicity, functional activity, and histologic appearance. Some resemble branchiomeric paragangliomas, whereas others may be virtually indistinguishable from adrenal pheochromocytomas.

The nomenclature of paragangliomas is confusing, and before the work of Glenner and Grimley[1] it was poorly standardized. Early authors classified paragangliomas according to the chromaffin reaction (i.e., chromaffin and nonchromaffin paragangliomas) on the assumption that catecholamine-secreting tumors such as pheochromocytomas would be chromaffin-positive and nonfunctional tumors chromaffin-negative. The chromaffin reaction is an unreliable procedure that does not always correspond to functional activity and is not specific for catecholamines. Moreover, nonfunctional tumors such as carotid body paragangliomas synthesize and store small amounts of catecholamine, further underscoring the fact that the chromaffin reaction is at best only a crude means of classifying this group of tumors. The most rational approach is that paragangliomas be named according to their anatomic site and further modified depending on whether functional activity is documented clinically. Thus, the common nonfunctioning carotid body tumor would be designated "carotid body paraganglioma, nonfunctional." This nomenclature is used herein.

CAROTID BODY PARAGANGLIOMA

The normal carotid body lies on the posterior aspect of the bifurcation of the common carotid artery, usually buried in the adventitia of the vessel.[2] It is a specialized chemoreceptor that monitors changes in the arterial oxygen tension and pH of the blood and, in turn,

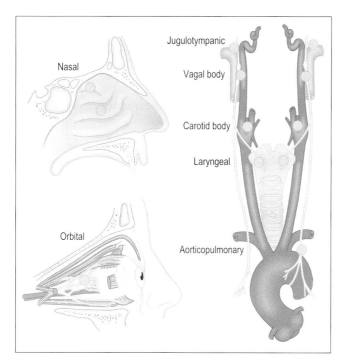

FIGURE 32–1 Distribution of branchiomeric paraganglia. (Modified from Lack EE, Cubilla AL, Woodruff JM, et al. Paragangliomas of the head and neck region: a clinical study of 69 patients. Cancer 1977; 39:397.)

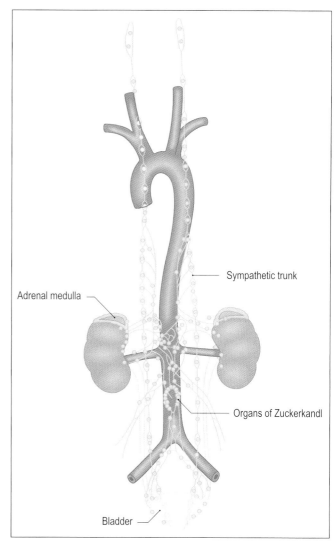

FIGURE 32–2 Distribution of aorticosympathetic paraganglia. (Modified from Glenner CG, Grimley PM. Tumors of the extra-adrenal paraganglion system [including chemoreceptors]. In: Atlas of tumor pathology, Fascicle 9, 2nd Series. Washington, DC: Armed Forces Institute of Pathology; 1974.)

influences in a reflex fashion the rate and depth of respiration and to a lesser extent the heart rate. It is among the largest of the paraganglia and can usually be identified during routine autopsy as a small red body approximately the size of a rice grain. It may assume a size of several millimeters in persons with chronic lung disease or those subjected to the chronic hypoxemia at high altitudes as a result of compensatory hyperplasia.

The carotid body receives its blood supply from the common or external carotid and its innervation primarily from sensory (afferent) fibers of the glossopharyngeal (IX) nerve, with lesser contributions from the vagus (X) nerve and superior cervical ganglion of the sympathetic nervous system. The organ is made up of round or polygonal cells (chief cells) surrounded by delicate sustentacular cells, an arrangement that creates the nest-like (zellballen) appearance. The chief cells have small dense-core granules measuring 100–200 nm, which are the sites of norepinephrine storage.

The exact function of the chief cells is unclear, although it is likely they influence the level of activity of the autonomic nerves in the organ. The sustentacular cells are modified Schwann cells that conduct nerves to their synaptic terminations on the chief cells. Although the chief cells and sustentacular cells are believed to be of neural crest origin, the supporting structures of the body are presumably of mesenchymal origin.

The carotid body tumor is the most common of the extra-adrenal paragangliomas, accounting for about 60% of all head and neck paragangliomas.[3–5] The overall incidence of these tumors is low, but paragangliomas are considerably more common in areas of high altitude such as Peru, Mexico, and Colorado, suggesting prolonged hyperplasia of the organ may eventually progress to neoplasia. Men are affected about twice as often as women in most series, except those reported at high altitudes, where women predominate.[3] Usually, the tumor occurs in patients between the ages of 40 and 60 years; occasional cases in children have been reported, and such cases may herald a germline mutation in the succinate dehydrogenase gene (SDH), especially *SDHB*.[6]

The most common sign is a painless, slowly enlarging mass located in the upper portion of the neck below the angle of the jaw. The tumor is usually movable from side to side but not in a vertical direction. A bruit may be

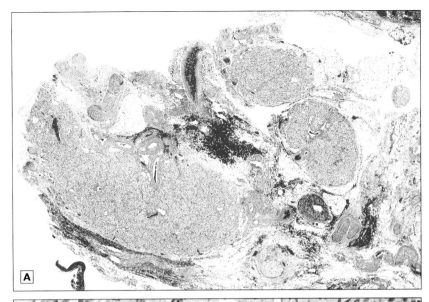

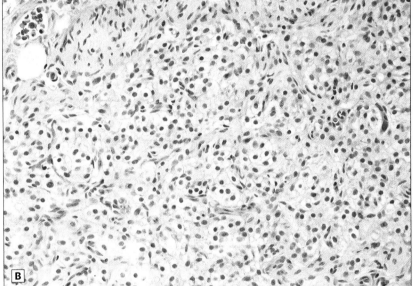

FIGURE 32–3 (A, B) Organ of Zuckerkandl (aorticosympathetic paraganglia) removed at autopsy from a child.

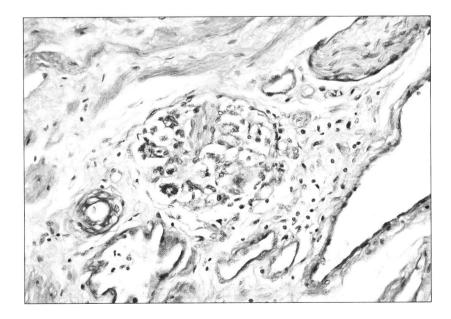

FIGURE 32–4 Normal paraganglion located in association with a small autonomic nerve in the retroperitoneum. Pigment, probably lipochrome, is present in some of the paraganglion cells.

audible over the tumor, and pressure on the tumor may cause an increase in the heart rate. Large tumors encroaching on nearby structures cause a variety of associated symptoms. Lesions impinging on the hypopharynx cause hoarseness, whereas involvement of the vagus or sympathetic nerve results in vocal cord paralysis or Horner syndrome. One to 3% of carotid body tumors are functional and result in clinical hypertension.[7] In the past, the level of accurate preoperative diagnosis was extremely low, and these tumors were often confused with tuberculous lymphadenitis, branchial cleft cyst, metastatic carcinoma, carotid artery aneurysm, schwannoma, or lymphoma. However, newer radiographic techniques have led to a more accurate preoperative diagnosis. Magnetic resonance imaging (MRI) represents the most important imaging technique for the evaluation and characterization of carotid body tumors.[5,8] This modality, along with angiography and functional imaging, allows for a thorough evaluation of the relationship of the tumor to the surrounding soft tissue and vascular structures. Arteriography assesses the vascular architecture of the tumor and may provide additional information on multicentric lesions not detectable by MRI.[5,8] Arteriography may also

be useful therapeutically since it allows for embolization of the dominant blood supply to the tumor prior to surgery, thus reducing the vascularity of the lesion and risk of hemorrhage (Fig. 32–5). Other techniques including indium pentetreotide scanning[9] and octreotide scintigraphy,[10] and color-coded Doppler sonography[11,12] may also be useful in the evaluation of these tumors.

Familial and multifocal tumors

Paragangliomas have a tendency to occur multifocally. Approximately 10% of sporadic tumors are multifocal, but up to 40% of familial lesions are multifocal.[13] Up to 10–20% of carotid body paragangliomas are familial, and such lesions are far more likely to be multifocal, bilateral, and present at an earlier age.[14] Most familial paragangliomas arise in the carotid bodies, but given the tendency of familial paragangliomas to be multifocal, some patients have tumors involving the carotid body, glomus jugulare, or other anatomic sites. Evaluation of numerous kindred suggests familial cases are inherited with an autosomal dominant pattern of inheritance with incomplete penetrance and genomic imprinting.[15,16] Germline mutations

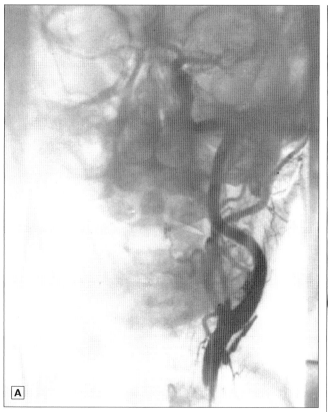
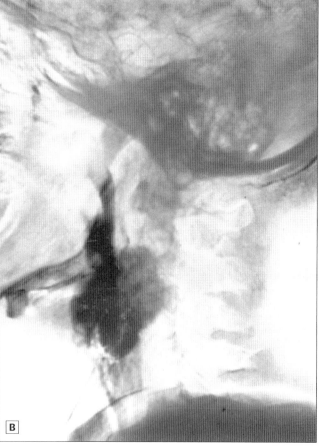

FIGURE 32–5 (A) Carotid angiography demonstrates widening and lateral displacement of the carotid bifurcation point caused by a carotid body tumor. **(B)** Tumor blush is evident during a later phase of the study.

of the succinate dehydrogenase family of genes, particularly *SDHD* and *SDHB*, are a major cause of familial paraganglioma and pheochromocytoma.[17-20] Mutations in these genes appear to play a minor role in sporadic head and neck paragangliomas.[20-22]

Paragangliomas may also arise in other hereditary settings, including patients with von Hippel-Lindau syndrome, multiple endocrine neoplasia type 2, neurofibromatosis type 1 and associated with gastrointestinal stromal tumors (Table 32–1).[23]

Gross and microscopic findings

Carotid body paragangliomas typically lie in the bifurcation of the common carotid artery and may be only partially attached to the vessel or may completely encase it. The intimacy of this relationship is a major factor in determining the surgical resectability of a given tumor. Most carotid body tumors have a lobular, beefy red to brown appearance and measure a few centimeters in diameter (Fig. 32–6). Hemorrhage and fibrosis are seen in some cases. The tumor is surrounded by a thin or incomplete capsule of connective tissue that is periodically penetrated by fine nerve branches. In the central portion of the neoplasm, the round or polygonal epithelioid cells are arranged in small nests (zellballen) around an elaborate vasculature (Fig. 32–7). In contrast to the normal gland, the zellballen of the carotid body tumor are larger and more irregular in shape, and the cells comprising the tumor are usually larger and more atypical than normal chief cells. Their centrally located nuclei have finely clumped chromatin, and the cytoplasm has either an amphophilic or granular eosinophilic

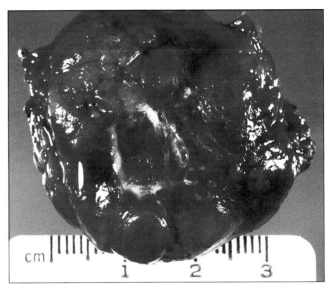

FIGURE 32–6 Cut section of a carotid body tumor. (Courtesy of Dr. Thomas J. Whelan, Honolulu, HI.)

TABLE 32–1	SYNDROMES WHICH INCLUDE PARAGANGLIOMA AS A COMPONENT	
Syndrome	**Gene locus/gene**	**Inheritance**
Familial paraganglioma	11q23 (*SDHD*)	Autosomal dominant
Familial paraganglioma	11q13.1 (*SDHC*)	Autosomal dominant
Familial paraganglioma	1q22-23 (*SDHB*)	Autosomal dominant
MEN 2A and 2B	10q11.2 (*RET*)	Autosomal dominant
von Hippel-Lindau disease	3p26 (*VAL*)	Autosomal dominant
Carney triad	unknown	Sporadic
Neurofibromatosis type 1	17q11.2 (*NF1*)	Autosomal dominant

Modified from: Perry CG, Young WF, McWhinney SR, et al. Am J Surg Pathol 2006; 30:42.

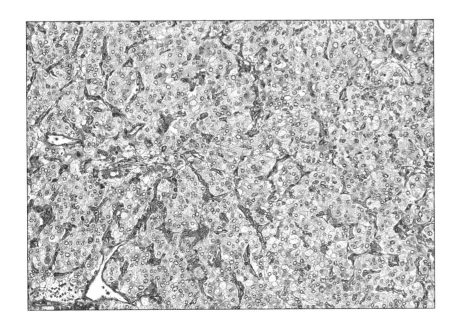

FIGURE 32–7 Medium-power view of a carotid body paraganglioma with a zellballen pattern.

appearance (Fig. 32–8). The cytoplasm of one cell occasionally envelops that of an adjacent cell, a phenomenon termed "cell embracing." Frequently, shrinkage or retraction of the cells away from the tiny vessels results in loss of the classic zellballen pattern. In these regions the cells seem to be arranged in short ribbons or cords similar to those in a carcinoid tumor, in pseudoglands as in an adenocarcinoma, or in pseudorosettes as in a neuroblastic tumor. Paragangliomas with these patterns are often misdiagnosed, a fact that emphasizes the need for ancillary diagnostic tests. Another peculiar but frequent artifact of the carotid body tumor is the foamy or vacuolar cytoplasmic change of the chief cell (Fig. 32–9). The cytoplasm contains one or more clear vacuoles that indent the small pyknotic nucleus in the same fashion that fat droplets displace or indent the nucleus of the lipoblast. It is possible to distinguish these cells from true lipoblasts by their close association with other cells having the conventional features of chief cells. Markedly sclerotic carotid body tumors have little or no nesting pattern, and small aggregates of cells lie isolated in the collagenized matrix (Fig. 32–10).[24] Spindling of the chief cell ("sarcomatoid" pattern) occurs in a small number of cases and does not appear to affect the prognosis adversely.[4] Occasionally, carotid body tumors are mistaken for vascular tumors (Fig. 32–11), specifically hemangiopericytomas, if the vessels become ectatic and compress the intervening chief cells (Figs 32–12, 32–13).

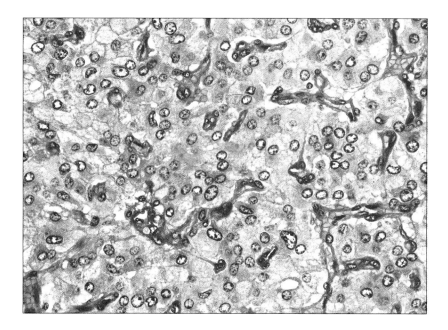

FIGURE 32–8 High-power view of a carotid body paraganglioma composed of nests of uniform round cells surrounding a delicate vasculature.

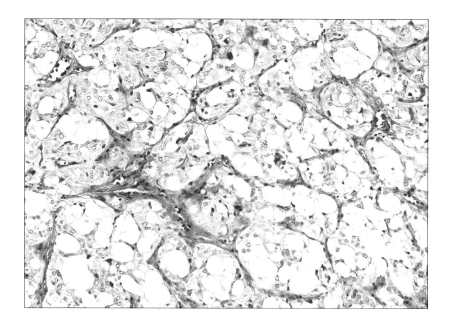

FIGURE 32–9 Vacuolated cells in a carotid body paraganglioma, some of which resemble lipoblasts.

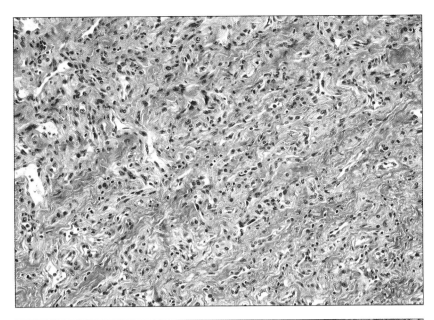

FIGURE 32–10 Hyalinized carotid body paraganglioma with isolated neoplastic cells surrounded by dense fibrous stroma.

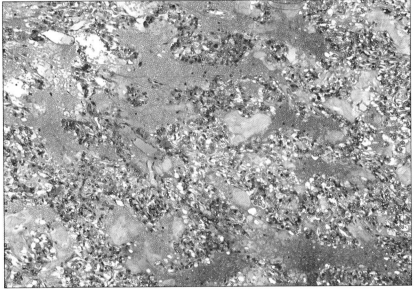

FIGURE 32–11 Carotid body paraganglioma with marked congestion of vessels simulating a vascular neoplasm.

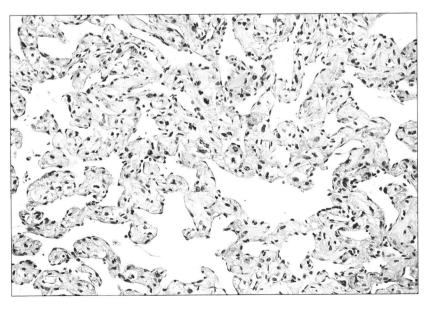

FIGURE 32–12 Paraganglioma with ectatic vasculature simulating the appearance of a hemangiopericytoma.

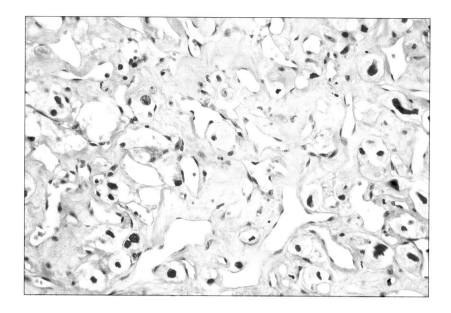

FIGURE 32–13 High-power view of a hyalinized carotid body paraganglioma with a hemangiopericytoma-like vasculature.

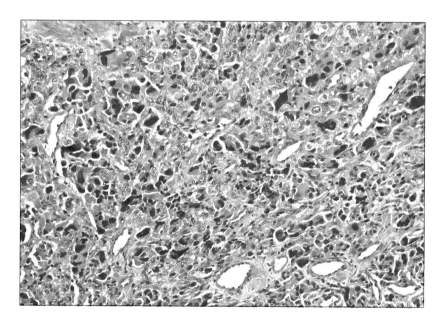

FIGURE 32–14 Malignant carotid body tumor composed of broad sheets of pleomorphic cells with rare mitotic figures.

Malignant carotid body tumors

It is usually difficult to recognize the potentially metastasizing carotid body tumor because many are virtually devoid of histologically malignant features. A few, however, have atypical features that we believe warrant a histologic diagnosis of malignancy. These tumors are characterized by extremely large zellballen, which blend into broad sheets composed of pleomorphic cells with mitotic figures (Fig. 32–14). Focal necrosis is usually present in the zellballen, and vascular invasion may also be documented. Tumors with these features are uncommon, so an outright diagnosis of malignancy is infrequent. It should be emphasized that nuclear pleomorphism ("random atypia") and giant cell formation are common findings in benign carotid body tumors (Figs 32–15,

32–16) and should not be regarded as evidence sufficient to declare the lesion malignant.

Special staining and other procedures

In the past, the chromaffin reaction, based on the observation that chromic acid oxidizes catecholamines (i.e., norepinephrine, epinephrine) and indoleamines (i.e., serotonin) to a brown polymer, was used to identify tissue containing catecholamines. As indicated by Glenner and Grimley,[1] it is an insensitive, non-specific, capricious method for demonstrating catecholamines. It is usually invalidated by prior formalin fixation, excessive washing, or dehydration of the tissue; and it fails to detect small amounts of catecholamine. Moreover, it does not invari-

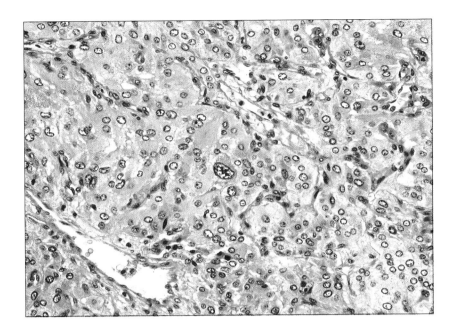

FIGURE 32-15 Rare atypical cell found in an otherwise typical carotid body paraganglioma.

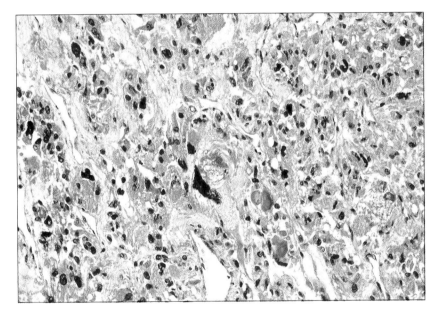

FIGURE 32-16 Carotid body paraganglioma containing scattered atypical cells with smudgy nuclear chromatin.

ably identify tissues that presumably have large amounts of this substance, possibly because of anoxic loss of the biogenic amine, low concentration of the substance in a given cell, or differences in the protein envelope surrounding the compound. Although both the normal carotid body and carotid body paraganglioma contain small amounts of catecholamines, the chromaffin reaction is not sensitive enough to detect these quantities. Consequently, with few exceptions, carotid body tumors are chromaffin-negative.

Immunohistochemical findings

With optimally fixed material, neuron-specific enolase, synaptophysin, neurofilament protein, and chromogranin (Fig. 32–17) can be demonstrated in the chief cells

of most, if not all, branchiomeric paragangliomas.[25,26] In addition, the delicate sustentacular network can be elegantly demonstrated using antibodies to S-100 protein (Fig. 32–18), and in a few instances these same cells coexpress glial fibrillary acidic protein. A variety of other polypeptides (enkephalin, neuropeptide Y, serotonin, gastrin, substance P, bombesin) can also be demonstrated in chief cells,[27] but the immunologic profile seems to vary slightly, depending on the type of paraganglioma (Table 32–2).

Ultrastructural findings

By electron microscopy, the predominant cell resembles the normal chief cell and is round or polyhedral and closely interdigitates with other cells by means of

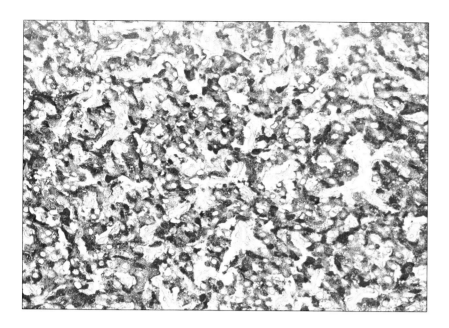

FIGURE 32–17 Diffuse immunostaining for chromogranin A in a carotid body paraganglioma.

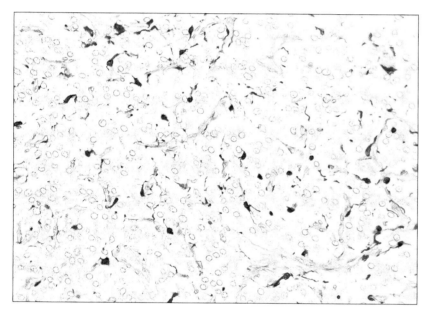

FIGURE 32–18 Paraganglioma with a delicate sustentacular network outlined by the immunostain for S-100 protein.

TABLE 32–2	IMMUNOHISTOCHEMICAL FINDINGS IN PARAGANGLIOMAS
Substance	**% positive (n = 99)**
Neuron-specific enolase	100
Leu-enkephalin	76
Met-enkephalin	75
Somatostatin	67
Pancreatic polypeptide	51
Vasoactive intestinal peptide	43
Substance P	31
Adrenocorticotropic hormone	28
Calcitonin	23
Bombesin	15
Neurotensin	12

From Linnoila RI, Lack EE, Steinberg SM, et al. Decreased expression of neuropeptides in malignant paragangliomas: an immunohistochemical study. Hum Pathol 1988; 19:47.

intercellular junctions.[28] The number of ribosomes and mitochondria vary from cell to cell. The hallmark of the cell is the presence of small dense-core granules measuring 100–200 nm in diameter (Fig. 32–19) that represent sites of catecholamine storage. Sustentacular cells, which have elongated cell processes, are usually not demonstrable by electron microscopy in carotid body tumors.[29] The number of nerve fibers is markedly reduced, compared to the normal carotid body and, if present, do not bear the normal relation to chief cells.

Behavior and treatment

Most carotid body tumors are clinically benign and are cured if total excision can be accomplished at the time of the initial surgery. A small number of patients develop

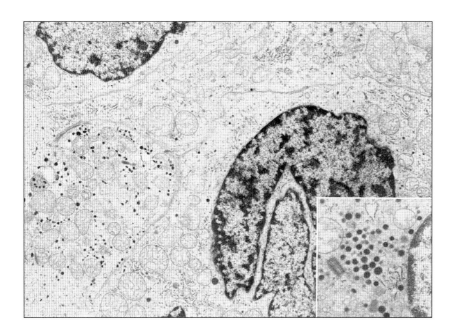

FIGURE 32–19 Electron micrograph of a paraganglioma illustrating closely apposed cells characterized by small dense-core granules **(inset)**. (From Taxy JB, Battifora H. The electron microscope in the diagnosis of soft tissue tumors. In: Trump B, Jones RT, eds. Diagnostic electron microscopy. New York: Wiley; 1980.)

metastases. Patients who develop local tumor recurrence or who have untreated tumors of long duration seem to be at greatest risk for this complication. The incidence of metastasis is estimated at 6–9%.[30] The incidence of "malignancy," reported as 50% from an early study at the Mayo Clinic, was based on an evaluation of histologic features alone and was not borne out by subsequent follow-up information.[31]

The most common site of metastasis is the regional lymph nodes, and the remainder occur at distant sites, particularly lung and bone. Of 51 cases of malignant head and neck paragangliomas extracted from the National Cancer Database diagnosed between 1985 and 1996, 68.6% had metastases confined to regional lymph nodes and 34.4% of patients had distant metastases.[32] Typically, there is a long interval between the time of diagnosis and the appearance of metastasis, and as such, extended follow-up care is advisable.

Technologic advances in vascular surgery and anesthesia now make it possible to resect more carotid body tumors with fewer complications than previously.[8,33] Bilateral carotid arteriography is advisable before surgery to document the extent of the lesion, determine the presence of a contralateral lesion, and assess the degree of collateral cerebral blood flow should ligation of the carotid artery become necessary. Functional activity should be excluded by means of preoperative catecholamine levels. Patients with functional tumors should be premedicated in the same fashion as patients with adrenal pheochromocytomas.[33]

Localized lesions are easily removed by subadventitial dissection of the carotid artery with preservation of the entire system. More extensive lesions that wrap themselves around the vessel may require resection of the

vessel with grafting.[34] Selection of patients for the latter procedure is usually based on several factors, including patient age, degree of histologic aggressiveness, and whether basic functions such as swallowing or breathing are compromised. The most common complication of surgery is damage to cranial nerves.[5,30] A small number of patients with bilateral tumors develop postoperative baroreceptor failure and hypertension secondary to bilateral loss of carotid sinus function.[35] Extensive intraoperative blood loss can be significantly reduced by preoperative tumor embolization.[36,37] Radiotherapy has been advocated for larger tumors where resection would result in significant morbidity and for metastases.[38]

JUGULOTYMPANIC PARAGANGLIOMA (GLOMUS JUGULARE TUMOR)

Paragangliomas involving the temporal bone and specifically the middle ear take their origin from the paraganglia that follow the auricular branch of the vagus nerve or the tympanic branch of the glossopharyngeal nerve or those related to the bulb of the jugular vein. Although it is conventional to refer to these tumors collectively as glomus jugulare tumors, some prefer to designate the tumors involving the middle ear as glomus tympanicum and to reserve the term glomus jugulare for those that grow upward from the jugular bulb,[39–41] given the differences in surgical approaches. In some cases, particularly those of long duration, it is difficult to define the origin of the tumor.

Paraganglioma is the most common neoplasm of the middle ear, and those in the temporal bone represent the second most common type of extra-adrenal paraganglioma. Most occur in women, and the peak incidence is during the fifth decade.[42] The manner of presentation depends on the rate of growth and the location. Those that arise in the temporal bone usually extend laterally, eventually presenting as a mass in the middle ear or the external auditory canal. In such patients the initial symptoms develop early and include dizziness, pulsating tinnitus, and conductive hearing loss. The degree of hearing loss is directly related to the extent of invasion of the labyrinth. Usually after several years, discoloration of the tympanic membrane or a friable hemorrhagic mass in the auditory canal appears. Often an aural polyp, cholesteatoma, or vascular tumor is erroneously diagnosed.[42] Tumors of the jugular bulb, in contrast, grow upward, enlarging the jugular foramen and producing radiographically characteristic crescentic erosions of the bone crest between the jugular vein and carotid artery.[43] Although these tumors also involve the middle ear, they often, in addition, extend to the base of the brain, causing palsies of the cranial nerves in almost 40% of patients.[33,44] Additional studies utilizing computed tomography (CT), MRI, and angiography are useful for determining the size and extent of the lesion, possible synchronous lesions, the extent of intracranial extension, and for assessing the relation of the tumor to major vessels.[45–47]

The incidence of overt functional activity is estimated at 1% in jugulotympanic paragangliomas.[48] One particularly striking case was reported in which the patient experienced cyclic changes in blood pressure at 10- to 17-minute intervals associated with increased norepinephrine levels.[49] Intraoperative manipulation can rarely give rise to a hypertensive crisis.[43] Jackson et al. reported an increased incidence of perioperative gastrointestinal complications, including cholecystitis and pancreatitis, possibly related to the production of cholecystokinin.[50]

Histologically, these tumors are virtually identical to carotid body tumors. They are usually arranged in a zellballen configuration, although the zellballen are smaller and less uniform than those of the carotid body tumor (Figs 32–20, 32–21). They are usually highly vascular tumors, a feature that has often led to the mistaken diagnosis of hemangioma when biopsy specimens of these tumors are obtained from the external auditory canal. Typically, the tumors are chromaffin-negative, although argyrophilic granules can be demonstrated by means of the Grimelius stain. The immunohistochemical and ultrastructural findings are identical to those seen in carotid body tumors.

The behavior and treatment of jugulotympanic paragangliomas can be most accurately assessed by clinical stage. The Fisch classification[51] combines glomus tympanicum and jugulare tumors (Table 32–3), whereas the Glascock/Jackson classification systems separate these two groups, given the differences in surgical approach depending on site (Tables 32–4, 32–5).[52,53] For patients with surgically curable tumors, the type of operation performed is in turn dependent on tumor site, tumor size, and the relation of the tumor to major vessels (transcanal tympanotomy, postauricular approach, skull base approach, infratemporal fossa approach).[54]

The clinical course of paragangliomas arising in these locations is usually benign, although some patients develop metastatic disease. In the study by Brown,[55] 138 of the 150 patients with low-stage tumors were alive without disease at 10 years. In contrast, 14 of 81 patients with higher-stage disease died as a direct result of their tumor. In only two of 231 patients did metastasis develop, one to the lung and one to the liver. Johnstone et al. reviewed 20 jugulare tympanic paragangliomas that produced metastasis and found the common metastatic sites to be the lung (nine cases), vertebra or bone (six cases),

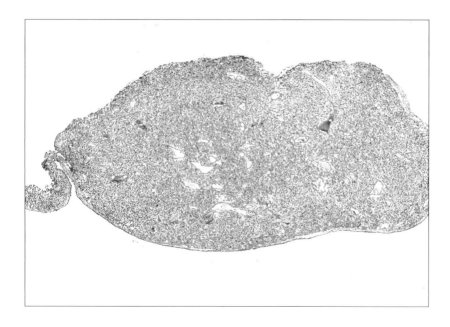

FIGURE 32–20 Low-power view of a jugulotympanic paraganglioma.

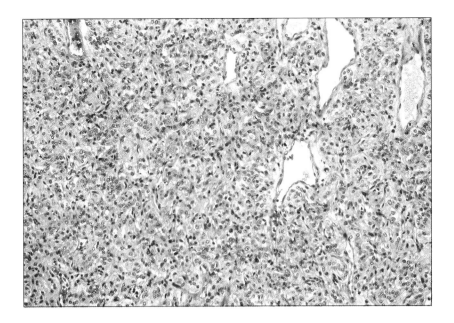

FIGURE 32–21 Jugulotympanic paraganglioma with the characteristic zellballen arrangement of cells similar to that seen in carotid body tumors.

TABLE 32–3	FISCH CLASSIFICATION FOR PARAGANGLIOMAS OF THE GLOMUS TYMPANICUM AND GLOMUS JUGULARE	
Type	**Criteria**	
A	Tumor limited to the middle ear cleft (typanicum)	
B	Tumor limited to the tympanomastoid area with no bone destruction in the infralabyrinthine compartment of the temporal bone	
C	Tumor involving the infralabyrinthine compartment of the temporal bone	
C1	Jugular foramen and jugular bulb involvement	
C2	Vertical portion of carotid canal	
C3	Horizontal portion of carotid canal	
D1	Tumor with intracranial extension <2 cm in diameter	
D2	Tumor with intracranial extension >2 cm in diameter	

From Oldring D, Fisch U. Glomus tumors of the temporal region: surgical therapy. Am J Otol 1979; 1:7.

TABLE 32–5	GLASCOCK/JACKSON CLASSIFICATION OF PARAGANGLIOMAS OF THE GLOMUS JUGULARE	
Type	**Criteria**	
I	Small tumor involving the jugular bulb, middle ear, and mastoid	
II	Tumor extending into the internal auditory canal (± intracranial extension)	
III	Tumor extending into the petrous apex (± intracranial extension)	
IV	Tumor extending beyond the petrous apex into the clivus or infratemporal fossa (± intracranial extension)	

From Jackson CG. Skull base surgery. Am J Otol 1981; 3:161.

and liver (four cases). Only three of the 20 tumors produced metastasis in regional lymph nodes.[56]

TABLE 32–4	GLASCOCK/JACKSON CLASSIFICATION FOR PARAGANGLIOMAS OF THE GLOMUS TYMPANICUM	
Type	**Criteria**	
I	Small mass limited to the promontory	
II	Tumor completely filling the middle ear space	
III	Tumor filling the middle ear and extending into the mastoid	
IV	Tumor filling the middle ear, extending into the mastoid or through the tympanic membrane to fill the external auditory canal; may also extend anteriorly to the internal carotid artery	

From Jackson CG. Skull base surgery. Am J Otol 1981; 3:161.

VAGAL PARAGANGLIOMA (VAGAL BODY TUMOR)

Vagal paragangliomas account for less than 5% of all head and neck paragangliomas, making it the third most common paraganglioma of the head and neck after carotid body and glomus jugulare tumors.[57,58] These tumors arise from small dispersed collections of paraganglia that follow the cervical course of the vagus nerve, particularly at the level of the jugular and nodose ganglia. These paraganglia usually lie just underneath the perineurium but occasionally are embedded in the substance of the nerve. Consequently, vagal body tumors develop as high cervical masses between the mastoid process and the angle of the jaw in the parapharyngeal space. The close relation with the nerves at the base of the brain results in neurologic symptoms, including weakness of the tongue, vocal cord paralysis, hoarseness, and in some cases Horner syndrome.[59,60] Rarely are these tumors functional.[61] Like glomus jugulare tumors, these lesions are more frequent in women than in men, and multifocal tumors are found in about 10–15% of patients. They can be clearly distinguished from carotid body tumors arteriographically because they usually lie above the carotid bifurcation, causing anterior displacement of the vessels without widening of the bifurcation point. At surgery the tumor is usually wrapped around the nerve. Occasionally, the nerve fibers are splayed over the tumor, presumably in cases where the lesion arises from intravagal paraganglia.[62]

Histologically, vagal body paragangliomas are similar to carotid body tumors, except they are often traversed by dense fibrous bands representing the residual vagal perineurium (Fig. 32–22). Ultrastructurally, the tumors contain chief cells that show a gradation in cytoplasmic density similar to the light and dark cells of the carotid body. They contain dense-core neurosecretory granules, some of which have a more elongated or "pleomorphic" appearance than those of the carotid body tumor.[63]

Approximately 10–20% of vagal body tumors metastasize, most commonly to regional lymph nodes, although distant metastasis to lung and bone also occurs.[64] Local infiltration of the internal carotid artery and extension into the cranial vault represent significant problems in disease control. Surgical resection is the treatment of choice, although it is usually not possible to excise these lesions without sacrificing the vagus nerve.[65]

MEDIASTINAL PARAGANGLIOMA

Mediastinal paragangliomas arise from paraganglia associated with the pulmonary artery and aortic arch or from the segmental paraganglia associated with the sympathetic chain. The former tumors are located in the anterior mediastinum and are termed "aortic body tumors," whereas the latter are located in the posterior mediastinum and are the mediastinal equivalent of retroperitoneal (extra-adrenal) paragangliomas.

Aortic body paragangliomas can originate at any site where the aortic body chemoreceptor has been identified: (1) anterolateral to the aortic arch; (2) lateral to the innominate artery; (3) at the angle of the ductus arteriosus and descending aorta; and (4) to the upper right of the main pulmonary artery. Most reported cases have occurred in persons over age 40 years, and they affect the genders equally. They may be associated with paragangliomas at other sites,[66,67] and occasionally arise in patients with Carney's triad.[68,69]

Clinically, although many of these tumors are found incidentally in asymptomatic patients, a significant number of patients present with symptoms related to catecholamine secretion, including headache, hypertension, and sweating.[70,71] Radiographically, the tumors are highly vascular masses of the anterior or superior mediastinum that are fed by vessels from the subclavian, internal mammary, or intercostal arteries, with early drainage into the superior vena cava.[72,73] Histologically and immunohistochemically, they are identical to the tumors of the carotid body.[74]

Mediastinal paragangliomas have a rather aggressive course. Although only about 10% of patients develop metastasis, many eventually die of the disease. Of the 41

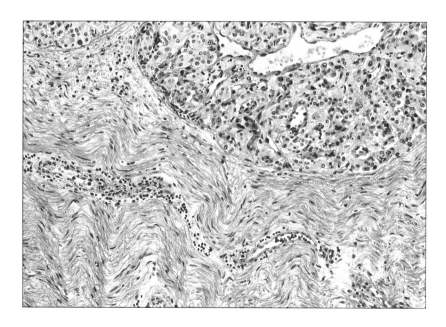

FIGURE 32–22 Vagal body paraganglioma embedded in the vagal nerve.

cases reported in the literature and reviewed by Olson and Salyer,[75] only 19 patients were alive and well without evidence of disease. Of the remainder, 14 had either inoperable disease or died as a result of the tumor. Three were alive with residual mediastinal tumor, four had tumor documented incidentally at autopsy, one was lost to follow-up, and one had multiple tumors. In a review of the literature of anterior and middle mediastinal paragangliomas, Lamy et al. found a high rate of local recurrence (56%) and documented metastasis in 21 of 79 (27%) reported cases.[76] Optimum therapy is complete surgical excision, using cardiopulmonary bypass if necessary.[77] When complete excision cannot be accomplished, the prognosis is guarded, as slow progression and death from tumor may ensue.

Posterior mediastinal paragangliomas are far less common than the foregoing type.[78] They occur in younger persons (average age 29 years) and in about half of cases are associated with symptoms referable to functional activity by the tumor. In the remainder of the patients, the mass, which is usually located in the costovertebral sulcus at the level of the fifth to seventh ribs, is discovered incidentally at the time of chest radiography.

The tumors are related to the sympathetic chain, and for this reason they can be considered histogenetically and embryologically similar to the extra-adrenal paragangliomas of the retroperitoneum. They may combine features of classic carotid body tumor or adrenal pheochromocytoma. In the study by Moran et al., 12 of 16 mediastinal paragangliomas were located in the posterior mediastinum.[79] Two patients in this series developed metastatic disease, both with posterior mediastinal paragangliomas. Complete surgical excision is the preferred treatment and is usually accomplished more readily than with paragangliomas in the anterior mediastinum.

RETROPERITONEAL PARAGANGLIOMA

Approximately 10–20% of paragangliomas of the retroperitoneum arise outside the adrenal from paraganglia that lie along the aortic axis in close association with the sympathetic chain. The largest collection of paraganglia includes the organs of Zuckerkandl (Figs 32–3, 32–4), paired structures overlying the aorta at the level of the inferior mesenteric artery. These structures are prominent during early infancy but gradually regress after 12–18 months of age, leaving behind only small microscopic residua. Although they are believed to serve chemoreceptor functions in animals, their physiologic role in humans is not well understood. Most extra-adrenal paragangliomas arise from this organ, whereas a smaller number are derived from the paraganglia lying at other points along the aortic or iliac vessels.

Retroperitoneal paragangliomas occur at a relatively earlier age than those of the head and neck. Most occur in persons 30–45 years of age, although the malignant forms may have an even younger median age.[80,81] Men and women are affected in approximately equal numbers in most series. Occasionally these tumors are multiple, or they may be associated with paragangliomas of other sites[82] or with other tumors such as gastrointestinal stromal tumors of the stomach and pulmonary chondromas as a component of Carney's triad.[83]

Back pain and a palpable mass are the two most common presenting symptoms. About 10% of patients present initially with metastatic disease, and about 20% of these tumors are discovered incidentally at the time of autopsy. Symptoms related to production of norepinephrine occur in 25–60% of patients with these tumors. Such patients develop chronic or intermittent hypertension, headaches, and palpitations. In contrast, functional adrenal paragangliomas (pheochromocytomas) may be associated with increased serum levels of epinephrine and norepinephrine, and the exact constellation of symptoms depends on the relative amounts of each. Hypertension predominates in norepinephrine-secreting tumors, whereas hypotension, hypovolemia, palpitations, and tachyarrhythmias are hallmarks of those producing large amounts of epinephrine.[84] The difference in secretory patterns is believed to be related to the presence of methyltransferase in some adrenal pheochromocytomas (which converts norepinephrine to epinephrine) and its absence in extra-adrenal paragangliomas. Rare retroperitoneal tumors induce hypertension by compressing renal vessels, resulting in renal ischemia.[85]

Extra-adrenal paragangliomas are rarely diagnosed preoperatively unless the lesion is functional. In the latter instance, the diagnosis can be established by measuring total urinary catecholamines, and the mass can be localized by means of angiography. Scintigraphic localization of both adrenal and extra-adrenal lesions has been accomplished by means of iodine 131(^{131}I) metaiodobenzylguanidine (MIBG), a structural analogue of norepinephrine.[86] Localization of these tumors has also been accomplished using the radiolabeled somatostatin analogue octreotide.[87] CT scans and MRI are also highly sensitive for detecting small tumors.[88]

Pathologic findings

These tumors are partially encapsulated brown masses that usually measure several centimeters in diameter (Fig. 32–23). Hemorrhage is a common finding. Histologically, retroperitoneal paragangliomas may resemble a branchiomeric paraganglioma or adrenal pheochromocytoma, or they may combine features of both. Most, however, are similar to the adrenal pheochromocytoma.

They are composed of small polygonal or slightly spindled cells with an amphophilic or eosinophilic cytoplasm. The cells are arranged in short, irregular anastomosing sheets around a delicate vasculature (Figs 32–24, 32–25). The cell outlines are often indistinct so the sheets have a syncytial quality. Eosinophilic globules may be identified in the cytoplasm of the cells and vary in size from a few micrometers to the size of a nucleus. These structures seem to represent remnants of dense-core granules, and their presence has been correlated with benignancy (see below). Rare tumors are composed of

cells with a melanin-like cytoplasmic pigment (neuromelanin).[89] Hemorrhage in these nests of cells is not infrequent (Fig. 32–26). Although few retroperitoneal paragangliomas resemble carotid body tumors in their entirety, it is often possible to find occasional areas in these lesions where the cells are round and grow in small nests. A few retroperitoneal paragangliomas are highly pleomorphic lesions made up of spindled or angular cells with deeply eosinophilic cytoplasm and large hyperchromatic nuclei. Such tumors grow in extremely large sheets and often lack the organization of the usual paraganglioma (Fig. 32–27).

On initial inspection these pleomorphic tumors are worrisome and may be mistaken for carcinomas, except that little mitotic activity accompanies the pleomorphic changes. In rare instances, areas of ganglioneuroma are encountered in retroperitoneal paragangliomas (Figs 32–28, 32–29).

Criteria of malignancy

The criteria of malignancy for paragangliomas have been controversial. In the opinion of some, the only definite criterion of malignancy is metastatic disease. Linnoila et al. analyzed various features in clinically benign and malignant paragangliomas and concluded that extra-adrenal location, coarse nodularity, confluent necrosis, and absence of hyaline globules may be predictive of malignancy (Table 32–6).[90] Altogether, 71% of malignant tumors had two or three of these features, whereas 89% of benign tumors had one or none. The same authors suggested that decreased expression of a variety of neuropeptides may also correlate with malignancy and may therefore serve as an adjunctive means of identifying aggressive behavior. Benign lesions typically express five or more neuropeptides and malignant lesions only two.[91]

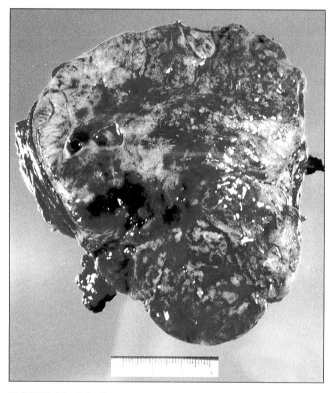

FIGURE 32–23 Gross appearance of a retroperitoneal paraganglioma with brown cut surface and focal hemorrhage.

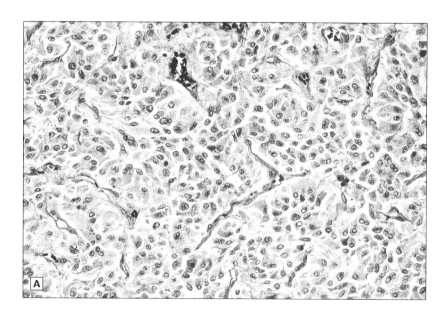

FIGURE 32–24 (A) Extra-adrenal paraganglioma with sheet-like growth of cells in one area.

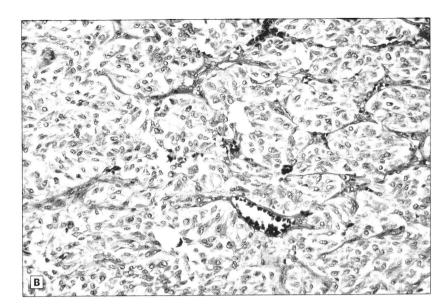

FIGURE 32–24 Continued. **(B)** In other areas cells have lost cohesion, with formation of clear spaces.

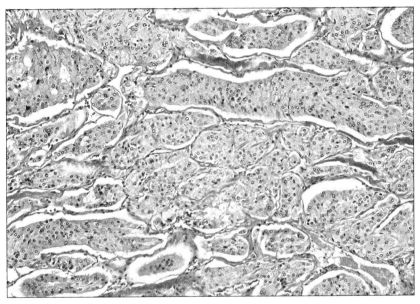

FIGURE 32–25 Carcinoid-like pattern in a retroperitoneal paraganglioma.

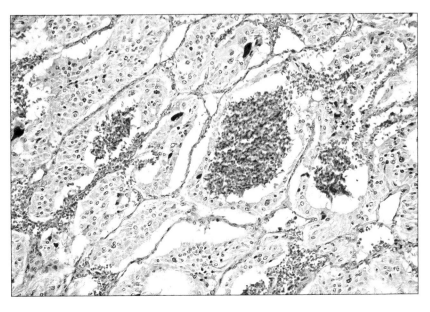

FIGURE 32–26 Paraganglioma with cystic hemorrhage.

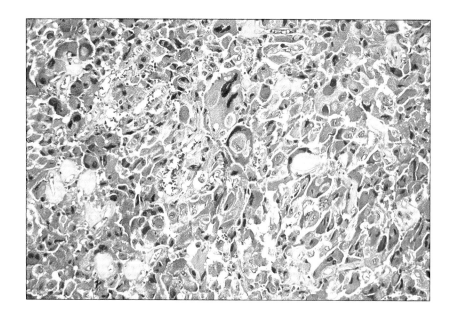

FIGURE 32–27 Pleomorphic form of a retroperitoneal paraganglioma. Cells are large and angular and have a deeply staining cytoplasm. Cell embracing, a general feature of paragangliomas, is evident in this tumor.

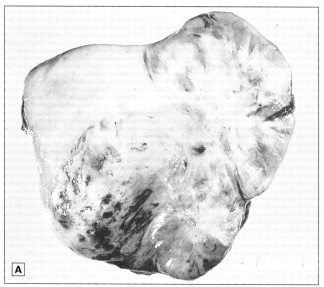

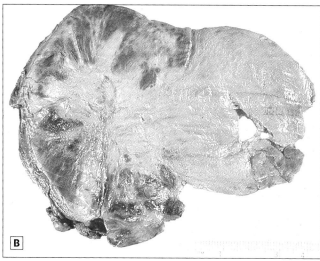

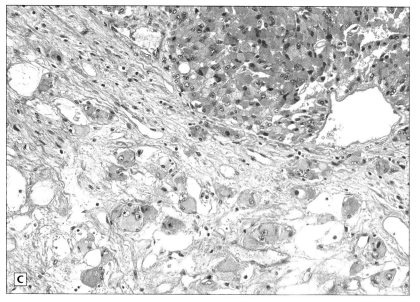

FIGURE 32–28 (A) Gross appearance of a retroperitoneal paraganglioma mixed with a ganglioneuroma. Most of the tumor was composed of ganglioneuromatous elements (white areas) with a lesser component of paraganglioma (brown areas). **(B)** Chromaffin reaction accentuates the paragangliomatous portions of this tumor. **(C)** Histologic appearance of a mixed retroperitoneal paraganglioma with ganglioneuromatous elements characterized by prominent ganglion cells.

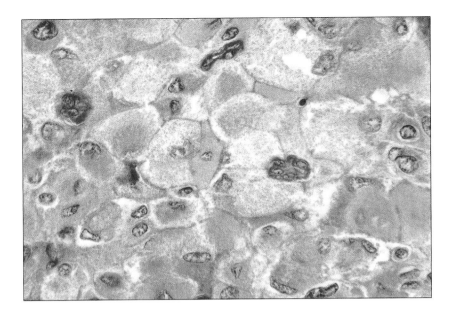

FIGURE 32–29 Chromaffin-positive granules in the cells of a retroperitoneal paraganglioma.

TABLE 32–6	HISTOLOGIC FEATURES OF CLINICALLY BENIGN AND MALIGNANT SYMPATHOADRENAL PARAGANGLIOMAS		
Histologic feature	**Malignant (n = 34)**	**Benign (n = 64)**	**p**
Zellballen pattern (%)	44	30	NS
Trabecular pattern (%)	21	30	NS
Mixed patterns (%)	33	38	NS
Diffuse (sold pattern) (%)	0	3	NS
Confluent tumor necrosis (%)	32	6	0.0023
Mitotic rate (mean/30 HPF)	3	1	NS
Hyaline globules (%)	32	59	0.013
Extensive local/vascular invasion (%)	32	11	0.022

NS, not significant; HPF, high-power fields.
Modified from Linnoila RI, Keiser HR, Steinberg SM, et al. Histopathology of benign versus malignant sympathoadrenal paragangliomas: clinicopathologic study of 120 cases including unusual histologic features. Hum Pathol 1990; 21:1168.

TABLE 32–7	CLINICAL AND PATHOLOGIC FEATURES OF CLINICALLY BENIGN AND MALIGNANT SYMPATHOADRENAL PARAGANGLIOMAS		
Parameter	**Malignant (n = 10)**	**Benign (n = 23)**	**p**
Male gender (%)	90	44	0.08
Mean age (years)	38	49	0.05
Neurofibromatosis (%)	0	100	0.04
Tumor weight, mean (g)	481	124	0.05
Ki-67 index, mean (%)	5	1	0.0009
Extra-adrenal site (%)	40	9	0.03

Modified from Clarke MR, Weyant RJ, Watson CG, et al. Prognostic markers in pheochromocytoma. Hum Pathol 1998; 28:522.

Clarke et al. found extra-adrenal location, male gender, young age, tumor weight, and Ki-67 labeling index to be predictive of malignancy (Table 32–7).[81] Several other studies have found a positive correlation between high proliferative index as measured with the MIB-1 antibody and malignant clinical behavior.[92,93] Analogous to the situation with neuroblastoma, the extent of S-100 protein staining of sustentacular cells has also been found to be of prognostic significance.[94]

Immunohistochemical findings

The immunologic profile of this form of paraganglioma is similar to that of the branchiomeric forms in that neuron-specific enolase, neurofilament protein, synaptophysin, and chromogranin can be identified in chief cells, which in turn are surrounded by a sustentacular network of cells that stain positively for S-100 protein.[95] Leu-

enkephalin, an opiate-like pentapeptide that comprises part of the β-endorphin molecule, can be identified in many adrenal and extra-adrenal paragangliomas.[96] This finding is to be expected in view of the fact that this pentapeptide is produced by normal and hyperplastic adrenal medullary cells. Insulin-like growth factor II, a polypeptide of 67 amino acids that is homologous to the β-chain of proinsulin, has been identified in adrenal tissues, the carotid body, and paraganglia and can also be localized to most chief cells in adrenal and extra-adrenal paragangliomas.[97] Its significance is unclear, but it is known to have a mitogenic influence on fibroblasts and can enhance differentiation in myoblasts and neuroblastoma cell lines. A variety of neuropeptides can be localized to the chief cells (detailed in Table 32–2).

Behavior and treatment

Early reports in the literature consistently indicated that extra-adrenal paragangliomas had a more aggressive course than those in the adrenal.[98] A study based on experience from Memorial Hospital offers evidence to the contrary.[99] Approximately 50% of both adrenal and extra-adrenal tumors were malignant, as evidenced by metastatic disease or locally aggressive behavior. The 5-year survival rate was 77% for patients with adrenal tumors and 82% for those with extra-adrenal tumors, figures that are not significantly different. When patients with malignant tumors were compared by site, there was still no statistical difference in disease-free survival rates. Similarly, Clarke et al. studied 66 pheochromocytomas and retroperitoneal paragangliomas, 10 of which metastasized. Of the 10 tumors that metastasized, four were extra-adrenal in origin.[81]

There is little correlation between the functional activity of the tumor and the degree of malignancy. Dissemination of this tumor occurs both lymphatically and hematogenously, and the most common sites of metastasis are the regional lymph nodes, bone, liver, and lung.[100]

If a retroperitoneal paraganglioma is suspected clinically, appropriate steps to document functional activity should be undertaken before surgery. Premedication of patients with β-adrenergic blocking agents is mandatory to avert intraoperative hypertensive crises or tachyarrhythmias during surgical manipulation of the tumor. Surgery should be aimed at complete removal, as adjunctive therapies including MIBG, radiotherapy and chemotherapy[101] can only be considered palliative. Because of the excellent localization of these tumors by modern radiographic techniques, some have advocated laparoscopic surgery as an alternative to laparotomy.[102]

MISCELLANEOUS PARAGANGLIOMAS

Paragangliomas may arise in numerous locations other than those already mentioned, including the nasopharynx,[103] larynx,[104] orbit,[105] gallbladder,[106] kidney,[107] thyroid,[108] bladder,[109] prostate,[110] lung,[111] pancreas,[112] and heart.[113] Although it has been claimed that they may also arise in the extremities from paraganglia that follow the arterial vessels, systematic microscopic search by Karnauchow[114] of 38 autopsy cases failed to reveal acceptable structures. Moreover, some cases reported as paragangliomas of the extremity seem in reality to be alveolar soft part sarcomas. In our opinion, paraganglioma of the extremity should be diagnosed with great reserve and only after alternative diagnoses such as carcinoma, melanoma, and alveolar soft part sarcoma have been excluded by appropriate staining procedures, clinical history, and electron microscopic studies.

Nasopharyngeal paraganglioma

Most paragangliomas involving the nasopharynx arise from adjacent structures, such as the glomus jugulare and vagal body, and extend secondarily into this region. Primary nasopharyngeal tumors arising from submucosal paraganglia are rare, and this diagnosis is an exclusionary one.[115-117] These tumors are pulsatile blue masses arising high in the nasopharynx. They produce symptoms of dysphonia, dysphagia, nasal obstruction, and epistaxis. Their appearance is similar to that of the carotid body tumor.

Laryngeal paraganglioma

Laryngeal paragangliomas arise from the paired paraganglia situated in the soft tissue of the larynx.[118] The superior pair are located at the level of the superior margin of the thyroid cartilage, whereas the inferior pair are located at the border of the thyroid and cricoid cartilage. Aberrant locations near the upper tracheal rings have also been identified. Most laryngeal paragangliomas occur in women, mainly during the fourth to sixth decades of life.[118-120] Most arise above the level of the vocal cords and involve the ipsilateral aryepiglottic fold, although some arise in a subglottic location.[121,122] Affected patients usually develop hoarseness, dysphagia, and dyspnea. These tumors are histologically similar to other branchiomeric paragangliomas. The relative malignancy of these tumors has been disputed.[123] Barnes and co-workers maintained that almost all are benign, with fewer than 2% exhibiting aggressive behavior.[124] The high incidence of metastasis, reported as 25% in a review of the literature by Gallivan et al.,[125] is most likely the result of misdiagnosis of laryngeal carcinomas or atypical carcinoids. Surgical removal is standard therapy although there has been limited success with laser excision.[126]

Orbital paraganglioma

Orbital paragangliomas are rare tumors that are presumed to arise from the paraganglia associated with the ciliary ganglion. They produce symptoms of visual loss and throbbing pain and deficits of one or more cranial nerves.[105] Unfortunately, many orbital paragangliomas reported in the past are, in fact, alveolar soft part sarcomas that have been misdiagnosed. Excluding 13 of the 29 cases reported at that time, Archer and colleagues found that the 16 acceptable orbital paragangliomas occurred at a wide range of ages (3–68 years) with an equal gender distribution.[127] Nearly 40% of those treated with exenteration recurred, but none of the tumors to date has produced metastatic disease.

Gangliocytic paraganglioma

Described in 1962 by Taylor and Helwig,[128] gangliocytic paraganglioma is an unusual tumor that combines features of paraganglioma, carcinoid, and ganglioneuroma. It almost always occurs in the second (periampullary) portion of the duodenum,[129–131] although rare cases have been described in other sites including the appendix,[132] lung,[133] nasopharynx,[134] bronchus,[135] mediastinum,[136] and even arising in an ovarian cystic teratoma.[137] The tumor predominantly affects men and makes its appearance during adult life, usually heralded by gastrointestinal tract bleeding. Most can be demonstrated on upper gastrointestinal tract series as pedunculated or sessile lesions that arise in the submucosa and deform the overlying mucosa. Rare examples of this tumor have occurred in patients with neurofibromatosis type 1, raising the possibility of a more than fortuitous association.[138]

Histologically, the tumors are quite distinctive. They are composed of epithelioid areas that may appear indistinguishable from conventional paraganglioma (Figs 32–30, 32–31) or may have a ribbon-like or trabecular arrangement similar to that of carcinoid (Fig. 32–32). The epithelioid areas are surrounded by a delicate network of Schwann cells and nerve axons (Fig. 32–33). Scattered among the epithelioid areas are variably differentiated ganglion cells. Although most do not appear fully differentiated, they can be easily recognized by their abundant cytoplasm, vesicular nuclei, and faint cytoplasmic basophilia. A prominent neuromatous stroma is seen in some gangliocytic paragangliomas and these resemble a ganglioneuroma.

By immunohistochemistry, the paraganglioma and carcinoid-like areas express both synaptophysin and chromogranin.[139] The ganglion cells express neuron-specific enolase, synaptophysin and neurofilament protein, whereas S-100 protein is easily demonstrated in the sustentacular network surrounding the epithelioid cells (Fig. 32–34). A variety of other antigens can be identified in the epithelioid cells of these tumors, including neuron-specific enolase, insulin, glucagon, leu-

enkephalin, pancreatic polypeptide, somatostatin, vasoactive intestinal peptide and serotonin.[140–143]

It has been postulated that this tumor arises from the primordium of the pancreas, which undergoes hyperplasia and recapitulates, in an exaggerated fashion, the endodermal-neuroectodermal complexes of van Campenout, which normally occur in the duodenum. However, it has become increasingly clear that this tumor is not restricted to the periampullary region, making this an untenable hypothesis. Almost all tumors have proved to be benign, with only rare reports of lymph node metastases, but even these seem to follow an indolent course.[143–145] Hence, simple excision, including endoscopic resection[146–148] to prevent recurrent gastrointestinal hemorrhage, is usually adequate therapy.

Paraganglioma of the cauda equina

Paraganglioma of the cauda equina has been recognized only recently as a distinct entity, with fewer than 100 cases having been reported in the literature.[149] Early cases were probably misdiagnosed as ependymomas or carcinomas. Men are affected slightly more often than women, and the tumor occurs most frequently in patients 50–60 years of age. Most present with "cauda equina syndrome," which includes lower back pain, weakness of the extremity, or urinary or fecal incontinence. Extreme elevations in cerebrospinal fluid protein can be documented in a significant proportion of cases.[150–152] The tumors are extramedullary, intradural masses that may or may not be attached to the cauda equina. They resemble other paragangliomas in all respects, although in almost one-half of tumors, ganglionic differentiation may be seen.[150] The chief cells stain for neuron-specific enolase, neurofilament protein, synaptophysin, and

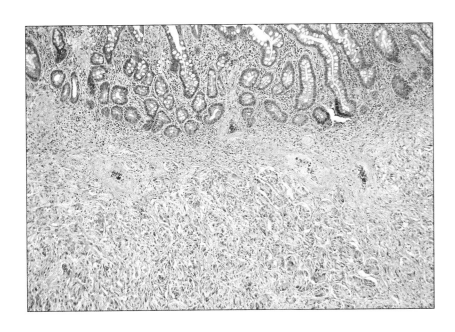

FIGURE 32–30 Low-power view of a gangliocytic paraganglioma.

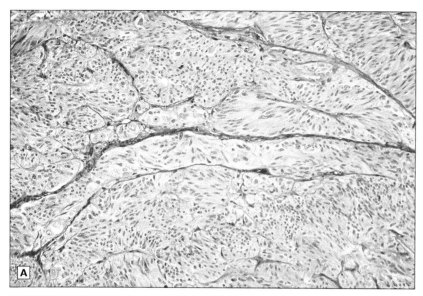

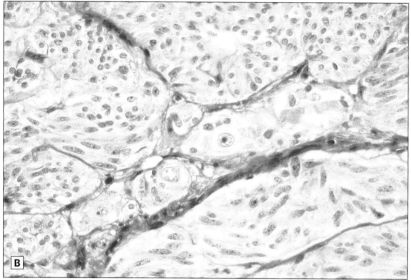

FIGURE 32–31 (A) Gangliocytic paraganglioma with a typical low-power appearance. (B) Focal differentiating ganglion cells are seen in epithelioid areas.

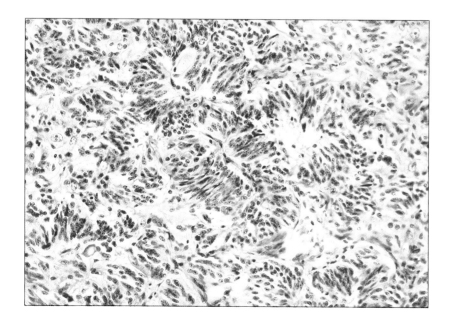

FIGURE 32–32 Carcinoid-like area in a gangliocytic paraganglioma.

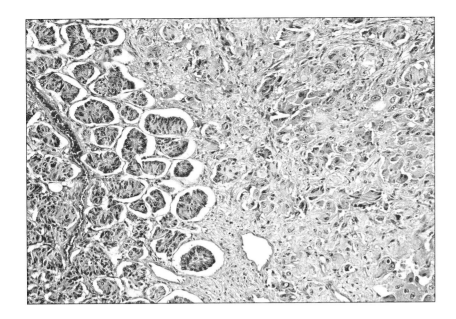

FIGURE 32–33 Gangliocytic paraganglioma consisting of an admixture of carcinoid-like areas and ganglion cells.

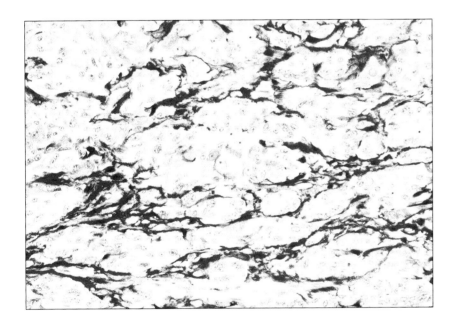

FIGURE 32–34 S-100 protein-positive sustentacular network surrounding epithelioid nests in a gangliocytic paraganglioma.

chromogranin, as well as other peptides including soma-tostatin and ACTH.[153,154] Unlike paragangliomas from other sites, cauda equina tumors often express cytokera-tins (Fig. 32–35), which correlates with the ultrastruc-tural finding of cytoplasmic intermediate filaments, in addition to dense-core neurosecretory granules.[155–157] Thus, the precise relation between these tumors and paragangliomas from other sites is somewhat obscure. Although most are benign, their location may complicate complete surgical excision, leading to local recurrence in about 10% of patients.[150,158] There are rare reports of intracranial and intraspinal metastasis.[159,160] Radiother-apy has been recommended for unencapsulated or incompletely excised tumors.[153]

Cardiac paraganglioma

Cardiac paraganglioma is one of the rarest forms of para-ganglioma, with fewer than 60 cases reported in the lit-erature.[113,161–163] Most have occurred in women at an average age of 45 years. The tumor arises primarily on the left atrium or in the interventricular groove at the aortic root and commonly gives rise to hypertensive symptoms. The lesions are histologically and immunohistochemi-cally similar to other forms of paraganglioma. Treatment of these inaccessible tumors usually requires resection of the posterior atrial wall with coronary artery bypass.[164] Although most are clinically benign, rare tumors have given rise to distant metastasis.

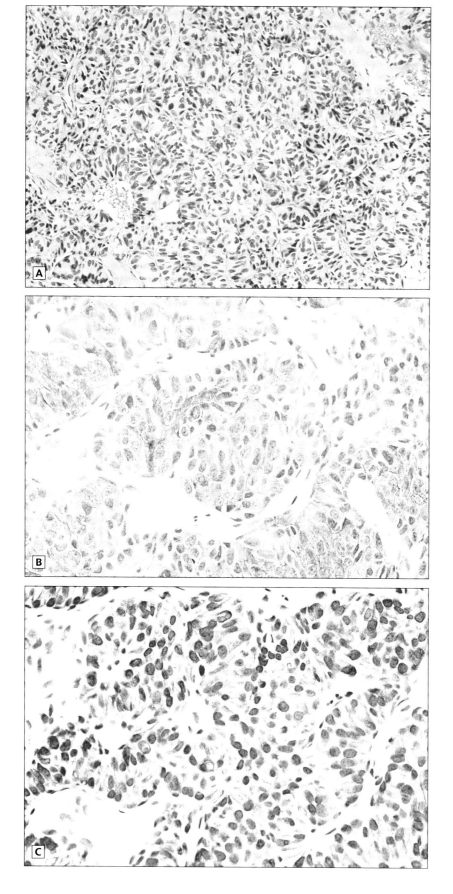

FIGURE 32–35 (A) Typical histologic appearance of a paraganglioma of the cauda equina. The same tumor was diffusely immunoreactive for synaptophysin **(B)** and cytokeratin **(C)**.

REFERENCES

1. Glenner GG, Grimley PM. Tumours of the extraadrenal paraganglion system (including chemoreceptors). In: Atlas of tumor pathology, Fascicle 9, 2nd Series. Washington, DC: Armed Forces Institute of Pathology; 1974.

Carotid body paraganglioma

2. Biscoe TJ. The carotid body. what next? Am Rev Respir Dis 1977; 115:189.
3. Saldana MJ, Salem LE, Travezan R. High altitude hypoxia and chemodectomas. Hum Pathol 1973; 4:251.
4. Lack EE, Cubilla AL, Woodruff JM, et al. Paragangliomas of the head and neck region: a clinical study of 69 patients. Cancer 1977; 39:397.
5. Pellitteri PK, Rinaldo A, Myssiorek D, et al. Paragangliomas of the head and neck. Oral Oncol 2004; 40:563.
6. Mora J, Cascon A, Robledo M, et al. Pediatric paraganglioma: An early manifestation of an adult disease secondary to germline mutations. Pediatr Blood Cancer 2005; 47:785.
7. Eisenhofer G, Goldstein DS, Sullivan P, et al. Biochemical and clinical manifestations of dopamine-producing paragangliomas: utility of plasma methoxytyramine. J Clin Endocrinol Metab 2005; 90:2068.
8. Gujrathi CS, Donald PJ. Current trends in the diagnosis and management of head and neck paragangliomas. Curr Opin Otolaryngol Head Neck Surg 2005; 13:339.
9. Myssiorek D. Head and neck paragangliomas: an overview. Otolaryngol Clin North Am 2001; 34:829.
10. Telischi FF, Bustillo A, Whiteman ML, et al. Octreotide scintigraphy for the detection of paragangliomas. Otolaryngol Head Neck Surg 2000; 122:358.
11. Alkadhi H, Schuknecht B, Stoeckli SJ, et al. Evaluation of topography and vascularization of cervical paragangliomas by magnetic resonance imaging and color duplex sonography. Neuroradiology 2002; 44:83.
12. Stoeckli SJ, Schuknecht B, Alkadhi H, et al. Evaluation of paragangliomas presenting as a cervical mass on color-coded Doppler sonography. Laryngoscope 2002; 112:143.
13. Bikhazi PH, Roeder E, Attaie A, et al. Familial paragangliomas: The emerging impact of molecular genetics on evaluation and management. Am J Otol 1999; 20:639.
14. Isik AC, Erem C, Imamoglu M, et al. Familial paraganglioma. Eur Arch Otorhinolaryngol 2006; 263:23.
15. Heutink P, van Schothorst EM, van der Mey AG, et al. Further localization of the gene for hereditary paragangliomas and evidence for linkage in unrelated families. Eur J Hum Genet 1994; 2:148.
16. Heutink P, van der Mey AG, Sandkuijl LA, et al. A gene subject to genomic imprinting and responsible for hereditary paragangliomas maps to chromosome 11q23-qter. Hum Mol Genet 1992; 1:7.
17. Bayley JP, van Minderhout I, Weiss MM, et al. Mutation analysis of SDHB and SDHC: novel germline mutations in sporadic head and neck paraganglioma and familial paraganglioma and/or pheochromocytoma. BMC Med Genet 2006; 7:1.
18. Eng C, Kiuru M, Fernandez MJ, et al. A role for mitochondrial enzymes in inherited neoplasia and beyond. Nat Rev Cancer 2003; 3:193.
19. Baysal BE. Genomic imprinting and environment in hereditary paraganglioma. Am J Med Genet C Semin Med Genet 2004; 129:85.
20. Braun S, Riemann K, Pusch CM, et al. Paraganglioma in the area of the head and neck. A review of molecular genetic research. HNO 2004; 52:11.
21. Benn DE, Croxson MS, Tucker K, et al. Novel succinate dehydrogenase subunit B (SDHB) mutations in familial phaeochromocytomas and paragangliomas, but an absence of somatic SDHB mutations in sporadic phaeochromocytomas. Oncogene 2003; 22:1358.
22. Braun S, Riemann K, Kupka S, et al. Active succinate dehydrogenase (SDH) and lack of SDHD mutations in sporadic paragangliomas. Anticancer Res 2005; 25:2809.
23. Perry CG, Young WF Jr, McWhinney SR, et al. Functioning paraganglioma and gastrointestinal stromal tumor of the jejunum in three women: syndrome or coincidence. Am J Surg Pathol 2006; 30:42.
24. Plaza JA, Wakely PE Jr, Moran C, et al. Sclerosing paraganglioma: report of 19 cases of an unusual variant of neuroendocrine tumor that may be mistaken for an aggressive malignant neoplasm. Am J Surg Pathol 2006; 30:7.
25. Kliewer KE, Cochran AJ. A review of the histology, ultrastructure, immunohistology, and molecular biology of extra-adrenal paragangliomas. Arch Pathol Lab Med 1989; 113:1209.
26. Kliewer KE, Wen DR, Cancilla PA, et al. Paragangliomas: assessment of prognosis by histologic, immunohistochemical, and ultrastructural techniques. Hum Pathol 1989; 20:29.
27. Fried G, Wikstrom LM, Hoog A, et al. Multiple neuropeptide immunoreactivities in a renin-producing human paraganglioma. Cancer 1994; 74:142.
28. Alpert LI, Bochetto JF Jr. Carotid body tumor: ultrastructural observations. Cancer 1974; 34:564.
29. Min KW. Diagnostic usefulness of sustentacular cells in paragangliomas: immunocytochemical and ultrastructural investigation. Ultrastruct Pathol 1998; 22:369.
30. Netterville JL, Reilly KM, Robertson D, et al. Carotid body tumors: a review of 30 patients with 46 tumors. Laryngoscope 1995; 105:115.
31. Harrington SW, Claggett OT, Dockerty MB. Tumors of the carotid body: clinical and pathologic considerations of 20 tumours affecting 19 patients (1 bilateral). Ann Surg 1941; 114:820.
32. Lee JH, Barich F, Karnell LH, et al. National cancer data base report on malignant paragangliomas of the head and neck. Cancer 2002; 94:730.
33. Sharma PK, Massey BL. Avoiding pitfalls in surgery of the neck, parapharyngeal space, and infratemporal fossa. Otolaryngol Clin North Am 2005; 38:795.
34. Fruhwirth J, Koch G, Hauser H, et al. Paragangliomas of the carotid bifurcation: oncological aspects of vascular surgery. Eur J Surg Oncol 1996; 22:88.
35. Sniezek JC, Sabri AN, Netterville JL. Paraganglioma surgery: complications and treatment. Otolaryngol Clin North Am 2001; 34:993.
36. Tikkakoski T, Luotonen J, Leinonen S, et al. Preoperative embolization in the management of neck paragangliomas. Laryngoscope 1997; 107:821.
37. Liu DG, Ma XC, Li BM, et al. Clinical study of preoperative angiography and embolization of hypervascular neoplasms in the oral and maxillofacial region. Oral Surg Oral Med Oral Pathol Oral Radiol Endod 2006; 101:102.
38. Davidovic LB, Djukic VB, Vasic DM, et al. Diagnosis and treatment of carotid body paraganglioma: 21 years of experience at a clinical center of Serbia. World J Surg Oncol 2005; 3:10.

Jugulotympanic paraganglioma

39. Brown S. Glomus tympanicum tumor. Ear Nose Throat J 2002; 81:608.
40. House JW, Fayad JN. Glomus tympanicum. Ear Nose Throat J 2005; 84:548.
41. Jackson CG. Glomus tympanicum and glomus jugulare tumors. Otolaryngol Clin North Am 2001; 34:941.
42. Nguyen DQ, Boulat E, Troussier J, et al. The jugulotympanic paragangliomas: 41 cases report. Rev Laryngol Otol Rhinol (Bord) 2005; 126:7.
43. Stewart KL. Paragangliomas of the temporal bone. Am J Otolaryngol 1993; 14:219.
44. Parhizkar N, Hiltzik DH, Selesnick SH. Facial nerve rerouting in skull base surgery. Otolaryngol Clin North Am 2005; 38:685.
45. Coulier B, Mailleux P, Lefrancq M. Images in clinical radiology. Glomus tympanicum: CT diagnosis. JBR-BTR 2003; 86:359.
46. Lowenheim H, Koerbel A, Ebner FH, et al. Differentiating imaging findings in primary and secondary tumors of the jugular foramen. Neurosurg Rev 2006; 29:1.
47. van den Berg R. Imaging and management of head and neck paragangliomas. Eur Radiol 2005; 15:1310.
48. Blumenfeld J, Cohen N, Anwar M, et al. Hypertension and a tumor of the glomus jugulare region. Evidence for epinephrine biosynthesis. Am J Hypertens 1993; 6:382.
49. Spector GJ, Sobol S, Thawley SE, et al. Panel discussion: glomus jugulare tumors of the temporal bone. Patterns of invasion in the temporal bone. Laryngoscope 1979; 89:1628.
50. Jackson CG, Gulya AJ, Knox GW, et al. A paraneoplastic syndrome associated with glomus tumors of the skull base? Early observations. Otolaryngol Head Neck Surg 1989; 100:583.
51. Oldring D, Fisch U. Glomus tumors of the temporal region: surgical therapy. Am J Otol 1979; 1:7.
52. Glasscock ME, Jackson CG. Temporal approach: surgical anatomy, difficulties and complications. Rev Laryngol Otol Rhinol (Bord) 1979; 100:21.
53. Glasscock ME, Jackson CG. Glomus tumors: diagnosis and surgery. Rev Laryngol Otol Rhinol (Bord) 1979; 100:131.
54. Forest JA 3rd, Jackson CG, McGrew BM. Long-term control of surgically treated glomus tympanicum tumors. Otol Neurotol 2001; 22:232.
55. Brown JS. Glomus jugulare tumors revisited: a ten-year statistical follow-up of 231 cases. Laryngoscope 1985; 95:284.
56. Johnstone PA, Foss RD, Desilets DJ. Malignant jugulotympanic paraganglioma. Arch Pathol Lab Med 1990; 114:976.

Vagal paraganglioma

57. Urquhart AC, Johnson JT, Myers EN, et al. Glomus vagale: paraganglioma of the vagus nerve. Laryngoscope 1994; 104:440.
58. Sniezek JC, Netterville JL, Sabri AN. Vagal paragangliomas. Otolaryngol Clin North Am 2001; 34:925.
59. Leonetti JP, Brackmann DE. Glomus vagale tumor: the significance of early vocal cord paralysis. Otolaryngol Head Neck Surg 1989; 100:533.
60. Borba LA, Al-Mefty O. Intravagal paragangliomas: report of four cases. Neurosurgery 1996; 38:569.
61. Groblewski JC, Thekdi A, Carrau RL. Secreting vagal paraganglioma. Am J Otolaryngol 2004; 25:295.
62. Miller RB, Boon MS, Atkins JP, et al. Vagal paraganglioma: the Jefferson experience. Otolaryngol Head Neck Surg 2000; 122:482.

63. Chaudhry AP, Haar JG, Koul A, et al. A nonfunctioning paraganglioma of vagus nerve: an ultrastructural study. Cancer 1979; 43:1689.
64. Netterville JL, Jackson CG, Miller FR, et al. Vagal paraganglioma: a review of 46 patients treated during a 20-year period. Arch Otolaryngol Head Neck Surg 1998; 124:1133.
65. Persky MS, Setton A, Niimi Y, et al. Combined endovascular and surgical treatment of head and neck paragangliomas – a team approach. Head Neck 2002; 24:423.

Mediastinal paraganglioma

66. Kwon HJ, Park JH, Jin GY, et al. Posterior mediastinal paraganglioma with bilateral adrenal pheochromocytoma. Respir Med 2004; 98:574.
67. Hann U, Geist-Barth B, Menon AK, et al. Aortico-pulmonary paraganglioma associated with bilateral carotid body tumors. Diagnostic presentation and clinical implications. J Cardiovasc Surg (Torino) 2001; 42:131.
68. Diment J, Tamborini E, Casali P, et al. Carney triad: case report and molecular analysis of gastric tumor. Hum Pathol 2005; 36:112.
69. Scopsi L, Collini P, Muscolino G. A new observation of the Carney's triad with long follow-up period and additional tumors. Cancer Detect Prev 1999; 23:435.
70. Bisignani G, Boncompagni E, Plastina F. Arterial hypertension caused by mediastinal paraganglioma. Description of a case and review of the literature. G Ital Cardiol 1985; 15:652.
71. Herrera MF, van Heerden JA, Puga FJ, et al. Mediastinal paraganglioma: a surgical experience. Ann Thorac Surg 1993; 56:1096.
72. Sahin-Akyar G, Erden I, Yagci C, et al. Magnetic resonance imaging findings of a nonfunctional mediastinal paraganglioma with an unusual presentation. Eur Radiol 1997; 7:1114.
73. Tanaka F, Kitano M, Tatsumi A, et al. Paraganglioma of the posterior mediastinum: value of magnetic resonance imaging. Ann Thorac Surg 1992; 53:517.
74. Assaf HM, al-Momen AA, Martin JG. Aorticopulmonary paraganglioma. A case report with immunohistochemical studies and literature review. Arch Pathol Lab Med 1992; 116:1085.
75. Olson JL, Salyer WR. Mediastinal paragangliomas (aortic body tumor): a report of four cases and a review of the literature. Cancer 1978; 41:2405.
76. Lamy AL, Fradet GJ, Luoma A, et al. Anterior and middle mediastinum paraganglioma: complete resection is the treatment of choice. Ann Thorac Surg 1994; 57:249.
77. Gopalakrishnan R, Ticzon AR, Cruz PA, et al. Cardiac paraganglioma (chemodectoma): a case report and review of the literature. J Thorac Cardiovasc Surg 1978; 76:183.
78. Spector JA, Willis DN, Ginsburg HB. Paraganglioma (pheochromocytoma) of the posterior mediastinum: a case report and review of the literature. J Pediatr Surg 2003; 38:1114.
79. Moran CA, Suster S, Fishback N, et al. Mediastinal paragangliomas. A clinicopathologic and immunohistochemical study of 16 cases. Cancer 1993; 72:2358.

Retroperitoneal paraganglioma

80. Barfield R, Hill DA, Hoffer FA, et al. Retroperitoneal paraganglioma. Med Pediatr Oncol 2002; 39:120.
81. Clarke MR, Weyant RJ, Watson CG, et al. Prognostic markers in pheochromocytoma. Hum Pathol 1998; 29:522.
82. Mena J, Bowen JC, Hollier LH. Metachronous bilateral nonfunctional intercarotid paraganglioma (carotid body tumor) and functional retroperitoneal paraganglioma: report of a case and review of the literature. Surgery 1993; 114:107.
83. Spatz A, Bressac-de-Paillerets B, Raymond E. Soft tissue sarcomas. Case 3. Gastrointestinal stromal tumor and Carney's triad. J Clin Oncol 2004; 22:2029.
84. Kimura N, Miura Y, Nagatsu I, et al. Catecholamine synthesizing enzymes in 70 cases of functioning and non-functioning phaeochromocytoma and extra-adrenal paraganglioma. Virchows Arch A Pathol Anat Histopathol 1992; 421:25.
85. Nakano S, Kigoshi T, Uchida K, et al. Hypertension and unilateral renal ischemia (Page kidney) due to compression of a retroperitoneal paraganglioma. Am J Nephrol 1996; 16:91.
86. d'Herbomez M, Gouze V, Huglo D, et al. Chromogranin A assay and (131)I-MIBG scintigraphy for diagnosis and follow-up of pheochromocytoma. J Nucl Med 2001; 42:993.
87. Kwekkeboom DJ, van Urk H, Pauw BK, et al. Octreotide scintigraphy for the detection of paragangliomas. J Nucl Med 1993; 34:873.
88. Sahdev A, Sohaib A, Monson JP, et al. CT and MR imaging of unusual locations of extra-adrenal paragangliomas (pheochromocytomas). Eur Radiol 2005; 15:85.
89. Lack EE, Kim H, Reed K. Pigmented ("black") extraadrenal paraganglioma. Am J Surg Pathol 1998; 22:265.
90. Linnoila RI, Keiser HR, Steinberg SM, et al. Histopathology of benign versus malignant sympathoadrenal paragangliomas: clinicopathologic study of 120 cases including unusual histologic features. Hum Pathol 1990; 21:1168.
91. Linnoila RI, Lack EE, Steinberg SM, et al. Decreased expression of neuropeptides in malignant paragangliomas: an immunohistochemical study. Hum Pathol 1988; 19:41.
92. Brown HM, Komorowski RA, Wilson SD, et al. Predicting metastasis of pheochromocytomas using DNA flow cytometry and immunohistochemical markers of cell proliferation: a positive correlation between MIB-1 staining and malignant tumor behavior. Cancer 1999; 86:1583.
93. Nagura S, Katoh R, Kawaoi A, et al. Immunohistochemical estimations of growth activity to predict biological behavior of pheochromocytomas. Mod Pathol 1999; 12:1107.
94. Montresor E, Iacono C, Nifosi F, et al. Retroperitoneal paragangliomas: role of immunohistochemistry in the diagnosis of malignancy and in assessment of prognosis. Eur J Surg 1994; 160:547.
95. Fraga M, Garcia-Caballero T, Antunez J, et al. A comparative immunohistochemical study of phaeochromocytomas and paragangliomas. Histol Histopathol 1993; 8:429.
96. Balog T, Marotti T, Sverko V, et al. Enkephalin degrading enzymes in pheochromocytoma patients. Oncol Rep 2003; 10:253.
97. Kontogeorgos G, Scheithauer BW, Kovacs K, et al. Growth factors and cytokines in paragangliomas and pheochromocytomas, with special reference to sustentacular cells. Endocr Pathol 2002; 13:197.
98. Lack EE, Cubilla AL, Woodruff JM, et al. Extra-adrenal paragangliomas of the retroperitoneum: A clinicopathologic study of 12 tumors. Am J Surg Pathol 1980; 4:109.
99. Pommier RF, Vetto JT, Billingsly K, et al. Comparison of adrenal and extraadrenal pheochromocytomas. Surgery 1993; 114:1160.
100. O'Riordain DS, Young WF Jr, Grant CS, et al. Clinical spectrum and outcome of functional extraadrenal paraganglioma. World J Surg 1996; 20:916.
101. Pitiakoudis M, Koukourakis M, Tsaroucha A, et al. Malignant retroperitoneal paraganglioma treated with concurrent radiotherapy and chemotherapy. Clin Oncol (R Coll Radiol) 2004; 16:580.
102. Whitson BA, Tuttle TM. Laparoscopic resection of periaortic paragangliomas. Am Surg 2005; 71:450.

Miscellaneous paragangliomas

103. Bijlenga P, Dulguerov P, Richter M, et al. Nasopharynx paraganglioma with extension in the clivus. Acta Neurochir (Wien) 2004; 146:1355.
104. Brown SM, Myssiorek D. Lateral thyrotomy for excision of laryngeal paragangliomas. Laryngoscope 2006; 116:157.
105. Sharma MC, Epari S, Gaikwad S, et al. Orbital paraganglioma: report of a rare case. Can J Ophthalmol 2005; 40:640.
106. Mehra S, Chung-Park M. Gallbladder paraganglioma: a case report with review of the literature. Arch Pathol Lab Med 2005; 129:523.
107. Takahashi M, Yang XJ, McWhinney S, et al. cDNA microarray analysis assists in diagnosis of malignant intrarenal pheochromocytoma originally masquerading as a renal cell carcinoma. J Med Genet 2005; 42:e48.
108. Foppiani L, Marugo A, Del Monte P, et al. Thyroid paraganglioma manifesting as hot toxic nodule. J Endocrinol Invest 2005; 28:479.
109. Zhou M, Epstein JI, Young RH. Paraganglioma of the urinary bladder: a lesion that may be misdiagnosed as urothelial carcinoma in transurethral resection specimens. Am J Surg Pathol 2004; 28:94.
110. Campodonico F, Bandelloni R, Maffezzini M. Paraganglioma of the prostate in a young adult. Urology 2005; 66:657.
111. Dahir KM, Gonzalez A, Revelo MP, et al. Ectopic adrenocorticotropic hormone hypersecretion due to a primary pulmonary paraganglioma. Endocr Pract 2004; 10:424.
112. Ohkawara T, Naruse H, Takeda H, et al. Primary paraganglioma of the head of pancreas: contribution of combinatorial image analyses to the diagnosis of disease. Intern Med 2005; 44:1195.
113. Turley AJ, Hunter S, Stewart MJ. A cardiac paraganglioma presenting with atypical chest pain. Eur J Cardiothorac Surg. 2005; 28:352
114. Karnauchow PN. Investigation into the occurrence of paraganglia in lower limbs. Lab Invest 1957; 6:368.
115. Kanoh N, Nishimura Y, Nakamura M, et al. Primary nasopharyngeal paraganglioma: a case report. Auris Nasus Larynx 1991; 18:307.
116. Kuhn JA, Aronoff BL. Nasal and nasopharyngeal paraganglioma. J Surg Oncol 1989; 40:38.
117. Schuller DE, Lucas JG. Nasopharyngeal paraganglioma. Report of a case and review of literature. Arch Otolaryngol 1982; 108:667.
118. Myssiorek D, Rinaldo A, Barnes L, et al. Laryngeal paraganglioma: an updated critical review. Acta Otolaryngol (Stockh) 2004; 124:995.
119. Del Gaudio JM, Muller S. Diagnosis and treatment of supraglottic laryngeal paraganglioma: report of a case. Head Neck 2004; 26:94.
120. Ferlito A, Barnes L, Wenig BM. Identification, classification, treatment, and prognosis of laryngeal paraganglioma. Review of the literature and eight new cases. Ann Otol Rhinol Laryngol 1994; 103:525.
121. Maisel R, Schmidt D, Pambuccian S. Subglottic laryngeal paraganglioma. Laryngoscope 2003; 113:401.
122. Aribas OK, Kanat F, Avunduk MC. Inferior laryngeal paraganglioma presenting as plunging goiter. Eur J Cardiothorac Surg 2004; 25:655.

123. Ferlito A, Milroy CM, Wenig BM, et al. Laryngeal paraganglioma versus atypical carcinoid tumor. Ann Otol Rhinol Laryngol 1995; 104:78.

124. Barnes L, Ferlito A, Wenig BM. Laryngeal paragangliomas. a review and report of a single case. J Laryngol Otol 1997; 111:197.

125. Gallivan MV, Chun B, Rowden G, et al. Laryngeal paraganglioma. Case report with ultrastructural analysis and literature review. Am J Surg Pathol 1979; 3:85.

126. Sesterhenn AM, Folz BJ, Lippert BM, et al. Laser surgical treatment of laryngeal paraganglioma. J Laryngol Otol 2003; 117:641.

127. Archer KF, Hurwitz JJ, Balogh JM, et al. Orbital nonchromaffin paraganglioma. A case report and review of the literature. Ophthalmology 1989; 96:1659.

128. Taylor HB, Helwig EB. Benign nonchromaffin paragangliomas of the duodenum. Virchows Arch Pathol Anat Physiol Klin Med 1962; 335:356.

129. El Idrissi-Lamghari A, Rioux-Leclercq N, Pagenault M, et al. Voluminous juxtapapillary gangliocytic paraganglioma. Gastrointest Endosc 2005; 62:445.

130. Plaza JA, Vitellas K, Marsh WL Jr. Duodenal gangliocytic paraganglioma: a radiological–pathological correlation. Ann Diagn Pathol 2005; 9:143.

131. Burke AP, Helwig EB. Gangliocytic paraganglioma. Am J Clin Pathol 1989; 92:1.

132. van Eeden S, Offerhaus GJ, Peterse HL, et al. Gangliocytic paraganglioma of the appendix. Histopathology 2000; 36:47.

133. Hironaka M, Fukayama M, Takayashiki N, et al. Pulmonary gangliocytic paraganglioma: case report and comparative immunohistochemical study of related neuroendocrine neoplasms. Am J Surg Pathol 2001; 25:688.

134. Sinkre P, Lindberg G, Albores-Saavedra J. Nasopharyngeal gangliocytic paraganglioma. Arch Pathol Lab Med 2001; 125:1098.

135. Kee AR, Forrest CH, Brennan BA, et al. Gangliocytic paraganglioma of the bronchus: a case report with follow-up and ultrastructural assessment. Am J Surg Pathol 2003; 27:1380.

136. Weinrach DM, Wang KL, Blum MG, et al. Multifocal presentation of gangliocytic paraganglioma in the mediastinum and esophagus. Hum Pathol 2004; 35:1288.

137. Mahdavi A, Silberberg B, Malviya VK, et al. Gangliocytic paraganglioma arising from mature cystic teratoma of the ovary. Gynecol Oncol 2003; 90:482.

138. Castoldi L, De Rai P, Marini A, et al. Neurofibromatosis-1 and ampullary gangliocytic paraganglioma causing biliary and pancreatic obstruction. Int J Pancreatol 2001; 29:93.

139. Altavilla G, Chiarelli S, Fassina A. Duodenal periampullary gangliocytic paraganglioma: report of two cases with immunohistochemical and ultrastructural study. Ultrastruct Pathol 2001; 25:137.

140. Scheithauer BW, Nora FE, LeChago J, et al. Duodenal gangliocytic paraganglioma. Clinicopathologic and immunocytochemical study of 11 cases. Am J Clin Pathol 1986; 86:559.

141. Perrone T. Duodenal gangliocytic paraganglioma and carcinoid. Am J Surg Pathol 1986; 10:147.

142. Perrone T, Sibley RK, Rosai J. Duodenal gangliocytic paraganglioma. An immunohistochemical and ultrastructural study and a hypothesis concerning its origin. Am J Surg Pathol 1985; 9:31.

143. Tomic S, Warner T. Pancreatic somatostatin-secreting gangliocytic paraganglioma with lymph node metastases. Am J Gastroenterol 1996; 91:607.

144. Sundararajan V, Robinson-Smith TM, Lowy AM. Duodenal gangliocytic paraganglioma with lymph node metastasis: a case report and review of the literature. Arch Pathol Lab Med 2003; 127:e139.

145. Dookhan DB, Miettinen M, Finkel G, et al. Recurrent duodenal gangliocytic paraganglioma with lymph node metastases. Histopathology 1993; 22:399.

146. Hengstler P, Binek J, Meyenberger C. Endoscopic resection of a juxtapapillary gangliocytic paraganglioma. Endoscopy 2003; 35:633.

147. Nagai T, Torishima R, Nakashima H, et al. Duodenal gangliocytic paraganglioma treated with endoscopic hemostasis and resection. J Gastroenterol 2004; 39:277.

148. Nakamura H, Kobayashi F, Itakura M, et al. A case of duodenal gangliocytic paraganglioma. Nippon Shokakibyo Gakkai Zasshi 2000; 97:905.

149. Gelabert-Gonzalez M. Paragangliomas of the lumbar region. Report of two cases and review of the literature. J Neurosurg Spine 2005; 2:354.

150. Sonneland PR, Scheithauer BW, LeChago J, et al. Paraganglioma of the cauda equina region. Clinicopathologic study of 31 cases with special reference to immunocytology and ultrastructure. Cancer 1986; 58:1720.

151. Haslbeck KM, Eberhardt KE, Nissen U, et al. Intracranial hypertension as a clinical manifestation of cauda equina paraganglioma. Neurology 1999; 52:1297.

152. Sankhla S, Khan GM. Cauda equina paraganglioma presenting with intracranial hypertension: case report and review of the literature. Neurol India 2004; 52:243.

153. Miliaras GC, Kyritsis AP, Polyzoidis KS. Cauda equina paraganglioma: a review. J Neurooncol 2003; 65:177.

154. Moran CA, Rush W, Mena H. Primary spinal paragangliomas: A clinicopathological and immunohistochemical study of 30 cases. Histopathology 1997; 31:167.

155. Pytel P, Krausz T, Wollmann R, et al. Ganglioneuromatous paraganglioma of the cauda equine – a pathological case study. Hum Pathol 2005; 36:444.

156. Chetty R. Cytokeratin expression in cauda equina paragangliomas. Am J Surg Pathol 1999; 23:491.

157. Labrousse F, Leboutet MJ, Petit B, et al. Cytokeratins expression in paragangliomas of the cauda equina. Clin Neuropathol 1999; 18:208.

158. Yang SY, Jin YJ, Park SH, et al. Paragangliomas in the cauda equina region: clinicopathoradiologic findings in four cases. J Neurooncol 2005; 72:49.

159. Strommer KN, Brandner S, Sarioglu AC, et al. Symptomatic cerebellar metastasis and late local recurrence of a cauda equina paraganglioma. Case report. J Neurosurg 1995; 83:166.

160. Roche PH, Figarella-Branger D, Regis J, et al. Cauda equina paraganglioma with subsequent intracranial and intraspinal metastases. Acta Neurochir (Wien) 1996; 138:475.

161. Lupinski RW, Shankar S, Agasthian T, et al. Primary cardiac paraganglioma. Ann Thorac Surg 2004; 78:e43.

162. McGann C, Tazelaar H, Cho SR, et al. In vivo detection of encapsulated intracardiac paraganglioma by delayed gadolinium enhancement magnetic resonance imaging. J Cardiovasc Magn Reson 2005; 7:371.

163. Orr LA, Pettigrew RI, Churchwell AL, et al. Gadolinium utilization in the MR evaluation of cardiac paraganglioma. Clin Imaging 1997; 21:404.

164. Abad C, Jimenez P, Santana C, et al. Primary cardiac paraganglioma. Case report and review of surgically treated cases. J Cardiovasc Surg (Torino) 1992; 33:768.

CARTILAGINOUS SOFT TISSUE TUMORS

CHAPTER CONTENTS

Benign extraosseous cartilaginous lesions are uncommon and usually present as tumor-like masses. Although still unclear as to whether most are neoplastic or metaplastic in origin, some have been shown to be clonal, suggesting a neoplastic process. In the past we arbitrarily employed the term *soft part* or *extraskeletal chondroma* for small, well-defined solitary nodules of hyaline cartilage that are unattached to bone and occur primarily in the distal extremities, especially the fingers and hand. We have used the same designation for the rare chondroma-like lesions that occur in the gastrointestinal and respiratory tracts. These lesions, however, must be distinguished from the cartilaginous rests of branchial origin that are usually found in the soft tissues of the lateral neck in infants and small children and from the metaplastic cartilage encountered in some benign lipomatous (chondroid lipoma) and fibromatous (calcifying aponeurotic fibroma) neoplasms; they must also be distinguished from multiple cartilaginous nodules in the synovium (synovial chondromatosis) and from the cartilage in myositis ossificans and its variants.

Malignant cartilaginous tumors also occur as primary soft tissue neoplasms, but they are much less common than primary chondrosarcomas of bone and are of two types: *myxoid chondrosarcoma* and *mesenchymal chondrosarcoma*.

Well-differentiated extraosseous chondrosarcomas resembling hyaline cartilage are rare. In fact, if such a tumor is encountered in soft tissue, it is more likely an extension or metastasis of a bone tumor than a primary soft tissue neoplasm. Well-differentiated chondrosarcomas do arise from the synovium, sometimes secondary to synovial chondromatosis, and from the periosteum (periosteal chondrosarcoma). They also appear following radiation therapy or injection of radioactive material, usually after a latent period of many years. For example, Ghalib et al. recorded a chondrosarcoma of the larynx that appeared 40 years after a course of irradiation for hyperthyroid-

ism.[1] Schajowicz and colleagues reported a chondrosarcoma of the axilla secondary to injection of Thorotrast for the diagnosis of hemangioma.[2] Rare examples of chondrosarcoma also occur in parenchymal organs. In some locations (e.g., bladder), they usually represent part of a carcinosarcoma.

EXTRASKELETAL CHONDROMA (CHONDROMA OF SOFT PARTS)

Extraskeletal chondroma is a benign cartilaginous tumor that occurs predominantly in the hands and feet. Its variable histologic appearance not infrequently leads to a mistaken diagnosis of chondrosarcoma. There are two large series of this entity, including a report of 70 cases from the Mayo Clinic[3] and 104 cases from the files of the Armed Forces Institute of Pathology (AFIP).[4]

Clinical findings

The tumor occurs primarily in the soft tissues of the hands and feet, usually with no connection to the underlying bone.[5,6] The single most common site is the fingers, where more than 80% are found. Less frequent sites include the hands, toes, feet, and trunk; unusual cases have been described in the dura,[7] larynx,[8] pharynx,[9] oral cavity,[10] skin,[11] parotid gland,[12] and fallopian tube.[13] Extraskeletal chondroma grows as a slowly enlarging nodule or mass that seldom causes pain or tenderness; the tumor mainly affects adults 30–60 years of age and is rare in children.[14] There is a slight male predominance. It is often associated with tendons, tendon sheaths, or joint capsules.[15] Nearly all of the tumors are solitary, although Dellon et al. described bilateral chondromas in the right index and left ring fingers of a patient with renal failure.[16] In addition, Humphreys and colleagues described an unusual case of multiple cutaneous chondromas of the face in a patient whose brother and nephew were similarly affected, suggesting an autosomal dominant mode of inheritance.[17] In general, however, multiple chondroid lesions are more likely forms of synovial chondromatosis. The association of pulmonary chondroma, gastric epithelioid stromal tumor, and extra-adrenal paraganglioma is known as *Carney's triad*.

Radiographically, the lesion is well demarcated and does not involve bone, although some tumors cause compression deformities or bone erosion. Discrete, irregular, ring-like or curvilinear calcifications are often demonstrable (Fig. 33–1).[15] Computed tomography (CT) scans and magnetic resonance imaging (MRI) are useful for determining the exact site of the tumor and its relation to the adjacent bone.[18]

Pathologic findings

Chondromas are firm, well-demarcated, oval-round masses. Occasional ones are soft or friable with focal cystic change. Nearly all are small, seldom exceeding 3 cm in greatest diameter. They may be attached to the tendon or tendon sheath. Microscopically, they vary in appearance. About two-thirds consist of mature hyaline cartilage arranged in distinct lobules with sharp borders (Fig. 33–2). Some are altered by focal fibrosis (*fibrochondroma*) or ossification (*osteochondroma*);[19,20] others show myxoid change (*myxochondroma*), sometimes together with focal hemorrhage. About one-third display focal or diffuse calcification, usually a late feature that may completely obscure the cartilaginous nature of the tumor and mimic tumoral calcinosis.[21] The calcified material is granular, floccular, or crystalline and often outlines the contours of the chondrocytes in a lace-like pattern (Figs 33–3 to 33–5). Calcification tends to be more pronounced in the center than at the periphery of the lobule. It is often accompanied by cellular degeneration and necrosis,

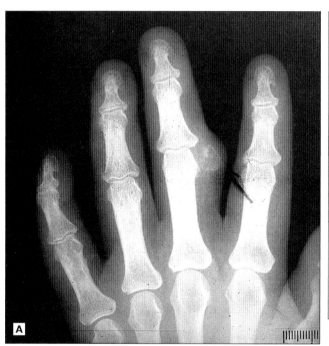

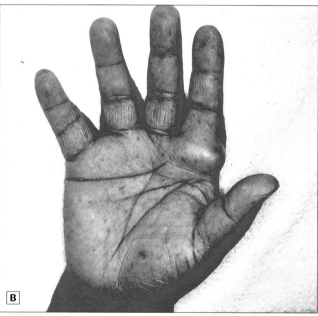

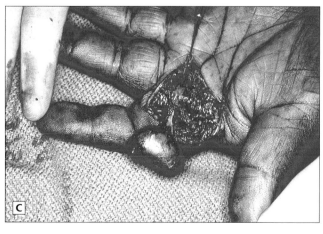

FIGURE 33–1 Chondroma of soft parts. **(A)** Radiograph of the left third finger showing a small soft tissue mass with foci of calcification. **(B)** Chondroma of soft parts at the base of the right second finger. **(C)** Intraoperative specimen of enucleated chondroma of soft parts.

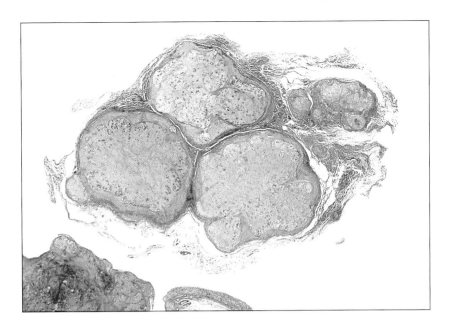

FIGURE 33–2 Cross-section of a chondroma of soft parts showing circumscription and a multinodular growth pattern.

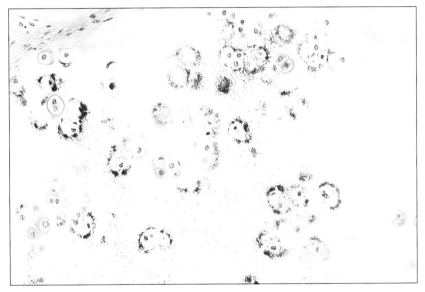

FIGURE 33–3 Chondroma of soft parts consisting of mature hyaline cartilage with nests of benign-appearing cells in lacunae.

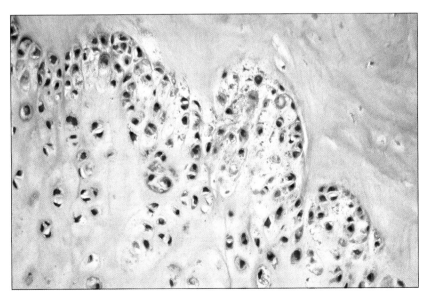

FIGURE 33–4 Chondroma of soft parts with a hypercellular zone at the periphery of a lobule.

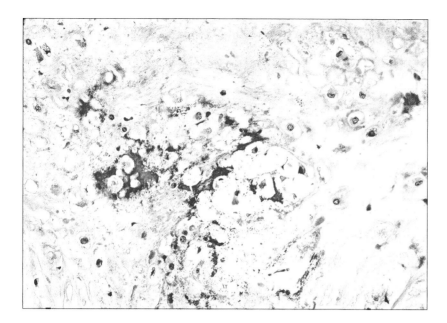

FIGURE 33–5 Calcified chondroma of soft parts. Calcium deposits surround and partly replace the cartilage cells.

which accounts for the softened gross appearance of some of these tumors. Cells with periodic acid-Schiff (PAS)-positive, diastase-resistant intracytoplasmic hyaline globules, possibly representing a glycoproteinaceous secretory product,[22] may be occasionally encountered.

A striking feature that occurs in about 15% of cases is a granuloma-like proliferation of epithelioid and multi-nucleated giant cells reminiscent of a fibroxanthoma or a giant cell tumor (Figs 33–6, 33–7).[23–25] This proliferation is most conspicuous at the tumor margin and along the interlobular vascular channels. There are also rare extraskeletal chondromas in which the presence of plump immature-appearing cells in a myxoid background simulates a chondrosarcoma. In general, however, these tumors can be recognized as chondromas by the presence of more mature, less cellular cartilaginous areas at the periphery. Other examples, such as the series of eight cases reported by Cates and colleagues, exhibit features that closely simulate those of chondroblastoma.[25]

Like normal chondrocytes, the cells of the extraskeletal chondroma are positive for vimentin and S-100 protein.[24] The matrix is rich in types I and III collagen, while there seems to be reduced amounts of types II and IV collagen. Ultrastructurally, the chondrocytes have large indented nuclei, abundant rough endoplasmic reticulum, and occasional membrane-bound vacuoles. Short microvil-lous processes, or filopodia, extend from the cytoplasmic surfaces into the surrounding intercellular matrix (Fig. 33–8). In calcified cases the latter contains variously sized aggregates of hydroxyapatite crystals.[4]

Clonal chromosomal abnormalities have been identified in some extraskeletal chondromas including monosomy 6, trisomy 5 and rearrangements of chromosome 11.[26–29]

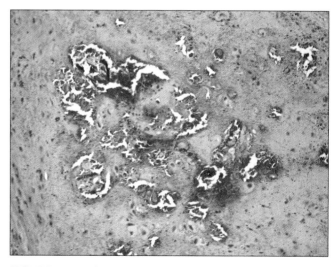

FIGURE 33–6 Calcified chondroma of soft parts. (Photograph courtesy of Dr. John X. O'Connell.)

Differential diagnosis

Distinction from other benign lesions should not be difficult. *Calcifying aponeurotic fibroma* is characterized by short bar-like foci of cartilaginous metaplasia in a dense, poorly circumscribed fibromatous background. It occurs in the hand rather than in the distal portion of the digits and almost always affects patients younger than 25 years. *Tumoral calcinosis* may mimic a heavily calcified chondroma, but it lacks cartilage and usually shows a distinct histiocytic response to the calcified material. *Giant cell tumor of tendon sheath* has a more uniform cellular pattern and rarely has metaplastic cartilage or bone. Radiography usually allows distinction from *periosteal* or *juxtacortical*

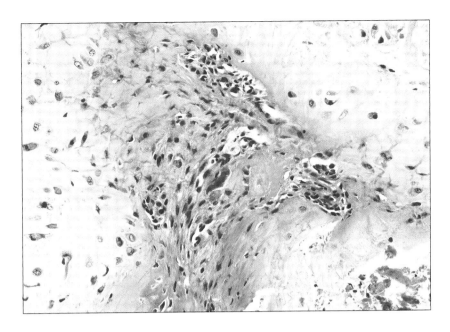

FIGURE 33–7 High-power view of interlobular septa in a chondroma of soft parts. Rare multinucleated giant cells are seen.

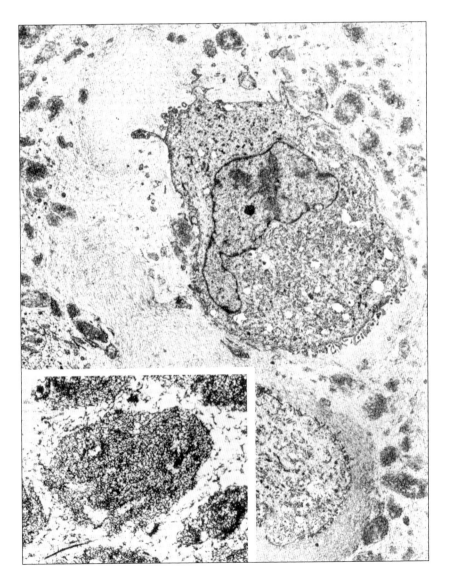

FIGURE 33–8 Electron micrograph of a calcified chondroma of soft parts showing loosely spaced cartilage cells with abundant rough endoplasmic reticulum, free ribosomes, and short irregular microvillous processes surrounded by aggregates of calcium crystals. **(Inset)** Aggregates of hydroxyapatite crystals under high magnification. (From Chung EB, Enzinger FM. Benign chondromas of soft parts. Cancer 1978; 41:1414.)

chondroma, a small well-circumscribed tumor located underneath the periosteum that causes erosion of the underlying cortex with "ledges" or "buttresses" at the margin of the tumor and from *subungual osteochondroma*, a lesion that has cartilage overlying well-developed bone.

Synovial chondromatosis differs from extraskeletal chondroma by its occurrence in large joints, such as the knee, hip, elbow, or shoulder joint and the formation of numerous, small, metaplastic cartilaginous or osteocartilaginous nodules of varying size attached to the synovial membrane of the joint, tendon sheath, or lining of the adjacent extra-articular bursa (Figs 33–9 to 33–11).[30] Rarely, it occurs in the surrounding soft tissues (extra-articular synovial chondromatosis).[31] These synovial nodules often become detached and are found as loose bodies in the joint space. Some are hypercellular with clustering of tumor cells and increased mitotic activity. Most become calcified or ossified and can be readily demonstrated by routine radiography as multiple, small, discrete radiopaque bodies (loose bodies or joint mice). *Nonmineralized "loose bodies"* are demonstrable on arthrograms, CT scans, bone scans or MRI as multiple filling defects outlined by contrast material.[32] As in extraskeletal chondromas, hypercellularity, binucleate cells, and nuclear atypia are compatible with a benign clinical course. However, rare instances of *chondrosarcoma* arising in synovial chondromatosis have been reported.[33,34]

Drawing a sharp line between *extraskeletal myxoid chondrosarcoma* and the *myxoid variant of chondroma* may be difficult, especially with those rare tumors that exhibit a moderate degree of cellular pleomorphism. Usually, however, the cartilage cells of chondromas are better differentiated, especially in the peripheral portion of the

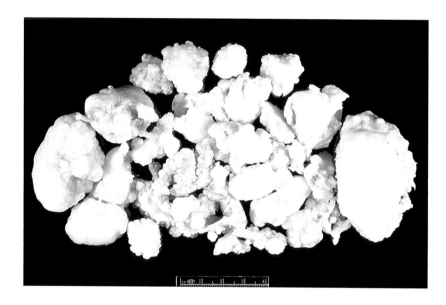

FIGURE 33–9 Conglomerate of variably sized nodules of synovial chondromatosis.

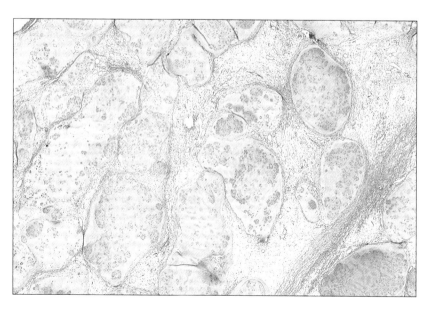

FIGURE 33–10 Synovial chondromatosis of the left knee.

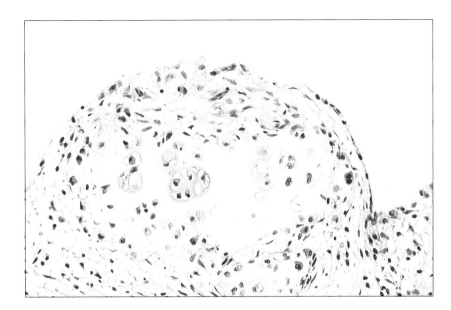

FIGURE 33–11 High-power view of synovial chondromatosis with a nodule of metaplastic cartilage underneath the synovium.

tumor; they tend to be less cellular and smaller; and as a rule they occur in the soft tissues of the hands and feet, unusual locations for myxoid chondrosarcoma. Finally, a significant subset of extraskeletal myxoid chondrosarcomas show evidence of a t(9;22) and analysis by FISH or RT-PCR for evidence of an aberration of the *EWS* gene can be helpful in difficult cases.

Discussion

Although some of the chondroblastic or myxoid forms of extraskeletal chondroma cause concern because of their atypical cellular features, there is no evidence that these tumors behave differently from the well-differentiated forms composed of adult-type hyaline cartilage. We have seen a few tumors that recurred locally, but all were treated effectively by reexcising the tumor. Overall, up to 15% of cases recur locally.[4] It is noteworthy that we have never encountered transformation of extraskeletal chondroma to chondrosarcoma, although this is by no means rare with chondroid lesions of bone. Local excision is the preferred mode of therapy.

EXTRASKELETAL MYXOID CHONDROSARCOMA

Extraskeletal myxoid chondrosarcoma is a morphologically distinctive neoplasm characterized by a multinodular architecture and cords or clusters of chondroblast-like cells deposited in an abundant myxoid matrix. It is categorized by the WHO as a tumor of uncertain differentiation since there is a paucity of convincing evidence of cartilaginous differentiation. However, given that it is classified as a chondrosarcoma, we have chosen to include the discussion of this entity in this chapter.

Extraskeletal myxoid chondrosarcoma has also been reported as "chordoid sarcoma"[35] and by Hajdu et al.[36] as *tendosynovial sarcoma*, a term coined for a group of neoplasms that have a close association with tendosynovial structures, including synovial sarcoma, epithelioid sarcoma, clear cell sarcoma, and extraskeletal myxoid chondrosarcoma. Myxoid chondrosarcoma occurs primarily in the deep tissues of the extremities, especially the musculature. Because a morphologically identical tumor also occurs in bone, radiographic examination, CT scan, or MRI is necessary to establish its soft tissue origin. It is a relatively slow-growing tumor but has a propensity for local recurrence and eventually pulmonary metastasis, sometimes years after the initial diagnosis.

Clinical findings

This tumor is quite uncommon and accounts for less than 3% of all soft tissue sarcomas.[37] It most commonly arises in patients older than 35 years, and only a few cases have been encountered in children and adolescents.[38,39] Most series have found a peak incidence during the fifth or sixth decades of life.[40,41] Men are affected about twice as often as women. The clinical signs and symptoms are non-specific. Most patients present with a slowly growing, deep-seated mass that causes pain and tenderness in approximately one-third of cases. Complications such as ulceration and intra-tumoral hemorrhage may be encountered with large tumors. The duration of symptoms varies considerably, ranging from a few weeks to several years. Some patients have a history of trauma prior to discovery of the tumor, but as with other sarcomas the significance of this finding remains uncertain and is in all likelihood coincidental.

More than two-thirds of the tumors occur in the proximal extremities and limb girdles, especially the thigh and popliteal fossa, similar to myxoid liposarcoma.[40,42-46] Most are deep-seated, although occasional tumors are confined to the subcutis; the latter may be difficult to distinguish from myxoid forms of chondroma. Rare examples have been described in unusual locations including the pleura,[47] mediastinum,[48] retroperitoneum,[49] abdomen,[50] vulva,[51] central nervous system,[52] and fingers.[53] Radiography, CT scans, and MRI show a soft tissue mass with no distinctive radiologic features that would set the tumor apart from other types of soft tissue sarcoma.[54]

Pathologic findings

Macroscopically, the neoplasm is a soft to firm, ovoid, lobulated to nodular, circumscribed mass surrounded by a dense fibrous pseudocapsule. On section, it has a gelatinous, gray to tan-brown surface, its color largely dependent on the extent of hemorrhage, a frequent feature of the tumor (Fig. 33–12). Occasionally, hemorrhage is so prominent the tumor is mistaken for a hematoma. Highly cellular higher-grade tumors often have a fleshy consistency.

The size of the tumor varies from a few centimeters to 15 cm or more; most, however, are 4–7 cm in greatest diameter at the time of excision. Meis-Kindblom et al. reported a size range from 1.1 to 25.0 cm and a median tumor size of 7 cm.[40]

Microscopically, a characteristic multinodular pattern is clearly evident at low magnification (Fig. 33–13). The individual tumor nodules consist of round or slightly elongated cells of uniform shape and size separated by variable amounts of mucoid material (Figs 33–14 to 33–18). The individual cells have small hyperchromatic nuclei and a narrow rim of deeply eosinophilic cytoplasm reminiscent of chondroblasts (Fig. 33–19). Occasional cells show cytoplasmic vacuolization. Unlike chondrosarcoma of bone, differentiated cartilage cells with distinct lacunae are rare; on careful and prolonged search of multiple sections they can be detected in about one-third of cases. Mitotic figures are rare in typical cases but may be numerous in less well differentiated and more cellular forms of the tumor.[55,56]

Characteristically, the individual cells are arranged in short anastomosing cords, strands, or pseudoacini, often creating a lace-like appearance. Less frequently, the cellular elements are disposed in small loosely textured whorls or aggregates, reminiscent of an epithelial neoplasm. Rarely, cellular foci composed of fibroblastic/myofibroblastic spindle-shaped cells are present.[42] Indeed, if these features prevail throughout the tumor, a definitive diagnosis of chondrosarcoma may not be possible. Although most extraskeletal myxoid chondrosarcomas are highly myxoid tumors, a distinct subset are hypercellular with less myxoid stroma between the neoplastic cells; they are composed of sheets of large cells with vesicular nuclei and prominent nucleoli and are referred to as the cellular variant of extraskeletal myxoid chondrosarcoma (Fig. 33–20).[40,56] These tumors are best diagnosed by identifying typical less-cellular areas of extraskeletal myxoid chondrosarcoma or by cytogenetics/molecular genetics (discussed below). Some tumors are composed of a cellular proliferation of relatively small round cells closely resembling extraskeletal Ewing's sarcoma/primitive neuroectodermal tumor (ES/PNET) (Fig. 33–21). Even more rarely, typical extraskeletal

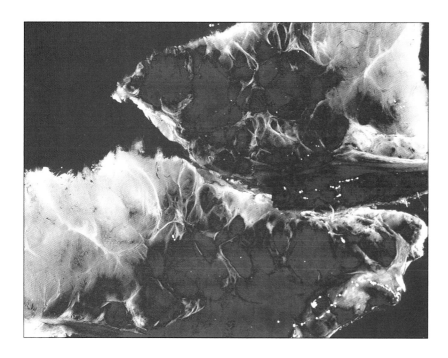

FIGURE 33–12 Gross appearance of an extraskeletal myxoid chondrosarcoma with a characteristic gelatinous appearance and a multinodular growth pattern. The dark appearance of some of the nodules is the result of hemorrhage.

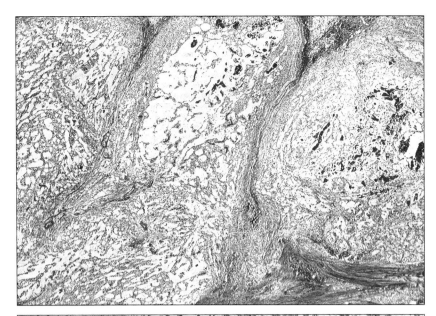

FIGURE 33–13 Low-power view of an extraskeletal myxoid chondrosarcoma with a characteristic nodular arrangement.

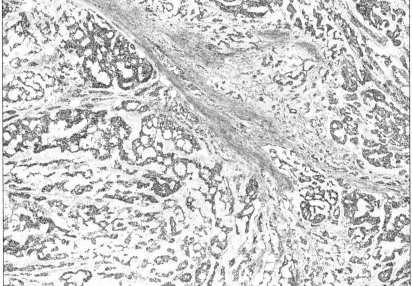

FIGURE 33–14 Extraskeletal myxoid chondrosarcoma. Cords of eosinophilic cells are deposited in an abundant myxoid stroma.

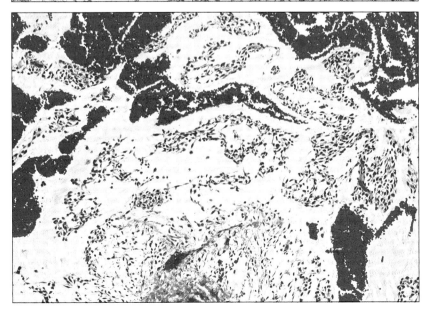

FIGURE 33–15 Characteristic alignment of tumor cells in strands and cords separated by large amounts of mucoid material in an extraskeletal myxoid chondrosarcoma. Note the areas of hemorrhage, a characteristic feature of this tumor.

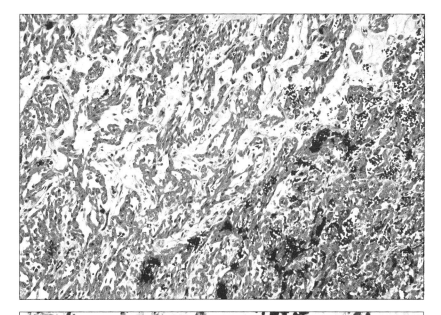

FIGURE 33–16 Extraskeletal myxoid chondrosarcoma. Cords of spindle-shaped cells with deeply eosinophilic cytoplasm are separated by mucoid material.

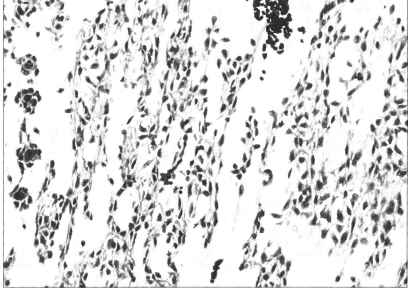

FIGURE 33–17 Extraskeletal myxoid chondrosarcoma with strands of small eosinophilic cells widely separated by mucoid material.

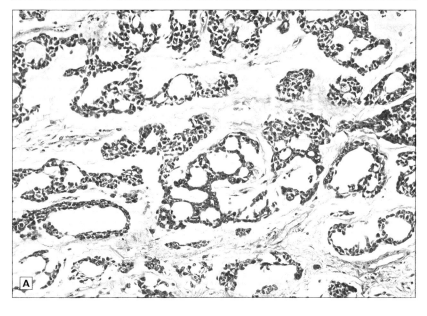

FIGURE 33–18 (A) Extraskeletal myxoid chondrosarcoma composed of cells arranged in a pseudoacinar pattern.

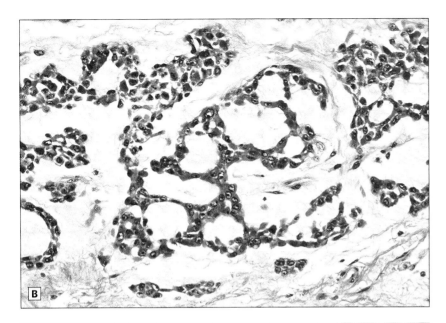

FIGURE 33–18 Continued. **(B)** High-power view of densely eosinophilic epithelioid cells arranged in pseudoacini.

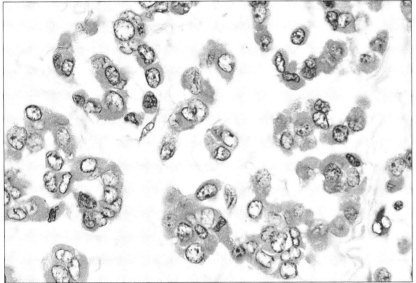

FIGURE 33–19 High-power view of chondroblasts in an extraskeletal myxoid chondrosarcoma. The cells are surrounded by a rim of deeply eosinophilic cytoplasm.

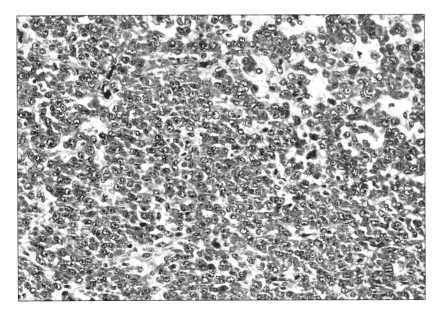

FIGURE 33–20 Cellular variant of an extraskeletal myxoid chondrosarcoma composed of large cells with vesicular nuclei and deeply eosinophilic cytoplasm. Other areas of typical myxoid chondrosarcoma were present in this tumor.

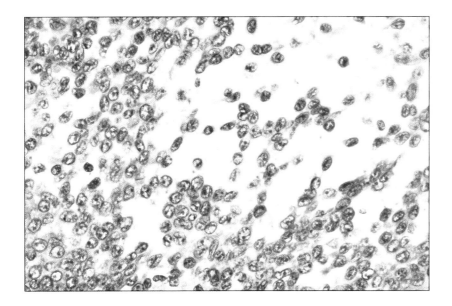

FIGURE 33–21 Cellular variant of extraskeletal myxoid chondrosarcoma composed of small round cells mimicking an extraskeletal Ewing's sarcoma/primitive neuroectodermal tumor.

myxoid chondrosarcomas are associated with or progress to a high-grade pleomorphic sarcoma (dedifferentiated extraskeletal myxoid chondrosarcoma),[57] and still others may have rhabdoid features characterized by cells with large paranuclear hyaline inclusions.[45,58,59] Secondary changes such as fibrosis and hemorrhage are common, but calcification or bone formation is rare.

In the more typical tumors, the extracellular mucinous material is abundant and consists largely of chondroitin 4-sulfate, chondroitin 6-sulfate, and keratan sulfate.[60] It stains deeply with the colloidal iron stain and the Alcian blue preparation; unlike other richly mucinous soft tissue tumors (with the exception of myxochondroma and chordoma), the staining reaction is not inhibited by pre-treating the sections with hyaluronidase. As in normal cartilage cells, intracellular PAS-positive and diastase-sensitive material (glycogen) is another typical feature of the tumor.

Immunohistochemical findings

The cells of myxoid chondrosarcoma stain strongly for vimentin, but this is the only marker that is consistently positive. Dei Tos and colleagues found that only seven of 39 (17.8%) myxoid chondrosarcomas stained for S-100 protein.[61] Given that most of the lesions in the differential diagnosis stain for this antigen, these authors argued that the absence of S-100 protein is diagnostically useful for recognizing myxoid chondrosarcoma. We have found that slightly fewer than one-half of extraskeletal myxoid chondrosarcomas stain for S-100 protein, often with rather focal and weak immunoreactivity. As with many other types of sarcoma, rare cases show focal immuno-reactivity for cytokeratins.[40] In addition, almost 30% of cases may show scattered cells that are EMA positive.[45]

Some authors have found evidence of neuroendocrine differentiation, as evidenced by staining for neuron-specific enolase, chromogranin, or synaptophysin and/or identification of dense-core granules on ultrastructural examination.[62-64] Interestingly, the presence of neuroendocrine features has been associated with the relatively uncommon t(9;17)(q22;q11).[64] Others have found these cells to express microtubule-associated proteins-2 and class III β-tubulin, which are components of microtubules and specifically localized in neurons and their derivatives.[65,66] This has been taken as further evidence of neural/neuroendocrine differentiation in at least some examples of extraskeletal myxoid chondrosarcoma.

Ultrastructural findings

The tumor is composed of fusiform, spindle-shaped or ovoid cells with round, often indented or clefted nuclei, distinct nucleoli, and abundant cytoplasm with a well-developed Golgi complex, numerous mitochondria, glycogen granules, microfilaments, and a prominent rough endoplasmic reticulum containing granular amorphous material (Fig. 33–22).[40,67,68] Densely packed bundles or parallel arrays of microtubules may also be present, a feature that has been observed in myxoid chondrosarcomas of bone and other neoplasms as well.[68,69] The cellular surfaces are slightly scalloped, and there are finger-like cytoplasmic projections (Fig. 33–23), but these features are less-well-pronounced than in normally developing chondroblasts.[70] There are also intracytoplasmic inclusions of matrix material and macular or desmosomal intercellular attachments without tonofilaments. The extracellular spaces contain copious amounts of an amorphous, granular or finely fibrillary matrix and a varying number of collagen fibers.[40] As mentioned previously, a

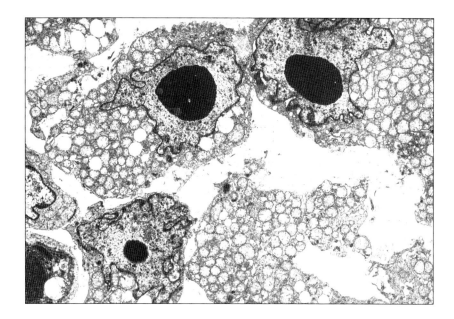

FIGURE 33–22 Electron micrograph of an extraskeletal myxoid chondrosarcoma with numerous mitochondria in chondroblasts.

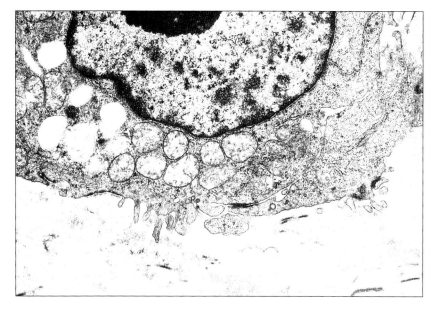

FIGURE 33–23 Electron micrograph of an extraskeletal myxoid chondrosarcoma with the finger-like cytoplasmic projections characteristic of this tumor.

minority of cases show clear-cut ultrastructural evidence of neuroendocrine differentiation in the form of neurosecretory granules.

Cytogenetic findings

Extraskeletal myxoid chondrosarcoma is characterized most commonly by a balanced translocation: t(9;22)(q22;q12), which fuses the *EWS* gene on 22q12 with the *NOR1* gene (variably known as *NR4A3*, *CHN*, *TEC*) on 9q22.[71] This fusion gene can be detected in approximately 70% of cases. Less commonly, extraskeletal myxoid chondrosarcoma is characterized by the presence of a t(9;17)(q22;q11), joining *NOR1* with *RBP56* (also known as *TAF2N*) on 17q11.[72–74] In a study of 18 cases of extraskeletal myxoid chondrosarcoma by Pana-

gopoulos and colleagues, one of these two translocations was detected in 16 of 18 cases, including 13 cases with a t(9;22) and three cases with t(9;17).[75] A third chromosomal variant, t(9;15)(q22;q21) has also been more recently described.[74,76,77] Interestingly, Brody and coworkers did not detect the *EWS/NOR1* fusion transcript in four cases of skeletal myxoid chondrosarcoma, suggesting this lesion is pathogenetically distinct from its extraskeletal counterpart.[78]

The molecular genetic consequences of these translocations is now being unraveled. Filion and Labelle found that the *EWS/NOR1* fusion is capable of inducing transformation of a CFK2 chondrogenic cell line.[79] Furthermore, this fusion down-regulates the *PLAGL1* gene, implicating a role for this gene in the development of extraskeletal myxoid chondrosarcoma.[80] *NOR1* is an

TABLE 33-1	**LIGHT MICROSCOPIC FEATURES OF EXTRASKELETAL MYXOID CHONDROSARCOMA AND DIFFERENTIAL DIAGNOSTIC CONSIDERATIONS**				
Diagnosis	**Cellularity**	**Vascularity**	**Pleomorphism**	**Matrix**	
Myxoma	1+	1+	0	HA	
Myxoid liposarcoma	1+	3+ (fine)	1+	HA	
Myxoid MFH	1+ to 2+	3+ (coarse)	2+ to 3+	HA	
Myxoid chondrosarcoma	1+ (cords)	1+	1+	CS	

MFH, malignant fibrous histiocytoma; HA, hyaluronic acid; CS, chondroitin sulfate.

orphan nuclear receptor that acts as a transcription factor by binding to its putative coactivator, *SIX3*.[81,82] In a gene expression analysis study, Subramanian and co-workers found a distinct pattern of gene expression in extraskeletal myxoid chondrosarcoma, with striking overexpression of the *PPARG* gene, suggesting activation of lipid metabolism pathways.[83]

Differential diagnosis

Extraskeletal myxoid chondrosarcoma may be difficult to distinguish from a number of benign or malignant chondroid-like or myxoid lesions, including the *myxoid variant of extraskeletal (soft part) chondroma*, as discussed previously in this chapter. *Chondromyxoid fibroma* rarely occurs as a periosteal tumor or in soft tissue as secondary tissue implantations. It can be recognized by its greater degree of cellular pleomorphism and condensation of the tumor cells underneath a narrow, richly vascularized fibrous band that borders the individual tumor nodules. In addition, there may be multinucleated giant cells and foci of calcification or ossification, features rarely seen in myxoid chondrosarcomas.

Juxtacortical (parosteal) chondrosarcoma lacks the myxoid component and shows a broad attachment to the perichondrium or periosteum of the involved bone, sometimes with invasion of the underlying cortex and cortical irregularities on radiographs. *Chordoma*, especially its myxoid form, enters the differential diagnosis, but this diagnosis is unlikely if the tumor occurs outside its usual location in the sacrococcygeal region, the base of the skull, or the cervical spine. Extraskeletal myxoid chondrosarcoma shows no radiographic evidence of bone involvement and lacks multivacuolated, physaliphorous tumor cells. Immunohistochemically, chordoma co-expresses S-100 protein and markers of epithelial differentiation (EMA and cytokeratins, particularly cytokeratins 8 and 19). Ultrastructurally, the cells show peculiar multilayered structures composed of rough endoplasmic reticulum and mitochondria in close juxtaposition.

Myxoma and myxoid liposarcoma must also be considered in the differential diagnosis (Table 33–1). *Myxoma* displays a similar paucity of vascular structures, but it is less cellular, as the cytologically bland cells are separated

TABLE 33-2	**MOLECULAR GENETIC ALTERATIONS IN EXTRASKELETAL MYXOID CHONDROSARCOMA AND OTHER MYXOID SARCOMAS IN THE DIFFERENTIAL DIAGNOSIS**	
Diagnosis	**Translocations**	**Genes**
Myxoid chondrosarcoma	t(9;22)(q22;q12)	*NOR1; EWS*
	t(9;17)(q22;q11)	*NOR1; RBP56*
Myxoid liposarcoma	t(12;16)(q13;p11)	*CHOP; FUS*
	t(12;22)(q13;q12)	*CHOP; EWS*
Myxoid MFH	None characteristic	

by abundant myxoid stroma. *Myxoid liposarcoma*, on the other hand, displays a striking plexiform vascular pattern and contains typical lipoblasts, especially at the margin of the tumor lobules. S-100 protein is found in approximately 40% of myxoid liposarcomas and does not help distinguish this tumor from extraskeletal myxoid chondrosarcoma. Both myxoma and myxoid liposarcoma can be clearly distinguished from myxoid chondrosarcoma by the absence of stainable mucin after treating the sections with hyaluronidase. In difficult cases, molecular genetic analysis (RT-PCR or FISH) evaluating for aberrations of *EWS*, *FUS*, and *CHOP* can be quite helpful (Table 33–2).

Still another problem is the distinction of extraskeletal myxoid chondrosarcoma from benign and malignant *mixed tumor/myoepithelioma* as well as *parachordoma*, which likely is related to the former. These tumors display a curious modulation between epithelioid and spindled areas. Although the immunophenotype of deeply situated myoepithelial lesions is incompletely defined, we reserve this diagnosis for lesions that clearly express epithelial and myoepithelial markers, including cytokeratin, S-100 protein, glial fibrillary acidic protein, p63, and calponin. Parachordoma is typically lobulated and contains nests of vacuolated cells deposited in a myxoid matrix, resembling the physaliphorous cells of chordoma. The tumor cells contain intracytoplasmic glycogen, and the stromal mucoid material is rich in hyaluronic acid, which stains positively with Alcian blue stain and is sensitive to predigestion with hyaluronidase. This tumor typically co-expresses S-100 protein and epithelial markers (keratin and EMA) (Table 33–3).

TABLE 33–3	IMMUNOHISTOCHEMICAL FEATURES OF EXTRASKELETAL MYXOID CHONDROSARCOMA AND DIFFERENTIAL DIAGNOSTIC CONSIDERATIONS						
Tumor	CAM5.2	CK7	CK19	EMA	S100	CEA	Actin
Myxoid chondrosarcoma	−	−	−	−	±	−	−
Chordoma	+	±	+	+	+	+	−
Myxoid liposarcoma	−	−	−	−	±	−	−
Mixed tumor/parachordoma	+	−	−	+	+	−	±

Myxopapillary ependymoma can be distinguished by its characteristic location in the sacrum, perivascular growth, positivity for glial fibrillary acidic protein, and the presence of glial-type microfilaments.

Discussion

Generally, extraskeletal myxoid chondrosarcoma is a relatively slow-growing tumor that recurs and eventually metastasizes in most cases. Of the 31 patients in the series by Enzinger and Shiraki, 20 were alive at last follow-up, but six of these patients developed recurrence and four died of metastatic disease.[41] In the more recent study by Meis-Kindblom and colleagues, local recurrences and metastasis developed in 48% and 16% of patients, respectively.[40] Estimated 5-, 10-, and 15-year survival rates were 90%, 70%, and 60%, respectively. Ten-year survival rates ranging from 78% to 88% have been reported in more recent studies, but 10-year disease-free survivals are much lower, ranging from 14% to 36%.[45,46,84]

Late recurrence and metastasis are common. In the series from the AFIP, one patient developed a recurrence 18 years after the initial excision; in another case pulmonary metastasis became evident 10 years after surgical removal of the tumor and 4 years after removal of a regional lymph node metastasis.[41] Tanaka and Asao observed a recurrence 30 years after initial presentation.[85] The most frequent metastatic sites are the lungs, soft tissues, and lymph nodes, although cases have been documented to metastasize to unusual sites such as the pancreas[86] and heart.[87]

Radical local excision with or without adjuvant radiotherapy seems to be the treatment of choice. Good results with high-dose irradiation (6000 cGy) have been reported,[46,88] but chemotherapy has not been found to be efficacious.[46,89]

Whereas there are some cases in which aggressive clinical behavior could be suggested by histologic features such as high cellularity associated with high nuclear grade,[56] the largest study published to date by Meis-Kindblom and colleagues found no association between cellularity and clinical outcome.[40] In a more recent study by Oliveira et al., tumor size of 10 cm or greater, high cellularity, mitotic activity greater than 2/10 high-power fields (HPF), MIB-1 index greater than 10%, and anapla-

sia or the presence of rhabdoid cells were associated with more aggressive behavior.[45] Meis-Kindblom et al. found increasing patient age, large tumor size, and proximal tumor location to be predictive of an adverse outcome.[40]

EXTRASKELETAL MESENCHYMAL CHONDROSARCOMA

First described as a distinct entity by Lichtenstein and Bernstein in 1959,[90] extraskeletal mesenchymal chondrosarcoma is a malignant cartilaginous tumor composed of two components: sheets of primitive mesenchymal cells and interspersed islands of well-differentiated hyaline cartilage. Because of the latter, extraskeletal mesenchymal chondrosarcoma has traditionally been considered a variant of chondrosarcoma, although cytogenetic data have raised the alternative idea that these lesions may be closely related to extraskeletal Ewing sarcoma/primitive neuroectodermal tumor (ES/PNET) (see below). Until more evidence is available, we have continued to classify this tumor as a variant of chondrosarcoma. Because of its prominent vascular pattern, several cases reported in the earlier literature were initially interpreted as hemangiopericytoma with cartilaginous differentiation.[91] Mesenchymal chondrosarcoma is a rare tumor that is two to three times more common in bone than in soft tissue.[92-94] Unlike myxoid chondrosarcoma, it is a rapidly growing tumor with a high incidence of metastasis.

Clinical findings

This neoplasm differs from other forms of chondrosarcoma by its preponderance in young adults 15–35 years of age and its slightly more frequent occurrence in females than in males. The tumor may also occur in young children,[95,96] and has even been described as a congenital lesion.[97] The principal anatomic sites of extraskeletal mesenchymal chondrosarcoma are the region of the head and neck, particularly the orbit, the cranial and spinal dura mater, and the occipital portion of the neck, followed by the lower extremities, especially the thigh (Table 33–4).[98,99] Rare examples of this tumor have been

TABLE 33–4	ANATOMIC DISTRIBUTION OF 51 EXTRASKELETAL MESENCHYMAL CHONDROSARCOMAS	
Anatomic location	**No. of patients**	**%**
Upper extremities	6	12
Lower extremities	18	35
Orbit	5	10
Trunk	8	16
Dura/meninges	11	21
Head and neck	3	6
Total	51	100

Data are from Guccion et al.,[99] Huvos et al.,[92] and Nakashima et al.[93]

TABLE 33–5	UNUSUAL LOCATIONS OF REPORTED CASES OF MESENCHYMAL CHONDROSARCOMA	
Site	**First author**	**Year**
Perineum	Morimura[124]	2004
Retroperitoneum	White[125]	2003
Heart	Nesi[126]	2000
Abdominal wall	Johnson[127]	1997
Labium majus	Lin[128]	1996
Pleura	Luppi[129]	1996
Cauda equina	Rushing[130]	1995
Parapharynx	Gomersall[131]	1990
Mediastinum	Chetty[132]	1990
Nasopharynx	Hamada[133]	2005
Sinonasal	Knott[134]	2003
Thyroid	Abbas[135]	2004
Cerebellum	Yassa[136]	2005

described in virtually every anatomic site and are summarized in Table 33–5.

Orbital lesions tend to produce exophthalmos, orbital pain, blurring of vision, and headaches;[98,100-102] intracranial and intraspinal tumors are accompanied by vomiting, headaches, and various motor and sensory defects.[103,104] Tumors in the extremities usually manifest as a painless, slowly enlarging mass situated in the musculature. We have reviewed cases in which a metastasis from a primary mesenchymal chondrosarcoma of bone mimicked a soft tissue tumor, and as such, a bone survey is essential, particularly when the tumor occurs in an unusual location. In most cases, radiography reveals a well-defined soft tissue mass, often with irregular radiopaque stipplings, arcs, flecks, or streaks as the result of focal calcification or bone formation in cartilaginous areas (Fig. 33–24).[95] CT scans, MRI, and angiography are helpful for outlining the tumor prior to surgical therapy.[105]

Pathologic findings

Grossly, mesenchymal chondrosarcoma presents as a multilobulated circumscribed mass that shows considerable variation in size. In the series from the AFIP, the smallest tumor was 2.5 cm and the largest 37 cm.[99] Cut sections show a mixture of fleshy soft gray-white tissue and scattered foci of irregularly sized cartilage and bone. At times there are also small areas of hemorrhage and necrosis, but hemorrhage is much less prominent than in myxoid chondrosarcoma.

Microscopically, mesenchymal chondrosarcoma exhibits a characteristic pattern composed of sheets of undifferentiated round, oval, or spindle-shaped cells with an abrupt transition with small well-defined nodules of well-differentiated, benign-appearing hyaline cartilage, frequently with central calcification and ossification (Figs 33–25 to 33–27). The undifferentiated cells have ovoid or elongated hyperchromatic nuclei and scanty, poorly outlined cytoplasm; they are arranged in small

aggregates or in a hemangiopericytoma-like pattern about sinusoidal vascular channels lined by a single layer of endothelium (Figs 33–28, 33–29). Solid cellular and richly vascular patterns may be present in different portions of the same neoplasm. The cartilaginous foci are usually well defined, but there are also poorly circumscribed cartilaginous areas that gradually blend with the undifferentiated tumor cells. Spindle cell areas, with or without collagen formation, are present in some cases but are rarely a prominent feature of the tumor. The staining characteristics of the cartilaginous areas are indistinguishable from those of other forms of chondrosarcoma.

Immunohistochemically, the cartilaginous portion of the tumor typically shows strong S-100 protein positivity, whereas only isolated cells in the undifferentiated areas stain for this antigen.[106,107] Moreover, as in other round cell tumors, the undifferentiated cells may stain for neuron-specific enolase and Leu-7. Actin, cytokeratin and EMA are typically negative, but according to several studies, rare examples show scattered cells that stain for desmin, myogenin, or myoD1, making distinction from alveolar rhabdomyosarcoma quite difficult.[108,109] Interestingly, divergent rhabdomyosarcomatous differentiation has been described in exceptional cases of mesenchymal chondrosarcoma.[110]

In the absence of the cartilaginous foci, the undifferentiated areas may closely resemble other round cell sarcomas, particularly ES/PNET. Although early reports on the product of the *MIC2* gene (CD99) indicated that the undifferentiated areas of extraskeletal mesenchymal chondrosarcoma were negative for this antigen,[111,112] a subsequent report by Granter et al.[113] found that all 11 of their cases showed strong membranous immunoreactivity for CD99 in these undifferentiated areas. Similarly, Hoang and colleagues found CD99 staining in 17 of 21 cases.[108] These divergent results are likely due to the use of different antibodies and different antigen retrieval

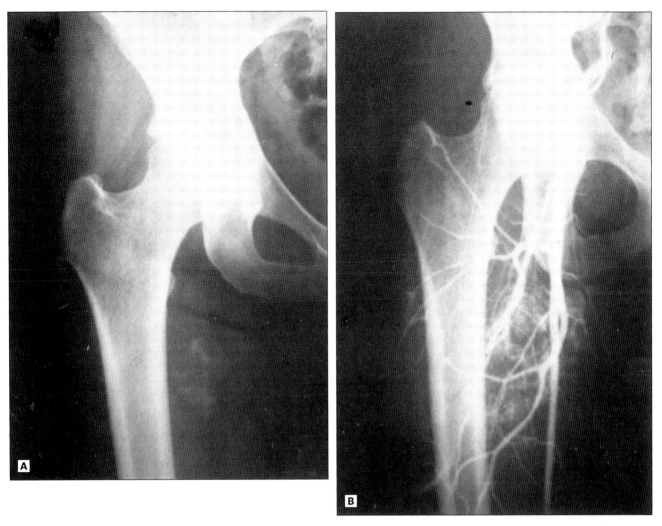

FIGURE 33–24 Extraskeletal mesenchymal chondrosarcoma of the right thigh. **(A)** Radiograph of a soft tissue mass with focal calcification. **(B)** Angiogram demonstrates the rich vascularity of the tumor.

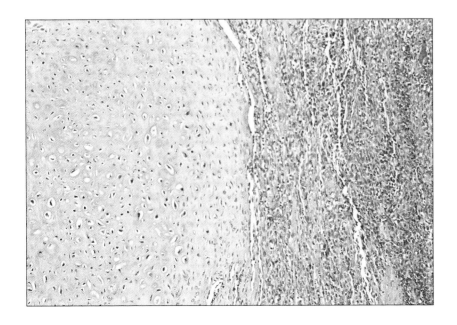

FIGURE 33–25 Low-power view of a mesenchymal chondrosarcoma with the characteristic bimorphic picture: islands of well-differentiated cartilage surrounded by sheets of small, undifferentiated tumor cells.

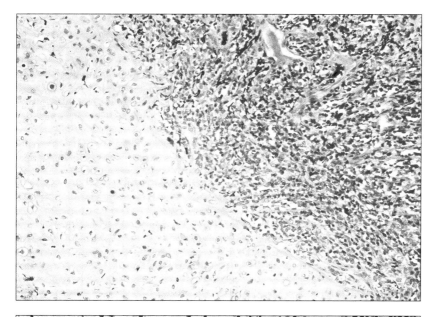

FIGURE 33–26 Sharp demarcation between small, undifferentiated tumor cells and well-differentiated cartilage in a mesenchymal chondrosarcoma.

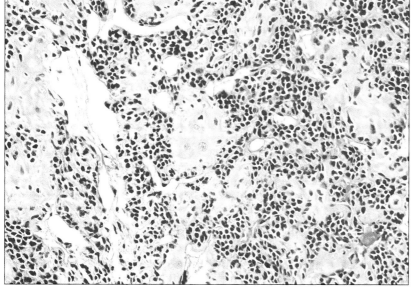

FIGURE 33–27 Extraskeletal mesenchymal chondrosarcoma with an intimate admixture of islands of cartilaginous tissue and small round cells.

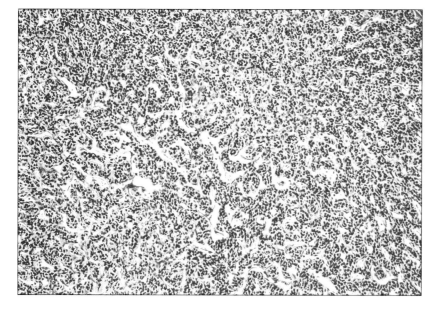

FIGURE 33–28 Small round cells surround a prominent hemangiopericytoma-like vasculature in an extraskeletal mesenchymal chondrosarcoma.

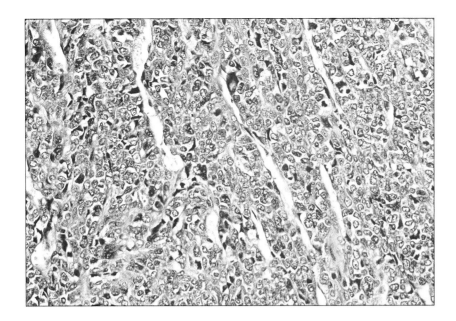

FIGURE 33–29 High-power view of small round cells surrounding hemangiopericytoma-like vessels in an extraskeletal mesenchymal chondrosarcoma.

techniques. We have found fairly consistent CD99 membranous immunoreactivity in mesenchymal chondrosarcoma and, therefore, we believe this marker does not allow distinction of extraskeletal mesenchymal chondrosarcoma from ES/PNET.

More recently, Wehrli and colleagues reported on the utility of Sox9, a transcription factor thought to be a master regulator of chondrogenesis, as helpful in distinguishing mesenchymal chondrosarcoma from other small round blue cell tumors.[114] Prior evidence has suggested that this tumor differentiates towards premesenchymal chondroprogenitor cells.[115] In this study, 21 of 22 mesenchymal chondrosarcomas showed nuclear staining in both the primitive mesenchymal cells and the cartilaginous component. All other types of small round blue cell tumors including neuroblastoma (n = 10), rhabdomyosarcoma (n = 11), ES/PNET (n = 9), desmoplastic small round cell tumor (n = 5), small cell carcinoma (n = 7), Merkel cell carcinoma (n = 6), small cell osteosarcoma (n = 6) and all lymphomas/leukemias (n = 14) were negative for this antigen.

Ultrastructural findings

The cells in well-differentiated cartilaginous areas have irregular round to stellate or scalloped configurations with short cytoplasmic processes, large ovoid nuclei, abundant rough endoplasmic reticulum with focal sac-like dilatations, a well-developed Golgi apparatus, and variable amounts of glycogen.[116–118] The extracellular spaces contain filamentous, finely granular material. In contrast, the undifferentiated, round, ovoid, or polygonal cells have large nuclei, prominent nucleoli, and inconspicuous cytoplasm with few organelles. The cellular elements are closely packed with cohesive cell membranes and desmosomes but without cytoplasmic projections. Fibroblast-like cells with increased rough endoplasmic reticulum and occasional desmosome-like junctions may also be present in the tumor.

Cytogenetic findings

There are relatively few cytogenetic studies of well-characterized examples of mesenchymal chondrosarcoma. Most of these tumors have been shown to harbor complex cytogenetic alterations.[117,119,120] Interestingly, Sainati et al. identified one case of osseous mesenchymal chondrosarcoma with t(11;22)(q24;q12), typical of the ES/PNET family of tumors, raising the possibility that mesenchymal chondrosarcoma may be histogenetically related to the aforementioned group of tumors.[121] However, confirmatory findings have not yet been reported by others. In two cases (one skeletal and one extraskeletal), a Robertsonian 13;21 translocation was detected.[122]

Differential diagnosis

Although typical mesenchymal chondrosarcomas pose no particular diagnostic problem, recognition of this tumor may be difficult with small biopsy or needle biopsy specimens that demonstrate only one of the two tissue elements. In particular, tumors without the cartilaginous element may be mistaken for *ES/PNET*, *malignant hemangiopericytoma*, or *poorly differentiated synovial sarcoma* with a prominent hemangiopericytoma-like pattern. Although we have observed well-differentiated cartilage in rare examples of typical hemangiopericytoma, as a rule the presence of cartilage makes a diagnosis of hemangiopericytoma highly unlikely. Metaplastic cartilage may also occur in poorly differentiated synovial sarcoma, but it is much less common than foci of calcification or bone. Careful search for a biphasic pattern or epithelial differentiation with antibodies against cytokeratin or EMA is indicated in difficult cases. Since CD99 does not allow distinction of mesenchymal chondrosarcoma from ES/PNET or even poorly differentiated synovial sarcoma, molecular analysis for evidence of *EWS* or *SYT* aberrations can be extremely useful. In our practice, paraffin-embedded tissue is routinely utilized for FISH analysis using dual-color, break-apart *EWS* and *SYT* probes.

Distinction from differentiated forms of *extraskeletal chondrosarcoma* may also cause some diagnostic difficulty. These rare tumors, however, always display a more uniform pattern and lack the contrasting differentiated and undifferentiated areas.

Discussion

Mesenchymal chondrosarcoma is a fully malignant tumor that pursues an aggressive clinical course and metastasizes in a high percentage of cases.[99] Nakashima et al. reported 5- and 10-year survival rates of 54.6% and 27.3%, respectively.[93] Earlier studies from Memorial Sloan-Kettering[92] and the Mayo Clinic[123] revealed similar 10-year survival rates.

The principal metastatic site is the lung. Lymph node metastasis is less common than with myxoid chondrosarcoma. Several of our patients followed a protracted clinical course with late metastases, but there seems to be no reliable prognostic relation to the patient's age or degree of cellular differentiation. Combined radical surgery and chemotherapy or radiotherapy appears to be the treatment of choice.

REFERENCES

1. Ghalib SH, Warner ED, DeGowin EL. Laryngeal chondrosarcoma after thyroid irradiation. JAMA 1969; 210:1762.
2. Schajowicz F, Defilippi-Novoa CA, Firpo CA. Thorotrast induced chondrosarcoma of the axilla. Am J Roentgenol Radium Ther Nucl Med 1967; 100:931.

Extraskeletal chondroma (chondroma of soft parts)

3. Dahlin C, Salvador H. Cartilaginous tumors of the soft tissues of the hands and feet. Mayo Clin Proc 1974; 49:721.
4. Chung EB, Enzinger FM. Chondroma of soft parts. Cancer 1978; 41:1414.
5. Anthouli-Anagnostopoulou FA, Papachristou G. Extraskeletal chondroma, a rare soft tissue tumor. Case report. Acta Orthop Belg 2000; 66:402.
6. DelSignore JL, Torre BA, Miller RJ. Extraskeletal chondroma of the hand. Case report and review of the literature. Clin Orthop 1990; 254:147.
7. Bergmann M, Pinz W, Blasius S, et al. Chondroid tumors arising from the meninges – report of 2 cases and review of the literature. Clin Neuropathol 2004; 23:149.
8. Lewis JE, Olsen KD, Inwards CY. Cartilaginous tumors of the larynx: clinicopathologic review of 47 cases. Ann Otol Rhinol Laryngol 1997; 106:94.
9. Wang DH, Guan XL, Xiao LF, et al. Soft tissue chondroma of the parapharyngeal space: a case report. J Laryngol Otol 1998; 112:294.
10. Tosios K, Laskaris G, Eveson J, et al. Benign cartilaginous tumor of the gingiva. A case report. Int J Oral Maxillofac Surg 1993; 22:231.
11. Ando K, Goto Y, Hirabayashi N, et al. Cutaneous cartilaginous tumor. Dermatol Surg 1995; 21:339.
12. Kostopoulos IS, Daniilidis I, Velegrakis G, et al. Chondroma of the parotid gland. Clinical–histologic–immunohistochemical findings of a rare case. Laryngorhinootologie 1993; 72:261.
13. Han JY, Han HS, Kim YB, et al. Extraskeletal chondroma of the fallopian tube. J Korean Med Sci 2002; 17:276.
14. Pollock L, Malone M, Shaw DG. Childhood soft tissue chondroma: A case report. Pediatr Pathol Lab Med 1995; 15:437.

15. Bansal M, Goldman AB, DiCarlo EF, et al. Soft tissue chondromas: diagnosis and differential diagnosis. Skeletal Radiol 1993; 22:309.
16. Dellon AL, Weiss SW, Mitch WE. Bilateral extraosseous chondromas of the hand in a patient with chronic renal failure. J Hand Surg 1978; 3:139.
17. Humphreys TR, Herzberg AJ, Elenitsas R, et al. Familial occurrence of multiple cutaneous chondromas. Am J Dermatopathol 1994; 16:56.
18. Hondar Wu HT, Chen W, Lee O, et al. Imaging and pathological correlation of soft-tissue chondroma: a serial five-case study and literature review. Clin Imaging 2006; 30:32.
19. Gulati Y, Maheshwari A, Sharma V, et al. Extraskeletal osteochondroma of the thigh: a case report. Acta Orthop Belg 2005; 71:115.
20. Sheff JS, Wang S. Extraskeletal osteochondroma of the foot. J Foot Ankle Surg 2005; 44:57.
21. Nakamura R, Ehara S, Nishida J, et al. Diffuse mineralization of extraskeletal chondroma: a case report. Radiat Med 1997; 15:51.
22. del Rosario AD, Bui HX, Singh J, et al. Intracytoplasmic eosinophilic hyaline globules in cartilaginous neoplasms: a surgical, pathological, ultrastructural, and electron probe X-ray microanalytic study. Hum Pathol 1994; 25:1283.
23. Isayama T, Iwasaki H, Kikuchi M. Chondroblastoma-like extraskeletal chondroma. Clin Orthop 1991; 268:214.
24. Yamada T, Irisa T, Nakano S, et al. Extraskeletal chondroma with chondroblastic and granuloma-like elements. Clin Orthop 1995; 315:257.
25. Cates JM, Rosenberg AE, O'Connell JX, et al. Chondroblastoma-like chondroma of soft tissue: an underrecognized variant and its differential diagnosis. Am J Surg Pathol 2001; 25:661.
26. Buddingh EP, Naumann S, Nelson M, et al. Cytogenetic findings in benign cartilaginous neoplasms. Cancer Genet Cytogenet 2003; 141:164.
27. Tallini G, Dorfman H, Brys P, et al. Correlation between clinicopathological features and karyotype in 100 cartilaginous and chordoid tumours. A report from the chromosomes and morphology (CHAMP) collaborative study group. J Pathol 2002; 196:194.
28. Dal Cin P, Qi H, Sciot R, et al. Involvement of chromosomes 6 and 11 in a soft tissue

chondroma. Cancer Genet Cytogenet 1997; 93:177.
29. Bridge JA, Bhatia PS, Anderson JR, et al. Biologic and clinical significance of cytogenetic and molecular cytogenetic abnormalities in benign and malignant cartilaginous lesions. Cancer Genet Cytogenet 1993; 69:79.
30. Polster JM, Evans P, Schils J, et al. Radiologic case study. Synovial chondromatosis of the pisotriquetral joint. Orthopedics 2005; 28:1130, 1205.
31. Robinson P, White LM, Kandel R, et al. Primary synovial osteochondromatosis of the hip: extracapsular patterns of spread. Skeletal Radiol 2004; 33:210.
32. Chung CB, Isaza IL, Angulo M, et al. MR arthrography of the knee: how, why, when. Radiol Clin North Am 2005; 43:733.
33. Hallam P, Ashwood N, Cobb J, et al. Malignant transformation in synovial chondromatosis of the knee? Knee 2001; 8:239.
34. Blokx WA, Rasing LA, Veth RP, et al. Late malignant transformation of biopsy proven benign synovial chondromatosis: an unexpected pitfall. Histopathology 2000; 36:564.

Extraskeletal myxoid chondrosarcoma

35. Martin RF, Melnick PJ, Warner NE, et al. Chordoid sarcoma. Am J Clin Pathol 1973; 59:623.
36. Hajdu SI, Shiu MH, Fortner JG. Tendosynovial sarcoma: a clinicopathological study of 136 cases. Cancer 1977; 39:1201.
37. Tsuneyoshi M, Enjoji M, Iwasaki H, et al. Extraskeletal myxoid chondrosarcoma – a clinicopathologic and electron microscopic study. Acta Pathol Jpn 1981; 31:439.
38. Hachitanda Y, Tsuneyoshi M, Daimaru Y, et al. Extraskeletal myxoid chondrosarcoma in young children. Cancer 1988; 61:2521.
39. Yi JW, Park YK, Choi YM, et al. Bulbous urethra involved in perineal extraskeletal myxoid chondrosarcoma in a child. Int J Urol 2004; 11:436.
40. Meis-Kindblom JM, Bergh P, Gunterberg B, et al. Extraskeletal myxoid chondrosarcoma: a reappraisal of its morphologic spectrum and prognostic factors based on 117 cases. Am J Surg Pathol 1999; 23:636.
41. Enzinger FM, Shiraki M. Extraskeletal myxoid chondrosarcoma. An analysis of 34 cases. Hum Pathol 1972; 3:421.

42. Abramovici LC, Steiner GC, Bonar F. Myxoid chondrosarcoma of soft tissue and bone: a retrospective study of 11 cases. Hum Pathol 1995; 26:1215.

43. Vaquero DH, Suarez MC, Contreras IR, et al. Extraosseous sarcoma. A case report. Int Orthop 1990; 14:367.

44. Okamoto S, Hisaoka M, Ishida T, et al. Extraskeletal myxoid chondrosarcoma: a clinicopathologic, immunohistochemical, and molecular analysis of 18 cases. Hum Pathol 2001; 32:1116.

45. Oliveira AM, Sebo TJ, McGrory JE, et al. Extraskeletal myxoid chondrosarcoma: a clinicopathologic, immunohistochemical, and ploidy analysis of 23 cases. Mod Pathol 2000; 13:900.

46. McGrory JE, Rock MG, Nascimento AG, et al. Extraskeletal myxoid chondrosarcoma. Clin Orthop 2001; 382:185.

47. Goetz SP, Robinson RA, Landas SK. Extraskeletal myxoid chondrosarcoma of the pleura. Report of a case clinically simulating mesothelioma. Am J Clin Pathol 1992; 97:498.

48. Suster S, Moran CA. Malignant cartilaginous tumors of the mediastinum: clinicopathological study of six cases presenting as extraskeletal soft tissue masses. Hum Pathol 1997; 28:588.

49. Fukuda T, Ishikawa H, Ohnishi Y, et al. Extraskeletal myxoid chondrosarcoma arising from the retroperitoneum. Am J Clin Pathol 1986; 85:514.

50. Gaudier F, Khurana JS, Dewan S, et al. Fine-needle aspiration cytology of intra-abdominal wall extraskeletal myxoid chondrosarcoma: a case report and review of the literature. Arch Pathol Lab Med 2003; 127:1211.

51. Santacruz MR, Proctor L, Thomas DB, et al. Extraskeletal myxoid chondrosarcoma: a report of a gynecologic case. Gynecol Oncol 2005; 98:498.

52. Gonzalez-Lois C, Cuevas C, Abdullah O, et al. Intracranial extraskeletal myxoid chondrosarcoma: case report and review of the literature. Acta Neurochir (Wien) 2002; 144:735.

53. Okamoto S, Hara K, Sumita S, et al. Extraskeletal myxoid chondrosarcoma arising in the finger. Skeletal Radiol 2002; 31:296.

54. Tateishi U, Hasegawa T, Nojima T, et al. MRI features of extraskeletal myxoid chondrosarcoma. Skeletal Radiol 2006; 35:27.

55. Reid R, de Silva MV, Paterson L. Poorly differentiated extraskeletal myxoid chondrosarcoma with t(9;22)(q22;q11) translocation presenting initially as a solid variant devoid of myxoid areas. Int J Surg Pathol 2003; 11:137.

56. Lucas DR, Fletcher CD, Adsay NV, et al. High-grade extraskeletal myxoid chondrosarcoma: a high-grade epithelioid malignancy. Histopathology 1999; 35:201.

57. Ramesh K, Gahukamble L, Sarma NH, et al. Extraskeletal myxoid chondrosarcoma with dedifferentiation. Histopathology 1995; 27:381.

58. Oshiro Y, Shiratsuchi H, Tamiya S, et al. Extraskeletal myxoid chondrosarcoma with rhabdoid features, with special reference to its aggressive behavior. Int J Surg Pathol 2000; 8:145.

59. Sigauke E, Rakheja D, Maddox DL, et al. Absence of expression of SMARCB1/INI1 in malignant rhabdoid tumors of the central nervous system, kidneys and soft tissue: an immunohistochemical study with implications for diagnosis. Mod Pathol 2006; 19:717.

60. Fletcher CD, Powell G, McKee PH. Extraskeletal myxoid chondrosarcoma: a histochemical and immunohistochemical study. Histopathology 1986; 10:489.

61. Dei Tos AP, Wadden C, Fletcher CDM. Extraskeletal myxoid chondrosarcoma: an immunohistochemical reappraisal of 39 cases. Appl Immunohistochem 1997; 5:73.

62. Domanski HA, Carlen B, Mertens F, et al. Extraskeletal myxoid chondrosarcoma with neuroendocrine differentiation: a case report with fine-needle aspiration biopsy, histopathology, electron microscopy, and cytogenetics. Ultrastruct Pathol 2003; 27:363.

63. Goh YW, Spagnolo DV, Platten M, et al. Extraskeletal myxoid chondrosarcoma: a light microscopic, immunohistochemical, ultrastructural and immuno-ultrastructural study indicating neuroendocrine differentiation. Histopathology 2001; 39:514.

64. Harris M, Coyne J, Tariq M, et al. Extraskeletal myxoid chondrosarcoma with neuroendocrine differentiation: a pathologic, cytogenetic, and molecular study of a case with a novel translocation t(9;17)(q22;q11.2). Am J Surg Pathol 2000; 24:1020.

65. Hu B, McPhaul L, Cornford M, et al. Expression of tau proteins and tubulin in extraskeletal myxoid chondrosarcoma, chordoma, and other chondroid tumors. Am J Clin Pathol 1999; 112:189.

66. Hisaoka M, Okamoto S, Koyama S, et al. Microtubule-associated protein-2 and class III beta-tubulin are expressed in extraskeletal myxoid chondrosarcoma. Mod Pathol 2003; 16:453.

67. Payne C, Dardick I, Mackay B. Extraskeletal myxoid chondrosarcoma with intracisternal microtubules. Ultrastruct Pathol 1994; 18:257.

68. Antonescu CR, Argani P, Erlandson RA, et al. Skeletal and extraskeletal myxoid chondrosarcoma: a comparative clinicopathologic, ultrastructural, and molecular study. Cancer 1998; 83:1504.

69. DeBlois G, Wang S, Kay S. Microtubular aggregates within rough endoplasmic reticulum: an unusual ultrastructural feature of extraskeletal myxoid chondrosarcoma. Hum Pathol 1986; 17:469.

70. Weiss SW. Ultrastructure of the so-called "chordoid sarcoma": evidence supporting cartilaginous differentiation. Cancer 1976; 37:300.

71. Sciot R, Dal Cin P, Fletcher C, et al. t(9;22)(q22-31;q11-12) is a consistent marker of extraskeletal myxoid chondrosarcoma: evaluation of three cases. Mod Pathol 1995; 8:765.

72. Bjerkehagen B, Dietrich C, Reed W, et al. Extraskeletal myxoid chondrosarcoma: multimodal diagnosis and identification of a new cytogenetic subgroup characterized by t(9;17)(q22;q11). Virchows Arch 1999; 435:524.

73. Sjogren H, Meis-Kindblom JM, Orndal C, et al. Studies on the molecular pathogenesis of extraskeletal myxoid chondrosarcoma – cytogenetic, molecular genetic, and cDNA microarray analyses. Am J Pathol 2003; 162:781.

74. Hisaoka M, Ishida T, Imamura T, et al. TFG is a novel fusion partner of NOR1 in extraskeletal myxoid chondrosarcoma. Genes Chromosomes Cancer 2004; 40:325.

75. Panagopoulos I, Mertens F, Isaksson M, et al. Molecular genetic characterization of the EWS/CHN and RBP56/CHN fusion genes in extraskeletal myxoid chondrosarcoma. Genes Chromosomes Cancer 2002; 35:340.

76. Gan TI, Rowen L, Nesbitt R, et al. Genomic organization of human TCF12 gene and spliced mRNA variants producing isoforms of transcription factor HTF4. Cytogenet Genome Res 2002; 98:245.

77. Sjogren H, Wedell B, Meis-Kindblom JM, et al. Fusion of the NH2-terminal domain of the basic helix-loop-helix protein TCF12 to TEC in extraskeletal myxoid chondrosarcoma with translocation t(9;15)(q22;q21). Cancer Res 2000; 60:6832.

78. Brody RI, Ueda T, Hamelin A, et al. Molecular analysis of the fusion of EWS to an orphan nuclear receptor gene in extraskeletal myxoid chondrosarcoma. Am J Pathol 1997; 150:1049.

79. Filion C, Labelle Y. The oncogenic fusion protein EWS/NOR-1 induces transformation of CFK2 chondrogenic cells. Exp Cell Res 2004; 297:585.

80. Poulin H, Labelle Y. The PLAGL1 gene is down-regulated in human extraskeletal myxoid chondrosarcoma tumors. Cancer Lett 2005; 227:185.

81. Hisaoka M, Okamoto S, Yokoyama K, et al. Coexpression of NOR1 and SIX3 proteins in extraskeletal myxoid chondrosarcomas without detectable NR4A3 fusion genes. Cancer Genet Cytogenet 2004; 152:101.

82. Laflamme C, Filion C, Bridge JA, et al. The homeotic protein Six3 is a coactivator of the nuclear receptor NOR-1 and a corepressor of the fusion protein EWS/NOR-1 in human extraskeletal myxoid chondrosarcomas. Cancer Res 2003; 63:449.

83. Subramanian S, West RB, Marinelli RJ, et al. The gene expression profile of extraskeletal myxoid chondrosarcoma. J Pathol 2005; 206:433.

84. Kawaguchi S, Wada T, Nagoya S, et al. Extraskeletal myxoid chondrosarcoma: a multi-institutional study of 42 cases in Japan. Cancer 2003; 97:1285.

85. Tanaka N, Asao T. Chordoid sarcoma of the soft tissue of the nape of the neck: a case with a 20 year follow-up. Virchows Arch A Pathol Anat Histol 1978; 379:261.

86. Fotiadis C, Charalampoulos A, Chatzikokolis S, et al. Extraskeletal myxoid chondrosarcoma metastatic to the pancreas: a case report. World J Gastroenterol 2005; 11:2203.

87. Banfic L, Jelic I, Jelasic D, et al. Heart metastasis of extraskeletal myxoid chondrosarcoma. Croat Med J 2001; 42:199.

88. Hitchon H, Nobler MP, Wohl M, et al. The radiotherapeutic management of chordoid sarcoma. Am J Clin Oncol 1990; 13:208.

89. Patel SR, Burgess MA, Papadopoulos NE, et al. Extraskeletal myxoid chondrosarcoma. Long-term experience with chemotherapy. Am J Clin Oncol 1995; 18:161.

Extraskeletal mesenchymal chondrosarcoma

90. Lichtenstein L, Bernstein D. Unusual benign and malignant chondroid tumors of bone: a survey of some mesenchymal cartilage tumors and malignant chondroblastic tumors including a few multicentric ones and chondromyxoid fibromas. Cancer 1959; 12:1142.

91. Reeh MJ. Hemangiopericytoma with cartilaginous differentiation involving orbit. Arch Ophthalmol 1966; 75:82.

92. Huvos AG, Rosen G, Dabska M, et al. Mesenchymal chondrosarcoma. a clinicopathologic analysis of 35 patients with emphasis on treatment. Cancer 1983; 51:1230.

93. Nakashima Y, Unni KK, Shives TC, et al. Mesenchymal chondrosarcoma of bone and soft tissue. A review of 111 cases. Cancer 1986; 57:2444.

94. Bertoni F, Picci P, Bacchini P, et al. Mesenchymal chondrosarcoma of bone and soft tissues. Cancer 1983; 52:533.

95. Shapeero LG, Vanel D, Couanet D, et al. Extraskeletal mesenchymal chondrosarcoma. Radiology 1993; 186:819.

96. Crosswell H, Buchino JJ, Sweetman R, et al. Intracranial mesenchymal chondrosarcoma in an infant. Med Pediatr Oncol 2000; 34:370.

97. Tuncer S, Kebudi R, Peksayar G, et al. Congenital mesenchymal chondrosarcoma of the orbit: case report and review of the literature. Ophthalmology 2004; 111:1016.

98. Rushing EJ, Armonda RA, Ansari Q, et al. Mesenchymal chondrosarcoma: a clinicopathologic and flow cytometric study of

13 cases presenting in the central nervous system. Cancer 1996; 77:1884.

99. Guccion JG, Font RL, Enzinger FM, et al. Extraskeletal mesenchymal chondrosarcoma. Arch Pathol 1973; 95:336.

100. Jacobs JL, Merriam JC, Chadburn A, et al. Mesenchymal chondrosarcoma of the orbit. Report of three new cases and review of the literature. Cancer 1994; 73:399.

101. Bagchi M, Husain N, Goel MM, et al. Extraskeletal mesenchymal chondrosarcoma of the orbit. Cancer 1993; 72:2224.

102. Khouja N, Ben Amor S, Jemel H, et al. Mesenchymal extraskeletal chondrosarcoma of the orbit. Report of a case and review of the literature. Surg Neurol 1999; 52:50.

103. Salvati M, Caroli E, Frati A, et al. Central nervous system mesenchymal chondrosarcoma. J Exp Clin Cancer Res 2005; 24:317.

104. Platania N, Nicoletti G, Lanzafame S, et al. Spinal meningeal mesenchymal chondrosarcoma. Report of a new case and review of the literature. J Neurosurg Sci 2003; 47:107.

105. Shinaver CN, Mafee MF, Choi KH. MRI of mesenchymal chondrosarcoma of the orbit: case report and review of the literature. Neuroradiology 1997; 39:296.

106. Devoe K, Weidner N. Immunohistochemistry of small round-cell tumors. Semin Diagn Pathol 2000; 17:216.

107. Swanson PE, Lillemoe TJ, Manivel JC, et al. Mesenchymal chondrosarcoma. An immunohistochemical study. Arch Pathol Lab Med 1990; 114:943.

108. Hoang MP, Suarez PA, Donner LR, et al. Mesenchymal chondrosarcoma: a small cell neoplasm with polyphenotypic differentiation. Int J Surg Pathol 2000; 8:291.

109. Gengler C, Letovanec I, Taminelli L, et al. Desmin and myogenin reactivity in mesenchymal chondrosarcoma: a potential diagnostic pitfall. Histopathology 2006; 48:201.

110. Marshman LA, Gunasekera L, Rose PE, et al. Primary intracerebral mesenchymal chondrosarcoma with rhabdomyosarcomatous differentiation: case report and literature review. Br J Neurosurg 2001; 15:419.

111. Ambros IM, Ambros PF, Strehl S, et al. MIC2 is a specific marker for Ewing's sarcoma and peripheral primitive neuroectodermal tumors. Evidence for a common histogenesis of Ewing's sarcoma and peripheral primitive neuroectodermal tumors from MIC2 expression and specific chromosome aberration. Cancer 1991; 67:1886.

112. Devaney K, Abbondanzo SL, Shekitka KM, et al. MIC2 detection in tumors of bone and adjacent soft tissues. Clin Orthop Relat Res 1995; 310:176.

113. Granter SR, Renshaw AA, Fletcher CD, et al. CD99 reactivity in mesenchymal chondrosarcoma. Hum Pathol 1996; 27:1273.

114. Wehrli BM, Huang W, De Crombrugghe B, et al. Sox9, a master regulator of chondrogenesis, distinguishes mesenchymal chondrosarcoma from other small blue round cell tumors. Hum Pathol 2003; 34:263.

115. Aigner T, Loos S, Muller S, et al. Cell differentiation and matrix gene expression in mesenchymal chondrosarcomas. Am J Pathol 2000; 156:1327.

116. Dickersin GR, Rosenberg AE. The ultrastructure of small-cell osteosarcoma, with a review of the light microscopy and differential diagnosis. Hum Pathol 1991; 22:267.

117. Dobin SM, Donner LR, Speights VO Jr. Mesenchymal chondrosarcoma. A cytogenetic, immunohistochemical and ultrastructural study. Cancer Genet Cytogenet 1995; 83:56.

118. Sato N, Minase T, Yoshida Y, et al. An ultrastructural study of extraskeletal mesenchymal chondrosarcoma. Acta Pathol Jpn 1984; 34:1355.

119. Szymanska J, Tarkkanen M, Wiklund T, et al. Cytogenetic study of extraskeletal mesenchymal chondrosarcoma. A case report. Cancer Genet Cytogenet 1996; 86:170.

120. Sjogren H, Orndal C, Tingby O, et al. Cytogenetic and spectral karyotype analyses of benign and malignant cartilage tumours. Int J Oncol 2004; 24:1385.

121. Sainati L, Scapinello A, Montaldi A, et al. A mesenchymal chondrosarcoma of a child with the reciprocal translocation (11;22)(q24;q12). Cancer Genet Cytogenet 1993; 71:144.

122. Naumann S, Krallman PA, Unni KK, et al. Translocation der(13;21)(q10;q10) in skeletal and extraskeletal mesenchymal chondrosarcoma. Mod Pathol 2002; 15:572.

123. Dahlin DC, Henderson ED. Mesenchymal chondrosarcoma. Further observations on a new entity. Cancer 1962; 15:410.

124. Morimura Y, Fujimori K, Sato T, et al. Imprint cytology of extraskeletal mesenchymal chondrosarcoma of the perineum: A case report. Acta Cytol 2004; 48:649.

125. White DW, Ly JQ, Beall DP, et al. Extraskeletal mesenchymal chondrosarcoma: case report. Clin Imaging 2003; 27:187.

126. Nesi G, Pedemonte E, Gori F. Extraskeletal mesenchymal chondrosarcoma involving the heart: report of a case. Ital Heart J 2000; 1:435.

127. Johnson DB, Breidahl W, Newman JS, et al. Extraskeletal mesenchymal chondrosarcoma of the rectus sheath. Skeletal Radiol 1997; 26:501.

128. Lin J, Yip KM, Maffulli N, et al. Extraskeletal mesenchymal chondrosarcoma of the labium majus. Gynecol Oncol 1996; 60:492.

129. Luppi G, Cesinaro AM, Zoboli A, et al. Mesenchymal chondrosarcoma of the pleura. Eur Respir J 1996; 9:840.

130. Rushing EJ, Mena H, Smirniotopoulos JG. Mesenchymal chondrosarcoma of the cauda equina. Clin Neuropathol 1995; 14:150.

131. Gomersall LN, Needham G. Case report: mesenchymal chondrosarcoma occurring in the parapharyngeal space. Clin Radiol 1990; 42:359.

132. Chetty R. Extraskeletal mesenchymal chondrosarcoma of the mediastinum. Histopathology 1990; 17:261.

133. Hamada H, Taskin Yucel O, Engin H, et al. Mesenchymal chondrosarcoma of the nasopharynx. Otolaryngol Head Neck Surg 2005; 133:639.

134. Knott PD, Gannon FH, Thompson LD. Mesenchymal chondrosarcoma of the sinonasal tract: a clinicopathological study of 13 cases with a review of the literature. Laryngoscope 2003; 113:783.

135. Abbas M, Ajrawi T, Tungekar MF. Mesenchymal chondrosarcoma of the thyroid – a rare tumour at an unusual site. APMIS 2004; 112:384.

136. Yassa M, Bahary JP, Bourguoin P, et al. Intra-parenchymal mesenchymal chondrosarcoma of the cerebellum: case report and review of the literature. J Neurooncol 2005; 74:329.

OSSEOUS SOFT TISSUE TUMORS

This chapter is principally concerned with the following extraskeletal bone-forming lesions: (1) myositis ossificans and related non-neoplastic, heterotopic ossifications, (2) fibrodysplasia (myositis) ossificans progressiva, and (3) extraskeletal osteosarcoma.

Myositis ossificans, by far the most common of the lesions, is a localized, self-limiting ossifying process that follows mechanical trauma in most cases. Identical lesions also occur in persons with no apparent history of preceding injury, and in some of these cases an infectious process has been suggested as a possible cause or initiating factor. Whereas most of these lesions originate in muscle tissue, morphologically similar proliferations also arise in the subcutis, tendons, fasciae, and periosteum. Depending on their location, these heterotopic ossifications have been variously classified as *panniculitis ossificans, fasciitis ossificans, florid reactive periostitis*, and *fibro-osseous pseudotumor of digits*.

Not further discussed in this chapter are other rare heterotopic ossifications that occur after various kinds of soft tissue injury. Such lesions have been described in surgical scars, particularly those of the abdomen,[1,2] in burns,[3] and in association with dislocations of the elbow and other joints, and total hip arthroplasty.[3] They have also been observed in patients with tetanus,[4] in hemophiliacs,[5] in paraplegics secondary to traumatic spinal injury,[6] following pharmacologically induced paralysis,[7] and in patients with spina bifida, myelomeningocele, syringomyelia, cerebral palsy, or poliomyelitis, probably induced by passive movement or forced exercise.[8] Repeated minor soft tissue trauma is also the cause of the "drill bone" or "shooter bone" in the deltoid and pectoralis muscles, the "rider bone" in the adductor muscles of the thigh, and the "shoemaker's bone" in the rectus muscle of the lower abdominal wall – all lesions that are rarely encountered today but have been repeatedly described in the earlier literature.

In addition to these more deeply seated lesions, localized bone formations in the dermis and subcutis are not particularly rare. They may be solitary or multiple, and they occur spontaneously or in connection with a variety of neoplastic (e.g., linear basal cell nevus, basal cell carcinoma, chondrosyringoma, calcifying epithelioma) and non-neoplastic (e.g., scars, acne, puncture wounds, injections, organizing hematomas, pseudohypoparathyroidism, dermatomyositis) processes. Many of these lesions have been reported as *osteoma cutis*, but they too seem to be products of metaplasia rather than neoplasia.[9]

Fibrodysplasia ossificans progressiva (myositis ossificans progressiva) is a heritable disorder in which massive crippling ossification occurs following diffuse fibroblastic proliferation in muscle and associated soft tissues, especially those of the back, shoulder, and neck. The process has its onset during early childhood and follows a relentless clinical course with total disability in its later stages. Microscopically, the early phase of the lesion may be confused with fibromatosis, but this process can be definitively identified radiographically in nearly all cases by the presence of microdactylia and other malformations of the hands and feet.

Extraskeletal osteosarcoma, the only true neoplasm discussed in this chapter, is a highly malignant tumor that afflicts a much older age group than osteosarcoma of bone. Occasionally it occurs in radiation-damaged tissues. With vanishingly rare exceptions, there is no convincing evidence that it ever occurs as a malignant transformation of heterotopic ossification, including myositis ossificans.[10]

NON-NEOPLASTIC HETEROTOPIC OSSIFICATIONS

Myositis ossificans

Myositis ossificans is a benign ossifying process that is generally solitary and well circumscribed. It is found most commonly in the musculature, but it may also occur in other tissues, including tendons, subcutaneous fat (sometimes referred to as *panniculitis ossificans*) and even within nerves.[11] Distinguishing between traumatic and nontraumatic forms of myositis ossificans serves little purpose, as both forms are morphologically identical and are assuredly secondary to some kind of injury.

Histologically, the early stage of myositis ossificans has immature and highly cellular zones that are often confused with extraskeletal osteosarcoma. The late stage of myositis ossificans, on the other hand, consists almost entirely of mature lamellar bone and is sometimes misinterpreted as an osteoma. As Ackerman and others have pointed out, the term *myositis ossificans* is a misnomer because the lesion is not necessarily confined to the musculature, is devoid of bone in its early proliferative phase, and lacks a significant degree of inflammation.[12] If inflammation is present, it is usually minimal and is mostly evident in the tissues surrounding the lesion. For these reasons, myositis ossificans and related processes have also been designated as "pseudomalignant osseous tumors of soft tissues"[12] and "extraosseous localized, non-neoplastic bone and cartilage formation."[12] Although undoubtedly these terms are more descriptively accurate and less confining, they are more cumbersome and have not been widely accepted in the literature. For this reason the conventional term *myositis ossificans* is retained for this chapter.

Clinical findings

The initial complaint, noted within hours or days after injury, is pain or tenderness, followed by a diffuse, doughy soft tissue swelling. Later, usually during the second or third week after onset, the swelling becomes more circumscribed and indurated and gradually changes into a mass that is distinctly outlined and firm to stony on palpation. The mass averages 3–6 cm in greatest diameter, but lesions measuring as large as 15 cm have been observed.

The condition chiefly affects young, vigorous, athletically active adolescents and adults, predominantly males,[13,14] but it may also be found in older persons and females. Myositis ossificans is rare in small children;[15] most ossifying soft tissue lesions in this age group are examples of fibrodysplasia ossificans progressiva. In about 80% of cases the lesion involves the limbs; the favored sites in the lower extremity are the quadriceps muscle and the gluteus muscle and in the upper extremity the flexor muscles, especially the brachialis muscle. Trauma-induced lesions have also been described in the head and neck, particularly in the masseter temporalis and sternocleidomastoid muscles. Rare examples of a histologically identical lesion may also arise within nerves.[11,16] Deep-seated lesions may involve both muscle and underlying periosteum. Rarely, similar lesions arise in the mesentery, usually in middle-aged to elderly men (median age 49 years) following significant abdominal surgery or trauma.[1,17] These patients usually present with bowel obstruction.

Laboratory findings in myositis ossificans are typically normal. There are no significant changes in serum calcium or phosphorus levels, but sometimes the erythrocyte sedimentation rate, white blood cell count, and alkaline phosphatase levels are slightly elevated; these changes return to normal after the lesion is removed.

Radiographic findings

At the initial stage, radiographs show merely a slight increase in soft tissue density. Calcification is rarely seen before the end of the third week after injury and initially presents as rather faint, irregular, floccular radiopacities, sometimes described as the "dotted veil" pattern of myositis ossificans. As the lesion progresses and becomes increasingly calcified, it presents as a well-outlined soft tissue mass that is most densely calcified at its periphery. Calcification becomes clearly apparent radiographically 4–6 weeks after the onset of the lesion; it proceeds from the periphery toward the center of the process, but even in late lesions the central core tends to remain uncalcified (Figs 34–1, 34–2). Angiograms reveal a diffuse blush and

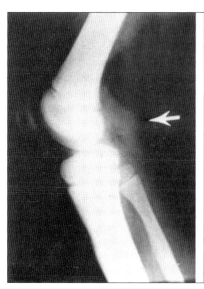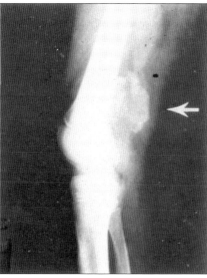

FIGURE 34–1 Myositis ossificans of the popliteal fossa showing evidence of progressive ossification within a 22-day period.

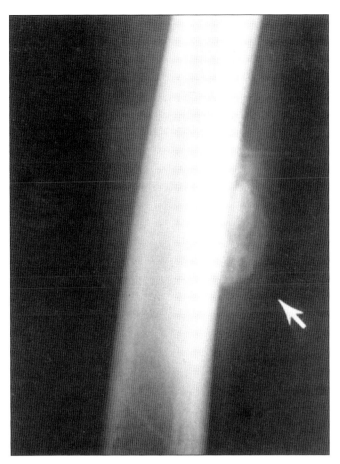

FIGURE 34-2 Radiograph of myositis ossificans (arrow) of the upper thigh. The lesion had been present for 5 weeks.

fine neovascularity during the early phase of the process. The appearance of myositis ossificans on computed tomography (CT) and magnetic resonance imaging (MRI) is quite characteristic and often leads to the correct diagnosis.[18-20]

Pathologic findings

Grossly, most of the lesions measure 3-6 cm in greatest diameter. They tend to be well circumscribed and cut with a gritty sensation; they are white, soft, and rather gelatinous (or hemorrhagic) in the center and yellow-gray with a rough granular surface at the periphery.

Histologically, myositis ossificans is characterized by the presence of a distinct zonal pattern that reflects different degrees of cellular maturation, a pattern that is most conspicuous in lesions of 3 weeks' or more duration. In these cases the innermost portion of the lesion is composed of immature, loosely textured, often richly vascular fibroblastic tissue bearing a close resemblance to nodular fasciitis or granulation tissue (Fig. 34-3). The constituent fibroblasts and myofibroblasts display a mild degree of cellular pleomorphism and rather prominent mitotic activity. They are intermingled with a varying number of macrophages, chronic inflammatory cells, fibrinous material, and not infrequently multinucleated giant cells. In addition, there may be prominent endothelial proliferation, focal hemorrhage, fibrin, and entrapped atrophic or necrotic muscle fibers.[21]

Peripheral to these areas is an intermediate zone in which the cells become condensed into ill-defined trabeculae consisting of a mixture of fibroblasts, osteoblasts, and varying amounts of osteoid separated by thin-walled, ectatic vascular channels (Figs 34-4 to 34-6). Farther toward the periphery the osteoid increasingly undergoes

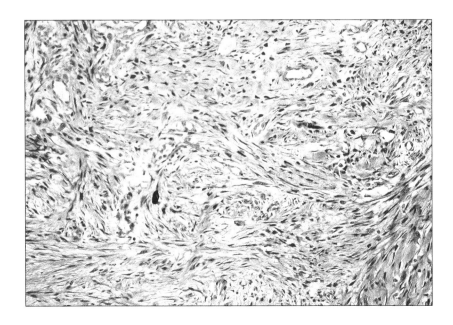

FIGURE 34-3 Central portion of myositis ossificans showing fibroblastic/myofibroblastic proliferation closely resembling nodular fasciitis.

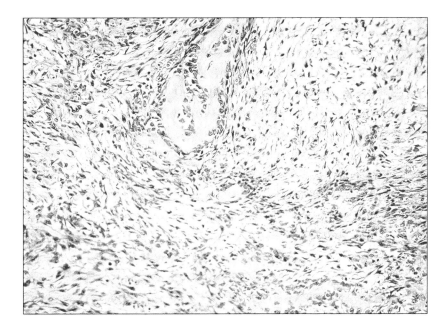

FIGURE 34–4 Intermediate portion of myositis ossificans with transition from proliferating spindle-shaped cells to trabeculae of osteoid lined by plump osteoblasts.

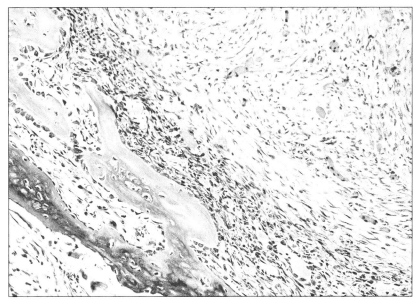

FIGURE 34–5 Osteoblast-lined osteoid adjacent to spindle cell proliferation resembling nodular fasciitis in a case of myositis ossificans.

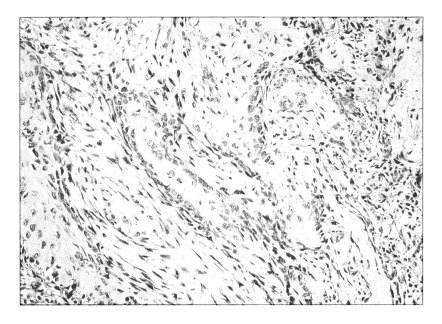

FIGURE 34–6 Myositis ossificans. Numerous osteoblasts are seen lining osteoid, surrounded by a cytologically bland proliferation of spindle-shaped cells.

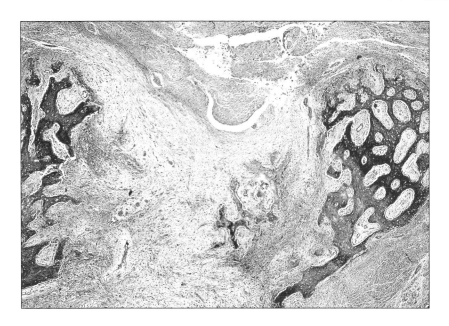

FIGURE 34–7 Low-magnification view of a peripheral portion of myositis ossificans displaying a zone of osteoid trabeculae rimmed by osteoblasts, underneath which is a proliferation of spindle-shaped cells.

TABLE 34–1	DIFFERENTIAL DIAGNOSTIC FEATURES OF MYOSITIS OSSIFICANS, FIBRO-OSSEOUS PSEUDOTUMOR OF THE DIGITS, AND EXTRASKELETAL OSTEOSARCOMA				
Lesion	**Peak age**	**Site**	**Zoning**	**Pleomorphism**	**Atypical mitoses**
Myositis ossificans	2nd–3rd decades	Muscles of lower or upper extremities	Immature central areas, mature lamellar bone at periphery	Absent to mild	Absent
Fibro-osseous pseudotumor	2nd–3rd decades	Digits	Usually absent	Absent to mild	Absent
Extraskeletal osteosarcoma	6th–7th decades	Muscles of lower or upper extremities	If present, has central osteoid or bone and atypical spindled cells at periphery	Moderate to severe	Present

calcification and evolves into mature lamellar bone (Fig. 34–7). Not infrequently, islets of immature or mature cartilage are present and precede bone formation. Characteristically, bone formation is most prominent at the margin of the lesion, often with rimming of the osteoid by a monolayer of osteoblasts showing little variation in size and shape. The bone is separated from the surrounding muscle tissue by a zone of loose, myxoid, or compressed fibrous tissue. The surrounding muscle often shows atrophic changes, sometimes together with a mild inflammatory infiltrate and focal sarcolemmal proliferation. In some lesions, particularly those arising in the subcutaneous fat, the zonal pattern is absent or inconspicuous. Older lesions consist only of mature lamellar bone together with interspersed fat cells, fibrous tissue, and thin-walled vascular spaces indistinguishable from osteoma. Ultrastructurally, myositis ossificans consists of fibroblasts and myofibroblasts with focally condensed myofilaments, macrophages, and preosteoblasts and osteoblasts with numerous mitochondria and prominent rough endoplasmic reticulum.

Malignant transformation of myositis ossificans

We have seen no convincing cases of malignant transformation of myositis ossificans, but there are several accounts in the literature in which transformation of myositis ossificans into extraskeletal osteosarcoma is claimed.[10] In most of these cases, the presence of myositis ossificans is poorly documented, and in only a few is the diagnosis based on biopsy. In some of the reported cases, long duration and dedifferentiation of a well-differentiated osteosarcoma may have simulated an origin in myositis ossificans. Regardless, for all practical purposes, myositis ossificans is a benign pseudosarcomatous lesion and should be treated as such.

Differential diagnosis

It is of paramount importance to distinguish this lesion from extraskeletal osteosarcoma (Table 34–1). This is best accomplished on the basis of the characteristic zoning phenomenon of myositis ossificans, that is, the presence of immature cellular areas in the center and more mature, ossifying areas with osteoblastic rimming at the periphery. In sharp contrast, osteosarcoma displays a more disorderly growth of hyperchromatic and often pleomorphic cells with lace-like rather than trabecular osteoid formation and sometimes a "reverse zoning effect" (i.e., osteoid or bone formation in the interior and older portion of the lesion and immature spindle cell formation at its margin). Moreover, unlike myositis ossificans, extraskeletal osteosarcoma shows a greater degree of cellular atypia, no subsidence of growth at the periphery, and infiltration of neighboring tissues in a destructive manner. Mitotic figures are present in the immature portions of myositis ossificans and osteosarcoma, but several clearly atypical or tripolar forms point toward malignancy. Confusion of myositis ossificans with osteosarcoma is most likely with small biopsy specimens obtained during the initial proliferative phase or obtained from the cellular center of an early lesion.

The differential diagnosis may also be a problem in cases in which the lesion lacks the characteristic zoning phenomenon and grows in an irregular multifocal or multilobulated fashion, as in most cases of fibro-osseous pseudotumor involving the distal portions of the fingers or toes (discussed below). Because extraskeletal osteosarcomas occur rarely in young persons, consideration of the age of the patient may help reach a correct diagnosis.

Rarely, a soft tissue metastasis of a silent osteoblastic carcinoma can masquerade as myositis ossificans. Benign lesions also may be confused with myositis ossificans, including purely reactive lesions such as nodular fasciitis, proliferative myositis, post-traumatic periostitis, and exuberant fracture callus. Proliferative myositis may have minute foci of osteoid or bone, but characteristically this feature is associated with a diffuse proliferation of plump fibroblasts resembling ganglion cells. Post-traumatic periostitis manifests as an ossified mass that is attached to bone with a broad base. Exuberant callus is usually associated with a discernible fracture line on standard radiographs.

Discussion

The pathogenesis of myositis ossificans is still poorly understood. In cases with a definite history of traumatic injury, it can be assumed that the process commences with tissue necrosis or hemorrhage, or both, followed by exuberant reparative fibroblastic/myofibroblastic and vascular proliferation, eventually leading to progressive ossification. The exact environmental or humoral conditions that favor ossification as opposed to a nonossifying reactive myofibroblastic proliferation are not understood. Detachment and intramuscular implantation of periosteal cells are not necessary prerequisites for ossification because this process also takes place in the subcutis and at other sites that are a considerable distance from bone.

Similarly, the occurrence of ectopic ossifications in paraplegics and patients with tetanus may be explained by trauma resulting from passive exercise rather than disturbed neurotrophic factors. The source of the osteoblasts remains an enigma. They may be transformed fibroblasts, or they may be derived from primitive perivascular mesenchymal cells secondary to injury and necrosis of muscle and other tissues.[22]

A satisfactory explanation for non-traumatic cases of myositis ossificans is even more problematic. It is likely that minor injury such as a spontaneous muscle tear or a similar disruptive lesion associated with heavy manual labor, weight lifting, or some other strenuous exercise or activity has been overlooked or forgotten; yet it is difficult to exclude the possibility that some of these cases are caused or initiated by an infectious process. Lagier and Cox reported a patient who had had an anti-influenza vaccination 15 days before the onset of the lesion.[23]

Because myositis ossificans is a benign, self-limiting process, the prognosis is excellent, and there is no need for further therapy once the diagnosis of myositis ossificans has been established. Although quite challenging, this lesion can occasionally be diagnosed by core biopsy[24] or even fine needle aspiration.[25] If the lesion is partly excised at an early phase of its growth, it may continue to grow for a limited period; in these cases repeated radiographic examinations should be obtained during the follow-up period to document the maturation of the lesion and the absence of destructive growth. Spontaneous regression of myositis ossificans has also been observed.[26]

Fibro-osseous pseudotumor of the digits

Fibro-osseous pseudotumor of the digits, a heterotopic ossification closely related to myositis ossificans, occurs in the subcutaneous tissue of the digits.[27] It has been described under various names, including *florid reactive periostitis of the tubular bones of hands and feet,*[28] *pseudomalignant osseous tumor of the soft tissues,*[29] and *parosteal fasciitis.*[30] This lesion appears to be closely related to bizarre parosteal osteochondromatous proliferation (Nora's lesion) and acquired osteochondroma. Clinically, this process presents as a painful, localized, fusiform, often erythematous swelling in the soft tissues of the fingers, especially the region of the proximal phalanx (Fig. 34–8)[27,28] and, less commonly, the toes.[31] It predominantly affects young adults and, unlike myositis ossificans, is more common in women.

Radiographically, fibro-osseous pseudotumor of the digits is usually an ill-defined soft tissue mass with focal calcification that lacks the typical zoning pattern of myositis ossificans.[32,33] There may be thickening of the adjacent periosteum, and rare cases erode adjacent bone.[34] Histologically, the lesion closely resembles myositis ossificans but lacks its orderly zonal pattern; it consists merely

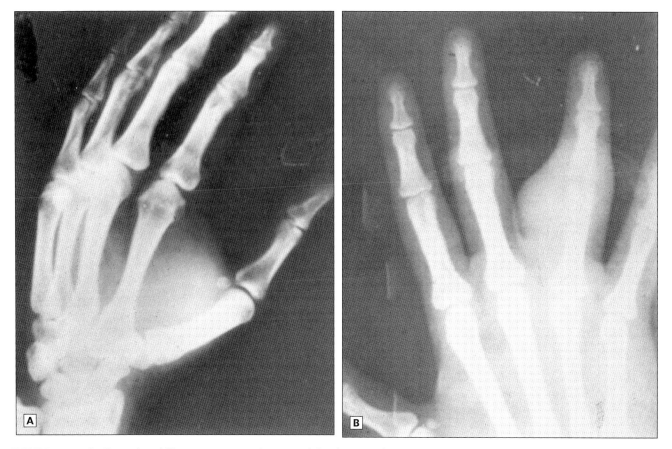

FIGURE 34–8 Radiographs of fibro-osseous pseudotumor of the thenar eminence **(A)** and the right ring finger **(B)**.

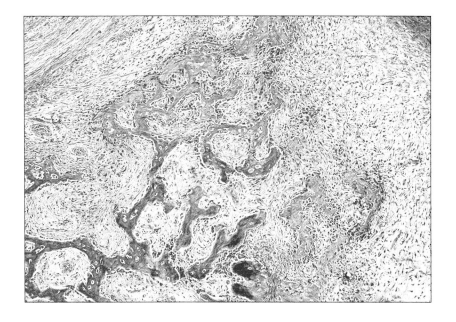

FIGURE 34–9 Fibro-osseous pseudotumor of the right index finger showing a peripheral zone of proliferating spindle cells and a central zone of osteoid.

of an irregular, often nodular mixture of loosely arranged fibroblasts, a prominent myxoid matrix, and deposits of osteoid rimmed by uniform osteoblasts (Figs 34–9 to 34–12).[21,27] Multinucleated giant cells may be seen, and in some cases there is a mild lymphoplasmacytic infiltrate. Immunohistochemically, the spindle-shaped cells express vimentin and actin, suggesting myofibroblastic differentiation.[35]

The major differential diagnosis is with *extraskeletal osteosarcoma*. The latter lesion typically occurs in older patients and rarely involves the digits. Furthermore, extraskeletal osteosarcoma is characterized by more

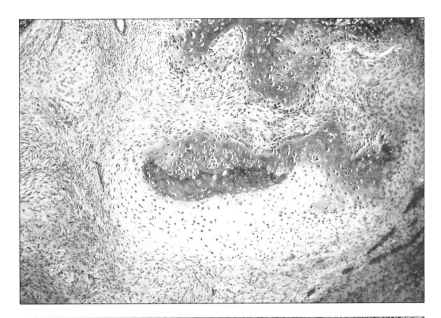

FIGURE 34–10 Fibro-osseous pseudotumor with osteoblast-rimmed osteoid material and a surrounding chondroid zone.

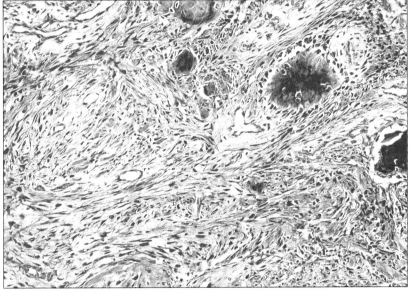

FIGURE 34–11 High-magnification view of fibro-osseous pseudotumor with proliferation of spindle-shaped cells adjacent to trabeculae of osteoid resembling myositis ossificans.

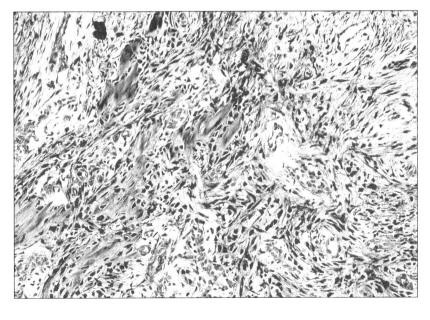

FIGURE 34–12 Fibro-osseous pseudotumor with an admixture of proliferating cytologically bland spindle-shaped cells and osteoid.

pleomorphic hyperchromatic cells and atypical mitotic figures. *Bizarre parosteal osteochondromatous proliferation* (*Nora's lesion*), similar to fibro-osseous pseudotumor, predominantly involves the short tubular bones of the hands and feet of young adults.[36-39] Given the overlapping clinical and histologic features, it has been proposed that Nora's lesion most likely represents an intermediate step between fibro-osseous pseudotumor of the digits and acquired osteochondroma (Turret exostosis).[40] Nora's lesion presents as a well-delineated mass attached to the bone surface. Histologically, a zonal architecture is apparent at low magnification with central or basally located new bone surrounded by a peripheral cap of cartilage. The cartilage often shows foci of hypercellularity with binucleated cells which may result in a misinterpretation of malignancy if the entire clinical and radiographic picture is not considered.

As with the conventional form of myositis ossificans, the exact pathogenetic mechanism of this process is not clear. In the series by Dupree and Enzinger,[27] a history of trauma was provided in only nine of 21 patients. Similarly, Spjut and Dorfman reported a history of trauma in five of 12 cases.[28] Most are cured by complete excision, and local recurrences are generally related to inadequate excision.[41,42] Of the seven cases with follow-up information in the series from the Armed Forces Institute of Pathology (AFIP), only one patient developed a local recurrence.[27] Spjut and Dorfman reported local recurrence in only one of 10 patients.[28]

FIBRODYSPLASIA (MYOSITIS) OSSIFICANS PROGRESSIVA

Fibrodysplasia (myositis) ossificans progressiva (FOP) is a rare, slowly progressive autosomal dominant disorder that principally affects children under the age of 10 years. It is characterized by progressive fibroblastic proliferation and subsequent calcification and ossification of subcutaneous fat, muscles, tendons, aponeuroses, and ligaments. The disorder is often associated with congenital symmetric malformations of the digits, especially microdactyly or adactyly of the thumbs and great toes, which precede onset of the fibroblastic proliferations and calcifications. Its prevalence in children, diffuse or multinodular soft tissue involvement, progressive clinical course, and increased familial incidence distinguish it from localized myositis ossificans.

Clinical findings

The disease has its onset between birth and 6 years of age, although in rare instances it arises in older children and even in young adults.[43] Males and females are about equally affected, and there is no predilection for any particular race. As in localized myositis ossificans, FOP presents as a painful, doughy soft tissue swelling that most commonly begins in the upper paraspinal muscles and spreads from the axial to the appendicular skeleton, typically from cranial to caudal and from the proximal to the distal extremities (Fig. 34–13).[44] This typical progression may be modified by injury, immunization, surgery,[21] and even following an influenza-like illness.[45] The preosseous lesion is a highly vascular fibroblastic proliferation that is histologically similar to that seen in the infantile forms of fibromatosis.[46,47] During the later stages the fibroblastic proliferation is replaced by endochondral ossification with mature lamellar bone having bone marrow elements that may involve an entire muscle from origin to insertion.[47] This causes progressive muscle stiffening, immobilization, and contraction deformities, leading to severe changes in posture and gait as well as increasing difficulties in respiration.[48] In fact, patients with FOP are much more likely to suffer a catastrophic fall resulting in traumatic brain injury, intracranial hemorrhage, or death than are those without this disease.[49] Involvement of the masseter muscle may impair normal mastication and result in severe weight loss.[50] Many patients die during early adult life from respiratory failure or pneumonia.[43,51,52]

Malformation or the absence of one or more digits is an almost constant finding that helps distinguish this disease from infantile forms of fibromatosis. The malformations are usually present at birth or appear soon thereafter; in the earliest stage they are best identified radiographically (Fig. 34–14); they consist mainly of bilateral shortening of the fingers (microdactyly), absence of both thumbs and great toes (adactyly), or digital deviations, particularly valgus position of the great toe (bilateral hallux valgus). Connor and Evans,[53] in a review of 34 affected patients, reported hallux valgus in 79%, short first metacarpals in 59%, and deviation (clinodactyly) of the fifth fingers in 42%. In 29 of the 34 cases, the skeletal alterations were present at birth. Sometimes the significance of these osseous malformations is not immediately recognized, and surgical correction is attempted, precipitating ectopic ossification. Additional radiographic changes, which appear at a later stage of the disease, consist of bony bridges in muscles and tendons; contractures and ankylosis of the shoulder, elbow, spine, and other joints;[54-56] exostosis of the tibia and other bones; metaphyseal widening of long bones;[57] and osteoporosis (Fig. 34–15). CT scans and MRI may help demonstrate early changes of the disease (Fig. 34–16);[54] bone scans reveal increased tracer uptake at the sites of ossification. Deformity of the ears, absence of teeth, deafness, and sexual infantilism may also be part of the clinical picture.[58] Laboratory findings are generally unremarkable, except for elevated alkaline phosphatase levels. Basic fibroblast growth factor, a potent stimulator of angiogenesis, has been found to be significantly elevated in the urine in patients with acute flare-ups of FOP but not during

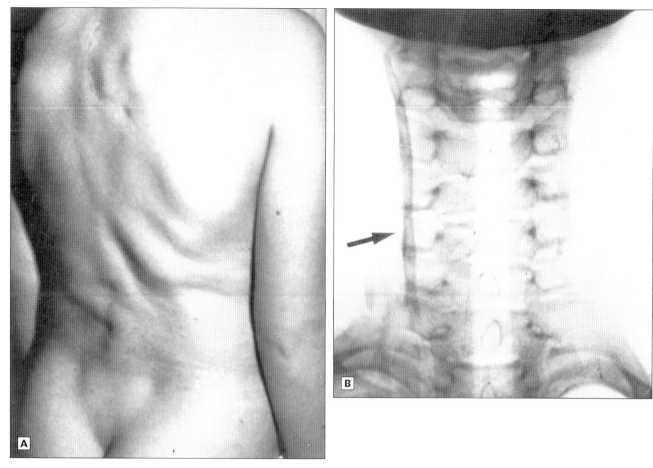

FIGURE 34–13 **(A)** Fibrodysplasia (myositis) ossificans progressiva involving the back of a child with ill-defined, indurated nodules caused by focal fibroblastic proliferation and ossification of the musculature. **(B)** Radiograph of linear ossification of paraspinal muscles (arrow). (Courtesy of Prof. Dr. Günther Möbius, Schwerin.)

disease quiescence.[59] Although the human leukocyte antigen HLA-B27 is common in patients with disorders of heterotopic bone formation,[60] this allele has not been found with increased prevalence in patients with FOP.[61]

Pathologic findings

There are essentially two stages of the disease. The first consists of nodular swelling of muscle and subcutis caused by interstitial edema, perivascular lymphocytic inflammation, and a loose proliferation of fibroblasts, usually in the endomysium and perimysium (Fig. 34–17).[62] During the second stage, collagen is laid down between the fibroblasts, followed by variable muscular atrophy, calcification, ossification of the collagenized fibrous tissue, and formation of mature bone and cartilage. Unlike localized myositis ossificans, the ossification occurs in the center of the nodules. The nodules often interconnect, leading eventually to the formation of bony bridges that replace muscles, tendons, and ligaments.

Gannon and colleagues found that the cells in the early preosseous fibroblastic stage are immunoreactive for bone morphogenetic protein 2/4 (BMP4, discussed below), whereas the cells of infantile fibromatosis do not stain for this antigen.[63]

Genetic aspects of fibrodysplasia ossificans progressiva

A rare disease, FOP is inherited in an autosomal dominant pattern,[64] and most cases appear to be due to new mutations, probably related to the low reproductive fitness of afflicted individuals.[65,66] In addition, there is variable expression of this disorder, as some patients have a milder form of the disease.[67,68] Janoff and colleagues reported a fascinating case in which this disease occurred in two half-sisters with the same unaffected mother and different unaffected fathers, suggesting that the mother had a mutant gene in numerous ova but that the mutant gene was present in few or no somatic cells (gonadal mosaicism).[69]

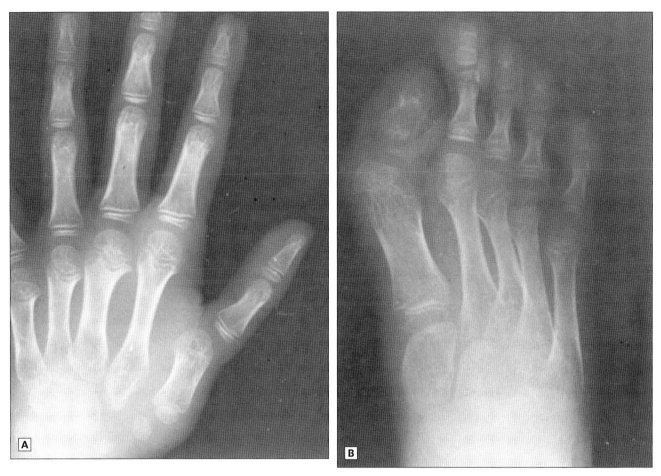

FIGURE 34–14 Fibrodysplasia (myositis) ossificans progressiva. **(A)** Radiograph shows shortening and deviation of the thumb. **(B)** Radiograph shows malformation of the great toe, a relatively common radiographic finding in this disease.

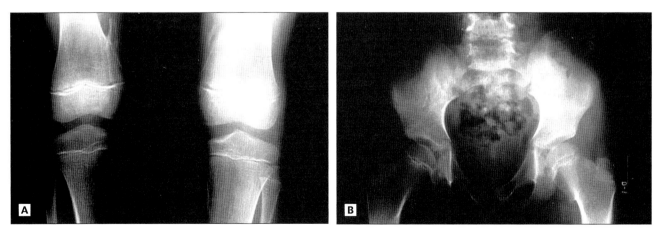

FIGURE 34–15 (A) Radiograph of both knees of a 7-year-old boy with fibrodysplasia (myositis) ossificans progressiva. Ossification is demonstrated along the medial femoral condyles bilaterally as well as the medial left tibial metaphysis along sites of ligamentous insertions producing pseudoexostoses. **(B)** Radiograph of the pelvis of the same patient showing bilateral broad, short femoral necks and small pseudoexostoses along the medial femoral metaphyses.

The gene or genes that are mutated in FOP are now being elucidated.[70] Genetic linkage studies are difficult given that most cases appear to arise from new mutations, but these studies have identified potential mutant genes at 4q27-31[71] and 17q21-22 (noggin gene).[72–74]

The underlying biochemical process is also becoming clearer, as there is overproduction of BMP4 in lesional lymphocytes, lesional proliferating fibroblasts, and lymphoblastoid cell lines from patients with this disease.[62,75–78] This gene is a member of the transforming growth factor β gene superfamily and has been mapped to chromosome 14q22-23.[79,80] The BMP genes have the ability to induce the complete cellular program of endochondral bone formation and likely play a critical role in the pathogenesis of this disease. However, Xu and Shore were unable to identify any mutations in the *BMP4* gene, suggesting an abnormality of a regulatory gene.[66]

A variety of other inflammatory and osteogenic mediators have also been implicated. Gannon and coworkers found a 40- to 150-fold increased density of mast cells at the periphery of early-stage highly vascular fibroproliferative lesions in these patients when compared to controls.[81] The osteogenic transcription factor Runx2 has been found to be expressed by the stromal cells, implicating its role as central to the ossification process.[82]

Discussion

The outlook is poor, and usually the disease proves fatal within a period of 10–15 years, frequently as the result of severe respiratory insufficiency caused by progressive immobilization of the thorax. Biopsy and trauma may lead to the development of new lesions and should be avoided. Unfortunately, this is a fairly common problem. In a study of 138 patients with well-documented FOP, Kitterman et al. reported an incorrect initial diagnosis in 87% of patients.[52] The mean duration between onset of symptoms and an established diagnosis was 4.1 years. Sixty-seven percent of patients had unnecessary diagnostic (biopsy) procedures, and 68% received inappropriate therapy. Most importantly, 49% of patients developed permanent loss of mobility secondary to invasive interventions resulting in post-traumatic ossification.

A variety of therapeutic modalities have been employed, with minimal success. Dietary measures, steroids, and agents binding minerals or blocking calcification (EDTA and EHDP) have been tried with disappointing results.[83]

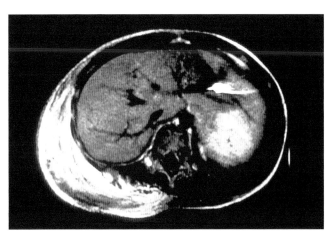

FIGURE 34–16 Fibrodysplasia (myositis) ossificans progressiva. MRI of the same patient depicted in Figure 34–15 reveals a large soft tissue mass that extends along the deep and superficial muscles of the back from the lower neck to the lower thoracic spine.

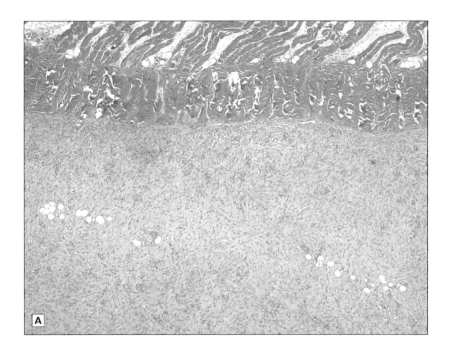

FIGURE 34–17 (A) Low-magnification view of fibrodysplasia (myositis) ossificans progressiva. A loosely textured fibroblastic proliferation superficially resembling nodular fasciitis is apparent.

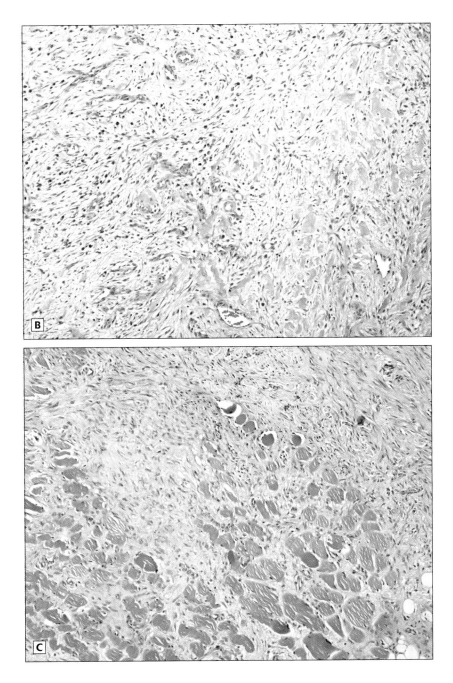

FIGURE 34–17 Continued. **(B)** Spindled to stellate-shaped cells are deposited in a myxoid matrix and associated with dense collagen. **(C)** The proliferation is seen interdigitating between skeletal muscle fibers.

High doses of intravenous disodium etidronate may be helpful for decreasing pain, swelling, and acute flare-ups of this disease,[84,85] but excessive use can result in rickets-like osseous abnormalities.[86] Isotretinoin, a retinoid capable of inhibiting differentiation of mesenchymal cells into cartilage and bone, is not an effective mode of therapy.[87,88] More recently, Altschuler proposed a potential role for rituximab, a monoclonal anti-CD20 antibody, given the apparent central role of BMP4 overexpression by B lymphocytes.[89]

The differential diagnosis includes the battered child syndrome, ectopic bone formation with multiple congenital anomalies, pseudohypoparathyroidism, and dermatomyositis with multiple calcifications. The latter entity is also associated with shortening of the metacarpal and metatarsal bones, exostoses, and multiple subcutaneous ossifications.[53] Finally, as mentioned earlier, the initial noncalcified fibrous proliferation of fibrodysplasia ossificans progressiva may be mistaken for an infantile form of fibromatosis.

EXTRASKELETAL OSTEOSARCOMA

Extraskeletal osteosarcoma is a malignant mesenchymal neoplasm that produces osteoid, bone, or chondroid material, and is located in the soft tissues without attachment to the skeleton. Compared with osteosarcoma of bone, extraskeletal osteosarcoma is rare, accounting for 1–2% of all soft tissue sarcomas.[90,91] Some occur following radiation for other malignancies.[92,93] Although there are some similarities with skeletal osteosarcomas, extraskeletal osteosarcomas are quite distinctive, particularly with respect to their morphologic appearance.

Excluded from this chapter are osteosarcomas arising in the breast, urinary bladder, prostate, and other visceral organs because in many of these tumors there is a participating epithelial component suggesting carcinosarcoma. We have also excluded malignant mesenchymomas, a rather nebulous entity that exhibits, by definition, two or more well-defined malignant mesenchymal components.

There are few reliable data in the literature as to the incidence of extraskeletal osteosarcoma. Allan and Soule[94] encountered 26 cases among 2100 soft tissue sarcomas, an incidence of 1.24%. Lorentzon et al.,[95] in a study of the Swedish Cancer Registry, found only four extraskeletal osteosarcomas (1.65%) among 242 osteosarcomas of bone. They calculated an annual incidence of two to three cases per million of population.

Clinical findings

Although osteosarcomas of bone occur chiefly during the first two decades of life, extraskeletal osteosarcomas are rarely encountered in patients under 40 years of age. In a series of 40 extraskeletal osteosarcomas reported from the Mayo Clinic,[96] the mean age was 50.7 years (range 23–81 years), and in a series of 25 cases from Denmark,[97] patients ranged in age from 35 to 82 years, with a mean age of 67 years. The data as to the gender incidence vary, and both male and female predominance has been reported. Lee and colleagues found a male/female ratio of 1.9:1.0.[96]

There are no specific signs or symptoms. Generally, the tumor presents as a progressively enlarging soft tissue mass that is painful in about one-third of patients. Large and late examples of the tumor may ulcerate through the skin but usually only after biopsy or some other surgical procedure. The duration of symptoms varies from a few weeks to many years, although most present within 6–8 months following the initiation of symptoms.[96–98]

Among the various anatomic sites, the muscles of the thigh are most commonly affected;[99,100] the large muscles of the pelvic and shoulder girdles and retroperitoneum are other relatively common sites.[101,102] Most of the tumors are deep-seated and fixed to the underlying tissues, but occasional lesions are freely movable and are confined to the subcutis or even the dermis.[103,104] There are also reports of extraskeletal osteosarcomas arising in unusual locations including the larynx,[105] tongue,[106] mediastinum,[107] spermatic cord,[108] penis,[109] pleura,[110]

lung,[111] heart,[112] colon,[113] and central nervous system.[114] The laboratory findings show no specific abnormalities. Alkaline phosphatase is usually normal with localized disease, but it is often elevated in the presence of metastases. With conventional radiographs, CT scan, and MRI, extraskeletal osteosarcoma manifests as a soft tissue mass with spotty to massive calcifications and no evidence of bone involvement (Figs 34–18 to 34–20A).[115,116]

Pathogenesis

Mechanical injury has been hypothesized to be a causative agent, but the etiologic significance of trauma is difficult to assess. Preceding trauma has been reported in 12.5%[99] to 23.0%[96] of patients. There are anecdotal reports of osteosarcoma arising at the sites of a previous injection and fracture. Extraskeletal osteosarcoma arising in myositis ossificans is exceedingly rare,[117] and most of these reports are poorly documented. Eckardt et al. reported an unusual case of an osteosarcoma of the thigh that developed in a heterotopic ossification of dermato-

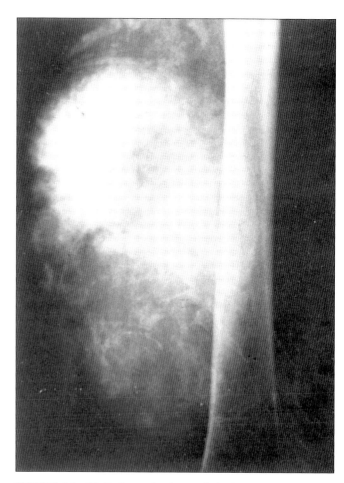

FIGURE 34–18 Radiograph of extraskeletal osteosarcoma of the mid-thigh demonstrating a soft tissue mass with extensive ossification. (From Chung EB, Enzinger FM. Extraskeletal osteosarcoma. Cancer 1987; 60:1132.)

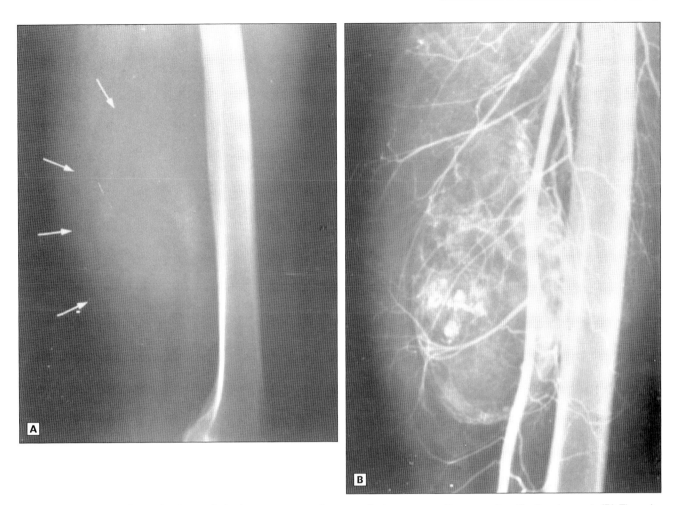

FIGURE 34–19 (A) Radiograph of extraskeletal osteosarcoma shows a soft tissue mass with areas of ossification (arrows). **(B)** There is a moderate degree of vascularization in the angiogram with focal neovascularity and stretching and displacement of arteries.

myositis 28 years after onset of the disease.[118] Unlike osteosarcoma of bone, the tumor has not been reported in siblings, but Mirra et al. reported a unique case of an extraskeletal osteosarcoma that arose in the mother of a daughter who had previously died of skeletal osteosarcoma.[119]

Radiation-induced extraskeletal osteosarcoma

Since Martland described the development of osteosarcoma in patients engaged in the manufacture of luminous watch dials,[120] numerous cases of osseous and extraosseous postradiation osteosarcomas have been reported in the literature.[121] Most of the extraskeletal osteosarcomas occurred in patients who underwent radiation therapy for a malignant neoplasm, most commonly breast carcinoma.[92,122] In most instances the tumor becomes apparent 4 years or more after radiotherapy. Assessment of these cases is facilitated by the presence of chronic radiodermatitis in the skin overlying the tumor or radiation change in the surrounding muscle tissue.[121]

There are also sporadic cases that developed following diagnostic procedures with radioactive thorium dioxide (Thorotrast). One of these, an extraskeletal osteosarcoma of the mandibular region in a 51-year-old man, appeared 30 years after a Thorotrast angiogram of the carotid artery.[123]

Pathologic findings

The tumor varies in its gross appearance from a well-circumscribed mass with a distinct pseudocapsule to an infiltrating tumor without discernible borders. Frequently, it is firm to stony on palpation. Less often, it presents as a soft or multicystic mass. On section it usually displays a granular white surface with yellow flecks and multiple foci of necrosis and hemorrhage. Most of the tumors measure 5–10 cm when excised (Fig. 34–20B).

Microscopically, extraskeletal osteosarcomas have in common the presence of neoplastic osteoid and bone, occasionally with neoplastic cartilage. There is a striking variation in the relative prominence of this material and

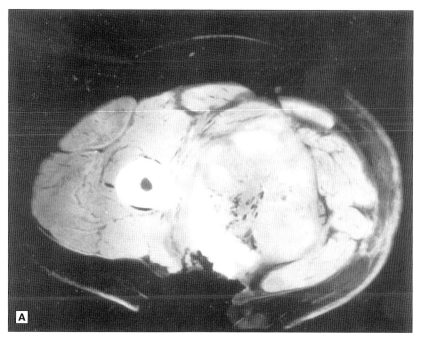

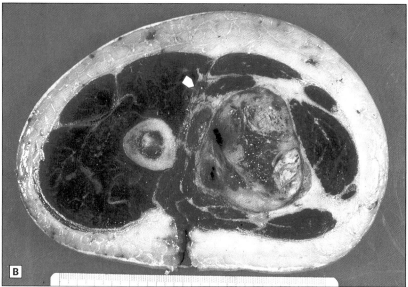

FIGURE 34-20 Computed tomography scan **(A)** and cross-section of extraskeletal osteosarcoma of the thigh **(B)**. Note the circumscription of the tumor, areas of hemorrhage, and the absence of bone involvement.

the associated osteoblastic and fibroblastic elements. Extraskeletal osteosarcomas, like osteosarcomas of bone, range from tumors that resemble fibrosarcoma or a high-grade pleomorphic sarcoma (*fibroblastic osteosarcoma*) to extremely cellular tumors with an irregular round or spindle cell pattern with considerable pleomorphism and mitotic activity (*osteoblastic osteosarcoma*). In our experience, the vast majority of extraskeletal osteosarcomas closely resemble a pleomorphic undifferentiated sarcoma ("MFH-like") except for the presence of osteoid deposition. Usually, the osteoid is deposited in a fine, ramifying, lace-like or coarsely trabecular pattern, occasionally showing transitions toward sheaths of osteoid or mature-appearing bone (Figs 34-21 to 34-23). Unlike myositis

ossificans in which the most mature portion is located at the periphery, there is often a "reverse zoning phenomenon" (i.e., central deposition of osteoid material and atypical spindle cell proliferation at the periphery). Atypical cartilage of variable cellularity, with or without myxoid areas or focal bone formation, is present in many cases (Fig. 34-24), but rarely predominates (*chondroblastic osteosarcoma*). There are also a varying number of benign and malignant multinucleated giant cells of the osteoclastic type that are often associated with hemorrhage (*osteoclastic* or *giant cell osteosarcoma*) (Fig. 34-25). The vascular pattern varies substantially. Very rarely, lesions with markedly dilated vascular spaces resembling a vascular tumor (*telangiectatic osteosarcoma*) occurs (Fig. 34-26),[124]

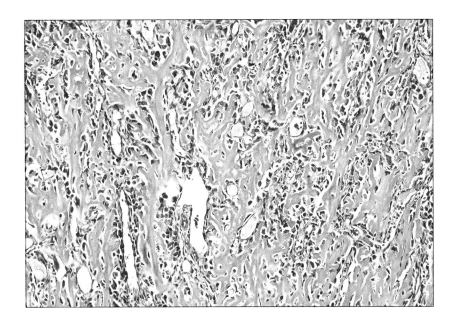

FIGURE 34–21 Extraskeletal osteosarcoma with large hyperchromatic cells separated by hyalinized collagen and osteoid.

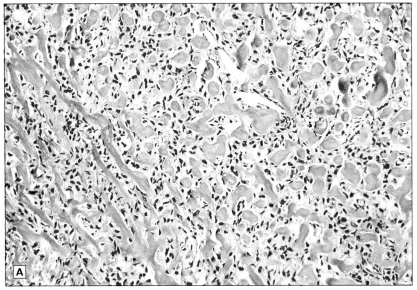

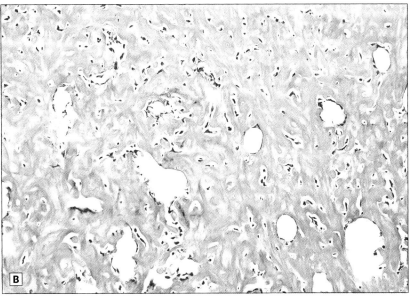

FIGURE 34–22 Extraskeletal osteosarcoma of the retroperitoneum. **(A)** Malignant cells are compressed by osteoid material. **(B)** In this portion of the tumor there is a broad expanse of osteoid with relatively few malignant cells.

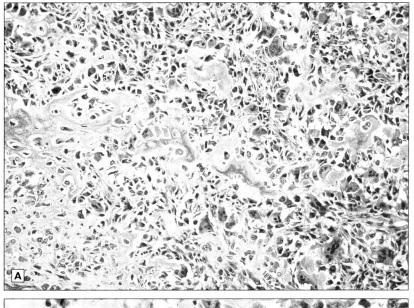

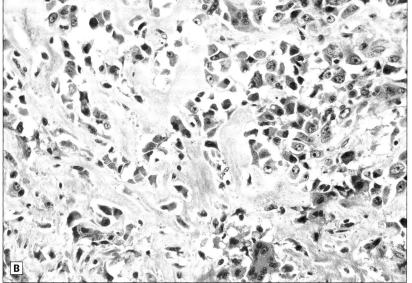

FIGURE 34–23 (A) Extraskeletal osteosarcoma of the thigh. Bands of osteoid material are seen between pleomorphic spindle-shaped and epithelioid cells. (B) High-magnification view of malignant cells depositing osteoid in an extraskeletal osteosarcoma.

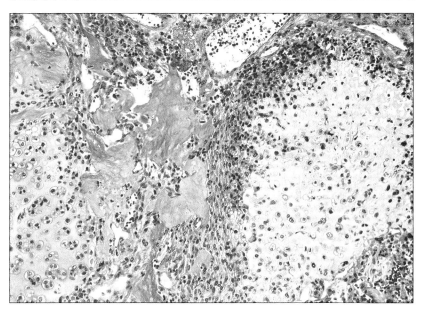

FIGURE 34–24 Osteoblastic osteosarcoma with chondroblastic and osteoblastic areas adjacent to one another.

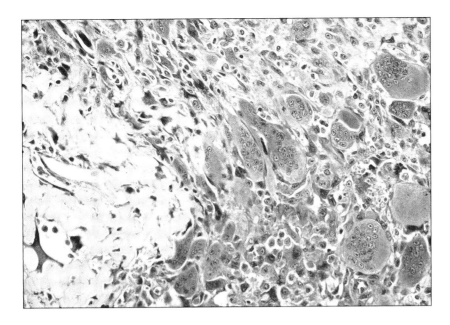

FIGURE 34–25 Osteoclast-like giant cells in an extraskeletal osteosarcoma.

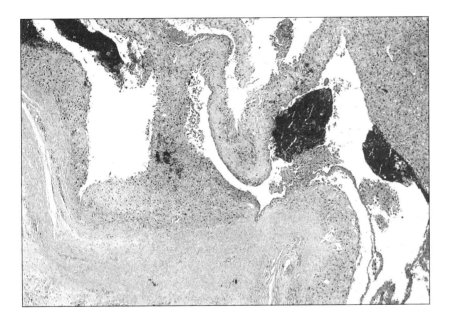

FIGURE 35–26 Telangiectatic extraskeletal osteosarcoma with markedly dilated blood-filled spaces lined by pleomorphic tumor cells.

although this variant is extremely uncommon in extraskeletal osteosarcomas. Well-differentiated forms resembling parosteal osteosarcoma,[125–127] and, even more rarely, tumors with a small cell pattern (*small cell osteosarcoma*) have also been described (Fig. 34–27).[100] Metastatic lesions closely resemble their primary neoplasms.

Immunohistochemical and ultrastructural findings

In recent years, monoclonal antibodies to osteocalcin and osteonectin have been utilized in an attempt to recognize skeletal and extraskeletal osteosarcoma.[128] Fanburg-Smith and colleagues found that an antibody to osteocalcin was 82% sensitive for extraskeletal osteosar-

coma neoplastic cells, with immunostaining of neoplastic cells away from bone in 91% of cases and in 75% for bony tumor matrix.[128] They reported 100% specificity for osteoblasts, as this antigen was nonreactive in all nonbone cells. However, an antibody to osteonectin was not specific for osteoblasts. Focal positivity for desmin, actin, S-100 protein, and cytokeratins may occasionally be found.[97]

There are only a few ultrastructural studies of extraskeletal osteosarcoma, but all indicate the cells are indistinguishable from those found in primary osteosarcoma of bone.[129] They have irregularly shaped, large nuclei with crenated or indented nuclear membranes. There is a prominent endoplasmic reticulum that ranges from narrow tubular to markedly dilated cisternae, often

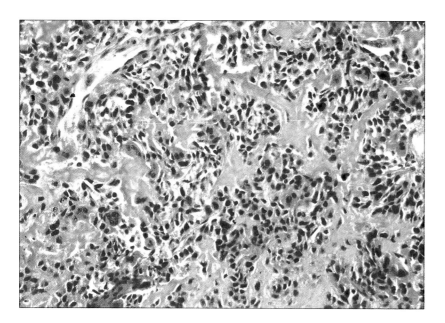

FIGURE 34–27 Extraskeletal osteosarcoma composed predominantly of small round cells adjacent to bands of osteoid.

enveloping mitochondria and having a finely granular content. There are also scattered free ribosomes, a well-developed Golgi complex, varying amounts of filamentous material, and occasional lysosomes and lipid inclusions. Pinocytotic vesicles and desmosomes or tight junctions are absent or rare. Occasionally, there are multinucleated osteoclast-like giant cells with numerous mitochondria and multiple cellular processes.[130] The extracellular spaces contain a feltwork of interlacing collagen fibers, sometimes with scattered delicate electron-dense particles and deposits of needle-shaped, crystalline hydroxyapatite.

Differential diagnosis

It is not always easy to distinguish extraskeletal osteosarcoma from other benign and malignant bone- and cartilage-forming soft tissue lesions. The differentiation from *myositis ossificans* and other reactive reparative processes has already been discussed in this chapter (Table 34–1). Among malignant tumors, metaplastic bone may be found in synovial sarcoma, epithelioid sarcoma, malignant melanoma, and other mesenchymal or epithelial neoplasms. In most of these neoplasms, osteoid or bone is confined to a small portion of the tumor and is relatively well differentiated without the disorderly pattern and cellular pleomorphism of osteosarcoma. For some of them, however, it is exceedingly difficult to reach a definitive diagnosis and to exclude osteosarcoma. In fact, at times the only distinguishing feature between extraskeletal osteosarcoma and other high-grade pleomorphic ("MFH-like") tumors with metaplastic bone is the relatively small amounts of neoplastic osteoid and bone in the latter tumor. According to Bhagavan and Dorfman,[131] the presence of the osseous and chondroid elements in the fibrous septa and pseudocapsule favor a pleomorphic sarcoma. Bane and colleagues, on the other hand, propose that the production of any neoplastic osteoid or bone in a pleomorphic sarcoma, no matter how focal, warrants a diagnosis of osteosarcoma.[100] Thus, the distinction between extraskeletal osteosarcoma and a high-grade pleomorphic sarcoma with bone is sometimes arbitrary, residing with the definitional criteria of the author.

Parosteal osteosarcoma may also make its appearance as a bulky lobulated densely ossified extraosseous mass focally indistinguishable from an extraskeletal osteosarcoma. In most cases this relatively low-grade tumor can be identified by its greater overall differentiation, its broad attachment to a thickened cortical bone, and its tendency to encircle the shaft of the bone and cause cortical erosion.[132] Differential diagnostic considerations must also include *periosteal osteosarcoma*,[133] a more aggressive and less-well-differentiated osteoblastic tumor that is often marked by a prominent chondroblastic component, and the rare *high-grade surface osteosarcoma*.[134]

Discussion

The outlook is grave, and most patients with this tumor succumb to metastatic disease within 2–3 years after the initial diagnosis. In the series by Bane et al.,[100] 13 (50%) of 26 tumors recurred locally and 16 (61.5%) metastasized; five patients had distant metastases at presentation. Similarly, Lee and colleagues[96] reported local recurrences and distant metastases in 45% and 65% of patients, respectively, with 33 of 40 (83%) patients dying of tumor during the follow-up period. The lungs constitute the most common metastatic site, followed by the liver, bones, regional lymph nodes, and soft tissue. Despite the dismal prognosis, combination therapy with radical surgery (possibly limb-sparing segmental resection as an alternative to amputation), radiotherapy, and sequential preoperative or postoperative multiagent chemotherapy should be carried out in the hope of improving survival.[98,135]

Tumor size, histologic subtype, and proliferation index have been proposed as prognostic variables. Bane and colleagues found that a tumor size of 5 cm or more was an unfavorable prognostic indicator,[100] although tumor size was not found to be of prognostic significance in other series.[97] Chung and Enzinger found that patients with the fibroblastic type of extraskeletal osteosarcoma had a slightly better prognosis than those with other histologic subtypes,[99] whereas Lee et al. reported that patients with the chondroblastic type fared slightly better.[96]

REFERENCES

1. Patel RM, Weiss SW, Folpe AL. Heterotopic mesenteric ossification: a distinctive pseudosarcoma commonly associated with intestinal obstruction. Am J Surg Pathol 2006; 30:119.
2. Wilson JD, Montague CJ, Salcuni P, et al. Heterotopic mesenteric ossification ("intraabdominal myositis ossificans"): report of five cases. Am J Surg Pathol 1999; 23:1464.
3. Vanden Bossche L, Vanderstraeten G. Heterotopic ossification: a review. J Rehabil Med 2005; 37:129.
4. Karapinar H, Yagdi S. A case of myositis ossificans as a complication of tetanus treated by surgical excision. Acta Orthop Belg 2003; 69:285.
5. Massey GV, Kuhn JG, Nogi J, et al. The spectrum of myositis ossificans in haemophilia. Haemophilia 2004; 10:189.
6. Wittenberg RH, Peschke U, Botel U. Heterotopic ossification after spinal cord injury. Epidemiology and risk factors. J Bone Joint Surg [Br] 1992; 74:215.
7. Ackman JB, Rosenthal DI. Generalized periarticular myositis ossificans as a complication of pharmacologically induced paralysis. Skeletal Radiol 1995; 24:395.
8. Brown H, Ehrlich HP, Newberne PM, et al. Paraosteoarthropathy – ectopic ossification of healing tendon about the rodent ankle joint: histologic and type V collagen changes. Proc Soc Exp Biol Med 1986; 183:214.
9. Sethuraman G, Malhotra AK, Khaitan BK, et al. Osteoma cutis in pseudohypoparathyroidism. Clin Exp Dermatol 2006; 31:225.
10. Konishi E, Kusuzaki K, Murata H, et al. Extraskeletal osteosarcoma arising in myositis ossificans. Skeletal Radiol 2001; 30:39.

Non-neoplastic heterotopic ossifications

11. George DH, Scheithauer BW, Spinner RJ, et al. Heterotopic ossification of peripheral nerve ("neuritis ossificans"): report of two cases. Neurosurgery 2002; 51:244.
12. Ackerman LV. Extra-osseous localized nonneoplastic bone and cartilage formation (so-called myositis ossificans): clinical and pathological confusion with malignant neoplasms. J Bone Joint Surg [Am] 1958; 40:279.
13. Jarvinen TA, Jarvinen TL, Kaariainen M, et al. Muscle injuries: biology and treatment. Am J Sports Med 2005; 33:745.
14. Beiner JM, Jokl P. Muscle contusion injury and myositis ossificans traumatica. Clin Orthop 2002; 403:S110.
15. Heifetz SA, Galliani CA, DeRosa GP. Myositis (fasciitis) ossificans in an infant. Pediatr Pathol 1992; 12:223.
16. Yoshida S, Taira H, Kataoka M, et al. Idiopathic heterotopic ossification within the tibial nerve. A case report. J Bone Joint Surg [Am] 2002; 84:1442.

17. Androulaki A, Chatzoulis G, Kalahanis N, et al. Heterotopic mesenteric ossification: a rare reactive process. J Gastroenterol Hepatol 2005; 20:664.
18. Laor T. MR imaging of soft tissue tumors and tumor-like lesions. Pediatr Radiol 2004; 34:24.
19. Parikh J, Hyare H, Saifuddin A. The imaging features of post-traumatic myositis ossificans, with emphasis on MRI. Clin Radiol 2002; 57:1058.
20. Boutin RD, Fritz RC, Steinbach LS. Imaging of sports-related muscle injuries. Radiol Clin North Am 2002; 40:333.
21. de Silva MV, Reid R. Myositis ossificans and fibro-osseous pseudotumor of digits: a clinicopathological review of 64 cases with emphasis on diagnostic pitfalls. Int J Surg Pathol 2003; 11:187.
22. Chalmers J, Gray DH, Rush J. Observations on the induction of bone in soft tissues. J Bone Joint Surg [Br] 1975; 57:36.
23. Lagier R, Cox JN. Pseudomalignant myositis ossificans. A pathological study of eight cases. Hum Pathol 1975; 6:653.
24. Issakov J, Flusser G, Kollender Y, et al. Computed tomography-guided core needle biopsy for bone and soft tissue tumors. Isr Med Assoc J 2003; 5:28.
25. Dodd LG, Martinez S. Fine-needle aspiration cytology of pseudosarcomatous lesions of soft tissue. Diagn Cytopathol 2001; 24:28.
26. Nisolle JF, Delaunois L, Trigaux JP. Myositis ossificans of the chest wall. Eur Respir J 1996; 9:178.
27. Dupree WB, Enzinger FM. Fibro-osseous pseudotumor of the digits. Cancer 1986; 58:2103.
28. Spjut HJ, Dorfman HD. Florid reactive periostitis of the tubular bones of the hands and feet. A benign lesion which may simulate osteosarcoma. Am J Surg Pathol 1981; 5:423.
29. Patel MR, Desai SS. Pseudomalignant osseous tumor of soft tissue: a case report and review of the literature. J Hand Surg [Am] 1986; 11:66.
30. McCarthy EF, Ireland DC, Sprague BL, et al. Parosteal (nodular) fasciitis of the hand. A case report. J Bone Joint Surg [Am] 1976; 58:714.
31. De Maeseneer M, Jaovisidha S, Lenchik L, et al. Myositis ossificans of the foot. J Foot Ankle Surg 1997; 36:290.
32. Sundaram M, Wang L, Rotman M, et al. Florid reactive periostitis and bizarre parosteal osteochondromatous proliferation: Pre-biopsy imaging evolution, treatment and outcome. Skeletal Radiol 2001; 30:192.
33. Kransdorf MJ, Meis JM. From the archives of the AFIP. Extraskeletal osseous and cartilaginous tumors of the extremities. Radiographics 1993; 13:853.
34. Howard RF, Slawski DP, Gilula LA. Florid reactive periostitis of the digit with cortical erosion: a case report and review of the literature. J Hand Surg [Am] 1996; 21:501.
35. Sleater J, Mullins D, Chun K, et al. Fibro-osseous pseudotumor of the digit: a comparison to myositis ossificans by light

microscopy and immunohistochemical methods. J Cutan Pathol 1996; 23:373.
36. Endo M, Hasegawa T, Tashiro T, et al. Bizarre parosteal osteochondromatous proliferation with a t(1;17) translocation. Virchows Arch 2005; 447:99.
37. Claude V, Couture C, Battin-Bertho R, et al. Unusual parosteal osteochondromatous proliferation or Nora's tumor. A clinicopathological analysis of 4 cases. Ann Pathol 2003; 23:258.
38. Zambrano E, Nose V, Perez-Atayde AR, et al. Distinct chromosomal rearrangements in subungual (Dupuytren) exostosis and bizarre parosteal osteochondromatous proliferation (Nora lesion). Am J Surg Pathol 2004; 28:1033.
39. Meneses MF, Unni KK, Swee RG. Bizarre parosteal osteochondromatous proliferation of bone (Nora's lesion). Am J Surg Pathol 1993; 17:691.
40. Dorfman HD, Czerniak B. Reactive and metabolic conditions simulating neoplasms of bone. In: Bone tumors. St. Louis: Mosby; 1998:1143.
41. Rogers GF, Brzezienski MA. Florid reactive periostitis of the middle phalanx: a case report and review of the literature. J Hand Surg [Am] 1999; 24:1014.
42. Craver RD, Correa-Gracian H, Heinrich S. Florid reactive periostitis. Hum Pathol 1997; 28:745.

Fibrodysplasia (myositis) ossificans progressive

43. Cohen RB, Hahn GV, Tabas JA, et al. The natural history of heterotopic ossification in patients who have fibrodysplasia ossificans progressiva. A study of forty-four patients. J Bone Joint Surg [Am] 1993; 75:215.
44. Rocke DM, Zasloff M, Peeper J, et al. Age- and joint-specific risk of initial heterotopic ossification in patients who have fibrodysplasia ossificans progressiva. Clin Orthop 1994. 301:243.
45. Scarlett RF, Rocke DM, Kantanie S, et al. Influenza-like viral illnesses and flare-ups of fibrodysplasia ossificans progressiva. Clin Orthop 2004; 423:275.
46. Kaplan FS, Strear CM, Zasloff MA. Radiographic and scintigraphic features of modeling and remodeling in the heterotopic skeleton of patients who have fibrodysplasia ossificans progressiva. Clin Orthop 1994; 304:238.
47. Kaplan FS, Tabas JA, Gannon FH, et al. The histopathology of fibrodysplasia ossificans progressiva. An endochondral process. J Bone Joint Surg [Am] 1993; 75:220.
48. Kussmaul WG, Esmail AN, Sagar Y, et al. Pulmonary and cardiac function in advanced fibrodysplasia ossificans progressiva. Clin Orthop 1998; 346:104.
49. Glaser DL, Rocke DM, Kaplan FS. Catastrophic falls in patients who have fibrodysplasia ossificans progressiva. Clin Orthop 1998; 346:110.
50. Herford AS, Boyne PJ. Ankylosis of the jaw in a patient with fibrodysplasia ossificans

progressiva. Oral Surg Oral Med Oral Pathol Oral Radiol Endod 2003; 96:680.

51. Smith R. Fibrodysplasia (myositis) ossificans progressiva. Clinical lessons from a rare disease. Clin Orthop 1998; 346:7.

52. Kitterman JA, Kantanie S, Rocke DM, et al. Iatrogenic harm caused by diagnostic errors in fibrodysplasia ossificans progressiva. Pediatrics 2005; 116:e654.

53. Connor JM, Evans DAP. Fibrodysplasia ossificans progressive: the clinical features and natural history of 34 patients. J Bone Joint Surg [Am] 1982; 64:76.

54. Hagiwara H, Aida N, Machida J, et al. Contrast-enhanced MRI of an early preosseous lesion of fibrodysplasia ossificans progressiva in a 21-month-old boy. Am J Roentgenol 2003; 181:1145.

55. Mahboubi S, Glaser DL, Shore EM, et al. Fibrodysplasia ossificans progressiva. Pediatr Radiol 2001; 31:307.

56. Baysal T, Elmali N, Kutlu R, et al. The stone man: myositis (fibrodysplasia) ossificans progressiva. Eur Radiol 1998; 8:479.

57. O'Reilly M, Renton P. Metaphyseal abnormalities in fibrodysplasia ossificans progressiva. Br J Radiol 1993; 66:112.

58. Gulaldi NC, Elahi N, Sasani J, et al. Tc-99m MDP scanning in a patient with extensive fibrodysplasia ossificans progressiva. Clin Nucl Med 1995; 20:188.

59. Kaplan F, Sawyer J, Connors S, et al. Urinary basic fibroblast growth factor. A biochemical marker for preosseous fibroproliferative lesions in patients with fibrodysplasia ossificans progressiva. Clin Orthop 1998; 346:59.

60. Lopez de Castro JA. Structural polymorphism and function of HLA-B27. Curr Opin Rheumatol 1995; 7:270.

61. Calvert GT, Shore EM. Human leukocyte antigen B27 allele is not correlated with fibrodysplasia ossificans progressiva. Clin Orthop 1998; 346:66.

62. Gannon FH, Valentine BA, Shore EM, et al. Acute lymphocytic infiltration in an extremely early lesion of fibrodysplasia ossificans progressiva. Clin Orthop 1998; 346:19.

63. Gannon FH, Kaplan FS, Olmsted E, et al. Bone morphogenetic protein 2/4 in early fibromatous lesions of fibrodysplasia ossificans progressiva. Hum Pathol 1997; 28:339.

64. Delatycki M, Rogers JG. The genetics of fibrodysplasia ossificans progressiva. Clin Orthop 1998; 346:15.

65. Kaplan FS, McCluskey W, Hahn G, et al. Genetic transmission of fibrodysplasia ossificans progressiva. Report of a family. J Bone Joint Surg [Am] 1993; 75:1214.

66. Xu M, Shore EM. Mutational screening of the bone morphogenetic protein 4 gene in a family with fibrodysplasia ossificans progressiva. Clin Orthop 1998; 346:53.

67. Janoff HB, Tabas JA, Shore EM, et al. Mild expression of fibrodysplasia ossificans progressiva: a report of 3 cases. J Rheumatol 1995; 22:976.

68. Connor JM, Skirton H, Lunt PW. A three generation family with fibrodysplasia ossificans progressiva. J Med Genet 1993; 30:687.

69. Janoff HB, Muenke M, Johnson LO, et al. Fibrodysplasia ossificans progressiva in two half-sisters: evidence for maternal mosaicism. Am J Med Genet 1996; 61:320.

70. Kaplan FS, Glaser DL, Hebela N, et al. Heterotopic ossification. J Am Acad Orthop Surg 2004; 12:116.

71. Feldman G, Li M, Martin S, et al. Fibrodysplasia ossificans progressiva, a heritable disorder of severe heterotopic ossification, maps to human chromosome 4q27-31. Am J Hum Genet 2000; 66:128.

72. Fontaine K, Semonin O, Legarde JP, et al. A new mutation of the noggin gene in a French

73. Semonin O, Fontaine K, Daviaud C, et al. Identification of three novel mutations of the noggin gene in patients with fibrodysplasia ossificans progressiva. Am J Med Genet 2001; 102:314.

74. Lucotte G, Bathelier C, Mercier G, et al. Localization of the gene for fibrodysplasia ossificans progressiva (FOP) to chromosome 17q21-22. Genet Couns 2000; 11:329.

75. Shafritz AB, Kaplan FS. Differential expression of bone and cartilage related genes in fibrodysplasia ossificans progressiva, myositis ossificans traumatica, and osteogenic sarcoma. Clin Orthop 1998; 346:46.

76. Lanchoney TF, Olmsted EA, Shore EM, et al. Characterization of bone morphogenetic protein 4 receptor in fibrodysplasia ossificans progressiva. Clin Orthop 1998; 346:38.

77. de la Pena LS, Billings PC, Fiori JL, et al. Fibrodysplasia ossificans progressiva (FOP), a disorder of ectopic osteogenesis, misregulates cell surface expression and trafficking of BMPRIA. J Bone Miner Res 2005; 20:1168.

78. Olmsted EA, Kaplan FS, Shore EM. Bone morphogenetic protein-4 regulation in fibrodysplasia ossificans progressiva. Clin Orthop 2003; 408:331.

79. Van den Wijngaard A, Pijpers MA, Joosten PH, et al. Functional characterization of two promoters in the human bone morphogenetic protein-4 gene. J Bone Miner Res 1999; 14:1432.

80. Shore EM, Xu M, Shah PB, et al. The human bone morphogenetic protein 4 (BMP-4) gene: molecular structure and transcriptional regulation. Calcif Tissue Int 1998; 63:221.

81. Gannon FH, Glaser D, Caron R, et al. Mast cell involvement in fibrodysplasia ossificans progressiva. Hum Pathol 2001; 32:842.

82. Hegyi L, Gannon FH, Glaser DL, et al. Stromal cells of fibrodysplasia ossificans progressiva lesions express smooth muscle lineage markers and the osteogenic transcription factor Runx2/ Cbfa-1: clues to a vascular origin of heterotopic ossification? J Pathol 2003; 201:141.

83. Francis MD, Valent DJ. Historical perspectives on the clinical development of bisphosphonates in the treatment of bone diseases. J Musculoskelet Neuronal Interact 2007; 7:2.

84. Dua T, Kabra M, Kalra V. Familial fibrodysplasia ossificans progressiva: trial with etidronate disodium. Indian Pediatr 2001; 38:1305.

85. Brantus JF, Meunier PJ. Effects of intravenous etidronate and oral corticosteroids in fibrodysplasia ossificans progressiva. Clin Orthop 1998; 346:117.

86. Pazzaglia UE, Beluffi G, Ravelli A, et al. Chronic intoxication by ethane-1-hydroxy-1,1-diphosphonate (EHDP) in a child with myositis ossificans progressiva. Pediatr Radiol 1993; 23:459.

87. Jones G, Rocke DM. Multivariate survival analysis with doubly-censored data: Application to the assessment of accutane treatment for fibrodysplasia ossificans progressiva. Stat Med 2002; 21:2547.

88. Zasloff MA, Rocke DM, Crofford LJ, et al. Treatment of patients who have fibrodysplasia ossificans progressiva with isotretinoin. Clin Orthop 1998; 346:121.

89. Altschuler EL. Consideration of rituximab for fibrodysplasia ossificans progressiva. Med Hypotheses 2004; 63:407.

Extraskeletal osteosarcoma

90. Sordillo PP, Hajdu SI, Magill GBea. Extraosseous osteogenic sarcoma: a review of 48 patients. Cancer 1983; 51:727.

91. Klein MJ, Siegal GP. Osteosarcoma: anatomic and histologic variants. Am J Clin Pathol 2006; 125:555.

92. Orta L, Suprun U, Goldfarb A, et al. Radiation-associated extraskeletal osteosarcoma of the chest wall. Arch Pathol Lab Med 2006; 130:198.

93. Fang Z, Yokoyama R, Mukai K, et al. Extraskeletal osteosarcoma: a clinicopathologic study of four cases. Jpn J Clin Oncol 1995; 25:55.

94. Allan CJ, Soule EH. Osteogenic sarcoma of the somatic soft tissues. Clinicopathologic study of 26 cases and review of literature. Cancer 1971; 27:1121.

95. Lorentzon R, Larsson SE, Boquist L. Extra-osseous osteosarcoma: a clinical and histopathological study of four cases. J Bone Joint Surg [Br] 1979; 61:205.

96. Lee JS, Fetsch JF, Wasdhal DA, et al. A review of 40 patients with extraskeletal osteosarcoma. Cancer 1995; 76:2253.

97. Lidang Jensen M, Schumacher B, Myhre Jensen O, et al. Extraskeletal osteosarcomas: a clinicopathologic study of 25 cases. Am J Surg Pathol 1998; 22:588.

98. Goldstein-Jackson SY, Gosheger G, Delling G, et al. Extraskeletal osteosarcoma has a favourable prognosis when treated like conventional osteosarcoma. J Cancer Res Clin Oncol 2005; 131:520.

99. Chung EB, Enzinger FM. Extraskeletal osteosarcoma. Cancer 1987; 60:1132.

100. Bane BL, Evans HL, Ro JY, et al. Extraskeletal osteosarcoma. A clinicopathologic review of 26 cases. Cancer 1990; 65:2762.

101. Secil M, Mungan U, Yorukoglu K, et al. Case 89: retroperitoneal extraskeletal osteosarcoma. Radiology 2005; 237:880.

102. Hamdan A, Toman J, Taylor S, et al. Nuclear imaging of an extraskeletal retroperitoneal osteosarcoma: respective contribution of 18FDG-PET and (99m)tc oxidronate (2005:1b). Eur Radiol 2005; 15:840.

103. Santos-Juanes J, Galache C, Miralles M, et al. Primary cutaneous extraskeletal osteosarcoma under a previous electrodessicated actinic keratosis. J Am Acad Dermatol 2004; 51:S166.

104. Pillay P, Simango S, Govender D. Extraskeletal osteosarcoma of the scalp. Pathology 2000; 32:154.

105. Athre RS, Vories A, Mudrovich S, et al. Osteosarcomas of the larynx. Laryngoscope 2005; 115:74.

106. Dubey SP, Murthy DP, Cooke RA, et al. Primary osteogenic sarcoma of the tongue. J Laryngol Otol 1999; 113:376.

107. Gladish GW, Sabloff BM, Munden RF, et al. Primary thoracic sarcomas. Radiographics 2002; 22:621.

108. Beiswanger JC, Woodruff RD, Savage PD, et al. Primary osteosarcoma of the spermatic cord with synchronous bilateral renal cell carcinoma. Urology 1997; 49:957.

109. Bacetic D, Knezevic M, Stojsic Z, et al. Primary extraskeletal osteosarcoma of the penis with a malignant fibrous histiocytoma-like component. Histopathology 1998; 33:185.

110. Sabloff B, Munden RF, Melhem AI, et al. Radiologic-pathologic conferences of the University of Texas M.D. Anderson Cancer Center: extraskeletal osteosarcoma of the pleura. Am J Roentgenol 2003; 180:972.

111. Chapman AD, Pritchard SC, Yap WW, et al. Primary pulmonary osteosarcoma: case report and molecular analysis. Cancer 2001; 91:779.

112. Minami H, Wakita N, Kawanishi Y, et al. Primary osteosarcoma of heart with severe congestive heart failure. Jpn J Thorac Cardiovasc Surg 2000; 48:607.

113. Shimazu K, Funata N, Yamamoto Y, et al. Primary osteosarcoma arising in the colon: report of a case. Dis Colon Rectum 2001; 44:1367.

114. Saesue P, Chankaew E, Chawalparit O, et al. Primary extraskeletal osteosarcoma in the

pineal region. Case report. J Neurosurg 2004; 101:1061.

115. Kajihara M, Sugawara Y, Miki H, et al. Tl-201 and tc-99m HMDP scintigraphic findings in extraskeletal osteosarcoma. Clin Nucl Med 2005; 30:356.

116. Murphey MD, Robbin MR, McRae GA, et al. The many faces of osteosarcoma. Radiographics 1997; 17:1205.

117. Konishi E, Kusuzaki K, Murata H, et al. Extraskeletal osteosarcoma arising in myositis ossificans. Skeletal Radiol 2001; 30:39.

118. Eckardt JJ, Ivins JC, Perry HO, et al. Osteosarcoma arising in heterotopic ossification of dermatomyositis: case report and review of the literature. Cancer 1981; 48:1256.

119. Mirra JM, Fain JS, Ward WG, et al. Extraskeletal telangiectatic osteosarcoma. Cancer 1993; 71:3014.

120. Martland HS. Occupational poisoning in manufacture of luminal watch dials. JAMA 1929; 92:466.

121. Laskin WB, Silverman TA, Enzinger FM. Postradiation soft tissue sarcomas. An analysis of 53 cases. Cancer 1988; 62:2330.

122. Fang Z, Matsumoto S, Ae K, et al. Postradiation soft tissue sarcoma: a multiinstitutional analysis of 14 cases in Japan. J Orthop Sci 2004; 9:242.

123. Hasson J, Hartman KS, Milikow E, et al. Thorotrast-induced extraskeletal osteosarcoma of the cervical region. Report of a case. Cancer 1975; 36:1827.

124. Dubec JJ, Munk PL, O'Connell JX, et al. Soft tissue osteosarcoma with telangiectatic features: MR imaging findings in two cases. Skeletal Radiol 1997; 26:732.

125. Okada K, Ito H, Miyakoshi N, et al. A low-grade extraskeletal osteosarcoma. [review] [23 refs]. Skeletal Radiol 2003; 32:165.

126. Abramovici LC, Hytiroglou P, Klein RM, et al. Well-differentiated extraskeletal osteosarcoma: report of 2 cases, 1 with dedifferentiation. Hum Pathol 2005; 36:439.

127. Fukunaga M. Extraskeletal osteosarcoma histologically mimicking parosteal osteosarcoma. Pathol Int 2002; 52:492.

128. Fanburg-Smith JC, Bratthauer GL, Miettinen M. Osteocalcin and osteonectin immunoreactivity in extraskeletal osteosarcoma: a study of 28 cases. Hum Pathol 1999; 30:32.

129. Reddick RL, Michelitch HJ, Levine AM, et al. Osteogenic sarcoma: a study of the ultrastructure. Cancer 1980; 45:64.

130. Waxman M, Vuletin JC, Saxe BI, et al. Extraskeletal osteosarcoma: light and electron microscopic study. Mt Sinai J Med 1981; 48:322.

131. Bhagavan BS, Dorfman HD. The significance of bone and cartilage formation in malignant fibrous histiocytoma of soft tissue. Cancer 1982; 49:480.

132. Unni KK, Dahlin DC, Beabout JW, et al. Parosteal osteogenic sarcoma. Cancer 1976; 37:2466.

133. Unni KK, Dahlin DC, Beabout JW. Periosteal osteogenic sarcoma. Cancer 1976; 37:2476.

134. Wold LE, Unni KK, Beabout JW, et al. High-grade surface osteosarcomas. Am J Surg Pathol 1984; 8:181.

135. Patel SR, Benjamin RS. Primary extraskeletal osteosarcoma – experience with chemotherapy. J Natl Cancer Inst 1995; 87:1331.

BENIGN SOFT TISSUE TUMORS AND PSEUDOTUMORS OF UNCERTAIN TYPE

CHAPTER CONTENTS

This chapter discusses a heterogeneous group of benign tumors or pseudotumors in which the line of differentiation remains in question. Many of the lesions are characterized by abundant myxoid stroma (intramuscular myxoma, juxta-articular myxoma, cutaneous myxoma, aggressive angiomyxoma, and ganglion, among others); there is evidence that the cells in these lesions are fibroblastic or have some features of myofibroblasts.

TUMORAL CALCINOSIS

Tumoral calcinosis is a distinct clinical and histologic entity that is characterized by tumor-like periarticular deposits of calcium that are found foremost in the regions of the hip, shoulder, and elbow. The disorder occurs predominantly in otherwise healthy children, adolescents, and young adults, is more often multiple than solitary, and not infrequently affects two or more siblings of the same family. Unlike similar calcifications associated with renal insufficiency, hypervitaminosis D, and milk-alkali syndrome, there are no demonstrable abnormalities in calcium metabolism.

The term *tumoral calcinosis* was coined by Inclan in 1943,[1] but this condition was recognized as an entity much earlier. In 1899, Duret observed this process in siblings: a 17-year-old girl and her younger brother who had multiple calcifications in the neighborhood of the hip and elbow joint.[2] Later, in 1935, Teutschlaender gave a detailed account of another typical case, an 11-year-old girl with multiple lesions in the shoulder and elbow regions which had their onset at age 2 years. He thought that this process was secondary to fat necrosis and used the term "lipid calcinosis."[3] Since these descriptions, numerous other acceptable examples of this growth have been reported under various names, including calcifying bursitis,[4] calcifying collagenolysis,[5] and Kikuyu bursa. In New Guinea the natives aptly refer to it as "hip stones."[6]

Clinical findings

The principal manifestation of the disease is the presence of a large, firm, subcutaneous calcified mass that is asymptomatic and slowly growing, often gradually enlarging over many years; it is usually located in the vicinity of a large joint, especially the trochanteric and gluteal regions of the hip, the lateral portion of the shoulder, and the posterior elbow (Table 35–1). It is less frequent in the hands, feet, and knees.[7] However, examples of tumoral calcinosis have been described in many sites, including the spine,[8] temporomandibular joint,[9] and skin.[10] The lesion is firmly attached to the underlying fascia, muscle, or tendon and may infiltrate these structures, but it is unrelated to bone. Approximately two-thirds of patients have multiple lesions, some of which are bilateral and symmetric. The underlying joints are unaffected, and with few exceptions patients with tumoral calcinosis are in good health. Small and more deep-seated lesions are frequently overlooked and are often incidental findings during examination for some other cause. Large lesions, measuring 20 cm or more in diameter, are not particularly rare.

Tumoral calcinosis typically has its onset during the first and second decades of life; it is rare in patients older than 50 years. Overall, males and females are about equally affected. In the series of Pakasa and Kalengayi,[11] males predominated over females at a ratio of 1.5:1.0 in patients who developed the disease during the first two decades of life; during adulthood, women were affected about twice as often. Approximately two-thirds of cases involve blacks, predominantly Africans and African-Americans.[11–13] About half affect siblings, and in some instances several generations of the same family are

TABLE 35–1	ANATOMIC LOCATIONS OF 105 CASES OF TUMORAL CALCINOSIS	
Site	**No. of cases**	**%**
Hips	33	31
Buttocks	27	26
Upper extremities	16	15
Lower extremities	12	11
Spine/sacrum	7	7
Miscellaneous	10	10
Total	105	100

Modified from Pakasa NM, Kalengayi RM. Tumoral calcinosis: a clinicopathological study of 111 cases with emphasis on the earliest changes. Histopathology 1997; 31:18.

involved.[14] These cases seem to be inherited in an autosomal recessive manner and have been associated with mutations in either the *GALNT3* gene[15,16] or the *FGF23* gene.[17,18] Complications of the disease are rare. Occasionally, there is ulceration of the overlying skin with secondary infection, fistula formation, and discharge of a yellow-white chalky fluid.[11] Larger lesions may also affect nearby joints or impinge on anatomic structures. For example, lesions arising near the wrist can cause carpal tunnel syndrome.[19]

Laboratory examinations show no evidence of increased calcium levels, but in many patients there is slight to moderate hyperphosphatemia.[20,21] Calcitriol (1,25-dihydroxyvitamin D_3) may also be elevated, but serum alkaline phosphatase and uric acid levels are normal.

Examination with radiography, computed tomography (CT) scan, or magnetic resonance imaging (MRI) reveals a subcutaneous conglomerate of multiple, rounded opacities separated by radiolucent lines (fibrous septa) imparting a "chicken-wire" pattern of lucencies with distinct fluid levels in some of the nodules (Figs 35–1, 35–2).[22] There are no associated bony abnormalities; despite the large amounts of calcium in the lesion, there is no evidence of osteoporosis in the skeleton as in patients with renal insufficiency and secondary hyperparathyroidism.

Pathologic findings

Study of the gross specimen discloses a firm, rubbery mass that is unencapsulated, extends into the adjacent muscles and tendons, and is usually 5–15 cm in greatest diameter. On sectioning, the mass consists of a framework of dense fibrous tissue containing spaces filled with yellow-gray, pasty, calcareous material or chalky, milky liquid that is easily washed out, resulting in irregular cystic cavities. Chemical analysis of the intra- and extracellular calcified material reveals hydroxyapatite.[23]

Microscopically, active and inactive phases of the disease can be distinguished, often together in the same lesion (Figs 35–3, 35–4). Slavin et al. proposed a three-stage classification scheme to describe these lesions, spanning from cellular lesions devoid of calcification to cellular cystic lesions with calcification, and finally hypocellular calcified lesions.[23] In the active (cellular) phase, a central mass of amorphous or granular calcified material is bordered by a florid proliferation of mono- or multinucleated macrophages, osteoclast-like giant cells, fibroblasts, and chronic inflammatory elements. Fibrohistiocytic nodules may be seen during the early proliferative phase and are characterized by fibroblast-like cells, foamy histiocytes, occasional mononuclear macrophages, and hemosiderin-laden macrophages. During the inactive phase there is merely calcified material surrounded by dense fibrous material extending into the adjacent tissues or a cystic space surrounded by calcium deposits. Sometimes the calcified material forms small psammoma body-like masses with concentric layering of calcium (calcospherites) that bear a superficial resemblance to ova of parasites. Examination with electron microscopy reveals histiocytes with and without lipid inclusions, needle-shaped hydroxyapatite crystals, crystalline aggregates with a dense central core, and laminated calcospherites.[24,25] Hydroxyapatite crystals and noncrystalline calcific deposits arise primarily in intracytoplasmic membrane-bound vesicles and mitochondria.

Differential diagnosis

Morphologically, identical periarticular lesions may be encountered in patients with chronic renal disease and secondary hyperparathyroidism, but most patients with these lesions are older than those with tumoral calcinosis, have additional calcifications in visceral organs such as the kidney, lung, heart, and stomach, and have abnormally low calcium levels.[26] There are also tumoral calcinosis-like lesions and vascular calcifications associated with hyperphosphatemia in patients with end-stage renal disease undergoing hemodialysis.[27] Similar calcifying soft tissue lesions, but associated with hypercalcemia, occur in patients with hypervitaminosis D,[28] primary hyperparathyroidism,[29] and milk-alkali syndrome (Burnett syndrome),[30] a rare condition associated with prolonged antacid therapy for peptic ulcer. Patients with excessive osteolysis and mobilization of calcium in destructive neoplastic and infectious lesions of bone may also develop lesions that can resemble tumoral calcinosis. More recently, Laskin and colleagues described a group of tumoral calcinosis-like lesions which arise in an acral location and are smaller in size and seem to be pathogenetically distinct from tumoral calcinosis.[30a] In all of these lesions a detailed clinical history and laboratory data aid in reaching a reliable diagnosis (Table 35–2).

Calcinosis universalis and *calcinosis circumscripta* likewise are located in the skin and subcutis and are associated with normal serum calcium and phosphorus levels. Calcinosis universalis forms multiple nodules or plaques

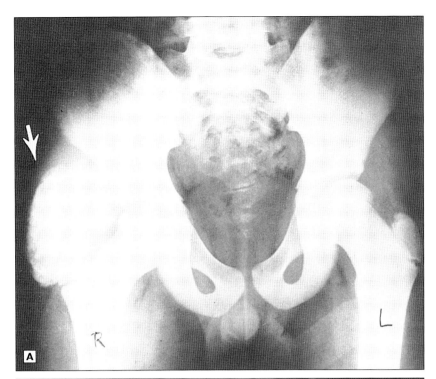

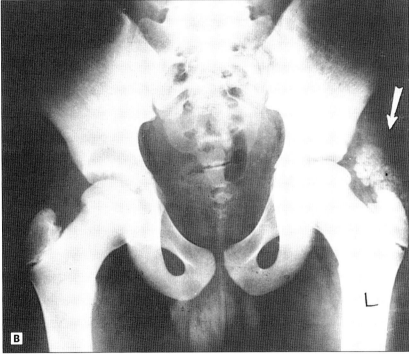

FIGURE 35–1 Radiograph of tumoral calcinosis involving the soft tissues of both hips (arrows). Nine months after the calcified mass in the right hip **(A)** was removed, a second mass developed in the left hip **(B)**.

that occur mainly in children and are associated in about half of the cases with manifestations of scleroderma or dermatomyositis.[31] It may ultimately lead to limited mobility, contractures, and ankylosis. Calcinosis circumscripta, on the other hand, chiefly affects middle-aged women and most commonly involves the hand and wrist, including tendon sheaths. It is associated in a large percentage of cases with Raynaud's disease or scleroderma, sclerodactyly, or polymyositis.[32] The CREST syndrome is a related condition involving *c*alcinosis cutis, *r*aynaud's phenomenon, *e*sophageal hypomotility, *s*clerodactyly, and *t*elangiectasis.

There are also dystrophic calcifications, as in calcareous tendinitis, that show an identical microscopic picture but are smaller and develop in damaged tissue secondary to minor injury, ischemic necrosis, or a necrotizing infectious process. Calcifications of tendons and ligaments have also been reported in patients undergoing long-term

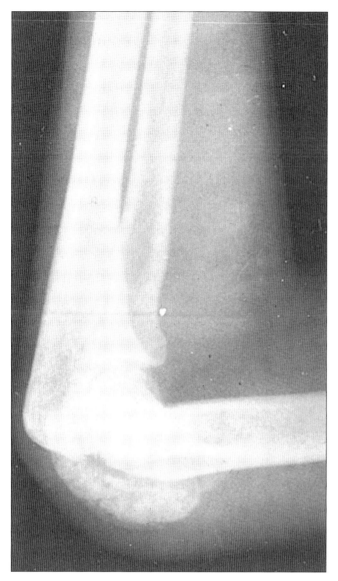

FIGURE 35–2 Tumoral calcinosis in the right elbow region of an 18-year-old man. The radiograph shows a calcified mass in the elbow region.

therapy with etretinate, a synthetic vitamin A derivative prescribed for acne, psoriasis, and various keratinization disorders.[33] Other forms of calcification, such as those of the scrotal skin, are not uncommon, but the exact cause is still not clear.[34]

Discussion

Tumoral calcinosis is an inborn error in calcium metabolism, which in most cases appears to be inherited in an autosomal recessive pattern. Laboratory studies reveal normal calcium levels, but in many cases there is elevation of serum phosphorus levels, probably the result of increased tubular reabsorption or reduced renal excretion of phosphorus. Slavin and colleagues described a family

in which seven of 13 siblings developed tumoral calcinosis.[23] All seven had hyperphosphatemia and normocalcemia. One had increased phosphorus levels prior to the onset of the calcification, but in the remaining six siblings without calcifications, phosphorus levels were normal. Subsequent studies over the past several years have implicated the *GALNT3* gene located on 2q24-31, which encodes for a glycosyltransferase responsible for initiating mucin-type O-glycosylation.[35,36] The *FGF23* gene, which encodes for a potent phosphaturic protein, has also been implicated as central to the pathogenesis of this disease.[17]

Trauma is rarely reported by patients with tumoral calcinosis, but minor repeated trauma and tissue injury seem to play a role in the calcifying process; it probably serves as a trigger mechanism in genetically susceptible individuals that leads to a chain of events, beginning with hemorrhage, fat necrosis, fibrosis, and collagenization and ending with collagenolysis and ultimately massive calcification.

Prognosis

The treatment of choice is surgical removal of the lesion as early as possible, when the lesion is still small and amenable to total resection.[11,37] Incomplete excision may lead to recurrence, secondary infection, or abscess formation. A number of other medical therapies have been attempted, but with limited success.

INTRAMUSCULAR MYXOMA

There is a dizzying array of benign mesenchymal lesions characterized by abundant myxoid matrix, a small number of inconspicuous stellate- or spindle-shaped cells, and a poorly developed vascular pattern. Most seem to be composed of modified fibroblasts that produce excessive amounts of glycosaminoglycans rich in hyaluronic acid and little collagen. Chief among them is the intramuscular myxoma, a benign mesenchymal lesion that is of particular importance because it is almost always cured by local excision yet is easily mistaken for a myxoid sarcoma.

Clinical findings

Intramuscular myxoma is a tumor of adult life that occurs primarily in patients 40–70 years of age.[38–40] In our experience it is rare in young adults and virtually nonexistent in children and adolescents. About two-thirds of the patients are women.[41–44] There is no evidence of increased familial incidence.

The clinical manifestations are non-specific, and it is difficult to diagnose this tumor before biopsy and microscopic examination. In most patients the sole presenting

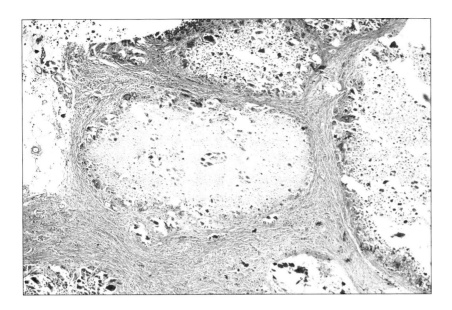

FIGURE 35–3 Tumoral calcinosis. Amorphous calcified material bordered by a florid proliferation of macrophages and multinucleated, osteoclast-like giant cells. The nodules are separated by bands of dense fibrous tissue.

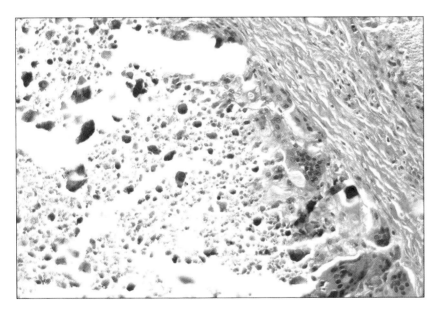

FIGURE 35–4 Tumoral calcinosis with a characteristic mixture of calcified material, histiocytes, and multinucleated giant cells.

TABLE 35–2	TUMOR-LIKE CALCIFIC LESIONS IN SOFT TISSUE

Tumoral calcinosis
Chronic renal failure with secondary hyperparathyroidism
Milk-alkali syndrome
Hypervitaminosis D
Bone destruction secondary to infection/neoplasm

Modified from McGregor DH, Mowry M, Cherian R, et al. Nonfamilial tumoral calcinosis associated with chronic renal failure and secondary hyperparathyroidism: report of two cases with clinicopathological, immunohistochemical, and electron microscopic findings. Hum Pathol 1995; 26:607.

sign is a painless, palpable mass that is firm, slightly movable, and often fluctuant. Pain or tenderness is present in fewer than one-fourth of patients.[38] As one would expect, pain and occasional numbness, paresthesia, and muscle weakness distal to the lesion are mostly associated with tumors of large size. Because of the relative lack of symptoms, most of the tumors are present for several months or even years before they are excised. The rate of growth varies, but there is no close relation between size and clinical duration. A history of trauma is rarely given, and the tumor is not etiologically related to thyroid dysfunction, as in myxedema.

By far the most frequent sites of the tumor are the large muscles of the thigh, shoulder, buttocks, and upper arm (Fig. 35–5). Unusual examples have been reported in the muscles of the head and neck,[45,46] the forearm,[47] and even the small muscles of the hand.[48] The exact location in the musculature varies: some tumors are completely surrounded by muscle tissue, and others are firmly attached on one side to muscle fascia. There are also myxomas of identical appearance that arise from the periosteum, subchondral epiphysis, and joint capsule. Angiographic

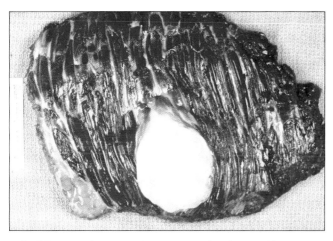

FIGURE 35–5 Intramuscular myxoma showing a uniform yellowish-white cut surface. The tumor characteristically appears well circumscribed.

examination reveals a poorly vascularized soft tissue mass surrounded by well-vascularized muscle tissue.[39] Magnetic resonance imaging reveals a well-defined, usually homogeneous tumor exhibiting low signal intensity relative to skeletal muscle on T1-weighted images and a hyperintense appearance relative to muscle on T2-weighted images.[49,50]

Multiple intramuscular myxomas and fibrous dysplasia

Although most intramuscular myxomas are solitary, there are occasional patients in whom two or more myxomas are present, usually in the same region of the body. Microscopically, these tumors are in no way different from the solitary intramuscular myxomas. Nearly all are associated with monostotic or polyostotic fibrous dysplasia of bone, generally in the same anatomic region where the myxomas are located (Fig. 35–6).[51–53] In this setting,

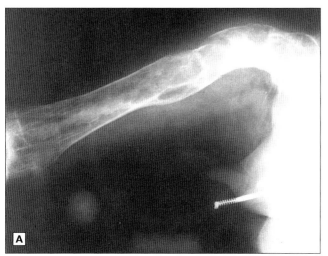

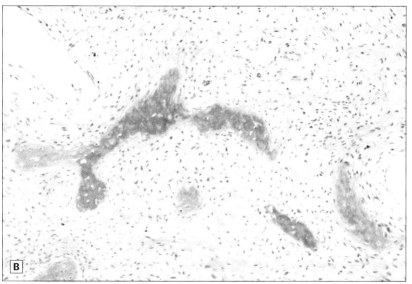

FIGURE 35–6 Patient with multiple intramuscular myxomas and fibrous dysplasia. **(A)** Characteristic radiographic features of fibrous dysplasia involving the humerus show a shepherd's crook deformity. **(B)** Histologic appearance of fibrous dysplasia. An intramuscular myxoma was found in the soft tissues adjacent to the humerus.

females are affected more commonly than males, even more so than in solitary cases. Often there is a long interval between the appearances of the two processes. In most cases the fibrous dysplasia is noted during the growth period, whereas the multiple myxomas, like their solitary forms, become apparent many years later, during adult life. On occasion, multiple intramuscular myxomas are detected before the osseous lesions. If specifically sought, radiologically evident bone abnormalities are seen in many patients with intramuscular myxomas.[43] In the case reported by Mazabraud and co-workers, an osteosarcoma developed in a patient with fibrous dysplasia and multiple myxomas,[54] a phenomenon that has been noted by others. Activating missense mutations in the Arg201 codon of the gene encoding the alpha subunit of G_S (*GNAS1*), the G protein that stimulates cAMP formation, have been recognized in fibrous dysplasia of bone and McCune-Albright syndrome, a syndrome consisting of polyostotic fibrous dysplasia, sexual precocity, and café-au-lait spots.[55,56] Recently, these same mutations have been identified in intramuscular myxomas with and without fibrous dysplasia.[57,58]

Pathologic findings

The gross appearance is characteristic and changes little from case to case. Most tumors are ovoid or globular and have a glistening gray-white or white appearance, depending on the relative amounts of collagen and myxoid material (Fig. 35–7). They consist of a mass of stringy, gelatinous material with occasional small fluid-filled, cyst-like spaces, and they are covered by bundles of skeletal muscle or fascial tissue (Fig. 35–8). Although on gross examination most of the tumors appear to be well circumscribed, many infiltrate the adjacent musculature or are surrounded by edematous muscle tissue, which may serve as a natural cleavage plane for the surgeon. The size varies greatly; the majority measure 5–10 cm in greatest diameter, but some lesions are 20 cm or larger.

On histologic examination, the tumor varies little in its appearance and is composed of relatively small numbers of inconspicuous cells, abundant mucoid material, and a loose meshwork of reticulin fibers (Figs 35–9 to 35–11). Characteristically, mature collagen fibers and vascular structures are sparse. Fluid-filled cystic spaces are seen occasionally (Figs 35–12, 35–13), but they are rarely a prominent feature.[59] The constituent cells have small, hyperchromatic, pyknotic-appearing nuclei and scanty cytoplasm that sometimes extends along the reticulin fibers with multiple processes, giving the cell a stellate appearance (Figs 35–14, 35–15). There is little cellular pleomorphism, and there are no multinucleated giant cells. In some cases there are also scattered macrophages with small intracellular droplets of lipid material (Fig. 35–16). The small size of these droplets and the absence of nuclear deformation or scalloping afford their distinc-

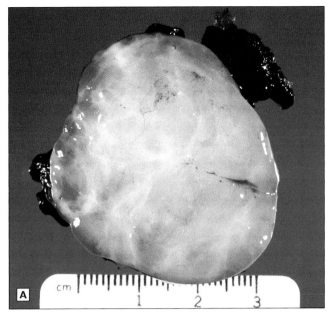

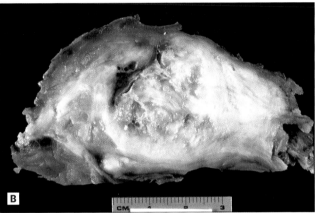

FIGURE 35–7 Gross appearances of intramuscular myxoma. **(A)** The tumor has a mucoid, gelatinous cut surface with thin fibrous septa. **(B)** Fibrous-appearing intramuscular myxoma.

tion from lipoblasts (Fig. 35–17). At the periphery, where the tumor merges with the surrounding muscle, fat cells and atrophic muscle fibers are occasionally scattered in the mucoid substance. These residual muscle fibers can be misinterpreted as evidence of rhabdomyoblastic differentiation, resulting in a misdiagnosis of rhabdomyosarcoma.

Some intramuscular myxomas show focal areas of hypercellularity and hypervascularity, which may cause further confusion with a myxoid sarcoma (so-called cellular myxoma) (Fig. 35–18).[60–62] In the study by Nielsen et al.,[60] 38 of 51 cases of intramuscular myxoma (76%) had hypercellular zones that comprised 10–80% of the tumor. However, even in these hypercellular zones, the cells lack nuclear atypia, and there is a paucity of mitotic figures and an absence of necrosis. Areas of more typical hypocellular intramuscular myxoma allow their definitive recognition.

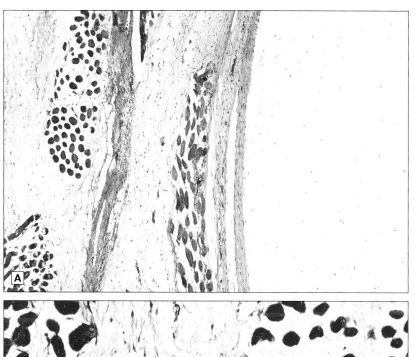

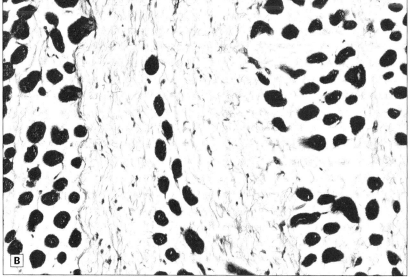

FIGURE 35–8 Intramuscular myxoma. Although grossly well circumscribed, the tumor infiltrates the surrounding skeletal muscle **(A)**. Higher-magnification appearance of the peripheral portion of an intramuscular myxoma with atrophy of the surrounding skeletal muscle **(B)**.

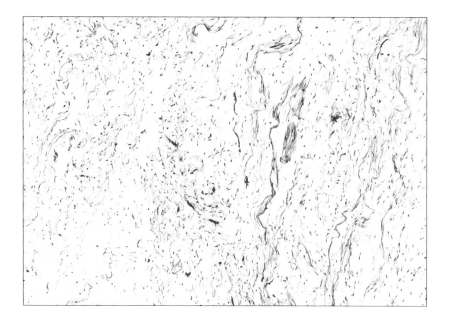

FIGURE 35–9 Low-magnification appearance of intramuscular myxoma characterized by a paucity of cells, abundance of mucoid material, and almost complete absence of vascular structures.

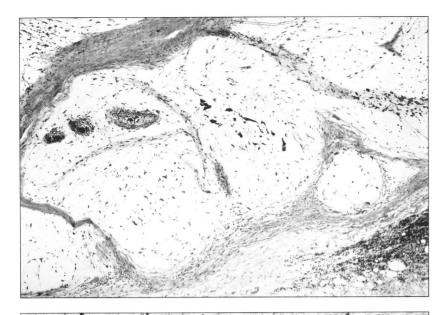

FIGURE 35–10 Intramuscular myxoma. Intersecting fibrous septa give the tumor a multilobular appearance.

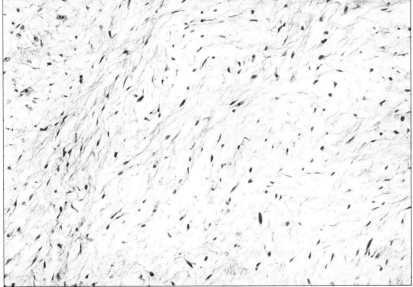

FIGURE 35–11 Intramuscular myxoma. The tumor cells are widely separated by abundant mucoid material and generally do not touch one another.

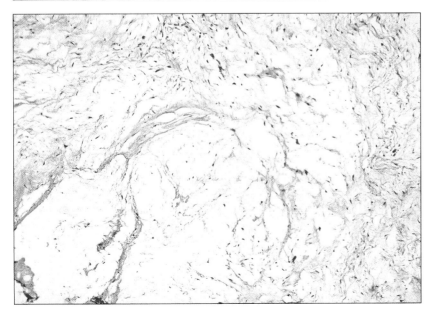

FIGURE 35–12 Intramuscular myxoma with prominent fluid-filled cystic spaces.

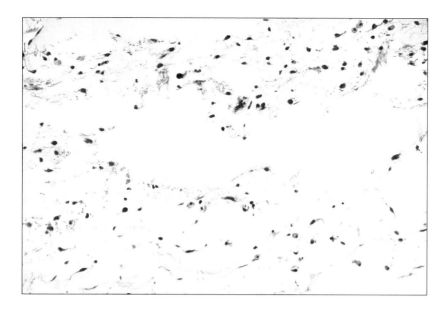

FIGURE 35–13 Cystic area in an intramuscular myxoma.

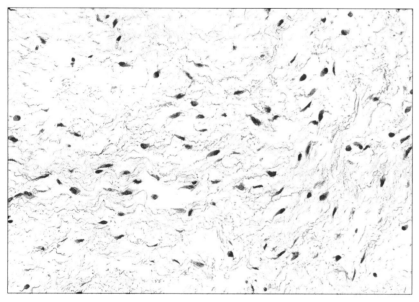

FIGURE 35–14 Intramuscular myxoma. The tumor is composed of cytologically bland spindled and stellate-shaped cells that are widely separated by myxoid stroma.

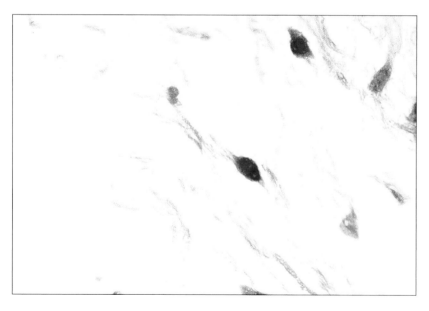

FIGURE 35–15 High-magnification appearance of pyknotic cells with tapered cytoplasm in an intramuscular myxoma.

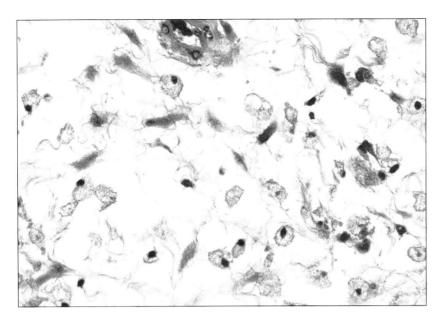

FIGURE 35–16 Intramuscular myxoma with collection of macrophages with small intracellular droplets of lipid material.

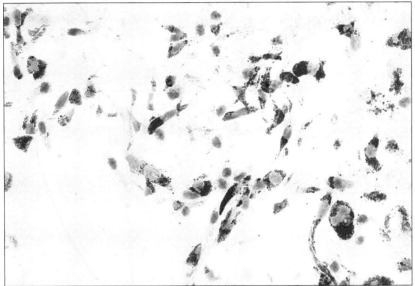

FIGURE 35–17 Frozen section of intramuscular myxoma with granular oil red O-positive intracellular lipid material mimicking a liposarcoma.

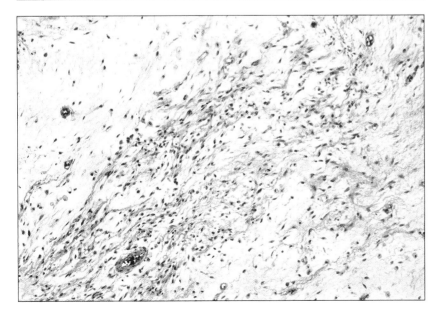

FIGURE 35–18 Hypercellular focus in an otherwise typical intramuscular myxoma.

Immunohistochemically, the cells stain positively for vimentin; unlike lipoblasts, they do not stain for S-100 protein. Rare cells may also stain for actins, suggesting focal myofibroblastic differentiation. The cells are suspended in large amounts of mucoid material that stains positively with Alcian blue and colloidal iron stains. The mucoid material is depolymerized by prior treatment of the sections with hyaluronidase.[40]

Ultrastructural examination discloses predominantly fibroblast- and myofibroblast-like cells with prominent rough endoplasmic reticulum, microfilamentous material, a prominent Golgi complex, and pinocytotic and secretory vesicles, together with a mixture of amorphous and granular material and collagen fibers in the extracellular spaces (Fig. 35–19A). There are also macrophage-like cells with small lipid droplets or secretory vacuoles and multiple cytoplasmic processes (Fig. 35–19B).[42]

Differential diagnosis

Numerous benign and low-grade malignant myxoid neoplasms are apt to be confused with intramuscular myxoma (Table 35–3). At times, the tumor is difficult to distinguish from myxolipoma, myxoid neurofibroma, neurothekeoma, myxochondroma, and nodular fasciitis, conditions discussed in previous chapters. More impor-

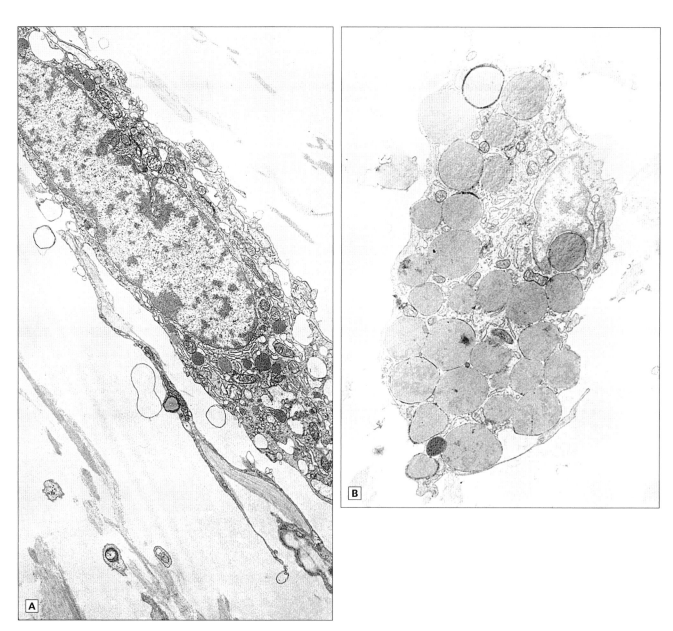

FIGURE 35–19 (A) Electron microscopy of an intramuscular myxoma with fibroblast-like cells; note the prominent rough endoplasmic reticulum and collagen fibers in the extracellular spaces. **(B)** Electron microscopy of an intramuscular myxoma. Macrophage-like cells with multiple membrane-bound lipid droplets. **(A, B:** Courtesy of Veterans Administration Hospital, Ann Arbor, MI.)

TABLE 35–3	DIFFERENTIAL DIAGNOSIS OF INTRAMUSCULAR MYXOMA		
Tumor type	Pleomorphism	Vascularity	Matrix
Intramuscular myxoma	–	Inconspicuous	Hyaluronic acid
Myxoid liposarcoma	+	Fine, plexiform	Hyaluronic acid
Myxoid chondrosarcoma	+	Irregular	Chondroitin sulfate
Myxoid MFH	+++	Coarse, curvilinear	Hyaluronic acid

MFH, malignant fibrous histiocytoma.

tantly, intramuscular myxoma may be confused with low-grade myxoid sarcomas of various types. *Low-grade myxofibrosarcoma*, similar to intramuscular myxoma, predominantly affects adults and may arise in either superficial or deep soft tissues. At the low end of the histologic spectrum, myxofibrosarcoma is a hypocellular neoplasm composed of spindle-shaped cells deposited in an abundant myxoid stroma. However, the cells always demonstrate a greater degree of nuclear hyperchromasia and cytologic atypia than those of intramuscular myxoma. Many of these neoplasms also have prominent curvilinear blood vessels, often with perivascular tumoral condensation. *Myxoid liposarcoma* is characterized by a regular plexiform vasculature with spindle-shaped or stellate cells with mild cytologic atypia deposited in a myxoid stroma. In addition, the identification of cells with adipocytic differentiation, including well-formed lipoblasts, is useful for this distinction. *Extraskeletal myxoid chondrosarcoma* is composed of nests and cords of cells with densely eosinophilic cytoplasm deposited in a chondroitin sulfate-rich stroma. Although blood vessels are often not conspicuous, these lesions frequently show areas of hemorrhage and hemosiderin deposition. Immunostaining for S-100 protein, when positive, is useful for recognizing this entity, although fewer than one-half of all cases stain for this antigen. Perhaps the most difficult distinction is from a *low-grade fibromyxoid sarcoma (Evans tumor)*, especially when dealing with a cellular intramuscular myxoma. Low-grade fibromyxoid sarcoma is an uncommon tumor that occurs in the deep soft tissues of young adults. Histologically, this tumor is composed of cytologically uniform spindle-shaped cells deposited in a variably collagenous and myxoid matrix, often with a swirling arrangement of tumor cells around thin-walled capillaries. The transition between fibrous and myxoid zones is often abrupt. In difficult cases, evaluation for evidence of a t(7;16) characteristic of this tumor can be extremely helpful. In our practice, we utilize paraffin-embedded tissue for evaluation by FISH using a probe to the *FUS* gene, which is characteristically altered in the Evans tumor.

Discussion

Despite their frequently large size and prominent myxoid appearance, intramuscular myxomas are benign and

TABLE 35–4	ANATOMIC LOCATION OF 65 JUXTA-ARTICULAR MYXOMAS	
Site	No. of cases	%
Knee	57	88.0
Shoulder	3	4.5
Elbow	3	4.5
Hip	1	1.5
Ankle	1	1.5
Total	65	100.0

Modified from Meis JM, Enzinger FM. Juxtaarticular myxoma: a clinical and pathological study of 65 cases. Hum Pathol 1992; 23:639

rarely recur locally. In the series by Nielsen and colleagues, none of the 32 patients for whom follow-up information was available developed a local recurrence, including those with hypercellular lesions.[60] In the rare examples that do recur, re-excision is typically curative.

JUXTA-ARTICULAR MYXOMA

Juxta-articular myxoma is an uncommon lesion marked by the accumulation of mucinous material in the vicinity of the large joints, most commonly the knee (almost 90% of cases) but occasionally near the shoulder, elbow, hip, or ankle (Table 35–4).[41,63–65] It almost always arises in adults, particularly men, with a predilection for the third through fifth decades of life. In the largest series to date, the patients ranged in age from 16 to 83 years, with a median age of 43 years.[65] The growth typically presents as a swelling or mass that is sometimes rapidly enlarging and is not infrequently associated with pain or tenderness.[64] These lesions may be associated with antecedent trauma and can arise adjacent to a joint with osteoarthritis. Some lesions are discovered incidentally during total knee or hip arthroplasty.[65] When in the region of the knee, they are frequently referred to as parameniscal cyst, cystic myxomatous tumor, or periarticular myxoma. The radiologic features are similar to those found with intramuscular myxoma.[66]

Grossly, most lesions are 2–6 cm, but some are as large as 12 cm at the time of excision. They typically have a mucoid cystic or multicystic appearance on cut section. Histologically, juxta-articular myxoma closely resembles intramuscular myxoma and is composed of scattered

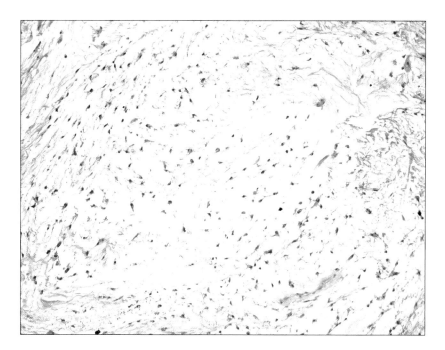

FIGURE 35-20 Juxta-articular myxoma composed of a hypocellular proliferation of bland spindled cells evenly deposited in a myxoid stroma. The histology is essentially identical to that seen in intramuscular myxoma.

small, spindled or stellate-shaped fibroblast-like cells deposited in a richly myxoid matrix that often contains variously sized thin- or thick-walled cystic spaces (Fig. 35–20). Occasionally, there are hypercellular areas with slight cellular pleomorphism, features that may arouse suspicion of a low-grade myxoid sarcoma. The process involves not only the periarticular soft tissues and the overlying cutaneous fat, but also the joint capsule, tendons, and rarely skeletal muscle. Some lesions have areas of hemorrhage and hemosiderin deposition with scattered chronic inflammation and reactive fibroblastic proliferation. This lesion has the same immunohisto-chemical and ultrastructural features as its intramuscular counterpart.

Juxta-articular myxoma is benign but is apt to recur after incomplete excision. In the series by Meis and Enzinger,[65] recurrences appeared in 10 of the 29 patients for whom follow-up information was available, including one lesion that recurred four times.

The pathogenesis of this condition is not clear, but it may represent an exuberant reactive fibroblastic proliferation with overproduction of mucin. On the other hand, Sciot et al. described a case with clonal chromosomal changes, including trisomy 7 and a translocation between chromosomes 8 and 22.[67] Unlike intramuscular myxoma, this lesion does not have mutations in the *GNAS1* gene.[58]

soft tissues as a myxomatous swelling or mass overlying a radiographically demonstrable osteolytic defect of the mandible or maxilla.[68-71] It may also displace and destroy teeth, extend into the adjacent maxillary sinus, and involve the soft tissues of the face.[70] It chiefly affects young adults, with a predilection for females; it is slightly more frequent in the mandible than in the maxilla.[70] Rare lesions have been described in infants and children.[72,73] These lesions have a fairly characteristic appearance on CT scans and MRI such that there is usually a high index of suspicion prior to surgery.[74]

Microscopically, myxomas of the jaw are poorly circumscribed myxoma-like masses that differ from other myxomatous lesions merely by a slightly greater degree of cellularity and cellular pleomorphism and a higher rate of mitotic activity. Rare lesions also have epithelial inclusions presumed to be of odontogenic origin.[75,76] The cells are immunoreactive with antibodies against vimentin and S-100 protein but not desmin or cytokeratin.[77] Similar to normal odontogenic epithelium, the epithelial inclusions stain for cytokeratin 19.[78] Electron microscopic examination reveals the presence of fibroblasts and myofibroblasts.[69] Surgical removal of the growth is often difficult, and the lesion is apt to recur, especially when it is treated by curettage rather than excision.[70] More cellular forms may be difficult to distinguish from fibrous dysplasia and ossifying fibroma.[69]

MYXOMA OF THE JAW (ODONTOGENIC MYXOMA)

Although myxoma of the jaw (odontogenic myxoma) is primarily a bone tumor, it occasionally manifests in the

CUTANEOUS MYXOMA (SUPERFICIAL ANGIOMYXOMA)

Cutaneous myxoma, also known as *superficial angiomyxoma*, was first described by Carney and colleagues in their 1986

study of the superficial myxoid tumors which occurred in the setting of Carney complex, which had been described one year earlier.[79,80] This lesion was later more fully characterized by Allen et al. in 1988[81] and Calonje and colleagues in 1999.[82] Cutaneous myxoma should be distinguished from the other cutaneous myxoid lesions with which it may be confused because it has a propensity for local recurrence.

Cutaneous myxoma arises slightly more commonly in males, predominantly middle-aged adults with a peak incidence between 20 and 40 years of age.[41,82] Rare congenital examples have been described.[83] These lesions can arise essentially anywhere in the superficial tissues but there is a predilection for the trunk, lower extremities, and head and neck; some arise in the genital region (vulva, mons pubis, scrotum/inguinal) of both males and females.[84] Histologically identical lesions may arise in the setting of Carney complex, particularly those that are multiple and arise in the eyelids and external ear.[85] Clinically, most appear as slowly growing polypoid or papulonodular cutaneous lesions which may be confused with a cyst, skin tag, or neurofibroma.[82]

Pathologic findings

Grossly, cutaneous myxomas are usually well circumscribed, but some are poorly demarcated. The majority are between 1 and 5 cm and have a gray to white, glistening, gelatinous cut surface. Thin fibrous septa traverse the neoplasm, resulting in a vaguely multinodular tumor. Cysts that are sometimes filled with keratinous debris may be identified grossly.

As seen by light microscopy, this lesion has a lobular or multinodular appearance at low magnification (Figs 35–21, 35–22); most are histologically poorly circumscribed with extension into the underlying subcutaneous tissue and rarely skeletal muscle. A sparse proliferation of spindled to stellate-shaped cells is deposited in an extensive myxoid stroma, sometimes forming cysts or irregular clefts, that is sensitive to hyaluronidase digestion (Figs 35–23, 35–24). The cells have indistinct cell borders and oval nuclei with inconspicuous nucleoli; mitotic figures are rare. Binucleated or multinucleated cells may be seen, as are scattered cells with intranuclear cytoplasmic pseudoinclusions. There is often a prominent vasculature that is focally arborizing, reminiscent of that seen in myxoid liposarcomas (Fig. 35–25). Other vascular alterations including perivascular hyalinization, perivascular lymphocytes, and fibrin thrombi may be seen. A mixed inflammatory infiltrate is common, particularly stromal neutrophils, a feature unique to this tumor when compared to other cutaneous myxoid lesions.[82] Up to one-quarter of these tumors have epithelial structures consisting of basaloid buds, epithelial strands, or epidermoid (keratin-filled) cysts, possibly as a result of entrapment of adnexal structures by the neoplasm (Figs 35–26 to 35–28).[81,82]

Immunohistochemically, the tumor cells consistently express vimentin and CD34 but rarely stain for cytokeratins or S-100 protein.[82] Some cells stain for smooth muscle actin, muscle-specific actin, or desmin, possibly indicating focal myofibroblastic differentiation.

Differential diagnosis

The differential diagnosis of cutaneous myxoma is extensive and includes many benign and low-grade malignant myxoid lesions including aggressive angiomyxoma, focal cutaneous mucinosis, cutaneous myxoid cyst, dermal nerve sheath myxoma (myxoid neurothekeoma), myxoid

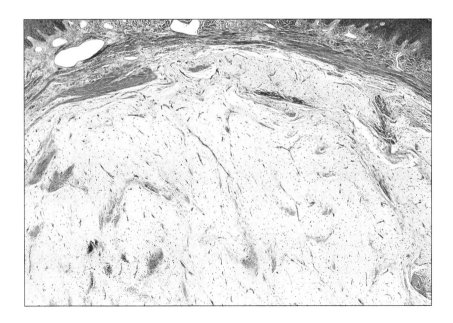

FIGURE 35–21 Cutaneous myxoma (superficial angiomyxoma). At low magnification, the tumor is hypocellular with prominent myxoid stroma; it appears fairly well circumscribed at its superficial aspect.

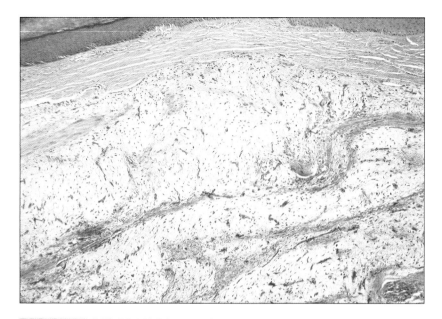

FIGURE 35–22 Multilobular appearance of a cutaneous myxoma.

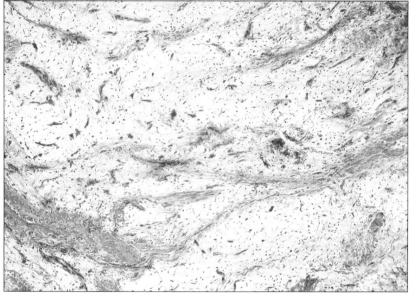

FIGURE 35–23 Cutaneous myxoma. Fibrous septa subdivide the tumor into ill-defined lobules.

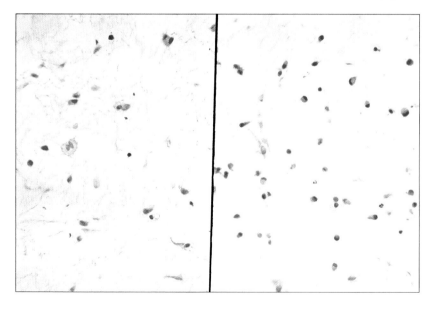

FIGURE 35–24 Cutaneous myxoma stained with Alcian blue stain without **(left)** and with **(right)** pretreatment with hyaluronidase.

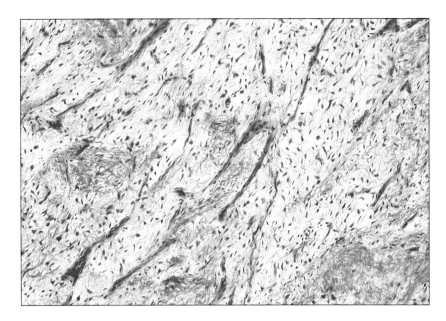

FIGURE 35–25 Cutaneous myxoma. A prominent arborizing vasculature is present, mimicking that found in myxoid liposarcoma.

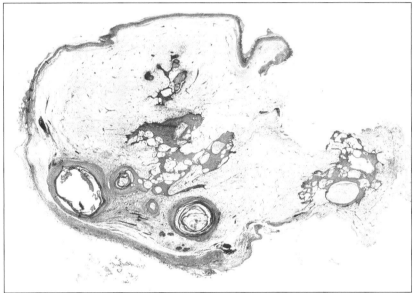

FIGURE 35–26 Cutaneous myxoma in a patient with Carney complex. Note the adnexal structures surrounded by myxoid matrix.

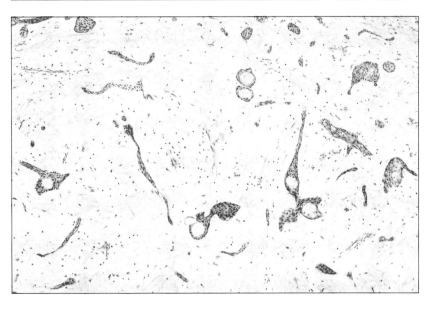

FIGURE 35–27 Cutaneous myxoma in a patient with Carney complex. Numerous epithelial strands are found in the substance of the neoplasm.

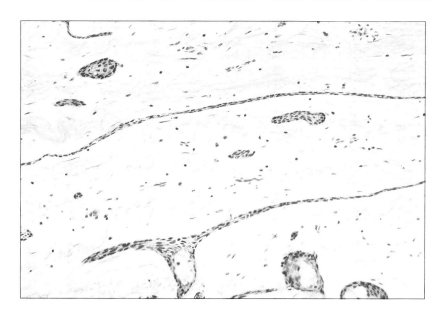

FIGURE 35–28 High-magnification view of elongated epithelial strands which appear to be compressed by the surrounding neoplasm in a cutaneous myxoma in a patient with Carney complex.

neurofibroma, superficial acral fibromyxoma, myxoid liposarcoma, and myxofibrosarcoma.

Some cutaneous myxomas arise in the genital region and so may be confused with *aggressive angiomyxoma*. The latter lesion, however, tends to be much larger, involves deeper structures, usually in the female pelvic region, and has a vascular pattern that differs from that of cutaneous myxoma. *Focal cutaneous mucinosis* lacks the lobular architecture, stromal neutrophils, and epithelial structures found in cutaneous myxoma. *Cutaneous myxoid cyst* is easily distinguished given its almost exclusive location on the fingers. Similarly, *superficial acral fibromyxoma* arises almost exclusively on the fingers and toes of middle-aged adults.[86] *Myxoid neurothekeoma* has a more pronounced lobular growth pattern and is characterized by plumper cells that are usually positive for S-100 protein. *Myxoid neurofibroma* is composed of cells with wavy or buckled nuclei that are also S-100 protein-positive.

Myxoid liposarcoma is usually more deeply located and larger than cutaneous myxoma and is characterized by a "chicken-wire" plexiform vasculature with scattered lipoblasts. *Myxofibrosarcoma* has a greater degree of nuclear atypia and hyperchromasia as well as curvilinear vessels often lined by hyperchromatic tumor cells.

Discussion

Cutaneous myxoma has a propensity for local recurrence if incompletely excised. In the series by Allen and colleagues, eight of 20 (40%) tumors recurred, including five of eight tumors with epithelial components.[81] Calonje et al. reported a recurrence rate of 30%, including one case that recurred three times.[82] In the latter series, recurrences developed a median of 12 months following initial excision. No cutaneous myxoma has been reported to metas-

tasize. Although Allen et al. noted that recurrences were more common in tumors with epithelial elements,[81] the smaller series of cases arising in the genital region reported by Fetsch et al. did not confirm this association.[84]

CARNEY COMPLEX

The triad of cutaneous and cardiac myxomas, spotty pigmentation, and endocrine overactivity was first described by Carney et al. in 1985 (Fig. 35–29).[79] The disorder is familial and is transmitted as an autosomal dominant trait and principally affects young adults.[87] Most individuals with the complex harbor a mutation of the *PRKAR1A* gene, which encodes for the regulatory R1 alpha subunit of protein kinase A.[88–90]

The cutaneous myxomas arising in this complex have a predilection for the eyelids and range from small sessile papules to large pedunculated, finger-like masses; they are multiple in most cases and are characterized by an appearance during early adulthood (mean age 18 years).[80] The lesions are found in the dermis or subcutaneous tissue, are usually sharply circumscribed, and are characterized by cytologically bland spindled and stellate-shaped cells deposited in an abundant myxoid stroma with a prominent capillary vasculature, identical to sporadic cutaneous myxomas discussed in the previous section. They are often associated with a basaloid proliferation of the surface epithelium, which may cause misclassification of some of these lesions as basal cell carcinoma or trichofolliculoma. In 1994, Ferreiro and Carney reported the association of myxomas of the external ear with Carney complex.[85] Of the 152 patients with this complex known to these authors, 22 (14%) had myxomas of the external ear. Furthermore, 22 of 26

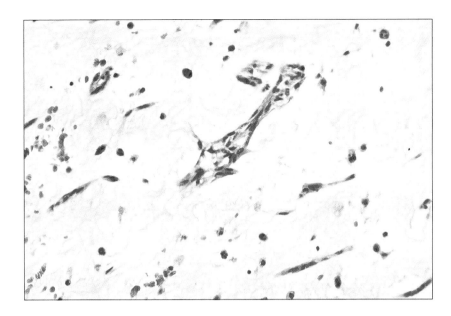

FIGURE 35–29 Cardiac myxoma in a patient with Carney complex.

patients (85%) with ear myxomas were found to have Carney complex. Multifocal myxoid fibroadenomas and myxomatosis of the breast are also occasional components of this complex.[91]

The most serious components of the syndrome are psammomatous melanotic schwannoma (see Chapter 29) and cardiac myxoma. Cardiac myxomas, regardless of their association with this syndrome, may be associated with peripheral tumor emboli, and up to 24% of all patients with cardiac myxomas die of its complications.[92]

The spotty skin pigmentation includes lentigines that predominantly affect the face, particularly the vermilion border of the lips, and blue nevi, including epithelioid blue nevi.[93–96] Endocrine overactivity may be due to the presence of primary pigmented nodular adrenocortical disease resulting in Cushing's syndrome,[97,98] pituitary adenoma resulting in acromegaly,[99] or sexual precocity associated with testicular lesions, particularly large-cell calcifying Sertoli cell tumor. Thyroid gland abnormalities ranging from follicular hyperplasia to cystic carcinoma have been associated with Carney complex.[100,101]

GANGLION (GANGLION CYST)

Ganglion is by far the most common and best known of the more superficially located myxoid lesions. It occurs as a unilocular or multilocular cystic or myxoid mass on the dorsal surface of the wrist in young persons, especially women, generally 25–45 years of age. Less often, it is found on the volar surface of the wrist or fingers and the dorsum of the foot and toes.[102–104] It is, in fact, the most common lesion of the hand and wrist, accounting for 50–70% of all masses in this location. In about half

of the cases the condition is associated with tenderness or mild pain and causes interference of function. A history of trauma is given by about half of the cases.

Ganglia usually measure 1.5–2.5 cm in diameter. They are frequently attached to the joint capsule and tendon sheaths and probably are due to excessive mucin production by fibroblasts rather than disintegration of preformed fibrous structures. There is no communication between the ganglion and the joint space. Some of these lesions are easily confused with myxomas, especially during the initial myxoid stage of development. Most, however, are readily recognized by their location and the presence of multiple thick-walled cystic spaces of variable size in association with myxoid areas. Focal myxoid change is noted in the earliest stage (Fig. 35–30). Subsequently, microscopic cysts develop and coalesce into larger ones until finally the lesion assumes its typical form of a dominant cyst (Fig. 35–31). Most of these lesions can be treated nonoperatively but a select group is surgically excised, with a very low rate of recurrence. Ganglion-like lesions may also arise in the subperiosteal region or bone.[105] Intraneural ganglion-like lesions (nerve sheath ganglion)[106] and myxoid neurothekeoma (nerve sheath myxoma) are discussed and illustrated in Chapter 29.

AGGRESSIVE ANGIOMYXOMA

The term *aggressive angiomyxoma* was coined by Steeper and Rosai in 1983 for a morphologically distinctive, slowly growing myxoid neoplasm that occurs chiefly in the genital, perineal, and pelvic regions of adult women.[107] Despite its bland histologic features, it has a propensity to recur locally.

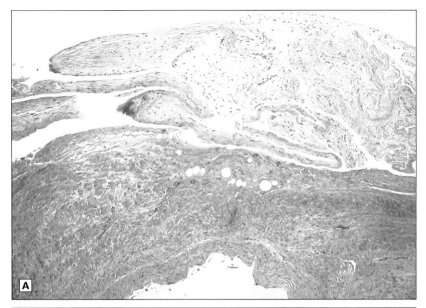

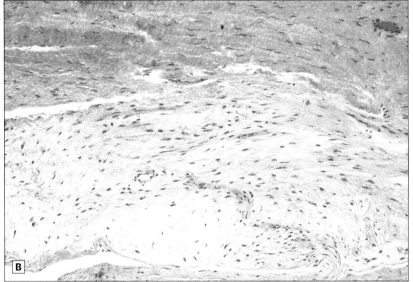

FIGURE 35–30 **(A)** Low-magnification view of a ganglion cyst with multiple irregular thick-walled cystic spaces and focal myxoid change in the surrounding matrix. **(B)** High-magnification view of focal myxoid change with bland spindle-shaped cells in a ganglion cyst.

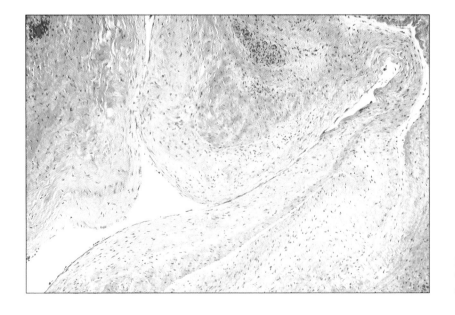

FIGURE 35–31 Ganglion. Dominant cyst with prominent myxoid change in the surrounding soft tissue.

Clinical and radiologic findings

The neoplasm predominantly affects reproductive-age females with a peak incidence during the third decade of life. The female/male ratio is more than 6 : 1,[108] but this tumor has been increasingly recognized as arising in the inguinal region, along the spermatic cord, or in the scrotum or pelvic cavity of men.[109-113] In women, the vulvar region is the most common site of involvement and may be initially misdiagnosed clinically as a Bartholin cyst, periurethral cyst, or hernia.[114] Although slowly growing, these lesions aggressively infiltrate the perivaginal and perirectal soft tissues.

The radiologic features of this tumor have been well described. MRI reveals a mass with high signal intensity on T2-weighted images with translevator extension and growth around perineal structures.[115]

Pathologic findings

Grossly, aggressive angiomyxomas are soft, partly circumscribed, or polypoid; on cross-section they have a glistening, homogeneous, gelatinous appearance and range in size from a few centimeters to 20 cm or more. Steeper and Rosai reported a pelvic/retroperitoneal tumor in a 34-year-old woman that measured 60 cm in greatest diameter.[107] In the series by Fetsch et al., 23 of 27 tumors were 10 cm or larger.[108] Most have a lobulated appearance. Although some areas of the tumor may be sharply marginated, others show adherence or infiltration into the surrounding soft tissues.

Microscopically, the tumor is composed of widely scattered spindled to stellate-shaped cells with ill-defined cytoplasm and variably sized, thin- or thick-walled vascular channels in a myxoid stroma that is rich in collagen fibers and, like other richly myxoid tumors, often contains foci of hemorrhage (Figs 35–32 to 35–35). Although the cellularity is usually low and uniform throughout the tumor, some lesions have focal areas of increased cellularity, particularly around large vessels and at the periphery of the tumor.[108,114] The cells have small round to oval hyperchromatic nuclei with small centrally located nucleoli (Fig. 35–36). Mitotic figures are rare or absent and are not atypical. The stroma is characterized by prominent myxoid change with fine collagen fibrils, often with areas of erythrocyte extravasation. A characteristic feature is the presence of variably sized vessels that range from small thin-walled capillaries to large vessels with secondary changes including perivascular hyalinization and medial hypertrophy (Fig. 35–37). Mast cells are often prominent, and some tumors have perivascular lymphoid aggregates. Small bundles of spindle-shaped cells with eosinophilic cytoplasm may be present, frequently appearing to spin off from blood vessels.[114] These cells have more conventional features of smooth muscle cells, with cigar-shaped nuclei and perinuclear vacuoles. Occasional aggressive angiomyxomas have features overlapping those seen in angiomyofibroblastomas, including epithelioid cells arranged in cords around blood vessels and multinucleated cells, suggesting that these two lesions are on a morphologic spectrum.[116,117]

Immunohistochemical and ultrastructural findings

Immunohistochemically, the cells of aggressive angiomyxoma show diffuse staining for vimentin. Although earlier reports of this entity noted an absence of desmin staining,[111] most recent studies have shown fairly consis-

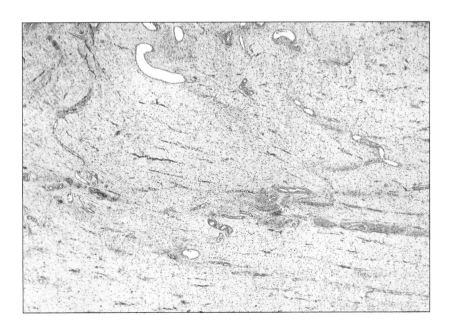

FIGURE 35–32 Aggressive angiomyxoma. The tumor is hypocellular and has prominent thin- and thick-walled vascular channels surrounded by a myxoid stroma.

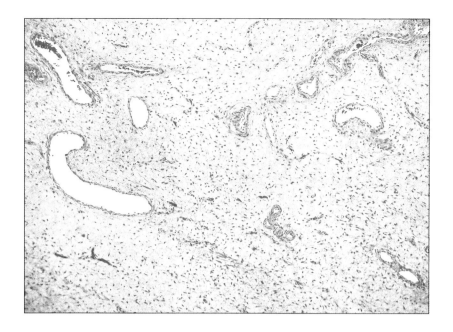

FIGURE 35–33 Aggressive angiomyxoma. Spindle-shaped cells are evenly distributed in a myxoid stroma. Prominent vessels are apparent.

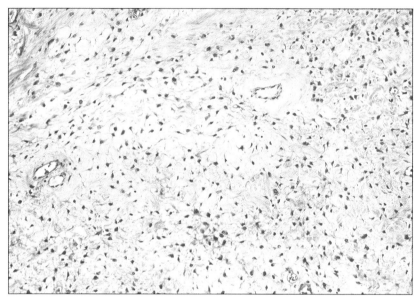

FIGURE 35–34 Aggressive angiomyxoma. Cytologically bland spindled and stellate-shaped cells are evenly distributed in a myxoid stroma.

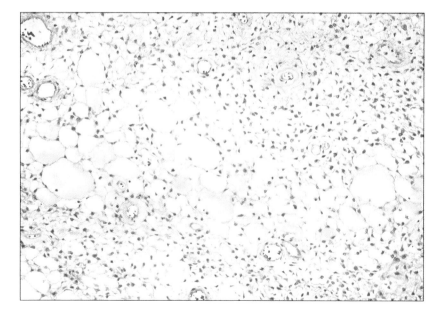

FIGURE 35–35 Microcystic change in an aggressive angiomyxoma.

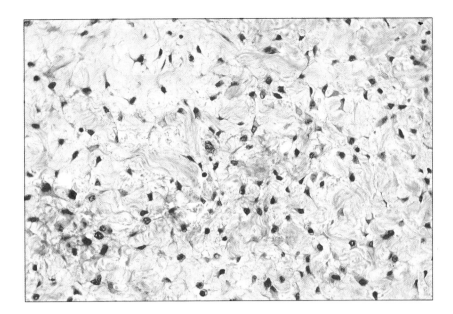

FIGURE 35–36 High-magnification view of bland spindled and stellate-shaped cells in an aggressive angiomyxoma.

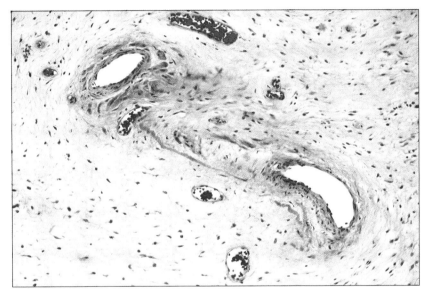

FIGURE 35–37 Characteristic thin- and thick-walled vascular channels in an aggressive angiomyxoma.

tent desmin immunoreactivity (Fig. 35–38; Table 35–5).[108,116] Immunostains for muscle-specific actin and smooth muscle actin are also positive in most cases, whereas S-100 protein and cytokeratins are not expressed by the neoplastic cells. A variable proportion of cells in some aggressive angiomyxomas also express CD34 and factor XIIIa.[118,119] The expression of both estrogen and progesterone receptors is a consistent finding in tumors from both genders, suggesting a hormonal role in the development or growth of these lesions.[120–122] Androgen receptors have been detected in tumors from males, but very few cases have been studied to determine if this is a consistent finding or if this is restricted to tumors in males.[109] As discussed in the section below, there may be some utility in staining for *HMGA2*, which is frequently overexpressed in this tumor.[123] Electron microscopic examination shows cells with fibroblastic, myofibroblastic, and smooth muscle differentiation.[124]

Cytogenetic findings

Relatively few examples of aggressive angiomyxoma have been studied cytogenetically. However, a consistent clonal aberration involving 12q13-15 has been identified.[125,126] Specifically, the *HMGA2* gene has been implicated. In one case report by Nucci and colleagues,[126] an aggressive angiomyxoma harbored a t(8;12) resulting in deregulation of *HMGA2*. Micci et al. reported a tumor with a t(11;12)(q23;q15) as the sole karyotypic aberration.[127]

Differential diagnosis

Aggressive angiomyxoma must be differentiated from other benign myxoid neoplasms given its propensity for local recurrence. *Angiomyofibroblastoma* is a neoplasm that arises in the subcutaneous tissues of the vulva, vagina, and rarely the scrotum. Most are small (less than 10 cm)

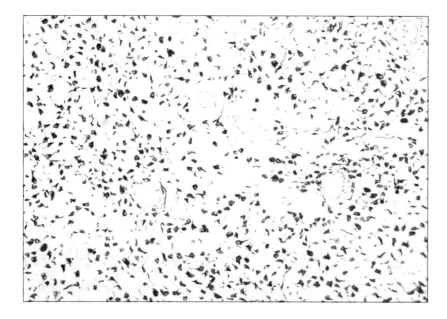

FIGURE 35–38 Diffuse desmin immunoreactivity in an aggressive angiomyxoma.

TABLE 35–5	IMMUNOHISTOCHEMICAL DATA IN SERIES OF AGGRESSIVE ANGIOMYXOMAS		
Marker	Fetsch et al.[108]	Granter et al.[114]	Total (%)
Desmin	22/22	13/14	35/36 (97)
Smooth muscle actin	19/20	10/11	29/31 (94)
Muscle-specific actin	16/19	11/12	27/31 (87)
CD34	8/16	–	8/16 (50)
Estrogen receptor	13/14	–	13/14 (93)
Progesterone receptor	9/10	–	9/10 (90)
S-100 protein	0/20	0/14	0/34 (0)

and well circumscribed; they are composed of plump epithelioid cells arranged in a striking perivascular distribution. Binucleated and multinucleated cells are commonly seen. The lesion rarely assumes a myxoid appearance, and there are typically numerous thin-walled vessels with perivascular hyalinization. As previously stated, aggressive angiomyxoma and angiomyofibroblastoma have overlapping histologic and immunohistochemical features. However, the distinction between these two entities is of clinical importance, as aggressive angiomyxoma has a much higher risk of recurrence than angiomyofibroblastoma, a lesion that is usually cured following simple excision (Table 35–6).

Aggressive angiomyxoma also shares histologic features with *intramuscular myxoma* and *juxta-articular myxoma*, but these tumors arise in different anatomic sites and are generally less cellular, less vascular, and have more abundant stromal mucin than the aggressive angiomyxoma.

Cutaneous myxoma (superficial angiomyxoma) is a relatively uncommon neoplasm that typically involves the dermis or subcutaneous tissue (or both) but it may arise in the vulvar or perineal region. This lesion is characteristically lobular or multinodular and is composed of a sparsely cellular proliferation of stellate and spindle-shaped cells deposited in an abundant myxoid matrix. Although this lesion has vascularity, it lacks the thick-walled large vessels of aggressive angiomyxoma, frequently has stromal neutrophils, and the neoplastic cells usually do not express desmin, estrogen, or progesterone receptors.

Myxoid neurofibroma may also closely resemble aggressive angiomyxoma but is composed of cells with wavy or buckled nuclei, occasionally with the formation of Wagner-Meissner bodies, and diffuse immunoreactivity for S1-00 protein. These lesions also lack the characteristic vascularity of aggressive angiomyxoma.

Myxoid leiomyoma, a tumor that may reach a large size and is frequently found in the pelvic region, differs from aggressive angiomyxoma by its less prominent vascular pattern and the presence of widely scattered smooth muscle cells in a myxoid matrix. The tumor cells are larger and have more abundant eosinophilic cytoplasm than those of aggressive angiomyxoma, and they tend to be arranged in small packets or loose fascicles.

Fibroepithelial stromal polyps of the vulvovaginal region have a wide spectrum of morphologic appearances and as such enter into the differential diagnosis. This lesion usually arises in young to middle-aged women, most commonly in the vagina. Histologically, fibroepithelial stromal polyps are polypoid with a central fibrovascular core. As part of this spectrum, this lesion can be hypocellular and myxoid. However, multinucleated stromal cells

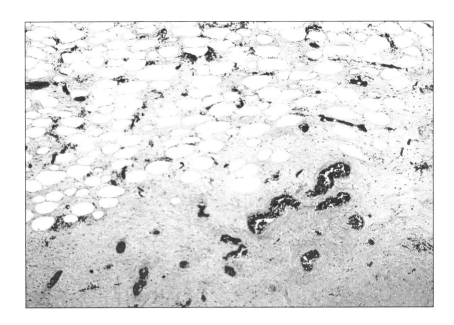

FIGURE 35–39 Infiltration of surrounding adipose tissue in an aggressive angiomyxoma. This pattern of infiltration likely accounts for the high rate of local recurrence of this tumor.

TABLE 35–6	DIFFERENTIAL DIAGNOSTIC FEATURES OF AGGRESSIVE ANGIOMYXOMA AND ANGIOMYOFIBROBLASTOMA	
Feature	**Aggressive angiomyxoma**	**Angiomyofibroblastoma**
Gross appearance	Poorly circumscribed, infiltrative	Circumscribed
Size	Large (many ≥10 cm)	Most ≤3 cm
Cellularity	Uniform	Perivascular hypercellularity
Cell shape	Spindled	Epithelioid
Vasculature	Variably sized, thick-walled	Numerous, thin-walled, often perivascular hyalinization
Multinucleation	Absent	Present
Recurrence	50%	Rare

are characteristic and are usually found near the epithelial–stromal interface. There is a great deal of immunophenotypic overlap with aggressive angiomyxoma since the stromal cells may express desmin, actin, estrogen, and progesterone receptors.

Like aggressive angiomyxoma, *pelvic fibromatosis* primarily affects women between the ages of 20 and 35 years and is an infiltrative process often entrapping surrounding soft tissue structures; it is composed of more elongated spindle-shaped cells separated by abundant collagen and arranged in sweeping fascicles. Some pelvic fibromatoses have striking myxoid change, but areas of more typical fibromatosis are invariably present. Although these lesions have a uniform distribution of small to medium-sized vessels, they lack the large-caliber thick-walled vessels characteristic of aggressive angiomyxoma.

Because aggressive angiomyxoma may become extremely large and has a tendency to infiltrate the surrounding soft tissues, a low-grade myxoid sarcoma is not infrequently considered. *Myxoid liposarcoma* arises only rarely in the pelvic region and can be distinguished by its characteristic fine plexiform vasculature and the identification of scattered lipoblasts. *Myxofibrosarcoma (low-grade myxoid malignant fibrous histiocytoma)* is distinguished from aggressive angiomyxoma by the presence of cells with more obvious cytologic atypia and hyperchromasia and its characteristic curvilinear vascular pattern.

Discussion

Aggressive angiomyxoma tends to locally recur, estimated in about 30% of patients (Fig. 35–39). Steeper and Rosai reported five cases with more than 12-months follow-up, four of which recurred locally, one as late as 14 years after local excision.[107] Begin et al. described six cases with follow-up data, all of which recurred within 9–84 months after excision.[111] A 36% rate of local recurrence was reported by both Fetsch et al.[108] and Granter et al.[114] More recent studies found a recurrence rate of less than 10% following aggressive surgical excision.[119,128] Neither size nor cellularity correlate with the risk of local recurrence. Because many of these tumors have infiltrative borders, complete excision is often difficult and likely accounts for the high rate of local recurrence.

More recently, some patients have been successfully treated with adjuvant hormonal therapy, including gonadotropic-releasing hormone agonists.[129–131] In 2003, an apparent histologically classic aggressive angiomyxoma that metastasized to the lung was reported.[132] Clearly, this event is exceedingly rare, and other metastasizing cases have not been documented. Although the line of differentiation has been debated since its initial description, most report features of fibroblastic, myofibroblastic, and/or smooth muscle differentiation by either immunohistochemistry or ultrastructural analysis. Tumors with composite features of aggressive angiomyxoma and angiomyofibroblastoma raise the possibility that these two lesions are related and possibly derived from a primitive mesenchymal cell (possibly a multipotential perivascular cell) normally found in the lower female genital tract that has the capability of differentiating along multiple lines. In our experience these two lesions are reasonably distinctive such that they can be reliably distinguished in virtually all cases.

AMYLOID TUMOR (AMYLOIDOMA)

Although systemic amyloid deposition is much more common, localized deposits of amyloid may result in a mass (amyloidoma), and such deposits have been reported in virtually every anatomic site. Amyloidomas may arise in association with immunocytic dyscrasias, including multiple myeloma and plasmacytoid lymphoma, but they may occur in patients on long-term hemodialysis, as well as those with chronic infectious or inflammatory diseases (tuberculosis, osteomyelitis, rheumatoid arthritis).[133] Some occur in patients with no clinical evidence of immunocytic dyscrasia or any other coexisting or preexisting disease; these lesions are rare and are found mainly in the soft tissues[134,135] or as solitary or multiple nodules in the respiratory,[136] urinary,[137,138] or gastrointestinal tracts.[139] There are also reports of localized amyloid tumors in the region of the head and neck,[140] breast,[141] heart,[142] liver,[143] bone,[144] nervous system,[145] and skin, where they are usually much smaller and occur as multiple macules or papules in the upper dermis.[146]

Grossly, amyloidomas consist of a lobulated nodule or mass with a white-yellow or pink-yellow waxy surface. Microscopic examination discloses amorphous faintly eosinophilic material that is PAS-positive and metachromatic with the crystal violet stain. The deposits are typically surrounded by histiocytes and multinucleated giant cells associated with a variable lymphoplasmacytic infiltrate. The plasma cells usually show no evidence of immaturity or cellular atypia (Figs 35–40, 35–41). In most cases the interspersed vessel walls are diffusely thickened by amyloid deposits. Rare lesions also show prominent areas of metaplastic bone or cartilage.[147] Elastic stains help distinguish the tumor from elastofibroma, and the absence of a fibroblastic proliferation distinguishes it from tumoral calcinosis. In addition, the deposited amyloid stains positively with the Congo red preparation, showing an "apple-green" birefringence under polarized light (Fig. 35–42). The Congo red affinity is abolished by prior treatment of the sections with potassium permanganate in most reactive or inflammatory forms of the disease characterized by amyloid A protein (AA).[148] The subtypes of amyloid can be further differentiated by immunohistochemical demonstration of the kappa and lambda light chains in AL amyloid, amyloid A protein in AA amyloid, and β_2-microglobulin in hemodialysis-associated amyloid.[149] Electron microscopy shows that the amyloid consists of fine, straight, nonbranching fibrils that measure 70–100 nm in diameter.

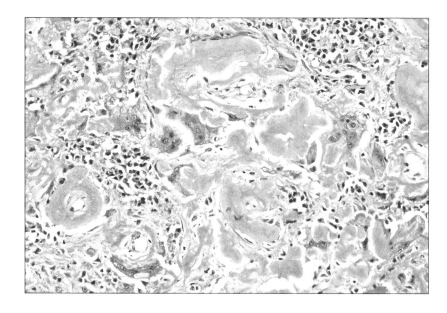

FIGURE 35–40 Amyloid tumor with amorphous deposits of amyloid associated with foreign body-type giant cells and plasma cells.

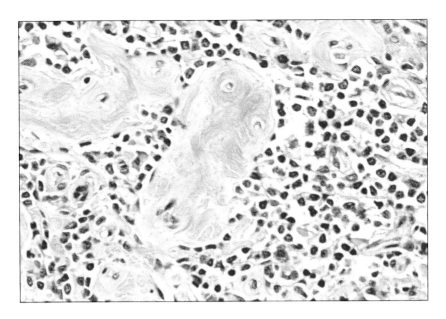

FIGURE 35–41 High magnification of amyloid tumor with prominent plasma cell infiltrates surrounding deposits of amyloid.

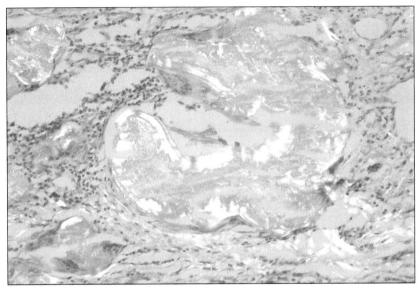

FIGURE 35–42 Apple-green birefringence under polarized light in an amyloid tumor.

Early reports often provided no information as to the type of amyloid comprising the tumor-like mass. More recent reports have described deposits of both the AA[150] and AL[144] types with few reports of β$_2$-microglobulin amyloid.[151] Laeng et al. detected monoclonal rearrangements of the heavy-chain immunoglobulin gene in amyloidomas of the nervous system, providing strong support for the concept that at least some of these lesions are composed of AL-producing B-cell clones capable of terminal differentiation.[145] Of the 14 soft tissue amyloidomas reported by Krishnan et al.,[150] 10 were associated with plasmacytoid lymphoma (nine cases) or myeloma (one case). In their review of the literature of amyloidoma of bone, Pambuccian et al. found all lesions to be composed of AL amyloid, with many patients progressing to generalized disease.[144]

REFERENCES

Tumoral calcinosis

1. Inclan A. Tumoral calcinosis. JAMA 1943; 121:490.
2. Duret MH. Tumeurs multiples et singulieres des bourses sereuses (endotheliomes peut etre d'origine parasitaire). Bull Mem Soc Anat (Paris) 1899; 74:725.
3. Teutschlaender O. Zur kenntnis der progressiven lipocalcinogranulomatose der muskulatur. Virchows Arch 1935; 295:424.
4. Stahnke M, Mangham DC, Davies AM. Calcific haemorrhagic bursitis anterior to the knee mimicking a soft tissue sarcoma: report of two cases. Skeletal Radiol 2004; 33:363.
5. Thomson JG. Calcifying collagenolysis (tumoural calcinosis). Br J Radiol 1966; 39:526.
6. Murthy DP. Tumoral calcinosis: a study of cases from Papua New Guinea. J Trop Med Hyg 1990; 93:403.
7. Kim HS, Suh JS, Kim YH, et al. Tumoral calcinosis of the hand: three unusual cases with painful swelling of small joints. Arch Pathol Lab Med 2006; 130:548.
8. Durant DM, Riley LH 3rd, Burger PC, et al. Tumoral calcinosis of the spine: a study of 21 cases. Spine 2001; 26:1673.

9. Dimitroulis G. Tumoral calcinosis of the articular disc of the temporomandibular joint: a rare entity. J Oral Maxillofac Surg 2004; 62:1551.

10. Inamadar AC, Palit A, Yelikar BR. Tumoral calcinosis with cutaneous involvement in an elderly man. Dermatology 2004; 209:246.

11. Pakasa NM, Kalengayi RM. Tumoral calcinosis: a clinicopathological study of 111 cases with emphasis on the earliest changes. Histopathology 1997; 31:18.

12. Jain SP. Tumoral calcinosis in Somalia and Ethiopia: a report of twenty-one cases and brief review of literature. East Afr Med J 1989; 66:476.

13. McKee PH, Liomba NG, Hutt MS. Tumoral calcinosis: a pathological study of fifty-six cases. Br J Dermatol 1982; 107:669.

14. Adams WM, Laitt RD, Davies M, et al. Familial tumoral calcinosis: association with cerebral and peripheral aneurysm formation. Neuroradiology 1999; 41:351.

15. Specktor P, Cooper JG, Indelman M, et al. Hyperphosphatemic familial tumoral calcinosis caused by a mutation in GALNT3 in a European kindred. J Hum Genet 2006; 51:487.

16. Campagnoli MF, Pucci A, Garelli E, et al. Familial tumoral calcinosis and testicular microlithiasis associated with a new mutation of GALNT3 in a white family. J Clin Pathol 2006; 59:440.

17. Chefetz I, Heller R, Galli-Tsinopoulou A, et al. A novel homozygous missense mutation in FGF23 causes familial tumoral calcinosis associated with disseminated visceral calcification. Hum Genet 2005; 118:261.

18. Larsson T, Davis SI, Garringer HJ, et al. Fibroblast growth factor-23 mutants causing familial tumoral calcinosis are differentially processed. Endocrinology 2005; 146:3883.

19. Cofan F, Garcia S, Combalia A, et al. Carpal tunnel syndrome secondary to uraemic tumoral calcinosis. Rheumatology (Oxford) 2002; 41:701.

20. Blay P, Fernandez-Martinez JM, Diaz-Lopez B. Vertebral involvement in hyperphosphatemic tumoral calcinosis. Bone 2001; 28:316.

21. de Beur SM. Tumoral calcinosis: a look into the metabolic mirror of phosphate homeostasis.[comment] J Clin Endocrinol Metab 2005; 90:2469.

22. Martinez S. Tumoral calcinosis: 12 years later. Semin Musculoskelet Radiol 2002; 6:331.

23. Slavin RE, Wen J, Kumar D, et al. Familial tumoral calcinosis. A clinical, histopathologic, and ultrastructural study with an analysis of its calcifying process and pathogenesis. Am J Surg Pathol 1993; 17:788.

24. Kindblom LG, Gunterberg B. Tumoral calcinosis. An ultrastructural analysis and consideration of pathogenesis. APMIS 1988; 96:368.

25. Arikawa J, Higaki Y, Mizushima J, et al. Tumoral calcinosis: a case report with an electron microscopic study. Eur J Dermatol 2000; 10:52.

26. Fujiyoshi A, Ng R, Bornemann M. Improved hypercalcemia after debulking of uremic tumoral calcinosis in a parathyroidectomized patient. Hawaii Med J 2005; 64:122.

27. Franco M, Albano L, Gaid H, et al. Resolution of tumoral calcinosis in a hemodialysis patient using low calcium dialysate. Joint Bone Spine 2005; 72:95.

28. Selby PL, Davies M, Marks JS, et al. Vitamin D intoxication causes hypercalcaemia by increased bone resorption which responds to pamidronate. Clin Endocrinol (Oxf) 1995; 43:531.

29. Sturdee SW, Bollen SR. Intra-articular calcification in primary hyperparathyroidism. Knee 2004; 11:323.

30. Randall RE Jr, Strauss MB, McNeely WF. The milk-alkali syndrome. Arch Intern Med 1961; 107:163.

30a. Laskin WB, Miettinen M, Fetsch JF. Calcarous lesions of the distal extremities resembling tumoral calcinosis (tumoral calcinosis like lesions): Clinicopathologic study of 43 cases emphasizing a pathogenesis-based approach to classification. Am J Surg Pathol 2007; 31:15.

31. Santili C, Akkari M, Waisberg G, et al. Calcinosis universalis: a rare diagnosis. J Pediatr Orthop 2005; 14:294.

32. Sehgal VN, Khandpur S, Sardana K, et al. Dystrophic calcinosis cutis circumscripta. J Eur Acad Dermatol Venereol 2003; 17:729.

33. Gollnick HP. Oral retinoids – efficacy and toxicity in psoriasis. Br J Dermatol 1996; 135(Suppl 49):6.

34. Hicheri J, Badri T, Fazaa B, et al. Scrotal calcinosis: pathogenesis and case report. Acta Dermatovenerol Alp Panonica Adriat 2005; 14:53.

35. Frishberg Y, Topaz O, Bergman R, et al. Identification of a recurrent mutation in GALNT3 demonstrates that hyperostosis-hyperphosphatemia syndrome and familial tumoral calcinosis are allelic disorders. J Mol Med 2005; 83:33.

36. Topaz O, Bergman R, Mandel U, et al. Absence of intraepidermal glycosyltransferase ppGalNac-T3 expression in familial tumoral calcinosis. Am J Dermatopathol 2005; 27:211.

37. Mockel G, Buttgereit F, Labs K, et al. Tumoral calcinosis revisited: pathophysiology and treatment. Rheumatol Int 2005; 25:55.

Intramuscular myxoma

38. Enzinger FM. Intramuscular myxoma: a review and follow-up study of 34 cases. Am J Clin Pathol 1965; 43:104.

39. Ireland DC, Soule EH, Ivins JC. Myxoma of somatic soft tissues. A report of 58 patients, 3 with multiple tumors and fibrous dysplasia of bone. Mayo Clin Proc 1973; 48:401.

40. Kindblom LG, Stener B, Angervall L. Intramuscular myxoma. Cancer 1974; 34:1737.

41. Allen PW. Myxoma is not a single entity: a review of the concept of myxoma. Ann Diagn Pathol 2000; 4:99.

42. Hashimoto H, Tsuneyoshi M, Daimaru Y, et al. Intramuscular myxoma. A clinicopathologic, immunohistochemical, and electron microscopic study. Cancer 1986; 58:740.

43. Miettinen M, Hockerstedt K, Reitamo J, et al. Intramuscular myxoma – a clinicopathological study of twenty-three cases. Am J Clin Pathol 1985; 84:265.

44. Silver WP, Harrelson JM, Scully SP. Intramuscular myxoma: a clinicopathologic study of 17 patients. Clin Orthop 2002; 403:191.

45. Ozawa H, Fujii M, Tomita T, et al. Intramuscular myxoma of scalene muscle: a case report. Auris Nasus Larynx 2004; 31:319.

46. Robin C, Bastidas JA, Boguslaw B. Case report: myxoma of the temporalis muscle. Oral Surg Oral Med Oral Pathol Oral Radiol Endod 2004; 97:620.

47. Ly JQ, Bau JL, Beall DP. Forearm intramuscular myxoma. AJR Am J Roentgenol 2003; 181:960.

48. Al-Qattan MM, El-Shayeb A, Rasool MN. An intramuscular myxoma of the hand. Hand Surg 2004; 9:97.

49. Luna A, Martinez S, Bossen E. Magnetic resonance imaging of intramuscular myxoma with histological comparison and a review of the literature. Skeletal Radiol 2005; 34:19.

50. Bancroft LW, Kransdorf MJ, Menke DM, et al. Intramuscular myxoma: characteristic MR imaging features. AJR Am J Roentgenol 2002; 178:1255.

51. Kabukcuoglu F, Kabukcuoglu Y, Yilmaz B, et al. Mazabraud's syndrome: intramuscular myxoma associated with fibrous dysplasia. Pathol Oncol Res 2004; 10:121.

52. Iwasko N, Steinbach LS, Disler D, et al. Imaging findings in Mazabraud's syndrome: seven new cases. Skeletal Radiol 2002; 31:81.

53. Pettersson H, Hudson TM, Springfield DS, et al. Cystic intramuscular myxoma: report of a case. Acta Radiol Diagn (Stockh) 1985; 26:425.

54. Mazabraud A, Semat P, Roze R. A propos de l'association de fibromyxomes des tissus mous a la dysplasie fibreuse des os. Presse Med 1967; 75:2223.

55. Lietman SA, Ding C, Levine MA. A highly sensitive polymerase chain reaction method detects activating mutations of the GNAS gene in peripheral blood cells in McCune-Albright syndrome or isolated fibrous dysplasia. J Bone Joint Surg [Am] 2005; 87:2489.

56. Lumbroso S, Paris F, Sultan C, et al. Activating Gs alpha mutations: analysis of 113 patients with signs of McCune-Albright syndrome – a European collaborative study. J Clin Endocrinol Metab 2004; 89:2107.

57. Okamoto S, Hisaoka M, Ushijima M, et al. Activating Gs (alpha) mutation in intramuscular myxomas with and without fibrous dysplasia of bone. Virchows Arch 2000; 437:133.

58. Okamoto S, Hisaoka M, Meis-Kindblom JM, et al. Juxta-articular myxoma and intramuscular myxoma are two distinct entities. Activating Gs alpha mutation at Arg 201 codon does not occur in juxta-articular myxoma. Virchows Arch 2002; 440:12.

59. Nishimoto K, Kusuzaki K, Matsumine A, et al. Surrounding muscle edema detected by MRI is valuable for diagnosis of intramuscular myxoma. Oncol Rep 2004; 11:143.

60. Nielsen GP, O'Connell JX, Rosenberg AE. Intramuscular myxoma: a clinicopathologic study of 51 cases with emphasis on hypercellular and hypervascular variants. Am J Surg Pathol 1998; 22:1222.

61. Catroppo JF, Olesnicky L, Ringer P, et al. Intramuscular low-grade myxoid neoplasm with recurrent potential (cellular myxoma) of the lower extremity: case report with cytohistologic correlation and review of the literature. Diagn Cytopathol 2002; 26:301.

62. van Roggen JF, McMenamin ME, Fletcher CD. Cellular myxoma of soft tissue: a clinicopathological study of 38 cases confirming indolent clinical behaviour. Histopathology 2001; 39:287.

Juxta-articular myxoma

63. Echols PG, Omer GE Jr, Crawford MK. Juxta-articular myxoma of the shoulder presenting as a cyst of the acromioclavicular joint: a case report. J Shoulder Elbow Surg 2000; 9:157.

64. Minkoff J, Stecker S, Irizarry J, et al. Juxta-articular myxoma: a rare cause of painful restricted motion of the knee. Arthroscopy 2003; 19:E6.

65. Meis JM, Enzinger FM. Juxta-articular myxoma: a clinical and pathologic study of 65 cases. Hum Pathol 1992; 23:639.

66. King DG, Saifuddin A, Preston HV, et al. Magnetic resonance imaging of juxta-articular myxoma. Skeletal Radiol 1995; 24:145.

67. Sciot R, Dal Cin P, Samson I, et al. Clonal chromosomal changes in juxta-articular myxoma. Virchows Arch 1999; 434:177.

Myxoma of the jaw

68. Barker BF. Odontogenic myxoma. Semin Diagn Pathol 1999; 16:297.

69. Regezi JA. Odontogenic cysts, odontogenic tumors, fibroosseous, and giant cell lesions of the jaws. Mod Pathol 2002; 15:331.

70. Simon EN, Merkx MA, Vuhahula E, et al. Odontogenic myxoma: a clinicopathological study of 33 cases. Int J Oral Maxillofac Surg 2004; 33:333.

71. Tamme T, Soots M, Kulla A, et al. Odontogenic tumours, a collaborative retrospective study of 75 cases covering more than 25 years from Estonia. J Craniomaxillofac Surg 2004; 32:161.

72. Wachter BG, Steinberg MJ, Darrow DH, et al. Odontogenic myxoma of the maxilla: a report of two pediatric cases. Int J Pediatr Otorhinolaryngol 2003; 67:389.

73. Fenton S, Slootweg PJ, Dunnebier EA, et al. Odontogenic myxoma in a 17-month-old child: a case report. J Oral Maxillofac Surg 2003; 61:734.

74. MacDonald-Jankowski DS, Yeung RW, Li T, et al. Computed tomography of odontogenic myxoma. Clin Radiol 2004; 59:281.

75. Kimura A, Hasegawa H, Satou K, et al. Odontogenic myxoma showing active epithelial islands with microcystic features. J Oral Maxillofac Surg 2001; 59:1226.

76. Hisatomi M, Asaumi J, Konouchi H, et al. Comparison of radiographic and MRI features of a root-diverging odontogenic myxoma, with discussion of the differential diagnosis of lesions likely to move roots. Oral Dis 2003; 9:152.

77. Lombardi T, Kuffer R, Bernard JP, et al. Immunohistochemical staining for vimentin filaments and S-100 protein in myxoma of the jaws. J Oral Pathol 1988; 17:175.

78. Lombardi T, Lock C, Samson J, et al. S100, alpha-smooth muscle actin and cytokeratin 19 immunohistochemistry in odontogenic and soft tissue myxomas. J Clin Pathol 1995; 48:759.

Cutaneous myxoma

79. Carney JA, Gordon H, Carpenter PC, et al. The complex of myxomas, spotty pigmentation, and endocrine overactivity. Medicine (Baltimore) 1985; 64:270.

80. Carney JA, Headington JT, Su WP. Cutaneous myxomas. A major component of the complex of myxomas, spotty pigmentation, and endocrine overactivity. Arch Dermatol 1986; 122:790.

81. Allen PW, Dymock RB, MacCormac LB. Superficial angiomyxomas with and without epithelial components. Report of 30 tumors in 28 patients. Am J Surg Pathol 1988; 12:519.

82. Calonje E, Guerin D, McCormick D, et al. Superficial angiomyxoma: clinicopathologic analysis of a series of distinctive but poorly recognized cutaneous tumors with tendency for recurrence. Am J Surg Pathol 1999; 23:910.

83. Bedlow AJ, Sampson SA, Holden CA. Congenital superficial angiomyxoma. Clin Exp Dermatol 1997; 22:237.

84. Fetsch JF, Laskin WB, Tavassoli FA. Superficial angiomyxoma (cutaneous myxoma): a clinicopathologic study of 17 cases arising in the genital region. Int J Gynecol Pathol 1997; 16:325.

85. Ferreiro JA, Carney JA. Myxomas of the external ear and their significance. Am J Surg Pathol 1994; 18:274.

86. Fetsch JF, Laskin WB, Miettinen M. Superficial acral fibromyxoma: a clinicopathologic and immunohistochemical analysis of 37 cases of a distinctive soft tissue tumor with a predilection for the fingers and toes. Hum Pathol 2001; 32:704.

Carney complex

87. Carney JA, Hruska LS, Beauchamp GD, et al. Dominant inheritance of the complex of myxomas, spotty pigmentation, and endocrine overactivity. Mayo Clin Proc 1986; 61:165.

88. Wilkes D, Charitakis K, Basson CT. Inherited disposition to cardiac myxoma development. Nat Rev Cancer 2006; 6:157.

89. Wilkes D, McDermott DA, Basson CT. Clinical phenotypes and molecular genetic mechanisms of Carney complex. Lancet Oncol 2005; 6:501.

90. Veugelers M, Wilkes D, Burton K, et al. Comparative PRKAR1A genotype-phenotype analyses in humans with Carney complex and prkar1a haploinsufficient mice. Proc Natl Acad Sci USA 2004; 101:14222.

91. Carney JA, Toorkey BC. Myxoid fibroadenoma and allied conditions (myxomatosis) of the breast. A heritable disorder with special associations including cardiac and cutaneous myxomas. Am J Surg Pathol 1991; 15:713.

92. Amano J, Kono T, Wada Y, et al. Cardiac myxoma: its origin and tumor characteristics. Ann Thorac Cardiovasc Surg 2003; 9:215.

93. Chrousos GP, Stratakis CA. Carney complex and the familial lentiginosis syndromes: link to inherited neoplasias and developmental disorders, and genetic loci. J Intern Med 1998; 243:573.

94. Carney JA. Carney complex: the complex of myxomas, spotty pigmentation, endocrine overactivity, and schwannomas. Semin Dermatol 1995; 14:90.

95. Carney JA, Ferreiro JA. The epithelioid blue nevus. A multicentric familial tumor with important associations, including cardiac myxoma and psammomatous melanotic schwannoma. Am J Surg Pathol 1996; 20:259.

96. Carney JA, Stratakis CA. Epithelioid blue nevus and psammomatous melanotic schwannoma: the unusual pigmented skin tumors of the Carney complex. Semin Diagn Pathol 1998; 15:216.

97. Groussin L, Horvath A, Jullian E, et al. A PRKAR1A mutation associated with primary pigmented nodular adrenocortical disease in 12 kindreds. J Clin Endocrinol Metab 2006; 91:1943.

98. Groussin L, Cazabat L, Rene-Corail F, et al. Adrenal pathophysiology: lessons from the Carney complex. Horm Res 2005; 64:132.

99. Daly AF, Jaffrain-Rea ML, Beckers A. Clinical and genetic features of familial pituitary adenomas. Horm Metab Res 2005; 37:347.

100. Jayasena SN, Ariyasinghe JT, Gunawardena DM, et al. Large-cell calcifying Sertoli cell tumour of the testis detected at screening of a family with Carney syndrome. Urol Int 2005; 75:365.

101. Stratakis CA, Kirschner LS, Carney JA. Clinical and molecular features of the Carney complex: diagnostic criteria and recommendations for patient evaluation. J Clin Endocrinol Metab 2001; 86:4041.

Ganglion (ganglion cyst)

102. Nahra ME, Bucchieri JS. Ganglion cysts and other tumor related conditions of the hand and wrist. Hand Clin 2004; 20:249.

103. Soren A. Pathogenesis, clinic, and treatment of ganglion. Arch Orthop Trauma Surg 1982; 99:247.

104. McAllister DR, Koh J, Bergfeld JA. Plantar ganglion cyst associated with stress fracture of the third metatarsal. Am J Orthop 2003; 32:35.

105. Tuzuner T. Penetrating type intraosseous ganglion cyst of the lunate bone. West Indian Med J 2005; 54:247.

106. Baldauf J, Junghans D, Schroeder HW. Endoscope-assisted microsurgical resection of an intraneural ganglion cyst of the hypoglossal nerve. J Neurosurg 2005; 103:920.

Aggressive angiomyxoma

107. Steeper TA, Rosai J. Aggressive angiomyxoma of the female pelvis and perineum. Report of nine cases of a distinctive type of gynecologic soft-tissue neoplasm. Am J Surg Pathol 1983; 7:463.

108. Fetsch JF, Laskin WB, Lefkowitz M, et al. Aggressive angiomyxoma: a clinicopathologic study of 29 female patients. Cancer 1996; 78:79.

109. Chihara Y, Fujimoto K, Takada S, et al. Aggressive angiomyxoma in the scrotum expressing androgen and progesterone receptors. Int J Urol 2003; 10:672.

110. Carlinfante G, De Marco L, Mori M, et al. Aggressive angiomyxoma of the spermatic cord. Two unusual cases occurring in childhood. Pathol Res Pract 2001; 197:139.

111. Begin LR, Clement PB, Kirk ME, et al. Aggressive angiomyxoma of pelvic soft parts: a clinicopathologic study of nine cases. Hum Pathol 1985; 16:621.

112. Iezzoni JC, Fechner RE, Wong LS, et al. Aggressive angiomyxoma in males. A report of four cases. Am J Clin Pathol 1995; 104:391.

113. Tsang WY, Chan JK, Lee KC, et al. Aggressive angiomyxoma. A report of four cases occurring in men. Am J Surg Pathol 1992; 16:1059.

114. Granter SR, Nucci MR, Fletcher CD. Aggressive angiomyxoma: reappraisal of its relationship to angiomyofibroblastoma in a series of 16 cases. Histopathology 1997; 30:3.

115. Jeyadevan NN, Sohaib SA, Thomas JM, et al. Imaging features of aggressive angiomyxoma. Clin Radiol 2003; 58:157.

116. Belge G, Caselitz J, Bonk U, et al. Genetic studies of differential fatty tissue diagnosis. Pathologe 1997; 18:160.

117. Zamecnik M, Michal M. Comparison of angiomyofibroblastoma and aggressive angiomyxoma in both sexes: four cases composed of bimodal CD34 and factor XIIIa positive dendritic cell subsets. Pathol Res Pract 1998; 194:736.

118. Silverman JS, Albukerk J, Tamsen A. Comparison of angiomyofibroblastoma and aggressive angiomyxoma in both sexes: four cases composed of bimodal CD34 and factor XIIIa positive dendritic cell subsets. Pathol Res Pract 1997; 193:673.

119. van Roggen JF, van Unnik JA, Briaire-de Bruijn IH, et al. Aggressive angiomyxoma: a clinicopathological and immunohistochemical study of 11 cases with long-term follow-up. Virchows Arch 2005; 446:157.

120. Abu JI, Bamford WM, Malin G, et al. Aggressive angiomyxoma of the perineum. Int J Gynecol Cancer 2005; 15:1097.

121. McCluggage WG, Patterson A, Maxwell P. Aggressive angiomyxoma of pelvic parts exhibits oestrogen and progesterone receptor positivity. J Clin Pathol 2000; 53:603.

122. McCluggage WG. Recent advances in immunohistochemistry in gynaecological pathology. Histopathology 2002; 40:309.

123. Nucci MR, Fletcher CD. Vulvovaginal soft tissue tumours: update and review. Histopathology 2000; 36:97.

124. Skalova A, Michal M, Husek K, et al. Aggressive angiomyxoma of the pelvioperineal region. Immunohistological and ultrastructural study of seven cases. Am J Dermatopathol 1993; 15:446.

125. Kazmierczak B, Dal Cin P, Wanschura S, et al. Cloning and molecular characterization of part of a new gene fused to HMGIC in mesenchymal tumors. Am J Pathol 1998; 152:431.

126. Nucci MR, Weremowicz S, Neskey DM, et al. Chromosomal translocation t(8;12) induces aberrant HMGIC expression in aggressive angiomyxoma of the vulva. Genes Chromosomes Cancer 2001; 32:172.

127. Micci F, Panagopoulos I, Bjerkehagen B, et al. Deregulation of HMGA2 in an aggressive angiomyxoma with t(11;12)(q23;q15). Virchows Arch 2006; 448:838.

128. Amezcua CA, Begley SJ, Mata N, et al. Aggressive angiomyxoma of the female genital tract: a clinicopathologic and immunohistochemical study of 12 cases. Int J Gynecol Cancer 2005; 15:140.

129. Shinohara N, Nonomura K, Ishikawa S, et al. Medical management of recurrent aggressive angiomyxoma with gonadotropin-releasing hormone agonist. Int J Urol 2004; 11:432.

130. Poirier M, Fraser R, Meterissian S. Case 1. Aggressive angiomyxoma of the pelvis: response to luteinizing hormone-releasing hormone agonist. J Clin Oncol 2003; 21:3535.

131. McCluggage WG, Jamieson T, Dobbs SP, et al. Aggressive angiomyxoma of the vulva: dramatic response to gonadotropin-releasing hormone agonist therapy. Gynecol Oncol 2006; 100:623.

132. Blandamura S, Cruz J, Faure Vergara L, et al. Aggressive angiomyxoma: a second case of metastasis with patient's death. Hum Pathol 2003; 34:1072.

Amyloid tumor (amyloidoma)

133. Glenner GG. Amyloid deposits and amyloidosis. The beta-fibrilloses (first of two parts). N Engl J Med 1980; 302:1283.

134. Romagnoli S, Braidotti P, Di Nuovo F, et al. Amyloid tumour (amyloidoma) of the leg: histology, immunohistochemistry and electron microscopy. Histopathology 1999; 35:188.

135. Sidoni A, Alberti PF, Bravi Sea. Amyloid tumours in the soft tissues of the legs: case report and review of the literature. Virchows Arch 1998; 432:563.

136. Ihling C, Weirich G, Gaa A, et al. Amyloid tumors of the lung: an immunocytoma? Pathol Res Pract 1996; 192:446.

137. Hamidi AK, Liepnieks JJ, Bihrle R, et al. Local synthesis of amyloid fibril precursor in AL amyloidosis of the urinary tract. Amyloid 1998; 5:49.

138. Khan SM, Birch PJ, Bass PS, et al. Localized amyloidosis of the lower genitourinary tract: a clinicopathologic and immunohistochemical study of nine cases. Histopathology 1992; 21:143.

139. Hemmer PR, Topazian MD, Gertz MA, et al. Globular amyloid deposits isolated to the small bowel: A rare associated with AL amyloidosis. Am J Surg Pathol 2007; 31:141.

140. Thompson LDR, Derringer GA, Wenig BM. Amyloidosis of the larynx: a clinicopathologic study of 11 cases. Mod Pathol 2000; 13:528.

141. Luo JH, Rotterdam H. Primary amyloid tumor of the breast: a case report and review of the literature. Mod Pathol 1997; 10:735.

142. Warner KJ, Blackwell GG, Herrera GA, et al. Cardiac amyloidoma with IgM-kappa gammopathy. Arch Pathol Lab Med 1994; 118:1148.

143. Yamamoto T, Maeda N, Kawasaki H. Hepatic failure in a case of multiple myeloma-associated amyloidosis (kappa-AL). J Gastroenterol 1995; 30:393.

144. Pambuccian SE, Horyd ID, Cawte T, et al. Amyloidoma of bone: a plasma cell/plasmacytoid neoplasm; report of three cases

and review of the literature. Am J Surg Pathol 1997; 21:179.

145. Laeng RH, Aftermatt HJ, Scheithauer BW, et al. Amyloidomas of the nervous system: a monoclonal B-cell disorder with monotypic amyloid light chain gamma amyloid production. Cancer 1998; 82:362.

146. Kibbi AG, Rubeiz NG, Zaynon ST, et al. Primary localized cutaneous amyloidosis. Int J Dermatol 1992; 31:95.

147. Yokoo H, Nakazato Y. Primary localized amyloid tumor of the breast with osseous metaplasia. Pathol Int 1998; 48:545.

148. Weiss SW. Tumoral amyloidosis of soft tissue (amyloidoma): new approaches to an old problem. Am J Clin Pathol 1993; 100:91.

149. Feiner HD. Pathology of dysproteinemia: light chain amyloidosis, non-amyloid immunoglobulin deposition disease, cryoglobulinemia syndromes, and macroglobulinemia of Waldenstriauom. Hum Pathol 1988; 19:1255.

150. Krishnan J, Chu WS, Elrod JP, et al. Tumoral presentation of amyloidosis (amyloidomas) in soft tissue: a report of 14 cases. Am J Clin Pathol 1993; 100:135.

151. Tomm Y, Htew M, Chandra R, et al. Bilateral beta 2-micro globulin amyloidomas of the buttocks in a long-term hemodialysis patient. Arch Pathol Lab Med 1994; 118:651.

SOFT TISSUE TUMORS OF INTERMEDIATE MALIGNANCY OF UNCERTAIN TYPE

CHAPTER CONTENTS

In previous editions of this textbook, several entities of uncertain type were placed into either benign or malignant categories. Although these entities still remain an enigma with regard to line of cellular differentiation, larger clinicopathologic studies of each of these entities have revealed a better understanding of their clinical behavior. While some of these entities were initially placed into the benign category (e.g., ossifying fibromyxoid tumor and pleomorphic hyalinizing angiectatic tumor of soft parts), it is clear these lesions have a significant risk for local recurrence and can even metastasize on occasion. Similarly, other entities of uncertain type were originally categorized among the malignant tumors (inflammatory myxohyaline tumor/acral myxoinflammatory fibroblastic sarcoma) but, given the lower risk for metastasis, especially with adequate therapy, behave less aggressively than the other lesions in this category. As such, we believe there is ample justification to categorize these tumors into those of intermediate malignancy, albeit of uncertain lineage.

OSSIFYING FIBROMYXOID TUMOR OF SOFT TISSUE

The ossifying fibromyxoid tumor of soft tissue, first described in a series of 59 cases from the Armed Forces Institute of Pathology (AFIP) in 1989,[1] is a rare tumor of uncertain differentiation which most commonly arises in the extremities. Close to 150 cases have been reported in the literature, mostly in the form of case reports or small series. Although the original description of this tumor by Enzinger and colleagues emphasized the bland morphologic appearance and typically benign clinical behavior, even in this series there was an indication that exceptional examples act in a clinically aggressive fashion. Several subsequent reports described tumors with typical features that unexpectedly metastasized, or tumors which had atypical or overtly malignant histologic features, some of which behaved aggressively.[2-5] As such, it seems reasonable to consider ossifying fibromyxoid tumor a neoplasm of uncertain differentiation that usually (but not always) acts in a clinically benign fashion.

Clinical findings

Ossifying fibromyxoid tumor almost exclusively affects adults (mean age near 50 years), with only rare examples documented in children.[6,7] Men are affected more commonly than women. Most patients present with a small, painless, well-defined, often lobulated subcutaneous mass which involves the extremities in approximately 70% of cases (Table 36-1). Less commonly involved sites include the trunk, head and neck, mediastinum, and retroperitoneum.[8-12] Radiographic studies usually reveal a well-circumscribed mass with an incomplete ring of peripheral calcification and scattered calcifications in the substance of the neoplasm (Fig. 36-1).[13] Erosion of underlying bone and periosteal reaction is rarely seen.[1]

TABLE 36–1	ANATOMIC LOCATION OF 59 CASES OF OSSIFYING FIBROMYXOID TUMOR	
Site		**No. of cases**
Upper extremity		20 (34%)
Shoulder/upper arm		10
Elbow/forearm		4
Hands/fingers		6
Lower extremity		20 (34%)
Buttock/thigh		11
Knee/lower leg		4
Foot		5
Trunk		11 (19%)
Chest wall		9
Abdomen		1
Flank		1
Head and neck		8 (13%)
Total		59 (100%)

Modified from Enzinger FM, Weiss SW, Liang CY. Ossifying fibromyxoid tumor of soft parts: a clinicopathological analysis of 59 cases. Am J Surg Pathol 1989; 13:817.

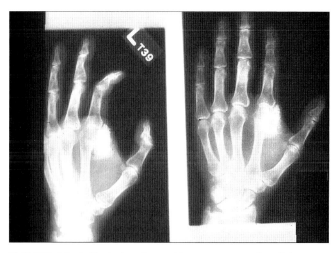

FIGURE 36–1 Typical radiographic appearance of ossifying fibromyxoid tumor of soft tissue. The tumor is well circumscribed and has extensive calcification.

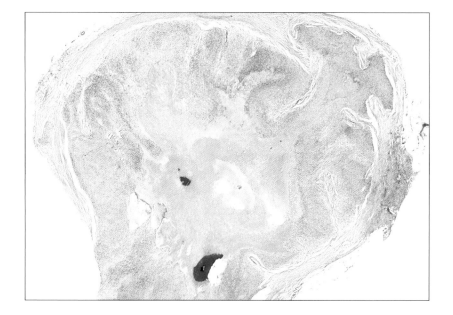

FIGURE 36–2 Ossifying fibromyxoid tumor of soft tissue. A pseudocapsule almost completely surrounds the neoplasm.

Pathologic findings

Grossly, ossifying fibromyxoid tumor is usually well circumscribed, spherical, and lobulated or multinodular, typically covered by a thick fibrous pseudocapsule (Fig. 36–2). Most measure 3–5 cm, but occasional lesions are 15 cm or larger. On cut section, the tumor is tan-white and often has a gritty texture, as one would expect in a tumor that frequently has calcifications.

Microscopically, the majority are located in the subcutaneous tissue, but some are attached to tendons, fascia, or involve the underlying skeletal muscle. A typical ossifying fibromyxoid tumor is composed of uniform round, ovoid, or spindle-shaped cells arranged in nests and cords and deposited in a variably myxoid and collagenous stroma (Figs 36–3 to 36–7). In approximately 80% of cases, there is an incomplete shell of lamellar bone found at the periphery of the nodules, either within or immediately beneath a dense fibrous pseudocapsule and sometimes extending into the substance of the tumor (Fig. 36–8). Despite extensive sampling, up to 20% of cases are nonossifying.[14,15]

The constituent cells, which vary little in size and shape, are characterized by pale-staining vesicular nuclei with minute nucleoli and small amounts of eosinophilic cytoplasm (Fig. 36–9). The cells may be deposited in a variety of patterns, including cords, nests, or sheets; or they may be randomly distributed in a fibromyxoid matrix. Some lesions are predominantly myxoid with an abundant stroma of Alcian blue-positive, hyaluronidase-

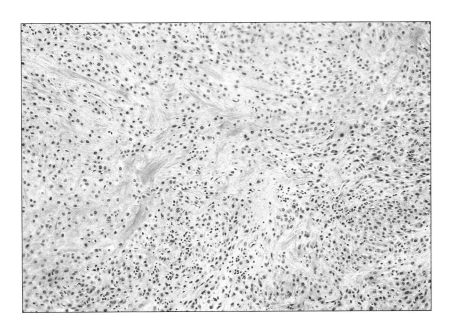

FIGURE 36–3 Low-magnification appearance of an ossifying fibromyxoid tumor. The cells are arranged in a variety of patterns and deposited in a variably hyalinized and myxoid matrix.

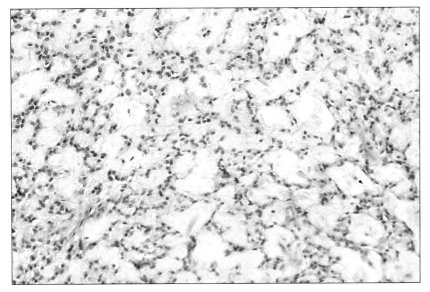

FIGURE 36–4 Ossifying fibromyxoid tumor. Cords of small tumor cells are suspended in a myxoid matrix.

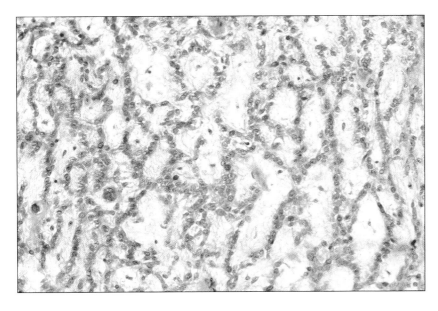

FIGURE 36–5 Thin cords of epithelioid tumor cells in an ossifying fibromyxoid tumor.

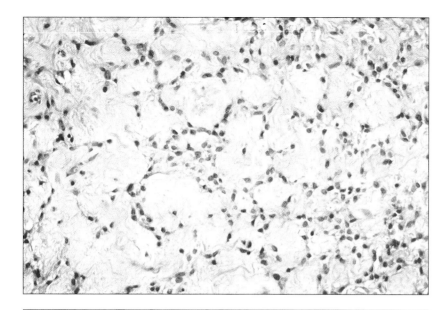

FIGURE 36–6 Less-cellular zone in an ossifying fibromyxoid tumor.

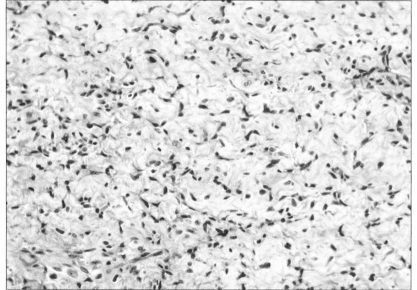

FIGURE 36–7 Fibrous zone in an ossifying fibromyxoid tumor, with compression of cords of tumor cells.

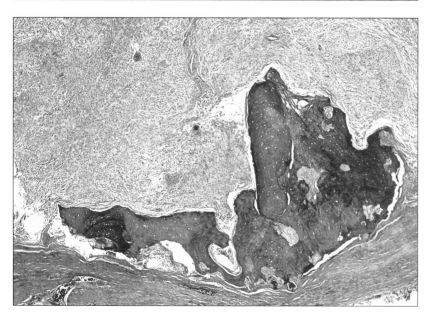

FIGURE 36–8 Ossifying fibromyxoid tumor with an incomplete rim of lamellar bone.

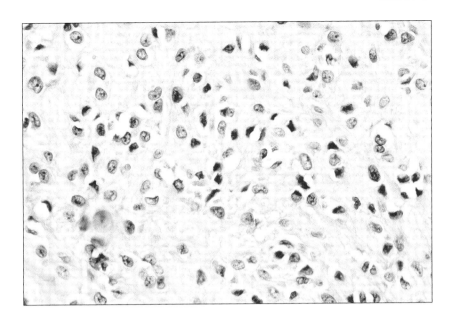

FIGURE 36–9 High-magnification view of bland epithelioid cells with vacuolated or eosinophilic cytoplasm in an ossifying fibromyxoid tumor.

sensitive acid mucopolysaccharides, occasionally forming microcysts.[4,15] Other tumors are predominantly collagenous, sometimes with a gradual transition between densely hyalinized collagen and osteoid. Such areas may be composed of epithelioid cells and resemble sclerosing epithelioid fibrosarcoma. Small foci of calcification and metaplastic cartilage may also be seen in the tumor nodules. Most have a rich vasculature, with many vessels exhibiting perivascular hyalinization and others subintimal fibrin deposition or thrombosis.

As thoroughly described by Folpe and Weiss[15] and others,[2] rare ossifying fibromyxoid tumors have atypical or overtly malignant features, usually consisting of some combination of high nuclear grade, high cellularity, or increased mitotic activity (>2 mitotic figures [MF]/50 high-power fields [HPF]). Most tumors with these features have areas of typical ossifying fibromyxoid tumor, but rarely the tumor is composed exclusively of such areas (Figs 36–10, 36–11). The significance of these areas will be discussed in detail below.

Immunohistochemical and ultrastructural findings

Immunohistochemically, the cells are positive for vimentin and express S-100 protein in about 70% of cases (Fig. 36–12), but immunoreactivity for the latter tends to be less intense than in schwannoma.[16,17] Atypical or malignant areas seem to express S-100 protein less often than typical areas.[15] The cells may also express Leu-7, neuron-specific enolase, and glial fibrillary acidic protein (GFAP). Up to 20% of cases stain focally for desmin; rare examples show scattered cells that stain for smooth muscle actin or cytokeratins.[15]

In their original series, Enzinger et al. noted ultrastructural features suggesting both cartilaginous and schwannian differentiation.[1] The cells have irregular cell borders with short processes and intracellular microfilaments. In addition, well-developed and occasionally reduplicated external lamina may be present (Fig. 36–13).[1,18] However, ossifying fibromyxoid tumor lacks certain characteristic ultrastructural features of both cartilaginous and Schwann cell tumors. Other features which have been noted include ribosome-lamellar complexes;[15] more recently, Min et al. suggested the cells have the ultrastructural features of myoepithelial cells.[19]

Cytogenetic findings

Very few cases of ossifying fibromyxoid tumor have been studied by cytogenetics. Nishio et al. reported a histologically and clinically malignant tumor that showed a complex karyotype demonstrating t(3;11)(p21;p15), t(5;13)(q13;q34), and deletions of 12q13, 9p22, and 8p21, among others.[20] Sovani and co-workers reported an ossifying fibromyxoid tumor with loss of chromosome 6, extra material of unknown origin attached to the long arm of chromosome 12, and an unbalanced translocation involving chromosomes 6 and 14.[21] Lastly, one of the cases reported by Folpe and Weiss showed a complex karyotype including a t(11;19)(q11;q13) and abnormalities of chromosomes 1 and 3.[15]

Differential diagnosis

The differential diagnosis includes benign and malignant epithelioid nerve sheath tumors (epithelioid neurofibroma, epithelioid schwannoma, epithelioid malignant peripheral nerve sheath tumor), chondroid syringoma (cutaneous mixed tumor), myxoid chondrosarcoma, and epithelioid smooth muscle tumors.

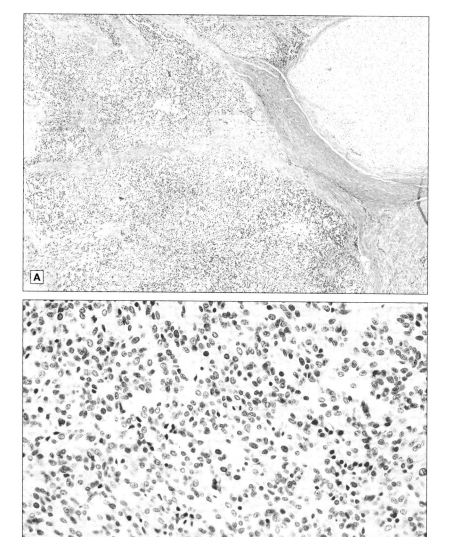

FIGURE 36–10 (A) Low-magnification view of a malignant ossifying fibromyxoid tumor showing the characteristic multilobular appearance. Some of the lobules are strikingly cellular. **(B)** High-magnification view of a cellular focus in a malignant ossifying fibromyxoid tumor.

The ossifying fibromyxoid tumor has many features in common with *nerve sheath tumors*. However, ossifying fibromyxoid tumor has not been documented to arise from a peripheral nerve, and the architectural and cytologic features are not typical of either epithelioid neurofibroma or epithelioid schwannoma. The cells lack the cytologic atypia characteristic of epithelioid malignant peripheral nerve sheath tumors.

The absence of epithelial markers in the ossifying fibromyxoid tumor helps exclude *chondroid syringoma* as a diagnostic consideration. The lobulated architecture and arrangement of the neoplastic cells into cord-like structures bears some resemblance to *myxoid chondrosarcoma*, but the stroma of ossifying fibromyxoid tumor varies between myxoid and collagenous, and the neoplastic cells have less eosinophilic cytoplasm than those of myxoid chondrosarcoma. Histochemically, periodic acid-Schiff (PAS) staining usually reveals abundant intra-cytoplasmic glycogen in the cells of myxoid chondrosarcoma, a feature lacking in ossifying fibromyxoid tumors. The ultrastructural characteristics of the two tumors are also quite distinctive. *Epithelioid smooth muscle tumors* usually express myoid antigens and lack S-100 protein, and they exhibit ultrastructural evidence of myoid differentiation.

Discussion

Behavior of the ossifying fibromyxoid tumor varies. The vast majority of these tumors are histologically benign and have the characteristic features described in the original series from the AFIP ("typical ossifying fibromyxoid tumor"). Not unexpectedly, most of these pursue a benign clinical course. However, it has been noted that on rare occasion even histologically typical tumors may locally recur and metastasize. For example, Yoshida and col-

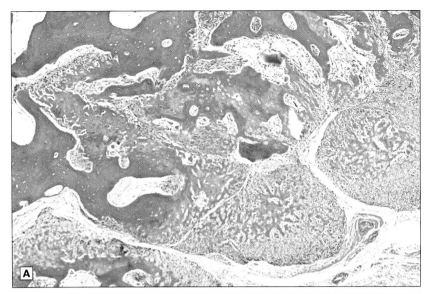

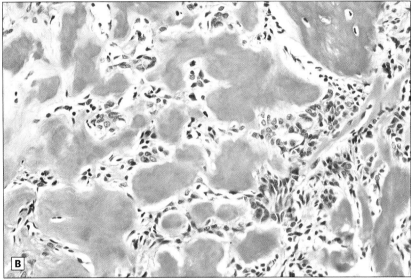

FIGURE 36–11 (A) Recurrent lesion in a 50-year-old man who had a typical ossifying fibromyxoid tumor resected 2 years earlier. **(B)** This lesion was more cellular than this patient's original tumor and showed areas reminiscent of a low-grade osteosarcoma with formation of abundant osteoid.

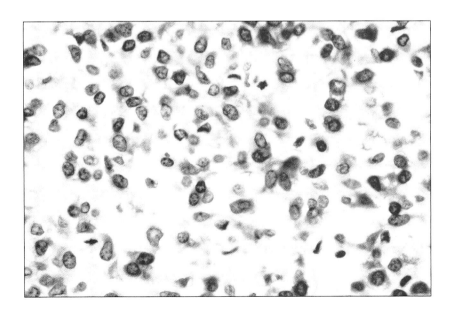

FIGURE 36–12 Ossifying fibromyxoid tumor with strong S-100 protein immunoreactivity.

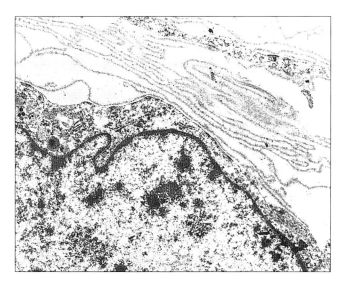

FIGURE 36–13 Electron micrograph of an ossifying fibromyxoid tumor with reduplication and scroll formation of external laminae, suggesting a tumor with neural differentiation. (From Enzinger FM, Weiss SW, Liang CY. Ossifying fibromyxoid tumor of soft parts: a clinicopathological analysis of 59 cases. Am J Surg Pathol 1989; 13:817.)

TABLE 36–2	PROPOSED CLASSIFICATION OF OSSIFYING FIBROMYXOID TUMORS
	Diagnostic criteria
Typical OFMT	Low nuclear grade and low cellularity with mitotic activity <2 MF/50 HPF
Atypical OFMT	Tumors deviating from typical OFMT but not meeting criteria for malignant OFMT
Malignant OFMT	High nuclear grade or high cellularity and mitotic activity ≥2 MF/50 HPF

Modified from: Folpe AL, Weiss SW. Ossifying fibromyxoid tumor of soft parts: a clinicopathologic study of 70 cases with emphasis on atypical and malignant variants. Am J Surg Pathol 2003; 27:421.

TABLE 36–3	RISK OF LOCAL RECURRENCE AND METASTASIS IN 45 CASES OF OSSIFYING FIBROMYXOID TUMOR WITH FOLLOW-UP		
	No. cases with follow-up	Local recurrences (%)	Metastases (%)
Typical OFMT	25	3 (12)	1 (4)
Atypical OFMT	16	2 (13)	1 (6)
Malignant OFMT	10	6 (60)	6 (60)

Modified from: Folpe AL, Weiss SW. Ossifying fibromyxoid tumor of soft parts: a clinicopathologic study of 70 cases with emphasis on atypical and malignant variants. Am J Surg Pathol 2003; 27:421.

leagues described a case lacking malignant features but which locally recurred, metastasized, and ultimately killed the patient.[3] In the original report of typical ossifying fibromyxoid tumors by Enzinger et al.,[1] 11 of 41 patients (27%) for whom follow-up information was available experienced one or more recurrences. In addition, one patient with three recurrences developed a similar tumor in the contralateral thigh that was presumed to be a metastasis. The patient committed suicide shortly after discovery of the contralateral lesion. One additional patient developed a recurrence that histologically progressed to a well-differentiated osteosarcoma. Combining the results of their study with those of the three largest previously published series,[1,4,17] Folpe and Weiss estimated the overall recurrence and metastatic rates of "typical ossifying fibromyxoid tumor" to be 17% and 5%, respectively, suggesting this tumor be considered a lesion of intermediate malignancy.[15]

As mentioned above, some of these tumors have atypical histologic features, including high nuclear grade, increased cellularity, and increased mitotic activity. Williams and co-workers described a series of nine head and neck tumors, one of which was histologically malignant (high cellularity, high nuclear grade, and a mitotic rate of 5 MF/10 HPF) and locally recurred within the 2-year follow-up period.[5] In 1995, Kilpatrick et al. reported six "atypical" and "malignant" ossifying fibromyxoid tumors.[2] All of the tumors in this report had histologic features of malignancy, including areas of increased cellularity, increased mitotic activity, or deposition of centrally placed osteoid. Although meaningful follow-up was not available in four of these cases, one patient, a

68-year-old man with a 9 cm deep soft tissue mass adjacent to the greater trochanter, developed a local recurrence and histologically proven pulmonary metastases.

More recently, Folpe and Weiss described 70 cases of ossifying fibromyxoid tumor with an emphasis on atypical and malignant variants.[15] Twenty cases (29%) were histologically "typical" and showed low cellularity, low nuclear grade, and fewer than 2 MF/50 HPF. Most of the cases in this series (45 cases; 64%) showed a mixture of typical and atypical areas, and five cases (7%) showed essentially no areas of typical ossifying fibromyxoid tumor. By univariate analysis, high cellularity, high nuclear grade, and mitotic activity of >2 MF/50 HPF were significantly associated with both local recurrence and metastasis. An infiltrative growth pattern was associated with local recurrence, but not metastasis. None of the other features evaluated showed any correlation with an adverse clinical outcome. Thus, the authors suggested that tumors with high nuclear grade or those with high cellularity and mitotic activity of >2 MF/50 HPF should be regarded as sarcomas with significant potential for metastasis. Of the 10 cases in this category with clinical follow-up, six developed metastatic disease. Since cases that deviated from "typical" ossifying fibromyxoid tumor had a metastatic rate (6%) that was similar to typical tumors (4%), Folpe and Weiss opted to avoid the term "atypical ossifying fibromyxoid tumor" and considered those cases within the general category of ossifying fibromyxoid tumor (Tables 36–2 and 36–3).[15]

The line of differentiation of this tumor has been disputed since its initial description, with cartilaginous, myoepithelial, osteogenic, and myoid origins suggested. The preponderance of published evidence is more suggestive of peripheral nerve sheath differentiation. The encapsulation and the immunohistochemical expression of "neural" antigens including S-100 protein, Leu-7, neuron-specific enolase, and GFAP are in keeping with this theory. Furthermore, at least some of the ultrastructural features suggest schwannian differentiation, albeit incomplete, prompting some to suggest that this lesion could be regarded as a low-grade malignant peripheral nerve sheath tumor.[14] The fact that malignant forms of this tumor have displayed clear-cut osteosarcomatous areas has led to an opposing view that they represent an unusual bone or cartilage-producing tumor. Folpe and Weiss conjectured that this tumor may ultimately prove to be a translocation-associated sarcoma, the result of which is a tumor with a "scrambled phenotype" due to the recombination of genes related to neural and chondroid differentiation.[15]

INFLAMMATORY MYXOHYALINE TUMOR OF THE DISTAL EXTREMITIES WITH VIROCYTE OR REED-STERNBERG-LIKE CELLS (ACRAL MYXOINFLAMMATORY FIBROBLASTIC SARCOMA)

In 1998, Montgomery and colleagues reported 49 cases of a previously undescribed tumor of the distal extremities with unusual histologic features often prompting a misdiagnosis of an inflammatory or infectious process.[22] Because of the presence of scattered bizarre cells with vesicular nuclei and macronucleoli and a prominent inflammatory background, the authors coined the term *inflammatory myxohyaline tumor of distal extremities with virocyte or Reed-Sternberg-like cells*. In this initial report, local recurrences occurred in almost one-fourth of the patients, although none developed metastatic disease. Shortly thereafter, Meis-Kindblom and Kindblom[23] reported a series describing the identical tumor, including one patient with biopsy-proven metastasis and used the term "acral myxoinflammatory fibroblastic sarcoma" to emphasize the occasionally aggressive clinical course.

Clinical findings

Although the age range is broad, most patients with this tumor are in the fourth and fifth decades of life.[22-24] Males and females are affected equally, and most patients present with a slowly growing, painless, ill-defined mass of the distal extremities. The upper extremities are affected more commonly than the lower extremities, with the single most common site being the soft tissues of the

TABLE 36-4	ANATOMIC DISTRIBUTION OF 95 INFLAMMATORY MYXOHYALINE TUMORS OF THE DISTAL EXTREMITIES	
Anatomic site		**No. of cases**
Upper extremities		65 (68%)
Fingers/hands		53
Wrist/lower arm		10
Miscellaneous		2
Lower extremities		30 (32%)
Toes/feet		16
Ankles/lower leg		13
Miscellaneous		1

Data are from references 22 and 23.

fingers and hand, although some lesions arise in the lower arm and wrist. On the lower extremities, these tumors may arise in the toes, feet, ankles, and lower legs (Table 36-4). There are few cases reported in the literature that have arisen in extra-acral sites.[25,26] Some patients report mild pain and decreased mobility of the affected site, and occasionally there is a history of antecedent trauma, which serves to bring the tumor to clinical attention. Given its location, the lesion is often thought to represent a ganglion cyst or some form of tenosynovitis. Magnetic resonance imaging (MRI) findings are not diagnostic but typically reveal a poorly circumscribed mass with involvement of the underlying tendon sheath.[27]

Pathologic findings

Grossly, the tumor is multinodular and poorly circumscribed, and it is often removed piecemeal by the surgeon (Fig. 36-14). Gelatinous-appearing areas are conspicuous in the lesions with extensive myxoid change. The tumors range in size from 1 to 8 cm (mean 3-4 cm).

At low magnification the tumor is multinodular and poorly circumscribed and frequently involves surrounding tendon sheaths and the synovium of adjacent joints (Fig. 36-15). Most arise in the subcutaneous tissue, but some involve the dermis and others focally infiltrate skeletal muscle. Destruction or invasion of underlying bony structures has not been reported.

The most striking feature at low magnification is that of a dense inflammatory infiltrate merging with myxoid or hyaline zones (Figs 36-16, 36-17). In most cases, leukocytes and plasma cells predominate, although neutrophils and eosinophils are conspicuous in some tumors (Fig. 36-18).[28] Germinal centers are occasionally encountered. The amount of myxoid and hyalinized stroma varies from case to case. Some tumors are composed predominantly of hypocellular myxoid zones (Fig. 36-19), whereas other tumors may have only focal myxoid change. Hyaline zones contain a sparse mixture of inflammatory and neoplastic cells and often resemble the hyalinized zones of inflammatory myofibroblastic tumor (Fig. 36–20). Hemosiderin deposition may be conspicuous.

Examination of more cellular zones reveals bizarre atypical cells deposited in a hyalinized or myxoid stroma and allows for recognition of this lesion as a neoplastic process. These atypical cells range in shape from plump spindled cells to histiocytoid or epithelioid cells (Fig. 36–21). The spindled cells have a moderate degree of nuclear atypia, whereas the larger epithelioid cells often have large vesicular nuclei with macronucleoli and prominent eosinophilic cytoplasm, imparting a close similarity to virocytes or Reed-Sternberg cells (Figs 36–22, 36–23)

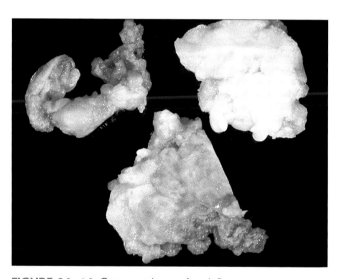

FIGURE 36–14 Gross specimen of an inflammatory myxohyaline tumor showing multinodular focally gelatinous mass. (From Montgomery EA, Devaney KO, Giordano TJ, et al. Inflammatory myxohyaline tumor of distal extremities with virocyte or Reed-Sternberg-like cells: a distinctive lesion with features simulating inflammatory conditions, Hodgkin's disease, and various sarcomas. Mod Pathol 1998; 11:384.)

Despite the marked degree of nuclear atypia, there is a paucity of mitotic figures, typically with fewer than 2 MF/50 HPF. Ganglion-like cells resembling those seen in proliferative fasciitis may be widely scattered throughout the neoplasm or form small nodular collections. Some bizarre cells have multivacuolated cytoplasm simulating lipoblasts (Fig. 36–24) and others appear to engulf inflammatory cells.[29] Multinucleated giant cells including Touton-type giant cells are occasionally encountered (Fig. 36–25). In addition, there is often an intermingling of round mononuclear cells with bland nuclear features and small amounts of amphophilic cytoplasm. Necrosis is rarely present.

Immunohistochemical and ultrastructural findings

The mononuclear and larger bizarre cells consistently stain for vimentin, with variable immunoreactivity for CD68, CD34, and smooth muscle actin (Table 36–5).[22,23] Immunostains for S-100 protein, HMB-45, desmin, epithelial membrane antigen (EMA), leukocyte common antigen, CD15 (Leu-M1), and CD30 (Ki-1) are typically negative. Focal immunoreactivity for cytokeratins is sometimes found. The lymphocytic infiltrate is predominantly composed of T cells with a smaller component of B cells.

The bizarre neoplastic cells characteristically have a single, often clefted nucleus with one or more large nucleoli and occasional intranuclear cytoplasmic inclusions.[23] There are abundant rough endoplasmic reticulum and mitochondria, as well as densely packed perinuclear whorls of intermediate filaments, although actin-type and thin filaments are not seen. Small lipid droplets, glycogen, and scattered lysosomes may also be seen in the cytoplasm. Overall, the ultrastructural features are

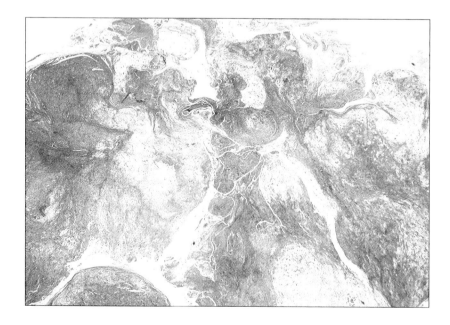

FIGURE 36–15 Low-power view of inflammatory myxohyaline tumor illustrating a mixture of myxoid, hyaline, and inflammatory zones.

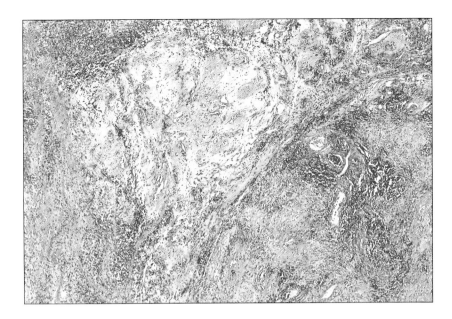

FIGURE 36–16 Admixture of myxoid, hyaline, and inflammatory zones in an inflammatory myxohyaline tumor.

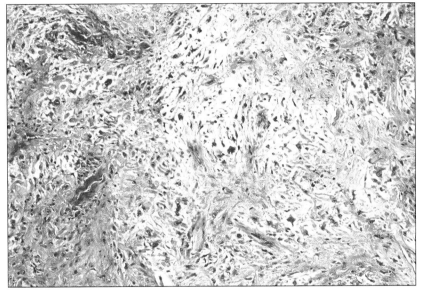

FIGURE 36–17 Inflammatory myxohyaline tumor. Note the transition between myxoid and hyaline zones.

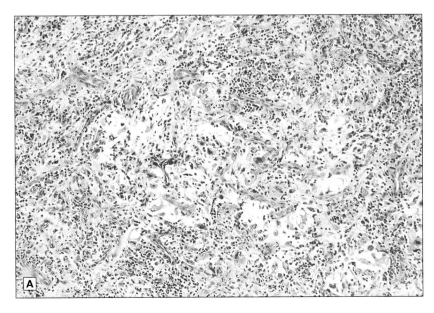

FIGURE 36–18 (A, B) Inflammatory myxohyaline tumor with prominent inflammatory zones.

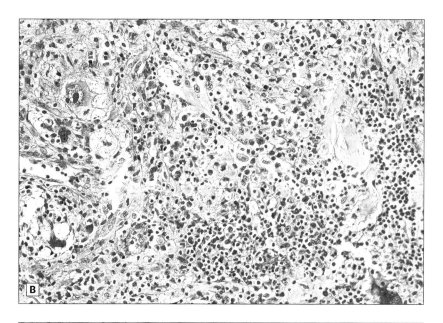

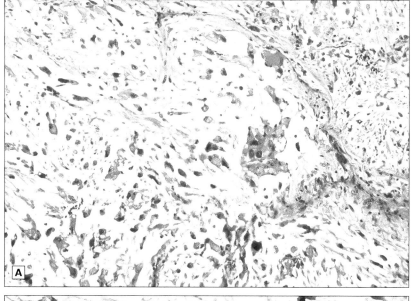

FIGURE 36–18 Continued.

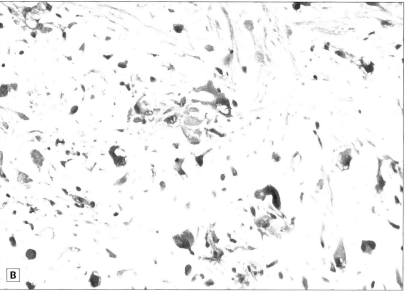

FIGURE 36–19 **(A)** Low-magnification view of a myxoid zone in an inflammatory myxohyaline tumor. **(B)** Higher-magnification view of cells with smudgy nuclei in a myxoid zone of an inflammatory myxohyaline tumor.

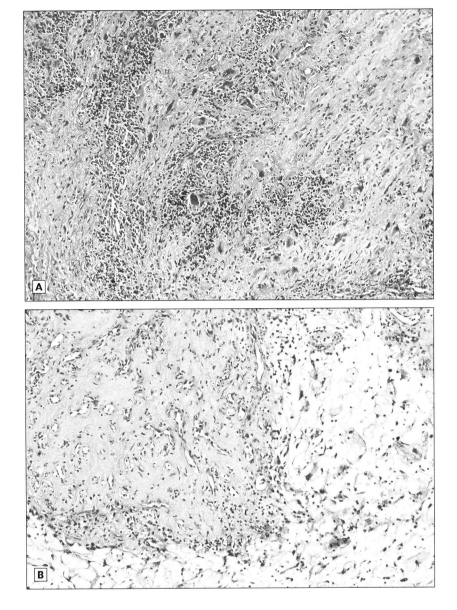

FIGURE 36–20 Inflammatory myxohyaline tumor. **(A)** Hyaline area with prominent inflammatory component. **(B)** Sharp transition between myxoid and hyaline zones.

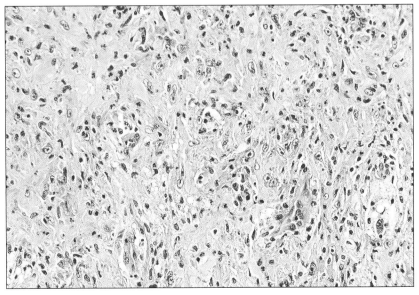

FIGURE 36–21 Inflammatory myxohyaline tumor. Neoplastic cells range from spindled to epithelioid.

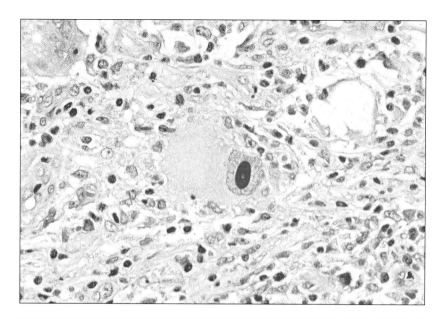

FIGURE 36–22 Enlarged tumor cell with a large eosinophilic nucleolus resembling a virocyte in an inflammatory myxohyaline tumor.

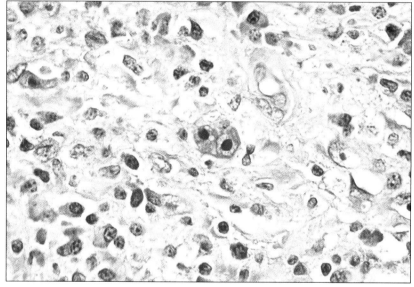

FIGURE 36–23 Inflammatory myxohyaline tumor with cells resembling Reed-Sternberg cells.

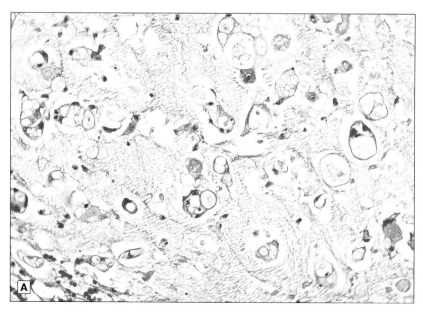

FIGURE 36–24 Myxoid zones in an inflammatory myxohyaline tumor. **(A)** Bizarre cells are distended with stromal mucin.

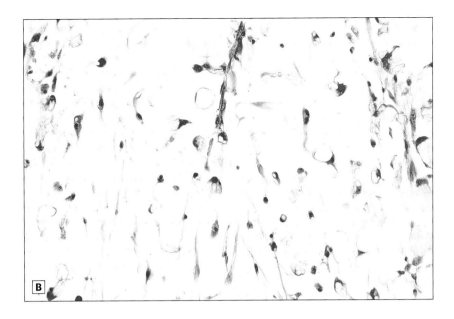

FIGURE 36–24 Continued. **(B)** Pseudo-lipoblasts are prominent in this tumor.

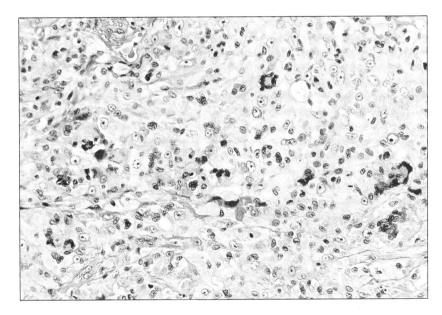

FIGURE 36–25 Scattered multinucleated giant cells in a cellular zone of inflammatory myxohyaline tumor.

	IMMUNOHISTOCHEMICAL DATA ON INFLAMMATORY MYXOHYALINE TUMORS OF THE DISTAL EXTREMITIES
TABLE 36–5	
Marker	**No. of cases stained**
Vimentin	35/35 (100%)
CD68	23/35 (66%)
CD34	7/25 (28%)
Cytokeratin	4/38 (11%)
Smooth muscle actin	2/33 (6%)
CD15	0/5
CD30	0/12
EMA	0/28
S-100 protein	0/44
Desmin	0/6

Data are from references 22 and 23.

most consistent with a tumor showing fibroblastic differentiation.[25]

Cytogenetic findings

No characteristic cytogenetic aberration has been identified. Lambert et al. reported a single case with a t(1;10)(p22;q24) and loss of chromosomes 3 and 13.[30] Another case showed complex supernumerary ring chromosomes composed of segments from chromosome 3 and a derivative chromosome 13.[31]

Differential diagnosis

Because of the wide array of appearances of this tumor, the differential diagnosis in part depends on the cellularity of the lesion and the relative amount of myxoid and hyaline stroma. An infectious or inflammatory process is often considered, given the prominent inflammatory background, cells with virocyte-like nuclei, and necrosis. Special stains for microbial organisms are invariably negative, as are immunohistochemical stains for cytomegalovirus. Montgomery et al. analyzed 10 cases by polymerase chain reaction (PCR) for the presence of Epstein-Barr virus (EBV);[22] four patients were found to harbor EBV, but the level of amplification was compatible with latent, rather than active, viral infection.

Giant cell tumor of the tendon sheath is often a diagnostic consideration given the location of the tumor, the prominent inflammatory component, and the presence of Touton-like giant cells and hemosiderin. Recognition of the large bizarre cells, which are widely scattered in some cases, is critical for distinguishing these lesions. This tumor also has histologic features that overlap with those found in *inflammatory myofibroblastic tumor*, although the cells of inflammatory myxohyaline tumor are more bizarre than those seen in the latter and lack the well-developed immunohistochemical and ultrastructural features of myofibroblasts. Moreover, the acral location of the inflammatory myxohyaline tumor is not characteristic of inflammatory myofibroblastic tumor. Finally, ALK-1 proven positivity is frequently found in inflammatory myofibroblastic tumor, particularly those arising in the abdomen.

For those tumors with prominent myxoid stroma, there are a number of benign and malignant myxoid lesions that could be considered. The large bizarre cells characteristic of inflammatory myxohyaline tumor would not be found in any benign myxoid soft tissue neoplasm. Distinction from *myxofibrosarcoma/myxoid malignant fibrous histiocytoma* (MFH) is the most difficult aspect of the differential diagnosis; both tumors have enough distinguishing characteristics to support the contention that they are distinct entities. Focal areas of high-grade pleomorphic sarcoma may be seen in myxofibrosarcoma/ myxoid MFH, whereas high-grade areas would not be found in inflammatory myxohyaline tumor. Additional differences include the alternating myxoid and hyalinized zones, a more striking inflammatory infiltrate, the presence of virocyte-like cells, and the acral location typical of inflammatory myxohyaline tumor.

The presence of Reed-Sternberg-like cells also raises the possibility of *Hodgkin's disease* in some cases. Immunohistochemically, the large atypical cells lack expression of CD15 and CD30 as one would expect to find in the Reed-Sternberg cells of Hodgkin's disease.

Discussion

In the series of 51 cases reported by Montgomery et al.,[22] follow-up information was obtained in 27 patients with a median follow-up period of 53 months. Of these 27 patients, six (22%) developed at least one local recurrence 15 months to 10 years after the initial excision, but none developed metastatic disease. In the subsequent study of 44 cases by Meis-Kindblom and Kindblom,[23] follow-up information obtained in 36 patients revealed a local recurrence rate of 67%, including eight patients who had two local recurrences and five who had at least three local recurrences. The rather striking difference in recurrence rates between these studies probably reflects a difference in the referral base. The cases reported from the AFIP were largely ascertained retrospectively,[23] and many were not originally diagnosed as sarcoma, whereas those reported by Montgomery et al. were ascertained prospectively and all were diagnosed as low-grade sarcomas and treated more aggressively.[22] One patient reported by Meis-Kindblom and Kindblom[23] developed a histologically documented inguinal lymph node metastasis 1.5 years after the initial excision. A second patient developed suspected pulmonary metastases 2 years after the first local recurrence and 5 years after the initial presentation, although the metastases were not documented histologically (Table 36–6). Sakaki and colleagues reported an acral tumor that metastasized only 3 months after initial excision.[32] We have reviewed exceptional cases that progressed to a high-grade pleomorphic (MFH-like) sarcoma. Wide local excision without adjuvant therapy appears to be adequate treatment for this tumor.

PARACHORDOMA/MIXED TUMOR/ MYOEPITHELIOMA OF SOFT TISSUE

The entity of parachordoma was first described by Laskowski in 1951 as "chordoma periphericum"[33] but was

TABLE 36–6	CLINICAL BEHAVIOR OF INFLAMMATORY MYXOHYALINE TUMORS OF THE DISTAL EXTREMITIES			
Study	No. of cases with follow-up	Follow-up interval (median)	Local recurrence	Metastasis
Meis-Kindblom et al.[23]	36	6 months to 45 years (5 years)	24/36 (67%)	2/36 (6%)
Montgomery et al.[22]	27	6 months to 10 years (53 months)	6/27 (22%)	0/27 (0%)

more fully described in a series of 10 cases by Dabska in 1977.[34] Since that time, fewer than 60 cases have been described in the literature, mostly in the form of case reports or small series.[35-42] However, the very existence of parachordoma has been questioned since its initial description, and in fact, there is some evidence to support the contention that parachordoma is part of a morphologic spectrum that includes mixed tumor and myoepithelioma of soft tissue,[43,44] as evidenced by the recent WHO classification of soft tissue tumors. The ensuing discussion will encompass the salient features of parachordoma and mixed tumor/myoepithelioma of soft tissue, summarizing the evidence both for and against the relationship between these unusual soft tissue neoplasms.

Clinical findings

Cases reported as parachordoma have arisen in patients of all ages, but there is a peak incidence in the second through fourth decades of life. In the series of 7 cases reported by Folpe and colleagues, patients ranged in age from 7 to 62 years, with a mean age of 35 years.[45] There is no significant gender predilection, and most patients present with a slowly enlarging, painless mass in the deep soft tissue of the extremities, usually in the muscles of the thigh, calf, upper arm, or forearm.

Mixed tumor/myoepithelioma is usually found in adults, although the age range is broad. In the largest series published to date (101 cases from Brigham and Women's Hospital),[44] patients ranged in age from 3 to 83 years with a mean age of 38 years, and no gender predilection. Similar to parachordoma, most patients present with a painless soft tissue mass, although pain and paresthesias are reported in a minority of patients. Most arise in the lower limb/limb girdle, especially the thigh and groin/inguinal region (Table 36–7).[44,46-48] Slightly less often, it arises in the upper limb/limb girdle, followed by the head and neck and trunk.[44,48] The tumor may be situated primarily in the subcutis or deep to the fascia; less often, the lesion may be centered in or secondarily involve the dermis.[48-50]

Pathologic findings

Grossly, parachordoma forms a nodular mass ranging in size from 1 to 12 cm in greatest dimension, but most are 3–7 cm (Fig. 36–26). Mixed tumor/myoepithelioma has a similar gross appearance. In the series from Brigham and Women's Hospital, tumor size ranged from slightly less than 1 cm to up to 20 cm (mean 4.7), although histologically benign tumors were significantly smaller than histologically malignant tumors (3.8 cm and 5.9 cm, respectively).[44] Most are grossly well circumscribed and have a yellow-white to tan cut surface that is glistening, myxoid, or gelatinous. Necrosis is rarely a prominent feature.

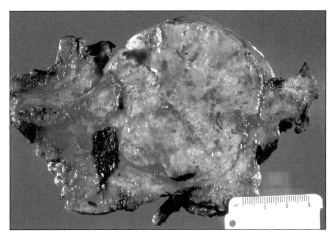

FIGURE 36–26 Gross appearance of a parachordoma arising in the chest wall of a 55-year-old man.

TABLE 36–7	ANATOMIC DISTRIBUTION OF 101 SOFT TISSUE MYOEPITHELIAL TUMORS	
Anatomic location		**No. of cases**
Lower limb/limb girdle		41
Upper limb/limb girdle		35
Head and neck		15
Trunk		10
Total		101

Modified from: Hornick JL, Fletcher CDM. Myoepithelial tumors of soft tissue: a clinicopathologic and immunohistochemical study of 101 cases with evaluation of prognostic parameters. Am J Surg Pathol 2003; 27:1183.

Microscopically, parachordoma consists of small nests of pale-staining cells resembling the cells of the notochord. Most of the cells are round, eosinophilic cells arranged in cords, chains, or pseudoacini reminiscent of myxoid chondrosarcoma (Figs 36–27 to 36–30). Not uncommonly, the cells show a transition to spindle-shaped cells (Fig. 36–31) or small, round glomoid cells (Fig. 36–32).[45] All lesions have a population of cells with vacuolated cytoplasm resembling physaliferous cells found in chordomas (Figs 36–33, 36–34). There is usually only a mild degree of nuclear atypia, and mitotic figures are inconspicuous, usually with less than 1 MF/20 HPF. The cells are deposited in a matrix that varies from myxoid to hyaline (Fig. 36–35) and contains a high concentration of hyaluronic acid, as evidenced by reduction of Alcian blue staining after hyaluronidase predigestion.[45] Although grossly well circumscribed, there are frequently small nests of cells that are separated from the main tumor and trail off into the surrounding soft tissue structures, sometimes evoking a desmoplastic stromal response (Fig. 36–36).

The histologic appearance of mixed tumor/myoepithelioma spans a morphologic spectrum similar to that observed in their counterparts in the salivary gland (Figs 36–37, 36–38). Myoepitheliomas show a

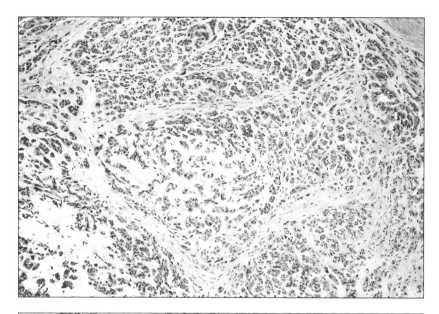

FIGURE 36–27 Parachordoma showing multinodular masses of epithelioid to spindle cells, with a variably myxochondroid matrix.

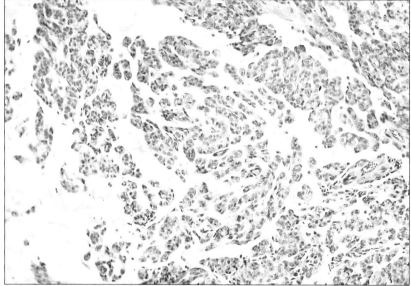

FIGURE 36–28 Parachordoma. Nests of epithelioid cells are suspended in a myxoid matrix.

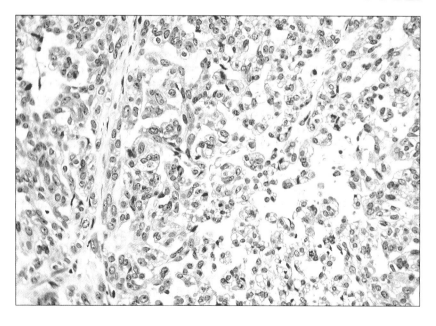

FIGURE 36–29 Parachordoma. Nests and cords of epithelioid to spindle-shaped cells are deposited in a myxochondroid matrix.

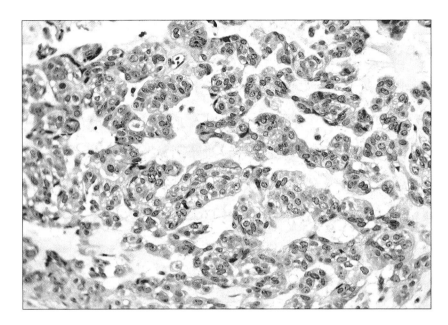

FIGURE 36–30 Nests of uniform-appearing epithelioid cells suspended in a myxochondroid matrix in a parachordoma.

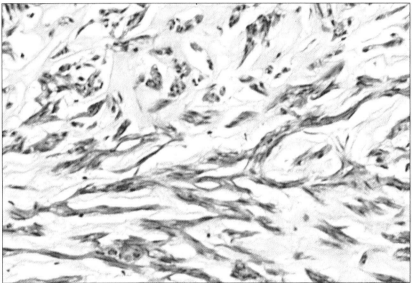

FIGURE 36–31 Focus of spindle cells in parachordoma.

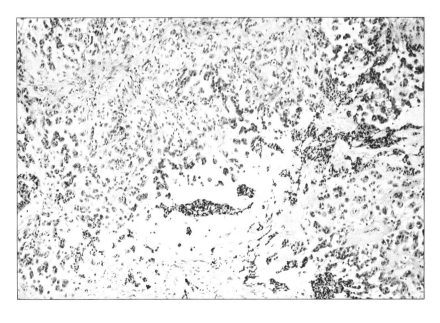

FIGURE 36–32 Transition from large epithelioid cells to small glomoid cells in a parachordoma.

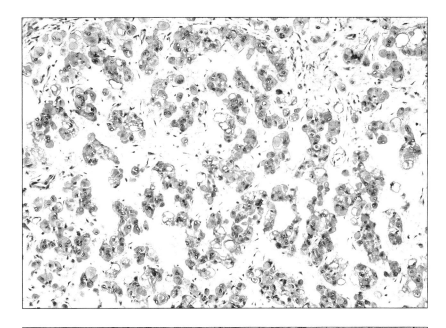

FIGURE 36–33 Chordoma-like area in a parachordoma. Nests of large cells with abundant eosinophilic and vacuolated cytoplasm are suspended in a myxochondroid matrix.

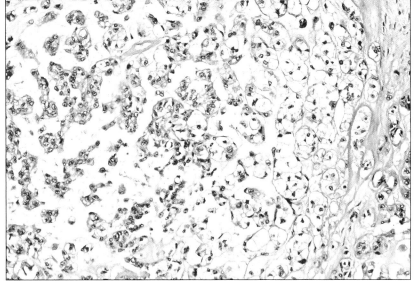

FIGURE 36–34 Parachordoma. Transition from eosinophilic cells to cells with clear, vacuolated cytoplasm.

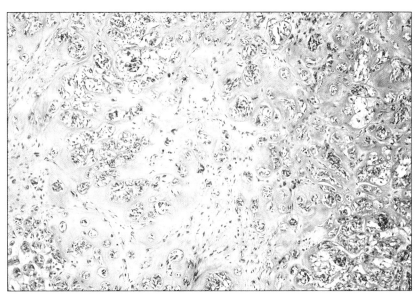

FIGURE 36–35 Parachordoma with a densely hyalinized matrix.

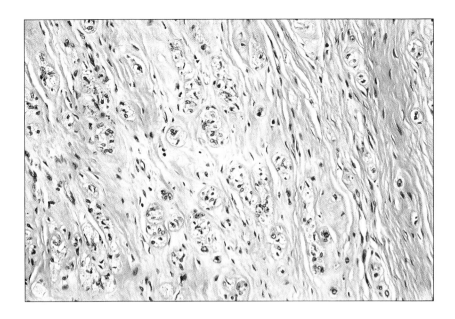

FIGURE 36–36 Periphery of a parachordoma with infiltrating small nests and single cells in a desmoplastic background.

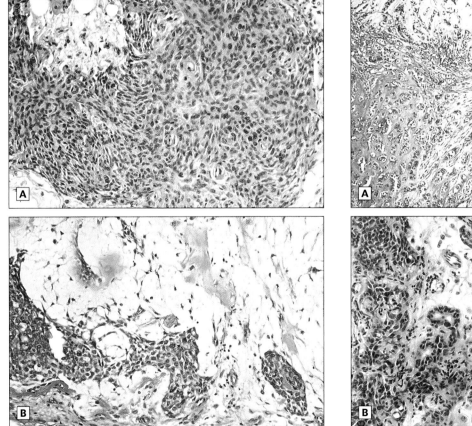

FIGURE 36–37 **(A)** Soft tissue myoepithelioma with a solidly cellular proliferation of spindled cells merging with epithelioid cells. **(B)** Nests of spindled cells deposited in an abundant myxoid stroma in a soft tissue myoepithelioma. (Case courtesy of Dr. Chris Fletcher, Brigham & Women's Hospital, Boston, Massachusetts.)

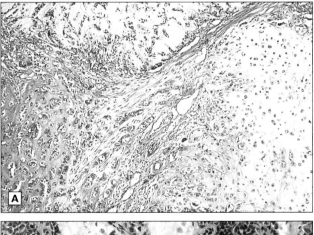

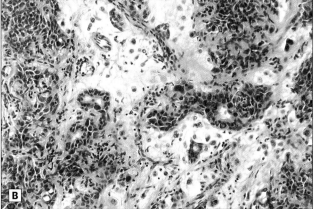

FIGURE 36–38 **(A)** Low-magnification view of a soft tissue mixed tumor showing an admixture of cords of epithelioid cells and metaplastic cartilage. **(B)** Ductal differentiation in a soft tissue mixed tumor. (Case courtesy of Dr. Chris Fletcher, Brigham & Women's Hospital, Boston, Massachusetts.)

predominantly reticular growth pattern with cords of epithelioid, ovoid, or spindled cells deposited in a variably collagenous or chondromyxoid stroma. In some cases, the cells are arranged in nests or large sheets, but mixed architectural patterns are common.[44] "Parachordoma-like" areas consisting of large epithelioid cells with eosinophilic to clear or vacuolated cytoplasm may be seen in a minority of cases which are otherwise typical for myoepithelioma. The stroma varies in character from case to case and in different areas of the same tumor. The cells themselves may be epithelioid, spindled, clear, or plasmacytoid. Similar to the stromal component, the cell type varies among cases and within the same tumor. While some tumors are composed exclusively of one cell type, most commonly there is a mixture of all cell types similar to that described in parachordoma. Cases that show clear-cut ductal differentiation are best classified as mixed tumors. Metaplastic cartilage, bone, or both can be seen in a small percentage of cases.

While most mixed tumor/myoepitheliomas have minimal or no atypia and are composed of uniform small nuclei with fine chromatin and inconspicuous nucleoli, some have cytologically malignant features and are composed of larger cells with vesicular or coarse chromatin and prominent nucleoli.[44] In the series by Hornick and Fletcher, 61 of 101 tumors were classified as histologically benign, whereas 40 tumors were felt to be histologically malignant based upon the cytologic features (malignant myoepithelioma, malignant mixed tumor, or myoepithelial carcinoma).[44] Some histologically malignant tumors show small foci of classic benign-appearing areas; others have foci of heterologous chondrosarcomatous or osteosarcomatous differentiation.[44]

Immunohistochemical and ultrastructural findings

By immunohistochemistry, the cells of parachordoma characteristically co-express cytokeratins (Fig. 36–39), including cytokeratin 8/18, EMA, S-100 protein, Leu-7, and vimentin.[45,51,52] The cells do not stain for cytokeratin 1/10, cytokeratin 7, or cytokeratin 20.[53] Type IV collagen surrounds groups of cells in a nest-like fashion.[45] Immunostains for CD34, actin, GFAP, and calponin are typically negative.

Mixed tumor/myoepitheliomas have a similar immunophenotype to that described for parachordoma, but there are some minor differences. Similar to parachordoma, mixed tumor/myoepitheliomas consistently co-express epithelial markers (cytokeratins and/or EMA) and S-100 protein.[44,47,48] Hornick and Fletcher found staining for AE1/AE3, CAM5.2, CK14, and EMA in 77%, 51%, 32%, and 63% of cases, respectively.[44] Cytokeratin staining can be seen in all cell types but is often focal. Among myogenic markers, most cases stain for calponin (reportedly negative in parachordoma), but staining for smooth muscle actin and desmin is found in approximately 35% and 15% of cases, respectively. Nuclear staining for the basal cell/myoepithelial marker p63 is not common, as fewer than 25% of cases show staining for this antigen.[44] GFAP is expressed in almost 50% of cases.

By electron microscopy, parachordoma is composed of cells showing incomplete epithelial differentiation, with primitive cell junctions, fragmented basal lamina, and microvillous projections.[51,52,54–57] Similar ultrastructural features are seen in the cells of mixed tumor/myoepithelioma, although the epithelial features are more well developed, with tumor cells surrounded by basal

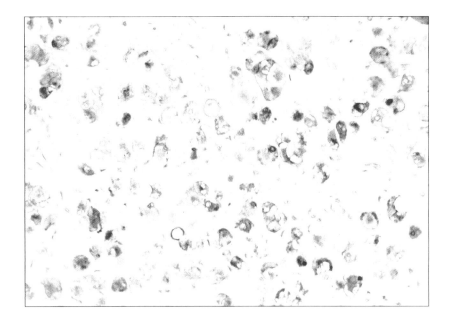

FIGURE 36–39 Parachordoma with strong immunoreactivity for high-molecular-weight cytokeratin.

lamina and containing cytoplasmic filaments and intercellular junctions.[46,58,59]

Cytogenetic findings

Not unexpectedly, few parachordomas have been studied by cytogenetics. In a series of seven parachordomas reported by Folpe and colleagues,[45] one patient had multiple cytogenetic aberrations including trisomy 15 and monosomies of chromosomes 1, 16, and 17. Tihy et al. reported a parachordoma with small der2(2)5(2;4),del (3q) and loss of chromosomes 9, 19, 20, and 22.[60] Limon et al. reported a tumor with a complex karyotype, although this tumor may actually represent an ossifying fibromyxoid tumor.[61] Additionally, Tong and colleagues described a parachordoma with a complex karyotype including loss of chromosomes 1, 2, and 6 and a small der(5)t(1p;5q).[62]

Similarly, very few cases of mixed tumor/myoepithelioma have been studied by cytogenetics. Pauwels et al. reported an intramuscular mixed tumor with a complex karyotype including a der(17)t(15;17)(q11;p12).[63] A recent report of a single histologically and clinically malignant myoepithelioma revealed a hypotetraploid karyotype with several chromosomal losses and complex structural changes.[64] Thus far, there is no conclusive cytogenetic evidence to link parachordoma with mixed tumor/myoepithelioma.

Differential diagnosis

Given the morphologic heterogeneity of this group of tumors, the differential diagnosis is quite broad and depends in large part upon the predominant cell type and stromal component. If ducts are present, the diagnosis of mixed tumor is straightforward. Most commonly, considerations include extraskeletal myxoid chondrosarcoma, ossifying fibromyxoid tumor, and chordoma.

Distinction from *extraskeletal myxoid chondrosarcoma* may be particularly challenging. This tumor typically shows a multinodular pattern with cords of eosinophilic spindled to ovoid cells deposited in a myxoid matrix. There is such a significant degree of morphologic overlap with parachordoma/mixed tumor/myoepithelioma that immunohistochemistry and/or molecular diagnostic testing is required. Myoepitheliomas typically co-express cytokeratin (or EMA) and S-100 protein, whereas extraskeletal myxoid chondrosarcoma expresses S-100 protein in a minority of cases and does not typically express cytokeratins. In addition, extraskeletal myxoid chondrosarcoma is characterized by a t(9;22) involving the *EWS* gene.

Ossifying fibromyxoid tumor also enters the differential diagnosis. This tumor is a lobulated neoplasm composed of cords or nests of uniform, pale-staining, ovoid cells deposited in a variably myxoid or hyalinized stroma with a rim of metaplastic bone at the periphery in 70% of cases. Most ossifying fibromyxoid tumors stain for S-100 protein, and about 50% stain for desmin. Focal cytokeratin positivity is very uncommon.

Chordoma is also a consideration, especially for tumors with a focal or predominant parachordoma-like pattern. Some authors even consider parachordoma to be the peripheral counterpart of axial chordoma, but we doubt this.[34] Both tumors are characterized by round cells with vacuolated cytoplasm (physalipherous-like) arranged in nests and cords. Unlike chordoma, parachordoma shows a blending of these vacuolated cells with spindled cells and small glomoid cells. In contrast to chordoma, the matrix of parachordoma is abolished by hyaluronidase predigestion. There is significant immunophenotypic overlap between these lesions, since both are characterized by expression of EMA, CAM5.2, S-100 protein, and vimentin. Chordomas express CK1/10 and CK19, both of which are absent in parachordoma.[40,45,51,53] Furthermore, type IV collagen is only rarely and focally expressed in chordoma, in contrast to the nest-like arrangement around groups of cells in parachordoma.[45]

Myoepithelial carcinoma (malignant myoepithelioma) may be confused with *metastatic carcinoma*, *metastatic melanoma*, and even *epithelioid sarcoma*, especially the proximal type. Obviously, knowledge of a history of a primary carcinoma or a melanoma elsewhere is of paramount importance. In the absence of such a history, immunohistochemistry can be extremely helpful in distinguishing among these lesions. Immunoreactivity for myogenic markers (e.g., calponin, desmin), S-100 protein, and GFAP support a diagnosis of myoepithelial carcinoma over metastatic carcinoma. Melanomas typically co-express S-100 protein and melanocytic antigens such as HMB-45 or Melan A, and they rarely express cytokeratins, GFAP, or myogenic markers. Epithelioid sarcoma frequently expresses cytokeratin and EMA, but not S-100 protein, GFAP, or myogenic markers.

Discussion

Given the small number of cases reported in the literature, it is difficult to know the true natural history of parachordoma. However, most cases behave in an indolent fashion, although it clearly has the potential for local recurrence. In a review of the literature by Folpe and colleagues in 1999,[45] six of 24 reported cases with clinical follow-up information had locally recurred, although there is very little information available pertaining to the adequacy of surgical excision of these cases. Some of these recurrences occurred many years after the initial excision. For example, Dabska reported a local recurrence 19 years after initial therapy.[34] There are several reports of parachordoma that have metastasized. Limon et al. reported metastasis of a tumor that originated in the palm that metastasized to an axillary lymph node after 7 years.[61] However, as previously mentioned, there is some doubt as to whether this tumor is in fact a parachordoma. Miettinen et al. reported a 67-year-old woman with a popliteal mass that metastasized to the lungs and resulted in the patient's death at 12 months.[65] In 2003, Abe and colleagues reported a parachordoma that arose in the calf of a 68-year-old male that metastasized to the lungs, bone, and skin after an amputation.[66]

Although most mixed tumor/myoepitheliomas of soft tissue are histologically and clinically benign, some cases locally recur, and others are either histologically malignant, clinically malignant, or both. In the series of 12 cutaneous and soft tissue myoepitheliomas by Michal and Miettinen,[48] one patient developed metastatic disease and died as a direct result of the tumor. Similarly, of the 10 patients with clinical follow-up information in the series by Kilpatrick et al.,[43] two patients developed local recurrence, and two additional patients developed lung and lymph node metastases and died of their tumor. In the much larger subsequent series reported by Hornick and Fletcher,[44] of the 33 histologically benign cases with follow-up, six locally recurred (18%), but none metastasized (mean follow-up of 36 months). Of the 31 histologically malignant cases with follow-up, 13 (42%) recurred and 10 (32%) metastasized (mean follow-up of 50 months). Four patients died of metastatic tumor with metastatic sites including lung, mediastinum, spine, orbit, bone, brain, and other unusual soft tissue sites (Table 36–8). There was no apparent correlation between margin status and risk of local recurrence, but local recurrence and metastasis were significantly more likely in patients with histologically malignant tumors. These authors suggested that the presence of at least moderate cytologic atypia (prominent nucleoli, vesicular or coarse chromatin, nuclear pleomorphism) warrants classification as a malignant myoepithelioma/myoepithelial carcinoma.[44]

As previously alluded to, there is no uniform agreement as to whether parachordoma is a distinct entity separate from mixed tumor/myoepithelioma, or whether it is simply a morphologic variant of a mixed tumor/myoepithelioma. Following the series of soft tissue myoepitheliomas reported by Kilpatrick et al. in 1997,[43] O'Connell and Berean suggested in a letter to the editor that some tumors reported as mixed tumor/myoepithelioma were likely examples of parachordoma.[67] In response

to that letter, Fletcher and Kilpatrick argued the point that parachordoma fits within the spectrum of mixed tumor/myoepithelioma,[68] focusing on the clinical, morphologic, and immunohistochemical overlap, as described above. Particularly compelling is the recognition of otherwise typical mixed tumor/myoepitheliomas with areas indistinguishable from parachordoma.[44] Further cytogenetic analysis of classic examples of parachordoma and mixed tumor/myoepithelioma will likely help to elucidate the histogenetic relationship between these tumors.

PLEOMORPHIC HYALINIZING ANGIECTATIC TUMOR OF SOFT PARTS

Initially described in 1996 in a series of 14 cases by Smith et al.,[69] pleomorphic hyalinizing angiectatic tumor of soft parts (PHAT) is a rare yet distinctive tumor of intermediate malignancy that differs in several respects from schwannoma on one hand and conventional "malignant fibrous histiocytoma" on the other. Since its initial description, fewer than 100 additional cases of PHAT have been reported in the literature,[70-77] and it is likely that this neoplasm continues to be mistaken for the above entities, among others. Accurate recognition of this neoplasm is of clinical importance given its propensity for local recurrence.

Clinical findings

Pleomorphic hyalinizing angiectatic tumor of soft parts characteristically arises in adults as a slowly enlarging mass that is often present for several years before coming to clinical attention. In the series of 41 cases reported by Folpe and Weiss, patients ranged in age from 10 to 79 years, with a median age of 51 years.[70] In most cases the clinical impression is that of a hematoma, a benign neoplasm, or even a Kaposi sarcoma. There may be a slight female predilection. The single most common site of the tumor is the subcutaneous tissue of the lower extremities. In the original series of 14 cases described by Smith et al.,[69] 11 tumors arose in the subcutaneous tissue, including eight in the lower extremities and one each in the buttock, chest wall, and arm. However, three tumors arose in skeletal muscle, one each in the shoulder, thigh, and chest wall. In the more recent and larger series by

TABLE 36–8	RISK OF LOCAL RECURRENCE AND METASTASIS IN 64 CASES OF SOFT TISSUE MYOEPITHELIOMA WITH FOLLOW-UP		
Histologic category	No. cases	Local recurrence (%)	Metastases (%)
Benign myoepithelial tumors	33	6 (18)	0 (0)
Malignant myoepithelial tumors	31	13 (42)	10 (32)

Modified from: Hornick JL, Fletcher CDM. Myoepithelial tumors of soft tissue: a clinicopathologic and immunohistochemical study of 101 cases with evaluation of prognostic parameters. Am J Surg Pathol 2003; 27:1183.

Folpe and Weiss,[70] the most common site was the lower extremity (ankle/foot in 15 cases and lower leg in 10 cases), followed by the thigh, perineum, buttock and arm (Table 36–9). Single cases arose in the axilla, back, and hand. The tumor ranges in size from less than 1 cm to up to 20 cm in greatest dimension, but most are in the range of 5–7 cm. Many patients have noted the presence of tumor for a significant period of time prior to seeking treatment.

Pathologic findings

Grossly, most tumors have a lobulated appearance with a cut surface that varies in color from white-tan to maroon (Fig. 36–40). Rare examples have a prominent cystic component, and others show conspicuous myxoid change. The tumors are not encapsulated; although some have fairly well-demarcated borders, most show diffusely infiltrative margins with trapping of normal tissues at the tumor periphery.

TABLE 36–9	ANATOMIC LOCATION OF 41 CASES OF PLEOMORPHIC HYALINIZING ANGIECTATIC TUMOR	
Anatomic location		**No. of cases**
Ankle/foot		15
Lower leg		10
Thigh		6
Perineum		3
Buttock		2
Arm		2
Axilla		1
Back		1
Hand		1
Total		41

Data from reference 70.

Microscopically, the most striking feature at low magnification is the presence of clusters of thin-walled ectatic blood vessels scattered throughout the lesion. The vessels range in size from small to macroscopic, and they tend to be distributed in small clusters (Figs 36–41, 36–42). Typically, the ectatic vessels are lined by endothelium with a thick subjacent rim of amorphous eosinophilic material that is often surrounded by lamellated collagen. Some vessels show organizing intraluminal thrombi with papillary endothelial hyperplasia. Hyaline material emanates from the vessels and extends into the stroma of the neoplasm, trapping neoplastic cells. The constituent cells are plump, spindled, and rounded with pleomorphic

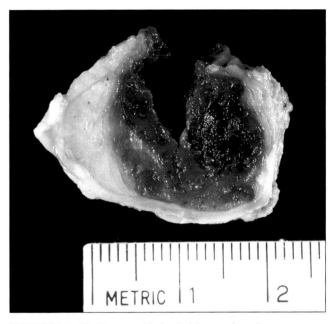

FIGURE 36–40 Pleomorphic hyalinizing angiectatic tumor. Gross specimen with a hemorrhagic appearance.

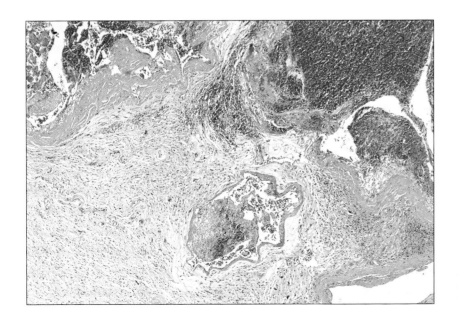

FIGURE 36–41 Pleomorphic hyalinizing angiectatic tumor with clusters of thin-walled ectatic vessels, a characteristic feature of this tumor.

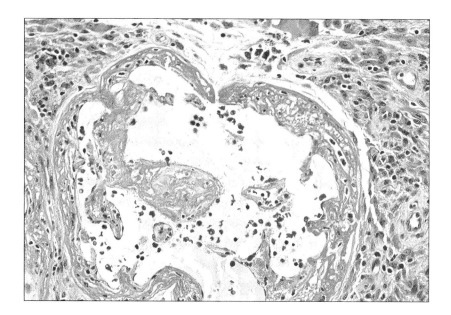

FIGURE 36–42 Characteristic high-power view of a vessel in a pleomorphic hyalinizing angiectatic tumor.

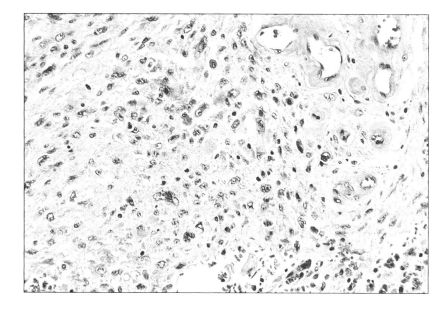

FIGURE 36–43 Pleomorphic nuclei in a pleomorphic hyalinizing angiectatic tumor. Despite the marked nuclear pleomorphism, mitotic figures are scarce.

nuclei arranged in sheets or occasionally in fascicles reminiscent of fibrosarcoma (Fig. 36–43). In general, the cells have hyperchromatic, pleomorphic nuclei lacking discernible cytoplasmic differentiation. Not uncommonly, intranuclear cytoplasmic inclusions are prominent (Fig. 36–44). Despite the striking degree of nuclear pleomorphism, mitotic figures are scarce (usually <1 MF/50 HPF). Occasional tumor cells, particularly those adjacent to ectatic vessels, contain intracytoplasmic hemosiderin. The tumors have a variable inflammatory infiltrate, most prominently mast cells, although in some lesions lymphocytes, plasma cells, and eosinophils are conspicuous. Foci of psammomatous calcification are occasionally present.

In the series reported by Folpe and Weiss, the authors emphasized the identification of a pattern at the periphery of some tumors, which they termed "early PHAT."[70] These areas are characterized by low to at most moderate cellularity composed of bland spindled cells with wavy nuclei arranged in fascicles (Fig. 36–45). The cells infiltrate the surrounding adipocytes in a manner reminiscent of dermatofibrosarcoma protuberans. Sometimes, these peripheral zones have clusters of abnormally arranged ectatic blood vessels with fibrin deposition, although the vascular changes are far less impressive than those found more centrally. Abundant, finely granular intracytoplasmic hemosiderin pigment is a conspicuous feature. Other features characteristic of PHAT including pleomorphic cells with intranuclear pseudoinclusions and a mixed inflammatory infiltrate may be found in early PHAT with careful searching.

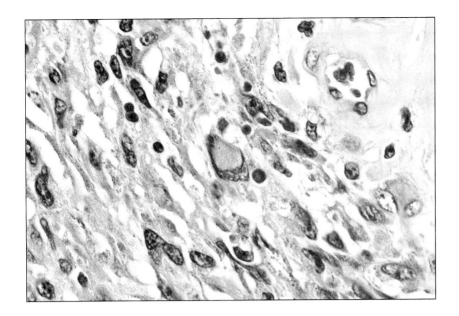

FIGURE 36–44 Pleomorphic hyalinizing angiectatic tumor with tumor cells that have prominent intranuclear cytoplasmic inclusions.

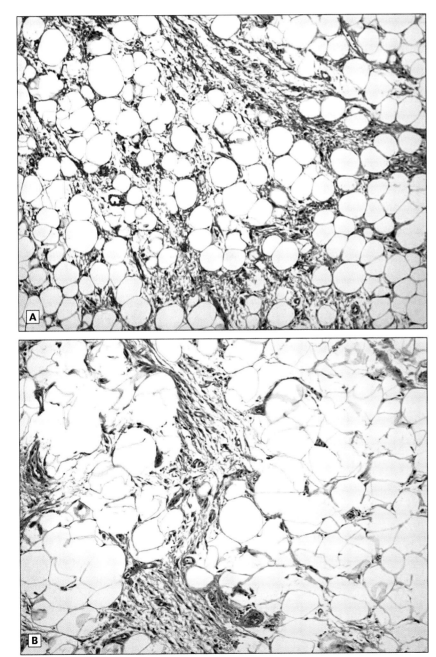

FIGURE 36–45 **(A)** "Early" PHAT characterized by a proliferation of bland spindled cells infiltrating mature adipose tissue. **(B)** Higher-magnification view of a more-cellular zone of "early" PHAT. Focal hemosiderin deposition is apparent.

Immunohistochemical and ultrastructural findings

Immunohistochemistry shows that the neoplastic cells do not stain for S-100 protein, thereby helping to exclude schwannoma as a diagnostic consideration. The cells consistently express vimentin, and most also stain for CD34.[78,79] Immunoreactivity for factor XIIIa may be present,[74] but the tumors generally do not express actin, desmin, cytokeratin, EMA, von Willebrand factor, or CD31. Groisman et al. reported immunoreactivity for vascular endothelial growth factor (VEGF), a secreted protein implicated in tumor-associated angiogenesis, in both tumoral and endothelial cells.[74]

Few PHATs have been evaluated by electron microscopy.[73] The neoplastic cells lack specific evidence of differentiation and generally contain large numbers of cytoplasmic filaments which have been confirmed to represent vimentin filaments by immunoelectron microscopy.[69] Overall, the cells have features suggesting fibroblastic differentiation.[73]

Differential diagnosis

Pleomorphic hyalinizing angiectatic tumor of soft parts bears a striking resemblance to *schwannoma*, although several light microscopic and immunohistochemical features allow their distinction. Unlike schwannoma, PHAT is not encapsulated and usually grows in an infiltrative manner. It lacks distinct Antoni A and B zones and does not express S-100 protein.

The tumor also resembles *psammomatous melanotic schwannoma*, as psammomatous calcifications are sometimes found in PHAT and intranuclear inclusions raise the possibility of a neural neoplasm. Unlike psammomatous melanotic schwannoma, which co-expresses S-100 protein and HMB-45, PHAT lacks these antigens.

The pronounced nuclear pleomorphism in the absence of specific features of differentiation also raises the possibility of a *pleomorphic sarcoma* ("MFH"). Despite the striking cellularity in many PHATs, this tumor lacks significant mitotic activity. In addition, intranuclear cytoplasmic inclusions are not a feature of pleomorphic sarcomas, nor is the expression of CD34.

Discussion

The clinical behavior of PHAT is characterized by local recurrence in up to 50% of cases, but metastases have not been documented. In the original study by Smith et al.,[69] follow-up information available for eight patients revealed that four (50%) developed local recurrence, including one patient with an aggressive recurrence necessitating amputation and another who suffered multiple recurrences over a 25-year period. In the larger and more recent study by Folpe and Weiss, six of 18 (33%) patients

with follow-up information developed local recurrences.[70] In addition, one case in their study showed histologic progression to a myxoid pleomorphic sarcoma in a recurrence. Wide local excision is recommended as the best therapeutic approach whenever possible.

Because of the paucity of reports of this neoplasm, its true nature has yet to be elucidated. The absence of S-100 protein immunoreactivity essentially negates the possibility that it is an unusual neural neoplasm. Some have suggested that PHAT is related to solitary fibrous tumor and giant cell angiofibroma given the overlapping histologic and immunohistochemical features,[71,72] but the expression of CD34 in PHAT seems to be a less consistent finding than in these other neoplasms.

The most striking histologic feature of PHAT is the hyalinizing angiectatic vasculature. This may reflect, in part, the slow growth of the tumor, as suggested by the low Ki-67 index and S-phase fraction.[69,71] It has also been suggested that deposition of hyaline material leads to progressive vascular obliteration and tumoral hypoxia, which in turn promotes vascular endothelial growth factor production by the neoplastic cells, resulting in active angiogenesis.[74]

The relationship of "early PHAT" to *hemosiderotic fibrohistiocytic lipomatous lesion* (HFLL) is intriguing. As originally described by Marshall-Taylor and Fanburg-Smith,[80] HFLL is a reactive lesion that typically occurs in the foot/ankle region of middle-aged patients and consists of an admixture of fat, moderately cellular fascicles of spindled cells with hemosiderin, macrophages, chronic inflammatory cells, and a focally myxoid stroma. This lesion also shows vascular hyalinization and scattered pleomorphic cells. Local recurrences were noted in 50% of cases, but none metastasized. Folpe and Weiss found a remarkable resemblance between "early PHAT" and HFLL, and suggested that HFLL is not a reactive lesion but rather a neoplastic one related to PHAT. These authors also hypothesized that the vascular changes were likely an early and pivotal event for the pathogenesis of PHAT since they were identified in the "early PHAT" lesions as well.[70]

HEMANGIOPERICYTOMA-SOLITARY FIBROUS TUMOR

The term hemangiopericytoma was first coined by Stout and Murray for tumors thought to originate from the pericytes, a modified dendritic-like smooth muscle cell encircling blood vessels (see Chapter 26). Unfortunately, the original descriptions by Stout were vague,[81–83] and it is clear that he included a number of lesions, such as myofibroma, under this rubric. It was not until the 1976 paper by Enzinger and Smith[84] that a more useful architectural and cytologic description of hemangiopericytoma was set forth. Their classic description emphasized the staghorn, partially hyalinized vessels surrounded by small rounded and fusiform cells which displayed no obvious light microscopic features of differentiation. Just as importantly, they made clear the importance of distinguishing hemangiopericytomas from other lesions that could have a pericytic vascular pattern, notably high-grade synovial sarcomas. In addition, they defined features that were associated with malignancy. The importance of this paper seemed forgotten over the years as the term hemangiopericytoma grew increasingly unpopular because pericytic differentiation could be confirmed in only a minority of cases ultrastructurally,[85-88] and actin, a marker of pericytes, was infrequently present in these lesions.[89-92] Moreover, as a diagnosis of exclusion, diagnostic reproducibility amongst pathologists was often poor.[93]

The waning popularity of the diagnosis of hemangiopericytoma also coincided with the increasing popularity of the diagnosis of solitary fibrous tumor (SFT), a pleural-based lesion first described by Klemperer and Rabin.[94] The observation that similar lesions occurred outside the pleura and had overlapping features with classic hemangiopericytoma, including CD34 immunoreactivity, paved the way for the popular belief that all hemangiopericytomas were, or should become, solitary fibrous tumors. This was not based on any quantum leap in the understanding of either tumor but rather observed histologic similarities between the two and a preference of one term over the other. Which term is better is debatable, and what lineage these lesions recapitulate is uncertain. Nevertheless, the acknowledgement that the two are similar, if not identical, is useful and has been endorsed by the World Health Organization.[95] A comparison of the two lesions, reflecting their similarity, is shown in Table 36–10.

Clinical features

Hemangiopericytoma-solitary fibrous tumor (HPC-SFT) is primarily a tumor of adult life which affects the sexes equally. It is located almost exclusively in deep soft tissue, particularly thigh, pelvic fossa, retroperitoneum, and serosal surfaces.[96] Although formerly believed to be restricted to the pleura, classic SFTs have been increasingly recognized in extrapulmonary sites.[97-100] Specific symptoms relate to the location of the tumor. Those in somatic soft tissue present as painless enlarging masses, whereas those within the abdominal cavity produce symptoms referable to impingement on specific organs. Serosal lesions are preferentially located on the pleura where they are usually discovered as incidental findings during work-up for another abnormality. Most are rounded, sharply outlined, homogeneous densities or masses on a pedicle which shifts with positional changes (Fig. 36–46). Less commonly, they grow endophytically into the lung[101] or as a plaque-like mass over the fissures.

Hypoglycemia has been reported in about 5% of HPC-SFTs, most often those located in the pelvis and retroperitoneum, and may lead to symptoms of sweating, headache, disorientation, convulsions, and even coma. It is mediated through production of insulin-like growth factors (IGFs) by the tumor.[102-104] IGFs and insulin-like growth factor receptor (IGF-R) mRNA can be identified in tumor cells even in the absence of clinical hypoglycemia.[105,106] Hypoglycemic symptoms abate with tumor removal. In addition, the IGFs stimulate proliferation of tumor cells through an autocrine loop that can be abolished when the receptors are inactivated.

Pathologic findings

Hemangiopericytoma-solitary fibrous tumors grow in deep soft tissue as a circumscribed mass (Fig. 36–47) or as exophytic lesions from the serosal surfaces (Fig. 36–48). Most measure 5–10 cm. in diameter and have a gray-white to red-brown color on cut section. Hemorrhage and cystic degeneration may be seen.

HPC-SFTs are highly variable in appearance depending on the relative proportion of cells and fibrous stroma. The cellular end of this spectrum corresponds to "classic hemangiopericytoma" (Figs 36–49 to 36–56) and the

TABLE 36–10	COMPARISON OF HEMANGIOPERICYTOMA AND SOLITARY FIBROUS TUMOR	
Parameter	**Hemangiopericytoma**	**Solitary fibrous tumor**
Location	Usually extremity	Usually body cavity, particularly pleura
Association with hypoglycemia	Yes	One-fourth[113]
Pericytic vascular pattern	+++ (definitional)	Focal
Spindling	Typically not	Yes
Broad zones of hyalinization	Variable to focal	Typical
Histologic malignant forms	Small number	Small number
CD34	Most positive	Virtually all positive
Cytogenetic abnormality	Abnormalities of 12q	Trisomy 21[130]
Comparative genomic hybridization	No gains/losses[129]	Frequent gains/losses[129]

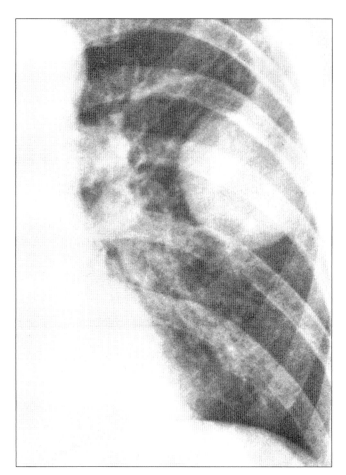

FIGURE 36–46 Radiograph of a solitary fibrous tumor of the pleura. Note the circumscribed mass in the left chest.

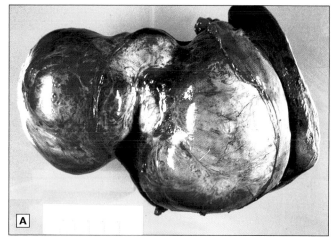

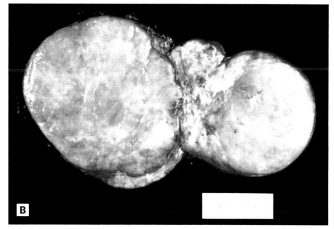

FIGURE 36–48 Solitary fibrous tumor growing as an exophytic mass from the surface of the liver **(A)**. Cut section shows a dense white interior **(B)**.

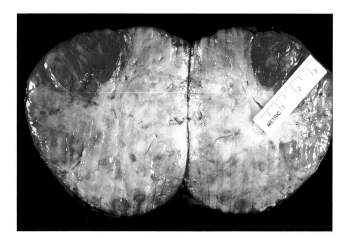

FIGURE 36–47 Gross specimen of a hemangiopericytoma.

hyalinized end to "classic solitary fibrous tumor." However, it should be emphasized that many cases have hybrid features (Fig. 36–57). Classic hemangiopericytoma consists of tightly packed round to fusiform cells with indistinct cytoplasmic borders which are arranged around an elaborate vasculature. The vessels form a con-

tinuous, ramifying vascular network which exhibits striking variation in caliber. As a rule, the dilated, branching vessels divide and communicate with small or minute vessels which may be partly compressed and obscured by the surrounding cellular proliferation. Typically, the dividing sinusoidal vessels have a "staghorn" or "antler-like" configuration (Fig. 36–49). Commonly, the vessels, particularly large ones, are invested with a thick coat of collagen which extends into the interstitium (Fig. 36–51). Myxoid change is common (Fig. 36–53) and, when extreme, may produce an appearance similar to a myxoid liposarcoma. However, the presence of coarse-walled vessels, interstitial hyalinization, and the absence of lipoblasts are important features that distinguish these hemangiopericytomas from myxoid liposarcomas. Similar changes have been observed in SFTs.[107]

In contrast, lesions having features of classic "solitary fibrous tumor" consist principally of spindle cells (Figs 36–58 to 36–62). The arrangement of the cells varies from area to area in the same tumor. In some zones the cells are arranged in short, ill-defined fascicles, whereas

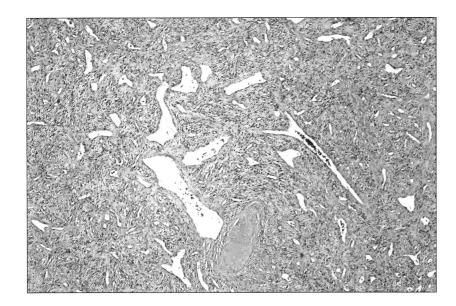

FIGURE 36-49 Hemangiopericytoma with a richly vascular pattern consisting of large and small vessels lined by a single layer of flattened endothelial cells.

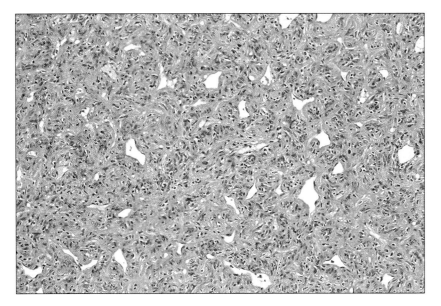

FIGURE 36-50 Hemangiopericytoma with predominantly small vessels.

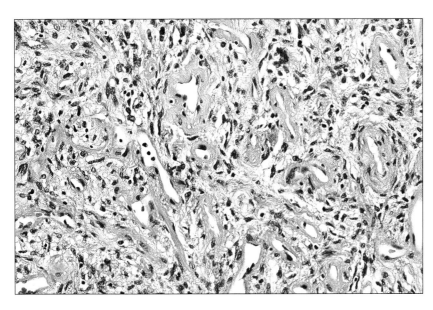

FIGURE 36-51 Hemangiopericytoma with perivascular hyalinization.

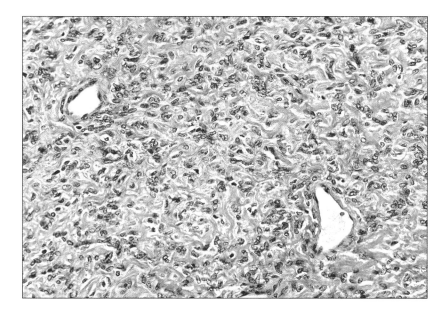

FIGURE 36–52 Hemangiopericytoma with interstitial hyalinization.

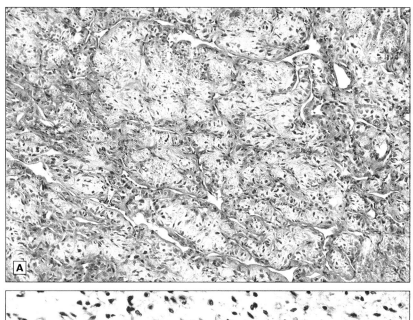

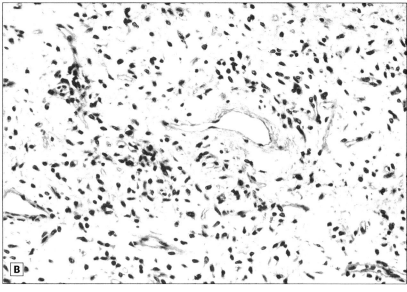

FIGURE 36–53 (A) Myoid change in a hemangiopericytoma. **(B)** At high power, vessels are seen to be thicker and less elaborate than those in a myxoid liposarcoma.

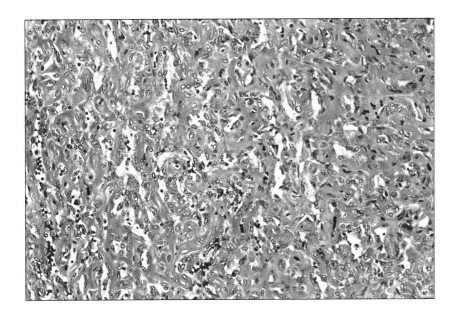

FIGURE 36–54 Pseudovascular pattern due to loss of cellular cohesion in a hemangiopericytoma.

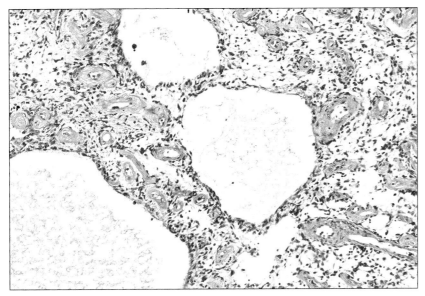

FIGURE 36–55 Cystic change in a hemangiopericytoma.

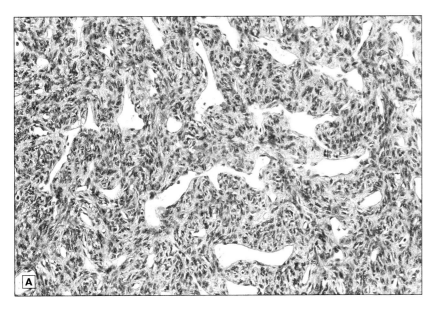

FIGURE 36–56 (A, B) The cells in hemangiopericytoma range from round/ovoid to slightly spindled.

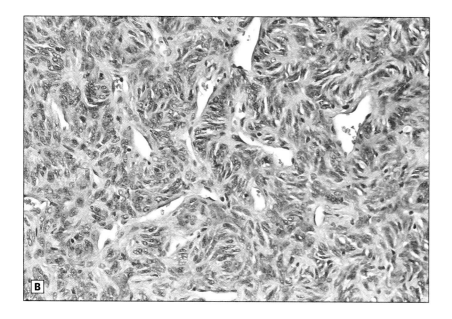

FIGURE 36–56 Continued.

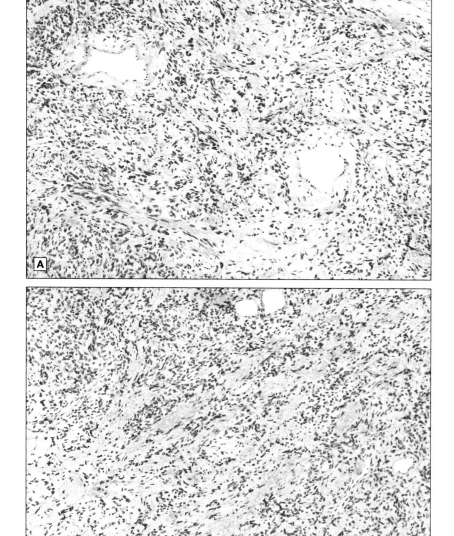

FIGURE 36–57 Tumor with features intermediate between a classic hemangiopericytoma and a classic solitary fibrous tumor. Tumor has a pericytic vascular pattern **(A)** but shows areas of interstitial hyalinization **(B)**, and more spindling of the tumor cells **(C)**.

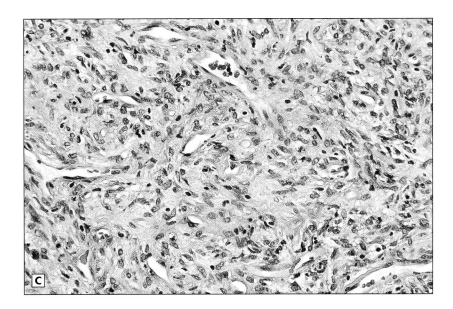

FIGURE 36–57 Continued.

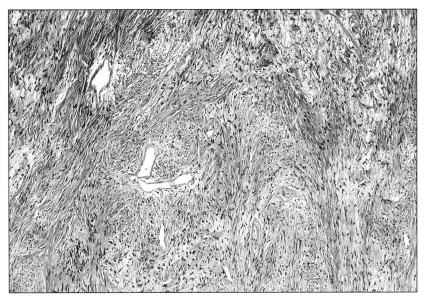

FIGURE 36–58 Solitary fibrous tumor with a heavily hyalinized area and focally prominent staghorn vessels.

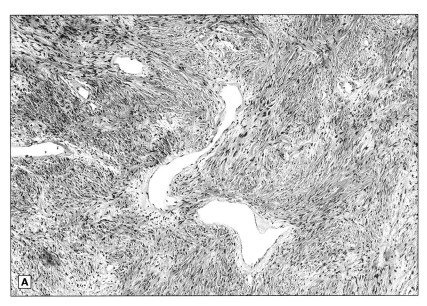

FIGURE 36–59 Solitary fibrous tumor showing a "pericytic" pattern **(A)** and "patternless pattern" **(B)** consisting of small fusiform cells randomly arranged between collagen bundles.

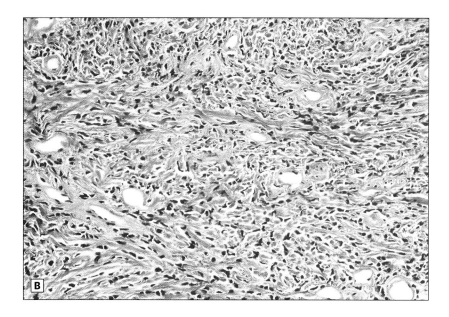

FIGURE 36–59 Continued.

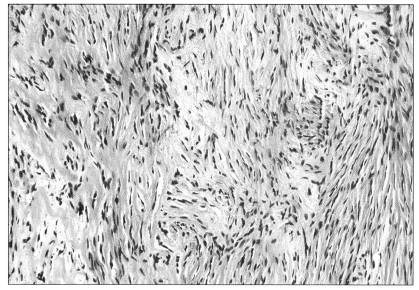

FIGURE 36–60 Solitary fibrous tumor with a characteristic cracking artifact between the cells and collagen.

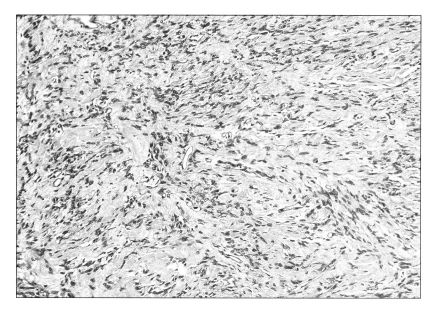

FIGURE 36–61 Solitary fibrous tumor with a staggered or grouped arrangement of cells in the collagen.

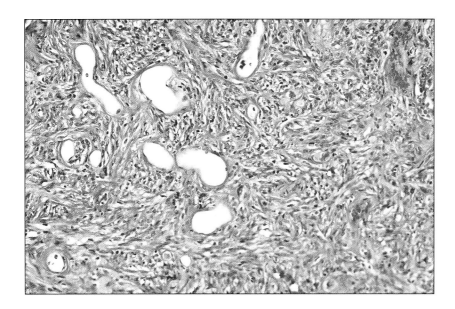

FIGURE 36–62 Solitary fibrous tumor with a hemangiopericytoma-like area.

in others they are arranged randomly in what has been described as a "patternless pattern." A characteristic feature of the lesion, which usually suggests the diagnosis even at low power, is the striking hyalinization. In these areas the cells are usually arranged singly or in small parallel clusters next to dense collagen. Artifactual "cracks" develop between the cells and collagen or between groups of collagen fibers (Fig. 36–60). Gaping staghorn vessels, while occasionally present, are not as striking as in classic hemangiopericytoma (Fig. 36–62).

A small subset of HPC-SFTs contain a variable amount of fat as an integral part of the tumor[108–109] and may be mistaken for well-differentiated or dedifferentiated liposarcomas (see below). Unusual features that can confuse the histologic picture of HPC-SFT are the presence of pseudovascular spaces created by the loss of cellular cohesion (Fig. 36–59), cystic change (Fig. 36–55), and giant cells (see below).

Malignancy in hemangiopericytoma-solitary fibrous tumor

The majority of HPC-SFTs are histologically benign. However, a small percentage of HPC-SFTs possess atypical features (Figs 36–63, 36–64). The criteria for malignancy in HPC vary from study to study. The criteria proposed by Enzinger and Smith for malignancy in classic hemangiopericytoma identify overtly malignant or high-grade lesions but fail to address low-grade lesions.[84] In their study, large size (>5 cm), increased mitotic rate (≥4 MF/10 HPF), high cellularity, presence of immature and pleomorphic tumor cells, and foci of hemorrhage and necrosis predicted a highly malignant course (Fig. 36–65). McMaster et al.,[96] in a review of 60 cases from the

Mayo Clinic, used similar but less stringent criteria for malignant behavior: either a slight degree of anaplasia and 1 MF/10 HPF or a moderate degree of cellular anaplasia and 1 MF/20 HPF. Most recently, Middleton et al.[91] associated recurrence or metastasis with a trabecular pattern, necrosis, mitoses, vascular invasion, and cellular atypia. In our practice, we identify lesions with the features reported by Enzinger and Smith as malignant, although we employ the term "low malignant potential" for lesions with lower levels of mitotic activity (1–3 MF/10 HPF), especially if they have any degree of atypia and cellularity. We do not use the term "malignant hemangiopericytoma" for round cell sarcomas which simply have a pericytic vascular pattern as most prove to be sarcomas of other types (e.g., synovial sarcoma). Malignancy in SFT has been assessed on very similar parameters as classic HPC and is defined by high cellularity, >4 MF/10HPF, and hemorrhage/necrosis.[110,112]

Immunohistochemical and ultrastructural findings

Many hemangiopericytomas express CD34 but usually in a smaller percentage of cases and to a lesser degree than solitary fibrous tumors (Fig. 36–66). SFT of pleural and extrapleural origin typically express CD34 (80–90%), CD99 (70%), bcl2 (30%),[88,110,113–117] EMA (30%), and actin (20%). Desmin (Fig. 36–67), cytokeratin, and S-100 protein are usually absent.[88] The high sensitivity of CD34 for solitary fibrous tumors has resulted in a more accurate and consistent diagnosis of the entity, undoubtedly accounting for the increasing number of solitary fibrous tumors now diagnosed at extrathoracic sites (Fig. 36–68).

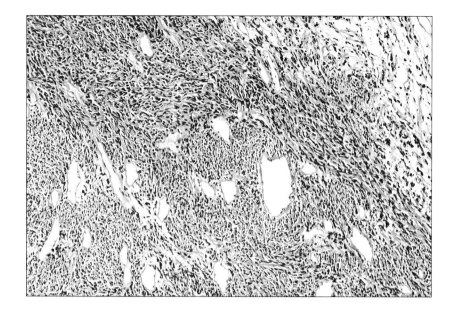

FIGURE 36–63 Malignant solitary fibrous tumor with heightened cellularity. Tumor also contained areas of histologically benign solitary fibrous tumor.

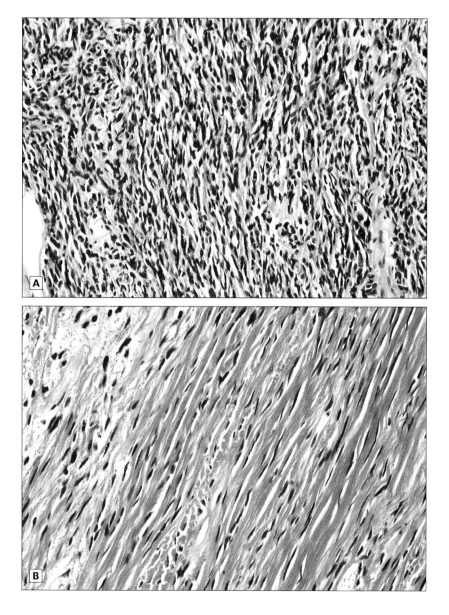

FIGURE 36–64 (A) Malignant area of a malignant solitary fibrous tumor. **(B)** High-power view of benign areas for comparison. Same case as in Figure 36–63.

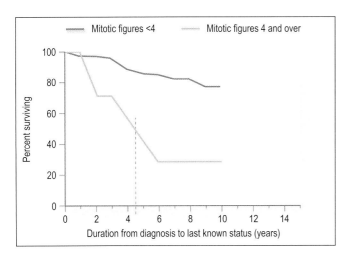

FIGURE 36-65 Actuarial survival rate of patients with hemangiopericytoma and relative survival based on the number of mitotic figures. Mitotic figures and necrosis are the two most important criteria when distinguishing benign from malignant hemangiopericytomas. (From Enzinger FM, Smith BH. Hemangiopericytoma: an analysis of 106 cases. Hum Pathol 1976; 7:61.)

Most early ultrastructural studies attempted to draw parallels between the cells of classic HPC and normal pericytes.[85,118] However, fewer than 30% of reported cases provided convincing evidence of pericytic differentiation.[88] Neoplastic cells are described as having rounded nuclei, an organelle-poor cytoplasm containing occasional arrays of microfilaments, cell processes, and poorly developed junctions. It has been pointed out that the cells comprising these tumors are fundamentally undifferentiated,[86] and it is only because of their topographic relation to blood vessels and their close association with periendothelial basement membrane that a relation to normal pericytes is inferred.[86] Moreover, mesenchymal cells that reside farther from the capillary may not display a close association with basement membrane.[85] SFTs seems to display considerable cellular heterogeneity. They contain fibroblasts, pericytes, undifferentiated perivascular cells and endothelial cells, leading some to conclude they arise from pluripotential perivascular cells.[119,120]

Differential diagnosis

The differential diagnosis of HPC-SFT is lengthy and includes both benign and malignant lesions having a prominent pericytic vascular pattern.

Fibrous histiocytoma, particularly its deep subcutaneous form, usually displays a more prominent, more uniform spindle-cell pattern than hemangiopericytoma, often with a distinct storiform arrangement of the tumor cells. There are, however, occasional examples of this tumor in which distinction may be exceedingly difficult and many such lesions seem to occur in the orbit.

Synovial sarcoma, in about 10–20% of cases, exhibits a distinctive but focal hemangiopericytoma-like pattern. This pattern usually occurs in high-grade round cell areas of the synovial sarcoma. The caliber of the vascular channels does not have a broad range as is seen in hemangiopericytomas. Synovial sarcomas are almost always associated with distinct spindle cells, hyalinized-calcified areas, glands, and expression of cytokeratin.

Mesenchymal chondrosarcoma simulates the features of hemangiopericytoma in the closely packed small-cell areas but is readily recognizable by the presence of islands of well-differentiated cartilage or, much less frequently, bone. Ill-defined foci of immature cartilage may also be present in the small-cell component (see Chapter 33).

Juxtaglomerular tumors that secrete renin and cause hypertension may also be misinterpreted as hemangiopericytomas,[121-124] especially those rare lesions that occur in extrarenal locations such as the retroperitoneum. In most of these neoplasms large epithelioid cells and thick-walled vessels are present, and some contain PAS-positive renin crystals.

Cytogenetic findings

Several balanced translocations have been observed in hemangiopericytomas, including t(12;19),[125,126] t(13;22),[127] and t(3;12).[128] The single most common abnormality are rearrangements of the long arm of chromosome 12, a site similar to those affected in lipomas and leiomyomas. Comparative genomic hybridization shows that hemangiopericytomas do not display any change in DNA copy numbers, unlike the solitary fibrous tumor.[129] However, trisomy 21 has been noted in a SFT.[130]

Discussion

The clinical behavior of HPC-SFT has traditionally been a problematic area, largely because of inclusional criteria. Studies often do not make clear whether classic HPC, classic SFT, or both were analyzed. Frequently the proportion of lesions with overtly malignant versus conventional features is not clear. Thus, there is pressing need to analyze the entire spectrum of lesions in a standard fashion to determine if there are inherent differences between the two ends of this spectrum.

The recent experience reported from Memorial Sloan-Kettering Cancer Center found a 93% and 80% 2- and 5-year survival rate, respectively, for classic hemangiopericytoma but made no mention if histologically malignant tumors were included.[131] It was noted that all patients undergoing complete surgical excision were alive at 5 years. Poorer survivals were reported from M.D. Anderson Cancer Center, possibly because of the

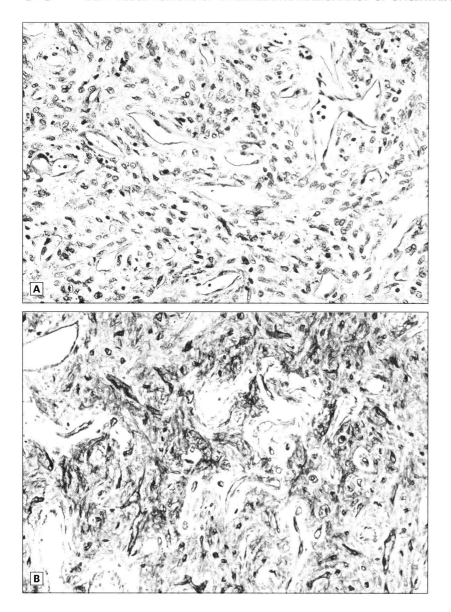

FIGURE 36–66 CD34 immunostain in hemangiopericytomas. Most tumors are positive, but staining may be relatively focal **(A)** or occasionally diffuse **(B)**.

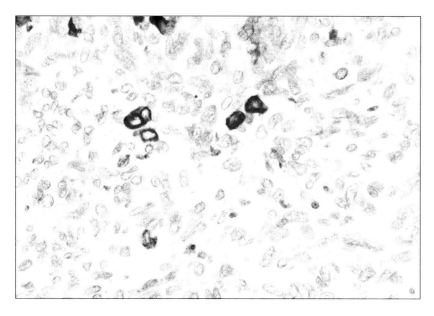

FIGURE 36–67 Rarely, tumor cells in hemangiopericytomas are desmin-positive.

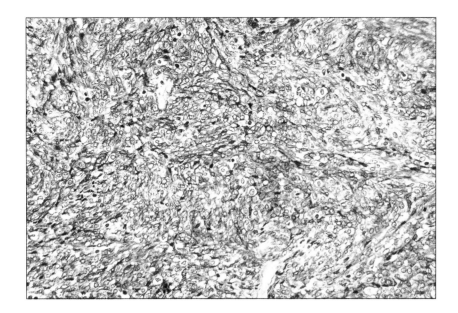

FIGURE 36–68 CD34 immunostain in a solitary fibrous tumor showing diffuse staining.

inclusion of histologically malignant cases. Metastases were noted in about 30% of patients with a 5-year actuarial survival of 71%.[132] Significantly higher disease-free survival and lower local recurrence rates were associated with extremity lesions versus meningeal and retroperitoneal lesions.

Overall, thoracic and extrathoracic SFTs are quite similar clinically and biologically.[111] The majority have rather banal or benign histologic features and pursue a favorable course. Those that have "malignant" areas, generally defined as areas of high cellularity, >4 MF/10 HPF, and hemorrhage/necrosis,[111,112] are at risk for metastasis. This principle is well illustrated by the following studies. In the most extensive series of thoracic solitary fibrous tumors reported from a single institution, two-thirds were judged benign on the basis of a number of histologic parameters.[133] All but two of the patients in this group were free of disease following simple excision or wedge resection of the lung. Malignant tumors had a more variable outcome. Approximately one-half of the patients were cured of their tumors following excision, whereas the remainder developed recurrences, metastases, or both (Table 36–11). Overall, the metastatic rate of solitary fibrous tumors was 9% (16 of 169 with follow-up information). In addition to the criteria mentioned above, nonpedunculated growth and an atypical location (e.g., parietal pleura, interlobar fissure, mediastinum, or endophytic growth into lung) was also correlated with more aggressive behavior (Table 36–12). Two other studies reaffirmed these observations. Vallat-Decouvelaere et al.[110] reported their experience from a large consultation service and indicated that approximately 10% of extrathoracic solitary fibrous tumors have atypical features (cellularity, atypia, >4 MF/10 HPF, necrosis) or a history of local recurrence. Eight of 10 patients in this category

TABLE 36–11	CLINICAL BEHAVIOR OF INTRATHORACIC SOLITARY FIBROUS TUMORS	
Histologic diagnosis*	**Recurrence (%)**	**Metastases (%)**
Benign	2	0
Malignant†	39	22

Data from England DM, Hochholzer L, McCarthy MJ. Localized benign and malignant fibrous tumors of the pleura: a clinicopathologic review of 223 cases. Am J Surg Pathol 1989; 13:640.
*There were 98 benign tumors with follow-up ranging from 1 to 317 months (median 57 months) and 71 malignant tumors with follow-up ranging from 2 to 372 months (median 31 months).
†Tumors were classified as malignant based on one or more of the following features in any portion of tumor: high cellularity with crowded overlapping nuclei, >4 mitoses/10 HPF, nuclear atypia, pleomorphic giant cells, and atypical mitoses.

TABLE 36–12	FEATURES ASSOCIATED WITH MALIGNANCY IN SOLITARY FIBROUS TUMORS	
Thoracic[133]		**Soft tissue[98]**
Histologic features		
Increased cellularity		Increased cellularity
Pleomorphism		Pleomorphism
Mitoses (>4/10 HPF)		Mitoses (>4/10 HPF)
Clinical/gross features		
Nonpedunculated		
Atypical location (parietal pleura, parenchyma)		
Size >10 cm		
Necrosis/hemorrhage		

developed local recurrences, and five died of distant metastasis. A more recent study of 79 cases of both thoracic and extrathoracic lesions also found that large size (>10 cm) and presence of malignant areas predicted metastasis.[111] However, size and malignant areas were not independent variables. Based on these data, it has been suggested that most SFTs with benign histologic features can be treated by surgery alone, whereas those with "malignant" areas require adjuvant therapy of some type.[111]

VARIANTS OF HEMANGIOPERICYTOMA-SOLITARY FIBROUS TUMOR

Lipomatous hemangiopericytoma-solitary fibrous tumor

Lipomatous HPC-SFT is a rare variant that contains a variable amount of mature fat as an integral part of the tumor[108,109] (Figs 36–69, 36–70). Microscopically, they consist of areas of histologically benign HPC-SFT admixed with microscopic or macroscopic areas of mature fat. In the typical case, about one-fourth to three-fourths of the tumor is mature fat. In some areas, spindling of the peri-

cytic areas creates a resemblance to a spindle cell lipoma. To date, all the lesions with follow-up information have behaved in a benign fashion, although a few have recurred. The principal significance of this variant is that it is easily mistaken for a well-differentiated liposarcoma, particularly when only a small biopsy specimen is available. In these situations it is helpful to be apprised of the clinical features that suggest a relatively circumscribed, rather than infiltrative, mass.

Meningeal (cranial and intraspinal) hemangiopericytoma-solitary fibrous tumor

Meningeal hemangiopericytomas are indistinguishable from HPC-SFTs at other sites and are no longer considered variants of meningioma.[92,134,135] Unlike conventional meningiomas, meningeal HPC-SFTs lack S-100 protein

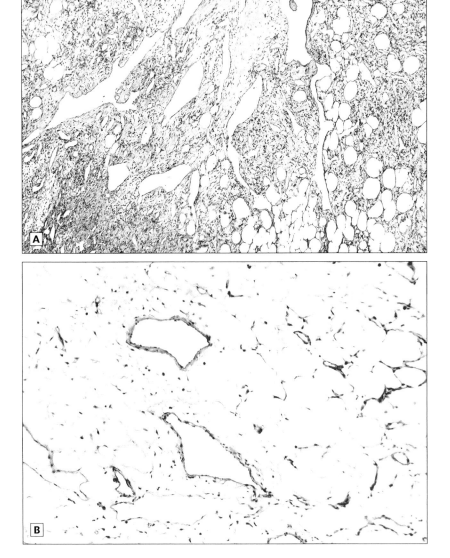

FIGURE 36–69 Lipomatous hemangiopericytoma, showing a range of appearances, from areas having only focal fat **(A)** to those that are predominantly fatty **(B)**.

and EMA, and they do not display mutations in the *NF2* locus on chromosome 22.[136,137] They express vimentin as the sole intermediate filament. They occur at a younger age than meningiomas, grow more often along the sinuses, bleed profusely at operation, and have a tendency to recur. They may metastasize to extracranial sites. Guthrie et al.,[138] in a review of 44 meningeal HPC-SFTs, reported 5- and 15-year survival rates of 67% and 23%, respectively. Mena et al.,[139] in another large series, noted a recurrence rate of 60.6% and a metastatic rate of 23.4%.

Hemangiopericytoma-solitary fibrous tumor with giant cells (giant cell angiofibroma)

A giant-cell-rich form of HPC-SFT was described by Dei Tos as "giant cell angiofibroma."[140] Although originally

identified in the orbital region, this tumor may occur in diverse locations.[141] It displays all the features of a classic SFT but is identified by pseudovascular spaces (resulting from a loss of cellular–stromal cohesion) lined by multinucleated stromal giant cell (Figs 36–71 to 36–74).

INFANTILE HEMANGIOPERICYTOMA

Infantile hemangiopericytoma deserves separate consideration because of its different histologic picture and clinical behavior from adult HPC-SFT. These lesions mostly occur in infants during the first year of life and, like juvenile hemangiomas, are mostly located in the subcutis and oral cavity.[142,143] Tumors in older children and deep-seated tumors in the muscle, mediastinum, and abdomen have also been described.[144,145] Alpers et al.[142]

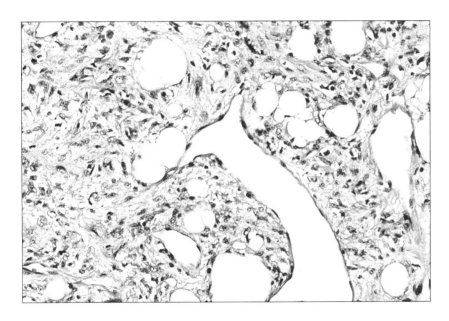

FIGURE 36–70 Lipomatous hemangiopericytoma.

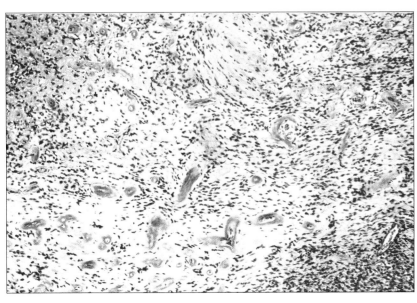

FIGURE 36–71 Giant cell angiofibroma with cellular proliferation of spindle-shaped cells between small blood vessels with marked perivascular hyalinization.

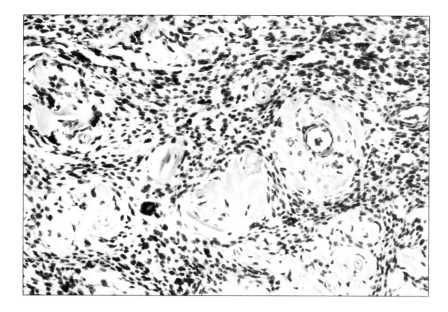

FIGURE 36–72 High-power view of a giant cell angiofibroma with cellular spindle cell proliferation between hyalinized blood vessels and scattered multinucleated floret-like giant cells.

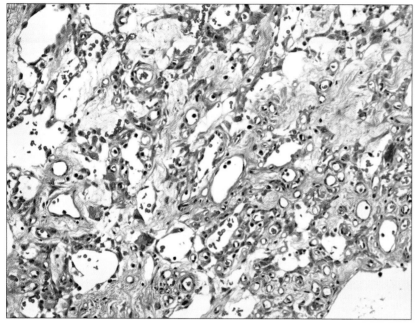

FIGURE 36–73 Scattered multinucleated giant cells in a giant cell angiofibroma.

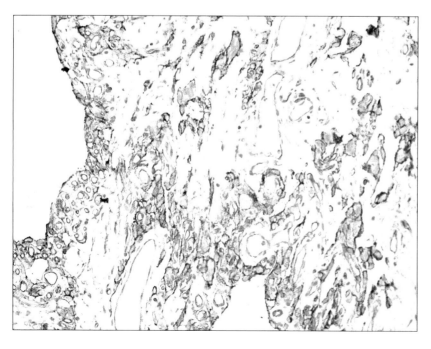

FIGURE 36–74 CD34 immunoreactivity in a giant cell angiofibroma.

reported an infantile hemangiopericytoma of the tongue and sublingual region that was discovered at birth, grew in an infiltrative manner, and recurred rapidly after local excision. After 30 months, the child was well with no evidence of further recurrence or metastasis. All lesions in our cases have been solitary, but there are rare accounts of patients with multiple tumors.[146] One was associated with Kasabach-Merritt syndrome.[146]

Microscopically, infantile hemangiopericytoma bears a close resemblance to the adult type, but many lesions, especially superficial ones, are multilobulated, often with distinct intravascular and perivascular satellite nodules outside the main tumor mass (Fig. 36–75A) and frequent endovascular growth (Fig. 36–75B). There is often increased mitotic activity and focal necrosis, features that indicate a poor prognosis for adult-type hemangiopericytomas but generally do not with the infantile form. Judging from our cases and the literature, most of these tumors tend to follow a benign clinical course; they are curable by local excision or may regress spontaneously.[146,147] In rare instances, however, there may be local infiltrative growth or recurrence and even

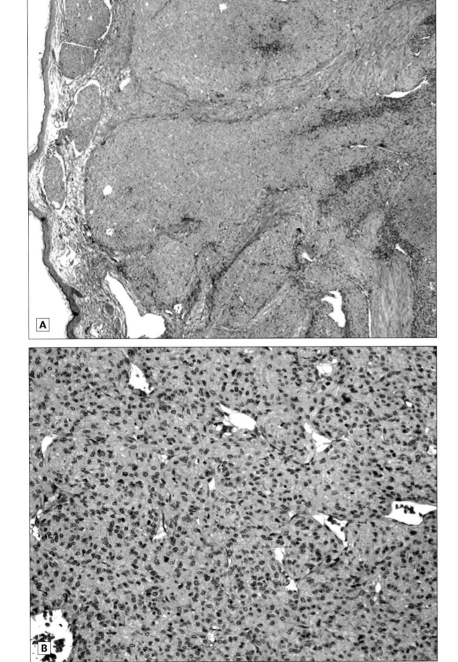

FIGURE 36–75 **(A)** Low-magnification view of infantile hemangiopericytoma with the typical multilobular arrangement of tumor cells. **(B)** Higher-magnification view of infantile hemangiopericytoma.

metastasis.[148] Deep-seated lesions and those occurring in older children seem to pursue a more aggressive clinical course than superficial ones that appear during the first years of life.

The hemangiopericytoma-like pattern found in the lobular or tufted hemangioma (a variant of lobular capillary hemangioma marked by dermal or subcutaneous capillary or vascular lobules), infantile myofibromatosis, and infantile fibrosarcoma must be distinguished from that of infantile hemangiopericytoma (see Chapters 10 and 22). Other benign and malignant neoplasms that may cause diagnostic difficulty include the juvenile hemangioma, glomus tumor, angiosarcoma, vascular forms of leiomyoma and leiomyosarcoma, endometrial stromal sarcoma, malignant peripheral nerve sheath tumor, mesothelioma, and liposarcoma.

PHOSPHATURIC MESENCHYMAL TUMOR, MIXED CONNECTIVE TISSUE TYPE

For over nearly 50 years, it has been known that tumors of various types could be associated with osteomalacia.[149] In 1987, Weidner and Santa Cruz[150] made a seminal observation that most osteomalacia-associated tumors had a very similar and distinctive appearance and proposed the term "phosphaturic mesenchymal tumor of the mixed connective tissue type" (PMTMCT) for this specific group of lesions. Their work was not fully appreciated, because tumors associated with oncogenic osteomalacia continued to be reported under a variety of terms including hemangiopericytoma, chondroblastoma, giant cell tumor, and osteosarcoma.[149] The most authoritative paper on the subject by Folpe et al.[151] has reaffirmed these findings in a large series of 32 cases accompanied by an analysis of the literature. Over 80% of osteomalacia-associated mesenchymal tumors conform to the PMTMCT, the features of which are so distinctive that the diagnosis can be made even in the absence of the clinical symptomatology.[151]

The majority of patients are adults who present with a long history of osteomalacia characterized by phosphaturia, hyperphosphatemia, decreased serum 1,25 dihydroxyvitamin D3 levels, and resistance to vitamin D treatment, all of which abate following removal of the tumor. The majority of these tumors occur in soft tissue with a lesser number in bone. They are composed of small, rounded, fusiform, or spindled cells embedded within a smudgy matrix containing a delicate capillary vascular pattern (Fig. 36–76). The matrix undergoes calcification which results in flocculent deposits of mineral salts encrusting the cells (Fig. 36–77). Bone may also be deposited. By immunohistochemistry, the tumor cells express fibroblast growth factor 23, the putative substance responsible for the renal phosphate wasting. Following

removal of these tumors the symptoms regress. There have been a few cases of histologically malignant PMTMCTs which metastasized.

PERIVASCULAR EPITHELIOID CELL FAMILY OF TUMORS

The term perivascular epithelioid cell neoplasm (PEComa) has been applied to a growing family of tumors composed of histologically and immunohistochemically distinctive perivascular epithelioid cells. This family includes renal and extrarenal angiomyolipoma (AML), lymphangiomyomatosis (LAM), clear cell "sugar" tumor of the lung (CCST), and a number of extrapulmonary spindled and epithelioid neoplasms that have been referred to by a variety of names including primary extrapulmonary sugar tumor (PEST),[152] clear cell myomelanocytic tumor,[153] and abdominopelvic sarcoma of perivascular epithelioid cells.[154]

The concept of a family of tumors composed of these distinctive perivascular epithelioid cells has evolved over the last century. Renal AML and its association with the tuberous sclerosis complex (TSC) has been recognized for many years.[155] In the late 1960s and early 1970s, LAM and CCST were formally described.[156,157] Valensi reported the association between LAM and TSC in 1973,[158] and the next year, Monteforte and Kohnen noted the association between AML and LAM.[159] A breakthrough observation occurred in 1991, when Pea et al. identified HMB-45 immunoreactivity and premelanosomes in renal AML.[160] Identical observations were made in hepatic AML,[161] pulmonary CCST,[162] and LAM,[163] thereby solidifying the concept that AML, LAM, and CCST were related to one another morphologically, immunohistochemically, and through their association with TSC. The PEComa family of tumors subsequently grew quickly following the 1996 report by Zamboni and colleagues of a pancreatic tumor that was morphologically identical to CCST.[164] PEComa of both epithelioid and spindle-cell type have been reported in a wide variety of intra-abdominal, bone, soft tissue, and visceral sites, including the falciform ligament/ligamentum teres, mesentery, uterus, heart, thigh, and gastrointestinal tract. The following discussion will focus on AML, LAM, and non-AML, non-LAM PEComas.

Angiomyolipoma

The term *angiomyolipoma (AML)* should be reserved for a specific lesion arising most commonly in one or both kidneys as a solitary or multicentric mass; rarely, the mass is a pedunculated growth or presents as a satellite nodule outside the renal capsule. Multiple and bilateral lesions are less common than solitary ones and are more often encountered in patients with tuberous sclerosis.[155]

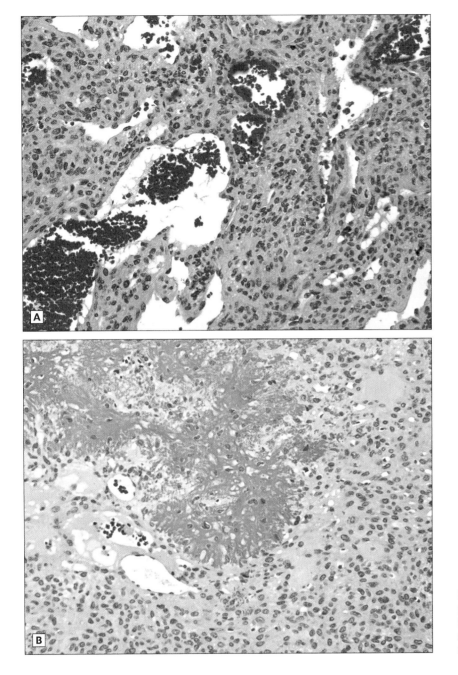

FIGURE 36–76 (A) Phosphaturic mesenchymal tumor, mixed connective tissue type, illustrating bland rounded cells situated around an intricate vasculature and **(B)** matrix containing the smudgy blue-gray material.

Clinical findings

Angiomyolipoma occurs more commonly in women than men, with a median age in the fifth decade of life. In about two-thirds of cases it causes symptoms such as abdominal or flank pain, hematuria, or chills and fever. Less commonly, it is asymptomatic and is discovered as an incidental finding at operation for some unrelated cause or at autopsy. Rarely, sudden, severe flank pain and shock are caused by rupture of the tumor and massive perirenal or retroperitoneal hemorrhage.[165] Rare instances of associated hypertension have been recorded.[166] Although most lesions occur in the kidney, extrarenal sites of AML include the liver,[167,168] nasal cavity,[169] oral cavity,[170] colon,[171] lung,[172] and skin.[173]

Approximately one-third of patients present with manifestations of the TSC, ranging from hyperpigmented spots, shagreen patches, periungual fibromas, and angiofibromas to renal cysts, cardiac rhabdomyoma, and gliosis and calcification of the cerebral cortex with mental deficiency.[174,175] There are also rare cases in which the tumor is associated with LAM[176,177] and renal cell carcinoma.[178] Computed tomography (CT) scans and MRI reveal a fatty mass with intermixed soft tissue densities, except in those cases in which the absence of fat or hemorrhage obscures the radiologic findings.[179]

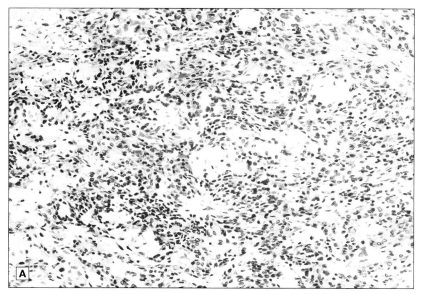

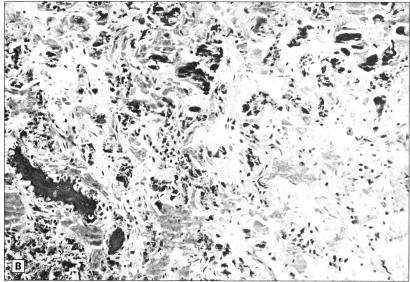

FIGURE 36–77 Phosphaturic mesenchymal tumor associated with osteomalacia. This distinctive subset of tumors is associated with oncogenic osteomalacia and consists of primitive mesencymal cells associated with a prominent vasculature **(A)** and calcification. **(B)** Some of these tumors have been labeled "hemangiopericytoma."

Pathologic findings

Grossly, the lesion presents as a yellow to gray mass, varying in size from a few centimeters to 20 cm or more (average 9 cm). Large lesions may become attached to the diaphragm or liver. Focal hemorrhage is present in about half of the cases. The tumor is usually well delineated from the surrounding renal parenchyma (Fig. 36–78). Some tumors extend into the inferior vena cava,[180] and others involve perirenal lymph nodes,[181] both of which may contribute to a presumed diagnosis of malignancy.

Microscopically, AML is composed of three tissue components that vary greatly in distribution: (1) mature adipose tissue with some variations in cellular size and nuclear appearance; (2) convoluted thick-walled blood vessels with little or no abnormal elastica and frequent hyalinization of the media; and (3) irregularly arranged sheets and interlacing bundles of smooth muscle often with a prominent perivascular arrangement (Figs 36–79, 36–80). In some cases the smooth muscle element displays a striking degree of cellular pleomorphism, with hyperchromatic nuclei, occasional multinucleated giant cells, and necrotic foci (Fig. 36–81). Additionally, there may be epithelioid smooth muscle cells containing spherical granules and dense PAS-positive, needle-shaped or rhomboid crystals similar to those in juxtaglomerular tumors, but the cells do not stain for renin (Fig. 36–82).[182–184] Some cases of AML show profound cystic change, which may obscure the recognition of this tumor.[185]

Immunohistochemically, the smooth muscle cells of AML are not only immunoreactive for actin and desmin but also, unlike other smooth muscle tumors, express the melanoma-associated antigen HMB-45 (Fig. 36–83).[160] In addition to HMB-45, other markers of melanocytic differentiation including Melan A, MiTF, and

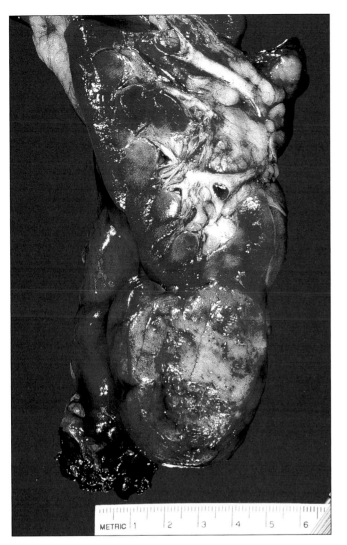

FIGURE 36–78 Angiomyolipoma of the kidney. The lesion, well circumscribed, is broadly attached to one pole of the kidney. Focal hemorrhage within the nodule is apparent.

tyrosinase have been identified in the majority of these lesions.[186-188] A significant percentage of cases stain for progesterone receptors and, less commonly, estrogen receptors.[189-191] CD117 (KIT) is also expressed in the majority of tumors.[192]

Ultrastructurally, many of these muscle cells contain myofilaments, glycogen particles, and electron-dense granules. As previously mentioned, premelanosomes are often identified.[155]

Cytogenetic findings

Although relatively few of these lesions have been studied by cytogenetics, some have been found to show trisomy 7 or 8,[193,194] and others reveal loss of heterozygosity of the TSC genes on chromosomes 9q34 (*TSC1*) and 16p13 (*TSC2*).[189,195] Loss of hamartin and tuberin expression, the products of *TSC1* and *TSC2* genes, respectively, can be detected in AML with *TSC1* and *TSC2* mutations.[196]

Differential diagnosis

Although the histologic appearance of the tumor is characteristic and should not cause difficulty with the diagnosis, rare cases of AML are mistaken for *sarcomas* or *carcinomas*. Those tumors that have a prominent fatty component may be mistaken for *liposarcoma*. The presence of convoluted thick-walled blood vessels and immunoreactivity for HMB-45 in the smooth muscle cells allows their distinction. AML with an inconspicuous fatty component may be confused with *leiomyosarcoma*, particularly those that are large, hypercellular, and pleomorphic. This distinction may be particularly challenging on a needle biopsy specimen. The smooth muscle cells of AML tend to be plumper and paler than those found in leiomyosarcoma, and HMB-45 immunoreactivity can be

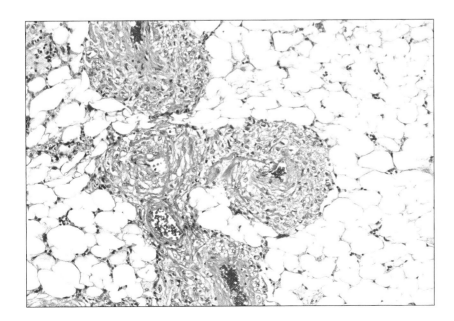

FIGURE 36–79 Angiomyolipoma with the basic components of the tumor: mature adipose tissue and smooth muscle surrounding thick-walled, medium-sized, vascular channels.

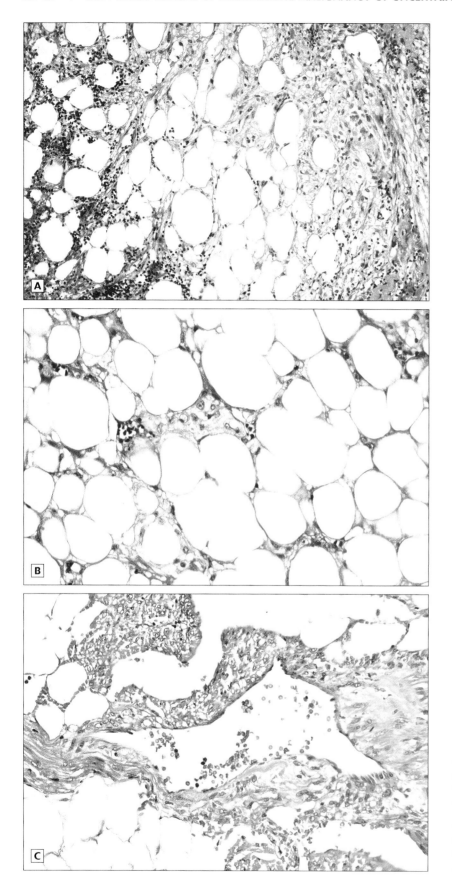

FIGURE 36–80 **(A)** Angiomyolipoma exhibiting an admixture of mature fat cells and vacuolated smooth muscle cells.
(B) Isolated vacuolated smooth muscle cells in an angiomyolipoma. Areas such as this could be mistaken for liposarcoma, particularly when the cells show cytologic atypia.
(C) Angiomyolipoma with collections of vacuolated smooth muscle cells arranged around dilated vascular spaces.

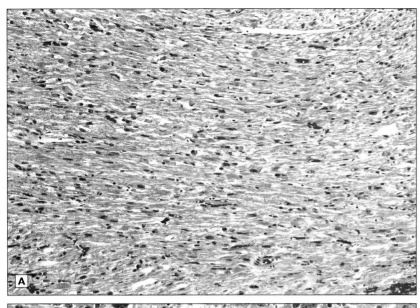

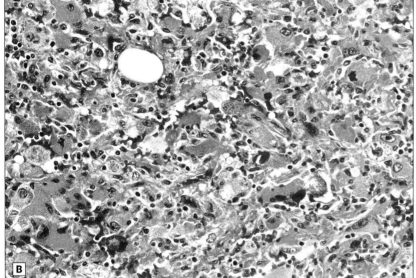

FIGURE 36–81 (A) Angiomyolipoma with an area composed of atypical spindle-shaped smooth muscle cells arranged in fascicles. Such areas could be confused for leiomyosarcoma or dedifferentiated liposarcoma with divergent leiomyosarcomatous differentiation. **(B)** Angiomyolipoma exhibiting striking variation in the size and shape of smooth muscle elements, with rare cells showing marked cytologic atypia, a feature that has been mistaken for evidence of malignancy.

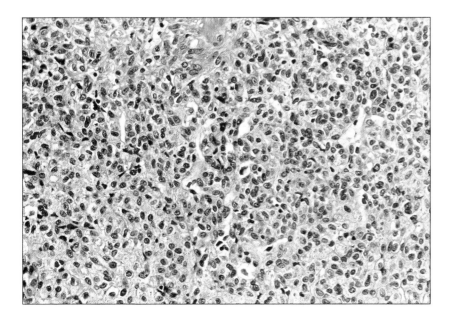

FIGURE 36–82 Angiomyolipoma composed of uniform small epithelioid smooth muscle cells, a feature that could be mistaken for renal cell carcinoma, particularly in patients with tuberous sclerosis.

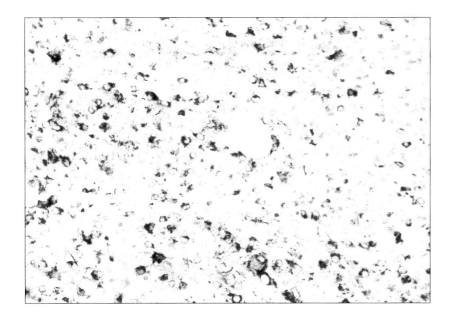

FIGURE 36-83 HMB-45 immunoreactivity in the smooth muscle cells of an angiomyolipoma.

extremely useful in this setting. Given that both renal cell carcinoma and AML are associated with the tuberous sclerosis complex, some epithelioid AML are confused with renal cell carcinoma, and vice versa. The use of EMA and HMB-45 immunostains should allow the distinction of these two lesions.

Discussion

Typical renal AML virtually always acts in a clinically benign fashion, even those with atypical features. There is no evidence that the presence of regional or systemic lymph node involvement, perirenal satellite tumors, or angiomyolipomatous growth in other organs reflect malignant potential.[155,197] There are, however, very rare examples of otherwise typical AML that have transformed to an overtly sarcomatous epithelioid or spindled neoplasm with subsequent malignant behavior.[198,199] On the other hand, epithelioid renal AML does harbor metastatic potential, especially those cases showing necrosis and/or marked nuclear atypia.[200-206] In their review of the literature, Hornick and Fletcher approximated that one-third of reported epithelioid AML have resulted in metastases, occasionally resulting in patient death.[200] Several of the cases reported by Pea et al. of "renal cell carcinoma," which they reclassified as monotypic epithelioid angiomyolipoma, were characterized by an aggressive clinical course.[201] Similarly, L'Hostis et al. reported a case of a "monophasic epithelioid pleomorphic" angiomyolipoma that metastasized to the liver and paravertebral region resulting in the patient's death 2 years after presentation.[207] For whatever reason, hepatic AML, including epithelioid variants, usually act in a clinically benign fashion, with rare exception.[208]

AML typically grows slowly and is adequately treated by partial nephrectomy. Small, asymptomatic tumors may require only careful follow-up, although total nephrectomy may be necessary for large tumors. Cases have also been treated successfully by therapeutic embolization or cryotherapy.[209]

Lymphangiomyoma and lymphangiomyomatosis

Lymphangiomyomatosis (LAM) is a rare disease characterized by a proliferation of perivascular epithelioid cells[210,211] around lymphatics and lymph nodes of the mediastinum, retroperitoneum, and the pulmonary interstitium.[212] Localized lesions are referred to as lymphangiomyoma, whereas extensive lesions involving large segments of the lymphatic chain with or without pulmonary involvement are designated lymphangiomyomatosis. LAM and tuberous sclerosis appear to be overlapping diseases. Patients with pulmonary LAM and tuberous sclerosis-associated renal angiomyolipomas share a common allelic loss of the *TSC2* gene.[213,214] In addition, 1% of patients with tuberous sclerosis have changes in the lung very similar to LAM. Conversely, 15% of patients with LAM have angiomyolipomas. However, pulmonary LAM, unlike tuberous sclerosis, affects only women.

Clinical findings

The disease occurs exclusively in women, usually during the reproductive years (mean age about 40 years). Progressive dyspnea, the most common symptom, can be related to the almost constant presence of chylous pleural effusion or to pulmonary involvement, which occurs in about half of patients.[215-218] Other symptoms include pneumothorax, hemoptysis, and rarely abdominal pain, chylous ascites, and chyluria.

Radiographic studies can be helpful for diagnosing this condition. Lymphangiography indicates obstruction in the major lymphatic ducts (Fig. 36–84A), ectatic lymph vessels distal to the obstruction, occasionally lymphatic–venous connections, and general loss of lymph node architecture (Fig. 36–84B). Chest radiographs demonstrate changes highly characteristic of this condition (Fig. 36–85). In the fully developed case there is a coarse reticular nodular infiltrate with bulla. Numerous thin-walled cysts are noted on high-resolution CT, and pulmonary function studies indicate severe diffusion impairment.

Pathologic findings

At surgery these lesions are red to gray spongy masses that preferentially replace the thoracic duct and mediastinal lymph nodes (Fig. 36–86). Less often, they involve the retroperitoneal lymph nodes only; in particularly dramatic cases the entire lymphatic chain from neck to inguinal region is transformed into multiple confluent masses. Chylous effusion is encountered in most cases, and in some instances the pleural surfaces are noted to "weep" fluid, suggesting the presence of numerous abnormal communications between the lymphatics and the pleural surface. When the process affects the lungs as well, the organ has a honeycomb appearance with formation of numerous blebs or bullae.

Histologically, the lymphangiomyoma has a remarkably uniform appearance. The perivascular epithelioid cells are arranged in short fascicles around a ramifying network of endothelium-lined spaces (Figs 36–87 to 36–90) and have an abundant grainy eosinophilic cytoplasm and nuclei devoid of pleomorphism and mitotic activity (Fig. 36–90). Occasionally, foci of lymphocytes are scattered between the muscle cells; in many instances they represent vestiges of preexisting lymph nodes. The vascular spaces are usually empty but are sometimes filled with eosinophilic material containing fat droplets and occasional lymphocytes.

In the lung, the pathologic changes are extensive and severe (Figs 36–91, 36–92). The primary lesion is a haphazard proliferation of smooth muscle cells that surround arterioles, venules, and lymphatics (Fig. 36–91A), and which diffusely thicken the alveolar septa. Secondary changes ensue, including bulla formation, as a result of air trapping by obstructed bronchioles, and hemorrhage and hemosiderin deposition as a result of venule destruction. Although the macroscopic appearance of honeycombing may initially suggest the diagnosis of end-stage interstitial fibrosis, the two lesions are quite different histologically. LAM is characterized by an exclusive proliferation of smooth muscle cells that can be identified after applying a trichrome stain by their cytoplasmic fuchsinophilia (Fig. 36–91B). The muscle proliferation that accompanies end-stage interstitial fibrosis (muscular cirrhosis) is less striking and is always associated with areas of fibrosis.

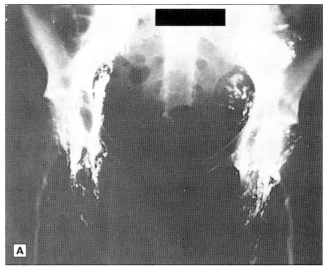

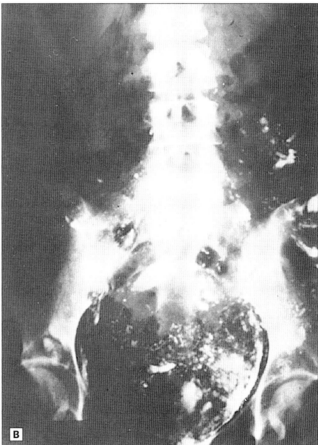

FIGURE 36–84 Lymphangiogram of a patient with lymphangiomyomatosis. **(A)** Initial film shows markedly dilated lymphatic vessels suggesting proximal obstruction. **(B)** Follow-up film (48 hours) shows amorphous collections of contrast material indicative of a loss of normal lymph node architecture. (Courtesy of Dr. Van Vliet, Grand Rapids, MI.)

Differential diagnosis

The full-blown case rarely presents diagnostic difficulty. Problems arise in limited forms of the disease when only one or two lymph nodes in the mediastinum or retroperitoneum are examined. Partial replacement of a lymph node might initially suggest the diagnosis of *metastatic leiomyosarcoma* (Fig. 36–93). The most helpful histologic

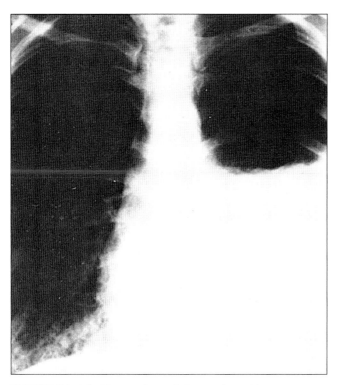

FIGURE 36–85 Chest radiograph in a patient with lymphangiomyomatosis. Lung volume is unaltered despite extensive interstitial disease. Massive (chylous) effusion is present on the left. (Courtesy of Dr. Van Vliet, Grand Rapids, MI.)

feature is the consistent orientation of the smooth muscle cells around endothelial spaces. Leiomyosarcomas show no predictable or consistent polarization toward vessels and, except in extremely well-differentiated cases, they usually have more pleomorphism and mitotic activity. The presence of lipid droplets in the fluid bathing the smooth muscle cells in lymphangiomyomas is also suggestive of the diagnosis. Because the smooth muscle cells of LAM react with the HMB-45 antibody and conventional smooth muscle cells rarely do, this antibody can be used to make this distinction as well.

Rarely, smooth muscle proliferations in the lung have features intermediate between those of LAM and metastatic well-differentiated leiomyosarcoma, or so-called benign metastasizing leiomyoma. One such case was reported by Banner et al.,[219] and we have reviewed a similar case. In our case, hundreds of microscopic smooth muscle nodules were present throughout the lung but bore no consistent relation to the lymphatics. They were composed of fusiform to spindled smooth muscle cells, only some of which had discernible linear striations. Follow-up information, indicating no apparent source for the tumor, strongly suggested a primary smooth muscle proliferation. Such cases deserve the closest scrutiny and careful clinical evaluation to rule out pulmonary metastasis of a well-differentiated smooth muscle tumor of gynecologic, gastrointestinal, or retroperitoneal origin.

Discussion

The clinical course of patients with this disease is variable. Those with localized lesions may survive for long periods following surgical excision, but patients with pulmonary involvement usually experience progressive pulmonary insufficiency. Approximately 30–70% of patients with pulmonary disease will die within 10 years

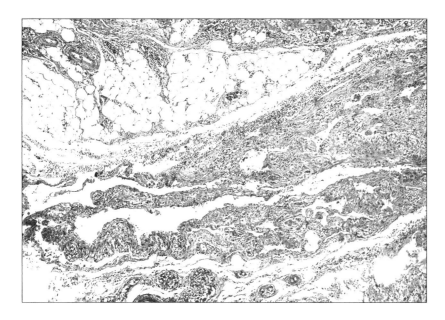

FIGURE 36–86 Lymphangiomyomatosis involving large lymphatic channels.

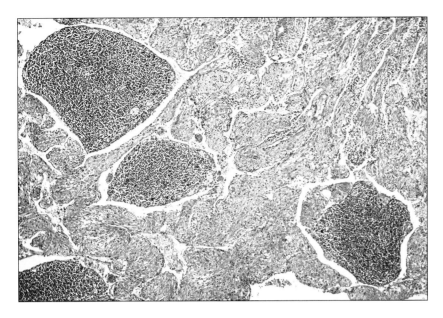

FIGURE 36–87 Lymphangiomyoma.

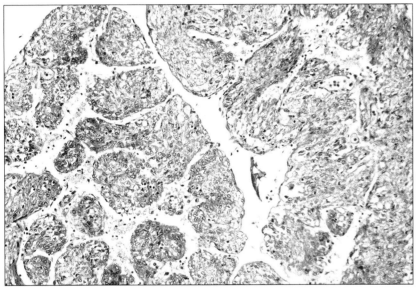

FIGURE 36–88 Lymphangiomyoma with the classic "pericytoma" pattern.

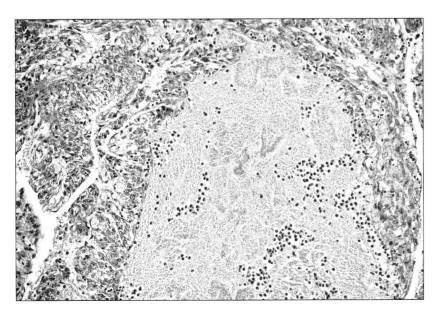

FIGURE 36–89 Lymphangiomyoma with lymph fluid in vascular spaces.

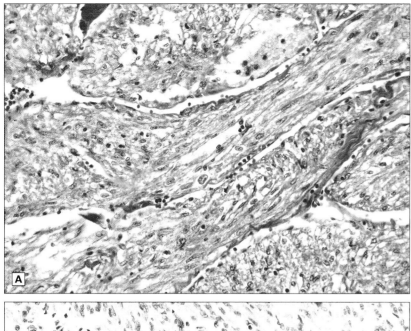

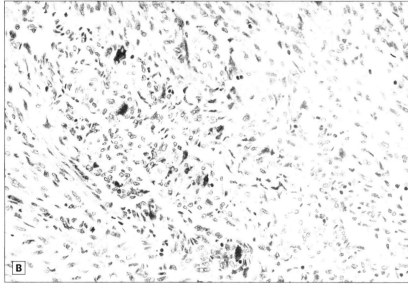

FIGURE 36–90 Lymphangiomyoma with distinctive partially vacuolated smooth muscle cells surrounding endothelium-lined spaces **(A)**. These "perivascular epithelioid clear cells" co-express smooth muscle and melanin markers. **(B)** This field shows focal positivity using HMB-45 antibody.

of diagnosis. Estrogen and progesterone receptor proteins have been detected in pulmonary or abdominal tissue in this disease, and some patients have responded to progesterone or antiestrogen treatment.[220-224] Recently, heart-lung transplantation has been employed as a definitive treatment, although recurrences of the disease have been noted in the transplanted lung.[225]

PEComa (excluding AML, LAM and pulmonary CCST)

Although AML, LAM, and pulmonary CCST are well described, relatively little is known about other members of the PEComa family, which includes lesions described under the rubrics of primary extrapulmonary sugar tumor (PEST), clear cell myomelanocytic tumor, abdominopelvic sarcoma of perivascular epithelioid cells, and PEComa

arising in visceral sites, bone, and soft tissue. Since the initial report of a PEST arising in the pancreas, similar lesions have been described in virtually every anatomic site. In 2005, Folpe et al. reported details of 26 PEComas of soft tissue and gynecologic origin and reviewed the literature on this topic.[226]

Clinical findings

These tumors can arise in patients of virtually any age, although the peak incidence is in the fourth decade of life.[226] There is a striking female predominance, even if one excludes those tumors that arise in gender-specific sites such as the uterus and prostate. Overall, the female-to-male ratio is approximately 7:1. Although a hormonal influence is possible, very few PEComas (aside from AML and LAM) have been evaluated for estrogen or progester-

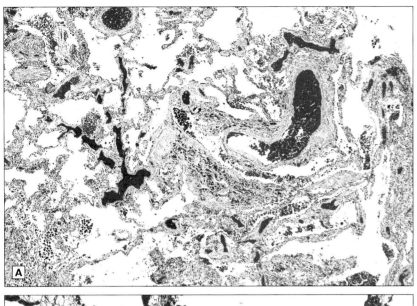

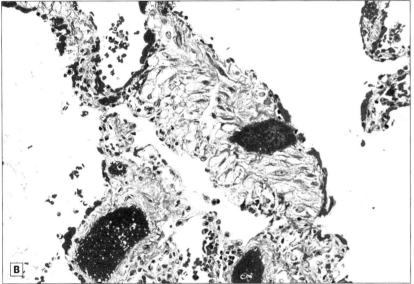

FIGURE 36–91 Lymphangiomyomatosis of the lung **(A)** with characteristic perivascular epithelioid cells (PEC) **(B)** (Trichrome stain).

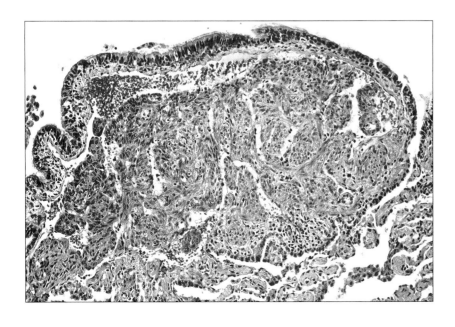

FIGURE 36–92 End-stage lung involved by lymphangiomyomatosis.

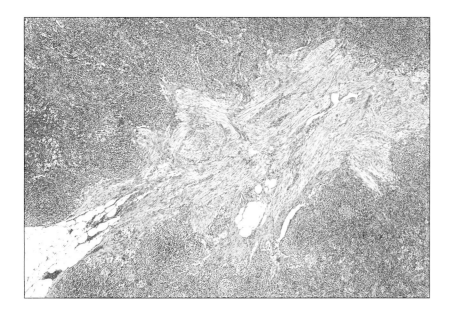

FIGURE 36–93 Lymph node partially involved by lymphangiomyomatosis.

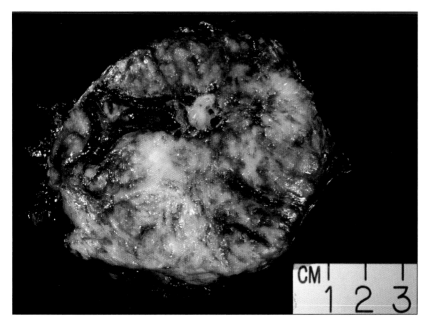

FIGURE 36–94 Gross appearance of a soft tissue PEComa. The cut surface has a variegated appearance, including focal areas of necrosis.

one receptor expression. Up to 40% of these tumors arise in gynecologic locations, most commonly the uterus.[227,228] An equivalent percentage of cases arise in the somatic soft tissues/skin;[226,229,230] visceral[231-233] and bone[234] PEComas are less common. Symptoms are related to the site of origin. Tumor size ranges widely, but most are between 4 and 6 cm at the time of excision. Very few patients with these tumors (<10%) show signs of the TSC.[226]

Pathologic findings

PEComas are generally grossly circumscribed, but some are histologically infiltrative into the surrounding soft tissue. The cut surface may be solid, firm, or even myxoid, and areas of hemorrhage or necrosis may be grossly appreciated (Fig. 36–94).

Histologically, PEComas are composed of clear to lightly eosinophilic cells that are arranged into nests, fascicles, and occasionally sheets, often with a radial arrangement around blood vessels (Figs 36–95 to 36–99). Overall cellularity is usually low to moderate, but some cases are highly cellular. An admixture of epithelioid and spindled cells is common; some cases are predominantly spindled, identical to so-called "clear cell myomelanocytic tumor,"[226] and some are predominantly epithelioid, identical to clear cell sugar tumor or monotypic epithelioid AML. Most tumors are composed of relatively uniform nuclei of low nuclear grade, but some have higher-grade nuclei and prominent nuclear pleomorphism that is identifiable at low magnification. Multinucleated giant cells are common, and occasionally one may encounter giant cells with a central eosinophilic

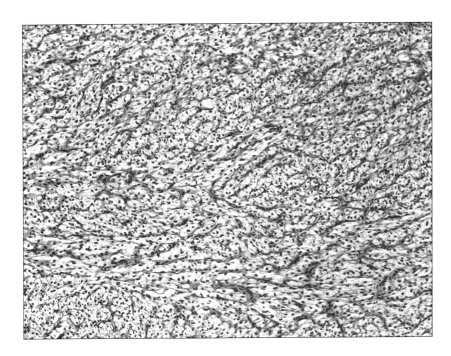

FIGURE 36–95 PEComa of soft tissue composed predominantly of nests of epithelioid cells with cleared-out cytoplasm.

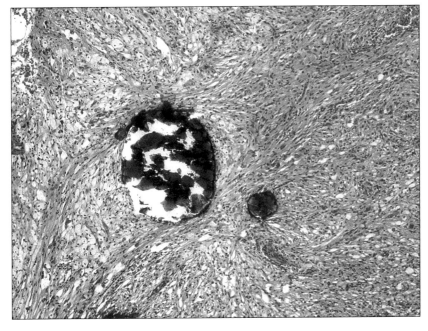

FIGURE 36–96 Higher-magnification view of nests of epithelioid cells in a PEComa of soft tissue.

zone surrounded by a peripheral clear zone, reminiscent of the "spider cells" seen in adult rhabdomyoma (Fig. 36–100). Most tumors have few, if any, mitotic figures, but some, especially those of higher nuclear grade, may have prominent mitotic activity (>5 MF/50 HPF), including atypical mitotic figures (Fig. 36–101). Coagulative necrosis and angiolymphatic invasion are uncommonly identified.

Immunohistochemical and ultrastructural findings

PEComas typically show immunohistochemical evidence of both smooth muscle and melanocytic differen-tiation. In the study by Folpe et al., HMB-45 was the most sensitive melanocytic marker (96% of cases) (Fig. 36–102), followed by Melan A (72%) and MiTF (50%) (Fig. 36–103).[226] All of their cases expressed at least one melanocytic marker. Smooth muscle actin was found in 80% of cases and was typically stronger in epithelioid cells. Desmin was expressed in 36% of cases. Overall, 20 of 24 cases (83%) co-expressed smooth muscle actin and HMB-45 and/or Melan A. Interestingly, this study found one-third of cases to stain for S-100 protein, a potential diagnostic pitfall in distinguishing this lesion from melanoma or clear cell sarcoma. However, all of the S-100 protein-positive tumors also stained for one

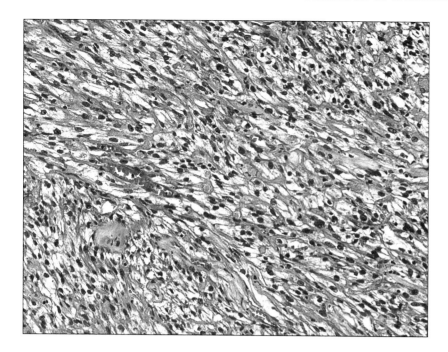

FIGURE 36–97 High-magnificent view of cells with a spindled morphology in a soft tissue PEComa.

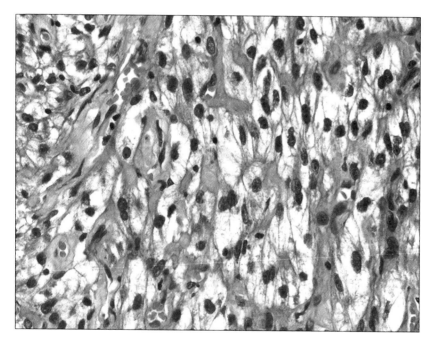

FIGURE 36–98 Soft tissue PEComa with uniform-appearing nuclei.

or more muscle markers. Although uncommon, rare cells may also stain for pancytokeratins. CD117 (KIT) expression is similarly uncommon. Ultrastructural analysis reveals evidence of both smooth muscle and melanocytic differentiation in the form of premelanosomes (Fig. 36–104).[152]

Cytogenetic findings

Relatively few cases of PEComa have been karyotyped, and a specific cytogenetic aberration has not been identified. The presence of a t(3;10) has been reported in one

clear cell myomelanocytic tumor.[153] Pan and colleagues performed comparative genomic hybridization (CGH) on a number of PEComas and found frequent losses on chromosomes 19, 16p, 17p, 1p, and 18p and gains on chromosomes X, 12q, 3q, 5, and 2q.[235]

Differential diagnosis

The differential diagnosis of PEComa is quite broad and dictated by the location of the tumor and predominant morphology (spindled versus epithelioid). Given the consistent expression of melanocytic markers, it is easy

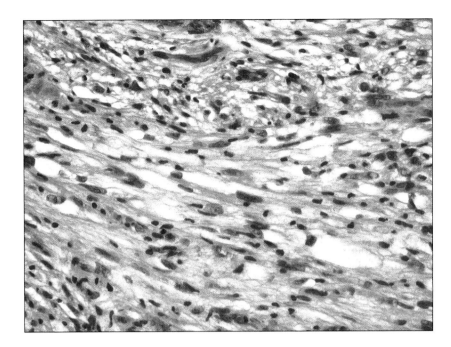

FIGURE 36–99 Bland-appearing spindled cells in soft tissue PEComa.

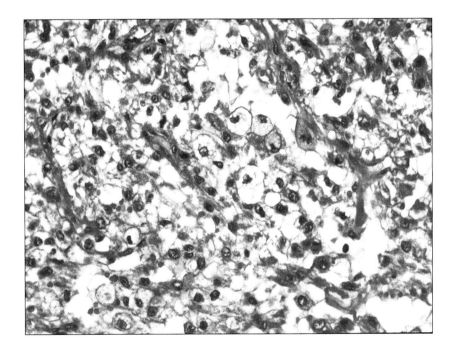

FIGURE 36–100 Cells reminiscent of "spider cells" seen in adult rhabdomyoma in a case of soft tissue PEComa.

to understand how this lesion could be confused with either a *melanoma* or *clear cell sarcoma*. In addition, up to one-third of PEComas stain for S-100 protein, although strong, diffuse S-100 protein staining is typical of melanoma and clear cell sarcoma. Expression of muscle markers usually allows for this distinction, although not all PEComas express these antigens. As noted by Folpe et al., one should be wary of diagnosing PEComa in an HMB-45-positive, S-100 protein-positive, actin-negative tumor.[226] Identification of the specific t(12;22) resulting in an *EWS/ATF-1* gene fusion can be

invaluable in distinguishing clear cell sarcoma from PEComa.

Intra-abdominal PEComas can be confused with a *gastrointestinal stromal tumor (GIST)* since both may show an admixture of spindled and epithelioid cells. PEComas are typified by their characteristic clear to lightly eosinophilic cytoplasm and elaborate capillary vasculature. CD117 is expressed in some PEComas, but is a far more consistent feature in GIST. CD34 is also expressed in the majority of GISTs, but is not charac-teristic of PEComa. Immunohistochemical demonstra-

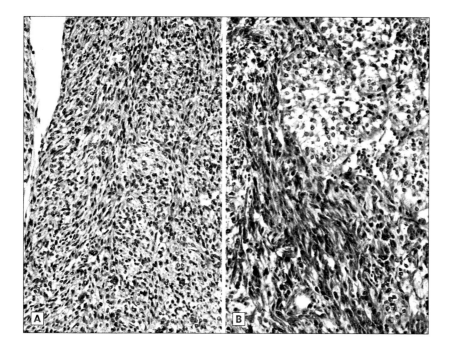

FIGURE 36–101 (A) Highly cellular focus in a malignant PEComa. **(B)** High-magnification view of highly cellular focus in a malignant PEComa.

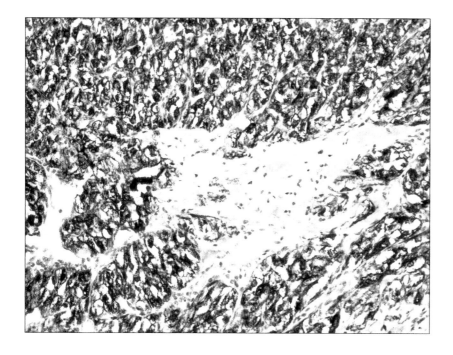

FIGURE 36–102 HMB-45 immunoreactivity in a soft tissue PEComa.

tion of melanocytic differentiation is the most reliable way to distinguish PEComa from GIST.

Clear cell carcinomas (e.g., cervix, vagina, renal cell carcinoma) also enter the differential diagnosis, especially for PEComas with an epithelioid morphology. Clear cell carcinomas strongly express cytokeratins and do not express melanocytic markers.

PEComas can also be confused with true smooth muscle tumors, either spindled or epithelioid, especially when they arise in the abdomen or uterus. In the original report of "clear cell myomelanocytic tumor" by Folpe and colleagues,[153] a number of cases had been previously published as leiomyosarcomas of the ligamentum teres. Silva et al. recently identified a subset of uterine smooth muscle tumors with mixed epithelioid and spindled features that harbored HMB-45-positive cells; these authors argued against designating such tumors as PEComas on the basis of simply identifying rare HMB-45-positive cells in an otherwise typical smooth muscle tumor.[236] Morphologically, true smooth muscle tumors are composed of cells

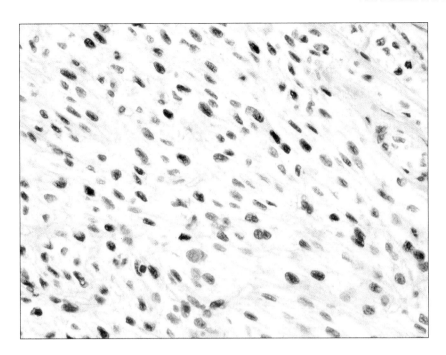

FIGURE 36–103 Nuclear immunoreactivity for MiTF in a soft tissue PEComa.

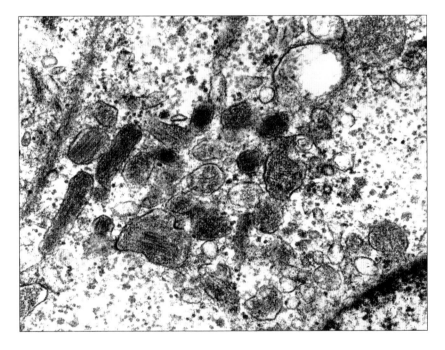

FIGURE 36–104 Ultrastructural appearance of a soft tissue PEComa characterized by the presence of premelanosomes.

with diffuse cytoplasmic eosinophilia, perinuclear vacuoles, and cigar-shaped nuclei, and they usually lack the delicate capillary network seen in most PEComas. Multinucleated giant cells and "spider-like" cells are characteristic of PEComa. Unfortunately, there is significant overlap in immunophenotype since, as mentioned above, morphologically typical uterine smooth muscle tumors occasionally express HMB-45, although they do not express Melan A. Thus, the co-expression of smooth muscle actin and Melan A or MiTF would strongly favor a PEComa.

Discussion

Given that this group of tumors was not even delineated until the mid-1990s and their relative rarity, it has not been possible to fully define criteria for malignancy in PEComas. In the study by Folpe et al., follow-up information in 26 patients (median follow-up period of 30 months) revealed local recurrence and metastases in 13% and 21% of patients, respectively.[226] The most common sites of metastasis included the liver, lung, and bone. Similarly, in their review of the literature, 7% of patients

TABLE 36–13	PROPOSED CLASSIFICATION OF PECOMAS
Category	**Histologic criteria**
Benign	No worrisome features (<5 cm, non-infiltrative, not high nuclear grade, not high cellularity, mitotic activity ≤1 MF/50HPF, no necrosis, no vascular invasion)
Uncertain malignant potential	Nuclear pleomorphism/multinucleated giant cells only OR size >5 cm only
Malignant	Two or more worrisome features (≥5 cm, infiltrative, high nuclear grade, high cellularity, mitotic activity >1 MF/50 HPF, necrosis, vascular invasion)

Modified from reference 226.

TABLE 36–14	RISK OF AGGRESSIVE CLINICAL BEHAVIOR OF PECOMA BASED UPON HISTOLOGIC CLASSIFICATION	
Category		**Aggressive behavior**
Benign		0/22 (0%)
Uncertain malignant potential		2/23 (7%)
Malignant		12/17 (71%)

Modified from reference 226.

were found to have local recurrence, and 20% developed metastatic disease. Overall, close to 80% of patients were alive with no evidence of disease as of last follow-up. Tumor size >8 cm, mitotic activity >1 MF/50 HPF and coagulative necrosis were found to be associated with aggressive clinical behavior. In their evaluation of previously published cases with sufficient morphologic detail, tumor size >5 cm, infiltrative growth pattern, high nuclear grade, coagulative necrosis, and mitotic activity >1 MF/50 HPF were associated with aggressive clinical behavior. As such, Folpe and colleagues proposed a provisional classification of PEComas into benign, uncertain malignant potential, and malignant categories (see Tables 36–13 and 36–14). Benign tumors had no worrisome features (i.e., <5 cm, non-infiltrative, low to moderate nuclear grade and cellularity, mitotic activity = 1 MF/50 HPF, no coagulative necrosis or vascular invasion). Tumors of uncertain malignant potential had either nuclear pleomorphism/multinucleated giant cells only or tumor size >5 cm. Tumors with two or more worrisome features were classified as malignant. There have been a number of case reports and small series of malignant PEComa;[154,237,238] some of these patients have been treated with adjuvant therapy (including Gleevec),[239] but the efficacy of such therapy is not known.

REFERENCES

Ossifying fibromyxoid tumor of soft tissue

1. Enzinger FM, Weiss SW, Liang CY. Ossifying fibromyxoid tumor of soft parts. A clinicopathological analysis of 59 cases. Am J Surg Pathol 1989; 13:817.
2. Kilpatrick SE, Ward WG, Mozes M, et al. Atypical and malignant variants of ossifying fibromyxoid tumor. Clinicopathologic analysis of six cases. Am J Surg Pathol 1995; 19:1039.
3. Yoshida H, Minamizaki T, Yumoto T, et al. Ossifying fibromyxoid tumor of soft parts. Acta Pathol Jpn 1991; 41:480.
4. Zamecnik M, Michal M, Simpson RH, et al. Ossifying fibromyxoid tumor of soft parts: a report of 17 cases with emphasis on unusual histological features. Ann Diagn Pathol 1997; 1:73.
5. Williams SB, Ellis GL, Meis JM, et al. Ossifying fibromyxoid tumour (of soft parts) of the head and neck: a clinicopathological and immunohistochemical study of nine cases. J Laryngol Otol 1993; 107:75.
6. Aminudin CA, Sharaf I, Hamzaini AH, et al. Ossifying fibromyxoid tumour in a child. Med J Malaysia 2004; 59:49.
7. Al-Mazrou KA, Mansoor A, Payne M, et al. Ossifying fibromyxoid tumor of the ethmoid sinus in a newborn: report of a case and literature review. Int J Pediatr Otorhinolaryngol 2004; 68:225.
8. Williams RW, Case CP, Irvine GH. Ossifying fibromyxoid tumour of soft parts – a new tumour of the parotid/zygomatic arch region. Br J Oral Maxillofac Surg 1994; 32:174.
9. Ijiri R, Tanaka Y, Misugi K, et al. Ossifying fibromyxoid tumor of soft parts in a child: a case report. J Pediatr Surg 1999; 34:1294.

10. Ekfors TO, Kulju T, Aaltonen M, et al. Ossifying fibromyxoid tumour of soft parts: report of four cases including one mediastinal and one infantile. APMIS. 1998; 106:1124
11. Nakayama F, Kuwahara T. Ossifying fibromyxoid tumor of soft parts of the back. J Cutan Pathol 1996; 23:385.
12. Thompson J, Castillo M, Reddick RL, et al. Nasopharyngeal nonossifying variant of ossifying fibromyxoid tumor: CT and MR findings. AJNR Am J Neuroradiol 1995; 16:1132.
13. Schaffler G, Raith J, Ranner G, et al. Radiographic appearance of an ossifying fibromyxoid tumor of soft parts. Skeletal Radiol 1997; 26:615.
14. Fisher C, Hedges M, Weiss SW. Ossifying fibromyxoid tumor of soft parts with stromal cyst formation and ribosome-lamella complexes. Ultrastruct Pathol 1994; 18:593.
15. Folpe AL, Weiss SW. Ossifying fibromyxoid tumor of soft parts: a clinicopathologic study of 70 cases with emphasis on atypical and malignant variants. Am J Surg Pathol 2003; 27:421.
16. Miettinen M. Ossifying fibromyxoid tumor of soft parts. Additional observations of a distinctive soft tissue tumor. Am J Clin Pathol 1991; 95:142.
17. Schofield JB, Krausz T, Stamp GW, et al. Ossifying fibromyxoid tumour of soft parts: immunohistochemical and ultrastructural analysis. Histopathology 1993; 22:101.
18. Donner LR. Ossifying fibromyxoid tumor of soft parts: evidence supporting Schwann cell origin. Hum Pathol 1992; 23:200.
19. Min KW, Seo IS, Pitha J. Ossifying fibromyxoid tumor: modified myoepithelial cell tumor? Report of three cases with immunohistochemical and electron microscopic studies. Ultrastruct Pathol 2005; 29:535.

20. Nishio J, Iwasaki H, Ohjimi Y, et al. Ossifying fibromyxoid tumour of soft parts. Cytogenetic findings. Cancer Genet Cytogenet 2002; 133:124.
21. Sovani V, Velagaleti GV, Filipowicz E, et al. Ossifying fibromyxoid tumor of soft parts: report of a case with novel cytogenetic findings. Cancer Genet Cytogenet 2001; 127:1.

Inflammatory myxohyaline tumor of the distal extremities with virocyte or Reed-Sternberg-like cells

22. Montgomery EA, Devaney KO, Giordano TJ, et al. Inflammatory myxohyaline tumor of distal extremities with virocyte or Reed-Sternberg-like cells: a distinctive lesion with features simulating inflammatory conditions, Hodgkin's disease, and various sarcomas. Mod Pathol 1998; 11:384.
23. Meis-Kindblom JM, Kindblom LG. Acral myxoinflammatory fibroblastic sarcoma: a low-grade tumor of the hands and feet. Am J Surg Pathol 1998; 22:911.
24. Michal M. Inflammatory myxoid tumor of the soft parts with bizarre giant cells. Pathol Res Pract 1998; 194:529.
25. Jurcic V, Zidar A, Montiel MD, et al. Myxoinflammatory fibroblastic sarcoma: a tumor not restricted to acral sites. Ann Diagn Pathol 2002; 6:272.
26. McFarlane R, Meyers AD, Golitz L. Myxoinflammatory fibroblastic sarcoma of the neck. J Cutan Pathol 2005; 32:375.
27. Tateishi U, Hasegawa T, Onaya H, et al. Myxoinflammatory fibroblastic sarcoma: MR appearance and pathologic correlation. AJR Am J Roentgenol 2005; 184:1749.
28. Alkuwari E, Gravel DH. A 30-year-old man with a soft tissue mass on the right elbow. Inflammatory myxohyaline tumor of the distal extremities with prominent eosinophilic

infiltrate. Arch Pathol Lab Med 2006; 130:e35.

29. Kinkor Z, Mukensnabl P, Michal M. Inflammatory myxohyaline tumor with massive emperipolesis. Pathol Res Pract 2002; 198:639.

30. Lambert I, Debiec-Rychter M, Guelinckx P, et al. Acral myxoinflammatory fibroblastic sarcoma with unique clonal chromosomal changes. Virchows Arch 2001; 438:509.

31. Mansoor A, Fidda N, Himoe E, et al. Myxoinflammatory fibroblastic sarcoma with complex supernumerary ring chromosomes composed of chromosome 3 segments. Cancer Genet Cytogenet 2004; 152:61.

32. Sakaki M, Hirokawa M, Wakatsuki S, et al. Acral myxoinflammatory fibroblastic sarcoma: a report of five cases and review of the literature. Virchows Arch 2003; 442:25.

Parachordoma/mixed tumor/myoepithelioma of soft tissue

33. Laskowski J. Zarys onkologii. In: Pathology of tumors. Warsaw: PZWL; 1995:91.

34. Dabska M. Parachordoma: a new clinicopathologic entity. Cancer 1977; 40:1586.

35. Gimferrer JM, Baldo X, Montero CA, et al. Chest wall parachordoma. Eur J Cardiothorac Surg 1999; 16:573.

36. Hemalatha AL, Srinivasa MR, Parshwanath HA. Parachordoma of tibia – a case report. Indian J Pathol Microbiol 2003; 46:454.

37. Hirokawa M, Manabe T, Sugihara K. Parachordoma of the buttock: an immunohistochemical case study and review. Jpn J Clin Oncol 1994; 24:336.

38. Karabela-Bouropoulou V, Skourtas C, Liapi-Avgeri G, et al. Parachordoma. A case report of a very rare soft tissue tumor. Pathol Res Pract 1996; 192:972.

39. Ishida T, Oda H, Oka T, et al. Parachordoma: an ultrastructural and immunohistochemical study. Virchows Arch A [Pathol Anat Histopathol] 1993; 422:239.

40. Imlay SP, Argenyi ZB, Stone MS, et al. Cutaneous parachordoma. A light microscopic and immunohistochemical report of two cases and review of the literature. J Cutan Pathol 1998; 25:279.

41. Koh JS, Chung JH, Lee SY, et al. Parachordoma of the tibia: report of a rare case. Pathol Res Pract 2000; 196:269.

42. Sanguela OP, White CR Jr. Parachordoma. Am J Dermatopathol 1994; 16:185.

43. Kilpatrick SE, Hitchcock MG, Kraus MD, et al. Mixed tumors and myoepitheliomas of soft tissue: a clinicopathologic study of 19 cases with a unifying concept. Am J Surg Pathol 1997; 21:13.

44. Hornick JL, Fletcher CD. Myoepithelial tumors of soft tissue: a clinicopathologic and immunohistochemical study of 101 cases with evaluation of prognostic parameters. Am J Surg Pathol 2003; 27:1183.

45. Folpe AL, Agoff SN, Willis J, et al. Parachordoma is immunohistochemically and cytogenetically distinct from axial chordoma and extraskeletal myxoid chondrosarcoma. Am J Surg Pathol 1999; 23:1059.

46. Kuhnen C, Herter P, Kasprzynski A, et al. Myoepithelioma of soft tissue – case report with clinicopathologic, ultrastructural, and cytogenetic findings. Pathologe 2005; 26:331.

47. Mentzel T. Myoepithelial neoplasms of skin and soft tissues. Pathologe 2005; 26:322.

48. Michal M, Miettinen M. Myoepitheliomas of the skin and soft tissues. Report of 12 cases. Virchows Arch 1999; 434:393.

49. Kutzner H, Mentzel T, Kaddu S, et al. Cutaneous myoepithelioma: an under-recognized cutaneous neoplasm composed of myoepithelial cells. Am J Surg Pathol 2001; 25:348.

50. Hornick JL, Fletcher CD. Cutaneous myoepithelioma: a clinicopathologic and immunohistochemical study of 14 cases. Hum Pathol 2004; 35:14.

51. Fisher C, Miettinen M. Parachordoma: a clinicopathologic and immunohistochemical study of four cases of an unusual soft tissue neoplasm. Ann Diagn Pathol 1997; 1:3.

52. Niezabitowski A, Limon J, Wasilewska A, et al. Parachordoma – a clinicopathologic, immunohistochemical, electron microscopic, flow cytometric, and cytogenetic study. Gen Diagn Pathol 1995; 141:49.

53. Scolyer RA, Bonar SF, Palmer AA, et al. Parachordoma is not distinguishable from axial chordoma using immunohistochemistry. Pathol Int 2004; 54:364.

54. Fisher C. Parachordoma exists – but what is it? Adv Anat Pathol 2000; 7:141.

55. Carstens PH. Chordoid tumor: a light, electron microscopic, and immunohistochemical study. Ultrastruct Pathol 1995; 19:291.

56. Shin HJ, Mackay B, Ichinose H, et al. Parachordoma. Ultrastruct Pathol 1994; 18:249.

57. Povysil C, Matejovsky Z. A comparative ultrastructural study of chondrosarcoma, chordoid sarcoma, chordoma and chordoma periphericum. Pathol Res Pract 1985; 179:546.

58. Colombat M, Lesourd A, Moughabghab M, et al. Soft tissue myoepithelioma, a rare tumor. A case report. Ann Pathol 2003; 23:55.

59. Bisceglia M, Cardone M, Fantasia L, et al. Mixed tumors, myoepitheliomas, and oncocytomas of the soft tissues are likely members of the same family: a clinicopathologic and ultrastructural study. Ultrastruct Pathol 2001; 25:399.

60. Tihy F, Scott P, Russo P, et al. Cytogenetic analysis of a parachordoma. Cancer Genet Cytogenet 1998; 105:14.

61. Limon J, Babinska M, Denis A, et al. Parachordoma: a rare sarcoma with clonal chromosomal changes. Cancer Genet Cytogenet 1998; 102:78.

62. Tong G, Perle MA, Desai P, et al. Parachordoma or chordoma periphericum? Case report of a tumor of the thoracic wall. Diagn Cytopathol 2003; 29:18.

63. Pauwels P, Dal Cin P, Roumen R, et al. Intramuscular mixed tumour with clonal chromosomal changes. Virchows Arch 1999; 434:167.

64. van den Berg E, Zorgdrager H, Hoekstra HJ, et al. Cytogenetics of a soft tissue malignant myoepithelioma. Cancer Genet Cytogenet 2004; 151:87.

65. Miettinen M, Karaharju E, Jarvinen E. Chordoma with a massive spindle-cell sarcomatous transformation: a light- and electron-microscopic and immunohistochemical study. Am J Surg Pathol 1987; 11:563.

66. Abe S, Imamura T, Harasawa A, et al. Parachordoma with multiple metastases. J Comput Assist Tomogr 27:634. 2003;

67. O'Connell JX, Berean KW. Parachordomas. Am J Surg Pathol 1997; 21:1120.

68. Fletcher CDM, Kilpatrick SE. Parachordoma (letter to the editor). Am J Surg Pathol 1997; 21:1120.

Pleomorphic hyalinizing angiectatic tumor of soft parts

69. Smith ME, Fisher C, Weiss SW. Pleomorphic hyalinizing angiectatic tumor of soft parts. A low-grade neoplasm resembling neurilemoma. Am J Surg Pathol 199620:21.;

70. Folpe AL, Weiss SW. Pleomorphic hyalinizing angiectatic tumor: analysis of 41 cases supporting evolution from a distinctive

precursor lesion. Am J Surg Pathol 2004; 28:1417.

71. Fukunaga M, Ushigome S. Pleomorphic hyalinizing angiectatic tumor of soft parts. Pathol Int 1997; 47:784.

72. Gallo C, Murer B, Roncaroli F. Pleomorphic hyalinizing angiectatic soft-tissue tumor. Description of a case. Pathologica 1997; 89:531.

73. Capovilla M, Birembaut P, Cucherousset J, et al. Pleomorphic hyalinizing angiectatic tumor of soft parts: ultrastructural analysis of a case with original features. Ultrastruct Pathol 2006; 30:59.

74. Groisman GM, Bejar J, Amar M, et al. Pleomorphic hyalinizing angiectatic tumor of soft parts: immunohistochemical study including the expression of vascular endothelial growth factor. Arch Pathol Lab Med 2000; 124:423.

75. Husek K, Vesely K. Pleomorphic hyalinizing angiectatic tumor. Cesk Patol 2001; 37:177.

76. Fujiwara M, Yuba Y, Wada A, et al. Pleomorphic hyalinizing angiectatic tumor of soft parts: report of a case and review of the literature. J Dermatol 2004; 31:419.

77. Lee JC, Jiang XY, Karpinski RH, et al. Pleomorphic hyalinizing angiectatic tumor of soft parts. Surgery 2005; 137:119.

78. Matsumoto K, Yamamoto T. Pleomorphic hyalinizing angiectatic tumor of soft parts: a case report and literature review. Pathol Int 2002; 52:664.

79. Silverman JS, Dana MM. Pleomorphic hyalinizing angiectatic tumor of soft parts: immunohistochemical case study shows cellular composition by CD34+ fibroblasts and factor XIIIa+ dendrophages. J Cutan Pathol 1997; 24:377.

80. Marshall-Taylor C, Fanburg-Smith JC. Hemosiderotic fibrohistiocytic lipomatous lesion: ten cases of a previously undescribed fatty lesion of the foot/ankle. Mod Pathol 2000; 13:1192.

Hemangiopericytoma-solitary fibrous tumor

81. Stout AP. Hemangiopericytoma: a study of 25 new cases. Cancer 1949; 2:1027.

82. Stout AP, Murray MR. Hemangiopericytoma: a vascular tumor featuring Zimmermann's pericytes. Ann Surg 1942; 116:26.

83. Stout AP. Tumors featuring pericytes: glomus tumor and hemangiopericytoma. Lab Invest 1956; 5:217.

84. Enzinger FM, Smith BH. Hemangiopericytoma: an analysis of 106 cases. Hum Pathol 1976; 7:61.

85. Battifora H. Hemangiopericytoma: ultrastructural study of five cases. Cancer 1973; 31:1418.

86. Erlandson RA, Woodruff JM. Role of electron microscopy in the evaluation of soft tissue neoplasms, with emphasis on spindle cell and pleomorphic tumors. Hum Pathol 1998; 29:1372.

87. Dardick I, Hammar SP, Scheithauer BW. Ultrastructural spectrum of hemangiopericytoma: a comparative study of fetal, adult and neoplastic pericytes. Ultrastruct Pathol 1989; 13:111.

88. Gengler C, Guillou L. Solitary fibrous tumour and haemangiopericytoma: evolution of a concept. Histopathology 2006; 48:63.

89. Schurch W, Skalli O, Lagace R, et al. Intermediate filament proteins and actin isoforms as markers for soft-tissue tumor differentiation and origin. III. Hemangiopericytomas and glomus tumors. Am J Pathol 1990; 136:771.

90. Nemes Z. Differentiation markers in hemangiopericytoma. Cancer 1992; 69:133.

91. Middleton LP, Duray PH, Merino MJ. The histological spectrum of hemangiopericytoma: application of immunohistochemical analysis including proliferative markers to facilitate diagnosis and predict prognosis. Hum Pathol 1998; 29:636.

92. D'Amore ESG, Manivel JG, Sung JH. Soft tissue and meningeal hemangiopericytomas: an immunohistochemical and ultrastructural study. Hum Pathol 1990; 21:414.

93. Fletcher CDM. Hemangiopericytoma – a dying breed? Reappraisal of an "entity" and its variant: a hypothesis. Curr Diagn Pathol 1994; 1:19.

94. Klemperer P, Rabin CB. Primary neoplasms of the pleura: a report of five cases. Arch Pathol 1931; 11:385.

95. Guillou L, Fletcher CDM, et al. Extrapleural solitary fibrous tumor and hemangiopericytoma. In: Fletcher CDM, Unni KK, Mertens F, eds. World Health Organization classification of tumours: pathology and genetics of tumours of soft tissue and bone. Pathology edn. Lyon: IARC Press; 2002:86–90.

96. McMaster MJ, Soule EH, Ivins JC. Hemangiopericytoma: a clinicopathologic study and long-term follow-up of 60 patients. Cancer 1975; 36:2232.

97. Brunnemann RB, Ro JY, Ordonez NG, et al. Extrapleural solitary fibrous tumor: a clinicopathologic study of 24 cases. Mod Pathol 1999; 12:1034.

98. Fukunaga M, Naganuma H, Nikaido T, et al. Extrapleural solitary fibrous tumor: a report of seven cases. Mod Pathol 1997; 10:443.

99. Hasegawa T, Matsuno Y, Shimoda T, et al. Extrathoracic solitary fibrous tumors: their histological variability and potentially aggressive behavior. Hum Pathol 1999; 30:1464.

100. Young RH, Clement PB, McCaughey WT. Solitary fibrous tumors ("fibrous mesotheliomas") and potentially aggressive behavior. Hum Pathol 1999; 114:493.

101. Yousem SA, Flynn SD. Intrapulmonary localized fibrous tumor: intraparenchymal so-called localized fibrous mesothelioma. Am J Clin Pathol 1988; 89:365.

102. Fukasawa Y, Takada A, Tateno M, et al. Solitary fibrous tumor of the pleura causing recurrent hypoglycemia by secretion of insulin-like growth factor II. Pathol Int 1998; 48:47.

103. Masson EA, MacFarland IA, Graham D, et al. Spontaneous hypoglycemia due to pleural fibroma: role of insulin-like growth factors. Thorax 1991; 46:930.

104. Benn JJ, Firth RG, Sonksen PH. Metabolic effect of an insulin-like factor causing hypoglycemia in a patient with haemangiopericytoma. Clin Endocrinol (Oxf) 1990; 32:769.

105. Hoog A, Sandberg Nordqvist AC, Hulting AL, et al. High molecular weight IGF-2 expression in a hemangiopericytoma associated with hypoglycaemia. APMIS 1997; 105:469.

106. Pavelic K, Spaventi S, Gluncic V, et al. The expression and role of insulin-like growth factor II in malignant hemangiopericytomas. J Mol Med 1999; 77:865.

107. De Saint Aubain Somerhausen N, Rubin BP, Fletcher CD. Myxoid solitary fibrous tumor: a study of seven cases with emphasis on differential diagnosis. Mod Pathol 1999; 12:463.

108. Ceballos KM, Munk PL, Masri BA, et al. Lipomatous hemangiopericytoma: a morphologically distinct soft tissue tumor. Arch Pathol Lab Med 1999; 123:941.

109. Folpe AL, Devaney K, Weiss SW. Lipomatous hemangiopericytoma: a rare variant of hemangiopericytoma that may be confused with liposarcoma. Am J Surg Pathol 1999; 23:1201.

110. Vallat-Decouvelaere AV, Dry SM, Fletcher CD. Atypical and malignant solitary fibrous tumors in extrathoracic locations: evidence of their comparability to intrathoracic tumors. Am J Surg Pathol 1998; 22:1501.

111. Gold JS, Antonescu CR, Hajdu C, et al. Clinicopathologic correlates of solitary fibrous tumour. Cancer 2002; 94:1057.

112. Nielsen GP, O'Connell JX, Dickersin GR, et al. Solitary fibrous tumor of soft tissue: a report of 15 cases including 5 malignant examples with light microscopic and ultrastructural data. Mod Pathol 1997; 10:1028.

113. Suster S, Nascimento AG, Miettinen M, et al. Solitary fibrous tumors of soft tissues: a clinicopathologic and immunohistochemical study of 12 cases. Am J Surg Pathol 1995; 19:1257.

114. Van de Rijn M, Lombard CM, Rouse RV. Expression of CD34 by solitary fibrous tumors of the pleura, mediastinum and lung. Am J Surg Pathol 1994; 18:814.

115. Chilosi M, Facchetti F, Dei Tos AP, et al. Bcl-2 expression in pleural and extrapleural solitary fibrous tumors. J Pathol 1997; 181:362.

116. Hanau CA, Miettinen M. Solitary fibrous tumor: histological and immunohistochemical spectrum of benign and malignant variants presenting at different sites. Hum Pathol 1995; 26:440.

117. Hasegawa T, Hirose T, Seki K, et al. Solitary fibrous tumor of the soft tissue: an immunohistochemical and ultrastructural study. Am J Clin Pathol 1996; 106:325.

118. Nunnery EW, Kahn LB, Reddick RL, et al. Hemangiopericytoma: a light microscopic and ultrastructural study. Cancer 1981; 47:906.

119. Ide F, Obara K, Mishima K, et al. Ultrastructural spectrum of solitary fibrous tumors: a unique perivascular tumor with alternative lines of differentiation. Virchows Archiv 2005; 446:646.

120. Bristelli M, Mark EJ, Dickersin GR. Solitary fibrous tumor of the pleura: eight new cases and review of 360 cases in the literature. Cancer 1981; 47:2678.

121. Gherardi G, Arya S, Hickler RB. Juxtaglomerular body tumor: a rare occult, but curable cause of lethal hypertension. Hum Pathol 1974; 5:236.

122. Robertson PW, Klidjian A, Hardin LK, et al. Hypertension due to renin-secreting renal tumor. Am J Med 1967; 43:963.

123. Warshaw BL, Anand SK, Olsen DL, et al. Hypertension secondary to a renin-producing juxtaglomerular tumor. J Pediatr 1979; 94:247.

124. Ohmori H, Motoi M, Sato H, et al. Extrarenal renin-secreting tumor associated with hypertension. Acta Pathol Jpn 1977; 27:567.

125. Henn W, Wullich B, Thoennes M, et al. Recurrent t(12;19)(q13;q13.3) in intracranial and extracranial hemangiopericytoma. Cancer Genet Cytogenet 1993; 71:3009.

126. Sreekantaiah C, Bridge JA, Rao UN, et al. Clonal chromosomal abnormalities in hemangiopericytoma. Cancer Genet Cytogenet 1991; 54:173.

127. Limon J, Rao U, Dal Cin P, et al. Translocation t(13;22) in hemangiopericytoma. Cancer Genet Cytogenet 1986; 21:309.

128. Mandahl N, Orndal C, Heim S, et al. Aberrations of chromosome segment 12q13–15 characterize a subgroup of hemangiopericytomas. Cancer 1993; 71:3009.

129. Miettinen MM, el-Rifai W, Sarlomo-Rikala M, et al. Tumor size-related DNA copy number changes occur in solitary fibrous tumors but not in hemangiopericytomas. Mod Pathol 1997; 10:1194.

130. Dal Cin P, Sciot R, Fletcher CD, et al. Trisomy 21 in solitary fibrous tumor. Cancer Genet Cytogenet 1996; 86:58.

131. Espat NJ, Lewis JJ, Keung D, et al. Conventional hemangiopericytoma: a modern analysis of outcome. Cancer 2002; 95:1746.

132. Spitz FR, Bouvet M, Pisters PW, et al. Hemangiopericytoma: a 20-year single-institution experience. Ann Surg Oncol 1998; 5:350.

133. England DM, Hochholzer L, McCarthy MJ. Localized benign and malignant fibrous tumors of the pleura: a clinicopathologic review of 223 cases. Am J Surg Pathol 1989; 13:640.

Variants of hemangiopericytoma-solitary fibrous tumor

134. Carneiro SS, Scheithauer BW, Nascimento AG, et al. Solitary fibrous tumor of the meninges: a lesion distinct from fibrous meningioma: a clinicopathologic and immunohistochemical study. Am J Clin Pathol 1996; 106:217.

135. Iwaki T, Fukui M, Takeshita I et al. Hemangiopericytoma of the meninges: a clinicopathologic and immunohistochemical study. Clin Neuropathol 1988; 7:93.

136. Joseph JT, Lisle DK, Jacoby LB, et al. NF2 gene analysis distinguishes hemangiopericytoma from meningioma. Am J Pathol 1995; 147:1450.

137. Perry A, Scheithauer BW, Nascimento AG. The immunophenotypic spectrum of meningeal hemangiopericytoma: a comparison with fibrous meningioma and solitary fibrous tumor of meninges. Am J Surg Pathol 1997; 21:1354.

138. Guthrie BL, Ebersold MJ, Scheithauer BW, et al. Meningeal hemangiopericytoma: histopathologic features, treatment and long-term follow-up of 44 cases. Neurosurgery 1989; 25:514.

139. Mena H, Ribas JL, Pezeshkppour GH, et al. Hemangiopericytoma of the central nervous system: a review of 94 cases. Hum Pathol 1991; 22:84.

140. Dei Tos AP, Seregard S, Calonje E, et al. Giant cell angiofibroma. A distinctive orbital tumor in adults. Am J Surg Pathol 1995; 19:1286.

141. Guillou L, Gebhard S, Coindre JM. Orbital and extraorbital giant cell angiofibroma: a giant cell-rich variant of solitary fibrous tumor? Clinicopathologic and immunohistochemical analysis of a series in favor of a unifying concept. Am J Surg Pathol 2000; 24:971.

Infantile hemangiopericytoma

142. Alpers CE, Rosenau W, Finkbeiner WE, et al. Congenital (infantile) hemangiopericytoma of the tongue and the sublingual region. Am J Clin Pathol 1984; 81:377.

143. Baker DL, Oda D, Myall RW. Intraoral infantile hemangiopericytoma: literature review and addition of a case. Oral Surg Oral Med Oral Pathol 1992; 73:596.

144. Eimoto T. Ultrastructure of an infantile hemangiopericytoma. Cancer 1977; 40:2161.

145. Kauffman SL, Stout AP. Hemangiopericytoma in children. Cancer 1960; 13:695.

146. Chung KC, Weiss SW, Kuzon WM. Multifocal congenital hemangiopericytomas associated with Kasabach-Merritt syndrome. Br J Past Surg 1995; 48:240.

147. Chen KT, Kassel SH, Medrano VA. Congenital hemangiopericytoma. J Surg Oncol 1986; 31:127.

148. Jakobiec FA, Howard GM, Jones IS, et al. Hemangiopericytoma of the orbit. Am J Ophthalmol 1974; 78:816.

Phosphaturic mesenchymal tumor, mixed connective tissue type

149. Park YK, Unni KK, Beabout JW, et al. Oncogenic osteomalacia: a clinicopathologic study of 17 bones lesions. J Korean Med Sci 1994; 9:289.

150. Weidner N, Santa Cruz D. Phosphaturic mesenchymal tumor: a polymorphous group

causing osteomalacia or rickets. Cancer 1987; 59:1442.

151. Folpe AL, Fanburg-Smith JC, Billings SD, et al. Most osteomalacia-associated mesenchymal tumors are a single histopathologic entity: an analysis of 32 cases and comprehensive review of the literature. Am J Surg Pathol 2004; 28:1.

Perivascular epithelioid cell family of tumors

152. Tazelaar HD, Batts KP, Srigley JR. Primary extrapulmonary sugar tumor (PEST): a report of four cases. Mod Pathol 2001; 14:615.

153. Folpe AL, Goodman ZD, Ishak KG, et al. Clear cell myomelanocytic tumor of the falciform ligament/ligamentum teres: a novel member of the perivascular epithelioid clear cell family of tumors with a predilection for children and young adults. Am J Surg Pathol 2000; 24:1239.

154. Bonetti F, Martignoni G, Colato C, et al. Abdominopelvic sarcoma of perivascular epithelioid cells. Report of four cases in young women, one with tuberous sclerosis. Mod Pathol 2001; 14:563.

155. Eble JN. Angiomyolipoma of kidney. Semin Diagn Pathol 1998; 15:21.

156. Frack MD, Simon L, Dawson BH. The lymphangiomyomatosis syndrome. Cancer 1968; 22:428.

157. Liebow AA, Castleman B. Benign clear cell ("sugar") tumors of the lung. Yale J Biol Med 1971; 43:213.

158. Valensi QJ. Pulmonary lymphangiomyoma, a probable forme frust of tuberous sclerosis. A case report and survey of the literature. Am Rev Respir Dis 1973; 108:1411.

159. Monteforte WJ Jr, Kohnen PW. Angiomyolipomas in a case of lymphangiomyomatosis syndrome: relationships to tuberous sclerosis. Cancer 1974; 34:317.

160. Pea M, Bonetti F, Zamboni G, et al. Melanocyte-marker-HMB-45 is regularly expressed in angiomyolipoma of the kidney. Pathology 1991; 23:185.

161. Weeks DA, Malott RL, Arnesen M, et al. Hepatic angiomyolipoma with striated granules and positivity with melanoma – specific antibody (HMB-45): a report of two cases. Ultrastruct Pathol 1991; 15:563.

162. Gaffey MJ, Mills SE, Askin FB, et al. Clear cell tumor of the lung. A clinicopathologic, immunohistochemical, and ultrastructural study of eight cases. Am J Surg Pathol 1990; 14:248.

163. Chan JK, Tsang WY, Pau MY, et al. Lymphangiomyomatosis and angiomyolipoma: closely related entities characterized by hamartomatous proliferation of HMB-45-positive smooth muscle. Histopathology 1993; 22:445.

164. Zamboni G, Pea M, Martignoni G, et al. Clear cell "sugar" tumor of the pancreas. A novel member of the family of lesions characterized by the presence of perivascular epithelioid cells. Am J Surg Pathol 1996; 20:722.

165. Unlu C, Lamme B, Nass P, et al. Retroperitoneal haemorrhage caused by a renal angiomyolipoma. Emerg Med J 2006; 23:464.

166. Springer AM, Saxena AK, Willital GH. Angiomyolipoma with hypertension mimicking a malignant renal tumor. Pediatr Surg Int 2002; 18:526.

167. Majid S, White D, Sarkar S. An unusual cause for the incidental finding of multiple liver lesions. Diagnosis: multiple fatty vascular lesions of angiomyolipomas. Gut 2006; 55:983, 1029.

168. Xu AM, Zhang SH, Zheng JM, et al. Pathological and molecular analysis of sporadic hepatic angiomyolipoma. Hum Pathol 2006; 37:735.

169. Erkilic S, Kocer NE, Mumbuc S, et al. Nasal angiomyolipoma. Acta Otolaryngol 2005; 125:446.

170. Piattelli A, Fioroni M, Rubini C, et al. Angiomyolipoma of the palate. Report of a case. Oral Oncol 2001; 37:323.

171. Sharara AI, Tawil A. Angiomyolipoma of the colon. Clin Gastroenterol Hepatol 2005; 3:A35.

172. Kasuno K, Ueda S, Tanaka A, et al. Pulmonary angiomyolipoma recurring 26 years after nephrectomy for angiomyolipoma: benign clinical course. Clin Nephrol 2004; 62:469.

173. Tsuruta D, Maekawa N, Ishii M. Cutaneous angiomyolipoma. Dermatology 2004; 208:231.

174. Patel U, Simpson E, Kingswood JC, et al. Tuberose sclerosis complex: analysis of growth rates aids differentiation of renal cell carcinoma from atypical or minimal-fat-containing angiomyolipoma. Clin Radiol 2005; 60:665.

175. Henske EP. Tuberous sclerosis and the kidney: from mesenchyme to epithelium, and beyond. Pediatr Nephrol 2005; 20:854.

176. De Pauw RA, Boelaert JR, Haenebalcke CW, et al. Renal angiomyolipoma in association with pulmonary lymphangioleiomyomatosis. Am J Kidney Dis 2003; 41:877.

177. Cohen MM, Pollock-BarZiv S, Johnson SR. Emerging clinical picture of lymphangioleiomyomatosis. Thorax 2005; 60:875.

178. Jimenez RE, Eble JN, Reuter VE, et al. Concurrent angiomyolipoma and renal cell neoplasia: a study of 36 cases. Mod Pathol 2001; 14:157.

179. Israel GM, Hindman N, Hecht E, et al. The use of opposed-phase chemical shift MRI in the diagnosis of renal angiomyolipomas. AJR Am J Roentgenol 2005; 184:1868.

180. Coumbaras M, Dahan H, Strauss C, et al. Renal angiomyolipoma complicated by extension to the renal vein and inferior vena cava. J Radiol 2006; 87:572.

181. Gogus C, Safak M, Erekul S, et al. Angiomyolipoma of the kidney with lymph node involvement in a 17-year old female mimicking renal cell carcinoma: a case report. Int Urol Nephrol 2001; 33:617.

182. Eble JN, Amin MB, Young RH. Epithelioid angiomyolipoma of the kidney: a report of five cases with a prominent and diagnostically confusing epithelioid smooth muscle component. Am J Surg Pathol 1997; 21:1123.

183. Belanger EC, Dhamanaskar PK, Mai KT. Epithelioid angiomyolipoma of the kidney mimicking renal sarcoma. Histopathology 2005; 47:433.

184. Mai KT, Perkins DG, Collins JP. Epithelioid cell variant of renal angiomyolipoma. Histopathology 1996; 28:277.

185. Davis CJ, Barton JH, Sesterhenn IA. Cystic angiomyolipoma of the kidney: a clinicopathologic description of 11 cases. Mod Pathol 2006; 19:669.

186. Makhlouf HR, Ishak KG, Shekar R, et al. Melanoma markers in angiomyolipoma of the liver and kidney: a comparative study. Arch Pathol Lab Med 2002; 126:49.

187. Jungbluth AA, King R, Fisher DE, et al. Immunohistochemical and reverse transcription-polymerase chain reaction expression analysis of tyrosinase and microphthalmia-associated transcription factor in angiomyolipomas. Appl Immunohistochem Mol Morphol 2001; 9:29.

188. Zavala-Pompa A, Folpe AL, Jimenez RE, et al. Immunohistochemical study of microphthalmia transcription factor and tyrosinase in angiomyolipoma of the kidney, renal cell carcinoma, and renal and retroperitoneal sarcomas: comparative evaluation with traditional diagnostic markers. Am J Surg Pathol 2001; 25:65.

189. Henske EP, Ao X, Short MP, et al. Frequent progesterone receptor immunoreactivity in tuberous sclerosis-associated renal angiomyolipomas. Mod Pathol 1998; 11:665.

190. Colombat M, Boccon-Gibod L, Carton S. An unusual renal angiomyolipoma with morphological lymphangioleiomyomatosis features and coexpression of oestrogen and progesterone receptors. Virchows Arch 2002; 440:102.

191. Logginidou H, Ao X, Russo I, et al. Frequent estrogen and progesterone receptor immunoreactivity in renal angiomyolipomas from women with pulmonary lymphangioleiomyomatosis. Chest 2000; 117:25.

192. Makhlouf HR, Remotti HE, Ishak KG. Expression of KIT (CD117) in angiomyolipoma. Am J Surg Pathol 2002; 26:493.

193. Wullich B, Henn W, Siemer S, et al. Clonal chromosome aberrations in three of five sporadic angiomyolipomas of the kidney. Cancer Genet Cytogenet 1997; 96:42.

194. Dal Cin P, Sciot R, Van Poppel H, et al. Chromosome analysis in angiomyolipoma. Cancer Genet Cytogenet 1997; 99:132.

195. El-Hashemite N, Zhang H, Henske EP, et al. Mutation in TSC2 and activation of mammalian target of rapamycin signaling pathway in renal angiomyolipoma. Lancet 2003; 361:1348.

196. Plank TL, Logginidou H, Klein-Szanto A, et al. The expression of hamartin, the product of the TSC1 gene, in normal human tissues and in TSC1- and TSC2-linked angiomyolipomas. Mod Pathol 1999; 12:539.

197. Brecher ME, Gill WB, Straus FH 2nd. Angiomyolipoma with regional lymph node involvement and long-term follow-up study. Hum Pathol 1986; 17:962.

198. Ferry JA, Malt RA, Young RH. Renal angiomyolipoma with sarcomatous transformation and pulmonary metastases. Am J Surg Pathol 1991; 15:1083.

199. Cibas ES, Goss GA, Kulke MH, et al. Malignant epithelioid angiomyolipoma ("sarcoma ex angiomyolipoma") of the kidney: a case report and review of the literature. Am J Surg Pathol 2001; 25:121.

200. Hornick JL, Fletcher CD. PEComa: what do we know so far? Histopathology 2006; 48:75.

201. Pea M, Bonetti F, Martignoni G, et al. Apparent renal cell carcinomas in tuberous sclerosis are heterogeneous: the identification of malignant epithelioid angiomyolipoma. Am J Surg Pathol 1998; 22:180.

202. Martignoni G, Pea M, Bonetti F, et al. Carcinoma-like monotypic epithelioid angiomyolipoma in patients without evidence of tuberous sclerosis: a clinicopathologic and genetic study. Am J Surg Pathol 1998; 22:663.

203. Christiano AP, Yang X, Gerber GS. Malignant transformation of renal angiomyolipoma. J Urol 1999; 161:1900.

204. Lowe BA, Brewer J, Houghton DC, et al. Malignant transformation of angiomyolipoma. J Urol 1992; 147:1356.

205. Yamamoto T, Ito K, Suzuki K, et al. Rapidly progressive malignant epithelioid angiomyolipoma of the kidney. J Urol 2002; 168:190.

206. Warakaulle DR, Phillips RR, Turner GD, et al. Malignant monotypic epithelioid angiomyolipoma of the kidney. Clin Radiol 2004; 59:849.

207. L'Hostis H, Deminiere C, Ferriere JM, et al. Renal angiomyolipoma: a clinicopathologic, immunohistochemical, and follow-up study of 46 cases. Am J Surg Pathol 1999; 23:1011.

208. Dalle I, Sciot R, de Vos R, et al. Malignant angiomyolipoma of the liver: a hitherto unreported variant. Histopathology 2000; 36:443.
209. Silverman SG, Tuncali K, vanSonnenberg E, et al. Renal tumors: MR imaging-guided percutaneous cryotherapy – initial experience in 23 patients. Radiology 2005; 236:716.
210. Bonetti F, Pea M, Martignoni G, et al. Clear cell ("sugar") tumor of the lung is a lesion strictly related to angiomyolipoma – the concept of a family of lesions characterized by the presence of the perivascular epithelioid cells (PEC). Pathology 1994; 26:230.
211. Bonetti F, Pea M, Martignoni G, et al. Cellular heterogeneity in lymphangiomyomatosis of the lung. Hum Pathol 1992; 22:727.
212. Taylor JR, Ryu J, Colby TV, et al. Lymphangioleiomyomatosis: clinical course in 32 patients. N Engl J Med 1990; 323:1254.
213. Carsillo T, Astrinidis Henske EP. Mutations in the tuberous sclerosis complex gene TSC2 are a cause of sporadic pulmonary lymphangioleiomyomatosis. Proc Natl Acad Sci USA 2000; 97:6085.
214. Strizheva GD, Carsillo T, Kruger WD, et al. The spectrum of mutations in TSC1 and TSC2 in women with tuberous sclerosis and lymphangiomatosis. Am J Respir Crit Care Med 2001; 163:253.
215. Cornog JL, Enterline HT. Lymphangiomyoma: a benign lesion of chyliferous lymphatics synonymous with lymphangiopericytoma. Cancer 1966; 19:1909.
216. Corrin B, Liebow AA, Friedman PJ. Pulmonary lymphangiomyomatosis. Am J Pathol 1975; 79:348.
217. Enterline HT, Roberts B. Lymphangiopericytoma. Cancer 1955; 8:582.
218. Wolff M. Lymphangiomyoma: clinicopathological study and ultrastructural confirmation of its histogenesis. Cancer 1973; 31:988.
219. Banner AS, Carrington CB, Emory WB, et al. Efficacy of oophorectomy in lymphangioleiomyomatosis and benign metastasizing leiomyoma. N Engl J Med 1981; 305:204.
220. Colley MH, Geppert E, Franklin WA. Immunohistochemical detection of steroid receptors in a case of pulmonary lymphangioleiomyomatosis. Am J Surg Pathol 1989; 13:803.
221. Brentani MM, Carvalho RR, Saldiva PH, et al. Steroid receptors in pulmonary lymphangiomyomatosis. Chest 1984; 85:96.
222. McCarty KS, Mossler JA, McLelland R, et al. Pulmonary lymphangiomyomatosis responsive to progesterone. N Engl J Med 1980; 303:1461.
223. Tomasian A, Greenberg MS, Rumerman H. Tamoxifen for lymphangioleiomyomatosis. N Engl J Med 1982; 306:745.
224. Ohori NP, Yousem SA, Sonmez-Alpan E, et al. Estrogen and progesterone receptors in lymphangioleiomyomatosis, epithelioid hemangioendothelioma and sclerosing hemangioma of the lung. Am J Clin Pathol 1991; 96:529.
225. Bittman I, Rolf B, Amann G, et al. Recurrence of lymphangioleiomyomatosis after single lung transplantation: new insights into pathogenesis. Hum Pathol 2003; 34:95.
226. Folpe AL, Mentzel T, Lehr HA, et al. Perivascular epithelioid cell neoplasms of soft tissue and gynecologic origin: a clinicopathologic study of 26 cases and review of the literature. Am J Surg Pathol 2005; 29:1558.
227. Vang R, Kempson RL. Perivascular epithelioid cell tumor ('PEComa') of the uterus: a subset of HMB-45-positive epithelioid mesenchymal neoplasms with an uncertain relationship to pure smooth muscle tumors. Am J Surg Pathol 2002; 26:1.
228. Bosincu L, Rocca PC, Martignoni G, et al. Perivascular epithelioid cell (PEC) tumors of the uterus: a clinicopathologic study of two cases with aggressive features. Mod Pathol 2005; 18:1336.
229. Mentzel T, Reisshauer S, Rutten A, et al. Cutaneous clear cell myomelanocytic tumour: a new member of the growing family of perivascular epithelioid cell tumours (PEComas). Clinicopathological and immunohistochemical analysis of seven cases. Histopathology 2005; 46:498.
230. de Saint Aubain Somerhausen N, Gomez Galdon M, Bouffioux B, et al. Clear cell "sugar" tumor (PEComa) of the skin: a case report. J Cutan Pathol 2005; 32:441.
231. Pan CC, Yu IT, Yang AH, et al. Clear cell myomelanocytic tumor of the urinary bladder. Am J Surg Pathol 2003; 27:689.
232. Pan CC, Yang AH, Chiang H. Malignant perivascular epithelioid cell tumor involving the prostate. Arch Pathol Lab Med 2003; 127:E96.
233. Yamamoto H, Oda Y, Yao T, et al. Malignant perivascular epithelioid cell tumor of the colon: report of a case with molecular analysis. Pathol Int 2006; 56:46.
234. Insabato L, De Rosa G, Terracciano LM, et al. Primary monotypic epithelioid angiomyolipoma of bone. Histopathology 2002; 40:286.
235. Pan CC, Jong YJ, Chai CY, et al. Comparative genomic hybridization study of perivascular epithelioid cell tumor: molecular genetic evidence of perivascular epithelioid cell tumor as a distinctive neoplasm. Hum Pathol 2006; 37:606.
236. Silva EG, Deavers MT, Bodurka DC, et al. Uterine epithelioid leiomyosarcomas with clear cells: reactivity with HMB-45 and the concept of PEComa. Am J Surg Pathol 2004; 28:244.
237. Dimmler A, Seitz G, Hohenberger W, et al. Late pulmonary metastasis in uterine PEComa. J Clin Pathol 2003; 56:627.
238. Greene LA, Mount SL, Schned AR, et al. Recurrent perivascular epithelioid cell tumor of the uterus (PEComa): an immunohistochemical study and review of the literature. Gynecol Oncol 2003; 90:677.
239. Rigby H, Yu W, Schmidt MH, et al. Lack of response of a metastatic renal perivascular epithelial cell tumor (PEComa) to successive courses of DTIC-based therapy and imatinib mesylate. Pediatr Blood Cancer 2005; 45:202.

MALIGNANT SOFT TISSUE TUMORS OF UNCERTAIN TYPE

CHAPTER CONTENTS

The neoplasms described in this chapter are a heterogeneous group of tumors that are considered to be of uncertain histogenesis because they have no precise normal tissue counterpart. Each is characterized by its own distinctive clinical and pathologic features.

SYNOVIAL SARCOMA

Synovial sarcoma is a clinically and morphologically well-defined entity that, despite its name, is extremely uncommon in joint cavities and is encountered in areas with no apparent relation to synovial structures. It occurs primarily in the para-articular regions of the extremities, usually in close association with tendon sheaths, bursae, and joint capsules.

Its microscopic resemblance to developing synovium was suggested early in the literature, but there is no evidence that this tumor arises from or differentiates toward synovium. Indeed, there are such significant immunophenotypic and ultrastructural differences between synovial sarcoma and normal synovium that most regard the label "synovial sarcoma" a fanciful designation that has its roots in the descriptive works of the earlier literature. In 1927, Smith used the term *synovioma*,[1] whereas Lejars and Rubens-Duval[2] preferred the term *synovial endothelioma*. It should be noted in passing that the term *tendosynovial sarcoma*, coined by Hajdu et al.,[3,4] is not restricted to synovial sarcoma but embraces a collection of sarcomas including epithelioid sarcoma, clear cell sarcoma, and extraskeletal myxoid chondrosarcoma. For this reason it has no diagnostic purpose. Although synovial sarcoma continues to be the term of choice, some have suggested that it be renamed carcinosarcoma or even spindle cell carcinoma of soft tissue, a term that more accurately captures the essence of this lesion. The reported data on the frequency of this tumor vary, but synovial sarcoma accounts for 5–10% of all soft tissue sarcomas.[5] In a recent review of over 6000 patients with soft tissue sarcomas seen at M.D. Anderson Cancer Center, approximately 6% were synovial sarcomas.[6]

Histologically, there are two major categories of synovial sarcoma: biphasic and monophasic types. *Biphasic synovial sarcoma* has distinct epithelial and spindle cell components, in varying proportions. Of the *monophasic synovial sarcomas*, the vast majority is of the *monophasic fibrous type*, which itself is the most common subtype of synovial sarcoma. There is also a *monophasic epithelial type*, but this tumor is not reliably recognized and distinguished from adenocarcinoma without cytogenetic or molecular genetic studies. In practice, predominantly epithelial forms of synovial sarcoma are diagnosed by recognizing small spindle cell sarcoma areas, having cytogenetic/molecular genetic data, or both. Synovial sarcoma may also present as a poorly differentiated round cell sarcoma often arranged in a pericytomatous pattern (*poorly differentiated synovial sarcoma*), but this is not really a distinct subtype of synovial sarcoma; rather, it represents a form of tumor progression that can occur in either monophasic or biphasic tumors.

Clinical findings

Age and gender incidence

Synovial sarcoma is most prevalent in adolescents and young adults 15–40 years of age. In the largest series published to date by Ladanyi and colleagues, the patients ranged in age from 6 to 82 years, with a mean age of 34 years.[7] Forty-four percent of patients were under age 30 at diagnosis. Other large clinicopathologic studies have also found a peak in the third decade of life.[8–10] The tumor may arise in children 10 years of age or younger, and there are several reports in the literature of this tumor arising in newborns.[11] Males are affected more often than females, with an average male/female ratio of 1.2:1.0. There does not appear to be a predilection for any particular race.

Clinical complaints

The most common presentation is that of a palpable, deep-seated swelling or mass associated with pain or tenderness in slightly more than half of cases. Less frequently, pain or tenderness is the only manifestation of the disease. There may be minor limitation of motion, but severe functional disturbance or weight loss is seldom encountered; when it does occur, it is nearly always associated with poorly differentiated, large tumors of long duration. The mechanism for the common symptoms of pain and tenderness is unknown. Other clinical complaints are related to the location of the tumor. Primary or secondary involvement of nerves may cause projected pain, numbness, and paresthesia.

The preoperative duration of symptoms varies considerably. Generally, the tumor grows slowly and insidiously, often giving a false impression as to the degree of malignancy, delaying diagnosis and therapy. In most cases the duration is 2–4 years, but there are also cases in which a slow-growing mass or pain at the tumor site has been noted for as long as 20 years prior to operation. Not infrequently, these cases are incorrectly diagnosed initially as arthritis, synovitis, or bursitis.

Trauma

Although most patients with synovial sarcoma fail to give a definitive history of antecedent trauma, there are patients with such a history in our cases and in the literature; most had sustained a minor or major injury during athletic or recreational activities. The interval between the episode of trauma and onset of the tumor varies considerably, ranging from a few weeks to as long as 40 years. It is likely that trauma is coincidental, since synovial sarcoma predominates in parts of the body (extremities) that are most prone to injury. There are rare reports of synovial sarcoma arising in the field of previous therapeutic irradiation[12-14] and one of a tumor associated with a metal implant used for hip replacement surgery.[15]

Anatomic location

Synovial sarcomas occur predominantly in the extremities, where they tend to arise in the vicinity of large joints, especially the knee region (Table 37–1). They are intimately related to tendons, tendon sheaths, and bursal structures, usually just beyond the confines of the joint capsule; less frequently, they are attached to fascial structures, ligaments, aponeuroses, and interosseous membranes. They are rare in joint cavities; according to our material and most reviews, intra-articular synovial sarcomas account for fewer than 5% of all cases.[16]

In most series, 85–95% of all synovial sarcomas arise in the extremities, with a predilection for the lower extremities. In the lower extremities, most occur in the vicinity of the knee, with fewer arising in the foot, lower leg-ankle region, and hip-groin. Tumors arising in the upper extremities, which account for approximately

TABLE 37–1	SYNOVIAL SARCOMA: AFIP, 345 CASES
Anatomic location	**No. of cases**
Head-neck	31 (9.0%)
Neck	12
Pharynx	7
Larynx	7
Other	5
Trunk	28 (8.1%)
Chest	10
Abdominal wall	9
Other	9
Upper extremities	80 (23.2%)
Forearm-wrist	24
Shoulder	22
Elbow-upper arm	20
Hand	14
Lower extremities	206 (59.7%)
Thigh-knee	102
Foot	45
Lower leg-ankle	33
Hip-groin	22
Other	4
Total	345 (100.0%)

AFIP, Armed Forces Institute of Pathology.

10–15% of all cases, are fairly evenly distributed among the forearm-wrist region, shoulder, elbow-upper arm region, and hand. Occasionally, one encounters minute (<1 cm) synovial sarcomas arising in the hands and feet; these tumors seem to follow a clinically favorable course.[16a]

Following the extremities, the head and neck region is the second most common site of synovial sarcoma, accounting for up to 5–10% of all cases. Most of these tumors seem to originate in the paravertebral connective tissue spaces and manifest as solitary retropharyngeal or parapharyngeal masses near the carotid bifurcation. Additional cases in this general area have been reported in the paranasal sinuses,[17] mandible,[18] parotid gland,[19] and tonsil.[20] Because of the unusual location, synovial sarcomas in this region are often misdiagnosed.

About 5% of synovial sarcomas arise in the trunk, including the chest wall and abdominal wall.[21] Like synovial sarcomas at other sites, these neoplasms are usually deep-seated. Fetsch and Meis, who reviewed 27 cases culled from the Armed Forces Institute of Pathology (AFIP) material, noted a large number of cystic tumors among their cases.[21] The age and gender incidence of these tumors and their behavior corresponds to that of synovial sarcomas at other sites.

Synovial sarcoma has been described at virtually every anatomic site including the heart,[22] pleuropulmonary region,[23,24] kidney,[25] prostate,[26] liver,[27] mediastinum,[28] retroperitoneum,[29] gastrointestinal tract,[30] and peripheral nerve,[31] among others. With tumors arising in these unusual sites, definitive recognition becomes more difficult and usually requires confirmation by molecular genetic techniques.

Radiographic findings

Radiographic studies may be extremely helpful for suggesting a preoperative diagnosis of synovial sarcoma, largely because of the presence of calcification. Most synovial sarcomas present on routine films as round or oval, more or less lobulated swellings or masses of moderate density, usually located in close proximity to a large joint. The underlying bone tends to be uninvolved, but in about 15–20% of the cases, there is a periosteal reaction, superficial bone erosion, or invasion. Massive bone destruction, which is rare, is mostly caused by poorly differentiated synovial sarcomas of long duration and large size.

The most striking radiologic characteristic, found in 15–20% of synovial sarcomas, is the presence of multiple small, spotty radiopacities caused by focal calcification and, less frequently, bone formation.[32] In most instances these changes consist merely of fine stippling, but in some cases large portions of the tumor are marked or even outlined by radiopaque masses (Figs 37–1 to 37–3). Confusion with other tumors is possible, but radiopacities are not observed in most other forms of sarcoma with the exception of extraskeletal osteosarcoma, a tumor that tends to occur in an older group of individuals.

Computed tomography (CT) and magnetic resonance imaging (MRI) are valuable tools for determining the site of origin and extent of the lesion. Like conventional radiographs, they show a para-articular heterogeneous septated mass, often with associated calcification or bone erosion, but they do not provide a specific or diagnostic picture.[33]

Gross findings

The gross appearance varies depending on the rate of growth and the location of the tumor. Slowly growing lesions tend to be sharply circumscribed, round, or multilobular; as a result of compression of adjacent tissues by the expansively growing tumor, they are completely or partially invested by a smooth, glistening pseudocapsule (Fig. 37–4). Cyst formation may be prominent, and occasional lesions present as multicystic masses (Fig. 37–5).[34] Most of the tumors are firmly attached to surrounding tendons, tendon sheaths, or the exterior wall of the joint capsule; not infrequently, portions of these structures adhere to the gross specimen. On palpation they are either soft or firm, depending on their collagen content. On section, they are yellow to gray-white. They may attain a size of 15 cm or more, but most are between 3 and 6 cm at the time of excision. Calcification is common but rarely a discernible macroscopic feature. Less well-differentiated and more rapidly growing

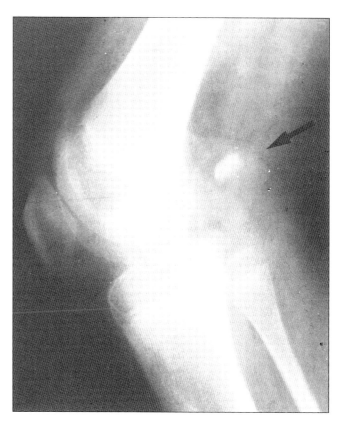

FIGURE 37–1 Radiograph of a synovial sarcoma originating in the popliteal fossa. Note the focal calcification in the tumor (arrow), a feature that is present in about 20% of these cases.

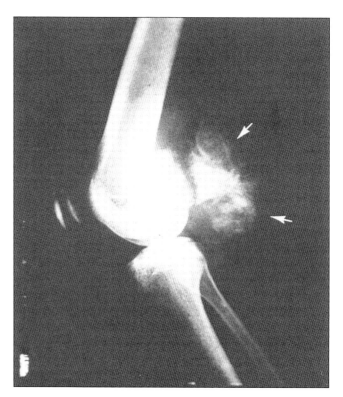

FIGURE 37–2 Massive calcification and ossification in a synovial sarcoma of the popliteal fossa (arrows). In general, tumors with extensive calcification carry a better prognosis than those without.

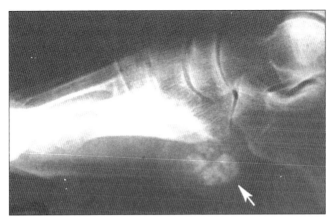

FIGURE 37–3 Radiograph of a synovial sarcoma of the planta pedis showing extensive calcification of the tumor (arrow).

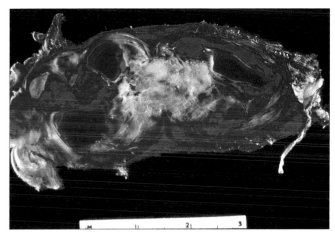

FIGURE 37–5 Multicystic synovial sarcoma of the knee region.

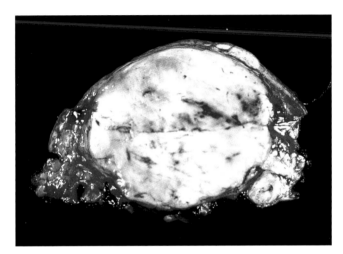

FIGURE 37–4 Photomicrograph of a high-grade monophasic fibrous synovial sarcoma. The tumor has a fleshy gray-tan appearance with focal hemorrhage.

synovial sarcomas tend to be poorly circumscribed and commonly exhibit a rather variegated and often friable or shaggy appearance, frequently with multiple areas of hemorrhage, necrosis, and cyst formation. Markedly hemorrhagic tumors may be confused with angiosarcomas or even organizing hematomas.

Microscopic findings

Unlike most other types of sarcoma, the tumor is composed of two morphologically different types of cells: *epithelial cells*, resembling those of carcinoma, and fibrosarcoma-like *spindle cells*, sometimes incorrectly designated as *stromal cells*. Transitional forms between epithelial and spindle cells suggest a close relation, which is also supported by tissue culture, ultrastructural, immunohistochemical, and molecular genetic findings. Depending on the relative prominence of the two cellular elements and the degree of differentiation, synovial sarcomas form

a continuous morphologic spectrum and can be broadly classified into the (1) *biphasic type*, with distinct epithelial and spindle cell components in varying proportions; (2) *monophasic fibrous type*; (3) rare *monophasic epithelial type*; and (4) *poorly differentiated (round cell) type*.

Biphasic synovial sarcoma

The classic synovial sarcoma – the biphasic type – is generally readily recognizable by the coexistence of morphologically different but histogenetically related epithelial cells and fibroblast-like spindle cells (Figs 37–6 to 37–8). The epithelial cells are characterized by large, round or oval, vesicular nuclei and abundant pale-staining cytoplasm with distinctly outlined cellular borders. The cells are cuboidal to tall and columnar; they are arranged in solid cords, nests or glandular structures that contain granular or homogeneous eosinophilic secretions (Figs 37–9, 37–10). The glandular spaces lined by epithelial cells must be distinguished from cleft-like artifacts that are the result of tissue shrinkage. Outpouchings of the cyst-like spaces into the surrounding uninvolved tissue may wrongly suggest an origin within a bursa, particularly because some of these spaces are lined by a single layer of epithelial cells bearing a resemblance to normal synovium.

Not infrequently, cuboidal or flattened epithelial cells also cover small villous or papillary structures often with spindle cells rather than connective tissue in the papillary core. A diagnosis of squamous cell carcinoma may also be suggested by focal squamous metaplasia, including the occasional formation of squamous pearls and keratohyaline granules.

The surrounding spindle cell component consists mostly of well-oriented, rather plump, spindle-shaped cells of uniform appearance with small amounts of indistinct cytoplasm and oval dark-staining nuclei. Generally, the cells form solid, compact sheets that are similar in many respects to fibrosarcoma (Figs 37–11, 37–12),

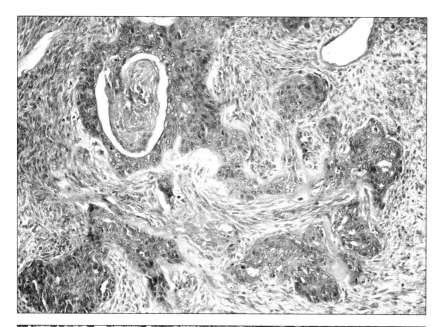

FIGURE 37–6 Biphasic synovial sarcoma showing close apposition of epithelial structures with malignant spindle cells.

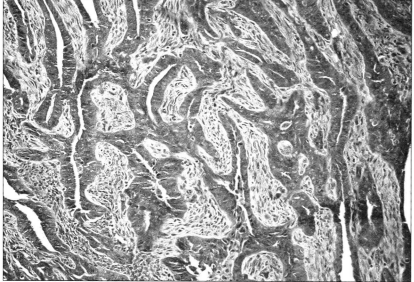

FIGURE 37–7 Typical biphasic synovial sarcoma with columnar epithelial cells surrounded by spindle cell elements.

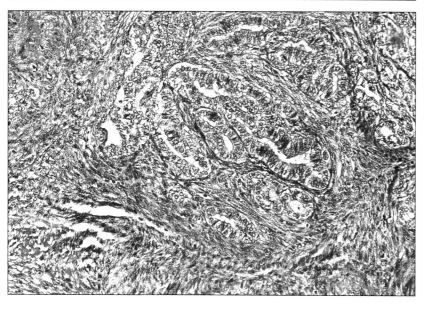

FIGURE 37–8 Biphasic synovial sarcoma with glandular epithelial structures adjacent to a malignant spindle cell component.

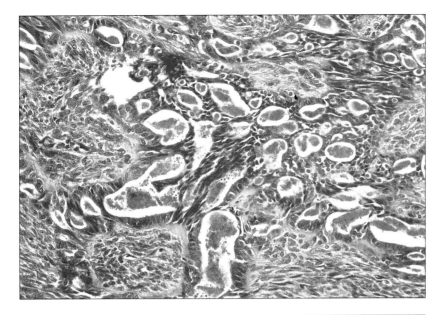

FIGURE 37–9 Biphasic synovial sarcoma. The epithelial structures have intraluminal eosinophilic secretions.

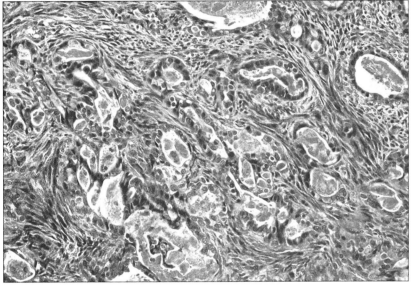

FIGURE 37–10 Biphasic synovial sarcoma with prominent intraluminal eosinophilic secretions in epithelial elements.

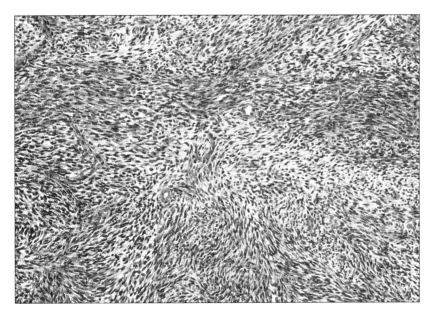

FIGURE 37–11 Fibrosarcoma-like area in a synovial sarcoma. Note the alternating darkly staining and lightly staining regions, imparting a marbled appearance.

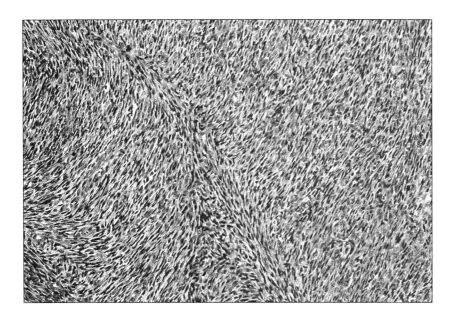

FIGURE 37–12 Fibrosarcoma-like area in a synovial sarcoma. The spindle cells are arranged in distinct fascicles.

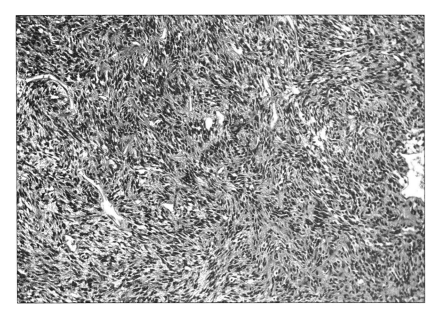

FIGURE 37–13 Synovial sarcoma with focal nuclear palisading reminiscent of a neural tumor.

except for the absence of long, sweeping fascicles or a herringbone pattern and a more irregular nodular arrangement. Mitotic figures in synovial sarcoma occur in both epithelial and spindle-shaped cells, but as a rule only the poorly differentiated forms of the tumor exhibit more than two mitotic figures (MFs) per high-power field (HPF). Occasionally there is nuclear palisading (Fig. 37–13); but in contrast to leiomyosarcomas and malignant peripheral nerve sheath tumors, this feature is confined to a small portion of the tumor.

Commonly, the cellular portions of synovial sarcoma alternate with less cellular areas displaying hyalinization, myxoid change, or calcification. The collagen in the hyalinized zones may be diffusely distributed or form narrow bands or plaque-like masses sometimes associated with a markedly thickened basement membrane separating epithelial and spindle-cell elements (Fig. 37–14). The myxoid areas are generally less conspicuous and tend to occupy only a small, ill-defined portion of the tumor, although some cases are predominantly myxoid (Fig. 37–15).[35]

Calcification with or without ossification is another diagnostically important and characteristic feature that is present to a varying degree in about 20% of synovial sarcomas. It may be inconspicuous and consist merely of a few small irregularly distributed spherical concretions, or it may be extensive and occupy a large portion of the neoplasm (Fig. 37–16).[32,36,37] In general, calcification is preceded by hyalinization and is more pronounced at the periphery of the tumor than at its center. Rarely, chondroid changes are present, nearly always together with focal calcification and ossification.

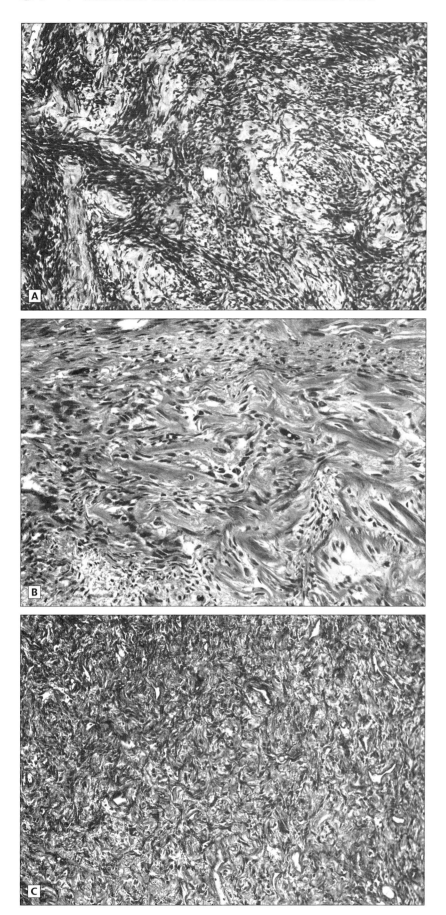

FIGURE 37–14 (A) Monophasic synovial sarcoma with prominent perivascular hyalinization. **(B)** Thick collagen bands separate malignant spindle cells in a monophasic synovial sarcoma. This pattern of hyalinization is characteristic of this tumor. **(C)** Extensive hyalinization in a synovial sarcoma with compression of neoplastic cells.

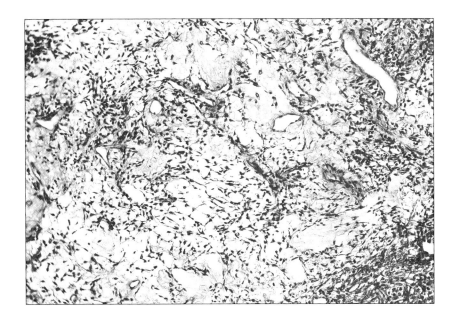

FIGURE 37–15 Prominent myxoid change in synovial sarcoma.

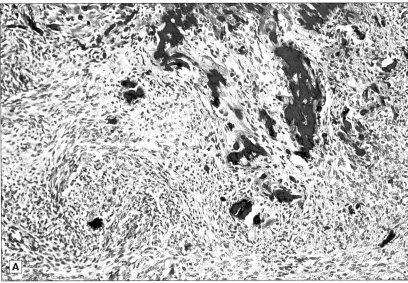

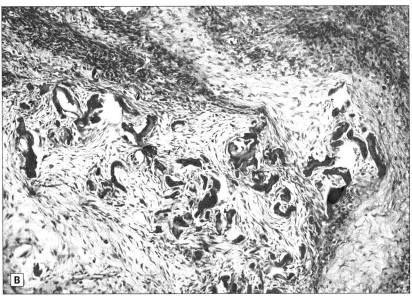

FIGURE 37–16 (A) Calcification in a synovial sarcoma, a common feature of this neoplasm. **(B)** Note the focus of calcification in this small monophasic fibrous synovial sarcoma of the foot.

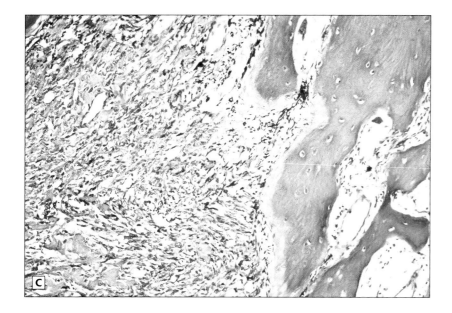

FIGURE 37–16 Continued. **(C)** Monophasic fibrous type of synovial sarcoma with osseous metaplasia.

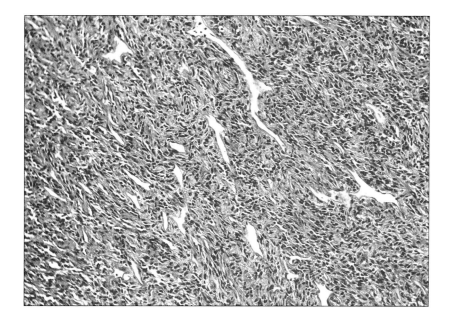

FIGURE 37–17 Prominent hemangiopericytomatous vasculature in a synovial sarcoma.

Mast cells are yet another conspicuous feature of synovial sarcoma; they show no particular arrangement but are more numerous in the spindle-cell than in the epithelial portions of the neoplasm. Inflammatory elements and multinucleated giant cells are rare.

The degree of vascularity varies. In some cases it is a dominant feature with numerous dilated vascular spaces resembling hemangiopericytoma (Fig. 37–17); in others there are merely a few scattered vascular structures. Some cases show prominent cystic changes (Fig. 37–18). Secondary changes such as hemorrhage are most prominent in poorly differentiated tumors. Scattered lipid macrophages, siderophages, multinucleated giant cells, and deposits of cholesterol may be present but are much less conspicuous in synovial sarcomas than in synovitis.

Monophasic fibrous synovial sarcoma

The monophasic fibrous form of synovial sarcoma is a relatively common neoplasm, the existence of which has been confirmed by positive immunostaining of some or most of the spindle cells for epithelial antigens, by ultrastructural features revealing epithelial differentiation, and by identical cytogenetic and molecular genetic abnormalities found in the biphasic type (discussed below). Because this type is closely related to the biphasic type and merely represents one extreme of its morphologic spectrum, the previously mentioned morphologic parameters of the spindle-cell portion of the biphasic type, such as cellular appearance, hyalinization, myxoid change, mast cell infiltrate, hemangiopericytomatous vasculature,

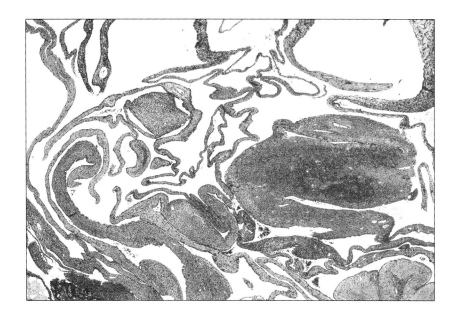

FIGURE 37–18 Cystic synovial sarcoma. Malignant spindle cells are seen in the thickened fibrous septa.

and focal calcification, apply equally to the monophasic fibrous type.

In some cases, an obvious epithelial component can be identified by extensive sampling, in which case the tumor is more appropriately designated as a biphasic synovial sarcoma. Even in those cases without obvious epithelial differentiation, however, many monophasic fibrous synovial sarcomas have foci in which the cells have a more epithelioid morphology and appear to be more cohesive than the surrounding spindle-shaped cells. The cells in these foci have more eosinophilic cytoplasm but otherwise have the same nuclear features as the surrounding spindle-shaped cells. Such areas often show immunohistochemical evidence of epithelial differentiation (Fig. 37–19).

Monophasic epithelial synovial sarcoma

What has been said about the diagnosis of the monophasic fibrous type of synovial sarcoma applies also to the monophasic epithelial synovial sarcoma, a rarely recognized neoplasm. In our experience, it is often difficult to render this diagnosis with any degree of certainty without corroborating cytogenetic or molecular genetic data. In fact, it might be argued that this variant exists only conceptually as a means of validating the entire (epithelial) biphasic spectrum of synovial sarcoma. However, with the ability to analyze tumors for the characteristic translocation and fusion transcript, it is now feasible to diagnose monophasic epithelial synovial sarcoma in tumors that otherwise would be misdiagnosed as other benign or malignant epithelial neoplasms. The most important differential considerations are metastatic carcinoma, melanoma, and adnexal tumors. However, other epithelioid mesenchymal tumors should also be considered, including epithelioid sarcoma and epithelioid malignant

peripheral nerve sheath tumor. We have encountered several tumors of this type, but all had minute foci of spindle-cell differentiation and, strictly speaking, were biphasic synovial sarcomas with an exceptionally prominent epithelial pattern (Figs 37–20 to 37–22).

Poorly differentiated synovial sarcoma

Poorly differentiated synovial sarcoma can be thought of as a form of tumor progression that can be superimposed on any of the other synovial sarcoma subtypes. Recognition of this subtype of synovial sarcoma is of practical importance not only because it poses a special problem in diagnosis but also because it behaves more aggressively and metastasizes in a significantly higher percentage of cases.[38-40] The incidence of the poorly differentiated type among synovial sarcomas is difficult to estimate, but in the study by Machen et al.,[41] 21 of 34 (62%) synovial sarcomas had poorly differentiated foci, in some cases accounting for up to 90% of the neoplasm. However, this pattern predominates in fewer than 20% of all cases of synovial sarcoma.

Histologically, poorly differentiated synovial sarcoma may have three patterns:[42] (1) a large-cell or epithelioid pattern composed of variably sized rounded nuclei with prominent nucleoli (Fig. 37–23); (2) a small-cell pattern with nuclear features similar to other small round cell tumors; and (3) a high-grade spindle-cell pattern composed of spindle-shaped cells with high-grade nuclear features and a high mitotic rate (Fig. 37–24) often accompanied by necrosis. Such tumors often have a richly vascular pattern with dilated thin-walled vascular spaces resembling those of malignant hemangiopericytoma. In fact, it appears that a high percentage of sarcomas interpreted as malignant hemangiopericytomas are actually examples of poorly differentiated synovial sarcoma.

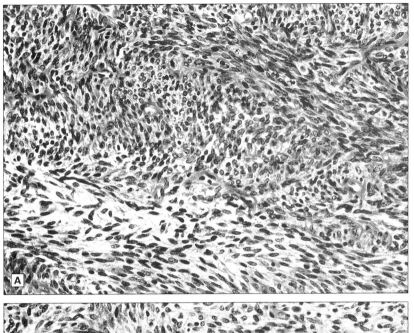

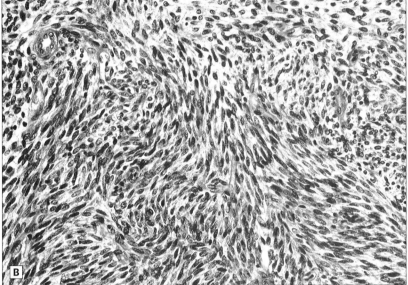

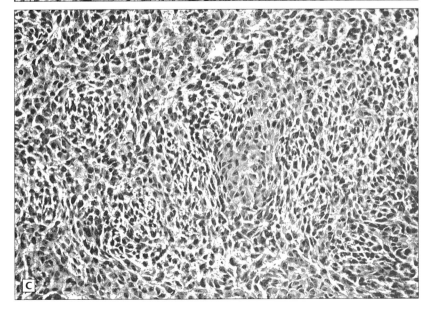

FIGURE 37–19 (A) High-magnification view of a monophasic fibrous synovial sarcoma. The malignant spindle cells are relatively uniform with respect to one another. **(B)** Uniform spindle cells in a monophasic fibrous synovial sarcoma. **(C)** Epithelioid area in a monophasic fibrous synovial sarcoma. A small group of cells have increased amounts of eosinophilic cytoplasm and appear more cohesive.

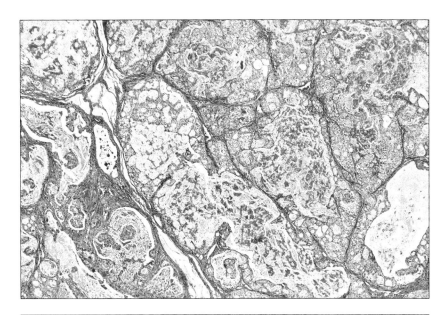

FIGURE 37–20 Monophasic epithelial-type synovial sarcoma. A cribriform glandular pattern was prominent throughout this neoplasm.

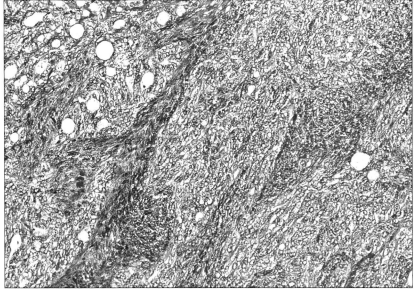

FIGURE 37–21 Predominantly epithelial-type synovial sarcoma. Small areas with a well-developed spindle cell pattern are present.

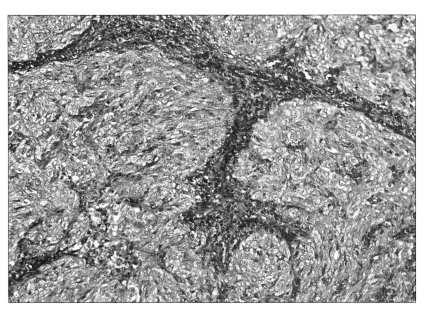

FIGURE 37–22 Predominantly epithelial-type synovial sarcoma. Most of this tumor was composed of sheets of cohesive epithelioid cells with only small foci of spindle-cell differentiation.

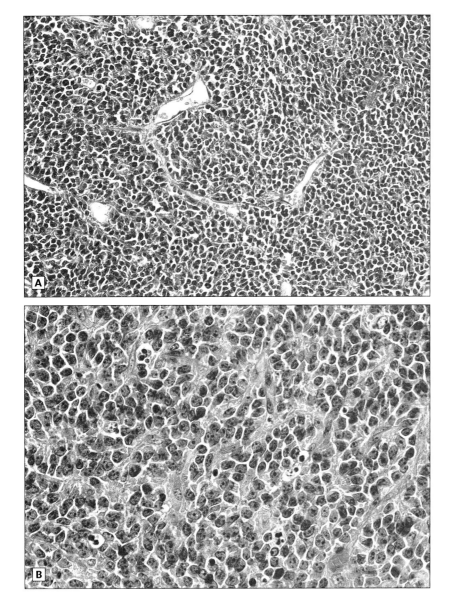

FIGURE 37–23 Poorly differentiated area of a synovial sarcoma. **(A)** Low-magnification view with a prominent hemangiopericytomatous vasculature. **(B)** Note the cytologic features of round cells in poorly differentiated synovial sarcoma.

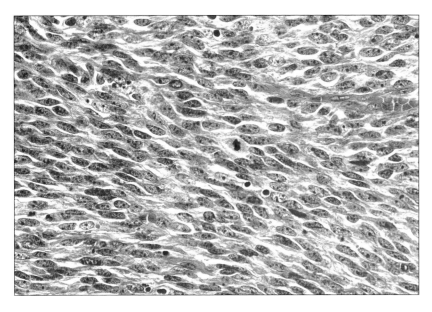

FIGURE 37–24 Poorly differentiated synovial sarcoma composed of spindle cells with high-grade nuclear features.

Occasionally, cells with intracytoplasmic hyaline inclusions imparting a rhabdoid morphology may be found in poorly differentiated areas.[43] Distinguishing this tumor from other round cell sarcomas such as the Ewing's sarcoma/primitive neuroectodermal tumor (ES/PNET) family may be exceedingly difficult and often requires ancillary immunohistochemical and/or molecular genetic techniques.[38,39]

Special staining procedures

Two distinctive types of mucinous material are present in synovial sarcomas. Secretions in the epithelial cells, intracellular clefts, and pseudoglandular spaces stain positively with the periodic acid-Schiff (PAS), colloidal iron, Alcian blue, and mucicarmine stains. The staining characteristics of the mucinous secretions remain unaltered after treatment of the secretions with diastase and hyaluronidase, but in general and in distinction to adenocarcinomas, the mucinous material is more conspicuous in the intracellular clefts and pseudoglandular spaces than in the secreting epithelial cells. This mucinous material is composed predominantly of chondroitin sulfate and hyaluronic acid.[44] In contrast to mesothelioma, granular intracellular glycogen that stains positively for PAS is never a striking feature of synovial sarcoma.

The second type of mucinous material, stromal or mesenchymal mucin, which is elaborated by the spindle cells, also stains positively for colloidal iron and Alcian blue stains, but it is weakly carminophilic and stains negatively with the PAS preparation. It is present in the interstices of the spindle-cell areas and the loosely textured myxoid portions of the tumor. This material is rich in hyaluronic acid and, like other mesenchymal mucins, is completely removed by prior treatment with hyaluronidase. PAS and Alcian blue preparations – as well as various metachromatic stains – are also useful for identifying the mast cell infiltrate, but are not necessary to perform.

Immunohistochemical findings

Most synovial sarcomas display immunoreactivity for cytokeratins and epithelial membrane antigen (Fig. 37–25). In an immunohistochemical study of 100 synovial sarcomas by Guillou et al.,[45] focal positivity for epithelial membrane antigen (EMA) and cytokeratin was found in 97% and 69% of cases, respectively. In this study, only 1 of 100 cases was negative for both of these epithelial markers. In our experience and that reported in the literature, approximately 90% of all synovial sarcomas are cytokeratin-positive. In general, the intensity of staining is more pronounced in the epithelial component than in the spindled component. In some lesions of the monophasic fibrous type, only a few isolated cells express these antigens, making it necessary to stain and examine multiple sections from different portions of the tumor (Fig. 37–26).[46] Poorly differentiated variants usually, but not always, express these epithelial markers. In the study by Folpe and colleagues,[38] all nine poorly differentiated synovial sarcomas stained for EMA, whereas only 30% and 50% stained for low- and high-molecular-weight cytokeratins, respectively. Similarly, van de Rijn et al. found staining for EMA and cytokeratin in 95% and 42% of poorly differentiated synovial sarcomas, respectively.[39] In contrast to other spindle cell sarcomas, the cells of synovial sarcoma express cytokeratins 7 and 19.[46,47] In fact, these markers often decorate a larger proportion of cells than either EMA or AE1/AE3. Miettinen et al. evaluated 110 synovial sarcomas of all subtypes and found fairly consistent expression of CK7, CK19, CK8/18, and CK14 in the epithelial cells of biphasic tumors.[46] However,

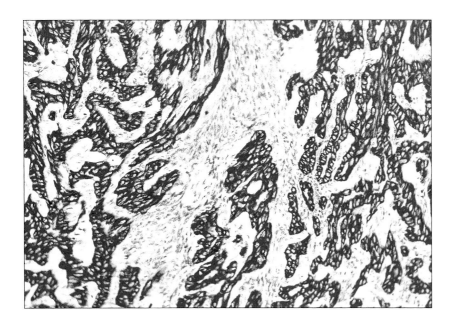

FIGURE 37–25 High-molecular-weight cytokeratin immunoreactivity highlights the epithelial elements in this biphasic synovial sarcoma.

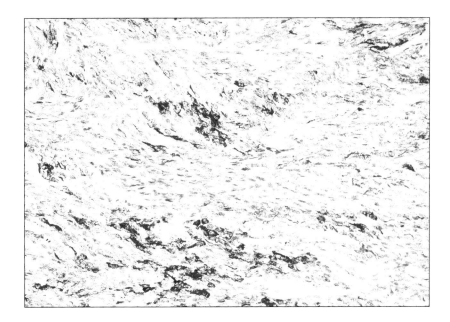

FIGURE 37–26 Focal immunoreactivity for cytokeratin 7 in a monophasic fibrous synovial sarcoma.

the cells of monophasic synovial sarcoma had a more limited cytokeratin repertory, with focal expression of CK7 (79%), CK19 (60%), and CK8/18 (45%). Poorly differentiated cells showed even more limited expression of CK7 (50%) and CK19 (61%). In a study of 60 t(X;18) *SYT-SSX*-positive cases, Pelmus and colleagues found EMA to be the most sensitive epithelial marker.[48]

Although not emphasized until recently, up to 30% of synovial sarcomas show focal immunoreactivity for S-100 protein.[45,47,48] Most of these S-100 protein-positive synovial sarcomas co-express epithelial markers, but the occasional synovial sarcoma expresses S-100 protein in the absence of EMA or AE1/AE3, thereby causing confusion with a malignant peripheral nerve sheath tumor. In such cases, the detection of CK7 and/or CK19 and/or molecular genetic studies may be useful for recognizing monophasic fibrous synovial sarcoma.

CD99, the product of the *MIC2* gene, can be immunohistochemically detected in the cytoplasm or cell membrane in 60–70% of synovial sarcomas.[48,49] BCL2 protein is diffusely expressed in virtually all synovial sarcomas, especially in the spindled cells,[50] but is of limited diagnostic value since many other tumors express this antigen. Unlike many other spindle cell tumors, synovial sarcoma is virtually always negative for CD34, although there are rare exceptions. Calponin has also been found to be frequently expressed in synovial sarcoma, which may be useful in recognizing poorly differentiated variants, since other round cell tumors are negative for this antigen.[51]

More recently, TLE1 has emerged as a potentially useful marker of synovial sarcoma.[51a] Gene expression profiling studies have consistently identified *TLE1* as an excellent discriminator of synovial sarcoma from other sarcomas. Terry et al. found the TLE protein to be

expressed in 91 of 94 molecularly confirmed synovial sarcomas while it was very rarely expressed in other mesenchymal neoplasms.[51a]

Ultrastructural findings

The biphasic tumors are composed of epithelial and spindle cells with transitional forms showing features of both cell types. The epithelial cells have sharply defined, ovoid nuclei with narrow, dense rims of chromatin and abundant cytoplasm containing mitochondria, a prominent Golgi complex, rare paranuclear aggregates of intermediate filaments, lysosomes, and smooth and rough endoplasmic reticulum, sometimes arranged in stacked arrays. On rare occasions, tonofilaments are found in the epithelial cells, especially in the areas of squamous metaplasia. Frequently, the epithelial cells are disposed in clusters or gland-like structures, with microvilli or villous filopodia on the surfaces facing the intercellular or pseudoglandular spaces. Many of the spaces contain electron-dense mucinous material. In contrast to the cells of normal synovium, the epithelial cells are interconnected by junctional complexes, zonulae adherens, or desmosome-like structures, a finding supported by the consistent expression of tight junction-related proteins including ZO-1, claudin, and occludin.[52] The fibroblast-like spindle cells have irregularly outlined nuclei, marginated chromatin, and small nucleoli. The cytoplasm contains mitochondria and a prominent Golgi apparatus, but there is less cytoplasm and a less well-developed rough endoplasmic reticulum than that of typical fibroblasts. A continuous basal lamina, a structure that is absent in normal synovium, often separates the epithelial clusters and gland-like structures from the surrounding spindle-shaped cells (Fig. 37–27).[53,54]

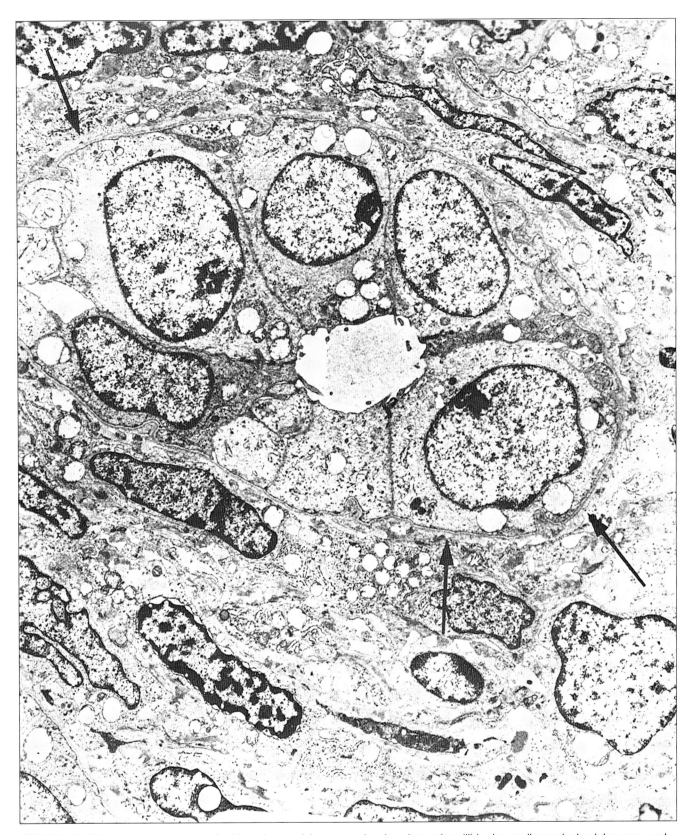

FIGURE 37–27 Electron micrograph of a biphasic synovial sarcoma showing short microvilli in the small pseudoglandular space and separation of the epithelial and fibroblast-like spindle-cell elements by a distinct basal lamina (arrows). (Courtesy of Dr. R.F. Armstrong, Victoria Hospital, London, Canada.)

The ultrastructural features of the monophasic fibrous type are indistinguishable from those of the spindle-cell areas of the biphasic type. There are, however, identifying features of early epithelial differentiation, such as intercellular or cleft-like spaces of varying size bordered by multiple microvilli, as well as poorly developed junctions or desmosome-like structures. In addition, there are occasional cell clusters similar to those seen in the biphasic type. There is no distinct basal lamina, but there are occasional fragments of basal lamina or condensed ground substance at the cell surfaces.[55]

Cytogenetic and molecular genetic findings

A consistent, specific translocation, most commonly a balanced reciprocal translocation, t(X;18)(p11;q11), is found in virtually all synovial sarcomas, regardless of subtype.[56] This translocation involves the fusion of the *SYT* gene on chromosome 18 and either the *SSX1* or *SSX2* gene on the *X* chromosome (both at Xp11), or rarely, with *SSX4* (also at Xp11).[57–59] The function of the SYT-SSX fusion protein has yet to be fully defined but fuses transcriptional activation (SYT) and repression (SSX) domains resulting in the dysregulation of gene expression.[57] DNA microarray expression profiling studies have shown upregulation of a number of genes including *IGFBP2*, *IGF2*, and *ELF3*. A consistent finding has been the up-regulation of genes involved with the Wnt signaling pathway, including *TLE1*.[60,61] *SYT-SSX1* and *SYT-SSX2* appear to be mutually exclusive gene fusions, and there is concordance of fusion type between primary tumors and their metastases.[62] Overall, approximately two-thirds of synovial sarcomas harbor an *SYT-SSX1* fusion and one-third reveal an *SYT-SSX2* fusion. Interestingly, several studies have found an association between fusion type and histology. The vast majority of tumors with *SYT-SSX2* are monophasic fibrous tumors, whereas almost all biphasic synovial sarcomas have an *SYT-SSX1* fusion.[7,63,64] The SYT-SSX fusion can be detected by real-time reverse transcriptase-polymerase chain reaction (RT-PCR)[65–67] or fluorescence in situ hybridization (FISH)[68] using frozen or paraffin-embedded tissue.[69,70,70a] These techniques are particularly useful for monophasic fibrous and poorly differentiated synovial sarcomas which may be difficult to distinguish from other spindle cell and round cell sarcomas, respectively, as discussed further below. It is also invaluable in distinguishing the rare monophasic epithelial type of synovial sarcoma from adenocarcinoma. In our own practice, we utilize paraffin-embedded tissue for analysis by FISH using a dual-color, breakapart SYT probe. In general, although we do not believe molecular testing is required in every case, if the diagnosis of synovial sarcoma is in question for any reason, we proceed with ancillary molecular diagnostic testing provided there is adequate tissue.

Differential diagnosis

Distinguishing synovial sarcoma from other neoplasms may be difficult, and in many instances a reliable diagnosis is not possible without ancillary diagnostic techniques. The differential diagnosis depends of course on the subtype of synovial sarcoma.

Differential diagnosis of biphasic synovial sarcoma

In general, biphasic synovial sarcoma causes few diagnostic problems, especially if the tumor is located in the extremities near a large joint and occurs in a young adult. However, when the tumor arises in an unusual site, *carcinosarcoma*, *glandular malignant peripheral nerve sheath tumor* (MPNST), and *malignant mesothelioma* enter the differential diagnosis. In carcinosarcomas of any site, the glandular element usually shows a significantly greater degree of nuclear pleomorphism than the epithelial component seen in biphasic synovial sarcoma. Similarly, the spindle-cell component of carcinosarcomas is usually more cytologically atypical. Glandular MPNST, a rare neoplasm, usually can be recognized by the presence of intestinal-type epithelium with goblet cells, the occasional association with rhabdomyosarcomatous elements (Triton tumor), and the occurrence in patients with manifestations of neurofibromatosis type 1.[71,72]

Synovial sarcoma may arise in the pleuropulmonary region or peritoneum and thus may cause confusion with malignant mesothelioma. However, the latter tumor typically presents in older patients, often male, usually with a history of significant asbestos exposure. Furthermore, malignant mesotheliomas involve the pleura or peritoneum diffusely and only rarely present as a localized mass. Histologically, malignant mesotheliomas with spindled and epithelial areas usually show a gradual transition between these two areas. Synovial sarcomas, on the other hand, have a sharp abutment of gland with stroma. There is some immunohistochemical overlap, since synovial sarcomas express calretinin in over 50% of cases.[73] However, synovial sarcomas frequently express Ber-Ep4 and are negative for WT1. Finally, identification of a t(X;18) or *SYT-SSX* fusion would confirm a diagnosis of synovial sarcoma in extremely difficult cases.

Differential diagnosis of monophasic fibrous synovial sarcoma

The monophasic fibrous synovial sarcoma may resemble a number of other spindle cell neoplasms including fibrosarcoma, leiomyosarcoma, MPNST, hemangiopericytoma, and spindle cell carcinoma. Often, an immunohistochemical panel is necessary to make this distinction, and in difficult cases, cytogenetic or molecular genetic techniques can confirm the diagnosis. This tumor can be distinguished from *fibrosarcoma* by its frequent location near large joints, its irregular and often multilobular growth pattern, the plump appearance of the nuclei, and the focal whorled arrangement of the spindle cells. In general, mitotic figures are less common than in fibrosarcomas. Additional factors that suggest a synovial sarcoma are the presence of mast cells, foci of calcification, the presence of a focal hemangiopericytoma-like vasculature, and, most importantly, the demonstration of cytokeratin or EMA in the neoplastic cells. It is likely that many so-called fibrosarcomas reported in the older literature are actually monophasic fibrous synovial sarcomas.

Some monophasic fibrous synovial sarcomas contain spindle cells with more eosinophilic cytoplasm, reminiscent of *leiomyosarcoma*. However, leiomyosarcomas typically have cells arranged in better-defined fascicles that intersect at right angles to each other. The nuclei are blunt-ended, often with a paranuclear vacuole, and the cytoplasm is more densely eosinophilic. Although some leiomyosarcomas express cytokeratins, particularly CK8/18, virtually all of these tumors stain strongly for smooth muscle actin, and many others express muscle-specific actin or desmin. The absence of bcl-2 protein in leiomyosarcoma may also be useful for this distinction.

The *malignant peripheral nerve sheath tumor* may bear a close resemblance to the monophasic fibrous type of synovial sarcoma (Table 37–2). Given the chemosensitivity of synovial sarcoma, this distinction is of more than academic interest. Obvious origin from a nerve suggests a diagnosis of MPNST, although rare examples of synovial sarcoma arise in peripheral nerves.[31] Synovial sarcomas do not arise from preexisting neurofibromas or in patients with neurofibromatosis type 1. Both MPNST and monophasic synovial sarcoma may have alternating areas of hyper- and hypocellularity, imparting a marbled appearance at low magnification. Neuroid-type whorls and perivascular or subintimal involvement of blood vessels by the neoplastic cells suggest a diagnosis of MPNST.

Cytologically, the cells of MPNST are often wavy or buckled and appear to have been pinched at one end, with bulbous protrusion of the opposite end of the nucleus. Immunohistochemically, approximately two-thirds of MPNSTs stain focally for S-100 protein. Because S-100 protein is found in up to 30% of synovial sarcomas, this marker alone cannot distinguish between these two neoplasms. Similarly, although up to 90% of synovial sarcomas express EMA or AE1/AE3, some examples of MPNST express these antigens as well. In this context, CK7 and CK19 may be useful in that virtually all synovial sarcomas express CK7, CK19, or both, whereas both of these antigens are rarely expressed in MPNST.[47] Recently, HMGA2 was found to be consistently expressed in MPNST and only rarely in synovial sarcoma, suggesting this marker may be a useful addition to the immunohistochemical panel.[74]

Finally, we believe detection of an *SYT-SSX* fusion allows for a definitive diagnosis of synovial sarcoma. Although one study suggested that up to 75% of MPNSTs had a t(X;18), subsequent studies by several groups have found the t(X;18) to be exclusive of synovial sarcoma.[75-77] Technical issues likely account for the false-positive cases in the study by O'Sullivan and colleagues.[59,78] Coindre and colleagues confirmed that MPNSTs are t(X;18)-negative sarcomas by analyzing 25 cases occurring in NF1 patients.[78a]

Many synovial sarcomas exhibit a prominent hemangiopericytoma-like vascular pattern, which can result in an erroneous diagnosis of *hemangiopericytoma*. The latter tumor is quite uncommon and by definition is a diagnosis of exclusion. Typically, this vascular pattern is present as a focal phenomenon in synovial sarcoma, whereas, by definition, hemangiopericytoma has this vasculature throughout the entire neoplasm, including myxoid and hyalinized zones. In addition, hemangiopericytoma lacks immunohistochemical evidence of epithelial differentiation and expresses CD34 in up to 80% of cases, a marker typically absent in synovial sarcomas.

Differential diagnosis of monophasic epithelial synovial sarcoma

Distinction of purely epithelial forms of synovial sarcoma from *adnexal* or *metastatic carcinoma* is virtually impossible in the absence of a focal biphasic pattern. Fortunately, most of these tumors, when carefully sampled, have focal spindle-cell areas that are sufficiently characteristic to allow a specific diagnosis. As previously mentioned, molecular diagnostic techniques should be utilized in suspected cases.[79]

Differential diagnosis of poorly differentiated synovial sarcoma

In most instances, poorly differentiated synovial sarcoma resembles a number of other small round cell neoplasms

TABLE 37–2	IMMUNOHISTOCHEMICAL AND MOLECULAR GENETIC FEATURES OF MONOPHASIC FIBROUS SYNOVIAL SARCOMA COMPARED TO MALIGNANT PERIPHERAL NERVE SHEATH TUMOR	
	MSS %	**MPNST %**
AE1/AE3	90	30
CK7	85	
CK19	85	
S-100 protein	30	60
CD99	60–70	Rare
SYT aberration	+	

MSS, monophasic synovial sarcoma; MPNST, malignant peripheral nerve sheath tumor.

TABLE 37–3	IMMUNOHISTOCHEMICAL AND MOLECULAR GENETIC FEATURES OF POORLY DIFFERENTIATED SYNOVIAL SARCOMA COMPARED TO EWING'S SARCOMA/ PRIMITIVE NEUROECTODERMAL TUMOR FAMILY	
	PDSS %	**ES/PNET %**
CD99	60–70	+
AE1/AE3	50–60	Rare
CAM5.2	50–60	30
CK7	70	
CK19	70	
SYT aberration	+	
EWS aberration		+

PDSS, poorly differentiated synovial sarcoma; ES/PNET, Ewing's sarcoma/primitive neuroectodermal tumor.

including the ES/PNET family of tumors, neuroblastoma, rhabdomyosarcoma, malignant hemangiopericytoma, mesenchymal chondrosarcoma, and lymphoma. A diagnosis of poorly differentiated synovial sarcoma is made simpler if one can identify a lower-grade component that is typical of either monophasic or biphasic synovial sarcoma. In the absence of such a component, or if only a small amount of tissue composed entirely of round cells is available, distinction from the aforementioned entities invariably requires ancillary diagnostic techniques.

Although CD99 is a highly sensitive marker of the ES/PNET family of tumors, this antigen is found in up to 70% of synovial sarcomas, including poorly differentiated variants (Table 37–3). Furthermore, epithelial markers may be absent in poorly differentiated synovial sarcoma and, although not well recognized, many ES/PNETs express cytokeratins, especially CAM5.2.[80-84] Machen et al. found CK7 and CK19 useful for this distinction in that most poorly differentiated synovial sarcomas, including those that lack AE1/AE3 and EMA, express CK7, CK19, or both, whereas these antigens are typically absent in the ES/PNET family of tumors.[85] Identification of the *EWS-FLI-1* or *SYT-SSX* fusions are useful for confirming diagnoses of ES/PNET and poorly differentiated synovial sarcoma, respectively.

Neuroblastoma arises from structures of the sympathetic nervous system during early childhood, characteristically has Homer Wright rosettes, and lacks expression of both CD99 and epithelial markers. *Rhabdomyosarcoma* can be excluded by the absence of desmin, myogenin, or MyoD1; appropriate T- and B-cell markers help exclude *lymphoma*. Distinction from *malignant hemangiopericytoma* may be exceedingly difficult given that some poorly differentiated synovial sarcomas lack immunohistochemical evidence of epithelial differentiation. In such cases, detection of an *SYT-SSX* fusion can confirm a diagnosis of poorly differentiated synovial sarcoma.

Some poorly differentiated synovial sarcomas are composed of large epithelioid cells, sometimes accompanied by cells with rhabdoid features. Such tumors may be difficult to distinguish from *metastatic carcinoma, epithelioid sarcoma,* and *malignant extrarenal rhabdoid tumor.* Recognition of a lower-grade area more typical of synovial sarcoma is the most useful way to distinguish these neoplasms. In the absence of such foci, a broad immunohistochemical panel (including antibodies to INI1/h SNFS, which characterizes malignant extrarenal rhabdoid tumor)[86] coupled with ultrastructural and molecular genetic data can usually resolve this dilemma.

Discussion

Recurrence and metastasis

Although traditionally considered to be a uniformly high-grade malignancy, advancements in therapy have lowered the incidence of recurrence and metastasis, with improved long-term survival. As one would expect, the prognosis is poorest in cases treated merely by local excision with inadequate margins and without any adjunctive therapy. In these cases recurrence rates as high as 80% are reported.[87] With adequate surgical excision or with adjunctive radiotherapy, the recurrence rate has been reported to be significantly lower (less than 40%). In most cases the recurrent growth manifests within the first 2 years after initial therapy.

Metastatic lesions develop in about half of cases, most commonly to the lung, followed by the lymph nodes and the bone marrow. In our series,[41] all patients who developed metastatic disease had involvement of one or both lungs; similarly, in the series of Ryan et al., the lung was affected in 94% of cases and the lymph nodes in 10%.[88]

There are numerous accounts of late metastasis and long periods of survival after metastasis. Thunold and Bang observed a woman who had a calcified synovial sarcoma removed at age 14 years and developed lung metastasis 26 years later.[89] On the other hand, there are rare instances in which pulmonary metastasis is already present at the time of or prior to the initial diagnosis. Microscopically, the metastatic lesions are usually similar to the primary neoplasm, but metastases of biphasic tumors often exhibit a more prominent spindle-cell pattern than the primary lesion, a lesser degree of cellular differentiation, and increased mitotic activity. Care should be exercised when interpreting pulmonary metastasis of any spindle cell sarcoma to avoid interpreting entrapped alveolar spaces as evidence of biphasic differentiation.

Prognosis

Reported 5-year survival rates for synovial sarcoma range from 36% to 76%,[7,8,90–93] and up to 82% in heavily calcified tumors.[36] Reported 10-year survival rates range from

TABLE 37–4	**FAVORABLE AND UNFAVORABLE PROGNOSTIC FACTORS BY MULTIVARIATE ANALYSIS FOR SYNOVIAL SARCOMA**

Low risk for metastasis
   Patient age <25 years
   Tumor size <5 cm
   Absence of poorly differentiated areas
High risk for metastasis
   Patient age >40 years
   Tumor size ≥5 cm
   Poorly differentiated areas

Modified from Bergh P, Meis-Kindblom JM, Gherlinzoni F, et al. Synovial sarcoma: identification of low and high risk groups. Cancer 1999; 85:2596.

20% to 63%.[91,94] The differences in the 5- and 10-year survival rates reflect the relatively high incidence of late metastases. Numerous clinical and microscopic factors have been reported to influence survival (Table 37–4). Major clinical factors associated with a more favorable clinical outcome include young age of the patient (15 years or younger),[8,95] tumor size smaller than 5 cm,[7,95–98] distal extremity location,[93,94] and low tumor stage.[7,93,99]

A wide array of histologic features has been reported to be of prognostic significance, but there is often disagreement among studies. There is still no agreement as to the prognostic significance of the microscopic subtype. Whereas some have found biphasic synovial sarcomas to behave in a more indolent fashion than monophasic tumors,[100] others have not found this to be so.[101] It is difficult to compare the results of these studies, however, because of great differences in the criteria used to distinguish the synovial sarcoma subtypes. In the study by Machen et al. the proportion of each tumor composed of spindled and epithelial areas was evaluated semiquantitatively and was not found to be of prognostic significance.[41]

Two histologic patterns of synovial sarcoma have special clinical significance. Extensively calcified synovial sarcomas appear to have a better long-term prognosis. In a series of extensively calcified synovial sarcomas by Varela-Duran and Enzinger,[36] local recurrence and pulmonary metastases were detected in 32% and 29% of patients, respectively. In our own study of extremity synovial sarcomas, 24% of cases had areas of calcification ranging from 5% to 20% of the tumors, but we did not find that the presence or extent of calcification had an impact on clinical behavior.[41] On the other hand, it is clear that tumors with poorly differentiated areas generally behave more aggressively and metastasize in a higher percentage of cases than those without such areas.[40,92,95,102] Thorough sampling of these tumors is required to determine the presence and extent of poorly differentiated areas. Other histologic features reported to have an adverse prognostic impact include the presence of rhabdoid cells,[94] extensive tumor necrosis,[103] high mitotic index (>10 mitoses/10 HPF),[41,93,96] and high nuclear grade.[41] Aneuploidy,[101] high

proliferative (PCNA, Ki-67) index,[104,105] and low p27[KIP1] expression[106,107] have also been reported to be adverse prognostic indicators, but it is not clear whether these techniques are more predictive than the mitotic index alone. Other potential biomarkers of poor prognosis include aberrant p53 expression,[108,109] aberrant β-catenin expression,[102,110] expression of dysadherin,[110a] expression of insulin-like growth factor 1 receptor,[111] or insulin-like growth factor 2 (IGF2),[112] and co-expression of hepatocyte growth factor and its receptor (c-MET).[108]

Although there is some disagreement, some have found *SYT-SSX* fusion subtype to be an independent prognostic indicator. In the study by Kawai and colleagues,[113] a longer metastasis-free survival period in those patients with localized tumors and *SYT-SSX2* was observed. This contention was strongly supported by the much larger study by Ladanyi et al. of 243 patients with synovial sarcoma.[7] In this study, the median overall survival for the *SYT-SSX2* group was about twice that of the *SYT-SSX1* group (13.7 versus 6.1 years), and the 5-year survival rates were 73% and 53%, respectively. However, the impact of fusion type on survival was not significant when stratified for disease status at presentation. Among patients with localized disease at diagnosis, median overall survival for the *SYT-SSX2* group was about 50% longer than those in the *SYT-SSX1* group (13.7 years versus 9.2 years). By multivariate analysis, fusion type was the only independent factor to significantly impact overall survival. Whereas other studies also found improved survival for those with *SYT-SSX2* fusion positive tumors,[114,115] a large study by Guillou and colleagues did not find this to be the case.[92] Nevertheless, analysis of fusion type by RT-PCR or even FISH[116] might become standard practice in order to provide powerful prognostic information.

Therapy

Local control of synovial sarcoma is clearly related to the adequacy of initial surgical excision. Simple local excision without ancillary therapy is incapable of checking the growth and spread of the tumor, and most reviewers recommend extensive surgery as the therapy of choice, including radical local excision, often with removal of an entire muscle or muscle group, and amputation, depending mainly on the size of the tumor and its location. Because radical local excision is often impossible with tumors situated near a large joint – the favored location of synovial sarcoma – adjunctive radiotherapy in addition to local excision of the tumor is favored over amputation.[96,117]

Synovial sarcoma is a chemosensitive sarcoma. In particular, regimens that include ifosfamide and doxorubicin or epirubicin are efficacious, resulting in a partial or complete response in about 50% of patients.[99,118–120] There is also strong interest in potential targeted therapies for synovial sarcoma. For example, BCL2 is overexpressed in the vast majority of synovial sarcomas. The increased expression of this anti-apoptotic protein is not due to gene amplification or rearrangement but rather is likely secondary to increased protein stability or transcriptional activation.[121] In vivo studies on synovial sarcoma cell lines have shown effective BCL2 blockade by G3139, an oligonucleotide that decreases BCL2 expression and induces apoptosis.[122] Several studies have shown overexpression of EGFR in up to 55% of synovial sarcomas.[60,123,124] Currently, a phase II trial of the EGFR inhibitor gefitinib for patients with locally advanced or metastatic synovial sarcomas that overexpress EGFR is ongoing in Europe.[125] Although not common, some synovial sarcomas overexpress Her2,[126-128] suggesting a possible role for trastuzumab in patients with recurrent or metastatic disease.

Line of differentiation

There is still considerable debate as to the exact line of differentiation of this neoplasm. This uncertainty is also reflected in the new edition of the World Health Organization Soft Tissue Classification in which synovial sarcoma is placed among the "tumors of uncertain differentiation." In the past, most discussion centered on whether synovial sarcomas arose from preformed synovium. The largely outdated concept that sarcomas arise from mature, preformed tissue has given way to a discussion as to whether these tumors have cellular features that resemble normal synovium. As previously mentioned, synovial sarcomas rarely arise in joint cavities, and these tumors may arise in locations in which normal synovial structures are rare or nonexistent, including the lung, heart, and abdominal wall. Furthermore, there are significant immunohistochemical and ultrastructural differences between the cells of synovial sarcoma and those of the synovial lining. Some reviewers believe that the term synovial sarcoma should be abandoned, but it is so well established in the literature that there seems little reason to alter it at present until there is a consensus as to the appropriate choice of alternate terms.

ALVEOLAR SOFT PART SARCOMA

Alveolar soft part sarcoma is a clinically and morphologically distinct soft tissue sarcoma first defined and named by Christopherson et al. in 1952.[129] Before this report, typical cases had been described under various designations including malignant myoblastoma, angioendothelioma, and even liposarcoma. Since 1952, numerous examples have been reported and studied immunohistochemically and electron microscopically; but there is still uncertainty as to its exact nature. However, recent advances have been made in understanding the molecular pathogenesis and even the nature of the characteristic PAS-positive crystals. Alveolar soft part sarcomas are uniformly malignant; there is no benign counterpart of the tumor.

Alveolar soft part sarcoma is an uncommon neoplasm; its frequency among our cases is estimated at 0.5–1.0% of all soft tissue sarcomas. It is even less common in other series. Ekfors et al.,[130] for example, found only one alveolar soft part sarcoma among 246 malignant soft tissue tumors in Finland, an incidence of 0.4%.

Clinical findings

This tumor occurs principally in adolescents and young adults and is most frequently encountered in patients 15–35 years of age (Table 37–5).[131-136] Female patients outnumber males, especially among patients under 25 years of age.[137] Infants and children are affected less frequently. There are two main locations of the tumor. When it occurs in adults, it is seen predominantly in the lower extremities, especially the anterior portion of the thigh. In a study of 102 alveolar soft part sarcomas by Lieberman et al.,[131] 39.5% involved the soft tissues of the buttock or thigh. The tumor has also been described in a variety of unusual locations including the female genital tract,[138] mediastinum,[139] breast,[140] urinary bladder,[140a] gastrointestinal tract,[141] and bone.[142] When the tumor affects infants and children, it is often located in the region of the head and neck, especially the orbit and tongue; tumors in the head and neck tend to be smaller, probably because of earlier detection (Table 37–6).[143,144]

Alveolar soft part sarcoma usually presents as a slowly growing, painless mass that almost never causes functional impairment. Because of the relative lack of symptoms it is easily overlooked; in a number of cases metastasis to the lung or brain is the first manifestation of the disease.[134,136,145] Headache, nausea, and visual changes are often associated with cerebral metastasis. As a rule, the tumor is richly vascular, causing pulsation or a distinctly audible bruit in some instances; massive hemorrhage may be encountered during surgical removal. In rare instances there is erosion or destruction of the underlying bone.[146] Hypervascularity with prominent draining

TABLE 37–5	AGE DISTRIBUTION OF 102 ALVEOLAR SOFT PART SARCOMAS	
Age (years)	No. of patients	%
0–9	12	12
10–19	17	17
20–29	42	41
≥30	31	30
Total	102	100

Modified from Lieberman PH, Brennan MF, Kimmel M, et al. Alveolar soft-part sarcoma: a clinicopathologic study of half a century. Cancer 1989; 63:1.

veins and prolonged capillary staining are usually demonstrable with angiography and CT scans. On MRI, the tumor typically demonstrates high signal intensity on both T2- and T1-weighted images.[147]

Pathologic findings

The gross specimen tends to be poorly circumscribed, soft, and friable; on section, it consists of yellow-white to gray-red tissue, often with large areas of necrosis and hemorrhage. Frequently, the tumor is surrounded by numerous tortuous vessels of large caliber.

The microscopic picture varies little from tumor to tumor, and the uniformity of the microscopic picture is one of its characteristic features. Dense fibrous trabeculae of varying thickness divide the tumor into compact groups or compartments of irregular size that in turn are subdivided into sharply defined nests or aggregates of tumor cells (Figs 37–28, 37–29). These cellular aggregates are separated from one another by thin-walled, sinusoi-

dal vascular channels lined by a single layer of flattened endothelial cells. In most instances, the cellular aggregates exhibit central degeneration, necrosis, and loss of cohesion resulting in a pseudoalveolar pattern (Fig. 37–30). This pattern should not be confused with the more irregular alveolar pattern of alveolar rhabdomyosarcoma. Less frequently, the nest-like pattern is inconspicuous or absent entirely, and the tumor is merely composed of uniform sheets of large granular cells with few or no discernible vascular channels (Fig. 37–31). This more solid, or compact type of alveolar soft part sarcoma occurs mainly in infants and children.

The individual cells are large, rounded, or more often polygonal and display little variation in size and shape. They have distinct cell borders and one or more vesicular nuclei with small nucleoli and abundant granular, eosinophilic, and sometimes vacuolated cytoplasm. Mitotic figures are scarce. Rare pleomorphic tumors have been reported in the literature (Fig. 37–32).[148]

At the margin of the tumor there are usually numerous dilated veins, probably the result of multiple arteriovenous shunts in the neoplasm similar to hemangiopericytoma and paraganglioma. Vascular invasion is a constant, striking finding that explains the tendency of the tumor to develop metastasis at an early stage of the disease (Fig. 37–33).

Histochemical stains are useful for establishing the diagnosis in that PAS preparation reveals varying amounts of intracellular glycogen and characteristically PAS-positive, diastase-resistant rhomboid or rod-shaped crystals (Fig. 37–34). These crystals vary greatly in number from case to case. In some cases, they can be identified in almost every cell whereas in others they are difficult to find or absent. Masson was the first to describe and depict these crystals as a diagnostic feature of alveolar soft part sarcoma.[149] In our experience, the typical crystalline

TABLE 37–6	ANATOMIC DISTRIBUTION OF 102 ALVEOLAR SOFT PART SARCOMAS		
Location		**No. of patients**	**%**
Buttock/thigh		40	39.5
Leg/popliteal		17	16.6
Chest wall/trunk		13	12.9
Forearm		10	9.7
Arm		8	8.5
Back/neck		6	6.4
Tongue		4	3.2
Retroperitoneum		4	3.2
Total		102	100.0

Modified from Lieberman PH, Brennan MF, Kimmel M, et al. Alveolar soft-part sarcoma: a clinicopathologic study of half a century. Cancer 1989; 63:1.

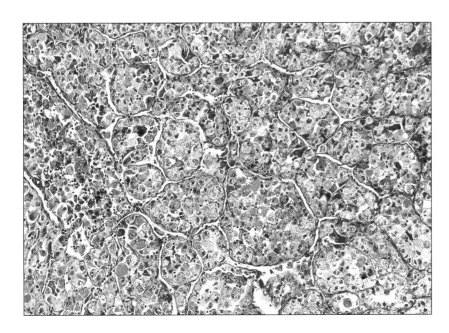

FIGURE 37–28 Alveolar soft part sarcoma with a typical organoid arrangement of tumor cells.

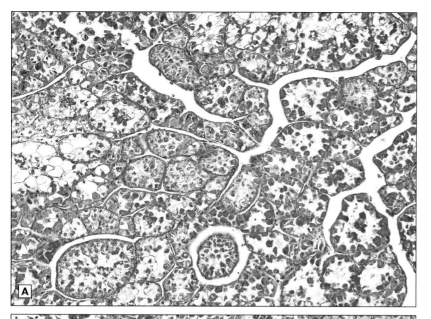

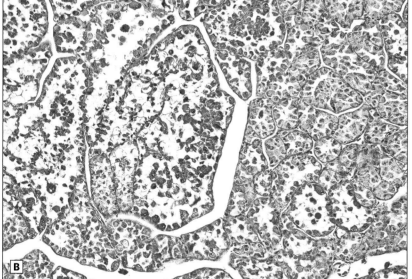

FIGURE 37–29 **(A)** Low-magnification view of alveolar soft part sarcoma composed of nests of large tumor cells with central loss of cellular cohesion resulting in a pseudoalveolar pattern. **(B)** Higher-power view revealing cell nests that are separated by thin-walled, sinusoidal vascular spaces.

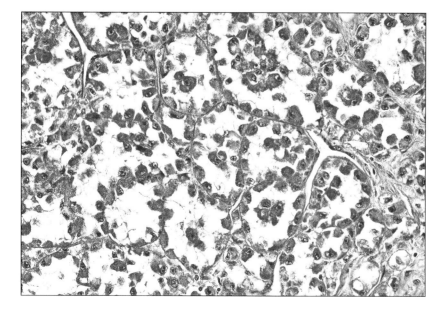

FIGURE 37–30 Prominent pseudoalveolar growth pattern in an alveolar soft part sarcoma.

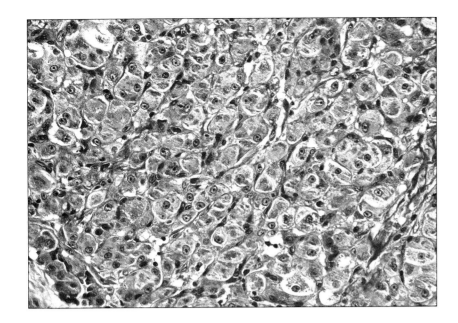

FIGURE 37–31 Alveolar soft part sarcoma arising in a child showing clustering and small nests of tumor cells.

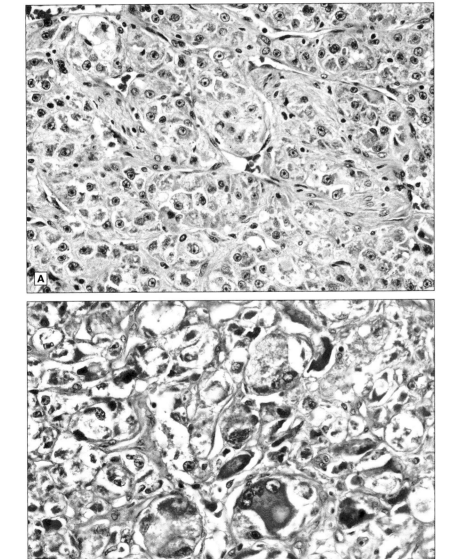

FIGURE 37–32 Range of cytologic atypia in alveolar soft part sarcomas. **(A)** This is the typical cytologic appearance of alveolar soft part sarcoma, with relatively uniform nuclei and prominent nucleoli. **(B)** Scattered atypical cells in an alveolar soft part sarcoma.

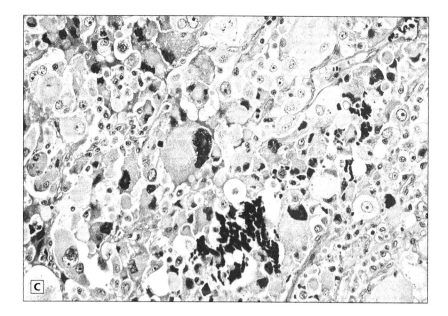

FIGURE 37–32 Continued. **(C)** Marked cytologic atypia in an alveolar soft part sarcoma.

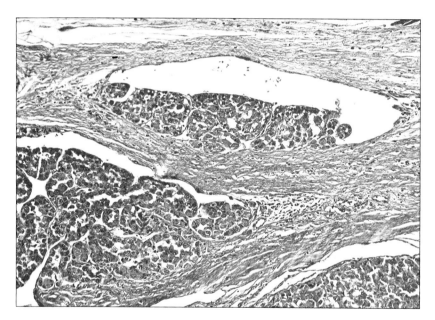

FIGURE 37–33 Dilated peripheral vein with tumor invasion.

material is present in at least 80% of the tumors; in the remainder there are merely PAS-positive granules, probably precursors of the crystals. The crystals are a feature of both primary and metastatic alveolar soft part sarcomas.

The nature of these crystals has become recently elucidated, albeit serendipitously. In the course of characterizing a monoclonal antibody to the monocarboxylate transporter 1 (MCT1) in a variety of tissues and tumors, Ladanyi and colleagues noted expression on the surface and in the cytoplasm of the cells in examples of alveolar soft part sarcoma.[150] MCT1 is one of a family of transporter proteins that catalyzes the rapid transport of monocarboxylates across plasma membranes. It is located ubiquitously but is prevalent in cardiac and skeletal muscle.[151] The protein is normally associated with the rough endoplasmic reticulin and is transported to the plasma membrane in association with its chaperone, CD147. Ladanyi et al. found an abundance of MCT1 and CD147 on the surface of the cells of alveolar soft part sarcoma, as well as within the cytoplasm in the region of the characteristic crystals.[150] Western blot analysis confirmed the nature of the protein and ultrastructural immunohistochemistry localized MCT1 and CD147 to the cytoplasmic crystals and their precursor granules.

Immunohistochemical findings

Numerous immunohistochemical studies have attempted to elucidate the histogenesis of this unusual tumor, often resulting in contradictory results.[152,153] The cells generally do not stain with antibodies against cytokeratin, EMA, neurofilaments, GFAP, serotonin, or synaptophysin; they

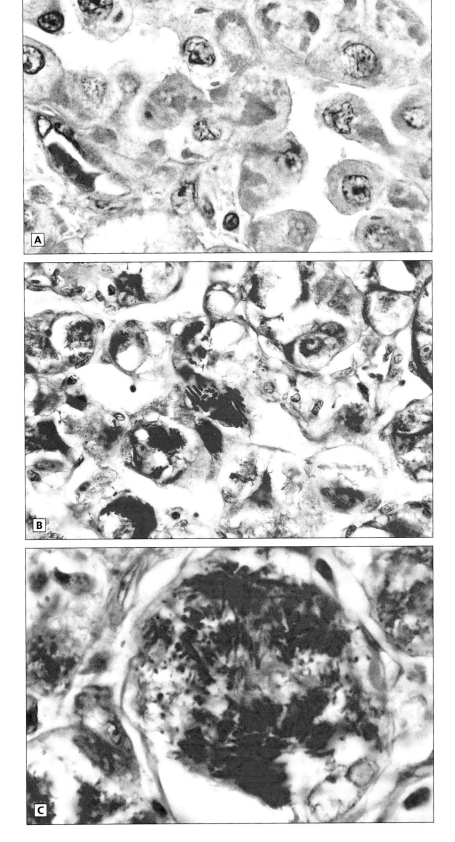

FIGURE 37–34 (A) High-magnification view of an alveolar soft part sarcoma. There is focal condensation of eosinophilic cytoplasm. **(B)** Periodic acid-Schiff (PAS) staining with diastase reveals varying amounts of intracellular crystalline material. **(C)** High-magnification view of crystalline material, diagnostic of alveolar soft part sarcoma.

occasionally express S-100 protein and neuron-specific enolase, but these markers are of no diagnostic value. The reports in regard to staining for muscle markers differ somewhat, but most have demonstrated muscle markers in less than 50% of tumors.[137,154]

In 1991, Rosai et al. detected the myogenic nuclear regulatory protein MyoD1 by immunohistochemistry (confirmed by Western blot analysis) and suggested this as confirmatory evidence of its skeletal muscle nature.[155] In contrast, Cullinane et al. were unable to detect MyoD1 by Northern blot analysis.[156] Using paraffin-embedded samples, Wang and colleagues were unable to detect nuclear expression of MyoD1 in 12 alveolar soft part sarcomas, although there was considerable granular cytoplasmic immunoreactivity.[157] Subsequent studies have failed to detect either MyoD1 or myogenin in alveolar soft part sarcoma,[158,159] effectively excluding classic skeletal muscle differentiation.

Ultrastructural findings

Electron microscopy shows the cells to contain numerous mitochondria, prominent smooth endoplasmic reticulum, glycogen, and a well-developed Golgi apparatus. Characteristically, there are rhomboid, rod-shaped, or spicular crystals with a regular lattice pattern and sparse electron-dense secretory granules (Fig. 37–35). Both the crystals and dense granules are membrane-bound and consist of crystallized and uncrystallized filaments that are 4–6 nm in diameter, suggesting transitions between the two structures. The filaments are arranged in a parallel fashion with a periodicity of 10 nm.[160-162] The large polygonal cells are separated from the intervening vascular channels by a discontinuous basal lamina. Rare desmosomes or hemidesmosomes are present between the individual cells and between cells and surrounding basal laminae.[162]

Cytogenetic findings

Cytogenetic studies of this tumor have identified a specific alteration, der(17)t(X;17)(p11.2q25).[163] This unbalanced translocation results in the fusion of the *TFE3* gene on Xp11.2 (a member of the basic-helix-loop-helix family of transcription factors) to a novel gene named *ASPL* (also known as *ASP-SCR1* or *RCC17* on 17q25). The resulting fusion gene encodes for a fusion protein that localizes to the nucleus and functions as an aberrant transcription factor.[163,164] Interestingly, this same gene fusion has been found in an unusual variant of pediatric renal cell carcinoma characterized by nested and pseudopapillary architecture, psammomatous calcifications, and epithelioid cells with abundant clear cytoplasm and well-defined cell borders.[165-167] However, among soft tissue sarcomas, the *ASPL-TFE3* fusion appears to be both sensitive and specific. Exactly how or even whether the *ASPL-*

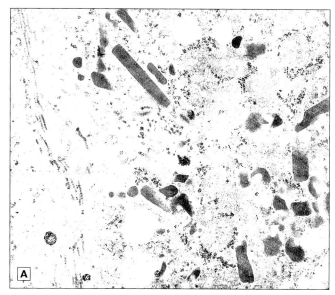

FIGURE 37–35 Electron micrographs depicting intracellular crystalline structures in an alveolar soft part sarcoma.

TFE3 fusion is related to the accumulation of crystalline deposits of MCT1 and CD147 is not known. Saito and colleagues suggested a role for DNA mismatch repair, since inactivation of *hMSH2* and *hMLH1* was detected in some *ASPL-TFE3*-positive alveolar soft part sarcomas.[168]

Differential diagnosis

The differential diagnosis chiefly includes metastatic *renal cell carcinoma, paraganglioma,* and *granular cell tumor* (Table 37-7). Alveolar rhabdomyosarcoma is sometimes confused with alveolar soft part sarcoma but more because of the similarity in name than in the microscopic picture.

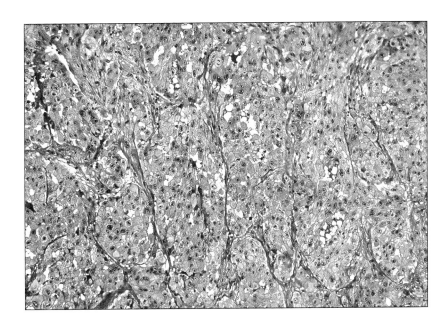

FIGURE 37–36 Metastatic renal cell carcinoma simulating an alveolar soft part sarcoma.

TABLE 37–7	DIFFERENTIAL DIAGNOSTIC FEATURES OF ALVEOLAR SOFT PART SARCOMA		
Lesion	**Glycogen**	**Crystals**	**Immunohistochemistry**
Alveolar soft part sarcoma	+	+	Variable muscle markers; TFE3
Renal cell carcinoma	+	–	Epithelial membrane antigen
Paraganglioma	–	–	Neuroendocrine markers (synaptophysin, chromogranin); S-100 protein in sustentacular cells
Granular cell tumor	–	–	S-100 protein

Renal cell carcinoma, primary or metastatic, often bears a striking resemblance to alveolar soft part sarcoma (Fig. 37–36), but in most cases it can be distinguished by the absence of the characteristic PAS-positive crystalline material. The pale-staining cytoplasm of its cells and the fat content of renal cell carcinoma are less reliable features because each may be encountered in degenerated forms of alveolar soft part sarcoma (Fig. 37–37). Immunoreactivity for EMA is useful for confirming a diagnosis of renal cell carcinoma, as this antigen is absent in alveolar soft part sarcoma. Staining for TFE3 can be helpful, although it must be kept in mind that some pediatric renal cell carcinomas and granular cell tumors also express this antigen.[165,167,169] Glycogen is present in both alveolar soft part sarcoma and renal cell carcinoma, but it is absent in *granular cell tumor* and *paraganglioma*. It is also noteworthy that the cells of granular cell tumor are less well defined, have a distinctly granular cytoplasm, and show strong S-100 protein staining.

The clinical features are also of value in the differential diagnosis. Primary renal cell carcinomas are usually demonstrable radiographically in the retroperitoneum. Renal cell carcinoma, paraganglioma, and malignant granular cell tumor chiefly affect patients over 40 years of age; they are rare in patients younger than 25 years. Moreover, as mentioned elsewhere, there is no record that a "bona fide" paraganglioma has ever occurred in the extremities.

Clinical behavior and therapy

The ultimate prognosis is poor despite the relatively slow growth of the tumor. Of the 91 patients with follow-up information in the study from Memorial Sloan-Kettering Cancer Center, only 15% of patients were alive after 20 years.[131] Portera and colleagues reported their experience in treating 74 patients with alveolar soft part sarcoma at M.D. Anderson Cancer Center.[134] Thirty-five percent of patients presented with AJCC stage III or IV, but 65% of patients presented with stage IV disease. Five-year local recurrence free, distant recurrence free, disease free, and overall survival for 22 patients with localized disease at presentation were 88%, 84%, 71%, and 87%, respectively. In contrast, the median survival for patients with metastases was 40 months with a 5-year overall survival of 20%. All patients who had brain metastases had evidence of metastatic disease at other sites. Metastases tend to occur early in the course of the disease, and there are many reports of patients who present with pulmonary or brain metastasis. On the other hand, metastasis may also be delayed for many years; Lillehei et al. reported a patient who developed brain metastases 33 years after the

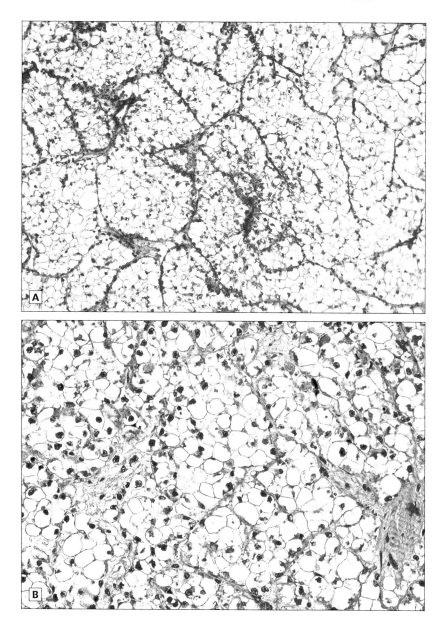

FIGURE 37–37 (A) Low-magnification view of alveolar soft part sarcoma simulating a renal cell carcinoma of clear cell type. The cytoplasmic clearing likely represents a degenerative feature of this tumor. **(B)** Higher-magnification view showing close simulation of a renal cell carcinoma by this alveolar soft part sarcoma.

initial presentation, emphasizing the need for long-term follow-up.[170]

The most important prognostic parameters appear to be age at diagnosis, tumor size, and the presence of metastasis at presentation.[131,136] In the study by Lieberman et al. there was an increased risk of metastasis at presentation with increasing age, as only 17% of patients who presented during the first decade of life had metastatic disease compared to 32% in patients older than 30 years of age.[131] Improved prognosis in children may in part be related to the location of the tumor, early clinical detection, small size, and better resectability.[135,143] In addition, patients who present with metastatic disease tend to have primary tumors that are larger than those in patients who do not have metastasis at presentation.[131,135] Although the development of metastatic disease clearly portends a grave prognosis, resection of solitary brain metastases may be of prognostic benefit.[171] The principal metastatic sites are the lungs, followed by the brain and skeleton. Metastases to lymph nodes are infrequent.

Treatment is not particularly promising, and the relatively slow growth of the tumor must be considered when one is assessing the effect of therapy. Most reviewers recommend radical surgical excision of primary and metastatic lesions combined with radiotherapy or chemotherapy (or both), although most report limited success with systemic therapies.[133,172]

Discussion

Despite numerous immunohistochemical and electron microscopic studies, the line of cellular differentiation of alveolar soft part sarcoma remains obscure. Over the years, several concepts concerning the nature of this tumor have been entertained. A variant of paraganglioma was first proposed by Smetana and Scott[173] who emphasized the morphologic resemblance of alveolar soft part sarcoma to paraganglioma and favored a chemoreceptor origin. They stressed the close ultrastructural resemblance between alveolar soft part sarcomas and carotid body tumors, including the presence of chief cells, peripheral spindle-shaped cells, and electron-dense secretory-like granules. Strong evidence against this concept, however, is not only the abundance of glycogen and PAS-positive, diastase-resistant crystalline material in the tumor cells but also that the cells of alveolar soft part sarcoma are not argyrophilic with Grimelius stain, do not stain with antibodies to neurofilaments, chromogranin, synaptophysin, serotonin, and met-enkephalin, and contain no intracellular catecholamines as indicated by the complete absence of formaldehyde vapor-induced fluorescence in the tumor cells.[174,175] Furthermore, alveolar soft part sarcomas differ in several clinical aspects from paragangliomas. They prevail in patients younger than 30 years, chiefly involve the extremities, and behave in a malignant manner with frequent metastasis to lung, brain, and bone. There is also some question as to the existence of paraganglionic structures in the muscles of the extremities. We have never encountered paraganglia or related structures in the soft tissues of the limbs, nor were they detected by Karnauchow and Magner[176] who carried out a systematic search for such structures in the thigh.

Skeletal muscle differentiation has been suggested by many over the years, but a number of studies have also detracted from this concept. Fisher and Reidbord first suggested the possibility of skeletal muscle differentiation on the basis of the resemblance of the membrane-bound crystals to those in nemaline myopathy and rhabdomyoma.[177] This concept was strengthened by immunohistochemical studies that demonstrated the potential of the tumor cells to express desmin and muscle-specific actin. Although the initial detection of MyoD1 in a case of alveolar soft part sarcoma reported by Rosai et al.[155] seemed to lend support to the concept of skeletal muscle differentiation, others have been unable to duplicate this finding and, thus, there is no convincing evidence that alveolar soft part sarcomas exhibit skeletal muscle differentiation.

Still another concept of the histogenesis was offered by DeSchryver-Kecskemeti et al., who contended that the cytoplasmic granules of alveolar soft part sarcomas are similar to the renin granules of juxtaglomerular tumors and proposed the name "angioreninoma."[178] There is, however, no sign of hyperreninism (e.g., hypertension, hypokalemia, aldosteronism) in patients with alveolar soft part sarcoma; according to Mukai et al.,[174] immunostaining for renin is negative and plasma renin levels are normal.

EPITHELIOID SARCOMA

The term *epithelioid sarcoma* has been applied to a morphologically distinctive neoplasm that is likely to be confused with a variety of benign and malignant conditions, especially a granulomatous process, a synovial sarcoma, or an ulcerating squamous cell carcinoma. The tumor mainly afflicts young adults; its principal sites are the fingers, hands, and forearms. In fact, epithelioid sarcoma is the most common soft tissue sarcoma in the hand and wrist, followed by alveolar rhabdomyosarcoma and synovial sarcoma.

Clinical findings

Epithelioid sarcoma is most prevalent in adolescents and young adults 10–35 years of age (median age 26 years).[179-181] It is uncommon in children and older persons,[182-184] but no age group is exempt. Male patients outnumber females by about 2:1,[180,181] and there is no predilection for any particular race. The tumor most commonly arises on the flexor surfaces of the fingers, hands and forearm, followed by the knee and lower leg, especially the pretibial region, the buttocks and thigh, the shoulder and arm, and the ankle, foot, and toe (Table 37–8). It is rare in the trunk and head and neck region[185] with the exception of the scalp. There are a number of reports in which epithelioid sarcoma arose on the penis and clinically mimicked Peyronie's disease.[186,187] Other uncommon sites include the vulva,[188] perineum,[189] cervix,[190] lung,[191] and dura.[192]

The tumor occurs in both the superficial and deep soft tissues. When located superficially, it usually presents as a firm nodule that may be solitary or multiple, has a callus-like consistency, and is often described as a "woody hard knot" or "firm lump" that is slowly growing and painless. Nodules situated in the dermis are often elevated above the skin surface and frequently become ulcerated weeks or months after they are first noted. Such lesions may be erroneously diagnosed as an "indurated ulcer," "draining abscess," or "infected wart" that fails to

TABLE 37–8	ANATOMIC DISTRIBUTION OF 215 EPITHELIOID SARCOMAS	
Location	No. of patients	%
Hand/fingers	65	30
Forearm/wrist	37	17
Knee/lower leg	31	15
Buttock/thigh	22	10
Shoulder/arm	20	9
Ankle/foot/toes	19	9
Trunk	12	6
Head and neck	9	4
Total	215	100

From Chase DR, Enzinger FM. Epithelioid sarcoma: diagnosis, prognostic indicators, and treatment. Am J Surg Pathol 1985; 9:241.

heal despite intensive therapy (Figs 37–38, 37–39). Deep-seated lesions are usually firmly attached to tendons, tendon sheaths, or fascial structures; they tend to be larger and less well defined and manifest as areas of induration or as multinodular lumpy masses, sometimes moving slightly with motion of the extremity (Fig. 37–40). Pain or tenderness is rarely a prominent symptom, with the exception of the tumors that encroach on large nerves. The size of the tumor varies substantially and ranges from a few millimeters to 15 cm or more, but most are 3–6 cm at the time of excision. Because many lesions are multinodular, determination of their exact size is often impossible.

Radiographic examination typically reveals a soft tissue mass with an occasional speckled pattern of calcification. Cortical thinning and erosion of underlying bone may be present, but invasion and destruction of adjacent bone are rare. MRI is useful for revealing the anatomic extent of the tumor and planning appropriate surgery.[193,194]

Pathologic findings

Gross inspection usually reveals the presence of one or more nodules measuring 0.5–5.0 cm in greatest diameter.

Deep-seated tumors, attached to tendons or fascia, tend to be larger and present as firm, multinodular masses with irregular outlines. The cut surface has a glistening gray-white or gray-tan mottled surface with focal yellow or brown areas caused by focal necrosis or hemorrhage.

There are two principal types of epithelioid sarcoma: the classic type (far more common), and the "proximal type." This discussion will focus on the former, as the latter has distinctive features and will be discussed separately.

Histologically, the classic type of epithelioid sarcoma has a distinct nodular arrangement of the tumor cells, a tendency to undergo central degeneration and necrosis, and an epithelioid appearance with cytoplasmic eosino-

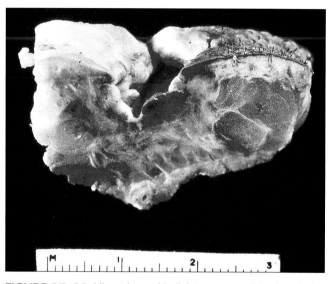

FIGURE 37–39 Ulcerating epithelioid sarcoma of the hand with indurated margins.

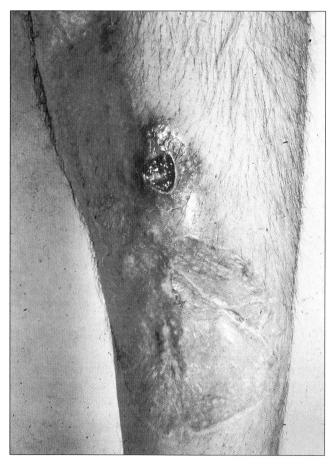

FIGURE 37–38 Recurrent ulcerating epithelioid sarcoma of the anterior tibial region in a 21-year-old man.

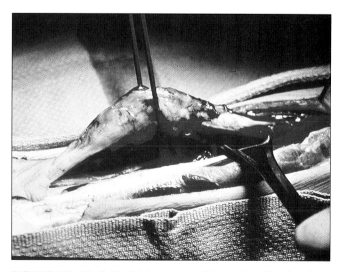

FIGURE 37–40 Epithelioid sarcoma of the wrist infiltrating the tendon of the flexor carpi ulnaris in a 28-year-old man. (From Enzinger FM. Epithelioid sarcoma: a sarcoma simulating a granuloma or a carcinoma. Cancer 1970; 26:1029.)

philia. The nodular pattern, probably the most conspicuous single feature of epithelioid sarcoma, varies somewhat. In some tumors the nodules are well circumscribed; in others they are less well defined and are often compacted into irregular multinodular masses (Figs 37–41, 37–42). Multiple nodules are less common in tissue obtained at the initial operation than in recurrent tumors. In rare cases the presence of multiple small superficial satellite nodules near the operative site may mimic a dermatologic disease.[195] Necrosis of the tumor nodules is a common finding (Fig. 37–43); it is most prominent in the center of the nodules and at times is associated with hemorrhage and cystic change. Fusion of several necrotizing nodules results in a "geographic" lesion with scalloped margins (Fig. 37–44). When the tumor spreads within a fascia or aponeurosis, it forms festoon-like or garland-like bands punctuated by areas of necrosis. Not infrequently, the tumor grows along the neurovascular bundle and invests large vessels or nerves. Vascular invasion may be present, but in our experience it is rarely a prominent feature.

Lesions located or extending into the dermis often ulcerate through the skin and may simulate an ulcerating squamous cell carcinoma, especially because of the pronounced epithelioid appearance and eosinophilia of the tumor cells. This process occurs mainly in areas with small amounts of subcutaneous fat such as the fingers and the prepatellar and pretibial regions.

The constituent cellular elements range from large ovoid or polygonal cells with deeply eosinophilic cytoplasm to plump spindle-shaped cells (Figs 37–45 to 37–47). In some cases, the spindle-cell pattern predomi-

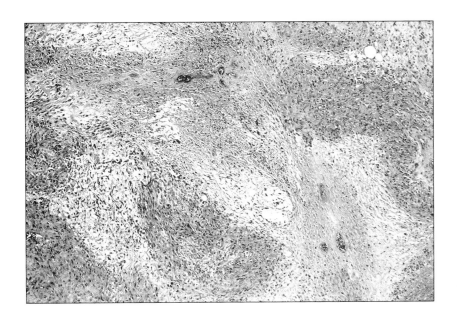

FIGURE 37–41 Typical low-magnification appearance of an epithelioid sarcoma with a pseudogranulomatous pattern.

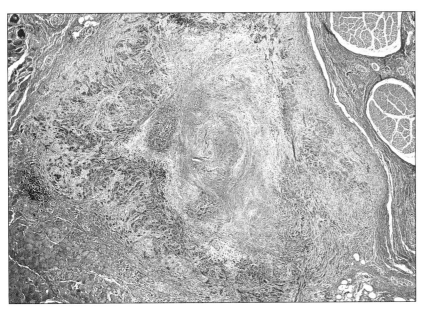

FIGURE 37–42 Epithelioid sarcoma. Note the nodules with central necrosis mimicking a necrotizing granulomatous process.

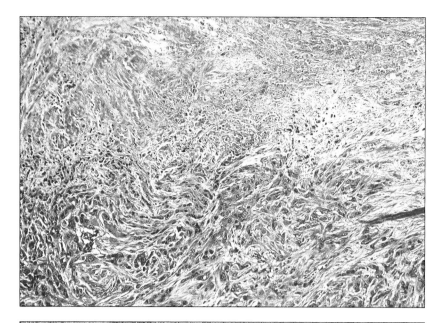

FIGURE 37–43 Epithelioid sarcoma with central necrosis of the tumor nodule.

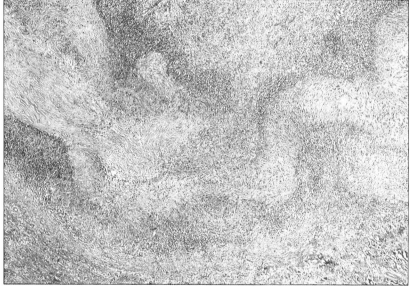

FIGURE 37–44 Epithelioid sarcoma. Fusion of several necrotizing nodules results in areas of geographic necrosis with scalloped margins.

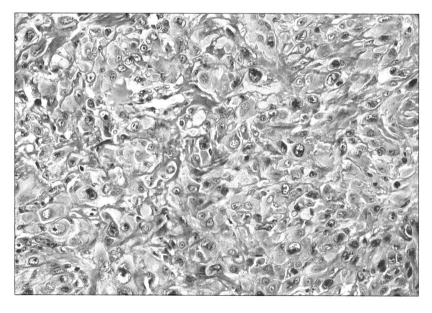

FIGURE 37–45 Cytologic features of malignant epithelioid cells in an epithelioid sarcoma.

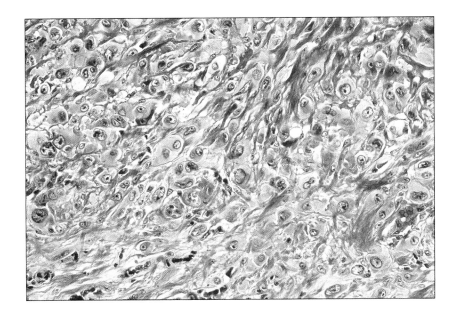

FIGURE 37–46 Close interplay between collagen and malignant epithelioid cells with densely eosinophilic cytoplasm in an epithelioid sarcoma.

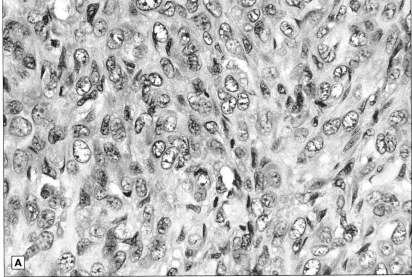

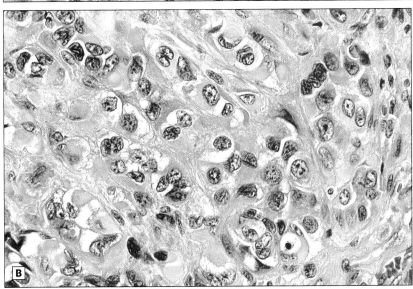

FIGURE 37–47 (A, B) Cytologic appearance of malignant epithelioid cells in epithelioid sarcoma. Most of the tumor cells have abundant deeply eosinophilic cytoplasm.

nates ("fibroma-like" variant) and obscures the characteristic epithelioid features and nodularity (Figs 37–48, 37–49).[196,197] In general, cellular pleomorphism is minimal. Usually, epithelioid and spindle-shaped cells merge imperceptibly, and there is never the distinct biphasic or pseudoglandular pattern that one encounters in biphasic synovial sarcoma (Fig. 37–50). In some tumors the loss of cellular cohesion and secondary hemorrhage may closely simulate an angiosarcoma; in others, the presence of intracellular lipid droplets suggests the incipient lumen formation of endothelial cells seen in epithelioid hemangioendotheliomas. Intercellular deposition of dense hyalinized collagen is common and, together with the eosinophilic cytoplasm, contributes to the deeply eosinophilic appearance of the tumor. Calcification and bone formation are found in 10–20% of cases, but carti-laginous metaplasia is rare (Fig. 37–51).[198] Aggregates of chronic inflammatory cells along the peripheral margin of the tumor nodules are present in most cases and may mimic a chronic inflammatory process (Fig. 37–52).

Histochemical staining techniques contribute little to the diagnosis. The cytoplasm stains a deep red-brown with the Masson trichrome stain. There is no stainable intracellular mucin, but Alcian blue-positive and hyaluronidase-sensitive mesenchymal mucin is often found in the surrounding matrix. There may also be some intracellular glycogen.

Immunohistochemical findings

Most epithelioid sarcomas stain for both low- and high-molecular weight cytokeratins (Fig. 37–53), EMA, and

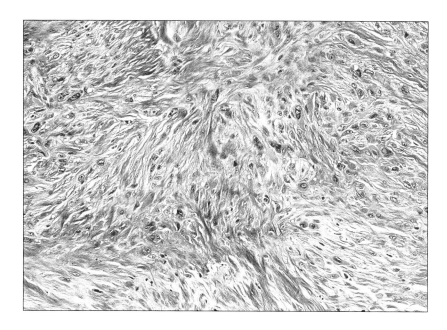

FIGURE 37–48 Epithelioid sarcoma with a predominantly spindle-cell pattern.

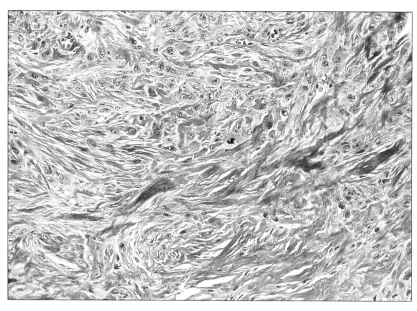

FIGURE 37–49 Interplay between dense collagen bundles and malignant spindle cells in an epithelioid sarcoma.

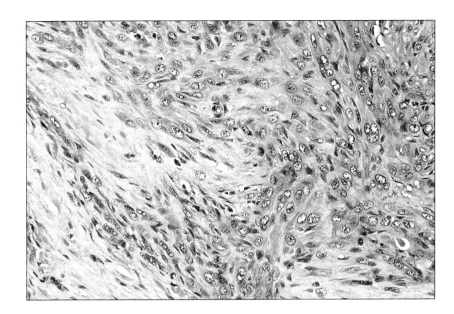

FIGURE 37–50 Transition from epithelioid to spindle cells and interdigitating collagen bundles in an epithelioid sarcoma.

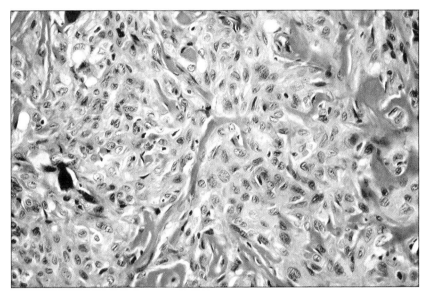

FIGURE 37–51 Focal calcifications in an epithelioid sarcoma, an unusual feature of this neoplasm.

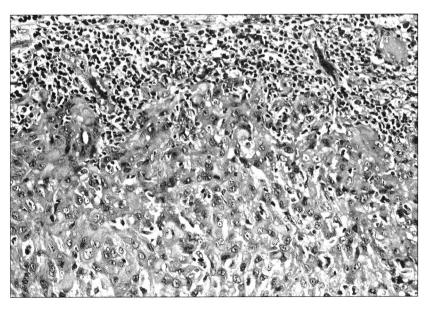

FIGURE 37–52 Aggregates of chronic inflammatory cells along the peripheral margin of a tumor nodule in an epithelioid sarcoma.

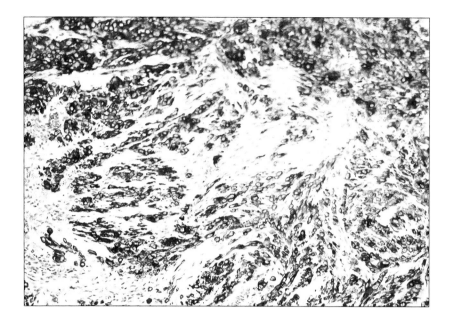

FIGURE 37–53 Strong cytokeratin immunoreactivity typical of epithelioid sarcoma.

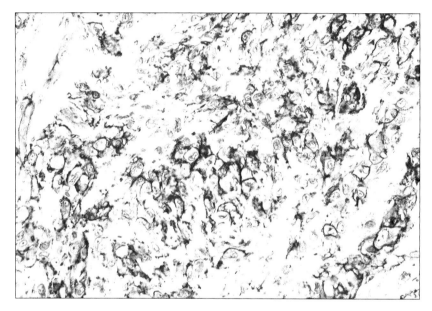

FIGURE 37–54 Membranous immunoreactivity for CD34 in an epithelioid sarcoma. This antigen is found in up to 70% of cases.

vimentin.[199-201] The degree of immunoreactivity, however, varies considerably from tumor to tumor and in different portions of the same neoplasm. In the large immunohistochemical study by Miettinen and colleagues, the tumors stained for vimentin, EMA, CK8, and CK19 in 100%, 96%, 94%, and 72% of cases, respectively.[200] Some cases also showed focal staining for CK7 and 34βH12. Usually, the presence of cytokeratin is more pronounced in epithelioid areas than in spindled areas. Up to 60% of cases stain for CD34 (Fig. 37–54).[200] Recently, Kato et al. found consistent strong CA-125 staining in this tumor;[202] some patients have elevated serum CA-125, raising the possibility that this could be used as a serum marker to monitor disease.[203] Antibodies directed against S-100 protein, neurofilament protein, carcinoembryonic antigen, von Willebrand factor, and CD31 are typically negative.

Ultrastructural findings

Most investigators report polygonal and spindle-shaped cells with ovoid, indented nuclei containing small amounts of marginally placed chromatin. The cytoplasm contains arrays of rough endoplasmic reticulum, a prominent Golgi apparatus, free ribosomes, and occasional mitochondria, lysosomes, and droplets of osmiophilic material. Intermediate filaments are a common, often striking feature. They may be arranged longitudinally as in myofibroblasts, but they more often form paranuclear masses or whorls, a feature that probably accounts for the voluminous cytoplasm and the striking epithelioid (and often rhabdoid) appearance of the tumor cells (Fig. 37–55).[204,205] There are occasionally interdigitating cellular processes with maculae adherens or intercellular

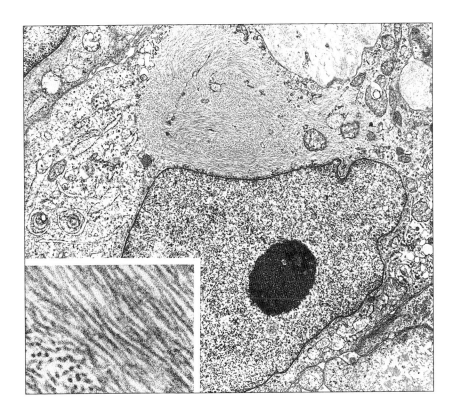

FIGURE 37–55 Ultrastructure of an epithelioid sarcoma showing polygonal cells with a paranuclear mass of intermediate filaments. **(Inset)** High-power view of intracytoplasmic bundles of intermediate filaments ranging in diameter from 7 to 12 nm. (From Mukai M, Torikata C, Iri H, et al. Cellular differentiation of epithelioid sarcoma: an electron-microscopic, enzyme histochemical, and immunohistochemical study. Am J Pathol 1985; 119:44.)

desmosome-like junctions and small intercellular cystic or cleft-like spaces surrounded by filopodia.

Cytogenetic findings

Cytogenetic data for epithelioid sarcomas are relatively limited, but these studies have not yet revealed a specific alteration characteristic of this tumor. Rearrangements of 8q, 18q11, and 22q11 have been noted on several occasions.[206–213] In particular, involvement of 22q11 is of interest since this is the site of the tumor suppressor gene *INI1*, which has been implicated as central to the pathogenesis of malignant extrarenal rhabdoid tumor (MERT). As discussed elsewhere in this chapter, this alteration links the "proximal-type" epithelioid sarcoma to MERT.

Differential diagnosis

The frequency with which epithelioid sarcoma is mistaken for a benign process is chiefly a result of its deceptively bland appearance during the initial stage of the disease. Small superficially located tumors with a nodular or multinodular pattern are likely to be mistaken for an inflammatory process, particularly a *necrotizing infectious granuloma, necrobiosis lipoidica, granuloma annulare*, or *rheumatoid nodule*. In contrast to the latter processes, the individual cells in epithelioid sarcoma tend to be more sharply defined, are larger and more eosinophilic, and stain positively for cytokeratins and EMA. The epithelioid features, nodularity, and immu-nostaining for cytokeratin also aid in differentiating epithelioid sarcoma from nodular fasciitis, fibrous histiocytoma, and fibromatosis.

Epithelioid sarcoma may also be mistaken for a wide array of epithelioid-appearing malignant soft tissue neoplasms (Fig. 37–56). The cytologic features of the constituent cells are reminiscent of those seen in both *epithelioid malignant peripheral nerve sheath tumor* (MPNST) and *melanoma*. Unlike epithelioid sarcoma, epithelioid MPNST tends to stain strongly for S-100 protein and virtually never expresses cytokeratins, although EMA may be rarely detected. Similarly, malignant melanoma virtually always expresses S-100 protein, and many lesions also stain for HMB-45, Melan A, or other specific melanocytic antigens.

Epithelioid sarcoma also has overlapping features with *epithelioid angiosarcoma*. Histologically, both are composed of large epithelioid cells with cytoplasmic vacuoles. Furthermore, epithelioid sarcoma may have a hemorrhagic pseudoangiosarcomatous pattern.[214] Confusion between these two entities is compounded by the fact that epithelioid angiosarcomas occasionally express cytokeratins and CD34. The absence of specific endothelial markers such as von Willebrand factor and CD31 in epithelioid sarcoma allows their distinction.

More recently, a variant of hemangioendothelioma has been reported which shows histologic features strikingly similar to those seen in epithelioid sarcoma (*epithelioid sarcoma-like hemangioendothelioma*).[184,215] This tumor arises in the superficial or deep soft tissues, often in the

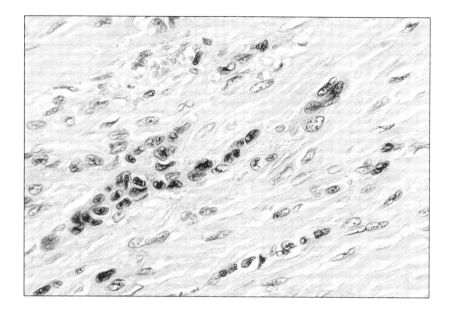

FIGURE 37–56 Peripheral portion of an epithelioid sarcoma with cording of epithelioid cells mimicking invasive lobular carcinoma of the breast.

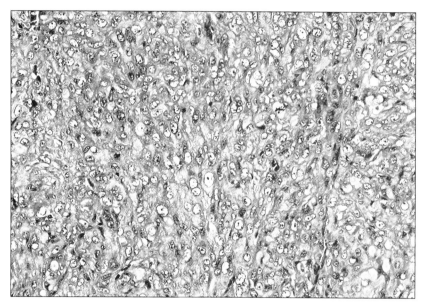

FIGURE 37–57 "Proximal-type" epithelioid sarcoma composed of sheets of large epithelioid cells with marked cytologic atypia.

extremities, of young to middle-aged adults. Histologically, it is characterized by solid sheets and nests of epithelioid to slightly spindled cells with cytoplasmic eosinophilia and only subtle evidence of vascular differentiation in the form of focal intracytoplasmic vacuolization. Like epithelioid sarcoma, the neoplastic cells consistently stain for cytokeratins and vimentin, but in addition they show clear-cut evidence of vascular endothelial differentiation by virtue of consistent expression of CD31 and FLI-1, although they are CD34-negative.

Some epithelioid sarcomas are difficult to distinguish from ulcerating *squamous cell carcinoma*. However, epithelioid sarcoma lacks keratin pearls and dyskeratosis in the adjacent epithelium. Immunohistochemically, most epithelioid sarcomas stain for cyclin D1 (nuclear) and are negative for CD5/6, whereas squamous cell carcinomas typically have the opposite immunophenotype.[216,217]

"Proximal-type" epithelioid sarcoma

In 1997, Guillou et al. described a "proximal-type" epithelioid sarcoma characterized by its propensity to arise in axial locations (pelvis, perineum, genital tract), its more aggressive behavior, and by its predominance of large epithelioid cells with marked cytologic atypia, frequently with intracytoplasmic hyaline inclusions, imparting a rhabdoid appearance to the tumor cells (Figs 37–57 to 37–59).[214] They were described as having an immunophenotype similar to that of classic epithelioid sarcoma, although some stained focally for desmin and smooth muscle actin.[214,218] As described, these tumors have many features overlapping those of malignant extrarenal rhabdoid tumor (MERT), discussed elsewhere in this chapter. Although Guillou et al. argued that a number of tumors reported as MERT arising in proximal

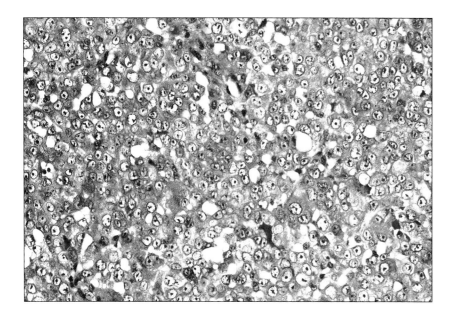

FIGURE 37–58 Sheets of large epithelioid cells with macronucleoli in a "proximal-type" epithelioid sarcoma.

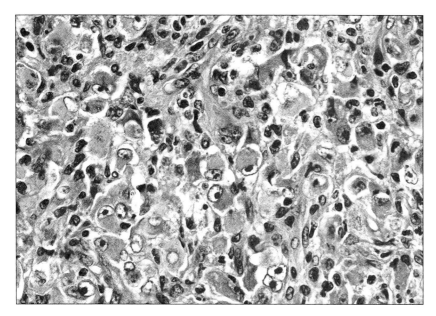

FIGURE 37–59 "Proximal-type" epithelioid sarcoma composed of large epithelioid cells with marked cytologic atypia and intracytoplasmic hyaline inclusions, imparting a rhabdoid appearance.

locations represent this unusual form of epithelioid sarcoma, we are not yet convinced that the "proximal-type" epithelioid sarcoma represents a distinct clinicopathologic entity. In fact, we believe it more likely represents a variant of MERT, as opposed to the opposite. In either case it should be distinguished from the classic form of epithelioid sarcoma.

Microscopically, proximal-type epithelioid sarcoma has a multinodular pattern of growth and is composed of large epithelioid cells with marked cytologic atypia, large vesicular nuclei, and prominent nucleoli. Paranuclear hyaline inclusions imparting a rhabdoid appearance are characteristic.[214,218-220] Although necrosis is common, the pseudogranulomatous pattern observed in classic epithelioid sarcoma is not present. The immunohistochemical and ultrastructural features are reportedly similar to those of classic epithelioid sarcoma.[199,200,218] Interestingly, aberrations of the *INI1* gene on 22q characteristic of MERT have also been reported in the proximal-type epithelioid sarcoma.[206 - 208] In the study by Modena et al., six of 11 epithelioid sarcomas had inactivating mutation of *INI1*; all six cases with this mutation were of the proximal type.[206]

Clinical course and therapy

Epithelioid sarcoma has a high risk for local recurrence and metastasis and requires long-term follow-up, given that recurrence or metastasis may occur many years after the initial diagnosis. For the classic type of epithelioid sarcoma, overall 5-year survival rates range from 50% to up to 85%,[180,215,221,222] and 10-year survival rates range

TABLE 37–9	SITE OF METASTATIC DISEASE IN 83 METASTASIZING EPITHELIOID SARCOMAS	
Location	No. of cases	%
Lung	42	51
Lymph nodes	28	34
Scalp	18	22
Bone	11	13
Brain	11	13
Liver	10	12
Pleura	9	11

Modified from Chase DR, Enzinger FM. Epithelioid sarcoma: diagnosis, prognostic indicators, and treatment. Am J Surg Pathol 1985; 9:241.

TABLE 37–10	REPORTED ADVERSE PROGNOSTIC FEATURES FOR EPITHELIOID SARCOMA
Male gender	
Non-distal extremity tumors	
Large tumor size ($\geq$5 cm)	
Increased tumor depth	
High mitotic index	
Hemorrhage	
Necrosis	
Vascular invasion	
Inadequate initial excision	

from 42% to 55%.[215,221,223] In the study from the AFIP,[180] follow-up data, available in 202 patients, showed recurrence and metastatic rates of 77% and 45%, respectively; 32% of patients died as a direct result of their tumor. The most common sites of metastasis were the lung (51%) and regional lymph nodes (34%) and less frequently the skin, central nervous system, and soft tissue (Table 37–9). The scalp was the site of metastasis in 22% of the cases.

Multiple recurrences, often as the result of marginal resection, are a characteristic feature of the tumor. One of the patients reported by Chase and Enzinger was treated for recurrent tumor growth in the left pretibial region on 11 occasions during a 16-year period.[180] Another patient had 20 surgical procedures for recurrent growth within a period of 10 years. Recurrent tumors are typically confluent nodules in the dermis or along tendons and fascial structures at or near the original tumor site. There are also cases where the skin adjacent and proximal to the tumor is studded with small, crater-like ulcerated nodules or plaques, a striking picture unlike that of any other recurrent soft tissue sarcoma.[195] In fact, the tendency for this tumor to track along an extremity some distance from the original scar suggests local "metastasis," rather than local "recurrence" in the strict sense of the word. Recurrence generally develops within the first year after diagnosis, but recurrence may be late; in one of the cases reported by Chase and Enzinger it became apparent 25 years after the primary tumor was removed by local excision.[180]

Intravascular growth and lymph node involvement are ominous features.[224] Metastasis may occur early in the course of disease (even before detection of the primary tumor), or it may occur many years following the initial diagnosis. One patient in the study from the AFIP developed metastatic disease 19 years after the initial diagnosis.[180] Prognosis therefore should be rendered with considerable caution, even if the patient appears to be well and free of tumor 5 years after the initial diagnosis.

Prognosis depends on various factors, including the gender of the patient, the site, size and depth of the tumor, the number of mitotic figures, the presence or absence of hemorrhage, necrosis, vascular invasion, and the adequacy of the initial excision (Table 37–10). In the series by Chase and Enzinger,[180] the survival rate for females was 78% compared to 64% for males. The improved outcome in females was even more pronounced in the series of Bos and colleagues, who reported a 5-year survival rate of 80% in females compared to 40% in males.[225]

Tumor site also appears to be prognostically important in that tumors arising in the distal extremities have a more favorable prognosis than those in the trunk and proximal portion of the limbs.[180,183,223] Tumor size greater than 5 cm is also associated with a more aggressive clinical course.[226,227] More recently, the expression of dysadherin, a membranous glycoprotein which downregulates E-adherin and promotes metastasis, has been found to be a significant poor prognostic factor.[227a]

Accurate assessment and comparison of the efficacy of treatment is difficult, especially if the cases are derived from multiple sources, as in the AFIP material. It is clearly evident, however, that inadequate therapy (marginal resection) is associated with a more aggressive clinical course.[227] Adequate treatment requires early radical local excision or amputation if the primary tumor is situated in the fingers or toes. Amputation should also be considered as treatment for recurrent growth but does not seem to offer any benefit to patients with distant metastasis.[228] Regional lymph node dissection should be included among the therapeutic modalities because lymph node metastasis is a fairly common occurrence in epithelioid sarcoma. Some have suggested that sentinel lymph node biopsy may be helpful in determining the need for a full dissection.[229] In all cases, surgical treatment should be combined with radiotherapy and multiagent chemotherapy over a prolonged period, similar to the chemotherapy given for other adult-type sarcomas. However, the true benefit of adjuvant therapy has yet to be fully shown.[230]

Discussion

There is still no consensus as to the line of cellular differentiation of epithelioid sarcoma. Not surprisingly, the relationship between epithelioid sarcoma and synovial sarcoma has been postulated in view of the intimate association of the tumor with tendons and aponeuroses, the mixture of epithelioid and spindled cellular elements, the immunoreactivity for epithelial markers, the ultrastructural demonstration of light and dark cells and microvilli in some of the cases, and the reported occurrence of a morphologically distinct epithelioid and synovial sarcoma that presented at two locations in the same knee.[231] There are, however, a number of contrasting features: the predominant location of epithelioid sarcoma in the hand, the consistent absence of pseudoglandular structures and intracellular mucin droplets, the lack of basal laminae ultrastructurally, and the absence of the t(X;18) characteristic of synovial sarcoma. Over the past years it has also been suggested that epithelioid sarcoma is a tumor of primitive mesenchymal cells with fibroblastic and histiocytic differentiation,[232] a primitive mesenchymal tumor with differentiation along histiocytic and synovial lines,[233] a variant of fibrosarcoma,[234] a tumor of myofibroblasts altered by massive production of intermediate filaments,[235] a malignant giant cell tumor of the tendon sheath,[205] and a tumor related to nodular tenosynovitis and arising from synovioblastic mesenchyme.[236]

Trauma to the site of the tumor may be a contributing factor and has been reported in a large number of cases. In the series by Chase and Enzinger,[180] for example, unsolicited reports of antecedent trauma were given in 20% of cases. Prat and colleagues reported a history of trauma in six of 22 patients, including one case in which an epithelioid sarcoma of the hand developed following exposure to plutonium.[181] Another example originated in the scar tissue of a caesarean section,[233] and Puissegur-Lupo et al. observed an epithelioid sarcoma that arose in scar tissue 17 months after traumatic amputation of three fingers of the right hand.[237] Several examples have also occurred in patients exposed to chemicals including Agent Orange[238] and hydrazine fuel.[239]

DESMOPLASTIC SMALL ROUND CELL TUMOR

Desmoplastic small round cell tumor (DSRCT) is a relatively uncommon entity that typically involves the abdominal or pelvic peritoneum (or both) of young males and pursues an aggressive clinical course. The lesion is characterized by a proliferation of small round cells deposited in an abundant desmoplastic stroma and multiphenotypic differentiation by immunohistochemistry. This lesion has had a variety of names, including undifferentiated malignant epithelial tumor involving serosal surfaces of the scrotum and abdomen in young males,[240] desmoplastic small cell tumor with divergent differentiation,[241] intra-abdominal desmoplastic small round cell tumor,[242] malignant small cell epithelial tumor of the peritoneum co-expressing mesenchymal-type intermediate filaments,[243] intra-abdominal neuroectodermal

tumor of childhood with divergent differentiation,[244] and desmoplastic small cell tumor with multiphenotypic differentiation.[245] Given the fact that this lesion clearly can occur in extra-abdominal locations as well as in adults, desmoplastic small round cell tumor is now the most commonly used name for this neoplasm.

Clinical findings

Most patients with this tumor are 15–35 years of age, although patients as young as 5 years[246] and as old as the seventh and eighth decades of life have been reported.[247,248] In a study of 109 patients with this tumor by Gerald et al.,[249] the patients ranged in age from 6 to 49 years (mean 22 years). Males far outnumber females at a ratio of approximately 4:1.[247,249-251]

Most present with a large abdominal and/or pelvic mass with extensive peritoneal involvement, usually without an identifiable visceral site of origin (Table 37–11). The most common complaint is abdominal distension, often associated with pain and constipation. Other signs and symptoms include intestinal or ureteral obstruction, ascites, difficulty with urination, and impotence.[252] Although most tumors arise in the abdomen/pelvis, this tumor has also been described in the paratesticular region,[253-255] ovary,[256] pleura,[257] central nervous system,[258] parotid gland,[247] sinonasal region,[259] bone,[260] lung,[261] kidney,[262] cervicovaginal region,[263] extremities,[264] and pancreas.[265]

Pathologic findings

Grossly, the tumor forms a solid, large multilobulated mass that is white or gray-white on cross-section, sometimes distorted by cystic change and areas of necrosis. Microscopically, most tumors are composed of sharply demarcated nests of varying size with small round or oval cells embedded in a hypervascular desmoplastic stroma (Figs 37–60 to 37–62). Large tumor cell nests often have central necrosis (Fig. 37–63). The neoplastic cells appear undifferentiated and have small hyperchromatic nuclei with inconspicuous nucleoli and scant

TABLE 37–11	ANATOMIC DISTRIBUTION OF 109 CASES OF DESMOPLASTIC SMALL ROUND CELL TUMOR	
Location	**No. of patients**	**%**
Abdominal cavity	103	94
Thoracic region	4	4
Posterior cranial fossa	1	1
Hand	1	1
Total	109	100

From Gerald WL, Ladanyi M, de Alava E, et al. Clinical, pathologic, and molecular spectrum of tumors associated with t(11;22)(p13;q12): desmoplastic small round-cell tumor and its variants. J Clin Oncol 1998; 16:3028.

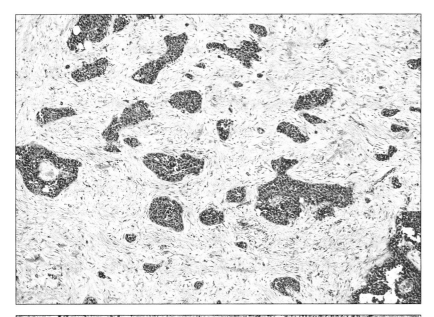

FIGURE 37–60 Desmoplastic small round cell tumor. Nests of undifferentiated tumor cells are surrounded by abundant fibrous stroma.

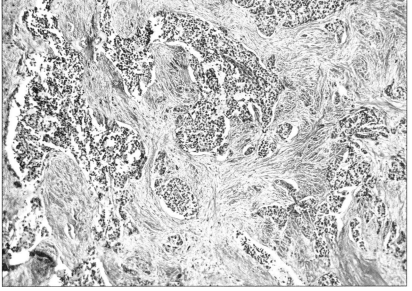

FIGURE 37–61 Nests of undifferentiated tumor cells are separated by a dense fibrous stroma in this desmoplastic small round cell tumor.

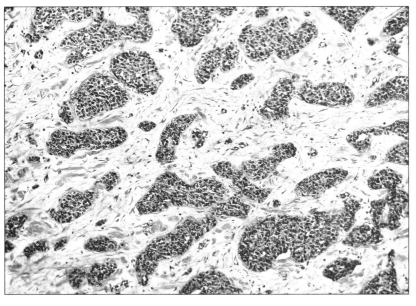

FIGURE 37–62 Prominent desmoplastic stroma surrounds varying-sized nests of tumor cells in a desmoplastic small round cell tumor.

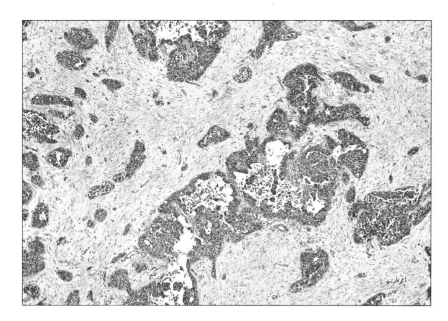

FIGURE 37-63 Desmoplastic small round cell tumor. Larger tumor nests show central necrosis.

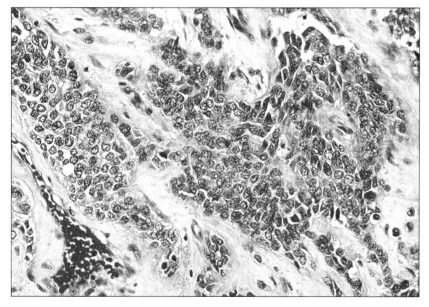

FIGURE 37-64 Desmoplastic small round cell tumor. The tumor cells appear undifferentiated and have small hyperchromatic nuclei with inconspicuous nucleoli.

amounts of eosinophilic cytoplasm (Fig. 37–64). In most cases the nuclei are relatively uniform, but some tumors show focal areas with increased nuclear atypia, and rare tumors are composed predominantly of markedly atypical cells.[251] The cells may be arranged in a variety of patterns including large nests with central necrosis, tubular-like structures, trabeculae separated by fibrovascular septa reminiscent of a "zellballen" pattern, and cords of single cells similar to lobular carcinoma of the breast (Fig. 37–65).[266] Typically, the cellular aggregates are surrounded and separated by abundant fibrous connective tissue with only a scattering of spindle-shaped fibroblasts and myofibroblasts. Occasionally, the tumor cells have more abundant cleared-out or vacuolated cytoplasm or even a signet ring-like appearance. A relatively common finding is the presence of rhabdoid-like foci in which the tumor cells have paranuclear intracytoplasmic

hyaline inclusions composed of aggregates of intermediate filaments (Fig. 37–66). Other unusual features include Homer Wright-like rosettes, papillary areas, zones that resemble transitional cell carcinoma, and areas composed predominantly of cells with a spindled morphology.[251]

Immunohistochemical findings

The tumor is characterized by a polyphenotypic profile with expression of epithelial, mesenchymal, and neural markers (Table 37–12). Virtually all tumors stain for epithelial markers, including cytokeratins and EMA. In the comprehensive study by Gerald and colleagues, cytokeratins and EMA were expressed in 86% and 93% of cases, respectively.[249] Occasionally, immunostains for cytokeratin reveal a dot-like pattern of cytoplasmic immunoreactivity. Stains for CK20 (positive in Merkel cell carcinoma)

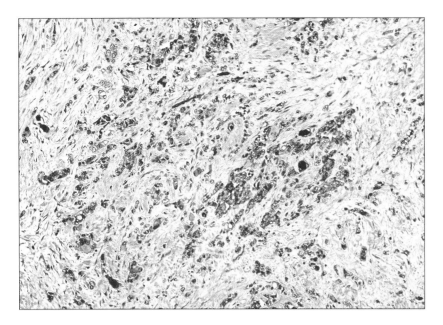

FIGURE 37–65 Desmoplastic small round cell tumor. Cords of cells are surrounded by a dense fibrous stroma mimicking lobular carcinoma of the breast.

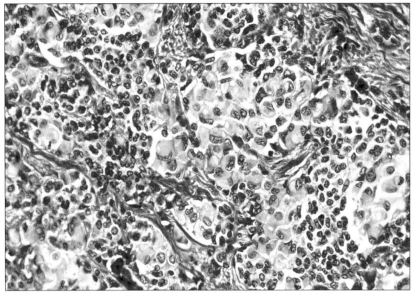

FIGURE 37–66 Focus of cells with a rhabdoid appearance in a desmoplastic small round cell tumor.

TABLE 37–12	SUMMARY OF IMMUNOHISTOCHEMICAL DATA ON DESMOPLASTIC SMALL ROUND CELL TUMORS REPORTED IN THE LITERATURE	
Marker	**No. positive**	**Cases %**
Cytokeratin	97/107	91
Desmin	107/117	91
EMA	64/73	88
Vimentin	87/103	84
NSE	88/107	82
Synaptophysin	11/43	26
S-100 protein	13/74	18
Neurofilament protein	6/50	12
CD99	4/33	12
Chromogranin	7/64	11

Modified from Ordóñez NG. Desmoplastic small round cell tumor. II. An ultrastructural and immunohistochemical study with emphasis on new immunohistochemical markers. Am J Surg Pathol 1998; 22:1314.

and CK5/6 (positive in malignant mesothelioma) are typically negative in DSRCT,[267] although epithelial markers including MOC-31 and Ber-Ep4 are commonly expressed.

Virtually all DSRCT stain for vimentin, but perhaps the most useful diagnostic marker is desmin. Up to 90% of cases stain for this antigen, typically with a perinuclear dot-like pattern, a unique pattern of desmin immunoreactivity peculiar to DSRCT (Fig. 37–67). Although often taken as evidence of myogenic differentiation, immunostains for nuclear myogenic regulatory proteins including MyoD1 and myogenin are negative; rare lesions express muscle-specific or smooth muscle actin.[267,268]

A variety of neural antigens have been detected in DSRCT, most commonly neuron-specific enolase and Leu-7, having been reported in 82% and 49% of cases, respectively.[267] However, immunoreactivity for

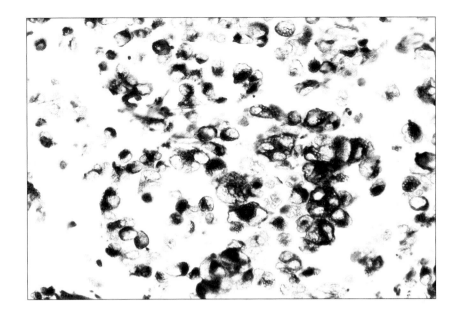

FIGURE 37–67 Typical perinuclear dot-like pattern of desmin immunoreactivity peculiar to desmoplastic small round cell tumors.

more specific markers of neuroendocrine differentiation including synaptophysin and chromogranin are uncommon.

CD99 and NB-84 are markers that have been utilized in the differential diagnosis of small round cell neoplasms. Although CD99 is a highly sensitive marker for the ES/PNET family, it is far from specific and has been detected in many other round cell neoplasms, including up to one-third of DSRCT.[250,267,269] Similarly, although NB-84 is a sensitive marker of neuroblastoma, it has been reported in other tumors, including up to 50% of DSRCT.[270,271]

As discussed below, the Wilms' tumor gene (*WT1*) on 11p13 is central to the pathogenesis of DSRCT. Nuclear expression of WT1 (using antibodies to the carboxy terminus) is a consistent feature of this tumor.[272,273] In the study by Hill et al.,[273] all 11 DSRCT tested showed strong and diffuse nuclear staining, whereas all 11 ES/PNET were negative for this antigen. Similar results were reported by Barnoud and colleagues.[272]

A high-molecular-weight glycoprotein, CA-125 is often present in mucinous carcinomas of the ovary and adenocarcinomas of the uterine cervix and endometrium.[274] It has also been found to be expressed by the tumor cells in DSRCT.[267] Interestingly, some patients with DSRCT have elevated serum levels of CA-125, which may return to normal levels following aggressive treatment, thereby suggesting some use to monitor disease status.[263,275,276]

Ultrastructural findings

The most striking ultrastructural feature of this tumor is the intracellular whorls and packets of microfilaments that are usually located near the nucleus, often compressing the nucleus or pushing it toward the periphery. There are a moderate number of mitochondria, free ribosomes, and small lakes of glycogen. Dense-core granules are infrequently found.[277] The cells are closely apposed with occasional filopodia, tight cell junctions, or small desmosomes with tonofilaments. Sometimes, the cell clusters are partly enveloped by a basal lamina.[267] Z-band material and thick or thin filaments suggesting myogenic differentiation are not seen.

Cytogenetic and molecular genetic findings

The identification of a unique cytogenetic abnormality t(11;22)(p13; q12) in this tumor has helped to establish the DSRCT as a distinct clinicopathologic entity.[278,279] The breakpoints involve the *EWS* gene on 22q12 and the Wilms' tumor gene (*WT1*) on 11p13.[280,281] *WT1* is a tumor suppressor gene that encodes a zinc-finger-type transcription factor that normally represses promoters that control expression of growth factors such as platelet-derived growth factor (PDGFA).[282] The fusion protein appears to induce expression of PDGFA, a potent mitogen and chemoattractant for fibroblasts and endothelial cells, thus serving as a potential link between the unique translocation and histologic characteristics of this tumor.[282,283]

The fusion transcript can be detected by RT-PCR or FISH using frozen or fixed tissue.[284–286] Most commonly, this fusion involves exon 7 of *EWS* and exon 8 of *WT1*; rare variant fusions have been described.[287,288] Although the *EWS-WT1* fusion has been described only in DSRCT, (Table 37–13) rare examples of DSRCT have been reported to have fusions characteristically identified in the ES/PNET family, including *EWS-ERG*[289] and *EWS-FLI1*.[290]

TABLE 37–13	SENSITIVITY AND SPECIFICITY OF THE *EWS-WT1* FUSION TRANSCRIPT FOR DESMOPLASTIC SMALL ROUND CELL TUMORS	
Diagnosis	***EWS-WT1*-positive**	**%**
DSRCT	11/12	92
Primitive neuroectodermal tumor family	0/8	0
Wilms' tumor	0/17	0
Alveolar rhabdomyosarcoma	0/13	0
Nonalveolar rhabdomyosarcoma	0/9	0

Modified from de Alava E, Ladanyi M, Rosai J, et al. Detection of chimeric transcripts in desmoplastic small round cell tumor and related developmental tumors by reverse transcriptase polymerase chain reaction: a specific diagnostic assay. Am J Pathol 1995; 147:1584.

Differential diagnosis

The DSRCT must be differentiated from other small round cell tumors including extraskeletal ES/PNET, alveolar rhabdomyosarcoma, neuroblastoma, lymphoma, poorly differentiated carcinoma, small cell carcinoma, Merkel cell carcinoma, and malignant mesothelioma. When arising in the typical clinicopathologic setting, DSRCT can be easily distinguished from these other entities, although ancillary techniques including immunohistochemistry and molecular genetics are invariably required. The immunohistochemical expression of epithelial, mesenchymal, and neural antigens, particularly the dot-like pattern of desmin staining, are useful for arriving at a diagnosis. Given that the immunophenotypic features overlap with many of the aforementioned tumors, a panel of immunostains is generally required. In questionable cases, RT-PCR or FISH analysis for evidence of an *EWS-WT1* fusion is indicated.

The differential diagnosis of DSRCT continues to broaden as its pathologic profile expands; neoplasms including sarcomatoid carcinoma, spindle cell sarcomas of various types, metastatic adenocarcinoma, and malignant extrarenal rhabdoid tumor may occasionally be entertained as diagnostic considerations. As above, a combination of immunohistochemical and molecular genetic analysis should allow for this distinction.

Discussion

The DSRCT is a highly aggressive neoplasm with an extremely poor prognosis. In the series reported by Ordóñez et al. in 1993,[291] 16 of 22 patients died of the disease within 8–50 months after the initial therapy. In a follow-up study published in 1998,[267] 25 of 35 patients for whom follow-up information was available died of widespread metastasis, and the remainder were alive with disease. In a study from the Memorial Sloan-Kettering Cancer Center,[292] 13 of 32 patients treated with an extensive debulking procedure (>90% of tumor removed) followed by systemic chemotherapy remained progression-free, although three of these patients died from toxicity related to treatment. Although the prognosis remains dismal, improved survival is correlated with a complete or good response to multimodality therapy, including extensive surgical debulking.[293,294] Complete excision is often impossible because of the irregular outline of the tumor and the presence of multiple implants in the peritoneum. Adamson et al. recently reported a case in which the patient's tumor showed a significant response to an inhibitor of PDGFR, raising the hope of more effective targeted therapy.[295]

The exact nature of this tumor is still uncertain. Some have speculated that the DSRCT is derived from mesothelial or submesothelial cells, given the predominant location of this tumor in mesothelial cell-lined cavities and the immunohistochemical expression of both epithelial and mesenchymal antigens. The cells of the DSRCT invariably express desmin, as do normal mesothelial cells, submesothelial mesenchymal cells, and some malignant mesotheliomas. However, there are a number of immunohistochemical differences between the DSRCT and mesothelioma such as the expression of MOC-31, Ber-Ep4, and Leu-M1 in DSRCT (usually absent in malignant mesotheliomas), and the absence of CK5/6 and thrombomodulin (usually present in malignant mesotheliomas). Furthermore, there is no ultrastructural evidence of mesothelial differentiation in DSRCT; as previously noted, some tumors arise in locations not lined by mesothelial cells.

MALIGNANT EXTRARENAL RHABDOID TUMOR

Malignant rhabdoid tumor of the kidney, initially described in 1978 and thought to be a "rhabdomyosarcomatoid variant of Wilms' tumor," has subsequently been defined as a distinct clinicopathologic entity different from Wilms' tumor.[296,297] Most tumors arising in the kidney occur in children less than 1 year of age and have an aggressive clinical course. The majority of patients die of widespread metastatic disease within a short time from the initial diagnosis.

Subsequently, tumors with a histologic appearance similar to that of tumors arising in the kidney have been described in virtually every extrarenal anatomic site including the skin,[298] soft tissues,[299,300] genitourinary tract,[301,302] gastrointestinal tract,[303] liver,[304] paratesticular region,[305] and most prominently the central nervous system, where they are referred to as atypical teratoid/rhabdoid tumors.[306,307] Lesions arising in the soft tissues most frequently occur in deep axial locations including the paraspinal region and neck.[299] It is often difficult to determine from the descriptions of these tumors whether they represent "pure" extrarenal rhabdoid tumors composed exclusively of cells with a rhabdoid morphology (malignant extrarenal rhabdoid tumor or MERT) or they represent focal rhabdoid areas within a "parent" neoplasm of recognizable phenotype (composite extrarenal rhabdoid tumor or CERT).[308] The term "MERT" as it pertains to soft tissue should be used for tumors with a predominant rhabdoid morphology in which no other clear line of differentiation can be documented. In this regard, it should be noted that carcinomas of various types may have rhabdoid features, most commonly renal cell carcinoma.[309,310] In addition, cells with rhabdoid features may be found in many types of sarcoma (e.g., epithelioid sarcoma,[219] DSRCT,[249] leiomyosarcoma,[311] synovial sarcoma,[43] rhabdomyosarcoma,[312] myxoid chondrosarcoma,[313] endometrial stromal sarcoma,[314] malignant mesothelioma,[315] meningioma,[316] and lymphoma. Clinically, MERTs occur over a much broader age range than those found in the kidney, although these lesions are still far more common in children, occasionally arising as widely disseminated congenital lesions.[317,318] Like their renal counterparts, MERTs are generally characterized by an aggressive clinical behavior, as fewer than 50% of patients survive more than 5 years regardless of the type of therapy employed.[297] As described in greater detail below, the histogenetic relationship between renal and extrarenal rhabdoid tumors (including those arising in the central nervous system) has been confirmed by the finding that they possess the same cytogenetic and molecular alterations.

Pathologic findings

Grossly, MERT is usually less than 5 cm in greatest dimension, although size varies considerably. The cut surface is usually soft, fleshy, and gray to tan in color, frequently with foci of hemorrhage and necrosis.

The histologic hallmark of MERT is the presence of "rhabdoid" cells – large polygonal cells with eccentric vesicular nuclei, prominent nucleoli, and abundant cytoplasm containing juxtanuclear eosinophilic, PAS-positive hyaline inclusions or globules (Figs 37–68 to 37–70). These inclusions correlate ultrastructurally to a paranuclear intracellular aggregate composed of compact bundles or whorls of intermediate filaments 10 nm in length (Figs 37–71 to 37–73).[319] Some benign tumors, including pleomorphic adenomas and myoepitheliomas of the salivary glands, have intracytoplasmic hyaline inclusions, but these tumors lack the nuclear cytologic atypia to designate them as having a rhabdoid morphology. Evaluation of multiple sections may be required to determine if the rhabdoid cells are a component of a "composite" extrarenal rhabdoid tumor (CERT) with a recognizable neoplastic phenotype (Fig. 37–74). In addition, ancillary techniques such as immunohistochemistry, electron microscopy, and molecular genetic analysis is necessary to recognize such a "parent" neoplasm, particularly if the rhabdoid cells comprise a substantial portion of the tumor, as well as to confirm the diagnosis of MERT.

Immunohistochemical and ultrastructural findings

A variety of antigens may be detected in the cells of MERT including epithelial (Fig. 37–75), mesenchymal, and neural antigens.[299,320] Vimentin is the most consistently expressed marked, followed by EMA and cytokeratin. Less commonly, the cells express muscle specific actin, smooth muscle actin, CD99, Leu-7, synaptophysin, and S-100 protein.

More recently, a monoclonal antibody to the *INI1* gene product has been found to be a valuable addition

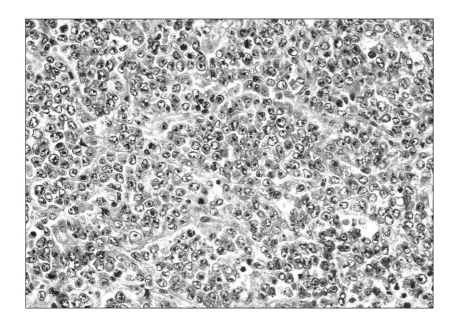

FIGURE 37–68 Malignant extrarenal rhabdoid tumor composed of nests of large epithelioid cells.

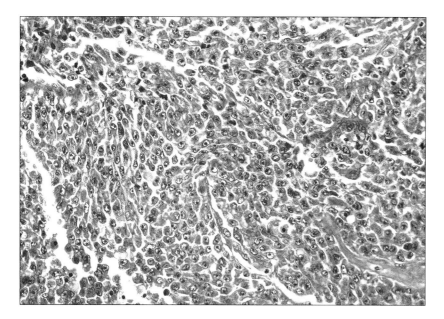

FIGURE 37–69 Sheets of large epithelioid cells with abundant eosinophilic cytoplasm in a malignant extrarenal rhabdoid tumor.

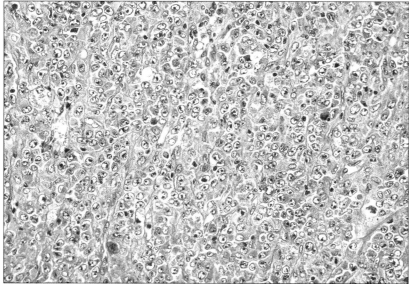

FIGURE 37–70 Malignant extrarenal rhabdoid tumor with a sheet of uniform large epithelioid cells having macronucleoli and abundant eosinophilic cytoplasm.

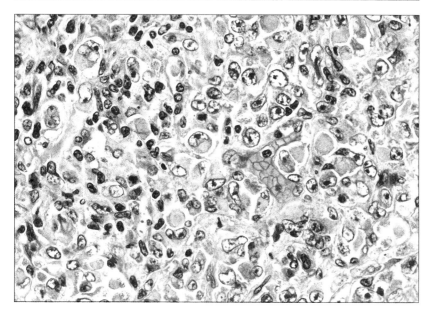

FIGURE 37–71 Malignant extrarenal rhabdoid tumor. The tumor cells have eccentric nuclei with macronucleoli.

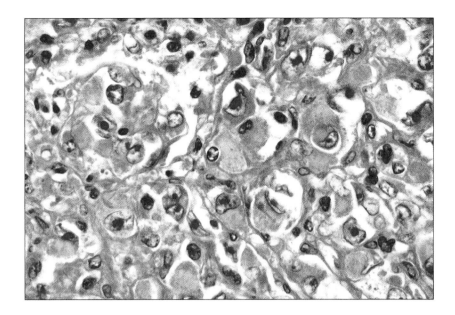

FIGURE 37–72 High-magnification view of paranuclear intracytoplasmic hyaline inclusions in a malignant extrarenal rhabdoid tumor.

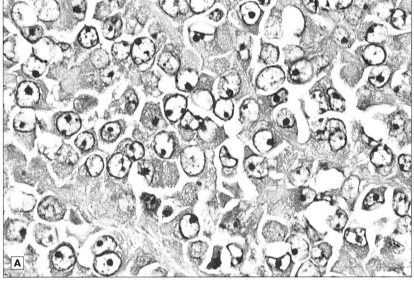

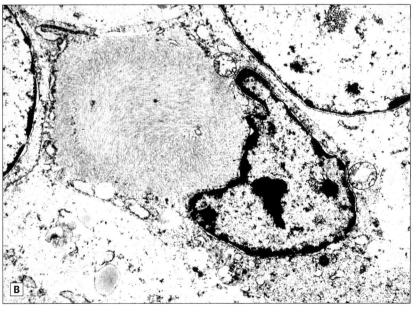

FIGURE 37–73 Malignant extrarenal rhabdoid tumor. **(A)** Cells with rhabdoid morphology. **(B)** Ultrastructural correlate, with a paranuclear whorl of intermediate filaments.

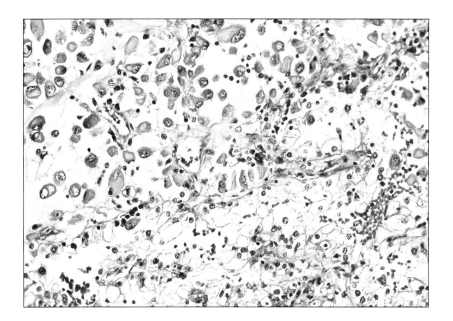

FIGURE 37–74 "Composite" extrarenal rhabdoid tumor with a typical clear cell renal cell carcinoma appearance at the bottom and cells with rhabdoid features near the top.

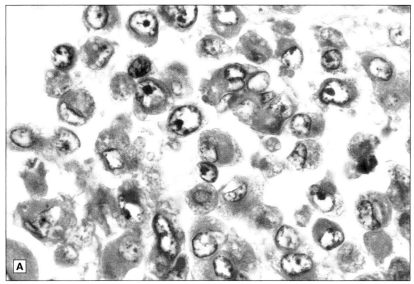

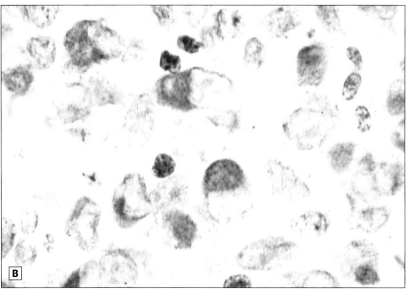

FIGURE 37–75 Malignant extrarenal rhabdoid tumor. **(A)** High-magnification view of rhabdoid cells. **(B)** Paranuclear immunoreactivity for CAM5.2 in rhabdoid cells.

TABLE 37–14	UTILITY OF IMMUNOHISTOCHEMICAL ANALYSIS OF HSNF5/INI1 IN DISTINGUISHING RENAL AND EXTRARENAL MALIGNANT RHABDOID TUMORS FROM OTHER PEDIATRIC SOFT TISSUE TUMORS

Tumor	INI staining
Renal rhabdoid tumor	0/19
Extrarenal rhabdoid tumor	0/8
ES/PNET	13/13
ARMS	3/3
ERMS	2/2
DSRCT	5/5
Clear cell sarcoma	4/4
Wilms' tumor	6/6

ES/PNET, Ewing sarcoma/primitive neuroectodermal tumor; ARMS, Alveolar rhabdomyosarcoma; ERMS, Embryonal rhabdomyosarcoma; DSRCT, Desmoplastic small round cell tumor.
Modified from Hoot A, Russo P, Judkins A, et al. Immunohistochemical analysis of hSNF5/ INI1 distinguishes renal and extrarenal malignant rhabdoid tumors from other pediatric soft tissue tumors. Am J Surg Pathol 2004; 22:1485.

to the immunohistochemical evaluation of these tumors (Table 37–14).[86,321,322] Judkins and colleagues first reported the sensitivity and specificity of this marker in recognizing atypical teratoid/rhabdoid tumors of the central nervous system.[322] Subsequently, Hoot et al. evaluated this marker in a large number of renal and extrarenal rhabdoid tumors as well as an array of other pediatric soft tissue tumors.[86] In all 27 cases of renal or extrarenal rhabdoid tumor, including 21 tumors with either a chromosome 22 deletion or an *INI1* mutation, there was no detectable expression of the INI1 protein in any of the tumor cells. In contrast, nuclear expression of INI1 protein was detected in all other tumors evaluated, including ES/PNET (13 cases), Wilms' tumor (six cases), DSRCT (five cases) and alveolar rhabdomyosarcoma (three cases). More recently, Sigauke and colleagues found an absence of expression of INI1 protein in a large number of malignant rhabdoid tumors of the central nervous system, kidney and soft tissue.[322a] Interestingly, all four cases of epithelial sarcomas tested were also negative for this antigen.

Ultrastructurally, rhabdoid cells are characterized by paranuclear aggregates or whorls of intermediate filaments 10 nm in size, predominantly composed of cytokeratin.[323,324] Additionally, the cytoplasm contains a moderate amount of dilated rough endoplasmic reticulum, few mitochondria, lysosomes, lipid droplets, and free ribosomes.[319]

Cytogenetic findings

The molecular alterations of renal and extrarenal rhabdoid tumors (including those arising in the central nervous system) have been recently elucidated. Earlier cytogenetic studies consistently found 22q aberrations including monosomy of chromosome 22 with or without partial deletion of the remaining chromosome 22.[325–327]

Schofield and colleagues reported loss of heterozygosity on 22q in 80% of renal rhabdoid tumors, suggesting the presence of a tumor suppressor gene at this locus.[328] Subsequent studies have consistently found deletions or mutations of the *INI1* gene (also known as *hSNF5/ SMARGB1/BAF47*) in the vast majority of renal and extrarenal rhabdoid tumors, and atypical teratoid/rhabdoid tumors of the central nervous system.[329–332] *INI1* is a member of the SWI/SNF chromatin-remodeling complex and is thought to have a direct role in activation and suppression of gene expression.[329] Germline and somatic mutations of the *INI1* gene have been found in murine knockout models[333] and in patients with multiple rhabdoid tumors (rhabdoid predisposition syndrome).[334,335] There is some variation in the genetic features, as central nervous system tumors are characterized by a high frequency of monosomy 22, whereas extrarenal tumors have a higher incidence of homozygous deletion of the entire *INI1* gene.[329] Overall, up to 20% of rhabdoid tumors of all sites show no evidence of *INI1* gene alterations. Genetic analysis of composite extrarenal rhabdoid tumors (CERT) by FISH has shown an absence of deletions of 22q11, indicating retained *INI1* function,[336] and these tumors retain nuclear expression of *INI1* protein.[337]

Discussion

Because of the definitional issues regarding MERT, it is difficult to cite meaningful studies from the literature. It has been proposed that the rhabdoid phenotype represents a "final common pathway" for the evolution of many tumors to a higher-grade, more clinically aggressive neoplasm[329,338] analogous to the tumor progression seen with dedifferentiated sarcomas. We believe there is ample evidence to support the existence of MERT as a clinico-pathologic entity, rather than simply a pattern of tumor progression, a contention firmly based in the recognition of mutations of the *INI1* gene, which are characteristic of this tumor.

MALIGNANT MESENCHYMOMA

The term malignant mesenchymoma has been applied to a large array of tumors utilizing a variety of diagnostic criteria. At present, this term serves little diagnostic use and should be abandoned altogether for the approach detailed below. From a historic point of view, Stout coined this term for nonepithelial malignant tumors "showing two or more unrelated, differentiated tissue types in addition to the fibrosarcomatous element."[339] He applied the term to a wide variety of neoplasms; after his initial report of eight cases in 1948 he had collected 355 cases by 1959.[340] Others, however, used this term in an entirely different setting. For example, Symmers and Nangle[341] and Ewing and Harrison[342] employed this term for a group of myxoid liposarcomas because of their lipoblastic, myxoid, and vascular components. Thomas and Kothare[343] applied it to a poorly differentiated sarcoma with "tissue similar to embryonal mesenchyme."

In 1991, Newman and Fletcher attempted to refine the criteria for this diagnosis by excluding a variety of morphologic patterns that were judged to show no specific differentiation, such as fibrosarcoma, hemangiopericytoma, myxofibrosarcoma, and pleomorphic malignant fibrous histiocytoma.[344] In addition, although the authors attempted to exclude "dedifferentiated" sarcomas, it appears as if some of these cases and some reported by Brady et al. are actually dedifferentiated liposarcomas with a minor low-grade component.[345]

There remain several neoplasms that would qualify as malignant mesenchymoma according to the definition stated above, but are frequently treated (rather arbitrarily) as distinct and separate entities. For example, malignant peripheral nerve sheath tumors may contain areas of rhabdomyosarcoma (malignant Triton tumor), yet these lesions have never been categorized as "malignant mesenchymoma." Likewise, osseous and cartilaginous differentiation has been accepted as a component of some atypical lipomatous tumors. Thus, there seem to be as many exceptions to the rules as there are rules themselves for the diagnosis of malignant mesenchymoma.

For all of these reasons, we believe the label "malignant mesenchymoma" is best deleted from classification schemes, a contention clearly supported by the WHO classification of soft tissue tumors published in 2002. Sarcomas displaying two or more lines of differentiation are best diagnosed by identifying the lines of differentiation, their approximate amounts, and the grade of the most aggressive component. To continue to use the term "malignant mesenchymoma" unites a diverse group of lesions while eclipsing far more important issues of histologic grade. The suggestion that "malignant mesenchymoma" behaves less aggressively than the level of differentiation suggests is based on six cases, four of which had less than 5 years of follow-up.[344]

REFERENCES

Synovial sarcoma

1. Smith LW. Synoviomata. Am J Pathol 1927; 3:355.
2. Lejars F, Rubens-Duval H. Les sarcomes primitifs des synoviales articulaires. Rev Chir (Paris) 1910; 41:751.
3. Brodsky JT, Burt ME, Hajdu SI, et al. Tendosynovial sarcoma. Clinicopathologic features, treatment, and prognosis. Cancer 1992; 70:484.
4. Hajdu SI, Shiu MH, Fortner JG. Tendosynovial sarcoma: a clinicopathological study of 136 cases. Cancer 1977; 39:1201.
5. Kransdorf MJ. Malignant soft-tissue tumors in a large referral population: distribution of diagnoses by age, sex, and location. AJR Am J Roentgenol 1995; 164:129.
6. Herzog CE. Overview of sarcomas in the adolescent and young adult population. J Pediatr Hematol Oncol 2005; 27:215.
7. Ladanyi M, Antonescu CR, Leung DH, et al. Impact of SYT-SSX fusion type on the clinical behavior of synovial sarcoma: a multi-institutional retrospective study of 243 patients. Cancer Res 2002; 62:135.
8. Spillane AJ, A'Hern R, Judson IR, et al. Synovial sarcoma: a clinicopathologic, staging, and prognostic assessment. J Clin Oncol 2000; 18:3794.
9. Campbell C, Gallagher J, Dickinson I. Synovial sarcoma – towards a simplified approach to prognosis. A NZ J Surg 2004; 74:727.
10. Paulino AC. Synovial sarcoma prognostic factors and patterns of failure. Am J Clin Oncol 2004; 27:122.
11. Raney RB. Synovial sarcoma in young people: background, prognostic factors, and therapeutic questions. J Pediatr Hematol Oncol 2005; 27:207.
12. Deraedt K, Debiec-Rychter M, Sciot R. Radiation-associated synovial sarcoma of the lung following radiotherapy for pulmonary metastasis of Wilms' tumour. Histopathology 2006; 48:473.
13. Egger JF, Coindre JM, Benhattar J, et al. Radiation-associated synovial sarcoma: clinicopathologic and molecular analysis of two cases. Mod Pathol 2002; 15:998.
14. van de Rijn M, Barr FG, Xiong QB, et al. Radiation-associated synovial sarcoma. Hum Pathol 1997; 28:1325.
15. Lamovec J, Zidar A, Cucek-Plenicar M. Synovial sarcoma associated with total hip replacement. A case report. J Bone Joint Surg [Am] 1988; 70:1558.
16. Namba Y, Kawai A, Naito N, et al. Intraarticular synovial sarcoma confirmed by SYT-SSX fusion transcript. Clin Orthop Relat Res 2002; 395:221.
16a. Michal M, Fanburg-Smith JC, Lasota J, et al. Minute synovial sarcomas of the hands and feet: a clinicopathologic study of 21 tumors less than 1 cm. Am J Surg Pathol 2006; 30:721.
17. Gallia GL, Sciubba DM, Hann CL, et al. Synovial sarcoma of the frontal sinus. Case report. J Neurosurg 2005; 103:1077.
18. Tilakaratne WM. Synovial sarcoma of the mandible. J Oral Pathol Med 2006; 35:61.
19. Barkan GA, El-Naggar AK. Primary synovial sarcoma of the parotid gland. Ann Diagn Pathol 2004; 8:233.
20. Rangheard AS, Vanel D, Viala J, et al. Synovial sarcomas of the head and neck: CT and MR imaging findings of eight patients. AJNR Am J Neuroradiol 2001; 22:851.
21. Fetsch JF, Meis JM. Synovial sarcoma of the abdominal wall. Cancer 1993; 72:469.
22. Hazelbag HM, Szuhai K, Tanke HJ, et al. Primary synovial sarcoma of the heart: a cytogenetic and molecular genetic analysis combining RT-PCR and COBRA-FISH of a case with a complex karyotype. Mod Pathol 2004; 17:1434.
23. Begueret H, Galateau-Salle F, Guillou L, et al. Primary intrathoracic synovial sarcoma: a clinicopathological study of 40 t(X;18)-positive cases from the French Sarcoma Group and the Mesopath Group. Am J Surg Pathol 2005; 29:339.
24. Frazier AA, Franks TJ, Pugatch RD, et al. From the archives of the AFIP: pleuropulmonary synovial sarcoma. Radiographics 2006; 26:923.
25. Taylor SM, Ha D, Elluru R, et al. Synovial sarcoma of the pericricoidal soft tissue. Otolaryngol Head Neck Surg 2002; 126:428.
26. Pan CC, Chang YH. Primary synovial sarcoma of the prostate. Histopathology 2006; 48:321.
27. Srivastava A, Nielsen PG, Dal Cin P, et al. Monophasic synovial sarcoma of the liver. Arch Pathol Lab Med 2005; 129:1047.
28. Suster S, Moran CA. Primary synovial sarcomas of the mediastinum: a clinicopathologic, immunohistochemical, and ultrastructural study of 15 cases. Am J Surg Pathol 2005; 29:569.
29. Ulusan S, Kizilkilic O, Yildirim T, et al. Radiological findings of primary retroperitoneal synovial sarcoma. Br J Radiol 2005; 78:166.
30. Billings SD, Meisner LF, Cummings OW, et al. Synovial sarcoma of the upper digestive tract: a report of two cases with demonstration of the X;18 translocation by fluorescence in situ hybridization. Mod Pathol 2000; 13:68.
31. Chu PG, Benhattar J, Weiss LM, et al. Intraneural synovial sarcoma: two cases. Mod Pathol 2004; 17:258.
32. Winnepenninckx V, De Vos R, Debiec-Rychter M, et al. Calcifying/ossifying synovial sarcoma shows t(X;18) with SSX2 involvement and mitochondrial calcifications. Histopathology 2001; 38:141.
33. Tateishi U, Hasegawa T, Beppu Y, et al. Synovial sarcoma of the soft tissues: prognostic significance of imaging features. J Comput Assist Tomogr 2004; 28:140.
34. Morrison C, Wakely PE Jr, Ashman CJ, et al. Cystic synovial sarcoma. Ann Diagn Pathol 2001; 5:48.
35. Krane JF, Bertoni F, Fletcher CD. Myxoid synovial sarcoma: an underappreciated morphologic subset. Mod Pathol 1999; 12:456.
36. Varela-Duran J, Enzinger FM. Calcifying synovial sarcoma. Cancer 1982; 50:345.
37. Milchgrub S, Ghandur-Mnaymneh L, Dorfman HD, et al. Synovial sarcoma with extensive

osteoid and bone formation. Am J Surg Pathol 1993; 17:357.

38. Folpe AL, Schmidt RA, Chapman D, et al. Poorly differentiated synovial sarcoma: immunohistochemical distinction from primitive neuroectodermal tumors and high-grade malignant peripheral nerve sheath tumors. Am J Surg Pathol 1998; 22:673.

39. van de Rijn M, Barr FG, Xiong QB, et al. Poorly differentiated synovial sarcoma: an analysis of clinical, pathologic, and molecular genetic features. Am J Surg Pathol 1999; 23:106.

40. de Silva MV, McMahon AD, Paterson L, et al. Identification of poorly differentiated synovial sarcoma: a comparison of clinicopathological and cytogenetic features with those of typical synovial sarcoma. Histopathology 2003; 43:220.

41. Machen SK, Easley KA, Goldblum JR. Synovial sarcoma of the extremities: a clinicopathologic study of 34 cases, including semi-quantitative analysis of spindled, epithelial, and poorly differentiated areas. Am J Surg Pathol 1999; 23:268.

42. Meis-Kindblom JM, Stenman G, Kindblom LG. Differential diagnosis of small round cell tumors. Semin Diagn Pathol 1996; 13:213.

43. Wen P, Prasad ML. Synovial sarcoma with rhabdoid features. Arch Pathol Lab Med 2003; 127:1391.

44. Nakamura T, Nakata K, Hata S, et al. Histochemical characterization of mucosubstances in synovial sarcoma. Am J Surg Pathol 1984; 8:429.

45. Guillou L, Wadden C, Kraus MD et al. S-100 protein reactivity in synovial sarcoma: a potentially frequent diagnostic pitfall; immunohistochemical analysis of 100 cases. Appl Immunohistochem 1996; 4:167.

46. Miettinen M, Limon J, Niezabitowski A, et al. Patterns of keratin polypeptides in 110 biphasic, monophasic, and poorly differentiated synovial sarcomas. Virchows Arch 2000; 437:275.

47. Smith TA, Machen SK, Fisher C, et al. Usefulness of cytokeratin subsets for distinguishing monophasic synovial sarcoma from malignant peripheral nerve sheath tumor. Am J Clin Pathol 1999; 112:641.

48. Pelmus M, Guillou L, Hostein I, et al. Monophasic fibrous and poorly differentiated synovial sarcoma: immunohistochemical reassessment of 60 t(X;18)(SYT-SSX)-positive cases. Am J Surg Pathol 2002; 26:1434.

49. Olsen SH, Thomas DG, Lucas DR. Cluster analysis of immunohistochemical profiles in synovial sarcoma, malignant peripheral nerve sheath tumor, and Ewing sarcoma. Mod Pathol 2006; 19:659.

50. Suster S, Fisher C, Moran CA. Expression of bcl-2 oncoprotein in benign and malignant spindle cell tumors of soft tissue, skin, serosal surfaces, and gastrointestinal tract. Am J Surg Pathol 1998; 22:863.

51. Fisher C, Montgomery E, Healy V. Calponin and h-caldesmon expression in synovial sarcoma; the use of calponin in diagnosis. Histopathology 2003; 42:588.

51a. Terry J, Saito T, Subramanian S, et al. TLE1 as a diagnostic immunohistochemical marker for synovial sarcoma emerging from gene expression profiling studies. Am J Surg Pathol 2007; 31:240.

52. Billings SD, Walsh SV, Fisher C, et al. Aberrant expression of tight junction-related proteins ZO-1, claudin-1 and occludin in synovial sarcoma: an immunohistochemical study with ultrastructural correlation. Mod Pathol 2004; 17:141.

53. Dardick I, Ho SP, McCaughey WT. Soft-tissue sarcoma of undetermined histogenesis: an ultrastructural study. Arch Pathol Lab Med 1981; 105:214.

54. Fisher C. The value of electron microscopy and immunohistochemistry in the diagnosis of soft tissue sarcomas: a study of 200 cases. Histopathology 1990; 16:441.

55. Dickersin GR. Synovial sarcoma: a review and update, with emphasis on the ultrastructural characterization of the nonglandular component. Ultrastruct Pathol 1991; 15:379.

56. Sandberg AA, Bridge JA. Updates on the cytogenetics and molecular genetics of bone and soft tissue tumors. Synovial sarcoma. Cancer Genet Cytogenet 2002; 133:1.

57. dos Santos NR, de Bruijn DR, Kater-Baats E, et al. Delineation of the protein domains responsible for SYT, SSX, and SYT-SSX nuclear localization. Exp Cell Res 2000; 256:192.

58. Brodin B, Haslam K, Yang K, et al. Cloning and characterization of spliced fusion transcript variants of synovial sarcoma: SYT/SSX4, SYT/SSX4v, and SYT/SSX2v. Possible regulatory role of the fusion gene product in wild type SYT expression. Gene 2001; 268:173.

59. Ladanyi M. Fusions of the SYT and SSX genes in synovial sarcoma. Oncogene 2001; 20:5755.

60. Nagayama S, Katagiri T, Tsunoda T, et al. Genome-wide analysis of gene expression in synovial sarcoma using a cDNA microarray. Cancer Res 2002; 62:5859.

61. Baird K, Davis S, Antonescu CR, et al. Gene expression profiling of human sarcomas: insights into sarcoma biology. Cancer Res 2005; 65:9226.

62. Panagopoulos I, Mertens F, Isaksson M, et al. Clinical impact of molecular and cytogenetic findings in synovial sarcoma. Genes Chromosomes Cancer 2001; 31:362.

63. Antonescu CR, Kawai A, Leung DH, et al. Strong association of SYT-SSX fusion type and morphologic epithelial differentiation in synovial sarcoma. Diagn Mol Pathol 2000; 9:1.

64. Kawai A, Woodruff J, Healey JH, et al. SYT-SSX gene fusion as a determinant of morphology and prognosis in synovial sarcoma. N Engl J Med 1998; 338:153.

65. Hill DA, Riedley SE, Patel AR, et al. Real-time polymerase chain reaction as an aid for the detection of SYT-SSX1 and SYT-SSX2 transcripts in fresh and archival pediatric synovial sarcoma specimens: report of 25 cases from St. Jude Children's Research Hospital. Pediatr Dev Pathol 2003; 6:24.

66. Jin L, Majerus J, Oliveira A, et al. Detection of fusion gene transcripts in fresh-frozen and formalin-fixed paraffin-embedded tissue sections of soft-tissue sarcomas after laser capture microdissection and RT-PCR. Diagn Mol Pathol 2003; 12:224.

67. Guillou L, Coindre J, Gallagher G, et al. Detection of the synovial sarcoma translocation t(X;18) (SYT;SSX) in paraffin-embedded tissues using reverse transcriptase-polymerase chain reaction: a reliable and powerful diagnostic tool for pathologists. A molecular analysis of 221 mesenchymal tumors fixed in different fixatives. Hum Pathol 2001; 32:105.

68. Terry J, Barry TS, Horsman DE, et al. Fluorescence in situ hybridization for the detection of t(X;18)(p11.2;q11.2) in a synovial sarcoma tissue microarray using a breakapart-style probe. Diagn Mol Pathol 2005; 14:77.

69. Argani P, Zakowski MF, Klimstra DS, et al. Detection of the SYT-SSX chimeric RNA of synovial sarcoma in paraffin-embedded tissue and its application in problematic cases. Mod Pathol 1998; 11:65.

70. Hostein I, Menard A, Bui BN, et al. Molecular detection of the synovial sarcoma translocation t(X;18) by real-time polymerase chain reaction in paraffin-embedded material. Diagn Mol Pathol 2002; 11:16.

70a. Amary MF, Berisha F, Bernardi Fdel C et al. Detection of SS18-SSX fusion transcripts in formalin-fixed paraffin-embedded neoplasms: analysis of conventional RT-PCR, qRT-PCR and dual color FISH as diagnostic tools for synovial sarcoma. Mod Pathol 2007; 20:482.

71. Huang L, Espinoza C, Welsh R. Malignant peripheral nerve sheath tumor with divergent differentiation. Arch Pathol Lab Med 2003; 127:e147.

72. Nagasaka T, Lai R, Sone M, et al. Glandular malignant peripheral nerve sheath tumor: an unusual case showing histologically malignant glands. Arch Pathol Lab Med 2000; 124:1364.

73. Miettinen M, Limon J, Niezabitowski A, et al. Calretinin and other mesothelioma markers in synovial sarcoma: analysis of antigenic similarities and differences with malignant mesothelioma. Am J Surg Pathol 2001; 25:610.

74. Hui P, Li N, Johnson C, et al. HMGA proteins in malignant peripheral nerve sheath tumor and synovial sarcoma: preferential expression of HMGA2 in malignant peripheral nerve sheath tumor. Mod Pathol 2005; 18:1519.

75. Coindre JM, Hostein I, Benhattar J, et al. Malignant peripheral nerve sheath tumors are t(X;18)-negative sarcomas. Molecular analysis of 25 cases occurring in neurofibromatosis type 1 patients, using two different RT-PCR-based methods of detection. Mod Pathol 2002; 15:589.

76. Tamborini E, Agus V, Perrone F, et al. Lack of SYT-SSX fusion transcripts in malignant peripheral nerve sheath tumors on RT-PCR analysis of 34 archival cases. Lab Invest 2002; 82:609.

77. van de Rijn M, Barr FG, Collins MH, et al. Absence of SYT-SSX fusion products in soft tissue tumors other than synovial sarcoma. Am J Clin Pathol 1999; 112:43.

78. O'Sullivan MJ, Kyriakos M, Zhu X, et al. Malignant peripheral nerve sheath tumors with t(X;18). A pathologic and molecular genetic study. Mod Pathol 2000; 13:1253.

78a. Coindre JM, Hostein I, Benhattar J, et al. Malignant peripheral nerve sheath tumors are t(X;18)-negative sarcomas. Molecular analysis of 25 cases occurring in neurofibromatosis type 1 patients, using two different RT-PCR-based methods of detection. Mod Pathol 2002; 15:589.

79. Sanders ME, van de Rijn M, Barr FG. Detection of a variant SYT-SSX1 fusion in a case of predominantly epithelioid synovial sarcoma. Mol Diagn 1999; 4:65.

80. Goldblum JR, Machen SK, Fisher C. Cytokeratins in round cell sarcomas. Am J Surg Pathol 2000; 24:1174.

81. Jimenez RE, Folpe AL, Lapham RL, et al. Primary Ewing's sarcoma/primitive neuroectodermal tumor of the kidney: a clinicopathologic and immunohistochemical analysis of 11 cases. Am J Surg Pathol 2002; 26:320.

82. Collini P, Sampietro G, Bertulli R, et al. Cytokeratin immunoreactivity in 41 cases of ES/PNET confirmed by molecular diagnostic studies. Am J Surg Pathol 2001; 25:273.

83. Gu M, Antonescu CR, Guiter G, et al. Cytokeratin immunoreactivity in Ewing's sarcoma: prevalence in 50 cases confirmed by molecular diagnostic studies. Am J Surg Pathol 2000; 24:410.

84. Folpe AL, Goldblum JR, Rubin BP, et al. Morphologic and immunophenotypic diversity in Ewing family tumors: a study of 66 genetically confirmed cases. Am J Surg Pathol 2005; 29:1025.

85. Machen SK, Fisher C, Gautam RS, et al. Utility of cytokeratin subsets for distinguishing poorly differentiated synovial sarcoma from

peripheral primitive neuroectodermal tumour. Histopathology 1998; 33:501.

86. Hoot AC, Russo P, Judkins AR, et al. Immunohistochemical analysis of hSNF5/INI1 distinguishes renal and extra-renal malignant rhabdoid tumors from other pediatric soft tissue tumors. Am J Surg Pathol 2004; 28:1485.

87. Menendez LR, Brien E, Brien WW. Synovial sarcoma. A clinicopathologic study. Orthop Rev 1992; 21:465.

88. Ryan JR, Baker LH, Benjamin RS. The natural history of metastatic synovial sarcoma: experience of the Southwest Oncology Group. Clin Orthop Relat Res 1982; 164:257.

89. Thunold J, Bang G. Synovial sarcoma: a case report. Acta Orthop Scand 1976; 47:231.

90. Lewis JJ, Antonescu CR, Leung DH, et al. Synovial sarcoma: a multivariate analysis of prognostic factors in 112 patients with primary localized tumors of the extremity. J Clin Oncol 2000; 18:2087.

91. Mullen JR, Zagars GK. Synovial sarcoma outcome following conservation surgery and radiotherapy. Radiother Oncol 1994; 33:23.

92. Guillou L, Benhattar J, Bonichon F, et al. Histologic grade, but not SYT-SSX fusion type, is an important prognostic factor in patients with synovial sarcoma: a multicenter, retrospective analysis. J Clin Oncol 2004; 22:4040.

93. Trassard M, Le Doussal V, Hacene K, et al. Prognostic factors in localized primary synovial sarcoma: a multicenter study of 128 adult patients. J Clin Oncol 2001; 19:525.

94. Oda Y, Hashimoto H, Takeshita S, et al. The prognostic value of immunohistochemical staining for proliferating cell nuclear antigen in synovial sarcoma. Cancer 1993; 72:478.

95. Bergh P, Meis-Kindblom JM, Gherlinzoni F, et al. Synovial sarcoma: identification of low and high risk groups. Cancer 1999; 85:2596.

96. Singer S, Baldini EH, Demetri GD, et al. Synovial sarcoma: prognostic significance of tumor size, margin of resection, and mitotic activity for survival. J Clin Oncol 1996; 14:1201.

97. Deshmukh R, Mankin HJ, Singer S. Synovial sarcoma: the importance of size and location for survival. Clin Orthop 2004; 419:155.

98. Brecht IB, Ferrari A, Int-Veen C, et al. Grossly-resected synovial sarcoma treated by the German and Italian Pediatric Soft Tissue Sarcoma Cooperative Groups: discussion on the role of adjuvant therapies. Pediatr Blood Cancer 2006; 46:11.

99. Spurrell EL, Fisher C, Thomas JM, et al. Prognostic factors in advanced synovial sarcoma: an analysis of 104 patients treated at the Royal Marsden Hospital. Ann Oncol 2005; 16:437.

100. Cagle LA, Mirra JM, Storm FK, et al. Histologic features relating to prognosis in synovial sarcoma. Cancer 1987; 59:1810.

101. el-Naggar AK, Ayala AG, Abdul-Karim FW, et al. Synovial sarcoma. A DNA flow cytometric study. Cancer 1990; 65:2295.

102. Hasegawa T, Yokoyama R, Matsuno Y, et al. Prognostic significance of histologic grade and nuclear expression of beta-catenin in synovial sarcoma. Hum Pathol 2001; 32:257.

103. Golouh R, Vuzevski V, Bracko M, et al. Synovial sarcoma: a clinicopathological study of 36 cases. J Surg Oncol 1990; 45:20.

104. Lopes JM, Nesland JM, Reis-Filho JS, et al. Differential Ki67 and bcl-2 immunoexpression in solid-glandular and spindle cell components of biphasic synovial sarcoma: a double immunostaining assessment with cytokeratin and vimentin. Histopathology 2002; 40:464.

105. Barbashina V, Benevenia J, Aviv H, et al. Oncoproteins and proliferation markers in synovial sarcomas: a clinicopathologic study of 19 cases. J Cancer Res Clin Oncol 2002; 128:610.

106. Kawauchi S, Fukuda T, Oda Y, et al. Prognostic significance of apoptosis in synovial sarcoma: correlation with clinicopathologic parameters, cell proliferative activity, and expression of apoptosis-related proteins. Mod Pathol 2000; 13:755.

107. Antonescu CR, Leung DH, Dudas M, et al. Alterations of cell cycle regulators in localized synovial sarcoma: a multifactorial study with prognostic implications. Am J Pathol 2000; 156:977.

108. Oda Y, Sakamoto A, Satio T, et al. Molecular abnormalities of p53, MDM2, and H-ras in synovial sarcoma. Mod Pathol 2000; 13:994.

109. Schneider-Stock R, Onnasch D, Haeckel C, et al. Prognostic significance of p53 gene mutations and p53 protein expression in synovial sarcomas. Virchows Arch 1999; 435:407.

110. Saito T, Oda Y, Sakamoto A, et al. Prognostic value of the preserved expression of the E-cadherin and catenin families of adhesion molecules and of beta-catenin mutations in synovial sarcoma. J Pathol 2000; 192:342.

110a. Izumi T, Oda Y, Hasegawa T, et al. Dysadherin expression as a significant prognostic factor and as a determinant of histologic features in synovial sarcoma: special reference to its inverse relationship with E-cadherin expression. Am J Surg Pathol 2007; 31:85.

111. Xie Y, Tornkvist M, Aalto Y, et al. Gene expression profile by blocking the SYT-SSX fusion gene in synovial sarcoma cells. Identification of XRCC4 as a putative SYT-SSX target gene. Oncogene 2003; 22:7628.

112. Sun Y, Gao D, Liu Y, et al. IGF2 is critical for tumorigenesis by synovial sarcoma oncoprotein SYT-SSX1. Oncogene 2006; 25:1042.

113. Kawai A, Naito N, Yoshida A, et al. Establishment and characterization of a biphasic synovial sarcoma cell line, SYO-1. Cancer Lett 2004; 204:105.

114. Mezzelani A, Mariani L, Tamborini E, et al. SYT-SSX fusion genes and prognosis in synovial sarcoma. Br J Cancer 2001; 85:1535.

115. Nilsson G, Skytting B, Xie Y, et al. The SYT-SSX1 variant of synovial sarcoma is associated with a high rate of tumor cell proliferation and poor clinical outcome. Cancer Res 1999; 59:3180.

116. Surace C, Panagopoulos I, Palsson E, et al. A novel FISH assay for SS18-SSX fusion type in synovial sarcoma. Lab Invest 2004; 84:1185.

117. Randall RL, Schabel KL, Hitchcock Y, et al. Diagnosis and management of synovial sarcoma. Curr Treat Options Oncol 2005; 6:449.

118. Albritton KH, Randall RL. Prospects for targeted therapy of synovial sarcoma. J Pediatr Hematol Oncol 2005; 27:219.

119. Okcu MF, Munsell M, Treuner J, et al. Synovial sarcoma of childhood and adolescence: a multicenter, multivariate analysis of outcome. J Clin Oncol 2003; 21:1602.

120. Ferrari A, Gronchi A, Casanova M, et al. Synovial sarcoma: a retrospective analysis of 271 patients of all ages treated at a single institution. Cancer 2004; 101:627.

121. Mancuso T, Mezzelani A, Riva C, et al. Analysis of SYT-SSX fusion transcripts and bcl-2 expression and phosphorylation status in synovial sarcoma. Lab Invest 2000; 80:805.

122. Joyner DE, Albritton KH, Bastar JD, et al. G3139 antisense oligonucleotide directed against antiapoptotic bcl-2 enhances doxorubicin cytotoxicity in the FU-SY-1 synovial sarcoma cell line. J Orthop Res 2006; 24:474.

123. Thomas DG, Giordano TJ, Sanders D, et al. Expression of receptor tyrosine kinases epidermal growth factor receptor and HER-2/neu in synovial sarcoma. Cancer 2005; 103:830.

124. Nielsen TO, Hsu FD, O'Connell JX, et al. Tissue microarray validation of epidermal growth factor receptor and SALL2 in synovial sarcoma with comparison to tumors of similar histology. Am J Pathol 2003; 163:1449.

125. Blay JY, Ray-Coquard I, Alberti L, et al. Targeting other abnormal signaling pathways in sarcoma: EGFR in synovial sarcomas, PPAR-gamma in liposarcomas. Cancer Treat Res 2004; 120:151.

126. Sapi Z, Papai Z, Hruska A, et al. Her-2 oncogene amplification, chromosome 17 and DNA ploidy status in synovial sarcoma. Pathol Oncol Res 2005; 11:133.

127. Olsen RJ, Lydiatt WM, Koepsell SA, et al. C-erb-B2 (HER2/neu) expression in synovial sarcoma of the head and neck. Head Neck 2005; 27:883.

128. Nuciforo PG, Pellegrini C, Fasani R, et al. Molecular and immunohistochemical analysis of HER2/neu oncogene in synovial sarcoma. Hum Pathol 2003; 34:639.

Alveolar soft part sarcoma

129. Christopherson WM, Foote FWJ, Stewart FW. Alveolar soft-part sarcoma: structurally characteristic tumors of uncertain histogenesis. Cancer 1952; 5:100.

130. Ekfors TO, Kalimo H, Rantakokko V, et al. Alveolar soft part sarcoma: a report of two cases with some histochemical and ultrastructural observations. Cancer 1979; 43:1672.

131. Lieberman PH, Brennan MF, Kimmel M, et al. Alveolar soft-part sarcoma. A clinico-pathologic study of half a century. Cancer 1989; 63:1.

132. Lieberman PH, Foote FW Jr, Stewart FW, et al. Alveolar soft-part sarcoma. JAMA 1966; 198:1047.

133. Anderson ME, Hornicek FJ, Gebhardt MC, et al. Alveolar soft part sarcoma: a rare and enigmatic entity. Clin Orthop 2005; 438:144.

134. Portera CA Jr, Ho V, Patel SR, et al. Alveolar soft part sarcoma: clinical course and patterns of metastasis in 70 patients treated at a single institution. Cancer 2001; 91:585.

135. Casanova M, Ferrari A, Bisogno G, et al. Alveolar soft part sarcoma in children and adolescents: a report from the Soft-Tissue Sarcoma Italian Cooperative Group. Ann Oncol 2000; 11:1445.

136. Ogose A, Yazawa Y, Ueda T, et al. Alveolar soft part sarcoma in Japan: multi-institutional study of 57 patients from the Japanese Musculoskeletal Oncology Group. Oncology 2003; 65:7.

137. Ordonez NG. Alveolar soft part sarcoma: a review and update. Adv Anat Pathol 1999; 6:125.

138. Roma AA, Yang B, Senior ME, et al. TFE3 immunoreactivity in alveolar soft part sarcoma of the uterine cervix: case report. Int J Gynecol Pathol 2005; 24:131.

139. Flieder DB, Moran CA, Suster S. Primary alveolar soft-part sarcoma of the mediastinum: a clinicopathological and immunohistochemical study of two cases. Histopathology 1997; 31:469.

140. Wu J, Brinker DA, Haas M, et al. Primary alveolar soft part sarcoma (ASPS) of the breast: report of a deceptive case with xanthomatous features confirmed by TFE3 immunohistochemistry and electron microscopy. Int J Surg Pathol 2005; 13:81.

140a. Amin MB, Patel RM, Oliveira P, et al. Alveolar soft-part sarcoma of the urinary bladder with urethral recurrence: a unique case with emphasis on differential diagnoses and diagnostic utility of an immunohistochemical panel including TFE3. Am J Surg Pathol 2006; 30:1322.

141. Yaziji H, Ranaldi R, Verdolini R, et al. Primary alveolar soft part sarcoma of the stomach: a case report and review. Pathol Res Pract 2000; 196:519.

142. Koguchi Y, Yamaguchi T, Yamato M, et al. Alveolar soft part sarcoma of bone. J Orthop Sci 2005; 10:652.

143. Fanburg-Smith JC, Miettinen M, Folpe AL, et al. Lingual alveolar soft part sarcoma; 14 cases: novel clinical and morphological observations. Histopathology 2004; 45:526.

144. Kim HS, Lee HK, Weon YC, et al. Alveolar soft-part sarcoma of the head and neck: clinical and imaging features in five cases. AJNR Am J Neuroradiol 2005; 26:1331.

145. Kebudi R, Ayan I, Gorgun O, et al. Brain metastasis in pediatric extracranial solid tumors: survey and literature review. J Neurooncol 2005; 71:43.

146. Pang LM, Roebuck DJ, Griffith JF, et al. Alveolar soft-part sarcoma: a rare soft-tissue malignancy with distinctive clinical and radiological features. Pediatr Radiol 2001; 31:196.

147. Suh JS, Cho J, Lee SH, et al. Alveolar soft part sarcoma: MR and angiographic findings. Skeletal Radiol 2000; 29:680.

148. Evans HL. Alveolar soft-part sarcoma. A study of 13 typical examples and one with a histologically atypical component. Cancer 1985; 55:912.

149. Masson P. Tumeurs humaines: histologie, diagnostics et techniques. 2nd edn. Paris: Librairie Maloine; 1959.

150. Ladanyi M, Antonescu CR, Drobnjak M, et al. The precrystalline cytoplasmic granules of alveolar soft part sarcoma contain monocarboxylate transporter 1 and CD147. Am J Pathol 2002; 160:1215.

151. Weiss SW. Alveolar soft part sarcoma: are we at the end or just the beginning of our quest? Am J Pathol 2002; 160:1197.

152. Foschini MP, Eusebi V. Alveolar soft-part sarcoma: a new type of rhabdomyosarcoma? Semin Diagn Pathol 1994; 11:58.

153. Jong R, Kandel R, Fornasier V, et al. Alveolar soft part sarcoma: review of nine cases including two cases with unusual histology. Histopathology 1998; 32:63.

154. Miettinen M, Ekfors T. Alveolar soft part sarcoma. Immunohistochemical evidence for muscle cell differentiation. Am J Clin Pathol 1990; 93:32.

155. Rosai J, Dias P, Parham MD. MyoD1 protein expression in alveolar soft part sarcoma as confirmatory evidence of its skeletal muscle nature. Am J Surg Pathol 1991; 15:974.

156. Cullinane C, Thorner PS, Greenberg ML, et al. Molecular genetic, cytogenetic, and immunohistochemical characterization of alveolar soft-part sarcoma. Implications for cell of origin. Cancer 1992; 70:2444.

157. Wang NP, Bacchi CE, Jiang JJ, et al. Does alveolar soft-part sarcoma exhibit skeletal muscle differentiation? An immunocytochemical and biochemical study of myogenic regulatory protein expression. Mod Pathol 1996; 9:496.

158. Gomez JA, Amin MB, Ro JY, et al. Immunohistochemical profile of myogenin and MyoD1 does not support skeletal muscle lineage in alveolar soft part sarcoma. Arch Pathol Lab Med 1999; 123:503.

159. Cessna MH, Zhou H, Perkins SL, et al. Are myogenin and MyoD1 expression specific for rhabdomyosarcoma? A study of 150 cases, with emphasis on spindle cell mimics. Am J Surg Pathol 2001; 25:1150.

160. Shipkey FJ, Lieberman PH, Foote FW Jr, et al. Ultrastructure of alveolar soft part sarcoma. Cancer 1964; 17:821.

161. Ordonez NG, Mackay B. Alveolar soft-part sarcoma: a review of the pathology and histogenesis. Ultrastruct Pathol 1998; 22:275.

162. Ordonez NG, Ro JY, Mackay B. Alveolar soft part sarcoma. An ultrastructural and immunocytochemical investigation of its histogenesis. Cancer 1989; 63:1721.

163. Ladanyi M, Lui MY, Antonescu CR, et al. The der(17)t(X;17)(p11;q25) of human alveolar soft part sarcoma fuses the TFE3 transcription factor gene to ASPL, a novel gene at 17q25. Oncogene 2001; 20:48.

164. Sandberg A, Bridge J. Updates on the cytogenetics and molecular genetics of bone and soft tissue tumors: alveolar soft part sarcoma. Cancer Genet Cytogenet 2002; 136:1.

165. Argani P, Antonescu CR, Illei PB, et al. Primary renal neoplasms with the ASPL-TFE3 gene fusion of alveolar soft part sarcoma: a distinctive tumor entity previously included among renal cell carcinomas of children and adolescents. Am J Pathol 2001; 159:179.

166. Argani P, Lal P, Hutchinson B, et al. Aberrant nuclear immunoreactivity for TFE3 in neoplasms with TFE3 gene fusions: a sensitive and specific immunohistochemical assay. Am J Surg Pathol 2003; 27:750.

167. Rakheja D, Kapur P, Tomlinson GE, et al. Pediatric renal cell carcinomas with Xp11.2 rearrangements are immunoreactive for hMLH1 and hMSH2 proteins. Pediatr Dev Pathol 2005; 8:615.

168. Saito T, Oda Y, Kawaguchi K, et al. Possible association between tumor-suppressor gene mutations and hMSH2/hMLH1 inactivation in alveolar soft part sarcoma. Hum Pathol 2003; 34:841.

169. Argani P, Ladanyi M. Recent advances in pediatric renal neoplasia. Adv Anat Pathol 2003; 10:243.

170. Lillehei KO, Kleinschmidt-DeMasters B, Mitchell DH, et al. Alveolar soft part sarcoma: an unusually long interval between presentation and brain metastasis. Hum Pathol 1993; 24:1030.

171. Wang CH, Lee N, Lee LS. Successful treatment for solitary brain metastasis from alveolar soft part sarcoma. J Neurooncol 1995; 25:161.

172. Reichardt P, Lindner T, Pink D, et al. Chemotherapy in alveolar soft part sarcomas. What do we know? Eur J Cancer 2003; 39:1511.

173. Smetana HF, Scott WF. Soft tissue tumors of peculiar character and uncertain origin (malignant tumors of nonchromaffin paraganglia). Milit Surg 1951; 109:330.

174. Mukai M, Iri H, Nakajima T, et al. Alveolar soft-part sarcoma. A review on its histogenesis and further studies based on electron microscopy, immunohistochemistry, and biochemistry. Am J Surg Pathol 1983; 7:679.

175. Mukai M, Torikata C, Iri H. Alveolar soft part sarcoma: an electron microscopic study especially of uncrystallized granules using a tannic acid-containing fixative. Ultrastruct Pathol 1990; 14:41.

176. Karnauchow N, Magner D. The histogenesis of alveolar soft part sarcoma. J Pathol Bacteriol 1963; 89:169.

177. Fisher ER, Reidbord H. Electron microscopic evidence suggesting myogenous derivation of the so-called alveolar soft part sarcoma. Cancer 1971; 27:150.

178. DeSchryver-Kecskemeti K, Kraus FT, Engleman W, et al. Alveolar soft-part sarcoma – a malignant angioreninoma: histochemical, immunocytochemical, and electron-microscopic study of four cases. Am J Surg Pathol 1982; 6:5.

Epithelioid sarcoma

179. Enzinger FM. Epithelioid sarcoma. A sarcoma simulating a granuloma or a carcinoma. Cancer 1970; 26:1029.

180. Chase DR, Enzinger FM. Epithelioid sarcoma. Diagnosis, prognostic indicators, and treatment. Am J Surg Pathol 1985; 9:241.

181. Prat J, Woodruff JM, Marcove RC. Epithelioid sarcoma: an analysis of 22 cases indicating the prognostic significance of vascular invasion and regional lymph node metastasis. Cancer 1978; 41:1472.

182. Kodet R, Smelhaus V, Newton WA Jr, et al. Epithelioid sarcoma in childhood: an immunohistochemical, electron microscopic, and clinicopathologic study of 11 cases under 15 years of age and review of the literature. Pediatr Pathol 1994; 14:433.

183. Casanova M, Ferrari A, Collini P, et al. Epithelioid sarcoma in children and adolescents: a report from the Italian Soft Tissue Sarcoma Committee. Cancer 2006; 106:708.

184. Billings SD, Folpe AL, Weiss SW. Epithelioid sarcoma-like hemangioendothelioma. Am J Surg Pathol 2003; 27:48.

185. Zimmer LA, Gillman G, Barnes L. Postauricular epithelioid sarcoma. Otolaryngol Head Neck Surg 2004; 131:1022.

186. Lowentritt B, Parsons JK, Argani P, et al. Pediatric epithelioid sarcoma of the penis. J Urol 2004; 172:296.

187. Ormsby AH, Liou LS, Oriba HA, et al. Epithelioid sarcoma of the penis: report of an unusual case and review of the literature. Ann Diagn Pathol 2000; 4:88.

188. Altundag K, Dikbas O, Oyan B, et al. Epithelioid sarcoma of vulva: a case report and review of the literature. Med Oncol 2004; 21:367.

189. Ikeda K, Tate G, Suzuki T, et al. Fine needle aspiration cytology of primary proximal-type epithelioid sarcoma of the perineum: a case report. Acta Cytol 2005; 49:314.

190. Jeney H, Heller DS, Hameed M, et al. Epithelioid sarcoma of the uterine cervix. Gynecol Oncol 2003; 89:536.

191. Etienne-Mastroianni B, Falchero L, Chalabreysse L, et al. Primary sarcomas of the lung: a clinicopathologic study of 12 cases. Lung Cancer 2002; 38:283.

192. Kurtkaya-Yapicier O, Scheithauer BW, Dedrick DJ, et al. Primary epithelioid sarcoma of the dura: case report. Neurosurgery 2002; 50:198.

193. Chao KC, Chen C, Hsieh SC, et al. MRI of epithelioid sarcoma of the thigh. Clin Imaging 2005; 29:60.

194. Hanna SL, Kaste S, Jenkins JJ, et al. Epithelioid sarcoma: clinical, MR imaging and pathologic findings. Skeletal Radiol 2002; 31:400.

195. Heenan PJ, Quirk CJ, Papadimitriou JM. Epithelioid sarcoma. A diagnostic problem. Am J Dermatopathol 1986; 8:95.

196. Tan SH, Ong BH. Spindle cell variant of epithelioid sarcoma: an easily misdiagnosed tumour. Australas J Dermatol 2001; 42:139.

197. Mirra JM, Kessler S, Bhuta S, et al. The fibroma-like variant of epithelioid sarcoma. A fibrohistiocytic/myoid cell lesion often confused with benign and malignant spindle cell tumors. Cancer 1992; 69:1382.

198. Chetty R, Slavin JL. Epithelioid sarcoma with extensive chondroid differentiation. Histopathology 1994; 24:400.

199. Laskin WB, Miettinen M. Epithelioid sarcoma: new insights based on an extended

immunohistochemical analysis. Arch Pathol Lab Med 2003; 127:1161.

200. Miettinen M, Fanburg-Smith JC, Virolainen M, et al. Epithelioid sarcoma: an immunohistochemical analysis of 112 classical and variant cases and a discussion of the differential diagnosis. Hum Pathol 1999; 30:934.

201. Chase DR, Enzinger FM, Weiss SW, et al. Keratin in epithelioid sarcoma. An immunohistochemical study. Am J Surg Pathol 1984; 8:435.

202. Kato H, Hatori M, Kokubun S, et al. CA125 expression in epithelioid sarcoma. Jpn J Clin Oncol 2004; 34:149.

203. Kato H, Hatori M, Watanabe M, et al. Epithelioid sarcomas with elevated serum CA125: report of two cases. Jpn J Clin Oncol 2003; 33:141.

204. Masunaga A, Ikeda K, Suzuki T, et al. Proximal-type epithelioid sarcoma in a 36-year-old man: closer immunoelectron-microscopic resemblance of the tumor cells to epithelial cells than to mesenchymal cells. Pathol Int 2004; 54:616.

205. Fisher C. Epithelioid sarcoma: the spectrum of ultrastructural differentiation in seven immunohistochemically defined cases. Hum Pathol 1988; 19:265.

206. Modena P, Lualdi E, Facchinetti F, et al. SMARCB1/INI1 tumor suppressor gene is frequently inactivated in epithelioid sarcomas. Cancer Res 2005; 65:4012.

207. Lee MW, Jee KJ, Han SS, et al. Comparative genomic hybridization in epithelioid sarcoma. Br J Dermatol 2004; 151:1054.

208. Lualdi E, Modena P, Debiec-Rychter M, et al. Molecular cytogenetic characterization of proximal-type epithelioid sarcoma. Genes Chromosomes Cancer 2004; 41:283.

209. Debiec-Rychter M, Sciot R, Hagemeijer A. Common chromosome aberrations in the proximal type of epithelioid sarcoma. Cancer Genet Cytogenet 2000; 123:133.

210. Feely MG, Fidler ME, Nelson M, et al. Cytogenetic findings in a case of epithelioid sarcoma and a review of the literature. Cancer Genet Cytogenet 2000; 119:155.

211. Lushnikova T, Knuutila S, Miettinen M. DNA copy number changes in epithelioid sarcoma and its variants: a comparative genomic hybridization study. Mod Pathol 2000; 13:1092.

212. Cordoba JC, Parham DM, Meyer WH, et al. A new cytogenetic finding in an epithelioid sarcoma, t(8;22)(q22;q11). Cancer Genet Cytogenet 1994; 72:151.

213. Dal Cin P, Van den Berghe H, Pauwels P. Epithelioid sarcoma of the proximal type with complex karyotype including i(8q). Cancer Genet Cytogenet 1999; 114:80.

214. Guillou L, Wadden C, Coindre JM, et al. "Proximal-type" epithelioid sarcoma, a distinctive aggressive neoplasm showing rhabdoid features. Clinicopathologic, immunohistochemical, and ultrastructural study of a series. Am J Surg Pathol 1997; 21:130.

215. Saito T, Oda Y, Itakura E, et al. Expression of intercellular adhesion molecules in epithelioid sarcoma and malignant rhabdoid tumor. Pathol Int 2001; 51:532.

216. Lin L, Skacel M, Sigel JE, et al. Epithelioid sarcoma: an immunohistochemical analysis evaluating the utility of cytokeratin 5/6 in distinguishing superficial epithelioid sarcoma from spindled squamous cell carcinoma. J Cutan Pathol 2003; 30:114.

217. Lin L, Hicks D, Xu B, et al. Expression profile and molecular genetic regulation of cyclin D1 expression in epithelioid sarcoma. Mod Pathol 2005; 18:705.

218. Hasegawa T, Matsuno Y, Shimoda T, et al. Proximal-type epithelioid sarcoma: a

clinicopathologic study of 20 cases. Mod Pathol 2001; 14:655.

219. Zevallos-Giampietri EA, Barrionuevo C. Proximal-type epithelioid sarcoma: report of two cases in the perineum: differential diagnosis and review of soft tissue tumors with epithelioid and/or rhabdoid features. Appl Immunohistochem Mol Morphol 2005; 13:221.

220. Shiratsuchi H, Oshiro Y, Saito T, et al. Cytokeratin subunits of inclusion bodies in rhabdoid cells: immunohistochemical and clinicopathological study of malignant rhabdoid tumor and epithelioid sarcoma. Int J Surg Pathol 2001; 9:37.

221. Spillane AJ, Thomas JM, Fisher C. Epithelioid sarcoma: the clinicopathological complexities of this rare soft tissue sarcoma. Ann Surg Oncol 2000; 7:218.

222. Herr MJ, Harmsen WS, Amadio PC, et al. Epithelioid sarcoma of the hand. Clin Orthop 2005; 431:193.

223. Callister MD, Ballo MT, Pisters PW, et al. Epithelioid sarcoma: results of conservative surgery and radiotherapy. Int J Radiat Oncol Biol Phys 2001; 51:384.

224. Behranwala KA, A'Hern R, Omar AM, et al. Prognosis of lymph node metastasis in soft tissue sarcoma. Ann Surg Oncol 2004; 11:714.

225. Bos GD, Pritchard DJ, Reiman HM, et al. Epithelioid sarcoma. An analysis of fifty-one cases. J Bone Joint Surg [Am] 1988; 70:862.

226. Evans HL, Baer SC. Epithelioid sarcoma: a clinicopathologic and prognostic study of 26 cases. Semin Diagn Pathol 1993; 10:286.

227. Halling AC, Wollan PC, Pritchard DJ, et al. Epithelioid sarcoma: a clinicopathologic review of 55 cases. Mayo Clin Proc 1996; 71:636.

227a. Izumi T, Oda Y, Hasegawa, et al. Prognostic significance of dysadherin expression in epithelioid sarcoma and its diagnostic utility in distinguishing epithelioid sarcoma from malignant rhabdoid tumor. Mod Pathol 2006; 19:820.

228. Whitworth PW, Pollock RE, Mansfield PF, et al. Extremity epithelioid sarcoma. Amputation vs local resection. Arch Surg 1991; 126:1485.

229. Blazer DG 3rd, Sabel MS, Sondak VK. Is there a role for sentinel lymph node biopsy in the management of sarcoma? Surg Oncol 2003; 12:201.

230. Murray PM. Soft tissue sarcoma of the upper extremity. Hand Clin 2004; 20:325.

231. Schiffman R. Epithelioid sarcoma and synovial sarcoma in the same knee. Cancer 1980; 45:158.

232. Soule EH, Enriquez P. Atypical fibrous histiocytoma, malignant fibrous histiocytoma, malignant histiocytoma, and epithelioid sarcoma. A comparative study of 65 tumors. Cancer 1972; 30:128.

233. Bloustein PA, Silverberg SG, Waddell WR. Epithelioid sarcoma: case report with ultrastructural review, histogenetic discussion, and chemotherapeutic data. Cancer 1976; 38:2390.

234. Fisher ER, Horvat B. The fibrocytic deprivation of the so-called epithelioid sarcoma. Cancer 1972; 30:1074.

235. Pisa R, Novelli P, Bonetti F. Epithelioid sarcoma: a tumor of myofibroblasts, or not? Histopathology 1984; 8:353.

236. Miettinen M, Lehto VP, Vartio T, et al. Epithelioid sarcoma. Ultrastructural and immunohistologic features suggesting a synovial origin. Arch Pathol Lab Med 1982; 106:620.

237. Puissegur-Lupo ML, Perret WJ, Millikan LE. Epithelioid sarcoma. Report of a case. Arch Dermatol 1985; 121:394.

238. Chaudhuri A, Harris MD. "Proximal-type" epithelioid sarcoma: is Agent Orange still at large? Ann R Coll Surg Engl 2003; 85:410.

239. Helmers S, Ruland RT, Jacob LN. Epithelioid sarcoma of the thumb associated with hydrazine fuel exposure: a case report. Mil Med 2004; 169:41.

Desmoplastic small round cell tumor

240. Sesterhenn I, Davis CJ, Mostofi K. Undifferentiated malignant epithelial tumors involving serosal surfaces of scrotum and abdomen in young males. J Urol 1987; 137:214.

241. Gerald WL, Rosai J. Desmoplastic small cell tumor with divergent differentiation. Pediatr Pathol 1989; 9:177.

242. Gerald WL, Miller HK, Battifora H, et al. Intra-abdominal desmoplastic small round-cell tumor. Report of 19 cases of a distinctive type of high-grade polyphenotypic malignancy affecting young individuals. Am J Surg Pathol 1991; 15:499.

243. Ordonez NG, Zirkin R, Bloom RE. Malignant small-cell epithelial tumor of the peritoneum coexpressing mesenchymal type intermediate filaments. Am J Surg Pathol 1989; 13:413.

244. Variend S, Gerrard M, Norris PD, et al. Intraabdominal neuroectodermal tumour of childhood with divergent differentiation. Histopathology 1991; 18:45.

245. Gerald WL, Rosai J. Desmoplastic small cell tumor with multi-phenotypic differentiation. Zentralbl Pathol 1993; 139:141.

246. Basade MM, Vege DS, Nair CN, et al. Intra-abdominal desmoplastic small round cell tumor in children: a clinicopathologic study. Pediatr Hematol Oncol 1996; 13:95.

247. Wolf AN, Ladanyi M, Paull G, et al. The expanding clinical spectrum of desmoplastic small round-cell tumor: a report of two cases with molecular confirmation. Hum Pathol 1999; 30:430.

248. Reich O, Justus J, Tamussino KF. Intra-abdominal desmoplastic small round cell tumor in a 68-year-old female. Eur J Gynaecol Oncol 2000; 21:126.

249. Gerald WL, Ladanyi M, de Alava E, et al. Clinical, pathologic, and molecular spectrum of tumors associated with t(11;22)(p13;q12): desmoplastic small round-cell tumor and its variants. J Clin Oncol 1998; 16:3028.

250. Lae ME, Roche PC, Jin L, et al. Desmoplastic small round cell tumor: a clinicopathologic, immunohistochemical, and molecular study of 32 tumors. Am J Surg Pathol 2002; 26:823.

251. Ordonez NG. Desmoplastic small round cell tumor: I: a histopathologic study of 39 cases with emphasis on unusual histological patterns. Am J Surg Pathol 1998; 22:1303.

252. Carroll JC, Klauber GT, Kretschmar CS, et al. Urological aspects of intra-abdominal desmoplastic small round cell tumor of childhood: a preliminary report. J Urol 1994; 151:172.

253. Cummings OW, Ulbright TM, Young RH, et al. Desmoplastic small round cell tumors of the paratesticular region. A report of six cases. Am J Surg Pathol 1997; 21:219.

254. Garcia-Gonzalez J, Villanueva C, Fernandez-Acenero MJ, et al. Paratesticular desmoplastic small round cell tumor: case report. Urol Oncol 2005; 23:132.

255. Thuret R, Renaudin K, Leclere J, et al. Uncommon malignancies: Case 3. Paratesticular desmoplastic small round-cell tumor. J Clin Oncol 2005; 23:6253.

256. Elhajj M, Mazurka J, Daya D. Desmoplastic small round cell tumor presenting in the ovaries: report of a case and review of the literature. Int J Gynecol Cancer 2002; 12:760.

257. Parkash V, Gerald WL, Parma A, et al. Desmoplastic small round cell tumor of the pleura. Am J Surg Pathol 1995; 19:659.

258. Tison V, Cerasoli S, Morigi F, et al. Intracranial desmoplastic small-cell tumor:

report of a case. Am J Surg Pathol 1996; 20:112.

259. Finke NM, Lae ME, Lloyd RV, et al. Sinonasal desmoplastic small round cell tumor: a case report. Am J Surg Pathol 2002; 26:799.

260. Murphy A, Stallings RL, Howard J, et al. Primary desmoplastic small round cell tumor of bone: report of a case with cytogenetic confirmation. Cancer Genet Cytogenet 2005; 156:167.

261. Syed S, Haque AK, Hawkins HK, et al. Desmoplastic small round cell tumor of the lung. Arch Pathol Lab Med 2002; 126:1226.

262. Wang LL, Perlman EJ, Vujanic GM, et al. Desmoplastic small round cell tumor of the kidney in childhood. Am J Surg Pathol 2007; 31:576.

263. Khalbuss WE, Bui M, Loya A. A 19-year-old woman with a cervicovaginal mass and elevated serum CA 125. Desmoplastic small round cell tumor. Arch Pathol Lab Med 2006; 130:59.

264. Adsay V, Cheng J, Athanasian E, et al. Primary desmoplastic small cell tumor of soft tissues and bone of the hand. Am J Surg Pathol 1999; 23:1408.

265. Bismar TA, Basturak O, Gerald WL, et al. Desmoplastic small cell tumor in the pancreas. Am J Surg Pathol 2004; 28:808.

266. Dorsey BV, Benjamin LE, Rauscher F 3rd, et al. Intra-abdominal desmoplastic small round-cell tumor: expansion of the pathologic profile. Mod Pathol 1996; 9:703.

267. Ordonez NG. Desmoplastic small round cell tumor: II: an ultrastructural and immunohistochemical study with emphasis on new immunohistochemical markers. Am J Surg Pathol 1998; 22:1314.

268. Lamovec J. Intra-abdominal desmoplastic small round-cell tumour with expression of muscle specific actin. Histopathology 1994; 24:577.

269. Zhang PJ, Goldblum JR, Pawel BR, et al. Immunophenotype of desmoplastic small round cell tumors as detected in cases with EWS-WT1 gene fusion product. Mod Pathol 2003; 16:229.

270. Miettinen M, Chatten J, Paetau A, et al. Monoclonal antibody NB84 in the differential diagnosis of neuroblastoma and other small round cell tumors. Am J Surg Pathol 1998; 22:327.

271. Folpe AL, Patterson K, Gown AM. Antineuroblastoma antibody NB-84 also identifies a significant subset of other small blue round cell tumors. Appl Immunohistochem 1997; 5:239.

272. Barnoud R, Sabourin JC, Pasquier D, et al. Immunohistochemical expression of WT1 by desmoplastic small round cell tumor: a comparative study with other small round cell tumors. Am J Surg Pathol 2000; 24:830.

273. Hill DA, Pfeifer JD, Marley EF, et al. WT1 staining reliably differentiates desmoplastic small round cell tumor from Ewing sarcoma/ primitive neuroectodermal tumor. An immunohistochemical and molecular diagnostic study. Am J Clin Pathol 2000; 114:345.

274. Loy TS, Quesenberry JT, Sharp SC. Distribution of CA125 in adenocarcinomas: an immunohistochemical study of 481 cases. Am J Clin Pathol 1992; 98:175.

275. Parker LP, Duong JL, Wharton JT, et al. Desmoplastic small round cell tumor: report of a case presenting as a primary ovarian neoplasm. Eur J Gynaecol Oncol 2002; 23:199.

276. Ordonez NG, Sahin AA. CA 125 production in desmoplastic small round cell tumor: report of a case with elevated serum levels and prominent signet ring morphology. Hum Pathol 1998; 29:294.

277. Wills EJ. Peritoneal desmoplastic small round cell tumors with divergent differentiation: a review. Ultrastruct Pathol 1993; 17:295.

278. Biegel JA, Conard K, Brooks JJ. Translocation (11;22)(p13;q12): primary change in intra-abdominal desmoplastic small round cell tumor. Genes Chromosomes Cancer 1993; 7:119.

279. Sawyer JR, Tryka AF, Lewis JM. A novel reciprocal chromosome translocation t(11;22)(p13;q12) in an intraabdominal desmoplastic small round-cell tumor. Am J Surg Pathol 1992; 16:411.

280. Gerald WL, Rosai J, Ladanyi M. Characterization of the genomic breakpoint and chimeric transcripts in the EWS-WT1 gene fusion of desmoplastic small round cell tumor. Proc Natl Acad Sci USA 1995; 92:1028.

281. Ladanyi M, Gerald W. Fusion of the EWS and WT1 genes in the desmoplastic small round cell tumor. Cancer Res 1994; 54:2837.

282. Lee SB, Haber DA. Wilms tumor and the WT1 gene. Exp Cell Res 2001; 264:74.

283. Zhang PJ, Goldblum JR, Pawel BR, et al. PDGF-A, PDGF-rbeta, TGFbeta3 and bone morphogenic protein-4 in desmoplastic small round cell tumors with EWS-WT1 gene fusion product and their role in stromal desmoplasia: an immunohistochemical study. Mod Pathol 2005; 18:382.

284. Hill DA, O'Sullivan MJ, Zhu X, et al. Practical application of molecular genetic testing as an aid to the surgical pathologic diagnosis of sarcomas: a prospective study. Am J Surg Pathol 2002; 26:965.

285. Fritsch MK, Bridge JA, Schuster AE, et al. Performance characteristics of a reverse transcriptase-polymerase chain reaction assay for the detection of tumor-specific fusion transcripts from archival tissue. Pediatr Dev Pathol 2003; 6:43.

286. de Alava E, Ladanyi M, Rosai J, et al. Detection of chimeric transcripts in desmoplastic small round cell tumor and related developmental tumors by reverse transcriptase polymerase chain reaction. A specific diagnostic assay. Am J Pathol 1995; 147:1584.

287. Antonescu CR, Gerald WL, Magid MS, et al. Molecular variants of the EWS-WT1 gene fusion in desmoplastic small round cell tumor. Diagn Mol Pathol 1998; 7:24.

288. Shimizu Y, Mitsui T, Kawakami T, et al. Novel breakpoints of the EWS gene and the WT1 gene in a desmoplastic small round cell tumor. Cancer Genet Cytogenet 1998; 106:156.

289. Ordi J, de Alava E, Torne A, et al. Intraabdominal desmoplastic small round cell tumor with EWS/ERG fusion transcript. Am J Surg Pathol 1998; 22:1026.

290. Katz RL, Quezado M, Senderowicz AM, et al. An intra-abdominal small round cell neoplasm with features of primitive neuroectodermal and desmoplastic round cell tumor and a EWS/FLI-1 fusion transcript. Hum Pathol 1997; 28:502.

291. Ordóñez NG, el-Naggar AK, Ro JY, et al. Intraabdominal desmoplastic small cell tumor: a light microscopic, immunocytochemical, ultrastructural, and flow cytometric study. Hum Pathol 1993; 24:850.

292. Schwarz RE, Gerald WL, Kushner BH, et al. Desmoplastic small round cell tumors: prognostic indicators and results of surgical management. Ann Surg Oncol 1998; 5:416.

293. Kushner BH, Cheung NK, Kramer K, et al. Topotecan combined with myeloablative doses of thiotepa and carboplatin for neuroblastoma, brain tumors, and other poor-risk solid tumors in children and young adults. Bone Marrow Transplant 2001; 28:551.

294. Quaglia MP, Brennan MF. The clinical approach to desmoplastic small round cell tumor. Surg Oncol 2000; 9:77.

295. Adamson PC, Blaney SM, Widemann BC, et al. Pediatric phase I trial and pharmacokinetic study of the platelet-derived growth factor (PDGF) receptor pathway inhibitor SU101. Cancer Chemother Pharmacol 2004; 53:482.

Malignant extrarenal rhabdoid tumor

296. Beckwith JB, Palmer NF. Histopathology and prognosis of Wilms' tumors: results from the first National Wilms' Tumor Study. Cancer 1978; 41:1937.

297. Weeks DA, Beckwith JB, Mierau GW, et al. Rhabdoid tumor of kidney. A report of 111 cases from the National Wilms' Tumor Study Pathology Center. Am J Surg Pathol 1989; 13:439.

298. Petitt M, Doeden K, Harris A, et al. Cutaneous extrarenal rhabdoid tumor with myogenic differentiation. J Cutan Pathol 2005; 32:690.

299. Fanburg-Smith JC, Hengge M, Hengge UR, et al. Extrarenal rhabdoid tumors of soft tissue: a clinicopathologic and immunohistochemical study of 18 cases. Ann Diagn Pathol 1998; 2:351.

300. Oda Y, Tsuneyoshi M. Extrarenal rhabdoid tumors of soft tissue: clinicopathological and molecular genetic review and distinction from other soft-tissue sarcomas with rhabdoid features. Pathol Int 2006; 56:287.

301. Chang JH, Dikranian AH, Johnston WH, et al. Malignant extrarenal rhabdoid tumor of the bladder: 9-year survival after chemotherapy and partial cystectomy. J Urol 2004; 171:820.

302. Leath CA 3rd, Huh WK, Conner M, et al. Primary extrarenal rhabdoid tumor of the ovary. A case report. J Reprod Med 2003; 48:283.

303. Marcus VA, Viloria J, Owen D, et al. Malignant rhabdoid tumor of the colon. Report of a case with molecular analysis. Dis Colon Rectum 1996; 39:1322.

304. Donner LR, Rao A, Truss LM, et al. Translocation (8;13)(q24.2;q33) in a malignant rhabdoid tumor of the liver. Cancer Genet Cytogenet 2000; 116:153.

305. Salamanca J, Rodriguez-Peralto JL, Azorin D, et al. Paratesticular congenital malignant rhabdoid tumor diagnosed by fine-needle aspiration cytology. A case report. Diagn Cytopathol 2004; 30:46.

306. Burger PC, Yu IT, Tihan T, et al. Atypical teratoid/rhabdoid tumor of the central nervous system: a highly malignant tumor of infancy and childhood frequently mistaken for medulloblastoma: a Pediatric Oncology Group study. Am J Surg Pathol 1998; 22:1083.

307. Hilden JM, Meerbaum S, Burger P, et al. Central nervous system atypical teratoid/ rhabdoid tumor: results of therapy in children enrolled in a registry. J Clin Oncol 2004; 22:2877.

308. Wick MR, Ritter JH, Dehner LP. Malignant rhabdoid tumors: a clinicopathologic review and conceptual discussion. Semin Diagn Pathol 1995; 12:233.

309. Gokden N, Nappi O, Swanson PE, et al. Renal cell carcinoma with rhabdoid features. Am J Surg Pathol 2000; 24:1329.

310. Weeks DA, Beckwith JB, Mierau GW, et al. Renal neoplasms mimicking rhabdoid tumor of kidney. A report from the National Wilms' Tumor Study Pathology Center. Am J Surg Pathol 1991; 15:1042.

311. Oshiro Y, Shiratsuchi H, Oda Y, et al. Rhabdoid features in leiomyosarcoma of soft tissue: with special reference to aggressive behavior. Mod Pathol 2000; 13:1211.

312. Suarez-Vilela D, Izquierdo-Garcia FM, Alonso-Orcajo N. Epithelioid and rhabdoid rhabdomyosarcoma in an adult patient: a diagnostic pitfall. Virchows Arch 2004; 445:323.

313. Oshiro Y, Shiratsuchi H, Tamiya S, et al. Extraskeletal myxoid chondrosarcoma with rhabdoid features, with special reference to its aggressive behavior. Int J Surg Pathol 2000; 8:145.

314. Knapik J, Yachnis AT, Ripley D, et al. Aggressive uterine sarcoma with rhabdoid features: diagnosis by peritoneal fluid cytology and absence of INI1 gene mutation. Hum Pathol 2001; 32:884.

315. Ordonez NG. Mesothelioma with rhabdoid features: an ultrastructural and immunohistochemical study of 10 cases. Mod Pathol 2006; 19:373.

316. Batoroev YK, Nguyen GK. Rhabdoid meningioma diagnosed by imprint cytology. Acta Cytol 2005; 49:464.

317. White FV, Dehner LP, Belchis DA, et al. Congenital disseminated malignant rhabdoid tumor: a distinct clinicopathologic entity demonstrating abnormalities of chromosome 22q11. Am J Surg Pathol 1999; 23:249.

318. Leader J, Carlan SJ, Blum J. Congenital malignant extrarenal rhabdoid tumor: prenatal ultrasound findings. Obstet Gynecol 2002; 99:949.

319. Haas JE, Palmer NF, Weinberg AG, et al. Ultrastructure of malignant rhabdoid tumor of the kidney. A distinctive renal tumor of children. Hum Pathol 1981; 12:646.

320. Perlman EJ. Pediatric renal tumors: practical updates for the pathologist. Pediatr Dev Pathol 2005; 8:320.

321. Sigauke E, Rakheja D, Maddox DL, et al. Absence of expression of SMARCB1/INI1 in malignant rhabdoid tumors of the central nervous system, kidneys and soft tissue: an immunohistochemical study with implications for diagnosis. Mod Pathol 2006; 19:717.

322. Judkins AR, Burger PC, Hamilton RL, et al. INI1 protein expression distinguishes atypical teratoid/rhabdoid tumor from choroid plexus carcinoma. J Neuropathol Exp Neurol 2005; 64:391.

322a. Sigauke E, Rakheja D, Maddox DL, et al. Absence of expression of SMARCB1/INI1 in malignant rhabdoid tumors of the central nervous system, kidneys and soft tissue: an immunohistochemical study with implications for diagnosis. Mod Pathol 2006; 19:717.

323. Itakura E, Tamiya S, Morita K, et al. Subcellular distribution of cytokeratin and vimentin in malignant rhabdoid tumor: three-dimensional imaging with confocal laser scanning microscopy and double immunofluorescence. Mod Pathol 2001; 14:854.

324. Shiratsuchi H, Saito T, Sakamoto A, et al. Mutation analysis of human cytokeratin 8 gene in malignant rhabdoid tumor: a possible association with intracytoplasmic inclusion body formation. Mod Pathol 2002; 15:146.

325. Biegel JA. Genetics of pediatric central nervous system tumors. J Pediatr Hematol Oncol 1997; 19:492.

326. Biegel JA, Allen CS, Kawasaki K, et al. Narrowing the critical region for a rhabdoid tumor locus in 22q11. Genes Chromosomes Cancer 1996; 16:94.

327. Biegel JA, Rorke LB, Emanuel BS. Monosomy 22 in rhabdoid or atypical teratoid tumors of the brain. N Engl J Med 1989; 321:906.

328. Schofield DE, Beckwith JB, Sklar J. Loss of heterozygosity at chromosome regions 22q11–12 and 11p15.5 in renal rhabdoid tumors. Genes Chromosomes Cancer 1996; 15:10.

329. Biegel JA, Tan L, Zhang F, et al. Alterations of the hSNF5/INI1 gene in central nervous system atypical teratoid/rhabdoid tumors and renal and extrarenal rhabdoid tumors. Clin Cancer Res 2002; 8:3461.

330. Biegel JA, Kalpana G, Knudsen ES, et al. The role of INI1 and the SWI/SNF complex in the development of rhabdoid tumors: meeting summary from the workshop on childhood atypical teratoid/rhabdoid tumors. Cancer Res 2002; 62:323.

331. Rousseau-Merck MF, Versteege I, Legrand I, et al. hSNF5/INI1 inactivation is mainly associated with homozygous deletions and mitotic recombinations in rhabdoid tumors. Cancer Res 1999; 59:3152.

332. Versteege I, Sevenet N, Lange J, et al. Truncating mutations of hSNF5/INI1 in aggressive paediatric cancer. Nature 1998; 394:203.

333. Roberts CW, Galusha SA, McMenamin ME, et al. Haploinsufficiency of Snf5 (integrase interactor 1) predisposes to malignant rhabdoid tumors in mice. Proc Natl Acad Sci USA 2000; 97:13796.

334. Janson K, Nedzi LA, David O, et al. Predisposition to atypical teratoid/rhabdoid tumor due to an inherited INI1 mutation. Pediatr Blood Cancer 2005; 47(3):279.

335. Roberts CW. Genetic causes of familial risk in rhabdoid tumors. Pediatr Blood Cancer 2006; 47(3):235.

336. Fuller CE, Pfeifer J, Humphrey P, et al. Chromosome 22q dosage in composite extrarenal rhabdoid tumors: clonal evolution or a phenotypic mimic? Hum Pathol 2001; 32:1102.

337. Perry A, Fuller CE, Judkins AR, et al. INI1 expression is retained in composite rhabdoid tumors, including rhabdoid meningiomas. Mod Pathol 2005; 18:951.

338. Parham DM, Weeks DA, Beckwith JB. The clinicopathologic spectrum of putative extrarenal rhabdoid tumors. An analysis of 42 cases studied with immunohistochemistry or electron microscopy. Am J Surg Pathol 1994; 18:1010.

Malignant mesenchymoma

339. Stout AP. Mesenchymoma: the mixed tumor of mesenchymal derivatives. Ann Surg 1948; 127:278.

340. Nash A, Stout AP. Malignant mesenchymomas in children. Cancer 1961; 14:524.

341. Symmers WS, Nangle EJ. An unusual recurring tumour formed of connective tissues of embryonic type (so called mesenchymoma). J Pathol Bacteriol 1951; 63:417.

342. Ewing MR, Harrison CV. Mesenchymoma. Br J Surg 1957; 44:408.

343. Thomas JA, Kothare SN. Malignant mesenchymomata of soft tissues. Indian J Cancer 1974; 11:227.

344. Newman PL, Fletcher CD. Malignant mesenchymoma. Clinicopathologic analysis of a series with evidence of low-grade behaviour. Am J Surg Pathol 1991; 15:607.

345. Brady MS, Perino G, Tallini G, et al. Malignant mesenchymoma. Cancer 1996; 77:467.

INDEX

Note: Page numbers in *italics* refer to illustrations; page numbers followed by t refer to tables.

A

A103 antibody. See *Melan-A*.
Abdominal cavity. See also *Intra-abdominal region*.
 desmoplastic small round cell tumor, 1203, 1203t
 fibromatosis, 246–247
 leiomyosarcoma. See *Leiomyosarcoma, retroperitoneal/abdominal*.
Abdominopelvic sarcoma of perivascular epithelioid cells, 1138, 1148
Abscess, radiologic features, 58, 58t
Achilles tendon xanthomas, 356, *356*, 357
Acinar growth pattern, 124t. See also *Pseudoacinar pattern*.
 mesothelioma, 794
Acne vulgaris, keloids and, 216
Acoustic neurofibromatosis, bilateral. See *Neurofibromatosis 2*.
Acquired immune deficiency syndrome. See *AIDS/HIV infection*.
Acral fibromyxoma, superficial, 1080
Acral myxoinflammatory fibroblastic sarcoma. See *Inflammatory myxohyaline tumor of distal extremities*.
Acromegaly, Carney syndrome, 871, 1081
ACTB-GLI fusion gene, 87
Actin, 130t, 138–140
 aggressive angiomyxoma, 1085, 1086t
 angiomyolipoma, 1140
 benign genital stromal tumors, 538, 539–540, 540t
 congenital/infantile fibrosarcoma, 281
 fibrosarcoma, 307
 fibrous hamartoma of infancy, 261
 filaments, 518, 583, *584*
  rhabdomyosarcoma, 622, *623*
 glomus tumor, 757, *758*, 763
 hemangiopericytoma-solitary fibrous tumor, 1129
 infantile digital fibromatosis, 262–263
 inflammatory myofibroblastic tumor, 284–285
 leiomyoma, 521
 leiomyosarcoma, 553, 554, 556
 low-grade fibromyxoid sarcoma, 322
 muscle-specific, 130t, 140
 myofibroma and myofibromatosis, 265, 266
 myofibrosarcoma, 326
 myxoma, 1074, 1077
 nasopharyngeal angiofibroma, 215
 nodular fasciitis, 185
 PEComas, 1151
 pediatric round cell tumors, 621t

 pleomorphic fibroma of skin, 206
 plexiform fibrohistiocytic tumor, 394
 proliferative fasciitis, 192
 pseudosarcomatous myofibroblastic proliferations, 199
 recommendations for use, 142–143
 rhabdomyoma, 585, 586, 591
 rhabdomyosarcoma, 140, 620, 620t
 sarcomeric, rhabdomyosarcoma, 620, 620t, 621t
 smooth muscle, 130t, 140
  diagnostic applications, 166t
  inflammatory myxohyaline tumor of distal extremities, 1102, 1107t
  nodular fasciitis, 185, *188*
  proliferative myositis, *196*
  rhabdomyosarcoma, 620, 620t
 smooth muscle cells, 518
 superficial fibromatoses, 230–231, 233
 "tram-track" pattern, 140, *141*, 326
Actinic-damaged skin, atypical fibroxanthoma, 404, *404*
Actinolite, 792
Adactyly, fibrodysplasia ossificans progressiva, 1047
Adamantinoma, melanotic, 895–897, *896*, *897*
Adenocarcinoma
 differentiation from mesothelioma, 807
  electron microscopy, 803–804, 804t
  immunohistochemistry, 157t, 157–158, 802–803, 802t
  special stains, 801–802, 801t
 pseudolipoblasts, *483*
Adenoma, microcystic, of pancreas. See *Pancreas, microcystic adenoma of*.
Adenomatoid tumor, 817–818
 classification, 789–790, 790t
 clinical findings, *817*, 818
 immunohistochemistry, 818, *819*
 multicystic peritoneal mesothelioma resembling, 811, *814*
 pathologic findings, 818, *818–819*
Adenomatous polyposis, familial. See *Familial adenomatous polyposis*.
Adenomatous polyposis coli gene. See *APC gene*.
Adenomatous polyps, intestinal, Gardner syndrome, 249
Adipocytes. See *Lipocytes*.
Adipose tissue. See *Fat*.
Adiposis dolorosa, 463
Adnexal carcinoma, differentiation from synovial sarcoma, 1179
Adnexal structures, cutaneous myxoma, 1077, *1079*

Adnexal tumors, differentiation from glomus tumors, 756–757, *757*
Adrenal gland
 ganglioneuroma, 960, 960t
 myelolipoma, 456
 neuroblastoma, 946
 paraganglioma, 1003, 1008
Adrenal medulla, 989
Adrenaline. See *Epinephrine*.
Adrenocorticotropic hormone (ACTH), 998t, 1011
Adult rhabdomyoma. See *Rhabdomyoma, adult*.
AE1/AE3 antibody staining
 Ewing sarcoma/primitive neuroectodermal tumor, 975
 pseudosarcomatous myofibroblastic proliferations, 199
Age
 -related incidence, 2, *2*
 diagnostic value, 47, 54t, 119
Agent Orange, 3
Aggressive angiomyxoma. See *Angiomyxoma, aggressive*.
Aicardi syndrome, angiosarcoma, 704
AIDS/HIV infection
 bacillary angiomatosis, 674
 Kaposi sarcoma, 722, 723, *723*, 730
 lipodystrophy, 465
 lymph node evaluation, 725–728
AJCC. See *American Joint Committee on Cancer*.
Alcian blue stain
 cutaneous myxoma, *1078*
 low-grade fibromyxoid sarcoma, 317–319
 mesothelioma, 801–802, 801t, 814
 myxoid chondrosarcoma, 1028
 myxoid liposarcoma, 499–503, *503*
 sclerosing rhabdomyosarcoma, 619
 synovial sarcoma, 1175
Alcoholism
 fibromatoses associated with, 229, 233
 symmetric lipomatosis and, 463
ALK-1 (activin receptor-like kinase 1) gene, 668
ALK (anaplastic lymphoma kinase) gene rearrangements, 161
 inflammatory myofibroblastic tumor, 87–88, 199t, 288
 pseudosarcomatous myofibroblastic proliferations, 193–194, 199, 199t
ALK (anaplastic lymphoma kinase) protein, 161
 calcifying fibrous pseudotumor, 295, 296
 inflammatory myofibroblastic tumor, 288
 pseudosarcomatous myofibroblastic proliferations, *198*, 199, 199t